Oncology Rehabilitation

A Comprehensive Guidebook for Clinicians

Oncology Rehabilitation

A Comprehensive Guidebook for Clinicians

Deborah J. Doherty, PT, PhD
Chairperson, Associate Professor
Human Movement Science
Oakland University, Rochester
Michigan
United States

Christopher M. Wilson, PT, DPT, DScPT, Board Certified Geriatric Clinical Specialist
Associate Professor and Director of Clinical Education
Human Movement Science
Oakland University, Rochester
Michigan
United States

Lori E. Boright, PT, DPT, DScPT
Assistant Professor
School of Health Sciences
Oakland University, Rochester
Michigan
United States

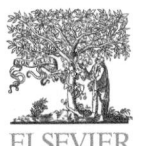

ELSEVIER

Elsevier
3251 Riverport Lane
St. Louis, Missouri 63043

ONCOLOGY REHABILITATION
A COMPREHENSIVE GUIDEBOOK FOR CLINICIANS

ISBN: 9780323810876

Content Strategist: Lauren Willis
Content Development Specialist: Ranjana Sharma
Publishing Services Manager: Deepthi Unni
Senior Project Manager: Kamatchi Madhavan
Design Direction: Patrick Ferguson

Printed in India

Last digit is the print number: 9 8 7 6 5 4 3 2 1

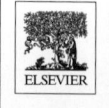

To all the beautiful souls who are on their cancer journey…I walk this journey with you. Thank you for your endless passion for life that ignited my yearning to share this collective wisdom and to my loving family—Del, Rick, Derek, Jacki, Miranna, Ricky, and Bryan— whose unconditional love gives me strength.
—Deb

To Amy, Emily, Jason, and my parents for their daily inspiration and support; to all my patients whose fight against cancer inspired this book.
—Chris

Dedicated to Jeff, Jamie, and Chloe for their ever-present support, as well as to my parents Duane and Susan Creviston, whose own cancer journeys inspire my work to improve cancer care for all survivors.
—Lori

Reviewers

Book Managers

Alyssa Logie, PT, DPT
Carly Pawlitz, BS, SPT
Morgan Shaw-Andrade, BS, SPT

Line Editors

Fadi Anwar, PT, DPT, OMPT
Nada Metti, MS, OTRL

Video Director and Photographer

John Krauss, PT, PhD, FAAOMPT, Board Certified in
     Orthopedic Physical Therapy
Oakland University, Rochester
Michigan
United States

Content Reviewers

Shelley Adams, PT, CLT
Retired Ascension St. John Providence, Southfield
Michigan
United States

Fadi Anwar, PT, DPT, OMPT
OMPT Specialists, Troy
Michigan
United States

Pamela Bartlo, PT, DPT, CCS
D'Youville College, Buffalo
New York
United States

Alethia Battles, JD, LMSW
University of Michigan, Ann Arbor
Michigan
United States

Emilee Bohde, PT, DPT
The Recovery Project, Clinton Township
Michigan
United States

Rich Briggs, PT, MA
Hospice Physical Therapy Associates, Chico
California
United States

Jennifer L. Bradt, PT, DPT, CLT-LANA
Mayo Clinic, Rochester
Minnesota
United States

Daniel D. Child, MD, PhD
University of Washington, Seattle
Washington
United States

Chad Compagner, PharmD
Beaumont Health, Royal Oak
Michigan
United States

Emily Companger, PT, DPT
Children's Hospital of Michigan, Detroit
Michigan
United States

Amy Compston, PT, DPT, CRT, CLT-LANA
The Ohio State University Comprehensive Cancer Center,
     Columbus
Ohio
United States

Nicole Dailey, PT, DPT
Henry Ford Outpatient Rehabilitation, Warren
Michigan
United States

Julie L. Derby, PT, MPT, tDPT, Graduate Certificate in
     Oncology Rehabilitation
Ascension Genesys Hospital and Ascension at Home, Grand Blanc
Michigan
United States

Saam Eslami, PT, MA, tDPT, GCOR
Private Practice, Tehran
Iran

April Gamble, PT DPT, CLT
ACR—The American Center for Rehabilitation
Kurdistan
Iraq

Scott Grumeretz, PT, DPT
Rush Hospital, Chicago
Illinois
United States

Alexandra Hill, PT, DPT, CLT-LANA, Board Certified Specialist in Women's Health Physical Therapy, Board Certified Specialist in Oncologic Physical Therapy
University of Florida Health, Jacksonville
Florida
United States

Shannon Kleinert, PT, DPT
Mary Free Bed at Covenant, Saginaw
Michigan
United States

Susan Lilly, PT, ScD
MD Anderson Cancer Center, Houston
Texas
United States

Christina Lombardi, PT, DPT
Good Shepherd Penn Partners, Yardley
Pennsylvania
United States

Brigido Mapili, PT
Beaumont Health, Royal Oak
Michigan
United States

Lauren McCloy, PT, DPT
Team Rehabilitation, St. Clair Shores
Michigan
United States

Nada Metti, MS, OTRL
The Recovery Project, Livonia
Michigan
United States

Sandy Moody
Turning Point, Atlanta
Georgia
United States

Alaina Newell, DPT, PT, CLT-LANA, Board Certified Specialist in Women's Health Physical Therapy, Board Certified Specialist in Oncologic Physical Therapy
ReVital Cancer Rehabilitation, Select Medical, Mechanicsburg
Pennsylvania
United States

Brianne Patton, PT, DPT
McLaren Health Care, Port Huron
Michigan
United States

Lorraine J. Pearl-Kraus, PhD, MSN, CS, FNP
LPK Healthcare Research, Policy, & Consulting Services, LLC, Grand Rapids
Michigan
United States

Janet Wiechec Seidell, PT, MPT, CLT
Beaumont Health, Troy
Michigan
United States

Laura Sheridan, PT, DPT
Memorial Sloan Kettering Cancer Center, New York
New York
United States

Jennifer Shifferd, PT, MPT, WCS, CLT
Michigan Medicine, Ann Arbor
Michigan
United States

Mike Shoemaker, PT, DPT, PhD, Board Certified Geriatric Clinical Specialist
Grand Valley State University, Grand Rapids
Michigan
United States

Lauren Sofen, PT, DPT, Board Certified Pediatric Clinical Specialist
Beaumont Health, Royal Oak
Michigan
United States

Zachary S. Tally, PT, DPT, Board-Certified Oncologic Clinical Specialist
Duke University Health System, Durham
North Carolina
United States

Rachel Tabak Tran, PT, DPT, Board-Certified Neurologic Clinical Specialist
Casa Colina Hospital and Centers for Healthcare, Pomona
California
United States

Emily Van Wasshenova, PhD
Oakland University, Rochester
Michigan
United States

Debbie Webster, BSN, RN, LMSW
Michigan Department of Health and Human Services, Lansing
Michigan
United States

Contributors

Allegra Ann Adams, PT, DPT, WCS
Physical Therapist
Physical Medicine & Rehabilitation
Michigan Medicine, Ann Arbor
Michigan
United States

Amani Awadh Aljohi, PT, MSc
Physical Therapist
Rehabilitation Hospital
Physical Therapy Department
King Fahad Medical City, Riyadh
Riyadh
Saudi Arabia

Sophia Andrews, PT, DPT
Physical Therapist
Rehabilitation
MD Anderson Cancer Center, Houston
Texas
United States

Sara Arena, PT, DScPT
Associate Professor
Human Movement Science
Oakland University, Rochester
Michigan
United States

Cynthia Barbe, PT, DPT, MS
Physical Therapist
Physical Medicine & Rehabilitation
The Johns Hopkins Hospital, Baltimore
Maryland
United States

Emil Berengut, PT, DPT, MSW
Manager
Physical Therapy Department
New York University, New York
New York
United States

Jill Binkley, PT, MSc, CLT, FAAOMPT
Program Director
Founder
TurningPoint Breast Cancer Rehabilitation, Atlanta
Georgia
United States

Lori E. Boright, PT, DPT, DScPT
Assistant Professor
School of Health Sciences
Oakland University, Rochester
Michigan
United States

Rochelle I. Brannan, MPT, CLT-LANA
Physical Therapist
Founder
West Cliff Physical Therapy and Lymphedema Care, Santa Cruz
   California
United States

**Megan Burkart, PT, DPT, CLT, Board Certified Clinical
   Specialist in Oncologic Physical Therapy**
Assistant Professor
Human Performance
West Virginia University, Morgantown
West Virginia
United States

Grace Burns, PT, DPT
Physical Therapist
Acute Rehabilitation
Beaumont Health, Troy
Michigan
United States

Steve Michael Burt, RN, MSN, NP-C
Nurse Practitioner
Radiation Oncology
Beaumont Health, Royal Oak
Michigan
United States;
Adjunct Professor
School of Nursing, Madonna University, Livonia
Michigan
United States

Scott J. Capozza, PT, MSPT
Physical Therapist
Rehabilitation Department
Yale New Haven Health, New Haven
Connecticut
United States;
Physical Therapist
Cancer Survivorship Clinic
Smilow Cancer Hospital at Yale Cancer Center, New Haven
Connecticut
United States

Grayson Stephen Chao, PT, DPT, OCS, CSCS
Adjunct Professor
Doctor of Physical Therapy Program
City University of New York—College of Staten Island,
    Willowbrook
New York
United States

Kelly Chaplin, PT, DPT, CLT
Physical Therapist
Northwestern Memorial Group
Northwestern Memorial Hospital, Chicago
Illinois
United States

Claire E. Child, PT, DPT, MPH, CCS
Teaching Associate
Rehabilitation Medicine, Division of Physical Therapy
University of Washington, Seattle
Washington
United States

**Andrew Chongaway, DPT, ACSM Certified Exercise
    Physiologist, ACSM/ACS Certified Cancer Exercise Trainer**
Physical Therapist
Rehab Services
Allegheny Health Network, Pittsburgh
Pennsylvania
United States

Reyna Colombo, MA, PT
Director
Rehabilitation
Beaumont Hospital Troy, Troy
Michigan
United States

Jena Colon, DPT, MBA
Manager
Rehab Services
MidMichigan Health, Midland
Michigan
United States

Emily Compagner, PT, DPT
Physical Therapist
Physical Therapy
Children's Hospital of Michigan, Detroit
Michigan
United States

Shara Creary-Yan, BSc, PT, GCOR, CLWT
Physical Therapist & Academic Staff (Lecturer & Research Assistant)
Mona Academy of Sport, Faculty of Sport
University of the West Indies, Kingston
Kingston
Jamaica

Erin Daiek, RD, RDN
Registered Dietitian
Clinical Dietitian
West Bloomfield Health and Rehabilitation Center,
    West Bloomfield
Michigan
United States

Sumi Dinda, PhD
Professor and Chair
Clinical Diagnostic Sciences
Oakland University, Rochester
Michigan
United States

Deborah J. Doherty, PT, PhD
Chairperson, Associate Professor
Human Movement Science
Oakland University, Rochester
Michigan
United States

April Gamble, PT, DPT, CLT
Founder and Director
ACR—American Center for Rehabilitation
Kurdistan
Iraq

Laura Gilchrist, PT, PhD
Professor
Physical Therapy Program
St. Catherine University, St. Paul
Minnesota
United States

Caroline S. Gwaltney, PT, DPT, CWS
Assistant Professor
Regional Clinical Coordinator
Physical Therapy Department
Central Michigan University, Mt. Pleasant
Michigan
United States

Shana Harrington, PT, PhD
Clinical Associate Professor
Exercise Science
University of South Carolina, Columbia
South Carolina
United States

**Mary Alice Hewelt, PT, MPT, Board Certified Oncologic
    Physical Therapy Specialist, Certified Lymphedema
    Therapist**
Physical Therapist
Beaumont Rehabilitation Services
Beaumont Health, St. Clair Shores
Michigan
United States

Meghan Huber, PT, DPT, ACSM Certified Exercise Physiologist
Physical Therapist
Physical Medicine and Rehabilitation
Mayo Clinic, Rochester
Minnesota
United States

Allison J. L'Hotta, OTD, OTR/L
Occupational Therapist and PhD Candidate
Occupational Therapy
Washington University School of Medicine, St. Louis
Missouri
United States

Hallie Lenker, PT, DPT
Pediatric Team Coordinator
Physical Medicine & Rehabilitation
Johns Hopkins Children's Center
Baltimore
United States

Sarah Lerchenfeldt, PharmD
Associate Professor
Foundational Medical Studies
Oakland University William Beaumont School of Medicine, Rochester Hills
Michigan
United States

Amy J. Litterini, PT, DPT
Survivorship Program Manager
MaineHealth Cancer Care Network, Scarborough
Maine
Associate Clinical Professor
University of New England, Portland
Maine
United States

Holly Lookabaugh-Deur, PT, DSc, GCS, CEEAA
Director of Clinical Services
Clinical Services
Ivy Rehab, Muskegon
Michigan
United States

Cynthia Marsili, PT, Board Certified Oncologic Physical Therapy Specialist, Certified Lymphedema Therapist
Physical Therapist
Rehab and Dialysis Center
Beaumont Health, Streling Heights
Michigan
United States

Mark A. Micale, PhD, FACMGG
Medical Director
Clinical Cytogenomics Laboratory
Associate Professor
Pathology and Laboratory Medicine and Obstetrics & Gynecology
Beaumont Health and Oakland University William Beaumont School of Medicine, Royal Oak
Michigan
United States

Laura Munger, LMSW
Certified in Mindfulness Meditation, Member of Association of Oncology Social Workers
Clinical Social Worker
Rise Counseling Service, Clarkston
Michigan
United States

Alaina Marie Newell, BS in Neuroscience, DPT
Director of Education
ReVital Cancer Rehabilitation
Select Medical, Mechanicsburg
Pennsylvania
United States;
Adjunct Faculty
Physical Therapy
Andrews University, Berrien Spring
Michigan
United States;
Adjunct Faculty
Physical Therapy
South College, Knoxville
Tennessee
United States

Julia C. Osborne, BSc (Hons) PT, CLT-LANA
Board Certified Specialist in Oncological Physical Therapy
Fulbright Specialist for World Learning
Founder and Director of Oncology Rehab and PORi
Oncology Rehabilitation, Centennial
Colorado
United States

Kirk Randall, PT
Physical Therapist and Manager
Outpatient
Mary Free Bed Rehabilitation Hospital, Grand Rapids
Michigan
United States

Sara Rivard, MA, RT(R)(CT)
Program Director and Special Instructor
Radiologic Technology—Clinical and Diagnostic Sciences
Oakland University, Rochester
Michigan
United States

Ursula M. Sansom-Daly, M.Psychol (Clin), PhD
Senior Research Fellow
Behavioural Sciences Unit, School of Women's and Children's Health
University of New South Wales (UNSW) Medicine, UNSW Sydney, Kensington
New South Wales
Australia;
Clinical Psychologist
Sydney Youth Cancer Service
Prince of Wales Hospital, Randwick
New South Wales
Australia

David Joseph Schwarz, PT, DPT, LMT, BBA, NCS
Physical Therapist
Dynamic Movement and Recovery, Grand Rapids
Michigan
United States
Instructor
Dynamic Principles, Grand Rapids
Michigan
United States

Kristina Sitarski, PT, MPT, CLT
Physical Therapist
RehabilitationTherapy Services
Beaumont Health, Dearborn
Michigan
United States

Suzette M. Smith, DPT, Board Certified Specialist in Oncologic Physical Therapy
Physical Therapist
Rehab, Beaumont Health, Troy
Michigan
United States

Bryan Spinelli, PT, PhD
Assistant Professor
Department of Physical Therapy
Thomas Jefferson University, Philadelphia
Pennsylvania
United States

Anne Swisher, PT, PhD, CCS, FAPTA
Professor
Division of Physical Therapy
West Virginia University, Morgantown
West Virginia
United States

Cynthia Tan, MPT, CLT-LANA
Physical Therapist
Outpatient clinic
Mary Free Bed Rehabilitation Hospital, Grand Rapids
Michigan
United States

Taire Thie, PT, DPT
Physical Therapist
Physical Medicine and Rehabilitation
University of Michigan, Ann Arbor
Michigan
United States

Rachel Tran, PT, DPT, NCS
Physical Therapy Manager
Department of Rehabilitation Services
Casa Colina Hospital and Centers for Healthcare, Pomona
California
United States

Frannie Westlake, DPT, Board Certified Neurologic and Oncologic Clinical Specialist
Physical Therapist
Oncology Rehab, Centennial
Colorado
United States

J. Lynne Williams, PhD, MT (ASCP)
Professor Emerita
Clinical & Diagnostic Sciences
Oakland University, Rochester
Michigan
United States

Christopher M. Wilson, PT, DPT, DScPT, Board Certified Geriatric Clinical Specialist
Associate Professor and Director of Clinical Education
Human Movement Science
Oakland University, Rochester
Michigan
United States;
Founding Residency Program Director
Oncology Residency
Beaumont Health, Troy
Michigan
United States

Karen M. Wiseman, PT, DPT, CLT-LANA, ABPTS Board Certified Oncology Rehabilitation Specialist
Physical Therapist
Physical Medicine and Rehabilitation
Beaumont Health, West Bloomfield
Michigan
United States

Courtney Witczak, PT, DPT, GCS
Supervisor of Physical Medicine and Rehabilitation
Physical Medicine and Rehabilitation
Beaumont Health, Troy
Michigan
United States

Biography

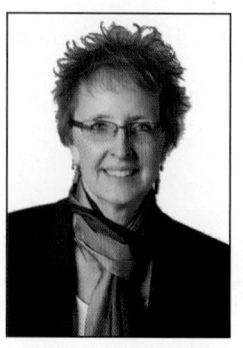

Deborah J. Doherty, PT, PhD

Deborah J. Doherty is the Chair of the Human Movement Science Department and Associate Professor in the Physical Therapy Program at Oakland University in Rochester, Michigan. She is an advanced practitioner in the treatment of patients diagnosed with cancer. Dr. Doherty co-developed the first international online Graduate Certificate for Oncology Rehabilitation Program at Oakland University for physical therapists, occupational therapists, speech language pathologists, and exercise scientists, which began fall of 2012. Her research focus is in Oncology Rehabilitation with an emphasis on Survivorship Programs and Prehabilitation. She is serving as the APTA-Michigan representative to the Michigan Cancer Consortium and has served as a co-chair for the Board of Directors, a member of the membership committee, and the Survivorship Workgroup Chairperson. Dr. Doherty championed the development of the Oncology Rehabilitation Special Interest Group for the APTA-Michigan and now serves as the Research Committee Chairperson. She was awarded the MPTA Oncology Rehabilitation Special Interest Group Honorary Excellence Award and the establishment of the Deborah J. Doherty Oncology Rehabilitation Excellence award. Dr. Doherty is the owner of a Physical Therapy Private Practice called Center for Survivorship. She treats patients diagnosed with cancer throughout the continuum of care. Dr. Doherty received her Bachelor in Science degree in Physical Therapy from Northwestern University, a Master of Arts degree in Health Care Administration from Central Michigan University and a Doctor of Philosophy degree in Anatomy from Michigan State University. She is a 16-year breast cancer survivor and a frequent lecturer on the topic of Oncology Rehabilitation to health care practitioners and survivors.

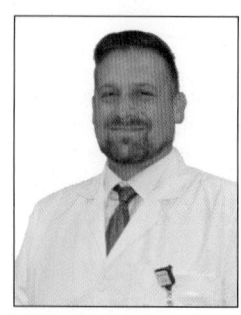

Chris Wilson, PT, DPT, DScPT

Dr. Wilson is an Associate Professor of physical therapy and Director of Clinical Education at Oakland University in Rochester, Michigan and was the founding residency program director for the Beaumont Health Oncology Residency in Troy, Michigan. His clinical focus is Geriatrics and Acute Care Palliative Care. He is active in clinical research in the areas of Oncology, Hospice/Palliative Care, and Geriatrics. Dr. Wilson received his Doctor of Science in Physical Therapy from Oakland University and also earned his Graduate Certificate in Oncology Rehabilitation from Oakland University. He received his transitional Doctor of Physical Therapy from University of St. Augustine with a Primary Care Certification and his Masters in PT from Oakland University. In 2008, Chris obtained his ABPTS Geriatric Clinical Specialist Certification (GCS). He is the author of the book entitled "Physical Activity and Rehabilitation in Life Threatening Illness" published by Routledge in 2021. In the past, Dr. Wilson has served as the Vice President of the Academy of Oncologic Physical Therapy and he was previously the Academy's Hospice Special Interest Group Chair. In addition, he has served as the global coordinator of the Hospice/Palliative Care subgroup for the World Confederation of Physical Therapy.

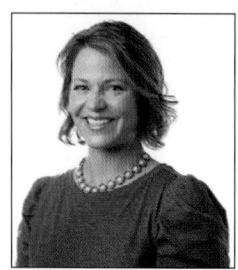

Lori E. Boright, PT, DPT, DScPT

Dr. Boright is an Assistant Professor at Oakland University in the Doctor of Physical Therapy Program. She received her DScPT and Graduate Certificate in Oncology Rehabilitation from Oakland University, transitional DPT from AT Still University, MPT from University of Michigan Flint, and BS in physiology from Michigan State University. She is a Clinical Cancer Exercise Specialist, credentialed by the University of Northern Colorado Cancer Rehabilitation Institute. Her research agenda focuses on primary and secondary disease prevention inclusive of prehabilitation for a variety of cancer diagnoses and upstreaming initiatives for community and population health promotion. Dr. Boright is a practicing physical therapist at Ascension South East Michigan, where she is responsible for leading clinical research initiatives and the development of the Oncology Rehabilitation service line across care settings. Dr. Boright currently serves the American Physical Therapy Association Michigan as Chair of the Oncology Rehabilitation Special Interest Group, the first state-level rehabilitation special interest group dedicated to advocacy and clinical best practice development for persons with oncology diagnoses.

Preface

We are overwhelmed with joy in bringing this important information to the world. Rehabilitation clinicians have been treating persons diagnosed and living with cancer (PDLWCs) for several decades, learning as we go along. The treatment of these persons has become more complex and has developed need as advancements in medical treatments are gratefully keeping persons alive longer; with this improved longevity comes more adverse effects to their functional, physical, social, emotional, and spiritual bodies. The body of knowledge in oncology rehabilitation (Onc R) has grown exponentially, and the editors of this book are thankful for the dedication, skills, and advocacy efforts of those professionals who came before us to expand this area of practice to such an extent that it requires a full-length book to define the depth and breadth of Onc R practice.

Onc R has had a very long and arduous evolution in the fields of physical therapy, occupational therapy, and speech-language pathology. For much of recorded human history, including late into the 20th century, the mortality rate from cancer remained high, long-term rehabilitation, therefore, was not considered a needed intervention. Onc R initially developed a solid foundation in the care of persons diagnosed with breast cancer—frequently focusing on major issues of lymphedema and shoulder joint mobility. As Onc R continued to develop, the field of physiatry or physical medicine and rehabilitation (PM&R) concurrently developed an Onc R specialty that aspires to fill that gap between the oncologists and the therapists. This medical specialty helped to bridge the gap in Onc R but at times may have resulted in a decreased awareness of the Onc R specialty skills of rehabilitation therapists themselves.

With the rapidly growing advancements in medical interventions for PDLWCs, survival rates have improved dramatically. This survival comes at a significant cost to quality of life (QOL). Medical interventions to treat primary or recurring cancer are most often accompanied by a plethora of adverse effects. These adverse effects can be short term but more often than not will last for years or a lifetime when left untreated. These consequential functional deficits and potential decline to a person's QOL can leave a person living with and beyond cancer (PLWBC, often commonly known as a cancer survivor) debating whether the treatments were worth it. For others, these adverse effects mean making substantial modifications to their work, family, and personal lives to accommodate the resultant functional, social, physical, and emotional changes. As therapists, we know that these potential lifetime changes are not inevitable and can frequently be prevented, mitigated, or managed, thereby allowing a person's QOL to be only temporarily compromised. This is a powerful skill of the Onc R therapist to help the person come through their journey recovered, revitalized, and renewed. Unfortunately, some individuals will experience severe challenges and may lose their battle with cancer. However, rehabilitation can provide these beautiful souls with optimized QOL during their journey. The advancement of the field of Onc R has not only provided best practice, and evidence-based treatments for each and every PDLWC but has also provided an avenue for professional growth through the initiation of 1) Onc R residency programs for physical therapists and occupational therapists; and 2) Board Certification as an Onc R Specialist, and with the associated recognition through national professional organizations.

The co-editors for this textbook have combined 86 years of experience in the field of physical therapy. We have witnessed firsthand the lack of rehabilitation services to PLWBCs, the lack of continuity in care, and the myriad barriers to access rehabilitation. The sadness comes from the fact that all PDLWCs can benefit from rehabilitation but due to the barriers in accessing Onc R services, these persons assume tragically that they must live with the functional, physical, social, and emotional deficits. We know that nothing could be farther from the truth. Rehabilitation professionals are the most qualified, knowledgeable, and well positioned clinicians to effectively treat the adverse effects caused from the treatments for cancer. Basic entry level education provides a solid foundation from which to begin. It was clear in our experiences, as well as the many therapists that came before us, that advanced training is the most beneficial to advance this field of study and provide the most evidence-based interventions. Specialization and/or residency is essential to build a level of confidence in Onc R clinicians to handle the complexity of issues that accompany a cancer diagnosis. The complexity of this population is not just within the medical domain but also impacts every social determinant of health, thereby requiring the Onc R clinician to have a depth and breadth of knowledge in a wide variety of cancer diagnoses and domains of health.

As co-editors, we recruited 56 authors from 17 states and 4 countries to walk this incredible journey with us. The overwhelming desire and commitment to participate in this epic journey along with the passion and dedication that accompanied these authors' chapters, brought us indescribable joy. We were all in universal agreement about the urgent need for this textbook to be completed. Many of these incredible authors powered through the writing and development of these chapters during a global pandemic while working on the front lines providing direct patient care in many hospitals and clinics. This truly demonstrates the overwhelming need for expanded access to Onc R services that all therapists believe exists. This is the first book written almost exclusively by Onc R therapists for Onc R therapists. However, the wisdom of these pages is beneficial to any health care practitioner, administrator, insurance company, or policymaker that truly has a desire to understand the needs of PLWBC and change their lives for the better.

The goals of this textbook are five-fold: (1) to serve as a guidebook that can be immediately put to use in the clinic by any rehabilitation professional; (2) to serve as a study guide for physical therapists writing for the American Board of Physical Therapy

Specialties Oncology Specialization Exam; (3) to provide guidance and resource to residents enrolled in Onc R Residency programs; (4) to provide administrators with the understanding of not only developing an Onc R program in the inpatient and outpatient settings, but to truly understand what benefits this programming can provide for PDLWCs and how it can develop Onc R clinicians to their highest levels of clinical expertise; and (5) to educate all other health care practitioners, especially physicians, physician extenders, nurses, social workers, and psychologists in the need for interdisciplinary, multidisciplinary, and interprofessional teams to work with this population.

The greatest challenge in writing this textbook was discerning what information to include as there is so much now available that has never been compiled in one location. Knowledge of the most common adverse effects caused from the treatments for cancer has grown tremendously in the last 20 years. Research has exponentially increased due to the palpable need for evidence but also the obvious and immense benefits achieved through Onc R. As clinicians, we have all looked into the faces of PLWBCs and heard their frustrations and cries of wanting a better life, closer to what they had before their cancer diagnosis. The common adverse effects, such as pain, muscle weakness, lymphedema, cardiotoxicity, cancer-related cognitive impairment, chemotherapy-induced polyneuropathy, and fatigue have become the foundational areas of Onc R. Although historically considered in only the most common cancers, these adverse effects have become recognized in all cancer diagnoses and are now also considered within the context of significant social and emotional challenges that can greatly impact the recovery and rehabilitation of each PLWBC. Again, historically rehabilitation professionals were only considered as

interventionists and would only be consulted to provide interventions after an issue or illness had already impacted a person's functional status. Now, rehabilitation has expanded into five levels of prevention (primordial, primary, secondary, tertiary, and quaternary). Onc R clinicians have a significant role to play in each area of prevention, making this complex area of study and clinical treatment one of the most challenging, demanding, and rewarding areas of clinical practice.

Crosswalk with Key American Physical Therapy Association Documents

This textbook has been carefully developed and is designed to be in line with key public documents for specialty practice and residency practice for physical therapists.

The American Physical Therapy Association has developed the Description of Specialty Practice (DSP) for those pursuing board certification as an oncologic specialist and the Description of Residency Practice (DRP) for those involved with oncologic residency programs.

To access this crosswalk, please visit the Evolve website at https://evolve.elsevier.com for the Crosswalk spreadsheet which will provide the location within this book where key content recommended by the oncologic DSP and DRP can be found. For the full versions of the DSP and DRP, visit www.apta.org.

The Description of Specialty Practice and Description of Residency Practice are copyright of the American Physical Therapy Association. All rights reserved. Excerpted with permission.

Foreword

As a clinician, academician, and researcher in the field of cancer and human immunodeficiency virus (HIV) rehabilitation for nearly four decades, I am pleased to witness the compilation of this text to guide clinicians to the highest level of oncology rehabilitation practice. When rehabilitation in this area was limited across the country during the early 1980s, my training at MD Anderson Cancer Center in Houston provided a strong foundation. Joining the *Oncology Section of the American Physical Therapy Association* (APTA), I found a small but mighty group of colleagues eager to advance this important aspect of rehabilitation. We thank our founding members who envisioned a world where individuals living with a cancer diagnosis encapsulated the spirit of *living life to the fullest*.

As the research chair of our Oncology Section for a decade, I have had the pleasure of leading committee members who are committed to advancing the science in this area and appreciating the magnitude of patient impact across all sections of the APTA. Thus, our national conference programming incorporated educational sessions that adroitly intersected all component sections of the APTA; severity of cancer stage, acute and chronic intervention management, multi-system impact, and age of the survivor. Cancer touches all who engage in clinical practice and we were determined to interrogate the available evidence and educate accordingly through our published work.

The formulation of the *Evaluation Database to Guide Effectiveness* (EDGE) dedicated Task Force teams for various cancer diagnoses, catapulted our members to research and publish systematic reviews for application across the cancer spectrum in clinical practice. Published clinical practice guidelines now foster translational evidence for high impact treatment for all cancer survivors. Through these formal efforts, we have created best practices to serve all cancer patients and all clinicians.

We are now on the global map of cancer recovery, because of the work of dedicated clinicians, researchers, member organizations, and policy makers who know that cancer recovery must go beyond physical rehabilitation. Because of this work, clinical practice guidelines are now incorporated into diagnosis and treatment to optimize care of cancer survivors. Our *Rehabilitation Oncology Journal* provides a forum for rehabilitation reach in high impact research and reporting. Collaborating with other colleagues further demonstrates the value of our care. Rehabilitation used to be necessary after life-saving procedures. Now we know that rehabilitation must encompass the mind and spirit as well as the body, often through targeted interventions through a lifetime. We know that every diagnosis and recovery has its challenges and every patient—no matter their age—needs specialized support. What was a privilege before is now a mandate, and this collection allows that mandated rehabilitation of mind, body, and spirit will be accomplished by interprofessional teams with the patient at the helm of their cancer journey.

From an international perspective, I witnessed through my Fulbright in South Africa the need for cancer rehabilitation education and program implementation and this guiding text will cultivate greater capacity to address the needs of cancer survivors globally. As the representative for the APTA Commission on Cancer (COC), I have been able to forge new accreditation standards for oncology rehabilitation and survivorship, enacted as of 2020. Such a change underscores the great urgency for this text. Oncology rehabilitation has evolved over the last four decades of my involvement with continued growth of membership and colleagues who forged a pathway to high impact care.

Our former "Section" and now "Academy" has cultivated specialization and momentum for emerging researcher and clinical experts. The practice of oncology rehabilitation presents unique challenges that make assessing and improving the patient experience especially complex yet invigorating. Those affected by a cancer diagnosis feel a compelling urgency to treat for cure, and if cure is not possible, ameliorate or address the side effects of treatment. Oncology rehabilitation fills those gaps and provides hope for reclamation of oneself through the journey with a cancer diagnosis.

Oftentimes, students arrive to oncology rehabilitation through a personal experience and receive varying information across DPT curriculum in accredited programs. The editors developed a collaborative cancer rehabilitation course track at Oakland University which serves as a model for other programs and this text complements teaching resources within a graduate curriculum. For the clinician, this text will open doors to guide students and enhance clinical decision and practice with various cancer populations. For the administrative aspects of oncology rehabilitation, this book will guide clinicians and proffer opportunities *"at the table"* to leverage rehabilitation services within COC accredited cancer centers across the United States.

As we know, a book like this is a labor of love. The editors of this book are dedicated to the highest level of clinical practice, research, and advocacy in the field of oncology rehabilitation from the point of diagnosis through survivorship. Kudos to the authors of this rich textbook, which is sorely needed to provide foundational education, a key resource for academicians teaching this important topic and clinicians in all types of clinical practice. This stellar effort has given us a detailed and illuminating picture of the myriad of challenges encountered in cancer survivorship. As the number of oncology rehabilitation specialists grow, we appreciate the richness of approaches to integrative cancer rehabilitation, continued development of clinical practice guidelines and knowledge translation ultimately for the highest good of all cancer survivors. It is the beginning of great things.

I view oncology rehabilitation through many lenses, as a clinician, researcher, breast cancer survivor and co-survivor, and am fortunate to be the recipient of my colleagues' exquisite care. Since my initial diagnosis, we have witnessed incredible advancement in cancer precision treatment and elevated the role of cancer rehabilitation. This book serves as a guide to entry level curriculum and clinicians with an eye toward critical future research needs, with guiding questions to test knowledge and case studies to illuminate complexities of care. This book brings together interprofessional experts from around the world to address rehabilitation from multiple perspectives. Through the presentation of five distinct units, the authors provide foundational concepts, effect of cancer treatments by systems, management of common cancer diagnosis, important considerations, and administrative aspects of oncology rehabilitation. The

editors' broad goals capture the value of oncology rehabilitation in a complete and nuanced way, and better inform decisions regarding developing, evaluating, prescribing, and advocating for cancer rehabilitation.

In the spirit of survivorship and continued momentum, I wish the reader a journey of impact, innovation, and an urge to join collaborative clinical and research efforts as you reap the pearls of knowledge through this text. Your impact on this inspiring population will lead you to an everlasting appreciation for determination, resilience, and capturing the fullness of life!

Mary Lou Galantino

Contents

Unit V: Administrative Aspects of Oncology Rehabilitation

Video Contents

UNIT I

Foundational Oncology Concepts

1

Fundamentals of Cancer

AMY J. LITTERINI, PT, DPT, ROCHELLE I. BRANNAN,
MPT, CLT-LANA, AND DEBORAH J. DOHERTY, PT, PhD

CHAPTER OUTLINE

What Is Cancer?

Cancer is a superordinate for a collection of diseases which share common characteristics. Some of these characteristics include uncontrolled cell proliferation, prevention of cells to self-destruct through normal cell triggers (apoptosis), spread of abnormal cells to other tissues in the body (metastasis) through the blood, lymph, transcoelomic, perineural invasion or direct extension, modification of the microenvironment, and evasion of immune surveillance.[1] Most carcinogens are believed to originate from a single cell that has become damaged or corrupted through a series of alterations to the DNA.[2] These mutations are the result of actual sequence changes in the DNA that may originate from exposure to carcinogens (e.g., physical or chemical carcinogens or oncogenic viruses). Some researchers categorize the DNA changes as occurring from genotoxic mechanisms and contrast that to nongenotoxic mechanisms that do not directly affect DNA, for example, immunosuppression-induced tissue inflammation.[2] While the most common theory for the development of cancer has been the progressive series of genetic aberrations and mutations of genes (including oncogenes and tumor suppressor genes), the evidence is building to suggest that epigenetic modifications are also responsible for a wide range of heritable changes in gene expression with no alteration in DNA sequence.[3] Most cancers are nonfamilial while a small percentage occur through certain family germline mutations. Cancers develop from the accumulation of genetic and epigenetic changes to the human body.[4] Genetic changes can result from aging, mutagenic chemicals, aflatoxins from fungus, radiation, smoking, ultraviolet light, and oxygen radicals. Epigenetic changes also include aging and smoking but to a larger extent chronic inflammation, ulcerative colitis, *Helicobacter pylori* infection-triggered gastritis, hepatitis B and hepatitis C infection triggered hepatitis, and estrogen.[4]

Field cancerization, also known as field defect or field effect, is another expanding area of study that should be considered when discussing cancer. Field cancerization is the process of transformation of an existing genetic and/or epigenetic precancerous lesion into a malignancy. For example, oral field cancerization causes the development of cancer at various rates in response to a carcinogen, such as tobacco. This leads to the development of abnormal tissues around a tumorigenic area, even after complete surgical removal which is considered the precursor for second primary tumors and recurrences.[5] Please see Chapter 4 for further information on pathology.

Epidemiology

The Burden of Cancer in the United States and Globally

Cancer is a leading cause of death in every country globally and cancer is considered a major barrier to increasing life expectancy.[6] Cancer is the second leading cause of death in the United States (US) and the leading cause of death worldwide. There were 1,806,590 new cases of cancer diagnosed in the US in 2020 and 18.1 million new cases (excluding nonmelanoma skin cancer) were diagnosed globally.[6-8] Deaths from cancer numbered 606,520 (US) and 9.5 million worldwide.[6-8] Sadly, 16,850 (US)[9] and 400,000 (global) children and adolescents (0–19 years) were diagnosed with cancer.[10] At the same time 1780 (US)[9] children died from cancer. Global data is not available, however the World Health Organization (WHO) reports more than 80% of children diagnosed with cancer are cured in high-income countries.[10] They also report that only about 15% to 45% are cured in low- and middle-income countries (LMICs).[9] The most common childhood cancers are leukemias, brain cancers, lymphomas, and solid tumors, such as neuroblastoma and Wilms tumor (see Chapter 25 for information on pediatric cancers).[9] The burden of cancer including both incidence and mortality are growing fast globally, secondary to aging, population growth as well as changes in risk factors, especially socioeconomic.[6]

The five most common adult cancers in descending order of cases in the US are breast, lung and bronchus, prostate, colon and rectum, and melanoma of the skin.[7] Globally they are lung, breast, colorectal, prostate, and skin (nonmelanoma).[6] The three most common cancers in men are prostate, lung, and colorectal and they account for an estimated 43% of all cancers diagnosed in men. Breast, lung, and colorectal cancers account for approximately 50% of all new cancer diagnoses in women in 2020.[6]

Based on 2013–2017 data, the cancer incidence or rate of new cases of cancer is currently 442.4 per 100,000 women and men annually and cancer mortality or cancer death rate is 158.3 per 100,000 women and men annually. Based on race/ethnicity and sex, cancer mortality is lowest in Asian/Pacific Islander women (85.6 per 100,000) and highest in African American men (227.3 per 100,000). The cancer mortality rate currently is higher among men (189.5 per 100,000) than women (135.7 per 100,000 women).[9]

Cancer survivorship is increasing rapidly with an estimated 16.9 million cancer survivors in the US[8] and 43.8 million globally.[11] It is estimated that roughly 39.5% of men and women will be diagnosed with cancer during their lifetime.[7] The number of new cancer cases annually is expected to increase to 29.5 million and the number of cancer-related deaths are expected to increase to 16.4 million by 2040.[7]

The statistics for the incidence and prevalence of cancers can be found in very reliable sources. See Table 1.1.

Hallmarks of Cancer

In 2000, Drs. Hanahan and Weinberg extensively studied the research and science of the development of cancer in the human animal. In their comprehensive review they describe the multistep progressive conversion of normal human cells into cancer cells. The authors suggest that the "vast catalog of cancer cell genotypes is a manifestation of six essential alterations in cell physiology that collectively dictate malignant growth."[12] Figure 1.1 illuminates the six characteristics that most, if not all, human tumors share.

The six characteristics depicted in Figure 1.1 are[13]:
1. Self-sufficiency in growth signals—tumor cells will grow even though they are not getting a message to grow.
2. Insensitivity to anti-growth signals—a cancer cell will ignore messages telling it to stop growing.
3. Evading apoptosis—a cancer cell will ignore a signal that is informing the cell that it is time to die.
4. Limitless replicative potential—all malignant cancer cells maintain the ability to replicate and eventually pick up more mutations.
5. Sustained angiogenesis or creation of blood supply—cells need nutrients to survive so they initiate the formation of new blood vessels that will provide for their growth via the process of "sustained angiogenesis."
6. Tissue invasion and metastasis—cancer cells invade nearby tissues or distant organs by leaving their original site to form new colonies and secondary tumors.

Most cancers acquire these six characteristics, however, the pathway to this acquisition is extremely variable. The mechanism of occurrence and the order in which they are achieved is very inconsistent and unpredictable.

TABLE 1.1 Cancer Statistic Resources	
Cancer Statistics	**Websites**
American Cancer Society (ACS)	https://www.cancer.org/research/cancer-facts-statistics/all-cancer-facts-figures/cancer-facts-figures-2020.html
Cancer Atlas by American Cancer Society (ACS), International Agency for Research on Cancer (IARC), and Union for International Cancer Control (UICC)	http://canceratlas.cancer.org/the-burden/
Cancer Stat Facts	https://seer.cancer.gov/statfacts/
Center for Disease Control (CDC)	https://www.youtube.com/watch?v=MJp4Ifboltw
IARC	https://gco.iarc.fr/
National Cancer Institute (NCI)	https://www.cancer.gov/about-cancer/understanding/statistics
SEER—Surveillance, Epidemiology and End Results Program	https://seer.cancer.gov/
Rare Cancers—NCI	https://www.youtube.com/watch?v=ES5KyIRT1qY
World Health Organization (WHO) Cancer	https://www.who.int/news-room/fact-sheets/detail/cancer

Created by Amy J. Litterini. Printed with permission.

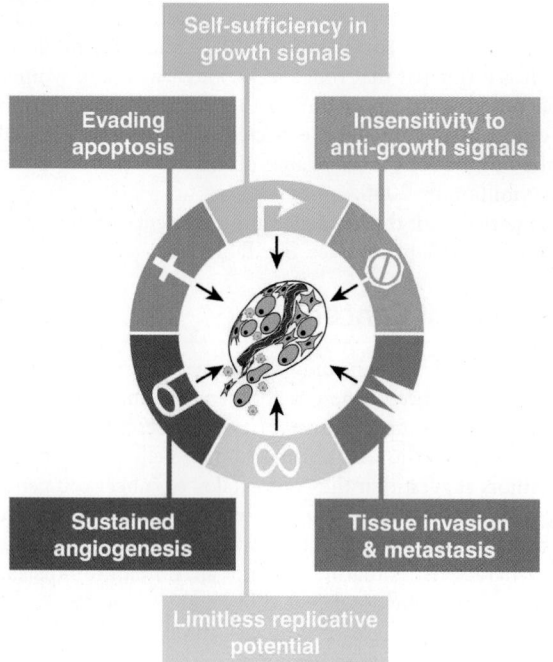

• **Fig. 1.1** Six Characteristics of Cancer Cells. (Reprinted with permission from Hanahan D, Weinberg RA. The hallmarks of cancer. *Cell.* 2000;100(1):57–70).

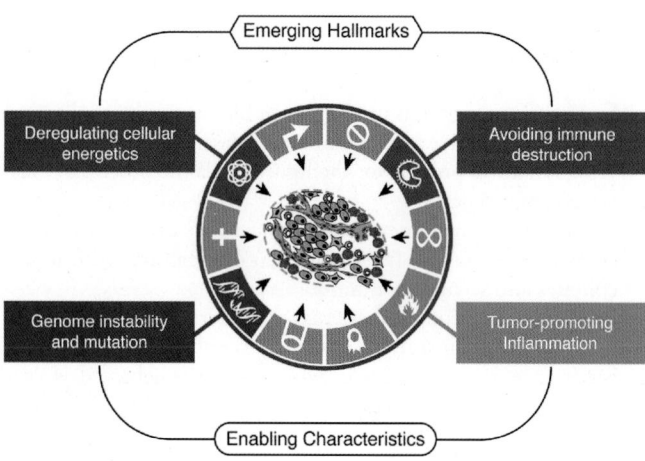

• **Fig. 1.2** Two Characteristics and Two Emerging Hallmarks. (Reprinted with permission from Hanahan D, Weinberg RA. Hallmarks of cancer: the next generation. *Cell.* 2011;144(5):646–674.)

After a decade of research, these same investigators proposed two more enabling characteristics underlying the ability of the original six hallmarks that allow cancer cells to survive, proliferate, and disseminate (Figure 1.2).[13] The first characteristic is genome instability and mutations which focus on the genetic diversity and the generation of random mutations including chromosomal rearrangements. The second characteristic is tumor-promoting inflammation of premalignant and malignant lesions that is driven by cells of the immune system. The authors have also added two emerging hallmarks. The first of which is deregulating cellular energetics that involves reprogramming of cellular energy metabolism to replace the normal metabolic program and support continuous cell growth and proliferation. The second emerging hallmark is avoiding immune destruction. This process protects cancer cells from attack and elimination by immune cells. Finally, the tumor

complexity does not end with the tumor itself; normal cells are recruited to create a tumor microenvironment that assists in the acquisition of the six hallmarks from the cells there.[13]

Cancer Classifications

Cancer has been classified utilizing various systems. Included below are four common classification methods: (1) histologic type; (2) tissue type; (3) amine precursor uptake and decarboxylation system (APUD); and (4) anatomic site.

Cancer Classification—Histologic Type[14]

Cancers can be broadly divided into six major classifications by histologic type: carcinoma, sarcoma, myeloma, leukemia, lymphoma, and mixed histological types. Table 1.2 provides a brief description of each histologic cancer type describing each cancer tissue origination. Subsequent chapters will describe each of these cancers in greater detail (see Table 1.2).

Cancer Classification—Tissue Type[15]

Cancers can also be classified by tissue type. This classification indicates the tissue where the cancer originates. Table 1.3 lists eight major histological types of cancer, the tissue subcategories, and the types of tumors that are found in each, including benign and malignant. Benign tumors are defined as an unusual growth or mass that is not cancerous, does not invade nearby tissue, and

TABLE 1.2	Cancer Classification by Histologic Type

Carcinoma
- Malignant neoplasm of epithelial origin
- Epithelial tissue covers body organs, the gastrointestinal tract and the skin
- Epithelial cancers account for 80%–90% of all cancer cases
  Two major carcinoma subtypes exist:
1. Adenocarcinoma
2. Squamous cell carcinoma
Generally, adenocarcinomas are found in the secreting organs and glands of the body. Common primary carcinoma sites include: breasts, lungs, colon, and prostate bladder.

Sarcoma
- Cancer originating in supportive and connective tissues
- Sarcoma tumors highly resemble the tissue in which it originates

Myeloma
- Cancer originating in the plasma cells of bone marrow
- The plasma cells produce some of the proteins found in blood

Leukemias
- Liquid cancer originating in the blood or bone marrow
- Both red and white blood cells can be affected by bone marrow diseases

Lymphomas
- Cancer originating in the lymphatic system—gland and nodes
- Lymphomas can occur in stomach, breast, and brain

Mixed histological types
- Cross-over between cancer types or within same histological type
- Examples include adenosquamous carcinoma, mixed mesodermal tumors, and gonadal tumors

Created by Rochelle I. Brannon. Printed with permission.

TABLE 1.3   Cancer Classification by Tissue Type

Tissue	Benign Tumors	Malignant Tumors
Bone and Cartilage		
Adult fibrous tissue	Fibroma	Fibrosarcoma
Embryonic myxomatous fibrous tissue	Myxoma	Myxosarcoma
Fat	Lipoma	Liposarcoma
Cartilage	Chondroma	Chondrosarcoma
Bone	Osteoma	Osteosarcoma
Notochord	—	Chordoma
Connective tissue, probably fibrous	Fibrous histiocytoma	Malignant fibrous histiocytoma
Endothelium and Mesothelium		
Blood vessels	Hemangioma Hemangiopericytoma	Hemangiosarcoma Angiosarcoma
Lymph vessels	Lymphangioma	Lymphangiosarcoma
Blood and Lymphoid Cells		
Hematopoietic cells	Pre-leukemias Myeloproliferative disorders	Leukemia, of various types; aleukemic leukemia
Lymphoid tissue	Plasmacytosis	Plasmacytoma Multiple myeloma Hodgkin lymphoma Non-Hodgkin lymphoma
Muscle		
Smooth muscle	Leiomyoma	Leiomyosarcoma
Straited muscle	Rhabdomyoma	Rhabdomyosarcoma
Epithelial Tissue		
Stratified squamous	Papilloma Seborrheic keratosis, some skin adnexal tumors	Squamous cell carcinoma Epidermoid carcinoma and some malignant skin adnexal tumors
Glandular epithelium	Adenoma	Adenocarcinoma
Liver	Hepatic adenoma	Hepatoma: hepatocellular carcinoma
Kidney	Renal tubular adenoma	Renal cell carcinoma Hypernephroma
Bile duct	Bile duct adenoma	Cholangiocarcinoma
Transitional epithelium	Transitional cell papilloma	Transitional cell carcinoma
Placenta	Hydatidiform mole	Choriocarcinoma
Testis	—	Seminoma Embryonal cell carcinoma
Neural		
Glial cells (several types)	—	Glioma, grades I–III Anaplastic Glioblastoma multiforme (grade IV)
Nerve cells	— — Ganglioneuroma	Ganglioneuroma Medulloblastoma
Meninges	Meningioma	Malignant meningioma
Nerve sheath	Schwannoma Neurilemmoma Neurofibroma	Malignant meningioma Malignant schwannoma Neurofibrosarcoma
Other Neural Crest-Derived Cell		
Pigment-producing cells in skin, eyes, and occasional other sites	Nevus	Melanoma
Schwann cells of peripheral nervous system	Schwannoma or Neurilemmoma	Malignant schwannoma
Merkel cells in squamous epithelium (unknown function)	—	Merkel cell neoplasm (similar to oat cell)

Created by Rochelle I. Brannon. Printed with permission.

does not spread to other parts of the body. Malignant tumors (neoplasms) are an abnormal growth of cells that can invade surrounding tissues and metastasize into other areas of the body. Not listed in Table 1.3 are gonadal tumors (tumors of the ovary or testis) which cannot be classified by tissue type since they involve a variety of tissue cell types.

Cancer Classification—Amine Precursor Uptake and Decarboxylation System[16]

A more recent classification of cancer is the APUD system. The APUD system is based on cells having an endocrine function which secrete small amine or polypeptide hormones (see Table 1.4).

Cancer Classification—Anatomic Site[17]

Another method for classification of cancer is by the anatomic site in which the cancer originates. Table 1.5 lists the common primary cancer sites along with typical associated histological tissue type and other characteristics.

Common Terms and Definitions

Common terminology is important for concise and accurate communication with other health care professionals, insurance companies, and in clinical documentation. The oncologic terminology is extensive. One reliable and comprehensive resource for this terminology is through the National Cancer Institute (NCI) at https://www.cancer.gov/publications/dictionaries/cancer-terms/. Other terms for cancer include malignant neoplasm, tumor, malignancy, and carcinoma. Most of the common terms will be defined throughout the text.

Dysplasia is defined as the presence of abnormal cells within a tissue or organ. Dysplasia is not cancer, but it may sometimes become cancer. Dysplasia can be mild, moderate, or severe, depending on how abnormal the cells look under a microscope

and how much of the tissue or organ is affected. *Hyperplasia* is an increase in the number of cells in an organ or tissue that appear normal under a microscope. Although they are not cancer, they may become cancer. *Metaplasia* is the next step where a change of cells occurs creating a form that does not normally occur in the tissue in which it is found. Finally, *neoplasia* is defined as abnormal and uncontrolled cell growth that can be classified as benign or malignant.

It is also important to be aware of the difference among the terms: Primary versus secondary, versus second primary tumors. *Primary tumor*—first or original cancerous cells located in a specific organ, structure, or region of the body. This specific cancer is diagnosed through microscopic biopsy. *Secondary tumor*—cancer cells that have metastasized to another area from primary site that can be diagnosed through microscopic biopsy. For example, a patient is found to have cancer cells in the prostate, bladder, and rectum. Cells from all three areas were examined under a microscope. It was determined that cells in all three areas were prostate cancer cells. Thus, the prostate was the primary tumor, while the bladder and the rectum were secondary tumors. *Second Primary tumor*—a new primary tumor determined by microscopic diagnosis that is unrelated to the first primary tumor. In the example above, if the prostate cancer cells were found in the prostate and bladder, and colon cancer cells were found in the colon, the colon cancer would be considered a second primary tumor.

This is an important concept to remember. The primary tumor diagnosed determines the medical treatment. Even if the primary tumor metastasizes to another location, the treatment is for the primary tumor. If a second primary tumor develops, then it has to be properly diagnosed and a treatment will be determined. For example, if a person is diagnosed with breast cancer, the chemotherapy treatment, if needed, is very specifically targeted to the breast cancer. If the breast cancer metastasizes to the lungs, it is still breast cancer cells in the lung so the treatment is based on the breast cancer diagnosis. However, if upon biopsy, it is found that there is a second primary cancer, as evidenced by lung cancer cells visible, there will also be an additional treatment provided

TABLE 1.4   APUD System (Amine Precursor Uptake and Decarboxylation)

Tissue	Benign Tumors	Malignant Tumors
Pituitary	Basophilic adenoma Eosinophilic adenoma Chromophobe adenoma	— — —
Parathyroid	Parathyroid adenoma	Parathyroid carcinoma
Thyroid (C cells)	C cell hyperplasia	Medullary carcinoma of thyroid
Bronchial lining (Kultschitzky cells)	—	Bronchial carcinoid; oat cell carcinoma
Adrenal medulla Pheochromocytoma	Pheochromocytoma	Malignant pheochromocytoma
Pancreas	Islet cell adenoma Insulinoma Gastrinoma	Islet cell carcinoma
Stomach and intestines	Carcinoid	Malignant carcinoid
Carotid body and chemo-receptor system	Chemodectoma Paraganglioma	Malignant carcinoid Malignant paraganglioma

Created by Rochelle I. Brannon. Printed with permission.

TABLE 1.5 Cancer Classification—Anatomic Site

Skin
Three main histological tissue types:
- Basalcell carcinoma
- Squamouscell carcinoma
- Melanoma

Lung
Two main histological tissue types:
- Non small cell lung cancer
- Small cell lung cancer

Breast
Female
Adenocarcinoma
- Most common breast cancer histological tissue classified as either noninvasive or invasive carcinoma

Noninvasive adenocarcinoma
- Ductal carcinoma in situ (DCIS)
- Lobular carcinoma in situ (LCIS)

Two most common invasive adenocarcinomas
- Invasive ductal carcinoma (IDC) 70%–80% of all women breast cancers
- Invasive lobular carcinoma (ILC)

Male
- Breast carcinoma, rare, less than 1% of all breast cancers

https://www.cancer.gov/types/breast/hp/male-breast-treatment-pdq#_1

Prostate
Adenocarcinoma
- Most common prostate histological tissue type
- Most common male cancer
- Second leading cause of male cancer deaths in the US

Colorectal
Adenocarcinoma
- Most common colorectal histological tissue type
- Fourth leading cancer diagnosed in the US

https://seer.cancer.gov/statfacts/html/colorect.html

Cervix and Uterus
Cervical
- Most commonly linked to Human papillomavirus (HPV)

Uterine
Two main histological tissue types
Adenocarcinoma
- Endometrial cancer
- 80% of uterine cancers

Sarcoma
- Uterine sarcoma
- 2%–4% of uterine cancers

https://www.cancer.net/cancer-types/uterine-cancer

Created by Rochelle I. Brannon. Printed with permission.

TABLE 1.6 Modifiable Risk Factor

A high proportion of deaths from common cancer types is attributable to one or more of the top risk factors for the worldwide burden of disease.[19]

Tobacco Usage
Cigarette smoking reduces life expectancy approximately 10 years.[20] Cigarette smoke is known to accelerate the aging process.[21]

Body Mass Index
Excess body weight is linked to the increased risk of many types of cancer such as esophagus; pancreas, thyroid, gallbladder, colon, and rectum; breast (postmenopausal), endometrium, and kidney.
Visceral adipose tissue produces cytokines that create chronic inflammation and promote tumor growth through multiple biologic mechanisms.[21]

Co-morbidities
Type 2 diabetes is associated with an increased risk of developing cancer of the colon; breast (postmenopausal) and pancreas.[21]

Poor Nutrition
Unhealthy diet is characterized by low intake of fruits and vegetables.
Low fruit and vegetable intake are linked to colon and stomach cancers.[19]
Consumption of red and processed meat is linked to colorectal cancers.[22]

Excessive Alcohol Consumption
Evidence exists to support a linear dose-response relationship between alcohol intake and increased cancer risk, with no safe level of consumption.[23]

Viral Infections
Unsafe sex, increases the transmission of infectious (human papillomaviruses, hepatitis B, hepatitis C viruses, and *Helicobacter pylori*) which are leading causes of cervical, liver, and stomach cancers, respectively.[19] Oncogenic HPV is associated with cervical, vulvar, vaginal, penile, anal, and oropharyngeal cancers with increasing incidence after age 50 years secondary to less condom use and healthcare professionals failing to ask about unsafe sexual behaviors. HIV infections are associated with increased risk of non-AIDS cancers (e.g., anal cancer, Hodgkin disease, liver cancer). Safe sex practices are needed throughout aging process to reduce cancer risk (HPV or HIV infection).[21]

Occupational Exposures
Chemical and physical agents: Environmental carcinogens and many known human carcinogens (e.g., asbestos, benzene, formaldehyde, radon, and ultraviolet (UV) radiation) are highly prevalent in the general environment, as consumer product, or the workplace.[21]

Ultraviolet Radiation Exposure
Meta-analysis of sunburns and melanoma concluded that sunburn at any age increases the risk of cutaneous melanoma, suggesting the importance of preventing excessive sun exposure not only among the young, but also across the life span. [22] UV radiation and indoor tanning was linked to 96.0% of melanoma diagnosis elicobacter in men and 93.7% of melanoma diagnosis of the skin in women. [24]

Created by Rochelle I. Brannon. Printed with permission.

specifically for the lung cancer diagnosis (i.e., surgery, chemotherapy, immunotherapy, etc).

Risk Factors

Only 5% to 10% of all cancers are considered a result of inherited genetic mutations.[18] The remainder of the risk factors are largely modifiable and/or epigenetic factors. There is increasing research on lifestyle behaviors that can decrease the risk for cancers. Onc R clinicians are well-positioned to be advocates and educators of healthy lifestyles to decrease the risk factors (see Table 1.6).

| TABLE 1.7 | Nonmodifiable Risk Factors |

Age

Cancer is considered an age-related disease. Cumulative risk for all cancers combined increases with age, up to age 70 years then decreases slightly.[21] In the complex aging process, epigenetic alterations such as DNA methylation is an emerging area of cancer research.[25] Genomic instability and epigenetic alteration are considered cancer hallmarks.

Genetic Make-up

Genetic testing is often recommended for a patient with a family cancer history to determine the inherited cancer risk. In the complex aging process, epigenetic alterations such as DNA methylation is an emerging area of cancer research.[26] Genomic instability and epigenetic alteration are considered cancer hallmarks. Inherited genetic mutations increase cancer risk:

1. Rare genetic mutations such as those causing neurofibromatosis, tuberous sclerosis, Li-Fraumeni syndrome and Von Hippel-Lindau (VHL) disease increase risk.[27]
2. BRCA1 or BRCA 2 breast cancer, ovarian cancer, male breast cancer, prostate cancer.
3. Colon and rectum cancer have an inherited risk factor when certain gene changes linked to familial adenomatous polyposis (FAP) or hereditary nonpolyposis colon cancer (HNPCC) (previously known as Lynch syndrome) are present.[28]
4. Inherited leukemia conditions present with increased cancer risk.

Gender

Lifetime probability of developing cancer is 44.85% for males, and 38.08% for females. The common cancers have the highest male-to-female (M:F) ratio: colorectal cancers: 1.35; lung and bronchus: 1.52; non-Hodgkin lymphoma (NHL): 1.44; (urinary) bladder: 4.0.[9] Other than breast cancer, which rarely occurs in males, only a few cancers are more common in females. Gall bladder, anus, and thyroid tumors consistently show an M:F ratio less than 1.0.[29]

Racial/Ethnic Groups

For all cancers and races/ethnicities combined, women are more likely to be diagnosed with cancer compared to men. Men are more likely to die from the disease.[30] African American men have the highest death rate for all combined cancer sites.[30] African Americans have higher incidence rates compared to Caucasians for colon and rectum; esophageal, kidney and renal pelvis; larynx; liver and intrahepatic bile duct; lung and bronchial; multiple myeloma; prostate; and stomach cancers.[27] Hispanic and American Indian/Alaska Native women have higher rates of cervical cancer compared to other racial/ethnic groups. African American women have the highest death rate from cervical cancer. African American women are almost twice as likely as Caucasian women to be diagnosed with triple-negative breast cancer.[31] Cancer disparities are an interplay of genetics, socioeconomic factors, insurance status, culture, diet, stress, and the environment.

Created by Rochelle I. Brannon. Printed with permission.

Nonmodifiable risk factors:

Risk factors that cannot be controlled or modified by the application of an intervention are termed nonmodifiable risk factors including: age, genetic make-up, gender, and race (see Table 1.7). Onc R clinicians educate their patients and the community on these risk factors.

Signs and Symptoms of Cancer

The diagnosis of cancer is confirmed with the identification of multiple different diseases, with the presentation of each specific cancer substantially varied based on factors such as location and tissue of origin, tumor size, adjacent anatomical structures involved, aggressiveness of cell type and grade, and the individual themselves. Theoretically, this variability could result in a multitude of *signs* (observed by others) and *symptoms* (experienced by the individual), with wide ranging levels of intensity.[32] General signs and symptoms of cancer include[33]:

1. Unexplained weight loss (associated with cancers of the esophagus, pancreas, stomach, and lung)
2. Fever (associated with leukemia and lymphoma)
3. Fatigue (associated with leukemia, colon, and gastric cancers)
4. Pain (associated with cancers of the bone and brain, as well as testicular, colorectal, and ovarian cancers)
5. Skin changes (e.g., hyperpigmentation, jaundice, erythema, and pruritis)

For the benefit of public health regarding education for cancer awareness, the presentation of commonly occurring cancers often provides classic warning signs. These include[34]:

1. Changes in bowel habits or bladder function
2. A lesion that does not heal
3. White patches or plaques in the mouth or on the tongue
4. Unusual bleeding or discharge
5. Thickening or lump in the breast or elsewhere
6. Indigestion or difficulty in swallowing
7. An obvious change in a wart or mole
8. A nagging cough or hoarseness

For the general public, the accurate recognition of well-documented warning signs and symptoms as indicative of a cancer diagnosis is often problematic. Global public health efforts have targeted awareness campaigns regarding the observation of cancer warnings, in an attempt to promote early detection via screening. From an educational standpoint, the WHO recommends consideration of primary prevention education strategies regarding the classic warning signs of cancer as early diagnosis of breast, cervix, head and neck, colorectal, and skin cancers as critical in reducing the global cancer burden with the early initiation of treatment.[35] Cultural and socioeconomic status influences associated with healthcare disparities have been observed and should be considered in the awareness of cancer signs and symptoms, as well as one's general attitude towards the initiation of early treatment.

In an attempt to address the disproportionate presentation of individuals with advanced cancer in the United Kingdom (UK), the Cancer Awareness Measure (CAM) was developed to identify the general ability to recall and/or recognize cancer warning signs, and identify barriers to seeking care for suspicious symptoms.[32] In a survey of 2216 adults in the UK (970 males, 1246 females), awareness of cancer warning signs was greater on open-ended/

recognition questions rather than closed/recall questions. Overall, the lowest levels of awareness were noted in men, younger respondents, individuals of lower socioeconomic status, and ethnic minorities.[32] Noted barriers to help-seeking behavior included logistical and practical difficulties such as making an appointment or being too busy, and emotional concerns such as worry regarding wasting the provider's time, and/or what might be found in an appointment.[32] One study investigated cancer suspicion associated with the experience of a cancer warning sign.[36] In a survey mailed to 9,771 healthy adults over the age of 50 in the UK, ten classic warning signs of cancer were provided. For those having experienced any of the warning signs identified (noted by 1732 of the 3756 respondents), suspicion for cancer as a potential causative factor was quite low (3.6%). Overall, suspicion for cancer was lowest in individuals with less educated backgrounds (odds ratio [OR] = 0.34, confidence interval [CI]: 0.20–0.59).[36] Additionally, lower socioeconomic status was correlated with delayed awareness of diagnosis, reduced engagement in help-seeking behaviors, and advanced stage disease at the time of presentation.[36]

Ideally, patients with a history of cancer are provided with appropriate education regarding the indicators of cancer recurrence and/or metastasis. The presentation of new physical symptoms such as unexplained pain (e.g., bone pain), neurologic symptoms, profound fatigue, abdominal distension, and/or changes in bowel or bladder habits should be triggers for communication with the medical team. Individuals participating in routine follow-up with their surgeon or oncologist should be screened with the appropriate tests to determine evidence of cancer metastasis to the anatomical locations most likely to present with distant spread. For example, in invasive cancers known to frequently metastasize first to the skeleton, bone scans are routinely ordered for regular follow-up monitoring in these survivors with higher grade tumors with the propensity for bony metastasis.[37] Comprehensive patient education following active treatment, and/or within a survivorship care plan, should be targeted towards awareness of the necessary routine follow-up plan and recognition of specific signs and symptoms of metastasis in cancer survivors.

Signs and symptoms of metastatic cancer vary depending on the location, size, and type of lesion. Aside from an obvious presentation of physical symptoms leading to further investigation with diagnostic imaging, some tumor biomarkers circulating within the bloodstream are used not only to assess responsiveness to treatment, but to also indicate cancer activity predictive of metastatic spread on a molecular level. For those individuals in which they are useful, tumor markers such as prostate specific antigen (PSA), cancer antigen (CA) 19-9 (pancreatic cancer), CA 15-3 (breast cancer), and CA 125 (ovarian cancer) are known predictors of cancer activity and/or progression. Circulating tumor DNA fragments are also under investigation for their role in assessment of tumor activity.[38]

Molecular and Clinical Analysis of Cancer

Staging

The majority of cancers are classified according to the American Joint Committee on Cancer (AJCC) TNM system, whereas **T** refers to *tumor* size in centimeters, **N** refers to the extent of regional lymph *nodal* involvement, and **M** refers to *metastasis* to distant tissues or organs.[39] The individual components or categories of T, N, and M contribute to staging as a whole, whereas the TNM is considered in combination to determine the actual stage of the cancer. Numbers following the **T** are indicative of the tumor size

ranges (measured in centimeters) with progressively higher numbers representing larger tumors, while numbers following the **N** are indicative of a greater number of nodes (representing ranges, i.e., N1 = 1–3; N2 = 4–9) containing cancer. The *clinical* staging of cancer (cTNM) involves the assessment of the malignancy based on the patient history and examination, laboratory testing, and diagnostic imaging. *Pathological* staging (pTNM, also known as the surgical stage) relies on the cTNM and results of tissue specimen histological analysis post-biopsy and/or surgical resection of tumor cells. For individuals receiving neoadjuvant therapy, staging is updated and referred to as ycTNM or ypTNM. For individuals receiving retreatment secondary to recurrence of cancer, staging is referred to as rTNM.[39]

Lower case letters following numbers (e.g., T4a [chest wall invasion] or N3c [cancer spread to the supraclavicular nodes]) are indicative of anatomical locations of tumor spread such as invasion into surrounding tissues. An "**X**" following the T, N, or M indicates the inability to measure, while a "**0**" indicates no findings of cancer in this category. A **T** followed by "is" indicates in situ disease (e.g., ductal carcinoma in situ).[39] The nodal status in the pathology report includes the total number of lymph nodes removed, the number of nodes found to be positive (+) for cancer cells, as well as the size of any cancerous deposits identified within the nodes (N*mic* = micrometastases [≤2 mm]; N*mac* = macrometastases; gross and/or extracapsular extension). *Lymphovascular invasion* (LVI), the presence of cancer cells in either a lymphatic vessel or the vasculature, is also noted within the pathology report following nodal dissection but is not considered to be a positive (+) lymph node finding.[40] For any Onc R clinician, it is critical to be aware of the lymph node status of each of their patients as it is not only indicative of cancer stage, but also the spectrum of risk of lymphedema (see Lymphedema in Chapter 9).

The TNM system leads to staging from 0 to IV, where for most solid tumors, stage 0 represents in situ disease, stages I to II represent local disease, stage III represents regional spread of disease, and stage IV represents distant spread of disease. Within the stages I to IV, further classification can occur (e.g., Stage IA or Stage IIB) based on individual tumor characteristics specific to different tumor types.[39]

Due to the nature of spread in hematological cancers, often presenting with systemic involvement at the time of diagnosis, the traditional TNM staging system is not utilized. However, staging is used to categorize extent of disease in liquid tumors (e.g., I–IV in lymphoma, 0–IV in leukemia, I–III in multiple myeloma). Additionally, central nervous system malignancies also deviate from the TNM classification system, and instead use grading systems (e.g., low-grade tumors [grades 1–2], and high-grade tumors [grades 3–4]).

Tumor Grading

Tumor grading is performed for characterization regarding the degree of differentiation, or deviation from the appearance of a normal, same type cell, as well as how rapidly they are dividing and reproducing (i.e., mitotic activity). According to the NCI,[37] tumor cell grades include: GX, or *undetermined grade*; G1, or *well differentiated / low-grade*; G2, or *moderately differentiated / intermediate grade*; G3, or *poorly differentiated / high-grade*; and G4, or *undifferentiated / high-grade*. Examples of dedicated grading systems by cancer type include the Nottingham Histological Grade for breast cancer (range grade I [score 3–5] to grade III [score 8–9]) and the Gleason score for prostate cancer (≤6 *low risk* to 9–10 *high risk*).[37,41]

Other reporting classifications for cancer include identification of hormone status (i.e., ± estrogen [ER] and/or progesterone receptors [PR] in breast cancer). Additionally, the identification of molecular genetic mutations within driver genes can be identified in the pathological staging of tumors (e.g., Human epidermal growth factor receptor-2 [HER2] status in breast cancer). In solid tumors such as non small cell lung cancer, identifying genetic mutations within histological subtypes (e.g., ALK, BRAF, KRAS, epidermal growth factor receptor [EGFR]) are indicative of overall prognosis and helps to guide the clinical decision-making process for treatment planning (see *Genetic Testing and Use of Genomics*).[42]

As the prognosis of invasive cancer is strongly influenced by the stage of the disease, accurate staging is critical in determining the recommended plan of care. Staging directs the provider in the clinical decision making of the type, sequencing, intensity, and duration of treatment recommended, and informs the patient and family how to best participate in shared decision-making. The staging work-up for individuals with invasive cancers also routinely involves lab studies (e.g., complete blood count [CBC], liver function tests [LFTs], and alkaline phosphatase [elevated levels can be indicative of liver or bone disease and raise suspicion for metastasis]), and diagnostic imaging such as computed tomography (CT) scanning of the chest, abdomen, and pelvis. For cancers likely to metastasize to the skeleton, bone scanning to assess for any metastatic spread of disease to the skeleton is frequently recommended.[43] For individuals at high risk for or suspected to have advanced disease, positron emission tomography (PET)/CT scanning is often added to further assess for metastasis. For cancers known to metastasize to the brain such as small cell lung carcinoma, magnetic resonance imaging (MRI) of the brain is generally recommended.[43]

Genetic Testing and Use of Genomics

The application of *genomics*, the molecular biology associated with the structure and mapping of genomes, has become deeply embedded in the field of oncology. The genetic profile of a tumor has now become, in many cases, at least equivalent if not more revealing than the actual size and location of a tumor. Therefore, genomics has become critical in the field of oncology care, and now frequently dictates the recommended cancer treatment prescription for many diagnoses.

Overexpression of Oncogenes

Normal cells have control mechanisms for division, or *mitosis*, and programmed cell death, or *apoptosis*, at regularly scheduled intervals. *Oncogenes* are genes which produce excessive growth factor receptor proteins involved with cell signaling pathways. These oncogenes essentially put the "brakes" on apoptosis and cause normal cells to reproduce relatively unchecked. If an oncogene is overexpressed, it can promote *carcinogenesis*, or the development of cancer. In breast cancer for example, overexpression of the HER2/neu oncogene is correlated with more aggressive cancers and a poorer prognosis. HER2 *positive* (+) breast cancers are treated with immunotherapy, specifically targeted monoclonal antibodies, which are designed to effectively deactivate the oncogene and help prevent it from promoting tumor growth (see Chapter 13).

Other notable oncogenes associated with carcinogenesis, as well as several additional syndromes, include the *Ras* family (i.e., KRAS, HRAS, and NRAS).[42] Most often these gene mutations are observed as a transposition at position 12 or 13 (i.e., Gly12 or

Gly13) of the amino acid glycine, or at position 61 (i.e., Gln61) of the amino acid glutamine, which result in the continual activation of the K-Ras protein. Specifically related to lung carcinoma, there are known to be a minimum of three acquired KRAS gene mutations associated with carcinogenesis. Overall, 15% to 25% of lung cancers are associated with KRAS mutations (25%–50% in Caucasians; 5%–15% in Asians), with the majority occurring in individuals with long-term tobacco use disorder.[42] Colon and pancreatic cancers have also been associated with Ras gene mutations.[44]

Inherited Genetic Mutations

Inherited genetic mutations are believed to be associated with 5% to 10% of cancer diagnoses and are associated with at least 50 different hereditary syndromes.[45] The most frequently identified mutation is in TP53, known to be associated with Li-Fraumeni syndrome, resulting in a higher risk for several types of cancers. Inherited BRCA1 and/or BRCA2 gene mutations, also known as hereditary breast and ovarian cancer syndrome (HBOC), increase the risk of developing breast cancer in both women and men, and ovarian cancer in women.[46] In addition, pancreatic cancer and melanoma risk in both sexes, and prostate cancer risk in men, also rises substantially in individuals with these mutations. Additionally, colorectal cancer risk is associated with the hereditary conditions of Lynch syndrome and familial adenomatous polyposis, resulting in higher levels of colonoscopy surveillance recommended at younger ages than the general population.[45]

Following a new diagnosis of cancer, assessment for genetic mutations is recommended for patients in specific at-risk categories, and for cancer diagnoses most frequently associated with genetic variants. In breast cancer for example, these include: cancer diagnosed before age 50; bilateral breast cancer; both breast and ovarian cancers in either the same woman or the same family; family history of multiple breast cancers (a close blood relative; 1st, 2nd, or 3rd degree in the maternal or paternal lineage); two or more primary types of BRCA1 or BRCA2-related cancers in a single family member; cases of male breast cancer; and/or Ashkenazi Jewish ethnicity.[46] For newly diagnosed female breast cancer survivors with BRCA1 and/or BRCA2 mutations, the immediate treatment options may include bilateral mastectomy, with or without reconstruction, as well as bilateral oophorectomy or salpingo-oophorectomy. The risk of the mutation in other family members, including siblings and offspring, must also be considered, and the risks and benefits of their genetic testing weighed through referral and consultation with a geneticist and/or genetic counselor.[45]

Patterns of Metastasis by Diagnosis

The biological and pathological processes of cancer metastasis are quite complex and complicated for a multitude of reasons. Cancers spread distantly by specific metastatic mechanisms with certain primary cancers having an affinity for particular distant host anatomical tissues. A sequence of several elaborate events are necessary for cancer cells to successfully metastasize, including: (1) detachment and escape from the primary tumor site; (2) invasion of surrounding tissues and penetration into circulatory or lymphatic channels and survival without detection; and (3) invasion and colonization at a distant site.[47] Once invasion of a new site occurs, persistent survival in this environment, and subsequent angiogenesis for further proliferation, require additional mechanisms and capabilities.[47] Several models of the metastatic mechanism have been proposed over the last many decades. The original progression model outlined the sequence of mutational events that occur to allow primary or disseminated cells to develop metastatic capabilities.[48] It is suspected that the metastatic mechanism begins early in the diagnostic process, with 60% to 70% of individuals estimated to have dormant metastatic colonies at the time of initial diagnosis.[49] Additionally, an estimated 5% of individuals presenting with solid tumors have a cancer of unknown primary (CUP) where the original tumor is clinically undetectable, which further complicates effective medical management.[49]

Cancer metastasis is a challenging scenario for both survivors and their providers. The multitude of considerations include, but are not limited to: (1) different types and stages of cancer metastasize at different rates; (2) the prognosis becomes poorer following metastasis; (3) individuals with a diagnosis of a primary cancer may experience cancer metastasis multiple years following their initial diagnosis; (4) individuals with metastatic disease may develop lesions in multiple distant sites simultaneously; and (5) effective treatment options for various types of metastatic lesions are limited.

Cancer Risk Prediction

Cancer risk prediction is an appealing concept for both healthcare providers and the individuals facing the psychosocial and emotional aspects of fear of the diagnosis of cancer. Additionally, the ability to recommend targeted surveillance strategies, specifically for individuals identified to be at higher risk for cancer development, increases the likelihood of early detection and better prognoses. Cancer risk prediction models have been developed for various cancers to selectively categorize levels of individual risk with the intent of appropriate follow-up protocols. Most statistical models (e.g., logistical regression, conditional regression, mixed recessive, multiplicative models) incorporate clinical and epidemiological variables with identified cancer-associated genetic variants to enhance risk prediction.[50] Cancer diagnoses frequently targeted for risk prediction models include: breast (e.g., Gail, Breast Cancer Risk Assessment Tool [BCRAT]), prostate, testicular, lung (e.g., The Liverpool Lung Project [LLP] Risk Model), bladder, and head and neck.[50] Colorectal cancer risk prediction was also recently modeled based on a familial risk profile (FRP) and familial history (FH) and compared to controls in the colon cancer family registry cohort.[51] The authors determined the FRP provided better risk stratification and risk discrimination than the FH-based model.[51]

In an individual with a known history of cancer, large datasets are available for certain diagnoses of cancer (e.g., breast and prostate), and predictive models exist to estimate extent of disease and risk level for recurrence. At the time of initial diagnosis, this information is most frequently used in clinical decision-making in the recommended level of aggressiveness in the cancer treatment plan (e.g., prostatectomy for prostate cancer, chemotherapy for breast cancer). A Partin table incorporates Gleason score, serum PSA level, and clinical cancer stage to predict the likelihood of organ-confined prostate cancer, extraprostatic extension of disease, seminal vesicle involvement, and/or lymph node invasion.[52] In contrast to the widespread use in prostate cancer treatment planning, a meta-analysis recently advised caution due to poor discriminative performance within different versions of Partin tables.[53]

Genomic Assays

Large data sets that have compiled cancer outcomes across specific patient populations can also be used to extrapolate risk of recurrence for individuals newly diagnosed with certain cancers. *Genomic assays*, or tests that analyze the genetic profile of tumors, have provided clear prognostic information for certain types of cancer, including both DCIS and invasive breast cancer, colon cancer, and prostate cancer.[54-56] These data are now used to compare the tumor biology of a new diagnosis of cancer with a database of other similar cancers, with the goals of providing informed clinical decision-making, including predicting the rate of local (e.g., DCIS) or distant (e.g., invasive) cancer recurrence, and determining adjuvant chemotherapy benefit. Genomic testing such as Oncotype Diagnosis (Genomic Health, Inc, Redwood City, CA) provides a Breast Recurrence Score, a Breast DCIS Score, a Colon Recurrence Score, and a Genomic Prostate Score which categorize cancer survivors at either low, intermediate, or high risk of recurrence within a 10-year time frame (https://www.oncotypeiq.com/en-US).

Other breast cancer-specific tumor genomic assays are available. The Breast Cancer Index test (Biotheranostics, San Diego, CA) has two outcomes: (1) it predicts recurrence risk of node-negative, hormone-receptor positive at 5 to 10 years post-diagnosis; and (2) it identifies the likely benefit of extending endocrine therapy from 5 to 10 years (http://www.biotheranostics.com/). The EndoPredict test (Myriad Genetics, Inc, Salt Lake City, UT) determines the risk for distant recurrence of newly diagnosed ER positive, HER2 negative, early-stage breast cancer within 10 years post-diagnosis (https://myriad.com/). The MammaPrint test (Agendia, Amsterdam, Nethlands) also predicts 10-year risk of recurrence in early-stage breast cancer (https://agendia.com/mammaprint/). Similarly, the Breast Cancer Prognostic Gene Signature Assay (Veracyte, South San Francisco, CA) provides risk of distant recurrence at 10 years in postmenopausal women with hormone-receptor positive, early-stage breast cancer (up to three positive lymph nodes) following 5 years of endocrine therapy (https://www.veracyte.com/our-products/prosigna).

To the best ability of the medical community, risk reduction of cancer recurrence, as well as early detection and treatment of metastatic lesions, are critical in effective long-term cancer survivorship care. Targeted attention and deliberate screening protocols help to guide the diagnostic workup for evidence of recurrence. The National Comprehensive Cancer Network (NCCN) publishes screening guidelines annually, by site of diagnosis, for all major cancers with recommended intervals and follow up by designated interdisciplinary team members.[57]

Other Considerations

Research is growing that identifies cancer's association with autoimmune disease, chronic inflammation, and the autonomic nervous system (ANS). These correlations are very important for Onc R clinicians. Each of these clinical considerations may increase the risk for cancer, as well as contribute to the severity of cancer treatment related adverse effects. Although these topics will be covered in more detail in subsequent chapters, it is particularly relevant to bring attention to the interrelationship of diseases with cancer and to highlight the need for Onc R clinicians to be vigilant in continuous observation and assessment to assist in differential diagnosis and early diagnosis.

Cancer and Autoimmune Diseases

There are well-documented bidirectional associations between cancer and autoimmune disorders. While an increased risk of malignancies, both hematological and nonhematological, have been observed in different autoimmune disorders, there are also some malignancies that increase the risk of developing an autoimmune disorder.[58] Investigators demonstrated how chronic inflammation and autoimmunity are associated with the development of malignancy.[59] Additionally, patients with a primary malignancy may develop an autoimmune-like disease. This cyclical model of autoimmunity and carcinogenesis creates an environment where a chronically overactive immune response can lead to cancer development, yet it can also be a marker of developing tumor immunity. For example, rheumatoid arthritis (RA) is associated with various types of cancers. Carcinomatous polyarthritis, an RA-like condition, has been documented to develop in patients with a preexisting gastrointestinal cancer or non-Hodgkin lymphoma.

Inflammation and Cancer

There is a plethora of evidence demonstrating the association between inflammation and cancer. C-reactive protein (inflammatory marker) is a risk factor for postmenopausal breast cancer among hormone therapy nonusers. The inflammatory mediators, together with insulin and estrogen, may play a role in the obesity–breast cancer relationship.[60] A meta-analysis also supported a significant association between serum ferritin and colorectal cancer.[61]

Autonomic Nervous System and Cancer

The ANS is known to regulate gene expression in primary tumors and their surrounding microenvironment. The activation of the sympathetic division of the ANS modulates gene expression programs that promote metastasis of solid tumors by stimulating macrophage infiltration, inflammation, angiogenesis, epithelial-mesenchymal transition, and tumor invasion, and by inhibiting cellular immune responses and programmed cell death.[62] One study revealed how the tumor behaves like an organ within which the tumorigenic microenvironment actually affects the gene expression as well as the phenotype of the cancer cells. This study also discussed the evidence for sympathetic and parasympathetic nerve fibers of the ANS infiltrating gastric and prostate tumors contributing to cancer development, invasion and metastasis. The hypothalamic-pituitary-adrenal (HPA) and sympathetic-adrenal-medullary (SAM) axis interplay in persons diagnosed with cancer where social factors or stressors might predict health outcomes among cancer survivors. The ANS can play a significant role in tumorigenesis and metastasis.[63]

Conclusion

Cancer is a complex disease that has the potential to affect every organ system of the body. To be effective Onc R clinicians, we are tasked with the cognizance and appreciation of the complexity and heterogeneity of cancer. This is essential for proper discernment of the disease and subsequent roles and responsibilities with reference to our scope of practice. To provide the highest level of quality care, the journey begins with understanding what cancer is.

Critical Research Needs

- Primary prevention—can education to the public on risk factors decrease the prevalence of cancer? (multicenter, public health included, longitudinal prospective or retrospective).

- Would exercise decrease inflammatory markers in patients before, during, and after treatment for cancer?
- Would annual check-up with PT including education, assessment of risk factors, and risk factor reduction decrease barriers to oncology rehabilitation (Onc R) treatment?
- Metastatic disease—testing the efficacy of physical therapy intervention at end of life with persons diagnosed with metastatic disease.

Case Study

At the time of her diagnosis of Stage I, ER+, PR+, HER2- invasive ductal carcinoma of the right breast at age of 42, Shaina had been running 25 miles a week and competing regularly in road races. The married elementary school teacher and mother of two adolescent sons was shocked to find herself thrust into cancer survivorship after leading such a healthy lifestyle and having no family history of breast cancer. She was treated with lumpectomy (tumor size 1.5 cm), sentinel lymph node biopsy (0/4 nodes involved), external beam radiation therapy, and a prescription for endocrine therapy with tamoxifen for 5 years.

Two years following her adjuvant treatment, Shaina presented with left shoulder pain which she attributed to increased miles of running in preparation for training for a marathon. She sought direct access care from her local outpatient orthopedic physical therapist (PT) who concluded that her physical therapy diagnosis was supraspinatus tendonitis, possibly complicated by subacromial bursitis, attributed to her upper extremity posture during distance running. Following 6 weeks of physical therapy twice-weekly including ultrasound, cross-friction massage and therapeutic exercise, Shaina saw no resolution of her shoulder pain. She sought care from her primary care physician and an x-ray was ordered. Mixed osteolytic and osteoblastic lesions in the left clavicle and the proximal left humerus were identified. A bone scan was ordered and revealed multiple skeletal lesions, not only in the left shoulder region, but also in multiple levels of the thoracic spine. A CT scan of the chest/abdomen/pelvis was negative for metastatic spread, as was an MRI of the brain. She was subsequently referred back to her medical oncologist for restaging of her cancer to stage IV and consideration of her medication options, as well as referral to her radiation oncologist for external beam radiation to the shoulder and spine.

Following the completion of radiation therapy and the initiation of a new endocrine therapy regimen and bisphosphonates, her posture had become guarded, and walking and transfers were painful. Due to profound fatigue, caring for her home and family had become difficult and the disease began to take an emotional toll. Her medical oncologist referred her to the Onc R clinician associated with the cancer center for an initial evaluation due to her functional mobility deficits, fatigue, and pain. At that time, she had stopped running completely.

After addressing body mechanics for functional mobility, and adaptive equipment training and pacing techniques for activities of daily living, Shaina and her Onc R clinician were able to focus on her as an athlete. Range of motion and strength deficits were addressed with both home- and gym-based therapeutic exercise prescription. Aquatic therapy was used to comfortably and safely initiate running, which was transitioned to an elliptical for progression to land to address endurance. Following discharge from physical therapy, Shaina continued in the cancer center's PT-prescribed, supervised exercise program for progression of her therapeutic exercise program to rebuild her endurance. After 4 months, and with physician approval, Shaina was able to resume road-running with an average of 10 to 12 miles per week.

Following the initiation of palliative chemotherapy due to liver metastases, Shaina continued to run for two additional years throughout her cancer care until 2 months prior to her death when her ascites became uncomfortable. She attributed her positive attitude and longevity with advanced disease, in part, to her ability to sustain herself as a runner in the way that she envisioned herself as an athlete. She was able to spend her remaining time traveling (several times to Hawaii) with her family, and watching her boys, by then teenagers, develop into fine young men. She was able to die at home peacefully, with the support of hospice and her family, surrounded by vases of beautiful tropical flowers.

Review Questions

Reader can find the correct answers and rationale in the back of the book.

1. According to the Hallmarks of Cancer, the ability of cancer cells to continue to pick up more mutations is most likely the result of the characteristic of:
   A. Evading apoptosis
   B. Limitless replicative potential
   C. Sustained angiogenesis
   D. Insensitivity to anti-growth signals
2. When defining the hallmarks of cancer, Drs. Hanahan and Weinberg identified two more enabling characteristics and two more emerging hallmarks. The body systems that have a **major responsibility** in these new considerations are:
   A. Immune, endocrine
   B. Neurological, muscular
   C. Muscular, integumentary
   D. Endocrine, autonomic
3. When a tumor invades surrounding tissue penetrating into the circulatory system without detection and colonizes at a distant site, it will then become classified as a:
   A. Primary tumor
   B. Secondary tumor
   C. Second primary tumor
   D. Tertiary tumor
4. A pathology report indicated that the breast cancer tumor grade was a G2. The most likely explanation for this grade is:
   A. Undetermined grade
   B. Well differentiated/low grade
   C. Moderately differentiated/moderate grade
   D. Poorly differentiated/high grade
5. A patient's breast cancer diagnosis TNM score was T4N2M1. The most likely explanation for that staging is:
   A. Small tumor with 4–9 lymph nodes involved and no distant metastases
   B. Large tumor with 1–3 lymph nodes involved and no distant metastases
   C. Small tumor with 1–3 lymph nodes involved and distant metastases
   D. Large tumor with 4–9 lymph nodes involved and distant metastases
6. Which statement is NOT paired correctly in terms of genetic mutations and which cancer type denotes an increased risk?
   A. TP53—Li-Fraumeni syndrome
   B. BRCA 1/BRCA2—breast cancer
   C. BRCA1/BRCA2—ovarian cancer
   D. TP53—Pancreatic cancer
7. The challenges of cancer metastasis include all of the following EXCEPT:
   A. The prognosis becomes poorer following metastasis
   B. Individuals with a diagnosis of a primary cancer will only develop metastasis within 1 to 10 years of the initial diagnosis
   C. Effective treatment options for various types of metastatic lesions are limited
   D. Individuals with metastatic disease may develop lesions in multiple distant sites simultaneously
8. An increase in the number of cells in an organ or tissue that appear normal under a microscope is termed as:
   A. Metaplasia
   B. Hyperplasia
   C. Neoplasia
   D. Dysplasia
9. Modifiable risks for cancer include all of the following EXCEPT:
   A. Alcohol consumption
   B. Body mass index
   C. Genetic makeup
   D. Viral infections
10. Common signs and symptoms of cancer include all of the following EXCEPT:
    A. Unexplained weight loss
    B. Unexplained pain
    C. Insomnia
    D. Skin changes (e.g., hyperpigmentation, jaundice, erythema, and pruritis)

References

1. The ICGC/TCGA Pan-Cancer Analysis of Whole Genomes Consortium. Pan-cancer analysis of whole genomes. *Nature.* 2020;578(7793):82–93. doi:10.1038/s41586-020.-1969-6.
2. Lee SJ, Yum YN, Kim SC, et al. Distinguishing between genotoxic and non-genotoxic hepatocarcinogens by gene expression profiling and bioinformatic pathway analysis. *Sci Rep.* 2013;3:2783, doi:10.1038/srep02783.
3. Park JW, Han JW. Targeting epigenetics for cancer therapy. *Arch Pharm Res.* 2019;42:159–170.
4. Takeshima H, Ushijima T. Accumulation of genetic and epigenetic alterations to cells and cancer risk. *NPJ Precis Oncol.* 2019;3:7. doi:10.1038/s41698-019-0079-0.

5. Mohan M, Jagannathan N. Oral field cancerization: an update on current concepts. *Oncol Rev*. 2014;8:244. doi:10.4081/oncol.2014.244.

6. Sung H, Ferlay J, Dielgel RL, et al. Global cancer statistics 2020: GLOBOCAN estimates of incidence and mortality worldwide for 36 cancers in 185 countries. *CA Cancer J Clin*. 2021;71(3):209–249.

7. National Cancer Institute. Cancer statistics; 2020. https://www.cancer.gov/about-cancer/understanding/statistics Accessed January 20, 2021.

8. Siegel RL, Miller KD. Cancer statistics. *CA Cancer J Clin*. 2020;70(1):7–30 2020.

9. National Cancer Institute. Cancer in children and adolescents; 2021. https://www.cancer.gov/types/childhood-cancers/child-adolescent-cancers-fact-sheet. Accessed April 25, 2021.

10. World Health Organization. Childhood cancer; 2021. https://www.who.int/news-room/fact-sheets/detail/cancer-in-children. Accessed February 21, 2021.

11. The Cancer Atlas. Cancer survivorship. https://canceratlas.cancer.org/the-burden/cancer-survivorship/. Accessed April 25, 2021.

12. Hanahan D, Weinberg RA. The hallmarks of cancer. *Cell*. 2000;100(1):57–70.

13. Hanahan D, Weinberg RA. Hallmarks of cancer: the next generation. *Cell*. 2011;144(5):646–674.

14. National Institute of Health. National Cancer Institute. SEER Training Modules. Cancer classification. https://training.seer.cancer.gov/disease/categories/classification.html. Accessed July 15, 2020.

15. National Institute of Health. National Cancer Institute. SEER Training Modules. Cancer classification. https://training.seer.cancer.gov/disease/categories/tumors.html. Accessed July 15, 2020.

16. National Institute of Health. National Cancer Institute. SEER Training Modules. Cancer classification. https://training.seer.cancer.gov/disease/categories/tumors.html. Accessed July 15, 2020.

17. National Institute of Health. National Cancer Institute. SEER Training Modules. Cancer types by site; 2020. https://training.seer.cancer.gov/disease/categories/site.html. Accessed July 15.

18. National Cancer Institute National Institute of Health. The genetics of cancer-hereditary cancer syndromes. https://www.cancer.gov/about-cancer/causes-prevention/genetics. Updated October 12, 2017. Accessed January 20, 2021.

19. Ott JJ, Ullrick A, Mascarenhas M, Stevens GA. Global cancer incidence and mortality caused by behavior and infection. *J Public Health*. 2011;33(2):223–233.

20. Peto R, Darby S, Deo, et al. Smoking, smoking cessation, and lung cancer in the UK since 1950: combination of national statistics with two case-control studies. *BMJ*. 2000;321(7257):323–329.

21. White MC, Hloman DM, Boehm JE, et al. Age and cancer risk: a potentially modifiable relationship. *Am J PreMed*. 2014;46(3S1):S7–S15.

22. Zhao Z, Feng Q, Yin Z, et al. Red and processed meat consumption and colorectal cancer risk: a systematic review and meta-analysis. *Oncotarget*. 2017;8(47):83306–83314.

23. Nelson DE, Jarman DW, Rehm J, et al. Alcohol-attributable cancer deaths and years of potential life lost in the U.S. *Am J Public Health*. 2013;103(4):641–648.

24. American Cancer Society. Ultra-Violet radiation. https://www.cancer.org/cancer/cancer-causes/radiation-exposure/uv-radiation.html. Accessed February 21, 2021.

25. Brooks-Wilson AR. Genetics of healthy aging and longevity. *Hum Genet*. 2013;132:1323–1338.

26. Ohio Department of Health. Non-modifiable, modifiable and environmental risk factors for cancer; 2015. https://odh.ohio.gov/wps/portal/gov/odh/know-our-programs/ohio-cancer-incidence-surveillance-system/resources/environment-risk-factors-for-cancer. Accessed July 20, 2020.

27. Dorak MT, Karpuzoglu K. Gender Differences in cancer susceptibility: an inadequately addressed issue. *Front Genet*. 2012;3:268 268.

28. Perdana NR, Mochtar CA, Umbas R, Hamid AR. The risk factors of prostate cancer and its prevention: a literature review. *Acta Med Indones*. 2016;48(3):228–238.

29. National Cancer Institute. Surveillance, Epidemiology, and End Results (SEER) Program. Reports on cancer. Cancer stat facts. *Cancer disparities*; 2020. https://seer.cancer.gov/statfacts/html/disparities.html. Accessed August 16.

30. National Cancer Institute. Understanding Cancer. *Cancer disparities*; 2019. https://www.cancer.gov/about-cancer/understanding/disparities#. Updated March 11, Accessed August 16, 2020.

31. Yedjou CG, Sims JN, Miele L, et al. Health and racial disparity in breast cancer. *Adv Exp Med Biol*. 2019;1152:31–49.

32. Robb K, Stubbings S, Ramirez A, et al. Public awareness of cancer in Britain: a population-based survey of adults. *Br J Cancer*. 2009;101(suppl 2):S18–S23.

33. Khawja SN, Mohammed S, Silberfein EJ, et al. Pancreatic cancer disparities in African Americans. *Pancreas*. 2015;44(4):522–527.

34. American Cancer Society. Signs and symptoms of cancer; 2020. https://www.cancer.org/cancer/cancer-basics/signs-and-symptoms-of-cancer.html. Accessed September 22, 2020.

35. World Health Organization. Early detection of cancer; 2020. https://www.who.int/cancer/detection/en/. Accessed September 22, 2020.

36. Whitaker KL, Winstanley K, Macleod U, Scott SE, Wardle J. Low cancer suspicion following experience of a cancer 'warning sign'. *Eur J Cancer*. 2015;51(16):2473–2479.

37. National Comprehensive Cancer Network. (a) Clinical practice guidelines in oncology. *Breast cancer*; 2020. V6.2020;BINV-1. https://www.nccn.org/professionals/physician_gls/pdf/breast.pdf. Accessed September 25, 2020.

38. Dawson SJ, Tsui DW, Murtaza M, et al. Analysis of circulating tumor DNA to monitor metastatic breast cancer. *N Engl J Med*. 2013;368(13):1199–1209.

39. Gress D, Edge S, Greene F, et al. Principles of cancer staging. In: Amin MB, Edge S, Greene F, et al, eds. *AJCC Cancer Staging Manual*. 8th ed., Springer, 2017:3–30.

40. Galimberti V, Cole BF, Viale G, et al. International Breast Cancer Study Group Trial 23-01. Axillary dissection versus no axillary dissection in patients with breast cancer and sentinel-node micrometastases (IBCSG 23-01): 10-year follow-up of a randomised, controlled phase 3 trial. *Lancet Oncol*. 2018;19(10):1385–1393.

41. Frkovic-Grazio S, Bracko M. Long term prognostic value of Nottingham histological grade and its components in early (pT1N0M0) breast carcinoma. *J Clin Pathol*. 2002;55(2):88–92.

42. US National Library of Medicine. KRAS gene; 2020. https://ghr.nlm.nih.gov/gene/KRAS#conditions. Accessed August 13, 2020.

43. National Comprehensive Cancer Network. NCCN guidelines for treatment of cancer by site; 2020. https://www.nccn.org/professionals/physician_gls/default.aspx#site. Accessed August 13, 2020.

44. Cox AD, Der CJ. Ras history: the saga continues. *Small GTPases*. 2010;1(1):2–27, doi: 10.4161/sgtp.1.1.12178.

45. National Cancer Institute. The genetics of cancer; 2020. https://www.cancer.gov/about-cancer/causes-prevention/genetics Updated July 24. Accessed August 13, 2020.

46. National Cancer Institute. Genetics of breast and gynecologic cancers (PDQ®)—health professional version. https://www.cancer.gov/types/breast/hp/breast-ovarian-genetics-pdq. Updated September 4, 2020. Accessed September 13, 2020.

47. Hunter KW, Crawford NP, Alsarraj J. Mechanisms of metastasis. *Breast Cancer Res*. 2008;10(suppl 1):S2, doi: 0.1186/bcr1988.

48. Nowell PC. The clonal evolution of tumor cell populations. *Science*. 1976;194:23–28.

49. Riethmuller G, Klein CA. Early cancer cell dissemination and late metastatic relapse: clinical reflections and biological approaches to the dormancy problem in patients. *Semin Cancer Biol*. 2001;11:307–311.

50. Wang X, Oldani MJ, Zhao X, Huang X, Qian D. A review of cancer risk prediction models with genetic variants. *Cancer Inform*. 2014;13(suppl 2):19–28.

51. Zheng Y, Hua X, Win AK, et al. A new comprehensive colorectal cancer risk prediction model incorporating family history, personal characteristics, and environmental factors. *Cancer Epidemiol Biomarkers Prev.* 2020;29(3):549–557.

52. Eifler JB, Feng Z, Lin BM, et al. An updated prostate cancer staging nomogram (Partin tables) based on cases from 2006 to 2011. *BJU Int.* 2013;111(1):22–29. doi:10.1111/j.1464-410X.2012.11324.x.

53. Eissa A, Elsherbiny A, Zoeir A, et al. Reliability of the different versions of Partin tables in predicting extraprostatic extension of prostate cancer: a systematic review and meta-analysis. *Minerva Urol Nefrol.* 2019;71(5):457–478. doi:10.23736/S0393-2249.19.03427-1.

54. Habel LA, Shak S, Jacobs MK, et al. A population-based study of tumor gene expression and risk of breast cancer death among lymph node-negative patients. *Breast Cancer Res.* 2006;8:R25. doi:10.1186/bcr1412.

55. Yothers G, O'Connell MJ, Lee M, et al. Validation of the 12-gene colon cancer recurrence score in NSABP C-07 as a predictor of recurrence in patients with stage II and III colon cancer treated with fluorouracil and leucovorin (FU/LV) and FU/LV plus oxaliplatin. *J Clin Oncol.* 2013;31(36):4512–4519. doi:10.1200/JCO.2012.47.3116.

56. Eggener S, Karsh LI, Richardson T, et al. A 17-gene panel for prediction of adverse prostate cancer pathologic features: prospective clinical validation and utility. *Urology.* 2019;126:76–82. doi:10.1016/j.urology.2018.11.050.

57. National Comprehensive Cancer Network. NCCN guidelines for treatment of cancer by site; 2020. https://www.nccn.org/professionals/physician_gls/default.aspx#site. Accessed August 13, 2020.

58. Giat E, Ehrenfeld M, Shoenfeld Y. Cancer and autoimmune diseases. *Autoimmun Rev.* 2017;16(10):1049–1057.

59. Frank AL, Slansky JE. Multiple associations between a broad spectrum of autoimmune diseases, chronic inflammatory diseases and cancer. *Anticancer Res.* 2012;32(4):1119–1136.

60. Gunter MJ, Wang T, Cushman M, et al. Circulating adipokines and inflammatory markers and postmenopausal breast cancer risk. *JNCI J Natl Cancer Inst.* 2015;107(9):169. doi:10.1093/jnci/djv169.

61. Feng Z, Chen JW, Feng JH, et al. The association between serum ferritin with colorectal cancer. *Int J Clin Exp Med.* 2015;8(12):22293–22299.

62. Cole SW, Nagaraja AS, Lutgendorf SK, Green PA, Sood AK. Sympathetic nervous system regulation of the tumour microenvironment. *Nat Rev Cancer.* 2015;15(9):563–572.

63. Magnon C. Role of the autonomic nervous system in tumorigenesis and metastasis. *Mol Cell Oncol.* 2015;2(2):e975643. doi:10.4161/23723556.2014.975643.

2

Foundations of Oncology Rehabilitation

AMY J. LITTERINI, PT, DPT, ROCHELLE I. BRANNAN, MPT CLT-LANA, AND
DEBORAH J. DOHERTY, PT, PhD

CHAPTER OUTLINE

What Is Oncology Rehabilitation?

Oncology rehabilitation (Onc R) is a clinical specialty practice that optimizes function, reduces symptom burden, maximizes independence, and improves quality of life (QOL) across the lifespan for persons diagnosed with cancer (PDWCs) as well as persons living with and beyond cancer (PLWBCs). Onc R is truly the education and empowerment of individuals throughout their lifetime. Onc R provides individuals with strategies and lifestyle behaviors

that may prevent some types of cancer and decrease the risk for cancer. Upon diagnosis, Onc R provides patient-centered services throughout the entire trajectory of diagnosis and treatment for cancer and then continues throughout the individual's lifetime as needed to mitigate and manage the adverse effects caused from the treatment for cancer. Onc R services encompass screening, consultation, and direct patient care including assessment and intervention, telerehabilitation, annual assessment and screening, as well as palliative and hospice care. Onc R interventions are individually designed to meet the specific needs of each PDWC. Every type of cancer and the treatments for that specific diagnosis affect a person's physical, mental, emotional, functional, and spiritual being in a very different way, thus individualized treatment programs and strategies for lifelong healing and QOL are essential. The Onc R clinician integrates the treatment program into the entire multidisciplinary cancer care journey with special emphasis on returning with renewed hope to flourish in the new version of them.

Four phases of rehabilitation were developed many years ago and have been the foundation for the practice of Onc R. They include preventative, restorative, supportive, and palliative care[1] (Table 2.1).

Onc R is continually evolving from these four phases through the work of many researchers. The next iteration of phases describes how Onc R ultimately aims to optimize health related quality of life (HRQOL) with each PLWBC that includes the following: 1)

pretreatment/surveillance to improve precancer treatment functional/physiologic status and reducing postoperative complications, 2) throughout treatment reducing adverse effects caused from treatments for cancer through long term optimization of health, and 3) the reduction of risks for other comorbid diseases via palliation. The focus of care changes through each phase with the identification of functional impairments and the prioritization of how to address these needs.[2] This aligns similarly with Dietz's cancer rehabilitation phases such that within each phase there may be a change in focus for rehabilitation depending on the past experiences of the PLWBC, and the potential limitations on QOL that they may be experiencing at the time.

We identified the need to combine the phases discussed with the models of prevention that were developed for public health and also evolved through the years.[3] The initial three levels of prevention (primary, secondary, and tertiary) have now progressed to five levels that includes two additional levels, primordial and quaternary[4] (Figure 2.1).

TABLE 2.1	Dietz's Four Phases of Rehabilitation
Rehabilitation	Definitions by Dietz
Preventative	Focuses on reducing the chance of developing impairments This phase can be started acutely after diagnosis, and continued through treatment (e.g., surgery, radiation therapy, systemic therapy)
Restorative	Addresses the functional impairments of each person living with and beyond cancer and aims to restore maximal function with minimal residual effects of treatment or disease
Supportive	Centers on optimizing function and performance status in the setting of progressive disease and further treatment(s) while reducing the decline in function and quality of life
Palliative	Emphasizes the maintenance of quality of life in the setting of terminal illness/disease

Created by Deborah Doherty. Adapted from Dietz JH Jr. Adaptive rehabilitation in cancer: a program to improve quality of survival. *Postgrad Med.* 1980;68(1):145–153. Printed with permission.

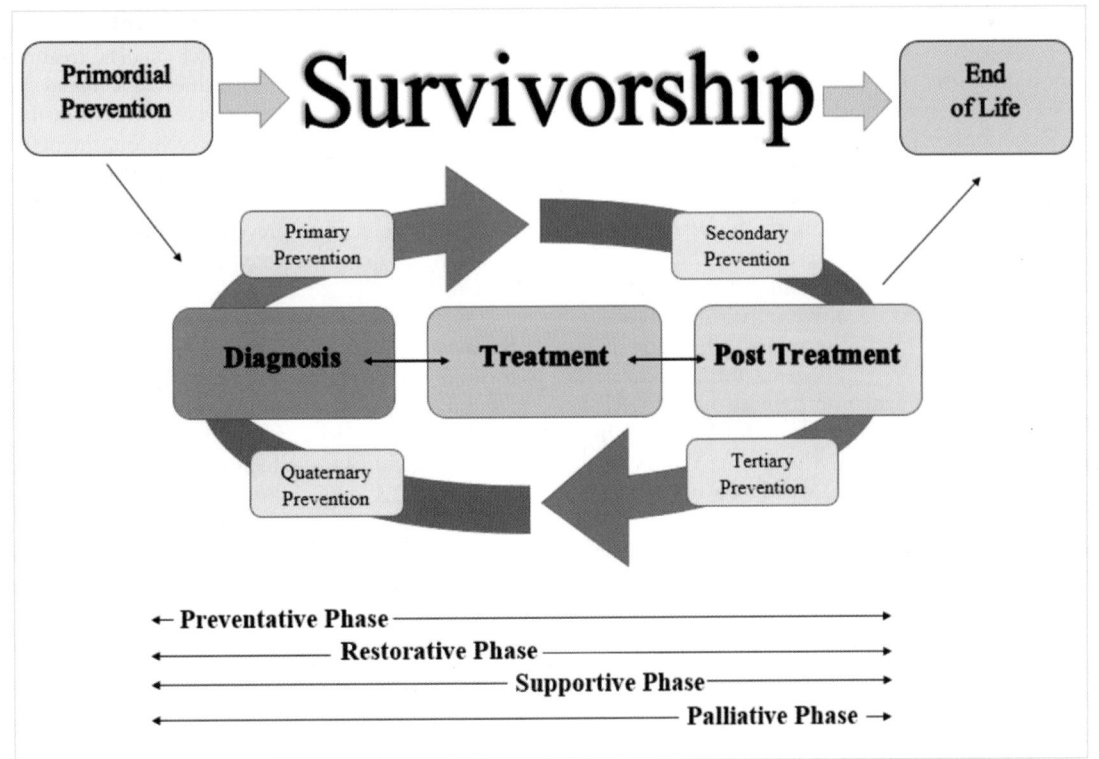

• **Fig. 2.1** Oncology Rehabilitation and Wellness Nexus Model. (Created by Andrew Chongaway, Amy J. Litterini, and Deborah Doherty 2021. Printed with permission.)

Primordial Prevention

Primordial prevention consists of risk reduction in population and community health targeting social and environmental conditions that improve access to increased physical activity. These community-based considerations not only decrease the risk factors for cancer but also decrease the risk factors for obesity and type 2 diabetes, which are also risk factors for cancer.

Primary Prevention

Primary prevention interventions aim to provide cancer risk reduction by altering individual behavior. Prevention involves reducing personal exposure to risk factors and behaviors that would increase the risk for cancer as well as addresses the broader social determinants of health. Lifestyle behaviors such as nutrition, sleep hygiene, stress reduction, social relationships, and spirituality are modifiable but often require guidance by a health professional.

Secondary Prevention

Secondary prevention focuses on identifying a disease or condition and providing intervention to reduce complications and limit disability. Secondary prevention refers to interventions for persons already diagnosed with cancer who either have not started treatment or have just started treatment but have not yet experienced any adverse effects. Onc R aims to prevent and/or decrease the severity from the adverse events that occur from cancer treatment. These interventions can be classified into two categories: (1) prehabilitation (see Chapter 27) provided before treatment, as well as, (2) rehabilitation provided from the moment of diagnosis throughout cancer treatment, which is discussed and evidenced in many chapters in this book.

Tertiary Prevention

Tertiary prevention prioritizes the promotion of an optimal QOL after disease/illness has occurred and maximizes function and wellness. Tertiary prevention focuses on interventions that help to manage the adverse events and effects of cancer treatment that impact function and QOL. The goal of this level of treatment is to reduce disability and restore function to the highest level possible. Common adverse effects that can result from the treatment for cancer may include axillary web syndrome (cording), balance impairment, cancer-related cognitive impairment (CRCI), cancer-related fatigue (CRF), cardiotoxicity, chemotherapy-induced polyneuropathy (CIPN), lymphedema, muscle weakness, pain, pelvic floor dysfunction, radiation-induced fibrosis (RIF)/radiation fibrosis syndrome (RFS), and more. Individualized and personalized Onc R care is essential to impact the physical, mental, emotional, social, and spiritual well-being of each individual. There is no test to determine what adverse effects someone will experience from cancer treatment, so education is imperative. These authors believe that every PLWBC has three fundamental needs: (1) understanding of the potential adverse effects of cancer treatment; (2) knowledge regarding the potential interventions for those adverse effects; and (3) access to the interventions through physician referral, direct access to Onc R, and financial support. Onc R clinicians work in partnership with the PLWBC to help preserve QOL by facilitating access to these three fundamental needs to gain control of their lives.

Quaternary Prevention

Quaternary prevention is defined as protecting persons from medical interventions that will likely do more harm than good.[5] The concept of quaternary prevention helps to identify the risk of over-medicalization and requires a dynamic balance between the assessment and health activities that achieve more benefit than harm. The concept of quaternary prevention is inter-related with the nonmaleficence principle of medical ethics known as *primum non nocere* (first, do no harm) by protecting PLWBCs from an excess of medical intervention. Examples in oncology of potential over-medicalization include radical prostatectomy for a low-grade prostate cancer resulting in incontinence and impotence or continuing aggressive chemotherapy at the end-of-life when the symptoms of treatment negatively impact QOL while providing a very low likelihood of improved survival. Onc R clinicians can educate the PLWBC and their family about the benefits of strategies such as active surveillance for prostate cancer rather than aggressive surgery, and services such as hospice care and its benefits to the patient and family, especially when patients continue devastating treatments for a disease that is untreatable. Onc R clinicians can also educate and empower PLWBCs about movement. Movement is essential across the continuum of care and throughout life in one form or another and is one of the few interventions that improve QOL and does no harm. However, it is important to have reassessment and modification of rehabilitation and/or physical activity programs to meet the needs of each person at each stage of their lifespan.

Within the levels of prevention described in Figure 2.1, it is clear to see that an Onc R clinician needs to be involved in all levels of prevention. It is important for each person to be involved in primordial and primary prevention and every PDWC will be part of each level of prevention, sometimes simultaneously throughout their lifetime. In this way, the person's illness can be considered psychological, physiological, and/or sociological, while the disease is the diagnosis towards which medical treatment is directed. With primary prevention, the illness and disease are not present. In secondary prevention, the disease will be present, but the illness may still be absent. In tertiary prevention, the person's illness and disease are both present. With quaternary prevention, the illness is present, but the disease may not be present in some cases. For this reason, quaternary prevention is often applicable to all levels of prevention to reduce potential over-medicalization through the care continuum.

While it may not seem as though the phases of rehabilitation and the five levels of prevention intertwine, there is significant crossover between the models that can lend to a broader scope of public health promotion, prospective surveillance, and timely use of Onc R services to prevent significant loss of function and provide individualized rehabilitation programs to optimize QOL. The Figure 2.1 depicts how these models can be correlated to cast a broader perspective in the world of Onc R and exercise/physical activity promotion (see Chapter 23). A focus on physical activity and function is crucial as research has demonstrated that roughly only one-third of PLWBCs are considered physically active,[2] and an even lower percentage of PDWCs who are actively going through treatment are meeting physical activity guidelines.[6] In addition, research has demonstrated that most people around the world are becoming less physically active, potentially increasing the risk for certain cancers such as colorectal and breast.[7] Lastly, health promotion and outreach within this population are extremely important as only a fraction of PLWBCs who could benefit from Onc R services actually receive care.[8] The focus and understanding of Onc R extends into assessing feasibility with more heterogenous groups and explores appropriate health promotion as well as accessibility for this population to be able to receive the services they need, want, or require.

Functional deficits resulting from the adverse effects of cancer treatment can be transient or persistent. They may occur immediately with the initiation of treatment or not present until months or years after cancer treatment has been completed.[9] Unmet physical and psychological needs are reported at moderate to high levels.[9] Ninety percent of women diagnosed with breast cancer will have one or more adverse treatment effects at 6 months and 62% at 6 years.[10] Twenty percent of children and 53% of adults living with and beyond cancer report limitations in function.[10] It is estimated that 92% of people living with metastatic cancer will have at least one physical impairment.[11]

Onc R is comprehensive and has the capability of improving cancer and treatment-related adverse effects and HRQOL. Currently, Onc R is not implemented as a standard of care for PDWCs Currently and is considered significantly underutilized among PLWBCs. It is estimated that less than 10% (possibly even as low as 1%–2%) of individuals with cancer-related impairments receive Onc R services even with easily remediable physical impairments.[9,11]

There is a critical need to strategically integrate rehabilitation into cancer care. The optimal introduction of Onc R is from the moment of diagnosis,[12] throughout the active treatment phase, and beyond. This will involve providing a systematic lifetime of screening to identify potential concerns that could lead to functional decline and providing interventions to mitigate issues and maintain the highest QOL. The slow implementation of Onc R as a standard of care is challenged by the well-defined Iron Triangle in Health Care[13] where quality, cost, and access are considered competing priorities so if one area is increased or improved, another area must be decreased or decline. Quality can be affected by the barriers to Onc R that have unnecessarily left many PLWBCs to "live with" their impairments and decreased function or figure out solutions on their own. These barriers include but are not limited to lack of referrals, impairments that go unidentified and unaddressed, services that are one-dimensional instead of comprehensive and coordinated, lack of insurance coverage, and more.[14] The cost priority can be influenced by the uncertainty regarding the roles of the multiple disciplines that provide care. There is currently a limited clinical workforce trained to work with PLWBCs[15] and many primary care providers lack training on the long-term and late effects of cancer treatment thus decreasing referrals.[16] Finally, the challenges of access to healthcare have been described as a fractured system where persons being treated for cancer may have to travel to multiple visits to several specialists just to treat one issue[15] or a person may not have the ability to travel due to cost of travel or distance to travel. The triangle needs to be reworked to add empowerment for PLWBCs PLWBCs plural through shared decision making, culturally responsible care, and the ability to become an equal partner in their cancer care. The real future of Onc R has been defined as sustainable programs that are innovative and include multidisciplinary and interprofessional models of care providing precision patient-centered rehabilitation with outcomes that will demonstrate the value of Onc R.[16]

Survivorship

Over the last several decades, the population of persons diagnosed with cancer (PDWCs) and persons living with and beyond cancer (PLWBCs) has grown along with their need for effective management of late and long-term cancer and cancer treatment-related adverse effects. In addition to the direct needs of the PDWC and PLWBC the need for accurate terminology was also born. The concept of *cancer survivorship* was thoughtfully described[17] in terms of three phases, or seasons, for a person with a cancer history (Table 2.2).

The term *cancer survivor* was defined in 1986 by the National Coalition for Cancer Survivorship (NCCS), in the deliberate attempt to replace the negative term *cancer victim*.[18] In the landmark 2006 publication *Cancer Patient to Cancer Survivor: Lost in Transition* by The Institute of Medicine (now the National Academy of Medicine), advocacy for improved recognition and access to survivorship care became a national initiative.[19] Further enhancement in *Seasons of Survivorship* occurred[20] including *acute* survivorship, adding *transitional* survivorship (the period immediately following intense treatment including careful observation), and expanding *extended* survivorship to include: "(1) alive and 'living with cancer' but requiring ongoing treatment for recurrent, active, and often advanced disease; (2) in a complete remission that requires ongoing therapy; or (3) in a complete remission and with a favorable prognosis."[20] Subsequently, the concept of long-term survivorship has developed to encompass those individuals living with cancer as a chronic disease due to the wide-ranging disease trajectories and cancer experiences from person to person.[21]

The current, accepted definition for a *cancer survivor* is an individual with a history of cancer "from the time of diagnosis throughout the balance of his or her life."[21] The concept of *cancer survivorship*, as a defined group, has subsequently been broadened to include family, friends, and caregivers. There is a debate in progress on the merits of the abandonment of war-time terminologies such as *battle*, the *fight*, and the term *survivor* itself. Some advocates are recommending the term *thriver* over survivor, however, that debate will likely continue for some time to come with a definitive terminology resolution yet to be determined. The authors of this text prefer to use the term Persons Living With and Beyond Cancer (PLWBCs) due to the controversy over the terminology of survivor. However, it is important to understand how the term is utilized in most United States (US) cancer literature.

TABLE 2.2	**Cancer Survivorship**	
	Medical stage, diagnostic, and therapeutic efforts	From diagnosis through the first year
Acute Survivorship[17]		
Extended Survivorship[17]	Remission, termination of treatment	End of the acute stage to 3-years postdiagnosis
Permanent Survivorship[17]	Considered cured, or the cancer being "permanently arrested"	Beyond 3-years postdiagnosis

Created by Amy J. Litterini. Printed with permission.

TABLE 2.3 Cancer Survivorship Standards and Resources

National Comprehensive Cancer Network	Survivorship. V2.2020. https://www.nccn.org/professionals/physician_gls/pdf/survivorship.pdf
American Cancer Society	Cancer Treatment and Survivorship Facts and Figures 2019–2021. https://www.cancer.org/content/dam/cancer-org/research/cancer-facts-and-statistics/cancer-treatment-and-survivorship-facts-and-figures/cancer-treatment-and-survivorship-facts-and-figures-2019-2021.pdf
National Cancer Institute	Facing Forward: Life After Cancer Treatment. https://www.cancer.gov/publications/patient-education/life-after-treatment.pdf
National Cancer Institute Office of Cancer Survivorship	For Healthcare Professionals. https://cancercontrol.cancer.gov/ocs/resources/health-care-professionals
American Society of Clinical Oncology	Survivorship Care Planning Tools. https://www.asco.org/practice-policy/cancer-care-initiatives/prevention-survivorship/survivorship-compendium
Centers for Disease Control and Prevention	Cancer Survivorship Care Plans. https://www.cdc.gov/cancer/survivors/life-after-cancer/survivorship-care-plans.htm
American College of Surgeons	2020 Standards and Resources. https://www.facs.org/quality-programs/cancer/coc/standards/2020

Created by Amy J. Litterini. Printed with permission.

Within the concept of cancer survivorship, formal groups have been categorized to best serve the needs of survivors. Formal survivor age groups include *pediatrics* (0–14 years of age), *adolescents* (15–19), *adolescent young adults* or AYA (15–39 years of age), *adults* (40–64 years of age), and *geriatric* (65 and older).[21,22] The largest age group of cancer survivors are geriatric, with an estimated 64% of all cancer survivors being 65 years or older. Due to improvements in survival rates (up to 84%–85% 5-year survival rate in the years 2008–2014), there is a growing population of adult survivors of childhood and adolescent cancers, estimated at 400,000 in the US in the year 2019. The largest groups of survivors by sex include breast cancer survivorship in women and prostate cancer survivorship in men.[21]

According to the American Cancer Society (ACS) estimates, within the US in 2021 there are over 17 million individuals with a history of cancer, with the vast majority (67%) being long-term survivors with at least 5 years since diagnosis. By the year 2030, an estimated 22.1 million Americans will be cancer survivors.[23] Several factors have resulted in the increasing number of survivors including improved early detection practices, more effective treatments, and the overall aging of the US population.

Associations such as the National Comprehensive Cancer Network (NCCN), the ACS, the NCI Office of Cancer Survivorship (OCS), the American Society of Clinical Oncology (ASCO), and the Centers for Disease Control and Prevention (CDC), have put forth recommendations for standards of care in cancer survivorship (Table 2.3). The American College of Surgeons' Commission on Cancer (CoC) has accreditation criteria associated with standards of survivorship care, as well as the utilization of survivorship care plans by community cancer centers.[24]

Onc R for Primary Prevention

As individuals begin their journey into cancer survivorship, cancer prevention often becomes more prominent in their healthcare focus. Certainly, immediate concerns, for both the PDWC and the provider, are often present in prevention of recurrent cancers; however, primary prevention also plays a vital role in life after an initial cancer diagnosis.

This critical component of cancer survivorship care involves the prevention and/or risk reduction of new, subsequent cancers.

A *subsequent* cancer is considered a new tumor with different morphology and pathology from the original, primary tumor (also called a *second primary*). Subsequent cancer diagnoses also referred to as *subsequent malignant neoplasms* (SMN), are often attributed to one's history of cancer and/or cancer treatment.[25] Particularly vulnerable are those PDWCs receiving treatment within younger age ranges (i.e., childhood cancer survivors, AYA survivors) (see Chapter 26 for an in-depth discussion on the AYA population). Exposure to radiotherapy increases the risk of SMNs in a dose-dependent way in the region of the treatment field, while anthracycline chemotherapies and alkylating agents are known to cause multiple solid and hematological cancers.[26] With an overall move toward a reduction in treatment exposure for most childhood cancers, a reduction in SMNs has been observed in recent decades. However, SMNs have been attributed to approximately 50% of the nonrelapse late mortality rate in pediatric cancer survivors beyond 5 years of survival.[27] In a large population-based cohort study of long-term AYA survivors (n = 200,945),[25] the diagnosis of subsequent cancers occurred most often in individuals with breast, cervical, and testicular cancers, as well as both female and male survivors of Hodgkin lymphoma. The absolute risk for the development of SMNs was also higher for individuals with a cancer diagnosis in the AYA category when compared to survivors of either childhood or adult cancers. The authors found lung cancer to be a frequent subsequent cancer in a large portion of cases,[25] with additional studies implicating chemotherapy and radiotherapy treatment for Hodgkin lymphoma as causative for lung carcinomas, which may be accelerated by the addition of tobacco use disorder.[28]

Patient Navigation

Due to the complex, interdisciplinary nature of cancer care, there are inherent challenges and difficulties for PDWCs and their loved ones when facing a cancer diagnosis. Patient navigation is an innovative and critical aspect of medical care, most frequently oncology care, designed to address these difficulties and improve the quality of care delivery across the cancer care continuum. Patient navigation was defined in 2011 as *"a community-based service delivery intervention designed to promote access to timely diagnosis and treatment of cancer and other chronic diseases by eliminating barriers to care."*[29] The first oncology-dedicated program in the US was founded in 1990 by surgeon Harold P. Freeman in Harlem, New York, which was motivated by patients with advanced breast cancers in his care. The initial program goals were to address socioeconomic disparities and ethnic, racial, and/or cultural barriers to screening, early detection, diagnosis, and treatment for underserved citizens from Harlem. Subsequent programs have expanded the scope of navigation and its reach across the healthcare system and continuum of care. According to outcomes including the stage of diagnosis and survival for women with breast cancer in Harlem, the 5-year survival rate was 39% in 1989 (Stage I disease at diagnosis: 49%; late-stage disease at diagnosis: 6%).[30] Following 5 years of patient navigation in Harlem, the 5-year survival rate increased to 70%, and for women with late stage disease at diagnosis, survival rose to 41%.[31] This, and subsequent evidence, has led to recognition, endorsement, and support of navigation services and sites by the ACS, the National Cancer Institute, the Community Health Centers, the Office of Rural Health Policy of the Health Resources and Services Administration (HRSA), the Indian Health Service, and the Centers for Medicare & Medicaid Services. By 2012, the CoC mandated patient navigation as a standard of care in accreditation by the American College of Surgeons.[32]

Additional roles in cancer patient navigation now include: reducing unnecessary delays between abnormal findings to diagnosis, and diagnosis to initiation of treatment; coordination of care by ensuring effective handoffs between providers; facilitating and scheduling second opinions and/or genetic testing; coordinating diagnosis-specific multi-disciplinary clinics; clinical trial enrollment; care transitions; referral to system and community support resources; and long-term survivorship care.[32] Barriers addressed by navigation may include: symptom management, distress levels, low health literacy, limited English proficiency, cultural concerns related to care, lack of transportation, substance use disorders, patient education needs, financial toxicity related to care, lack of social and emotional support, food insecurity, lack of adequate housing or homelessness, and lack of adequate insurance coverage.[32]

Formalized cancer navigation programs vary widely in format model, scope, and type from facility to facility. To date, there is no absolute standard as to which PDWCs should receive navigation services, and when and for how long they should receive them. The types of navigators and their training also vary widely from trained, nonprofessional lay navigation (e.g., peers, volunteers) to professional/clinical navigation (e.g., nurses, social workers), and are often dependent on geographical location, patient volumes, and facility resources and funding. From the perspective of Onc R, establishing a collegial relationship with local navigation teams is a critical step to advocating for timely referrals for appropriate rehabilitation care and establishing a clear line of communication.

Treatment Summaries and Survivorship Care Plans

Since a diagnosis of cancer and subsequent cancer treatment can leave survivors with a multitude of residual deficits, comprehensive education, diligent surveillance, and appropriate management are key. A multidisciplinary approach to long-term survivorship care requires several providers' expertise and aims to meet each survivor's unique medical, physical, psychosocial, and spiritual needs. Due to the complex and individualized nature of cancer care, a complete *treatment summary* is ideal to provide the individual with an accurate record of the care they received from all oncology disciplines, most specifically surgical, medical, and radiation oncology. This record informs the survivor of their history, and all future medical providers of the potential late effects of treatment or adverse sequelae for which the patient may be at risk (e.g., cardiac health, bone health, SMNs). Should an individual move, either geographically or to a new health system or provider, a cancer treatment summary helps to facilitate a smooth, informed transition with accurate documentation of past care.

Many cancer survivors will present with late effects of cancer treatment, associated with either cancer itself, or the treatment modalities used for management. Physical, psychological, social, functional/occupational, and spiritual distress and/or deficits are frequently noted in cancer survivors; however, they may go unaddressed for the sake of the demands of acute cancer care. Distress in cancer survivors has been strongly associated with levels of disability.[33] Therefore, distress screening by oncology providers has been strongly advocated for by national associations such as the NCCN.[34] Literature review examined the symptom burden in cancer survivorship and identified fatigue as not only the most reported symptom but also the most severe. Sleep disturbance was also identified as a frequently reported symptom and often occurred concurrently with symptoms of fatigue.[35] Additionally, pain, cognitive disturbance, and depression are found to be persistent well into post-treatment cancer survivorship.[35] For periods extending well beyond active cancer care, the effects of treatment often present with unmet needs. These deficits ultimately threaten HRQOL well into survivorship unless specific screening strategies and referral protocols are enacted, and the appropriate care is received. Data from the 2010 National Health Interview Survey was examined and found decreased physical and mental HRQOL in cancer survivors (n = 1822) when compared to the general population of US adults without a history of cancer (n = 24,804).[36] The multi-system late effects of cancer care can include, but are not limited to: cardiac toxicity (following anthracycline chemotherapy, certain targeted therapies, or chest radiation), neurotoxicities (e.g., peripheral neuropathy, cognitive deficits), myalgias and arthralgias (secondary to endocrine therapy or chemotherapy), bone fragility (associated with endocrine therapy and/or treatment-induced menopause), lymphedema (secondary to surgery and/or radiation), and conditions associated with radiation (e.g., fibrosis).[37] In breast cancer, for example, research has revealed that up to two-thirds of PLWBCs experience at least one long-term late effect from cancer treatment.[38] Due to the multitude of potential adverse effects faced by PLWBCs, screening for physical impairments such as general performance, mobility/balance, pain, fatigue, and distress are recommended and should result in appropriate referrals for rehabilitation.[39,40]

In the absence of obvious warning signs, generally healthy long-term cancer survivors should follow the recommended cancer screening protocols for new, primary cancers (e.g., breast, prostate, colorectal) based on the age and sex of the individual. Standardized screening guidelines should be accompanied by conversations with one's primary care provider, including the risks and benefits of screening as well as the influence of personal risk factors (e.g., tobacco use disorder, alcohol use disorder, elevated body mass index), family history (e.g., genetic mutations), and known environmental and/or occupational exposures (e.g., asbestos, radon, air, or water pollution).

In the era of extended survivorship and greater overall numbers of survivors, the push for improved after-care for people with cancer has become substantial. Developments in recent years have included survivorship appointments, survivorship clinics, guidance from survivorship navigators, and survivorship care plans. *Survivorship care plans* are intended to complement treatment summaries by emphasizing what follow-up tests should be done, when they should be done, and ordered by whom. The plans also encourage healthy lifestyle choices, behavioral modifications for risk reduction, and provide appropriate resources and referrals to specialists. Please see Table 2.3 for links to survivorship resources, and care plan and treatment summary templates.

Health Promotion

Like the general population, cancer survivors are recommended to follow guidelines for healthy eating, maintaining ideal body weight, and engaging in regular physical activity. In addition to regular physical activity, cancer survivors are advised to deliberately reduce sedentary behavior (e.g., sitting to watch television, excessive screen time on electronic devices). Beyond consuming a healthy diet, the literature also supports the reduction and/or elimination of the consumption of alcoholic beverages. The ACS publishes guidelines for diet and physical activity for health promotion and cancer risk reduction, both for the public and cancer survivors, with regular updates to maintain relevance and currency with the available literature.[41] Other healthy behaviors such as smoking cessation and/or the elimination of the use of any tobacco products (e.g., loose-leaf tobacco) or vaping devices are recommended. The utilization of sunscreen, and recommended practices for the protection from excessive ultraviolet exposure, are recommended not only for cancer survivors but also for the general population. Regular engagement with primary care and oncology care providers for health promotion and risk reduction, routine screening, and management of chronic conditions is advised.

Survivorship With Advanced Cancer

For PLWBCs with an ongoing disease that is not curative, maintenance regimens are usually prescribed to control, or slow, disease progression and mitigate symptoms. As first-line regimens often become ineffective over time, patients are most often switched to second-, third-, fourth-line regimens, or beyond as tolerated. For these individuals, a treatment summary is not possible, and a survivorship care plan is not always feasible or appropriate. Ongoing cancer treatment in the presence of advanced disease leads to greater disablement.[11] Of 163 individuals with metastatic breast cancer, 92% had at least one impairment (mean = 3.3 impairments). For individuals with disease progression, there is a need for the reduction of symptoms and a greater demand for Onc R to safely manage declines in function.[42]

Cancer Wellness/Integrative Oncology

In addition to addressing long-term physical adverse effects, Onc R clinicians can also help to address the social and emotional effects for cancer survivors. Practitioners who have demonstrated competency and received proper training can utilize various integrative medicine approaches, which are known to increase well-being, physical and psychological health, and QOL in cancer survivorship. The holistic approach of integrative medicine, which combines complementary and alternative approaches with traditional medicine, complements many of the innate values of Onc R. Techniques such as guided imagery, progressive relaxation, yoga, massage, Pilates, tai chi, Feldenkrais, Rolfing, acupuncture/acupressure, and craniosacral

therapy are examples of commonly used approaches within Onc R. Many cancer centers have established *cancer wellness* or *integrative oncology* programs offering a variety of additional integrative medicine services such as nutrition education, herbal and botanical consultations, various physical activity offerings, meditation, art therapy, music therapy, and pet therapy interventions.

A systematic review of integrative medicine strategies specifically in breast cancer survivorship was conducted for the development of a clinical practice guideline. The authors determined that: (1) meditation, yoga, and relaxation with imagery are recommended for routine use for anxiety and mood disorders; and (2) stress management, yoga, massage, music therapy, energy conservation, and meditation are recommended for stress reduction, anxiety, depression, fatigue, and QOL.[43] Onc R clinicians are trained to use a variety of techniques, interventions, and approaches to holistically address limitations and deficits across the continuum of care and recovery for PDWCs. Ideally, clinicians who do not themselves provide integrative therapies as part of their own personal or professional scope of practice would collaborate with local and regional integrative therapy practitioners experienced in treating PDWCs. Collegial discussions about indications and contraindications help to ensure the safe application of these interventions and smooth handoffs in cancer care.

Patient-Centered Care

Shared Decision-Making

Patient-centered care is based on several core principles including effective communication and shared decision-making.[44] The ability for an individual to make decisions about their course of healthcare treatment, although stressful, is also empowering and helps a person maintain some locus of control over their life. Although having options is perceived by many as a luxury in most ordinary circumstances, for a PDWC it is often perceived as an added burden in an already difficult situation during treatment planning. For persons diagnosed of breast or prostate cancer, the need to make definitive, time-dependent decisions about a selected course of care when there are several options is often a stress-inducing necessity (e.g., mastectomy vs. lumpectomy + radiation; active surveillance vs. prostatectomy vs. external beam radiation vs. brachytherapy). Patient education, effective communication, and patient navigation as described earlier in the chapter, become critical components of informed, shared decision-making.

The concept of shared decision-making across the continuum of cancer care ensures that the patient and their caregivers are properly informed of their situation and options, sufficiently educated about their choices, and engaged, empowered, and actively involved throughout the decision-making process with their clinicians.[44] The model of shared decision-making is unique in the bi-directional nature of the flow of information which allows for the final decision to be made jointly between the clinician and patient.[45] For newly diagnosed patients presenting with a decisional conflict, tools such as decision aids can provide the necessary decisional support. A decision aid is defined as "a tool that provides patients with evidence-based, objective information on all treatment options for a given condition."[46] Decision aids present the risks and benefits of all options and help patients understand how likely it is that those benefits or harms will affect them.[46] Examples of decision aids include written or electronic/web-based materials, or multimedia sources, often designed to illustrate the risks and statistical likelihood for certain outcomes (e.g., initial diagnoses, cancer recurrences, mortality). For the Onc

R professional caring for PLWBCs, recognizing decisional conflict, providing decisional support, and making necessary referrals to promote shared decision-making is necessary throughout the therapeutic relationship.

Communication

The ability for clinicians to use effective communication strategies with their patients and their caregivers is critical for the successful outcomes of interventions. Both patient education and informed, shared decision-making rely heavily on effective communication between the clinician and the individual who is the recipient of care. Effective communication centers on the awareness and recognition of cues in both verbal and nonverbal communication from patients through *receptive* communication, and the ability to deliver messages in return through *expressive* communication. Communication barriers that should be determined early and often, include: cultural differences, language barriers, vision or hearing impairments, cognitive deficits (e.g., dementia, delirium), medical conditions (e.g., aphasia), polypharmacy, and/or pain. To effectively "meet the patient where they are" at the onset of care is vital, and an initial assessment should include their perception of their condition (e.g., cause, effect). Utilization of standardized questions, such as Kleinmann's questions,[47] can assist the clinician in identifying personal and/or cultural influences on the individual's perception of their condition, and their health beliefs. It is the responsibility of the Onc R clinician to develop an awareness of the expectation of a typical presentation in patients within a particular population, as well as the presentation of patients within settings. Should a lack of awareness exist, gaining knowledge through continuing education, peer support, and/or mentorship are necessary to improve the future effectiveness of the clinician for the care of individuals within that setting.

The use of communication guides for difficult conversations can also be helpful for both the novice and experienced Onc R clinician, alike. Developed by clinicians from the Dana-Farber Cancer Institute and Harvard Medical School through Ariadne Labs (https://www.ariadnelabs.org/), the Serious Illness Conversation Guide (SICG) was designed as a learning tool to help facilitate early person-centered communication between clinicians and their patients facing serious illnesses using best practices for conversation flow (i.e., *set up, assess, share, explore,* and *close*) and proven patient-tested language (e.g., "I wish...," "I hope...," "I'm worried that..."). The goal of the tool is to discover their values, goals, and preferences within the context of their prognosis. A qualitative study of 118 advanced cancer survivors and 41 clinicians revealed the SICG to be feasible and associated with positive experiences for both the patients and the Onc R clinicians.[48] The SICG can be accessed here: https://www.ariadnelabs.org/wp-content/uploads/sites/2/2017/05/SI-CG-2017-04-21_FINAL.pdf. Other helpful conversation guides include those provided by VitalTalk (https://www.vitaltalk.org/), and from the Institute of Healthcare Improvement (https://theconversationproject.org/starter-kits/).

Teaching and Learning

There are numerous opportunities for teaching and learning experiences for Onc R clinicians. Topics include benefits across all five levels of prevention regarding Onc R, specifics about assessments and interventions, information about the actual cancer and its adverse effects need to be shared, discussed, and debated. Across several different environments, from the clinic to professional conferences, Onc R clinicians have both formal and informal teaching opportunities. One-on-one teaching occurs to patients, caregivers, students, peers, one's self, healthcare professionals, healthcare administrators, policymakers, and insurance company representatives. Group teaching can occur to patients, community members, advocacy groups, student and peer groups, and interprofessional groups. Being cognizant of the teacher's role in addressing a specific audience, and ensuring one meets their needs within the learner's role, are critical steps in selecting the appropriate educational techniques.[49]

The concepts of motor learning and motor control dictate the appropriate teaching style and method of feedback for the right patient at the right time. Motor learning occurs in three stages: the *cognitive* stage (the individual is working to understand the requirements of performing a task); *associative* stage (performance of the task becomes more coordinated and organized); and the *autonomous* stage (the individual can predictably perform the task with a little to no cognitive effort). The clinician must tailor their patient education to not only the stage of motor learning but also the type of task at hand (e.g., open vs. closed; discrete vs. continuous; stability vs. mobility). Barriers to motor learning, including challenges to attention and information processing, should be identified, and appropriately addressed in advance, when possible.[50] Patient education spans the patient-client management model in every phase from the examination (by history taking, systems review, and tests and measures), through the evaluation (diagnosis, prognosis, and plan of care [POC]) as well as with the prescription of interventions. Furthermore, discussions regarding changes to the POC, subsequent referral for condition management, and discharge planning with an emphasis on health and wellness initiatives following skilled intervention, become necessary throughout the episode of care. The ability to assess an individual's readiness for learning also involves several components. The determination of patient *literacy*, *health literacy*, and *health numeracy*, is essential before attempting any aspect of education[51] (see Table 2.4 for definitions).

The use of plain language by Onc R clinicians, and the development of patient education tools at the fifth-grade reading level, are recommended to universally account for varying literacy levels.[52] Assessing the patient's preferred type of learning method first (e.g., auditory, visual/spatial, kinesthetic/physical, verbal) allows the clinician to tailor the form of education to each patient. Ensuring understanding of the educational components delivered can be aided by techniques such as the *Teach-Back Method* (i.e., asking the patient to reiterate in their own words the information learned).[53]

Facilitating change often requires the consideration of the individual's readiness for the proposed change. Conceptual frameworks such as the Transtheoretical Model Stages of Change (precontemplative, contemplative, preparation, action, and maintenance) help to determine the level of patient readiness.[54] Patient education methods and prescribed interventions should be in alignment with the stage of change identified by a particular person at the time.

TABLE 2.4	**Literacy Definitions**
	Literacy Definitions
Literacy	Ability to understand basic verbal and written instructions
Health Literacy	Ability to process health-related information
Health Numeracy	Ability to interpret numerical health information

Created by Amy J. Litterini. Printed with permission.

Techniques such as the strength-based *Appreciative Inquiry* (promotes change through positive affirmation and appreciation) and *Motivational Interviewing* (guided communication intended to empower and strengthen personal commitments to change) with the use of Readiness Rulers (to assess importance and confidence on a 0–10 scale), can assist the patient-client interaction in a positive direction for effective change.[55–57] Finding a shared meaning between the patient and the clinician is the ideal (or desired) outcome that often requires some level of dialogue and negotiation.[58]

Models of Oncology Rehabilitation

Onc R clinicians are primary care clinicians who need to be integrated into cancer care from the moment of diagnosis. PLWBCs would greatly benefit from baseline screening to set goals for return to function postcancer treatment. There are many models of cancer care delivery. There is currently not a standard model of Onc R within cancer care. The authors are encouraging Onc R programs to include multimodal prehabilitation, prospective surveillance, and comprehensive Onc R treatment as indicated by the adverse occurrence of events during cancer treatment (perioperative, postoperative, during chemotherapy, radiation, immunotherapy), following cancer treatment, and annual screening and assessment with treatment as needed for continuous empowerment and improvement of QOL. Delivery of Onc R needs to be on an individualized basis depending on the stage of cancer and treatment as well as sociodemographic characteristics and personal preferences. Risk stratification is supported as one method of delivery.[59]

Prehabilitation

The evidence for prehabilitation is growing rapidly. The greatest challenge of including prehabilitation is timing, as there is often a small window of time between diagnosis and initiation of treatment. However, studies show that prehabilitation is well tolerated and patients who are stronger and have more endurance before they begin treatments for cancer will do much better postsurgery, radiation, and chemotherapy than patients that have a poor functional status.[60] Prehabilitation will be discussed in Chapter 27.

Prospective Surveillance Model

The Prospective Surveillance Model (PSM) is a comprehensive model of care that begins with an initial evaluation at the time of diagnosis to determine functional status before any cancer treatment. Although originally created for persons with breast cancer, the PSM has the potential to be developed for persons diagnosed with any cancer type. This model includes a prehabilitation assessment by an Onc R clinician before surgery for breast cancer and then every three months for the first year. This care model is based on determining baseline function, monitoring potential toxicities from the cancer treatments, and providing preventive and early intervention to mitigate the potential severity of late and long-term adverse events. The PSM has been shown to improve outcomes for reduced incidence of lymphedema and shoulder contractures.[61] Although this model would not be feasible for all PLWBCs due to time and financial commitment,[59] it does provide one model that proposes a definitive intervention of early detection and early treatment with the goal of decreasing adverse events, optimizing QOL, and improving exercise and functional capacity. This model of care, which is currently focused on impairment-driven rehabilitation, could also include mental health and palliative care as needed.[16] The PSM allows for triaging PLWBCs to five levels of care depending on their needs[16] (Table 2.5).

TABLE 2.5 Five Levels of Onc R Stepped Care

Five Levels[16]	Oncology Rehabilitation Stepped Care[16]	Description of Each Level
Level I	General conditioning activities	• This level is a basic exercise conditioning program for persons living with and beyond cancer (PLWBCs) who have a history of exercise participation and lack any specific impairments as most will have some aerobic fitness and muscle quality and also challenges includes psychosocial counseling.
Level II	General conditioning activities–specialized	• This level requires the expertise of oncology rehabilitation-trained clinicians that can provide an exercise prescription for PLWBCs who are vulnerable to potential impairments secondary to their specific diagnosis even if they currently do not have any.
Level III	Impairment directed care, uncomplicated	• Persons requiring this level of care are experiencing cancer-related adverse events and impairments that are challenging function. • These can include radiation induced fibrosis, axillary web syndrome, contractures from graft versus host disease, etc. • Specialized training by the clinician is necessary to treat in this level.
Level IV	Impairment directed care, complicated	• This Onc R level is focused on treating the severity of impairments as well as ongoing symptoms, increasing activity levels, and safely improving independence.
Level V	Inpatient cancer rehabilitation	• Treating all complications through multidisciplinary teams provides care for the multiple system deficits and impairments that are present. • This approach aims to keep the person functioning at the highest level of independence as possible while working to discharge the person home with a caregiver and potential homecare clinicians as needed.

Created by Deborah Doherty. Printed with permission. Adapted from Alfano CM, Pergolotti M. Next-generation cancer rehabilitation: a giant step forward for patient care. *Rehabil Nurs.* 2018;43(4):186–194.

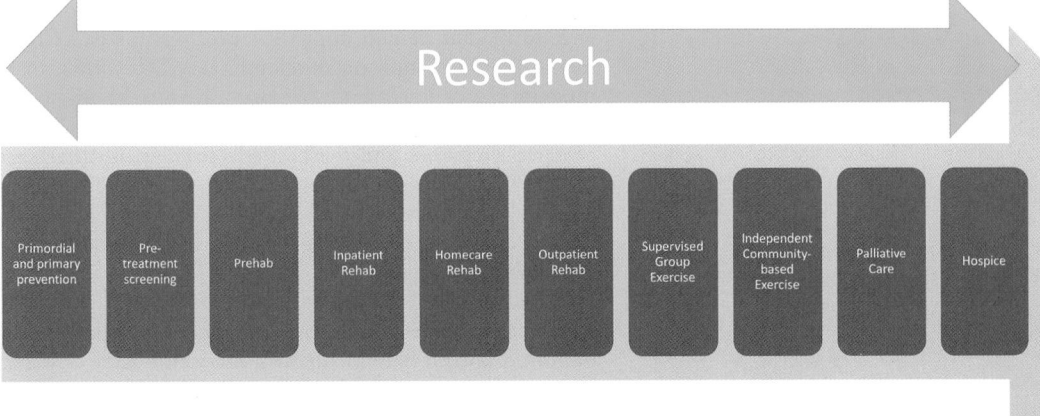

• **Fig. 2.2** Comprehensive Oncology Rehabilitation (Onc R) Model of Care. (Created by Deborah Doherty. Printed with permission.)

Comprehensive Onc R Model of Care

These authors have developed a figure to represent the goals of comprehensive Onc R which includes Onc R clinicians (Figure 2.2).

This model of care was built to integrate Onc R throughout a person's lifetime. Prevention includes primordial and primary prevention of education on lifestyle behaviors that will prevent cancer from ever occurring. *Prehabilitation* involves a structured, individual assessment to determine baseline function of the body systems including the neuromusculoskeletal, fascial, cardiopulmonary, and integumentary systems before the initiation of cancer treatment. This patient-centered intervention provides a foundation for setting goals to work towards upon completion of cancer treatment and it prepares the individual for potential adverse effects experienced during treatment. *Pretreatment screening* can also identify financial and mental health resources that may be needed. Some healthcare organizations choose to implement an Onc R screening program. Through an interview or targeted questions and a quick scan of the musculoskeletal system, potential deficits requiring rehabilitation intervention are identified. Screening can be completed in a radiation clinic, during preoperative education, or during chemotherapy visits. One study demonstrated that >30% of persons being treated for cancer (all diagnoses and stages of treatment) screened in a radiation clinic met the criteria for traditional physical therapy intervention and had not been referred.[62] *Inpatient Onc R* focuses on the person's movement function and independence in mobility during a hospitalization or an inpatient stay in order to transition to a lesser care environment. The Onc R clinician can provide a home exercise program that addresses cancer-specific impairments. Onc R is also provided in inpatient rehabilitation (IPR) centers or in skilled nursing facilities. Both settings provide intensive Onc R intending to build strength, function, and confidence in self-care. *Outpatient (OP) Onc R* after a transition to home continues to focus on the functional mobility of the PLWBC and allows for the time to educate the person on self-care strategies to continue treating the adverse effects from cancer treatments. *Supervised group exercises* can be very successful within a healthcare system or OP clinic providing a bridge between the medical setting and the community where *Independent Community-Based Exercise* can

continue. This will then allow the person to eventually integrate back into the community and participate in local group exercise programs. Finally, Onc R is an essential component of *Palliative Care* and *Hospice Care* to provide the highest QOL throughout the duration of a person's lifetime. *Research* is needed in all of the stages of cancer care. It is only with Onc R research that we can provide the evidence for practice to provide the value of this incredible service to PDWCs and PLWBCs.

Biopsychosocial Model of Cancer Care

The biopsychosocial model is both a philosophy of clinical care and a practical clinical guide. Philosophically, it is a way of understanding how suffering, disease, and illness are affected by multiple levels of organization, from the societal to the molecular… At the practical level, it is a way of understanding the patient's subjective experience as an essential contributor to accurate diagnosis, health outcomes, and humane care.[63]

Patient-centered care cannot be achieved without the due diligence of considering the biopsychosocial needs of every person dealing with cancer anywhere along the continuum of care. In the 2018 American Physical Therapy Association (APTA) 23rd Maley Lecture, Robert Palisano, PT, ScD, FAPTA, eloquently discussed the need for "healthcare systems to evolve from a medical to a biopsychosocial model." His vision for the future encompassed what he termed as "Lifecourse Health Development" as a progression and evolution of person-to-environment and environment-to-person transactions to address the physical, mental, and emotional well-being of each person throughout their lifetime to achieve personal goals. This philosophy crosses all ages and is very important for people with chronic conditions, including cancer, transforming the philosophy of care into a comprehensive and hopeful model.[64]

The biopsychosocial model includes biological, psychological, and social aspects of care (Figure 2.3). The biological components encompass genetics, epigenetics, tissue damage, stress reactivity, disease process, adverse events of treatment, and the changes that can occur with rehabilitation. Psychological components may include: health beliefs, coping abilities, locus of control,

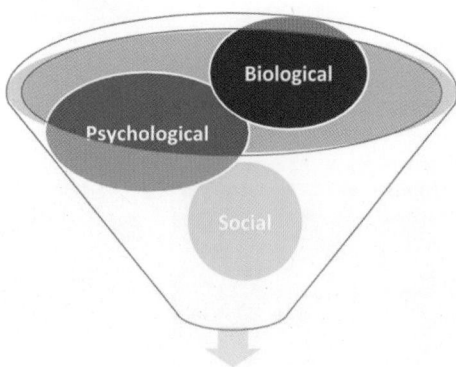

Biopsychosocial Model of Care

• **Fig. 2.3** Biopsychosocial Model of Care. (Created by Chris Wilson. Printed with permission.)

self-efficacy, and/or emotional response. Finally, the social aspects of care consider education, cultural influence, learning mechanisms, social relationships, spirituality, and the impact of the cancer treatment. Rehabilitation can influence all three of these areas of well-being.

The biopsychosocial model of care is optimally achieved with a multidisciplinary, interdisciplinary, and/or interprofessional approach to care. Traditionally these approaches have very different definitions: multidisciplinary encourages the expertise and skills of individual healthcare professionals from different disciplines to provide consultation for a specific patient, often in the same location to increase access to patients. Team meetings may be a component of care where cases are discussed. In contrast, interdisciplinary teams (IDTs) provide a consultation that integrates and intermeshes separate disciplines' assessments together with the patient and caregiver to create a POC. This patient-centered approach aims to empower the patient, so that they play an equal role in shared decision making.[65] It is noteworthy to understand that these terms are often used interchangeably in research and commentaries. Multidisciplinary teams (MDTs) aim to be an effective and efficient decision-making tool. Even though MDTs have been recommended internationally for over 25 years, it is not a standard of practice. There is a strong case for the value of the MDT and the best way to advance patient-centered care with the evolution of molecular pathology, informatics, clinical trials, patient engagement, and patient-reported outcomes.[66] The most important factors impacting team success are personal and team skills, the environment, and patient-centeredness, led by clinically feasible, observational methodology, and adequate training for all.[67]

A conceptual framework was developed to measure the intensity of the interdisciplinary teamwork (ITW) which is correlated to quality cancer care and positive patient-reported experience measures.[68] This framework describes teamwork as an "alliance of all medical and healthcare professionals related to a specific tumor site." The novelty of this framework not only includes team structure (team composition and meeting attendance) but converges team process (shared philosophy of care, intra-team coordination, leadership, and quality assessment activities) and triangulates these components with patient-reported experience measures. There was evidence that high intensity ITW reported positive perceptions to prompt access to care, good person-centered responses to patient-professional communication, and continuity of care compared to low ITW. This highlights the need for a positive

association between teamwork and patient self-reported experience to modernize and improve cancer services (see Chapter 31 for more information on developing a MDT within an Onc R program).

Two major goals of this team philosophy are to improve patient-centered outcomes and the cost-effectiveness of care. Interdisciplinary Onc R services bring together cancer care experts (e.g., nurses, physiatrists, exercise physiologists, rehabilitation therapists, social workers) and provides the structure for these teams to collaborate, agree on mutual goals for the PLWBC, addressing each person's individualized goals, while working individually within their scope of practice. This approach has demonstrated improved outcomes compared to interventions by a single discipline.[9] Interdisciplinary rehab teams have been shown to provide benefits in terms of decreased fatigue and physical outcomes. In one study when inpatient rehabilitation was combined with cognitive behavioral therapy and psychological education, there were a significantly better physical outcomes including increases in muscle strength, physical functioning, and energy levels. Onc R is considered a cost-effective means of utilizing resources to produce health gains.[9]

Interprofessional collaborative practice can be defined as multiple health workers from different professional backgrounds working together with patients, families, caregivers, and communities to deliver the highest quality of care across settings.[69] Using this concept, interprofessional patient-centered practice (IPPC) has been studied and aims to uphold the importance and power of the participation of the patient within the healthcare team[70] (Figure 2.4). This figure illustrates the desired IPPC components based on patients', caregivers', and professionals' perspectives on the most effective oncology teams. This patient-centered approach reflects the shared decision making of the patient, caregivers and team, as well as the respect for the patient's treatment objectives and goals while not imposing the health care professionals' values and goals, and consistency in team collaboration.

Globally, MDTs are composed of a multitude of healthcare professionals and do not always include Onc R. The ASCO includes Onc R as part of the oncology team,[71] demonstrating that progress is being made for the inclusion of Onc R clinicians, however more work is needed to ensure the inclusion of rehabilitation on every MDT for cancer care. The optimal cancer care team is displayed in Figure 2.5.

Standard Setting for Oncology Rehabilitation Services

A cancer rehabilitation specialty program is a patient-centered cancer model utilizing an interdisciplinary team approach. Interdisciplinary team members achieve professional competencies and incorporate evidence-based practices for preventive, restorative, supportive, and palliative needs for the patients served. Setting standards for comprehensive oncology care promotes the highest quality of care for people diagnosed with cancer. A commitment to the attainment of these standards is a commitment to quality services and continuous improvement assuring the public of a commitment to excellence in oncology care. Four organizations are discussed here including CoC and National Accreditation Program for Breast Cancer (NAPBC), the National Cancer Policy Forum (NCPF) and Rehabilitation, and the Commission on Accreditation of Rehabilitation Facilities (CARF) (Table 2.6).

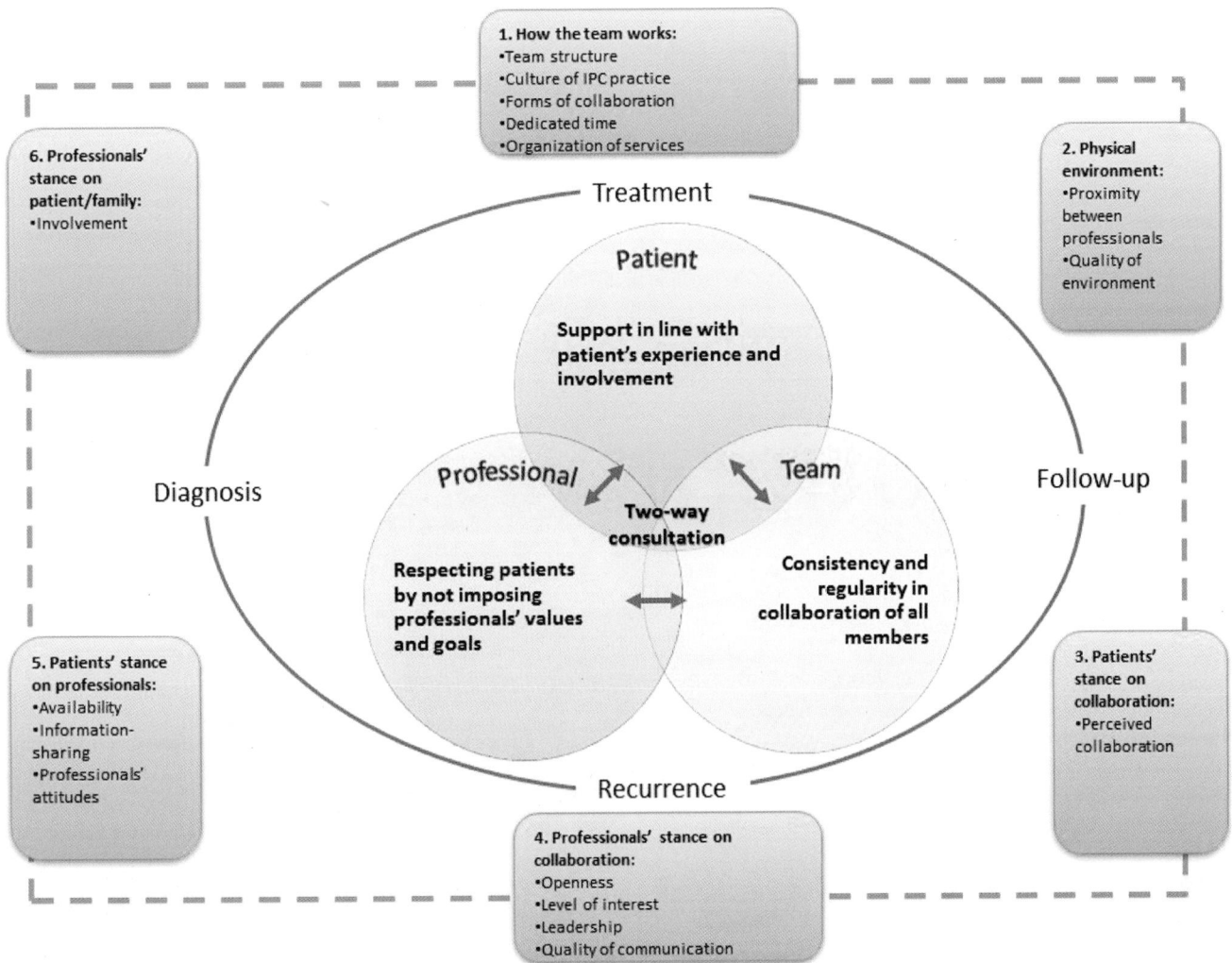

• **Fig. 2.4** Interprofessional Patient Centered Practice. (Printed with permission from Bilodeau K, Dubois S, Pepin J. Interprofessional patient-centred practice in oncology teams: utopia or reality? *J Interprof Care*. 2015;29(2):106–112. doi:10.3109/13561820.2014.942838.)

Commission on Cancer

The 2020 standards require each CoC facility to report what rehab services available, how these services are accessed, and how each institution will improve delivery based on quality improvement processes. The standards identify that rehabilitation care is an essential component of cancer care that optimizes patients' functional status and QOL through preventive, restorative, supportive, and palliative interventions. The availability of rehabilitation care services is an essential component of comprehensive cancer care, beginning at the time of diagnosis and being continuously available throughout treatment, surveillance, and, when applicable, through the end of life.[72]

National Accreditation Program for Breast Cancer Standards[73]

The NAPBC states on page 48 of the 2018 National Accreditation Program for Breast Cancer Standards Manual (NAPBC) 2018:
"Comprehensive breast cancer care is multidisciplinary and includes medical health professionals addressing patient needs identified along the breast cancer continuum from diagnosis through survivorship. Supportive services help patients and their families cope with the day-to-day details of a breast cancer diagnosis. These resources address emotional, physical, financial, and other needs of the breast cancer patient. Supportive services address the needs of the majority of patients, as well as provide for special populations or needs." It is important to note that, it also states: "The supportive services offered on-site will vary depending upon the scope of the facility, local staff expertise, and patient population" and "Supportive services not provided on-site are provided through referral to other facilities and/or local agencies." This is evidence that Onc R clinicians still have substantial and urgent opportunities to to advocate for all PDWCs and PLWBCs to assure that Onc R services are mandatory at every single healthcare facility where cancer surgery, chemotherapy and radiation are provided. Breast cancer is the most commonly diagnosed type of cancer globally and yet Onc R is not mandated as an essential part of cancer care.

National Cancer Policy Forum[74]

The NCPF under the auspices of the National Academies of Sciences, Engineering, and Medicine provides experts to identify

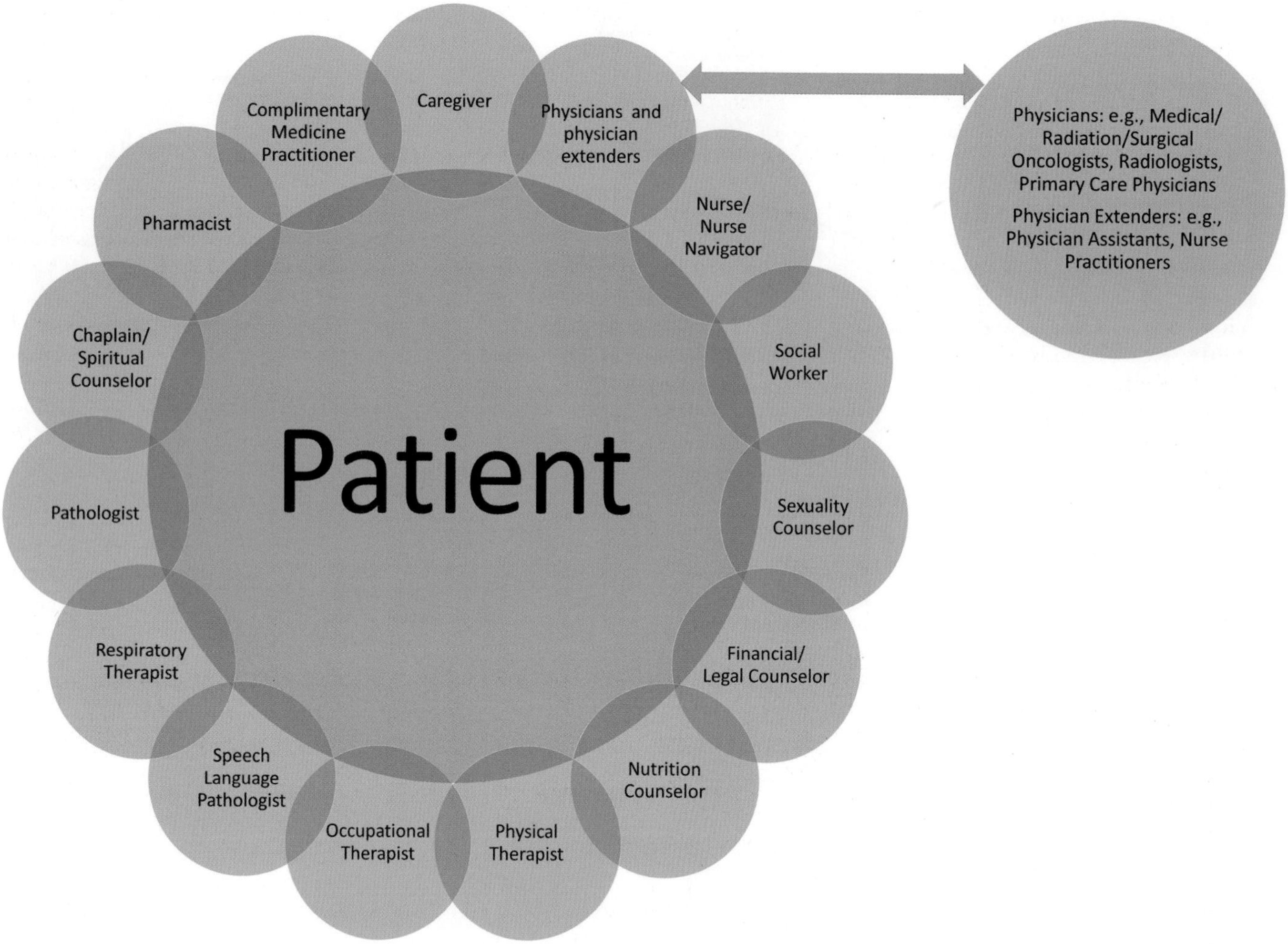

• **Fig. 2.5** Comprehensive Cancer Care Team. (Created by Deborah Doherty. Printed with permission.)

TABLE 2.6   **Standard Setting Organizations for Cancer Centers and Oncology Rehabilitation Services**

Organization	Mission
Commission on Cancer https://www.facs.org/quality-programs/cancer/coc	Directed by the American College of Surgeons, this consortium is involved in standard setting to ensure comprehensive, multidisciplinary quality cancer care as well as education, prevention, research, and monitoring quality care.
National Accreditation Program for Breast Cancer https://www.facs.org/quality-programs/napbc/about	Directed by the American College of Surgeons, this accrediting agency provides the structure and resources for organizations to develop a quality multidisciplinary, integrated, comprehensive breast cancer center.
National Cancer Policy Forum (NCPF) https://www.nationalacademies.org/our-work/national-cancer-policy-forum#sectionWebFriendlym	Working within the National Academies of Sciences, Engineering and Medicine, this organization of experts identifies emerging high-priority policy issues related to decreasing the burden of cancer. Evidence and information is gathered and shared through consensus committee studies and cancer research, (both basic and translational) and prevention.
Oncology Rehabilitation Centers	
Commission on Accreditation of Rehabilitation Facilities (CARF) http://www.carf.org/home/	An independent, nonprofit organization to provide global accreditation for rehabilitation facilities in multiple facilities and programs focused on advancing the quality of services. Cancer Rehabilitation is one of 15 medical rehabilitation programs accredited through CARF. Each program has a separate accreditation. CARF offers organizations a roadmap for continuous improvement. CARF accredited programs with Cancer Rehabilitation Specialty Programs in US can be located using http://www.carf.org/providerSearch.aspx.

Created by Amy J. Litterini. Printed with permission.

emerging high-priority policy issues in cancer research and cancer care. The NCPF convened in 2018 and provided a report emphasizing the importance of Onc R. In summary, the report stated that "survivorship care that lacks appropriate rehabilitation services could lead to unnecessary long-term physical and psychological suffering. Better integration of both prehabilitation and rehabilitation services was recommended and is essential for survivorship."[12] Since NCPF's first published report in 1999, clinical care pathways, cancer care delivery standards, and payment models have produced significant changes for patients with cancer. Although advances in cancer science and treatment continue, Onc R services remain elusive in the spectrum of cancer care. In May 2018, NCPF published the most specific recommendations for Onc R services. A summary of the forum's *Long-Term Survivorship Care After Cancer Treatment: Proceedings of a Workshop*[74] for rehabilitation clinicians include the five following domains as described below:

Improving the Delivery of Cancer Survivorship Care

- Expand the care team to include Onc R clinicians.
- Facilitate uptake of lifestyle interventions to reduce recurrence, second cancers, comorbidity, adverse changes in body composition, and functional decline.
- Adhere to professional and institutional performance and accreditation standards.
- Incorporate survivor and caregiver-reported outcomes in quality measurement.

Addressing Employment- and Work-Related Concerns

- Promote multidisciplinary approaches to address employment, education, and financial needs of cancer survivors.

Improving Symptom Management and Rehabilitation

- Disseminate evidence-based practice guidelines to manage cancer symptoms and treatment adverse effects.
- Provide evidence-based interventions for persistent fatigue or sleep problems.
- Implement cancer rehabilitation to maintain and restore function, reduce symptom burden, maximize independence, and improve QOL.
- Before initiating cancer treatment, refer cancer rehabilitation services to certain patients for minimizing toxicity and morbidity.

Expanding Education and Training Opportunities

- Include cancer survivorship content in education and training for entire cancer care teams, including rehabilitation specialists.
- Implement professional self-regulation to help oncology clinicians maintain and document relevant competencies.
- Extend the capacity to deliver survivorship care via internet-based interventions and telehealth, to support surveillance, patient self-management, and communication.

Addressing Research Needs

- Assess the physical and psychosocial well-being of patients during return to work.

Weight Management and Physical Activity

The NCPF created special recommendations on weight management in cancer care, which deserve some attention. This deserves some attention here. One of the most difficult topics to discuss with PDWC and PLWBCs is weight management especially when they are physically, emotionally, and mentally challenged dealing with the diagnosis of cancer, the treatments for cancer, and the changes in their QOL at all levels. Because weight management is essential in the primordial, primary, secondary, and tertiary prevention of cancer, Onc R clinicians need to work towards the integration of education and intervention of weight management with every PLWBC as a mandatory component of all Onc R programs across the continuum of care. When compared to adult populations of the same age, cancer survivors are more obese, experience greater fatigue, and have reduced muscle mass and strength. Because of these factors, PLWBCs have a higher risk for developing heart disease, stroke, osteoporosis, and metabolic syndrome.[75–77]

The NCPF addressed this topic in 2018 with the publication: *Incorporating Weight Management and Physical Activity Throughout the Cancer Care Continuum: Proceedings of a Workshop*.[78] Research concludes that obesity and excess weight is linked to the development of 13 cancers: breast (postmenopausal), colorectal, endometrial, esophageal (adenocarcinoma), gallbladder, gastric, kidney (renal cell), liver, meningioma, multiple myeloma, ovarian, pancreatic, and thyroid cancers.[76] The NCPF included rehabilitation specialists in the published workshop recommendations. Onc R clinicians are the experts in the assessment of a person's physical activity, functional, and mobility impairments and should be included in weight management treatment programs. The NCPF's recommendations with specific criteria are described below.

Advising Cancer Survivors About Improving Weight Management and Physical Activity

- Emphasize how weight management and physical activity interventions improve cancer survivors' QOL, reduce fatigue, and improve outcomes from comorbid conditions.
- Tailor interventions to fit the needs of the patient's interests and experiences and ensure that interventions are patient-centered.
- Increase public messaging about the importance of diet, weight management, and physical activity for people at risk for cancer, as well as for cancer survivors.
- Acknowledge the difficulty of losing weight and provide cancer survivors with the tools and support to help them succeed.

Improving Screening, Assessment, and Referral to Weight Management and Physical Activity Interventions

- Consider how a cancer survivor's co-morbidities and adverse effects of cancer and its treatment may affect the ability to perform various kinds of physical activity.
- Ensure weight management and physical activity interventions encompass a patient's preferences and experiences.
- Establish a list of local weight management and physical activity resources for clinicians to refer patients.

Delivering Weight Management and Physical Activity Interventions to Cancer Survivors

- Tailor interventions to the unique needs of different populations, including racial/ethnic minorities, childhood and older adult cancer survivors, and rural populations.
- Develop interventions to address the health risks common among older adult and childhood cancer survivors.
- Integrate clinical and community services to improve weight management and physical activity interventions for cancer survivors.

Improving Quality Measurement and Insurance Coverage of Lifestyle Interventions

- Assess the physical and psychosocial well-being of patients preparing to return to work.
- For a long-term path, all stakeholders must play a role to ensure cancer survivors have support to engage in a healthful dietary, physically active, and weight management lifestyle.

Incorporating Weight Management and Physical Activity Throughout Cancer Care

- A triage model for population-based screening of cancer survivors for weight management and physical activity interventions.

Weight management and physical activity screening can address adverse effects of primary cancer and prevent recurrence. Screening identifies unmet needs for the PLWBC in order to direct appropriate follow up care and referral. Beginning in 2019, programs will need to have a structured survivorship program, including a survivorship coordinator and team, to provide the care necessary to optimally support these patients.

The Commission on Accreditation of Rehabilitation Facilities[79]

Founded in 1966, CARF International is an independent, nonprofit accreditation and standards-setting organization Internationally, there are greater than 50,000 CARF-accredited programs. Every year, CARF publishes updated standard manuals (including quality standards for business practices, service-delivery processes, and specific program services) for each program accreditation area. Onc R is one of 15 settings and specialty areas in the program of medical rehabilitation (one of eight programs areas). Each program and area has its own CARF accreditation. CARF standards offer organizations a roadmap for continuous improvement while expanding on existing accredited programs. Because accreditation is an ongoing process, the health care organization is committed to continuously upgrading patients' services and supports leadership vision for the future while serving community needs.

The primary purpose of a CARF accredited cancer rehabilitation program is to focus on strategies to optimize outcomes from the time of a patient's cancer diagnosis through the trajectory of the cancer journey. CARF accredited programs with Cancer Rehabilitation Specialty Programs in the US can be located using http://www.carf.org/providerSearch.aspx. The benefits of CARF accreditation are provided in Figure 2.6.

Onc R Tools for Plan of Care Development

There is a multitude of measurement tools for performance and function validated in the oncology population. Several will be discussed throughout the text. Three common tools that are very helpful in all oncology settings include the International Classification of Function (ICF), Karnofsky Performance Status (KPS), and the Eastern Cooperative Oncology Group (ECOG) Performance Status.

The ICF Model

The ICF model provides a comprehensive, universally accepted biopsychosocial model and taxonomy for describing function.[80,81] The ICF model can be found at who.int/classifications/icf/en/.

The ICF model changes the healthcare system's perception and understanding of a person's disability. The ICF model transitions away from classifying a disabled person as one who has limited functional abilities in society. Instead, the ICF model describes how people live with their health condition and perform daily life activities.

Part I: Universal Language of ICF Functioning and Disability
The ICF model uses functioning as an umbrella term for body functions, body structures, activities, and participation. *Functioning* denotes the positive aspects of how an individual with a health condition interacts within their environment and personal context.

The first domain of the ICF model includes body functions and body structures. *Body function* identifies the physiological functions of all body systems including psychosocial function. In contrast, *body structure* describes the anatomical structures of the body (organs, extremities, neurovascular, etc.). The goal of enablement models such as ICF is to provide a common language. The ICF model defines impairments as causing deviations in body functions and body structures. Impairments within the ICF model include deviations from generally accepted societal standards. Functional deviations can be temporary or permanent.[79]

The second domain of the ICF model includes activity and participation. *Activity* is defined as the execution of a task at any complexity level. *Activity limitation* encompasses difficulties an individual may face in completing the activity. *Participation* refers to the person's involvement in everyday situations and social interactions. *Participation restrictions* are the problems an individual may encounter with involvement in life situations.[80]

Part II: Universal Language of ICF Environment and Personal Contextual Factors
The ICF model considers the dynamic interaction between a patient's health condition and the environment and personal factors that impact functioning and disability. *External environmental factors* include social attitudes and legal and social structures.

Personal factors, exclusive of the person's health condition or disability, encompass the background of an individual's lived experiences such as age, race, gender, educational background, and life experiences. Fitness level, lifestyle, coping strategies, social background, and professional career are other personal factors influencing how a person's health condition is experienced.[82] The ICF Model of Functioning and Disability is designed to provide a framework for evaluation and assessment as well as a coherent view of various dimensions of health at biological, individual, and social levels. An ICF Checklist can be found at: https://www.who.int/classifications/icf/icfchecklist.pdf. Components of the ICF Checklist are listed in Table 2.7.

In 2008, the APTA House of Delegates endorsed the ICF model for implementation into physical therapy.[82] Functional mobility is an essential physical ability categorized within the activities and participation domains of the ICF.[83] Integrating the ICF model as a framework within Onc R improves the accuracy for a comprehensive upper extremity functional mobility[84] evaluation and assessment as depicted by the following breast cancer example.

Example: Breast Carcinoma Profile With ICF Integration
A 62-year-old woman is referred to outpatient physical therapy for shoulder pain. She was diagnosed with right ductal carcinoma in situ (DCIS), and underwent a mastectomy with a sentinel lymph

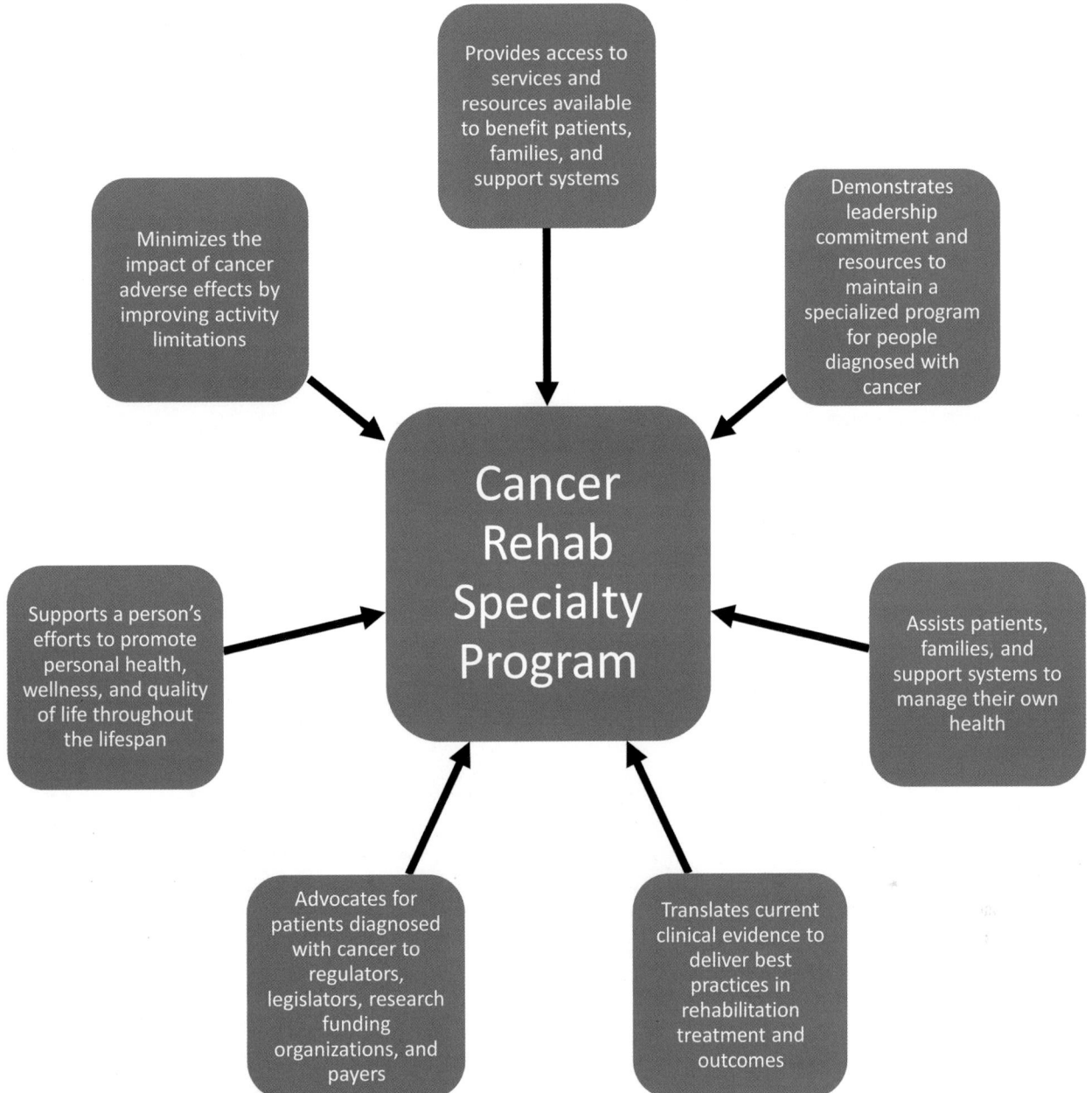

Provides access to services and resources available to benefit patients, families, and support systems

Minimizes the impact of cancer adverse effects by improving activity limitations

Demonstrates leadership commitment and resources to maintain a specialized program for people diagnosed with cancer

Supports a person's efforts to promote personal health, wellness, and quality of life throughout the lifespan

Cancer Rehab Specialty Program

Assists patients, families, and support systems to manage their own health

Advocates for patients diagnosed with cancer to regulators, legislators, research funding organizations, and payers

Translates current clinical evidence to deliver best practices in rehabilitation treatment and outcomes

• **Fig. 2.6** Benefits of CARF Accreditation Cancer Rehabilitation Specialty Program. *CARF*, Commission on Accreditation of Rehabilitation Facilities. (Created by Rochelle I. Brannon. Printed with permission.)

node dissection (SLND) (0/3 positive nodes). She completed an accelerated dose of radiation therapy (5 treatments over 1 week) to the chest wall. She has no pre-existing co-morbidities but has a body mass index (BMI) of 35 kg/m.[2]

The patient's primary complaint includes right shoulder pain with fear of moving her right arm. She notes difficulty reaching overhead for kitchen tasks, and she is unable to wash her back, carry a laundry basket, or make her bed. She has not been able to garden in 3 months and acknowledges experiencing increased bouts of fatigue. The patient describes a strong family support system and a caring husband. Before her medical leave, she worked full-time as a senior marketing analyst.

In supine, right active shoulder range of motion (AROM): flexion 120 (normal = 180°), abduction 110 (normal = 150°), and internal rotation 40 (normal = 90 °). A hand-held dynamometer

strength test was deferred. Palpation findings: absent sensation to light-touch surrounding the surgical mastectomy incision and absent sensation to light-touch around the two postoperative drain incisions. Irradiation changes are noted on the right chest wall hyperpigmentation with fibrosis of the tissues in the radiated field and tissue pain during end-range stretching of the shoulder.

For determining self-reported disabilities in the ICF model of activity and participation, the patient completed three surveys and risk factors were identified.
1. Disability of Arm, Shoulder, and Hand (Quick DASH) is a self-report questionnaire that describes ability and challenges of upper extremity function and activities.
2. Functional Assessment of Cancer Therapy-Breast (FACT-B +4) was utilized to capture the psychosocial, emotional, and physical impairments caused by cancer and its treatments.

TABLE 2.7	Components of International Classification of Function Checklist

Body Function	Body Structure	Activity Limitations and Participation Restriction	Environmental Factors	Personal Factors
Mental	Nervous systems	Learning and applying knowledge	Products and technology	Lifestyle habits
Sensory and pain	Eye, ear, and related structures	General tasks and demands	Natural environment	Social background
Voice and speech functions	Speech and voice	Communication	Human-built changes to environment	Education
Digestive, metabolic, and endocrine systems	Digestive, metabolic, and endocrine systems	Self-care	Attitudes	Race/ethnicity
Genitourinary and reproductive systems	Genitourinary and reproductive systems	Domestic life	Services, systems, policies	Sexual orientation
Neuromusculoskeletal and movement-related	Movement	Interpersonal interactions and relationships		Assets of the individual
Functions of the skin and related structures	Skin and related structures	Major life areas		
		Community, social, and civic life		
Other body functions	Other body structures	Other activity participation	Other environmental factors	

Created by Rochelle I. Brannon. Printed with permission.

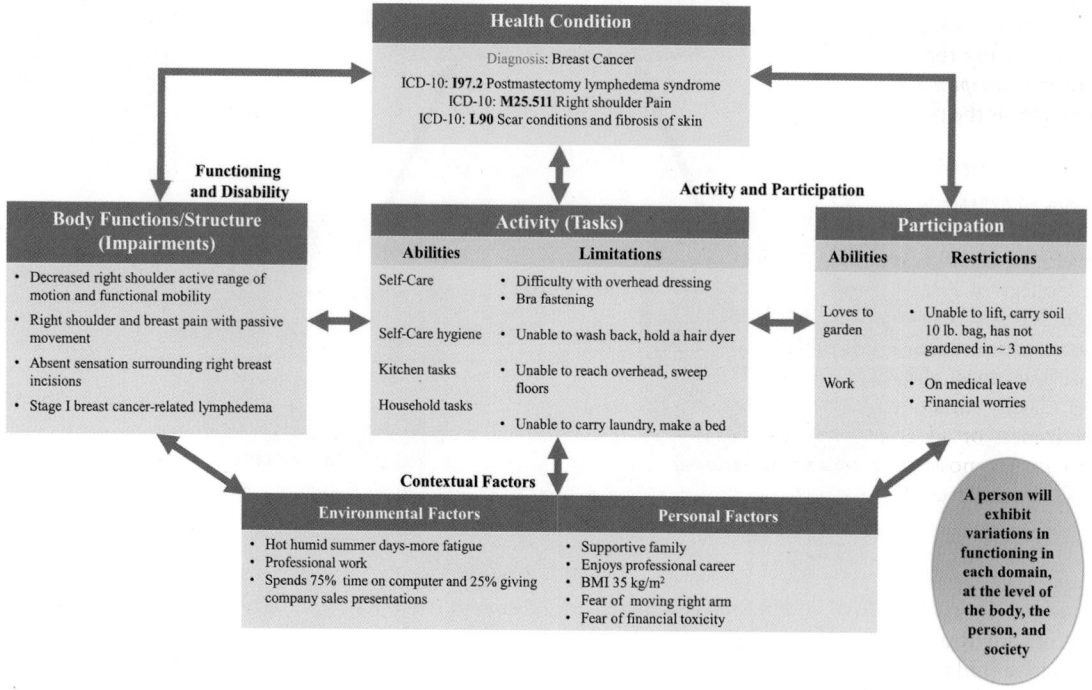

• **Fig. 2.7** ICF Evaluation. *AROM,* Active range of motion; *ICF,* International Classification of Function. (Created by Rochelle I. Brannon. Printed with permission.)

3. Modified Brief Fatigue Inventory (mBFI) which examines the severity and effect of fatigue on daily functioning in the previous 24 hours through a 9-item questionnaire.

Breast cancer-related lymphedema risk factors for this patient included high BMI, sentinel lymph node dissection (SLND), radiation therapy to the chest wall, and a sedentary lifestyle. The integration of this oncology case profile within the ICF model is illustrated in Figure 2.7.

Karnofsky Performance Status

The KPS was developed to evaluate the ability of a person diagnosed with cancer to tolerate chemotherapy. KPS covers 11 categories ranging from normal health (100) to death (0). A KPS score between 80 and 100 indicates a person remains functionally independent. Scores between 50 and 70 describe the patient as functionally unable to work but able to continue to reside at

Percentage (%)	Karnofsky Performance Scale	Score	ECOG Performance Scale
100	Normal, no complaints, no evidence of disease	0	Normal activity; asymptomatic
90	Able to carry on normal activity; minor signs or symptoms of disease	1	Symptomatic; fully ambulatory
80	Normal activity with effort; some signs or symptoms of disease		
70	Cares for self, unable to carry on normal activity or to do active work	2	Symptomatic; in bed <50% of time
60	Requires occasional assistance, but is able to care for most of his/her needs		
50	Requires considerable assistance and frequent medical care	3	Symptomatic; in bed 50% of time; not bedridden
40	Disabled, requires special care and assistance		
30	Severely disabled, hospitalization indicated; death not imminent		
20	Very sick, hospitalization indicated; death not imminent	4	100% bedridden
10	Moribund, fatal processes, progressing rapidly		
0	Dead	5	Dead

Karnofsky and Eastern Cooperative Group Performance Scales

• **Fig. 2.8** Combined Karnofsky Scale and ECOG. *ECOG*, Eastern Cooperative Oncology Group. (Reprinted with permission from Mariano J, Min, LC. *Management of Cancer in the Older Patient*. Elsevier; January 1, 2012.)

home while requiring some personal care assistance. With a score between 10 and 40, the person transitions to a dependent level of care. KPS is one performance tool an oncologist may use to determine candidacy for a cancer treatment regimen as well as how chemotherapy is affecting their patient's functional abilities. KPS also serves as an *interdisciplinary* communication tool for selecting appropriate resources as the person's baseline of function declines.[85]

The Eastern Cooperative Oncology Group Performance Status

Originally developed in 1981 by the ECOG who joined with the American College of Radiology Imaging Network (ACRIN) becoming the ECOG-ACRIN Cancer Research Group, this tool provides standardization among researchers to evaluate performance status during cancer clinical research.[86]

These tools classify functional impairments to help determine the effectiveness or adverse effects from cancer treatment as well as assist in prognosis. It is helpful to compare the KPS with the ECOG to understand how they correlate to each other (Figure 2.8).

Annual Rehab Screening

A future model of Onc R care is theorized by the authors of this chapter. This model would provide an annual Onc R assessment to assist in monitoring and identifying adverse effects as well as late and long-term effects to provide intervention as needed to mitigate functional impairments as well as maintain and improve QOL.

The authors of this chapter believe that an annual Onc R assessment for PLWBCs is the next step in true patient-centered comprehensive cancer care. Advocating for this follow-up care is the responsibility of Onc R clinicians. Due to documented late and long-term adverse events (see Chapter 28) and their sustained impact on QOL, it is important to promptly identify early red flags that may lead to adverse events, and to provide early intervention. Table 2.8 provides an example of a proposed annual breast cancer-specific Onc R assessment. Please note that each cancer

diagnosis has special considerations related to the functional deficits common to each cancer treatment protocol. Thus, this assessment is only one example and would include persons diagnosed and treated for breast cancer with surgery and chemotherapy. Ultimately, we are advocating for annual assessments specific to each cancer diagnosis that could be integrated into the electronic medical records system to prompt referrals. Figure 2.9 provides an example of an algorithm for a person diagnosed with breast cancer utilizing the annual assessment philosophy.

Conclusion

Onc R is one of the fastest growing specialties in the medical arena. Due to the substantial number of survivors, every health care practitioner needs to be familiar with the benefits of Onc R to participate in prevention, treatment, management, or referral. Individuals that seek medical care for any reason may have a cancer diagnosis and treatment in their history that may impact the current treatment they seek. Understanding the five levels of prevention and how Onc R clinicians can work in any or all of those domains or refer to clinicians to seek help at whatever level of prevention is needed. To provide patient-centered comprehensive cancer care, this knowledge is critical. Onc R is recognized as very beneficial by oncology organizations. This chapter serves as a call to action for to all Onc R clinicians to advocate for Onc R services in all settings. When properly provided and integrated, Onc R can provide PLWBCs with hope for sustained QOL throughout their lifetime.

Critical Research Needs

- Rehabilitation navigation–application with various cancer diagnoses, development of rehabilitation navigation programs, utilization of rehabilitation navigators, the difference in nurse versus physical therapist navigation, feasibility, and cost variable determination.
- Prospective surveillance programs for prostate, head and neck, leukemia, lymphoma, and colorectal cancers with or without telerehabilitation.

TABLE 2.8	Annual Oncology Rehabilitation Assessment for Persons Diagnosed With Breast Cancer

1. Review Prehabilitation (if available) and Post-Treatment Rehabilitation Medical Records
2. Subjective screening questions: Annual breast cancer rehabilitation assessment
   A. Chemotherapy and Chemotherapy Pain
      - Have you had any changes to your chemotherapy medications?
      - Are you experiencing any hand, finger, or foot pain, numbness, or tingling? Are the symptoms bilateral? Or unilateral?
      - Are there any other unexplained symptoms you may be experiencing, i.e., sharp, burning, shooting, electrical pain?
      - Are you having or have you had any joint pain?
   B. Breast Cancer-Related Lymphedema Secondary
      - Have you experienced any difficulty removing jewelry, i.e., rings, necklaces, a wristwatch?
      - Have you noticed any upper arm clothing feeling tighter on one side compared to the other side?
      - Have you noticed any intermittent numbness and tingling above or below the elbow?
   C. Exercise/Hobbies
      - What is your favorite exercise? How often do you engage in your favorite exercise?
      - Do you have a walking workout routine? What is your average walking time?
      - Are you participating in any available virtual online classes or community cancer group exercise classes?
      - Describe what you do for fun?
   D. Fatigue
      - Describe your daily energy level? Normal, good, fair, poor, always tired.
      - Are you easily fatigued after reading a newspaper? Would reading a book cause you fatigue?
      - Have you experienced shortness of breath during climbing stairs? Are you walking slower now compared to last year?
      - When you walk fast, are you easily out of breath?
      - Describe your sleep routine or regimen?
      - Overall, are your sleep patterns improving, staying the same, or worsening?
   E. Balance
      - Have you experienced any falls or near falls in your house or in the community?
      - Have you had any episodes of unexpected tripping in your house, yard, or in the community?
   F. Vestibular
      - Have you experienced any altered sensations of smell or taste?
      - Have you experienced any episodes of dizziness when you turn your head?
      - Have you had any episodes of dizziness?
      - Do you ever feel like you are on a ship swaying back and forth while standing still?
      - Do you ever need to hold onto household furniture to steady yourself?
   G. Fine Motor Control (peripheral neuropathy)
      - Do you have any difficulties with holding a kitchen knife when prepping vegetables?
      - Do you have any difficulties with twisting off the toothpaste cap?
      - Do you struggle with buttoning up your blouse?
   H. Pelvic Floor
      - If you cough or sneeze, do you notice any urinary leakage?
      - Do you experience pain with urination?
      - Does this urinary leakage bother you?
      - Do you have any questions regarding your bowel or bladder behaviors?
      - Have you noticed any changes to your sexual arousal patterns?
      - Any episodes of painful intercourse?
   I. Cognitive: Memory, attention, executive function, language memory, problem-solving
      - Attention: Do you have difficulties concentrating on one thing at a time?
      - Sustained and alternating/divided attention: Do you have trouble attending to two tasks at the same time such as following directions while driving?
      - Memory: Do you struggle with recalling appointments? Do you forget to bring things to appointments? Do you ever forget to take your medications?
      - Language memory: Do you have trouble finding the word you want to say? How often does this occur? (ask the patient to name as many animals as possible within 1 minute (15 + is considered within normal limits)
      - Executive function: Do you have trouble making a plan and sticking to it?
      - Problem-solving: Do you have trouble managing your finances?
   J. Nutrition
      - Describe your daily hydration intake.
      - Has your weight changed in the last year? If yes, was this change intentional?
      - Would you describe your diet as excellent, good, fair, or poor?
      - Do you experience any weekly episodes of constipation? Or diarrhea?
      - Describe your understanding of inflammatory foods and this food relationship to secondary lymphedema.
   K. Return to work
      - Have you returned to work?
      - Any work activities you cannot perform as well as you did before your breast cancer treatments started?
      - If you are returning to work soon, are you excited to go back to work?

TABLE 2.8 **Annual Oncology Rehabilitation Assessment for Persons Diagnosed With Breast Cancer—cont'd**

3. Objective Assessment
   A. Musculoskeletal (compare to prehab baseline or previous objective discharge documentation)
      1. Postural Assessment–Anterior Observation
         - In sitting, observation of the resting position of head and shoulders.
         - Does a dropped shoulder exist?
         - Does the patient present with exaggerated internal rotation of the humerus?
         - Compare pectoralis muscle symmetry: Is there muscle atrophy?
         - Do the breasts appear symmetrical or asymmetrical?
      2. Postural Assessment–Posterior Observation
         - Is scapular winging present?
         - Do you notice any lateral chest wall pockets of breast cancer-related lymphedema?
         - During the lateral thoracic palpation, did you detect any secondary lymphedema concerns?
   B. Range of Motion
      - Screen and clear cervical spine.
      - Perform bilateral upper extremity range of motion.
      - During movement testing, does the patient complain of musculoskeletal tissue discomforts with movement?
      - Does the patient complain of any musculoskeletal pain with movement?
   C. Strength
      - Grip: Perform grip strength assessment by using a handheld dynamometer.[87]
      - Manual Muscle Test (MMT): Perform upper extremity strength testing using a Handheld Isometric Dynamometry (HHD). These devices are now the MMT standard, have high accuracy, and have shown high levels of inter-rater and intra-rater reliability.[88,89]
   D. Neurological-Neurosensory
      - Cranial nerves–CN VIII, vestibular nerve (subject complaint of dizziness); CN V, trigeminal nerve (motor).
      - Motor reflex: Perform bilateral upper extremity deep tendon reflexes C5-6, C-7.
      - Sensation testing: Semmes-Weinstein Monofilaments Test on the great toe and index finger. The mechanical test quantifies touch thresholds (*subjective complaint is numbness or tingling of the fingers or toes*).
      - Vibration assessment–Perform based on the subjective exam: Numbness/tingling in hands and feet; Chemotherapy induced polyneuropathy impairments.
      - Dermatomes: Upper body levels based on subjective exam findings.
   E. Integumentary
      1. Surgical Incisional Tissue Mobility Assessment
         - Perform palpation assessment on adherent scars. Is there any subjective complaint of sensitive skin issues?
         - Does the patient complain of integumentary itchiness around surgical incisions?
         - Bilateral breast tissue mobility: Are there mobility palpation differences between the breast tissues? Is there subjective compliant of breast pains during mobility assessment?
         - Assessment and palpation around the surgical drain incision: Is sensation present or absent around the drain incisions? Is there any subjective complaint regarding tenderness or pain around the drain incisions?
   F. Inframammary Region:
      - Bilateral palpation assessment to inferior breast tissue: Are there any inframammary tissue differences between the breast tissues?
      - Is the compression bra fitting too tight leaving residual indurations?
      - Is there any breast cancer-related lymphedema present from a poorly fitting bra?
   G. Radiation Tissue Assessment:
      - Perform bilateral palpation between the sternum intercostals: Are there any radiation fibrosis changes between the sternum intercostals?
      - Complete palpation assessment around the radiation tattoos: Is there any subjective complaint of tissue discomfort around the radiation tattoos?
   H. Circumferential Measurement
      - Obtain previous prehabilitation baseline or previous status-post measurements: Performed annual bioimpedance assessment.
      - Perform standard 10.0 cm arm tape measurement and compare to prior baseline findings (Stout NL, Pfalzer LA, Levy E, et al. Segmental limb volume change as a predictor of the onset of lymphedema in women with early breast cancer. *PM R.* 2011;3(12):1098–1105. doi:10.1016/j.pmrj.2011.07.021).
   I. Self-Care Education
      1. Breast Cancer-Related Lymphedema (BCRL) Education
         - Review and explain the patient's previous known breast cancer-related lymphedema (BCRL) risk factors: BMI, the number of lymph nodes dissected, radiation therapy, exercise baseline, and nondominant hand.
         - Expand and review BCRL clinical signs and symptoms to maintain Stage I reversible BCRL.
         - Perform and review manual lymphatic drainage sequencing for continued independent daily home program compliance.
         - Education and instruction on signs and symptoms of arm cellulitis presentation. Stress critical importance to call PCP or go to an urgent care center for appropriate medical care.
      2. Compression Garment(s)
         - Review compression garment replacement protocol: If worn daily, is recommended to replace the compression garments every 6 months.
         - If the compression sleeve and gauntlet/glove are too small, a tourniquet effect may develop causing an episode of BCRL.
         - Explain and share newer compression materials for arm compression sleeve and gauntlet/glove products.
         - Share the newest compression bra products available on market.
      3. Education on Bone Health
         - Osteoporosis education on bone health risks from chemotherapy adverse effects.
         - Fracture Risk Assessment Tool (FRAX): Analyzes osteoporosis risk for postmenopausal women. (https://www.sheffield.ac.uk/FRAX/tool.aspx)
         - Educate on latest exercise recommendations: APTA, An Executive Summary of Reports (Campbell KL, Winters-Stone KM, Patel AV, et al. An Executive Summary of Reports From an International Multidisciplinary Roundtable on Exercise and Cancer: Evidence, Guidelines, and Implementation. Rehabil Oncol. 2019;37(4):144–152. doi:10.1097/01.REO.0000000000000186).

(Continued)

TABLE
2.8
Annual Oncology Rehabilitation Assessment for Persons Diagnosed With Breast Cancer—cont'd

J. Cardiovascular-Pulmonary
- Endurance: Functional assessment recommended–6-minute walk test (Fisher MI, Lee J, Davies CC, et al. Oncology Section EDGE Task Force on Breast Cancer Outcomes: A Systematic Review of Outcome Measures for Functional Mobility. Rehabil Oncol. 2015; 33(3): 19–31.).
- Expand updated exercises guidelines: APTA, An Executive Summary of Reports (Campbell KL, Winters-Stone KM, Patel AV, et al. An Executive Summary of Reports From an International Multidisciplinary Roundtable on Exercise and Cancer: Evidence, Guidelines, and Implementation. Rehabil Oncol. 2019;37(4):144–152. doi:10.1097/01.REO.0000000000000186).

K. Updated Treatment Summary and Follow-Up Care Plan
- Return in 1 year for annual rehabilitation breast cancer assessment: Schedule the annual assessment around your birthday for easier advanced planning.
- If you notice a change from today's functional assessment, it is important to return to your rehabilitation provider or your physician.
- As a courtesy, the rehabilitation provider should consider mailing the patient a completed annual breast cancer assessment. Encourage the patient to add the annual rehabilitation assessment into the survivorship medical records.
- Advise discussion with oncologist about cardiac screening with prior exposure to cardiotoxic cancer treatment regimes?

APTA American Physical Therapy Association Created by Rochelle I. Brannon. Printed with permission.

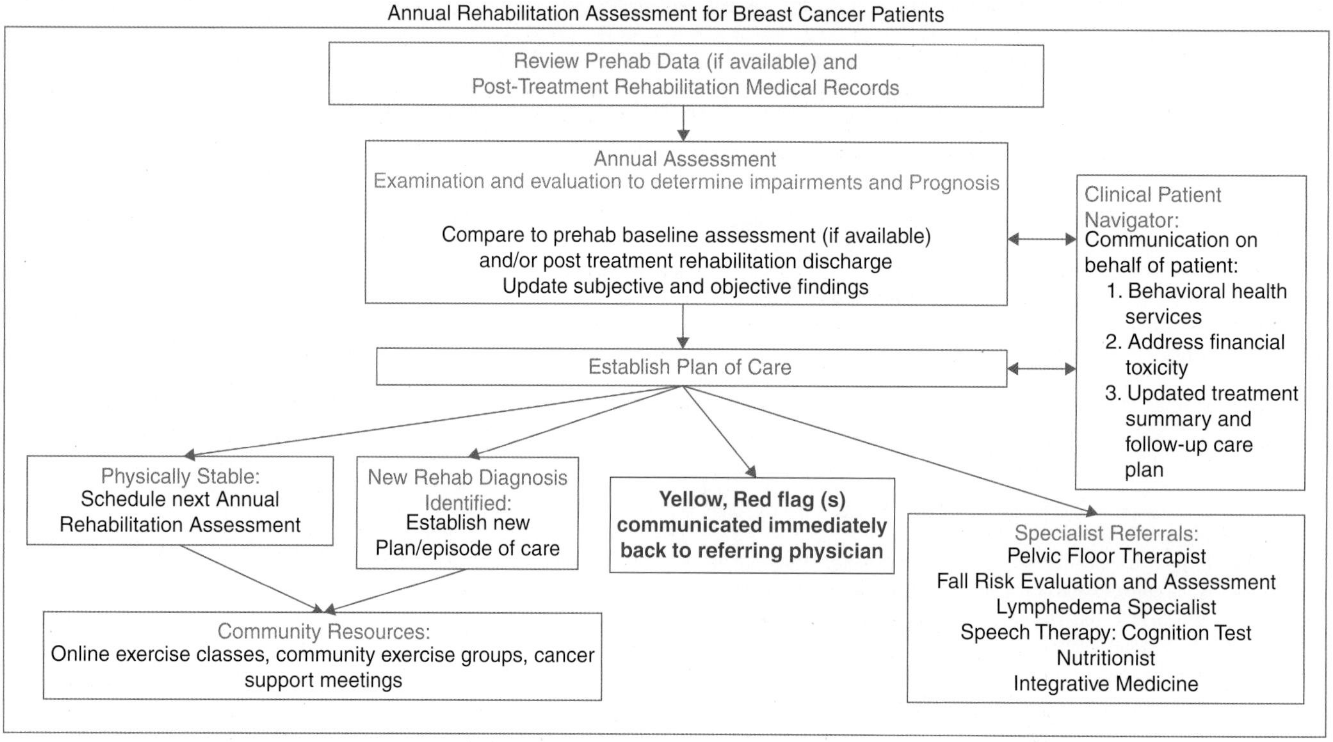

• **Fig. 2.9** Annual Oncology Rehabilitation Assessment for Persons Diagnosed With Breast Cancer. (Created by Rochelle I. Brannon. Printed with permission.)

- Can annual rehabilitation screening decrease the prevalence of late and long-term effects of cancer treatment?
- Development of the survivorship care plan including risk reduction for lymphedema, the American College of Sports Medicine (ACSM) physical activity recommendations, exercise prescription, self-treatment strategies provided at end of treatment course, feasibility of care plans, and benefits of care plans.

Case Studies

Case Study #1: Patient Navigation

A 37-year-old woman had palpated her own breast mass and requested her first mammogram through her primary care physician. Following mammography which revealed a suspicious 1.5cm lesion, the breast care nurse navigator scheduled an ultrasound which demonstrated a solid mass within the left breast which correlated with the mammography findings. Subsequently, a needle biopsy of the left breast was positive for the diagnosis of an estrogen receptor (ER) positive, progesterone receptor (PR) positive, and human epidermal growth factor receptor 2 (HER2) negative invasive ductal carcinoma. She was seen at a multidisciplinary breast cancer clinic, which she attended with her then-fiancé on Valentine's Day. Their plan was to be married approximately 6 months from the clinic date and start a family. A cheek swab for genetic testing was obtained at that time and was sent out for screening for BRCA1 and 2 mutations.

The multidisciplinary breast cancer care team included the medical oncologist, radiation oncologist, breast surgeon, research nurse, social worker, physical therapist, and clinical navigator. Before the patient arrived at the clinic, the care team met with the pathologist and radiologist to review imaging and slides. Her recommended treatment plan included lumpectomy with sentinel lymph node biopsy, followed by adjuvant dose-dense doxorubicin (Adriamycin) and cyclophosphamide (Cytoxan) followed by external beam radiation therapy. The long-term treatment included the recommendation of endocrine therapy with tamoxifen (Nolvadex) for 5 years. The navigator coordinated a second opinion at a tertiary care center in a large city for confirmation of the recommended treatment plan. The results of her genetic testing were returned, and she was negative for BRCA1 and 2 mutations. To address the patient's distress and anxiety associated with her new diagnosis and transition to illness, she was referred to the clinical social worker for individual and couples counseling.

For prospective surveillance, the patient was assessed for baseline measurements of her upper extremity with bioelectrical impedance preoperatively through the Onc R department. There, she was also educated on lymphedema risk reduction and the benefits of regular physical activity. The merits of maintaining an ideal body weight were also discussed for both cancer risk reduction and the benefits of a lowered risk of lymphedema. Recommendations were made for supervised moderate-to-vigorous physical activity preoperatively for prehabilitation, throughout her active cancer treatment, and into long-term survivorship to help combat CRF.

Her surgical recovery was uneventful, but her final pathology report revealed a Grade 2 lesion with lymphovascular invasion. Oncotype DX testing (a 21-gene test to estimate recurrence of breast cancer) revealed an intermediate risk for recurrence at 10 years. Subsequently, her chemotherapy regimen was expanded to include paclitaxel (Taxol) for four cycles. Her chemotherapy caused nausea and chemotherapy-induced peripheral neuropathy in her hands and feet. Her navigator scheduled her to see a registered dietitian to discuss options for management of her nausea, and to the physical therapist for balance screening and education on fall risk reduction. The patient was also referred for integrative oncology services for symptom management including massage therapy, Reiki, and acupuncture. Her radiation therapy resulted in minor fatigue and radiation dermatitis within the treatment field at the end of her course of radiation. After her active phase of treatment, her medical oncologist recommended the initiation of tamoxifen for endocrine therapy. However, the patient and her new husband wanted to start a family, and therefore she declined. The navigator scheduled the patient to see an endocrinologist/fertility specialist at a local fertility clinic to assess the feasibility of her hope for a successful pregnancy due to her recent exposure to chemotherapy which induced temporary, chemical menopause.

The patient received a treatment summary and a survivorship care plan after her active treatment from her navigator. Ongoing medical oncology appointments were recommended for follow-up screening for cardiac health, bone health, and signs and symptoms of recurrence. Additionally, bioimpedance measurements were repeated at scheduled intervals for prospective surveillance purposes for lymphedema screening. She was advised to maintain a physically active lifestyle including her prescribed aerobic and resistance exercise and yoga, initially through the cancer center's supervised exercise program, to be followed by an independent gym membership for ongoing access to physical activity opportunities.

The patient and her husband went on to conceive and deliver a healthy baby girl 2 years after the conclusion of her active cancer treatment. Her cancer treatment team came to visit her in the obstetrics ward, and her physical therapist made recommendations for the safe performance of activities of daily living to help her manage childcare in her new role as a mother.

Case Study #2: Untreated Stage IV Right Breast Carcinoma With Secondary Lymphedema

A 71-year-old woman was admitted to a hospital for ongoing right arm swelling. During her hospital stay, she was diagnosed with Stage IV carcinoma of the right breast. The pathology report revealed the breast tissue markers were ER positive, PR positive, with a negative HER2 status. The computed tomography (CT) findings confirmed a fungating right breast mass with metastatic disease to the bone, as well as metastasis within the three right axillary lymph node levels and into the mediastinal lymph nodes. The patient's metastatic disease continued with tiny nonspecific lung nodules, thickening tissue around the diaphragm crux and around her left adrenal gland. Upon hospital discharge, the patient followed hospital medical advice by completing an outpatient oncology consult.

An outpatient positron emission tomography (PET) scan confirmed a large right breast mass, extensive metastatic disease with a large retroperitoneal mass encircling the upper abdominal aorta, bony disease, and lymphadenopathy at multiple levels of the neck, chest, and abdomen. A brain magnetic resonance imaging (MRI) scan showed the left occipital lobe with a questionable enhancement area of concern. Radiation therapy was not recommended.

Although the medical oncologist recommended a palliative adjuvant regime, the patient declined any medical care for several weeks. Ten weeks later the patient agreed to a trial of anastrozole (Arimidex), an aromatase inhibitor hormone therapy drug.

A few weeks later, the patient experienced a deterioration in her medical condition requiring a second hospital admission. In addition to requiring a blood transfusion for severe anemia, the patient's creatine level of 5.28 mg/L was considered as medically alarming. Normal adult female creatine levels range from 0.5 mg/L to 1.1 mg/L. An abdominal ultrasound showed bilateral hydronephrosis and abnormal bladder thickening. The medical care team explained that the retroperitoneal lymphadenopathy compression was the likely cause of the bilateral acute kidney failure. One month later, the patient underwent a bilateral ureteral stent surgery. Unfortunately, the surgery was unsuccessful and an emergency surgery for bilateral nephrostomy tubes was completed three days later.

Prior to her hospital discharge, the medical care team gave the patient a prognosis of less than 6 months to live. Five days later the patient transitioned to hospice services for right breast medical wound dressing care, nephrostomy drain monitoring, and metastatic cancer symptom management.

Physical Therapy Hospice Lymphedema Evaluation: The hospice agency authorized a physical therapy lymphedema evaluation for worsening right arm swelling. At the time of the homecare physical therapy evaluation, the patient was 72-years-old and lived alone. Her functional baseline was independent with household activities except bathing and wound care.

Subjective Exam: The patient denied any physical pain. With a friend, she was continuing her 2 to 3 miles daily walking program. She also reported adhering to a healthy organic diet. The patient stated her lymphedema evaluation goals as: (1) wanting to decrease swelling in her right hand and fingers to hold a pen for writing checks; (2) continue holding utensils with her right hand

Right
Posterior
Upper
Quadrant

Isolated dermal
nodule with
discoloration

Cancer
Erysipelatoides

Malignant
lymphatic
fibrotic tissue

Wound
dressing

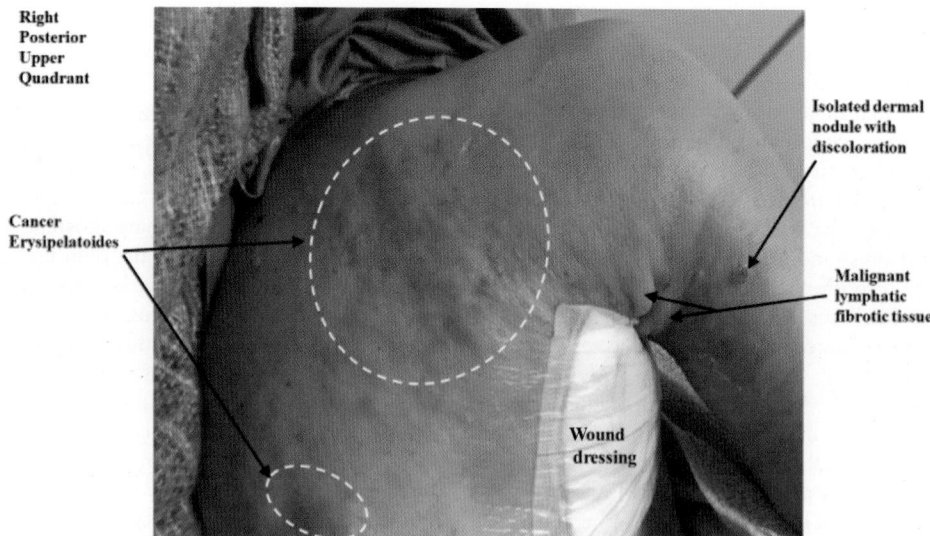

• **Fig. 2.10** Right Posterior Upper Quadrant. (Photo provided by Rochelle I. Brannon. Printed with permission.)

Right elbow with
joint contracture

Proximal tissue
softer than distally,
Erythema without
tissue warmth

Distal forearm
indurated thick
fibrotic tissue

Dorsomedial
lymphatic
territory

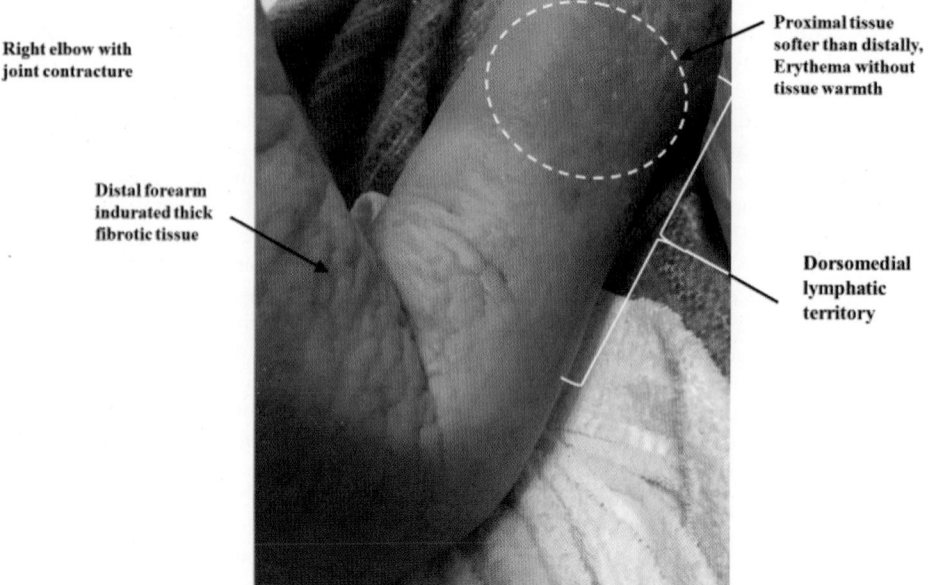

• **Fig. 2.11** Right Elbow With Joint Contracture. (Photo provided by Rochelle I. Brannon, Printed with permission.)

Right Anterior Shoulder

Cutaneous
nodules

Skin thickening
and multiple
well-defined
cutaneous
nodules

Malignant
lymphatic
fibrotic tissue

Indurated papules

Necrotic
tissue from
right
fungating
breast
tumor

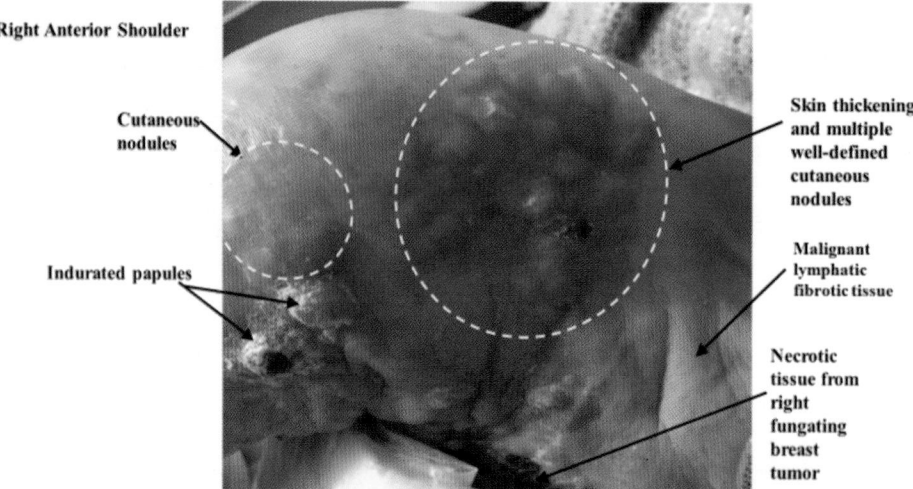

• **Fig. 2.12** Right Anterior Shoulder. (Photo provided by Rochelle I. Brannon. Printed with permission.)

for eating; and (3) improve right arm mobility for brushing her teeth and hair.

Objective Findings:

Posture: The patient presented with a severe thoracic kyphosis combined with a dropped forward head posture. During upright activities, the patient rested her right elbow flexed at 90 degrees across her chest. The patient used her left hand to lift the weight of her edematous right forearm and hand during ambulation.

Integumentary System: The right fungating breast tumor extended from the mediastinal area to the lateral breast/axillary region. The right supraclavicular region presented with multiple well-defined nodules and malignant lymphatic fluid (Figure 2.10). Numerous metastatic cutaneous nodules were clustered in the patient's mid thoracic spine and scapula.

Palpation: In bedside sitting, the right shoulder and hand were supported by pillows. Palpation revealed severe indurated lymphedema fibrosis from the right elbow to the patient's hand. Her fingers were severely edematous with 3+ pitting edema (Figure 2.11). Proximal right upper arm palpation revealed softer tissue quality as compared to the distal arm. The right upper arm presented with circumferential erythema and less stagnant edema compared to the distal forearm (Figure 2.12). The patient's left medial inguinal basin presented with a palpable nontender soft tissue mass measuring about 3.0 cm.

Musculoskeletal System: Passive movement of the right elbow beyond a 90 degrees flexed joint contracture was deferred. Passive shoulder abduction was minimal and limited by shearing risks to the friable right breast wound bed. Passive shoulder flexion ranged from neutral to 30 degrees. The right finger mobility and wrist flexion and extension, provided enough functional active range of movement for daily tasks.

Circumferential Limb Volume: Right arm standard lymphedema tape measurements were documented following the standard 4-centimeter protocol.

Assessment: The patient presented with cutaneous metastasis of a primary adenocarcinoma of the right breast. Her osseous metastatic disease presentation included the right anterior and posterior upper quadrant and left proximal medial thigh. Because metastatic disease included right axillary lymph node levels and supraclavicular lymph nodes, normal lymphatic fluid drainage into the right subclavian vein was prevented. The patient's functional impairments included limited right shoulder mobility, an elbow joint contracture and severe forearm indurated fibrotic tissue restrictions. The size and weight of the right forearm created donning and doffing dressing challenges.

Prognosis: Metastatic breast cancer, regardless of the metastatic site, remains incurable. The hospice rehabilitation therapeutic goals focused on maintaining present functional mobility baseline and comfort care.

Interventions (Table 2.9): Maintaining the functional mobility of the right fingers and wrist were critical for the patient to remain independent in her home. Expanded lymphedema education was provided to minimize patient's disappointment or unrealistic goal expectations. A lengthy patient education exchange occurred regarding risks related to moving the forearm's lymphatic fluid towards her upper arm. Moving the stagnant forearm

TABLE 2.9 71-Year-Old Female With Untreated Stage IV Breast Cancer

1st Hospital Admission: Right arm swelling	**Year One**	
Hospital Diagnostic Testing: CT Scan chest, abdomen, and pelvis Right breast biopsy MRI brain	2 days later	
Outpatient Oncology Consult: PET scan MRI brain	**Year Two** 2 weeks later	
Palliative Adjuvant Trial: Arimidex	2 months later	
2nd Hospital Admission: Diagnosis severe anemia and acute kidney failure	1 month later	
S/P bilateral ureteral stent placement	2 days later	
Emergency Surgery: S/P bilateral nephrostomy drain placement	3 days later	
Hospital Discharge: **Hospice services**	5 days later	
	Year Three 14 months later	**Hospice Physical Therapy Lymphedema Evaluation**
Hospice Wound dressing twice per week	2 weeks later	2nd Lymphedema visit
Hospice Wound dressing three times per week	1 week later; 1 month later	3rd Lymphedema visit Pro bono visit
Patient expired	2 months later	

CT, computed tomography; *PET*, positron emission tomography; *MRI*, magnetic resonance imaging; *S/P*, status post. Created by Rochelle I. Brannon. Printed with permission.

TABLE 2.10	Hospice Lymphedema Skilled Intervention and Patient Home Program	
Intervention	Description	Frequency
HEP: Exercises	Diaphragmatic breathing	As often as possibile
Prayer hands	Wrist extension, stretching-hold 30 secs	Wrist extension, stretching-hold 30 secs
Phalen's Test	Wrist flexion stretch 10 secs x 3 reps	5x before meals
Passive range	Right wrist radial/ulnar deviation	5x before meals
Active assist range	Forearm supination and pronation	10 reps each direction
Active range	Right hand make a fist, then extended fingers wide and long	5x hourly

HEP, home exercise program; *secs*, seconds; *reps*, repetitions Created by Rochelle I. Brannon. Printed with permission.
Modified compression bandages intervention:
Elastomull on fingers.
Artiflex soft, used as protective buffering layer on right hand to elbow.
4 cm x 5 m short stretch compression bandage, lightly applied to fingers and wrist,
15 cm width Isoband short stretch bandage, wrist to elbow.
Progression: FarrowWrapLITE compression garment and 15–20 mmHg compression glove
for 3 hours on and off as tolerated.

lymphatic fluid towards the supraclavicular region risks included possible exudate into the breast wound bed and tissue changes of right arm. Exercises to maintain the mobility of the right fingers, wrist, and elbow were given (Table 2.10). The application of intensive complete decongestive therapy may be modified among patients with advanced cancer. Modified short stretch compression bandages were applied to the fingers, wrist, and forearm for initial treatment (see Table 2.10. The patient was instructed to remove the compression bandages after 6 hours. If well tolerated a 15 to 20 mmHg compression glove was to be worn the following morning for 3 hours on and off during waking hours. The patient progressed to independent daily donning and doffing a compression garment with the compression glove for three hours on and off as tolerated.

Outcomes: Applying a modified compression bandage system resulted in decreased circumferential measurements in her forearm, hand, and fingers. However, lymphatic drainage of dorso-medial territory significantly altered the right upper arm tissue quality from "softness" to a tissue quality of firmness. Upper arm circumferential girth also increased from the limited superficial

and deep lymphatic pathways for normal lymphatic drainage decongestion.

Progression to arm wrap and compression glove provided the patient flexibility for daily donning and doffing. On average patient reported wearing the compression garments about 4 to 5 hours a day and compliancy to exercises was questionable. The off-the-shelf compression garments allowed the patient to hold utensils for eating and writing checks for several more weeks. The patient's goal using her right hand for hair grooming and brushing teeth remained unrealistic.

Although the patient maintained functional use of her right fingers and wrist, increased exudate into the wound bed required increased hospice wound care management. One month later, the right upper arm tissue was as severely fibrotic as the forearm and severity of the cutaneous metastasis worsened. Daily independent donning of the compression wrap became too challenging. During daytime hours, the patient intermittently wore the compression glove. Within two months, the patient required daily home assistance and her decline was rapid.

Review Questions

Reader can find the correct answers and rationale in the back of the book.

1. Onc R clinicians who educate a PLWBC and their family about the benefits of strategies such as active surveillance for prostate cancer rather than aggressive surgery is what form of prevention?
   A. Primary
   B. Secondary
   C. Tertiary
   D. Quaternary

2. What percent of women diagnosed with breast cancer will have one or more adverse treatment effects at 6 months?
   A. 50%
   B. 75%
   C. 80%
   D. 90%

3. *Seasons of Survivorship* include all of the following except:
   A. Acute
   B. Sustaining
   C. Transitional
   D. Extended

4. Asking the patient to reiterate in their own words the information learned is referred to as:
   A. Teach-Back method
   B. Auditory method
   C. Kinesthetic method
   D. Talk-Back method

5. Which organization is directed by the American College of Surgeons, this consortium is involved in standard setting to ensure comprehensive, multidisciplinary quality cancer care as well as education, prevention, research and monitoring quality care.

A. CARF
B. CoC
C. NAPBC
D. NCPF

6. A patient is being treated for RIF. The patient is able to drive themselves to therapy 3 times per week. This would be an example of what level of Onc R Stepped Care?
   A. General conditioning activities–specialized
   B. Impairment directed care, uncomplicated
   C. Impairment directed care, complicated
   D. General conditioning activities

7. The Prospective Surveillance Model of care is:
   A. Determining baseline function and monitoring potential toxicities from cancer treatment, then providing preventive and early intervention as needed
   B. Determining baseline function and providing education and exercise before cancer treatment
   C. Monitoring potential adverse effects from the time of diagnosis throughout survivorship, and providing all intervention needed through hospice care
   D. Monitoring potential adverse effects and reporting back to physician or social worker as needed

8. In the ICF's model of care, the topic of "learning and applying knowledge" would be a component of what category?
   A. Body function
   B. Activity limitations and participation
   C. Environmental factors
   D. Personal factors

9. In the ICF's model of care, support and relationships would be categorized as:
   A. Body structure
   B. Activity limitations and participation
   C. Environmental factors
   D. Personal factors

10. Rehab that centers on optimizing function and performance status in the setting of progressive disease and further treatments while reducing the decline in function and QOL is classified as:
    A. Palliative
    B. Supportive
    C. Restorative
    D. Preventative

References

1. Dietz JH Jr. Adaptive rehabilitation in cancer: a program to improve quality of survival. *Postgrad Med*. 1980;68(1):145–153. doi:10.1080/00325481.1980.11715495.
2. Suderman K, McIntyre C, Sellar C, McNeely ML. Implementing cancer exercise rehabilitation: an update on recommendations for clinical practice. *Current Cancer Ther Rev*. 2019;15(2):100–109.
3. Baumann LC, Karel A. Prevention: primary, secondary, tertiary. In: Gellman MD, Turner JR, eds. *Encyclopedia of Behavioral Medicine*: Springer; 2013. doi:10.1007/978-1-4419-1005-9_135.
4. Kisling LA, Das JM. Prevention strategies [Updated June 7, 2020]. In: StatPearls [Internet]: StatPearls Publishing; 2021. January. https://www.ncbi.nlm.nih.gov/books/NBK537222/.
5. Martins C, Godycki-Cwirko M, Heleno B, Brodersen J. Quaternary prevention: reviewing the concept. *Eur J Gen Pract*. 2018;24(1):106–111.
6. Courneya KS, Karvinen KH, Vallance JK. Exercise motivation and behavior change. In: Feuerstein M, ed. *Handbook of Cancer Survivorship*: Springer; 2007. https://doi.org/10.1007/978-0-387-34562-8_7.
7. Bull FC, Al-Ansari SS, Biddle S, et al. World Health Organization 2020 guidelines on physical activity and sedentary behaviour. *Br J Sports Med*. 2020;54(24):1451–1462.
8. Silver JK, Baima J, Mayer RS. Impairment-driven cancer rehabilitation: an essential component of quality care and survivorship. *CA Cancer J Clin*. 2013;63(5):295–317. doi:10.3322/caac.21186.
9. Raj VS, Pugh TM, Yaguda SI, Mitchell CH, Mullan SS, Garces NS. The who, what, why, when, where, and how of team-based interdisciplinary cancer rehabilitation. *Semin Oncol Nurs*. 2020;36(1):150974. doi:10.1016/j.soncn.2019.150974.
10. Stubblefield MD. The underutilization of rehabilitation to treat impairments in breast cancer survivors. *PM R*. 2017;9:5317–5323.
11. Cheville AL, Troxel AB, Basford JR, Kornblith AB. Prevalence and treatment patterns of physical impairments in patients with metastatic breast cancer. *J Clin Oncol*. 2008;26(16):2621–2629.
12. Stout NL, Silver JK, Alfano CM, Ness KK, Gilchrist LS. Long-term survivorship care after cancer treatment: a new emphasis on the role of rehabilitation services. *Phys Ther*. 2019;99(1):10–13.
13. van der Goes DN, Edwardson N, Rayamajhee V, Hollis C, Hunter D. An iron triangle ROI model for health care. *Clinicoecon Outcomes Res*. 2019;11:335–348.
14. Alfano CM, Cheville AL, Mustian K. Developing high-quality cancer rehabilitation programs: a timely need. *Am Soc Clin Oncol Educ Book*. 2016;35:241–249.
15. Cheville AL, Mustian K, Winters-Stone K, Zucker DS, Gamble GL, Alfano CM. Cancer rehabilitation: an overview of current need, delivery models and levels of care. *Phys Med Rehabil Clin N Am*. 2017;28:1–17.
16. Alfano CM, Pergolotti M. Next-generation cancer rehabilitation: a giant step forward for patient care. *Rehabil Nurs*. 2018;43(4):186–194.
17. Mullan F. Seasons of survival: reflection of a physician with cancer. *N Engl J Med*. 1985;313:270–273.
18. The National Coalition for Cancer Survivorship. History of NCCS; 2020. https://www.canceradvocacy.org/about-us/our-history/ Accessed July 20, 2020.
19. Hewitt M, Greenfield S, Stovall E. *From Cancer Patient to Cancer Survivor: Lost in Transition*: National Academies Press; 2006.
20. Miller K, Merry B, Miller J. Seasons of survivorship revisited. *Cancer J*. 2008;14(6):369–374.
21. American Cancer Society. *Cancer treatment & survivorship facts & figures 2019–2021*. https://www.cancer.org/research/cancer-facts-statistics/survivor-facts-figures.html. Accessed May 31, 2021.
22. National Cancer Institute. stat facts: cancer among adolescents and young adults (AYAs) (Ages 15–39). https://seer.cancer.gov/statfacts/html/aya.html. Accessed October 1, 2020.
23. American Cancer Society. Cancer facts and figures; 2021. https://www.cancer.org/research/cancer-facts-statistics/all-cancer-facts-figures/cancer-facts-figures-2021.html. Accessed May 30, 2021.
24. American College of Surgeons. Optimal resources for cancer care (2020 Standards); 2021. https://www.facs.org/quality-programs/cancer/coc/standards/2020.
25. Bright CJ, Reulen RC, Winter DL, et al. Risk of subsequent primary neoplasms in survivors of adolescent and young adult cancer (Teenage and Young Adult Cancer+Survivor Study): a population-based, cohort study. *Lancet Oncol*. 2019;20(4):531–545.
26. Turcotte LM, Neglia JP, Reulen RC, et al. Risk, risk factors, and surveillance of subsequent malignant neoplasms in survivors of childhood cancer: a review. *J Clin Oncol*. 2018;36(21):2145–2152.

27. Armstrong GT, Chen Y, Yasui Y, et al. Reduction in late mortality among 5-year survivors of childhood cancer. *N Engl J Med.* 2016;374(9):833–842.

28. Schaapveld M, Aleman BM, van Eggermond AM. Second cancer risk up to 40 years after treatment for Hodgkin's lymphoma. *N Engl J Med.* 2015;373:2499–2511.

29. Freeman HP, Rodriguez RL. The history and principles of patient navigation. *Cancer.* 2011;117(15):3539–3542.

30. Freeman HP, Wasfie TJ. Cancer of the breast in poor black women. *Cancer.* 1989;63(12):2562–2569.

31. Freeman HP, Muth BJ, Kerner JF. Expanding access to cancer screening and clinical follow-up among the medically underserved. *Cancer Pract.* 1995;3(1):19–30.

32. National Academies of Sciences, Engineering, and Medicine. *Longterm survivorship care after cancer treatment: proceedings of a workshop:* The National Academies Press; 2018. doi:10.17226/25043.

33. Banks E, Byles JE, Gibson RE, et al. Is psychological distress in people living with cancer related to the fact of diagnosis, current treatment or level of disability? Findings from a large Australian study. *Med J Aust.* 2010;193(suppl 5)):S62–S67.

34. National Comprehensive Cancer Network. NCCN distress thermometer and problem list for patients; 2020. https://www.nccn.org/patients/resources/life_with_cancer/pdf/nccn_distress_thermometer.pdf. Accessed October 13, 2020.

35. Wu HS, Harden JK. Symptom burden and quality of life in survivorship: a review of the literature. *Cancer Nurs.* 2015;38(1):E29–E54.

36. Weaver KE, Forsythe LP, Reeve BB, et al. Mental and physical health-related quality of life among U.S. cancer survivors: population estimates from the 2010 National Health Interview Survey. *Cancer Epidemiol Biomarkers Prev.* 2012;21(11):2108–2117. doi:10.1158/1055-9965.EPI-12-0740.

37. Leclerc AF, Jerusalem G, Devos M, Crielaard JM, Maquet D. Multidisciplinary management of breast cancer. *Arch Public Health.* 2016;74:50. doi:10.1186/s13690-016-0163-7.

38. Schmitz KH, Speck RM, Rye SA, DiSipio T, Hayes SC. Prevalence of breast cancer treatment sequelae over 6 years of follow-up: the Pulling Through Study. *Cancer.* 2012;118(suppl 8):2217–2225.

39. Stout NL, Santa Mina D, Lyons KD, Robb K, Silver JK. A systematic review of rehabilitation and exercise recommendations in oncology guidelines. *CA Cancer J Clin.* 2021;71(2):149–175. doi:10.3322/caac.21639.

40. Silver JK, Baima J, Mayer RS. Impairment-driven cancer rehabilitation: an essential component of quality care and survivorship: impairment-driven cancer rehabilitation. *CA Cancer J Clin.* 2013;63(5):295–317.

41. American Cancer Society. American cancer society guideline for diet and physical activity; 2020. https://www.cancer.org/healthy/eat-healthy-get-active/acs-guidelines-nutrition-physical-activity-cancer-prevention/guidelines.html. Accessed October 15, 2020.

42. Santiago-Palma J, Payne R. Palliative care and rehabilitation. *Cancer.* 2001;92(S4):1049–1052. doi:10.1002/1097-0142(20010815)92:4+<1049::AID-CNCR1418>3.0.CO;2-H.

43. Greenlee H, Balneaves LG, Carlson LE, et al. Clinical practice guidelines on the use of integrative therapies as supportive care in patients treated for breast. *J Natl Cancer Inst Monogr.* 2014;2014(50):346–358. doi:10.1093/jncimonographs/lgu041.

44. Institute of Medicine. *Delivering high-quality cancer care: charting a new course for a system in crisis:* The National Academies Press; 2013.

45. Schrager SB, Phillips G, Burnside E. A simple approach to shared decision making in cancer screening. *Fam Pract Manag.* 2017;24(3):5–10.

46. MedPAC (Medicare Payment Advisory Commission). *Report to the congress: aligning incentives in medicare;* 2010. http://www.medpac.gov/documents/jun10_entirereport.pdf. Accessed January 13, 2021.

47. Berlin E, Fowkes W. A teaching framework for cross-cultural health care. *Western J Med.* 1983;139:934–938.

48. Paladino J, Koritsanszky L, Nisotel L, et al. Patient and clinician experience of a serious illness conversation guide in oncology: a descriptive analysis. *Cancer Med.* 2020;9(13):4550–4560. doi:10.1002/cam4.3102.

49. Plack M, Driscoll M. Design considerations. In: Plack M, Driscoll M, eds. *Teaching and Learning in Physical Therapy: From Classroom to Clinic*: Slack, Inc.; 2011:121.

50. Plack M, Driscoll M. The learning triad. In: Plack M, Driscoll M, eds. *Teaching and Learning in Physical Therapy: From Classroom to Clinic*: Slack, Inc.; 2011:190.

51. Health Resources and Services Administration. Health literacy. https://www.hrsa.gov/about/organization/bureaus/ohe/health-literacy/index.html#:~:text=Health%20literacy%20is%20the%20degree,who%20have%20low%20socioeconomic%20status. Updated August 2019. Accessed October 21, 2020.

52. The Joint Commission. *Advancing effective communication, cultural competence, and patient- and family-centered care: a roadmap for hospitals.* The Joint Commission: Oakbrook Terrace, IL; 2010.

53. Agency for Healthcare Research and Quality. Use the teach back method. Tool #5. https://www.ahrq.gov/health-literacy/improve/precautions/tool5.html. Updated September 2020. Accessed October 21, 2020.

54. Prochaska JO. Transtheoretical model of behavior change. In: Gellman MD, Turner JR, eds. *Encyclopedia of Behavioral Medicine*: Springer; 2013. doi:10.1007/978-1-4419-1005-9_70.

55. Cooperrider DL, Srivastva S. Appreciative inquiry in organizational life. In: Woodman RW, Pasmore WA, eds. *Research in Organizational Change and Development.* Vol. 1: JAI Press; 1987:129–169.

56. Lundahl BW, Kunz C, Brownell C, Tollefson D, Burke BL. A meta-analysis of motivational interviewing: twenty-five years of empirical studies. *Res Soc Work Pract.* 2010;20(2):137–160.

57. Moyers TB, Martin T, Houck JM, Christopher PJ, Tonigan JS. From in-session behaviors to drinking outcomes: a causal chain for motivational interviewing. *J Consult Clin Psychol.* 2009;77(6):1113–1124. doi:10.1037/a0017189.

58. Plack M, Driscoll M. In: Plack M, Driscoll M, eds. *Teaching and Learning in Physical Therapy: From Classroom to Clinic*: Slack, Inc.; 2011:203.

59. Cheville AL, Mclaughlin SA, Haddad TC, Lyons KD, Newman R, Ruddy KJ. Integrated rehabilitation for breast cancer survivors. *Am J Phys Med Rehabil.* 2019;98(2):154–164.

60. Lukez A, Baima J. The role and scope of prehabilitation in cancer care. *Semin Oncol Nurs.* 2020;36(1):150976. doi:10.1016/j.soncn.2019.150976.

61. Stout NL, Binkley JM, Schmitz KH, et al. A prospective surveillance model for rehabilitation for women with breast cancer. *Cancer.* 2012;118(suppl 8):2191–2200.

62. Doherty D, Lahrman M, Linn S, Drouin JS. Prevalence of functional deficits and rehabilitation needs among individuals receiving radiation therapy for cancer: a descriptive study. *Rehabil Oncol.* 2013;31(4):23–31.

63. Borrell-Carrio F, Suchman AL, Epstein RM. The biopsychosocial model 25 years later: principles, practice, and scientific inquiry. *Ann Fam Med.* 2004;2(6):576–582.

64. APTA. Maley lecture 2018. https://www.apta.org/news/2018/07/02/next-2018-maley-lecture-health-care-must-adopt-a-biopsychosocial-model. Accessed December 27, 2020.

65. Jessup RL. Interdisciplinary versus multidisciplinary cancer teams: care do we understand the difference? *Aust Health Rev.* 2007;32(3):331.

66. Selby P, Popescu R, Lawler M, Butcher H, Costa A. The value and future developments of multidisciplinary team cancer care. *Am Soc Clin Oncol Educ Book.* 2019;39:332–340.

67. Soukup T, Labm BW, Arora S, Darzi A, Sevdalis N, Green JSA. Successful strategies in implementing a multidisciplinary team working in the care of patients with cancer: an overview and synthesis of available literature. *J Multidiscip Healthcare.* 2018;11:49–61.

68. Tremblay D, Roberge D, Touati N, Maunsell E, Berbiche D. Effects of interdisciplinary teamwork on patient-reported experience of cancer care. *BMC Health Services Res*. 2017;17:218. doi:10.1186/s12913-017-2166-7.

69. World Health Organization. Framework for action on interprofessional education and collaborative practice. https://www.who.int/hrh/resources/framework_action/en/. Accessed May 15, 2021.

70. Bilodeau K, Dubois S, Pepin J. Interprofessional patient-centred practice in oncology teams: utopia or reality? *J Interprofess Care*. 2015;29(2):106–112.

71. The Oncology Team. Cancer.net. https://www.cancer.net/navigating-cancer-care/cancer-basics/cancer-care-team/oncology-team. Updated August 2020. Accessed May 28, 2022.

72. 2020 Standards and Resources. Chapter 4. Personnel and services resources. Commission on cancer. https://www.facs.org/-/media/files/quality-programs/cancer/coc/2020-standards/chapter_4.ashx. Updated February 2021. Accessed February 21, 2021.

73. National Accreditation Program for Breast Centers Standards Manual. 2018 edition. https://www.facs.org/quality-programs/cancer-programs/national-accreditation-program-for-breast-centers/standards-and-resources/. Updated December 2020. Accessed June 16, 2022.

74. National Academies of Sciences, Engineering, and Medicine. *Long-term Survivorship Care after Cancer Treatment: Proceedings of a Workshop*: The National Academies Press; 2018. doi:10.17226/25043.

75. Greenlee H, Shi Z, Sardo Molmenti CL, Rundle A, Tsai WY. Trends in obesity prevalence in adults with a history of cancer: results from the U.S. National Health Interview Survey, 1997 to 2014. *J Clin Oncol*. 2016;34(26):3133–3140.

76. Henderson TO, Ness KK, Cohen HJ. Accelerated aging among cancer survivors: from pediatrics to geriatrics. *Am Soc Clin Oncol Educ Book*. 2014:e423–e430. doi:10.14694/EdBook_AM.2014.34.e423.

77. Lauby-Secretan B, Scoccianti C, Loomis D, et al. Body fatness and cancer: viewpoint of the IARC Working Group. *N Engl J Med*. 2016;375(8):794–798. doi:10.1056/NEJMsr1606602.

78. National Academies of Sciences, Engineering, and Medicine; Health and Medicine Division. Board on Health Care Services; National Cancer Policy Forum. *Incorporating Weight Management and Physical Activity Throughout the Cancer Care Continuum: Proceedings of a Workshop*: National Academies Press; 2018 January 12.

79. Accreditation CARF International. http://www.carf.org/Accreditation/. Accessed October 19, 2020.

80. World Health Organization. *Towards a Common Language for Functioning, Disability and Health*: ICF. World Health Organization; 2002. http://www.who.int/classifications/icf/training/icfbeginnersguide.pdf. Accessed September 15, 2020.

81. World Health Organization. ICF checklist. https://www.who.int/classifications/icf/icfchecklist.pdf. Updated September 2003. Accessed December 11, 2020.

82. Jette A. Toward a common language for function, disability, and health. *Phys Ther*. 2006;86(5):726–734.

83. Williams A. APTA endorses ICF model. *PT Magazine*. 2008;16(9):54.

84. Fisher MI, Lee J, Davies C, Geyer H, Colon G, Pfalzer L. Oncology section EDGE task force on breast cancer outcomes: a systematic review of outcome measures for functional mobility. *Rehabil Oncol*. 2015;33(3):19–31.

85. Goodman CC, Fuller KS. *Pathology: Implications for the Physical Therapist*. 4th ed. WB Saunders Company; 2015:5, figure 1-1.

86. ECOG-ACRIN Cancer Research Group. Eastern cooperative oncology group performance status. https://ecog-acrin.org/resources/ecog-performance-status. Accessed January 1, 2021.

87. Fisher MI, Davies C, Beuthin C, Colon G, Zoll B, Pfalzer L. Breast cancer EDGE task force outcomes: clinical measures of strength and muscular endurance: a systematic review. *Rehabil Oncol*. 2014;32(4):6–15.

88. Jackson SM, Cheng MS, Smith AR, Kolber MJ. Intrarater reliability of hand-held dynamometry in measuring lower extremity isometric strength using a portable stabilization device. *Musculoskel Sci Pract*. 2017;27:137–141.

89. Kim SG, Lim DH, Cho YH. Analysis of the reliability of the make test in young adults by using a hand-held dynamometer. *J Phys Ther Sci*. 2016;28(8):2238–2240.

3

Evidence-Based Practice in Oncology Rehabilitation

SHANA E. HARRINGTON, PT, PhD, BOARD-CERTIFIED CLINICAL SPECIALIST IN SPORTS PHYSICAL THERAPY, MANUAL THERAPY CERTIFIED

CHAPTER OUTLINE

Evidence-Based Practice Background

Evidence-based practice (EBP) should affect how oncology rehabilitation (Onc R) clinicians make clinical decisions but locating and interpreting research is often difficult for many.[1] Acquiring these skills is imperative since interpreting treatment outcomes is important to clinicians because it influences clinical decision-making which affects patient safety and efficacy.[1] The term EBP dates back to 1972 when Archie Cochrane, a British physician and epidemiologist, challenged medical providers to enhance their efficiency and effectiveness in clinical practice by integrating the current best evidence into their decision making.[2,3] In 1996, Dr. David Sackett defined evidence-based medicine as "the conscientious, explicit and judicious use of current best evidence in making decisions about the care of individual patients."[4,5] This definition was redefined by Sackett in 2000 as "the integration of best available evidence, clinical expertise, and patient preferences and values."[6] It was during this same year that the American Physical Therapy Association (APTA) House of Delegates adopted *Vision 2020* which included six elements that the leadership hoped to achieve by 2020, one of those elements was further instilling concepts of EBP.[7] To effectively understand, apply, and interpret EBP, a variety of skills necessary will be discussed in this chapter.

Sackett and colleagues proposed five steps for incorporating evidence-based medicine into clinical practice: (1) defining a clinically relevant question; (2) searching for the best evidence; (3) appraising evidence quality; (4) integrating the evidence in clinical practice; and (5) evaluating the process.[4,8] To pose a clear clinical question, four components, often referred to as PICO, need to be identified.[8] These components include (1) Patient population; (2) Intervention/treatment; (3) Comparison; and (4) Outcome of interest.[8] Let us now apply a PICO to a clinical scenario, a woman

who is currently receiving radiation for her breast cancer diagnosis. She has been referred to Onc R due to complaints of difficulty reaching overhead on her affected shoulder. The Onc R clinician wants to know if active shoulder flexion range of motion on the affected side will improve her self-reported upper extremity function using the Disabilities of Arm, Shoulder and Hand (DASH) outcome measure, while the woman is receiving radiation treatment compared to usual care, which is rest. The following is how the clinician would apply the PICO to this clinical scenario: the "P" = the woman with breast cancer, the "I" = active shoulder flexion range of motion on the affected side, the "C" = usual care (rest), and the "O" = patient-reported function on the DASH. Quality research begins with a sound clinical question and without this, supporting evidence will likely be lacking.

Once a focused and clinically relevant question has been developed, the next step is to search for the best evidence. Often, this step can seem daunting to Onc R clinicians who searched the literature back in the day looking through hard copies of journals or textbooks in a library. This is a stark contrast to now where electronic databases, which house journals, can be accessed more easily using the internet. No single database provides access to every article published. Fortunately, due to advances in technology, a variety of databases can be searched to look for relevant articles about Onc R from a computer. The most common databases can be viewed in Table 3.1. Another challenge is that not everyone can get access to full-text articles. There are a few resources that can help with this problem. Google Scholar provides an easy way to broadly search for scholarly literature and often the full-text articles can be downloaded from the site: https://scholar.google.com/. Included in American Physical Therapy Association (APTA) membership is access to the *APTA Article Search*, which provides full-text resources to explore articles through the EBSCO discovery service from over 4500 academic

TABLE 3.1	Common Databases
Name	**Web Address**
PubMed/MEDLINE	https://pubmed.ncbi.nlm.nih.gov/
PMC–US National Library of Medicine, National Institutes of Health (formerly PubMed Central)	https://www.ncbi.nlm.nih.gov/pmc/
CINAHL Database/EBSCO	https://www.ebsco.com/ products/research-databases?f%5B0%5D=database_ full_text%3Afull%20text
Cochrane	https://www.cochrane.org/
Cochrane Rehabilitation	https://rehabilitation.cochrane.org/

and clinical publications.[9] Additionally, membership in the APTA's Academy of Oncologic Physical Therapy will include access to the Academy's journal *Rehabilitation Oncology,* which allows for full-text access of articles including archives. *Rehabilitation Oncology* is an indexed resource for the dissemination of peer-reviewed research-based evidence related to oncologic physical therapy and cancer rehabilitation.[10]

Once the relevant articles have been retrieved, the next step is to determine the validity and usefulness through critically appraising the evidence.[11] This is often the most difficult task in applying evidence-based medicine because the skills in evaluating research and research methods may be unfamiliar to many.[11] One of the first things to identify in a research article is knowing what type of study design was conducted. A variety of study designs exist, and it is vital to understand the differences between these designs as well as how they relate to the quality of evidence. One way to compare and contrast the different types of study designs used in EBP is understanding the *levels of evidence pyramid* (Figure 3.1). This pyramid provides a way to visualize the quality of evidence based on the study design. For example, the top of the pyramid (meta-analyses) means that it is both the highest level of evidence and typically the least common, whereas as you go down the pyramid, the amount of evidence will increase as the quality of evidence decreases. It is essential to explain, that just because a study design is not on the higher portion of the pyramid, it does not mean there is no value in the findings. Many case reports and case series provide an abundance of information with regards to interventions that are often personalized to the participants and missing in detail in publications that utilize a randomized control trial design.

Statistics and Psychometrics

It is worthwhile to mention that publication in a peer-reviewed journal does not automatically mean the proper statistics and study design were used or that the author's explanation of the data was appropriate.[1] Basic knowledge of statistics and interpretation is essential to effectively translate research findings into practice as well as critically appraise the evidence. Statistical tests, validity, significance, effect sizes, and confidence intervals are aspects of research that clinicians should understand to critically appraise the evidence, which in turn improves clinical decision-making skills.[1] A basic understanding of statistical designs commonly used in Onc R can assist Onc R clinicians with critically appraising the evidence. One of the first steps in evaluating the appropriateness of a statistical test used in a study is to classify the purpose of the statistical analysis, which often falls into one of these three categories: (1) to determine the significance of the difference among group means; (2) to evaluate the relationship between two variables; or (3) to predict one variable based on another. Another appropriate next step is to determine if a parametric or nonparametric test has been used. When examining differences between group means, data that is parametric would be characterized as ratio or interval whereas nonparametric data would be nominal or ordinal.[12] Figure 3.2 shows the characteristics and examples of

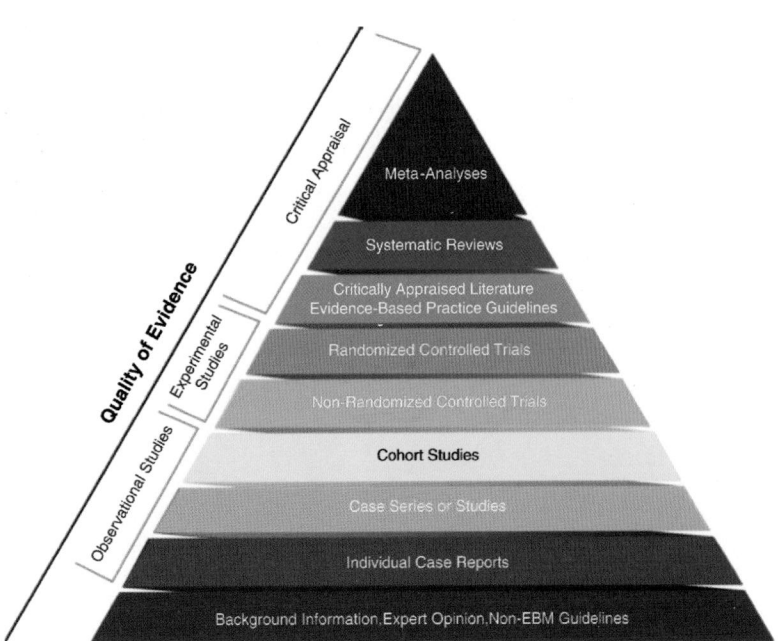

• **Fig. 3.1** The Evidence Pyramid. (Reprinted with permission from Elizabeth L, Whitlock EL, Chen CL. Chapter 90: Interpreting the medical literature. In: Gropper MA, ed. *Miller's Anesthesia.* Elsevier; 2020:2813–2824.e2.)

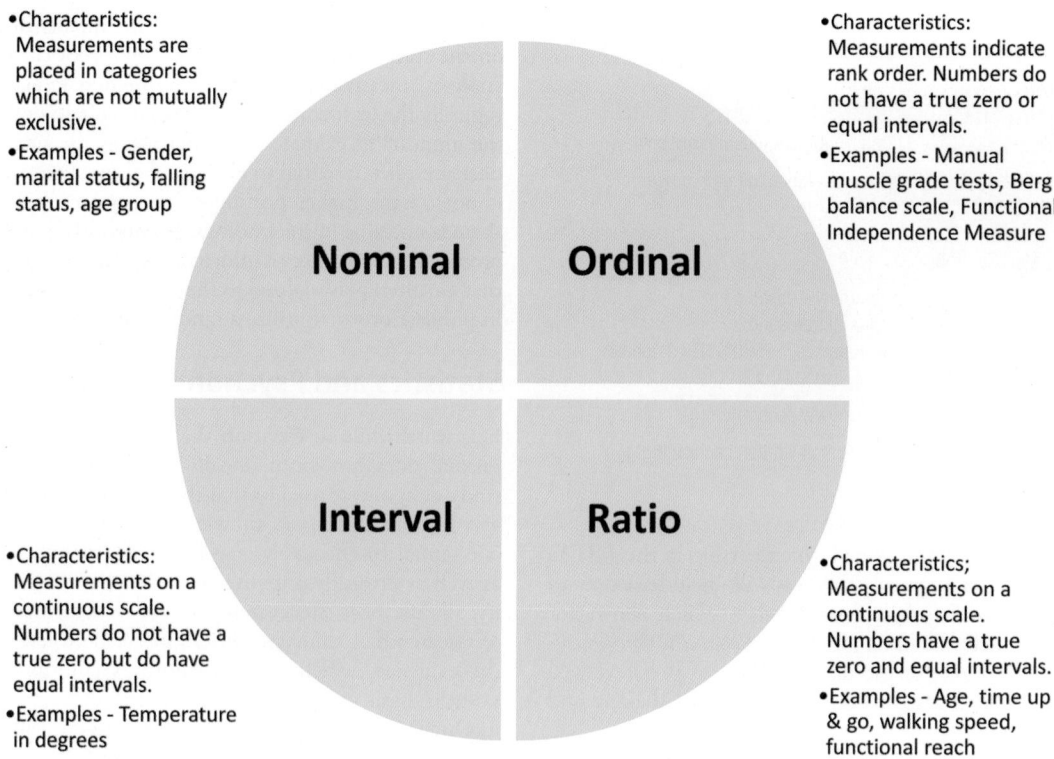

• **Fig. 3.2** Characteristics of Measurement Scales. (Created by Shana Harrington. Printed with permission.)

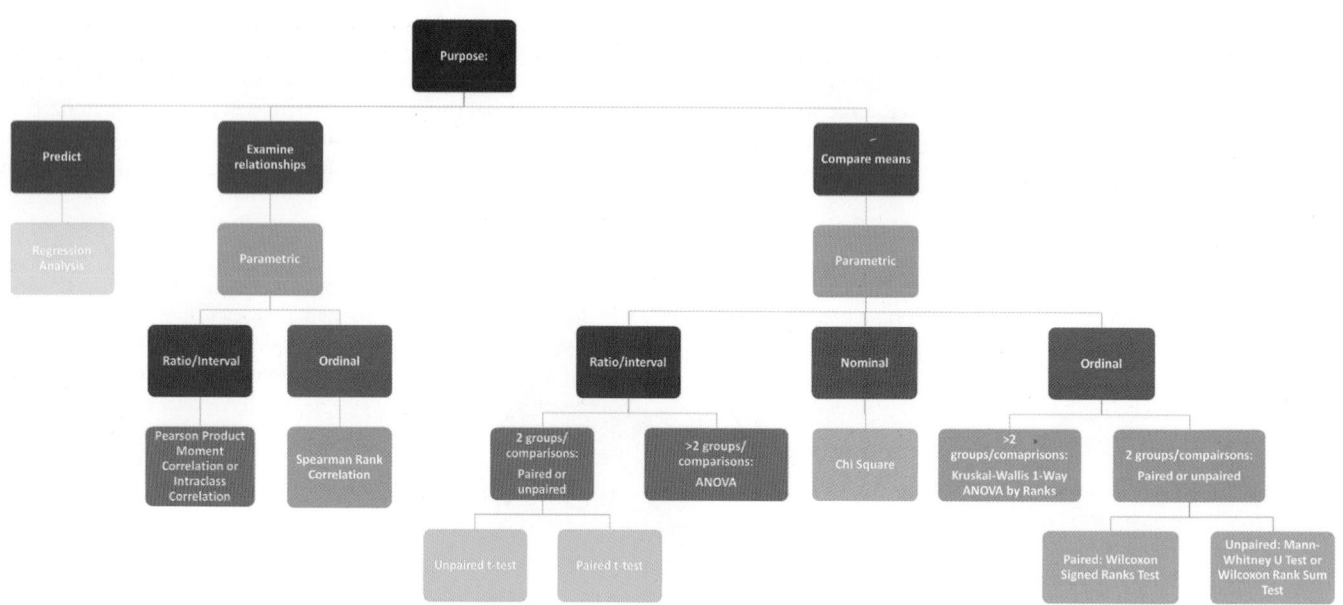

• **Fig. 3.3** Decision-Making Process for Statistical Analysis. (Created by Shana Harrington. Printed with permission.)

measurement scales. Discussing each statistical test falls outside the scope of this chapter; however, Figure 3.3 shows the decision-making process for selecting and evaluating statistical tests that are commonly used in rehabilitation research.

With the greater focus on evidence-based medicine, understanding the concepts of *P*-values, confidence intervals, and effect sizes are of importance for clinicians.[13] Study results that report

P-values and confidence intervals are becoming more frequently reported in the literature. These provide a slightly different estimate of statistical truth.[14] To understand *P*-values, the concept of null hypothesis is important. A null hypothesis assumes that there is no difference between groups or that the experimental variable being examined has no effect. *P*-values represent the likelihood that a perceived difference is because of random chance when the null hypothesis is true, which is known as a type I error.[14,15] This is in opposition to a type II error when the null hypothesis is false. A *P*-value is an "index for the strength of the evidence for the tested hypothesis, against the null hypothesis," it is not the likelihood that the null hypothesis is true.[14] Today, "statistical significance" is oftentimes set at a *P*-value of <.05, meaning that the null hypothesis is fittingly rejected if the probability of a type I error is <5%.[14]

While *P*-values help determine the reliability by which the null hypothesis can be rejected and consequently the strength of the observed result, *P*-values do not provide evidence about the accuracy of the result.[14] To address this, confidence intervals are calculated around the point estimate of the result to offer a range of values within which the true value is assured to exist with a specified level of confidence.[15] Often, confidence intervals are used to help better understand the clinical significance of the findings. For example, a wide confidence interval suggests an inexact result and specifies that the results should be interpreted with caution regarding statistical significance.[14] It is important to note that what is considered "wide" is often a subjective interpretation by the reader. Confidence intervals are most often calculated at a confidence level of 95%. If results are statistically significant with a *P*-value of 0.05 (or 5%), then the null hypothesis should not fall inside the 95% confidence interval.[14] In other words, if the same study was conducted over and over with a different sample of subjects, but with the same characteristics of the original sample, 95% of the means from those repeated measures would fall within this range.[13] For example, if a reported mean value = 0.4 (95% CI, –0.1 to 0.67), this can be interpreted that the between-group difference in the study sample was 0.4, with the true value represented in a range of –0.1 to 0.67 in the population.

From a clinical perspective, the absence or presence of statistically significant differences can be of limited value.[1] A nonsignificant outcome does not always imply that an intervention was not clinically effective because measurement variability and small sample sizes can influence statistical results.[16] Effect size is an important indicator of clinical significance and in recent years is more frequently reported in the literature.[1] An effect size demonstrates the magnitude of differences between groups, where larger effect sizes indicate a greater difference between groups.[1] Cohen[17] developed the traditional calculation of effect values based on group differences (change score), divided by the pooled standard deviation in the following equation:

$$\frac{\text{Change in Experimental Group vs. Control}}{\text{Standard Deviation of both groups}} = \frac{8}{10} = 0.8 \text{ Cohen}$$

Effect sizes have been operationally described and interpreted in the following ranges by Cohen[17]: <0.2 = trivial effect, 0.2–0.5 = small effect, 0.5–0.8 = moderate effect, >0.8 = large effect.

These effect sizes can be negative or positive, indicating the direction of the effect.[1] For example, an effect size of 0.45, would be a "small positive effect." A recent study wanted to determine if there were active range of motion differences in flexion and external rotation at 90 degrees between women who had recently completed their primary breast cancer treatment and healthy controls.[18] The study reported an effect size of 1.1 for flexion and 0.6 for external rotation at 90 degrees.[18] This can be interpreted using the ranges described by Cohen as a large effect for flexion and a moderate effect for external rotation at 90 degrees. There are other outcomes, such as minimal clinically important differences (MCID), which can help to further interpret and understand the clinical significance that will be discussed later in this chapter.

When deciding upon the best outcome or test to use during an Onc R clinician's initial evaluation and/or to measure the change of an intervention, it is important to understand a variety of psychometric properties. Psychometric properties are characteristics of measures and tests that describe and identify the attributes of a test or measure.[19] These include reliability, validity, minimal detectable change (MDC), MCID, sensitivity, specificity, and responsiveness. Satisfactory reliability and validity of an outcome or test is needed to be used in clinical practice and research according to EBP guidelines.[20] Figure 3.4 graphically represents reliability and validity.

Reliability is the potential to replicate a result consistently.[21] When examining reliability, stability and internal consistency of a measure are important.[21] Reliability coefficients range from 0 to +1.0, and in general, the higher the statistic, the measure is likely to be more consistent.[22] Test-retest reliability examines the stability of an outcome or test over a period of time.[23] Intraclass correlation coefficient (ICC) is used to estimate stability in test-retest reliability because it considers measurement errors.[23] ICC values greater than 0.90 are suggestive of excellent reliability, whereas values less than 0.50, between 0.50 and 0.75, and between 0.75 and 0.90 are suggestive of poor, moderate, and good reliability, respectively.[24] Internal consistency is another important reliability criterion that examines if all subparts of an instrument measure have the same characteristic.[25] Cronbach's alpha coefficient is used by most researchers to assess internal consistency.[26] There is no consensus on the interpretation of Cronbach's alpha coefficient although some studies establish that values higher than 0.70 are ideal, whereas others consider values under 0.70 but close to 0.60 as satisfactory.[21,25] It is noteworthy that internal consistency reliability coefficients are believed to be a generous estimate of reliability which may result in higher coefficients compared to others such as test-retest reliability coefficients,[22] Onc R clinicians should be aware of these limitations when interpreting reliability. Another form of reliability, known as inter-rater reliability, uses the indices' ICC for interpretation and compares consistency between two or

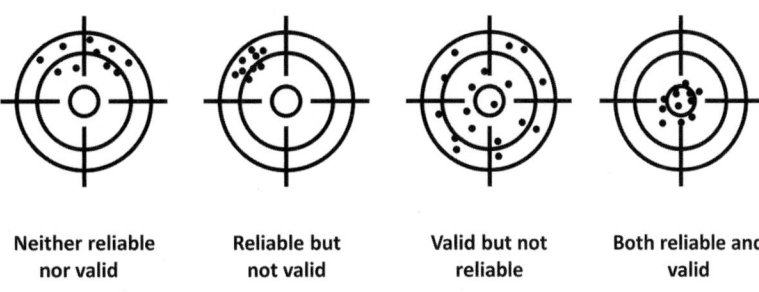

| Neither reliable nor valid | Reliable but not valid | Valid but not reliable | Both reliable and valid |

• **Fig. 3.4** Reliability and Validity. (Created by Chris Wilson. Printed with permission.)

more test observers. In contrast, intra-rater reliability compares consistency between the same people on a repeated attempt.

A clinical example of interpreting reliability for an assessment technique was reported by Harrington and colleagues when measuring pectoralis minor length in 29 women diagnosed with breast cancer using a palpation meter.[27] Bilateral pectoralis minor length was assessed by two licensed physical therapists (PTs) who were blinded to the measures.[27] Intratester ($ICC_{3,k}$ = 0.97) and intertester reliability ($ICC_{3,k}$ = 0.92) were excellent on the affected side and the unaffected side (intratester $ICC_{3,k}$ = 0.95 and intertester $ICC_{3,k}$ = 0.95).[27] Clinically, this means using a palpation meter to examine resting pectoralis minor length in women who have received treatment for breast cancer is a sound clinical option based on psychometric properties of reliability.

Validity refers to the property of an instrument to measure what it proposes.[21] Specifically, the "…..validity of a test concerns *what* the test measures and *how well* it does so."[28] While there are several different types of validity, for this chapter we will focus on content, criterion-related, and construct validity. These three forms of validity are important in determining the usefulness and limitations of specific outcomes and tests.[22] Content validity is how a measure reproduces the proposed domain or area of content.[22] For example, for a test to demonstrate content validity, the items of the test should be a representative sample of the set of abilities and skills the test is wanting to measure.[22] Typically, qualitative research through the assessment of subject matter experts is done to establish content validity.[22]

Criterion-related validity is used to establish the precision of a measure or test by comparing it with the gold standard, or criterion measure, that reflects the variable being tested.[22] Relative to assessment, there are two forms of criterion validity: concurrent and predictive. Concurrent validity deals with present time and when being established, test developers examine the correlation between a new instrument and an accepted measure of the construct.[22] In contrast, predictive validity is involved with the strength and direction of the relationship between an instrument score and a context-relevant, external criterion that is examined at some time later in the process.[29] Correlations, often reported as *r*, between the accepted measure (or gold standard) and the new measure is used to establish concurrent validity.[22] Referring back to the study by Harrington and colleagues, concurrent validity was examined comparing pectoralis minor length using the palpation meter (new measure) with a motion capture system (gold standard).[27] Significant correlations were found between the motion capture system and the palpation meter on the affected (*r* = 0.87) and unaffected (*r* = 0.81) side meaning the palpation meter is efficient and can be used instead of the gold standard motion capture system.[27]

Construct validity is when a test accurately and thoroughly measures a particular trait or construct.[28] Construct validity is a method of gathering information and assembling evidence in support of a test's accurate representation of a particular construct, rather than a single step.[22] Construct validity is typically verified through convergent and discriminant validities.[30] Convergent validity is when the same construct is measured between two different methods.[31] Whereas, discriminant validity is when different constructs are found between two different measures.[31]

Another measurement property that is important to understand for EBP purposes is sensitivity and specificity. Onc R clinicians should know how accurate a diagnostic tool of interest is in identifying the absence or presence of the target condition. Sensitivity is defined as a test's ability to correctly identify the target condition when the target condition is present, often referred to as the "true positive rate."[32] Having high sensitivity for a tool of interest (where 1.0 is perfect) is desirable as it will rarely miss someone who has the target condition. Whereas, specificity, referred to as a "true negative rate" is a test's ability to identify those without the target condition who truly do not have that condition. When a tool has a high specificity, it will rarely test positive when a person does not have the impairment of interest (e.g., a low chance of false-positive predictions). For example, the one-item fatigue scale had adequate sensitivity (>0.85) and specificity (>0.61) to screen for fatigue in individuals who were seeking care in a thoracic oncology clinic, with scores between 3 and 5 found to be optimal.[33] It is important to note that since the reported specificity of the one-item fatigue scale is >0.61, more people might get diagnosed with fatigue that might not truly have it clinically, which may result in unwarranted tests or treatments.

Outcome Measures

Outcome measures are used frequently in Onc R. An outcome measure is a tool administered to assess a patient's present-day status and may offer a score, a reading of results, and occasionally a risk categorization of the patient.[34] Outcome measures can provide baseline data that may help determine an appropriate intervention. Additionally, an outcome may be re-administered after a specified period and/or at the end of treatment to establish whether a patient has demonstrated change. With the emphasis on EBP in the Onc R professions, outcome measures offer reliable and credible explanation for intervention on an individual patient level.

Outcome measures used in clinical practice can be divided into four categories: (1) self-report (or patient-report) measures; (2) performance-based measures; (3) observer-reported measures; and (4) clinician-reported measures. Patient-reported outcome (PRO) measures are typically captured as a questionnaire. Although PROs seem subjective, they help to report the status of an individual's health condition that originates from the patient without any influence from a clinician.[35] Examples of PROs used in the oncology population include Functional Assessment of Cancer Therapy–General (FACT-G) and the DASH. Performance-based measures require an individual to perform a task or a series of movements. These measures are either based on an objective measure such as time to finish a task or a qualitative assessment that is allocated a score such as normal or abnormal.[36] Examples of performance-based measures commonly used in Onc R include the timed up and go, five times sit to stand, and 6-minute walk test.[37] Observer-reported measures are reports made by a proxy (e.g., a parent or caregiver) who is in direct contact with a patient when self-report is not an option (e.g., too young, too sick, or has cognitive impairments).[38] An example of an observer-reported measure includes the use of the parent proxy for the Pediatric Quality of Life Inventory (PedsQL V.4) in children 2 to 4 years who have diffuse intrinsic pontine gliomas.[39] Clinician-reported measures are done by a healthcare professional by using clinical judgment through observation of patient behaviors or signs.[36] Similar to observer-reported measures this might be used if a patient is too young, too sick, has cognitive impairments, and a parent or caregiver is not present or able to assist.

Before discussing other important attributes of outcome measures, understanding the difference between a screening and an assessment tool is paramount.[40] When selecting outcomes and tests, along with understanding terms related to psychometrics, all providers must be speaking the same language and understand the difference between a screening and an assessment tool.[40] Appropriate screening for individuals with cancer can trigger referrals to Onc R to address unmet needs. Onc R clinicians can then appropriately assess and identify impairments that many of these individuals face. A recent summary comparing and contrasting these terms and how many times they are misused is provided.[40] Screening tools are typically unidimensional, easy to interpret, and easy to administer.[41] Often, a screening tool can be answered with a simple "yes" or "no."[40] Examples of screening tools used in Onc R include the one-item fatigue scale and the National Comprehensive Cancer Network (NCCN) distress thermometer and problem list.[40–42] In contrast, an assessment tool by nature is more in-depth, multidimensional, and more comprehensive to identify not just that a problem exists but what the extent and source of the problem may be as well as how it impacts other parts of life such as function. The Piper Fatigue Scale-Revised is an assessment tool that looks at the multidimensional construct of cancer-related fatigue.[43]

Changes in outcome measures can be difficult to interpret. This is often because the statistical significance of a treatment effect is partially dependent on sample size; clinical relevance does not always correspond to the effect. Statistical significance does not always translate to clinical significance. Statistically significant effects are those that occur beyond some level of chance,[44] whereas clinical significance refers to the benefits derived from the treatment, its implications for clinical management, and its impact on the patient.[45,46]

Understanding responsiveness, defined as "the ability of an outcome measure to detect changes over time in the construct measured," is an important concept to appreciate regarding PROs.[47] This is imperative when an Onc R clinician is interested in measuring the change from an intervention. Responsiveness includes the minimal important change (MIC) (also known MCID), which is the smallest change in a score that would likely be important from the patient's perspective.[48] To ensure that MIC can be distinguished from measurement error, ideally, the MIC should exceed the MDC.[49] MDC is defined as the minimal amount of change in a test or score of an outcome measure that is unlikely due to measurement error and within-subject variability.[50] In other words, MDC is the amount that a patient needs to improve on an outcome for there to be a true change.

The MDC[95] was studied on three commonly used balance assessment tools in older individuals diagnosed with cancer.[51] The authors found that MDC was 6.86, 2.39, and 2.55 for the Balance Evaluation System Test (BESTest), Mini-Balance Evaluation Systems Test (Mini-BESTest), and the Brief Balance Evaluation Systems Test (Brief-BESTest), respectively.[51] Clinically, this means if a clinician administers one of the balance tools like the BESTest, at baseline and again after a specified timeframe or several sessions (e.g., week 4) of rehabilitation intervention, and the change score exceeds the MDC of 6.86, they can be 95% confident that the change in test scores reflects a true change of a person's status as opposed to normal variability or measurement error.

Several challenges should be noted while using PROs. First, it is difficult to find the responsiveness of an outcome reporting both the MIC and MDC for outcomes specific to individuals diagnosed with cancer. Often in Onc R, we will "borrow" tools from other populations. It should be understood that responsiveness applies to the population of interest that was studied. For example, the DASH is often used to examine upper extremity function in women with breast cancer. However, the DASH was developed

in adults with orthopedic problems of the upper extremity (e.g., glenohumeral arthritis). While there is a reported MIC of 10.83 and an MDC of 10.81, it should be understood that these only apply to adults with upper-limb musculoskeletal disorders, and those who had a history of tumor malignancy were excluded.[52] Second, PROs provide the patient's perspective; although this is important, a score on a PRO should be compared with objective clinical findings. It was found that in women who recently completed their treatment for breast cancer, scores on the DASH would be considered acceptable (representing low disability and high function); however, objective measures such as active range of motion were limited.[18,53] For example, one question on the DASH asks about how much difficulty a respondent has washing or blow-drying their hair. Many women would report no difficulty; however, their affected shoulder active flexion was not greater than 100 degrees. In this case, the women perceive that they can do the task, and in fact, they can, however, the quality in which they do it is poor which still may require intervention by rehabilitation professionals.

Evidence-Based Practice Oncology Rehabilitation Resources

There are several resources for clinicians to help support EBP in Onc R (Table 3.2). These resources include oncology/cancer rehabilitation journals, outcomes recommendations, clinical practice guidelines, guidelines for supportive care including survivorship, published standards for survivorship programs, and cancer exercise guidelines. Additionally, several organizations will be discussed below that support evidence-based Onc R. Understanding that these resources exist, their context and how to access them is imperative for each Onc R clinician. These resources are updated frequently with the changing needs of patients with cancer due to new advancements in treatment and detection.

EDGE Task Force and Academy of Oncologic Physical Therapy

Within the APTA is the Academy of Oncologic Physical Therapy. Its membership consists of PTs, physical therapist assistants (PTAs), student PTs, and student PTAs who manage the multifactorial needs of persons living with and beyond cancer (PLWBCs).[54] Their mission is to "advance PT practice for persons affected by cancer and chronic illness by maximizing movement and wellness across the lifespan."[54] Its members are involved in a variety of areas related to EBP. The Academy has an official quarterly journal, *Rehabilitation Oncology*, which is a peer-reviewed, indexed resource for advancing physical therapy practice and Onc R. This journal houses collections of published literature relevant to Onc R. Collections are based on impairments including balance and falls, cognition, fatigue, functional mobility, incontinence, and lymphedema to name a few. Collections are also grouped by type of cancer. The Evaluation Database to Guide Effectiveness (EDGE) Task Force Outcomes is housed within these collections. To foster standardization of outcome measures for PLWBCs, the Academy of Oncologic Physical Therapy formed its first EDGE Task Force in 2010. The Task Force members were charged with determining the relative merits of available assessment and outcome tools published in the literature by reviewing psychometric properties and clinical utility (cost, ease of use, ease of scoring).[55] Based on the conclusions in the literature, recommendations were

TABLE 3.2   Evidence-Based Practice Resources in Oncology Rehabilitation

Name	Description	Discipline of Focus	Web Address
Organizations			
ACRM–American Congress of Rehabilitation Medicine	A global community of researchers and consumers of research in the field of rehabilitation.	Multidisciplinary	https://acrm.org/about/about-acrm/
ACSM–American College of Sports Medicine	Organized a roundtable and published exercise guidelines for people living with and beyond cancer.	Multidisciplinary	https://www.acsm.org/
AOTA–American Occupational Therapy Association	AOTA is a national professional association established to represent the interests and concerns of occupational therapy practitioners and students of occupational therapy and to improve the quality of occupational therapy services.	Occupational Therapy	https://www.aota.org/
APTA–Academy of Oncologic Physical Therapy	Consists of PTs. PTAs and student physical therapists managing the rehabilitative needs of patients living with and beyond cancer and other chronic illnesses including HIV.	Physical Therapy	https://oncologypt.org/about-us/
ASHA–American Speech-Language-Hearing Association	ASHA is the national professional, scientific, and credentialing association.	Speech-Language Pathology	https://www.asha.org/
CoC–American College of Surgeons Commission on Cancer	CoC accreditation standards.	Multidisciplinary	https://www.facs.org/-/media/files/quality-programs/cancer/coc/optimal_resources_for_cancer_care_2020_standards.ashx
NCCN–National Comprehensive Cancer Network	Alliance of leading cancer centers devoted to patient care, research, and education. Has core NCCN Guidelines (clinical practice guidelines) resources available.	Multidisciplinary	https://www.nccn.org/patients/about/what.aspx https://www.nccn.org/patients/clinical/default.aspx
Journals			
American Journal of Occupational Therapy	The official publication of AOTA.	Occupational Therapy	https://ajot.aota.org/index.aspx
American Journal of Speech-Language Pathology (AJSLP)	One of the four journals of ASHA	Speech-Language Pathology	https://pubs.asha.org/journal/ajslp
Archives of Physical Medicine and Rehabilitation	The official journal of ACRM.	Multidisciplinary	https://www.archives-pmr.org
Journal of Cancer Survivorship–Research and Practice (JCSU)	The journal publishes peer-reviewed papers related to improving the understanding, prevention, and management of multiple areas related to cancer survivorship that can affect quality care, symptom management, function, and well-being.	Multidisciplinary	https://www.springer.com/journal/11764/
Physical Therapy & Rehabilitation Journal (PTJ)	The official journal of the APTA. Has published two recent oncology Clinical Practice Guidelines related to lymphedema.	Physical Therapy	https://academic.oup.com/ptj/pages/About
Rehabilitation Oncology	The official journal of the APTA–Academy of Oncologic Physical Therapy. Has collections including the EDGE Task Force Outcomes.	Physical Therapy	https://journals.lww.com/rehabonc/pages/default.aspx

APTA, American Physical Therapy Association; *PTs*, physical therapists; *PTAs*, physical therapist assistants; *EDGE*, Evaluation Database to Guide Effectiveness.

made for each outcome using the EDGE rating scale. Up to the year 2016, the EDGE rating scale used the following numbers and descriptors: 4—highly recommend, 3—recommend, 2A—unable to recommend at this time (the measure has been used in research in cancer; however, there is insufficient evidence to support a recommendation), 2B—unable to recommend at this time (there is no published evidence that the measure has been applied to individuals with cancer and there is insufficient evidence to support a recommendation), 1—do not recommend.[56] After using this scale

for several years, it was revised to provide clearer definitions.[56] The recommendation levels were reworked and adopted the following new wording and grades: 4—highly recommend, 3—recommend, 2—reasonable to use, and 1—not recommended.[56] Since its inception, the Oncology EDGE Task Force has published over 28 articles in *Rehabilitation Oncology* across the lifespan and for a variety of cancer diagnoses including colon, urogenital, prostate, head and neck, and breast. Additionally, five EDGE investigations focused on impairments across all cancers including pain in children, sexual dysfunction, clinical measures for pain, measures of cancer-related fatigue, and measures of balance in adult survivors of cancer.[57]

Clinical Practice Guidelines

Clinical practice guidelines (CPGs) are recommendations describing current best practices for a specific condition and are increasing in value to direct clinical practice in recent years.[58] The National Academy of Sciences (formerly the Institute of Medicine) defines a CPG as "statements that include recommendations, intended to optimize patient care that is informed by a systematic review of evidence and an assessment of the benefits and harms of alternative care options."[59,60] CPGs are based on the best available research evidence as well as the practice experience of expert Onc R clinicians.[58] A focused clinical question is developed before a systematic review of the evidence. Articles that meet defined inclusion criteria are then rated for quality and then overall evidence for the CPG topic area of interest.[58] The first CPG sponsored by the Academy of Oncologic Physical Therapy was published in 2017 on Diagnosis of Upper Quadrant Lymphedema Secondary to Cancer.[61] In 2020, a working group published an additional CPG for Interventions for Breast Cancer-Related Lymphedema.[62] Another working group has been developing a CPG related to Screening and Assessment of Cancer-Related Fatigue that is intended for publication in the peer-reviewed journal *Physical Therapy* in 2021. *Physical Therapy* is another resource for Onc R clinicians who work with those diagnosed with cancer. It is the authorized scientific journal of the APTA and publishes highly relevant and innovative content for scientists and clinicians.[63] The entire March 2020 issue 3 (volume 100) was devoted to work documenting rehabilitation practitioners' involvement with persons with oncologic diagnoses.[64] Included in the issue are a variety of studies, a scoping review, and a systematic review related to cancer survivorship and Onc R.

The NCCN is "an alliance of leading cancer centers devoted to patient care, research, and education."[65] Their mission is to "improve and facilitate quality, efficient, effective, and accessible cancer care so patients can live better lives."[65] A core resource created by NCCN is the NCCN Clinical Practice Guidelines in Oncology (NCCN Guidelines®). According to NCCN, these guidelines "are the recognized standard for clinical policy in oncology and are the most comprehensive and most frequently updated CPGs available in any area of medicine."[65] The CPGs developed by the NCCN are decision tools that are created by doctors to explain a disease and determine the best way to treat a patient.[65] Currently, there are 73 NCCN Guidelines free of charge and available on NCCN.org. One of the guidelines is devoted to Survivorship (Version 1.2021), which applies to survivors across the continuum of care, including those on endocrine therapy, with metastatic disease, and long-term survivors,[66] and was most recently updated in February 2021.[66] In the guideline, several standards for survivorship care are outlined, including assessment of late psychosocial and physical effects, intervention for consequences of cancer and treatment, and planning for ongoing survivorship care. A variety of late effects/long-term psychosocial and physical problems are discussed, including but not limited to distress, anxiety, depression, cognitive function, fatigue, lymphedema, hormone-related symptoms, pain, and sexual function. This guideline serves as a valuable evidence-based resource for Onc R professionals.

The American Congress of Rehabilitation Medicine (ACRM) is "a global community of both researchers and consumers of research in the field of rehabilitation."[67] Promoting EBP and practice-based research is a goal of ACRM and it is the only professional organization that has representation of the interdisciplinary rehabilitation team.[67] Within ACRM are networking groups, including the Measurement Networking Group and the Cancer Rehabilitation Networking Group (CRNG).[68] The Measurement Networking Group's mission is to "produce and synthesize evidence of psychometrically advanced and improved measurement that enhances patient care and influences healthcare policy."[68,69] Their goal is "to build the capacity of rehabilitation providers to select, use, and interpret outcome measures to inform EBP and policy."[68,69] The CRNG is comprised of interdisciplinary professionals who desire to improve the educational and networking opportunities in Onc R research, education, clinical care, and policy to improve the lives of people who have been diagnosed with cancer.[68] The mission of the CRNG is to advance the field of cancer rehabilitation by providing opportunities for education and professional development, advocating for standards in clinical practice and research, and supporting a forum for interdisciplinary and international exchange.[68] The ACRM annual conference, held each fall has several education sessions and posters related to Onc R. Within the CRNG, five task forces are currently active: Education, Research and Outcomes, Integrative Cancer Rehabilitation, Quality of Life and Person-Centered, Oncology Cognitive Rehabilitation, and Pediatric.[68]

Accreditation Standards

The American College of Surgeons' Commission on Cancer (CoC) recently released its CoC accreditation standards, Optimal Resources for Cancer Care (2020), and was updated February 2021.[70] There are several new additions including Standard 4.8 which calls for the establishment of a Survivorship Program, combining elements from the previous Survivorship Care Plan standard and recommendations from CoC and other member organizations including a representative from the APTA, who is also a member of the Oncology Academy.[70,71] This new standard necessitates accredited organizations to establish a Survivorship Program under the direction of a cancer committee.[71] A survivorship program provides criteria to develop a team that includes specialties such as rehabilitation services.[72] Each year, the committee must monitor, evaluate, and make recommendations for improvements, as needed, to rehabilitation care services and/or referrals.[73] This updated standard lists a variety of services that may be included in the survivorship program including survivorship care plans, Onc R services, and physical activity programs. Onc R professionals can play a vital role in any of these services and in doing so should bring evidence to support the care that is being implemented or is recommended to be implemented.

Expert Consensus Groups and Roundtables

In 2010, the American College of Sports Medicine (ACSM) organized a Roundtable meeting comprised of research experts and clinicians in the field of cancer and exercise to develop the first set of exercise guidelines for individuals diagnosed with and surviving cancer.[74] This guideline was updated recently in 2019 by convening an International Multidisciplinary Roundtable to update recommendations based on current evidence on the role exercise and physical activity have in cancer survivorship and prevention.[75] This Roundtable provides practical, evidence-based information for implementing exercise as a treatment strategy and models for implementation for PTs.[75] The findings again concluded that exercise testing and training were generally safe for people diagnosed with and surviving cancer and that every survivor should "avoid inactivity."[74] Evidence found that precise amounts of aerobic, combined aerobic and resistance training, and/or resistance training could ameliorate a variety of cancer-related health outcomes including anxiety, depression, fatigue, physical function, and health-related quality of life.[74] Evidence for other outcomes such as cognitive functioning and chemotherapy-induced peripheral neuropathy (CIPN) is emerging but there are too few high-quality trials to interpret the potential of the benefits of exercise for managing and/or preventing cognitive functioning and CIPN.[74] For PLWBCs, a moderate-intensity aerobic and/or resistance exercise program at least three times per week, 30 minutes a session, for at least 8 to 12 weeks may consistently improve treatment-related adverse effects and symptoms.[75]

Additional Resources

There are several other organizations and research journals involved in Onc R including the American Occupational Therapy Association, American Speech-Language Hearing Association, *American Journal of Occupational Therapy, American Journal* of *Speech-Language Pathology, Archives of Physical Medicine and Rehabilitation,* and *Journal of Cancer Survivorship—Research and Practice* (see Table 3.2).

Conclusion

To be a good consumer of the literature, understanding the components of EBP and how to apply them to clinical practice is necessary. To begin, it is important to understand the five steps for incorporating evidence-based medicine into clinical practice: (1) Defining a clinically relevant question; (2) searching for the best evidence; (3) appraising the quality of the evidence; (4) applying the evidence to clinical practice; and (5) evaluating the process.[4] Additionally, interpreting treatment outcomes through the application of EBP steps is important to clinicians because it influences clinical decision-making which affects patient safety and efficacy. Along with understanding the components and steps of EBP, clinicians need to be cognizant of what resources are available to support their assessment and interventions related to Onc R. Fortunately, there are a variety of resources available that are discussed in this chapter to support clinicians in this endeavor.

Review Questions

Reader can find the correct answers and rationale in the back of the book.

1. To pose a clear clinical question, what four components need to be identified?
   A. Patient population, intervention/treatment, comparison, and outcome of interest
   B. Participation, intervention/treatment, comparison, and outcome of interest
   C. Patient population, intervention/treatment, comparison, and observation
   D. Participation, intervention/treatment, comparison, and observation

2. Which of the following would be considered the outcome in the following clinical example: In a woman with breast cancer, does early active range of motion on the affected side improve upper extremity function on the Disabilities of Arm, Shoulder and Hand (DASH) when compared to usual care?
   A. Women with breast cancer
   B. Disabilities of Arm, Shoulder and Hand (DASH)
   C. Usual Care
   D. Early active range of motion

3. Which of the following journals is the official journal of APTA Oncology and is an indexed resource for the dissemination of peer-reviewed research-based evidence related to oncologic physical therapy and Onc R?
   A. Rehabilitation Oncology
   B. Physical Therapy Journal
   C. Archives of Physical Medicine and Rehabilitation
   D. Journal of Cancer Survivorship—Research and Practice

4. According to the Evidence Pyramid, which of the following types of study designs is considered observational?
   A. Meta-analysis
   B. Systematic review
   C. Randomized controlled trial
   D. Case study

5. Which of the following is considered a nominal variable?
   A. Manual muscle testing grade
   B. Functional independence measure
   C. Gender
   D. Age

6. Which statistic helps to determine the reliability by which the null hypothesis can be rejected and consequently the strength of the observed result?
   A. *P*-value
   B. Confidence interval
   C. Effect size
   D. Minimal clinically important difference

7. Which statistic provides evidence about the accuracy of a test result?
   A. Confidence interval
   B. Effect size
   C. Minimal clinically important difference
   D. *P*-value

8. According to Cohen, which of the following represents a moderate effect size?
   A. 0.3
   B. 0.6
   C. 0.9
   D. 1.2

9. Which of the following intraclass correlation coefficient suggests a measure has good reliability?
   A. 0.2
   B. 0.4
   C. 0.6
   D. 0.8

10. Which of the following type of validity is used to establish the precision of a measure or test by comparing it to a gold standard?
    A. Content
    B. Criterion-related
    C. Construct
    D. Predictive

References

1. Page P. Beyond statistical significance: clinical interpretation of rehabilitation research literature. *Int J Sports Phys Ther.* 2014;9(5):726–736.
2. Bernhardsson S, Lynch E, Dizon JM, et al. Advancing evidence-based practice in physical therapy settings: multinational perspectives on implementation strategies and interventions. *Phys Ther.* 2017;97(1):51–60.
3. Cochrane AL. Archie Cochrane in his own words: selections arranged from his 1972 introduction to "effectiveness and efficiency: random reflections on the health services. *Control Clin Trials.* 1989;10(4):428–433.
4. Sackett DL, Rosenberg WM, Gray JM, Haynes RB, Richardson WS. Evidence based medicine: what it is and what it isn't. *BMJ.* 1996;312(7023):71–72.
5. Timmermans S, Mauck A. The promises and pitfalls of evidence-based medicine. *Health Aff.* 2005;24(1):18–28.
6. Sackett DL, Straus SE, Richardson WS, Rosenberg W, Haynes RB. Evidence-based medicine: How to practice and teach EBM. 2nd ed. *Churchill Livingstone;* 2000.
7. American Physical Therapy Association. Vision Statement for the Physical Therapy Profession Established; 2000. https://centennial.apta.org/timeline/vision-statement-for-the-physical-therapy-profession-established/#:~:text=The%20vision%20included%20six%20elements,practice%2C%20and%20practitioner%20of%20choice. Accessed August 27, 2020.
8. Straus SE, Sackett DL. Using research findings in clinical practice. *BMJ.* 1998;317(7154):339–342.
9. American Physical Therapy Association. *APTA Article Search;* 2021. https://www.apta.org/patient-care/evidence-based-practice-resources/article-search.
10. APTA Oncology. Rehabilitation Oncology. https://journals.lww.com/rehabonc/Pages/aboutthejournal.aspx; 2021.
11. Steves R, Hootman JM. Evidence-based medicine: what is it and how does it apply to athletic training? *J Athl Train.* 2004;39(1):83–87.
12. LaPier T, Donovan C. Statistical case scenarios in geriatric physical therapy research. *Geriatr Notes.* 2000;7(1):11–17.
13. Wang EW, Ghogomu N, Voelker CC, et al. A practical guide for understanding confidence intervals and P values. *Otolaryngol Head Neck Surg.* 2009;140(6):794–799.
14. Flechner L, Tseng TY. Understanding results: P-values, confidence intervals, and number need to treat. *Indian J Urol.* 2011;27(4):532–535.
15. Altman DG, Gore SM, Gardner MJ, Pocock SJ. Statistical guidelines for contributors to medical journals. *Br Med J (Clin Res Ed).* 1983;286(6376):1489–1493.
16. Batterham AM, Hopkins WG. Making meaningful inferences about magnitudes. *Int J Sports Physiol Perf.* 2006;1(1):50–57.
17. Cohen J. *Statistical Power Analysis for the Behavioral Sciences.* Academic Press; 2013.
18. Harrington S, Padua D, Battaglini C, et al. Comparison of shoulder flexibility, strength, and function between breast cancer survivors and healthy participants. *J Cancer Surviv.* 2011;5(2):167–174.
19. Psychometric properties. http://psychology.iresearchnet.com/counseling-psychology/personality-assessment/psychometric-properties/. Accessed August 13, 2020.
20. Law M. Measurement in occupational therapy: scientific criteria for evaluation. *Can J Occup Ther.* 1987;54(3):133–138.
21. Souza ACd, Alexandre NMC, Guirardello EdB. Psychometric properties in instruments evaluation of reliability and validity. *Epidemiol Serv Saúde.* 2017;26:649–659.
22. McGoey KE, Cowan RJ, Rumrill PP, LaVogue C. Understanding the psychometric properties of reliability and validity in assessment. *Work.* 2010;36(1):105–111.
23. de Vet HC, Terwee CB, Knol DL, Bouter LM. When to use agreement versus reliability measures. *J Clin Epidemiol.* 2006;59(10):1033–1039.
24. Koo TK, Li MY. A guideline of selecting and reporting intraclass correlation coefficients for reliability research. *J Chiropr Med.* 2016;15(2):155–163.
25. Streiner DL. Starting at the beginning: an introduction to coefficient alpha and internal consistency. *J Pers Assess.* 2003;80(1):99–103.
26. Keszei AP, Novak M, Streiner DL. Introduction to health measurement scales. *J Psychosom Res.* 2010;68(4):319–323.
27. Harrington SE, Hoffman J, Katsavelis D. Measurement of pectoralis minor muscle length in women diagnosed with breast cancer: reliability, validity, and clinical application. *Phys Ther.* 2020;100(3):429–437.
28. Anastasi A, Urbina S. *Psychological Testing:* Prentice Hall/Pearson Education; 1997.
29. Bellini J, Rumrill J, Phillip D, Cook B, Fitzgerald S. Measurement and statistics in special education research. In: *Research in Special Education: Designs, Methods, and Applications.* Charles C Thomas; 2001.
30. Polit DF, Beck CT. The content validity index: are you sure you know what's being reported? Critique and recommendations. *Res Nurs Health.* 2006;29(5):489–497.
31. Peter JP. Construct validity: a review of basic issues and marketing practices. *J Mark Res.* 1981;18(2):133–145.
32. Gilchrist LS, Galantino ML, Wampler M, Marchese VG, Morris GS, Ness KK. A framework for assessment in oncology rehabilitation. *Phys Ther.* 2009;89(3):286–306.
33. Temel JS, Pirl WF, Recklitis CJ, Cashavelly B, Lynch TJ. Feasibility and validity of a one-item fatigue screen in a thoracic oncology clinic. *J Thorac Oncol.* 2006;1(5):454–459.
34. Fetters L, Tilson J. *Evidence Based Physical Therapy.* FA Davis; 2018.
35. Kluetz PG, Slagle A, Papadopoulos EJ, et al. Focusing on core patient-reported outcomes in cancer clinical trials: symptomatic adverse events, physical function, and disease-related symptoms. *Clin Cancer Res.* 2016;22(7):1553–1558.
36. Physiopedia. Outcome measures; 2020. https://www.physio-pedia.com/Outcome_Measures; Accessed August 25, 2020.
37. Harrington SE, Stout NL, Hile E, et al. Cancer rehabilitation publications (2008–2018) with a focus on physical function: a scoping review. *Phys Ther.* 2020;100(3):363–415.
38. Basch E, Bennett AV. Patient-reported outcomes in clinical trials of rare diseases. *J Gen Intern Med.* 2014;29(3):801–803.
39. Mandrell BN, Baker J, Levine D, et al. Children with minimal chance for cure: parent proxy of the child's health-related quality of life and the effect on parental physical and mental health during treatment. *J Neuro-oncol.* 2016;129(2):373–381.
40. Harrington SE, Fisher MI. Screening and assessment for cancer rehabilitation. *Rehabil Oncol.* 2018;36(2):141–142.
41. Gilchrist LS, Harrington S, Fisher MI. Oncology Section EDGE Task Force: clinical measures of pain and fatigue. Paper presented at APTA Combined Sections Meeting: San Antonio; 2017.
42. Fulcher CD, Gosselin-Acomb TK. Distress assessment: practice change through guideline implementation. *Clin J Oncol Nurs.* 2007;11(6):817–821.
43. Fisher MI HS, Cohn JC, Lee J, Malone D. A clinical practice guideline for the screening and assessment of cancer-related fatigue for healthcare providers. Paper presented at American Congress of Rehabilitation Medicine: Virtual; October 2020.
44. de Vet HC, Terwee CB, Ostelo RW, Beckerman H, Knol DL, Bouter LM. Minimal changes in health status questionnaires: distinction between minimally detectable change and minimally important change. *Health Qual Life Outcomes.* 2006;4(1):54.
45. Jacobson NS, Truax P. Clinical significance: a statistical approach to defining meaningful change in psychotherapy research. *J Consult Clin Psychol.* 1991;59(1):12–19.

46. Jaeschke R, Singer J, Guyatt GH. Measurement of health status: ascertaining the minimal clinically important difference. *Control Clin Trials.* 1989;10(4):407–415.

47. Mokkink LB, Terwee CB, Patrick DL, et al. The COSMIN study reached international consensus on taxonomy, terminology, and definitions of measurement properties for health-related patient-reported outcomes. *J Clin Epidemiol.* 2010;63(7):737–745.

48. Revicki D, Hays RD, Cella D, Sloan J. Recommended methods for determining responsiveness and minimally important differences for patient-reported outcomes. *J Clin Epidemiol.* 2008;61(2):102–109.

49. Budtz CR, Andersen JH, de Vos Andersen N-B, Christiansen DH. Responsiveness and minimal important change for the quick-DASH in patients with shoulder disorders. *Health Qual Life Outcomes.* 2018;16(1):1–6.

50. Portney LG, Watkins MP. *Foundations of Clinical Research: Applications to Practice.* Vol. 892: Pearson/Prentice Hall; 2009.

51. Huang MH, Miller K, Smith K, Fredrickson K, Shilling T. Reliability, validity, and minimal detectable change of Balance Evaluation Systems Test and its short versions in older cancer survivors: a pilot study. *J Geriatr Phys Ther.* 2016;39(2):58–63.

52. Franchignoni F, Vercelli S, Giordano A, Sartorio F, Bravini E, Ferriero G. Minimal clinically important difference of the disabilities of the arm, shoulder and hand outcome measure (DASH) and its shortened version (QuickDASH). *J Orthopa Sports Phys Ther.* 2014;44(1):30–39.

53. Harrington S, Padua D, Battaglini C, Michener LA. Upper extremity strength and range of motion and their relationship to function in breast cancer survivors. *Physiother Theory Pract.* 2013;29(7):513–520.

54. Oncology A. About Us; 2020. https://oncologypt.org/about-us/. Accessed August 20, 2020.

55. Hile E, Levangie P, Ryans K, Gilchrist L. Oncology Section Task Force on Breast Cancer Outcomes: clinical measures of chemotherapy-induced peripheral neuropathy—a systematic review. *Rehabil Oncol.* 2015;33(3):32–41.

56. Harrington S, Gilchrist L. Evolution of the EDGE rating scale. *Rehabil Oncol.* 2016;34(4):156–157.

57. Oncology A. Academy of Oncologic Physical Therapy EDGE Task Force Report Summaries; 2019. https://oncologypt.org/wp-content/uploads/2019/10/EDGE-Annotated-Bibliography-8.19-update.pdf. Accessed August 25, 2020.

58. Davies C, Levenhagen K, Ryans K, Perdomo M, Gilchrist L. How can a clinical practice guideline enhance my practice? *Rehabil Oncol.* 2017;35(3):111–113.

59. Quality AfHRa. Guidelines and Measures; 2020. https://www.ahrq.gov/gam/index.html.

60. Steinberg E, Greenfield S, Wolman DM, Mancher M, Graham R. *Clinical Practice Guidelines We Can Trust.* National Academies Press; 2011.

61. Levenhagen K, Davies C, Perdomo M, Ryans K, Gilchrist L. Diagnosis of upper quadrant lymphedema secondary to cancer: clinical practice guideline from the oncology section of the American Physical Therapy Association. *Phys Ther.* 2017;97(7):729–745.

62. Davies C, Levenhagen K, Ryans K, Perdomo M, Gilchrist L. Interventions for breast cancer–related lymphedema: clinical practice guideline from the academy of oncologic physical therapy of APTA. *Phys Ther.* 2020;100(7):1163–1179.

63. American Physical Therapy Association. About PTJ; 2020. https://academic.oup.com/ptj/pages/About.

64. Ness KK, Gilchrist L. Innovations in rehabilitation for people who have cancer or who have survived cancer. *Phys Ther.* 2020;100(3):361–362.

65. Network NCC. About; 2021. https://www.nccn.org/home/about. Accessed May 11, 2021.

66. Network NCC. NCCN Guidelines – Survivorship. https://www.nccn.org/guidelines/guidelines-detail?category=3&id=1466; https://www.nccn.org/professionals/physician_gls/pdf/survivorship.pdf; 2021. Accessed May 11, 2021.

67. Medicine ACoR. Who is ACRM?; 2020. https://acrm.org/about/about-acrm/. Accessed August 25, 2020.

68. Medicine ACoR. Cancer Rehabilitation Networking Group. https://acrm.org/acrm-communities/cancer/; 2020. Accessed August 20, 2020.

69. Medicine ACoR. Measurement interdisciplinary special interest group; 2020. https://acrm.org/acrm-communities/measurement/. Accessed August 25, 2020.

70. Cancer ACeS-Co. 2020 standards and resources; 2021. https://www.facs.org/quality-programs/cancer/coc/standards/2020. Accessed May 11, 2021.

71. Center GWC. Commission on cancer releases updated standards for 2020; 2020. https://cancercenter.gwu.edu/news/commission-cancer-releases-updated-standards-2020. Accessed August 25, 2020.

72. Cancer Co. Optimal Resources for Cancer Care; 2021. https://www.facs.org/2020standards.

73. Oncolens. What cancer centers need to know about the changing CoC accreditation standards; 2019. https://www.oncolens.com/blog/Changes_to_CoC_Accreditation_Standards/. Accessed August 20, 2020.

74. Campbell KL, Winters-Stone KM, Wiskemann J, et al. Exercise guidelines for cancer survivors: consensus statement from international multidisciplinary roundtable. *Med Sci Sports Exerc.* 2019;51(11):2375–2390.

75. Campbell KL, Winters-Stone KM, Patel AV, et al. An executive summary of reports from an international multidisciplinary roundtable on exercise and cancer: evidence, guidelines, and implementation. *Rehabil Oncol.* 2019;37(4):144–152.

4

The Biological Basis and Diagnostic Evaluation of Cancer

MARK A. MICALE, PhD, (ASCP)CG, FACMGG[a], J. LYNNE WILLIAMS, PhD, MT(ASCP)[b], SUMI DINDA, PhD[c], AND SARA RIVARD, MA, RT(R)(CT)[d]

CHAPTER OUTLINE

Introduction to the Pathophysiology of Cancer

Cancer is the second leading cause of death in the United States, surpassed only by cardiovascular disease.[1] However, cancer is not a single unique disease entity, but rather a group of diseases that share the characteristic of unregulated, excessive cellular growth. To understand the mechanisms behind the development of a cancer, one must first understand the normal processes that regulate cell proliferation, differentiation, and tissue homeostasis.

The term *neoplasia* means "new growth." Neoplasms typically develop when cells of a tissue replicate autonomously without being constrained by the regulatory influences that normally control cell growth. Such cells are described as "transformed" and display a degree of proliferative autonomy that results in formation of a neoplastic clone. Neoplasms are often referred to as *tumors* and can be divided into *benign* and *malignant* (Table 4.1). Both categories of tumors consist of transformed neoplastic cells and depend on the support of non-neoplastic stromal tissue as well as nutrients supplied by the host.

[a]Medical Director, Clinical Cytogenomics Laboratory and Associate Professor, Pathology and Laboratory Medicine and Obstetrics & Gynecology, Beaumont Health and Oakland University William Beaumont School of Medicine, MI, USA
[b]Professor Emerita Clinical & Diagnostic Sciences, Oakland University, MI, USA
[c]Professor and Chair Clinical Diagnostic Sciences, Oakland University, MI, USA
[d]Program Director and Special Instructor Radiologic Technology- Clinical and Diagnostic Sciences, Oakland University, MI, USA

TABLE 4.1   Characteristics of Benign and Malignant Tumors

Benign	Malignant
Cells are well differentiated and resemble tissue of origin	Cells are less to poorly differentiated and may not resemble tissue of origin or may be undifferentiated
Tend to be slow growing	Tend to be faster growing
Well circumscribed, may be encapsulated	Poorly circumscribed, often unencapsulated
Localized to site of origin	Locally invasive, may metastasize to distant sites

Created by Mark Micale PhD, (ASCP)CG, FACMGG. Printed with permission.

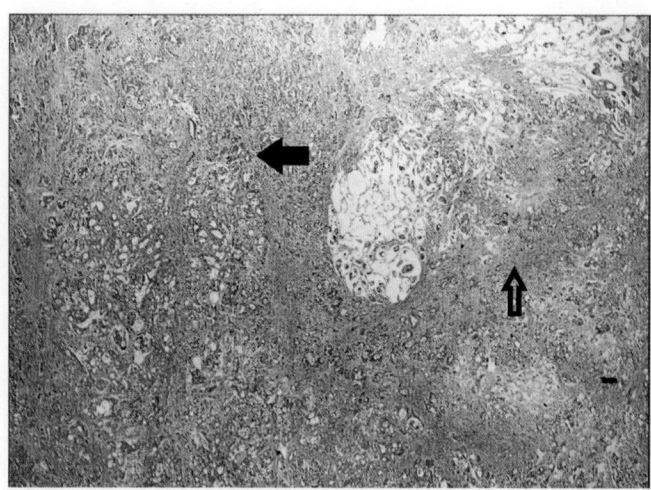

• **Fig. 4.2** Poorly Differentiated Pancreatic Adenocarcinoma, Infiltrating Cells (*Hollow Arrow*); and Poorly Formed Glandular Structures (*Solid Arrow*) Surrounded by Desmoplastic Stroma. (Photo courtesy of Mustafa Deebajah, MD, Beaumont Health Department of Pathology and Laboratory Medicine.)

A benign tumor is generally considered to be relatively innocuous, although it may sometimes produce significant morbidity and occasionally can be lethal. Benign neoplasms are composed mostly of well-differentiated cells, in that they resemble their normal tissue counterparts both morphologically and functionally. They tend to have slower growth patterns and grow as cohesive masses that remain localized to their site of origin. Thus, benign tumors characteristically do not undergo infiltration or invasion of surrounding tissue or metastasize to distant tissue sites. Often, they are encapsulated in a rim of fibrous tissue. This capsule makes the tumor discrete and easily excisable surgically. However, the lack of a capsule does not mean the tumor is malignant.

Malignant neoplasms may show a wide range of differentiation (referring to the extent to which the cells resemble their cells of origin). They may be subclassified as well-differentiated more closely resembling their normal counterparts (Figure 4.1), or poorly differentiated showing characteristics of primitive or immature cells (Figure 4.2).

A complete lack of differentiation is termed *anaplasia*. Malignant cells often show characteristic morphologic changes such as

pleomorphism (variation in size and shape), nuclear abnormalities (variation in nuclear shape and size, chromatin condensation, and enlarged nucleoli), and atypical mitoses (cell divisions). Malignant neoplasms tend to be faster growing tumors and are characterized by progressive infiltration as well as invasion and destruction of surrounding tissues. They usually lack a well-defined capsule and microscopic evaluation reveals malignant cells penetrating and infiltrating adjacent normal tissue structures (Figure 4.3).

The surgical pathologist during an intraoperative consultation ("frozen section") will comment on the presence or absence of clear margins when evaluating an excised tissue sample, providing the surgeon some idea as to whether the tumor has been completely excised (Figure 4.4A and B).

In addition, many cancers have the capacity to metastasize, or spread to tissues distant from the primary tumor site. The invasiveness of cancers allows them to penetrate blood vessels, lymphatics, and body cavities, facilitating spread throughout the body. While all malignant tumors have the capability to be invasive and to

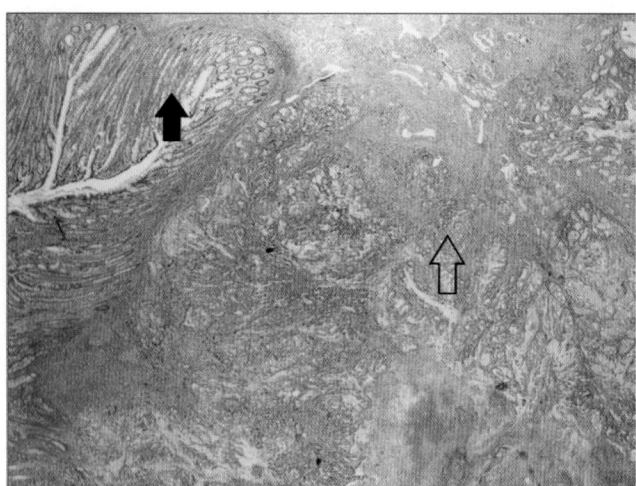

• **Fig. 4.1** Well-Differentiated Colonic Adenocarcinoma, Normal Colon (*Solid Arrow*) Adjacent to Well Differentiated Gland-Forming Carcinoma (*Hollow Arrow*). (Photo courtesy of Mustafa Deebajah, MD, Beaumont Health Department of Pathology and Laboratory Medicine.)

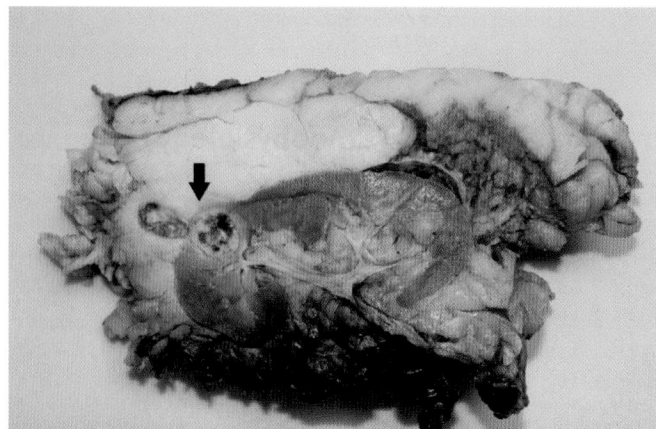

• **Fig. 4.3** Gross Appearance of Clear Cell Renal Cell Carcinoma With Focal Peri-Renal Fat Invasion (*Arrow*). (Photo courtesy of Mustafa Deebajah, MD, Beaumont Health Department of Pathology and Laboratory Medicine.)

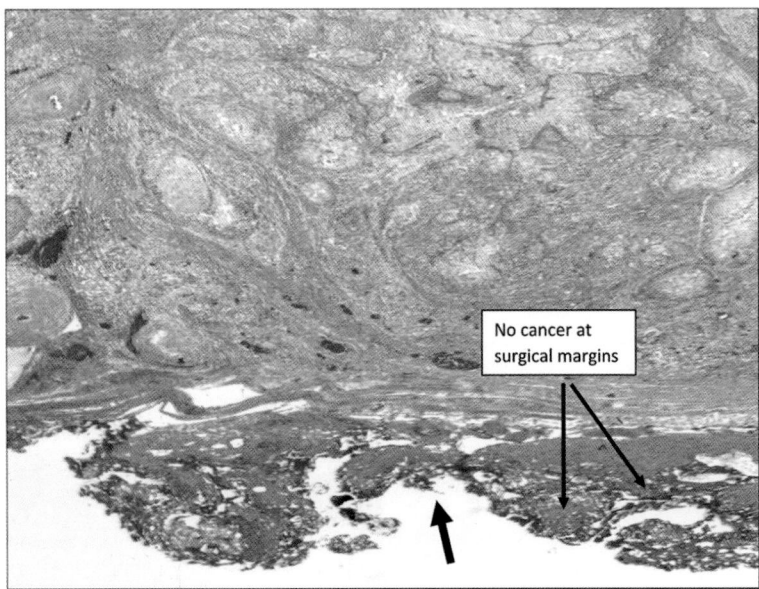

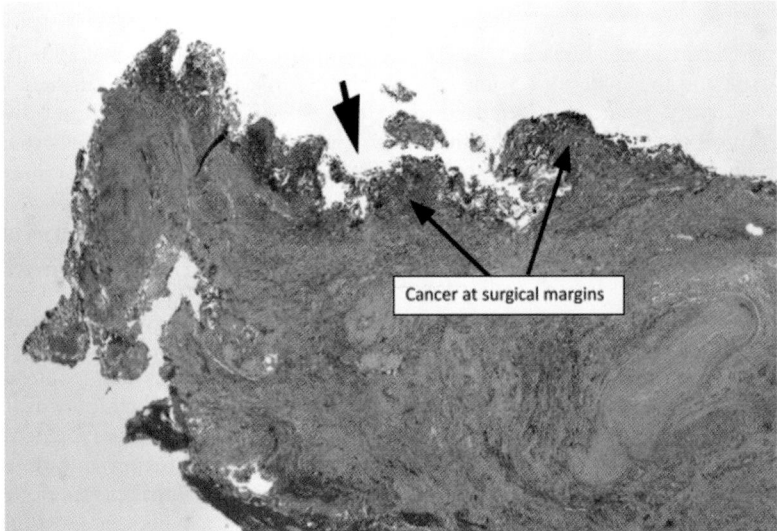

• **Fig. 4.4** Moderately Differentiated Squamous Cell Carcinoma of Cervix (Surgical Margins Are Inked Blue). Top Picture—Carcinoma Does Not Extend to the Inked Surgical Margin ("Negative Margins"). Bottom Picture—Carcinoma Extends and Touches the Inked Surgical Margin ("Positive Margins") Indicating that the Tumor Was Not Completely Excised, Necessitating Further Tissue Excision Until Negative Margins Are Achieved. (Photos courtesy of Mustafa Deebajah, MD, Beaumont Health Department of Pathology and Laboratory Medicine.)

metastasize, some do so very infrequently (e.g., basal cell carcinomas of the skin). In addition, while for many tumors, metastasis is a late-stage event in the tumor's life span, some malignancies are "genetically programmed" to metastasize at an earlier stage in development making them more difficult to treat.

Role of the Cell Cycle in Normal Tissue Homeostasis and Malignant Transformation

The ability of a tissue to maintain an adequate number of cells to carry out its functions is called *tissue homeostasis,* which depends on a balance between cell proliferation (mitotic cell division), cellular differentiation (acquisition of specialized functions and morphology), and cell death (elimination of damaged, unwanted, or excess cells from the tissue). Cancer is, by definition, a disruption of tissue homeostasis (i.e., unregulated, excessive growth of cells).

Cell proliferation is a fundamental necessity for the maintenance of steady-state tissue homeostasis which necessitates the replacement of dead or damaged cells. In multicellular organisms, normal cells will proliferate only when they receive a signal from their environment, usually in the form of a growth factor or endocrine signal. When a cell receives a signal to proliferate, it undergoes a series of events which have been well-defined both biochemically and morphologically, collectively referred to as the *cell cycle.* The cell cycle is divided into four phases, G_1 (Gap-1; Pre-synthetic growth), S (DNA synthesis), G_2 (Gap-2; Pre-mitotic growth), and M (mitosis) (Figure 4.5).

If a cell is not actively undergoing proliferation (i.e., is not in the cell cycle) it enters a dormant or quiescent state called G_0.

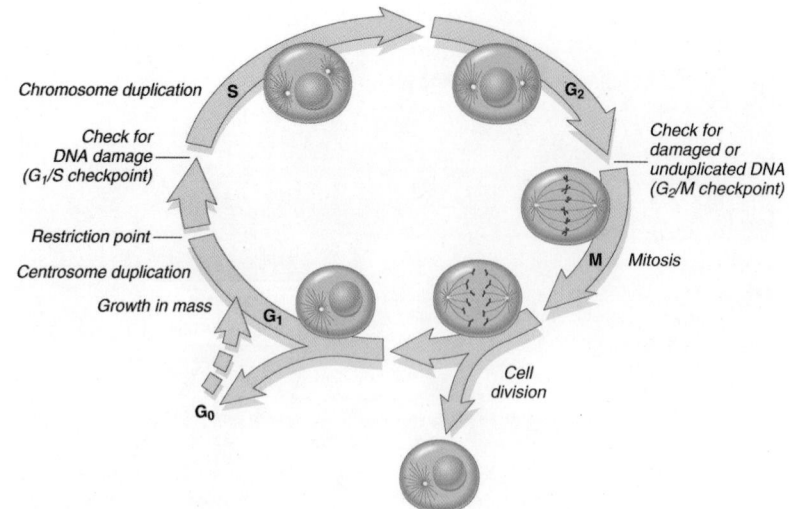

• **Fig. 4.5** Cell Cycle Landmarks. (Reprinted with permission from Kumar V, Abbas A, Aster J. *Robbins and Cotran Pathological Basis of Disease*. 10th ed. Elsevier; 2021: Figure 1.18.)

Some cells cycle continuously (referred to as labile cells), including cells lining the intestinal tract and the epidermis. Stable cells are those that are generally quiescent (G_0) but can be induced to reenter the cell cycle at G_1 and proliferate if appropriately stimulated (hepatocytes, mature lymphocytes). Permanent cells such as neurons and cardiac myocytes are terminally differentiated and have lost the capacity to proliferate (permanently in G_0).

During G_1, the cell increases in mass, duplicates its centrosome, and synthesizes components necessary for cell replication. During late G_1, the cell passes through a restriction point, which is the point at which the cell is committed to completion of the cell cycle and is no longer dependent on external growth signals (i.e., movement through the remainder of the cycle is autonomous). For cell replication to be effective, the cell must ensure that there is adequate synthesis of all cellular components, the DNA is replicated accurately, and both are equally apportioned to the two daughter cells. To safeguard the process, the cell cycle is regulated by checkpoints and cell cycle inhibitors.

Before the cell can progress to S phase, the cell must "pass" the G_1/S checkpoint, which checks for DNA damage before allowing DNA synthesis to occur. S phase is the period during which chromosome duplication occurs, followed by the second gap period (G2) and then mitosis, when karyokinesis (nuclear division) and cytokinesis (cytoplasmic separation) occur. The G_2/M checkpoint checks for damaged or unduplicated DNA. If the cell fails to pass either checkpoint, it will attempt to correct the damaged DNA. If DNA repair is unsuccessful, the cell will trigger apoptosis and die, thus ensuring the fidelity of the genetic material in the newly created cells. The cell cycle is regulated by a variety of activators and inhibitors (Figure 4.6).

Cyclins, proteins named because of the cyclic nature of their production and degradation, associate with enzymes called cyclin-dependent kinases (CDKs). Different cyclin/CDK complexes regulate movement through the cell cycle. The transient increase of a particular cyclin, and its binding to its appropriate CDK partner activates the kinase to phosphorylate protein substrates. After phosphorylation by the CDK kinase is complete, the cyclin is degraded, and the kinase activity ceases. Although more than 15 cyclins have been identified, cyclins A, B, D, and E. are the major ones regulating progression through the cell cycle. Each phase of the cell cycle is regulated by different cyclin/CDK

complexes. CDK inhibitors (CDKI) regulate the kinase activity of the cyclin/CDK complex. If the CDKIs are defective, cells with damaged DNA can survive and divide, resulting in propagation of mutations to daughter cells that increase risk for malignant transformation.

The Role of Apoptosis in Tissue Homeostasis and Its Dysregulation in Tumorigenesis

The other aspect of maintaining an appropriate number of cells for tissue homeostasis is cell death. The two major pathways of cell death are necrosis and apoptosis, which are morphologically, functionally, and biochemically distinct (Table 4.2).

When cells encounter potentially injurious insults such as hypoxia/ischemia, toxins, infectious agents, immunologic reactions, nutritional imbalances, or physical agents (trauma, temperature extremes, changes in atmospheric pressure), they generally die by the process of necrosis. Necrosis is generally considered the inevitable result of severe damage and is the "accidental" result of an injury too severe to be repaired.

When cells need to be eliminated during normal physiologic processes to maintain tissue homeostasis, they die by the process of apoptosis (also referred to as programmed cell death). This occurs by the activation of precise molecular pathways and is said to be a "regulated" form of cell death that occurs in healthy tissues. However, it can also be seen in some pathologic conditions (Table 4.3). In apoptosis, a series of enzymes are activated that degrade the cell's nuclear DNA along with nuclear and cytoplasmic proteins while maintaining an intact cellular membrane.

Apoptosis is controlled by specific biochemical pathways that regulate the balance of survival-inducing and death-inducing signals. Major players in this process are enzymes called caspases. Their activation results in the orderly degradation of cellular components during apoptosis. Other important contributors include pro-apoptotic and anti-apoptotic regulatory proteins. The cell is constantly evaluating its integrity by balancing these various pro- and anti-apoptotic signals. Major contributors to this process are the BCL2 family of proteins which are encoded by anti-apoptotic genes including *BCL2*, pro-apoptotic genes such as *BAX*, and the BH3-only proteins encoded by genes including *BAD* that promote apoptosis by

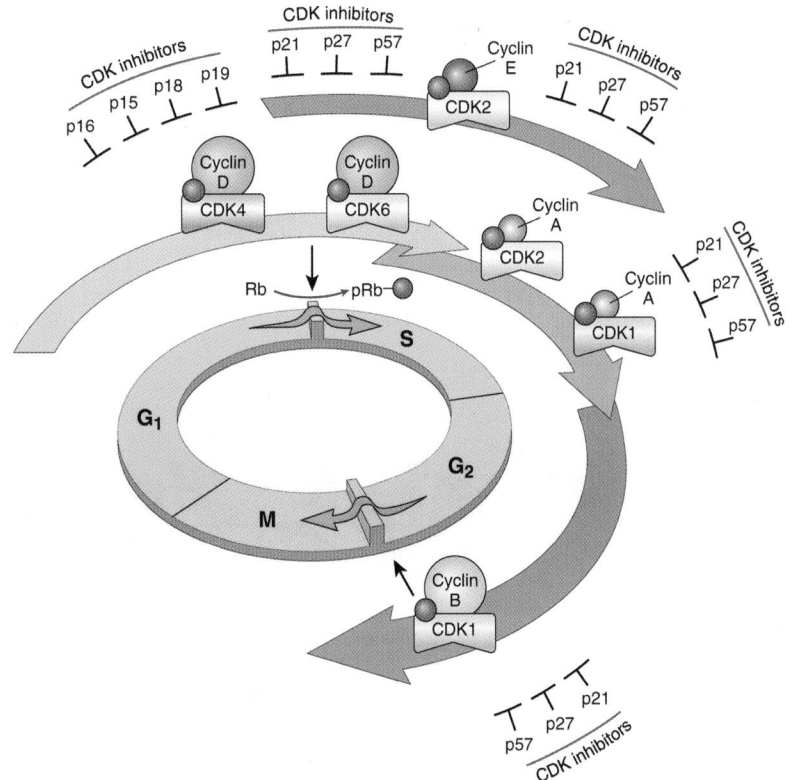

• **Fig. 4.6** Role of Cyclins, Cyclin-Dependent Kinases (CDKs), and Cyclin-Dependent Kinase Inhibitors (CDKIs) in Cell Cycle Regulation. (Reprinted with permission from Kumar V, Abbas A, Aster J. *Robbins and Cotran Pathological Basis of Disease*. 10th ed. Elsevier; 2021: Figure 1.19.)

TABLE 4.2   A Comparison of Cellular Necrosis and Apoptosis

Feature	Necrosis	Apoptosis
Cell size	Enlarged (swelling)	Reduced (shrinkage)
Nucleus	Chromatin condensation, nuclear fragmentation, dissolution of chromatin	Fragmentation into nucleosome-sized fragments
Plasma membrane	Disrupted	Intact, altered structure
Cellular contents	Enzymatic digestion, may leak out of cell	Intact, may be released in apoptotic bodies
Adjacent inflammation	Frequent	No
Physiologic or pathologic role	Usually pathologic (irreversible cell injury)	Usually physiologic (elimination of unwanted cells), can be pathologic after some forms of cell injury (e.g., DNA damage)

Created by Mark Micale, PhD (ASCP) CG, FACMGG. Printed with permission.

TABLE 4.3   Causes of Apoptosis

Normal Physiological Process	Pathological Conditions
During embryogenesis-involution of primordial structures or tissue remodeling	DNA damage
Turnover of proliferative tissues (e.g., intestinal epithelium, bone marrow, and thymic lymphocytes)	Accumulation of misfolded proteins
Involution of hormone-dependent tissues (e.g., endometrium)	Infections, particularly certain viral infections
Reduction of leukocytes at end of immune and inflammatory responses	Atrophy of parenchymal organs after duct obstruction (e.g., pancreas, parotid gland)
Elimination of potentially harmful self-reactive lymphocytes	

Adapted by Mark Micale, PhD, (ASCP) CG, FACMGG. Adapted with permission from Kumar V, Abbas A, Aster J. *Robbins and Cotran Pathological Basis of Disease*. 10th ed. Elsevier; 2021: Table 2.2.

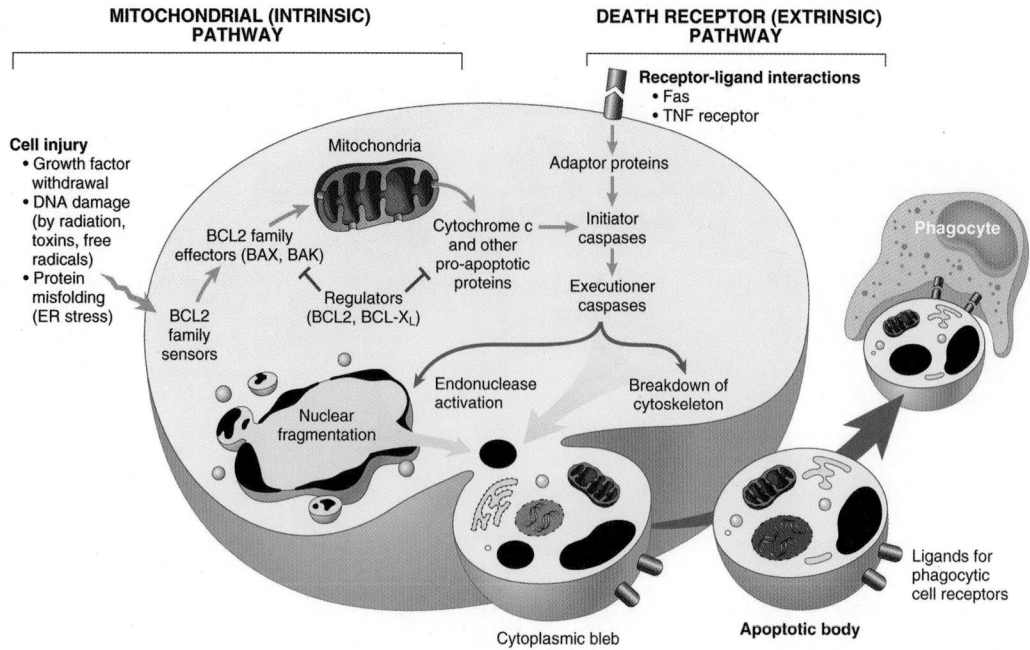

• **Fig. 4.7** Mechanisms of Apoptosis. *ER,* endoplasmic reticulum; *TNF,* tumor necrosis factor. (Reprinted with permission from Kumar V, Abbas A, Aster J. *Robbins and Cotran Pathological Basis of Disease.* 10th ed. Elsevier; 2021: Figure 2.13.)

neutralizing anti-apoptotic proteins. Finally, there are negative regulators of apoptosis, known as *inhibitor of apoptosis proteins* (IAPs), which can bind to activated caspase enzymes and prevent apoptosis.

There are two pathways for activation of apoptosis (Figure 4.7). The first involves the binding of "death-promoting" cytokines from the environment (Fas ligand/FasL or TNF) to death receptors on the cell surface (Fas or TNFR), referred to as the *extrinsic pathway.* The second, referred to as the *intrinsic pathway* or *mitochondrial pathway,* is responsible for apoptosis in most physiologic or pathologic situations. This pathway involves release of cytochrome C into the cytosol in response to changes in permeability of mitochondrial membranes when the cell is exposed to DNA-damaging agents or accumulates misfolded proteins. This activates a cascade of caspase enzymes to initiate apoptosis. When the normal processes that facilitate apoptosis become dysregulated through mutation of apoptosis regulatory genes, cells that should normally be eliminated (such as those that contain DNA damage) will instead be allowed to survive and proliferate, thus propagating their DNA damage which can be a transformative (tumorigenic) event.

The Cellular Hallmarks of Cancer

Cancers display fundamental changes that are considered the hallmarks of cancer, including self-sufficiency in growth signals, insensitivity to growth inhibitory signals, evasion of apoptosis, limitless replicative potential, sustained angiogenesis, invasion and metastasis, evasion of immune surveillance, altered cellular metabolism, tumor promoting inflammation, and genomic instability.[2]

Self-Sufficiency in Growth Signals

The dysregulation of cell/tissue growth that defines cancer is partly due to a *self-sufficiency in growth signals.* As indicated above, normal cells in multicellular organisms do not spontaneously proliferate, but do so only when they receive signals from their environment, generally growth factors that activate the cell cycle. Cancer cells

bypass this regulatory mechanism by providing their own growth signals, thus promoting autonomous proliferation. Cancer cells will typically demonstrate mutation or activation of the genes encoding the proteins that signal proliferation. The first step in proliferation is the binding of a growth factor to its specific receptor in the cell membrane. Cancer cells typically secrete their own growth factors or induce stromal cells in their environment to produce growth factors, thus acquiring growth self-sufficiency. Normally the growth factor receptor is dormant or inactive unless its specific growth factor binds. Upon binding of a growth factor, the receptor activates a series of signaling transduction pathways in the cytoplasm which communicate (transduce) events at the cell surface to the nucleus where specific nuclear transcription factors are activated to begin the transcription of the genes encoding the proteins needed to drive the cell through the cell cycle. Each step in this sequence is dormant until activated by the preceding step in a cascade of activation. Additional ways in which a cell can acquire self-sufficiency in growth is by mutating genes which code for proteins involved in this process so that they are constitutively active, bypassing the need for activation via the preceding step. Thus, a mutation in a gene for a growth factor receptor may result in a membrane protein that is always active, driving continuous proliferation in the absence of growth factor binding. Likewise, an activating mutation in one of the cytoplasmic signaling molecules can drive proliferation in the absence of growth factor binding to its receptor. An activating mutation of a pertinent transcription factor may result in ongoing proliferation, bypassing the first three steps (growth factor, activation of receptor, activation of signaling molecules). Any of the above would contribute to self-sufficiency in growth.

Mutations in many of the genes that encode the proteins that drive the cell cycle have been identified in various cancers. Excessive, unregulated cell proliferation may be associated with an increase in one or more of the cell cycle activators (cyclins, CDKs) or loss of activity of one or more of the cell cycle regulators (failure of checkpoint surveillance or loss of activity of a CDKI). Defects in the G_1/S cell cycle checkpoint are particularly notable in cancers, as the majority appears to have a mutation in a regulatory gene that disables the checkpoint, allowing cells to continually reenter S phase despite DNA damage. It is important to note that an increase of growth-promoting signals by itself is not sufficient to result in sustained proliferation of cancer cells. In otherwise normal tissue, the increased proliferation is limited by cell senescence and apoptosis.

Insensitivity to Growth Inhibitory Signals

In addition to growth-promoting proteins or cytokines, there are growth-inhibiting cytokines such as transforming growth factor β (e.g., TGFb) which plays a role in regulating tissue homeostasis. In many cancers, the growth-inhibiting effects of this cytokine are impaired by mutations in genes that encode proteins involved in TGFb signaling. Additionally, there are internal signals within the cell itself that have growth inhibitory actions. These anti-growth signals may prevent proliferation by inducing the cell to enter G_0 (quiescence). Alternatively, the cell may become senescent (a post-mitotic state in which the cell has lost replicative potential). The genes encoding these growth-inhibitory signals are often referred to as *tumor-suppressor genes (TSG)*. For a cancer cell to effectively become insensitive to these inhibitory signals, both alleles of the gene (one on each chromosome) must be mutated or silenced.

One of the most important tumor suppressor genes is the retinoblastoma (*RB*) gene on chromosome 13q14.2 that encodes the Rb protein (to be discussed later). One of the main functions of RB is to regulate the G_1/S cell cycle checkpoint. As mentioned above, this checkpoint must be by-passed for the malignant phenotype to be established. A second significant tumor suppressor is the *TP53 gene* which codes for the p53 protein. The p53 protein is an important growth inhibitory signal for tissue homeostasis, as it can activate temporary cell cycle arrest (quiescence), permanent cell cycle arrest (senescence) or can trigger apoptosis. It monitors internal cell stress, as well as DNA damage, and thus pays a central role in maintaining the integrity of the genome.

Evasion of Cell Death

Cancer cells frequently contain mutations in the genes that regulate apoptosis, making the cells resistant to cell death. This can allow for the propagation of mutation(s) inherent in older cells, thereby increasing the risk of malignant transformation. Most commonly these are mutations that affect the proteins involved in the intrinsic pathway of apoptosis. As the p53 protein plays an essential role in apoptosis, it is not surprising that *TP53* gene mutations would enable cancer cells to avoid apoptosis. In addition, many tumors show over-expression of the anti-apoptotic members of the BCL2 family proteins. For example, in follicular lymphoma, upregulation of BCL2 protein occurs thereby allowing the cells to survive for abnormally long periods.

Limitless Replicative Potential (Immortality)

Normal cells have a limited capacity for replication; after a fixed number of divisions, they enter what is called *replicative senescence* (a terminally nondividing state). Replicative senescence in cells is caused by the progressive shortening of structures called *telomeres* (short repeated sequences of DNA at the ends of chromosomes) which results in cell cycle arrest. The function of telomeres is to provide protection from enzymatic degradation of the ends of chromosomes to maintain chromosome and genomic stability. With each mitotic division an individual cell undergoes, a small section of the telomere is not replicated, resulting in the progressive

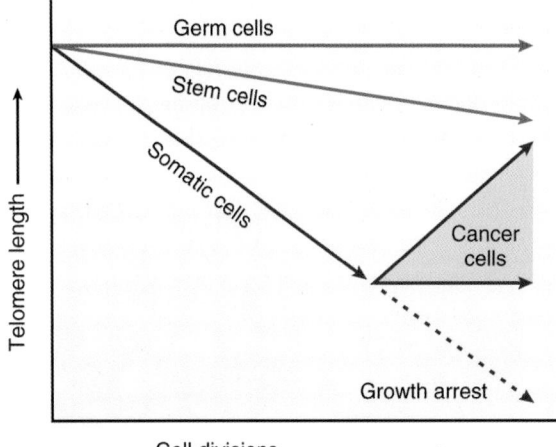

• **Fig. 4.8** The Role of Telomeres and Telomerase in Replicative Senescence of Cells. Telomere Length is Plotted Against the Number of Cell Divisions. In Most Somatic Cells There is No Telomerase Activity, Resulting in Progressive Telomere Shortening With Increasing Cell Divisions Until Growth Arrest or Senescence Occurs. Germ Cells and Stem Cells Both Contain Telomerase, but Only Germ Cells Have Sufficient Levels of the Enzyme to Stabilize Telomere Length Completely. In Cancer Cells, Telomerase is Often Reactivated, Resulting in Failure to Arrest Cell Division. (Reprinted with permission from Kumar V, Abbas A, Aster J. *Robbins and Cotran Pathological Basis of Disease.* 10th ed. Elsevier; 2021: Figure 2.36.)

shortening of telomeres. As they shorten, telomeres are sensed in cells as broken DNA, which eventually signals cell cycle arrest. To an extent, telomere length can be maintained by the action of the enzyme *telomerase*, which functions to add nucleotides to the ends of chromosomes. Telomerase is expressed in germ cells and stem cells but is absent in most somatic cells. As mature somatic cells age, they exit the cell cycle due to the progressive shortening of their telomeres. However, virtually all types of cancer cells become immortalized due to reactivation of telomerase and stabilization of their telomeres. The result is limitless replicative potential or immortality (Figure 4.8).

Sustained Angiogenesis

Even though a cell may have acquired all the genetic mutations it needs to undergo malignant transformation, additional factors are required to establish a malignancy. Solid tumors require the delivery of oxygen and nutrients and the removal of waste by a functional circulation. It has been estimated that a 1 to 2 mm zone is the maximal distance across which nutrients and oxygen can diffuse. To grow beyond this size, a cancer must stimulate neovascularization (development of new blood vessels, or neoangiogenesis). These new blood vessels are, however, leaky and dilated, an abnormal structure that contributes to metastasis.

Angiogenesis is controlled by a balance between angiogenic promoters and inhibitors. Early in development, most tumors do not induce angiogenesis, and thus remain small. At some point, a growing tumor initiates an angiogenic switch associated with increased production of angiogenic factors (basic fibroblast growth factor/bFGF, vascular endothelial growth factor/VEGF) and/or loss of angiogenic inhibitors (angiostatin and endostatin). Angiogenesis is essential if a solid tumor is to grow to a clinically significant size.

Invasion and Metastasis

Invasion and metastasis are major causes of cancer-related morbidity and mortality. Tumor cells frequently escape their site of origin and enter the circulation because of their invasive properties. Invasion and metastasis result from a series of steps starting with loosening of cell-cell contacts and invasion of tumor cells into blood and lymph vessels (invasion of the extracellular matrix), movement of the tumor cells through the vasculature (vascular dissemination), extravasation from the vessels ("homing" of tumor cells), formation of small foci of tumor cells in distal tissues (termed micrometastases), and their growth into macroscopic tumors (Figure 4.9). As discussed previously, in most cases metastasis occurs at a later stage of tumor development; however, it has

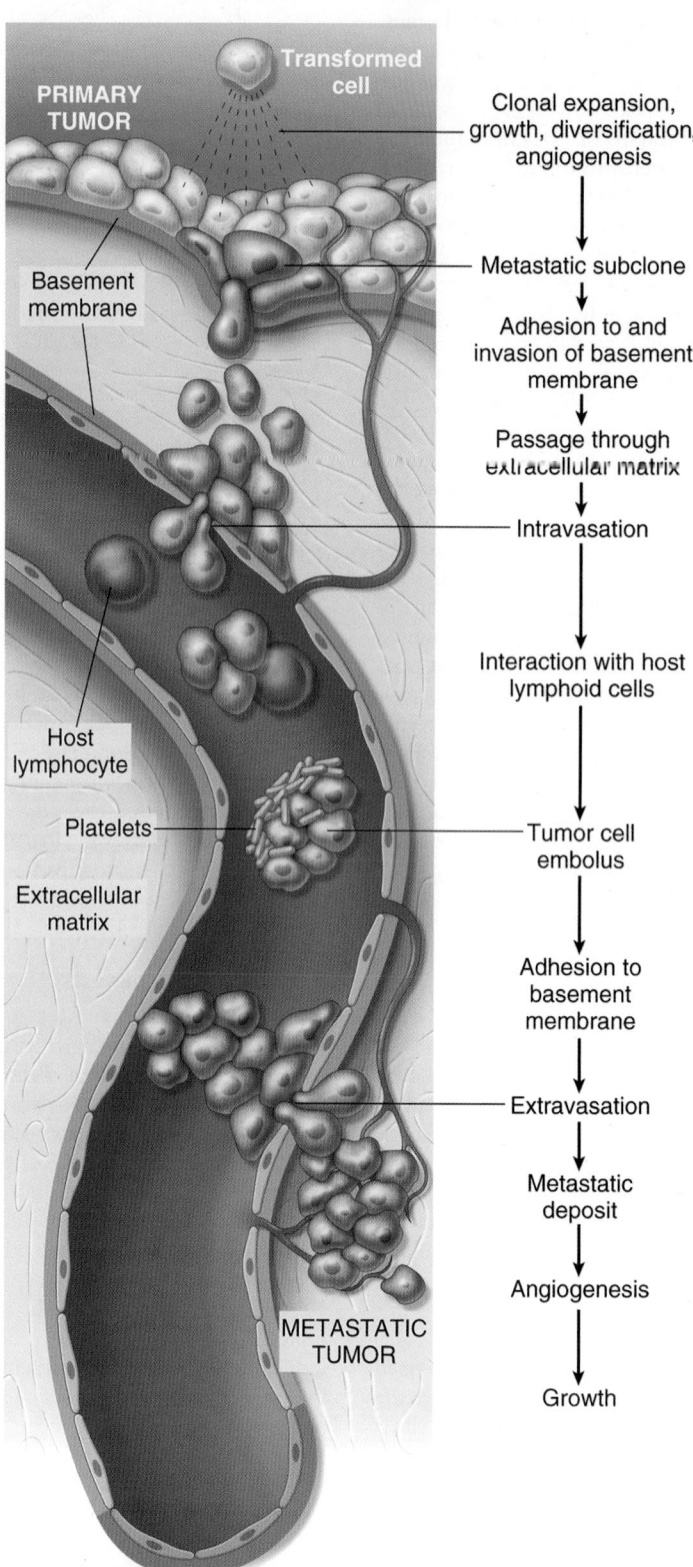

• **Fig. 4.9** The Metastatic Cascade. (Reprinted with permission from Kumar V, Abbas A, Aster J. *Robbins and Cotran Pathological Basis of Disease*. 10th ed. Elsevier; 2021: Figure 7.34.)

been known for some time that in certain tumors, the ability to invade and metastasize is an earlier event. This makes such tumors difficult to treat because the tumor is often no longer confined to the primary site of origin at the time of diagnosis.

Many, if not most, solid tumors routinely shed tumor cells into the circulation, and tumor-derived DNA can be detected in the patient's circulation (this forms the basis for the "liquid biopsy" which will be discussed in greater detail later in the chapter). The ability of tumor cells, however, to leave the circulation, invade, and grow to clinically significant sizes is inefficient, which limits the metastatic potential of circulating tumor cells. This may be due to destruction of the circulating tumor cells by the patient's immune cells (such as NK cells), or difficulty for the escaped tumor cells to adhere to vascular beds and invade normal distant tissues. Even if extravasation is successful, the tumor cells may not be able to grow in the secondary site due to lack of essential stromal support. The site at which metastases eventually develop is related to the anatomic location and vascular drainage of the primary tumor as well as the tropism of a particular tumor for specific tissues. Organ tropism describes the preference that many cancers have to establish a metastatic lesion in a particular tissue, for example, how prostate cancer preferentially metastasizes to adrenal gland, bone, liver, or lung.[3] In many cases, metastases occur in the first vascular bed available to the circulating tumor cells.

When cancers infiltrate tissues, they provoke a chronic inflammatory reaction. In patients with advanced cancers the inflammatory reaction can be extensive, causing a variety of systemic signs and symptoms. Patients may develop an anemia ("anemia of chronic disease" or "anemia of inflammatory disease"), fatigue, and cachexia. The inflammatory cells also modify the tumor microenvironment by: (1) releasing factors that promote proliferation; (2) removing growth suppressors; (3) enhancing resistance to cell death; (4) releasing factors that stimulate angiogenesis; (5) releasing proteases that promote tissue invasion and metastasis; and (6) facilitating the evasion of immune destruction.

Evasion of Immune Surveillance

It has been postulated for over a hundred years that tumor cells can be recognized as "foreign" and eliminated by the immune system (a process referred to as *immune surveillance*). This is based on the premise that one function of the immune system is to continuously scan the body for malignant cells and to destroy them. Supporting this is the recognition of both tumor-specific T-cells (NK cells) and antibodies in cancer patients. Also supporting this proposition is the observation of the increased incidence of certain cancers in immunodeficient people as well as the recent successful introduction of a variety of immunotherapies such as chimeric antigen receptor T-cell (CAR-T) therapy in the treatment of some cancers (see Chapter 5 for more on CAR-T).

Cancer cells express a variety of tumor-specific antigens that can potentially stimulate the host immune system. Despite this antigenicity, the patient's immune response to the tumor is often ineffective, possibly because cancer cells acquire the ability to evade anti-tumor responses. Since the immune system is capable of recognizing cancer cells, the lack of response must be due to the fact that either the tumor cells are invisible to the host immune system or the tumor produces factors that actively suppress the host's immunity. Some tumor cells acquire a mutation in antigen-presenting machinery (*APM*) genes that result in the inability for T-cells to react to the antigens presented to them.[4] If the tumor cell does not "present itself" to the T-lymphocytes, they will not be able to respond. Other tumors produce a variety

of proteins that inhibit cytotoxic T-lymphocyte (CTL) function. This latter process is believed to involve activating *immune checkpoints*, which are inhibitory pathways that maintain self-tolerance and control the size and duration of immune responses under normal circumstances. One example of this is the protein PD-L1 (programmed cell death ligand 1), which is often expressed on the surface of tumor cells. When PD-L1 binds to its receptor on CTL (PD-L1), it causes the CTL to become unresponsive and to lose its ability to kill tumor cells.

Altered Cellular Metabolism

Cancer cells typically demonstrate a distinctive form of cellular metabolism characterized by a high level of glucose uptake and increased conversion of glucose to lactose via the anaerobic glycolysis pathway (called the Warburg effect). The Warburg effect is not specific to tumor cells but is a general property of normal proliferative cells involved in immunity, angiogenesis, pluripotency, and infection by pathogens.[5] While anaerobic glycolysis is an inefficient process for producing ATP, it generates metabolic intermediates that are needed for the synthesis of cellular components (proteins, lipids, nucleic acids) needed by cells undergoing rapid proliferation. The recognition of this phenomenon has led to the development of an imaging modality that identifies disseminated malignancies utilizing fluorodeoxyglucose (a glucose analog) and positron emission tomography (PET) scanning.

The Molecular Basis of Cancer

Cancer is one of the most common genetic diseases, in that genetic mutations are required for the development of malignancy. These mutations can occur in either somatic tissues resulting in a sporadic cancer or can be inherited through the germ line, resulting in an increased risk of one or more cancers over the lifetime of the individual. Agents that cause DNA damage include chemicals, radiation, and viruses. This damaged DNA under normal circumstances is repaired or the cell with the damage is eliminated; however, some somatic mutations may permit propagation of the mutation or inherited mutations may affect the cell's ability to repair DNA or to undergo apoptosis, resulting in tumor formation. Researchers at the Wellcome Trust Sanger Institute determined that 1 to 10 mutations in so-called driver mutations (described below) are needed for cancer to develop.[6] As a mutated cell passes through the cell cycle and replicates, the clone can acquire additional mutations through development of genomic and/or chromosome instability. As the clone acquires additional mutations, it reaches a threshold when transformation occurs. This section describes the molecular mechanisms that underlie this process and describes how the identification of such mutations can guide medical management and inform choice of therapy. A flowchart to describe the molecular basis of cancer is provided in Figure 4.10.

Classification of Cancer Genes and Their Mutations

Oncogenes and Tumor Suppressor Genes

Proto-oncogenes are normal cellular genes that provide positive signals that lead to cell division and DNA transcription. Mutated proto-oncogenes are called oncogenes and are dominantly acting, meaning that only one mutation is needed for uncontrolled cell growth. Mutations in these genes are considered gain-of-function, in that the mutation confers new or enhanced activity to the protein

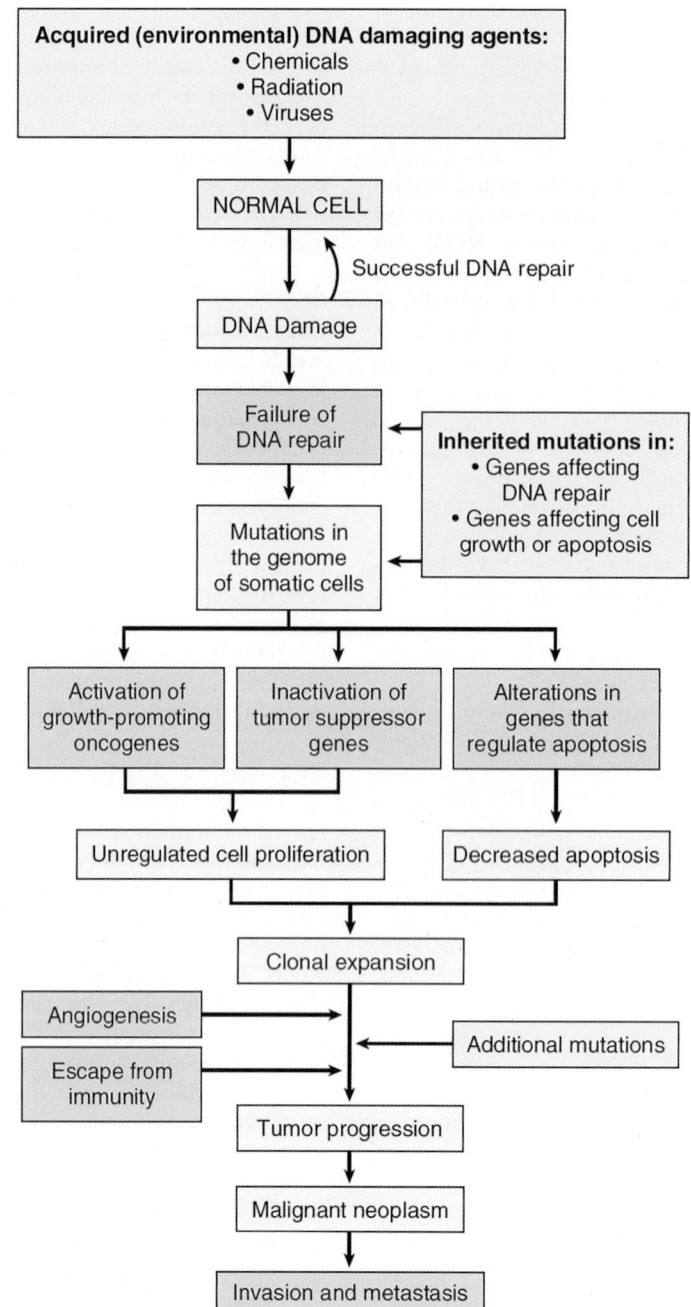

• **Fig. 4.10** Simplified Scheme of the Molecular Basis of Cancer. (Reprinted with permission from Kumar V, Abbas A, Fausto N, Aster J. *Robbins and Cotran Pathological Basis of Disease*. 8th ed. Saunders; 2010: Figure 7.25.)

because of continuous activation. Neoplastic transformation of oncogenes leads to: (1) increased production of secreted growth factors; (2) qualitative or quantitative abnormalities of growth factor receptors; (3) aberrant signal transduction; (4) dysregulated transcription factors causing activation of proliferation genes; (5) overproduction of factors which prevent apoptosis; and (6) dysregulation of cell cycle regulator proteins. Oncogenes are activated by chromosome translocation that relocates a gene to a new genomic location, gene amplification, mutation within the gene, or mutation in a region that controls expression of the gene. Examples of common oncogenes include *HER2/neu*, *RAS*, *MYC*, and *SRC*.

The *HER2 (Her2/neu or ERBB2)* gene encodes a receptor for human epidermal growth factor receptor type 2 which is found in normal cells and is involved in cell division. Extra copies of *HER2* are found in about 15% to 30% of breast cancers, with gene amplification driving protein receptor overexpression leading to proliferation and a more aggressive clinical course; however, therapy utilizing humanized monoclonal antibodies that target cells with HER2 overexpression (such as trastuzumab [Herceptin]) can be effective in preventing excessive cell proliferation. Such drugs can be used as a standalone treatment or in conjunction with other chemotherapeutic agents.[7]

Approximately 15% to 20% of all human tumors have *RAS* mutations (*KRAS, NRAS, HRAS*), with some tumors having much higher frequencies. *RAS* controls the transcription of different genes that are involved in kinase signaling pathways to regulate cell growth and differentiation. Binding of growth factor to its growth factor receptor activates inactive *RAS* which leads to subsequent activation of the second messenger system mitogen-activated protein (MAP)-kinase. This transduces the signal from the cell membrane to the nucleus to activate transcription and start cell cycle progression. Inactivation occurs through hydrolysis of guanosine triphosphate (GTP) to guanosine diphosphate (GDP) at a location on the inner cell membrane associated with the growth factor/growth factor receptor complex. Alterations in *RAS* protein by point mutation will result in the pathway being stuck in the "on" position, leading to continuous cell division and proliferation in the developing cancer.

The *SRC* protein belongs to the tyrosine kinase family. These proteins are involved in the phosphorylation/dephosphorylation processes which act as on/off switches for cell regulation. There are at least nine different *SRC* genes present in humans. *C-SRC* is normally found in low levels in cells; however, overexpression has been found in breast and other cancers.

The *MYC* proto-oncogene is a master transcriptional regulator of cell growth which is expressed in nearly all eukaryotic cells and plays an important role in many cellular processes including cell cycle progression, metabolism, and assembly of ribosomes for protein synthesis. Its deregulation in cancer occurs through a variety of mechanisms including gene amplification, transcriptional dysregulation through chromosome translocation, mutation within the *MYC* gene itself, or by epigenetic reprogramming. These lead to overexpression of the MYC protein, aberrant cellular signaling, and cellular transformation. *MYC* gene amplification is common in lung, breast, colon, and prostate tumors. In the common non-Hodgkin B-cell lymphoma called Burkitt lymphoma, a chromosome translocation involving the long arm of chromosomes 8 and 14 juxtaposes the *MYC* gene on chromosome 8 next to the constitutively active promoter of the *IGH* gene on chromosome 14, thus resulting in dysregulated overexpression of the MYC protein.

Tumor suppressor genes (TSGs) provide negative (inhibitory) signals that lead to the cessation of cell division and DNA transcription. TSGs are recessively acting, meaning that both copies of a TSG need to be mutated for initiation of the tumorigenic process. Mutations in these genes are considered loss-of-function, in that the mutation results in decreased production of a protein with impaired function. TSGs are involved in different cellular processes including regulation of transcription, restraining of cell division, DNA repair, apoptosis, and cellular communication. One useful functional classification of TSGs is either as a gatekeeper or as a caretaker of the genome. Gatekeeper genes such as *APC*, *RB*, and *NF1* directly regulate tumor growth by controlling cell cycling and cell death while caretaker genes such as *BRCA1* and *TP53* are involved in the maintenance of genome stability. Inactivation of both genes contributes directly to cancer development and progression. One general scheme for development of a tumor could be that mutation in one or a few caretaker genes occurs first, resulting in genomic instability and mutation in a gatekeeper gene. Mutation of additional gatekeepers with increasing genomic instability eventually leads to cancer initiation.

While a few oncogenes can be inherited in a mutated form, including MET (associated with hereditary papillary renal cell carcinoma) and RET (associated with increased risk for multiple endocrine neoplasia type 2), most familial cancer syndromes involve inherited mutations of TSGs. Mutations in important TSGs such as tumor protein 53 (*TP53*), breast cancer susceptibility genes 1 and 2 (*BRCA1 and BRCA2*), and *APC* result in common hereditary cancers including in breast and ovarian, prostate, and colon cancers. The TSG *TP53* codes for the p53 protein, which is an important growth inhibitory signal for tissue homeostasis, as it can activate temporary cell cycle arrest (quiescence), permanent cell cycle arrest (senescence), or can trigger apoptosis. With virtually every tumor type demonstrating a *TP53* gene mutation, and with its incidence in more than 50% of all human cancers, it is no wonder it is called the "Guardian of the Genome." The activities of *TP53* are regulated by many genes, with *p21* being one of the most important regulators involved in the cell cycle (Figure 4.11). The p21 protein is a negative regulator of cyclin dependent kinases responsible for cell cycle. Expression of p53 activates both *p21* resulting in arrest of the cell in G_1 and *GADD45* to start the process of DNA repair which involves many other genes. If successful, the cell completes its journey through the cell cycle; however, failure to repair DNA results in upregulation of pro-apoptotic genes including *BAX* and *PUMA*. Alteration of p53 can occur by mutations in the regulatory or protein coding regions of the gene, a decrease in transcriptional activity, or destabilization of p53 protein which is easily degradable. If *TP53* is mutated, then the cell cannot repair DNA damage resulting in propagation and expansion of a mutant clone along with the acquisition of additional mutations leading to formation of a malignancy.

To further demonstrate the role of p53 in cancer suppression, Abegglen and colleagues demonstrated that African elephants have at least 20 copies of the *TP53* gene (compared with one copy/two alleles in humans). As elephants mount an increased apoptotic response following DNA damage compared to humans, the authors speculated that the elephant's relative cancer resistance might be related to their increased ability to repair DNA damage because of multiple copies of *TP53*.[8]

Genomic evaluation of the p53 gene has diagnostic and prognostic significance. *TP53* mutations are associated with a poorer prognosis while nonmutated p53 in some cancers leads to a more favorable outcome, as tumor cells with nonmutated *TP53* are more sensitive to the effects of chemotherapy and radiation. Luckily, given the incidence of *TP53* mutation in cancer, recent evidence suggests that certain mutations may serve as antigens in cancer immunotherapy with some success.[9] Considering the role p53 plays in normal cellular function, it is no wonder that an inherited mutation in *TP53* can have devastating consequences. Such a mutation results in Li-Fraumeni syndrome, an inherited cancer predisposition syndrome resulting in a wide range of cancers including, but not limited to, cancers of the bone, blood (leukemia), breast, brain, stomach, colon, and pancreas.

The retinoblastoma (*RB*) tumor suppressor gene encodes a protein which normally acts as a negative growth inhibitor of the cell cycle. It inhibits transcription of genes that encode proteins necessary for DNA synthesis when the cell is in S phase. When activated by growth factors, the Rb protein allows for transcription of S phase genes needed by the cell to pass through the G_1/S cell cycle checkpoint. The antiproliferative effect of Rb is inhibited by *RB* gene mutation itself or by dysregulation of other important cell cycle regulators that interact with Rb.

Recent studies have revealed additional functions for *RB* including regulation of inflammation, mitochondria and metabolism, autophagy (the process of cells degrading unnecessary or damaged components to maintain cellular homeostasis), apoptosis, and

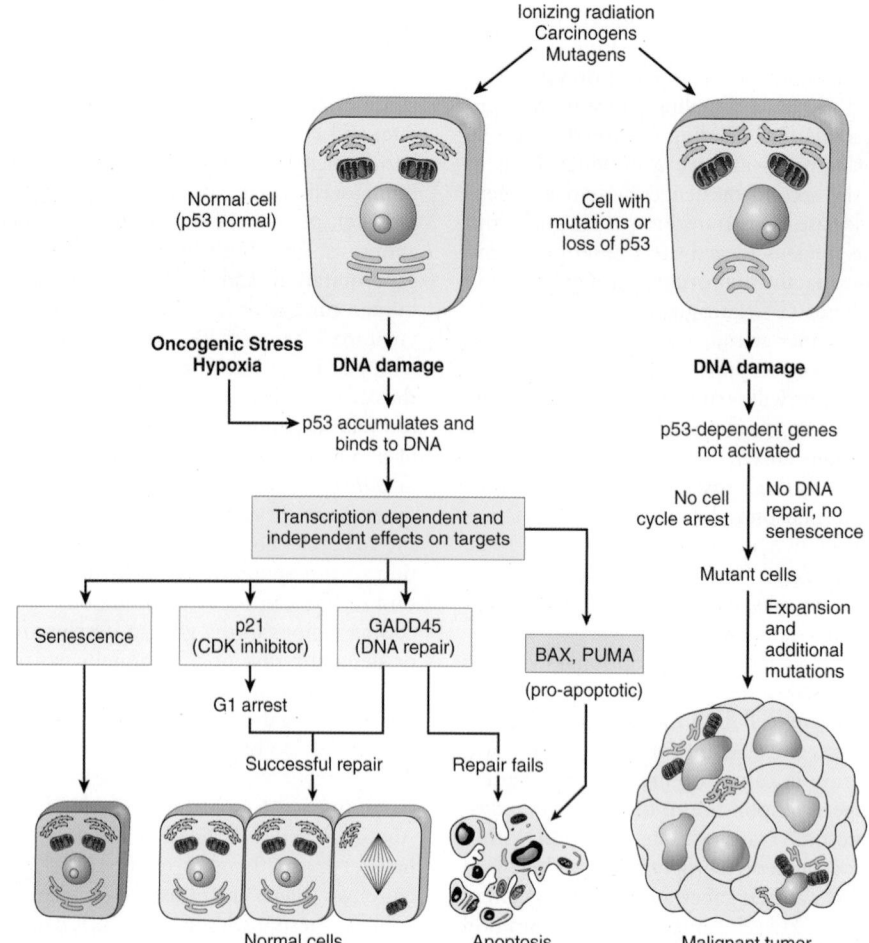

• **Fig. 4.11** Role of the *TP53* Gene in Maintaining the Integrity of the Human Genome. *CDK,* Cyclin-dependent kinases. (Reprinted with permission from Kumar V, Abbas A, Aster J. *Robbins and Cotran Pathological Basis of Disease.* 10th ed. Elsevier; 2021: Figure 7.27.)

stemness (the process in stem cells of self-renewal and generation of differentiated daughter cells).[10]

An inherited *RB* mutation results in an increased risk for development of a childhood retinal tumor called retinoblastoma and for other tumors later in life including osteosarcoma. The paradigm of Knudson's Two-Hit hypothesis is demonstrated in the pathogenesis of retinoblastoma, a scheme which applies to virtually all tumor suppressor genes and inherited cancer syndromes.[11] Inheritance of an *RB* mutation is the "first-hit" which is present in every cell in the body. In this case, only loss of the other *RB* allele ("second-hit") in any cell is needed for malignant transformation (a statistically more probable event). For this reason, inherited *RB* mutations are often associated with earlier age of onset, bilateral tumors, and increased incidence of certain sarcomas later in life. The reason why children with an inherited RB mutation initially develop retinoblastoma and no other tumors is unknown. Sporadic retinoblastoma is also observed, but in this case both "hits" must occur in the same cell (a statistically less probable event without an inherited *RB* mutation). In this case, unilateral tumors are far more common and there is no substantially increased risk for developing other malignancies (Figure 4.12). Such a scheme applies to virtually all tumor suppressor genes and their role in inherited versus sporadic cancer.

Mutations in the tumor suppressor genes *BRCA1* and *BRCA2* result in increased risk for development of several cancers. Recent studies demonstrate that 55% to 65% of *BRCA1* mutation carriers (those with an inherited mutation) and 45% of *BRCA2* mutation carriers will develop breast cancer by age 70. Mutations in *BRCA1* and *BRCA2* are found in 20% of familial breast and ovarian cancers. Specific germline mutations in these genes are also associated with an increased risk for prostate, colorectal, stomach, pancreatic, and other cancers. More than 1600 mutations have been documented in *BRCA1* while over 1800 mutations have been found in *BRCA2*, some occurring in high frequency in isolated groups such as Ashkenazi Jews (so called founder mutations).[12]

The main role for *BRCA1* and *BRCA2* is in maintaining genome integrity through the process of DNA repair. Loss of function of these genes results in genomic instability and the transformation of normal cells into cancer-initiating cells. Genomic instability drives the tumorigenic process and is critical for tumor evolution. Other roles for these genes more recently elucidated include transcriptional regulation, regulation of cell cycle progression, autophagy, chromatin remodeling and epigenetic regulation of gene expression (described later), and cancer stem cell development and evolution.[12]

Clues that should raise concern for the potential of an inherited *BRCA1* or *BRCA2* mutation include a diagnosis of breast or ovarian cancer before age 50, bilateral tumors, presence of breast and ovarian cancer in the same women or within the same pedigree, and family history of *BRCA1-* or *BRCA2-*associated tumors

PATHOGENESIS OF RETINOBLASTOMA

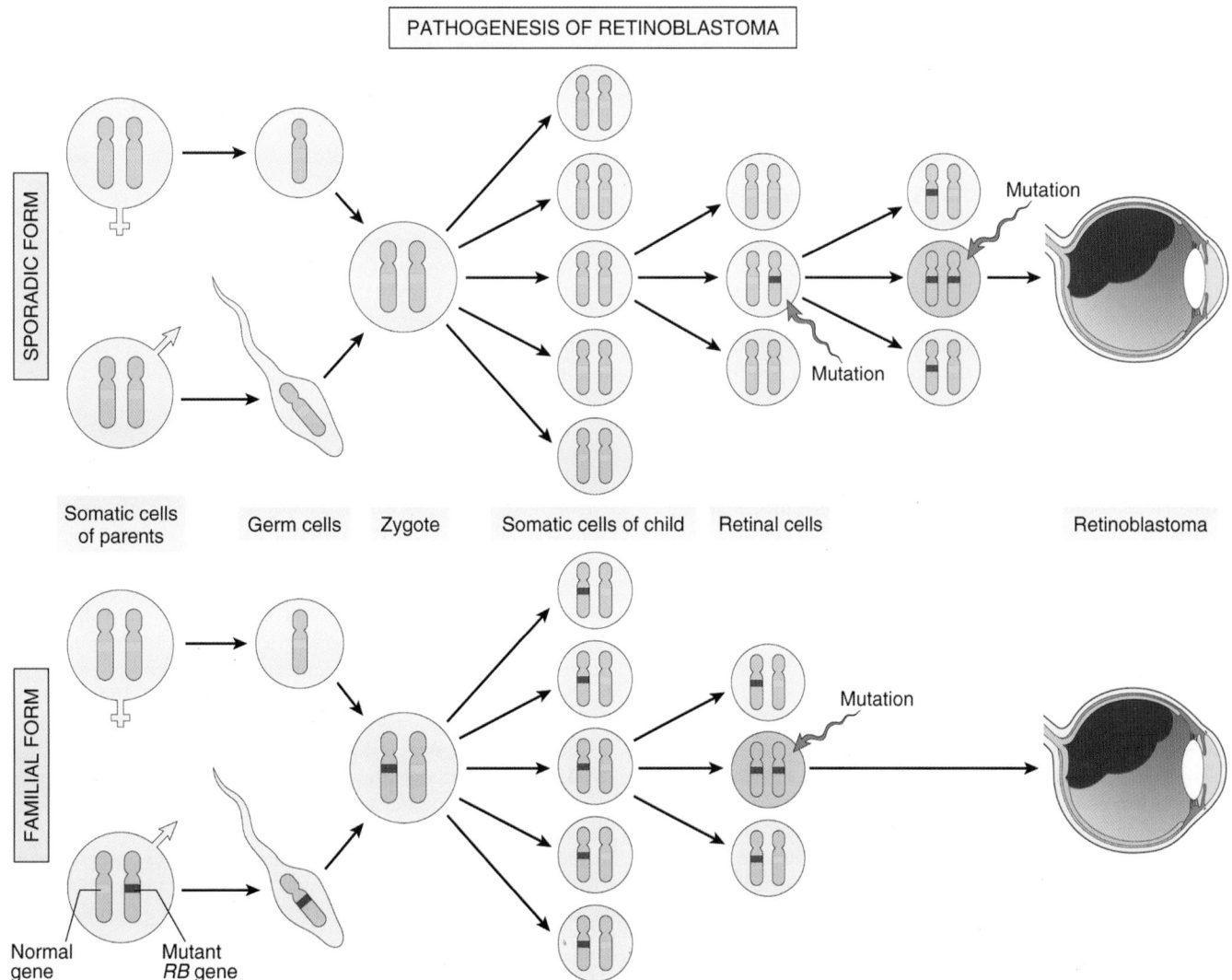

SPORADIC FORM

FAMILIAL FORM

Somatic cells of parents   Germ cells   Zygote   Somatic cells of child   Retinal cells   Retinoblastoma

Mutation

Mutation

Mutation

Normal gene

Mutant *RB* gene

• **Fig. 4.12** Pathogenesis of Retinoblastoma Demonstrating Knudson's Two-Hit Hypothesis. This Scheme Applies to Virtually All Tumor Suppressor Genes and Explains the Genesis of Sporadic Versus Familial Forms of Cancer. (Reprinted with permission from Kumar V, Abbas A, Aster J. *Robbins and Cotran Pathological Basis of Disease*. 10th ed. Elsevier; 2021: Figure 7.25.)

especially in first- or second-degree relatives. While *BRCA1* and *BRCA2* mutations are often associated with tumor aggressiveness and poor response to cancer treatment in most tumors, the results are more conflicting for breast cancer. *BRCA1* carriers are more likely to develop triple negative breast cancer (TNBC), in which there is a lack of expression of HER-2, estrogen receptors, and progesterone receptors. Such tumors do not respond to conventional treatments such as hormone therapy or drugs that target HER-2, estrogen, and progesterone receptors; however, cancer immunotherapy has been shown to be effective in both early and advanced TNBC. PARP (poly [ADP-ribose] polymerase) inhibitor drugs have shown promise in treating *BRCA*-mutated breast and ovarian cancer. PARP is an important enzyme responsible for repairing DNA damage. PARP inhibitors block the repair of DNA damage in *BRCA*-mutated cells leading to their death. The Food and Drug Administration (FDA) approved PARP inhibitors include olaparib (Lynparza) and rucaparib (Rubraca).[12]

The adenomatous polyposis coli (*APC*) gene is considered the gatekeeper of colonic neoplasia. Germline (inherited) *APC* mutations are identified in familial adenomatous polyposis, a syndrome whereby a carrier develops hundreds or thousands of adenomatous polyps in their colon during their second and third decades of life, resulting in a very high risk of colon cancer. In addition to hereditary forms of colon cancer, 70% to 80% of nonfamilial (sporadic) colon tumors also demonstrate *APC* mutations. *APC* is a component of the wingless-related integration site (WNT) signaling pathway which plays a major role during embryonic development by controlling cell growth and differentiation.

Driver and Passenger Mutations in Cancer Genes

In addition to classifying cancer genes by their function and genetic mechanism of action (gain or loss of function), it is also instructive to classify the mutations within those genes to develop a more thorough understanding of the tumorigenic process. Mutations within cancer genes can be classified as either driver or passenger mutations. Driver mutations confer a growth advantage to a cell through the alteration of fundamental cellular processes. These mutations are essential for tumor growth and comprise the smallest number of total mutations in any tumor. Different tumor types have different and characteristic sets of driver mutations which can serve as important targets for cancer therapies (see below). Passenger mutations are not essential for tumor growth and survival. These mutations, which number the largest in any tumor, occur over the course of a lifetime of exposure to mutagens or during the deregulated mitoses of malignant transformation.

Other Important Factors in Tumorigenesis— Epigenetics and Noncoding RNAs

The critical role of the epigenome in gene expression during fetal development, to maintain cellular homeostasis, and in the development of cancer is becoming increasingly appreciated. The epigenome refers to heritable factors that control gene expression without a change in DNA sequence. These factors primarily represent methylation of DNA that serves to turn genes "on" and "off." This is a common cellular process, as not every one of our 26,425 genes (as of May 20, 2022[13]) is active all the time. Genes are turned on and off throughout our lifetime as their protein products are needed. An example is alpha-fetoprotein (AFP) encoded by the *AFP* gene. AFP is a major plasma protein produced by the yolk sac and the liver during fetal life but is not usually found in adults. AFP expression in adults is often associated with hepatocarcinoma and teratoma and has prognostic value for managing advanced gastric cancer; however, hereditary persistence of AFP may also be found in individuals with no obvious pathology.

Epigenetic alterations can include DNA methylation, histone modification, noncoding RNAs, and changes in chromatin composition and/or organization. While epigenetics refers to what is happening in a single gene, epigenomics is the study of what is happening across the entire genome. The pattern of DNA "marking" across the genome is influenced by lifestyle and environmental factors. The initial discovery that the cytosine base in DNA can be methylated to become 5-methylcytosine (5mC) was important to understanding how DNA methylation contributes to the tumorigenic process. Much research over the last 40 years has elucidated genomic methylation patterns that can distinguish cancer cells from normal cells. The most prominent and earliest recognized change in DNA methylation patterns in cancer cells was regional decreases in DNA methylation, now recognized as global DNA hypomethylation. However, abnormal hypermethylation of cytosine-phosphate-guanine (CpG) islands found in or near the transcription site of cancer-related genes is also a common finding in tumor genomes. This change is associated with transcriptional silencing. Thus, dysregulated hypermethylation (turning off) of tumor suppressor genes results in their silencing while aberrant hypomethylation (turning on) of proto-oncogenes can lead to their inappropriate expression, both resulting in cancer initiation.[14]

Lifestyle behaviors such as smoking, ultraviolet light exposure, and alcohol consumption, along with diet can cause oxidative stress which can lead to epigenome modification. This pattern of epigenetic modification can be inherited, so the lifestyle of the mother can have profound influences on her developing fetus. It is well documented that folic acid, vitamins B_6 and B_{12}, and polyphenols found in vegetables and green tea can modulate DNA methylation and may aid in cancer prevention. Nasir and colleagues published a review of *nutrigenomics*, a new discipline that explores how diet influences the genome and epigenome in health and disease, and how diet modification can aid in cancer prevention.[15] While omega 3 fatty acids are the best example of nutrients and gene interaction not involving DNA methylation,

certain bioactive food compounds have a proven role in cancer prevention through an epigenetic mechanism. There is substantial evidence that zinc, selenium, and folate have anticancer properties.[16] Dietary polyphenols can help prevent many types of cancers including oral, breast, skin, esophageal, colorectal, prostate, pancreatic, and lung cancers. Physical activity and exercise have also been shown to modulate gene expression through changes in the epigenome. Grazioli and colleagues reviewed studies that demonstrated the effects of physical activity and exercise in modifying gene expression. Their review identified the positive results of exercise in inhibiting tumor progression by lowering DNA methylation of tumor suppressor genes. They also described research that revealed how brief, intense exercise significantly altered gene expression in 986 genes and 23 micro RNAs (miRNAs) associated with cancer.[17]

Micro RNAs are noncoding RNAs that post-transcriptionally regulate genes involved in critical cellular processes. As such, their up- or down-regulation influences protein expression of many genes with different functions. In cancer, aberrant up-or down-regulation of miRNAs result in dysregulation of signaling pathways involved in cell proliferation, apoptosis and survival, metastasis, cancer recurrence, and chemoresistance. For example, deletion of miRNAs miR-15 and miR-16 are found in chronic lymphocytic leukemia, a common leukemia in older adults. Loss of these miRNAs results in upregulation of the anti-apoptotic gene *BCL2*. Conversely, overexpression of miR-155 found in many B-cell lymphomas indirectly upregulates many proliferation genes, including *MYC*. Researchers are evaluating whether miR-NAs can be used as biomarkers to detect cancer at an early stage or can identify drug resistance during therapy, as abnormal levels of miRNA expression have been linked to drug insensitivity in cancer. In addition, the role of miRNAs in tumorigenesis makes them attractive targets for therapy. Current strategies in miRNA therapeutics include either inhibiting or replacing miRNAs.[18]

The Multistep Nature of Carcinogenesis

Nearly 30 years ago, Burt Vogelstein and his colleagues at Johns Hopkins University introduced the concept of the multistep nature of carcinogenesis.[19] The concept was that cancer is a genetic disease that requires several mutations to develop a malignancy. While cancer is clonal, in that one mutation in one gene in one cell can begin the process of transformation, additional genes are required for a tumor to form. Each mutation serves to destabilize the genome a little more which increases the risk of additional mutations, a process described by Vogelstein and Kinzler as a "wave of cellular multiplication" which can take many years to complete. Along the way the tumor gradually increases in size, cellular disorganization, and malignancy. They theorized that at least three to six such mutations appear to be required to complete this process. They used colon cancer as a model, describing how an APC mutation transforms the colonic epithelium into a "mucosa at risk," followed by acquisition of additional mutations that histologically and functionally transform the colonic mucosa in a morphologically identifiable sequence ending with carcinoma (Figure 4.13).

While this scheme may not apply to every subset of colon adenocarcinoma, some variation of it can be observed in most colon tumors. Since its description, genomic/histological progression schemes have been elucidated for many malignancies. A more generalized scheme applicable to all cancers illustrating the development of cancer through a series of complementary driver and

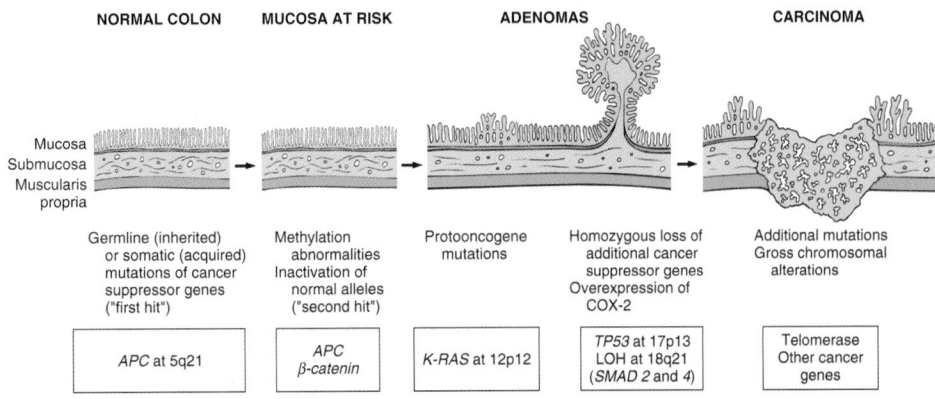

• **Fig. 4.13** Morphologic and Molecular Changes in Adeno-Carcinoma Sequence. (Reprinted with permission from Kumar V, Abbas A, Aster J. *Robbins and Cotran Pathological Basis of Disease*. 10th ed. Elsevier; 2021: Figure 17.49.)

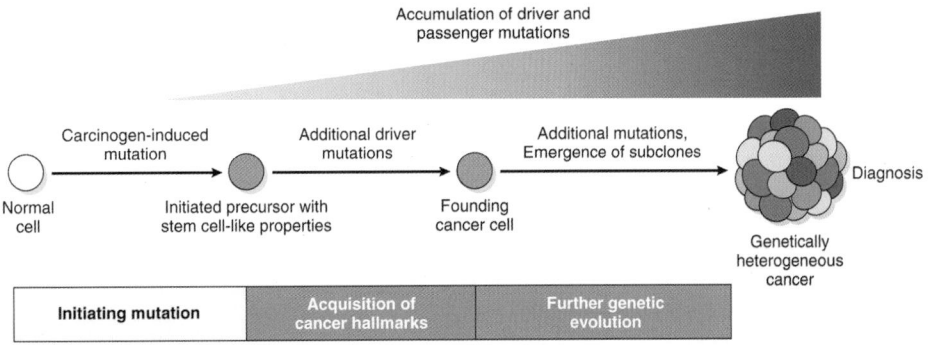

• **Fig. 4.14** Development of Cancer Through Stepwise Acquisition of Complementary Mutations. (Reprinted with permission from Kumar V, Abbas A, Aster J. *Robbins and Cotran Pathological Basis of Disease*. 10th ed. Elsevier; 2021: Figure 7.19.)

passenger mutations is given in Figure 4.14. Different malignancies are associated quantitatively with different numbers of driver and passenger mutations, with leukemias demonstrating the fewest number of passenger mutations compared with driver mutations, brain tumors revealing a mixture of driver and passenger mutations, and solid tumors showing the greatest number of passenger mutations, possibly because the heterogenous environment inherent in a solid tumor dictates that it become very genetically diverse for survival.

The Reality of Precision Cancer Medicine

With the development of sophisticated molecular genetic techniques such as next-generation sequencing (NGS) that can interrogate the genomes of individual cancers and populations of patients with the same malignancy, new diagnostic tools and therapeutic interventions are changing the course and prognosis, and even providing a cure, for some cancer patients. Precision cancer medicine describes the utilization of molecular biomarkers to prevent, diagnose, and treat cancer. Using massively-parallel sequencing techniques (collectively known as NGS), enormous amounts of tumor DNA sequence data can now be acquired in a relatively short period of time and at a reasonable cost for the purpose of informing the use of novel therapies that target only those cells with specific mutations (cancer cells), thereby sparing normal cells which are too often collaterally damaged when traditional cytotoxic chemotherapeutic agents are used, leading to

significant morbidity. It is believed that in the near future, a multidimensional approach utilizing tumor DNA and RNA sequencing (to identify the tumor's gene expression profile), along with epigenetic and proteomic (the sum total of proteins expressed by the tumor) analysis, will provide a real opportunity to identify specific cellular targets for small molecule drugs and monoclonal antibodies that may lead to either a complete cure for many cancers, or at least make many cancers chronic diseases without significantly reduced lifespan. The first molecularly targeted therapy drug that gained FDA-approval in 2001 is called imatinib mesylate (Gleevec) used to treat chronic myelogenous leukemia. Since then many other signal-transduction inhibitors such as gefitinib (Iressa) and erlotinib (Tarceva) and proteasome inhibitors such as bortezomib (Velcade) have come on the market and changed the disease course for many cancer patients. Monoclonal antibodies bind specific antigens on cancer cells, providing another mechanism for targeted therapy. Such drugs include rituximab (Rituxan) which targets B-lymphocyte-restricted antigen CD20, trastuzamab (Herceptin) which targets breast cancer cells overexpressing HER2, and pembrolizumab (Keytruda) which targets nonsmall cell lung carcinoma cells that express programmed-death ligand 1 (PD-L1).[20] The most comprehensive targeted NGS panel, called TruSight Oncology 500 from Illumina (San Diego, CA) analyzes 523 cancer genes to interrogate for pathogenic mutations that can guide the appropriate choice of therapy and/or inform prognosis. This test is used routinely today in many large academic medical centers to guide treatment. In addition to diagnostic assays, predictive assays are also important tools the oncologist can utilize to choose the best cancer treatments. Common molecular assays of this type include Oncotype DX and MammaPrint that establish the relative risk/benefit of adjuvant chemotherapy in women with early-stage breast cancer.

Another milestone in the development of precision cancer medicine was the identification of circulating tumor cells (CTCs) in peripheral blood, first described by Thomas Ashworth in 1869,[21] along with the ability to genomically analyze circulating tumor DNA (ctDNA). CTCs are intact cells which have broken off from a primary tumor and entered the bloodstream, while ctDNA is fragmented cell-free DNA also found in blood that was released from a primary tumor following tumor cell apoptosis or necrosis. The ability to perform serial mutational or protein-based molecular profiling not only at diagnosis (to develop a baseline and identify potential predictive biomarkers), but also during treatment (as a means of monitoring treatment efficacy), at tumor progression, and after treatment, all from a routine noninvasive blood specimen provides a real-time assessment of the tumor and its evolving biology. The early identification of CTCs is also a powerful method for early detection of malignancy in otherwise healthy people long before they would have otherwise been diagnosed with cancer.

With continued advances in genomic and proteomic cancer profiling along with the exponential development of targeted therapies, it is interesting to consider whether the most important part of the diagnostic work-up of a malignancy might be the identification of targetable mutations instead of histopathological and immunohistochemical characterization. For some biopsies with equivocal histology, much time and effort are needed to confirm the cell of origin of the tumor, including batteries of immunohistochemical stains and both internal and external consultations with pathology subspecialists. At times, all this effort provides only a "best guess" diagnosis, and possibly even worse, the dreaded diagnosis of "carcinoma of unknown origin" which has limited treatment options. With continued advances in genomic and proteomic profiling, tumor-specific patterns might be elucidated that could revolutionize cancer pathology evaluation. In addition, serial sequencing of primary and metastatic tumors in a patient can provide real-time data leading to informed treatment alterations. In terms of therapy, identifying drug-able targets in a tumor may be more important than determining its origin (e.g., lung, breast, prostate) (Figure 4.15).

On the other hand, while we know that very different tumor types may share similar driver mutations and molecular mechanisms, and thus may be potentially treated with the same drug or class of drugs, in practice variability in response does exist. For example, it is known that diverse tumors such as melanoma, colon adenocarcinoma, papillary thyroid cancer, hairy cell leukemia, and Langerhans cell histiocytosis all have a gain-of-function mutation in the *BRAF* gene, a component of the RAS signaling pathway. As such, utilization of BRAF inhibitors could theoretically be used to treat all these malignancies. In practice, however, these cancers all respond differently and with variable efficacy to BRAF inhibitors. So, while advanced genomic analysis of tumors promises to make pathological diagnosis much more accurate and informative, there will still be a place for traditional histopathologic analysis in the diagnostic work-up of a malignancy in the near future, albeit with the decreased necessity to perform ancillary testing. The knowledge gained from the tools of precision cancer diagnostics have already changed the role of the pathologist, and their role in the care of the cancer patient will need to evolve as new diagnostic tools come on-line. While a cure for all cancers may still not be on

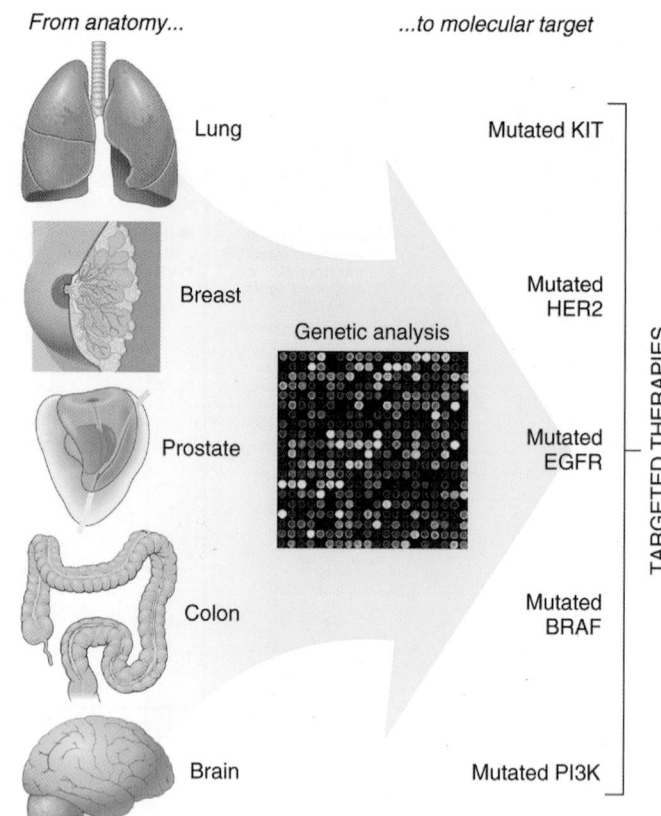

From anatomy...   ...to molecular target

Lung   Mutated KIT

Breast

Genetic analysis   Mutated HER2

Prostate   Mutated EGFR

Colon   Mutated BRAF

Brain   Mutated PI3K

TARGETED THERAPIES

• **Fig. 4.15** A Paradigm Shift: Classification of Cancer According to Therapeutic Targets Rather Than Cell of Origin and Morphology. (Reprinted with permission from Kumar V, Abbas A, Aster J. *Robbins and Cotran Pathological Basis of Disease.* 10th ed. Elsevier; 2021: Figure 7.47.)

the horizon, the significant advances described here provide great hope for many cancer patients to "beat" their disease, or at least be "long-term" survivors.

Diagnostic Imaging

The medical radiation sciences play an important part in the diagnosis, prognosis, and treatment of cancer. The term radiation sciences is a broad term used to describe many different types of diagnostic testing which may include ionizing or nonionizing radiation. Ionizing radiation can be damaging to human tissue, while nonionizing radiation is not. Other terms used synonymously to describe the medical radiation sciences are imaging sciences, diagnostic radiology, or radiologic technology.

Most cancer patients undergo multiple diagnostic exams ordered to confirm diagnosis and staging, and they may continue undergoing some of these tests while they are receiving treatment to determine if the treatment is efficacious (Table 4.4). Following treatment, patients may be required to have testing at certain time increments to look for signs that a cancer has returned, or to discover if it has spread to another location in the body. Discovering if the cancer has spread to other parts of the body is an important part of determining the stage of the cancer. Hematologic cancers such as leukemia do not often include imaging exams to visualize the leukemia itself, but physicians may still order exams to check for other abnormalities within the organs of the body (Figure 4.16).

Imaging also plays an important role during the biopsies of many types of tumors. Physicians perform biopsies under the

TABLE 4.4	Commonly Performed Radiographic Exams for Diagnosing Cancers
Cancer	**Common Radiographic Exams**
Adrenal	CT, MRI
Bladder	IVU, CT urogram
Bone	X-rays, CT, MRI, PET
Brain	MRI, CT/CTA, PET
Breast	Mammography, sonography, MRI
Colorectal	CT, endorectal MRI
Endometrial, Ovarian, Uterine	Sonography
Esophageal	Barium swallow/UGI radiography, CT
Gallbladder	Sonography, CT, MRI, cholangiogram
Kidney	CT, sonography
Liver	Sonography, CT, MRI
Lung	Chest X-ray, CT
Lymphoma	Chest X-ray, CT
Neuroblastoma, Wilms Tumor	Sonography, MRI, CT
Pancreatic	CT, MRI, sonography (EUS)
Prostate	Sonography, MRI
Stomach	UGI radiography, CT
Testicular	Sonography
Thyroid	Sonography, radioiodine scan (nuclear medicine)

CT, Computed tomography; *CTA,* computed tomography angiography; *EUS,* endoscopic ultrasound; *IVU,* intravenous urogram; *MRI,* magnetic resonance imaging; *PET,* positron emission tomography; *UGI,* upper gastrointestinal.
American Cancer Society. Find a Cancer Type. https://www.cancer.org/cancer/all-cancer-types.html. Accessed May 22, 2021.

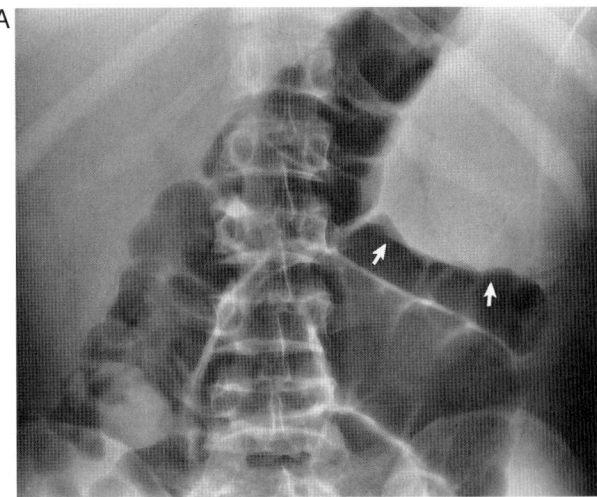

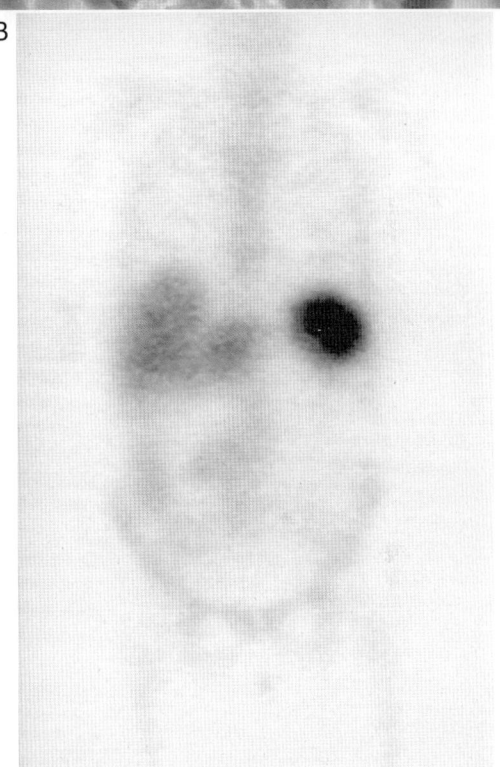

• **Fig. 4.16** Chronic Leukemia. (A) Massive Splenomegaly Has Caused Downward Displacement of the Colonic Splenic Flexure on This Upper Abdomen Image. *Arrows* Point to the Inferior Margin of the Spleen. (B) A Whole-Body Scan Where Indium Has Been Tagged to White Blood Cells, Showing a Grossly Enlarged Spleen on Images Taken 27 Hours After Injection. (Reprinted with permission from Eisenberg R, Johnson N. *Comprehensive Radiographic Pathology*. 7th ed. Mosby; 2020: Figure 9-13A. X-Ray; and Figure 9-13B. Body Scan.)

guidance of various imaging modalities such as sonography, computed tomography (CT), magnetic resonance imaging (MRI), or fluoroscopy. These various imaging techniques are used to help visualize the biopsy needles during the procedure (Figure 4.17). This also helps to avoid damaging other organs that may be near the tumor during the biopsy procedure.

These images and diagnostic tests are ordered by general practitioners or specialists through a prescription, and the exams are then performed by radiologic technologists. A radiologic technologist can be educated and certified in multiple areas within radiology, or they may choose to specialize and work in just one modality. The images are then interpreted by a radiologist, which is a doctor who completes their internship and residency in radiology. Radiologists can also complete fellowships and choose to specialize in one area of radiology. Many biopsies are performed by radiologists, with the assistance of radiologic technologists who perform the imaging during the procedure.

General Radiography (X-Ray) and Fluoroscopy

General radiography, more commonly described as X-ray, involves creating a radiograph using ionizing radiation. Tissues within the body show up on X-rays as shades of white, black, and gray with the color depending on the type of tissue and the X-ray's ability to penetrate it. Bone is very dense, making it difficult to penetrate, so

it appears on the X-ray as white; while air in the lungs and intestines shows as black. Other tissues, organs, fat, and muscles appear as different shades of gray. These X-rays, or radiographs, are most often visualized and stored digitally, as opposed to an older method of acquiring and storing which required a special radiographic film. X-rays were discovered in 1895, and the rapid advancement in technology and computers have greatly improved the quality of the imaging available today. Some of the advantages of general radiography over other imaging modalities are that they can be acquired fast, use low doses of radiation, are less expensive, and are not invasive.

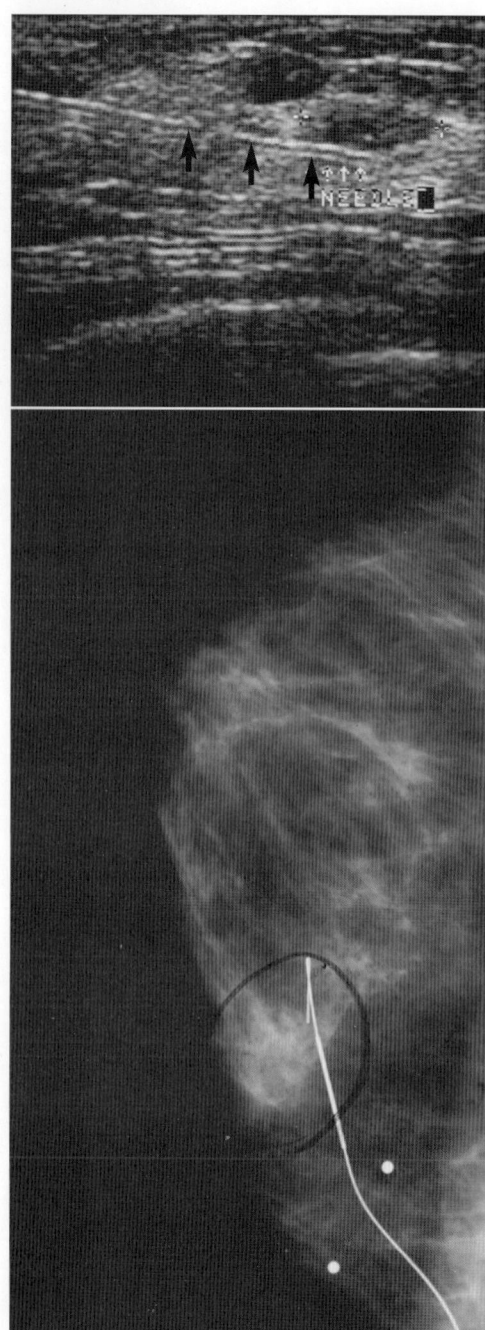

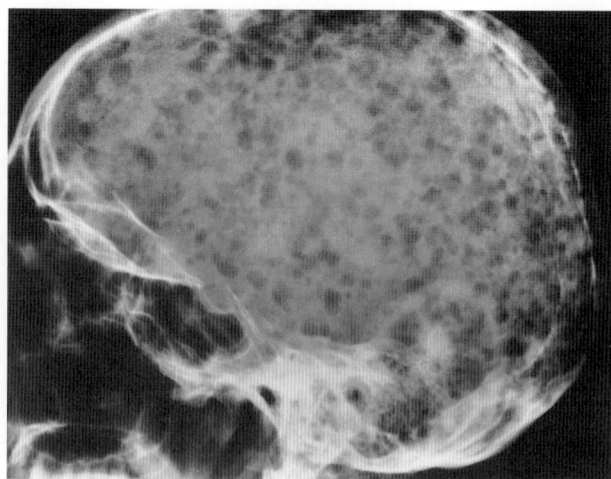

• **Fig. 4.18** Multiple Myeloma Diffuse Punched-Out Osteolytic Lesions Scattered Throughout the Skull. (Reprinted with permission from Eisenberg R, Johnson N. *Comprehensive Radiographic Pathology*. 7th ed. Mosby; 2020: Figure 4-77. Multiple Myeloma.)

• **Fig. 4.17** Ultrasound-Guided Localization. (A) Ultrasound Needle Localization for Surgical Biopsy of the Breast. *Black Arrows* Identify a White Line Indicating the Needle Location. (B) Mammography Image Verifying Needle Localization. (Reprinted with permission from Eisenberg R, Johnson N. *Comprehensive Radiographic Pathology*. 7th ed. Mosby; 2020: Figure 2-6. Ultrasound Guided Breast Biopsy.)

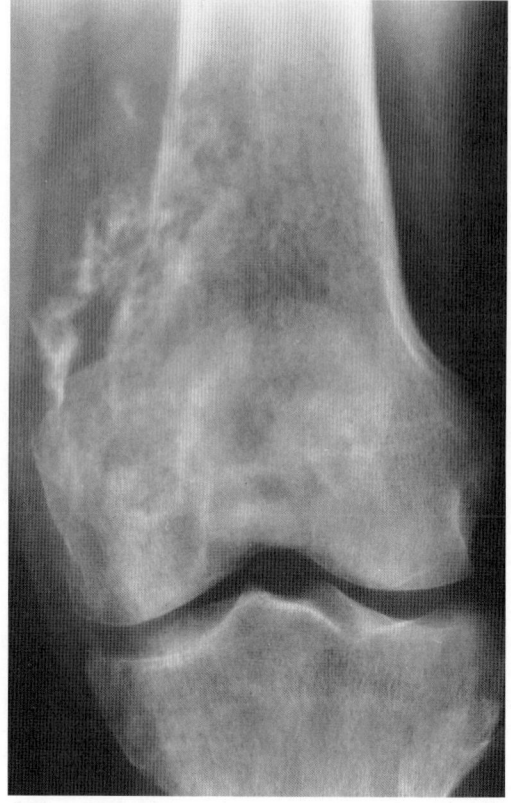

• **Fig. 4.19** Osteogenic Sarcoma (A) A Predominantly Destructive Lesion with an Irregular Periosteal Reaction. (Reprinted with permission from Eisenberg R, Johnson N. *Comprehensive Radiographic Pathology*. 7th ed. Mosby; 2020: Figure 4-73A. Osteogenic Sarcoma.)

The largest disadvantage is that they are limited in what they visualize because of superimposing structures, inability to differentiate small differences in density, and inability to penetrate bone.

General X-rays can be ordered for any part of the body. A practitioner may order X-rays of a patient when they are experiencing pain in a certain area, or for patients who have a known primary cancer—when a PET scan has already revealed an area of concern to examine the presence or extent of metastasis. Skeletal

X-rays may show various bone cancers, which can include multiple myeloma (Figure 4.18), osteogenic sarcoma (Figure 4.19), Ewing sarcoma (Figure 4.20), and chondrosarcoma (Figure 4.21). Cancer of the bone may appear as radiodense (bright) spots or radiolucent (dark) spots on a radiographic image. The appearance and size will depend on the type and stage of the tumor. When a patient has a known cancer that is suspected to have spread to

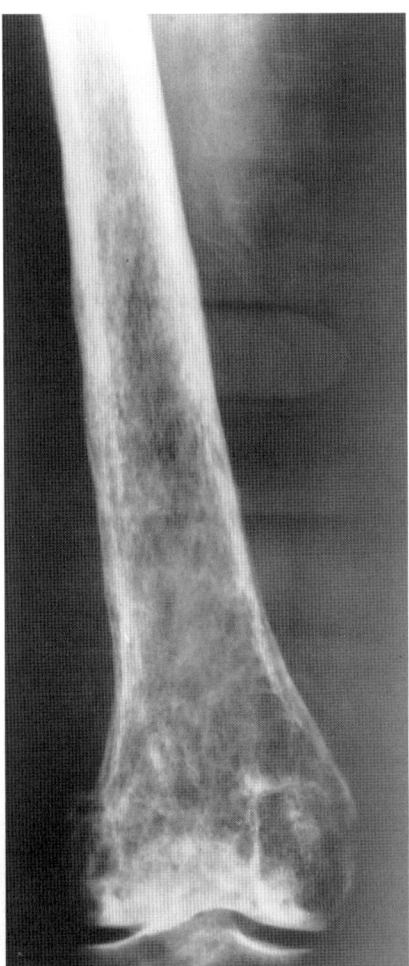

• **Fig. 4.20** Ewing Sarcoma Diffuse Permeative Destruction With a Mild Periosteal Response Involving the Distal Half of the Femur. (Reprinted with permission from Eisenberg R, Johnson N. Comprehensive Radiographic Pathology. 7th ed. Mosby; 2020: Figure 4-76. Ewing Sarcoma.)

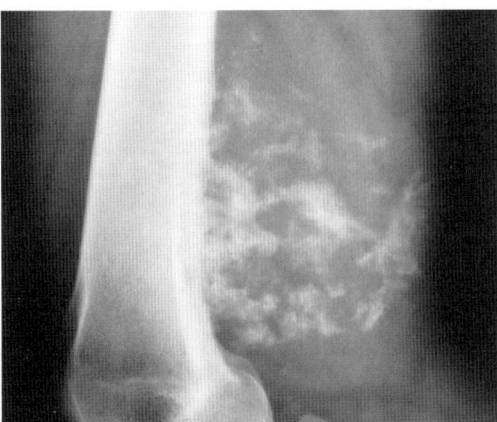

• **Fig. 4.21** Chondrosarcoma. A Prominent Dense Calcification in a Large Neoplastic Mass. (Reprinted with permission from Eisenberg R, Johnson N. *Comprehensive Radiographic Pathology*. 7th ed. Mosby; 2020: Figure 4-75. Chondrosarcoma.)

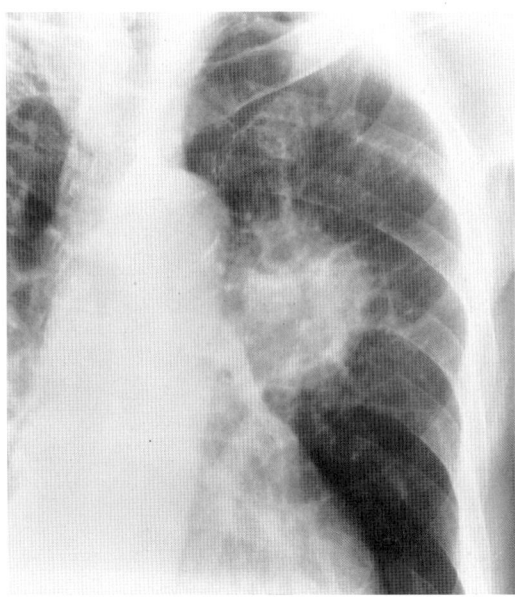

• **Fig. 4.22** Malignant Solitary Pulmonary Nodule (Bronchogenic Carcinoma) on X-Ray. Note Fuzzy, Ill-Defined (Spiculated) Margins. (Reprinted with permission from Eisenberg R, Johnson N. *Comprehensive Radiographic Pathology*. 7th ed. Mosby; 2020: Figure 3-54. Malignant Solitary Pulmonary Nodule [Bronchogenic Carcinoma].)

Chest X-rays are performed often in general radiography for a multitude of indications—cough, fever, difficulty breathing, asthma, heart failure, pain, etc. For cancers of the lung, whether primary or metastatic, CT is more sensitive in visualizing small nodules in early stages; however, if they are large enough, they can also be seen on a chest X-ray. They present as radiodensities and become more radiopaque (brighter) and larger in the later stages of malignancy. Lung tumors which are large enough to be detected on a chest X-ray are more difficult to treat (Figure 4.22). According to the National Lung Screening Trial, a clinical trial sponsored by the National Cancer Institute, patients who are screened with CT scans as opposed to chest X-rays have about a 20% lower risk of dying from lung cancer.

Fluoroscopy is a type of "live X-ray" which visualizes the imaging in "real-time." Fluoroscopy is capable of exposing the patient to higher amounts of radiation and should be utilized carefully. Fluoroscopy is commonly used for general radiography exams of the gastrointestinal (GI) tract and the urinary system. To visualize these specific body systems well on radiographs, it is necessary to administer a contrast medium which will appear very white on X-ray images because it is dense enough to block the X-rays from penetrating through it. There are many different types and brands of contrast media used in general radiography, but the contrast of choice for the GI tract is barium sulfate, $BaSO_4$, combined with air. Contrast for exams of the GI system can be ingested or administered orally, which is the case for upper GI (UGI) and esophagram procedures; or it can be administered rectally through the use of an enema tip, most often for barium enema procedures (BE or LGI). Rarely, barium sulfate and air may be contraindicated, and the use of a water-soluble contrast medium can usually be substituted (Figures 4.23 and 4.24).

Fluoroscopy exams of the upper and lower GI tracts can visualize abnormalities throughout the digestive system. Carcinomas of the digestive tract may present as strictures, filling defects, mucosa atrophy, or there may be polyps or lesions visualized. A stricture

bones, a practitioner may order an exam called a Metastatic Long Bone Survey. This will include X-rays of all of the bones of the body which are frequently affected by bone cancers or bone metastasis including the skull, spine, pelvis, and long bones.

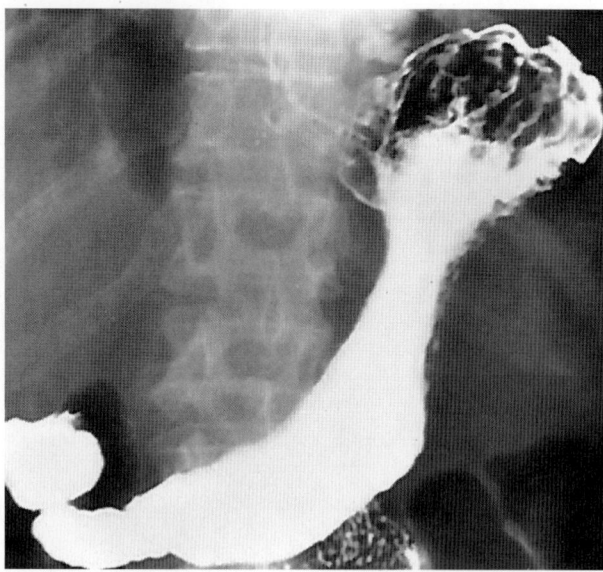

• **Fig. 4.23** Gastric Carcinoma. A Linitis Plastica Pattern is Demonstrated. (Reprinted with permission from Eisenberg R, Johnson N. *Comprehensive Radiographic Pathology.* 7th ed. Mosby; 2020: Figure 5-40. Gastric Carcinoma; and Figure 5-72 Carcinoma of the Colon.)

known as a "napkin-ring" or "apple core" sign on a radiograph is evidence of damage to the lumen of the intestine and is often caused by malignancy. These types of imaging studies can be helpful in detecting some cancers of the esophagus, stomach, or intestines; but are not always necessary to aid in the cancer diagnosis. It is more common for endoscopy or colonoscopy to be performed for the initial diagnosis of these cancers.

The contrast of choice for the urinary tract is a water-soluble contrast that contains small amounts of iodine which is safe to be injected into the vascular system. The kidneys quickly filter the contrast from the bloodstream, which then enables it to be seen on X-ray images, highlighting the kidneys, ureters, and eventually

making its way to the bladder. Radiographs can be performed following the administration of this contrast media, which is an exam called an intravenous urogram (IVU). Contrast can also be administered retrograde, through the urethra, for some exams of the urinary system, which includes cystography and retrograde urography, which are usually performed during fluoroscopy. These types of general radiography exams of the urinary system are performed infrequently, as CT has become the exam of choice in recent years as it provides the practitioner with higher quality images and more diagnostic information when it comes to diagnosing abnormalities of the kidneys, ureters, and bladder. Water-soluble contrast medium may be contraindicated if the patient has an allergy to iodinated contrast, or if the patient's kidneys are not functioning adequately. Although rare, there is a small risk of serious allergy to this type of contrast media.

Computed Tomography

CT involves the use of X-rays and computers to create images of the patient in sectional planes. The first CT scan was performed on a patient in 1971 and took several hours to complete images of the brain. Today, CT scanners are capable of acquiring hundreds of images in seconds. Once the images are acquired, most often in a transverse plane, CT images can be manipulated and viewed in multiple planes as well as three-dimensionally. The largest advantage of CT is its ability to provide very detailed images in a short amount of time. Some of the disadvantages include the large radiation doses associated with CT scans and limitations in visualizing soft tissues.

CT often requires the use of contrast media, similar to general radiography, however the contrast used for the GI tract is slightly different. This contrast has a higher ratio of water to the barium sulfate, which makes it less dense on the images. This is important in CT because the barium sulfate that is utilized in general radiography to visualize the digestive tract results in a streaking artifact on a CT image which degrades the image quality (Figure 4.25).

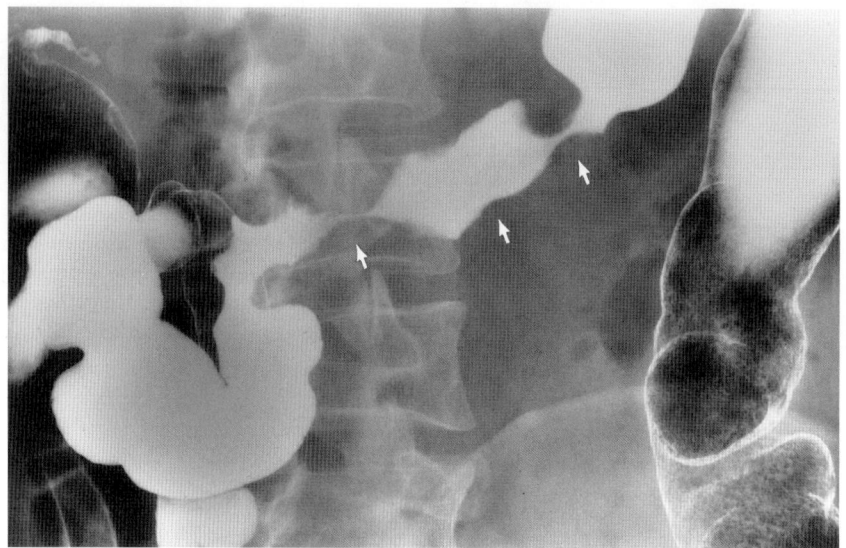

• **Fig. 4.24** Carcinoma of the Colon Developing in a Patient With Long-Standing Chronic Ulcerative Colitis. A Long, Irregular Lesion With a Bizarre Pattern is Visible in the Transverse Colon *(Arrows).* (Reprinted with permission from Eisenberg R, Johnson N. *Comprehensive Radiographic Pathology.* 7th ed. Mosby; 2020: Figure 5-72. Carcinoma of the Colon Developing in a Patient With Long-Standing Chronic Ulcerative Colitis.)

Iodinated contrast media is used often in CT via injection into a vein, and helps to visualize the urinary tract, but also highlights all of the other vessels in the body. CT technologists can use timing protocols that are very specific to the region or organ of interest during exams which utilize contrast media. The contrast helps to identify masses and areas which appear vascularly abnormal (Figure 4.26). As in general radiography, this contrast is sometimes contraindicated, which can be problematic when attempting to visualize certain pathologies.

CT is used in the diagnosis and staging of many cancers and is also used to look for metastasis throughout the body. Practitioners often order CTs of the neck, chest, abdomen, and pelvis which can help to visualize many common areas of metastatic disease which include the liver, lungs, lymph nodes, and bones (Figure 4.27). Similar to X-ray, cancers may be visualized on CT images as abnormal densities or irregular masses.

Head CTs can detect some lesions in the brain and are performed frequently as part of the initial diagnosis and staging; however, MRI is the best exam to visualize abnormalities of the brain and spinal cord (Figure 4.28).

CT exposes the patient to higher doses of ionizing radiation than what is used in general radiography. Practitioners are careful to order these exams only when the benefits outweigh the risks. It has been suggested that CT be used for cancer screening purposes in asymptomatic patients; however, this is not currently considered to be a safe practice for the majority of cancers. CT screening is sometimes performed specifically for the lungs, particularly in patients who have a history of smoking. CT scans of the lungs without contrast media can visualize nodules which are often too small to be seen on a chest X-ray in the early stages of lung cancer (Figure 4.29). As mentioned previously, low dose helical lung CT scans are proven to reduce mortality rates associated with lung cancer; however, they can also increase the risk of a false positive, which leads to unnecessary invasive procedures, such as biopsies.

Another CT exam which is sometimes used for screening purposes is the "virtual colonoscopy" for colorectal cancer (Figure 4.30).

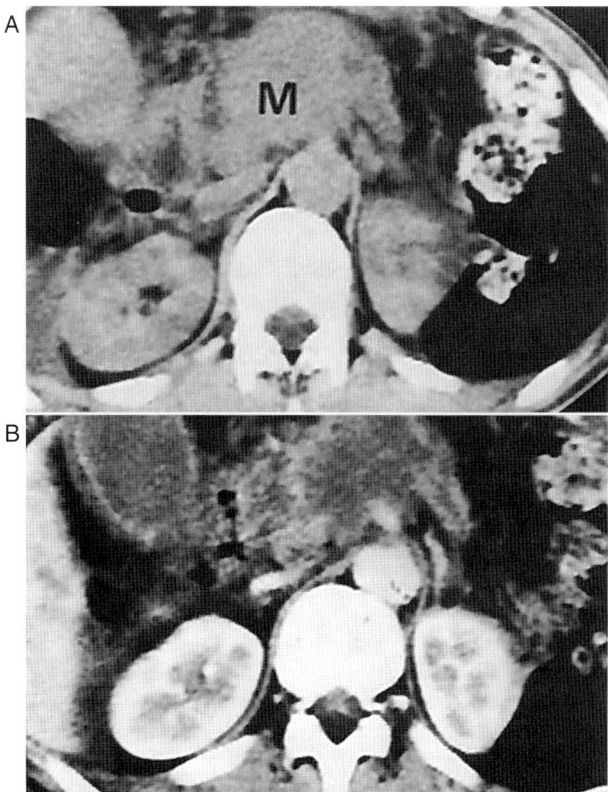

• **Fig. 4.26** Carcinoma of the Pancreas (A) Noncontrast Computed Tomography Scan Demonstrates a Homogeneous Mass (M) in the Body of the Pancreas. (B) After Intravenous Injection of a Bolus of Contrast Material, There is Enhancement of the Normal Pancreatic Parenchyma and the Surrounding Vascular Structures. The Pancreatic Carcinoma Remains Unchanged and Thus Appears as a Low-Density Mass. (Reprinted with permission from Eisenberg R, Johnson N. *Comprehensive Radiographic Pathology*. 7th ed. Mosby; 2020: Figure 5-109A and B. CT—Carcinoma of the Pancreas.)

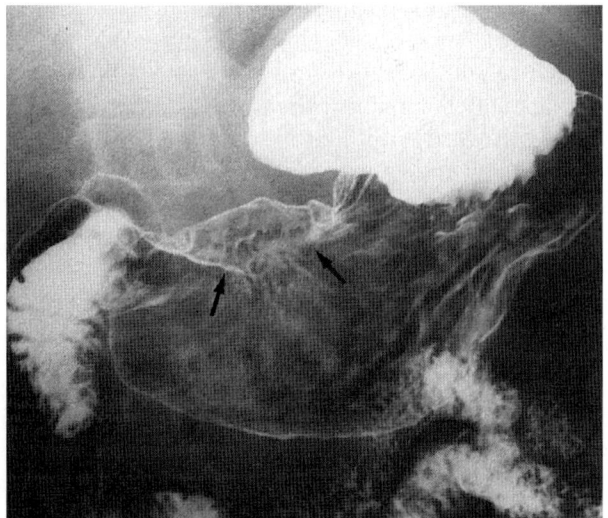

• **Fig. 4.25** Computed Tomography (CT) Staging of Gastric Carcinoma (A) Double-Contrast Study Demonstrates Large Lesser-Curvature Mass (*Arrows*) With a Thickened Wall. (B) CT Scan Shows a Thickened Gastric Wall; The Contrast Agent Demonstrates the Lumen of the Stomach. (Reprinted with permission from Eisenberg R, Johnson N. *Comprehensive Radiographic Pathology*. 7th ed. Mosby; 2020: Figure 5-42B. Computed Tomography (CT) Staging of Gastric Carcinoma.)

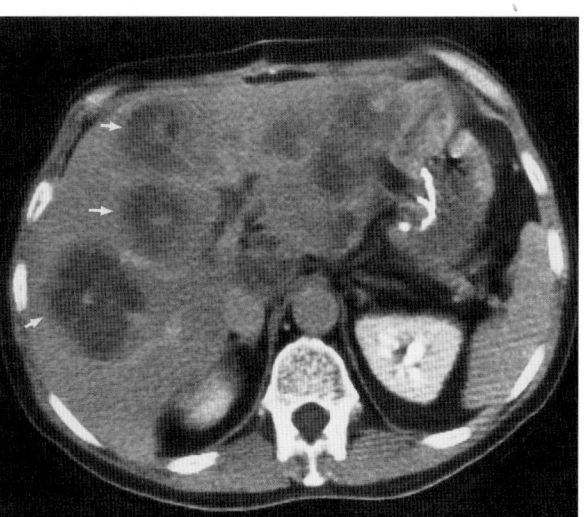

• **Fig. 4.27** Hepatic Metastases Computed Tomography Scan Shows Multiple Low-Density Metastases With High-Density Centers (*Arrows*). (Reprinted with permission from Eisenberg R, Johnson N. *Comprehensive Radiographic Pathology*. 7th ed. Mosby; 2020: Figure 5-100A. CT—Hepatic Metastases.)

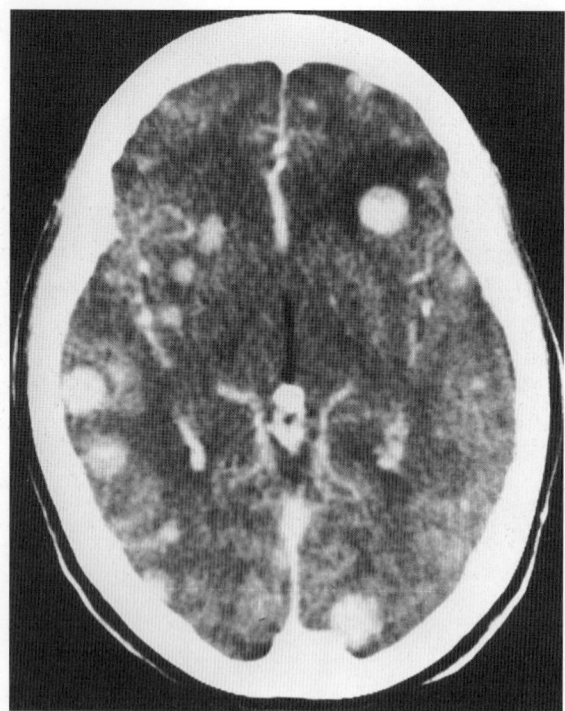

• **Fig. 4.28** Brain Metastases Computed Tomography Scan Shows Multiple Enhancing Masses of Various Shapes and Sizes Representing Hematogenous Metastases From Carcinoma of the Breast. (Reprinted with permission from Eisenberg R, Johnson N. *Comprehensive Radiographic Pathology*. 7th ed. Mosby; 2020: Figure 8-31. CT—Brain Metastases from Breast Cancer.)

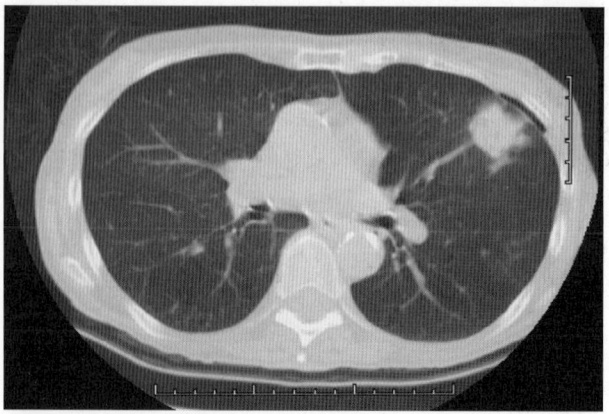

• **Fig. 4.29** Malignant Solitary Pulmonary Nodule (Adenocarcinoma) Computed Tomography Scan Demonstrates Spiculated Mass With Ill-Defined Contour. (Reprinted with permission from Eisenberg R, Johnson N. *Comprehensive Radiographic Pathology*. 7th ed. Mosby; 2020: Figure 3-57. CT—Malignant Solitary Pulmonary Nodule-Adenocarcinoma.)

This exam is comparable to a traditional colonoscopy regarding the extent to what it visualizes in the colon and is less invasive; however, the associated radiation exposure is of concern.

Magnetic Resonance Imaging

MRI also involves creating images of the patient in sectional planes, however the technology used is much different. MRI utilizes a type of nonionizing radiation that involves the use of radio waves and a very strong magnetic field to create images of the

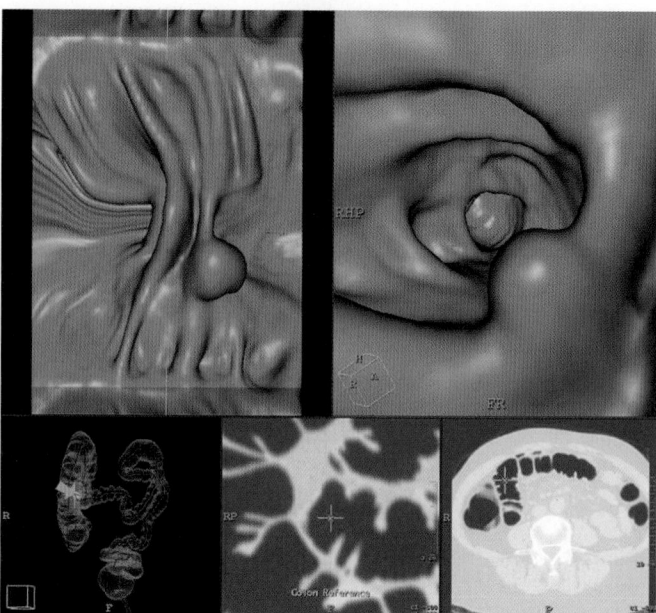

• **Fig. 4.30** CT colonography. Note: Polyp localized on intestinal wall. (Courtesy Philips Medical Systems.) (Reprinted with permission from Lampignano JP, Kendrick LE. *Bontrager's Textbook of Radiographic Positioning and Related Anatomy*. 9th ed. Elsevier; 2018: Figure 18.70. CT—Colonography.)

body. The first human MRI image was produced in 1977, and the first patient was scanned in 1978. MRI scanners are capable of scanning data in any plane and images can also be manipulated in order to view them in other planes or in 3D. Each exam performed in MRI includes various pulse sequences. These sequences may refer to the various projections that are obtained, but also may refer to contrast weighting. Contrast weighting refers to the difference in tissue brightness on the MRI images. The two most common MRI sequences are T1-weighted and T2-weighted scans, which are both acquired for each MRI exam. The appearance of the various tissues in the body will present differently on these two sequences, thus providing the radiologist with more information, which will enable them to provide the most accurate diagnosis. For example, cerebrospinal fluid will appear as dark on a T1-weighted image, and will appear bright on a T2-weighted image. T1-weighted images with contrast are best to detect and characterize brain lesions, while T2-weighted images are best to demonstrate bony tumors of the limbs.

The major advantage of MRI is its ability to provide high quality, detailed images of most soft tissues and organs of the body, including the brain and central nervous system, while not utilizing ionizing radiation (Figures 4.31 and 4.32). The disadvantages of MRI include safety concerns, high costs, and the length of time needed for each scan. The average MRI scan takes about 20 to 40 minutes and requires the patient to lie very still, which is often a problem for young children and patients who are claustrophobic. Many of these patients need sedation when undergoing an MRI. Patients who need an MRI scan also need to be screened thoroughly to ensure they do not have any metal in their body due to the magnetic field. Patients with pacemakers or other metal in the body that is not "MRI safe," and patients who are very obese may not be able to have MRI scans due to their body habitus being a limiting factor for the MRI machine opening.

Contrast media is also used in MRI; however, it is different from the contrast mentioned previously for general radiography and

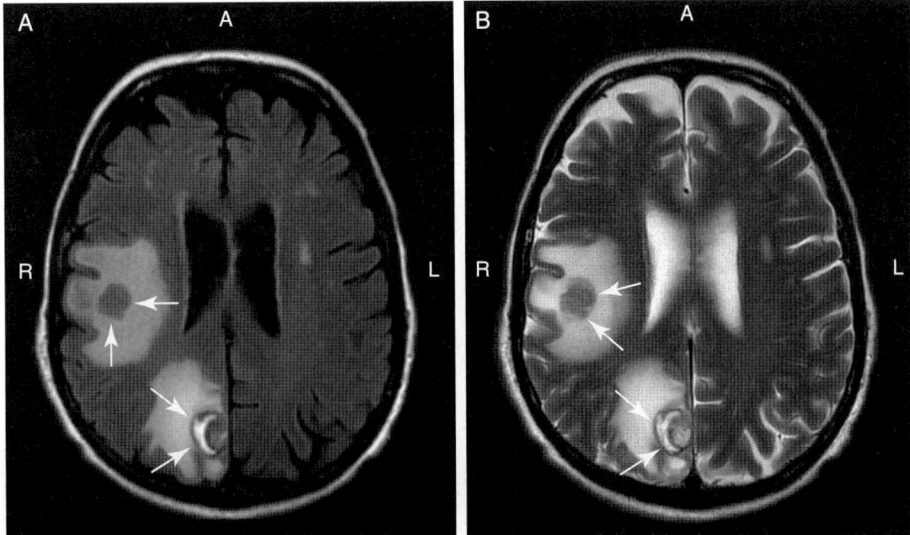

• **Fig. 4.31** Brain Metastases Axial T2-Weighted (A) and Fluid-Attenuated Inversion Recovery (B) Magnetic Resonance Images Demonstrate Two Large Masses (*Arrows*) Surrounded by Extensive High-Signal Intensity Edema. (Reprinted with permission from Eisenberg R, Johnson N. *Comprehensive Radiographic Pathology*. 7th ed. Mosby; 2020: Figure 8-30A and B. MRI Brain Metastases.)

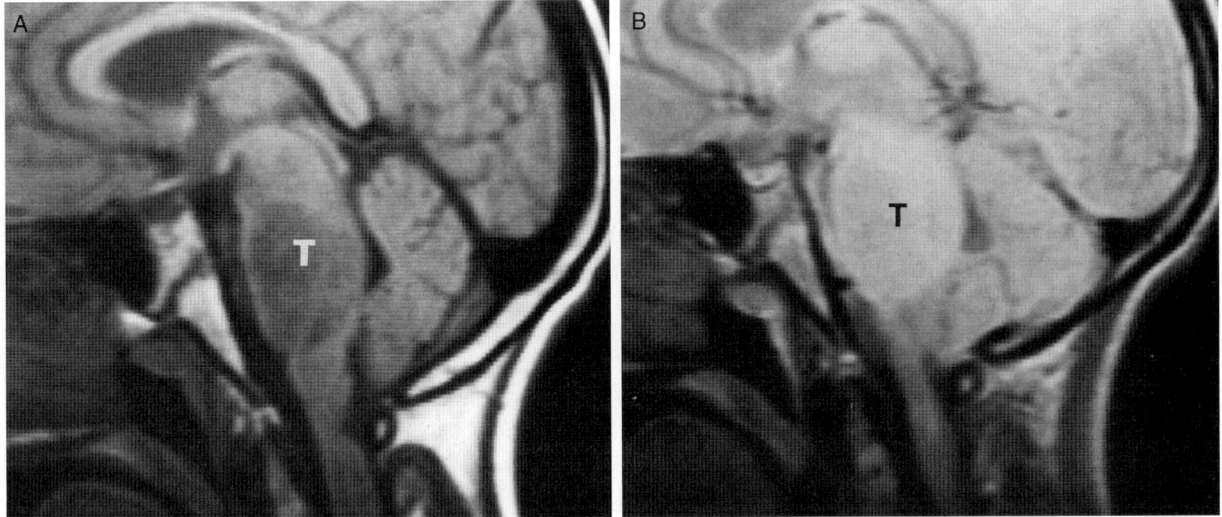

• **Fig. 4.32** Brainstem Glioma Sagittal Magnetic Resonance Images Show Enlargement of Brainstem Involving the Pons and Midbrain. Note that Various Imaging Techniques Alter the Appearance of the Tumor (T). (A) On a T1-Weighted Image, the Tumor is Gray (Low-Intensity Signal). (B) On a T2-Weighted Image, the Tumor Appears White (High-Intensity Signal). (Reprinted with permission from Eisenberg R, Johnson N. *Comprehensive Radiographic Pathology*. 7th ed. Mosby; 2020: Figure 8-12A and B. MRI Brainstem Glioma.)

CT. The most popular contrast media used in MRI is gadolinium-diethylenetriaminepentaacetic acid (Gd-DTPA)-Magnevist. It is metallic and magnetic and leads to an increase of brightness in certain tissues. The contrast used in MRI has fewer side effects than iodinated contrast, and for oncology patients, it can help to better detect primary tumors and metastatic disease on the MRI images (Figures 4.33–4.35).

As in CT, neoplasms may be visualized on MRI images as abnormalities in density or irregular masses. Since MRI is particularly useful when imaging soft tissues of the body, it does provide superior visualization of many different types of cancers including neoplasms of the brain, breast, prostate, uterus, adrenal glands, liver, pancreas, gallbladder, and colon. Although CT is usually the

exam of choice when bone needs to be evaluated, especially in cases of trauma, MRI is the better exam for determining the extent of bone tumors.

Diagnostic Medical Sonography

Diagnostic medical sonography (DMS/ultrasound or sonography) uses sound waves, or ultrasound, to create images. The concept of echolocation, which is the basis of ultrasound, was discovered in 1794; however, the first medical image was not performed until the 1940s. It is often the exam of choice in pregnancy and pediatrics because it utilizes nonionizing radiation, can be performed quickly, and usually painlessly. Sonography

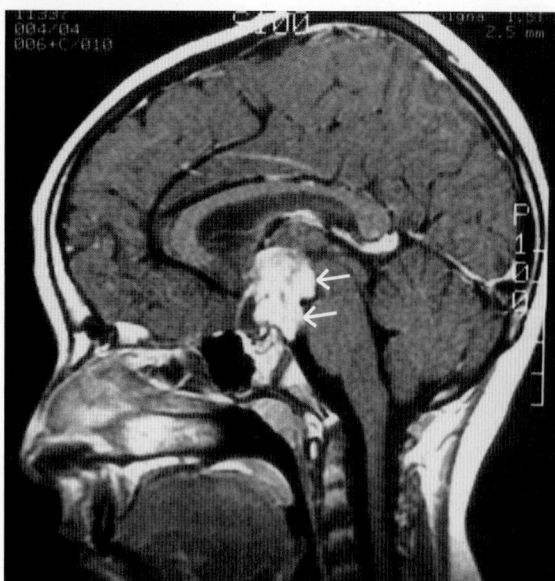

• **Fig. 4.33** With contrast agent, Gd-DTPA (T1-weighted image). Pathology appears as bright areas in the central brain; see arrows. *Gd-DTPA*, Gadolinium-diethylenetriaminepentaacetic acid. (Reprinted with permission from Lampignano JP, Kendrick LE. *Bontrager's Textbook of Radiographic Positioning and Related Anatomy*. 9th ed. Elsevier; 2018.)

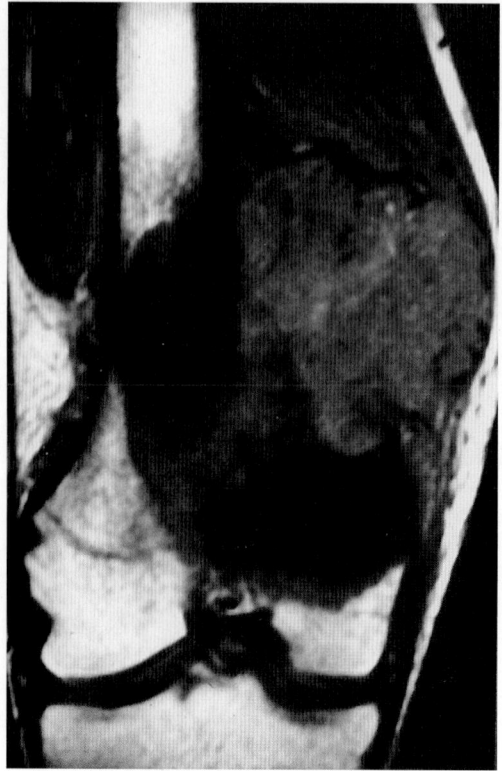

• **Fig. 4.34** MRI of Osteogenic Sarcoma. A Coronal Image Shows Destruction of the Intramedullary Bone and the Soft Tissue Extent of the Mass. (Reprinted with permission from Eisenberg R, Johnson N. *Comprehensive Radiographic Pathology*. 7th ed. Mosby; 2020: Figure 4-72. MRI of Osteogenic Sarcoma.)

is limited when bone or air superimpose the area of interest but has many applications including brain, cardiac, vascular imaging, abdominal imaging, and the ability to image joints, muscles, and tendons (Figure 4.36).

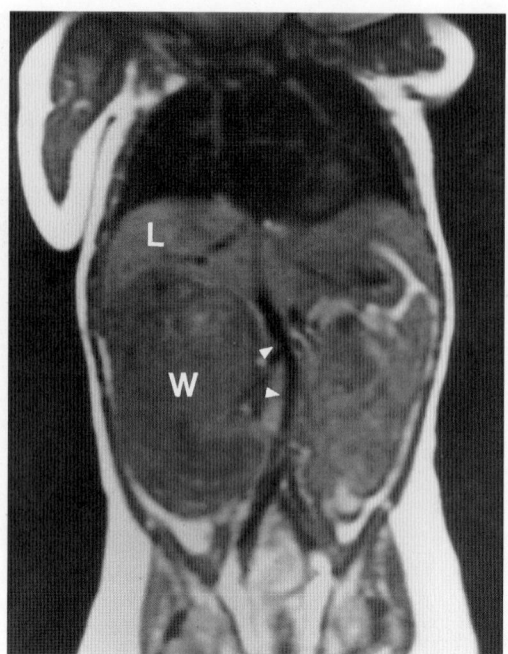

• **Fig. 4.35** Wilms Tumor T1-Weighted Coronal MRI Shows Sharply Marginated Infrahepatic Mass (W) That is Clearly Distinct from the Liver (L). The Inferior Vena Cava (*Arrowheads*), Although Displaced by the Mass, Shows No Evidence of Tumor Extension Into It. (Reprinted with permission from Eisenberg R, Johnson N. *Comprehensive Radiographic Pathology*. 7th ed. Mosby; 2020: Figure 6-52. MRI Wilms Tumor.)

Sonography is commonly used to examine the fetus and uterus during pregnancy, but it is also beneficial for visualizing fluid filled structures like cysts and other abdominal organs. Sonography can help to determine whether a mass is a solid structure or fluid filled, which helps to aid in the diagnosis of cancer, but it is not typically used to provide a definitive diagnosis. Solid masses on sonography images usually appear lighter than surrounding structures. It is best used on organs where there is not bone or air obscuring the images such as the liver, kidneys, gallbladder, uterus, thyroid, testicles, prostate, blood vessels, some areas of the GI tract and breasts (Figures 4.37 and 4.38).

Nuclear Medicine

Nuclear medicine includes all exams that require the injection of a radioactive material, called a radiopharmaceutical or radiotracer, before acquiring the images ordered of the specified body part. Radiopharmaceuticals are radioactive drugs which can be used in the diagnosis and treatment of disease. The radionuclide emits a gamma ray, and the pharmaceutical is formulated to carry the radionuclide to a specific organ. Images are performed using a nuclear medicine gamma camera, and may involve the use of a hybrid imaging system which combines the technology of nuclear medicine and another modality, such as CT or MRI, to then produce images of two modalities at the same time.

One clinical application of nuclear medicine with regards to oncology patients is the bone scan. Bone scans can detect abnormalities in the skeletal system such as metastasis or stress fractures. If there are "hot spots" detected on a bone during a bone scan, practitioners may order radiographs of that bone to determine the exact pathology.

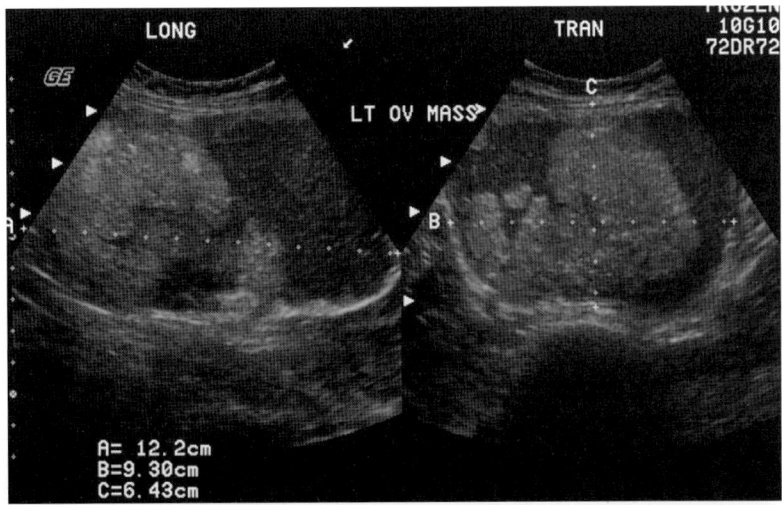

• **Fig. 4.36** A Sagittal and Transverse Sonographic Image of an Ovarian Mass. (Reprinted with permission from Kowalczyk N. *Radiographic Pathology for Technologists*. 7th ed. Mosby; 2018: Figure 10-18. US Ovarian Mass.)

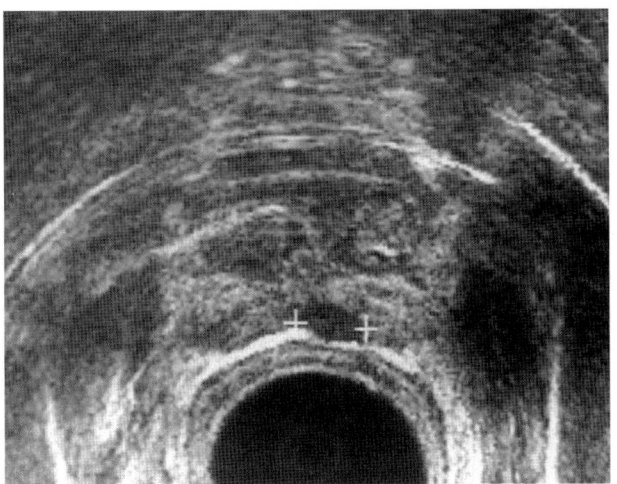

• **Fig. 4.37** Cancer of the Prostate Transrectal Ultrasound Image Demonstrates a Hypoechoic Mass (Between Cursors) With the Capsule Still Intact. (Reprinted with permission from Eisenberg R, Johnson N. *Comprehensive Radiographic Pathology*. 7th ed. Mosby; 2020: Figure 11-11. Transrectal US—Cancer of the Prostate and Figure 2-2A. Renal Cell Carcinoma.)

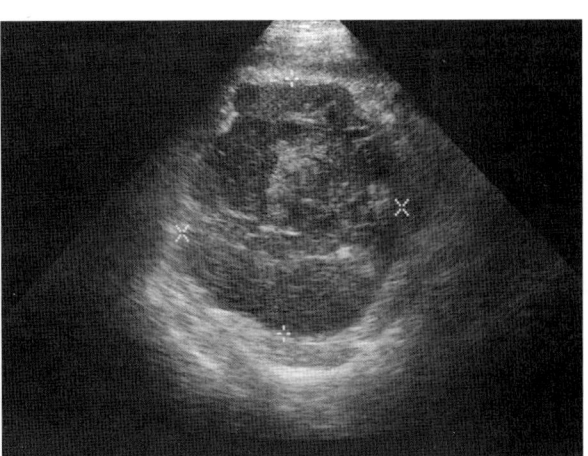

• **Fig. 4.38** Renal Cell Carcinoma Ultrasound Images of the Abdomen. Transverse Right Kidney Demonstrates a Hyperechoic Area (White) Within the Mass Caused by Renal Cell Carcinoma. (Reprinted with permission from Eisenberg R, Johnson N. *Comprehensive Radiographic Pathology*. 7th ed. Mosby; 2020: Figure 2-2A. Renal Cell Carcinoma.)

Positron Emission Tomography

PET is considered to be a branch of nuclear medicine, because the patient receives an injection of a positron-emitting radioisotope before having a PET scan performed. PET scans are often used in combination with CT or MRI utilizing a hybrid imaging technique. PET is a valuable tool in the diagnosis, staging, and follow-up of cancer and has the ability to detect functional changes in the body before the patient exhibits symptoms.

When PET imaging is performed on cancer patients, the radiopharmaceutical which is injected is ^{18}F-fluorodeoxyglucose (^{18}F-FDG). Malignant cells have an advanced glucose metabolism and they use sugar as an energy source. Glycolysis is the increased use of sugar by the cells and is a sign of malignancy. The glucose analog FDG will be absorbed easily by active tumors and will be visualized as a darker area on PET scan images. The brain will appear dark on PET images because it naturally utilizes a large amount of glucose. It is also normal for the kidneys and bladder to appear dark because the tracer

is excreted from the body through the urinary system (Figure 4.39). PET scans are useful in the diagnosis of cancer but are often ordered by practitioners to help stage cancer by identifying areas of metastasis. PET scans may also be requested following or during treatments to assess the effectiveness of the treatment (Figure 4.40).

Breast Imaging

Mammography

Mammography is a type of low dose X-ray used specifically for the breast. Unlike most other diagnostic exams, mammograms are frequently performed as screening tests, which means they are often ordered and performed before a person ever exhibits symptoms of the disease. According to the American Cancer Society, all women should begin having annual mammograms regardless of their risk or family history, at the age of 45.[22] These annual screening mammograms increase the odds of early detection, which improves breast

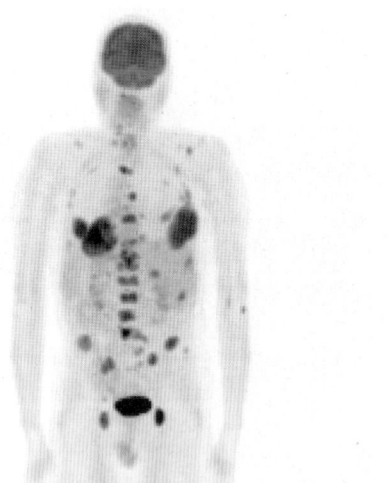

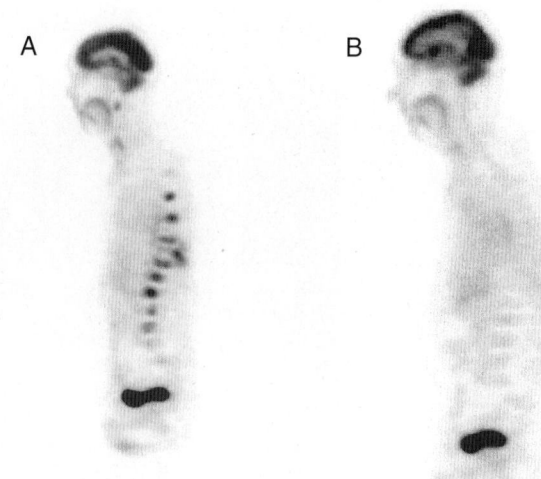

• **Fig. 4.39** Coronal view of a whole-body PET scan. Darker areas indicate increased uptake of F-FDG. It is normal to see activity in the brain because this organ naturally consumes a great deal of glucose. It is also normal to see activity in the collecting system of the kidneys or in the bladder as the tracer is excreted into the urinary system. The two focal areas in the liver are indicative of metastatic spread of breast cancer. *F-FDG,* F-fluorodeoxyglucose; *PET,* positron emission tomography. (Reprinted with permission from Lampignano JP, Kendrick LE. *Bontrager's Textbook of Radiographic Positioning and Related Anatomy.* 9th ed. Elsevier; 2018: Figure 20.8.)

• **Fig. 4.40** Positron Emission Tomography Used to Assess Effectiveness of Chemotherapy (A) Image Before Therapy. (B) After Chemotherapy, the Image Demonstrates Decreased Uptake of ^{18}F-fluorodeoxyglucose. (Reprinted with permission from Eisenberg R, Johnson N. *Comprehensive Radiographic Pathology.* 7th ed. Mosby; 2020: Figure 2-23A and B. Positron Emission Tomography Used to Assess Effectiveness of Chemotherapy.)

cancer treatment options and survival rates. Using X-rays to detect breast cancer was first documented in 1913, but modern mammography techniques were developed in the 1960s and have since been the gold standard for detecting breast cancer (Figure 4.41). Some disadvantages of mammography include the radiation dose (although, it is a very low dose), and its difficulty with imaging dense breast tissue.

This type of breast tissue is most often found in younger patients (up to age 30), and patients who have not had children.

Digital breast tomosynthesis (DBT) is a newer technique used during a mammogram that provides 3D imaging of the breast. This technology requires multiple images to be acquired at different angles and reconstructed into thin slices—allowing the

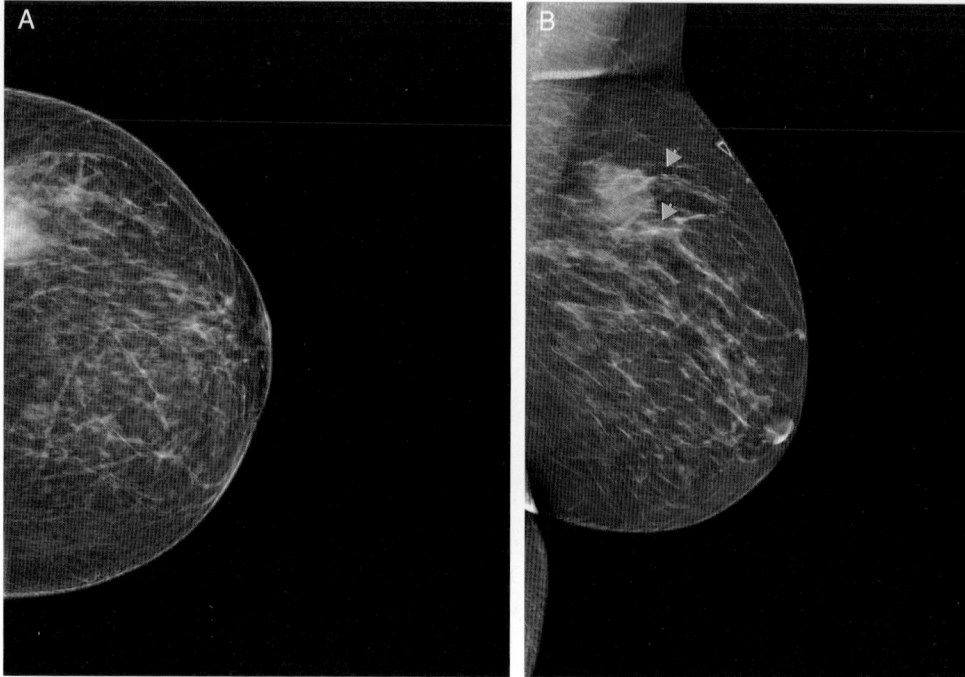

• **Fig. 4.41** Breast Cancer (A) Craniocaudal and (B) 90-Degree Mediolateral Projections on a Full-Field Digital Mammography System Demonstrating an Ill-Defined Irregular Lesion With Radiating Spicules *(Arrowheads).* (Reprinted with permission from Eisenberg R, Johnson N. *Comprehensive Radiographic Pathology.* 7th ed. Mosby; 2020: Figures 11-59A and B. Mammography.)

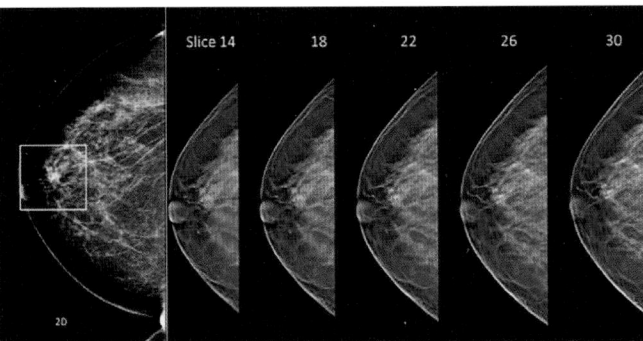

• **Fig. 4.42** The 2D image on the left shows a potential lesion in the sub-areolar region of the breast. However, the 3D breast tomosynthesis image on the right shows that in fact, there is no lesion present. Individual structures can be picked out on the separate slices, which summate to form the potential lesion seen on the 2D projection image. (Courtesy Hologic Inc. Bedford, Massachusetts.) (Reprinted with permission from Lampignano JP, Kendrick LE. *Bontrager's Textbook of Radiographic Positioning and Related Anatomy*. 9th ed. Elsevier; 2018: Figure 20.60.)

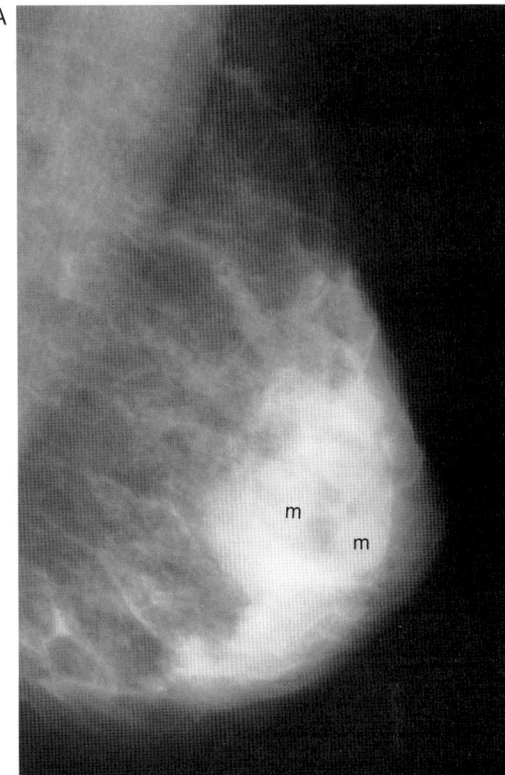

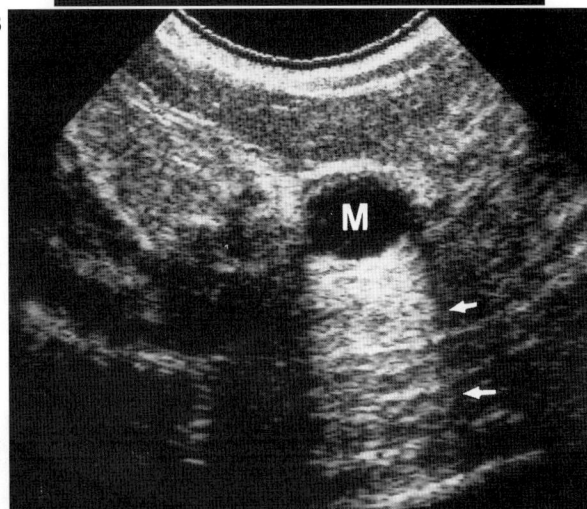

• **Fig. 4.43** Sonography for Breast Disease. (A) Mammogram Showing Several Rounded Masses (M) that Could Be Solid or Cystic in a Breast That is Very Dense Anteriorly. (B) Sonogram Clearly Shows That the Largest Mass (M) is Cystic Because It Contains No Internal Echoes and Shows Considerable Posterior Enhancement (*Arrows*). (Reprinted with permission from Eisenberg R, Johnson N. *Comprehensive Radiographic Pathology*. 7th ed. Mosby; 2020: Figures 11-62A and B. Mammogram and Sonography.)

interpreter to visualize structures that would have been overlapping with traditional mammography (Figure 4.42).

Breast Sonography

Breast sonography is very useful in aiding in a breast cancer diagnosis because it can easily distinguish between a cyst and a solid lesion. It is also useful in imaging dense breasts. Sonography is used following a mammogram to investigate specific findings and is not sufficient to replace a mammogram (Figure 4.43).

Breast Magnetic Resonance Imaging

The use of MRI in breast imaging increases annually. While the general disadvantages of MRI mentioned previously are still of concern, it has been effective in some applications of detecting breast cancer (Figures 4.44 and 4.45). MRI is more sensitive in detecting lesions in dense breasts, making it more suitable for younger patients who are high risk because of a family history or a positive *BRCA1* and *BRCA2* genes. It may also be used to visualize a palpable mass that could not be seen on mammography or sonography. One specific disadvantage of breast MRI is its high false-positive rate, which may lead to unnecessary invasive procedures for the patient.

Nuclear Breast Imaging

Nuclear medicine plays an important role in diagnosing breast cancer by helping physicians visualize small changes in cell metabolism that may be the result of malignancy. These changes may often be present before the disease has manifested physically. There are several nuclear medicine procedures which are helpful in imaging the breast.

Scintimammography (Sestamibi)
- Uses the radionuclide ^{99m}Tc sestamibi to help confirm breast cancer diagnosis
- Not used often because of a high false-positive rate
- Unreliable for lesions less than 1 cm

Sentinel Node Studies
- Injects sulfur colloid around the lesion subcutaneously
- Uses the lymph vessels to help localize before removing the node

Positron Emission Tomography Mammography
- Combines the use of ^{18}F-FDG with the same projections used during a mammogram, using the compression technique to stabilize the breast and prevent motion
- Capable of detecting lesions as small as 1.5 mm
- Disadvantages include high cost and more radiation exposure (exposes whole body to radiation)
- Being studied as a tool to determine extent of cancer

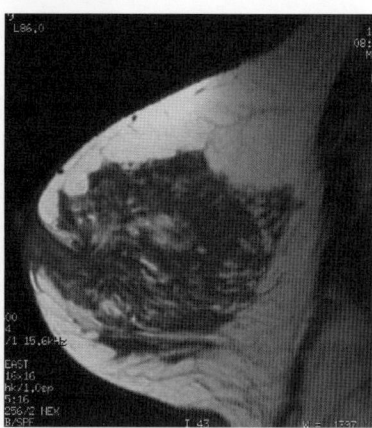

• **Fig. 4.44** T1-weighted MRI image of dense breast. (Reprinted with permission from Lampignano JP, Kendrick LE. *Bontrager's Textbook of Radiographic Positioning and Related Anatomy.* 9th ed. Elsevier; 2018: Figure 20.54.)

Breast-Specific Gamma Imaging (BSGI) or Molecular Breast Imaging (MBI)

- Newer version of sestamibi but the gamma camera is smaller and closer to the patient's breast
- Uses sestamibi as the imaging agent
- Clinical trials are still being done, may be helpful in imaging dense breasts
- Disadvantage of exposing the whole body to radiation

Thermography

Thermograms are currently being studied as a diagnostic tool in the detection of breast cancer. Thermography uses an infrared camera to produce images using the body's heat energy and can detect changes in the body's blood flow. This means that it may have the ability to detect functional changes in the breast tissue before a nodule can be palpated. The advantage to this procedure is it may have the ability to detect breast cancer and breast cancer risk sooner than other exams, which would increase the chance of survival, especially in younger women with dense breast tissue. The disadvantage is that it has a high number of false positives which leads to other unnecessary procedures for those patients. Further improvements and research are needed before the use of thermography is accepted as a screening tool for breast cancer.

Conclusion

Cancer, as the most common "genetic" disease, has been the recipient of a substantial amount of National Institutes of Health grant funding over the last 20 years. This effort, along with recent advances in genomic analysis of tumors, has significantly increased our understanding of the biological and molecular basis of the single greatest cause of death worldwide. Yet, we still have much to learn before we can cure many cancers, or at least make them chronic treatable diseases without significant mortality or morbidity. While still a scary diagnosis, the prognosis for most cancer patients for either long-term survival or cure is far better today than in the past. This is due, in large measure, to the technological advances in both Radiology and Pathology (especially in Molecular Pathology) which permits earlier diagnosis and far more extensive characterization of a tumor than was possible previously. Knowledge of this process will not only help the oncology rehabilitation clinician develop a more precise and effective plan of care, but will also help support the person with cancer with emotional and psychosocial aspects of their disease journey.

Critical Research Needs

- Impact of interpretation of a pathology report upon oncology rehabilitation diagnoses and treatment.
- Quantifying the molecular changes in cancer cells secondary to exercise (low, moderate, vigorous)
- Define the educational requirements needed for oncology rehabilitation professionals pursuing specialization as it relates to the diagnostic process
- Identify the cellular changes to cancer cells with therapeutic ultrasound or electrical stimulation

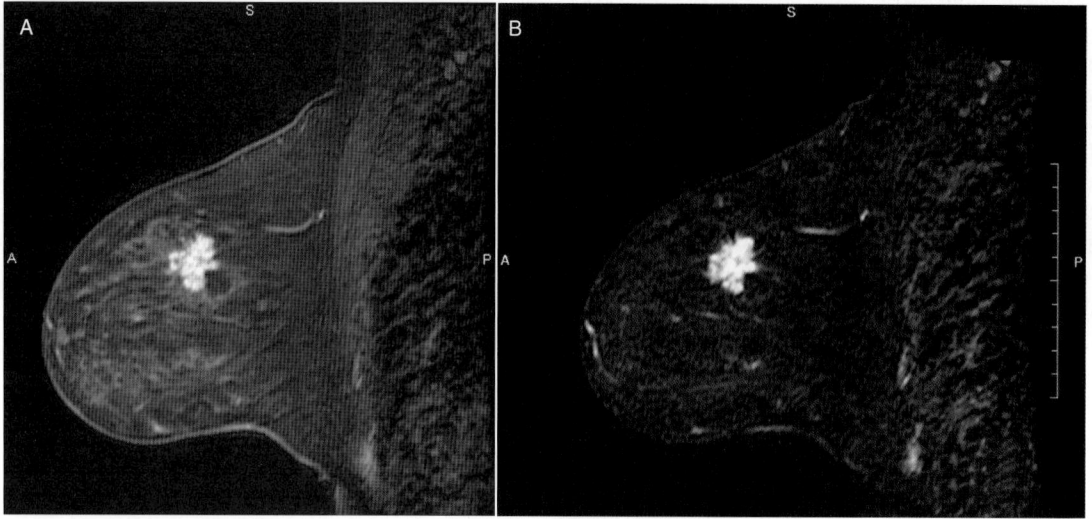

• **Fig. 4.45** Breast Carcinoma. (A) Unilateral Sagittal T1-Weighted Fat-Saturated Postcontrast Magnetic Resonance (MR) Image Demonstrates a Single Mass. (B) Postcontrast MR Subtraction Image Illustrates a Spiculated Mass. (Reprinted with permission from Eisenberg R, Johnson N. *Comprehensive Radiographic Pathology.* 7th ed. Mosby; 2020: Figures 11-65A and B. MRI—Breast Carcinoma.)

Case Study

A 50-year-old female presents to the clinic after finding a mass on the upper outer quadrant of her left breast. Her subjective history reveals the following: (1) her mother died from breast cancer at 68 years of age; (2) her maternal aunt was also diagnosed with breast cancer at an early age; (3) her menstruation began at age 11; (4) she is nullipara; (5) she is postmenopausal. On physical exam, she is markedly obese, and there is visual retraction of the skin and the nipple on her left breast. Mass is palpable during the breast exam and is described as fixed, hard, and nontender. The mass was not present in her last mammogram, completed 2 years ago. Axillary lymph nodes are also palpable. The patient is scheduled for an immediate mammography and needle biopsy to confirm suspicions of breast carcinoma. Blood test reveals the presence of BRCA1. The biopsy confirms that the cancer started in the ductal region and had broken through the ducts. Stage and grade: Stage-2A;T-2 cm;N-2; M-0. Pathology revealed HER-2-neu (–), estrogen, progesterone receptors (–) (Figure 4.46).

Diagnosis: Invasive ductal carcinoma: medullary pattern.

Treatment: mastectomy, radiation, and chemotherapy. Possible option of drug therapy with Lynparza.

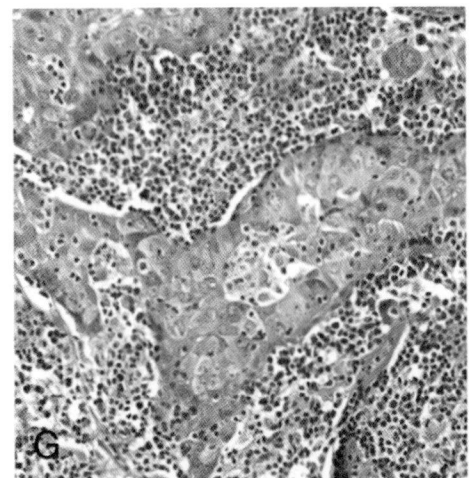

Fig. 4.46 Histologic features include (1) solid sheets of large cells with pleomorphic nuclei and prominent nucleoli, (2) frequent mitotic figures, (3) a moderate to marked lymphoplasmacytic infiltrate surrounding and within the tumor, and (4) a pushing (noninfiltrative) border (Fig. 23.22G).

Review Questions

Reader can find the correct answers and rationale in the back of the book.

1. Which of the following statements correctly states the role of the *RB* and p53 genes in tumorigenesis?
   A. The transcription complex E2F, which is required for progression from G₁ to S phase of the cell cycle, is inactivated by binding with the retinoblastoma gene protein
   B. The product of the p53 gene binds to pRb and prevents it from binding E2F
   C. The p53 gene prevents cells with DNA damage from proceeding to M phase of the cell cycle
   D. The p53 gene suppresses apoptosis in cells detected to have oncogenic changes
2. Which of the following correctly identifies an important event in tumorigenesis?
   A. Progressive shortening of telomeric sequences
   B. Up-regulation of genes which promote apoptosis
   C. Activation of telomerase enzyme
   D. Activating immune system cells such as T-cells
3. Epigenetic changes have been identified in many tumor types and are now proposed to be a fundamental mechanism involved in tumorigenesis. These changes include:
   A. Hypomethylation of tumor suppressor gene promoter regions.
   B. Global hypermethylation of oncogene sequences.
   C. Increasing levels of genomic instability in the tumor.
   D. Activation of microRNA genes
4. Which statement about driver mutations and passenger mutations is true?
   A. Driver mutations account for the largest number of mutations identified in any tumor
   B. Passenger mutations confer a growth advantage to a cell through the alteration of fundamental processes
   C. Driver mutations are essential for tumor transformation/growth

D. Passenger mutations are acquired over a short period of time prior to tumor formation
5. The chromosome translocation in follicular lymphoma involving chromosomes 14q and 18q leads to rearrangement of the *IGH* and *BCL2* genes resulting in overexpression of the *BCL2* gene. This overexpression of *BCL2*:
   A. Causes cancer cells to die
   B. Prevents apoptosis
   C. Causes chromosome telomeres to shorten
   D. Causes global hypomethylation of the tumor genome
6. Which medical imaging modality utilizes nonionizing radiation?
   A. Diagnostic medical sonography
   B. Computed tomography
   C. General radiography
   D. Fluoroscopy
7. Which medical imaging modality is capable of detecting functional changes in the body, often before the patient exhibits symptoms?
   A. Computed tomography
   B. Magnetic resonance imaging
   C. Diagnostic medical sonography
   D. Positron emission tomography
8. A 56-year-old woman sees her physician for a routine health examination. There are no remarkable findings on physical examination. A mammogram shows a 0.5 cm irregular area of increased density with scattered micro calcifications in the upper outer quadrant of the left breast. Excisional biopsy shows atypical lobular hyperplasia. The patient has been on postmenopausal estrogen-progesterone therapy for past 10 years. She has smoked 1 pack of cigarettes for the past 35 years. Which of the following conclusions is most pertinent to these findings?
   A. She has the *BRCA1* gene mutation
   B. The postmenopausal estrogen replacement therapy should be stopped

C. Her risk of breast carcinoma is increased

D. She should stop smoking

9. A mutation in *p53* that causes a loss of its function can result in a(n)

A. Ability of cells to arrest in G, phase after DNA damage

B. Increase in the production of an angiogenesis inhibitor

C. Decrease in induction of apoptosis of damaged cells

D. Increase in DNA repair

10. A 68-year-old female, recently diagnosed with breast cancer, is undergoing chemotherapy treatment. Two weeks following his first treatment, the patient presents with weakness, hair loss, and oral ulcers. Which of the following best explains the mechanism underlying these signs and symptoms?

A. Actively cycling normal cells are destroyed by the drug

B. Cell cycle-nonspecific effects of the drug damage normal cells

C. Present signs and symptoms likely result from an undiagnosed pathology

D. Tumor cell lysis results in damage to normal body cells

References

1. Center for Disease Control and Prevention. Leading Causes of Death. www.cdc.gov/nchs/fastats/leading-causes-of-death.htm; Updated March 1, 2021. Accessed May 22, 2021.

2. Hanahan D, Weinberg RA. Hallmarks of cancer: the next generation. *Cell*. 2011;144:646–674.

3. National Cancer Institute. Metastatic Cancer: When Cancer Spreads. National Cancer Institute website; Updated November 10, 2020. Accessed May 22, 2021.

4. Leone P, Shin EC, Perosa F, Vacca A, Dammacco F, Racanelli V. MHC class I antigen processing and presenting machinery: organization, function, and defects in tumor cells. *J Natl Cancer Inst*. 2013;105(16):1172–1187. doi:10.3389/fendo.2017.00279.

5. Abdel-Haleem Lewis NE, Jamshidi N, Mineta K, Gao X, Gojobori T. The emerging facets of non-cancerous Warburg effect. *Front Endocrinol (Lausanne)*. 2017;8:279.

6. Martincorena I, Raine KM, Gerstung M, et al. Universal patterns of selection in cancer and somatic tissues. *Cell*. 2018;173(7):1029–1041.

7. Iqbal N, Iqbal N. Human epidermal growth factor recepter (HER2) in cancers: overexpression and therapeutic implications. *Mol Biol Int*. 2014:852748. doi:10.1155/2014/852748.

8. Abegglen LM, Caulin AF, Chan A, et al. potential mechanisms for cancer resistance in elephants and comparative cellular response to DNA damage in humans. *JAMA*. 2015;314(17):1850–1860.

9. Sobhani N, D'Angelo A, Wang X, Young KH, Generali D, Li Y. Mutant p53 as an antigen in cancer immunotherapy. *Int J Mol Sci*. 2020;21(11):4087. doi:10.3390/ijms21114087.

10. Dick FA, Goodrich DW, Sage J, Dyson NJ. Non-canonical functions of the RB protein in cancer. *Nat Rev Cancer*. 2018;18(7):442–451.

11. Knudson AG. Mutation and cancer: statistical study of retinoblastoma. *Proc Natl Acad Sci USA*. 1971;68(4):820–823.

12. Gorodetska I, Kozeretska I, Dubrovska A. BRCA genes: the role in genome stability, cancer stemness, and therapy resistance. *J Cancer*. 2019;10(9):2109–2127.

13. Online Mendelian Inheritance in Man. OMIM Entry Statistics. https://omim.org/statistics/entry; Updated May 6, 2021. Accessed May 6, 2021.

14. Baylin SB, Jones PA. Epigenetic determinants in cancer. *Cold Spring Harb Perspect Biol*. 2016;8:a019505. doi:10.1101/cshperspect.a019505.

15. Nasir A, Hassan Bullo MM, Ahmed Z, Imtiaz A, Yaqoob E, Jadoon M. Nutrigenomics: epigenetics and cancer prevention: a comparative review. *Crit Rev Food Sci Nutr*. 2020;60(8):1375–1387.

16. Gröber U, Holzhauer P, Kisters K, Holick MF, Adamietz IA. Micronutrients in oncological intervention. *Nutrients*. 2016;8(3):163. doi:10.3390/nu8030163.

17. Grzioli E, Dimauro I, Mecatelli N, et al. Physical activity in the prevention of human diseases: role of epigenetic modifications. *BMC Genom*. 2017;18(suppl 8):802. doi:10.1186/s12864-017-4193-5.

18. Wong JS, Kqueen-Cheah Y. Potential miRNAs for miRNA-based therapeutics in breast cancer. *Non-coding RNA*. 2020;6(3):29. doi:10.3390/ncrna6030029.

19. Vogelstein B, Kinzler K. The multistep nature of carcinogenesis. *Trends Genet*. 1993;9(4):138–141.

20. Baldo BA, Pham NH. Targeted drugs for cancer therapy: small molecules and monoclonal antibodies. *Drug Allergy*.2020:59–137.

21. Ashworth TR. A case of cancer in which cells similar to those in the tumours were seen in the blood after death. *Aust Med J*. 1869;14:146.

22. Adler AM, Carlton R. *Introduction to Radiologic & Imaging Sciences & Patient Care*. 7th ed.: Elsevier; 2019.

5

Medical Management and Cancer Treatments

STEVEN M. BURT, RN, MSN, NP-C, JULIA C. OSBORNE, BSC (HONS) PT, CLT-LANA

CHAPTER OUTLINE

Introduction

Establishing a cancer treatment regimen requires complex analysis and an in-depth consideration of the pathology and histology of the presenting cancer. Each diagnosis has its staging and grading set, requiring each cancer to be viewed independently for their overall prognosis and survivability. In conjunction with staging and grading, the diagnostic process also takes into consideration numerous factors such as protein biomarkers, genetic biomarkers, hormone receptor status of the cancer cells, oncotype testing, recurrence scores, and any comorbidity at diagnosis. There is a substantial body of evidence that diagnosis at an earlier stage improves the response to treatment and likelihood of a curative outcome.

History and Background of Cancer Treatment

The disease that we now know as cancer emerged in the late 1700s and was often treated surgically. Following a hundred years of exploration and cell classification, radiation was first used as a cancer treatment in the late 19th century. The first chemotherapy was discovered as a result of mustard gas causing toxic changes to bone marrow cells of soldiers in World War II. Billions of dollars have been invested in the ongoing development of cancer treatment options over subsequent decades, and still today, research continues with ever-advancing sophistication and ever improving outcomes. With so many treatment options available, there needed to be an international system of prioritization of treatment options for all cancer types. This resulted in the formation of the National Comprehensive Cancer Network (NCCN), announced on January 31, 1995. Today, the NCCN is "dedicated to improving and facilitating quality, effective, efficient, and accessible cancer care so patients can live better lives."[1] The NCCN has developed guidelines for treatment by cancer type, including systemic and localized chemotherapy, radiation, surgery, hematopoietic stem cell transplantation, as well as new and innovative treatments.

Overview of Cancer Treatment

The treatment of cancer requires a multidisciplinary approach, often involving a combination of surgery, chemotherapy, biologic agents, and radiation. An episode of treatment can vary widely in terms of duration and mode (unimodal vs. multimodal). The National Cancer Database reviewed all cancer sites from 2008 to 2017 to estimate percent of patients who received single versus combinations of multimodal treatment. With respect to unimodal treatment, it was estimated that 35% of patients required surgery only, 4.9% required radiation only, and 5.1% required chemotherapy only. When combining multimodal forms of treatment, the numbers of options became numerous. The number of patients requiring a combination of surgery, radiation, and chemotherapy was 4.7%, with 6.0% requiring surgery and chemotherapy, and 4.8% requiring radiation and chemotherapy.[2]

The NCCN uses current Food and Drug Association (FDA)-approved research findings to provide disease-site algorithms for medical treatment planning and intervention. For example, in the pathway of breast cancer treatment, all patients will require an initial biopsy evaluated by the pathology team (Figure 5.1). Decisions are then made by the medical team based on a combination of clinical trial results and NCCN guidelines for treating the breast cancer disease site.

The degree and extent of a treatment regimen is based upon the stage, histologic grade, tumor pathology, receptor status, genetic abnormalities, and the patient's performance status at the time of diagnosis and throughout the treatment calendar.

Cancer Staging and Determining a Treatment Regimen

Cancer staging refers to the extent of the size and spread of the tumor. There are many staging systems; the most familiar is the TNM staging system (Tumor, Node, and Metastases). The American Joint Committee on Cancer (AJCC) published the 8th edition of the AJCC Cancer Staging Manual in October 2016.[3] This manual is commonly used by physicians to classify cancer patients, estimate a prognosis, and establish treatment approaches.

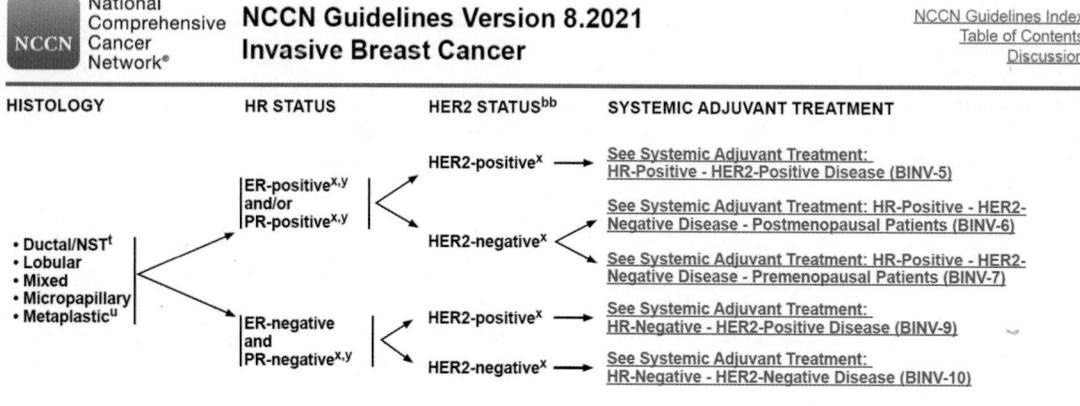

• **Fig. 5.1** Breast Cancer Treatment Algorithm.
t, According to the WHO carcinoma of no special type (NST) encompasses multiple patterns including medullary pattern, cancers with neuroendocrine expression, and other rare patterns.
u, There are rare subtypes of metaplastic carcinoma (e.g., low-grade adenosquamous and low-grade fibromatosis-like carcinoma) that are considered to have a favorable prognosis without adjuvant systemic therapies).
x, Correlation of histology, hormone receptor (HR), and HER2 status should always be done with awareness of unusual/discordant or borderline results.
y, Although patients with cancers with 1%-100% ER IHC staining are considered ER-positive and eligible for endocrine therapies, there are more limited data on the subgroup of cancers with ER-low-positive (1%-10%) results. The ER-low-positive group is heterogenous with reported biologic behavior often similar to ER-negative cancers; thus, individualized consideration of risks versus benefits of endocrine therapy and additional adjuvant therapies should be incorporated into decision making.
bb, footnote discontinued by NCCN in 2021 version of guidelines.

To date, with recent revisions, they have 104 printable staging forms for different cancers. It is important to note that there are other disease-specific staging classification systems, such as FIGO (International Federation of Gynecology and Obstetrics) for gynecological malignancies and Duke's Classification for colon cancer.[4] Hematological cancers have staging systems that are specific to each disease. Leukemias do not utilize the TNM system; instead, each subset has a unique system. Some additional cancers that do not use the TNM system include select childhood cancers, other hematological cancers, cancers of the female reproductive organs (FIGO), or central nervous system tumors (e.g., primary brain cancers). See Chapter 1 for background on cancer staging and grading.

Cancer Protein Biomarkers

Further specification of cancer and its treatment employs the identification of cancer protein biomarkers. These are also known as tumor markers and cytogenetic markers. Tumor markers and cytogenic markers are either released by tumor cells into the blood stream or released by surrounding tissues in response to the tumor cells. These allow further specification of the tumor and how it might behave. Tumor and cytogenic markers are also used as a form of disease surveillance over time.

Genetics and Molecular Genetic Studies

Genetics and molecular genetic studies contribute to the diagnosis and management of cancers. Genetic markers can also be tools for following a tumor's response to therapy, monitoring responses, and providing a sensitive means to detect relapse.[5] For example, in order to diagnose a person with chronic myeloid leukemia, the mutated gene BCR-ABL must be present. The additional genetic test can establish the degree of gene mutation present that guides treatment initiation and anticipated response to treatment. Also, gene expression tools for diagnoses such as breast, colon, and prostate cancers allow for the prediction of prognosis and outcomes. Genetic testing for inherited cancer genes allows for the identification of susceptibility genes within family trees. This provides opportunity for early or more frequent cancer screenings, prophylactic treatment options, and ongoing surveillance. The overall result is that increasing numbers of patients are being diagnosed earlier, providing greater opportunity for long-term survivorship.

Cancer Surgery

Cancer surgery is the oldest form of cancer treatment. Today, approximately 60% of people diagnosed with cancer will undergo some type of surgery. In some cases, this will be the only treatment required.[6] Cancer-related surgery is unique in that with the removal of the tumor, adjacent local-regional lymph nodes are often concurrently removed for biopsy and cancer staging purposes. This acute trauma to the local-regional lymphatic system can impact fluid equilibrium locally, thereby slowing down tissue healing times. This needs to be taken into consideration when managing acute surgical patients and their functional recovery. Other factors that impact the rate of tissue healing in patients recovering from cancer-related surgery include residual disease itself, pre-existing co-morbidities, and any multimodal treatments that the patient may have undergone prior to surgery, including radiation therapy and chemotherapy.

Intent of Surgery

Curative Surgery

Curative surgery is intended to remove all malignant (cancerous) tissue. It works best on localized cancers that have not demonstrated evidence of metastatic spread.[6] This includes removing part or all cancerous tissue and a small margin of the surrounding tissue with the likelihood of removal of local-regional lymph nodes for biopsy to determine the extent of local invasion, or absence thereof.[7]

Upon review of the pathology, the extent of the surgical margins is measured. If cancer extends beyond or close to the obtained specimen's margin, the treatment team will consider additional surgery—a re-excision of the tumor bed. Once surgery is completed, the patient may be offered radiation and/or chemotherapy. Many cancer forms have curative options with surgery alone, including cancers of the colon, prostate, breast, skin, cranial-based, head and neck, and lung.

Many times, there is a need to remove local lymph nodes adjacent to the surgical bed. It is typically a select sample, known as a sentinel lymph node biopsy (SNLB), or where applicable, a more aggressive lymph node dissection (LND) in which several nodes are removed. The sentinel lymph nodes are typically the first few lymph nodes in the lymph node bed to which the primary tumor drains. During SNLB, a substance, often a radioactive blue dye, is injected at the tumor site. The local lymphatic system will recognize the dye as a foreign substance and absorb it into its vessels and transport the dye to the apical or sentinel (first) lymph node in the nearest regional local lymph node bed. The pathway of the blue dye represents the exact same pathway in which the local lymphatic system will absorb invasive cancer cells and transport them to the apical or sentinel lymph node in the same regional local lymph node bed. This allows for the identification of the "first" lymph nodes that would most likely receive invasive cancer cells. If, after excision and analysis, the sentinel lymph node has no clear evidence of cancer cells, it improves confidence that the cancer has not locally metastasized.

The use of the sentinel lymph node procedure allows the surgeon to remove one to three apical/sentinel nodes that have proven to be an accurate route of migration for invasive cancer cells. An additional benefit of this type of procedure is that it precludes the need for a more extensive removal of lymph nodes, as well as decreasing postsurgical complications such as lymphedema. A SLNB may require transition into a LND, also known as a lymphadenectomy, when the sentinel lymph node has a high level of invasive cancer cells or there is a high level of suspicion that most of the remaining local lymph node bed is positive for cancer. This procedure has many more potential complications such as lymphedema, numbness, or tingling in the surgical area, and skin sloughing or breakdown, to name just a few.[8]

Debulking Surgery

A debulking surgery includes the removal of a substantial amount of the tumor, but some cancerous tissue will remain. This approach is employed when the removal of all cancerous tissue may result in unacceptable damage to surrounding organs or would be life threatening.[9] Many patients will require additional chemotherapy and/or radiation before or after this form of surgery. Debulking is more common in gynecological or genitourinary cancers prior to adjuvant (subsequent) treatments.

Palliative Surgery

In cases where the cancer disease process has progressed beyond the controls of combination therapies (multiple forms of chemotherapy and radiation therapy), palliative surgery can be used to manage a person's cancer symptoms. Palliative surgery is performed to control the cancer and its symptoms, not cure it. These surgeries incorporate the removal of cancerous tissue that is causing pain or dysfunction. It can also include surgeries such as the placement of a nerve block for pain control, or stent placement to alleviate obstructions in major blood vessels or along the gastrointestinal (GI) tract.[10] Kyphoplasty or internal fixation for bone metastases is also considered a palliative surgery.

Surgery for Device Implantation

In addition to the significant surgeries that many patients require for tumor management, there are additional surgical procedures that one may need to undergo to support other cancer treatments. For example, patients who receive systemic chemotherapy will have the option for placement of a peripherally inserted central line (PICC) or Mediport for safe and effective chemotherapy delivery. The surgical placement of an intraventricular access device (Ommaya reservoir) for the delivery of intrathecal chemotherapy is another example of device implantation (Figure 5.2).

Surgery for Pain Management

For patients actively receiving anticancer treatment, 59% report pain and one-third of patients even have pain after completing curative treatment.[11] The World Health Organizations' Analgesic Ladder has four steps that escalate to meet the pain management needs of patients. Ladder steps 1 to 3 require a combination of oral and transdermal agents with varying duration. The 4th and final level endorses nerve blocks, epidurals, neurolytic block therapies, and spinal stimulators. All are surgically implanted for the safe delivery of effective pain medication.[11]

Restorative Surgery

Restorative surgery is performed to improve cosmesis or improve functioning of a body part. These surgeries are often performed after curative surgery has taken place and once healing is completed or recovery from adjuvant treatments has occurred. Typical examples include breast reconstruction to restore shape and volume, oral surgery to restore the mouth's function, and rectal

surgery to implant artificial sphincters following treatment. One unique example is rotationplasty, which may be utilized in cases of osteosarcoma around the knee. After surgical excision and removal of the knee joint, the lower leg is moved up and fused to the distal femur after being rotated 180 degrees (Figure 5.3). A key component of this procedure is preservation of the nervous and vascular structures to allow for sensation and ankle plantarflexion (serving as "knee extension") and dorsiflexion (serving as "knee flexion") (Figure 5.4). After appropriate healing, a custom prosthesis can be applied to the newly rotated foot to restore gait function.

Surgical Approaches

The last section discussed the intent of the surgery for patients diagnosed with cancer. This section will focus on the types of surgical interventions available to patients with cancer.

Open Surgery

From the earliest days of surgery, the favored procedure was an open surgery. This type of surgery is known for making an incision in the skin using a scalpel with a typically sizeable surgical field, allowing the surgeon to view the intended tumor and its surrounding tissue. An open field is beneficial in surgeries with a known large tumor bed, local spread, or metastatic disease. Disadvantages of this approach may include a more extended recovery period, a greater potential for infection, a decrease in normal function, and additional scar tissue development.

Minimally Invasive Surgeries

The trend for the past 30 years has been a transition from the traditional "open surgery" to minimally invasive surgery. Substantial evidence has shown superior patient outcomes for this type of surgery over traditional open surgery for many standard procedures.[12]

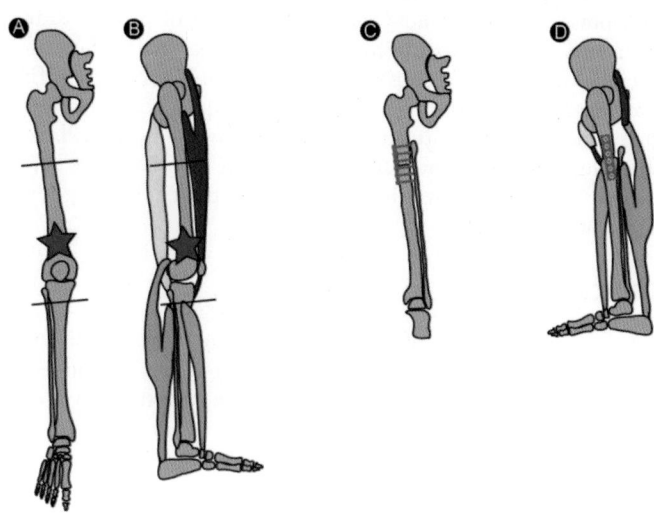

• **Fig. 5.3** Rotationplasty After Sarcoma Excision. (Reprinted with permission from Bernthal NM, Monument MJ, Randall RL, Jones KB. Rotationplasty: beauty is in the eye of the beholder. *Oper Tech Orthop.* 2014;24(2):103–110.)
A: Surgical planning for excision of diseased bone
B: Visualization of muscle structures to be preserved or transposed during excision
C: Internal fixation connecting the rotated tibia to the femoral shaft.
D: Muscular connections and transpositions after tumor excision.

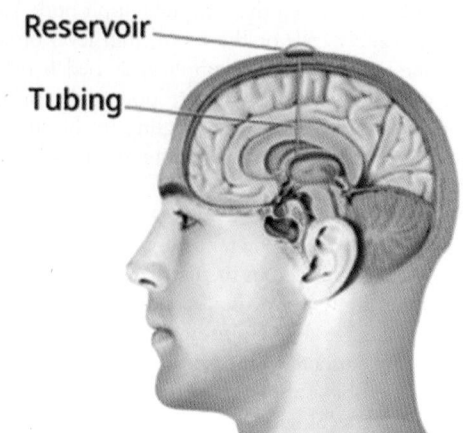

Reservoir
Tubing

• **Fig. 5.2** Intraventricular Access Device Placement. (Reprinted with permission from Elsevier Patient Handouts. Intraventricular Access Device Placement. https://www.clinicalkey.com/#!/content/patient_handout/5-s2.0-pe_66cad1fc-b1b0-4292-8e82-6c4e0b9a0f2c. Accessed April 17, 2021.)

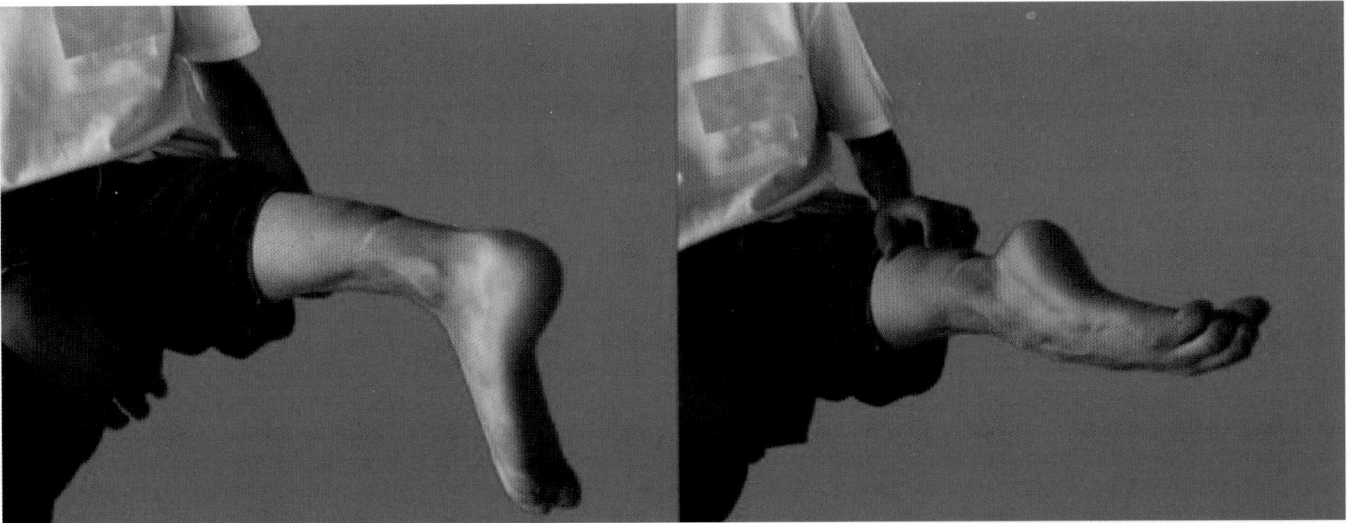

• **Fig. 5.4** Rotationplasty Which Uses Ankle Dorsiflexion to Replicate Knee Flexion. (Reprinted with permission from Bernthal NM, Monument MJ, Randall RL, Jones KB. Rotationplasty: beauty is in the eye of the beholder. *Oper Tech Orthop.* 2014;24(2):103–110.)

Laparoscopy

The most common of the minimally invasive surgeries is laparoscopic surgery. Laparoscopic surgery is often utilized for abdominal or pelvic cancers via small incisions with the procedure being guided with a small camera inserted into the cavity. In laparoscopic surgeries, the surgeon holds and directly places the instruments through the incisions and manually directs the probes to complete the procedure. Initially laparoscopic surgery was used for benign conditions such as splenectomy, pancreatectomy, gastrectomy, and hepatectomy. However, these were found to be safe and effective for oncologic diagnoses as well. Once validated, its use has expanded to many of the standard gastric and gynecological cancers. In 2008, a randomized trial comparing laparoscopy-assisted colectomy (LAC) versus open colectomy (OC) for colon cancer revealed a tendency of higher cancer-related survival ($P = .07$) and overall survival ($P = .06$) for the LAC. The probability of cancer-related survival was higher in the LAC group ($P = .02$) when compared with the OC.[13] Today it is the preferred method of surgery for colon, kidney, as well as many gynecologic cancers.

Robotic Surgery

Similar to laparoscopic surgery, robotic surgery utilizes probes placed in the body via a small incision. However, with robotic surgery, the surgeon sits at a control console some distance away from the patient, leaving the scrub nurse and surgical assistant at the bedside. The surgeon performs the surgery utilizing a finger control or joystick that directs the probes in the patient's cavity. The first robotic surgery was introduced to the theater of surgery about 25 years ago.[14] The benefits of robotic surgery have been well documented, including decreased blood loss, shorter hospital stays, and faster recovery.[15]

Cryosurgery

Cryosurgery (also known as cryotherapy) uses extreme cold to damage and destroy cancerous tissue. The cold is produced by liquid nitrogen or argon gas delivered directly to the cancerous tissue. Cryosurgery is used to treat superficial tumors such as skin cancers but it can also be implemented for internal and bone-based tumors. For internal tumors, cryotherapy can be applied to the tumor via a special probe called the cryoprobe. This allows contact and application directly to the tumor.[16]

Laser Surgery

Lasers are used for a variety of surgical intents including cutting, coagulating, or ablating tissues. Lasers utilize the emission of a single, coherent wavelength of light. Laser surgery can be supported by computer-based imaging and guidance systems to improve precision, control, and efficiency of surgery. In addition to their ability to cut or burn tissue, laser irritation alters cellular metabolism and cellular functions at the tumor site.[17] The primary clinical applications of lasers are external structures with easy accessibility, such as skin and the cornea, however, minimally invasive procedures can be utilized to treat deeper structures such as GI mucosa and bronchial structures.[18] Laser surgery is currently used to treat active cancers of the esophagus, lung, penis, and numerous cancers of the skin. The procedure is well-tolerated, with the adverse effects localized to the area of treatment. Patients often experience pain, slight bleeding, and potential for infection.[19]

Chemotherapy

During World War II in Bari Harbor, Italy, sulfur mustards were accidently spilled onto troops. The bone marrow and lymph nodes were found to be markedly depleted in those men that were exposed to the mustard gas.[20] This mishap led to the development and first administration of nitrogen mustard, the first documented chemotherapy drug for lymphoma in the 1940s. The 1940s and 1950s subsequently saw the development of chemotherapeutic agents such as methotrexate, vincristine, and vinblastine, all of which are still used today. Advances in anticancer drug discovery has resulted in the development of more than 100 anticancer drugs approved by the FDA between 1949 and 2014.[21] From 2015 to 2020 there has been a significant upswing in approved antineoplastic agents with approximately 40+ oncology drugs approved yearly. The report indicates that 44 new oncology drugs are expected to be approved in 2020, the most releases of oncologic agents in a given year by far.[22]

"First-line" chemotherapy is generally considered to be the evidence-based first choice to attempt to cure or control a cancer.[23] The current first-line therapies range from a single dose administration to weeks (if not months) of chemotherapy dosing to treat many different cancer types. The standard of care is an established course of treatment that is evidence-based and is inclusive of clinical practice guidelines provided by the Agency for Healthcare Research and Quality (AHRQ) and the NCCN. Before selecting and administering the regimens, many factors need to be considered, such as age, comorbidities, quality of life (QOL) considerations, and internal organ health. The choice of a chemotherapy regimen is not a "one size fits all" situation. Many regimens will be made up of multiple chemotherapy agents as well as other medications to control acute adverse effects such as nausea, anaphylactic shock, GI distress (i.e., vomiting and diarrhea), immunosuppression, and organ compromise. See Chapter 6 for further discussion on the variety of chemotherapy medications, pharmacologic effects, and adverse effects.

Cancer treatments can be as simple as a chemotherapy regimen; however, they may include additional surgery and radiation to produce the best outcomes. The timing and selection of which therapy drugs are administered initially versus secondarily or, in some instances, delivered together, has been studied for decades. Chemotherapy can be prescribed as induction chemotherapy, neoadjuvant chemotherapy, or adjuvant chemotherapy. This refers to the timing of treatment delivery as well as the desired function of chemotherapy treatment.

Induction Chemotherapy

Induction chemotherapy is considered the first line treatment of cancer using chemotherapeutic drugs with a curative intent. The goal and function of induction chemotherapy is to induce a cure. It is beneficial in the control of malignant lymphomas and squamous cell carcinomas (SCCs) of the head and neck when followed by surgery and/or radiation therapy or when treated concurrently with chemoradiotherapy.

Neoadjuvant Chemotherapy

Neoadjuvant chemotherapy is the administration of chemotherapy drugs with an intent to shrink the primary tumor and any potential distant micro-metastases before the use of surgery and/or radiation.[24] The desired effect of the neoadjuvant chemotherapy is to improve the chance of cure for a patient with an aggressive, fast growing cancer or a cancer with significant depth of invasion by achieving a *pathological complete response* (pCR). A pCR is determined when subsequent surgical excision of the primary tumor and associated apical/sentinel lymph nodes reveals pathology that is clear of any live cancer cells. Should any live cancer cells be located in the primary tumor site or associated apical/sentinel lymph nodes, the pathologist determines that there is a *pathological incomplete response* (pIR).

Adjuvant Chemotherapy

Adjuvant chemotherapy is typically used after all visible cancer has been removed with surgery and/or radiation.[24] Common aims of adjuvant chemotherapy are to attempt to treat any remaining cancer cells that may have remained in the local surgical area or micro-metastases that may have entered the systemic circulation or lymphatic tracts.

Administration of Chemotherapy

The delivery of chemotherapy occurs in many methods. It ranges from localized administration to systemic administration. The most common route of administration is systemic chemotherapy. Systemic treatment refers to drugs or therapies that potentially affect the entire body.[24] Although the advantages of systemic therapy is that it will reach cancer cells in distant areas of the body, it also concurrently affects healthy, noncancer cells, resulting in a wide variety of adverse effects. While intravenous (IV) and oral methods of administration are most common, examples of additional methods include topical, intrathecal, and subcutaneous administration.

Intravenous Administration

Chemotherapy is most frequently delivered via the peripheral IV system. The administration can be a peripheral IV, a peripherally inserted central catheter (PICC) line, an implanted venous access port ("port" or "mediport"), or a central line catheter. The advantages of IV chemotherapy are that there is an immediate therapeutic effect on cancer, the ability to administer several agents simultaneously, and the ability to reach distant sites, all with greater bioavailability. Many persons living with an acute cancer diagnosis have the aforementioned micro-metastases—a small collection of cancer cells shed from the original tumor that will metastasize to a distant site via blood or lymph nodes. They group to form a second tumor that is too small to be seen with imaging tests until such time that they reach a critical mass that is detectable by imaging tests.[25]

The disadvantages of IV chemotherapy include the potential for collateral damage that includes extravasation (when the chemotherapeutic agents leaks outside of the vein to the surrounding tissue), bruising or hematoma, clots at the IV site, or vein irritation/phlebitis. Some oncologists choose to give the patient a *dose-dense* chemotherapy when indicated. This involves delivery of a normal dose of chemotherapy; however, it is delivered at a higher frequency to aggressively treat the cancer before it has a chance to recover or develop drug resistance. As this is a quite aggressive cancer treatment, the adverse effects of dose-dense treatment can be more pronounced and more acute; however, there is early evidence showing that if the patient can handle dose-dense chemotherapy, the outcomes may be better.[26]

Oral Chemotherapy

Oral chemotherapy is another option for the systemic treatment of cancer. Oral neoplastic agents can provide a more accessible, more affordable modality for cancer than parenteral chemotherapy and are also used as supplements to traditional chemotherapy.[27] Of the 69 new drugs approved by the FDA between 2015 and 2020, 44 are oral chemotherapy drugs.[28] The delivery can be via pill, capsule, or liquid form.

The primary advantage of oral chemotherapy is rooted in patient convenience. Patients also cite a greater sense of control over their treatment.[29] QOL is especially important in the palliative setting, and oral treatment can reduce home/life disruption for both the patient and their family.[30] The administration of oral agents leads to less time in the oncologist's office and infusion rooms. Oral therapy, combined with ease of use and typically an adverse effect profile less than IV chemotherapies, makes it an attractive option for active patients.

One of the main considerations of oral chemotherapy is the bioavailability of the drug, this being the portion of the drug that enters the circulation, which may be highly variable for some drugs. One major cause of the limited or variable bioavailability is the drugs susceptibility to chemical breakdown in GI fluids.[31] This variable bioavailability can lead to an unpredictable amount of drug that achieves systemic distribution to eventually reach the target tissue.[32] Where the range of bioavailability for cancer drugs extends from low to virtually zero, it seems that a simple solution would be to increase oral doses.[32] However, with certain drugs, increasing oral doses can lead to prohibitive patient toxicities. To this end, low or uncertain bioavailability has directed many oral regimens to be daily, weekly, every other week, or three weeks on and one week off cycles to assure adequate dosing for effective treatment.

Adherence is defined as the extent to which individuals take medications prescribed by their physicians.[27] Compliance can occur in both directions of adherence. Many patients attempt to manage their adverse effects by "taking a day off" to improve their current situation. On the other hand, in rare cases, some patients will take more than the prescribed dose to be more aggressive in their treatment. Both choices may have substantial implications on outcomes and adverse events.

Additional Routes of Administration

In addition to IV and oral chemotherapy delivery, there are additional delivery forms that all have their advantages and disadvantages.

Cancer that has invaded the brain or spinal cord may benefit from intrathecal administration of chemotherapy. This is advantageous as a smaller dose may be needed with intrathecal administration as compared to systemic chemotherapy where the blood-brain barrier limits the amount of drug that will reach the intended central nervous system tissue. The two main access routes for intrathecal are via a lumbar puncture or the aforementioned Ommaya reservoir (Figure 5.2). After administration, the cerebrospinal fluid distributes the drug to the target tissue. In the case of a lumbar puncture, the patient is often expected to lay supine for a few hours to allow for proper closure of the punctured dura.

Intra-arterial or arterial chemotherapy is the delivery of concentrated doses of chemotherapy via the arterial blood system directly to the tumor. The chemotherapy can cause additional adverse effects to the specific delivery area before being absorbed and disseminated to the entire body. Many of the symptoms typically associated with chemotherapy (e.g., anemia, weakening of the immune system, loss of hair, nausea) may be decreased when this method is used.[33] A drawback to this method includes artery irritation, damage to muscles, and skin damage. This is a standard delivery mechanism for liver cancer and can also be used in cancers of the brain and head and neck.

Intracavitary chemotherapy is the administration of concentrated chemotherapy into a body cavity. This form of delivery will allow for the treatment of bladder cancer (intravesical), abdominal cavity cancers (intraperitoneal), and chest cavity (intrapleural).[34] The benefits of this delivery include the direct application to the tumor site. Adverse effects could include pressure or bloating of the cavity, feeling of a full bladder or the urge to urinate, nausea and vomiting, anorexia, and cavity irritation.

Hyperthermic intraperitoneal chemotherapy (HIPEC) is a cancer treatment that involves filling the abdominal cavity with chemotherapy drugs that have been heated and then subsequently drained in the abdomen (Figure 5.5). Also known as "hot chemotherapy", HIPEC is performed after surgical excision or tumor debulking from the abdomen. HIPEC is used to treat cancers that have invaded the lining of the abdominal cavity, such as those of the appendix, colon, stomach, and ovaries.

Topical chemotherapy is applying the chemotherapeutic medication to the skin as a lotion, cream, or ointment. These typically treat cancers of the skin. The advantages are the ease of use and

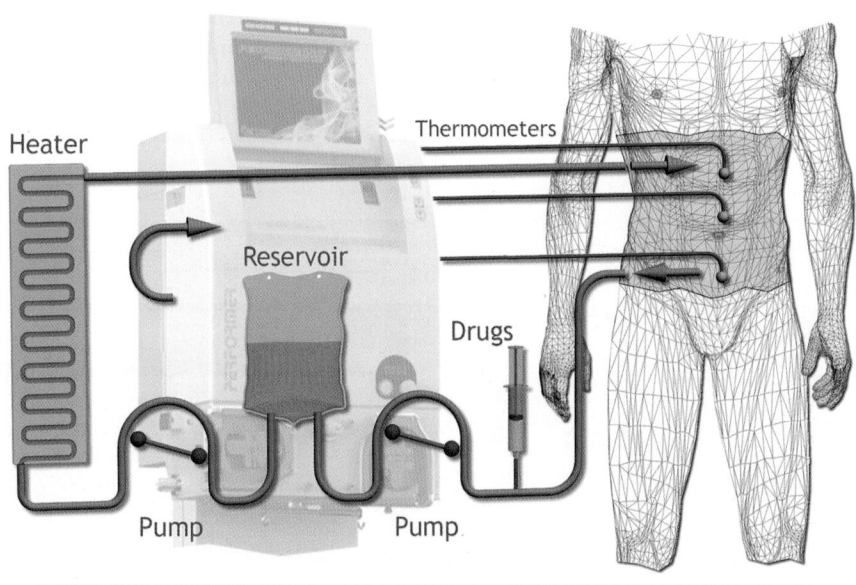

Hyperthermic Intra-Peritoneal Chemotherapy (HIPEC)

• **Fig. 5.5** Hyperthermic Intraperitoneal Chemotherapy. (Reprinted with permission from Corrado Bellini— Own work, CC BY-SA 4.0.)

quick application. The disadvantages include sensitive and red skin that burns, discharges fluid, itches, and changes color.[35]

Additional routes of administration of chemotherapeutic agents include intramuscular chemotherapy, subcutaneous chemotherapy, electrochemotherapy, and intralesional/intratumor chemotherapy.

Considerations During Exposure to Hazardous Drugs

The United States Pharmacopeial Convention (USP) is an organization that disseminates quality standards for medications. This is published in a compendium called US Pharmacopeia and National Formulary (USP-NF). The focus of USP Chapter <800> is the handling of hazardous drugs (HDs) in healthcare settings (https://www.usp.org/compounding/general-chapter-hazardous-drugs-handling-healthcare).[36] The aim is to promote worker safety, patient safety, and environmental protection, especially as it relates to long-term, low level exposures such as those experienced by oncology rehabilitation (Onc R) clinicians over a long career. The National Institute for Occupational Safety and Health (NIOSH) maintains a list of antineoplastic and other hazardous drugs.[37] Although most of Chapter <800> relates to preparing and administering hazardous drugs, as Onc R clinicians are going to be providing direct hands-on care, there is a risk for potential exposure. As an example, Chapter <800> identifies that patient-care activities such as "Handling body fluids (e.g., urine, feces, sweat, or vomit) or body-fluid contaminated clothing, dressings, linens, and other materials" is a potential route of exposure, including with those who have received antineoplastic therapy.[36p4] Patients on HDs can continue to excrete HDs and metabolites for days after administration. Clinicians are advised to utilize universal precautions vigilantly when there is a potential exposure to body fluids for a person using hazardous drugs according to NIOSH (which includes many antineoplastic drugs), (See https://www.cdc.gov/niosh/topics/hazdrug/default.html for a regularly updated list and resources.)[37] Depending on the situation and rehabilitation task to be undertaken, gloves, gown, eyewear, and/or masks would be warranted. In some HD situations where exposure risk is high, two pairs of gloves are advocated.[36] Any healthcare facility working with persons who are using one of these HDs should have a policy or procedure based on Chapter <800> standards which

should provide specific examples based upon the task and which precautions are necessary.[36]

Radiation Therapy

In 1896, Wilhelm Conrad Roentgen, a German physics professor presented a groundbreaking finding entitled "On a New Kind of Ray."[38] Within months of this publication, X-rays would be used for diagnosis and only 3 years later, radiation therapy consisting of X-rays and gamma rays began to be applied to treat cancer.[39] Unfortunately, early on, the researchers discovered that radiation could not only treat cancer, but it could also cause cancer. The focus of research rapidly shifted to controlling the amount of radiation delivered to an area treated. In the early 1950s the linear accelerator (Figure 5.6) was developed which allowed for increased precision and reduced adverse effects. Today the variety of delivery mechanisms for radiation for cancer treatment allow for highly precise and effective treatments.

Radiation is a treatment modality that delivers energy to kill malignant cells in the area targeted explicitly by clinicians. The radiation damages the DNA of the cancer cells by ionizing atoms, thereby causing breaks in the DNA strands.[40] This mechanism is considered the dominant factor that causes cellular death.[40] As with chemotherapy, the treatment affects both malignant and normal tissue in the field of treatment. However, in many cases, normal cells have the ability to withstand treatment and repair faster than malignant cells. The success of radiation therapy is dependent on dividing up the delivery of the total dose via fractionation or therapeutic ratio, which provides a risk-benefit approach to planning radiation. Radiotherapy is measured in the units Gray (Gy) and is divided into fractions. Fractionation, or dividing of the total doses into small daily fractions delivered over days to weeks, takes advantage of normal and malignant tissue's differential repair abilities.

In its essence, radiation is the acceleration of high-energy radiation beams used to damage the patients' DNA to prevent replication or induce cell death. In the field of radiation, there are many different beams utilized for treatments. Radiation beams come from three different particles: photons, protons, and electrons. The most commonly utilized particles are photons. Photons, in low dose forms, are used in X-rays. In radiation oncology, their benefit at higher doses is reaching tumors deep in the body. The photon beam's disadvantage is their inability to stop at the tumor

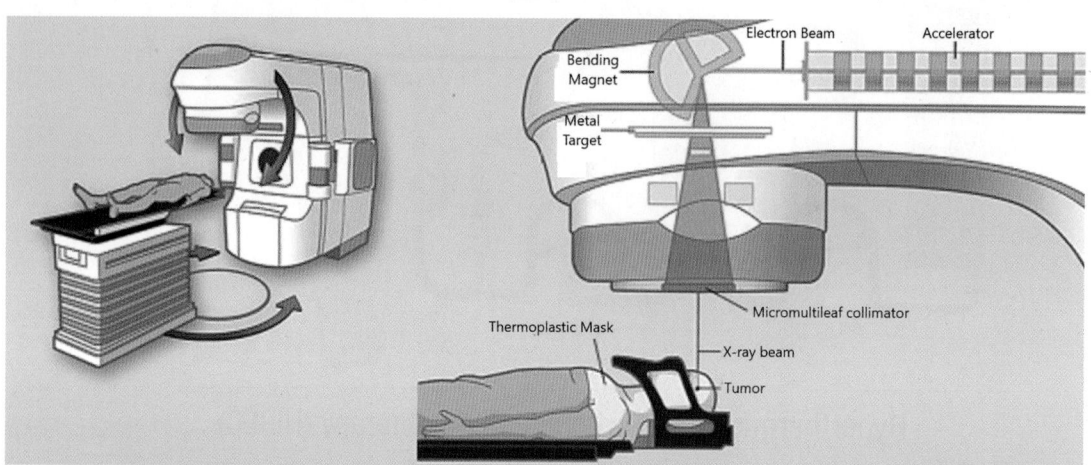

• **Fig. 5.6** Linear Accelerator. (Adapted with permission from D'Ambrosio AL, DeYoung C, Isaacson SR. Radiosurgical management of brain. *Neurosurg Clin N Am.* 2011;22(1):45–51.)

site, thus emitting their beam distal to the tumor. This exposure to surrounding tissue produces additional adverse effects such as radiation-induced fibrosis in soft tissue structures, and osteoradionecrosis in local boney tissue.

The most common delivery of photon radiation is from a linear accelerator which delivers external beam radiation therapy (EBRT) to a specified area of treatment. In a linear accelerator, the electrons accelerate to high energy which will exit the machine or strike a target to produce X-rays (a.k.a. photons). They can generate either photon or electron beams of various energies, and their output is managed with sophisticated computer controls (Figure 5.6).[40]

The primary difference between photons and electrons is the depth of the treatment that they can deliver. Photons are commonly used when the tumor is positioned deeper in the body. Electrons are utilized when the tumor is superficial, such as skin and breast tissue, allowing for a minimal degree of deeper tissue and organ damage. A typical comprehensive radiation plan utilizes a combination of the two types of beams.

One of the key clinical implications for Onc R professionals is that radiation does not have an immediate effect on tissue integrity. It generally takes approximately 1 to 2 weeks before tissue damage becomes apparent. After 7 to 14 days there can be substantial pain and skin burning which may require adaptations to a rehabilitation regimen (Figure 5.7). In some cases, late-effect radiation fibrosis may occur months to years after completion of radiation and requires the skills of an Onc R clinician to address (see Chapter 7).

Figure 5.8 depicts the amount of cells that survive based on radiation dosage. As depicted on the red line in the Figure 5.8, there is no consistent cell death over time when the radiation is completed in small dosages. After the radiation therapy regimen is completed, cancer cells and normal cells in the radiation field will continue to experience cell death.

As with any type of cancer treatment, radiotherapy is a delicate balance between killing the tumor cells as aggressively as possible without causing substantial damage to normal cells and adverse

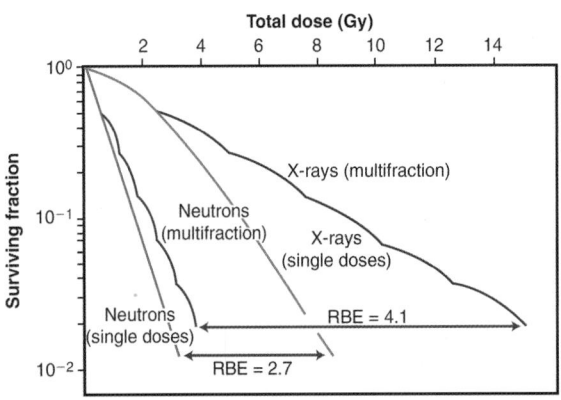

• **Fig. 5.8** Cellular Survival Curve With Fractionation Proportions of Surviving Cells to Radiation as a Function of its Severity (in Gy). Relative biological effectiveness (RBE) is defined as the ratio of the doses required by two radiations to cause the same level of effect (e.g., neutrons vs. X-rays). (Reprinted with permission from Zeman EM. Chapter 1: The biological basis of radiation oncology. In: *Gunderson & Tepper's Clinical Radiation Oncology.* 5th ed. Elsevier; 2020:20.)

effects such as skin breakdown, wounds, or organ failure that could threaten the person's health further. Therefore, the dosages are often done for small amounts of time daily with a break in between (usually aligned with weekends) over the course of weeks.

Simulation and Immobilization During Radiation Therapy

One of the key steps prior to initiating a radiation therapy regimen is the treatment planning process. The radiation oncologist will use sophisticated imaging software from computerized tomography to outline the tumor and minimize the impact to surrounding tissues—termed a *simulation*. Then the dosage in Gy is determined, and a treatment plan is established. In some cases, a permanent or temporary tattoo will be placed to assure consistent alignment of the radiation therapy beam. Patient set-up for treatment planning includes custom immobilization devices made for each individual patient in the treatment position.

Once a patient is "simulated" or "simmed" on one specific machine, generally that is their machine for the entire treatment dose delivery. In some cases, if the patient has substantial change in body structure, re-simulating may be necessary as the tumor's position may have changed anatomically. This might occur, for example, in the case of a substantial weight loss during treatment post head and neck cancer surgery.

Figure 5.9 depicts a blue bag immobilization, where the bag is filled with a conforming foam to the person's specific body habitus to allow them to get exactly into the position needed for repeated sessions. Most patients can be positioned in supine, but in some cases a different position such as prone or sidelying may be necessary. One key component for Onc R clinicians to consider is that some patients diagnosed with thoracic or breast cancers may need to be positioned with their arms above their head, and may require rehabilitation to improve range of motion to achieve this position prior to initiating radiation therapy. In addition to bluebag immobilization, individuals who have brain, or head and neck cancer may be positioned using an Aquaplast mask (Figure 5.10). It is important that this mask is fastened to the table to assure that the patient's head position remains stable during the treatment and from session to session. Many patients report claustrophobia from this device,

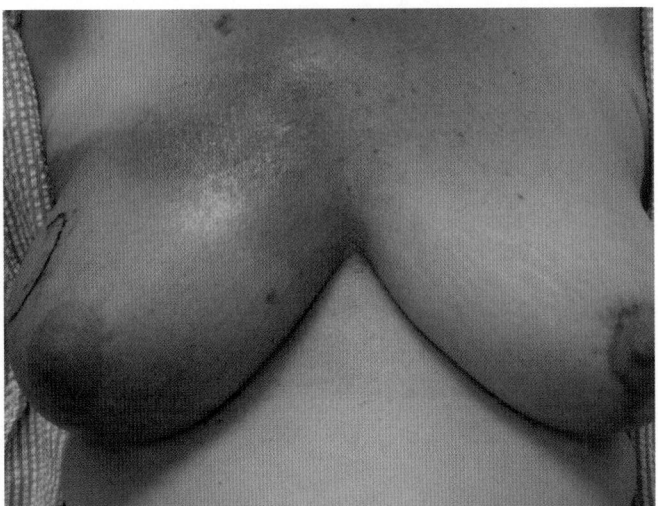

• **Fig. 5.7** Delayed Skin Changes After Radiation. Example of a patient treated with the standard 6-week radiation therapy with a sequential boost regimen demonstrating grade 2 erythema during the final week of treatment (2 Gy × 23 in 39 days). (Reprinted with permission from Raza S, Lymberis SC, Ciervide R, et al. Comparison of acute and late toxicity of two regimens of 3- and 5-week concomitant boost prone IMRT to standard 6-week breast radiotherapy. *Front Oncol.* 2012;2:44. doi:10.3389/fonc.2012.00044. Reprinted under CC BY 4.0 license.)

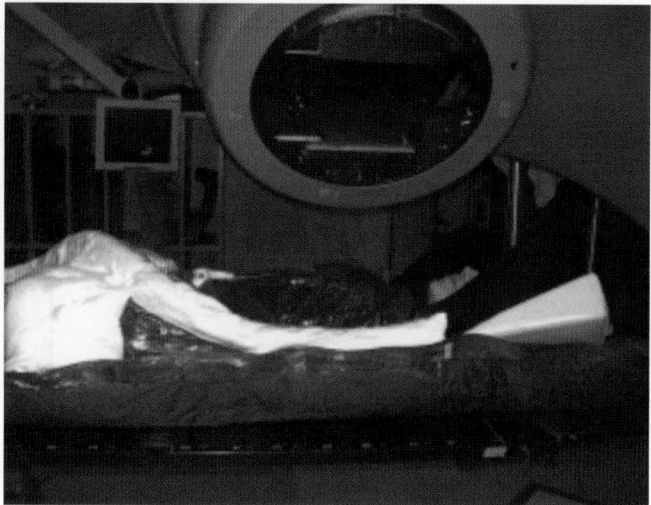

• **Fig. 5.9** Patient Immobilization With BodyFix System (Medical Intelligence). (Reprinted with permission from Swift PS. Radiation for spinal metastatic tumors. *Orthop Clin North Am.* 2009;40(1):133–144.)

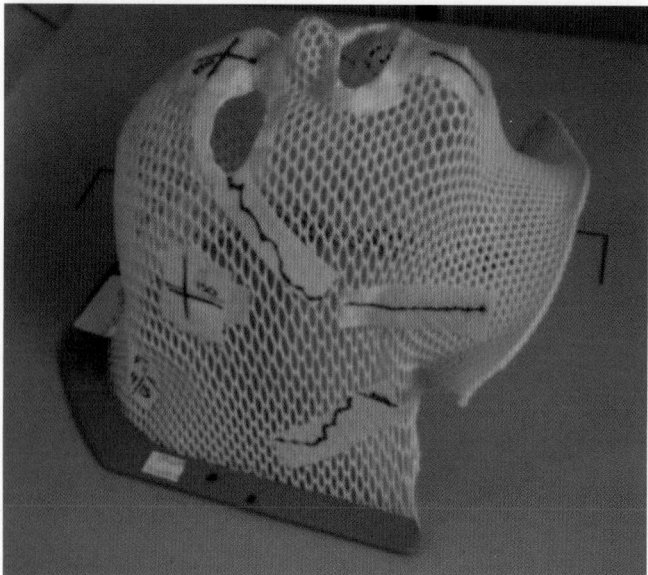

• **Fig. 5.10** Immobilization Mask That Fastens to Radiation Table. (Reprinted with permission from Kane GM, Dhami G. Chapter 26: Principles of radiation. In: Gurtner GC, ed. *Plastic Surgery. Volume 1: Principles.* 4th ed. Elsevier; 2018.)

illustrating one of the psychological stressors and trauma of the cancer journey that Onc R clinicians must be aware of.

Types of Radiotherapy

3D Conformal Radiation Therapy

In 3D conformal radiation therapy, a computed tomography (CT) scan, combined with special computer software, creates a 3D model of the area to be treated. This highly specific plan delivers precisely targeted doses to the tumor, sparing the surrounding tissue.[41] The most recent development is the use of magnetic resonance imaging (MRI) which provides ongoing accuracy to specifically target the tumor.

Intensity-Modulated Radiation Therapy

Intensity-modulated radiation therapy (IMRT) is an advanced form of 3D conformal radiation. IMRT allows the radiation intensity to be adjusted at different portions of the beams while the treatment is delivered. Also, it allows the tumor to be treated from many different angles in the body. The ability to adjust the dose of radiation within each beam enables IMRT to concurrently treat several areas while also "boosting" the tumor or the tumor bed postsurgery.[40]

Proton Beam Therapy

The first proposal for the use of protons in cancer treatment was in 1946; less than 10 years later, it was used to treat certain cancers. Over the past 30 years, research and laboratory applications have led to the United States' (US) FDA approval of proton therapy in 1988, and the first patient treatments in 1991. As of 2021, there are currently 34 proton radiation treatment centers in the US, with an additional 10 under construction.

The heavy particles used in proton therapy allows for more precise dose delivery while minimizing delivery of the dosage to proximate healthy tissue (Figure 5.11). After transmission through other tissues, the protons' energy is deposited in the target tissue in a sharp peak, termed the *Bragg peak*. The ability to precisely control the dosage of the protons' initial energy allows for the ability to minimize delivery of dosage to nearby normal tissue by a factor of two to three (Figure 5.12).[42] Because proton beams can be delivered at higher doses and are far more accurate than IMRT, ultimately fewer treatments are required. The pinpoint accuracy of the proton beam also allows for fewer long-term adverse effects. The patient treated with proton therapy is more likely to have a higher QOL while also having a better overall response to the treatment.[43] Proton beam therapy offers the most advanced radiation

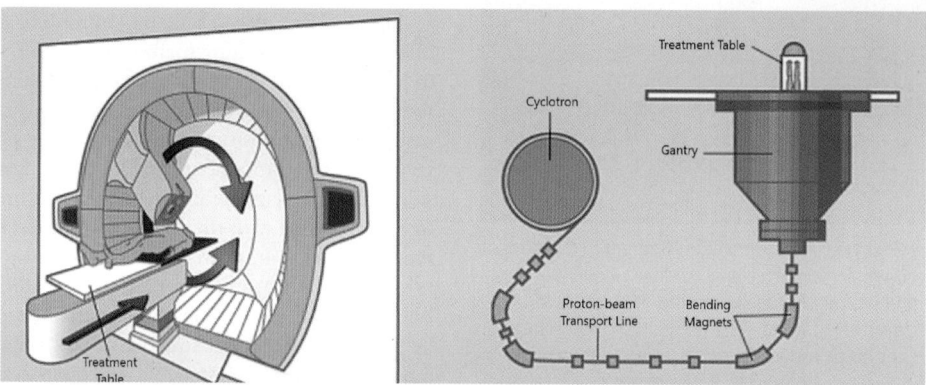

• **Fig. 5.11** Proton Beam Therapy. (Reprinted with permission from D'Ambrosio AL, DeYoung C, Isaacson SR. Radiosurgical management of brain. *Neurosurg Clin N Am.* 2011;22(1):45–51.)

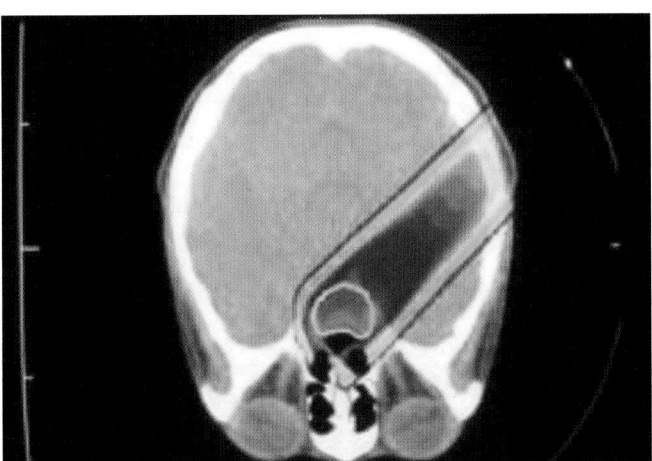

• **Fig. 5.12** Dose Delivery of Proton Beam Therapy. (Reprinted with permission from National Cancer Institute Visuals online. https://visualsonline.cancer.gov/details.cfm?imageid=2421. In the public domain.)

form to treat prostate, lung, head and neck, liver, esophagus, and brain cancers. Also, it is the preferred form of radiation for many pediatric cancers, especially primary brain tumors.

Image Guided Radiation Therapy

Image guided radiation therapy (IGRT) is used for treatment of cancers located near critical structures including nerves, blood vessels, and organs. In addition, IGRT is useful for tumors that are likely to move during treatment or between treatments such as tumors of the lung which may move during breathing. The linear accelerator is equipped with scanning abilities that include positron emission tomography (PET), CT, and MRI technologies. Prior to radiation delivery, a scan will be taken to determine the exact location of the tumor. Over the course of therapy, each time the scan is performed, computer programming allows for an updated delivery of the radiation based on changes in tumor size or location. In general, IGRT involves a series of sessions, generally 5 days a week for several weeks. The total dosage and frequency of treatments will be dependent on variables such as the type, location, and size of the tumor.

Stereotactic Radiotherapy

Stereotactic radiotherapy (SRT) employs several precisely focused radiation beams to treat a variety of cancers, including head and neck, spinal, brain, and liver cancers. 3D imaging is able to precisely deliver a high dosage of radiation to the tumor while minimizing the impact on surrounding healthy tissue. Treatment of the brain and spine with SRT generally requires only one session. SRT can be used to treat soft tissue tumors including those of the lung, liver, or adrenal gland and often require three to five sessions.

Gamma knife therapy is a form of stereotactic radiosurgery (SRS) that utilizes specialized gamma rays to treat tumors (benign or malignant), vascular malformations, trigeminal neuralgia, and other abnormalities of the brain. Gamma knife involves the administration of many radiation beams delivered from multiple angles to target one specific area of the brain (Figure 5.13). Each of the individual beams is not strong enough to negatively affect healthy tissue but when the beams meet, the combined energy is enough to treat the tumor.[44] The procedure is typically performed in one day and is well tolerated by patients. The downside is the need for a stabilizing head frame to be temporarily attached to the patient's head with four pins. This frame placement is then followed by imaging, treatment planning, and treatment. All are performed on the same day.

Brachytherapy

Radiation therapy can be delivered internally as well as the previously discussed external delivery methods. Brachytherapy is a form of internal radiation that allows for the delivery of more intense doses of radiation to small, localized areas that may not be feasible to treat via external radiation. Many types of implants conform to the organ or tumor that is to be treated. The radiation can be in the form of radioactive seeds, capsules, or pellets but can also be delivered by wires, needles, or tubes (Figure 5.14).[45] Brachytherapy comes in many forms and procedures and is most commonly utilized for gynecological malignancies and prostate cancer; however, is also applicable with breast, head and neck, and rectal cancers. The primary advantage of brachytherapy is the localized treatment, decreasing the amount of radiation that spills over to adjacent healthy tissue. That, combined with the radiation's focused application, makes it an excellent choice for many patients.

Brachytherapy radiation is delivered in a low dose rate (LDR) or high dose rate (HDR). The International Commission on Radiation Units (ICRU) defines LDR brachytherapy as 0.4 to 5 Gy per hour with HDR being delivered at greater than 12 Gy per hour. The typical source of radiation implant is iridium-192 for LDR and cesium-137 and iridium-192 for HDR treatment. Historically, LDR implants were inserted twice over 48 to 72 hours. Previously the patient

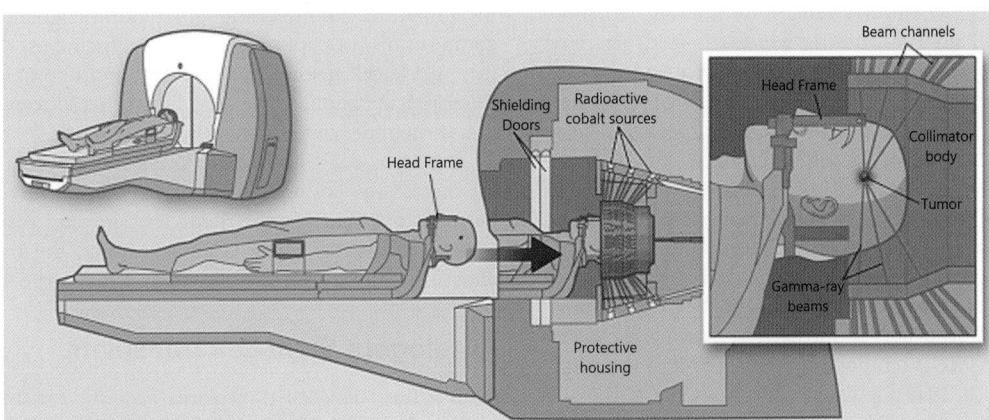

• **Fig. 5.13** Gamma Knife for Brain Tumor. (Reprinted with permission from D'Ambrosio AL, DeYoung C, Isaacson SR. Radiosurgical management of brain. *Neurosurg Clin N Am.* 2011;22(1):45–51.)

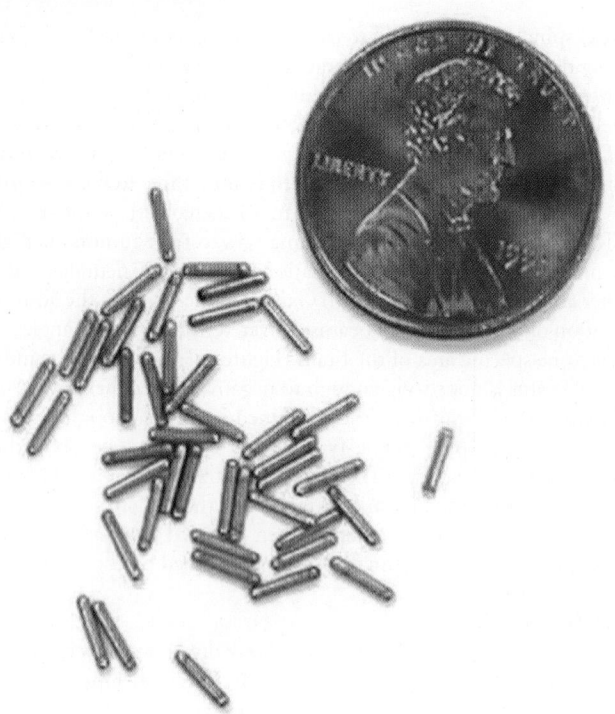

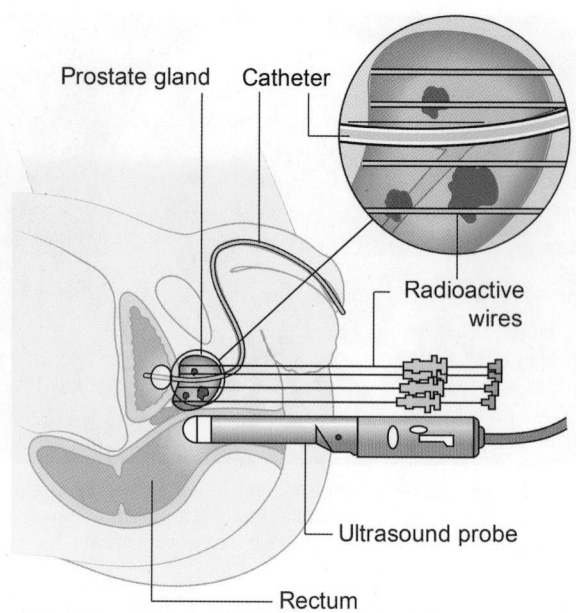

would typically remain inpatient for 1 to 3 days, no visitors were allowed, and the patient was cared for behind a lead drape. Today, technological advances have made HDR brachytherapy feasible with the convenience of outpatient treatment, decreased radiation exposure for healthcare workers, and better dosimetric treatment of the tumors.[40] When considering brachytherapy as a treatment option, the advantages of brachytherapy must be weighed against the potential complications of the invasive procedure. A person diagnosed with prostate cancer receiving HDR brachytherapy typically requires two treatments (Figure 5.15). These procedures are separated by 1 to 2 weeks with an overnight stay after each treatment.

Accelerated partial breast irradiation (APBI) is an approach focused on the lumpectomy bed with an extended margin of 1 to 2 cm of healthy tissue. This procedure allows accelerated delivery of radiation from a typical 16- to 20-day schedule to an accelerated 4- to 5-day schedule. The procedure includes the insertion of a device into the lumpectomy bed. The radiation seeds are transported into the device, where they remain for a calculated time, generally less than 30 minutes, during which the seeds irradiate the breast tissue. The percentage of local recurrence and the cosmetic results are an essential argument for the APBI brachytherapy technique. Based on available results from prospective clinical trials, excellent results in a selected patient group were achieved.[46]

Intraoperative radiation therapy (IORT) is the delivery of radiation during the initial cancer surgery. IORT is applicable for breast cancer but also is used for head and neck, pelvis, and GI cancers. Recent studies have provided evidence that IORT provides superior cancer control as compared to surgery and adjuvant radiation.[47] The delivery of radiation occurs immediately following excisional surgery. The IORT device is temporarily implanted into the surgical cavity. The device is then populated with HDR brachytherapy seeds, and the patient receives the treatment that typically lasts less than 30 minutes. The benefits to the patient are the convenience of surgery and radiation the same day. In addition, there are relatively fewer adverse effects to the tissues within the radiation field and reduced damage to surrounding tissues and vital structures. This procedure will be minimal and requires specific planning to incorporate preoperative imaging to determine that the surgical site would likely result in a positive or close margin, reduced risk to surrounding organs such as the bladder or bowel, and the estimation that IORT can be as effective as EBRT.[48]

Bone Marrow Transplant

Bone marrow transplant (BMT; hematopoietic stem cell transplant) involves the delivery of healthy hematopoietic stem cells in a patient with a cancerous or depleted marrow. The purpose of BMT is to improve bone marrow function and allows the transplanted cells to either destroy cancer cells or generate new bone marrow to replace the cancerous blood cells produced by the dysfunctional bone marrow cells.[49]

Stem cell transplant is not an option available to all cancers, and its use is typically limited to hematological malignancies. The common diseases treated with transplant include blood and marrow cancers such as select leukemias and lymphomas, multiple myeloma, amyloidosis, and other nonmalignant disorders. Less common diseases approved for BMT include severe aplastic anemia, sickle cell disease, thalassemia, immune deficiency diseases, inherited metabolic disorders, and other diseases and disorders currently under investigation in clinical trials.[50]

The stem cell transplant process initially requires identifying the disease and consideration such as current disease state, patient performance status, prior therapies, age, and insurance approval for the treatment. Once criteria are met, the transplant type is chosen that is best for the patient and their type of cancer.

Autologous Stem Cell Transplant

Autologous stem cell transplants account for the most hematological stem cell transplants, with approximately 60% of all transplants performed being autologous.[51] In autologous stem cell transplantation, the patient's own hematopoietic cells are infused to re-establish bone marrow function after myeloablation. The process involves harvesting of the patients' stem cells, followed by myeloablation and then infusion, or transplantation of the cells. Myeloablation can occur via administering high-dose chemotherapy, with or without total body irradiation.[52] Before administering the high-dose chemotherapy, the patient's stem cells are collected via peripheral stem cell collection or directly from their bone marrow. The harvest of these cells often occurs weeks to years ahead of the actual transplant. In the meantime, the harvested cells are preserved by being frozen in liquid nitrogen. Autologous stem cell transplant is the least risky due to the absence of graft-versus-host disease (GvHD) and the short engraftment time for the stem cells. It is considered a treatment option for the elderly and those with comorbidities. However, primary concerns related to autologous transplant include the risk of contaminating the graft (stem cells) with viable tumor cells and the lack of graft versus tumor effects.[52]

Allogeneic Stem Cell Transplant

Allogeneic stem cell transplantation is the transplantation of stem cells from a healthy donor to the recipient. This is often completed after myeloablative high-intensity chemotherapy and in some cases also includes total body irradiation. The donor can be a relative (typically first-degree brother or sister), an identical twin (syngeneic donor), or an unrelated donor (matched unrelated donor) via the international donor pool.

The selection of a stem cell donor initiates with identifying the major histocompatibility complex (MHC). This complex is found on chromosome 6 which encodes human leukocyte antigens (HLA).[49] Each individual's immunological identity is expressed in cell-surface proteins encoded in the HLA system, located on chromosome 6, and containing over 200 genes forming the MHC.[53] Additional considerations when choosing a potential donor include the donor age, past medical history, and past infectious disease history.

An additional stem cell source is that of an umbilical cord blood unit. As imperative as the HLA match is for an unrelated adult donor, it is less critical with a cord blood transplant. As compared to allogenic HCT, cord blood demonstrates increased engraftment rates, and a close HLA match appears to be less necessary during the transplantation process.[54] The primary criteria for use are based upon an adequate cord blood unit quantity. The minimum required total nucleated cell is the highest priority, followed by the CD34+ count, with the HLA match being the third priority. The extension of cord blood availability for SCT has extended these options a difficult time finding adequate HLA matches.[54]

The Transplant Procedure

Upon selecting the transplant type, the patient is admitted to the transplant unit ranging from 2 to 6 weeks. Before that actual transplantation of the stem cells, the patient undergoes a conditioning regimen to destroy any remaining cancer cells in their body. The treatment is typically an administration of high dose chemotherapy with or without total body irradiation. This regimen will also obliterate the bone marrow and weaken the immune system to keep the body from rejecting the transplanted stem cells. The weakened immune system is much more of a concern when the source of the stem cells is allogenic as opposed to autologous. The period between the stem cell infusion and the patient's reconstitution of their marrow (termed *engraftment*) is primarily based upon the marrow source type. In an allogeneic or donor marrow

infusion, the engraftment period is longer due to stem cells not being from "self" and is further delayed with immunosuppression medication. In an autologous stem cell, the source is harvested from the patient weeks to years before the transplant and the engraftment period is shorter due to the cell originating from the patient. The length of the engraftment period is associated with the risk of prolonged immunosuppression.

Following the initial treatment and engraftment period, the patient is discharged home. They are often quarantined for approximately 90 days to allow the stem cells to seed and take root in the patient's bone marrow. This time period is much less for an autologous transplant as compared to an allogeneic transplant. The ultimate goal of this form of treatment is a cure for the patient from their cancer disease.

Graft-Versus-Host Disease

After allogenic transplantation, a condition called GvHD may occur, especially in those who did not have a strong HLA match. In GvHD, the transplanted bone marrow or stem cells (graft) identify the cells in the recipient's body (host) as a foreign substance and generate an immune response toward the host body's cells. GvHD develops in connective tissues in the body, affecting skin, liver, or the GI tract.

Treatment usually includes increased immunosuppression in the form of oral or IV corticosteroids. In treating GvHD, the new immune system is suppressed, thereby increasing the risk of opportunistic infections including bacterial, viral, or fungal diseases, further complicating the transplantation and recovery process. This might also require antibiotics, antivirals, antifungals, or other supportive drugs to address these infections.

Biologic Therapies

A fourth and rapidly evolving component of cancer treatment is biologic therapies, which have three categories: immunotherapy, targeted therapy, and hormone therapy. These agents are a substantial area of innovation in cancer care and are often difficult for many cancer clinicians to grasp. These therapies are generally targeted to specific actions in the body, and therefore there are fewer adverse effects as compared to chemotherapy. Unlike chemotherapy, many targeted and hormonal therapies are considered cytostatic. They do not kill tumor cells, but they stop their growth and/or replication. This is done by altering the hormonal or biological environment that the cancer cell thrives in.

Immunotherapy

This type of treatment uses the body's own immune system to attack cancer cells by facilitating the targeting of these cells. Some of these agents include immune checkpoint inhibitors, cell-based immunotherapy, monoclonal antibodies, vaccinations, and immune system modulators. The most commonly encountered immunotherapies are monoclonal antibodies acting as immune checkpoint inhibitors.

Monoclonal Antibodies
Monoclonal antibodies often have the suffix "-mab" and work by up-regulating the body's immune response to be more sensitive and thereby kill cancer cells.[53] These affect both the B lymphocytes and T lymphocytes. Current monoclonal antibodies target checkpoint proteins called programmed cell death-1 (PD-1),

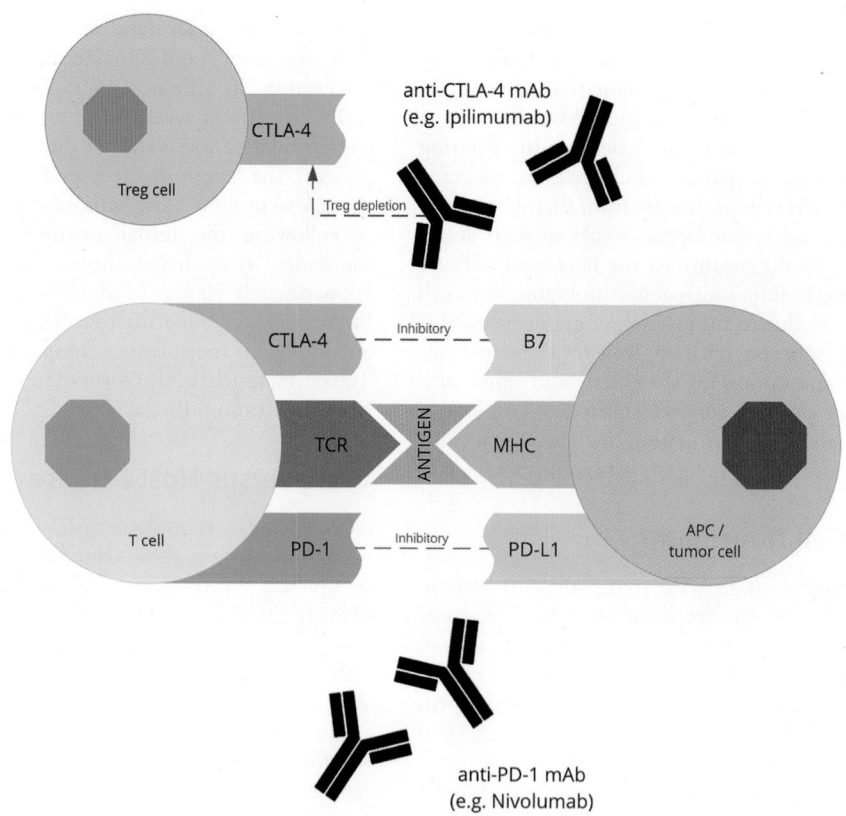

• **Fig. 5.16** Monoclonal Antibodies and Their Mechanism of Action. *CTLA-4*, Cytotoxic T-lymphocyte-associated protein-4; *MHC*, major histocompatibility complex; *PD-1*, programmed cell death-1; *PD-L1*, programmed cell death-ligand 1. (Reprinted with permission from Sanghera C, Sanghera R. Immunotherapy—strategies for expanding its role in the treatment of all major tumor sites. *Cureus.* 2019;11(10):e5938. doi:10.7759/cureus.5938.)

programmed cell death-ligand 1 (PD-L1), and cytotoxic T-lymphocyte-associated protein-4 (CTLA-4) (Figure 5.16).

Some monoclonal antibodies bind to PD-1 on the T cell side, while others bind to PD-L1 on the tumor side. This allows the tumor cell to be identified by the T cell as a foreign threat and subsequently be destroyed. Since some cancer cells have PD-L1, they are not identified as foreign cells and therefore are left alone. Monoclonal antibodies targeting PD-1 or PD-L1 are used to block the binding, therefore improving the chances of generating an immune response against the cancer cells.

There is another option for monoclonal antibodies to act as an immune checkpoint inhibitor. On the same T cell, there is a CTLA-4 receptor that acts as an "off-switch."[55] When inhibited, CTLA-4 allows the T cell to attack cancer cells as well. For example, the monoclonal antibody ipilimumab (Yervoy) attaches to CTLA-4 to deactivate it, thereby turning it "on" to attack cancer cells. Ipilimumab is used to treat melanoma but is also being researched for use in other cancers.

Chimeric Antigen Receptor T Cell Therapy

An increasingly common immunotherapy treatment for hematologic cancers (e.g., leukemia, lymphoma, multiple myeloma) is chimeric antigen receptor T (CAR-T) cell therapy, which results in modification of T-cells that can identify and attack the cancer cells (Figure 5.17).[56] First, T cells are extracted from the patient's bloodstream via IV access. After extraction, genetic information for the specific antigen of the cancer cells is encoded into the T cells which generates specific chimeric antigen receptors. These new chimeric

antigen receptors are found on the surface of the T cells. These new receptors will help the T cells identify and fight the hematologic cancer. Once coding is successful, these modified T cells are replicated outside of the patient's body. The patient then receives an infusion of these modified cells to identify and attack the cancer cells.

Targeted Therapy

Targeted therapies can affect cancer cells in a number of different ways. As their name suggests, they are targeted to specific functional behaviors of cancer cells. They may alter the cancer cell growth by modifying the actions of normal cells in the area. In addition, some may also increase the vulnerability of cancer cells to the body's own immune system.[57] Some may also alter pathways by in which normal cells transform into malignant cells. Because of their ability to cease or slow growth, these targeted therapies can prevent cancer cells from spreading, or enhancing repair of normal tissues that are damaged by treatment. There are a wide variety of uses and applications of the broad category of targeted therapies.

One of the most commonly known types of targeted therapy addresses the overexpression of the human epidermal growth factor (EGF)/human epidermal growth factor receptor (EGFR) pathway, which is a major factor in cancer growth across the spectrum of the disease.[57] An example of this pathway is EDG/EGFR pathway on SCC in head and neck cancer. The development of the targeted drug cetuximab (Erbitux) allows for the drug to act as a receptor blocker by landing on the over expressed EGFRs on the SCC surfaces. When the receptors are blocked by the Erbitux, the EGF/EGFR pathway is

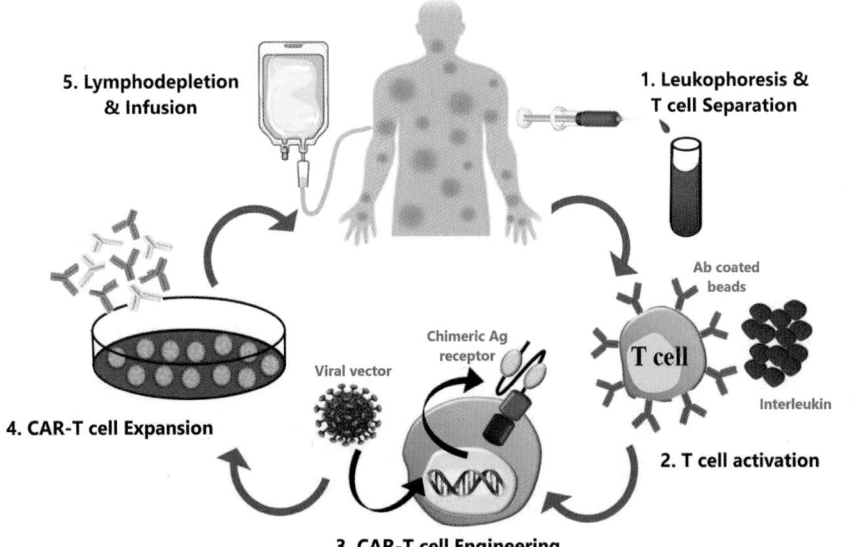

• **Fig. 5.17** Chimeric Antigen Receptor T (CAR-T) Cell Application Process. Separation, design, harvest, and administration of CAR-T cell for human diseases. Firstly, T cells are separated from patients (leukopheresis), harvested, and activated. The chimeric antigen receptor is designed and then engineered and produced in T cells. After expansion of produced CAR-T cell, the cells are administrated to the patients. (Reprinted with permission from Esmaeilzadeh A, Tahmasebi S, Athari SS. Chimeric antigen receptor-T cell therapy: applications and challenges in treatment of allergy and asthma. *Biomed Pharmacother.* 2020;123:109685.)

destroyed, and the SCC growth is inhibited. Another example of this pathway is the human epidermal growth factor receptor 2 (HER2) or HER2/neu receptor on breast cancer cells. Approximately 15% to 20% of all breast cancers are HER2-positive.[57] The overexpression of the HER2 receptors on cancer cell surfaces results in the cancer cells receiving increased concentrations of growth hormone, which promotes a more aggressive behavioral characteristic of breast cancer. This increases the disease recurrence as well as metastatic spread to the bone and the brain. The identification of the HER2 receptor results in the development of HER2-targeted therapies, including trastuzumab (Herceptin) which act to block the HER2 receptor and have substantially improved patient survival.[58]

Hormone Therapy

The growth of some tumors is facilitated by the presence of certain androgens. For example, a subset of breast tumors is positive for estrogen receptors (ERs) and/or progesterone receptors (PRs). This means that, in this case, breast cancer cells have two growth pathways, one being the EGF/EGFR pathway, and the second being the ER+/PR+ pathway.[59]

A common hormone therapy drug for treating premenopausal patients diagnosed with ER+/PR+ breast cancer is tamoxifen (Nolvadex, Soltamox). Tamoxifen blocks ERs and thereby prevents estrogen from entering the breast cancer cell.[59] Tamoxifen does have some potential adverse effects, which are similar to estrogen replacement therapy including endometrial cancer risk, stroke, deep vein thrombosis, and pulmonary embolus. In addition, the patient may also experience increased hot flashes.

Hormone therapy drugs for treating postmenopausal patients diagnosed with ER+/PR+ breast cancer are aromatase inhibitors. These inhibit the production of estrogen by blocking the enzyme aromatase and preventing the conversion of androgens into circulating estrogens in the patient's body.[59] Aromatase inhibitors have adverse effects resulting in arthralgias and myalgias as well as hot flashes,

osteoporosis, and fatigue. In some cases, the myalgias and arthralgias might be so severe that the patient may not be able to remain on the medication and an alternate means of treatment may be required.

The concept of androgen deprivation therapy should be considered and is used in some cases of prostate cancer and other androgen sensitive cancers. Testosterone and dihydrotestosterone stimulate prostate cancer cells to grow. Therefore, if the prostate is deprived of these androgens, it can slow or temporarily shrink a tumor.[59] When depriving or modifying the body's use of hormones, there are a number of different adverse effects. For prostate cancer, some of them include reduced bone mineral density and metabolic changes, a decreased libido and sexual dysfunction, as well as gynecomastia and testicular atrophy and in some cases anemia and fatigue.[59] For women who have hormone deprivation for breast cancer or endometrial cancer, the adverse effects are highly dependent on the treatment. In some cases, this may involve removing or ablating the ovaries, which are important in producing these hormones. Hot flashes, night sweats, and vaginal dryness are common adverse effects, as well as menstrual cycle disruption in premenopausal women.

For the treatment of prostate cancer, there is a gonadotrophin releasing hormone receptor agonist (e.g., oserelin, leuprorelin) that can slow or stop the growth of the prostate cancer, but this may cause osteoporosis, fatigue, impotence, hot flashes, and arthralgias as noted previously.[59]

Conclusion

This chapter has addressed the four main areas of treatment for persons diagnosed with cancer, namely surgery, chemotherapy, radiation therapy, and biologic therapies. The word "cancer" reflects more than 200 diseases, each with its own trajectory of experiences and treatment requirements and responses. Research in cancer treatment is an ever-evolving science of accelerating sophistication and success. As Onc R clinicians, it is our responsibility to stay abreast of the research updates and treatment methodologies of this very complex disease process. To do this, it is important that clinicians stay connected with each other, as well as to the entire medical team, and always remain focused on the standards of cancer treatment stated by the Commission on Cancer, the American College of Surgeons, and the NCCN. Onc R clinicians must understand not only cancer as a health condition, but also cancer treatment and its related effects to best help our patients across the cancer continuum and to help them live as well as possible for as long as possible.

Critical Research Needs

- Onc R clinicians' ability to screen for and identify adverse effects of targeted therapies
- Development and implementation of entry level guidelines for oncology in rehabilitation professionals' programs
- Development and effectiveness of a continuing education overview course for Onc R professionals on common cancer treatments and adverse effects

Case Study

A 59-year-old female was diagnosed with Stage IIIA, Grade III ER+, PR+, HER2+ left-sided invasive lobular breast cancer (BC). Prior to being diagnosed with BC and undergoing treatment for it, the patient enjoyed walking 2 miles a day, biking with her family over weekends, and attending Zumba classes. She has been unable to return to these activities since chemotherapy. She has difficulty completing all of her activities of daily living (ADL) and felt depressed that her QOL was so reduced. Thirteen months after diagnosis, the patient was referred to physical therapy with complaints of significant fatigue, arthralgic joint pain, reduced physical endurance, and poor balance resulting in a recent fall. Physical therapy interventions consisted of cardiovascular testing, balance re-education, generalized strengthening, core stabilization exercises, endurance training, and fall prevention.

Initial Diagnosis

- Cancer Tissue Type: Carcinoma—the cancer originated within the epithelial cells lining a lobule in the left breast.
- Cancer Grade: Grade III—high-grade tumor—aggressive, fast growing poorly differentiated tumor cells.
- Cancer Stage: T3N3M0 (AJCC) Stage IIIA—advanced disease with potential for distal micro-metastases (Figure 5.18).
- Hormone Receptor Status: Positive for ER signaling and PR signaling, and positive for HER2 signaling (sometimes termed *triple positive*).

Diagnostics Discussion

The patient presented with high-stage, high-grade lobular carcinoma in her left breast 13 months after diagnosis. The disease burden was further compounded by hormone receptor signaling which, in this case, was harnessing circulating estrogen, progesterone, and growth hormone from the endocrine environment surrounding the cancer to increase cancer cell proliferation, migration, adhesion, and apoptosis. From a physical therapy perspective, the Onc R clinician must understand these clinical implications for rehabilitation with respect to cancer diagnostics for any cancer treatments during the disease process. While scientific advancements in the

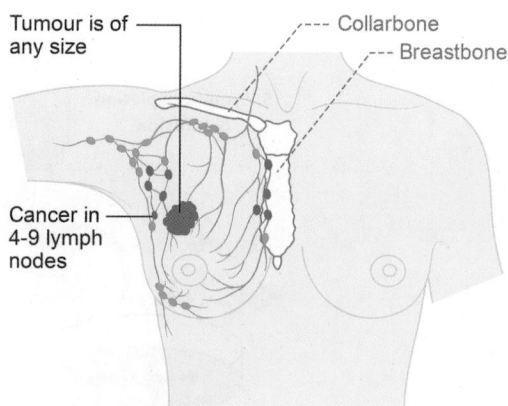

• **Fig. 5.18** Stage IIIA Breast Cancer. (Reprinted with permission from Cancer Research UK. CC 4.0.)

field of oncology have resulted in the successful response to medical treatment of patients diagnosed with cancer, despite treatment success, many patients experience significant functional impairments over time, resulting from their body systems' response to surgery,[60] chemotherapy,[61] and radiation therapy.[62]

Cancer Treatment Regimen

Figure 5.19 illustrates the timeline of this patient's cancer journey.

Neoadjuvant Chemotherapy: High dose chemotherapy treatment combining targeted and systemic chemotherapy agents is indicated to treat high grade triple positive invasive, micro-metastatic disease progression.[63] The patient received neoadjuvant chemotherapy that included both trastuzumab (Herceptin) and pertuzumab (Perjeta),[64] which are both monoclonal antibodies, as well as carboplatin and paclitaxel (Taxol) which are both neurotoxic forms of systemic chemotherapy. The desired effect of the neoadjuvant chemotherapy was to improve the curative opportunity for this patient given the aggressive, fast growing nature of her cancer. The goal was to achieve a pCR.

Surgery: Approximately 3 weeks after completion of neoadjuvant chemotherapy, given the size and invasive behavior of the tumor, the patient underwent a modified radical mastectomy. Once the tumor and the associated sentinel lymph nodes were excised, the pathologist determined the patient had a pCR resulting from the neoadjuvant chemotherapy treatment.

Radiation Therapy: Approximately 3 weeks post surgery the patient received photon-based EBRT to the left chest and supraclavicular areas. Radiation therapy is a local treatment form used to eradicate any remaining invasive cancer cells in the local region of the primary disease site. Radiation treatment was done consecutively for 5 days a week (with weekends off) for a total of 35 treatments (7 weeks).

Adjuvant Therapy: Three weeks after completion of radiation therapy, the patient resumed her Herceptin infusions and initiated an aromatase inhibitor to address the ER+ signaling of the cancer cells. Adjuvant therapy would be administered over an extended period to keep the patient in successful remission.

Chemotherapy Drugs

The physical therapist considered the adverse effects of each chemotherapy drug individually as well as compounded by combination regimens and their clinical implications on the patient's performance and symptoms to establish a plan of care (Figures 5.20, 5.21, 5.22).

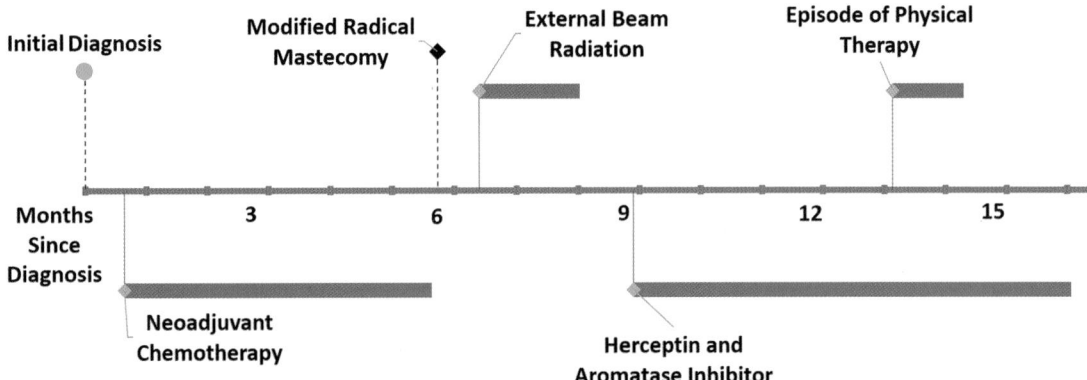

• **Fig. 5.19** Timeline of Cancer Journey for Case Study. (Created by Julia C. Osborne, BSc (Hons) PT, CLT-LANA. Printed with permission.)

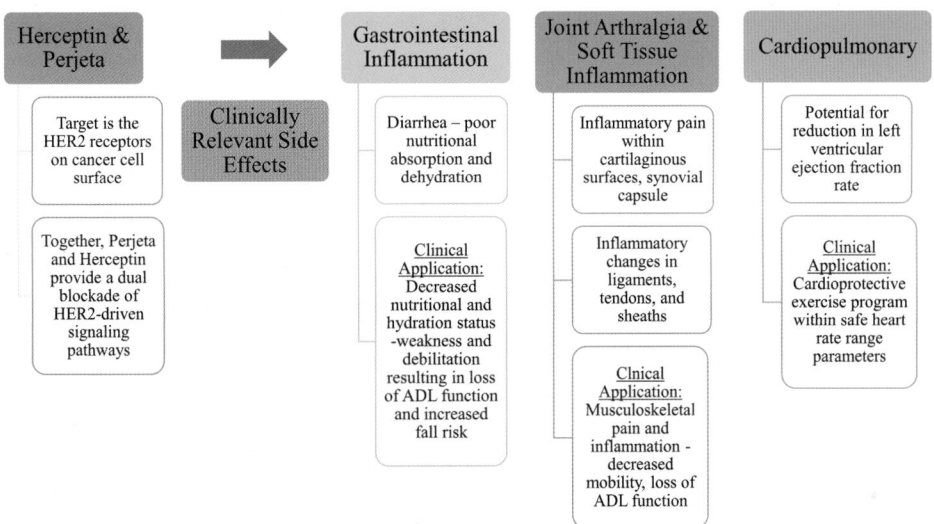

• **Fig. 5.20** Neoadjuvant Targeted Therapy and Clinically Relevant Adverse Effects. *ADL*, Activities of daily living; *HER2*, human epidermal growth factor receptor 2. (Created by Julia C. Osborne, BSc (Hons) PT, CLT-LANA. Printed with permission.)

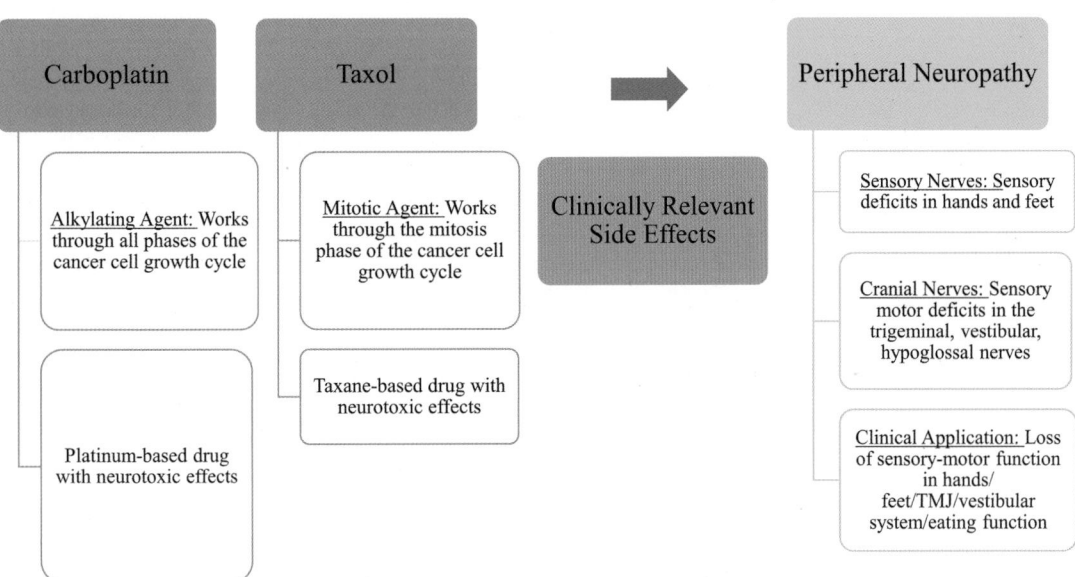

• **Fig. 5.21** Neoadjuvant Systemic Chemotherapy and Clinically Relevant Adverse Effects. (Created by Julia C. Osborne, BSc (Hons) PT, CLT-LANA. Printed with permission.)

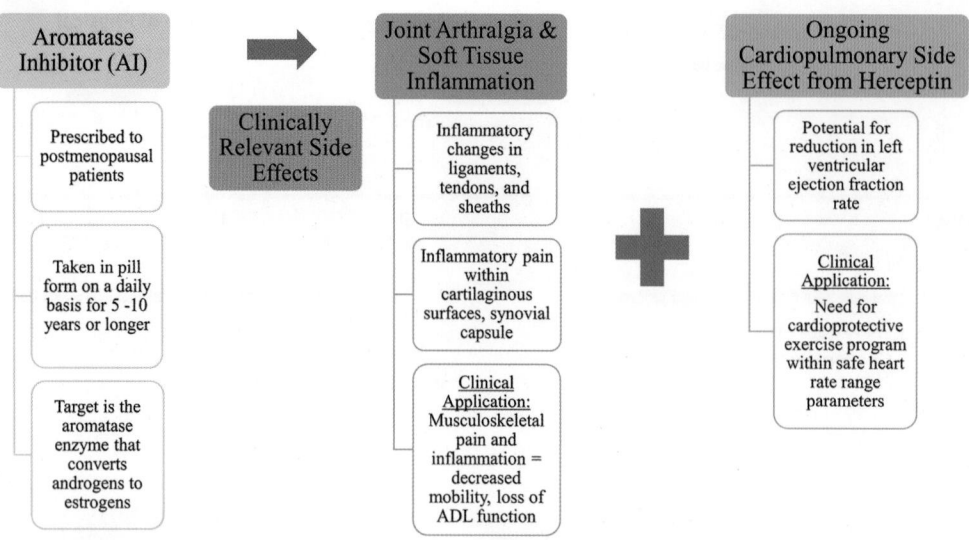

• **Fig. 5.22** Adjuvant Targeted Chemotherapy and Clinically Relevant Adverse effects. *ADL,* Activities of daily living. (Created by Julia C. Osborne, BSc (Hons) PT, CLT-LANA. Printed with permission.)

Physical Findings and Evaluation

Physical therapy initial examination took place 13 months after her initial diagnosis and 7 months after her mastectomy. Select outcome measures and their interpretation can be found on Table 5.1. Additional descriptions of these measures can be found in eAppendix 5.1 in the eBook. In addition, the therapist interpreted the findings based on the International Classification of Function (Figure 5.23).[74]

Summary Discussion

As illustrated in the table of outcome measures (Table 5.2) from initial evaluation to reassessment, she made progress in both her patient-reported and functional measures. These improvements made a difference in that patient's overall perspective of her QOL and her functional abilities. She was discharged from therapy after 15 visits.

TABLE 5.1	Review of Systems Consisted of Cardiovascular, Pulmonary, and Musculoskeletal Systems
Clinical Findings at Initial Evaluation	**Clinical Interpretation**
Left Ventricular Ejection Fraction Rate (LVEFR) = 51% Resting HR = 73	Medical records indicate she retained LVEFR > 50% during both neoadjuvant chemotherapy and adjuvant chemotherapy. Research shows that the cellular effects on cardiac function during Herceptin and Perjeta treatment are generally asymptomatic.[63] It is important therefore to implement an exercise program that prescribes aerobic exercise within a safe HR range for the patient.
FACIT-F[64] = 124/160	This scale has 5 domains: physical, emotional, social, and functional well-being as well as fatigue. This is a good gauge of the patient's perception of fatigue, and it provides insight into the quality of life (QOL) of the patient. The higher the score implies a better QOL.
The Modified Borg Scale[65] for Dyspnea and Shortness of Breath (SOB) = 7/10	The scale provides a tangible measure of how the patient experiences their SOB during functional activities.
Lower Extremity Functional Scale[66] (LEFS) = 47/80	The scale includes a variety of daily tasks that provides insight into how the patient is experiencing lower extremity function during all ADLs.
mCTSIB[67] = Loss of Balance With Eyes Open After 17 seconds	Patient has increased fall risk during and after chemotherapy secondary to the neurotoxic adverse effects of carboplatin and Taxol[68] as well as weakness and debilitation secondary to musculoskeletal pain and inflammation, SOB, and decreased endurance.
6-Minute Walk Test[69] = 483 m	Normative value for age matched females = 700 m Patient is well below norm. This is likely secondary to the neurotoxic adverse effects of carboplatin and Taxol, musculoskeletal pain and inflammation, SOB, significant fatigue, and decreased endurance.
TUG[70] = 38 seconds (Moderate to High Fall Risk)	A score of 30 seconds or more suggests that the person may be prone to falls. Alternatively, a recommended practical cut-off value for the TUG to indicate normal versus below normal performance is 12 seconds. The score is indicative of impairment secondary to the above listed adverse effects.

ADLs, Activities of daily living; *FACIT-F,* Functional Assessment of Chronic Illness Therapy—Fatigue; *HR,* heart rate; *mCTSIB,* modified clinical test of sensory interaction in balance; *TUG,* Timed-Up-and-Go.
(Created by Julia C. Osborne, BSc (Hons) PT, CLT-LANA. Printed with permission.)

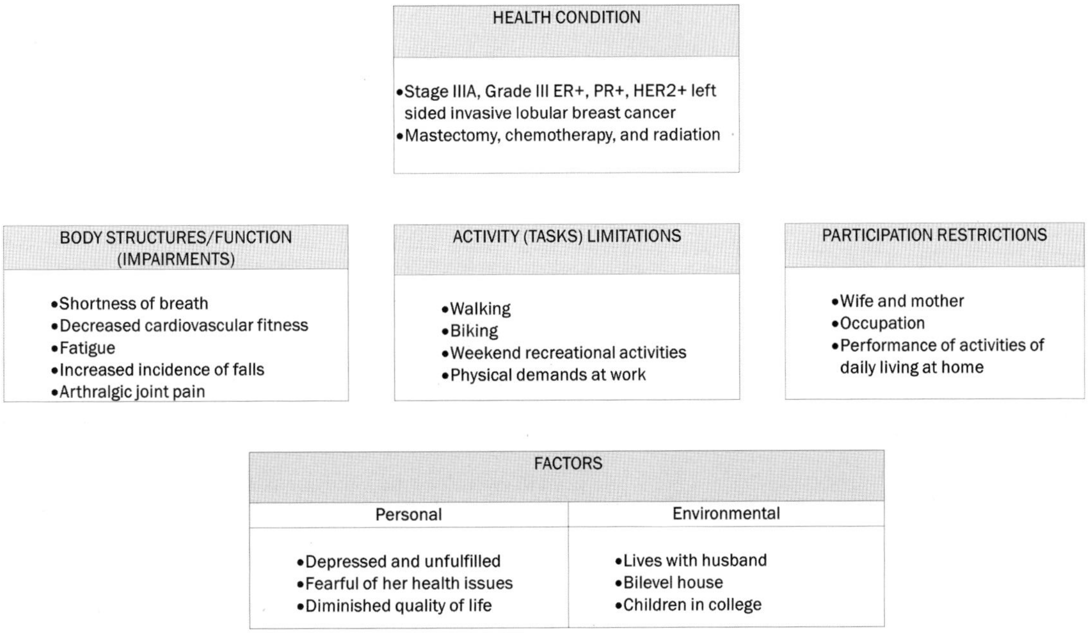

HEALTH CONDITION

- Stage IIIA, Grade III ER+, PR+, HER2+ left sided invasive lobular breast cancer
- Mastectomy, chemotherapy, and radiation

BODY STRUCTURES/FUNCTION (IMPAIRMENTS)

- Shortness of breath
- Decreased cardiovascular fitness
- Fatigue
- Increased incidence of falls
- Arthralgic joint pain

ACTIVITY (TASKS) LIMITATIONS

- Walking
- Biking
- Weekend recreational activities
- Physical demands at work

PARTICIPATION RESTRICTIONS

- Wife and mother
- Occupation
- Performance of activities of daily living at home

FACTORS

Personal	Environmental
• Depressed and unfulfilled • Fearful of her health issues • Diminished quality of life	• Lives with husband • Bilevel house • Children in college

• **Fig. 5.23** Application of the International Classification of Function. (Created by Julia C. Osborne, BSc (Hons) PT, CLT-LANA. Printed with permission.)

TABLE 5.2   Clinical Outcomes After 15 Sessions of Physical Therapy

Test and Measure During Physical Therapy	Initial Evaluation	Reassessment After 5th Visit	Reassessment After 10th Visit	Discharge Assessment After 15th Visit
FACIT-F	124/160	132/160	141/160	147/160
Modified Borg Scale for Dyspnea	7/10	7/10	5/10	4/10
LEFS	47/80	55/80	62/80	67/80
mCTSIB (seconds) Eyes Open (EO) Eyes Closed (EC)	EO = 17[a]	EO = 25[a]	EO = 30 EC = 22[a]	EO = 30 EC = 27[a]
6-Minute Walk Test	483 m (1584 ft)	492 m (1614 ft)	508 m (1666 ft)	587 m (1925 ft)
TUG (seconds)	38	32	24	21

[a]Unable to complete remainder of test. *FACIT-F,* Functional Assessment of Chronic Illness Therapy—Fatigue; *LEFS,* lower extremity functional scale; *mCTSIB,* modified clinical test of sensory interaction in balance; *TUG,* Timed-Up-and-Go. (Created by Julia C. Osborne, BSc (Hons) PT, CLT-LANA. Printed with permission.)

Review Questions

Reader can find the correct answers and rationale in the back of the book.

1. The most appropriate description of systemic chemotherapy drugs is that they:
   A. Are targeted
   B. Always have a cardiotoxic effect
   C. Always have a myelosuppressive effect
   D. Predominantly work during the mitosis phase of the cell cycle
2. "Invasive cancer"—implies that the cancer cells are:
   A. Locally invasive in the tissue of origin and into regional lymph nodes
   B. Invasive to distal sites such as bone, brain, liver, or lung
   C. Invasive in the tissue of origin only
   D. Invasive into tissue of origin and local surrounding tissues
3. Induction chemotherapy is prescribed to patients:
   A. After surgery and radiation to induce a pCR
   B. As a first line of treatment for curative intent
   C. In combination with radiation to induce a pCR
   D. As a form of neoadjuvant chemotherapy
4. Neoadjuvant chemotherapy is prescribed to patients:
   A. To treat early stage, low grade cancers
   B. To treat small lesions to induce a pCR

C.   To treat high grade aggressive lesions to induce a pCR

D. To treat late stage lesions, no matter the tumor size, to induce and pCR

5. If a tumor is Grade III, this means that:
   A. Cells are well differentiated and have low mitotic counts
   B. Cells are poorly differentiated and have high mitotic counts
   C. Cells have low mitotic counts and are poorly differentiated
   D. Cells have high mitotic counts and are well differentiated

6. Constant, unrelenting cancer-related pain in a patient who is still functional in ADLs, would most likely have their pain managed medically by:
   A. Rapid release opioids
   B. Slow release opioids
   C. NSAIDs
   D. Morphine

7. Radiation affects:
   A. Soft tissue structures
   B. Soft tissue and organ surfaces
   C. Soft tissue, organ surfaces, nerves, and bones
   D. Soft tissue, organ surfaces, nerves, bones, and lympho-vascular structures

8. Graft-versus-host disease
   A. Can occur after an autologous transplant and will affect connective tissues
   B. Can occur after an allogeneic transplant and will affect connective tissues
   C. Can occur secondary to failure of tissue grafting in surgical procedures
   D. Can occur secondary to a stem cell transplant versus a bone marrow transplant

9. HER2 receptors in HER2+ breast cancer respond to which type of chemotherapy?
   A. Immunotherapy
   B. Systemic chemotherapy
   C. Targeted chemotherapy
   D. Hormone therapy

10. Which of the following statements best describes proton therapy?
   A. Protons are a type of X-ray that can be used to carefully target specific tissue
   B. One of the advantages of proton therapy is that it has almost no exit dose
   C. Due to the wide beam of proton therapy, it is rarely utilized for brain tumors
   D. Proton therapy involves the insertion of radioactive seeds into the tumor tissue to treat it from the inside out

eAppendix 5.1

Physical Therapy Tests and Measures

FACIT-Fatigue[66]: This scale was created to measure the impact and severity of symptoms of cancer related fatigue over the past 7 days. The FACIT-F is a validated scale that has 5 domains: physical, emotional, social, and functional well-being as well as fatigue. This test was chosen to quantify the patient's self-report of quality of life in all domains. The higher the score on this test, the better the quality of life.

The Modified Borg Scale for Dyspnea[67]: This is a validated reliable tool used for assessing the patient's perception of dyspnea during activities such as walking short to moderate distances.

Lower Extremity Functional Scale (LEFS)[68]: The LEFS scale is a 20-item instrument that looks at a person's ability to perform everyday tasks. It is scaled from 0 to 80 with 80 being no disability. The minimal detectable change and the minimally clinically important difference is 9 points in someone with various lower extremity injuries. This test is typically used in the orthopedic population, but it is useful with the oncology patient population as well as it provides insight into the patient's perception of how they are functioning in all ADL including occupational and recreational ADLs.

Modified Clinical Test of Sensory Interaction in Balance (mCTSIB)[69]: The mCTSIB evaluates postural stability under four balance conditions to assess the influence of the visual, somatosensory, and vestibular systems on standing balance. Of the three procedure options described by Shumway-Cook et al., the therapist chose to measure time.[71] This test was chosen to assess the various domains of balance given that there is potential for several different causative factors for loss of balance in this patient—weakness, debilitation, poor endurance, and possible chemotherapy-induced peripheral neuropathy (CIPN) from her chemotherapy regimen.

6-Minute Walk Test[72]: The purpose of this test is to determine how far the patient can walk in 6 minutes, going at their own pace. Normative performance for healthy adults ranges from 400 to 700 m but there are no normative data for this test in the oncology population. This test was chosen to look at the patient's overall walking speed and to use as a measure of cardiovascular endurance and fall risk.

Timed-Up-and-Go (TUG)[73]: The TUG test evaluates the patient's ability to rise from a sitting position, walk a specified distance, turn around, and return to seated starting position. This test has been well validated to measure strength, balance, ability to co-ordinate movements, ability to turn while in motion, and ability to follow instructions. As with the 6-minute walk test, there are no normative data for this test in the oncology population. This test was chosen to quantify the patient's overall activity endurance, cardiovascular endurance, and fall risk.

References

1. National Comprehensive Cancer Network. About. https://www.nccn.org/about/default.aspx. Accessed April 15, 2021.
2. American College of Surgeons. National Cancer Database. https://www.facs.org/quality-programs/cancer/ncdb. Accessed April 15, 2021.
3. American Joint Committee on Cancer. *AJCC Cancer Staging Manual*. 8th ed. Springer; 2016.
4. Gross JJ. *Handbook of Oncology Nursing*. Vol. 1: Jones and Bartlett; 1994.
5. Korf BR, Mikhail FM. Overview of genetic diagnosis in cancer. *Curr Protoc Hum Genet*. 2017;93:10.1.1–10.1.9. doi:10.1002/cphg.36.

6. The University of Texas MD Anderson Cancer Center. Surgery. https://www.mdanderson.org/treatment-options/surgery.html. Accessed April 15, 2021.

7. National Cancer Institute. Curative surgery. https://www.cancer.gov/publications/dictionaries/cancer-terms/def/curative-surgery. Accessed April 15, 2021.

8. UCSF Department of Surgery. Lymphadenopathy. https://surgery.ucsf.edu/conditions–procedures/lymphadenectomy.aspx. Accessed April 15, 2021.

9. Stanford Health Care. Types of surgery for cancer treatment. https://stanfordhealthcare.org/medical-treatments/c/cancer-surgery/types.html. Accessed April 15, 2021.

10. National Cancer Institute: SEER Training Modules. Palliative and reconstructive surgeries. https://training.seer.cancer.gov/treatment/surgery/types/palliative.html. Accessed April 15, 2021.

11. Scarborough BM, Smith CB. Optimal pain management for patients with cancer in the modern era. *CA Cancer J Clin.* 2018;68(3):182–196.

12. Cooper MA, Hutfless S, Segev DL, et al. Hospital level under-utilization of minimally invasive surgery in the United States: retrospective review. *Br Med J.* 2014;349:g4198. doi:10.1136/bmj.g4198.

13. Lacy AM, Delgado S, Castells A, et al. The long-term results of a randomized clinical trial of laparoscopy-assisted versus open surgery for colon cancer. *Ann Surg.* 2008;248(1):1–7. doi:10.1097/SLA.0b013e31816a9d65.

14. Shah J, Vyas A, Vyas D. The history of robotics in surgical specialties. *Am J Robot Surg.* 2014;1(1):12–20.

15. Arms RG 3rd, Sun CC, Burzawa JK, et al. Improvement in quality of life after robotic surgery results in patient satisfaction. *Gynecol Oncol.* 2015;138(3):727–730.

16. NIH: National Cancer Institute. Cryosurgery in cancer treatment; 2003. http://www.cancer.gov/about-cancer/treatment/types/surgery/cryosurgery-fact-sheet. Accessed April 15, 2021

17. Khalkhal E, Razzaghi M, Rostami-Nejad M, et al. Evaluation of laser effects on the human body after laser therapy. *J Lasers Med Sci.* 2020;11(1):91–97.

18. Colt HG. Basic principles of medical lasers. UpToDate. https://www.uptodate.com/contents/basic-principles-of-medical-lasers. Updated October 26, 2020. Accessed April 15, 2021.

19. Canadian Cancer Society. Laser surgery. www.cancer.ca/en/cancer-information/diagnosis-and-treatment/tests-and-procedures/laser-surgery. Accessed April 15, 2021.

20. DeVita VT, Jr Chu E. A history of cancer chemotherapy. *Cancer Res.* 2008;68(21):8643–8653. doi:10.1158/0008-5472.CAN-07-6611.

21. Sun J, Wei Q, Zhou Y, Wang J, Liu Q, Xu H. A systematic analysis of FDA-approved anticancer drugs. *BMC Syst Biol.* 2017;11(5):1–7.

22. Wooldridge S. Oncology drugs lead the way for new approvals in 2020. BenefitsPro. https://www.benefitspro.com/2020/02/06/oncology-drugs-lead-the-way-for-new-approvals-in-2020/. Published February 6, 2020. Accessed April 16, 2021.

23. National Cancer Institute, Dictionary of Terms. First-line therapy. https://www.cancer.gov/publications/dictionaries/cancer-terms/def/first-line-therapy. Accessed May 23, 2021.

24. Chemocare. Chemotherapy terms. http://chemocare.com/chemotherapy/what-is-chemotherapy/chemotherapy-terms.aspx. Accessed April 16, 2021.

25. National Cancer Institute. Metastatic cancer: when cancer spreads. https://www.cancer.gov/types/metastatic-cancer. Updated November 10, 2020. Accessed April 16, 2021.

26. Blondeaux E, Poggio F, Del Mastro L. Role of dose-dense chemotherapy in high-risk early breast cancer. *Curr Opin Oncol.* 2019;31(6):480–485.

27. Krikorian S, Pories S, Tataronis G, et al. Adherence to oral chemotherapy: challenges and opportunities. *J Oncol Pharm Pract.* 2019;25(7):1590–1598.

28. National Cancer Institute, Dictionary of Terms. Oral chemotherapy. https://www.cancer.gov/publications/dictionaries/cancer-terms/def/oral-chemotherapy. Accessed May 23, 2021.

29. Ciruelos EM, Díaz MN, Isla MD, et al. Patient preference for oral chemotherapy in the treatment of metastatic breast and lung cancer. *Eur J Cancer Care.* 2019;28:e13164. doi:10.1111/ecc.13164.

30. Eek D, Krohe M, Mazar I, et al. Patient-reported preferences for oral versus intravenous administration for the treatment of cancer: a review of the literature. *Patient Prefer Adherence.* 2016;10:1609–1621. doi:10.2147/PPA.S106629.

31. Stuurman FE, Nuijen B, Beijnen JH, Schellens JH. Oral anticancer drugs: mechanisms of low bioavailability and strategies for improvement. *Clin Pharmacokinet.* 2013;52(6):399–414.

32. Tucker G. Pharmacokinetic considerations and challenges in oral anticancer drugs. *Clin Pharmacist.* 2019;11(6). doi:10.1211/PJ.2019.20206478.

33. Huang R, Boltze J, Li S. Strategies for improved intra-arterial treatments targeting brain tumors: a systematic review. *Front Oncol.* 2020;10:1443. doi:10.3389/fonc.2020.01443.

34. DeVita VT, Lawrence, TS Rosenberg SA. *Cancer: Principles and Practice of Oncology.* 11th ed. Wolters Kluwer; 2019.

35. MedlinePlus. Fluorouracil topical. https://medlineplus.gov/druginfo/meds/a605010.html. Accessed April 16, 2021.

36. United States Pharmacopeial Convention. USP general chapter <800>: hazardous drugs—handling in healthcare settings. USP 43-NF 38. https://www.usp.org/compounding/general-chapter-hazardous-drugs-handling-healthcare. Updated July 20, 2020. Accessed May 15, 2021.

37. Hazardous drug exposure in healthcare. National Institute for Occupational Safety and Health website. https://www.cdc.gov/niosh/topics/hazdrug/default.html. Updated May 4, 2020. Accessed May 15, 2021.

38. Rontgen WC. On a New Kind of Ray. *Science.* 1896; 3(59): 227-231. doi: 10.1126/science.3.59.227.

39. American Cancer Society. Evolution of cancer treatments: radiation. www.cancer.org/cancer/cancer-basics/history-of-cancer/cancer-treatment-radiation.html. Updated June 12, 2014. Accessed April 16, 2021.

40. Mitin T. Radiation therapy techniques in cancer treatment. UpToDate. https://www.uptodate.com/contents/radiation-therapy-techniques-in-cancer-treatment. Updated September 8, 2020. Accessed April 16, 2021.

41. Hoskin P, Choudhury A, Kenny LM, Andreas A. Chapter 67: Imaging for radiotherapy planning. In: *Grainger & Allison's Diagnostic Radiology.* 7th ed. Elsevier; 2021:1737–1751.

42. Delaney KH. *Protons and Charged-Particle Radiotherapy.* 1st ed. Lippincott Williams & Wilkins; 2008.

43. Riley B. Peaking into the future with proton therapy. *J Radiol Nurs.* 2007;26(4):115–120.

44. University of Virginia. Gamma knife: history and technical overview. https://med.virginia.edu/neurosurgery/services/gamma-knife/for-physicians/history-and-technical-overview/. Accessed April 16, 2021.

45. American Cancer Society. Getting internal radiation therapy (brachytherapy). https://www.cancer.org/treatment/treatments-and-side-effects/treatment-types/radiation/internal-radiation-therapy-brachytherapy.html. Updated February 10, 2017. Accessed April 16, 2021.

46. Skowronek J, Wawrzyniak-Hojczyk M, Ambrochowicz K. Brachytherapy in accelerated partial breast irradiation (APBI)—review of treatment methods. *J Contemp Bbrachytherapy.* 2012;4(3):152–164.

47. Willett CG, Czito BG, Tyler DS. Intraoperative radiation therapy. *J Clin Oncol.* 2007;25(8):971–977.

48. Moningi S, Armour EP, Terezakis SA, et al. High-dose-rate intraoperative radiation therapy: the nuts and bolts of starting a program. *J Contemp Brachytherapy.* 2014;6(1):99–105.

49. Khaddour KH. *Hematopoietic Stem Cell Transplantation (Bone Marrow Transplant).* StatPearls Publishing; 2020.

50. National Marrow Donor Program. Disease specific HCT indications and outcomes data. https://bethematchclinical.org/transplant-indi-

cations-and-outcomes/disease/specific-indications-and-outcomes/. Accessed April 16, 2021.

51. Health Resources and Services Administration. Transplant activity report. https://bloodstemcell.hrsa.gov/data/donation-and-transplantation-statistics-activity-report. Updated November 18, 2019. Accessed April 16, 2021.

52. Vose JM. Hematopoietic stem cell transplantation. In: Goldman LS, ed. *Goldmans Cecil Medicine*: Saunders; 2012:1158–1162.

53. Singh AM. Allogenic stem cell transplantation: a historical and a scientific review. *Cancer Res.* 2016;76(22):6445–6451.

54. Dehn J, Spellman S, Hurley CK, et al. Selection of unrelated donors and cord blood units for hematopoietic cell transplantation: guidelines from the NMDP/CIBMTR. *Blood.* 2019;134(12):924–934.

55. Lewis R, Plowman PN, Samash PN. Chapter 6: Malignant disease. In: Feather A, Randall D, Waterhouse M, eds. *Kumar and Clark's Clinical Medicine.* 10th ed. Elsevier; 2021:95–135.

56. Dinner S, Gurbuxani S, Jain N, Stock W, et al. Chapter 66: Acute lymphoblastic leukemia in adults. In: Hoffman R, Benz EJ, Silberstein LE et al, eds. *Hematology: Basic Principles and Practice.* 7th ed. Elsevier; 2018:1029–1054. e2.

57. Park BH. Chapter 171: Cancer biology and genetics. In: Goldman L, Schafer AI, eds. *Goldman-Cecil Medicine.* 26th ed. Elsevier; 2020:1199–1204. e2.

58. Wilson FR, Coombes ME, Wylie Q, et al. Herceptin® (trastuzumab) in HER2-positive early breast cancer: protocol for a systematic review and cumulative network meta-analysis. *Syst Rev.* 2017;6(1):196. doi:10.1186/s13643-017-0588-2.

59. Gallagher CJ, Smith M, Samash J. Chapter 17: Malignant disease. In: Kumar P, Clark M, eds. *Kumar and Clark's Clinical Medicine*: Elsevier; 2017:583–644.

60. Kootstra JJ, Dijkstra PU, Rietman H, et al. A longitudinal study of shoulder and arm morbidity in breast cancer survivors 7 years after sentinel lymph node biopsy or axillary lymph node dissection. *Breast Cancer Res Treat.* 2013;139(1):125–134.

61. Nelson-Veniard M, Thambo JB. Chemotherapy-induced cardiotoxicity: incidence, diagnosis and prevention. *Bull Cancer.* 2015;102(7–8):622–626.

62. Classen J, Nitzsche S, Wallwiener D, et al. Fibrotic changes after postmastectomy radiotherapy and reconstructive surgery in breast cancer. A retrospective analysis in 109 patients. *Strahlenther Onkol.* 2010;186(11):630–636.

63. Vici P, Pizzuti L, Natoli C, et al. Triple positive breast cancer: a distinct subtype? *Cancer Treat Rev.* 20151;41(2):69–76.

64. Scheuer W, Friess T, Burtscher H, Bossenmaier B, Endl J, Hasmann M. Strongly enhanced antitumor activity of trastuzumab and pertuzumab combination treatment on HER2-positive human xenograft tumor models. *Cancer Res.* 2009;69:9330–9336.

65. Jerusalem G, Lancellotti P, Kim SB. HER2+ breast cancer treatment and cardiotoxicity: monitoring and management. *Breast Cancer Res Treat.* 2019;177(2):237–250.

66. Butt Z, Lai JS, Rao D, Heinemann AW, Bill A, Cella D. Measurement of fatigue in cancer, stroke, and HIV using the Functional Assessment of Chronic Illness Therapy—Fatigue (FACIT-F) scale. *J Psychosom Res.* 2013;74(1):64–68.

67. Kendrick KR, Baxi SC, Smith RM. Usefulness of the modified 0–10 Borg scale in assessing the degree of dyspnea in patients with COPD and asthma. *J Emerg Nurs.* 2000;26(3):216–222.

68. Dingemans SA, Kleipool SC, Mulders MAM, et al. Normative data for the Lower Extremity Functional Scale (LEFS). *Acta Orthop.* 2017;88(4):422–426.

69. Huang MH, Blackwood J, Croarkin E. Oncology section task force on breast cancer outcomes: clinical measures of balance a systematic review. *Rehabil Oncol.* 2015;33(1):18–27.

70. Miltenburg NC, Boogerd W. Chemotherapy-induced neuropathy: a comprehensive survey. *Cancer Treat Rev.* 2014;40(7):872–882.

71. Shumway-Cook A, Horak FB. Assessing the influence of sensory integration on balance: Suggestions from the field. *Phys Ther.* 1986;66:1548–1549.

72. Casanova C, Celli BR, Barria P, et al. The 6-min walk distance in healthy subjects: reference standards from seven countries. *Eur Respir J.* 2011;37(1):150–156.

73. Sprint G, Cook D, Weeks D. Towards automating clinical assessments: a survey of the Timed Up and Go (TUG). *IEEE Rev Biomed Eng.* 2015;8:64–77.

74. World Health Organization. International Classification of Functioning, Disability and Health (ICF); 2001. https://www.who.int/standards/classifications/international-classification-of-functioning-disability-and-health. Accessed May 23, 2021.

6

Pharmacological Principles in Cancer Care

SARAH LERCHENFELDT, PHARMD, BCPS, CHRISTOPHER M. WILSON, PT, DPT, DSCPT, BOARD CERTIFIED GERIATRIC CLINICAL SPECIALIST

CHAPTER OUTLINE

Introduction

For many oncology rehabilitation (Onc R) clinicians who may not administer or prescribe medications, a clear understanding of the complex and ever-changing use of chemotherapeutics and supportive medications is often one of the most challenging parts of working with people with cancer (PWC). An overarching understanding of the clinical aims, mechanism of action, and adverse effects of antineoplastic agents is a skill that can not only help Onc R clinicians to provide better care but to also more effectively integrate care with the interdisciplinary cancer team. Furthermore, an

Onc R clinician can utilize their skills and interventions to facilitate optimal outcomes for chemotherapy or medical management. For example, one of the key concepts in treatment decisions for selection of a treatment regimen is a patient's performance status (e.g., Karnofsky Performance Scale) and if rehabilitative procedures can improve performance status, the individual may be a better candidate for the first line treatment regimen.[1] In addition, a comprehensive, safe Onc R program can improve a person's ability to tolerate a more aggressive first line chemotherapy regimen with less adverse effects, thereby improving the likelihood of survival or remission.[2] Finally, as pain, nausea, vomiting, or weakness are often adverse effects of chemotherapy, nonpharmacologic interventions for these issues may be useful adjuncts to the person's comprehensive care. The strategic balance between judicious use of pharmacologic and nonpharmacologic interventions is key to successful outcomes within cancer care and optimizing quality of life (QOL).

Overview of Important Pharmacological Principles

Pharmacology can be defined as the study of the interactions between drugs and the body. There are two broad divisions of pharmacology known as pharmacokinetics and pharmacodynamics. Pharmacokinetics (PK) refers to the movement of drugs through the body, whereas pharmacodynamics (PD) refers to the body's biological response to these drugs (Figure 6.1). Although therapists do not generally prescribe or administer drugs, it is important to consider pharmacokinetic and pharmacodynamic principles to help individualize Onc R regimens or identify certain adverse drug reactions if a body system is negatively affected by the cancer or its treatment.[3] In many cases, the Onc R clinician may be the first to observe or identify a clinical manifestation of an adverse drug effect, such as pain, ataxia, weakness, or abdominal distress. For this section, a variety of sources were utilized to develop and synthesize the content.[3–9]

Drug absorption, distribution, metabolism, and elimination are the basic principles of pharmacokinetics (Figure 6.2). These four properties determine the onset, intensity, and duration of action for different drugs. Once a drug is absorbed into the plasma it is distributed in systems within the body, such as the blood and lymphatic vessels, to reach its target organ. The drug may be metabolized, where the body typically inactivates the drug through enzymatic degradation (primarily in the liver), and

excreted, in which the drug is eliminated from the body (primarily by the kidneys, liver, and feces).

Each of these four principles will now be reviewed in more detail.

Pharmacokinetics

Absorption

Absorption is the transfer of a drug from the site of administration to the bloodstream. The rate and efficiency of absorption depends on several factors, including the drug's route of administration and its physico-chemical properties. Bioavailability is an important concept to consider when thinking about drug absorption. It can be defined as the proportion of the administered drug that reaches the systemic circulation in an unchanged form. Understanding bioavailability is important for multiple reasons. It can help Onc R clinicians determine a drug's most appropriate route and frequency. It is also important when determining an appropriate loading and maintenance dose.

Variations in bioavailability are often seen with different routes of administration. Parenteral administration includes the intravenous, intramuscular, and subcutaneous routes. This type of drug administration can be useful for drugs that are poorly absorbed or unstable in the gastrointestinal tract. They can also be used when patients are unable to take oral medications or when rapid onset of action is required. The intravenous route is considered to result in 100% bioavailability. With enteral administration, a drug can be swallowed, placed under the tongue (sublingual), or in between the gums (buccal). Whereas drugs that are swallowed must go through the digestive tract, sublingual and buccal administration allows drugs to be absorbed directly into the bloodstream. Enteral administration is often the most convenient and economical method. Some drugs can also be dispersed in an aerosol and are administered via inhalation, which may be most effective for individuals with respiratory disorders. In this case, the drug is delivered directly to the site of action, thereby minimizing systemic adverse effects. It is important to keep in mind that when a drug is given by routes other than intravenous, the bioavailability is generally reduced due to incomplete absorption. Drugs can also be introduced into the body by other routes of administration, including, but not limited to, transdermal or rectal routes.

Another important factor to consider when thinking about absorption is first-pass metabolism. After a drug is swallowed, a drug must pass through the gut lumen, gut wall, and then through the liver before reaching the general circulation. During its first pass through the liver the drug may be metabolized. In some cases, the liver enzymes inactivate large amounts of the drug and only limited amounts of active drug escape the process, thereby reducing bioavailability. First-pass metabolism principally affects drugs that are swallowed, in which parenteral administration of drugs avoids first-pass metabolism.

Distribution

In the process of distribution, drugs can reversibly leave the bloodstream and distribute into organs and tissues. Usually, a drug moves along a concentration gradient until equilibrium is established. One important concept to consider during drug distribution is protein binding. When drugs are bound to plasma proteins, like albumin, they cannot be distributed into tissues or eliminated and are considered pharmacologically inactive. Only free drugs are active and can exert an effect.

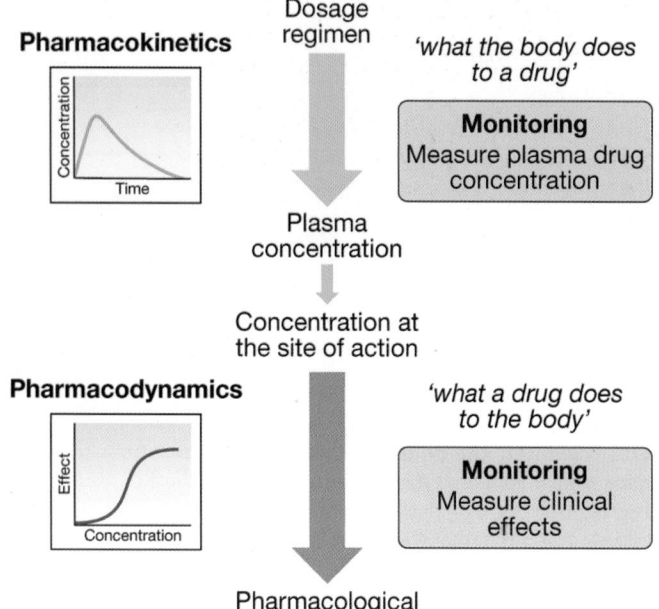

Pharmacokinetics

Concentration / Time

Dosage regimen

'what the body does to a drug'

Monitoring
Measure plasma drug concentration

Plasma concentration

Concentration at the site of action

Pharmacodynamics

Effect / Concentration

'what a drug does to the body'

Monitoring
Measure clinical effects

Pharmacological effects

• **Fig. 6.1** Pharmacokinetics and Pharmacodynamics. (Reprinted with permission from SRJ Maxwell. Chapter 2: Clinical therapeutics and good prescribing. In: Ralston SH, Penman ID, Strachan MWJ, Hobson RP, eds. *Davidson's Principles and Practice of Medicine.* 23rd ed. Elsevier; 2018.)

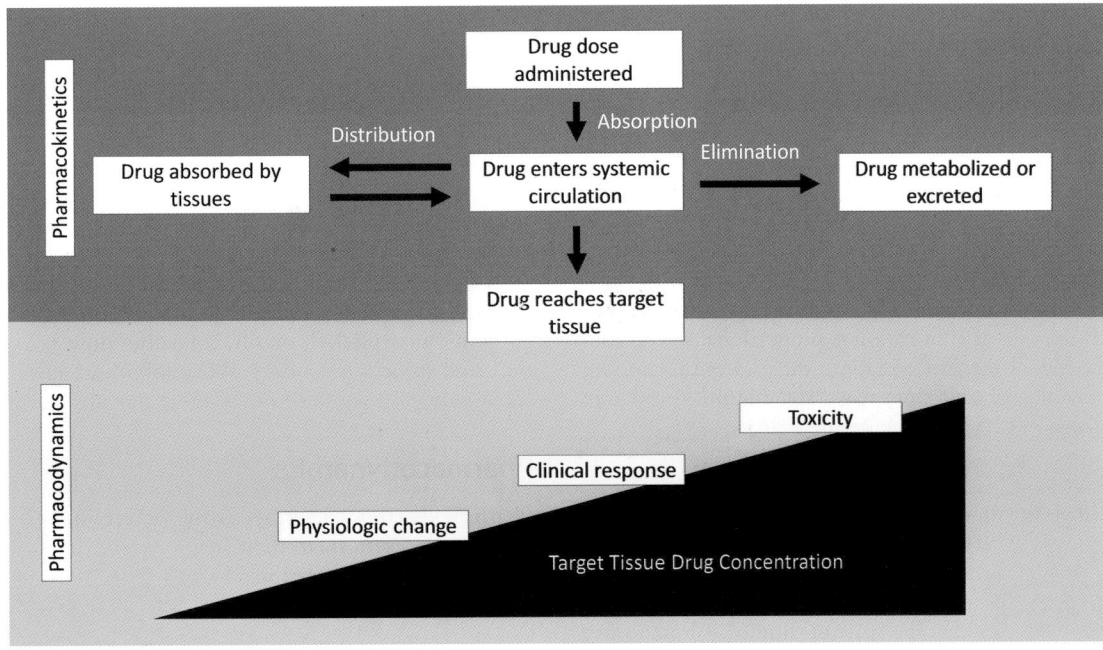

• **Fig. 6.2** Administration to Elimination of Drugs. (Created by Chris Wilson. Printed with permission.)

Clinically, there are important considerations for drugs that are highly bound to albumin. For example, the concentration of albumin falls in many conditions related to cancer, including liver disease, certain inflammatory states, or malnutrition. When this occurs, there is less albumin available to bind to the drug; this leaves more free or active drug to exert its effect. Since there is more active drug available in conditions with low albumin, an individual may be at an increased risk for adverse effects and toxicity if the dose is not adjusted. Another important consideration regarding protein binding is when there is competition among two drugs with high affinity for binding. In this case, there is the potential for a drug interaction which can increase the plasma free-drug concentration and lead to increased adverse effects or toxicity.

In addition to protein binding, there are some barriers to consider when evaluating drug distribution. One example is the blood–brain barrier, which is generally only permeable to lipid-soluble drugs, or those with a low molecular weight. This barrier must be considered when treating certain types of brain tumors or infections like meningitis.

The volume of distribution (Vd) is defined as the volume in which a drug would need to be distributed to produce the same concentration throughout the body as found in plasma. This should not be thought of as an actual physical volume of fluid, but is simply an abstract value that is useful when comparing the relative concentration of the drug in plasma with the rest of the body. In general, drugs with a high Vd are more likely to leave the plasma and enter the extravascular compartments of the body. For this reason, a higher dose of a drug may be required to achieve a given plasma concentration to achieve the intended clinical effect.

Metabolism

Drugs may be metabolized by the liver or other tissues, like the kidneys, gastrointestinal tract, and lungs. Drugs are generally converted to more water-soluble metabolites that can be excreted or eliminated from the body. Most drugs are metabolized to less active or inactive metabolites, although some drugs are metabolized to

active metabolites that can prolong the drug's duration of action. Prodrugs are medications that must be activated via metabolism before they can exert an effect. In some cases, the drug may be metabolized to a toxic metabolite.

To make drugs easier to excrete, there are two main pathways of biotransformation known as Phase 1 and Phase 2 metabolism. These are not sequential processes; some drugs only undergo phase 1 metabolism, whereas others only undergo phase 2 metabolism.

Phase 1 reactions utilize enzymes to transform the drug, which is often converted to a more water-soluble compound by introducing molecules to make the drug more polar. This often occurs via oxidation, reduction, and hydrolysis reactions. Cytochrome P450 enzymes are the most common enzymes catalyzing phase I reactions. These enzymes are essential for the metabolism of many medications. It is important to keep in mind that they are the source for many significant drug interactions, in which the cytochrome P450 enzymes can be inhibited or induced by drugs, resulting in adverse reactions or therapeutic failure. In phase 2, conjugation reactions occur. Often, the metabolic product of phase 1 reactions is combined with another compound that causes it to be more water-soluble. This allows for improved transport through the bloodstream to the kidneys where it can be excreted in the urine.

Elimination

Drug elimination is the process of removing an administered drug and its metabolites from the body. Modes of elimination include biotransformation to inactive metabolites and excretion via the kidney, bile duct, lungs, sweat, or feces. Renal excretion of unchanged drugs is a major route of elimination. Enhancing blood flow, increasing glomerular filtration rate, and decreasing plasma protein binding can help a drug be excreted more rapidly by causing increased filtration of the drug at the glomerulus. Kidney dysfunction may lead to higher plasma drug concentrations in which the dosing regimen may need to be adjusted to prevent drug toxicity.

Zero-order Elimination

With zero-order elimination, the rate of elimination is constant regardless of concentration. The concentrations of these drugs in plasma decrease in a linear fashion over time (e.g., 100 mg/mL → 75 mg/mL → 50 mg/mL → 25 mg/mL) (Figure 6.3B). This occurs with drugs that demonstrate saturation kinetics, in which the clearance mechanisms become saturated at or near the therapeutic concentration of the drug.

First-order Elimination

First-order elimination is more common than zero-order elimination, in which the rate of elimination is proportional to the concentration; the higher the concentration, the greater the amount of drug eliminated per unit time (e.g., 100 mg/mL → 50 mg/mL → 25 mg/mL →12.5 mg/mL) (Figure 6.3A).

Half-Life

A drug's half-life is the time it takes for the plasma drug concentration to be reduced by 50%. Drugs that display zero-order elimination do not have a constant half-life, whereas with first-order elimination, the elimination half-life is constant regardless of the amount of drug in the body. The "rule of thumb" is four to five half-lives must elapse after starting a drug-dosing regimen before steady state is reached. Additionally, after discontinuing the drug, over 95% of the drug will be eliminated in a time interval equal to five half-lives. The effects from a drug with a long half-life may last for several days, even after the drug is discontinued. Knowledge of a drug's elimination half-life allows the clinician to estimate the frequency of dosing required to maintain the plasma concentration of the drug within the therapeutic range.

Considerations in Drug Dosing

Drugs are generally administered to maintain a steady state concentration within the therapeutic window. The therapeutic window is the dosage range between the minimum effective therapeutic concentration and the minimum toxic concentration. A safe and effective dosing regimen will achieve therapeutic levels of the drug without exceeding the minimum toxic concentration that leads to a higher risk of adverse effects. More

information about therapeutic window can be found later in the chapter.

The steady state concentration is achieved when the "rate in" is equal to the "rate out," in which it usually takes about four to five half-lives to reach steady state. Once steady-state drug concentrations are achieved, subsequent doses should only replace the amount of drug that is lost through metabolism and excretion (Figure 6.4). This is known as the maintenance dose, in which the drug is dosed to maintain a steady state concentration within the therapeutic window. In some cases, a loading dose of a drug may be needed to achieve steady-state blood levels more rapidly (e.g., antibiotic in sepsis). Typically, a loading dose is only given one time and to help get a drug above minimum effective level and achieve the target concentration more quickly.

Pharmacodynamics

Pharmacodynamics describes a drug's effect on the body, in which most drugs exert their therapeutic effects and cause potential adverse effects through their interaction with target molecules, such as receptors.

Dose Response Relationships

A dose–response curve describes the relationship between an effect of a drug and the amount of drug given over a period of time (Figure 6.5). These are helpful for determining the safe and effective dosage range of a drug. When evaluating dose–response curves, affinity, potency, and efficacy can be considered. Affinity is the ability of a drug to bind to a receptor. Potency can be defined as the amount of drug required to produce an effect. Efficacy is the magnitude of response a drug causes when it interacts with a receptor. Efficacy is a more clinically useful characteristic than potency since greater efficacy means a drug is more therapeutically beneficial.

Therapeutic Window

The therapeutic window is the range of drug concentrations that elicits a therapeutic response without unacceptable adverse effects

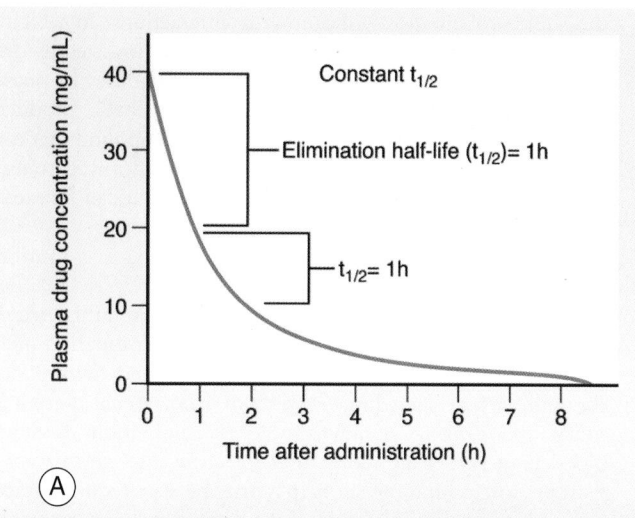

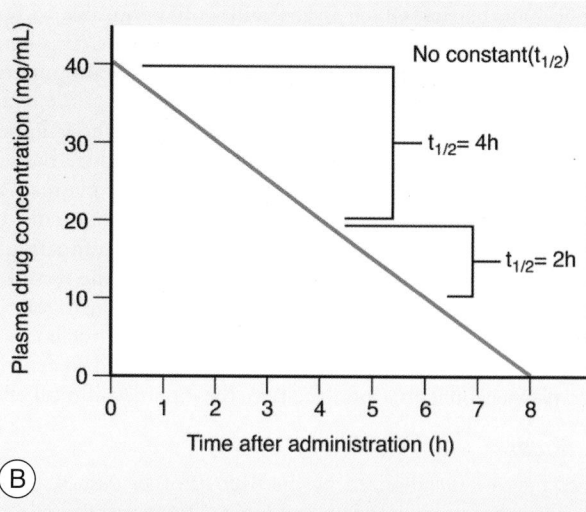

• **Fig. 6.3** Drug Plasma Elimination Pharmacokinetics (A) First Order Elimination. (B) Zero Order Elimination. (Reprinted with permission from Chapter 2: Pharmacokinetics. In: Brenner GM, Stevens CW, eds. *Brenner and Stevens' Pharmacology.* 5th ed. Elsevier; 2018.)

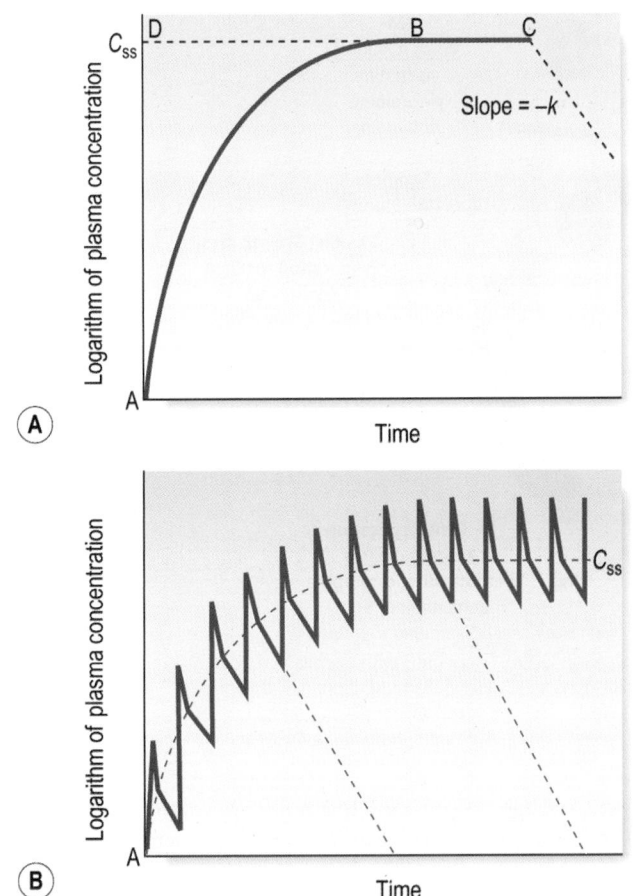

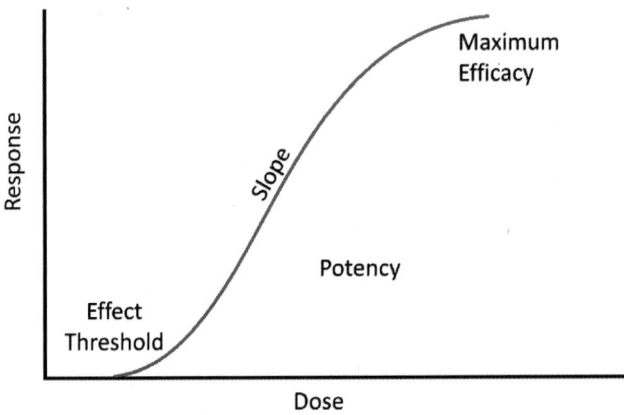

• **Fig. 6.4** Plasma Concentrations IV Versus Pill. Plasma Concentration via IV Administration (A) and Pill Administration (B). (Reprinted with permission from Page C. Chapter 4: Pharmacology. *Medical Sciences*. Elsevier; 2019.)

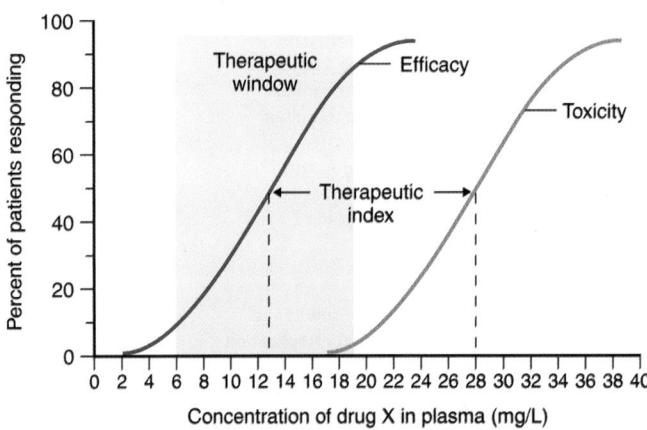

• **Fig. 6.6** Therapeutic Window and Therapeutic Index. (Reprinted with permission from Diasio RB. Chapter 26: Principles of drug therapy. In: Goldman L, Schafer AI, eds. *Goldman-Cecil Medicine*. 26th ed. Elsevier; 2020.)

• **Fig. 6.5** Dose-Response Curve. (Created by Chris Wilson. Printed with permission.)

or toxicity. Therapeutic window is often quantified by a Therapeutic Index (TI) (Figure 6.6). A large therapeutic window is preferred because there is a wider margin between an effective and potentially hazardous dose. For drugs with a small therapeutic window, the drug levels must be monitored closely as there is a small margin between an effective and potentially toxic dose. For example, warfarin is a drug in which the drug levels must be monitored very

closely because it has a narrow therapeutic window. If the dose is too low, the blood level will fall below the therapeutic range and may not be effective. This could lead to a potentially lethal blood clot. If the dose is too high, the blood level will be above the therapeutic range. In this case, the individual is at a higher risk for bleeding, such as a potentially dangerous cerebral hemorrhage.

Drug Classification Based on Interaction With Receptors

Agonists

Generally, when a drug favors the active receptor conformation upon binding it is called an agonist. Full agonists and partial agonists bind to the same receptor, but while a full agonist produces the maximal response, a partial agonist produces a less-than-maximal response, even when all receptors are occupied. In some cases, a partial agonist can even act as an antagonist, by reducing the response produced by a full agonist. For example, the opioid drug buprenorphine, a partial agonist, can bind with high affinity to the opioid receptor, and displace morphine, a full agonist, from the receptor. Since buprenorphine has less intrinsic activity than morphine, it may lead to opioid withdrawal symptoms.

Antagonists

Antagonists favor the inactive conformation of a receptor. When they bind to a receptor, they do not produce a response. They prevent receptor activation and block the effects of agonists. Some drugs cause functional antagonism, in which they act on a downstream receptor and inhibit the ability of an agonist to initiate a response. Drugs can modify or sequester an agonist, so that it is no longer capable of activating the receptor (e.g., heparin and protamine). A physiologic antagonist causes a physiologic effect opposite to that induced by the agonist (e.g., insulin and glucagon).

Targeting Specific Cell Cycle Phases With Chemotherapy

Chemotherapy agents can be classified based on their activity in the cell cycle, in which they can be cell cycle specific or nonspecific. Many cytotoxic chemotherapeutic agents are cell cycle specific

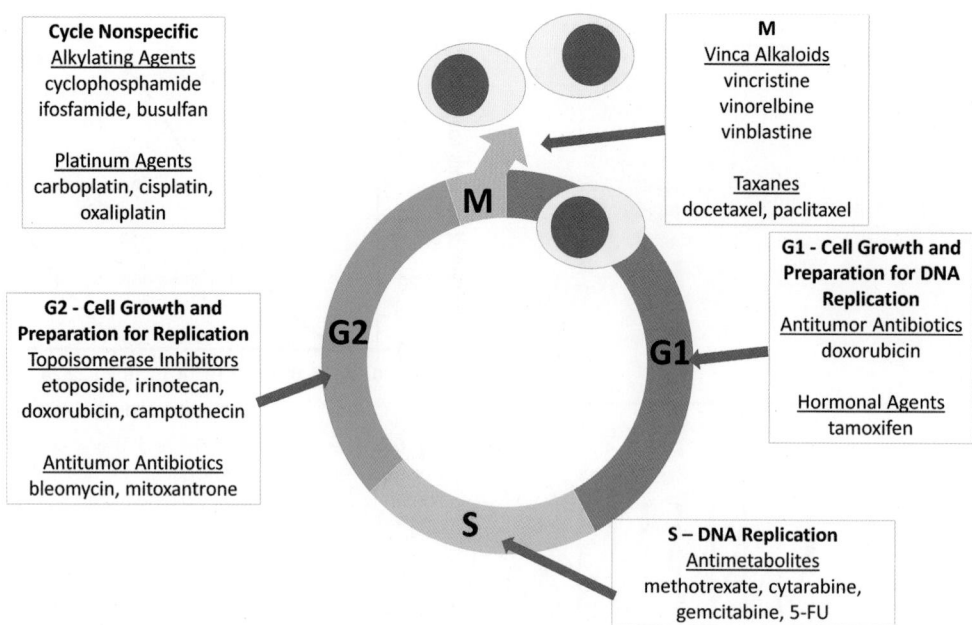

Cycle Nonspecific
Alkylating Agents
cyclophosphamide
ifosfamide, busulfan

Platinum Agents
carboplatin, cisplatin,
oxaliplatin

M
Vinca Alkaloids
vincristine
vinorelbine
vinblastine

Taxanes
docetaxel, paclitaxel

G1 - Cell Growth and
Preparation for DNA
Replication
Antitumor Antibiotics
doxorubicin

Hormonal Agents
tamoxifen

G2 - Cell Growth and
Preparation for Replication
Topoisomerase Inhibitors
etoposide, irinotecan,
doxorubicin, camptothecin

Antitumor Antibiotics
bleomycin, mitoxantrone

S – DNA Replication
Antimetabolites
methotrexate, cytarabine,
gemcitabine, 5-FU

• **Fig. 6.7** Chemotherapeutic Agents and the Cellular Replication Cycle. (Reprinted with permission from Principles of chemotherapy. In: Hoffman BL, Schorge JO, Bradshaw KD, Halvorson LM, Schaffer JI, Corton MM, eds. *Williams Gynecology.* 3rd ed. McGraw Hill; 2016.)

and work by attacking cells in a particular phase of the cell cycle (Figure 6.7). This means they exert their effect on the proportion of cells in the stage of the cycle in which the agent is active. Examples of these drugs include the antimetabolites, taxanes, and vinca alkaloids. Some drugs, like the alkylating agents, are cell cycle nonspecific, in which they exert their cytotoxic effect throughout the cell cycle. Cell cycle nonspecific drugs are more effective than cell cycle specific drugs in resting phase. Both types of agents are more effective when a large proportion of the tumor cells are proliferating. Generally, cancer cells divide more rapidly than noncancerous cells as neoplastic cells are resistant to the normal cellular replication controls. Theoretically, by combining drugs that act in different phases of the cell cycle, the overall cell kill rate should be improved.

The cell cycle is a sequence of events that a cell undergoes to replicate and divide into two daughter cells. During cell division, each cell progresses through a series of steps. In the first phase of growth, known as gap 1 (G_1), the cell increases in size and its cellular contents are duplicated. In the synthesis (S) phase, the DNA is replicated, and in the gap 2 (G_2) phase, the cell continues to grow and prepares to split into two cells. Together, these three phases are known as interphase. During the mitotic (M) phase, the cell, which contains a double complement of DNA, divides into two new identical cells. Following these steps, the cells return to the resting phase (G_0), where they remain until they receive a signal to divide. Through this process there is a series of checkpoints to ensure correct replication.

General Principles for Antineoplastic Therapy

Chemotherapy, also known as antineoplastic therapy, is a type of powerful drug treatment that is used to kill cancer cells. It works by stopping or slowing the growth of cancer cells which have lost normal growth controls.[4] The growth fraction can be defined as the proportion of cells in a tumor population that are actively dividing. Usually, human cancers are clinically detectable when the primary mass is at least 1 cm in diameter (consists of about 10^9 cells).[5] The growth fraction decreases as the tumor size increases,

due to factors such as blood supply limitations.[6] Cell destruction caused by chemotherapy is a first order process, in which the *log-cell kill model* states that each dose of chemotherapy kills a constant fraction of cells, rather than a constant number of cells.[6]

A variety of sources were utilized to develop and synthesize the content of the remaining portion of the chapter and complete references are available for the medication classes and individual drugs via accessible databases and texts.[3–9] It should be noted that the field of medical oncology is ever changing and is highly complex. This section of the text is designed to provide a broad overview of some key effects of chemotherapeutic agents but does not represent a comprehensive list of chemotherapeutic agents, their uses, or adverse effects. Refer to Box 6.1 for additional online resources for clinicians which were also used for synthesizing this section. See Appendix 6.1 for a quick reference guide for common chemotherapy medications and clinical implications.

Alkylating Agents

Alkylating agents are one class of chemotherapy agents. Cytotoxicity results from directly damaging DNA, in which these agents cause cell death through transfer of their alkyl groups to various cellular constituents. They may cause inhibition of DNA replication and transcription, mispairing of DNA, or DNA strand breakage. Alkylating agents work in all phases of the cell cycle. The dose limiting toxicity of alkylating agents is myelosuppression. Other potential adverse effects include nausea/vomiting, alopecia, infertility, and secondary leukemia.

• **BOX 6.1** **Online Resources for Cancer Medications**

Chemocare.com www.chemocare.com
Lexicomp https://online.lexi.com/ (Paid subscription)
UpToDate www.uptodate.com (Paid subscription)
Macromedex https://www.micromedexsolutions.com/home/dispatch (Paid subscription)

• APPENDIX 6.1 Chemotherapy Adverse Effects Quick Reference Guide

Drug	Drug Class	Cancer Types*	Adverse Effects*
Anastrozole (Arimidex)	Nonsteroidal aromatase inhibitor	Breast	Hot flashes, muscle/joint pain, nausea, mood disturbances, osteoporosis, insomnia, edema, dyspnea
Bevacizumab (Avastin)	Anti-VEGF monoclonal antibody	Cervical, colorectal, glioblastoma, NSCLC, hepatocellular, ovarian, renal cell	Nausea, vomiting, diarrhea neutropenia, thrombocytopenia, joint pain, hypertension, fatigue, bleeding, hemorrhage, thromboembolism, impaired wound healing
Capecitabine (Xeloda)	Antimetabolite (pyrimidine analog)	Colorectal, breast, esophageal, gastric, head and neck	Low blood counts, hand-foot syndrome, nausea, vomiting, constipation, mouth sores, numbness/polyneuropathy
Carboplatin (Paraplatin)	Alkylating agent (platinum analog)	Ovarian, head and neck, lung, esophageal, bladder, breast	Low blood counts, electrolyte abnormalities, nausea, vomiting, polyneuropathy, ototoxicity
Cisplatin (Platinol; Platinol-AQ)	Alkylating agent (platinum analog)	Testicular, ovarian, bladder, head and neck, esophageal, NSCLC, SCLC, breast, gastric, lymphoma, MM, osteosarcoma	Low blood counts, nausea, vomiting, nephrotoxicity, ototoxicity, polyneuropathy
Cyclophosphamide (Cytoxan)	Alkylating agent (nitrogen mustard)	HL, NHL, CLL, ALL CML, AML, MM, breast, ovarian	Leukopenia/neutropenia, nausea, vomiting, diarrhea, mouth sores
Docetaxel (Taxotere)	Antimicrotubular agent (Taxane)	Breast, gastric, NSCLC, SCLC, head and neck, prostate, stomach, ovarian	Low blood counts, polyneuropathy, nausea, vomiting, diarrhea, weakness, muscle pain
Doxorubicin (Adriamycin)	Anthracycline (topoisomerase II inhibitor)	ALL, AML, bladder, breast, bone/soft tissue sarcoma, head and neck, lymphoma, liver, kidney, MM, ovarian, SCLC, renal	Weakness, nausea, vomiting, low blood counts, mouth sores, cardiotoxicity
Exemestane (Aromasin)	Aromatase inhibitor	Breast	Hot flashes, bone/joint pain, hypertension, fatigue, depression, pain, insomnia
Etoposide (Vepesid, VP-16)	Topoisomerase II inhibitor	ALL, AML, NHL, HL, MM, testicular, bladder, prostate, lung, stomach, lymphoma, uterine, sarcoma	Low blood counts, menopause, nausea, vomiting, low blood pressure, mouth sores, diarrhea, polyneuropathy
Fluorouracil (5-FU; Adrucil)	Antimetabolite (pyrimidine analog)	Colorectal, gastric, esophageal, pancreatic, breast, head and neck, bladder, cervical, thymic	Diarrhea, nausea, low blood counts, hand-foot syndrome, mouth sores
Gemcitabine (Gemzar)	Antimetabolite (pyrimidine analog)	Pancreas, NSCLC, bladder, soft tissue sarcoma, breast, ovarian, head and neck	Low blood counts, fever, nausea, vomiting, mouth sores, dyspnea, peripheral edema
Leuprolide (Lupron)	Gonadotropin releasing hormone agonist	Breast, prostate	Hot flashes, decreased libido, weakness, mood changes, muscle/joint pain, weight gain, edema
Methotrexate (MTX, Otrexup, Trexall)	Antimetabolite (antifolate)	ALL, osteosarcoma, NHL, breast, head and neck, lung, gastric	Low blood counts, mouth sores, nephrotoxicity, diarrhea, nausea, vomiting, hepatotoxicity, central neurotoxicity
Oxaliplatin (Eloxatin)	Alkylating agent (platinum analog)	Colorectal, pancreatic, ovarian, testicular	Polyneuropathy, nausea, vomiting, diarrhea, mouth sores, low blood counts, back pain, join pain
Paclitaxel (Taxol)	Antimicrotubule agent (Taxane)	Breast, cervical, NSCLC, ovarian, lung, esophageal	Low blood counts, muscle/joint pain, polyneuropathy, edema, low blood pressure, nausea, vomiting, diarrhea
Tamoxifen (Nolvadex)	Selective estrogen receptor modulator (Antiestrogen)	Breast	Hot flashes, hypertension, edema, mood changes, nausea, thromboembolism
Trastuzumab (Herceptin)	Anti-HER2/Neu monoclonal antibody	HER2/neu+ breast, gastric cancer	Weakness, nausea, vomiting, diarrhea, muscle/joint pain, dyspnea, edema, dizziness, cardiotoxicity
Vinblastine (Velban)	Antimicrotubular agent (Vinca alkaloid)	Lymphoma, testicular, NSCLC, head and neck, bladder, soft tissue sarcoma	Low blood counts, weakness, nausea, vomiting, hypertension, muscle/joint pain, constipation, dyspnea
Vincristine (Oncovin)	Antimicrotubular agent (Vinca alkaloid)	ALL, chronic leukemias, lymphoma, MM, testicular, Ewing's sarcoma, intracranial tumors	Constipation, nausea, vomiting, polyneuropathy

*Not an all-inclusive list.

ALL, Acute lymphoblastic leukemia; *AML*, acute myeloid leukemia; *CLL*, chronic lymphocytic leukemia; *CML*, chronic myeloid leukemia; *DVT*, deep vein thrombosis; *GBM*, glioblastoma multiforme; *MM*, multiple myeloma; *NHL*, non-Hodgkin's lymphoma; *NSCLC*, non-small cell lung cancer; *SCLC*, small cell lung cancer; *WBC*, white blood count.

By Andrew Chongaway, PT, DPT.

The nitrogen mustard agents are one type of alkylating agent. Cyclophosphamide (Cytoxan) may be used as a conditioning regimen prior to a hematopoietic stem cell transplant, in the treatment of non-Hodgkin lymphoma (NHL), testicular cancer, and sarcoma. Ifosfamide (Ifex) may be used in the treatment of NHL, ovarian cancer, breast cancer, and neuroblastoma. Both agents are prodrugs that have the potential to cause hemorrhagic cystitis (hematuria, urinary urgency/frequency) due to acrolein, a toxic metabolite that is formed during metabolism to the active drug. The incidence can be reduced with the drug called mesna (Mesnex), which is often classified as a chemoprotectant or a cytoprotectant drug. Mesna inactivates acrolein thereby reducing the risk of the hemorrhagic cystitis. Ifosfamide also has the potential to cause neurologic toxicity.[10]

The nitrosoureas, another type of alkylating agent, includes carmustine (BiCNU, Gliadel Wafer) and lomustine (Gleostine). These drugs are highly lipid soluble and can cross the blood brain barrier. For this reason, they are used in the management of brain tumors. Hematologic toxicity may be delayed, therefore counts must be monitored for 6 weeks. They may also cause ataxia, dizziness, and pulmonary toxicity.

Platinum Analogs

The platinum analogs are commonly classified as alkylating agents, but do not technically alkylate DNA. The activated forms of these drugs react with nucleophilic sites on DNA to form cross-links and decrease replication, very similar to alkylating reactions. Cisplatin (Platinol; Platinol AQ) and carboplatin (Paraplatin) are used in the treatment of various cancers including lung, ovarian, bladder, and testicular. Cisplatin can cause neurotoxicity, including polyneuropathy, which is termed chemotherapy-induced polyneuropathy (CIPN). Neurologic complications may also include cognitive impairment as well as vestibulopathy, which can lead to ataxia and vertigo. Cisplatin can also cause nephrotoxicity. Carboplatin causes hematologic toxicity. Oxaliplatin (Eloxatin) is used in the management of colorectal cancer. It may also cause polyneuropathy. Finally, platinum analogs are known to cause ototoxicity and associated hearing loss. A baseline hearing test is often performed prior to the decision to administer certain platinum analogs.

Antimetabolites

The antimetabolites are structural analogs of naturally occurring substances in the body. They exert damage by incorporating directly into DNA or RNA or competing for binding sites on enzymes. They inhibit cell growth and proliferation in the S phase of the cell cycle. Common adverse effects include myelosuppression, mucositis, and neurotoxicity.

Methotrexate (Trexall) is a commonly used antimetabolite. It is a folic acid analog that competitively inhibits dihydrofolate reductase and interferes with DNA synthesis, repair, and cellular replication. It is used for various types of cancer, including leukemias, lymphomas, and osteosarcomas. Methotrexate has the potential to cause many adverse effects, including mucositis, acute renal failure, bone marrow suppression, gastrointestinal toxicity, and neurotoxicity. The elimination of methotrexate is reduced in patients with ascites and pleural effusions, which may prolong the effects of the drug and increase the risk of toxicity. Leucovorin (folinic acid) rescue is required with high-dose methotrexate to help limit toxicity to normal tissue. Leucovorin is a reduced form of folic acid that helps restore the folate required for DNA/RNA synthesis.[11]

5-Fluorouracil (5-FU) (Adrucil) and capecitabine (Xeloda) are antimetabolites used in the treatment of colorectal cancer and pancreatic cancer. They inhibit thymidylate synthetase which interferes with DNA synthesis. These agents may cause hand-and-foot syndrome, also known as palmar-plantar erythrodysesthesia or chemotherapy-induced acral erythema (Figure 6.8). This syndrome is characterized by numbness, tingling, paresthesia, and swelling. It may lead to erythema, desquamation, blistering, and severe pain.[12]

Cytarabine (Cytosar-U) is a pyrimidine analog that inhibits DNA polymerase resulting in decreased DNA synthesis and repair. It can cause myelosuppression and gastrointestinal toxicity (nausea, vomiting, diarrhea). Neurotoxicity can occur with high-dose treatment, including acute cerebellar toxicity. Individuals may also experience symptoms such as ataxia or personality changes. More severe cases may cause seizures, coma, or death.[13] Gemcitabine (Gemzar), which is utilized with various cancers (e.g., breast, ovarian, and pancreatic), is also a pyrimidine analog that inhibits DNA synthesis by inhibition of DNA polymerase and ribonucleotide reductase. Myelosuppression is the main adverse effect. Additionally, it causes gastrointestinal toxicity and may also cause a flu-like syndrome, including fever, malaise, headache, and chills.[14]

6-Mercaptopurine (6-MP) (Purixan) is a purine analog used in the treatment of acute lymphoblastic leukemia that inhibits *de novo* purine synthesis (via the ribose monophosphate metabolite)

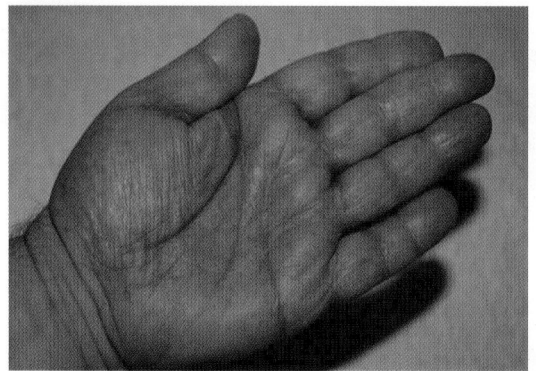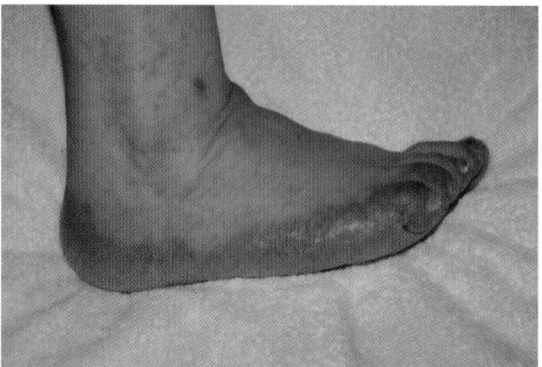

• **Fig. 6.8** Hand-and-Foot Syndrome. (Reprinted with permission from Webster-Gandy JD, How C, Harrold K. Palmar–plantar erythrodysesthesia (PPE): a literature review with commentary on experience in a cancer centre. *Eur J Oncol Nurs*. 2007;11(3):238–246.)

and DNA synthesis (via the deoxyribose triphosphate metabolite). It causes dose-limiting myelosuppression and hepatotoxicity. Since it is metabolized to an inactive metabolite by xanthine oxidase, significant dose reductions are required if given concomitantly with xanthine oxidase inhibitors like allopurinol (Aloprim, Zyloprim) or febuxostat (Uloric).

Microtubule Damaging Agents

Microtubules are intracellular structures that form part of the cell's cytoskeleton. They play a major part in many cellular processes, including cell division. Microtubules are the major components of mitotic spindles, which are used to pull chromosomes apart and move them to opposite sides of the dividing cell. This process ensures that newly formed daughter cells inherit a copy of each of the parent cell's chromosomes. Some drugs classes, including the vinca alkaloids and taxanes, exert their cytotoxic effect by damaging the microtubules.

The vinca alkaloids include vinblastine (Alkaban-AQ, Velban), vincristine (Oncovin, Vincasar PFS), and vinorelbine (Navelbine). They are used to treat different types of cancer like lymphoma and non-small cell lung cancer (NSCLC). These drugs work in the M phase of the cell cycle by inhibiting microtubule polymerization. They bind to the building blocks of tubulin and inhibit the microtubule formation that is necessary for cell division. Vinblastine and vinorelbine are known to cause dose-limiting myelosuppression. Vincristine can cause dose-limiting neurotoxicity. Most individuals receiving this agent will experience some degree of neuropathy. The earliest symptoms are usually paresthesias in the fingertips or feet (with or without pain), muscle cramps, or mild distal weakness. These symptoms often develop after several weeks of treatment and after cumulative doses. Occasionally, there may be profound weakness, with bilateral foot drop, wrist drop, and loss of all sensory modalities. Autonomic neuropathy may also occur with vincristine, leading to constipation and paralytic ileus.

The taxanes, which include paclitaxel (Taxol, Onxal) and docetaxel (Taxotere), are commonly used in the management of breast, ovarian, and lung cancers. They interfere with the late G_2 phase of the cell cycle. These agents work by promoting microtubule assembly. They stabilize the microtubules, preventing microtubule depolymerization, and arrest the cells that are in mitosis. Both agents can cause leukopenia and polyneuropathy. Treatment with paclitaxel may cause hypersensitivity reactions to the agent (Cremophor) used to solubilize the drug. Docetaxel may cause fluid retention and peripheral edema.

Topoisomerase Inhibitors

The topoisomerase family of enzymes alter the supercoiling of double-stranded DNA. A transient cut is formed in one or both strands of the DNA, allowing the supercoiled DNA to relax ahead of the replication fork as replication progresses. Regulation of DNA supercoiling is essential to transcription and replication. Topoisomerase inhibitors bind to topoisomerase I or topoisomerase II and limit the ability of DNA to repair itself resulting in cell death.

The camptothecins are topoisomerase I inhibitors and include topotecan (Hycamtin) and irinotecan (Camptosar). Topotecan is often used in the treatment of ovarian cancer and is known to cause myelosuppression. Irinotecan, a prodrug, is often used in the treatment of colorectal cancer. Its use is limited by severe gastrointestinal toxicity. An acute form of diarrhea may occur within 24 hours of administration due to cholinergic activity and can be treated with atropine. A delayed form of diarrhea may also occur about 2 to 10 days after treatment. As irinotecan is a prodrug, many of these toxic effects are due to an active metabolite (SN-38) that causes direct mucosal damage with water and electrolyte malabsorption and mucous hypersecretion. This form of diarrhea is very dangerous and can be life-threatening. It is treated with loperamide (Imodium). Persons with conditions such as Gilbert's syndrome are highly susceptible to irinotecan toxicity.

Etoposide (VP-16) (Toposar) is a topoisomerase II inhibitor. It is used in the management of small cell lung cancer (SCLC), testicular cancer, and lymphoma. The dose limiting toxicity for etoposide is myelosuppression, primarily leukopenia. Hypotension may occur due to rapid administration therefore it must be infused slowly.

The anthracyclines have multiple mechanisms of action. They inhibit topoisomerase II and prevent repair of DNA during replication causing DNA strand breaks. In addition, they have a high affinity for binding to DNA and insert themselves between DNA base pairs causing additional DNA breaks. Lastly, these agents are metabolized in the liver to form reactive oxygen species (e.g., oxygen free radicals), adding to both the cytotoxicity and adverse effect profile. The anthracyclines include doxorubicin (Adriamycin), daunorubicin (Cerubidine), idarubicin (Idamycin PFS), and epirubicin (Ellence). They can cause dose-limiting myelosuppression and dose-limiting cardiotoxicity. The risk of cardiotoxicity increases with cumulative doses and close monitoring of cardiac function with video imaging is required. A chronic form of cardiotoxicity may result from an increased production of free radicals within the myocardium leading to progressive injury and loss of cardiomyocytes. It can lead to dilated cardiomyopathy associated with heart failure. An acute form of cardiotoxicity may also occur, in which symptoms may include arrhythmias, myocarditis, and pericarditis. Acute cardiotoxicity is often considered transient and most individuals are usually asymptomatic.

Targeted Therapies

Monoclonal Antibodies

Monoclonal antibody drugs are commonly used in cancer treatment. They affect a number of different cell surface and soluble target proteins and function in many different ways. Some of their mechanisms of action include blocking an activation signal that is necessary for continued cell growth, antibody-dependent cellular cytotoxicity (ADCC), complement-dependent cytotoxicity (CDC), and induction of apoptosis. In some cases, the therapeutic effects are due to multiple mechanisms.[15]

Rituximab (Rituxan) is a mainstay in the therapy for a broad variety of B-cell malignancies. It is directed against the CD20 antigen on B-lymphocytes. Rituximab binds to antigen on the cell surface and activates complement-dependent B-cell cytotoxicity. It causes cell killing through antibody-dependent cellular toxicity and apoptosis. It has many indications, including CD20-positive NHL and CD20-positive chronic lymphocytic leukemia. Although all monoclonal antibodies have the potential to cause infusion-related reactions, rituximab has a high-risk for these reactions, which include fever, chills, and hypotension. For this reason, special precautions must be taken, in which premedication, such as acetaminophen (Tylenol) and diphenhydramine (Benadryl) can be administered to help attenuate or prevent infusion-related reactions.[16]

CD30 is a tumor marker elevated in many kinds of lymphoma. Brentuximab vedotin (Adcetris) is an antibody drug that is directed at CD30. It is conjugated with a synthetic antineoplastic agent that inhibits microtubule polymerization and causes cell death upon its release. Brentuximab is used for Hodgkin lymphoma and anaplastic large cell lymphoma. It can cause infusion-related reactions and neutropenia. In addition, this agent may cause polyneuropathy that is predominantly sensory. Persons living with and beyond cancer (PLWBCs) should be monitored for symptoms of neuropathy, including paresthesia, discomfort, neuropathic pain, and weakness.

Trastuzumab (Herceptin) is used in the treatment of human epidermal growth factor receptor 2 positive (HER-2+) breast cancer and gastric cancer. It binds to the HER-2 protein and causes ADCC, inhibiting the proliferation of cells which overexpress the HER-2 protein. Treatment of breast cancer with trastuzumab may be complicated by cardiotoxicity. In most PLWBCs, trastuzumab-induced cardiotoxicity is reversible, where left ventricular ejection fraction improves after trastuzumab withdrawal. Trastuzumab may also lead to pulmonary toxicity and infusion-related reactions.

Bevacizumab (Avastin) is a monoclonal antibody that prevents vascular endothelial growth factor-A (VEGF-A) from interacting with the target VEGF receptors, inhibiting microvascular growth. VEGF is an important angiogenic growth factor and its inhibition prevents tumors from being able to create new blood vessels, limiting the supply of nutrients, and slowing tumor growth. Bevacizumab is used in the management of many cancers, including colorectal cancer, NSCLC, and renal cancer. Unfortunately, it has several potential toxicities. It may cause or worsen hypertension; therefore, blood pressure must be monitored closely and caution must be used in patients with preexisting hypertension. Permanent discontinuation is recommended in individuals who experience a hypertensive crisis or hypertensive encephalopathy. Blocking VEGF increases risk of arterial thromboembolism and may lead to cerebral infarction, stroke, or myocardial infarction. It may also increase the risk of deep vein thrombosis. Gastrointestinal perforation and severe or fatal hemorrhage may occur. Additionally, the incidence of wound healing and surgical complications is increased in patients who have received bevacizumab. This agent should be discontinued at least 28 days prior to surgery and should not be reinitiated for at least 28 days after surgery and until the wound is fully healed.

Ipilimumab (Yervoy) is a monoclonal antibody which binds to the cytotoxic T-lymphocyte associated antigen 4 (CTLA-4) and may indirectly mediate T-cell immune responses against tumors and boost the immune response against melanoma cells in the body. Severe and fatal immune-mediated adverse effects due to T-cell activation and proliferation may occur, in which any organ system may be involved. Potential toxicities include enterocolitis, hepatitis, dermatitis (including toxic epidermal necrolysis), neuropathy, and endocrinopathy.

Immunomodulatory Drugs

Thalidomide (Thalomid) is an antineoplastic agent with a complex mechanism of action that includes immunomodulatory and antiangiogenic properties. Effects may include inhibition of tumor necrosis factor-alpha (TNF-α), increase in natural killer cells, altered adhesion molecule expression, enhanced cell-mediated cytotoxic effects, and suppression of angiogenesis. It is approved for the treatment of multiple myeloma in combination with dexamethasone. Adverse effects of thalidomide include bone marrow suppression, polyneuropathy, constipation, weakness, and fatigue. It causes an increased risk of thrombotic complications, including deep-vein thrombosis, especially in persons with hematologic

malignancy. For this reason, most patients are placed on anticoagulation when thalidomide is initiated. Due to the potential for severe and potentially life-threatening birth defects, thalidomide is contraindicated in pregnancy and extreme caution must be used in women of reproductive age. Lenalidomide (Revlimid), an analog of thalidomide, has similar actions in which it also has immunomodulatory, antiangiogenic, and antineoplastic properties. It also increases the risk of hematologic toxicity, thrombotic complications, and embryo-fetal toxicity. Lenalidomide is approved for use in the treatment of multiple myeloma, myelodysplastic syndrome, and lymphoma.

Tyrosine Kinase Inhibitors

Receptor tyrosine kinases (RTKs) are proteins responsible for the activation of signaling cascades important for many cellular functions, such as cell signaling and growth. In some cases, RTKs become dysregulated and lead to cancer. Drugs known as tyrosine kinase inhibitors are a type of targeted therapy that can block the actions of RTKs to help in the management of certain types of cancer. Unlike monoclonal antibodies, which are generally too large to penetrate the cell and often target the extracellular domain, tyrosine kinase inhibitors are considered small molecule drugs and can more easily enter the cell to reach their target. Due to these differences in mechanism, monoclonal antibodies and tyrosine kinase inhibitors that target the same receptor may have synergistic effects when used together.

One example is the BCR-ABL tyrosine kinase inhibitors, which includes imatinib (Gleevec), dasatinib (Sprycel), nilotinib (Tasigna), and ponatinib (Iclusig). BCR-ABL is a mutation formed by the combination of two genes that is found in certain types of cancer, including Philadelphia chromosome positive (Ph+) chronic myeloid leukemia. This mutation leads to uncontrolled cell proliferation. The BCR-ABL tyrosine kinase inhibitors inhibit proliferation and promote apoptosis in BCR-ABL positive cell lines. They can also be used in Ph+ acute lymphoblastic leukemia and other types of cancer. Adverse effects include cytopenia, fluid retention, edema, rash, and gastrointestinal distress. Nilotinib may cause pancreatitis. Dasatinib may cause QT-prolongation cardiac rhythm abnormalities.

Another example of tyrosine kinase inhibitors is that those inhibit the activity of the epidermal growth factor receptor (EGFR) to prevent growth and proliferation of cancer cells. Two drugs with this activity, gefitinib (Iressa) and erlotinib (Tarceva), are used in the treatment of specific types of NSCLC. Adverse effects may include dermatological reactions, such as skin rash, gastrointestinal distress, and increased liver enzymes.

Hormone Therapy

Some types of cancer are hormone-sensitive, including breast, ovarian, and prostate. These types of cancers can be treated with hormone therapy which can either prevent or slow the production of hormones or interfere with their effect in the body. For example, blocking the effects of estrogen in breast tissue can help in the management of breast cancer, whereas androgen deprivation therapy can prevent the effect of testosterone in the growth and spread of prostate cancer.

Depending on the tissue, estrogen can have desirable or undesirable effects. It displays agonist activity in bone, where it can help in the management of osteoporosis. In breast and endometrial tissues, it displays antagonist activity, where estrogenic actions might be deleterious and potentially lead to cancer. The selective estrogen receptor modulators (SERMs) were developed to have tissue-selective actions, including estrogen agonist effects in some tissues and antagonist effects in other tissues. Tamoxifen (Nolvadex, Soltamox) is a SERM that is commonly used in the treatment of hormone-responsive breast cancer. It acts as an antagonist in breast tissue to prevent receptor activation by endogenous estrogens. Unfortunately, tamoxifen also acts as an agonist in endometrial tissue and increases the risk of endometrial cancer. Other potential adverse effects include hot flashes and an increased risk of thromboembolic events. Toremifene (Fareston), which is also used in breast cancer treatment, has a similar mechanism of action and adverse effects.

Unlike the SERMs, fulvestrant (Faslodex) is a pure estrogen receptor antagonist. It competitively binds to estrogen receptors to block the actions of estrogen and inhibit tumor growth. It is approved for postmenopausal women with disease progression following an antiestrogen therapy, such as tamoxifen. Adverse effects may include nausea, injection site reactions, hot flashes, and abnormal liver enzymes.

Aromatase is an enzyme that converts androgens to estrogen in many tissues. The aromatase inhibitors (AIs), anastrozole (Arimidex), letrozole (Femara), and exemestane (Aromasin), work by blocking aromatase, reducing the levels of estrogen thereby delaying tumor progression. These drugs are approved for breast cancer treatment. Since they do not prevent the ovaries from making estrogen, they are primarily used in postmenopausal women. Adverse effects of AIs may include nausea, hot flashes, and decreased bone mineral density. A notable effect of AIs for Onc R clinicians is arthralgias and myalgias; these may be so severe that cessation of the medication may be considered or necessary due to their deleterious effect on overall QOL.

Under normal physiological conditions, the hypothalamus releases gonadotropin-releasing hormone (GnRH) in an intermittent, pulsatile manner. GnRH agonists are potent inhibitors of gonadotropin secretion, in which continuous administration desensitizes the pituitary to the activity of GnRH, resulting in suppression of luteinizing hormone (LH) and follicle-stimulating hormone (FSH). This leads to a decrease in estrogen and testosterone levels after about 1 week of therapy. In cancer treatment, these agents are used in hormone-responsive tumors, including prostate and breast cancer. Examples of GnRH agonists include leuprolide (Eligard, Lupron) and goserelin (Zoladex). They are often combined with medications that block steroid biosynthesis to prevent a tumor flare marked by a transient increase in symptoms from the initial rise in hormone levels. Adverse effects of GnRH agonists are related to the decreased hormone levels including hot flashes, decreased bone density, vaginal dryness (in women), and erectile dysfunction (in men). Firmagon is a GnRH antagonist used in the treatment of advanced prostate cancer. It blocks the GnRH receptor resulting in decreased secretion of LH and FSH, which results in a rapid decrease in testosterone production. Although it has similar adverse effects to GnRH agonists, it does not cause the initial tumor flare associated with GnRH agonists.

Anti-androgens inhibit testosterone from binding to its receptor, blocking its effects in the body and preventing the stimulation of cell growth in prostate cancer. The first-generation agents include flutamide (Eulexin) and bicalutamide (Casodex). The second-generation agents include enzalutamide (Xtandi), apalutamide (Erleada), and darolutamide (Nubeqa). Since they do not block androgen production, they are rarely used as monotherapy. In many cases, they are combined with GnRH agonists for the first few weeks of therapy to prevent tumor flare. Adverse effects

may include hot flashes, gastrointestinal distress, and decreased liver function. Overall, the adverse effects are similar to those of GnRH agonists, with fewer sexual adverse effects.

Abiraterone (Zytiga) is an androgen synthesis inhibitor that selectively inhibits CYP17. This enzyme is required for androgen biosynthesis and inhibition leads to decreased formation of testosterone precursors. It can be used in the management of metastatic prostate cancer. Hypertension, hypokalemia, and fluid retention may occur due to mineralocorticoid excess from CYP17 inhibition. Administration with prednisone can help decrease these effects. In addition, abiraterone has the potential to cause hepatotoxicity.

Combination Therapies

Although antineoplastic agents may be administered individually as a single drug, they are often delivered in combination with other medications. There are a wide variety of combination therapies, but in general, these are often medications from different classes with their own antineoplastic effects. Some combination therapies are intended to impact different parts of the cell cycle. A key consideration in use of combination therapies is mitigating or reducing the development of drug resistance that may occur from the use of a single agent. In addition, combining certain medications also can reduce the need for a larger dose of a single medication thereby reducing the likelihood of adverse effects which may delay or require cessation of chemotherapy. For example, a commonly used combination regimen in the treatment of breast cancer is AC-T. This regimen includes the administration of doxorubicin (Adriamycin) and cyclophosphamide (Cytoxan), an anthracycline topoisomerase inhibitor and a nitrogen mustard alkylating agent, respectively, followed by paclitaxel (Taxol) which is a taxane microtubule damaging agent.

A key strategy in considering how to mitigate and anticipate the adverse effects of these combination therapies is to examine each of the individual medications in the combination. After this, the Onc R clinician should screen for the most commonly encountered adverse effect, especially those adverse effects that may be elicited by multiple medications in the combination.

The list of combination therapies is lengthy and is frequently changing as new innovations are rapidly being developed. As such, the reader is presented with selected additional commonly encountered combination therapies in Table 6.1. In addition, Chemocare.com also maintains an index of common chemotherapy combination regimens and their acronyms. (http://chemocare.com/chemotherapy/acronyms/default.aspx).

Supportive Therapy

In addition to antineoplastic agents, there are pharmacologic agents commonly utilized to mitigate symptoms and adverse effects of cancer and its treatments. This section provides an overview of the most commonly used medications that a clinician may encounter during their Onc R practice.

Pain Management

Pain has been established as a common and disconcerting adverse effect of cancer and its treatments. It has been identified by the World Health Organization (WHO) as a critical concern.[17] See Chapter 22 for nonpharmacologic management of pain. A key consideration with treatment of cancer pain is identifying the

TABLE 6.1	Commonly Encountered Combination Chemotherapy Medications	
Combination Therapy Acronym	**Active Drugs in the Combination**	**Examples of Targeted Cancers**
AC-T	• doxorubicin (Adriamycin) (anthracycline topoisomerase inhibitor) • cyclophosphamide (Cytoxan) (nitrogen mustard alkylating agent) • Followed by paclitaxel (Taxol) (taxane microtubule damaging agent)	Breast cancer
EP	• etoposide (Toposar) (topoisomerase inhibitor) • cisplatin (Platinol) (platinum-based medication)	Testicular cancer, small cell lung cancer
VIP	• etoposide (VePsid) (topoisomerase inhibitor) • ifosfamide (Ifex) (nitrogen mustard alkylating agent) • cisplatin (Platinol) (platinum-based medication)	Advanced testicular cancer
FOLFOX	• leucovorin (folinic acid) (chemoprotectant) • 5-FU (Adrucil) (antimetabolite) • oxaliplatin (Eloxatin) (platinum-based medication)	Colorectal cancer and gastric cancers
CapeOx	• capecitabine (Xeloda) (antimetabolite) • oxaliplatin (Eloxatin) (platinum-based medication)	Colorectal cancer

root cause of pain which will help to properly address it. Some examples are nociceptive pain (e.g., from viscera or bone lesions), neuropathic pain, or nonphysiologic sources of pain (existential pain or spiritual distress). Pharmacologic management of pain can be discussed in three main categories: (1) nonopioid analgesics; (2) opioid analgesics; and (3) adjuvant analgesics, which are drugs with a primary indication other than pain that also demonstrate analgesic properties.

In general, nonopioid analgesics are preferred to opioids due to their lower adverse effect profile and decreased risk of dependence. In palliative situations and in severe pain situations, nonopioid medications are not often sufficient to manage the extent and duration of pain. In addition, in palliative situations, the concerns related to addiction are not considered relevant due to an impending end of life.[18] As opioids also have a sedating effect and may cause constipation, NSAIDs may be preferred over opioids in some situations. In order to achieve optimum pain control, patients may be on a combination of NSAIDs, opioids (long- and short-acting), and adjuvant medications.

Nonopioid Analgesics

Nonsteroidal anti-inflammatory drugs (NSAIDs): These medications inhibit the cyclooxygenase-1 (COX-1) and the COX-2 enzymes to prevent prostaglandin synthesis. COX-1 is considered the housekeeping enzyme that helps regulate many important processes, including gastric cytoprotection. The COX-2 enzyme is increased at sites of inflammation, in which it leads to the production of prostaglandins that promote pain, inflammation, and fever. As NSAIDs and aspirin are nonselective COX inhibitors, they inhibit both COX-1 and COX-2 enzymes. Inhibition of the COX-2 enzyme leads to the beneficial antipyretic, analgesic, and anti-inflammatory effects. Unfortunately, inhibition of the COX-1 enzyme prevents the production of prostaglandins necessary for many important functions. For example, inhibition of COX-1 may lead to a reduction in the gastrointestinal protective mucous, thereby increasing the risk of acid damage to the gastrointestinal (GI) pathway. One of the main adverse effects of NSAIDs is from GI distress or GI bleeding. Medications such as proton pump inhibitors may be given to reduce the risk of GI issues. In addition to their anti-inflammatory pain reduction, there appears to be direct influence on the nociception of pain at the peripheral and central nervous system. However, there is

not clear understanding of this mechanism. In addition, NSAIDs increase the risk of adverse cardiovascular events such as myocardial infarction, heart failure, stroke, and death. Other potentially serious adverse reactions include neurologic effects and renal dysfunction.

Aspirin: Aspirin (acetylsalicylic acid) is also considered an NSAID and inhibits both COX-1 and COX-2 pathways. At low doses, aspirin inhibits platelet aggregation, which is a significant consideration for those undergoing cancer treatments as many individuals also experience thrombocytopenia. In these cases, aspirin may be contraindicated, especially as aspirin's effects on platelets are irreversible and remain for the life of the platelet. At moderate doses, aspirin also has antipyretic (fever reducing) and analgesic effects. At high doses, aspirin has been shown to have anti-inflammatory properties. However as there are other anti-inflammatory medications that are more effective, aspirin is rarely used for its anti-inflammatory effects.

COX-2 Inhibitors: Finally, one class of NSAIDs, the COX-2 inhibitors are more selective for the COX-2 pathway. Since the COX-1 pathway that mediates protective secretions of the GI system is not inhibited, the more selective COX-2 inhibitors are thought to provide increased protection to the GI system as compared to the nonselective agents. For this reason, a potential advantage of the COX-2 inhibitor class is effective management of pain and inflammation with reduced risk of GI distress. Currently, celecoxib (Celebrex) is the only COX-2 inhibitor available in the United States (US).

Acetaminophen: Acetaminophen (Tylenol) is a nonopioid analgesic with centrally acting analgesic and antipyretic activity. While it plays an important role in the reduction of fever and moderate pain, it does not have anti-inflammatory properties. Acetaminophen inhibits prostaglandin synthesis in the central nervous system. It also inhibits endogenous pyrogens and stimulates pathways that block the transmission of nociceptive signals. Overall, acetaminophen is considered a safe and effective analgesic. It is important to keep in mind that high doses have been shown to cause significant liver damage, which may result in liver necrosis and even death. For this reason, it is important not to exceed the recommended daily dose. This is especially important to consider in individuals with cancer with liver metastases or impaired liver function, in which a reduced daily dose may be warranted. Acetaminophen may even be contraindicated in severe cases.

Opioid Analgesics

In general, opioids have their effect on receptors of the CNS nerves to mitigate the nociception and transmission of pain. Opioid analgesics are known for causing drowsiness or sleepiness, and in some cases delirium and psychosis. In addition, another common adverse effect of opioid administration is reduced GI motility and constipation. This class of medication has garnered a substantial amount of attention recently (especially in the US) due to the opioid crisis and the public campaigns by several governmental and professional organizations.[19] In addition to the public health issues of abuse and criminal trade of opioids, a major issue has been related to opioid overdoses even when prescribed by a medical professional.[19] The clinical manifestations of opioid overdose include lethargy, respiratory suppression, and anoxia. If not treated promptly, this anoxia may result in death. Due to the extensive clinical application of opioids in the cancer population, therapists and other healthcare providers should consider the availability of an emergency opioid antagonist such as naloxone (Narcan) (see below for more information on opioid antagonists).

In less severe cases, individuals who are taking a controlled dose of opioids may require supplemental oxygen, especially during rest due to the respiratory suppression. This may cause confusion to the patient or the Onc R clinician who notes new supplemental oxygen use in an asymptomatic patient who did not require it previously. As most Onc R clinicians are not often involved in the prescription or dosing of supplemental oxygen, the rationale for new oxygen use may not be immediately clear, therefore clinicians should endeavor to gather whether this new oxygen use is from a worsening or evolving cardiopulmonary condition or prophylactic use during exogenous opioid administration.

Although there are a wide variety of opioids beyond which can be covered in this chapter, a few of the most commonly utilized medications will be discussed including their uses and unique adverse effects if they vary from above (Table 6.2). The most commonly considered opioid is morphine (especially in palliative care), and it is considered to be a strong agonist, resulting in a substantial reduction in pain. In addition, morphine has been used clinically for addressing "oxygen hunger" or dyspnea in palliative care in those with inadequate cardiopulmonary systems to provide sufficient oxygenation. For cancer pain, pure opioid agonists are recommended.

When working with individuals taking opioids, providers should be screening for signs and symptoms of over-medication or overdose. The WHO offers the opioid overdose triad which includes constricted pupils, unconsciousness, and/or respiratory depression.[20] Respiratory depression may be appreciated clinically by observation of more shallow breathing or a reduction in pulse oximetry, especially during sleep or quiet resting. There are several forms of opioid reversal agents (antagonists) available that work quickly to reverse the symptoms of opioid overdose. There are injectable or nasally administered versions of the opioid-antagonist naloxone. Within the US, these are known by the trade name Narcan. Especially in practice settings where patients do not have easy access to nurses or physicians (e.g., outpatient clinic or homecare), an Onc R clinician should consider becoming trained in naloxone administration and have the medication available in the event that a person demonstrates symptoms of opioid overdose.[21] As administration of medications is not always within an Onc R clinician's scope of practice, a therapist preparing to be trained to administer naloxone should consult with their local licensing board or professional association for specific regulations related to this emergency lifesaving procedure.

Adjuvant Analgesics

As pain is a multifaceted, complex clinical problem, there are additional medication classes that may be utilized in management or mitigation of pain.[22] In fact, many of these adjuvant analgesics are utilized for treating symptoms beyond their commonly accepted use. For example, some agents have been found to be beneficial in the treatment of CIPN. These may include antidepressants (duloxetine [Cymbalta], venlafaxine [Effexor XR, Effexor], or tricyclic antidepressants) and anticonvulsants (gabapentin [Neurontin],

TABLE 6.2	Selected Opioids Used in Cancer Care
Morphine	• Can be administered as a solution or as an extended release a tablet or pill • Considered to be gold standard; potency of other opiates are measured against morphine • Can be used for oxygen hunger or dyspnea at rest
Codeine	• Used to treat mild to moderate pain (rarely used in cancer pain) • Is an antitussive which can help with coughing
Hydrocodone	• A synthetic opioid derivative of codeine • Often utilized in combination with acetaminophen as a tablet or pill to control moderate pain
Hydromorphone	• Commonly known as Dilaudid in the US and is often delivered via tablet or intravenously. • Applicable for individuals with strong acute or chronic pain, or those who need stronger or longer lasting agents
Fentanyl patch	• Provides a long duration of analgesia via a transdermal patch • An extremely potent synthetic analgesic and if inappropriately utilized, may result in overdose. • Fentanyl patches are generally changed every 72 hours. • Unlike a lidocaine patch which would be placed over a specific painful area (e.g., an arthritic joint), the fentanyl patch delivers systemic analgesia and can be placed in an easily accessible area • As with any pain patch, care should be taken by therapists to avoid dislodging or removing a pain patch during therapeutic exercise or other mobility task.
Methadone	• Strong opioid used for severe pain • Known for its use in management of opioid use disorder • Generally, the effects of methadone lasts 8-12 hours

Created by Christopher Wilson, PT, DPT, DScPT. Printed with permission.

pregabalin [Lyrica]). In some palliative scenarios or at the end of life, sedative hypnotic agents may be utilized to manage symptoms and improve comfort. However, these are not often a standard of care for nonpalliative PWCs due to their large adverse effect profile. Finally, more invasive procedures such as nerve blocks or epidural or intrathecal analgesic administration may assist in managing more severe pain and can be complemented by other enteral or parenteral pain medications.

Supportive Medications

In addition to chemotherapeutics and medications to manage pain, a PWC may also be on an assortment of different medications to treat the symptoms caused by chemotherapy, other medical treatments, the disease itself, or comorbid conditions. Although not a comprehensive listing, this section highlights some common drug classes that Onc R clinicians may encounter during cancer care.

Corticosteroids

This class of medications is a staple for use in combination with a variety of antineoplastic treatment regimens. Commonly utilized examples of corticosteroids include prednisone (Deltasone, Prednicot, Sterapred, Rayos), dexamethasone (Decadron), and methylprednisolone (Medrol). As some individuals may experience a variety of adverse effects of cancer and its treatments, corticosteroids have been utilized for a wide variety of symptoms and for prevention of some medical sequelae, including prevention of hypersensitivity reactions. Additionally, corticosteroids are used for chemotherapy-induced inflammatory reactions, treatment of brain metastases, pain, fatigue, dyspnea, or anorexia. In addition, PWC may also utilize corticosteroids for noncancer-related conditions including autoimmune disorders or arthritic conditions. Corticosteroids, also known as glucocorticoids, are strong immune modulators and act upon glucocorticoid receptors, which are found in a wide variety of cells throughout the body. Due to its efficacy, it is a very commonly utilized class of drugs, however long-term use can result in glucocorticoid resistance. A notable effect of long-term corticosteroid use is its catabolic effects on bone, skin, and structural tissues such as cartilage, tendons, and ligaments, which may delay healing times and result in increased risk of fracture or soft tissue injuries.[23] In addition, corticosteroids have the adverse effects of increased risk of infections, increased fasting blood glucose levels, or psychosis with large doses.[24] Finally, corticosteroids have been found to have negative effects on executive functioning and memory as well as have been associated with delirium, depression, manic episodes, and psychosis.[25]

Anticoagulants

One commonly encountered class of medications is anticoagulants, commonly referred to as blood thinners. Due to their use in preventing and treating venous thromboembolisms (VTEs), their use and administration may be familiar to many experienced Onc R clinicians. The most concerning adverse effects of anticoagulants is excessive or spontaneous bleeding which could be internal or external. Anticoagulants may be delivered parenterally (often via subcutaneous injection) or orally. Parenteral anticoagulants include heparin (UFH, unfractionated heparin) which is delivered via injection and inhibits coagulation by inactivating clotting factors, specifically thrombin and factor Xa. The laboratory test that is used to monitor heparin delivery is the activated partial thromboplastin time (aPTT) and with heparin administration, an increase in the aPTT will be noted from its baseline.[26] A related

medication class to heparin is low molecular weight heparins (LMWH) which includes enoxaparin (Lovenox) and dalteparin (Fragmin). In general, LMWH medications are easier to administer as they can be delivered on a fixed dose and are often more effective in stabilizing an acute VTE, with the commencement of physical mobility being allowed in 2 to 6 hours as opposed to UFH which may take 24 to 72 hours until mobility is safely indicated.[27] Finally, a synthetic medication, fondaparinux (Arixtra), is similar in structure and function to UFH and LMWH however only inhibits factor Xa as opposed to direct inhibition of thrombin.

Closely related to parenteral anticoagulants are oral anticoagulants which include direct Factor Xa inhibitors such as rivaroxaban (Xarelto), apixaban (Eliquis), edoxaban (Savaysa), and betrixaban (Bevyxxa) as well as direct thrombin inhibitors such as dabigatran (Pradaxa). Warfarin (Coumadin) is another oral anticoagulant with a different mechanism of action. It blocks the function of the vitamin K epoxide reductase complex in the liver, which is needed for activating the vitamin K available in the body. It decreases the reserves of functional vitamin K and reduces the synthesis of active clotting factors. Unlike UFH, warfarin levels are monitored by the international normalized ratio (INR) which is calculated based on the prothrombin time (PT) lab test. See Chapter 24 for additional information about VTE management and clinical implications of anticoagulant therapies.

Antiemetics

As some chemotherapeutic agents are known to cause nausea and vomiting (N/V), often termed chemotherapy-induced nausea or vomiting (CINV), a key medication class that will be encountered by Onc R clinicians are antiemetics, or anti-nausea medications. In the authors' experience, CINV is a common barrier to participation in rehabilitation, and proactive and aggressive treatment of CINV may be warranted if the person's nausea or vomiting symptoms become problematic. In addition, as uncontrolled N/V can result in dehydration, electrolyte imbalances, malnutrition and GI system tissue damage, management of N/V is a high priority. Some PWC may consider discontinuing a chemotherapy regimen due to severe N/V, which may have implications on survival outcomes of cancer. Almost all PWCs who receive chemotherapy will also be prescribed an antiemetic, also known as an anti-nausea agent. One relevant adverse effect of some antiemetics is drowsiness which may adversely affect rehabilitation participation. There are a wide variety of antiemetic classes and each has their own physiologic mechanisms of action which is important as N/V is a complex system of physiologic, emotional, and psychological factors. This provides physicians with a wide range of options to proactively manage or mitigate N/V symptoms. As antiemetics are more effective at preventing N/V than treating it, many medical oncologists often administer antiemetics prophylactically. See Box 6.2 for commonly utilized antiemetics.

Cannabinoids and Medical Marijuana

Over several years, the use of marijuana/cannabis and its derivatives have been growing in popularity and acceptance, however, the use of marijuana derivatives is not a novel concept in cancer care.[28] For example, dronabinol (Marinol, Syndros), a marijuana derivative, has been approved by the US Food and Drug Administration (FDA) since 1985 for cancer chemotherapy as an appetite stimulant and an antiemetic. In some cases, marijuana or its derivatives may be available via prescription

- Muscarinic M_1-receptor antagonists: scopolamine
- Histamine H_1-receptor antagonists: meclizine
- Dopamine receptor antagonists: prochlorperazine, promethazine, metoclopramide
- Selective $5\text{-}HT_3$ receptor antagonists: ondansetron, dolasetron, granisetron, and palonosetron
- Benzodiazepines: lorazepam
- Neurokinin 1 (NK_1) receptor antagonists: aprepitant, fosaprepitant
- Cannabinoids: dronabinol, nabilone

for medical use or even available recreationally without a prescription however it continues to be upheld as illegal at the US federal level. Within marijuana, there are two known active cannabinoid compounds, delta-9-tetrahydrocannabinol (THC) and cannabidiol (CBD) commonly applied to medical care.[28] As investigations into these compounds are ongoing, comprehensive knowledge of their full physiologic effects and efficacy remains incomplete. In general, THC is known for its psychoactive properties as well as its application as an appetite stimulant (e.g., dronabinol). Conversely, CBD is generally considered to lack psychoactive effects while it has demonstrated efficacy in reducing spasticity, cancer-related pain, and neuropathic pain.[29,30] Due to medical marijuana's increased popularity and availability, Onc R clinicians should be performing a thorough medical history including specifically asking about these products.[28] In the medical use of cannabis, there are concerns about monitoring dosing which may be a challenge if not administered via a controlled means. For example, some individuals may intake cannabis via inhalation as a marijuana cigarette that may result in lung irritation or an unpredictable amount of THC delivery, which may be especially relevant in those with underlying lung issues such as lung cancer. There are many consumer-oriented products that are advertised to have THC and/or CBD within them. As these are not regulated by a central agency (e.g., FDA), their efficacy or safety cannot be assumed. As with any psychoactive substance, clinicians need to take care to assure safety during rehabilitation which may include cessation or modification of activities that may increase fall risk or those that depend on quick reaction times (balance retraining). Finally, in scenarios where cancer pain or symptoms are not adequately controlled, or in palliative scenarios, the Onc R clinician may need to be a proactive advocate for the PLWBC to discuss cannabis as an option for symptom management with the rest of the interdisciplinary care team.

Medications for Neutropenia and Leukopenia

As many chemotherapeutic agents may cause leukopenia and neutropenia (reduced white blood cells and neutrophils), medications to increase neutrophils are often a staple in cancer care. Leukopenia and neutropenia are a result of the effects of the chemotherapeutic agents on the bone marrow and its ability to produce neutrophils. This results in an increased risk of infection in the immunocompromised individual. There are two commonly utilized colony-stimulating factors used in cancer care—filgrastim (Neupogen) and pegfilgrastim (Neulasta). In general, pegfilgrastim has a longer half-life than filgrastim; therefore, it is easier to use and administer. A common adverse effect of these agents is bone pain which has been shown to occur in 25% of patients.[31] This drug-induced bone pain may be treated by an NSAID or

nonpharmacologic means (see Chapter 22); some cases may require opioid medications.

Bone Modifying Agents

Persons with a cancer diagnosis are at risk for decreased bone mineral density or metastatic bone disease. Medications that inhibit osteoclast-mediated bone resorption may be utilized to treat or manage osteoporosis and some mixed or lytic bone metastases. A commonly encountered medication class for osteoporosis is bisphosphonates. Examples of these medications include alendronate (Fosamax), bandronate (Boniva), pamidronate (Aredia), risedronate (Actonel, Atelvia), and zoledronic acid (Reclast, Zometa).

Adverse effects of bisphosphonate use may include myalgias, arthralgias, or bone pain. In addition, oral intake (tablets) may also cause GI (N/V or heartburn). One key consideration for Onc R clinicians is that bisphosphonates may rarely cause osteonecrosis of the jaw as well as atypical bone fractures. In addition, calcium and vitamin D supplementation may be used in cases of specific nutritional deficiencies. Finally, denosumab (Prolia) is a human monoclonal antibody that has been utilized for the treatment of osteoporosis, treatment-induced bone loss, metastases to bone, and giant cell tumors of bone. As with some of the other bone modifying agents, the main adverse effects are achiness, discomfort, and skin irritation. As with bisphosphonates, osteonecrosis of the jaw is a risk. For any PLWBC on any of these medications, it is important to be cognizant that they are at risk of fractures. These medications may not be effective, and therapy interventions may need to be modified.

Agents to Prevent/Treat Gastrointestinal Dysfunction

Cancer and its treatments may result in constipation or diarrhea. In addition to the rehabilitative interventions and recommendations for these commonly encountered issues, pharmacological agents are often prescribed to assist with preventing or treating GI issues. For treatment of constipation, there are bulk-forming laxatives, osmotic laxatives, and irritant (stimulant) laxatives (cathartics). In addition, stool softeners and lubricating agents may also be prescribed. Finally, due to the well-known constipation effect of opioids, an appropriate bowel regimen should be started prophylactically. Often, stimulant laxatives and stool softeners are used concurrently during long-term opioid use. In some cases, opioid receptor antagonists may assist in reducing constipation in cases where opioids cannot be replaced or substituted. Conversely, for the treatment of diarrhea, loperamide (an opioid receptor agonist whose effects are confined to the GI tract) or bismuth subsalicylate may be utilized and are widely available over the counter. As GI irregularities may be significant barriers to rehabilitation, these issues should be addressed and mitigated promptly to optimize clinical outcomes.

Conclusion

As chemotherapeutic agents and supportive pharmacologic therapies are a staple of cancer treatment, Onc R clinicians are faced with the challenge of not only being experts in the provision of rehabilitative interventions but must also have a broad understanding of the adverse effects of these drugs. In addition, it behooves the clinician to incorporate the rationale behind the choices in chemotherapeutic agents in order to best develop their own plan of care and provide holistic, patient-centered care. For example, in some cases, neoadjuvant chemotherapy strategies may be utilized to shrink a neoplasm prior to surgical excision to facilitate achieving clean margins. At the other end of the spectrum, a person with widespread metastatic disease may receive chemotherapy for palliative or supportive measures. In this case, a key consideration must be whether the palliative chemotherapy will improve QOL (as opposed to just quantity of life). Finally, the person's age, comorbidities, and performance status also all play a key role. All of these considerations, in addition to patient preference, are incorporated into a final decision as to when, how, and which antineoplastic agents are administered. As rehabilitation is holistic, patient-centered, and may be able to mitigate the adverse effects of many of these medications, Onc R clinicians have the professional duty to learn as much as possible about how their services can affect or be affected by any medication.

Critical Research Needs

- Impact of predictable extent and duration of cardiotoxic chemotherapies on physical activity, rehabilitation, and QOL
- Efficacy of rehabilitative treatment interventions for managing chemotherapy-induced peripheral neuropathy
- Effect of aerobic exercise during treatment with chemotherapy infusions on pancytopenia and vital sign responses
- Best practices for Onc R clinician incorporation of chemotherapy medication information into an Onc R plan of care, including adverse effects and drug interactions.

Case Studies

CASE STUDY

Case Study 1

By Scott Grumeretz PT, DPT

A 32-year-old female with stage 2, grade 3, triple negative (ER, PR, HER2 negative) breast cancer of left breast and positive for BRCA1 mutation undergoes a regimen of chemotherapy. The patient begins with neoadjuvant chemotherapy regimen of dose-dense doxorubicin (Adriamycin [topoisomerase inhibitor antineoplastic agent]) and cyclophosphamide (Cytoxan [bidentate alkylating antineoplastic agent]), one dose every two weeks for a total of eight weeks following lumpectomy. A dose of pegfilgrastim (Neulasta [colony stimulating factor]) was given via injection the day following the completion of each cycle. During this time, the patient contracts a minor upper respiratory tract infection that left her bedridden for 5 days due to a low white blood cell count.

Following neoadjuvant therapy, the patient begins a new chemotherapy regimen of weekly doses of paclitaxel (Taxol [taxane]) and one dose of carboplatin (Paraplatin [alkylating agent]) every 3 weeks for a total of 12 weeks. A dose of filgrastim (Neupogen [colony stimulating factor]) was given via self-injection starting off at twice a week and increasing to four times a week as her white blood cell count decreased.

Including the above-mentioned changes in her white blood cell count, the primary adverse effects were general body aches, nausea and vomiting, and a minor amount of polyneuropathy. While no formal rehabilitation was

completed during her chemotherapy regimen, she regularly exercised via walking. Depending on the day, she would be limited to walking no further than her own mailbox or she would be able to walk upwards of one mile. She would go in for IV fluids due to dehydration and was given prochlorperazine (an antipsychotic and anti-emetic) and lorazepam (Ativan) to control the nausea. The lorazepam caused anterograde amnesia. The polyneuropathy and body aches steadily resolved following the end of her chemotherapy regimen. Based on the chemotherapy regimen, some other adverse effects that should be monitored during therapy would be shortness of breath, signs of cardiotoxicity, and balance impairments or instability with increased fall risk.

CASE STUDY

Case Study 2

By Brianne Patton PT, DPT

A 29-year-old female who was referred to a physical therapist by her medical oncologist for generalized weakness. She was diagnosed with Stage IIIB Hodgkin lymphoma 3 years prior to therapy referral. Her chemotherapy regimen began with ABVD (adriamycin, bleomycin, vinblastine, dacarbazine) twice monthly for 6 months, followed by ICE (ifosfamide, carboplatin, etoposide) three times a week for 3 months, and then received brentuximab every other week for 6 months. Each of these chemotherapy regimens began when the current treatment was no longer giving the desired response, and each came with their own set of adverse effects. While the patient states she felt "the best" on brentuximab, she was forced to discontinue this drug secondary to abdominal pain and increased CIPN in her hands and feet.

When the initial rounds of chemotherapy were deemed unsuccessful, she began the BEAM regimen (biCNU, etoposide, ara-C, melphalan) in preparation for a stem cell transplant. She underwent an autologous stem cell transplant and began maintenance lenalidomide (Revlimid) once daily for 6 months post-transplant, and later completed ten spinal radiation treatments over the course of 2 weeks. Unfortunately, the stem cell transplant failed.

She began total body irradiation for six treatments, followed by an allogeneic stem cell transplant. A few weeks later, she developed graft versus host disease (GvHD). This was treated with high dose prednisone resulting in more adverse effects including weight gain, fluid retention, muscle cramping, and weakness.

She presented for a physical therapy initial evaluation approximately 5 months after her allogeneic stem cell transplant. During the evaluation, she disclosed she was experiencing cancer related fatigue, hand tremors, neuropathy in hands and feet, generalized weakness, and "chemo brain," in which she was unable to remember certain things and had trouble finishing tasks and concentrating. The physical therapy plan of care included dynamic balance training, upper and lower extremity strengthening exercises, soft tissue mobilization for decreasing muscle spasms in her lower legs and feet, and aerobic endurance training. While she responded well to physical therapy treatment through several episodes of care over the course of the 12 months, the physical therapist recommended continued observation and monitoring, as well as an annual physical therapy evaluation and treatment as needed to combat the adverse effect resulting from chemotherapy and cancer related treatments.

Review Questions

Reader can find the correct answers and rationale in the back of the book.

1. A 42-year-old man presents to his primary care physician for the management of back pain. He is started on a new medication that binds to the mu opioid receptor to cause the maximum response. How would this drug be classified based on its interaction with the mu receptor?
   A. Competitive antagonist
   B. Full agonist
   C. Partial agonist
   D. Physiologic antagonist

2. A 22-year-old male presents to the infusion center for his third cycle of chemotherapy for the treatment of testicular cancer. At his appointment, he complains of numbness and tingling in his fingers which makes it difficult to perform simple activities such as buttoning a shirt. The clinician believes his symptoms are likely due to an adverse effect of his chemotherapy. What drug most likely caused his symptoms?
   A. Capecitabine
   B. Carmustine
   C. Cisplatin
   D. Cyclophosphamide

3. A 56-year-old female presents to the emergency department with complaints of severe diarrhea. She has a history of colorectal cancer and received her last cycle of chemotherapy 3 days before her symptoms started. Her past medical history is also significant for Gilbert's syndrome, hypothyroidism, and migraine headaches. The patient is diagnosed with severe gastrointestinal toxicity due to chemotherapy and promptly started on loperamide and admitted to the hospital for further evaluation. What is the mechanism of action for the drug that most likely caused this patient presentation?
   A. Activate xanthine oxidase
   B. Bind to HER2 protein
   C. Induce microtubule polymerization
   D. Inhibit topoisomerase

4. A 57-year-old male is being treated in the outpatient physical therapy clinic for pain, weakness, and fatigue. He is currently receiving IV chemotherapy for Stage IV colorectal cancer, but does not remember the medications included in the chemotherapy regimen. He notes that he is achy all over "in his bones" and says the doctors have noticed his blood levels are dropping. Which of the following would be the MOST appropriate course of action?
   A. Tell the patient to take some aspirin to address the inflammation
   B. Communicate with the physician to see if any colony stimulating factors are being provided
   C. Call for an ambulance as the patient may be experiencing micro-embolisms in the vasculature around his bones
   D. Tell the patient he may need radiation therapy to his bones to treat his metastatic bone disease

5. A 68-year-old female is undergoing chemotherapy in the acute care setting. She has been experiencing nausea and vomiting which has impacted her rehabilitation program. The oncologist increased the dose of her antiemetic medications including prochlorperazine (an antiemetic and anti-psychotic) as well as adding diphenhydramine (Benadryl). Which of the following is MOST likely to be an adverse effect of this medication that might impact rehabilitation?
   A. Polyneuropathy
   B. Drowsiness
   C. Tachycardia
   D. Agitation

6. A 56-year-old female is diagnosed with breast cancer and recently started AC-T combination chemotherapy (doxorubicin [Adriamycin] and cyclophosphamide followed by paclitaxel [Taxol]). The patient is very motivated to continue her exercise regimen which includes running. Which of the following considerations is MOST relevant when considering her exercise regimen?
   A. She should have an exercise test and have close monitoring of vital signs for cardiotoxicity
   B. She should exercise in large groups to make sure she is staying engaged and has a good support network
   C. She should not do any exercise or activity until her chemotherapy is done
   D. She is at high risk of falls and should use a walker

7. A 73-year-old male is being treated with cisplatin as adjuvant therapy after radiation for bladder cancer. A cystectomy was not an option due to his other underlying health issues, but he was active and golfed three times a week while walking the course. Recently, the patient noticed that his balance is worse and he is fearful of falling. He does not want to do any of his own ADLs or cook meals for himself so as to not make things worse. In addition, he is reporting fatigue. Which of the following is the least likely cause of his new onset symptoms?
   A. Polyneuropathy
   B. Neurotoxicity affecting the vestibular system
   C. Age related changes
   D. An infection from neutropenia

8. A 63-year-old male was newly diagnosed with colorectal cancer. The medical oncologist recommends a combination therapy called FOLFOX. He is being screened for rehabilitation needs and a prehabilitation program by the Onc R clinician. The patient is very anxious and asks the screening clinician why he cannot just get one chemotherapy medication and has to take all of these medications in combination. Which of the following is the MOST appropriate initial response?
   A. Explain that different chemotherapy medications have different effects on cancer cells to be more effective
   B. Tell him that his doctors know best and not to worry about it
   C. Tell him this is not your area and you are only here to talk about exercise
   D. Explain the exact cellular mechanisms and list of adverse effects of each of the medications included in FOLFOX

9. An Onc R clinician is mentoring a new colleague on the role of Onc R clinicians and what they should know and consider when working with a patient with cancer who has had chemotherapy. Which of the following is the

MOST appropriate method as it relates to how an Onc R clinician should approach working with this patient population?

A. Memorize each and every chemotherapy medication and their adverse effects

B. It is enough to know that chemotherapy was given but pursuing the details of the chemotherapy regimen is unnecessary

C. A detailed chemotherapeutic history should be obtained to allow the clinician to screen for any chemotherapy-induced adverse effects

D. A personal call to the medical oncologist is important for every patient to make sure the oncologic history is accurate

10. An Onc R clinician has a student with them who is shadowing and assisting with treatments. The student does not have very much cancer rehabilitation experience. The student asks the clinician, "What is the difference between chemotherapy and targeted therapy, I thought they tried to target the cancer with chemotherapy too?" Which of the following is the LEAST appropriate answer?

A. The student is right, targeted therapies affect cancer cells through the same mechanisms as many traditional chemotherapy agents.

B. Targeted therapies include monoclonal antibodies that have a variety of effects such as targeting the cancer cells for destruction by the immune system

C. Although targeted therapies generally have less adverse effects than chemotherapy, there are still adverse effects to watch out for.

D. Hormone therapies may also be used to slow the growth of certain cancers but are not chemotherapy

Appendix 6.1

References

1. Silver JK, Baima J, Mayer RS. Impairment-driven cancer rehabilitation: an essential component of quality care and survivorship. *CA Cancer J Clin*. 2013;63(5):295–317.

2. Lukez A, Baima J. The role and scope of prehabilitation in cancer care. *Seminar Oncol Nurs*. 2020;36(1):150976. doi:10.1016/j.soncn.2019.150976.

3. Ciccone C. *Pharmacology in Rehabilitation*. 4th ed.: FA Davis; 2007.

4. Chemotherapy to Treat Cancer. National Cancer Institute website. https://www.cancer.gov/about-cancer/treatment/types/chemotherapy; April 29, 2015. Accessed November 7, 2020.

5. Jameson JL, Fauci AS, Kasper DL, Hauser SL, Longo DL, Loscalzo J. *Harrison's Principles of Internal Medicine*. 20th ed.: McGraw-Hill Medical; 2018.

6. Katzung BG. *Basic and Clinical Pharmacology*. 14th ed.: McGraw Hill Professional; 2017.

7. Golan DE, Tashjian AH, Armstrong EJ, eds. *Principles of Pharmacology: The Pathophysiologic Basis of Drug Therapy*. 4th ed.: Lippincott Williams & Wilkins; 2011.

8. Brunton LL, Hilal-Dandan R, Knollmann BC. *Goodman & Gilman's: The Pharmacological Basis of Therapeutics*. 13th ed.: McGraw-Hill Education; 2018.

9. Whalen K. *Lippincott Illustrated Reviews: Pharmacology*. Lippincott Williams & Wilkins; 2018.

10. Linder BJ, Chao NJ, Gounder MM. Hemorrhagic cystitis in cancer patients. In: Drews RE, Schild SE, eds. *UpToDate*; 2020. UpToDate. https://www.uptodate.com/contents/hemorrhagic-cystitis-in-cancer-patients. Updated October 17, 2019. Accessed November 11, 2020.

11. LaCasce AS. Therapeutic use and toxicity of high-dose methotrexate. In: Maki R, Freedman AS, Pappo AS, eds. *UpToDate*, 2020. UpToDate;. https://www.uptodate.com/contents/therapeutic-use-and-toxicity-of-high-dose-methotrexate. Accessed November 11, 2020.

12. UpToDate. Capecitabine: drug information. *UpToDate*; 2020. www.uptodate.com. Accessed November 11, 2020.

13. UpToDate. Cytarabine: drug information. *UpToDate*; 2020. www.uptodate.com. Accessed November 11, 2020.

14. UpToDate. Gemcitabine: drug information. *UpToDate*; 2020. www.uptodate.com. Accessed November 11, 2020.

15. Glassman PM, Balthasar JP. Mechanistic considerations for the use of monoclonal antibodies for cancer therapy. *Cancer Biol Med*. 2014;11(1):20–33. doi:10.7497/j.issn.2095-3941.2014.01.002.

16. LaCasce AS, Castells MC, Burstein HJ, Meyerhardt JA. Infusion-related reactions to therapeutic monoclonal antibodies used for cancer therapy. In: Reed E, Drews RE, Adkinson NF, eds. *UpToDate*; 2020. UpToDate. www.uptodate.com. Updated October 13, 2020. Accessed November 11, 2020.

17. WHO revision of pain management guidelines. World Health Organization website. https://www.who.int/news/item/27-08-2019-who-revision-of-pain-management-guidelines. Updated August 27, 2019. Accessed February 11, 2021.

18. Wilson CM, Briggs R. Physical therapy's role in opioid use and management during palliative and hospice care. *Phys Ther*. 2018;98(2):83–85.

19. Vadivelu N, Kai AM, Kodumudi V, Sramcik J, Kaye AD. The opioid crisis: a comprehensive overview. *Curr Pain Headache Rep*. 2018;22(3):1–6.

20. Opioid overdose. World Health Organization website. https://www.who.int/news-room/fact-sheets/detail/opioid-overdose. Updated August 19, 2020. Accessed February 12, 2021.

21. Wilson C. Naloxone accessibility and use by rehabilitation therapists for opioid overdoses. *Home Healthc Now*. 2020;38(1):50–51.

22. Scarborough BM, Smith CB. Optimal pain management for patients with cancer in the modern era. *CA Cancer J Clin*. 2018;68(3):182–196.

23. Ramamoorthy S, Cidlowski JA. Corticosteroids: mechanisms of action in health and disease. *Rheum Dis Clin*. 2016;42(1):15–31.

24. Yasir M, Goyal A, Bansal P, et al. Corticosteroid adverse effects. In: StatPearls [Internet]. StatPearls Publishing; 2020. https://www.ncbi.nlm.nih.gov/books/NBK531462/.

25. Prado CE, Crowe SF. Corticosteroids and cognition: a meta-analysis. *Neuropsychol Rev*. 2019;29:288–312. https://doi.org/10.1007/s11065-019-09405-8.

26. Burchum J, Rosenthal L. Chapter 51: Drugs for angina pectoris*Lehne's Pharmacology for Nursing Care*. 10th ed.: Elsevier; 2019.

27. APTA Task Force on lab values. Laboratory values interpretation resource. APTA Acute Care Physical Therapy website. https://www.aptaacutecare.org/page/ResourceGuides. Updated 2019. Accessed February 12, 2021.

28. Ciccone CD. Medical marijuana: just the beginning of a long, strange trip? *Phys Ther*. 2017;97(2):239–248.

29. Rudroff T, Sosnoff J. Cannabidiol to improve mobility in people with multiple sclerosis. *Front Neurol*. 2018;9:183. doi:10.3389/fneur.2018.00183.

30. Blake A, Wan BA, Malek L, et al. A selective review of medical cannabis in cancer pain management. *Ann Palliat Med*. 2017;6(suppl 2):s215–s222.

31. Lambertini M, Del Mastro L, Bellodi A, Pronzato P. The five "Ws" for bone pain due to the administration of granulocyte-colony stimulating factors (G-CSFs). *Crit Rev Oncol Hematol*. 2014;89(1):112–128.

UNIT II

Adverse Effects of Oncologic Treatment by System

7

Musculoskeletal System

KRISTINA SITARSKI, PT, CLT, KAREN M. WISEMAN, PT, DPT, CLT-LANA, BOARD CERTIFIED ONCOLOGIC CLINICAL SPECIALIST

CHAPTER OUTLINE

Introduction

Cancer and the treatments for cancer can have many deleterious effects on the musculoskeletal (MSK) system that globally change the way a person living with cancer (PLWC) or a person living beyond cancer (PLBC) moves their body and performs everyday tasks. After a cancer diagnosis, there may be alterations in muscles, bones, joints, and tissues attributed to surgeries, radiation, and chemotherapy. Surgery causes scars of the superficial and deep fascial and muscle layers. Additionally, surgeries may disrupt muscles, joints, and nerves causing changes in movement patterns. Radiotherapy can cause acute and chronic dysfunction of the bone, soft tissue, and skin in the radiation field. These disruptions contribute to tightness and pain. Chemotherapy and other systemic treatments such as hormone therapies and steroids can disrupt bone health, muscle strength, and endurance. The systemic therapies may affect the nervous system with adverse effects including peripheral neuropathies that impact balance and ambulation. See Table 7.1 for adverse effects from medications and systemic treatments that impact the MSK system.[1-8] In this chapter, cancer effects related to bone, tissue, muscle, and joints will be identified. How the MSK changes from cancer and its treatments relate to posture and body mechanics are examined. Finally, assessment and treatment of the MSK system and how cancer may relate to rehabilitative care will be discussed.

Effects on Bone

Bone pain is the number one cause of cancer-related pain.[9] Cancer treatment can cause irreversible and long-lasting effects on the body of a person living with and beyond cancer (PLWBC), including the osseous structures. In addition, we see these effects worsen as the PLBC ages. For the oncology rehabilitation (Onc R) clinician, differential diagnosis is complicated by normal aging effects, cancer treatment related effects, and/or a new onset of cancer recurrence.

The stability of the skeletal system relies on three bone cells: osteoclasts, osteoblasts, and osteocytes. See Figure 7.1 for a cellular

TABLE 7.1 Medications/Treatments and Their Effects on the Musculoskeletal System[1-8]

Common Medications in Cancer	Adverse Effects on Musculoskeletal System
Corticosteroids	Avascular necrosis, Myopathy, Osteoporosis
Methotrexate	Arthralgia, Myalgia, Osteoporosis
Taxanes, Vinca alkaloids	Arthralgia, Myalgia, Sensorimotor polyneuropathy, Weakness, Decreased deep tendon reflexes, Foot drop
Platinum-based agents	Rhabdomyolysis, Sensory polyneuropathy, Weakness, Arthralgias and myalgias
Cyclophosphamide (Cytoxan, Neosar), ifosfamide (Ifex)	Avascular necrosis
Anti-androgens	Muscle wasting, Osteoporosis
Aromatase inhibitors	Arthralgias, Back pain, Osteopenia/osteoporosis, Weakness, Tendinopathy
Tamoxifen (SERM) (Soltamox) (selective estrogen receptor modulators)	Arthralgia, Bone pain, Myalgia
Alkylating agents	Joint arthralgia

TABLE 7.1 Medications/Treatments and their Effects on the Musculoskeletal System—cont'd

Common Medications in Cancer	Adverse Effects on Musculoskeletal System
Gonadotropin-releasing hormone agonist	Osteoporosis
Luteinizing hormone agonist	Bone pain
Bortezomib (Velcade) (targeted therapy)	Myalgias and muscle cramps, Polyneuropathy, Weakness
Thalidomide (immunomodulatory agents)	Sensorimotor polyneuropathy
Cetuximab (Erbitux), bevacizumab (Avastin), trastuzumab (Herceptin) (monoclonal antibodies)	Arthralgias, Myalgias, Abdominal and back pain (trastuzumab), Weakness, Polyneuropathy
Pertuzumab (monoclonal antibodies)	Polyneuropathy
Pembrolizumab (Keytruda) (monoclonal antibody PDL-1)	Arthralgia, Pain in extremities
Nivolumab (Opdivo) (targeted therapy PD-1 blocking antibody)	Musculoskeletal pain, Myasthenia gravis
Atezolizumab (Tecentriq) (Anti PD-L1 monoclonal antibody)	Arthralgia, Neck and back pain
Eribulin (Halaven) (Nontaxane microtubule inhibitor)	Polyneuropathy, Weakness
Ixabepilone (Ixempra) (antimicrotubule agent)	Arthralgias, Myalgias, Polyneuropathy, Weakness
5-Fluorouracil (5-FU) (pyrimidine antimetabolite)	Polyneuropathy
Oral bisphosphonates (bone modifying agent): Alendronate (Fosamax), Risedronate (Actonel), Ibandronate (Boniva)	Risedronate: Bone pain, Ibandronate: Atypical fractures, Asymptomatic hypocalcemia, Headache, Musculoskeletal pain
IV bisphosphonates (bone modifying agent): Zoledronic acid (Reclast)	Myalgia, Bone Pain, Headaches, Atypical fractures, Hypocalcemia, Osteonecrosis of jaw
Denosumab (Prolia, Xgeva) (monoclonal anti-body bone modifying agent)	Arthralgia, Back/extremity pain, Asymptomatic hypocalcemia, Osteonecrosis of jaw

Created by Kristina Sitarski and Karen Wiseman. Printed with permission.

depiction of bone function. Osteoclasts resorb bone and osteoblasts form new bone. Osteocytes communicate signals to begin or end the remodeling sequence. The interaction of osteoclasts and osteoblasts allow for normal bone remodeling to maintain the structure and function of every bone in the body. Multiple factors influence bone remodeling including hormonal, environmental, and nutritional factors.[10] For this reason, the normal bone remodeling process is impacted by a cancer diagnosis either at the point of diagnosis

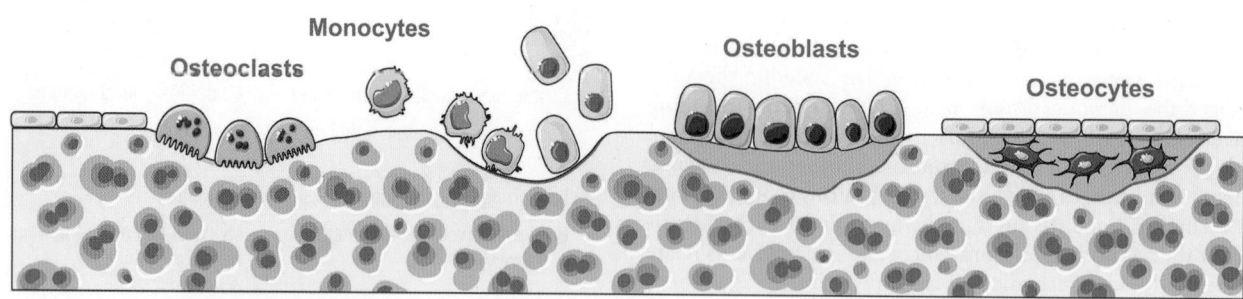

• **Fig. 7.1** Bone Cell Function. Osteoclasts resorb bone. Osteoblasts form new bone. Osteocytes communicate signals to begin or end the remodeling sequence. (Reprinted with permission from Laboratoires Servier, licensed under CC BY-SA 3.0: "Bone regeneration - Bone remodeling cycle III - Osteoclasts Monocytes Pre-osteoblasts etc – Smart-Servier (cropped).jpg".)

or years after remission. When this is disrupted, in the case of bony lesions, tumors, sarcomas, metastasis, osteoporosis, or osteonecrosis, the integrity of the bone is diminished. This leads to risk of fracture and/or spinal cord compression (SCC). Compromised bone has been shown to significantly increase morbidity and mortality.

The most common cancers that metastasize to the bone are breast, lung, prostate, thyroid, and renal cancers.[11–13] Common locations for metastases are seen in Table 7.2.[11,14,15] Metastases can have osteoblastic effects such as in prostate cancers or breast cancers (BCs). Metastases can also have osteolytic effects such as in renal, lung, and thyroid cancers. Osteolytic lesions result in degradation of the bone cortex whereas osteoblastic lesions increase activation of bone growth. Mixed lesions can also occur. Both osteoblastic and osteolytic tumor metastasis can weaken the bone. There are some key differences in the subjective and objective findings of pain in the spine, hip, and shoulder to assist with differential diagnosis of a malignant cause.

Physical Exam for Bone Pain of Neoplastic Origin

In any case of MSK pain in a PLWBC, recurrence or metastatic spread should be considered as a possible source of the symptoms. Back pain associated with cancer can present with specific symptoms. Back pain that is not relieved with rest or lying down, commonly in the thoracic spine, and is worse at night and may awaken the person from sleep should be further investigated for malignant cause. Furthermore, the quality of pain is usually dull, constant, and gradually progressive. There may be worsening neurologic deficits without a history of trauma or injury. Differential diagnosis includes mechanical back pain, spine infection, treatment-related arthralgias/myalgias, compression fracture, and SCC.[16]

An abnormal joint end feel should give an Onc R clinician suspicion for a more serious condition such as neoplasm.[14,15,17] An empty

end feel, such as pain that limits further range of motion (ROM), would be considered abnormal. Hip pain associated with cancer will have abnormal signs that include pain with weight bearing (WB), pain with resisted manual muscle testing (MMT), and a positive sign of the buttock. A positive sign of the buttock includes an empty end feel during passive range of motion (PROM) of the hip with a flexed knee, limited and painful straight leg raise (SLR), and noncapsular restriction patterns. Differential diagnosis includes bursitis, muscle abscess, septic arthritis, osteoarthritis (OA), arterial insufficiency, metastatic plexopathy, and radiation plexopathy.[14,17]

Upper extremity bony metastasis has a specific pain presentation demonstrating localized pain that is severe, insidious, and unremitting. Furthermore, glenohumeral joint testing is abnormal with an empty end feel and noncapsular restricted patterns if the lesion is located in the proximal humerus. Painful PROM and active range of motion (AROM), pain with resisted MMT, and pain with WB through the extremity can support a concern for malignancy. These findings warrant further referral to rule out an oncologic source of pain, especially in the absence of a precipitating cause or trauma.[11]

Pain with WB is a key indicator of bone metastasis, especially with a history of cancer and osteoporosis. This finding would require urgent consultation with the oncology team to perform diagnostic studies. If the patient has confirmed bone metastasis, oncologist clearance with updated WB status that considers fragility of the bone structure is important prior to initiating or resuming Onc R. A modified treatment plan can include education on assistive devices, positioning, energy conservation, activities of daily living (ADL) training, and an exercise program that addresses patient-specific goals.

Osteopenia and Osteoporosis

Osteopenia and the progression to osteoporosis has a significant long-term impact on fracture risk and morbidity in the cancer population. There are multiple causes of decreased bone density in PLWC. Risk factors for loss of bone density include prolonged glucocorticoid exposure, radiation, chemotherapy treatments (methotrexate, cyclophosphamide, 5-florauracil [FU]), untreated hormonal deficiencies (growth hormone, sex steroids, thyroid hormone), prolonged use of gonadotropin-releasing hormone (leuprolide acetate, goserelin), aromatase inhibitors (anastrozole, letrozole), and tamoxifen.[18] Furthermore, indirect complications such as the development of chronic kidney disease can increase the risk of osteoporosis.[19,20]

The criterion standard for diagnosing osteopenia or osteoporosis is a dual-energy X-ray absorptiometry (DEXA) scan. A DEXA scan reports objective measures called T score and Z score. These are used to diagnose osteopenia and osteoporosis. A T score compares

TABLE 7.2	Common Metastasis Site by Cancer[11,14,15]
Cancer	Common Metastasis Site
Breast	Spine, pelvis, femur, upper extremity
Lung	Spine, pelvis, femur, upper extremity
Prostate	Spine, pelvis, femur
Thyroid	Upper extremity
Renal	Upper extremity

Created by Kristina Sitarski and Karen Wiseman. Printed with permission.

the person being tested to healthy sex-matched young adults aged 25 to 30 years. The Z score compares the person to normal subjects of similar age, sex, and ethnicity. Risk prediction tools such as the University of Sheffields Fracture Risk Assessment Tool (FRAX) uses clinical data of risk factors to determine 10-year probability of both hip fracture and of a major osteoporotic fracture of the spine, forearm, hip, or shoulder (https://www.sheffield.ac.uk/FRAX/tool.aspx).[20] This can be used by the Onc R team for education in the prevention or management of osteopenia and osteoporosis. This education should include information about future fracture risk, importance of fall prevention, home safety and assistive device use.

Changes in bone density can also occur from hypercalcemia or hypocalcemia. Hypercalcemia is caused as the tumor dissolves and resorption of bone occurs. For this reason, it is more common with osteoclastic lesions. Hypercalcemia is common in pediatric cancers (e.g., acute lymphoblastic leukemia [ALL], neuroblastoma, rhabdomyosarcoma, rhabdoid tumors, Ewing sarcoma), and adult cancers (e.g., T cell leukemia/lymphoma, myeloma, solid tumors of the lung, head and neck, breast, ovary, kidney, and bladder). If moderate to severe hypercalcemia is present, immediate medical attention is needed.[18,21] Symptoms of hypercalcemia include generalized weakness, constipation, anorexia, polyuria, nausea, vomiting, dehydration, renal calculi, and encephalopathy. The patient will present with a history of malignancy with decreased bone density, and potentially compression or pathologic fractures. Hypercalcemia can be improved with immediate medical attention, bringing calcium levels to normal, and increasing bone deposition with the use of calcitonin and bisphosphonates.[18]

Hypocalcemia is caused by damage to parathyroid glands (during surgery for head and neck cancer [HNC]), extensive skeletal metastatic lesions, chemotherapies (cisplatin, 5-FU, leucovorin), hyperphosphatemia (tumor lysis syndrome, rhabdomyolysis, renal failure), hungry bone syndrome, and acute pancreatitis. It is more common with osteoblastic metastatic lesions such as those seen in prostate cancer. Hypocalcemia is also an adverse effect of denosumab and zoledronic acid, which are bone modifying agents that prevent osteoporosis.[1] Symptoms can include emotional instability and anxiety. Immediate medical attention is advised. Treatment includes receiving calcium gluconate through a central line while on continuous heart monitoring and supplementation of oral vitamin D and calcium.[18,20]

Bone Metastases

The cancers that are most likely to metastasize to the spine include breast, lung, prostate, thyroid, colon, and renal cancers. Some cancers are more likely to have osteoblastic metastasis. These include prostate cancer, carcinoid, small cell lung cancer, Hodgkin lymphoma (HL), or medulloblastoma. Other cancers are more likely to have osteolytic metastasis. These include multiple myeloma, (MM). renal cell carcinoma, melanoma, non-small cell lung cancer, non-Hodgkin lymphoma, thyroid cancer, and the majority of BC. Mixed lesions can also occur with both osteolytic and osteoblastic components which can be present with BC, gastrointestinal cancers, and squamous cancers.[21,22]

The primary symptom in malignancy of the spine is pain, weakness is the second most common symptom. Common sites of cancer-related pain are in the axial skeleton (with thoracic metastases being most common), femur, pelvis, humerus, ribs, and the skull. Subjective reports can include pain with movement, pain at night, radicular symptoms, changes of bowel and bladder, notable loss of function, significant reduction in quality of life (QOL) and depression. Objectively, the patient may demonstrate weakness, numbness or tingling,

TABLE 7.3 Findings Warranting Referral[15,16]

Finding	Indication
Inability to perform active straight leg raise due to pain in groin	Impending pathologic hip fracture
Back pain with radicular symptoms	Nerve root compression secondary to epidural tumor extension
Back pain with bending or twisting, relieved by lying down	Vertebral fractures and spinal instability
Disturbances in bowel and bladder	Cauda equina syndrome from tumor extension

Created by Kristina Sitarski and Karen Wiseman. Printed with permission.

changes in deep tendon reflexes, impaired balance, and an inability to perform AROM tests such as a SLR.[14–16,23] See Table 7.3 for findings and indications for potential diagnoses warranting further testing from the medical team.[15,16] Regular imaging is indicated to monitor bone density and/or bone metastases. Imaging may include bone scan, computed tomography (CT), magnetic resonance imaging (MRI), positron emission tomography (PET), or bone biopsy.[9]

Pathologic Fracture From Bone Metastasis

There are many risk factors that can lead to pathologic fracture in PLWC. Pathologic fractures are likely to occur in either the hip or spine. Spinal fractures occurring due to metastases are most likely to occur in the thoracic spine above the level of T7, whereas fractures due to osteoporosis alone are often below T7.[15,16] More risk factors that can lead to pathologic fracture in the cancer population are listed in Table 7.4.[20]

Diagnostic prediction scales have been developed to assess the risk of fracture and need for surgical intervention. These scales are based on imaging of the affected area and various clinical and structural features. Though these scales are comprehensive, there are multiple loading demands and other factors that are not synthesized within these decision-making scales. These include the

TABLE 7.4 Risk Factors for Pathologic Fracture in a PLWC[20]

Modifiable	Low vitamin D and calcium intake, smoking, >2 alcoholic beverages per day, sedentary without weight bearing exercise, household fall risks, weight loss, caffeine
Nonmodifiable	Age, history of prior fragility fractures, biochemical markers of bone resorption and formation above premenopausal range to be independent risk factors for fracture and low bone density to predict fracture risk
Reproductive	Age of menarche, amenorrhea, age of menopause, hypogonadism
Comorbidities	Celiac disease, rheumatoid arthritis, hyperparathyroidism
Medications	Glucocorticoids, antiepileptics, immunosuppressive agents, long-term heparin, total parenteral nutrition, cytotoxic drugs, proton pump inhibitors, and medication to induce hypogonadal state (aromatase inhibitors, luteinizing hormone releasing hormone agonists)

Created by Kristina Sitarski and Karen Wiseman. Printed with permission.

person's height, weight, activity level, loading regimen and factors that have weakened the strength of the bone including radiation, chemotherapy, immobilization, weight loss, sarcopenia, and other cancer-related factors.[24] For this reason, decisions regarding fracture risk should also include individualized clinical decision-making considering the comprehensive patient presentation, the patient's individual performance, medical history, and a thorough multidisciplinary discussion.

The Mirels scale, as seen in Table 7.5, is used to assess the risk of extremity fracture. A score of 9 or more is an indication for prophylactic surgical fixation. The sensitivity of the Mirels scale was 91% and specificity was 35%, which results in the tendency of the scale to over-predict the risk of fracture.[25] Studies have shown that axial cortical involvement >30 mm or circumferential cortical involvement >50% to be predictive of fracture.[2,26] The Spinal Instability Neoplastic Score (SINS) as seen in Table 7.6 is used to assess spinal instability based on imaging and clinical factors.[23,26] A score of 7 to 12 indicates impending instability and 13 to 18 suggests current instability. This can also be used as an indicator for surgical referral. Surgical consultation is recommended if the score is greater than 7. The SINS score has a sensitivity of 95.7% and specificity of 79.5%.[23] These scales have been used clinically for their ease of scoring and are useful for interdisciplinary communication. However, both the Mirels score and SINS scale tend to oversimplify and can overestimate fracture risk.[25,27] Therefore, use of these scales is best in combination with a multidisciplinary discussion. The Onc R clinician may see either of these classification scales in the medical chart and use the score to assist with exercise prescription, discharge planning, Onc R potential, and assistive device education.

SCC is an emergency and requires immediate medical attention. Tumor growth in the spine or pathologic fracture of spinal segments can compress the spinal cord and surrounding neural structures. SCC can create debilitating and permanent damage. Symptoms of metastatic SCC can be seen in Table 7.7.[28,29]

Two main pathologic fracture patterns are seen in the spine, including compression wedge fractures (Figure 7.2) or burst fractures (Figure 7.3). With a wedge fracture, the anterior of the vertebra collapses but the posterior wall is intact. In burst fractures, the

TABLE 7.5 Mirels Classification[2,26]

Location	
Peri-trochanter	3
Lower limb	2
Upper limb	1
Pain	
Severe	3
Moderate	2
Mild	1
Bone Lesion	
Lytic	3
Mixed	2
Blastic	1
Size (Bony Cortex)	
>2/3	3
1/3–2/3	2
<1/3	1
Total Score	
Requires prophylactic surgical fixation	>9

Created by Kristina Sitarski and Karen Wiseman. Printed with permission.

TABLE 7.6 Spinal Instability Neoplastic Score[23,26]

Location	
Junctional (occiput-C2, C7-T2, T11-L1, L5-S1)	3
Mobile spine (C3-C6, L2-4)	2
Semirigid (T3-T10)	1
Rigid (S2-S5)	0
Pain	
Yes	3
Occasional pain but not mechanical	1
Pain-free lesion	0
Bone Lesion	
Lytic	2
Mixed	1
Blastic	0
Radiographic Spinal Alignment	
Subluxation/translation present	4
De novo deformity (kyphosis, scoliosis)	2
Normal alignment	0
Vertebral Body Collapse	
>50% collapse	3
<50% collapse	2
No collapse with >50% body involvement	1
None of these	0
Posterolateral Involvement of Spinal Elements	
Bilateral	3
Unilateral	1
None of these	0
Total Score	
Impending instability	7–12
Current instability	13–18

Created by Kristina Sitarski and Karen Wiseman. Printed with permission.

TABLE 7.7 Symptoms of Metastatic Spinal Cord Compression[28,29]

Back or neck pain	Progressive weakness in lower extremities
Numbness or tingling in toes, fingers, buttocks	Unsteadiness on feet
Bowel and bladder changes	Pain radiating in a band-like fashion around chest or abdomen

Created by Kristina Sitarski and Karen Wiseman. Printed with permission.

anterior and middle column of the vertebrae collapse causing retropulsion of bone fragments or the tumor mass which can pierce or compress the surrounding regions.[23]

Medical Treatment of Pathologic Fracture

Treatment must be immediate within 48 hours of onset to alleviate pressure and stabilize spine and may include kyphoplasty, local radiation, and high dose steroids.[30,31] Surgical stabilization of the spine can be done prophylactically for those with spinal metastases or urgently for those with impending instability leading to SCC. Less invasive surgical techniques include vertebroplasty and kyphoplasty. These surgeries are shown to be effective methods for providing mechanical stability to the anterior spinal column while controlling pain and improving disability in both osteolytic,

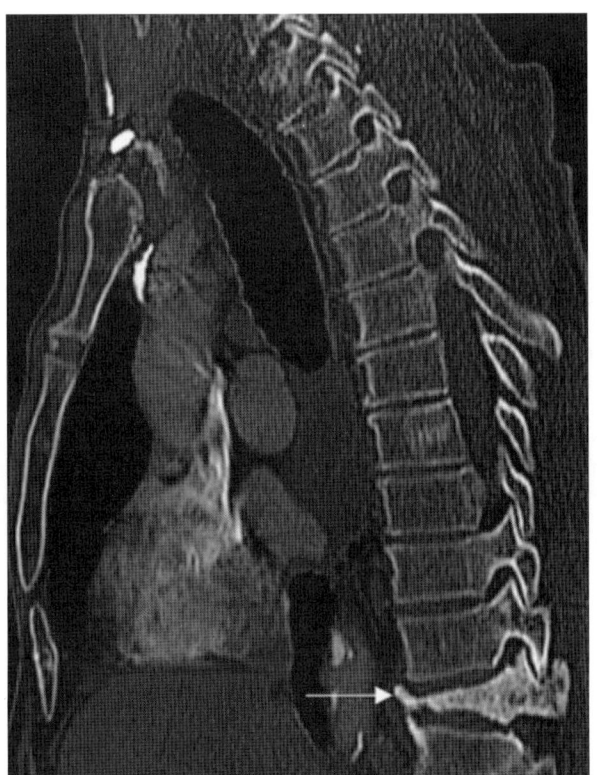

• **Fig. 7.2** Wedge Fracture of Thoracic Spine. A grade 3 wedge fracture of the thoracic spine with metastatic infiltration. (Reprinted with permission from Woo EK, Mansoubi H, Alyas F. Incidental vertebral fractures on multidetector CT images of the chest: prevalence and recognition. *Clin Radiol*. 2008;63(2):160–164.)

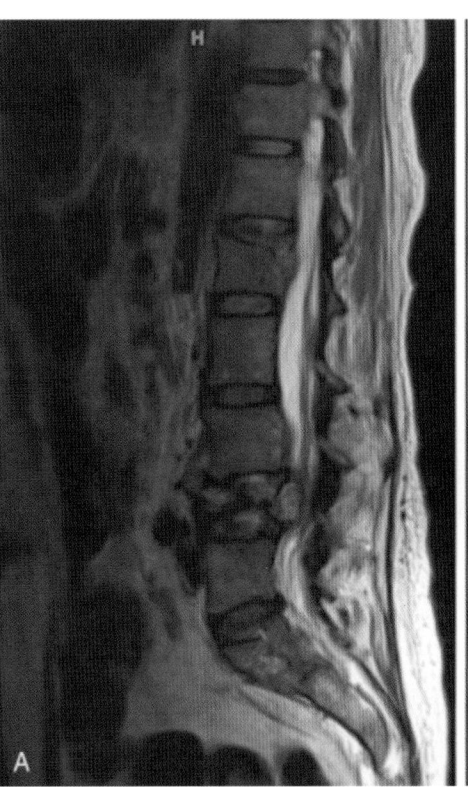

• **Fig. 7.3** Burst Fracture of Lumbar Spine. Burst fracture of L4 from metastatic disease. (Reprinted with permission from Quinones-Hinojosa A. *Schmidek & Sweet: Indications, Methods and Results. Operative Neurosurgical Techniques E-Book* (Expert Consult-Online and Print). Elsevier Health Sciences; 2012.)

osteoblastic, or mixed spinal metastases.[23] Surgery, combined with postoperative radiation therapy (RTx), is the best practice for SCC or spinal instability in patients with high performance status and longer life expectancy.[32] Those not receiving surgical fixation for spinal metastases may be given radiation to reduce other debilitating symptoms such as pain. In fact, radiation such as stereotactic body radiation therapy (SBRT) may be especially effective (see Chapter 5 for more on SBRT). One study demonstrated improved pain relief from SBRT when compared to conventional external beam radiotherapy for spinal metastases; 51% to 54% of patients reported complete relief within 7 days as well as 1 year from beginning SBRT versus 0% to 20% with external beam radiation.[23]

Surgical fixation may also be utilized to stabilize other areas of bony metastases such as the femur. Depending on the severity and amount of cortex involvement, the PLWC may undergo a total hip arthroplasty, hemiarthroplasty, intramedullary nailing, or plate and screw fixation. If the integrity of the bone is not compromised, the primary treatment may be RTx alone.

Other medical interventions for pathologic fracture from bone metastases include systemic therapies including chemotherapy, targeted therapies, and immunotherapy. Medications may assist with bone metabolism. These medications include calcium, vitamin D, and bisphosphonates that induce osteoclast apoptosis and decrease pain. Another medication, denosumab is a monoclonal antibody that reduces osteoclast maturation and reduces tumor bone destruction. Medications such as bisphosphonates are commonly used to reduce skeletal related events (SREs) and can improve bone pain and QOL once metastases have been found,

but are less often used as a prevention measure for SREs.[33] Furthermore, a variety of pain-specific interventions can be used such as corticosteroids, tricyclic antidepressants, morphine, cutaneous stimulation, spine cryoablation, and regional nerve blocks.[32]

Healing time from pathologic fracture can vary. Bone remodeling in a healthy adult takes 120 days with bone being completely remodeled in adults every 10 years.[34] In a PLWC, bone healing may be delayed or may not fully occur if the metastatic lesion continues to grow. Imaging at intervals along the healing process will assist the medical team to determine when to progress WB (if currently restricted), as well as assess for further spread of bone metastases.

Modifications in activity, WB and exercise will need to be made for the PLWC who has experienced a pathologic fracture from bone metastasis. As mentioned previously, the amount of cortical involvement determines the WB and activity restrictions. In spinal fractures, WB status of the extremities does not apply as much as lifting restrictions (typically less than 5 pounds/2–3 kg). Durable medical equipment (DME) needs should be identified. This can include a walker instead of a cane to off-weight the lower extremity or spine or use of a thoracic lumbar sacral orthosis (TLSO) brace to support the spine. In these cases, retraining in ADL performance will be needed to ensure safety and independence with necessary daily activities. For example, a tub transfer bench will be helpful to reduce fall risk and maintain spinal precautions. Overall, the focus of Onc R should be to maximize QOL, provide pain reduction techniques, education on pain science, and prescribe the correct assistive devices and braces.

Bone Lesions

Bone lesions or osteolytic lesions are spots of bone damage from cancerous plasma cells building in the bone marrow. This area of the lesion ceases to break down and regrow making it thin and fragile and likely to fracture. This is most common in MM. Many people learn they have MM after they break a bone. In many persons, these lesions can cause fractures, SCC, vertebral collapse, severe bone pain, and hypercalcemia. Onc R clinicians working with clients diagnosed with MM should have a high suspicion and concern for fracture.

Avascular Necrosis/Osteonecrosis

The presentation of avascular necrosis (or osteonecrosis) is most common in the femur, humerus, knee, shoulder, and ankle. In the affected bone, the blood supply may be disrupted causing the bone to die and break down without being able to remodel as it would in healthy areas. There can be many causes including alcohol, bisphosphonates, medical treatments (e.g., RTx, chemotherapy, organ transplants, steroid drugs), diabetes mellitus (DM), pancreatitis, autoimmune diseases, sickle cell disease, human immunodeficiency virus (HIV), smoking, gout, OA, and osteoporosis. Diagnostic imaging includes bone scan, MRI, CT scan, or plain film radiography. Medical treatments to improve vascularization and pain to the area include blood thinners, non-steroidal anti-inflammatory drugs (NSAIDs), and statins. In some cases, surgeries such as bone grafts, core decompression, or a total hip replacement may be required. Core decompression is utilized to remove osteonecrosis, improve blood flow, and preserve viable tissue. It was found in one study to have longer success than a total hip replacement.[35]

Osteoradionecrosis

Osteoradionecrosis is caused by localized radiation damage to blood vessels that leads to bone death. It occurs in 5% to 8% of HNC with radiation to the mandible.[36] The mandible is susceptible secondary to the limited blood supply. Osteoradionecrosis can develop years after RTx for HNC. Risk for osteoradionecrosis of the jaw significantly increases with RTx, exposed bone during RTx, poor oral hygiene, dry mouth, and if a dental exam and necessary dental work was not completed before RTx began.[37] A PLWC that is at risk should be monitored for the following symptoms: increase in pain, swelling, sores/ulcers in the mouth or jaw, trismus, decreased sensation in the mouth or jaw, infection, malocclusion, or a new onset of jaw fracture not related to any trauma. Given the necrosis to the area, it is important to preserve healthy tissue and revascularize the area if possible. Surgical interventions include debridement, microvascular reconstructive surgery, bone and/or soft tissue grafts, and dental implants. Lastly, hyperbaric oxygen therapy has been found beneficial for healing and revascularization to the affected area.[38]

Though osteoradionecrosis of the jaw is most common in HNC it can also occur in other areas of the body. Radiation-induced osteonecrosis is the potential mechanism underlying SBRT-induced vertebral compression fractures. A compression fracture rate of 65% has been reported 4 months after SBRT.[23] While radiation can provide benefit, bony degradation can occur in the acute or late effects for a PLWBC and the radiation oncology team has to weigh the potential adverse effects of this treatment.

Osteosarcoma

See Chapter 20 for more details on osteosarcoma.

Effects on Tissue

Cancer treatments can have direct effects on connective tissues such as ligaments, tendons, and fascia. This can occur after surgery, RTx, stem cell transplant, or as an adverse effect of systemic therapies. Changes to this area of the MSK system, as with others, can occur in varying time frames up to years after cancer remission.

In a recent review, the presence of shoulder and/or arm pain at 6 to 56 months after breast surgery was reported to be between 9% and 68% and the prevalence of breast and or scar pain was between 15% and 72%.[39] This is a wide range but shows the longevity of dysfunction related to cancer treatment. Even a well-healed scar without complications can cause shoulder dysfunction months or years from the surgery. Muscle manipulation during surgery, scar tissue formation, soft tissue adhesions, and adaptive postures (e.g., slouching or guarding) following surgery can cause myofascial dysfunctions.[40,41] Moreover, radiation has an impact on skin healing and can cause radiation fibrosis syndrome (RFS) that leads to further soft tissue adhesions, compensatory postures, and impaired joint mechanics. Onc R clinicians can assist with scar massage, myofascial release, and desensitization to improve pain, ROM, function, and cosmesis.

Surgical Tissue Changes

In most healthy individuals, it takes about 2 weeks for full closure of the wound with remodeling continuing for up to 2 years. Following surgery, scar massage may begin with approximation at 2 weeks postoperatively with caution to avoid shear forces that could cause wound dehiscence. Based on appearance and clinical judgment, it is often appropriate to progress to scar massage in vertical, horizontal, and circular directions after 4 to 6 weeks. Research into mechanical scar mobilization in hypertrophic burn scars found that scar massage may effectively decrease scar height and pain while improving vascularity and pliability.[42] Additionally, incorporating scar massage and lymphatic drainage techniques will help to create new pathways around this "road block" for lymphatic flow. Extreme caution is needed with any soft tissue techniques of recently radiated tissues. If the PLWC is undergoing radiation treatment to the area, it is necessary to avoid manual therapy, especially frictional forces to the affected region until well healed. Once healed and manual therapy is initiated, it is important to continually monitor for redness and irritation that may require treatment modification.

In addition to general surgical complications such as infections or wound dehiscence, cancer surgeries can have specific complications. Commonly seen complications to the tissue in the Onc R of persons with BC include axillary web syndrome (AWS), seroma, and lymphedema. A study of 964 women with BC found that 62.6% of them had a seroma, 35.9% had AWS, and 31.4% had lymphedema at 10 year follow up.[40,41] AWS incidence is higher in surgery with axillary lymph node dissection (ALND) (36%–72%) than sentinel lymph node biopsy (SLNB) (11%–58%).[43] AWS presents with pain down the medial arm that can extend from the axilla to the wrist with limitations in abduction with elbow extension and wrist dorsiflexion. There are often palpable and visible taut bands in the axilla and or antecubital regions. AWS frequently becomes symptomatic between 2 and 8 weeks postoperatively but can also develop and recur months to years after surgery.[44] AWS can be significantly improved with Onc R via myofascial release, ROM, and stretching exercises into the direction of restriction.

A seroma is a collection of serous fluid in a surgical cavity. Seroma incidence increases by applying whole breast radiation after intra-operative radiation.[44] Seroma may be avoided with closed-suction drains such as those routinely used after ALND, mastectomies, and plastic surgery procedures. When drains have been removed, a seroma can form in the cavity. More recent articles have studied drain-free postmastectomy flap fixation closure techniques for improved closure of the dead space to prevent seroma formation with good success.[45,46] However, if a seroma becomes tense and painful, or if infection is suspected, further medical intervention should be initiated to drain the seroma if necessary.[39,43] After surgical reduction of seroma, Onc R can assist with compression over the area to help reduce reoccurrence. This can be completed with use of foam padding and short stretch bandages and/or use of a compression bra. It is crucial for the Onc R provider to monitor for signs of infection, increased pain, or onset of seroma and regularly assess for any change in swelling that could suggest lymphedema.

Radiation Fibrosis

Many PLWCs will require RTx as a part of their treatment plan. Radiation has both short-term and long-term effects on tissues within the radiation field. Acute effects (typically during or immediately after treatment) are seen in the skin and mucosa because these cells replicate at a high rate. This can present as skin burns with or without desquamation. Redness of the skin frequently occurs. Depending on the location of radiation, dryness of the mucosal linings, such as in the mouth or perineal area, may significantly affect comfort. In the later stages (more than 3 months following completion of treatment), radiation can continue to affect the tissue due to the abnormal accumulation of fibrin in intravascular and extravascular compartments causing connective tissue fibrosis, nerve damage, and microvascular damage. See Table 7.8 for phases of radiation fibrosis.[47]

A common term used in this late phase is RFS. RFS is directly correlated with an increased radiation dose, greater dose per fraction, increased radiation field size, and prolonged therapy. Additionally, RFS is correlated with concurrent chemotherapy and prior surgery to the area as well as pre-existing connective tissue disease such as systemic scleroderma, systemic lupus, or Marfan's syndrome.

Due to the difference in cellular and microvascular anatomy of tissues and organs, radiation can impact each tissue differently in the late stages. For example, while late effects to the skin include dermatitis, ulceration, and infection, the late effects to muscles are myopathies. Myopathy in the muscles can cause weakness, fatigability, muscle spasms, and trigger points. Tensile strength of the tendons and ligaments can also be compromised. This leads to joint restrictions and contractures. Similarly, radiation to the lymphatic system can cause lymphedema. RFS can occur from direct exposure to the radiation field or indirectly due to compromise of the surrounding tissues. While radiation and the progressive fibrosis that occurs cannot be reversed, the specific diagnoses that become the sequelae such as frozen shoulder, dropped head syndrome (DHS), or lymphedema can be optimized individually with Onc R.[48]

TABLE 7.8	Phases of Radiation Fibrosis[47]	
Prefibrotic phase	• Asymptomatic • Endothelial cell dysfunction • Chronic local inflammation • Necrosis of microvasculature and local ischemia
Constitutive organized phase	• Symptomatic • Patchy areas of active fibrosis in a disorganized extracellular matrix with high density of myofibroblasts • Damage to endothelial cells and action of cytokines perpetuates fibrosis
Late fibroatrophic phase	• This stage may develop and progress years or decades following radiation therapy • Residual fibroblasts are locked in a dense extracellular matrix • Tissues then remain rigid, fragile, and poorly vascularized

Created by Kristina Sitarski and Karen Wiseman. Printed with permission.

Effects on Nervous Tissues

Cancer treatments can affect connective tissue, nerve tissue, muscle tissue, and fascial structures. Cancer treatments can cause microvascular injury to these tissues. This may cause scars and fibrosis in the region. In addition, nerves may be transected or damaged during cancer surgery causing a loss of that nerve's functional performance. A nerve that is commonly impacted with HNC during neck dissection surgery is the spinal accessory nerve (SAN). The SAN innervates the sternocleidomastoid and trapezius muscles. This presents as an inability to shrug or retract the scapula and loss of sensation that will lead to shoulder dysfunction. The frequency of postoperative morbidity of the SAN in one study was 46.7% for radical neck dissections, 42.5% for selective neck dissections, and 25% for modified neck dissections.[49] Even with nerve sparing techniques, devascularization and manipulation of the nerve during surgery to access the lymph nodes can cause SAN palsy. Body positioning during surgery can also have an impact. For example, to access and dissect the left side of the neck, the patient is placed in cervical extension, right lateral flexion, and right rotation with an outstretched arm. This positioning can result in significant nerve and fascial tension to the area potentially increasing nerve complications during prolonged surgical procedures.[36,48]

Peripheral nerve impairments are common after cancer treatments, especially chemotherapy-induced polyneuropathy (CIPN). CIPN can cause abnormal sensation, numbness and tingling, decreased touch thresholds, decreased vibration threshold, and reduced deep tendon reflexes. More information about CIPN can be found in Chapter 8 Neurological System.

Radiation plexopathies can occur leading to painful and debilitating conditions. Some of the conditions related to radiation plexopathies are thoracic outlet syndrome, nerve entrapments, radiculopathies, and neuropathies. Although plexopathies continue to occur, improved radiation techniques are reducing the impact of this treatment modality on nerve tissue. See Table 7.9 for a list of risk factors for radiation-induced poly neuropathies.[48,50]

Nerve symptoms should always be investigated through specific questioning for quality of symptoms. These are especially important to consider if findings are not reproducible or provokable

TABLE 7.9	Risk Factors for Radiation-Induced Polyneuropathy[48,50]	
Radiation Therapy (RTx) Factors	**Combined Treatment Factors**	**Patient-Related Factors**
• >50 Gy to plexus • >60 Gy to cranial nerves • Large doses per fraction • RTx volume including large portion of nerve fibers, high dose distribution, hot spot high dose • Salvage RTx or previously treated areas • Intracavitary radium source • After intraoperative radiation boost	• Surgery in the case of hematoma or chronic infection and extended lymph node dissection • Concomitant or previous neurotoxic chemotherapy (cisplatin, vinca alkaloids, taxanes) • Concomitant chemotherapy with intrathecal methotrexate	• Young or advanced age • Obesity • Comorbidity factors such as high blood pressure, diabetes mellitus, dyslipidemia, combined polyneuropathy (diabetic, alcoholic, genetic) or arteritis (smoking, multiple sclerosis) • Pre-existing collagen vascular disease • Hypersensitive patients

Created by Kristina Sitarski and Karen Wiseman. Printed with permission.

via MSK testing. Abnormal symptoms with concern for neural compression from tumor include unrelenting pain, especially at night with focal sensory disturbances or weakness in the distribution of the regional plexus or spinal segment. In the case of breast and lung tumors, the brachial plexus can be compressed by tumor progression. Likewise, the lumbosacral plexus can be compressed by colorectal tumors, gynecologic tumors, sarcomas, and lymphomas. These findings require an urgent referral to the oncologist or primary care physician for further testing.[48,50]

Once a thorough evaluation rules out tumor progression or cancer recurrence, Onc R interventions should include pain reduction and improving the function of the affected area. Investigators have noted the importance of avoiding stretching a plexus that has been immobilized by fibrosis.[50] An example of this is avoiding carrying heavy loads or extensive movements. This can cause sudden neurological decompensation. Modifying risk factors is also beneficial to Onc R management of neurologic symptoms. This includes controlling hypertension (HTN), DM, and smoking.[50]

Additional Tissue Effects

Another cancer treatment affecting tissues of the body is chronic graft-versus-host disease (C-GvHD). C-GvHD is a complication of stem cell transplant. It occurs in approximately 50% of transplant survivors and is the leading cause of morbidity that compromises QOL and function.[51] This occurs when the donor's immune system recognizes recipient tissues as a foreign substance. The immune response causes inflammation and fibrosis. MSK effects can be rare, but they are often combined with symptoms from long-term steroid use in GvHD such as myopathy, avascular necrosis, compression fractures, and osteopenia. Symptoms include joint stiffness, edema, decreased ROM, arthralgia, fasciitis, and rarely arthritis or synovitis. Usually, the overlying skin remains mobile but notable stiffness or edema is present in the extremities. In deep sclerosis or fasciitis, the skin and underlying tissue is severely hardened and fibrotic. It is important to provide education about potential joint or fascia manifestations among patients who are more than one year after transplantation, those who received high-dose total body irradiation conditioning, or those who had skin involvement or sclerosis with GvHD.[51,52]

Other tissue effects can be from systemic therapy such as chemotherapies. One such diagnosis is hand-foot syndrome (HFS), also known as palmar-plantar erythrodysesthesia. Concentration and administration of these chemotherapies can affect incidence and severity of HFS. Chemotherapy permeates into the small vessels, interstitial space, integumentary cells, and small fiber nerves. This can present with pain, numbness, and tingling in the palms and feet. It can progress to changes in skin color, blistering, ulcers,

ischemic necrosis, and desquamation. Chemotherapy dose modification can significantly reduce these symptoms and improve QOL. In the first 4 weeks, it is important to avoid activities that cause too much friction on the feet/hands due to blistering/ulcerations that occurs in severe cases. Education on the use of padded gloves and open shoes to avoid pressure points will be necessary to decrease shear forces and maintain ADL performance.[53]

Effects on Muscles and Joints

Cancer and the treatment continuum have many effects on muscles and joints. Chemotherapy and other treatment medications can affect muscles and joints creating pain and weakness. Additionally, those treatments may contribute to cancer related fatigue (CRF) creating a cycle of fatigue and weakness that increases morbidity. Cancer treatment may cause hospitalization and contribute to cachexia and sarcopenia. Older people make up a large proportion of PLWCs who are at risk for frailty. A diagnosis of cancer increases risk of morbidity and mortality associated with frailty. Onc R professionals can provide interventions and support in managing many of the muscle and joint side-effects associated with these cancer related issues.

Cancer Treatments

Taxane-based chemotherapy regimens are widely used in the treatment of breast, gynecologic, lung, and genitourinary cancers.[54] Myalgias and arthralgias are possible adverse effect of these drugs. Pain is usually generalized and typically appears within 48 hours of infusion.[55] This pain can be quite debilitating for the PLWC and may lead to chemotherapy dose reductions, treatment delays, and/or discontinuation of treatment.[54,55] The mechanism for this pain is not well understood but studies show that exercise training during chemotherapy is safe and effective to minimize symptom burden.[56] Onc R clinicians can provide education and guidance on exercise to help improve the pain experience and allow for fewer changes in treatment regimen.

Aromatase inhibitors (AIs) are a class of drugs used in the adjuvant phase of cancer treatment to treat hormone-positive BC. AI use has been shown to improve disease-free survival, local recurrence, and distant cancer recurrence. AI users frequently experience pain of the muscles and joints. A meta-analysis showed a pooled prevalence rate of 46% of PLBCs on this drug therapy reported AI-induced arthralgia.[57] AI-induced arthralgias and myalgias, which are often grouped together in research studies, are a significant contributor to nonadherence and discontinuation of the drug therapy.[58,59] Additionally, AI users with arthralgia are at risk for falls. A recent study showed that one in three AI users experienced a fall and about 10% of those required medical treatment for the fall.[60]

Onc R should be aimed at reducing the risk of falls, improving balance, and a comprehensive exercise program should be provided to improve arthralgias and myalgias. Education in pain science and management techniques will empower the PLBCs to manage their medication adverse effects. More information about the use of AI in persons diagnosed with BC can be found in Chapter 15.

Androgen deprivation therapy (ADT) is commonly used in the treatment of prostate cancer to improve survival.[61,62] ADT therapy is associated with decreased bone mineral density (BMD) and increased risk for bone fracture.[62] ADT therapy is also associated with changes in muscle mass causing loss of lean muscle.[63,64] Education in bone and muscle health is valuable for PLBCs taking ADT. Adhering to an exercise program, especially resistive or WB activities, may influence the changes that occur in the muscles and joints caused by ADT. In a recent systematic review and meta-analysis, exercise significantly improved upper and lower body muscle strength, increased exercise tolerance, and controlled body mass idnex (BMI) in prostate cancer patients taking ADT.[65] Men who are treated with ADT should receive education on the treatment effects and ways to manage the morbidity associated with ADT treatment. More information about the use of ADT can be found in Chapter 16.

Steroid Myopathy

Steroids are used in the oncology setting to help control the negative effects of the disease and treatment. Immune checkpoint inhibitors (ICIs) are a treatment where steroids may be used to support the treatment. ICIs work by blocking the checkpoints or "stops" of the immune system which will then enhance the body's immune response to the cancer.[66] Toxicities associated with ICI treatment can range from dermatologic to life threatening adverse reactions. Corticosteroids are prescribed to manage some of the adverse reactions and are recommended in the treatment for ICI-related toxicity.[66,67] However, there is still some question as to how steroids should be utilized in metastatic disease as there may be a detrimental effect on survival.[67]

Additionally, corticosteroid use is common in palliative care. Steroids have a role in the treatment of edema, anorexia, dyspnea, nausea, and pain. Adverse reactions from the use of steroids are dose- and duration-dependent. Therefore, the lowest effective dose should be used. Steroid myopathy is an adverse reaction to steroid use and often presents as proximal limb weakness. If a PLWC develops new-onset muscle fatigue and weakness of any muscle group while taking steroids, there is a high suspicion for steroid myopathy.[68] Treatment includes cessation of steroid therapy and exercise to strengthen the affected muscle groups.

Sedentary Effects on Muscles and Joints

Physical activity and sedentary behaviors are shown to have significant effect on mortality. The American College of Sports Medicine recommends that everyone, including PLWCs, get 150 minutes per week of moderate exercise or 75 minutes per week of vigorous exercise. Many people do not get the recommended amount of exercise but in addition to that they live a sedentary lifestyle. The amount of the day spent moving matters. Higher levels of physical activity (at any intensity) and less time spent sedentary are associated with substantially reduced risk for premature death.[69,70] Strong evidence exists to support an association between physical activity and cancer risk, as well as survival of many types of cancer.[71]

Sedentary behavior contributes to weakness. Muscle mass and muscle strength losses are associated with poorer QOL and overall

increased mortality.[72] PLWBCs are at risk for these health consequences. Although increased physical activity is a modifiable risk factor for cancer recurrence and mortality, studies show that physical activity decreases with a diagnosis of cancer.[73,74] Patients with BC who received chemotherapy treatment had the greatest impact on muscle strength.[70] Furthermore, prostate cancer survivors who had modest increases in physical activity and decreases in sedentary behavior were associated with clinically important improvement in QOL measurements.[75] PLBC should be educated on the health and QOL benefits of physical activity on muscle strengthening.

Hospital-Acquired Weakness

Hospitalization is a necessary part of the treatment plan for many PLWCs. Some hospitalizations may be planned for administration of chemotherapies, surgeries, and other treatments. Additionally, a PLWC may require hospitalization for adverse-effect management including pain and nausea. In advanced cancer, periods of hospitalization are nearly inevitable; a study reported that 71% of persons with advanced cancer required a hospitalization within the year following diagnosis.[76] Muscle weakness is a frequent complication of critical illness and hospitalization that can have short- and long-term effects.[77] Individualized physical exercise provided during hospitalization with an emphasis on progressive resistance training, seems to be an effective strategy to improve muscle strength of upper and lower limbs and to reverse the loss of muscle strength often associated with hospitalization in older patients.[78] Onc R should be a key component in the treatment strategy for hospitalized PLWCs. For more on acute management of PLWCs refer Chapter 24.

Frailty

Frailty is a clinical syndrome characterized by reduced physical function including weakness and reduced endurance. It is typically associated with advanced age but younger individuals can also become frail, especially if they have cancer or another disease that impacts their physiological reserve.[79] Frailty results in vulnerability, decreased resiliency to stressors, and reduced adaptive capacity.[79] Persons with frailty are at increased risk of morbidity and mortality from cancer, surgical complications, and chemotherapy intolerance.[79] Frailty should be considered when directing cancer treatment to optimize outcomes.

Assessment of frailty can be complex. A *comprehensive geriatric assessment* is considered best practice for older adults at risk for frailty. A comprehensive geriatric assessment battery of tests may include medical, functional, psychological, social, environmental, spiritual well-being, sexuality, and advanced care planning. However, assessment can be time consuming and consensus is lacking relative to the criteria that define frailty.[80]

Two scales that are commonly used clinically in oncology to assess global performance status and determine patient fitness for treatment include the Karnofsky Performance Scale and the Eastern Cooperative Oncology Group (ECOG) scale. These scales are clinician-rated tools and have considerable rater bias.[80] A study conducted at multiple health centers concluded that geriatric assessment was superior to oncologists' clinical judgment in identifying frailty.[80] Frailty is often underdiagnosed by oncologists in PLWCs.[80] This influences treatment decisions. A better understanding of frailty and the influence it has on treatment outcomes is necessary to optimize QOL.

One tool that may be useful in identifying those at risk for frailty in the clinical environment is the Fried phenotype from the Cardiovascular Health Study. The Fried phenotype has five criteria to identify the presence of frailty that provides a basis for clinical assessment of frail individuals and those at risk for frailty.[81] This phenotype includes both objective criteria and self-reported criteria. The five criteria are weight loss, exhaustion, physical activity, gait speed, and grip strength.

Exercise is one of the most effective interventions to reduce frailty.[81,82] There is no consensus on the duration and type of exercise to reverse frailty. Generally, exercise incorporating functional strengthening and balance should be included. An individualized home exercise program (HEP) that considers patient and family goals should be emphasized. Additionally, group exercise interventions can be valuable to this population with improvement of grip strength, gait speed, and a reduced fear of falling was noted in a systematic review of data.[81] See Chapter 23 for more details.

Sarcopenia and Cachexia

The terms sarcopenia and cachexia are used to describe disorders of muscle deficiency. Figure 7.4 shows that frailty, sarcopenia, and cachexia can be interrelated. The terms share similar characteristics, but they are distinct. See Table 7.10 for a comparison of cachexia and sarcopenia.[79–91] Cancer cachexia is defined by consensus as greater than 5% weight loss in the previous 6 months or 2% to 5% weight loss with either a BMI of <20 kg/m^2 or reduced muscle mass.[83] Sarcopenia is defined as a progressive and generalized skeletal muscle disorder that is associated with increased likelihood of adverse

outcomes including falls, fractures, physical disability and mortality.[84] People with cancer may have both cachexia and sarcopenia.

Cachexia can occur in a variety of chronic diseases including cancer, chronic obstructive pulmonary disorder, cardiac disease, and HIV/AIDS. It is very relevant in cancer patients where it occurs in up to 80% of cancer types and is a major cause of death in advanced cancer.[85] Characteristics of cancer cachexia include anorexia, metabolic changes, excess catabolism, and the presence of inflammatory cytokines.[85] The importance of body composition is being realized with the loss of skeletal muscle developing as a key factor in functional and QOL limitations of cachexia. Because of that, more specific identification of skeletal muscle mass is being assessed through the use of a DEXA scan, which measures lean mass, or through CT and MRI.[86] The advantage of CT or MRI is that they may already be a part of routine cancer care. Early diagnosis and treatment of cachexia may lead to improved management with better outcomes.

Sarcopenia has two defining parameters: decreased muscle mass and low muscle function. After age 40, healthy adults lose approximately 8% of their muscle mass every 10 years.[87] Additionally, conditions that reduce muscle activity can result in decreased muscle mass. These include chronic illness, sedentary lifestyle, hospitalization, immobilization and bed rest.[87] Individuals lose muscle mass through aging, illness, and inactivity. Identification of sarcopenia is similar to that of cachexia with imaging exams being the criterion standard to objectify muscle mass. DEXA, CT, and MRI are useful exams to perform. Additionally, bio-electrical impedance analysis (BIA), a method which estimates the volume of fat and lean body mass, and anthropometric measurements (arm or calf circumference) may be used.[88] Assessment of physical performance can be done using grip strength, walking speed, short physical performance battery (SPPB), and SARC-F (Strength, Assistance in walking, Rise from chair, Climb stairs and Falls) questionnaire.[88]

Physical activity interventions are shown to improve outcomes for sarcopenia and cachexia. A systematic review found that physical exercise has a beneficial impact on muscle mass, muscle strength, and physical performance in healthy subjects aged 60 years and older.[89] Another systematic review suggests that resistance training of large muscles of the body and the inclusion of high intensity training is a beneficial intervention for sarcopenia.[90] Additionally, exercise may have the ability to improve metabolism, function, and reduce muscle mass loss in those with cachexia.[91]

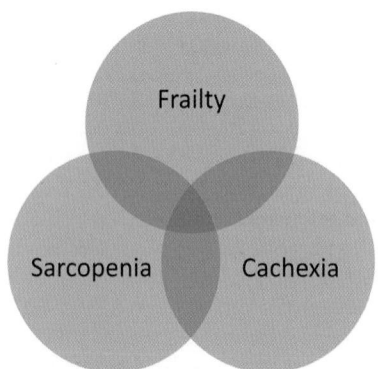

• **Fig. 7.4** Interrelated Muscle Deficiencies. Frailty, sarcopenia and cachexia are their own entities but can also be interrelated. (Created by Kristina Sitarski and Karen Wiseman. Printed with permission.)

TABLE 7.10	Contrasting Frailty, Cachexia, and Sarcopenia[79–91]		
	Frailty	**Cachexia**	**Sarcopenia**
Characteristics	↓function ↓strength ↓endurance ≥3 of 5 Fried criteria	5% weight loss in 6 months or 2%–5% weight loss in BMI <20. ↓strength, fatigue, anorexia, +metabolic changes, +inflammation	↓muscle mass ↓function
Evaluation	CGA, Fried phenotype	Imaging to assess skeletal muscle mass, weight loss assessment, hand grip assessment, biochemistry test (CRP >5.0 mg/L, Hgb <12 g/dL, albumin <3.2 g/dL)	Imaging to assess skeletal muscle mass, grip strength, walking speed, short physical performance battery (SPPB) and SARC-F (screening index for sarcopenia)
Treatment	Functional exercise, home exercise program, group exercise	Nutritional support, exercise, investigations underway into drug therapies	Exercise and possible dietary intervention

BMI, Body mass index; *CGA,* comprehensive geriatric assessment; *CRP,* c-reactive protein; *Hgb,* hemoglobin; *SARC-F,* strength, assistance in walking, rise from chair, climb stairs, and falls.
Created by Kristina Sitarski and Karen Wiseman. Printed with permission.

Therefore, because of the clear benefits that exercise training has for PLWCs, exercise should be considered an important intervention for sarcopenia and cachexia.

It is important to note that exercise should be dosed with consideration for the PLWC's energy demands and caloric intake; for example, energy demands should not exceed energy intake. Without the necessary energy intake to balance physical activity, cachexia can worsen. Nutritional strategies such as use of appetite stimulants and use of high calorie, small, frequent meals or oral supplements can be utilized. A consultation with a registered dietician can be helpful for a PLWC to assist with malnutrition.

Neuromuscular Junction Disorders

Myasthenia gravis (MG) can be triggered by an abnormal immune response to a cancerous tumor. MG is a disorder of acetylcholine receptors at the neuromuscular junction or of tyrosine kinase, which targets proteins in the muscle cells. This autoimmune disorder leads to muscle weakness and commonly presents as weakness of the ocular muscles causing diplopia (double vision) or ptosis (drooping eyelids). It may also affect the muscles of respiration. About 10% of those affected have thymoma.[92] Thymoma is a tumor of the thymus gland that may, or may not, be malignant. The thymus gland is located behind the sternum and plays a role in the immune system. Thymectomy is shown to improve outcomes in MG.[93] Additional treatments include immunotherapy, symptomatic treatment with acetylcholinesterase inhibition, and corticosteroids.[92,93] Early data suggests that physical exercise and strength training is safe and effective in the management of stable MG.[94]

Lambert-Eaton myasthenic syndrome (LEMS) is a rare disorder of the voltage-gated calcium channels, which disrupts the release of acetylcholine. The clinical features include proximal muscle weakness, autonomic features, and areflexia.[95] The paraneoplastic form of LEMS frequently occurs with small cell lung cancer (SCLC).[95] This connection is so strong that it is recommended that if cancer is not identified at the time of LEMS diagnosis, cancer screening should continue at regular intervals. A 2017 study compared drug therapy with 3,4-diaminopyridine base versus placebo. The study used a series of three timed up and go (TUG) tests to measure proximal weakness and assessed for neuromuscular fatigue, which is a clinical sign of LEMS.[96] The TUG scores were more than 30% slower without the drug therapy, demonstrating that 3,4-diaminopyridine base is an effective treatment to maintain functional strength in patients with LEMS.[96]

Effect on Body Mechanics and Posture

Breast Cancer

Patients with a history of BC can present with common dysfunctions in posture and body mechanics related to cancer treatment. Surgery for BC and RTx of the anterior chest and axilla can cause tightening of the skin and muscles of the upper quadrant. PLBCs commonly present with postural dysfunction from tight pectoral muscles causing rounding of the shoulder and increased thoracic kyphosis. Tightness of the pectoralis minor contributes to shortening and tension of the upper trapezius muscle. Along with this, a forward head position and increased upper cervical extension contribute to cervical radiculopathies. Limitations in shoulder ROM are also common in this patient population. These limitations and the resultant weakness will change how the patient dresses, grooms their hair, and performs overhead lifting tasks.

A recent study was performed to identify changes in posture after unilateral mastectomy with implant reconstruction. Women after mastectomy and reconstruction demonstrated statistically significant changes in sagittal spine alignment for anterior–posterior flexion of the trunk and lumbosacral inversion point when compared to controls.[97] Additionally, these changes caused greater energy expenditure to maintain an upright posture.[97] After mastectomy, posture and alignment should be assessed and early intervention initiated. This may prevent acute postural changes from becoming chronic MSK pain or dysfunction.

Reconstruction after mastectomy may include muscle and tissue transfers. These surgical procedures take tissue from autologous donor sites to re-create a breast. Patients may experience weakness from the harvest of the muscle and myofascial restrictions from the resulting scar. Reconstructive tissues harvested from the abdomen can create weakness of the abdominal and core muscles.[98] In these instances, it is important to provide education and interventions on core muscle strength, ergonomic retraining, and body mechanics. Interventions, with consideration for surgical precautions and tissue healing time, aimed at improving functional movement patterns for lifting and bending should emphasize back protection strategies utilizing lumbar stabilization concepts. More information about BC surgery including surgical precautions can be found in Chapter 15.

The treatment for a person with BC can change the way in which they use their upper extremities. Patients who underwent BC surgery showed a reduction in all directions of shoulder ROM. Patients who underwent modified radical mastectomy showed greater reduction in flexion and abduction ROM compared to those who underwent breast conserving surgery. The K-DASH (Korean version of Disability Arm and Shoulder Questionnaire) percentage of disability rose significantly over time with no significant difference between type of surgery, SLNB versus ALND, or whether the patient received radiation.[99] These changes could contribute to shoulder dysfunction in reaching and overhead lifting mechanics required for ADLs such as dressing and grooming.

Limitations in shoulder biomechanics can affect the way a person performs many activities. A recent study found that 10.3% of patients had adhesive capsulitis 13 months after BC surgery.[100] AWS may result in a loss of shoulder abduction but limitations are commonly reported in all directions of shoulder ROM and in elbow extension.[44] Assessment of shoulder biomechanics during overhead and functional reaching should guide intervention to avoid complications such as rotator cuff tendinopathy, shoulder impingement, brachial plexopathies, and thoracic outlet syndrome.

Hodgkin Lymphoma

HL is most commonly diagnosed in people aged 20 to 34 with a relative survival rate of 90% depending on stage.[101] HL is sensitive to radiation treatment and historical protocols for the disease involved high dose radiation to large areas of the body with the purpose of targeting lymph nodes throughout the area. These techniques were effective in treating HL but caused morbidity including secondary cancers and myelo-radiculo-plexo-neuro-myopathies. Modern radiation techniques have improved which has resulted in decreasing morbidity; however, late complications are still seen in this population. A retrospective study by Oishi et al.[102] of 189 patients diagnosed with HL found the mean time for medical evaluation for neuromuscular complications was about 24 years after diagnosis. This makes it important for Onc R clinicians to be aware of the potential for treatment complications long after the initial cancer.

DHS is one of the most common and debilitating disorders associated with mantle field radiation for HL. Mild cases of DHS present with complaints of weakness and fatigue of the neck. Severe cases of DHS can present with cervical dystonia, inability to lift the head to the neutral position, and pain (Figure 7.5). The cause of DHS is likely multifactorial and due to the late effects of radiation treatment on several neuromuscular structures.[48,103]

Similarly to the etiology seen in DHS, thoracic kyphosis is a commonly seen postural impairment in HL. In HL, radiculo-plexopathy of the upper cervical nerve roots of C5, C6 and the upper plexus causes weakness of the rhomboids, rotator cuff muscles, deltoids, and biceps.[48] These weaknesses allow for kyphotic changes to occur in the thoracic spine. Additional chronic conditions can arise from thoracic kyphosis include shoulder dysfunction and spinal compression fractures. Additional neuromuscular morbidities reported by Oishi and colleagues included myopathy (39%), plexopathy (29%), myelopathy (27%), and polyradiculopathy (13%).[102]

An Onc R intervention to address strength of the cervical extensors, parascapular muscles, and core, as well as flexibility of the anterior neck and chest structures is important. Long-term participation in a HEP emphasizing posture and body mechanics to improve functional movement patterns is valuable. Bracing can be used intermittently to assist with energy conservation and improve functional positioning however long-term bracing may not be advisable as the immobilization may accelerate disuse atrophy (Figure 7.6).[48,103]

Head and Neck Cancer

HNC is a complex group of cancers that develop in the oral cavity, pharynx, larynx, salivary glands, and paranasal sinuses. Treatment for HNC can include surgery, radiation, and chemotherapy. The neck contains a large number of lymph nodes and most surgical interventions for HNC will involve dissection of one or more layers of these nodes. Reduction in function of these muscles can change posture and movement patterns for the neck and shoulder girdle.[36] For more information on HNC, refer to Chapter 19. Modern procedures for neck dissection surgery have improved with an increased emphasis on preservation of surrounding structures. Two nerves that are commonly manipulated during neck

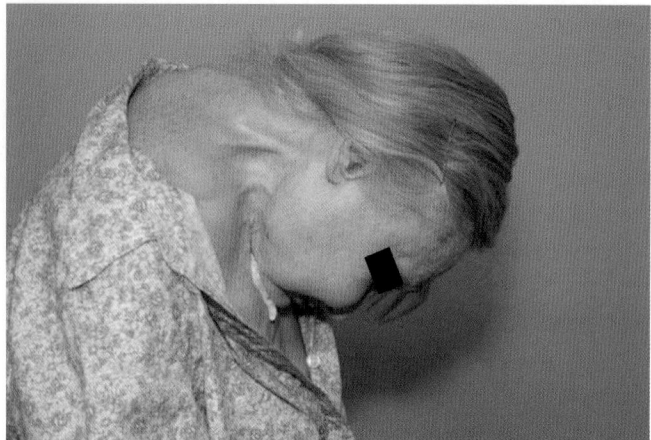

• **Fig. 7.5** Dropped Head Syndrome. A person living beyond cancer with radiation fibrosis and dropped head syndrome following radical neck dissection and radiation therapy for submental squamous cell carcinoma. (Reprinted with permission from DiFrancesco T, Khanna A, Stubblefield MD. Clinical evaluation and management of cancer survivors with radiation fibrosis syndrome. *Semin Oncol Nurs*. 2020;36(1):150982.)

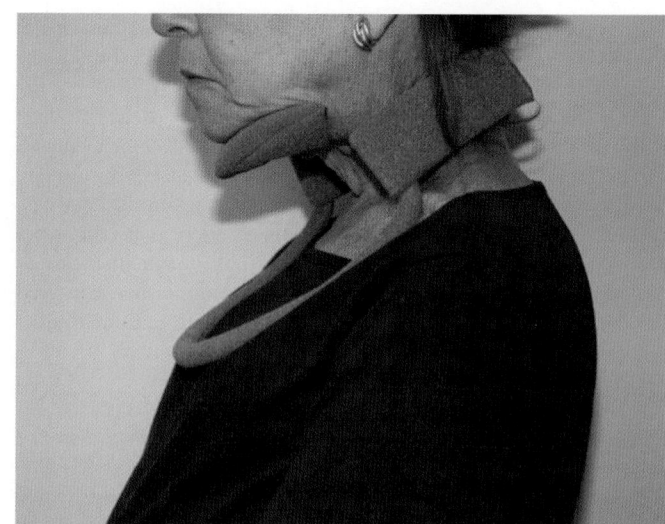

• **Fig. 7.6** Dropped Head Syndrome With Use of Cervical Collar. A person living beyond cancer with dropped head syndrome after treatment for Hodgkin lymphoma using a Headmaster cervical collar. (Reprinted with permission from DiFrancesco T, Khanna A, Stubblefield MD. Clinical evaluation and management of cancer survivors with radiation fibrosis syndrome. *Semin Oncol Nurs*. 2020;36(1):150982.)

dissection surgery are the marginal mandibular branch of the facial nerve and cranial nerve XI (SAN). Injury to the SAN during surgery can result in temporary or permanent loss of function affecting the sternocleidomastoid and trapezius muscle. A systematic review concluded that physical therapy is beneficial in the treatment of shoulder dysfunction following neck dissection. The evidence in this review was in favor of supervised, progressive resistance activities.[104]

RTx HNC can have similar effects as those seen in HL. Neuromuscular tissues receiving radiation demonstrate acute and late effects that impact posture, body mechanics, and function. These can include damage to the SAN, cervical nerve roots, and the cervical plexus. Spasm of the muscles and tissue fibrosis can lead to tightness of the neck resulting in difficulty turning the head for driving and performing common tasks. Additional radiation-induced morbidity seen in HNC is trismus, weakness of facial and swallowing muscles, and bone necrosis that may change the mechanics for speaking and eating. A 2017 systematic review found that beginning therapeutic exercises and stretching for the prevention of trismus related to HNC treatment was important for good results, although the authors were unable to recommend an optimal exercise protocol based on the literature.[105] For additional information related to assessment and intervention for PLWCs of the head and neck, see Chapter 19.

Multiple Myeloma

MM cancer presents with bone lesions that incur high fracture risk, especially of the spine. The Onc R clinician should understand the risk for fractures in MM using pathological fracture prediction scoring systems and chart review including review of available imaging. See Tables 7.5 and 7.6 for metastatic bone fracture scales. With consideration given to contraindications for fracture risk and in collaboration with the oncologist, regular physical activity is beneficial in tolerating treatment related adverse effects for patients with bone lesions.[106] Onc R focusing on body mechanics and postural strengthening are important interventions to decrease the risk of a bone related injury. Education in proper body mechanics to avoid twisting and shear forces in the presence of metastatic bone lesions will prevent pain and protect from fracture.

Assessment of the Musculoskeletal System

An Onc R evaluation for a PLWC or PLBC should be comprehensive and should include thorough history and systems review including integument, MSK, neurological, and cardiopulmonary systems. Furthermore, the Onc R clinician should also be vigilant for abnormal symptoms that could be an oncologic emergency. For example, a complaint of bone pain in a PLWC or PLBC should raise suspicion to the oncology practitioner. This can be a sign of cancer recurrence, metastases, fracture, or impending fracture which require urgent attention and communication with the oncologist.

Chart Review

A thorough chart review and patient history is necessary to screen for red flags. Above and beyond a normal chart review, it is imperative to look at the medical oncologist's assessment and most recent examination. The pertinent information includes the cancer diagnosis, prognosis, and staging. A review of cancer treatments includes time frame, recent imaging, and lab values. Lab values to assess are: (1) the complete blood count (CBC; including platelets, hemoglobin, hematocrit, white blood cells, and red blood cells), and (2) the complete metabolic panel (CMP; including creatinine, glucose, calcium, sodium and potassium levels), and an anticoagulant therapeutic range (international normalized ratio [INR] or partial thromboplastin time [PTT] level). A helpful reference is the American Physical Therapy Association's (APTA) Academy of Acute Care Physical Therapy Lab Values chart.[107] A knowledge of recent lab values will give the provider a sense of the PLWC's tolerance to activity, precautions with activity and prognosis for improvement with Onc R interventions.

Review of surgical documents and possible consultation with the surgeon will allow the Onc R clinician to appreciate the MSK changes caused by cancer surgery. For example, in a patient with a history of reconstructive or limb sparing surgery, noting which structures were removed or reconstructed and current precautions will be necessary before completing the evaluation and treatment. Furthermore, it is important to find out the sequence of the post operative care including any drains that were placed and if there were any wound complications or infections that occurred. The patient's subjective report will supplement the chart review by adding any complications and difficulties with cancer treatments, modified past and future treatment plans, current and prior level of function, and symptoms related to mobility. The examination of a PLWC may need to be adapted due to precautions, WB status,

vital signs, mobility status, and level of pain. Resistance testing, special tests, and joint mobility testing may need to be deferred secondary to impaired tissue healing. Instead, the Onc R clinician is advised to use functional movement assessments in the person's available ROM, assessment of strength by holding the limb against gravity, or by completing a functional outcome measure.

Precautions for the Initial Evaluation

Modification to the initial evaluation should be based on the prior chart review as well as concerns that arise through taking the subjective history. Of note, there are certain activity and WB restrictions for a PLWC with a concern for bone metastasis or confirmed bone metastases. These restrictions should be based on current imaging identifying cortical involvement as well as discussion with the medical team. A summary can be seen in Table 7.11.[28] A PLWC diagnosed with bone metastases frequently requires modification in examination and intervention procedures as highlighted in Table 7.12.[2,26,28] These should be considered when completing the initial evaluation and when prescribing assistive devices and an HEP.

Screening for Red Flags

During the examination, the practitioner should perform a thorough line of inquiry regarding the pain or dysfunction, especially when there are multiple pain sites and varied factors that aggravate the pain. The concordant sign, or primary reason for seeking rehabilitative care, should be distinguished from nonconcordant signs. Nonconcordant signs are other pain, problems, or issues that the person is experiencing. Specific tests or movements added to the examination will help the practitioner determine if their symptoms can be reproduced or changed. An example is a patient who presents with shoulder dysfunction after primary treatment for melanoma with positive regional lymph node disease. The patient had concordant signs of shoulder pain for 2 months, a forward head posture with thoracic kyphosis, limited shoulder AROM, and decreased strength. The concordant sign is expected based on the history of modified radical neck dissection and radiotherapy of the area with impact on cranial nerve XI (SAN that innervates sternocleidomastoid and trapezius muscles). The patient also had recent onset of contralateral rib pain that developed insidiously 7 days prior. Upon examination, the patient demonstrated decreased arm swing bilaterally and a stiff trunk posture when walking to the examination room. The quality and quantity of the contralateral rib pain is a nonconcordant sign. The nonconcordant signs may be due to a muscle strain from poor body mechanics or related to another medical issue, including cancer recurrence. In this case, evaluation of the

TABLE 7.11 Activity and Weight Bearing Restrictions Based on Cortical Bone Metastases[28]

Metastatic Involvement	Weight Bearing Status	Recommended Activity Restrictions
>50% cortex involved	TDWB or NWB with crutch (es) or walker	No resistance training or stretching, AROM (no twisting)
25%–50% cortex involved	PWB	Continue AROM, no stretching, light aerobics, avoid lifting/straining activity
0%–25% cortex involved	FWB	None Monitor pain

AROM, Active range of motion; FWB, full weight bearing; NWB, non-weight bearing; PWB, partial weight bearing; TDWB, touch down weight bearing.
Created by Kristina Sitarski and Karen Wiseman. Printed with permission.

TABLE 7.12	Rehabilitation Specific Precautions and Contraindications With Bone Metastases[2,26,28]

1. No MMT on involved limb. Focus on functional strength assessments and pain free ROM assessments.

2. Take precautions with open kinetic chain resistive exercises and multiplanar movements.

3. Avoiding shearing or torque forces on bone with bone at high risk of fracture or with healing fracture. This includes using hip and spine precautions.

4. If surgically stabilized, follow surgical recovery pattern with gradual loading and strengthening with focus on functional motions and pain as guide.

5. Modify exercises and ADLs to accommodate spinal stenosis, spondylolisthesis, THA, lymphedema, bone metastases, avascular necrosis, post-radiation avoid shearing forces of skin and clothing, aspiration risk post-esophagectomy (e.g., supine position), colostomy precautions, and core engagement to avoid hernia.

6. No joint mobilization or manipulation.

ADL, Activities of daily living; *MMT*, manual muscle test; *ROM*, range of motion; *THA*, total hip arthroplasty.
Created by Kristina Sitarski and Karen Wiseman. Printed with permission.

nonconcordant sign is warranted and may be a red flag. Red flags to be aware of are listed in Table 7.13.[2,14,15,20,28]

Objective Measurements and Special Tests

In addition to subjective questioning for red flags, it is important to get baseline measurements of ROM, muscle length, muscle strength, and joint play. Special tests related to specific joint pain may assist with determining concordant pain versus nonconcordant pain and assist with screening for malignant causes of pain. For example, in the case of hip pain, a hip scour test for pain in the hip joint or significant joint limitation with abnormal end feel may warrant further imaging before beginning Onc R. Another example can include special tests for shoulder pain to decipher if the cause of pain is from impingement, damage to the rotator cuff, thoracic outlet syndrome, or damage to the labrum. There is a good description of the scapular repositioning test that is beneficial to assess for reduced shoulder pain and improved shoulder elevation strength once scapula is manually repositioned into external rotation and posterior tilt. This test is positive if it provides symptom relief indicating scapular dyskinesis.[108] Upper and lower motor nerve testing, sensory testing, neurologic or vascular claudication tests, and upper or lower limb tension tests can be completed to confirm or rule out neurologic changes.[13]

TABLE 7.13	Red Flags for Oncology Rehabilitation Evaluation[2,14,15,20,28]

Subjective Red Flags	Objective Red Flags
Back pain (usually thoracic) not relieved with rest or lying down	Pain with weight bearing, resisted MMT, or joint ROM
Pain that is worse at night	Empty end feel during PROM
Progressive weakness in LE	Noncapsular restriction patterns in ROM
Bowel and bladder changes	Radicular symptoms in UE and LE, chest or abdomen
Increase in swelling, redness, heat/warmth to skin or scar specifically	Limited straight leg raise due to pain in groin
Change in mental status	Positive *sign of the buttock*

LE, Lower extremity; *MMT*, manual muscle test; *PROM*, passive range of motion; *ROM*, range of motion; *UE*, upper extremity.
Created by Kristina Sitarski and Karen Wiseman. Printed with permission.

Scar and integumentary assessment including fascial mobility is important to monitor at rest and throughout available ROM. The cause of limitations should be identified if possible (RFS, AWS, scar adhesions, muscle length issues, or postural deficits).[99] Scar and integumentary assessments can be described subjectively, measured for length, circumference, or depth, or via use of an objective scar assessment measure. One useful measurement tool is the Myofascial Adhesions in Patients after Breast Cancer (MAP-BC) assessment.[41] This assessment is comprehensive but can be lengthy to complete. See the case study at the end of this chapter for an example on scoring elements. Another potential scar scale that is more clinically efficient is the Patient and Observer Scar Assessment Scale (POSAS); however, its validity and reliability have only been established with burn scars versus linear surgical scars.[109]

Due to the scar's disruption of skin mobility and concurrent disruption to the lymphatic drainage in a body region, it is important to assess and monitor the area for lymphedema. A photograph comparing affected limb to unaffected limb or a simple baseline circumferential measurement is beneficial to monitor for change over time. For further information on lymphedema assessment and management, see Chapter 9.

The PLWC may also benefit from postural assessment either visually or objectively with use of a flexicurve ruler or inclinometer.[110] Farooki and Ukena suggested that vertebral fractures with kyphosis can be diagnosed with tests such the inability to touch the occiput to the wall and the presence of a gap less than three fingerbreadths between costal margin and iliac crest.[20] A finding of increased kyphosis increases the likelihood of past or future vertebral fractures. Moreover, it can lead to an anterior displacement of the person's center of gravity and may predispose the patient to balance disturbances and a fall. A finding of a fixed kyphosis in a person with a history of thoracic radiation should lead the Onc R clinician to a discussion of bone health with concern for osteoporosis of the thoracic spine.[20] Further assessment of breathing, muscle length testing, and balance assessment would be warranted. Other specific tests may be beneficial to have at baseline. These tests include quantifying muscle length for the pectoralis and hip flexors as these largely contribute to postural changes in the body.

Outcome Measures

In addition to MSK assessments, key measures to quantify include balance, gait, functional mobility, and aerobic capacity.[13] Even without subjective complaints of dysfunction in these areas, they are important to screen in all PLWCs. The PLWC may have a combination of these impairments from their cancer or cancer treatment that significantly increases their risk of falls and subsequent risk of fracture. The measures in Table 7.14 have been recommended by the APTA Oncology EDGE Task Force to capture the severity of subjective cancer-related pain, fatigue, or disability as well as objective deficits such as strength, balance, and gait issues.[111]

Common Treatments for Musculoskeletal System

Exercise is safe and feasible in the cancer population and can improve cardiovascular fitness, strength, bone health, and QOL.[112–116] It can also improve tolerance for cancer treatments.[114] In this population,

TABLE 7.14   EDGE Task Force Recommended Outcome Measures[111]

Neck dysfunction—head and neck cancers	Neck Disability Index, Northwick Park Neck Pain Questionnaire, Neck Pain and Disability Scale
Upper extremity dysfunction—breast and head and neck cancers	Disability of Arm Shoulder and Hand questionnaire, Shoulder Pain and Disability Index, Shoulder Rating Questionnaire, Penn Shoulder Score, Neck Dissection Impairment Index, University of Washington Quality of Life shoulder sub-scale
Temporomandibular dysfunction—head and neck cancers	The Graded Chronic Pain Scale, 8 and 20-item Jaw functional limitation scale, Temporomandibular Disorder Pain Screener
Health related quality of life and functional outcome measures for secondary lymphedema—breast cancer	Functional Assessment of Cancer Therapy-Breast +4, Disability of Arm Shoulder and Hand questionnaire
Health related quality of life—prostate cancer	European Organization for Research and Treatment of Cancer Quality of Life Questionnaire, Expanded Prostate Cancer Index, Functional Assessment of Cancer Therapy-Prostate, University of California Los Angeles-Prostate Cancer Index, European Organization for Research and Treatment of Cancer-Cancer 30, Functional Assessment of Cancer Therapy-General, Short Forms (SF-36, SF-12, SF-8).
Health related quality of life—breast cancer	European Organization for Research and Treatment of Cancer Quality of Life Questionnaire-Breast 23, BREAST-Q, Functional Assessment of Cancer Therapy-Breast, Functional Assessment of Cancer Therapy-Breast +4, European Organization for Research and Treatment of Cancer Quality of Life Questionnaire-Cancer 30, Functional Assessment of Cancer Therapy-General, Functional Living Index-Cancer, Ferrans and Powers Quality of Life Index-Cancer Version, Psychological Adjustment
Incontinence—urogenital cancers	American Urological Association Symptom Index, Pelvic Floor Distress Inventory-Short Form, Pelvic Floor Impact Questionnaire-Short Form, Incontinence Quality of Life Questionnaire and International Consultation on Incontinence Questionnaire-Short Form
Sexual dysfunction—various cancers	Sexual Function-Vaginal Changes Questionnaire, International Index of Erectile Function, Erection Hardness Score, Sexual Health Inventory for Men, Sexual Interest and Desire Inventory
Cancer related fatigue—various cancers	Modified Brief Fatigue Inventory, Cancer-Related Fatigue Distress Scale, 10-Point Rating Scale for Fatigue, MD Anderson Symptom Inventory, WU Cancer Fatigue Scale, Multidimensional Fatigue Symptom Inventory, Bidimensional Fatigue Scale, Cancer Fatigue Scale, Fatigue Symptom Inventory, Multidimensional Fatigue Inventory, Piper/Quick Piper, Profile of Mood States, Patient Reported Outcome Measure Information System Cancer Fatigue Short Form, Schwartz Cancer Fatigue Scale Brief fatigue inventory and Functional Assessment of Cancer Therapy-Breast
Pain—adult cancers	McGill Pain Questionnaire-Short Form, Numeric Rating Scale, Visual Analog Scale, Brief Pain Inventory, Brief Pain Inventory-Short Form, McGill Pain Questionnaire, Pain Disability Index, Pressure Pain Threshold (breast)
Pain—pediatrics	The Wong-Baker FACES Pain Rating Scale, The Oucher Pain Scale, Adolescent Pediatric Pain Tool, Pieces of Hurt Assessment Tool Poler Chip Tool
Chemotherapy-induced polyneuropathy	Functional Assessment of Cancer Therapy Gynecologic Oncology Group-Neurotoxicity Scale
Shoulder and glenohumeral outcome measures—breast cancer	Goniometry passive and active range of motion, inclinometer passive and active range of motion, joint play assessment, pectoralis major muscle length assessment
Scapular assessment—breast cancer	Dynamic motion assessment
Strength—breast, colon, and prostate cancer	Handheld dynamometry, hand grip strength with dynamometry
Functional mobility—prostate and breast cancer	Two Minute Walk Test, Six Minute Walk Test, 10 Meter Timed Walk Test, Timed Up and Go, Five Times Sit to Stand, Short Performance Physical Battery, Physical Performance Battery for Patients With Cancer, Assessment of Life Habits, Functional Independence Measure, Activity Measure for Post-Acute Care
Balance	Fullerton Advanced Balance Scale, Timed Up and Go, Balance Evaluation Systems Test, Five Times Sit to Stand, gait speed
Lymphedema—urogenital cancer and breast cancer	Water displacement, circumferential measurement by tape measure, Bioelectric Impedance Analysis

Listed from APTA Oncology EDGE Task Force Annotated. Bibliography from those listed as highly recommended and in areas where none were highly recommended utilized recommended for clinical use.[111]
Created by Kristina Sitarski and Karen Wiseman. Printed with permission.

the Onc R clinician should consider the past disease journey as well as the person's anticipated disease trajectory. PLBCs may experience treatment-related adverse effects months, years, and decades after cancer treatment. Additionally, PLWCs can experience progressive impairments as treatment continues or disease progresses. Understanding the common impairments encountered with different cancer diagnoses and treatment protocols will guide the Onc R clinician in prescribing appropriate therapeutic intervention.

Maintaining functional mobility is the key to improving QOL in PLWC. Onc R specialists must focus on multimodal interventions to assist with person-specific impairments. Physical Onc R interventions may include targeted aerobic training, resistance training, stretching, manual therapy, biophysical agents (a.k.a. modalities), balance and gait training, postural and body mechanics training, and education.

Aerobic Training

Aerobic training is beneficial for nearly all individuals. Moderate to vigorous intensity exercise appears to provide the most benefit compared to low intensity exercise.[114] However, even low intensity exercise will benefit deconditioned PLWBCs and should be encouraged based on individual tolerance. Aerobic training has been shown to reduce anxiety and depressive symptoms, improve fatigue, promote better QOL, and improve perceived physical function in PLWBCs.[115] A 2019 roundtable consensus statement found that moderate-intensity aerobic training at least three times per week, for a duration of 30 minutes, is an effective exercise prescription for PLWBCs.[113]

WB exercise is advocated for bone health. New research is studying the type of exercise promoting the best outcomes for BMD. A recent study compared various exercise routines in prostate cancer survivors undergoing ADT and found that impact-loading exercise in combination with resistance exercise should be recommended to counteract bone loss. The impact exercise examined in this study included a series of bounding, skipping, drop

jumping, hopping, and leaping activities that produced ground reaction forces of 3 to 5 times body weight, and was progressive in nature.[117] One investigator studied female cancer survivors participating in a 26 week exercise program consisting of aerobic training, circuit style resistance training, core training, and stretching in an hour format three times per week and found significant improvements in BMD at the spine, hip, and whole body.[118]

Resistance Training

Resistance training can take on many forms and be customized to meet patient goals. In PLBCs, resistance training has been shown to improve fatigue and QOL as well as one's perception of physical function.[118] PLWCs can benefit from resistance training to increase their lower-limb muscular strength, prevent the loss of lean body mass, and reduce body fat in those undergoing neoadjuvant and adjuvant therapy regardless of the type of treatment.[119] This may help protect against treatment related adverse effects on the MSK system.

PLWCs may experience changes in posture and the way they move their bodies secondary to cancer and treatment related adverse effects. They should be taught strengthening exercises to assist in maintaining posture and proper body mechanics. Proprioceptive neuromuscular facilitation (PNF) patterns with emphasis on posture and function should be taught. Additionally, functional strengthening allows a person with cancer to maintain better QOL. An example is focusing on strengthening of the gluteals, quadriceps, and hamstrings via a sit-to-stand or squat exercise, as seen in Figure 7.7, with concurrent education on proper body mechanics to assist with getting on and off the toilet. This is especially important because strength and confidence with toilet transfers are important for safety in the home.

A strong foundation in kinesiology and applying that knowledge in the presence of cancer-related changes in posture and body mechanics is important for Onc R professionals to have when working with PLWC. Figure 7.8 demonstrates a forward

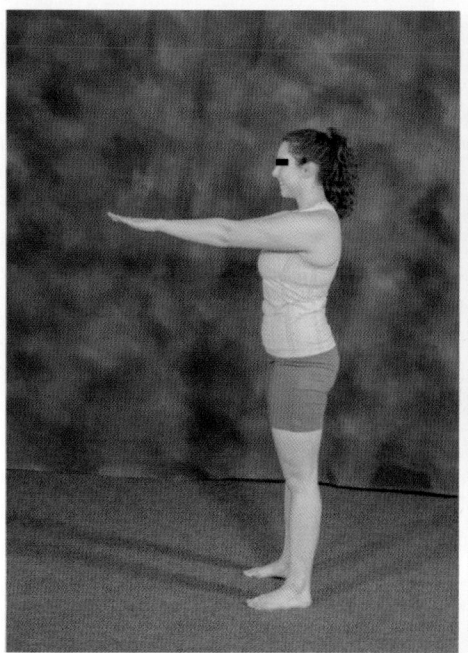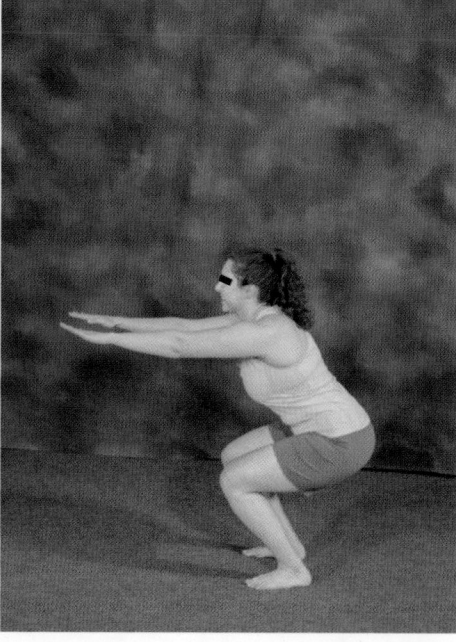

• **Fig. 7.7** Squat Exercise. Squat exercise where the exerciser squats for strengthening of legs. Exercise can be varied and made more functional by performing off a toilet height chair. (Photograph printed with permission from John Krauss.)

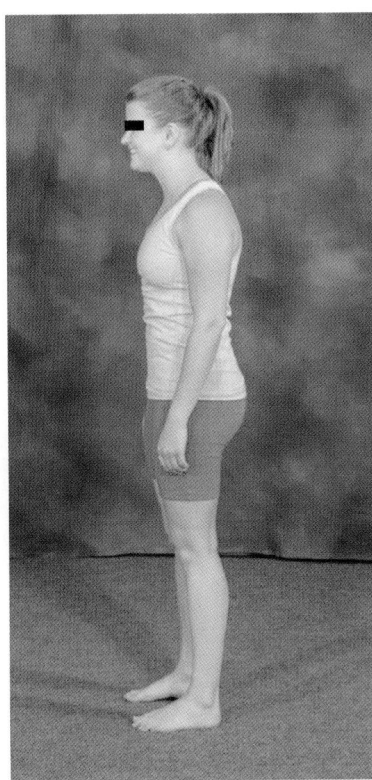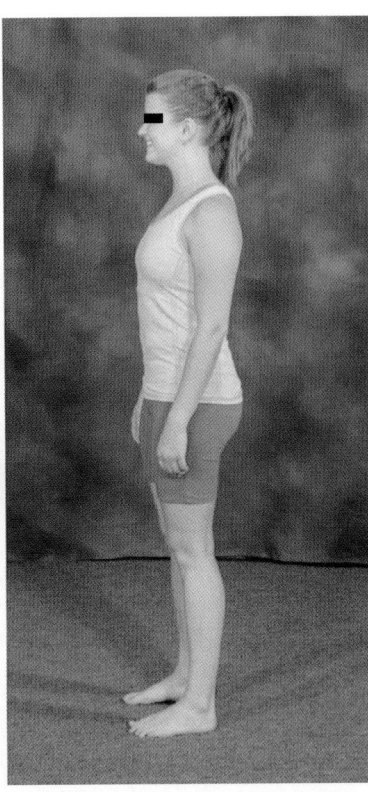

• **Fig. 7.8** Forward Head Position and Neutral Head Position. (Photograph printed with permission of John Krauss.)

head position and an example of a better head position. A forward head position is a common impairment with surgery and radiation to the anterior chest. Strengthening exercises to antagonist muscle groups help to improve postural symmetry and prevent injury or chronic pain conditions such as shoulder impingement. Figures 7.9 and 7.10 demonstrate a series of exercises to strengthen the parascapular and back muscles in various positions. Combining stretching and antagonist strengthening can effect changes resulting in overall improvement in biomechanical function. Exercise with this focus may also help the person to attune to their body and overall movement patterns.

Resistance training is beneficial in maintaining bone health and has been found to be safe and feasible in patients with and without bone metastasis. Bone is highly adaptive to its environment and is especially sensitive to mechanical forces including muscular contractions, gravitational forces, and loading forces. A study showed that guided resistance training to the paravertebral muscles of people with stable spinal bone metastasis had no negative impact on bone integrity. Therefore, careful resistance training may be practiced without fear of damaging the bone and such activity was shown to improve pain, reduce fatigue, and enhance QOL.[120] Figures 7.11 and 7.12 demonstrate additional upper body resistance training exercises that can be utilized.

Recent work examined the performance of spinal isometric exercises in supine, prone, quadruped, seated, and standing positions for participants with bone metastases of the spine. They found no SREs, worsening pain, or progression of metastases. In fact, they found up-regulation of osteoblastic activity through exercise which counteracted tumor-driven metabolic dysregulations which may preserve bone strength and slow tumor growth.[121] Most studies, up until recently, prescribed large

muscle group resistance training to all other areas of the body that would not affect the site of metastases. Table 7.15 discusses use of caution when completing exercises in areas of metastases and ultimately it is an Onc R clinician's judgment based on the presentation and pain reports of the PLWC and the patient's preference in collaboration with the patient's oncologists.[122,123] This is an adapted guideline.

Resistance training guidelines for PLWCs and PLBCs advise the addition of resistance training to aerobic training. Consensus prescription is at least two times per week, with at least two sets of 8 to 15 repetitions of at least 60% of one repetition maximum.[121–123] Focus should be given to large muscle groups such as parascapular muscles, gluteals, quadriceps, and abdominals.

Stretching

Stretching muscles to improve posture is an important part of the treatment for PLBC who are experiencing limitations in ROM of joints or muscles and changes in posture. There are various types of stretching that may be beneficial for the PLWC but consistency is key. Most evidence shows improvement in muscle length after 6 to 8-week programs. Both static and dynamic stretching have been shown to improve muscle length. Recommendations specifically promote dynamic stretching to improve power for jumping and running performance.[124] Furthermore, precontraction stretching such as PNF-type stretching (contract-relax, hold-relax, or contract-relax-agonist contract) has been shown to be beneficial. The recommended duration of hold for static stretching is between 15 and 30 seconds in two to four sets. However, older adults seem to benefit from longer duration static stretching of greater than 60 seconds. Furthermore, studies show that men 65 and older

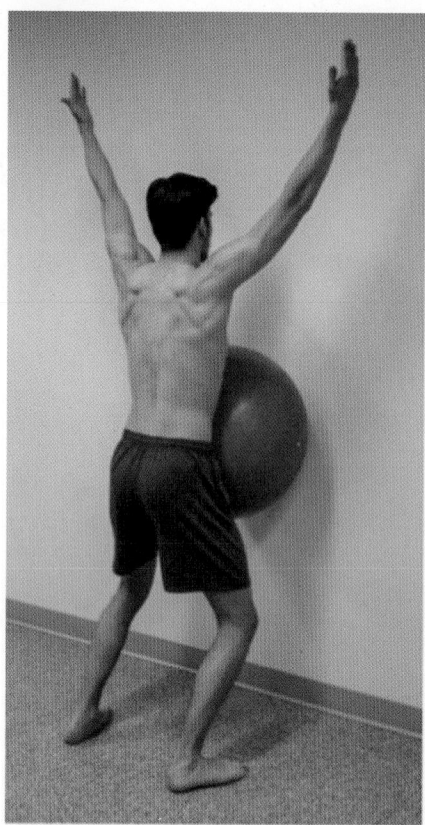
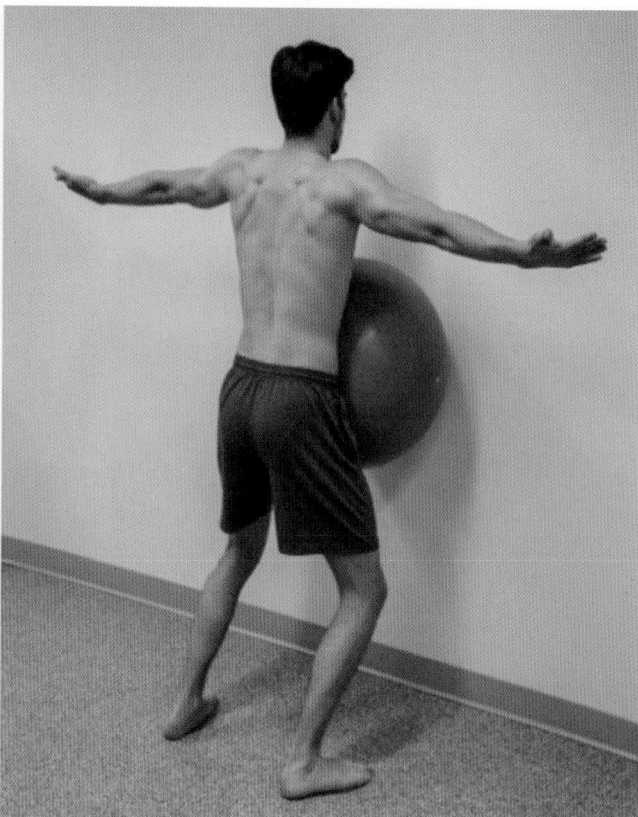
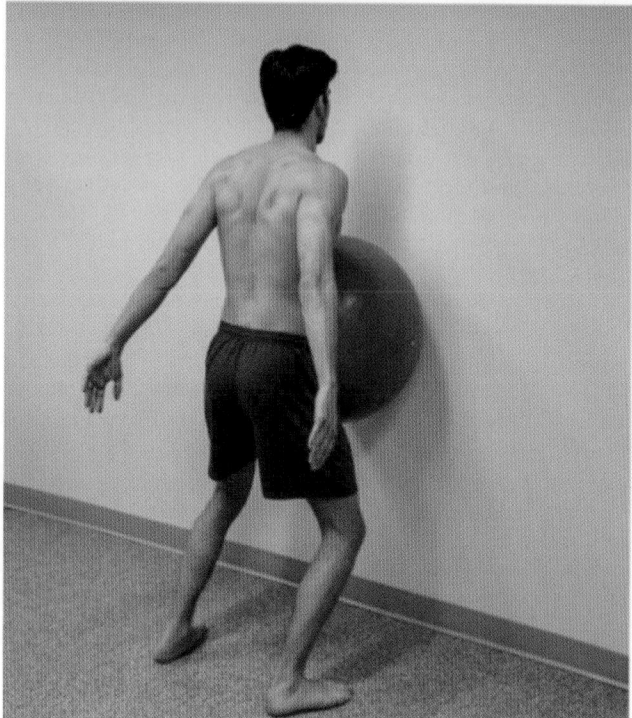

• **Fig. 7.9** Parascapular and Back Muscle Training With Ball-Beginner. Parascapular and back strengthening exercise where the exerciser forms a V with their arms moving the arms toward the wall and then back for a number of repetitions. Repeat with arm position in T and inverted V. (Photograph printed with permission from John Krauss.)

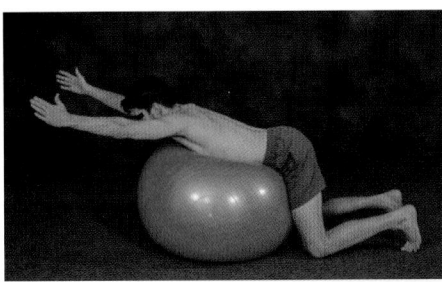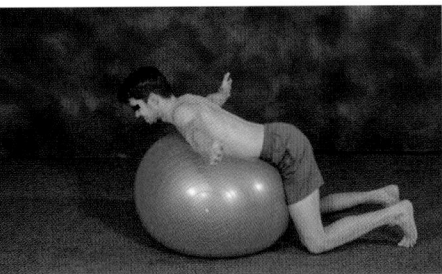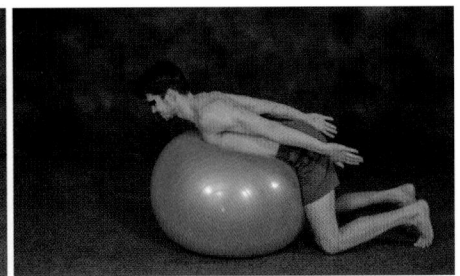

• **Fig. 7.10** Parascapular and Back Muscle Training With Ball-Progression. Parascapular and back strengthening exercise where the exerciser forms a V with their arms moving the arms toward the floor and then back for a number of repetitions. Repeat with arm position in T and inverted V. (Photograph printed with permission from John Krauss.)

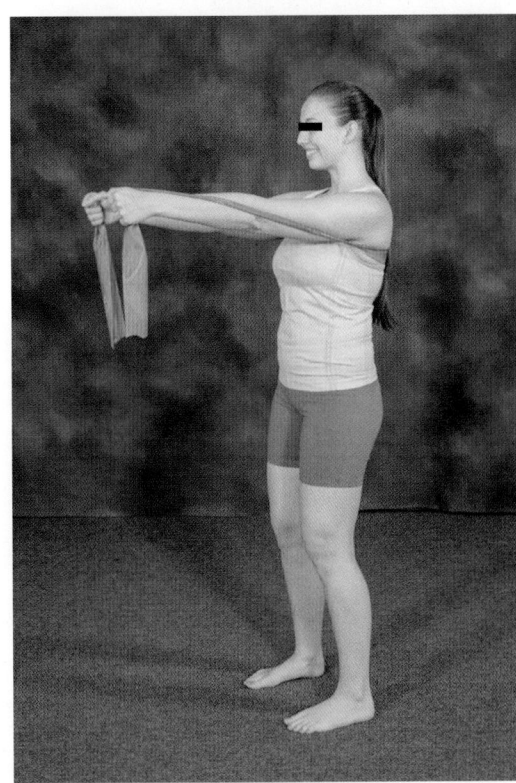

• **Fig. 7.11** Resisted Scapular Protraction. Resistance band protraction where the exerciser uses the resistance band to punch the fists out individually or together. The exerciser should stabilize with core muscles and utilize appropriate breathing patterns for maximum exercise effectiveness. (Photograph printed with permission from John Krauss.)

Stretching devices can be used at home to achieve the prolonged, low load stretch necessary for improved ROM. For example, use of a Dynasplint Trismus System (DTS) incorporates dynamic opening of the jaw with low-load prolonged stretch for up to 30 minutes used three times daily to improve jaw ROM.[36] The time consuming guidelines for use of these devices create a high burden of treatment on a PLBC and attrition rates are high. Though ongoing research into the usefulness of devices such as the Dynasplint or Therabite systems (alone and in conjunction with exercise) is being done, there is no consistent protocol for their use as an intervention for PLBC experiencing trismus or TMJ issues.[125,126] More research is needed to determine the optimal timing for use including whether patients benefit most from these devices before, during, or after RTx for HNCs. This adverse effect of treatment creates a great burden on PLBC and effective treatments need to be identified.

Yoga has been widely studied in the cancer population. Yoga appears to help with a variety of cancer-related symptoms including MSK symptoms.[127] Restorative yoga is a gentle and slow style of yoga that may benefit PLBCs who have tightness of the body. Many of the positions are held for long periods at end range creating the benefits of the prolonged, low load stretching described previously. Yoga positions also promote improved posture and body awareness. Additionally, yoga is widely recommended for improvements in health-related QOL with benefits shown in both physical and psychosocial aspects.[128] Figure 7.15 demonstrates a lower trunk rotation stretch that can improve trunk mobility.

Stretches focusing on the anterior chest and neck can help support healthy posture and are great for PLBCs who had upper body surgeries or radiation treatment. Dysfunction in the anterior chest and neck muscles are common after treatment for BC and HNC. Pectoral stretches (Figure 7.16), along with strengthening to parascapular postural muscles such as the rhomboids, will encourage upright and improved posture. This improvement in posture and scapular alignment, as well as strengthening of the parascapular muscles (Figure 7.17), that act as anchor muscles for shoulder mechanics, may prevent chronic pathology like rotator cuff tendonitis and biceps tendinopathy.

Early AROM after breast surgery can help improve shoulder function and pain during recovery. One study examined the outcomes of allowing free shoulder ROM after mastectomy with an implant or tissue expander reconstruction at 15 days versus 30 days postoperatively. No differences were noted in surgical complications and the group who performed earlier free shoulder ROM had better outcomes in ROM, pain, and fuction.[129] Care should always be given to stay within ROM restrictions provided by the

responded better to contract-relax stretching while women over 65 benefit more from static stretching.[124] Aside from improving muscle length, implementing early stretching programs in PLWCs can improve mobility of the affected joints. There are known benefits to increasing ROM using low load, prolonged stretching that maximizes total end range time.[48] This will help stretch the joint capsule and improve joint flexibility and tissue length. Figure 7.13 shows an active stretch that is beneficial for after surgery or radiation of the upper body to regain functional mobility of the arms. The exerciser may not be able to perform full ROM initially. Figure 7.14 demonstrates one way to stretch the hamstring muscles. Hamstring stretching is beneficial for many people especially those with surgery to the lower body and those with back pain.

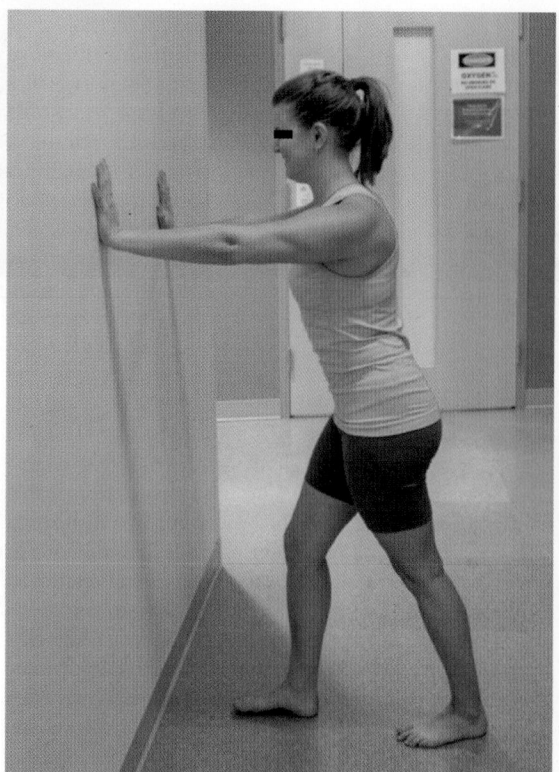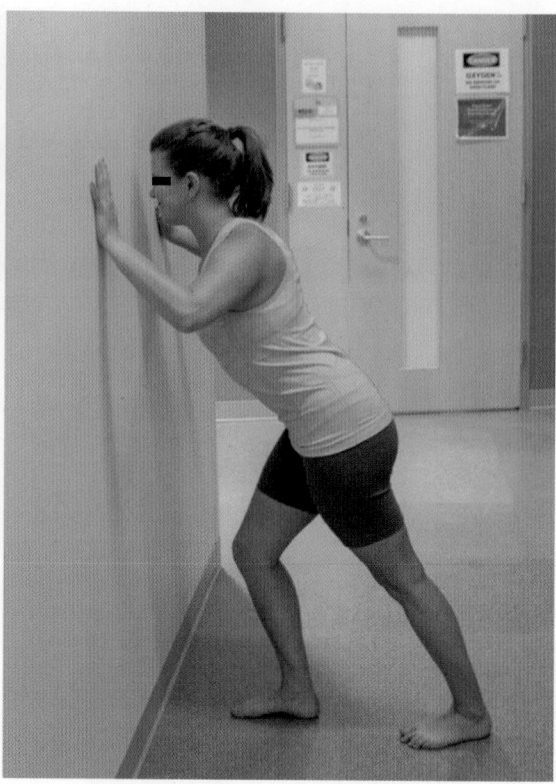

• **Fig. 7.12** Wall Push-Up. Wall push-up where the exerciser strengthens arm and back stabilizers by doing push-up against the wall. The exerciser should stabilize with core muscles and utilize appropriate breathing patterns for maximum exercise effectiveness. (Photograph printed with permission from John Krauss.)

TABLE 7.15 Guide to Exercise Prescription in Bone Metastases[122,123]

| Site Affected by Metastases | Exercise Mode | | | | | Stretching |
| | Resistance | | | Aerobic | | |
	Upper	Trunk	Lower	WB	NWB	Static
Pelvis	G	G	R	Y	G	G
Axial skeleton (lumbar)	G	Y	G	Y	G	R
Axial skeleton (thoracic/rib)	R	Y	R	G	G	R
Proximal femur	G	G	R	Y	G	G
All regions	R	Y	R	Y	G	R

Adapted from multiple sources. Rief H, Ackbar M, Keller M, et al. Quality of life and fatigue of patients with spinal bone metastases under combined treatment with resistance training and radiation therapy- a randomized pilot trial. *Radiat Oncol.* 2014;119(1): doi:10.1186/1748-717X-9-151; Sheill G, Guinan EM, Peat N, Hussey J. Considerations for exercise prescription in patients with bone metastases: a comprehensive narrative review. PMR. 2018;10(8):843–864. doi:10.1016/j.pmrj.2018.02.006; Hart NH, Galvão DA, Saunders C, et al. Mechanical suppression of osteolytic bone metastases in advanced breast cancer patients: a randomised controlled study protocol evaluating safety, feasibility and preliminary efficacy of exercise as a targeted medicine. *Trials.* 2018;19(1):695. doi:10.1186/s13063-018-3091-8.
Not an absolute guide as patient symptoms and goals should be the primary guide to exercise prescription.
Created by Kristina Sitarski and Karen Wiseman. Printed with permission.
Examples: Weight bearing (WB) aerobic = walking; non-weight bearing (NWB) aerobic such as cycling.
G = This exercise is safe and beneficial with this area of metastases.
Y = Indicates areas this author added due to new evidence marking isometric resistance training as safe in areas of bone metastases, with caution as outlined in this chapter. Furthermore, aerobic WB activities in patients with metastases such as a walking program is not contraindicated but should be symptom limited and supported with assistive devices to decrease any pain.
R = Avoid or use extreme caution over the end range of motions at proximal joint (e.g., hip and shoulder; however, no caution at knee or elbow unless otherwise warranted.) With static stretching, should practice spine precautions with axial stretching.

surgeon, but early ROM appears to be beneficial. Figure 7.18 demonstrates a rotational stretch that can be used to improve pectoral tightness. This stretch also identifies areas of tightness in the abdomen, spine and hips and will help stretch myofascial planes of tissue. Manual techniques such as muscle trigger point releases and spinal mobilizations can be used on areas of restriction and then rotational ROM retested to demonstrate improvement in tightness and motion. This stretch should not be performed immediately after breast mastectomy as it may be too aggressive for the pectoral muscle.

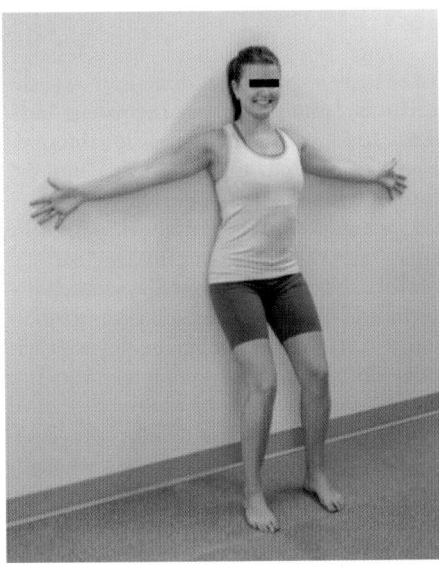
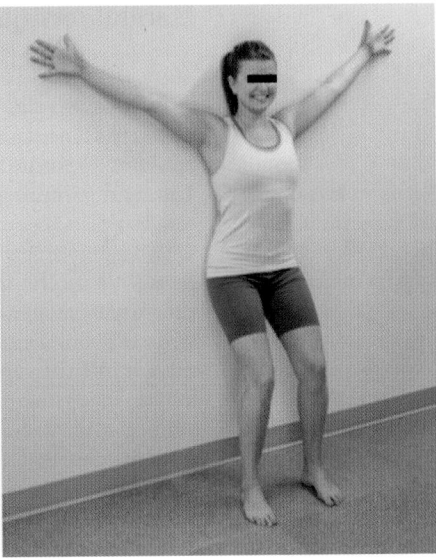
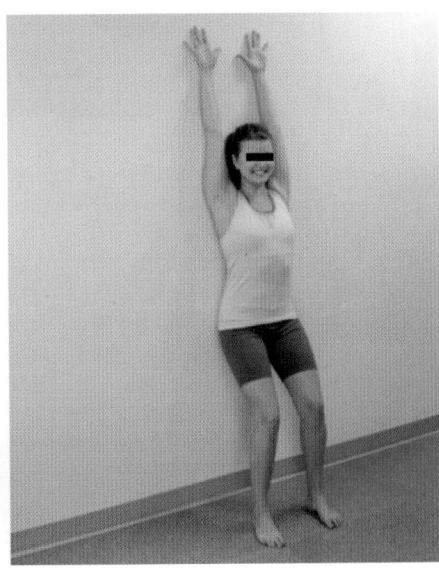

• **Fig. 7.13** Shoulder Abduction Against a Wall. Shoulder abduction stretch against the wall improves shoulder ROM. The exerciser can stop at their end range of motion and perform a static stretch. (Photograph printed with permission from John Krauss.)

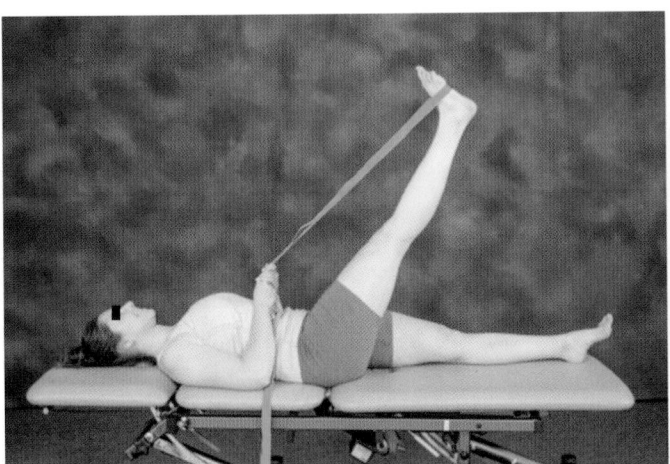
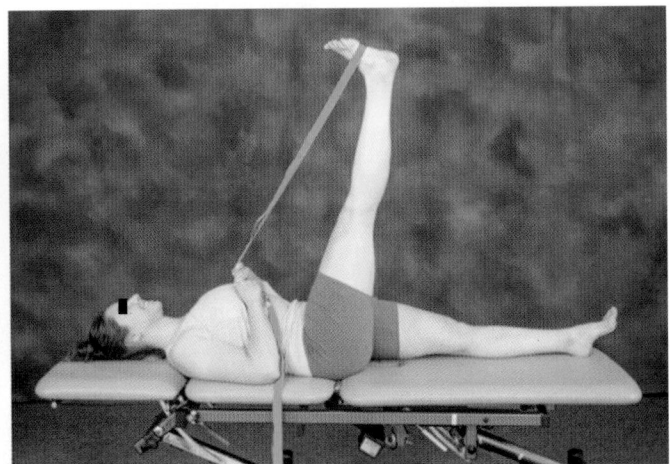

• **Fig. 7.14** Hamstring Stretching Resistance Band Assist. Hamstring stretching to improve muscle length. The exerciser should stop at their end range of motion and perform a static stretch. The exerciser can also perform a contract-relax stretch with resistance band assist. (Photograph printed with permission from John Krauss.)

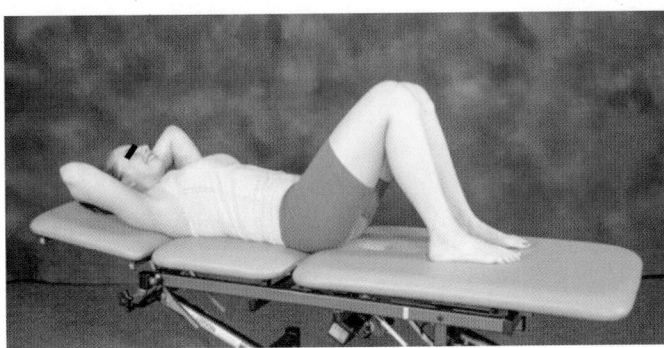
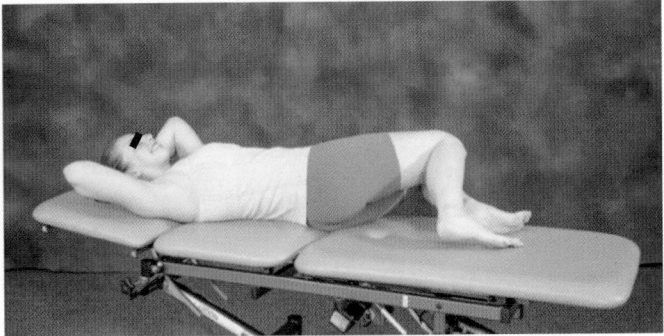

• **Fig. 7.15** Lower Trunk Rotation Stretch. Lower trunk rotation stretch to improve trunk and spine mobility. (Photograph printed with permission from John Krauss.)

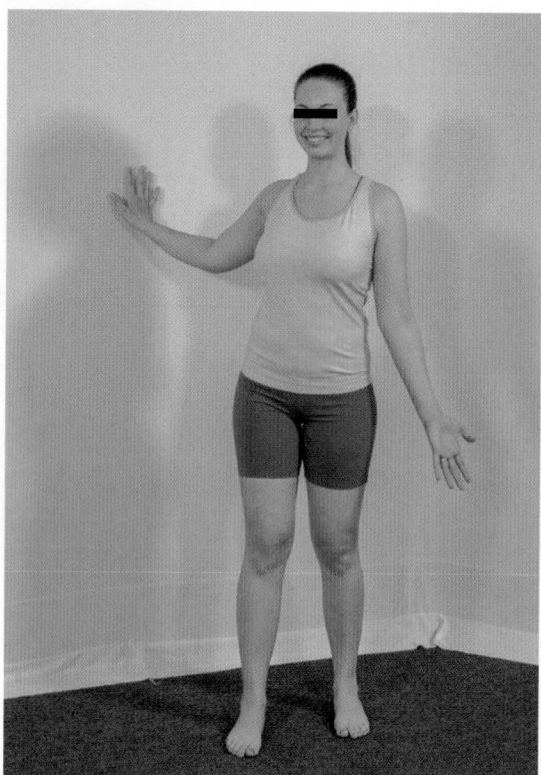

• **Fig. 7.16** Pectoral Muscle Stretching. Pectoral muscle stretching to improve muscle length. (Photograph printed with permission from John Krauss.)

Manual Techniques

There are several manual therapy techniques utilized in the Onc R of PLWCs. Myofascial release techniques are gentle manual techniques to reduce connective tissue restriction by applying sustained pressure. These techniques are used to elongate fascia, improve pain, and reduce motion restriction. Myofascial techniques compared to placebo manual techniques have been shown to improve shoulder movement, function, and pain in women after BC surgery.[130] The techniques are generally well tolerated. Additionally, self-myofascial release techniques can be taught and performed.

Strain-counterstrain techniques are utilized in the manual therapy treatment for people with tightness and MSK pain. In this technique, dysfunctional muscles are positioned in the shortened position and held for 90 seconds until tension eases and spasm reduces. This technique moves muscles and joints out of painful and restricted positions and is generally comfortable and well tolerated. Once the muscle is relaxed, the muscle and joint can be moved toward full ROM with less tension. Studies have shown that strain-counterstrain techniques reduce pain and disability and improve ROM.[131]

Trigger point release techniques can be implemented in many ways. Manual trigger point release is generally performed by delivering sustained pressure to an area of muscular tension within the tissue from a taut band of skeletal muscle or an area of hypersensitivity to pressure. Usually a thumb or fingertip is used and pressure is maintained to the shortened sarcomeres until release is appreciated or pain is decreased. Trigger point release techniques studied in subjects with neck disability and mechanical pain due to upper trapezius trigger points showed decrease in pain intensity

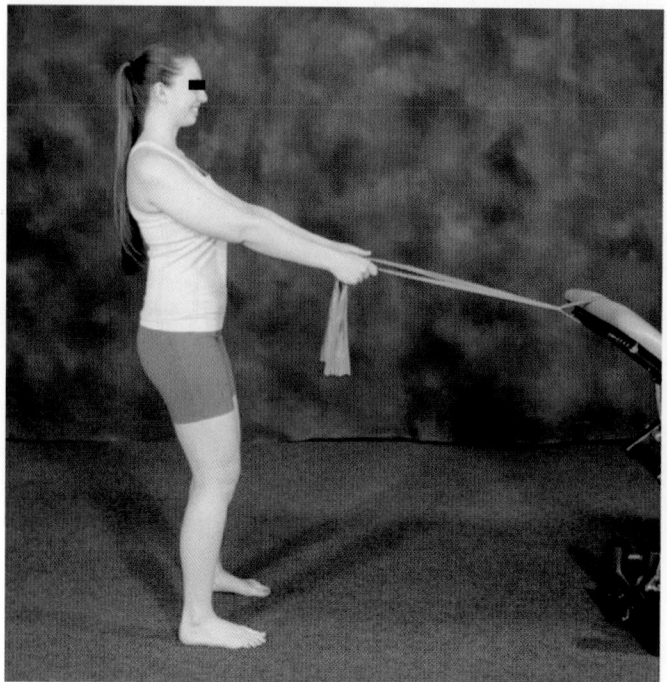
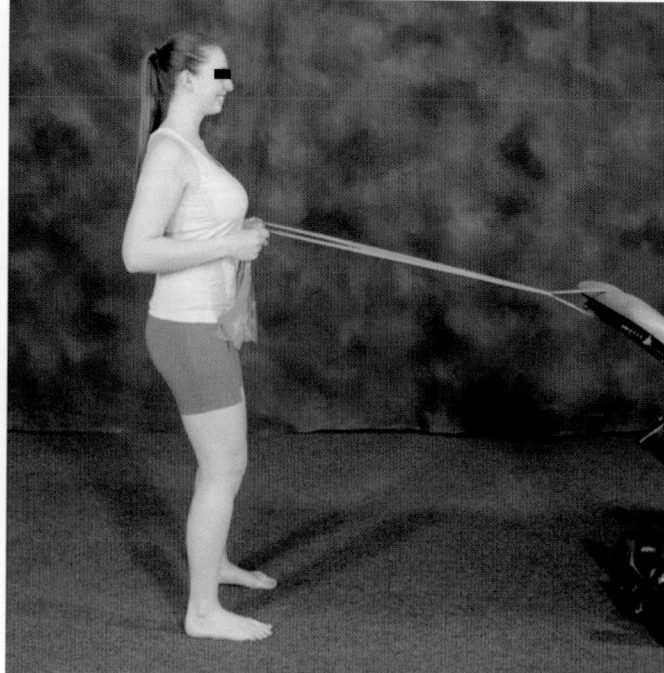

• **Fig. 7.17** Resistance Band Row. Resistance band row where the exerciser uses the resistance band to pull back in a rowing motion for a number of repetitions. The exerciser should stabilize with core muscles and utilize appropriate breathing patterns for maximum exercise effectiveness. (Photograph printed with permission from John Krauss.)

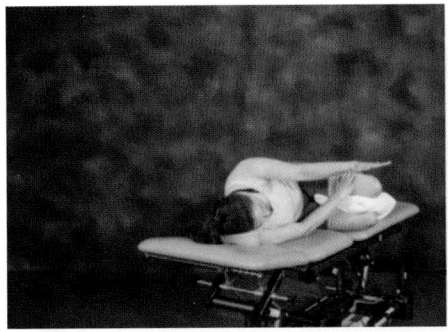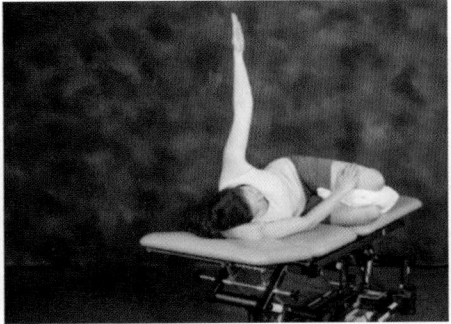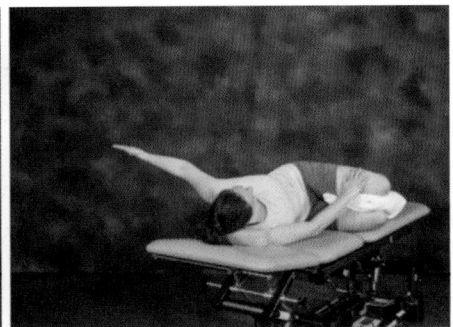

• **Fig. 7.18** Rotational Stretch. Rotational stretch can be performed to create even more rotation through the thoracic spine than is shown. This stretch is beneficial for myofascial planes, muscles, and joints. (Photograph printed with permission from John Krauss.)

and functional disability of the neck and an increased in cervical ROM.[132] Self trigger point release can be taught and may be assisted by the use of tools including Theracanes, foam rollers, and tennis balls. See Figure 7.19 for self trigger point release and Figures 7.20 and 7.21 for tool assisted trigger point release.

Kinesiology taping is the common term for the application of elastic, noninvasive therapeutic tape. Kinesiotape brand claims that application of their tape in the treatment for MSK conditions can re-educate muscle through the cutaneous mechanoreceptor stimulation or inhibition, improve edema, decrease pain through neurological suppression and the gate control theory of pain management and reposition subluxed joints through tension of the tape.[133] Some studies suggest that kinesiology taping can have positive effects on edema and pain, whereas, another meta-analysis did not find MSK benefits with taping.[133–136] The use of tape seems to be a versatile adjunct treatment but overall has little definitive supporting evidence. Figure 7.22 shows the application of therapeutic tape to the knee, upper back and lumbar spine. Figure 7.23 shows the application of therapeutic tape as an adjunct in lymphedema treatment.

Scar mobilization is performed using a variety of manual techniques. Physical scar management has been shown to provide improvement in pain, pigmentation, pliability, pruritus, scar area, and thickness in adults suffering from any type of scar tissue.[137] The most effective manual therapies for scar management after cancer treatment are not yet known. The use of silicone gel sheets has demonstrated effectiveness in the management of hypertrophic scars.[137] PLBC can be taught how to perform scar massage and how to use silicone gel sheets to achieve good outcomes for remodeling their surgical scars.

Balance and Gait Training

PLBCs can experience changes in balance and walking secondary to cancer treatment effects.[138] Taxane chemotherapy is known to cause CIPN which puts people at risk for falls and other disability.[138–140] Balance training can help ameliorate some of the negative effects of cancer treatment on PLBCs.[141] A comprehensive balance program including static and dynamic training, as well as, functional training is indicated for PLBCs. One example of this, the Otago Exercise Program (OEP) has been shown to reduce falls by 35% in frail older adults.[142] The OEP is a comprehensive exercise program that includes warm up exercises and a series of strength and balance exercises that are selected then progressed as the client improves. It has been modified in the United States to be completed in a "clinical management phase" in home or outpatient setting followed by "self-management phase" completed independently at home. A community model is also available

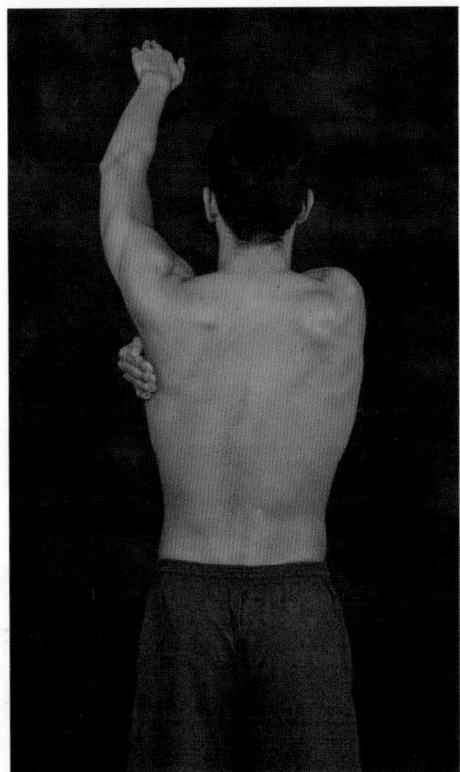

• **Fig. 7.19** Self Trigger Point Release. Self trigger point release to teres major and teres minor. (Photograph printed with permission from John Krauss.)

where participants are referred by local organizations such as the Area Agency on Aging, community members, or caseworkers, as opposed to the traditional model of referral by a physician or an Onc R clinician. The outcomes between a community-based OEP versus a clinic-based OEP have been studied and no significant differences in outcomes between the two models were found with both groups having significant improvement in self-perceived functional mobility and fall risk measures.[142]

A focus on gait training and safety is paramount. Onc R clinicians should assess for the need of an assistive device for PLWCs. The need for assistive devices may change, especially in the case of advanced cancer where a decline in function is expected. In addition, occupational therapists should consider the range of DME to facilitate safe ADL performance. Training and use of an assistive device early may help to reduce energy expenditure and improve

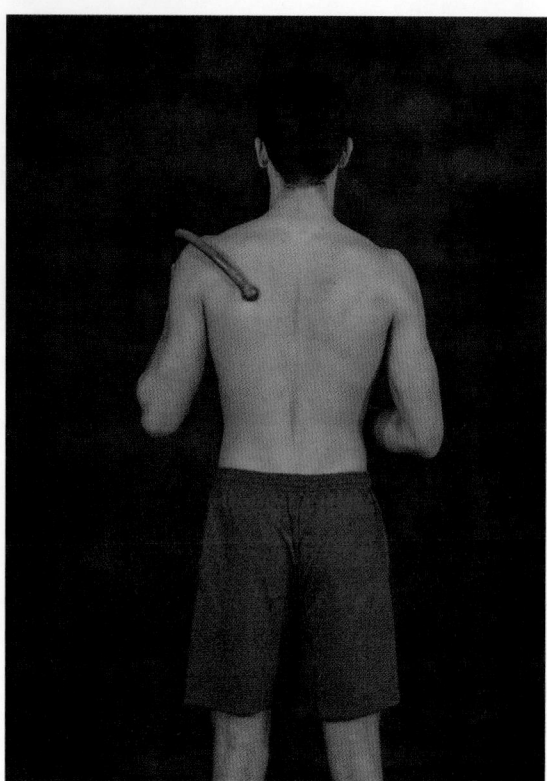

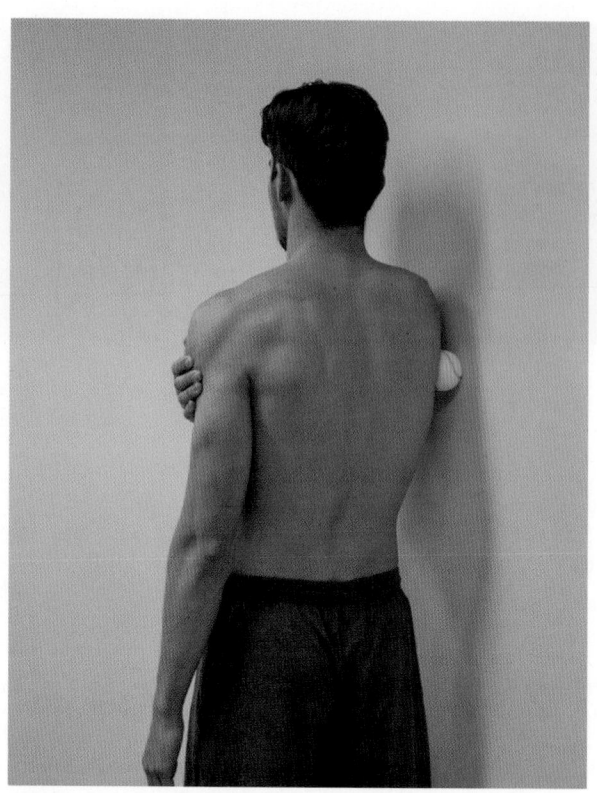

• **Fig. 7.20** Tool Assisted Trigger Point Release–Theracane. Trigger point release of teres major with assistance of Theracane. (Photograph printed with permission from John Krauss.)

• **Fig. 7.21** Tool Assisted Trigger Point Release–Tennis Ball. Trigger point release of teres major with assistance of a tennis ball against the wall. (Photograph printed with permission from John Krauss.)

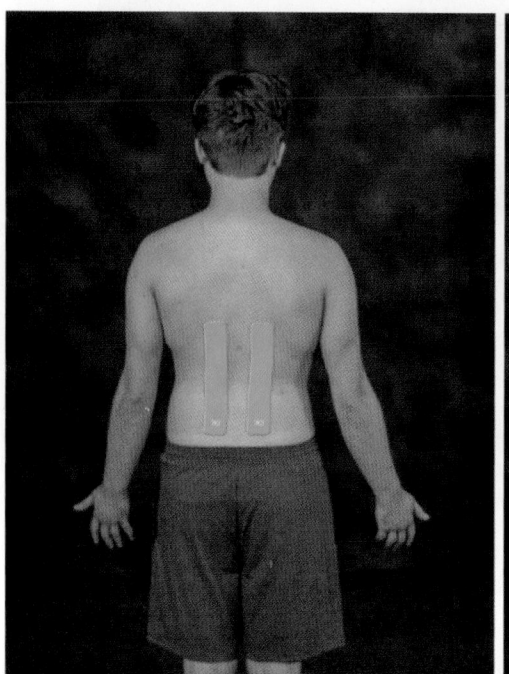

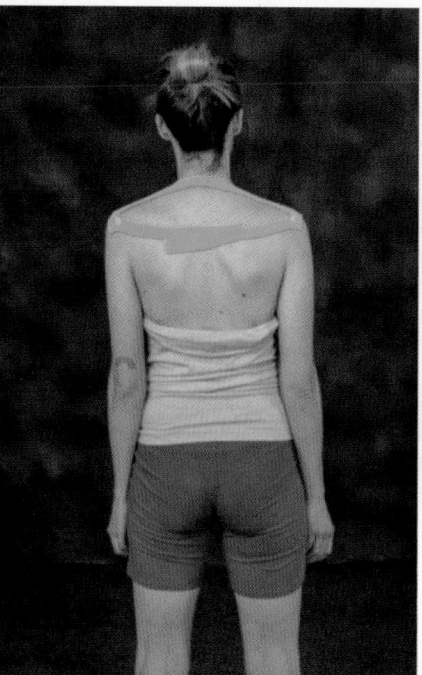

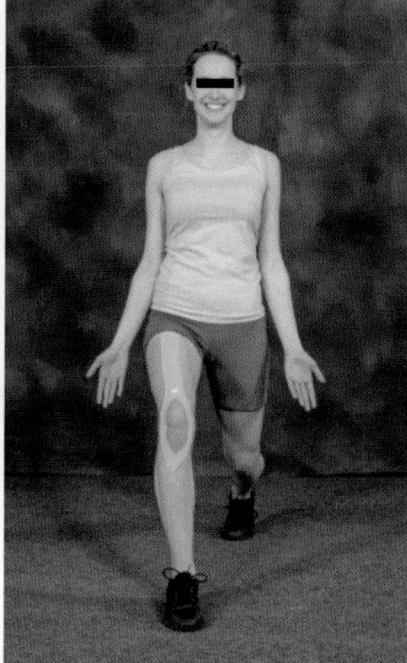

• **Fig. 7.22** Kinesiology Tape Application. Therapeutic application of kinesiology tape to the lumbar spine to reduce low back pain. Application to upper trapezius muscle to inhibit spasm. Application to the anterior knee and quadriceps to facilitate the muscle. (Photograph printed with permission from John Krauss.)

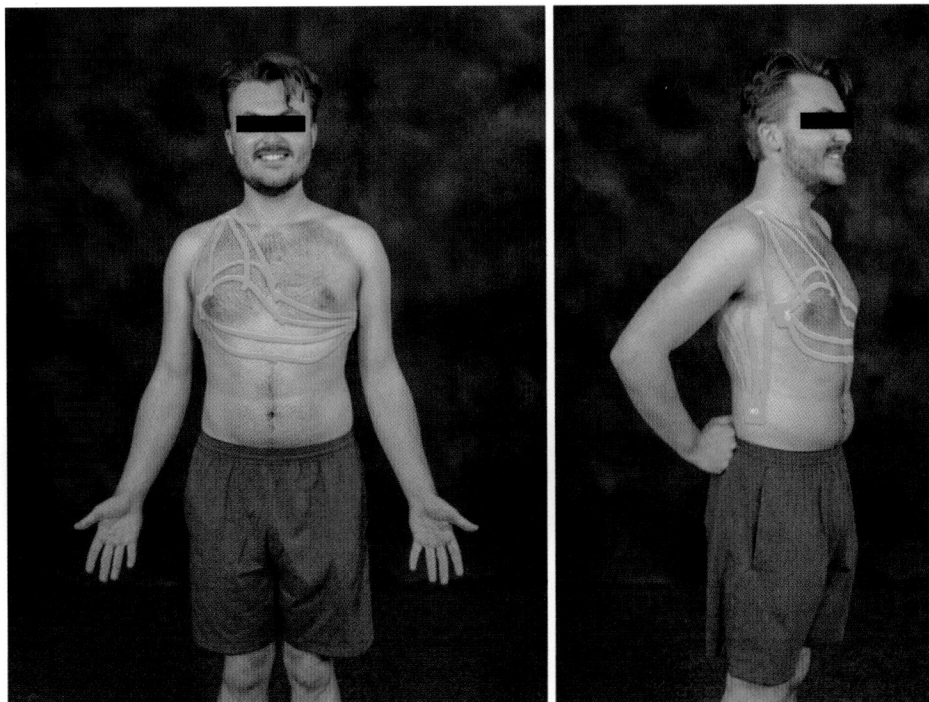

• **Fig. 7.23** Therapeutic Kinesiology Tape Application for the Treatment of Lymphedema. Therapeutic application of kinesiology tape as an adjunct treatment for lymphedema. The tape is anchored at the site of desired flow of lymphatic fluid. (Photograph printed with permission from John Krauss.)

safety allowing the PLWC to maintain QOL. Additionally, patient and caregiver training will make health transitions during the progression of advancing cancer easier to navigate.

Biophysical Agents

Several biophysical agents (modalities) can be safely applied to PLBCs. Caution should always be practiced in the use of modalities for PLWCs as some modalities are untested in this population and may interfere with cancer treatments (Table 7.16).[2]

Postural Training

The application of foundational kinesiology concepts in the presence of cancer-related changes in posture and body mechanics is important to support the PLWC. In the presence of spinal metastasis, postural training to prevent injury to the lumbar spine is essential, especially as most spinal metastases occur in the vertebral body. One of the most important strategies for preventing low back injury is to minimize lumbar spine flexion.[143] The Onc R clinician should educate on lifting and bending techniques to minimize lumbar spine flexion. Use of assistive devices for dressing or modification of clothing can be useful. Additionally, orthotics and bracing are helpful to support postural training and allow the patient to maximize function.

Common uses of braces include spinal braces that provide support or protected motion, neck braces to support individuals with DHS, bracing to support bones and joints with metastasis, and orthotics to enhance stability of foot mechanics.[48,103] A variety of orthoses and equipment are utilized to assist in functional movement in the case of nerve or motor impairments. These may include ankle-foot orthotics and upper extremity orthotics that help with eating and grooming.

In some cases, braces and orthotics may provide temporary assistance while the body recovers from cancer treatment. In all instances, the Onc R clinician should provide education on the equipment used and anticipated future needs.

Overtraining and Fatigue

CRF is the most common and disabling adverse effect for PLWBCs.[143] The pathophysiology for CRF is not entirely known. Current hypotheses behind CRF include dysregulation of cytokines, serotonin, and/or cortisol caused by the effects that chemotherapy or radiation have in the body. Additionally, disruption in circadian rhythms and/or peripheral neurotransmitter release which activate the vagal afferent nerves have been theorized as possible mechanisms of CRF. Activation of vagal afferent nerves can reduce somatic motor activity and muscle tone. Another mechanism hypothesized to play a role in CRF is the disruption of adenosine triphosphate (ATP) at the neuromuscular junction. ATP disruption changes the energy metabolism of skeletal muscle precipitating fatigue. CRF remains difficult to study secondary to it being expressed in a variety of ways with comorbidities such as pain, obesity, and sedentary behavior playing a part in symptom manifestation. The cause is likely multifactorial with proinflammatory cytokines playing a crucial role in many of the proposed mechanisms of CRF.

MSK management for CRF include both aerobic and resistance training exercises.[144] Systematic reviews have shown the benefit of moderate intensity exercise to improve outcomes in PLBCs with CRF.[145] These benefits may be the result of the ability of exercise to modulate some of the probable mechanisms such as improved inflammatory markers in the body and also the result of improved physiologic reserve. Guidelines for the prescription

TABLE 7.16	**Modality/Biophysical Agents Indications, Precautions and Contraindications for Cancer Survivors[2]**		
Modality/Biophysical Agents	**Indication**	**Precaution**	**Contraindication**
Heat	Pain relief, muscle relaxation, tissue extensibility	Impaired lymphatic function, scar tissue, open wounds, or skin fragility	Unmanaged tumor/active disease, peripheral vascular disease, severely impaired sensation, irradiated tissue
Ultrasound	Tissue extensibility, inflammation management	Impaired sensation, opens wounds or skin fragility	Individuals with cancer or with a history of cancer
Cryotherapy	Pain relief, acute management of inflammation, hair loss management	Impaired sensation, open wounds or skin fragility	Ischemic tissue, peripheral vascular disease, Raynaud's syndrome
Transcutaneous electrical nerve stimulation (TENS)	Sensory pain management, scar desensitization	Insensate tissue	Unmanaged tumor/active disease, over pacemaker, open wounds
Needle electromyography (EMG)	Measures muscle response to nerve stimulation	Thrombocytopenia	None
Functional electrical stimulation (FES)	Restoration of muscle firing when nerve conduction is intact (e.g., ambulation, limb function, swallowing, pelvic floor retraining)	Poor skin condition or indurated tissue	Unmanaged tumor/active disease
Low level light laser	Oral mucositis, scar tissue extensibility, lymphedema	Open wounds or skin fragility	Acute radiation dermatitis, unmanaged tumor/active disease
Manual therapy	Pain relief, tissue extensibility, joint mobility, soft tissue and radiation fibrosis management, lymphatic stimulation	Impaired sensation, dysvascular tissue, open wounds or skin fragility	Acute radiation dermatitis, unmanaged tumor/active disease, bone fragility due to metastasis or osteoporosis
Spinal manipulation	Spinal mobility and alignment, pain relief	Open wounds or skin fragility	Bone fragility due to metastasis or osteoporosis, radiculopathy, spinal stenosis, myelopathy, spinal cord compromise from tumor or lesion

Created by Kristina Sitarski and Karen Wiseman. Printed with permission.

of aerobic exercise were previously discussed and focus should be given to functional exercise like walking and exercise that the person enjoys to promote adherence. Specific resistance exercise for the treatment of CRF remain unknown. Resistance exercise that focuses on function are likely beneficial for those with CRF because they improve strength, performance at home and safety in the community. Training may include squats, step ups, core exercises, and wall push-ups.

It is important to monitor for overtraining and fatigue because PLWCs are at risk for cachexia. A discussion on changes in energy levels that happen while undergoing treatment will help explain perceived setbacks during treatment cycles when fatigue limits exercise ability. Also, recognition of the changes in energy consumption of an exercising body may help them to understand how exercise and nutrition go hand in hand to promote wellness. Energy demands should not exceed energy intake.

Education Topics in Rehabilitation

A PLWC may have many questions that can and should be brought up in the Onc R treatment sessions. Education can be focused on prevention of injury to the MSK system with information on exercise dosing for improved safety and function to meet the person's performance goals. Common issues that need to be explored are how current MSK impairments may change the PLBC's ability to participate optimally in the prescribed exercise. For example, issues like knee OA or back pain may make it difficult for a PLBC

to confidently begin a walking program. In cases such as these, a Onc R setting might prove most beneficial for problem solving and modification of exercise prescription.

There are many resources available for those PLWCs to learn about their cancer and the treatments they have undergone. One thorough resource for patient education materials is OncoLink from Penn Medicine under the "Build My Patient Treatment Binder" link that allows free downloaded materials on a large variety of topics that is both general and cancer specific (https://www.oncolink.org/treatment-binder).[112] Topics on this website include surgical procedures, radiation skin changes, chemotherapy adverse effects, medication adverse effects, bone health, nutrition during and after treatment, medical leave resources, financial assistance programs, and more.

Providing a PLWC with an understanding of the common impairments encountered with different cancer diagnoses and treatment protocols will help to ease concerns of the PLWC that what they are experiencing is an adverse effect. For example, this education may help a PLWC understand that the pain they feel in their neck after surgical intervention can be managed with MSK treatments (once cleared by their oncology team) like joint mobilization, self-stretching, and parascapular strengthening. This should empower them to manage these adverse effects.

Education can be very valuable to help a PLWC and their caregivers to find realistic options to maintain QOL, reduce risk factors for cancer recurrence, and to optimize their health. Below are a few MSK-focused education topics in Onc R.

Exercise Benefits and Prescription

PLWCs should be informed of the benefits of exercise and encouraged to be as active as possible within their capabilities and in accordance with their values and goals. This includes education to improve self-efficacy and modifications needed to safely perform exercise. First they should receive training on how to self-monitor signs and symptoms. They should be educated on when to stop or modify exercise and when to contact their healthcare team. They should also be educated in safe exercise progression including frequency, intensity, time, and type of exercise. It will be imperative to maintain open communication about symptoms related to movement and ADLs that may indicate a change in health status or need stop exercise.

Fall Prevention

Fall prevention education is important given the PLBC's significant risk of SREs such as fractures and osteoporosis. In fact, one study showed that breast cancer survivors had a 68% higher risk of osteopenia and osteoporosis compared to cancer-free women.[146] Furthermore, PLWBC expereinced falls at a 25% to 30% higher rate than the general population.[138] Often, the risk of falls increases beyond their first or second year post diagnosis. As described earlier, the late effects of cancer treatment can affect this even further as the PLBC ages. Thinking ahead to devices they may need intermittently during their treatment process such as a walker, transport chair, or a tub transfer bench can be helpful to ensure the PLWC has the necessary equipment for their "good" and "bad" days. Regular check-up appointments with the Onc R team can help to monitor changes needed to assistive devices or DME and progress or regress a HEP as the patient goes through various stages of treatment and survivorship. The person can also be encouraged to join community balance and fall prevention exercises groups such as the OEP.

Caregiver Education

Caregiver training is a crucial part of education in the Onc R setting. Consistency and carryover of surgical restrictions or WB restrictions is important to prevent falls and fractures and to improve healing. Caregivers may need to help with wound care, postoperative dressing changes, reminding them of lifting or movement restrictions, and helping with symptom management on their bad days.

Positioning and postural education precautions can include spinal precautions such as avoiding bending, lifting, or twisting. This is especially important in loaded positions in those with suspected or known spinal metastases or low bone density. Also, it is important to educate the patient on correct posture in functional positions and activities such as sitting, standing, and sleeping positions. Practice of lifting techniques such as the *hip hinge* or *golfer's lift* is useful in bending ADLs. Use of spinal orthoses for postural cueing may be beneficial for pain relief and maintaining QOL in ADLs.

Adverse Reactions or Red Flags

A PLWC and their caregiver should be educated on the signs of infection, especially postoperatively. With a body region at risk for lymphedema, it is important to avoid scrapes, cuts or burns, and avoid unnecessary blood pressure cuffs and venipuncture on the affected limb. More lymphedema risk reduction education can be found in Chapter 9. Reinforcement of education from radiation oncology for postradiation skin care topics is beneficial. These topics include patting skin dry without rubbing as well as avoiding perfumes, scented lotions, excessive sun exposure, hot tubs, saunas, or heavily chlorinated water. In addition, recommendations include using mild detergents, wearing loose fitting clothing, as well as providing education on fatigue after radiation. Furthermore, the patient may have postoperative surgical restrictions. For example, after breast surgery some surgeons restrict the arm ROM above 90 degrees for several weeks. Likewise, there are specific postostomy precautions and care guidelines. Many other cancer-specific surgery precautions exist and reinforcement of those precautions are necessary in the Onc R setting. It is important to be familiar with the precautions so the PLWC can have guidance throughout the healing process.

Nutrition

Nutritional counseling for PLWBCs is beneficial at any stage of cancer to meet the appropriate level of nutrients needed through food to sustain the person's energy level and assist with healing. This will help combat adverse effects to the MSK system from cancer treatments such as sarcopenia and cachexia. The Onc R team is well suited to reinforce and educate patients on nutrition. Education is valuable on how their food intake relates to the body's recovery and energy levels with exercise. Protein intake is essential to recover and heal after exercise or when healing from a fracture. More information on nutrition can be found in Chapter 30.

Education on water intake to the recommended 64 ounces per day is also important and can be used as a bridge to education on bladder habits and pelvic floor dysfunction.[147] Aside from a dietician, the PLWC may also benefit from referrals to speech language pathologists or naturopathic medicine for further testing and recommendations.

Pain

The Onc R team can provide invaluable education on pain science and ways to help manage pain. Furthermore, explaining the cause of pain and adverse effects of various cancer drugs may help the PLWC to understand and differentiate atypical from typical pain that they are feeling. For example, many medications, such as AIs, can cause arthralgias or myalgias. See Table 7.1. The Onc R clinician can educate a PLWC to manage pain and psychological distress with the use of exercise, yoga, breathing techniques, meditation, guided imagery, relaxation, and body scanning.

Many impairments previously discussed can affect breathing. Education on breathing and relaxation techniques is essential. Breathing and relaxation techniques decrease muscle tension and provide positive pain free movement patterns that reduce fear avoidance behaviors and improve overall pain.

Referrals can also be made to medical integrative medicine centers that offer naturopathic doctors, oncology massage, acupuncture, cupping, or Reiki therapy. These modalities can be a great adjunct to traditional medicine. See Chapter 22 for more information on managing cancer-related pain.

Conclusion

Bone pain is the number one cause of cancer-related pain and the differential diagnosis is complicated by normal aging effects, cancer treatment related effects, or a new onset of cancer recurrence. The most common cancers that metastasize to the bone include breast, lung, prostate, thyroid, and renal cancers. Pathologic fractures are likely to occur in either the hip or spine. Spinal fractures occurring due to metastases are most likely to occur in the thoracic spine above the level of T7, whereas fractures due to osteoporosis alone are often below T7.

Overall, the focus of Onc R should be to maximize QOL, provide pain reduction techniques and education on pain science as well as prescribing the correct assistive devices and braces. Radiation has an impact on skin healing and can cause RFS that leads to further soft tissue adhesions and compensatory posture and joint mechanics. Onc R providers can assist with scar massage, myofascial release and desensitization to improve pain, ROM, function, and even cosmesis.

Commonly seen complications to the tissue in of patients with BC include AWS, seroma, and lymphedema. Myalgia and arthralgias are an adverse effect of AI, ADT, and taxane based chemotherapy regimens. Exercise has been shown to improve these adverse effects. The terms sarcopenia and cachexia are used to describe disorders of muscle deficiency. People with cancer may have both cachexia, sarcopenia, as well as frailty. Exercise should be considered an important intervention for sarcopenia, cachexia and frailty.

Acute or late effects of cancer and/or its treatments can affect posture and body mechanics. Participation in a HEP emphasizing posture and body mechanics to improve functional movement patterns is valuable. Bracing can be used intermittently to assist with energy conservation and improve functional positioning. The Onc R clinician should have an index of suspicion for abnormal symptoms that could be an oncologic emergency. Red flags including night pain that is not relieved with rest, pain with WB, abnormal joint end feel, changes in bowel and bladder, progressive weakness and other nonreproducible pain responses should warrant referral to their physician. This can be a sign of cancer recurrence, metastases, fracture, or impending fracture which require urgent attention and communication with the oncologist. Finally, strength training is beneficial in maintaining bone health and has been found safe and feasible in patients with and without bone metastasis. Multiple studies have found no SREs, worsening pain, or progression of metastases with careful exercise prescription.

Critical Research Needs

- Prescription of impact/WB exercise to improve bone density in a person with cancer-related osteoporosis/osteopenia.
- Virtual versus in-person prehabilitation programs on adherence and outcomes.
- Validated and reliable functional outcome tools in multiple types of cancers and advanced cancers.
- Functional strengthening interventions on QOL measures in people with MM.
- Prehabilitation education and prescription of video-based stretching program in HNC to prevent kyphosis and neck ROM deficits.

Case Study

Patient History

A 52-year-old female presented to an outpatient physical therapy clinic with a history of stage 2A invasive ductal carcinoma (IDC) of the left breast (T2N0M0) ER/PR+, HER2-. She had undergone a lumpectomy with a total of 9 axillary lymph nodes removed (2 SLN + 7 ALND) followed by whole breast radiation to doses of 4256 cGy and 1000 cGy boost to the lumpectomy cavity. Her Oncotype

DX score was 31 indicating need for chemotherapy, however she declined chemotherapy. Due to the hormone-positive cancer and her postmenopausal status, the patient was placed on letrozole (Femara), an aromatase inhibitor post radiation. She had a series of drains and aspirations to a seroma that developed multiple infections in the left chest. Treatment included the oral antibiotic cefalexin (Keflex) and later IV antibiotics to better control the infection.

Chart Review

Past medical history: DM, hyperlipidemia, tachycardia, asthma, HTN, anxiety, depression, dizziness.

Surgical history: Left carpal tunnel release, cholecystectomy, two C-sections, six right arm surgeries from a traumatic injury 20 years prior.

Imaging: Breast mammogram showed IDC of left breast at 2 o'clock position.

Lab values: CBC within normal limits, lipid panel demonstrates controlled cholesterol, hemoglobin A1c was 6.2.

Subjective

She presented to physical therapy with complaints of left shoulder and arm pain and limited left shoulder ROM that impaired her functional independence. At the time of presentation to therapy, she was 17 months post breast surgery, and 14 months post completion of RTx. Initial patient-reported outcomes include: Disability of Arm Shoulder Hand (DASH) score of 70%, Modified Brief Fatigue Inventory score 4/10, and the Functional Assessment of Cancer Therapy-Breast (FACT-B) showed significant areas of concern were functional well-being as well as social/family well-being. Her pain was rated at 6/10 on Numeric Pain Rating Scale.

Examination Findings

Resting vitals: Blood pressure 118/75, heart rate 72, pulse oximetry 98% on room air.

Precautions or contraindications (if any): Due to prior complications with infection, monitoring and patient self-monitoring of scar were completed during each session and by patient semi-regularly. No red flags for mobility. No need to modify testing or interventions.

Special tests: Upper limb tension tests were negative. The Neer and Hawkins Kennedy tests for shoulder impingement were negative. A Dix-Hallpike test was performed secondary to dizziness, symptoms were not reproducible. Patient was referred to an Ear Nose and Throat specialist who ruled out vertigo.

Sensation: Her sensation was intact throughout the breast and axilla. She was highly sensitive to light-to-medium palpation throughout the chest and axilla.

Integument: A left breast and axillary scar was noted. Scar mobility was moderately limited over her breast and axilla, especially with abduction and flexion end ROM. Radiation tattoos were observed. Mild radiation fibrosis was limiting fascial and skin mobility over her left chest compared to the right. Her MAP-BC myofascial adhesion score (0 = least restricted, 9 = most restricted) showed the highest score in her axillary scar 4/9, breast scar 3/9, axilla 3/9, and lateral chest wall 3/9, while all other regions scored 2/9. See Table 7.17 for MAP-BC score example.

Edema: Referral to a lymphedema therapist was required as the patient had a greater than 2 cm circumferential difference in the involved arm compared to her uninvolved arm, though comparison was difficult due to scarring and past surgeries on right arm that could impact edema and potential atrophy. She was fitted for a compression glove and sleeve.

Palpation: Tenderness to palpation over pectoralis major and minor insertion, teres major, teres minor, and subscapularis. She was also sensitive to palpation in her axilla and lateral chest wall, as well as over the chest and axillary scar.

Joint play: Empty end feel due to pain and guarding.

ROM: Left shoulder ROM flexion limited to 118 degrees and abduction limited to 135 degrees. Shoulder ROM was moderately limited by pain and fascial and joint restrictions. Neck AROM limited in rotation, side bending, and extension.

Strength: Hand grip dynamometry left 30 lb (13.6 kg), right 43 lb (19.5 kg). Strength in the left shoulder was limited to between 4- and 4 out of 5.

Postural assessment tests: Flexicurve measure was taken from cervical to lumbar spine demonstrating exaggerated thoracic kyphosis and lumbar lordosis. Kyphosis index was 12.3%, lumbar lordosis index was 9.2%. Visual assessment demonstrated a protracted and elevated left shoulder.

Muscle length tests: In supine position, pectoral muscle tightness was observed with 4-inch height of left acromion from the table compared to 3-inch height of right acromion.

Balance and functional mobility assessment: Timed Up and Go score was 10 seconds without an assistive device. Six Minute Walk Test was 563 meters with the exercise heart rate 112, blood pressure 134/85, oxygen saturation 98%, and rating of perceived exertion 5/10 on the modified Borg CR10 scale.

TABLE 7.17	Case Example MAP-BC Myofascial Adhesions		
Region	Level	Fibrosis Score: 0 (No Adhesions) −3 (Very Stiff Adhesions)	Total Score Per Region
Axillary scar	Skin	2	4
	Superficial	2	
	Deep	0	
Breast scar	Skin	2	3
	Superficial	1	
	Deep	0	
Pectoralis muscle (anterior axillary fold)	Skin	1	2
	Superficial	1	
	Deep	0	
Axilla	Skin	2	3
	Superficial	1	
	Deep	0	
Frontal chest wall (sternum)	Skin	1	2
	Superficial	1	
	Deep	0	
Lateral chest wall (drain site)	Skin	2	3
	Superficial	1	
	Deep	0	
Inframammary fold	Skin	1	2
	Superficial	1	
	Deep	0	
Summary of fibrosis scores			19

Created by Kristina Sitarski and Karen Wiseman. Printed with permission.

Summary of Assessment

Upon completion of the physical therapy examination and evaluation of her past medical history, the patient was determined to have muscle and soft tissue imbalances, fear avoidance behavior causing left upper extremity guarding with resultant postural changes, ROM limitations, and lymphedema. It was determined that the patient would benefit from skilled outpatient physical therapy to address these deficits.

Differential Diagnosis

Upper extremity and breast lymphedema, complex regional pain syndrome, neck radiculopathy, radiation fibrosis and psychological factors, influencing pain experience.

Treatment

Twice per week for 45 to 60 minute sessions; 12 sessions of therapy were completed.

Therapeutic exercise: Exercise treatment included stretching of bilateral upper extremities and strengthening of the shoulder girdle; she requested not to complete neck ROM exercises secondary to fear of dizziness. The patient was instructed in postural facilitation exercises including optimal scapular position and activation of abdominal muscles. She was given verbal guidance and manual cueing during exercise performance for optimal posture and core activation. Examples of exercises completed in this case are seen in Table 7.18.

Manual therapy: The treatment included soft tissue mobilization of pectoralis major, teres major and minor, subscapularis, and upper arm. Myofascial and trigger point release manual techniques were selected on each treatment session according to patient's tolerance for such treatments with areas of focus including frontal and lateral chest wall, pectoralis region, axillary scar, and axilla, breast scar and inframammary fold.

Education

Topics that the Onc R clinician educated her on included red flags/warning signs, risk reduction for lymphedema, pain science for shoulder pain, a skin care regimen and avoiding infections, nutrition, hydration, an HEP, and various adverse effects that can cause arthralgias and myalgias. As an aspect of stress management, she was encouraged to engage in regular walking outside and perform diaphragmatic breathing. She was also introduced to meditation and educated on the value of mindfulness meditation for her mental well-being. Throughout the sessions, she would ask multiple questions related to fatigue that led to education about sleep habits and energy conservation techniques. Resources such as support groups were given to the patient to assist with coping and discussing her cancer journey with others.

Outcomes

Pain: Pain reduced from 6/10 to 4/10 on Numeric Pain Rating Scale.

Function: Improved dressing, cooking, cleaning with DASH score 40%, FACT-B demonstrated improvement in functional well-being and social/family well-being. Patient reported that she was actively participating in a support group.

TABLE 7.18 **Case Example Exercise Interventions**

Strengthening 2 Sets of 15	Stretching 3 Sets, 20 to 30 Second Hold	Postural Exercise 10 Sets, 5 Second Hold
Shoulder row with exercise bands	Wall angels	Shoulder retraction
Shoulder internal and external rotation with exercise bands	Pectoral stretch on wall, single side	Neck retraction
Serratus punches/protraction	Hooklying trunk rotation arms at a T	Abdominal isometric
Shoulder flexion with 2 pounds in standing	Behind head butterfly stretch for pectorals	Shoulder Y and T standing

Created by Kristina Sitarski and Karen Wiseman. Printed with permission.

AROM: Improved from flexion 118 to 145 degrees, and abduction 135 to 155 degrees.

Strength: Handgrip dynamometry left 38 lb, right 45 lb. Strength in the left shoulder was limited to between 4 and 4+ out of 5 with no pain to manual muscle testing.

Outcome measures: Timed Up and Go score was 8.5 seconds without an assistive device. Six Minute Walk Test was 620 meters. Exercise vital signs as follows: heart rate 108, blood pressure 130/85, pulse oximetry 98%, rating of perceived exertion 4/10 on the modified Borg CR10 scale.

Review Questions

Reader can find the correct answers and rationale in the back of the book.

1. Which of the following is the the BEST choice to complete the following sentence? A PLWC who is diagnosed with bone metastasis
   A. Should not perform exercise
   B. Should not perform lifting or bending functional tasks
   C. Should continue to run for exercise
   D. Should consult the multidisciplinary team for safety guidance

2. The risk of fracture can be assessed by diagnostic prediction scales. These scales are based on which information?
   A. Loading demands such as body weight
   B. Imaging and clinical features
   C. Factors that weaken the bone such as radiation
   D. Sarcopenia and frailty index

3. Radiation fibrosis syndrome is correlated with:
   A. Smaller radiation field size
   B. Short course of therapy
   C. Neo adjuvant chemotherapy
   D. Pre-existing connective tissue disorders (scleroderma, lupus, or Marfan syndrome)

4. Aromatase Inhibitors are a class of drug that may cause myalgias and arthralgias. This medication's adverse effects put PLBC at risk for:
   A. Hand foot syndrome
   B. Myasthenia gravis
   C. CIPN
   D. Risk of falls

5. Two scales that are commonly used clinically in oncology to assess global performance status and determine patient fitness for treatment include the Karnofsky Performance Scale and the ECOG scale. Which of the following is the the BEST choice to complete the following sentence? These scales
   A. Accurately assess patients for frailty
   B. Do not influence treatment decision making
   C. Are clinician rated tools and have considerable bias
   D. Over diagnosis of frailty

6. Cachexia is a disorder of muscle deficiency. Characteristics include anorexia, metabolic changes, excess catabolism, and the presence of inflammatory cytokines. Which of the following BEST describes additional characteristics of cachexia?
   A. Identified by plain film radiographs
   B. Assessed using the Fried frailty phenotype
   C. Treated with exercise and nutritional support
   D. Common in young cancer survivors

7. Cancer treatments can affect body mechanics and posture. Which of the following common treatments is MOST LIKELY to affect body mechanics?
   A. Checkpoint inhibitors
   B. Vitamin D supplementation
   C. Steroid therapy
   D. Radiation therapy

8. A PLW has a bone metastasis with 0% to 25% cortex involvement. Which of the following precautions would be MOST appropriate in this case based on the information provided?
   A. None, monitor for pain
   B. Partial weight bearing
   C. No resistance exercises
   D. AROM only, without twisting

9. PLBCs should be carefully monitored for red flags during an Onc R examination. Which of the following is LEAST likely to be a red flag of concern?
   A. Redness or swelling in the tissue
   B. Restricted shoulder ROM in capsular pattern
   C. Limited SLR secondary to groin pain
   D. Changes in mental status

10. PLBCs who were treated for breast cancer can have treatment related adverse effects that negatively impact posture. Which of the following is LEAST LIKELY to contribute to impaired posture?
    A. Rotator cuff tendinopathy
    B. Brachial plexopathies
    C. Lymphedema
    D. Shoulder impingement

References

1. Shapiro CL, Van Poznak C, Lacchetti C, et al. Management of osteoporosis in survivors of adult cancers with nonmetastatic disease: ASCO clinical practice guideline. *J Clin Oncol*. 2019;37:2916–2946.

2. Maltser S, Cristian A, Silver JK, Morris GS, Stout NL. A focused review of safety considerations in cancer rehabilitation. *PM R*. 2017;9(9):S415–S428.

3. Pruitt DW, Bolikal P. Rehabilitation of the pediatric cancer patient. In: Stubblefield MD, ed. *Cancer Rehabilitation: Principles and Practice*. 2nd ed. Springer; 2019:898–899.

4. Wampler M. Chemotherapy induced peripheral neuropathy fact sheet for professionals. *Acad Am Phys Ther Assoc (APTA Oncology)*. 2018:1–12.

5. Dang N, Yamada K. Head and neck cancer fact sheet for professionals. *Acad Am Phys Ther Assoc (APTA Oncology)*:1–4. doi:10.1093/annonc/mdh937.

6. Smoot B, Wampler M, Topp K. Breast cancer treatments and complications: implications for rehabilitation. *Rehabil Oncol*. 2009;27(3):21.

7. Stout N. Hormonal adjuvant therapy and its impact on function. Medbridge. 1–48.

8. Dicato MA. *Side Effects of Medical Cancer Therapy: Prevention and Treatment*: Springer; 2013. doi:10.1007/978-0-85729-787-7.

9. Kane CM, Hoskin P, Bennett MI. Cancer induced bone pain. *BMJ*. 2015;350:h315. doi:10.1136/bmj.h315.

10. Lee WC, Guntur AR, Long F, Rosen CJ. Energy metabolism of the osteoblast: implications for osteoporosis. *Endocr Rev*. 2017;38(3):255–266. doi:10.1210/er.2017-00064.

11. Wisotzky E, Khanna A. Upper extremity disorders in cancer. In: Stubblefield MD, ed. *Cancer Rehabilitation: Principles and Practice*. 2nd ed. Springer; 2019:737–751.

12. DePompolo RW, Cheville AL, Schmidt KD, Strick DM. Lower extremity disorders in cancer. In: Stubblefield MD, ed. *Cancer Rehabilitation: Principles and Practice*. 2nd ed. Springer; 2019:751–763.

13. Gilchrist LS, Galantino ML, Wampler M, Marchese VG, Morris GS, Ness KK. A framework for assessment in oncology rehabilitation. *Phys Ther*. 2009;89(3):286–306. doi:10.2522/ptj.20070309.

14. DePompolo RW, Cheville AL, Schmidt KD, Strick DM. Lower extremity disorders in cancer. In: Stubblefield MD, ed. *Cancer Rehabilitation: Principles and Practice*. 2nd ed. Springer; 2019:751–763.

15. Morris J, Belzarena AC, Boland P. Bone metastases. In: Stubblefield MD, ed. *Cancer Rehabilitation: Principles and Practice*. 2nd ed. Springer; 2019:780–789.

16. Money SR, Smith SR. Spine disorders in cancer. In: Stubblefield MD, ed. *Cancer Rehabilitation: Principles and Practice*. 2nd ed. Springer; 2019:729–737.

17. Vanwye WR. Patient screening by a physical therapist for nonmusculoskeletal hip pain. *Phys Ther*. 2009;89:248–256, doi:10.2522/ptj.20070366.

18. Raman S, Broussard JR. Endocrine complications of cancer and their treatment. In: Stubblefield MD, ed. *Cancer Rehabilitation: Principles and Practice*. 2nd ed. Springer; 2019:470–482.

19. Gutgarts V, Latcha S. Renal complications of cancer and their treatment. In: Stubblefield MD, ed. *Cancer Rehabilitation: Principles and Practice*. 2nd ed. Springer; 2019:464–470.

20. Farooki A, Ukena J. Osteoporosis in cancer. In: Stubblefield MD, ed. *Cancer Rehabilitation: Principles and Practice*. 2nd ed. Springer; 2019:763–780.

21. Macedo F, Ladeira K, Pinho F, et al. Bone metastases: an overview. *Oncol Rev*. 2017;11(1). doi:10.4081/oncol.2017.321.

22. Ibrahim T, Mercatali L, Amadori D. A new emergency in oncology: bone metastases in breast cancer patients (review). *Oncol Lett*. 2013;6(2):306–310.

23. Leone A, Cianfoni A, Zecchi V, Cortese MC, Rumi N, Colosimo C. Instability and impending instability in patients with vertebral metastatic disease. *Skeletal Radiol*. 2019;48(2):195–207. doi:10.1007/s00256-018-3032-3.

24. Benca E, Patsch JM, Mayr W, Pahr DH, Windhager R. The insufficiencies of risk analysis of impending pathological fractures in patients with femoral metastases: a literature review. *Bone Reports*. 2016;5:51–56.

25. Damron TA, Morgan H, Prakash D, Grant W, Aronowitz J, Heiner J. Critical evaluation of Mirels rating system for impending pathologic fractures. *Clin Orthop Relat Res*. 2003;415(415 suppl.):S201–S207.

26. Vargo MM. Precautions in cancer rehabilitation. In: Stubblefield MD, ed. *Cancer Rehabilitation: Principles and Practice*. 2nd ed. Springer; 2019:789–799.

27. Eggermont F, van der Wal G, Westhoff P, et al. Patient-specific finite element computer models improve fracture risk assessments in cancer patients with femoral bone metastases compared to clinical guidelines. *Bone*. 2020;130:115101. doi:10.1016/j.bone.2019.115101.

28. Macmillan Cancer Support. Physical activity for people with metastatic bone disease: guidance for healthcare professionals. https://www.macmillan.org.uk/healthcare-professionals/news-and-resources/guides/physical-activity-for-people-with-metastatic-bone-disease. Published November 30, 2020. Accessed March 27, 2022.

29. New PW. Rehabilitation of patients with spinal cord dysfunction in the cancer setting. In: Stubblefield MD, ed. *Cancer Rehabilitation: Principles and Practice*. 2nd ed. Springer; 2016:601–623.

30. Sodji Q, Kaminski J, Willey C, Al E. Management of metastatic spinal cord compression. *South Med J*. 2017;110(9):586–593.

31. Al-Qurainy R, Collis E. Metastatic spinal cord compression diagnosis and management. *BMJ*. 2016;353:i2539.

32. Curtin M, Piggott RP, Murphy EP, et al. Spinal metastatic disease: a review of the role of the multidisciplinary team. *Orthop Surg*. 2017;9(2):145–151. doi:10.1111/os.12334.

33. Hernandez RK, Wade SW, Reich A, Pirolli M, Liede A, Lyman GH. Incidence of bone metastases in patients with solid tumors: analysis of oncology electronic medical records in the United States. *BMC Cancer*. 2018;18(1):1–11. doi:10.1186/s12885-017-3922-0.

34. Langdahl B, Ferrari S, Dempster DW. Bone modeling and remodeling: potential as therapeutic targets for the treatment of osteoporosis. *Ther Adv Musculoskelet Dis*. 2016;8(6):225–235. doi:10.1177/1759720X16670154.

35. Andriolo L, Merli G, Tobar C, Altamura SA, Kon E, Filardo G. Regenerative therapies increase survivorship of avascular necrosis of the femoral head: a systematic review and meta-analysis. *Int Orthop*. 2018;42(7):1689–1704. doi:10.1007/s00264-018-3787-0.

36. Murphy BA, Mannion K, Lang Kuhs K, Castellanos EH, Twork GJ, Niermann K. Evaluation and management of head and neck cancer. In: Stubblefield MD, ed. *Cancer Rehabilitation: Principles and Practice*. 2nd ed. Springer; 2019:304–318.

37. Khan AA, Morrison A, Hanley DA, et al. Diagnosis and management of osteonecrosis of the jaw: a systematic review and international consensus. *J Bone Miner Res*. 2015;30(1):3–23. doi:10.1002/jbmr.2405.

38. Jenwitheesuk K, Mahakkanukrauh A, Punjaruk W, et al. Efficacy of adjunctive hyperbaric oxygen therapy in osteoradionecrosis. *Biores Open Access*. 2018;7(1):145–149. doi:10.1089/biores.2018.0019.

39. McNeely ML, Binkley JM, Pusic AL, Campbell KL, Gabram S, Soballe PW. A prospective model of care for breast cancer rehabilitation: postoperative and postreconstructive issues. *Cancer*. 2012;118(suppl 8):2226–2236. doi:10.1002/cncr.27468.

40. Jare SN, Shinde S, Patil S. Prevalence of myofascial dysfunctions in breast cancer survivors. *Int J Physiother*. 2019;6(6). doi:10.15621/ijphy/2019/v6i6/190227.

41. De Groef A, M Van Kampen, Vervloesem N, et al. An evaluation tool for myofascial adhesions in patients after breast cancer (MAP-BC evaluation tool): development and interrater reliability. *PLoS ONE*. 2017;12(6). doi:10.1371/journal.pone.0179116.

42. Ault P, Plaza A, Paratz J. Scar massage for hypertrophic burns scarring: a systematic review. *Burns*. 2018;44(1):24–38. doi:10.1016/j.burns.2017.05.006.

43. Jacob T, Bracha J. Identification of signs and symptoms of axillary web syndrome and breast seroma during a course of physical therapy 7 months after lumpectomy: a case report. *Phys Ther*. 2019;99(2):229–239.

44. Koehler LA, Haddad TC, Hunter DW, Tuttle TM. Axillary web syndrome following breast cancer surgery: symptoms, complications, and management strategies. *Breast Cancer Targets Ther*. 2019;11:13–19.

45. De Rooij L, Bosmans J, van Kuijk S, Vissers Y, Beets G, van Bastelaar J. A systematic review of seroma formation following drain-free mastectomy. *Eur J Surg Oncol*. 2021;47(4):757–763. doi:10.1016/j.ejso.2020.10.010.

46. van Bastelaar J, Granzier R, van Roozendaal LM, Beets G, Dirksen CD, Vissers Y. A multi-center, double blind randomized controlled trial evaluating flap fixation after mastectomy using sutures or tissue glue versus conventional closure: protocol for the Seroma reduction After Mastectomy (SAM) trial. *BMC Cancer*. 2018;18(1):830. doi:10.1186/s12885-018-4740-8.

47. Stubblefield MD. Clinical evaluation and management of RFS. *Phys Med Rehabil Clin N Am*. 2017;27:89–100.

48. Stubblefield MD. Radiation fibrosis syndrome. In: Stubblefield MD, ed. *Cancer Rehabilitation: Principles and Practice*. 2nd ed. Springer; 2016:989–1011.

49. Popovski V, Benedetti A, Popovic-Monevska D, Grcev A, Stamatoski A, Zhivadinovik J. Spinal accessory nerve preservation in modified neck dissections: surgical and functional outcomes. *Acta Otorhinolaryngol Ital*. 2017;37(5):368–374.

50. Delanian S, Lefaix JL, Pradat PF. Radiation-induced neuropathy in cancer survivors. *Radiother Oncol*. 2012;105(3):273–282. doi:10.1016/j.radonc.2012.10.012.

51. Andrews CC, Smith SR. Graft-versus-host disease. In: Stubblefield MD, ed. *Cancer Rehabilitation: Principles and Practice*. 2nd ed. Springer; 2019:980–989.

52. Inamoto Y, Pidala J, Chai X, et al. Assessment of joint and fascia manifestations in chronic graft-versus-host disease. *Arthritis Rheumatol*. 2014;66(4):1044–1052.

53. Dhawan M, Nagel MP, Lilker R, Lacouture ME. Dermatologic complications of cancer and their treatment. In: Stubblefield MD, ed. *Cancer Rehabilitation: Principles and Practice*. 2nd ed. Springer; 2019:516–525.

54. Fernandes R, Mazzarello S, Hutton B, et al. Taxane acute pain syndrome (TAPS) in patients receiving taxane-based chemotherapy for breast cancer—a systematic review. *Support Care Cancer*. 2016;24(8):3633–3650. doi:10.1007/s00520-016-3256-5.

55. Seguin C, Kovacevich N, Voutsadakis IA. Docetaxel-associated myalgia-arthralgia syndrome in patients with breast cancer. *Breast Cancer Targets Ther*. 2017;9:39–44. doi:10.2147/BCTT.S124646.

56. Mijwel S, Backman M, Bolam KA, et al. Adding high-intensity interval training to conventional training modalities: optimizing health-related outcomes during chemotherapy for breast cancer: the OptiTrain randomized controlled trial. *Breast Cancer Res Treat*. 2018;168(1):79–93.

57. Beckwée, L Leysen, K Meuwis, N Adriaenssens, Prevalence of aromatase inhibitor-induced arthralgia in breast cancer: a systematic review and meta-analysis, *Support Care Cancer* 25 (5) (2017) 1673–1686, doi: 10.1007/s00520-017-3613-z.

58. Suskin J, Shapiro CL. Osteoporosis and musculoskeletal complications related to therapy of breast cancer. *Gland Surg*. 2018;7(4):411–423.

59. Seber S, Solmaz D, Yetisyigit T. Antihormonal treatment associated musculoskeletal pain in women with breast cancer in the adjuvant setting. *Onco Targets Ther*. 2016;9:4929–4935.

60. Basal C, Vertosick E, Gillis TA, et al. Joint pain and falls among women with breast cancer on aromatase inhibitors. *Support Care Cancer*. 2019;27(6):2195–2202.

61. Tzortzis V, Samarinas M, Zachos I, Oeconomou A, Pisters LL, Bargiota A. Adverse effects of androgen deprivation therapy in patients with prostate cancer: focus on metabolic complications. *Hormones*. 2017(2):115–123.

62. Nguyen C, Lairson DR, Swartz MD, Du XL. Risks of major long-term side effects associated with androgen-deprivation therapy in men with prostate cancer. *Pharmacother J Hum Pharmacol Drug Ther*. 2018;38(10):999–1009.

63. Russell N, Grossmann M. Management of bone and metabolic effects of androgen deprivation therapy. *Urol Oncol*. 2021;39(10):704–712. doi:10.1016/j.urolonc.2018.10.007.

64. Saylor PJ, Smith MR. Adverse effects of androgen deprivation therapy: defining the problem and promoting health among men with prostate cancer. *JNCCN J Natl Compr Cancer Netw*. 2010;8(2):211–223.

65. Yunfeng G, Weiyang H, Xueyang H, Yilong H, Xin G. Exercise overcome adverse effects among prostate cancer patients receiving androgen deprivation therapy. *Medicine (Baltimore)*. 2017;96(27):e7368. doi:10.1097/MD.0000000000007368.

66. Brahmer JR, Lacchetti C, Schneider BJ, et al. Management of immune-related adverse events in patients treated with immune checkpoint inhibitor therapy: American Society of Clinical Oncology Clinical Practice guideline. *J Clin Oncol*. 2018;36(17):1714–1768.

67. Petrelli F, Signorelli D, Ghidini M, et al. Association of steroids use with survival in patients treated with immune checkpoint inhibitors: a systematic review and meta-analysis. *Cancers (Basel)*. 2020;12(3):546. doi:10.3390/cancers12030546.

68. Haran M, Schattner A, Kozak N, Mate A, Berrebi A, Shvidel L. Acute steroid myopathy: a highly overlooked entity. *QJM*. 2018;111(5):307–311.

69. Ekelund U, Tarp J, Steene-Johannessen J, et al. Dose-response associations between accelerometry measured physical activity and sedentary time and all cause mortality: systematic review and harmonised meta-analysis. *BMJ*. 2019;366. doi:10.1136/bmj.l4570.

70. Klassen O, Schmidt ME, Ulrich CM, et al. Muscle strength in breast cancer patients receiving different treatment regimes. *J Cachexia Sarcopenia Muscle*. 2017;8(2):305–316.

71. Patel A V, Friedenreich CM, Moore SC, et al. Introduction: the American College of Sports Medicine convened an International Multidisciplinary Roundtable on Exercise. *Med Roundtable Rep Phys Act*. 2019;51(11):2391–2402.

72. Li R, Xia J, Zhang X, et al. Associations of muscle mass and strength with all-cause mortality among US older adults. *Med Sci Sports Exerc*. 2018;50(3):458–467. doi:10.1249/MSS.0000000000001448.

73. Borch KB, Braaten T, Lund E, Weiderpass E. Physical activity before and after breast cancer diagnosis and survival - the Norwegian women and cancer cohort study. BMC Cancer. 2015;15:967. doi:10.1186/s12885-015-1971-9.

74. Fassier P, Zelek L, Partula V, et al. Variations of physical activity and sedentary behavior between before and after cancer diagnosis: results from the prospective population-based NutriNet-Santé cohort. *Medicine (Baltimore)*. 2016;95(40):e4629. doi:10.1097/MD.0000000000004629.

75. Gaskin CJ, Craike M, Mohebbi M, et al. Associations of objectively measured moderate-to-vigorous physical activity and sedentary behavior with quality of life and psychological well-being in prostate cancer survivors. *Cancer Causes Control*. 2016;27(9):1093–1103.

76. Whitney RL, Bell JF, Tancredi DJ, Romano PS, Bold RJ, Joseph JG. Hospitalization rates and predictors of rehospitalization among individuals with advanced cancer in the year after diagnosis. *J Clin Oncol*. 2017;35(31):3610–3617.

77. Vanhorebeek I, Latronico N. Van den Berghe G. ICU-acquired weakness. *Intensive Care Med*. 2020;46(4):637–653.

78. Sáez de Asteasu ML, Martínez-Velilla N, Zambom-Ferraresi F, et al. Changes in muscle power after usual care or early structured exercise intervention in acutely hospitalized older adults. *J Cachexia Sarcopenia Muscle*. 2020;11(4):997–1006. doi:10.1002/jcsm.12564.

79. Ethun CG, Bilen MA, Jani AB, Maithel SK, Ogan K, Master VA. Frailty and cancer: implications for oncology surgery, medical oncology, and radiation oncology. *CA Cancer J Clin*. 2017;67(5):362–377. doi:10.3322/caac.21406.

80. Kirkhus L, Benth JŠ, Rostoft S, et al. Geriatric assessment is superior to oncologists' clinical judgement in identifying frailty. *Br J Cancer.* 2017;117(4):470–477. doi:10.1038/bjc.2017.202.

81. Apóstolo J, Cooke R, Bobrowicz-Campos E, et al. Effectiveness of interventions to prevent pre-frailty and frailty progression in older adults: a systematic review. *JBI Database Syst Rev Implement Rep.* 2018;16(1):140–232.

82. Kidd T, Mold F, Jones C, et al. What are the most effective interventions to improve physical performance in pre-frail and frail adults? A systematic review of randomised control trials. *BMC Geriatr.* 2019;19(1):184.

83. Fearon K, Strasser F, Anker SD, et al. Definition and classification of cancer cachexia: an international consensus. *Lancet Oncol.* 2011;12(5):489–495.

84. Cruz-Jentoft AJ, Bahat G, Bauer J, et al. Sarcopenia: revised European consensus on definition and diagnosis. *Age Ageing.* 2019;48(1):16–31.

85. Porporato PE. Understanding cachexia as a cancer metabolism syndrome. *Oncogenesis.* 2016;5(2):200. doi:10.1038/oncsis.2016.3.

86. Bruggeman AR, Kamal AH, LeBlanc TW, Ma JD, Baracos VE, Roeland EJ. Cancer cachexia: beyond weight loss. *J Oncol Pract.* 2016;12(11):1163–1171. doi:10.1200/JOP.2016.016832.

87. Marzetti E, Calvani R, Tosato M, et al. Sarcopenia: an overview. *Aging Clin Exp Res.* 2017;29(1):11–17. doi:10.1007/s40520-016-0704-5.

88. Beaudart C, McCloskey E, Bruyère O, et al. Sarcopenia in daily practice: assessment and management. *BMC Geriatr.* 2016;16(1):1–10. doi:10.1186/s12877-016-0349-4.

89. Beaudart C, Dawson A, Shaw SC, et al. Nutrition and physical activity in the prevention and treatment of sarcopenia: systematic review. *Osteoporos Int.* 2017;28(6):1817–1833.

90. Beckwée D, Delaere A, Aelbrecht S, et al. Exercise interventions for the prevention and treatment of sarcopenia. A systematic umbrella review. *J Nutr Heal Aging.* 2019;23(6):494–502.

91. Hardee JP, Counts BR, Carson JA. Understanding the role of exercise in cancer cachexia therapy. *Am J Lifestyle Med.* 2019;13(1):46–60.

92. Gilhus NE. Myasthenia gravis. *N Engl J Med.* 2016;375(26):2570–2581.

93. Farmakidis C, Pasnoor M, Dimachkie MM, Barohn RJ. Treatment of myasthenia gravis. *Neurol Clin.* 2018;36(2):311–337.

94. Westerberg E, Molin CJ, Lindblad I, Emtner M, Punga AR. Physical exercise in myasthenia gravis is safe and improves neuromuscular parameters and physical performance-based measures: a pilot study. *Muscle Nerve.* 2017;56(2):207–214.

95. Kesner VG, Oh SJ, Dimachkie MM, Barohn RJ. Lambert-Eaton myasthenic syndrome. *Neurol Clin.* 2018;36(2):379–394.

96. Sanders DB, Juel VC, Harati Y, et al. 3,4-diaminopyridine base effectively treats the weakness of Lambert-Eaton myasthenia. *Muscle Nerve.* 2018;57(4):561–568.

97. Mangone M, Bernetti A, Agostini F, et al. Changes in spine alignment and postural balance after breast cancer surgery: a rehabilitative point of view. *Biores Open Access.* 2019;8(1):121–128.

98. Seidenstuecker K, Legler U, Munder B, Andree C, Mahajan A, Witzel C. Myosonographic study of abdominal wall dynamics to assess donor site morbidity after microsurgical breast reconstruction with a DIEP or an ms-2 TRAM flap. *J Plast Reconstr Aesthet Surg.* 2016;69(5):598–603. doi:10.1016/j.bjps.2015.11.007.

99. Lee CH, Chung SY, Kim WY, Yang SN. Effect of breast cancer surgery on chest tightness and upper limb dysfunction. *Medicine (Baltimore).* 2019;98(19):e15524. doi:10.1097/MD.0000000000015524.

100. Yang S, Hwan Park D, Hyun Ahn S, et al. Prevalence and risk factors of adhesive capsulitis of the shoulder after breast cancer treatment. *Support Care Cancer.* 2017;25(4):1317–1322. doi:10.1007/s00520-016-3532-4.

101. Howlader N, Noone A, Krapcho MSEER. *Cancer Statistics Review, 1975–2016.* Bethesda, MD: National Cancer Institute; 2019.

102. Oishi T, Kogelschatz CJ, Young NP, et al. Expanded neuromuscular morbidity in Hodgkin lymphoma after radiotherapy. *Brain Commun.* 2020;2(1):fcaa050. doi:10.1093/braincomms/fcaa050.

103. DiFrancesco T, Khanna A, Stubblefield MD. Clinical evaluation and management of cancer survivors with radiation fibrosis syndrome. *Semin Oncol Nurs.* 2020;36(1):150982. doi:10.1016/j.soncn.2019.150982.

104. Harris AS. Do patients benefit from physiotherapy for shoulder dysfunction following neck dissection? A systematic review. *J Laryngol Otol.* 2020;134(2):104–108.

105. Kamstra JI, van Leeuwen M, Roodenburg JLN, Dijkstra PU. Exercise therapy for trismus secondary to head and neck cancer: a systematic review. *Head Neck.* 2017;39(11):2352–2362.

106. Keilani M, Kainberger F, Pataraia A, et al. Typical aspects in the rehabilitation of cancer patients suffering from metastatic bone disease or multiple myeloma. *Wien Klin Wochenschr.* 2019;131(21–22):567–575.

107. Academy of Acute Physical Therapy. Laboratory values interpretation resource; 2017. https://www.aptaacutecare.org/page/ResourceGuides.

108. Lee I-G, Im S-C, Kim K. Effects of pectoralis minor length on strength improvement and pain reduction during scapular reposition test. *J Phys Ther Sci.* 2020;32:42–47.

109. Fearmonti R, Bond J, Erdmann D, Levinson H. A review of scar scales and scar measuring devices. *Eplasty.* 2010;10:e43.

110. Azadinia F, Kamyab M, Behtash H, Saleh Ganjavian M, Javaheri MR. The validity and reliability of noninvasive methods for measuring kyphosis. *J Spinal Disord Tech.* 2014;27(6):E212–E218. doi:10.1097/BSD.0b013e31829a3574.

111. Academy of Oncologic Physical Therapy. Academy of Oncologic Physical Therapy EDGE Task Force Report Summaries; 2019.

112. Segal R, Zwaal C, Green E, Tomasone JR, Loblaw A, Petrella T. Exercise for people with cancer: a clinical practice guideline. *Curr Oncol.* 2017;24(1):40–46.

113. Campbell KL, Winters-stone KM, Wiskemann J, et al. Exercise guidelines for cancer survivors: consensus statement from international multidisciplinary roundtable. *Med Sci Sport Exerc.* 2019;51(11):2375–2390.

114. Mustian KM, Cole CL, Lin PJ, et al. Exercise recommendations for the management of symptoms clusters resulting from cancer and cancer treatments. *Semin Oncol Nurs.* 2016;32(4):383–393.

115. Stout NL, Baima J, Swisher AK, Winters-Stone KM, Welsh J. A systematic review of exercise systematic reviews in the cancer literature (2005–2017). *PM R.* 2017;9(9):S347–S384..

116. Cormie P, Zopf EM, Zhang X, Schmitz KH. The impact of exercise on cancer mortality, recurrence, and treatment-related adverse effects. *Epidemiol Rev.* 2017;39(1):71–92.

117. Newton RU, Galvão DA, Galvao G, et al. Exercise mode specificity for preserving spine and hip bone mineral density in prostate cancer patients. *Med Sci Sport Exerc.* 2019;51(4):607–614.

118. Almstedt HC, Grote S, Korte JR, et al. Combined aerobic and resistance training improves bone health of female cancer survivors. *Bone Rep.* 2016;5:274–279.

119. Padilha CS, Poliana PC, Marinello C, et al. Evaluation of resistance training to improve muscular strength and body composition in cancer patients undergoing neoadjuvant and adjuvant therapy: a meta-analysis. *J Cancer Surviv.* 2017;11(3):339–349. doi:10.1007/s11764-016-0592-x.

120. Rief H, Bruckner T, Schlampp I, et al. Quality of life and fatigue of patients with spinal bone metastases under combined treatment with resistance training and radiation therapy—a randomized pilot trial. *Radiat Oncol.* 2014;9(1). doi:10.1186/s13014-016-0675-x.

121. Rief H, Ackbar M, Keller M, et al. Quality of life and fatigue of patients with spinal bone metastases under combined treatment with resistance training and radiation therapy—a randomized pilot trial. *Radiat Oncol.* 2014;9(1):151. doi:10.1186/1748-717X-9-151.

122. Sheill G, Guinan EM, Peat N, Hussey J. Considerations for exercise prescription in patients with bone metastases: a comprehensive narrative review. *PM R*. 2018;10(8):843–864. doi:10.1016/j.pmrj.2018.02.006.

123. Hart NH, Galvão DA, Saunders C, et al. Mechanical suppression of osteolytic bone metastases in advanced breast cancer patients: a randomised controlled study protocol evaluating safety, feasibility and preliminary efficacy of exercise as a targeted medicine. *Trials*. 2018;19(1):695. doi:10.1186/s13063-018-3091-8.

124. Page P. Clinical Commentary: current concepts in muscle stretching for exercise and rehabilitation. *Int J Sports Phys Ther*. 2012;7(1):109–119.

125. Lee R, Yeo ST, Rogers SN, et al. Randomised feasibility study to compare the use of Therabite® with wooden spatulas to relieve and prevent trismus in patients with cancer of the head and neck. *Br J Oral Maxillofac Surg*. 2018;56(4):283–291.

126. van der Geer SJ, Reintsema H, Kamstra JI, Roodenburg JLN, Dijkstra PU. The use of stretching devices for treatment of trismus in head and neck cancer patients: a randomized controlled trial. *Support Care Cancer*. 2020;28(1):9–11.

127. Lin PJ, Peppone LJ, Janelsins MC, et al. Yoga for the management of cancer treatment-related toxicities. *Curr Oncol Rep*. 2018;20(1):5. doi:10.1007/s11912-018-0657-2.

128. Narayanan S, Francisco R, Lopez G, et al. Role of yoga across the cancer care continuum: from diagnosis through survivorship. *J Clin Outcomes Manag*. 2019;26(5):219–228.

129. de Almeida Rizzi SKL, Haddad CAS, Giron PS, et al. Early free range-of-motion upper limb exercises after mastectomy and immediate implant-based reconstruction are safe and beneficial: a randomized trial. *Ann Surg Oncol*. 2020;27(12):4750–4759.

130. Serra-Añó P, Inglés M, Bou-Catalá C, Iraola-Lliso A, Espí-López GV. Effectiveness of myofascial release after breast cancer surgery in women undergoing conservative surgery and radiotherapy: a randomized controlled trial. *Support Care Cancer*. 2019;27(7):2633–2641. doi:10.1007/s00520-018-4544-z.

131. Fereira OA, Satralkar A. Effectiveness of strain counterstrain technique and neural tissue mobilisation on cervicogenic headache. *Indian J Physiother Occup Ther*. 2017;11(3):57. doi:10.5958/0973-5674.2017.00073.9.

132. Kashyap R, Iqbal A, Alghadir AH. Controlled intervention to compare the efficacies of manual pressure release and the muscle energy technique for treating mechanical neck pain due to upper trapezius trigger points. *J Pain Res*. 2018;11:3151–3160.

133. Ferreira R, Resende R, Roriz P. The effects of Kinesio Taping® in lower limb musculoskeletal disorders: a systematic review. *Int J Ther Rehabil Res*. 2017;6(3):1–13. doi:10.5455/ijtrr.000000266.

134. Sheng Y, Duan Z, Qu Q, Chen W, Yu B. Kinesio taping in treatment of chronic non-specific low back pain: a systematic review and meta-analysis. *J Rehabil Med*. 2019;51(10):734–740.

135. Ouyang JH, Chang KH, Hsu WY, Cho YT, Liou TH, Lin YN. Non-elastic taping, but not elastic taping, provides benefits for patients with knee osteoarthritis: systemic review and meta-analysis. *Clin Rehabil*. 2018;32(1):3–17.

136. Ghozy S, Minh Dung N, Ebraheem Morra M, et al. Systematic review efficacy of kinesio taping in treatment of shoulder pain and disability: a systematic review and meta-analysis of randomised controlled trials. *Physiotherapy*. 2020;107:176–188.

137. Deflorin C, Hohenauer E, Stoop R, Van Daele U, Clijsen R, Taeymans J. Physical management of scar tissue: a systematic review and meta-analysis. *J Altern Complement Med*. 2020;26(10):854–865. doi:10.1089/acm.2020.0109.

138. Morris R, Lewis A. Falls and cancer. *Clin Oncol*. 2020;32(9):569–578. doi:10.1016/j.clon.2020.03.011.

139. Monfort SM, Pan X, Patrick R, et al. Gait, balance, and patient-reported outcomes during taxane-based chemotherapy in early-stage breast cancer patients. *Breast Cancer Res Treat*. 2017;164(1):69–77.

140. Schmitt AC, Repka CP, Heise GD, Challis JH, Smith JD. Comparison of posture and balance in cancer survivors and age-matched controls. *Clin Biomech (Bristol, Avon)*. 2017;50:1–6. doi:10.1016/j.clinbiomech.2017.09.010.

141. Dhawan S, Andrews R, Kumar L, Wadhwa S, Shukla G. A Randomized controlled trial to assess the effectiveness of muscle strengthening and balancing exercises on chemotherapy-induced peripheral neuropathic pain and quality of life among cancer patients. *Cancer Nurs*. 2020;43(4):269–280.

142. Shubert TE, Smith ML, Goto L, Luohua J, Ory MG. Otago exercise program in the United States: comparison of 2 implemented models. *Phys Ther*. 2017;97(2):187–197.

143. Guo Y, Ngo-Huang AT, Fu JB. Perspectives on spinal precautions in patients who have cancer and spinal metastasis. *Phys Ther*. 2020;100(3):554–563.

144. Mustian KM, Alfano CM, Heckler C, et al. Comparison of pharmaceutical, psychological, and exercise treatments for cancer-related fatigue: a meta-analysis supplemental content. *JAMA Oncol*. 2017;3(7):961–968.

145. Kessels E, Husson O, van der Feltz-Cornelis CM. The effect of exercise on cancer-related fatigue in cancer survivors: a systematic review and meta-analysis. *Neuropsychiatr Dis Treat*. 2018;14:479–494.

146. Ramin C, May BJ, Roden RBS, et al. Evaluation of osteopenia and osteoporosis in younger breast cancer survivors compared with cancer-free women: a prospective cohort study. *Breast Cancer Res*. 2018;20(1):1–10.

147. McLymont V. Nutritional care of the cancer patient. In: Stubblefield MD, ed. *Cancer Rehabilitation: Principles and Practice*. 2nd ed. Springer; 2016:847–852.

8

Neurological System

FRANNIE WESTLAKE, PT, DPT, BOARD CERTIFIED NEUROLOGIC AND ONCOLOGIC CLINICAL SPECIALIST

CHAPTER OUTLINE

Introduction

The neurological system is the true center for communication among every organ and structure within the body; it also provides communication from the external world to the internal body. Whether primary cancer or adverse effects from cancer treatment, the changes to this system undesirably impacts one's whole being and greatly affects their quality of life (QOL). All other systems of the body are regulated and powered by the neurological system and will be negatively influenced. It is estimated that in 2021 about 24,530 malignant tumors of the brain or spinal cord (13,840 in males and 10,690 in females) will be diagnosed in the United States (US). Approximately 18,600 people (10,500 males and 8100 females) will die from brain and spinal cord tumors during this same year.[1]

Anatomy of the Central Nervous System and Peripheral Nervous System (PNS)

The neurological system is composed of two systems: the central nervous system (CNS) and peripheral nervous system (PNS). The CNS is composed of the brain and spinal cord, while the PNS includes all of the peripheral nerves extending from the spinal cord, including the cranial and autonomic nerves (Figure 8.1).

Central Nervous System

The brain plays a central role in the control of bodily functions which include movements, sensation, thoughts, memory, and speech. The spinal cord is connected to the brain via the brain stem and helps to provide input and output signals to allow for participation in the environment.[2] The brain is surrounded by the blood–brain barrier (BBB) while the spinal cord is surrounded by the blood–spinal cord barrier (BSCB), both help to separate blood and the cerebrospinal fluid (Figure 8.2).

The BBB and the BSCB are similar in function and morphology which includes protecting the brain and spinal cord from toxic substances but still allows for molecules to cross for the purpose of maintaining brain and spinal cord activities. One of the key differences is that the BSCB is more easily penetrable than the BBB. This can lead to more inflammation and susceptibility to CNS disorders.[3]

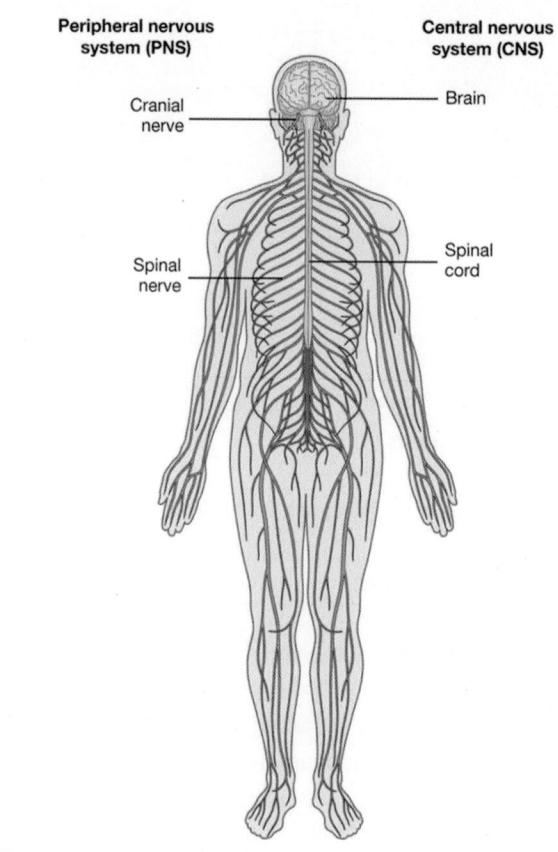

• **Fig. 8.1** Central and Peripheral Nervous System. (Reprinted with permission from Drake RL, Wayne Vogl A, Mitchell AWM. *Gray's Basic Anatomy*. 2nd ed. Elsevier; 2018:1–31.)

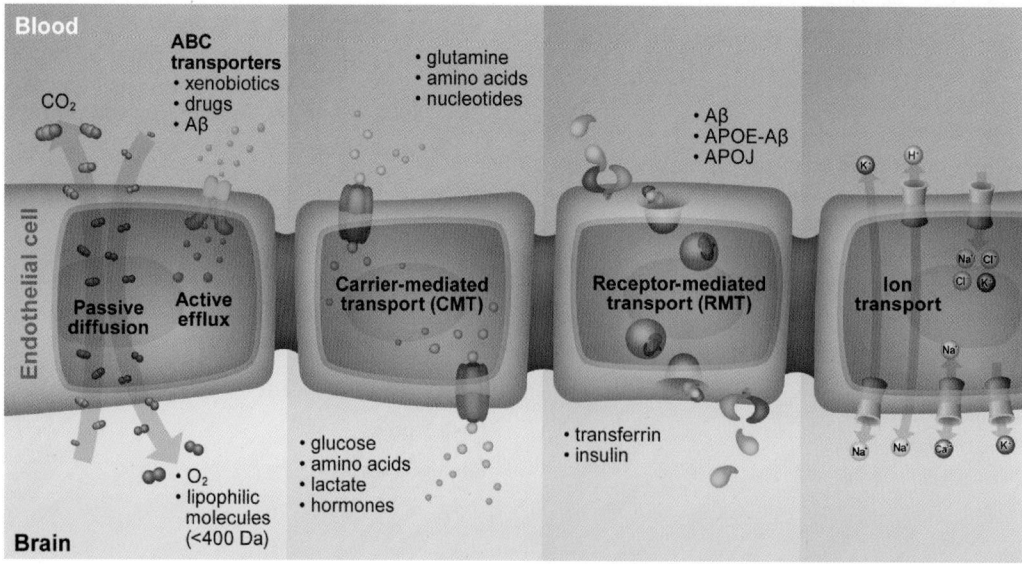

• **Fig. 8.2** Blood Brain Barrier and Blood Spinal Cord. (Reprinted with permission from Chen Y, Liu L. Modern methods for delivery of drugs across the blood-brain barrier. *Adv Drug Deliv Rev*. 2012;64(7):26.)

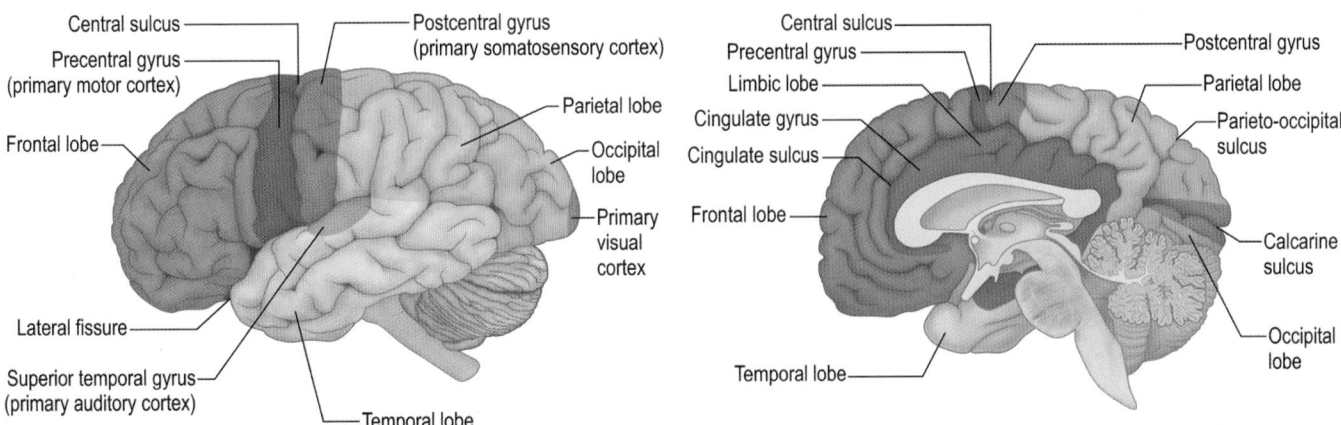

• **Fig. 8.3** Lobes of the Brain. (Reprinted with permission from Crossman AR, Neary D. *Neuroanatomy: An Illustrated Colour Text.* 6th ed. Elsevier; 2020:31.)

TABLE 8.1 Four Major Lobes of the Brain and Their Function

Frontal lobe	Responsible for voluntary movement and interacts with other lobes to participate in execution of sequential tasks, speech output, and aspects of behavior, mood, and memory.
Parietal lobe	Responsible for processing information such as pain, temperature, touch, and taste. It also interacts with other lobes to process information such as information about numbers, attention to the body's position, the space around the body and the relationship to this space.
Temporal lobe	Responsible for processing memory and auditory information. Also, performs speech and language functions.
Occipital lobe	Responsible for processing visual information.

Created by Frannie Westlake. Printed with permission.

TABLE 8.2 Central Structures of the Brain and Their Function

Thalamus	Integrates and relays sensory information to the cortex of the parietal, temporal, and occipital lobes. Located in the upper part of the brainstem and medially to the basal ganglia. It is also responsible for motor and memory control.
Hypothalamus	Located below the thalamus, and is responsible for regulating automatic functions (appetite, thirst, and body temperature). It also secretes hormones that stimulate or suppress the release of hormones in the pituitary gland.
Pituitary gland	Produces hormones that control functions of endocrine glands. It regulates the production of hormones that are responsible for growth, metabolism, sexual response, fluid/mineral balance, and stress response.
Cerebellum	Responsible for controlling equilibrium and coordination. It contributes to the generation of muscle tone.
Brainstem	Connects the brain and spinal cord. Includes the midbrain, pons and medulla oblongata. Allows for pathways to travel between the brain and spinal cord so there is response to input/output.

Created by Frannie Westlake. Printed with permission.

The brain has two hemispheres, right and left; and four lobes, the frontal, parietal, temporal, and occipital (Figure 8.3 and Table 8.1).

These lobes are connected by the corpus callosum. Among other functions, the right hemisphere controls movements on the left side of the body while the left hemisphere controls movements on the right side of the body. The cortex is made up of gray matter and is the external layer of the brain and contains neuronal cell bodies which contain DNA. This gray matter performs the storage and processing of information. The cells within the gray matter extend projections (axons) into other areas of the brain. There are other central structures of the brain (Table 8.2) that are important with the daily activities and performance of our bodies and response to various stimuli.[2]

Nerve fibers that exit the brain and spinal cord are classified as the peripheral nervous system. This includes all motor and sensory nerves, cranial nerves (Figure 8.4), and the autonomic nervous system, all of which are responsible for many functions and can be affected by cancer and cancer treatments. The cranial nerves are a part of the peripheral nervous system and can significantly be affected by chemotherapy (Figure 8.5 and Table 8.3 for detailed information on their functions).

Nerve roots that exit the spinal cord are named for the spinal cord segment for which they arise. Nerve roots that are anterior to the cord are called efferent (input towards limbs) and posterior are called afferent (input to spinal cord). The spinal cord has 30 segments that belong to four sections: cervical (8), thoracic (12), lumbar (5), sacral (5), coccygeal (1) (Table 8.4).[2]

Brain and Spinal Tumors

This section of the text will discuss primary brain and spinal cord tumors, metastatic disease to the brain and spinal cord, and other considerations for the CNS, for example, paraneoplastic syndrome and cerebrovascular complications of cancer.

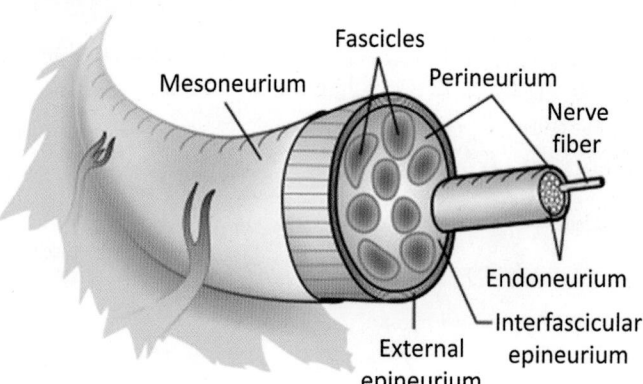

Mesoneurium · Fascicles · Perineurium · Nerve fiber · Endoneurium · Interfascicular epineurium · External epineurium

• **Fig. 8.4** Nerve Anatomy. (Reprinted with permission from Frost C, Rossonry GD. *Current Surgical Therapy.* 13th ed. Elsevier; 2020:854.)

TABLE 8.3 Cranial Nerves and Their Function

CN I: Olfactory	Sensory: Smell
CN II: Optic	Sensory: Vision
CN III: Oculomotor	Motor: 4 extrinsic eye muscles and pupillary response
CN IV: Trochlear	Motor: Superior oblique muscle
CN V: Trigeminal	Sensory: Ophthalmic: Scalp, forehead, and nose Maxillary: Cheeks, lower eye lid, nasal mucosa, upper lip, upper teeth, and palate Mandibular: Anterior 2/3 of tongue, skin over mandible and lower teeth Motor: Muscles of mastication
CN VI: Abducens	Motor: Lateral rectus muscle
CN VII: Facial	Sensory: External ear, taste from anterior 2/3 tongue, hard and soft palate Motor: Muscles of facial expression, lacrimal/submandibular/sublingual glands and mucous glands of nose and mouth
CN VIII: Vestibulocochlear	Sensory: Hearing and balance
CN IX: Glossopharyngeal	Sensory: Posterior 1/3 of tongue, external ear and middle ear cavity, carotid body and sinus, taste from posterior 1/3 tongue Motor: Parotid gland, stylopharyngeus
CN X: Vagus	Sensory: External ear, larynx, pharynx, thoracic/abdominal viscera, taste from epiglottis region of tongue Motor: Smooth muscles of pharynx and larynx
CN XI: Spinal Accessory	Motor: Trapezius and sternocleidomastoid
CN XII: Hypoglossal	Motor: Intrinsic and extrinsic tongue muscles

Created by Frannie Westlake. Printed with permission.

TABLE 8.4 Segments of the Spine and Their Function

Cervical Segments (8)	Transmit signals from or to areas of the head, neck, shoulders, arms, and hands
Thoracic Segments (12)	Transmit signals from or to areas of the arms, anterior/posterior chest, and abdomen.
Lumbar Segments (5)	Transmit signals from or to areas of the legs, feet, and pelvic organs
Sacral Segments (5)	Transmit signals from or to areas of the lower back, buttocks, pelvic organs, genital areas, and legs and feet

Created by Frannie Westlake. Printed with permission.

TABLE 8.5 World Health Organization Tumor Grade Descriptions

Grade I Tumor	Benign, slow growing, associated with long term survival
Grade II Tumor	Relatively slow growing, Cells look abnormal under microscope, can come back as higher grades
Grade III Tumor	Malignant, spreads into nearby normal parts of the brain
Grade IV Tumor	Most malignant, grows rapidly, forms new blood vessels to maintain rapid growth

Louis DN, Perry A, Wesseling P, et al. The 2021 WHO Classification of Tumors of the Central Nervous System: a summary. Neuro Oncol. 2021;23(8):1231–1251. doi:10.1093/neuonc/noab106.

Brain Tumors

The American Brain Tumor Association (ABTA) defines a brain tumor as "a growth of abnormal cells that have formed in the brain."[1] Tumors can be either benign or malignant. A benign tumor does not contain cancerous cells, but they often cause similar symptoms due to the size or pressure exerted on nearby structures and may require treatment including surgical or radiotherapy intervention. Malignant tumors contain cancerous cells, generally grow faster and more aggressively, and will invade other areas of the brain and spinal cord. Brain tumors are graded differently than other cancerous tumors (Table 8.5), as many times they do not grow outside of the primary lesion site. Brain tumors are classified as primary and metastatic.

A primary brain tumor originates from tissues of the brain or immediate surrounding areas. They are categorized as glial or non-glial cells (Figure 8.6), which develop on structures of the brain like nerves, blood vessels, and glands (Table 8.6).

Gliomas are the most prevalent brain tumor and account for 78% of malignant brain tumors.[1] They arise from the glia which are the supporting cells of the brain. Glial cells are subdivided into astrocytes, ependymal cells, and oligodendroglia cells. Astrocytes perform many functions in the brain and are known for their star shapes. Their functions include: (1) maintenance of the extracellular balance; (2) a role in the repair and scarring process after brain and spinal cord injuries; (3) biochemical support of the endothelial cells that form the BBB; and (4) provision of nutrients to the nervous tissue.[4] Astrocytes are the dominant glial cell in the brain and numerous studies indicate they are essential to the intracerebral immune response to *Toxoplasma gondii*, a parasite, in the brain. Ependymal cells line the ventricles and the central canal of the spinal cord.[5,6] Oligodendroglial cells provide support and insulation to axons in the CNS. They create the myelin sheath in the CNS and are similar to Schwann cells in the PNS.[6]

Metastatic tumors originate elsewhere in the body and then migrate to the brain through the circulatory system. The most common source of brain metastases is from lung cancer in males

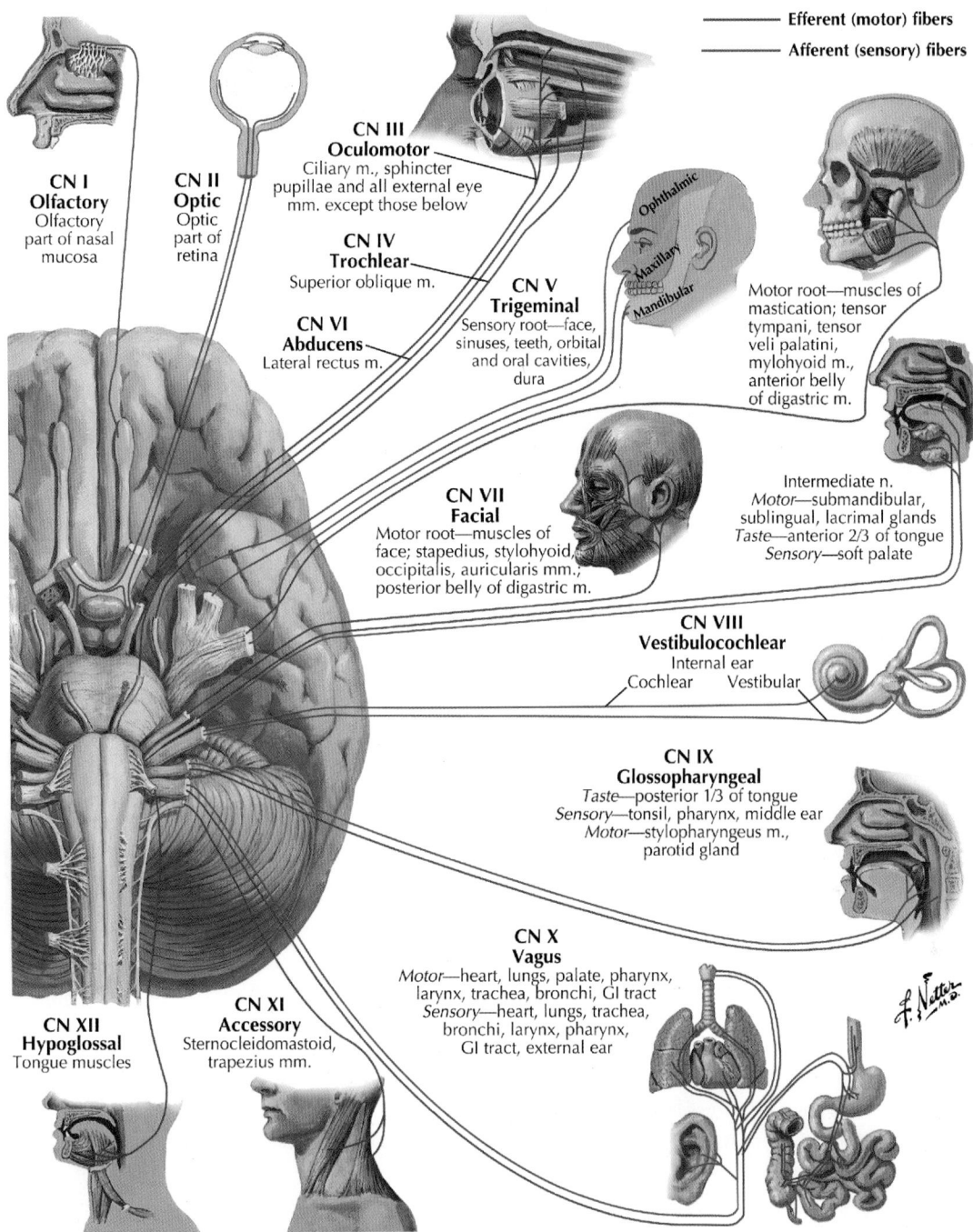

Efferent (motor) fibers
Afferent (sensory) fibers

CN I
Olfactory
Olfactory
part of nasal
mucosa

CN II
Optic
Optic
part of
retina

CN III
Oculomotor
Ciliary m., sphincter
pupillae and all external eye
mm. except those below

CN IV
Trochlear
Superior oblique m.

CN V
Trigeminal
Sensory root—face,
sinuses, teeth, orbital
and oral cavities,
dura

CN VI
Abducens
Lateral rectus m.

Ophthalmic
Maxillary
Mandibular

Motor root—muscles of
mastication; tensor
tympani, tensor
veli palatini,
mylohyoid m.,
anterior belly
of digastric m.

CN VII
Facial
Motor root—muscles of
face; stapedius, stylohyoid,
occipitalis, auricularis mm.;
posterior belly of digastric m.

Intermediate n.
Motor—submandibular,
sublingual, lacrimal glands
Taste—anterior 2/3 of tongue
Sensory—soft palate

CN VIII
Vestibulocochlear
Internal ear
Cochlear   Vestibular

CN IX
Glossopharyngeal
Taste—posterior 1/3 of tongue
Sensory—tonsil, pharynx, middle ear
Motor—stylopharyngeus m.,
parotid gland

CN X
Vagus
Motor—heart, lungs, palate, pharynx,
larynx, trachea, bronchi, GI tract
Sensory—heart, lungs, trachea,
bronchi, larynx, pharynx,
GI tract, external ear

CN XI
Accessory
Sternocleidomastoid,
trapezius mm.

CN XII
Hypoglossal
Tongue muscles

• **Fig. 8.5** Cranial Nerve. (Reprinted with permission from Frank H. Netter. Head and neck. In: *Atlas of Human Anatomy—3E*. 112. https://netterimages.com/cranial-nerves-distribution-of-motor-and-sensory-fibers-unlabeled-general-anatomy-frank-h-netter-3014.html.)

and breast cancer in females.[7] Other cancers that can metastasize to the brain include melanoma, colon, kidney, and thyroid gland.

Common Symptoms of Gliomas

Further description of glioma symptoms was established by the European Association for Neuro-Oncology (EANO) Guidelines for Palliative Care. They discuss in further detail headaches, epilepsy, venous thromboembolism, intracranial hemorrhage, anticoagulation, fatigue, and mood/behavior disorders. Below is an

example of each of these symptoms and how they present if a patient is diagnosed with a glioma.[8]

Headache

This is the primary pain reported by people diagnosed with a brain tumor. The pain typically presents from the tumor growth itself or the surrounding edema and can be a sign of intracranial pressure. Traditional medical management includes the use of corticosteroids (e.g., dexamethasone) given once a day but can increase to a higher dose and longer duration depending upon the person's

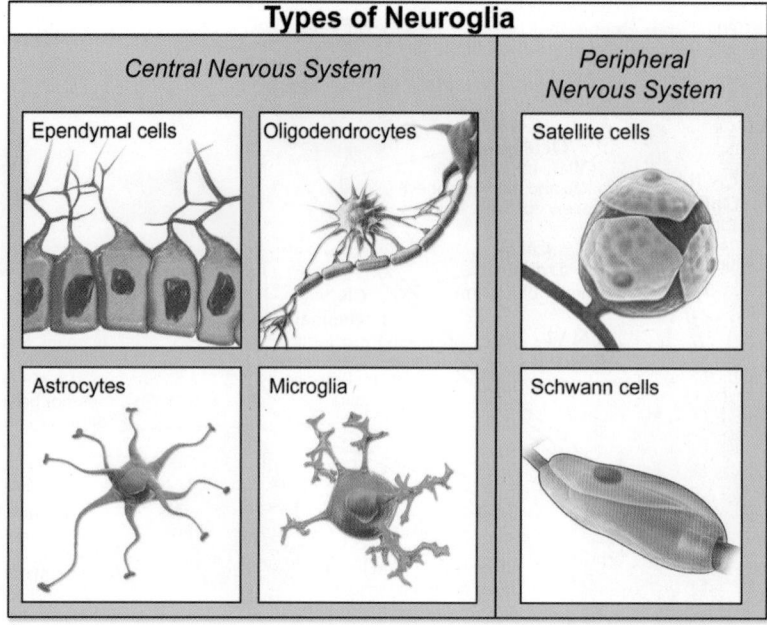

• **Fig. 8.6** Type of Neuroglia Cells. (Reprinted with permission from Medical gallery of Blausen Medical 2014. *WikiJournal Med.* 1(2).doi:10.15347/wjm/2014.010. ISSN 2002-4436.)

TABLE 8.6   Types of Brain Tumors

Chordomas	Benign	Prevalent between the ages of 50 and 60, most common location is base of skull and lower portion of spine.
Meningiomas	Benign	Most common benign intracranial tumor comprising of 10%–15% of all brain neoplasms. These tumors originate from the meninges.
Schwannomas	Benign	These tumors arise along the nerves and are comprised of cells that normally provide the electrical insulation of a nerve. Acoustic neuromas are the most common and they invade cranial nerve VIII.
Astrocytoma	Malignant	Most common glioma, accounts for almost half of all primary brain and spinal cord tumors. They occur most commonly in the cerebrum in adults and in the base of the brain in children. In children the tumors are mostly low grade and in adults they are high grade.
Glioblastoma multiforme (GBM)	Malignant	Most invasive type of glial tumor. They grow rapidly, spread to other tissues and have a poor prognosis. Most common in adults aged 50–70, are more prevalent in men than women.
Oligodendroglioma	Malignant	Derived from cells that make myelin which is the insulation for the wiring of the brain.
Ependymomas	Malignant	Derived from a neoplastic transformation of the ependymal cells lining the ventricular system and account for 2%–3% of all brain tumors.

Created by Frannie Westlake. Printed with permission.

needs. As a patient progresses in palliative care management, the use of opioids may be considered.

Epilepsy

Ninety percent of individuals diagnosed with a glioma will be treated for seizures at some point along their disease continuum.[8] This will be dependent upon the glioma subtype, tumor location, proximity to the brain cortex, and genetic factors. It is important to have adequate seizure control especially with the end-of-life process in these individuals. There have been studies to show an increase in the prevalence of seizures prior to death.[8] Swallowing function must be considered when selecting medication to manage a seizure.

Venous Thromboembolism

Any person with a history of cancer is at an increased risk of venous thromboembolism. In a person diagnosed with a glioma, the risk of venous thromboembolism peaks within the first 6 months after surgery especially in limbs that have impaired mobility, though there is an increase of intracranial hemorrhage when prophylaxis is started before induction of anesthesia. In cases where the tumor is bleeding, the duration of anticoagulation has to be weighed against the risk of intracranial hemorrhage.[8]

Fatigue

This is a common symptom and there are potential mechanisms that have been studied but primarily in rodent models or in human

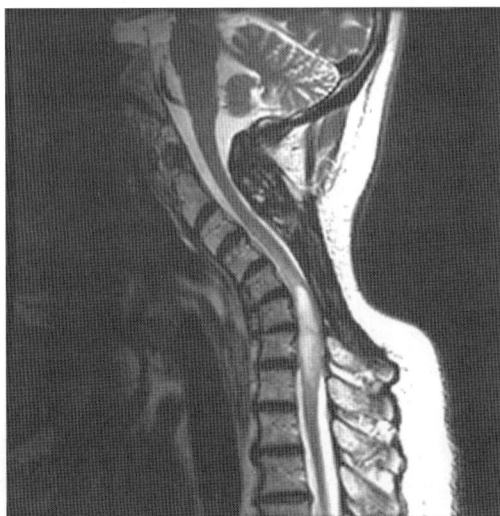

• **Fig. 8.7** Astrocytoma. (Reprinted with permission from DeAngelis LM. *Goldman-Cecil Medicine, 2-Volume Set.* Elsevier; 2020:1260–1270.e2.)

TABLE 8.7	Common Symptoms of a Brain Tumor[7]

- alteration in consciousness
- behavior changes
- focal neurological symptoms including changes in sensation or motor weakness
- headache
- hearing loss
- increased intracranial pressure
- personality changes
- seizures
- speech disturbance
- vomiting

American Association of Neurological Surgeons. Brain tumors. https://www.aans.org/en/Patients/Neurosurgical-Conditions-and-Treatments/Brain-Tumors. September 23, 2020. Accessed October 1, 2020.
Created by Frannie Westlake. Printed with permission.

studies of solid tumors of breast or lung cancer. In gliomas, the mechanisms considered as contributors to fatigue are the increase in blood levels of inflammatory cytokines, as well as decreased levels of glutamine and tryptophan in the brain which may disturb the circadian rhythms.[8] A recent study did not find strong evidence to support any pharmacological or nonpharmacological treatment for fatigue in persons diagnosed with brain tumors.[9] Despite this finding, it is important to remember that although nonpharmacological management has not been specifically studied in all aspects of cancer, it can be beneficial for the overall QOL for the person diagnosed with a glioma.

Mood and Behavioral Disorders

These are a major comorbidity for these individuals and their families. During a 6-month prevalence study, there was approximately a 20% prevalence of clinical depression and 60% prevalence of a new occurrence of a personality change dependent on the location of the tumor.[8] Treatment for these mood disorders need to be medically managed closely as there is minimal evidence of the effects of drug treatments in persons diagnosed with a primary brain tumor. The ABTA provides comprehensive statistics about the incidence of brain tumors (Table 8.8).

Spinal Tumors

Spinal tumors are categorized in two ways: by the region in which they occur (cervical, thoracic, lumbar, and sacral) and by their location in the spine (intradural-extramedullary, intramedullary, and extradural) (Figure 8.11 and 8.12).[10]

Intradural-extramedullary tumors are located inside the thick covering of the spinal cord but outside the actual spinal cord, which accounts for 40% of spinal tumors.[10] The common tumors in this area are meningiomas, schwannomas, neurofibromas, and ependymomas. Meningiomas that develop in the arachnoid membrane are benign but can be difficult to surgically remove. Schwannomas and neurofibromas, which are benign nerve root tumors, can become malignant over time if they are not treated.

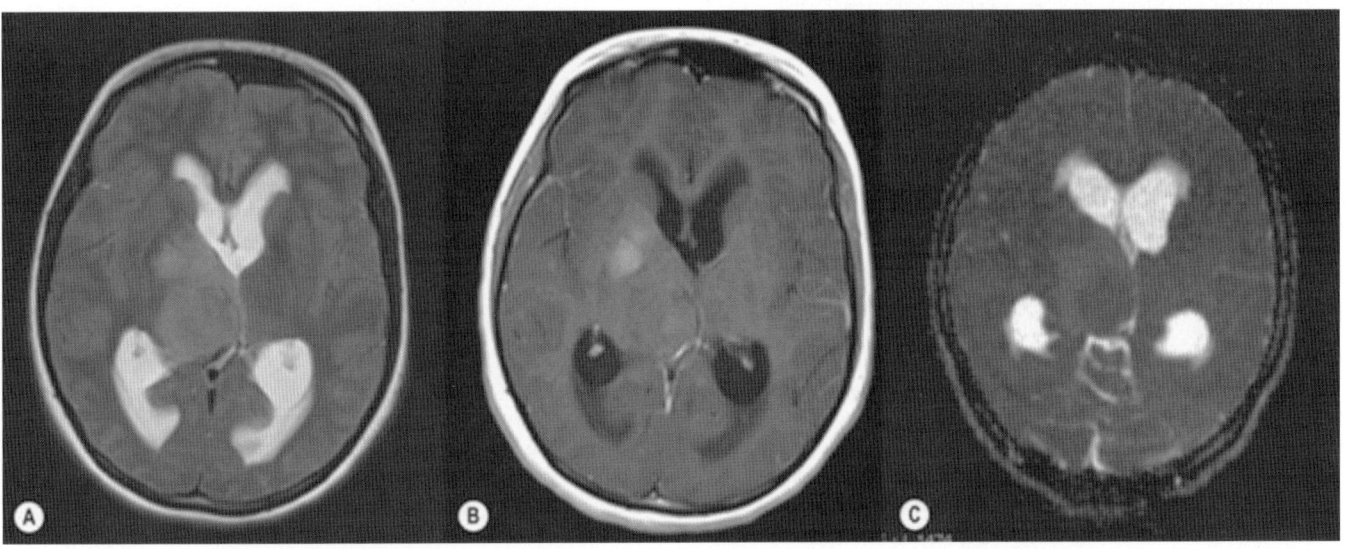

• **Fig. 8.8** Glioma. (Reprinted with permission from Jin Y, Peng H, Peng J. Brain glioma localization diagnosis based on magnetic resonance imaging. *World Neurosurg.* 2021;149:325–332.)

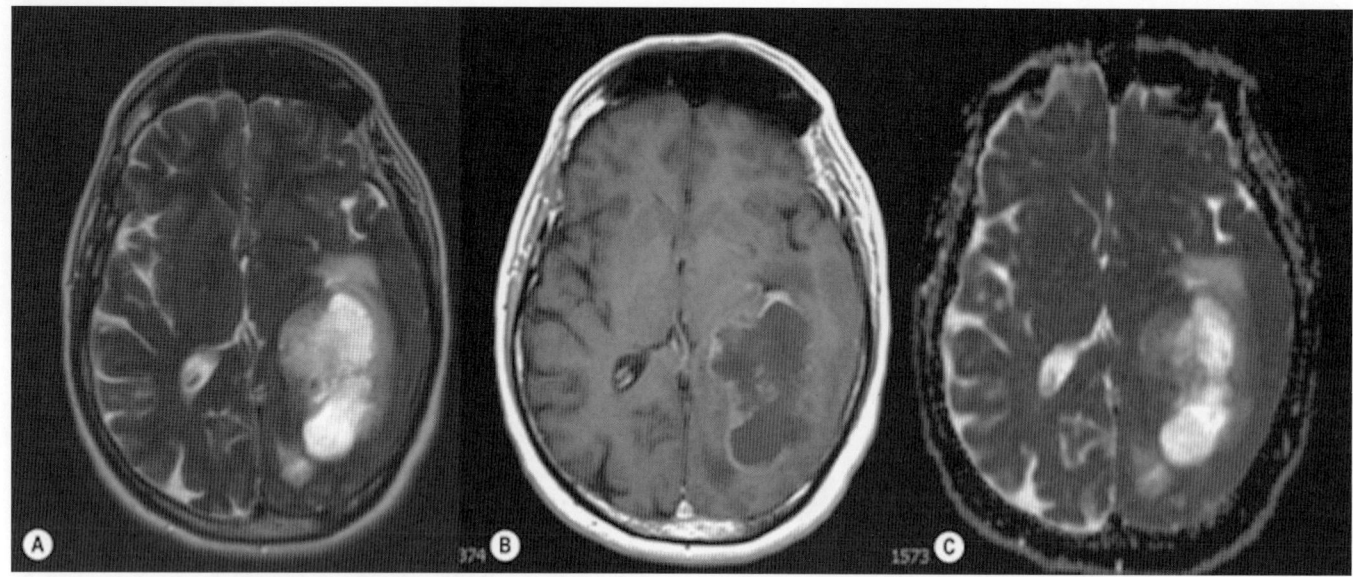

• **Fig. 8.9** Glioblastoma. (Reprinted with permission from Masdeu JC, Ajtai B, Faridar A. Bradley and Daroff's Neurology in Clinical Practice, 2-Volume Set. Elsevier; 2021:53.)

TABLE 8.8	**Brain Tumor Statistics**[1]

- Over 700,000 Americans are living with a brain tumor
- Nearly 80,000 people are diagnosed with a primary brain tumor every year
- 1/3 of brain and CNS tumors are malignant
- 28,000 children in the United States are diagnosed with brain tumors
- In 2020, nearly 16,000 people will die as a result of a brain tumor.
- The median age at diagnosis for all primary brain tumors is 60 years old
- Brain tumors are the second most common cancer among children 0–14, and they are the leading cause of cancer-related deaths in this age group
- Metastatic tumors affect nearly one in four patients with cancer
- Metastatic brain tumors are five times more common than primary brain tumors
- Up to 40% of patients with lung cancer will develop metastatic brain tumors

American Brain Tumor Association. Brain tumor education. https://www.abta.org/about-brain-tumors/brain-tumor-education/. June 28, 2020.
Created by Frannie Westlake. Printed with permission.

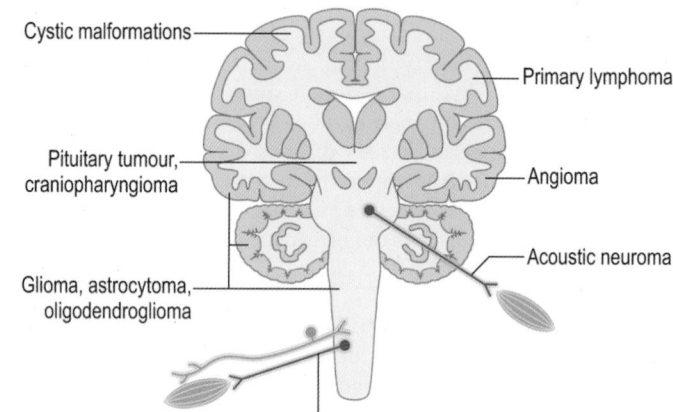

• **Fig. 8.10** Common Locations of Brain Tumors. (Reprinted with permission from Crossman AR, Neary D. *Neuroanatomy: An Illustrated Colour Text.* 6th ed. Elsevier; 2020.)

Ependymomas are typically large, benign tumors found at the base of the spinal cord. They can be difficult to remove due to the proximity to delicate neural structures in this area.

Intramedullary tumors grow inside the spinal cord. These typically derive from glial or ependymal cells. They are rare, comprising only 5% of all spinal tumors.[10] Astrocytomas (arising from glial cells) most commonly occur in the thoracic region followed by the cervical region. Ependymomas are most common in the filum terminale, which is the inferior most portion of the spinal cord, located at approximately the second lumbar vertebrae region of the spinal canal. Intramedullary ependymomas are typically benign or low grade as compared to intracranial ependymomas, but they can be difficult to remove.[10]

Extradural tumors are located outside the dura. The largest majority of spinal tumors develop in this extradural location at a frequency of 55%.[10] These lesions are often attributed to metastatic cancer and on occasion, can be located both within and outside of the spinal canal. The most common primary spinal tumor that originates in the bony spine is vertebral hemangiomas. These are benign and typically asymptotic. Table 8.9 lists the common signs and symptoms of spinal cancer.[10]

Metastasis to the Brain and Spinal Cord

Metastatic tumors originate elsewhere in the body and then migrate to the brain through the circulatory system. Between 30% and 70% of patients with metastatic cancer will experience spread of cancer to their spine. In spinal cord metastasis, the bony spinal column is the most common site of metastasis.[10] The most common primary cancers to spread to the spine are lung, breast, and prostate. Other cancers that can spread to the brain and spinal

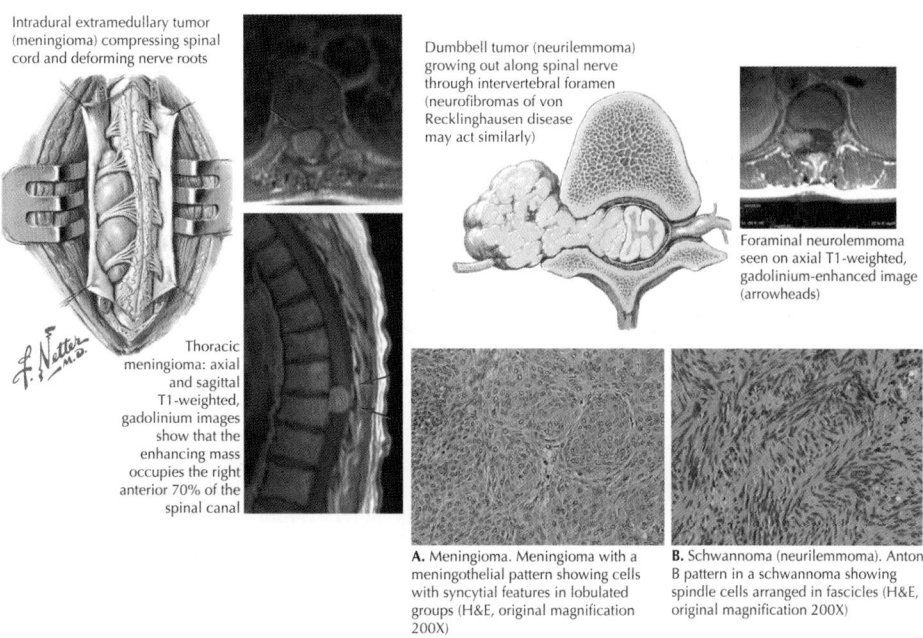

A. Meningioma. Meningioma with a meningothelial pattern showing cells with syncytial features in lobulated groups (H&E, original magnification 200X)

B. Schwannoma (neurilemmoma). Antoni B pattern in a schwannoma showing spindle cells arranged in fascicles (H&E, original magnification 200X)

• **Fig. 8.11** Intradural Extramedullary Tumor. (Reprinted with permission from Royden Jones H. Spinal cord tumors. In: *Netter's Neurology 2E*. 488. Netterimages.com.)

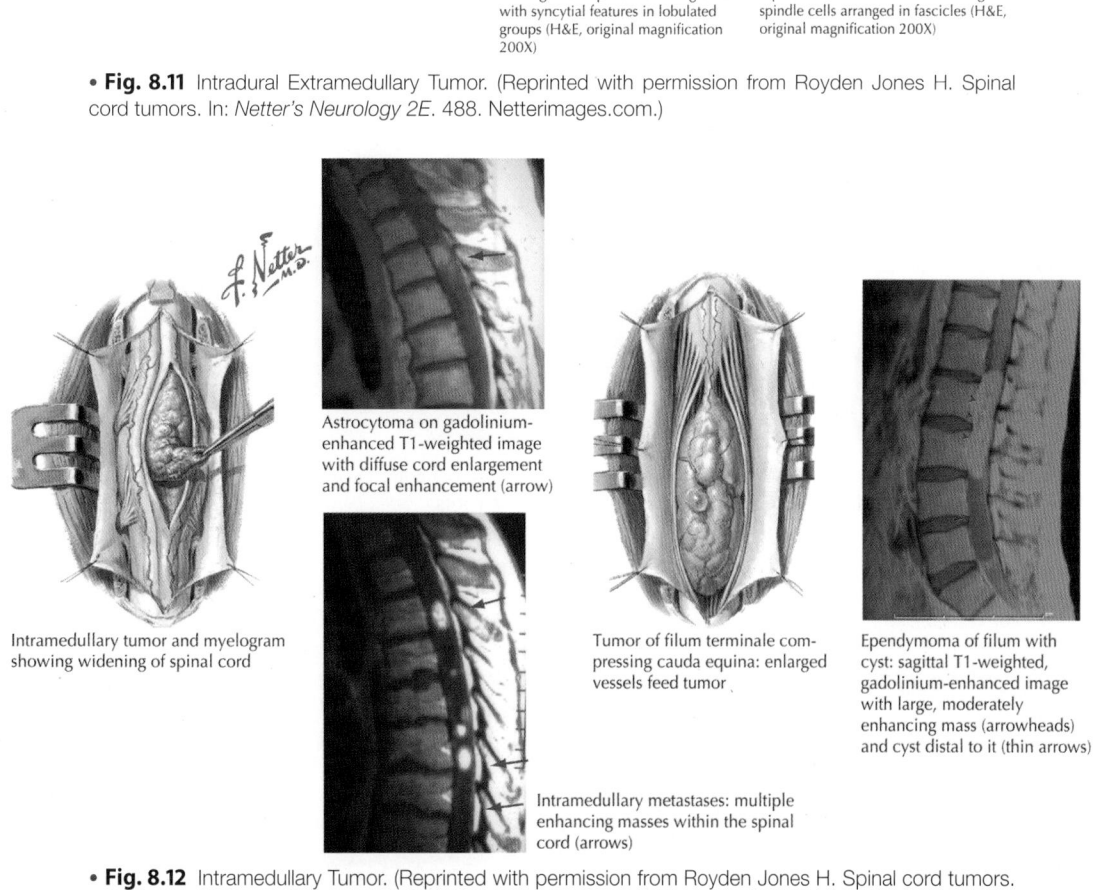

• **Fig. 8.12** Intramedullary Tumor. (Reprinted with permission from Royden Jones H. Spinal cord tumors. In: *Netter's Neurology 2E*. 490. https://netterimages.com/intradural-intramedullary-primary-spinal-cord-tumors-unlabeled-neurology-frank-h-netter-63077.html.)

cord include multiple myeloma, lymphoma, melanoma, sarcoma, gastrointestinal, kidney, and thyroid.

Other Considerations of CNS Syndromes

Paraneoplastic Neurological Syndromes

Paraneoplastic neurological syndromes are defined as remote effects of cancer that are not caused by the tumor and its metastasis, or by metabolic distributions, ischemia, or infections. These syndromes are rare and can affect 1 in 10,000 patients with cancer.[11] They can affect any part of the CNS and PNS, the neuromuscular junction or muscle. Currently it is thought that most or all paraneoplastic neurologic disorders are immune mediated.[12] These syndromes are caused by autoimmune processes triggered by the cancer and directed against antigens common to both the cancer and the nervous system. Many times, the patients with paraneoplastic neurological syndromes will exhibit changes in their neurological

| TABLE 8.9 | Common Signs and Symptoms of Spinal Cancer[10] |

- nonmechanical back pain
- loss of sensation or muscle weakness in legs, arms, and chest
- pain and/or neurologic symptoms that increase with a Valsalva maneuver
- difficulty walking
- decreased sensitivity to pain, heat, or cold
- loss of bowel or bladder function

American Association of Neurological Surgeons. Spinal tumors. https://www.aans.org/en/Patients/Neurosurgical-Conditions-and-Treatments/Spinal-Tumors. Accessed October 1, 2020. Created by Frannie Westlake. Printed with permission.

system prior to the cancer being clinically overt, such as encephalitis, ataxia, neuropathy, myoclonus, and psychiatric disturbances. Diagnosis is commonly made through presence of onconeural protein antibodies in blood. About 1/3 of persons diagnosed with paraneoplastic neurological syndromes have detectable antibodies and 5% to 10% will have an atypical antibody that is not well characterized.[11]

The best way to stabilize paraneoplastic neurological syndromes is to stabilize the cancer, though it is important to note that not all individuals with a paraneoplastic neurological syndrome will be diagnosed with cancer. The incidence of cancer can range from 5% to 60%.[11] In 80% of individuals, the diagnosis of the paraneoplastic neurological syndrome antedates that diagnosis of cancer by several months to several years.[11] If the person does have positive antibodies, the search for the cancerous tumor begins, typically

Extradural tumors

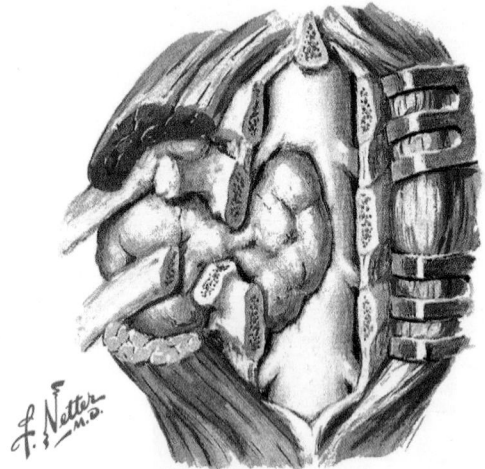

Lymphoma invading spinal canal via intervertebral foramen, compressing dura mater and spinal cord

Intradural extramedullary tumors

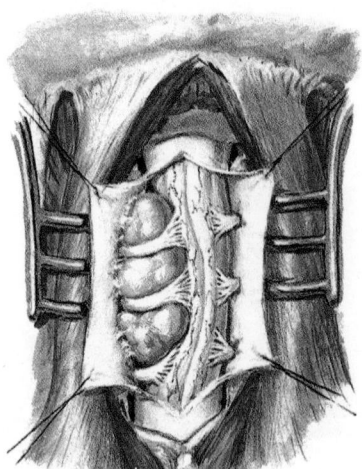

Meningioma compressing spinal cord and distorting nerve roots

Intramedullary tumors

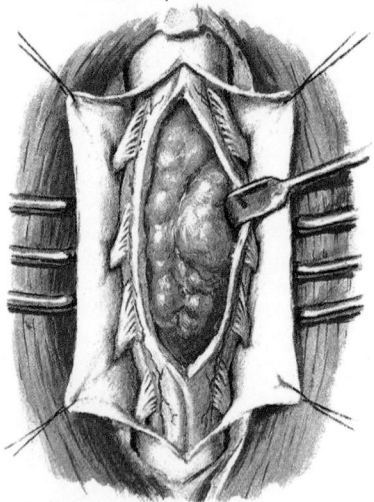

Astrocytoma exposed by longitudinal incision in bulging spinal cord

• **Fig. 8.13** Types of Spinal Tumors. (Reprinted with permission from Royden Jones H. Brain tumors. In: *Netter's Neurology 2E*. 484. https://netterimages.com/myelographic-and-ct-characteristics-of-spinal-tumors-labeled-jones-2e-neurology-neurosciences-frank-h-netter-63313.html.)

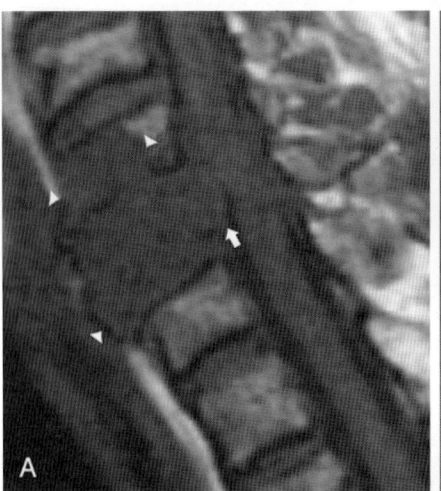

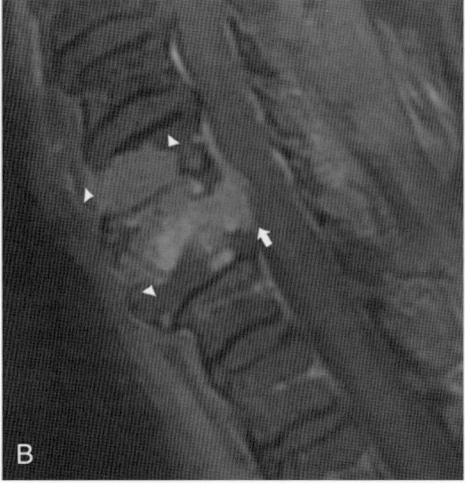

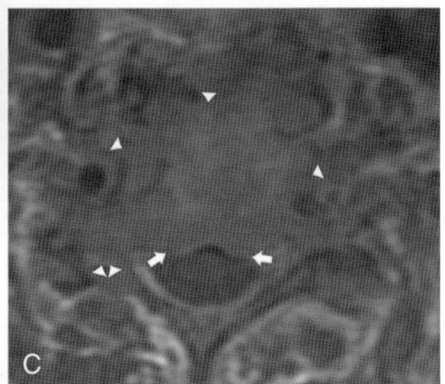

• **Fig. 8.14** Images of Brain and Spinal Metastatic Cancer. (Reprinted with permission from Hong B, Nakamura M, Brandis A, Becker H, Krauss JK. Spinal metastasis of papillary tumor of the pineal region. *Clin Neurol Neurosurg*. 2011;113(3):235–238.)

with a computerized tomography (CT) scan if lung cancer is suspected or a breast/pelvic exam with mammography and pelvic CT, if a gynecological tumor is anticipated. Primarily treatment or at least stabilization of a paraneoplastic neurological syndrome is to treat the cancer. Paraneoplastic neurological syndrome treated by itself rarely improves with immunomodulatory treatment. The use of intravenous immunoglobulins, steroids, or plasmapheresis has been found to be helpful.[11]

Lambert-Eaton Myasthenic Syndrome

LEMS occurs in about 1% of persons diagnosed with small cell lung cancer (SCLC).[11] LEMS is defined as an autoimmune disorder at the neuromuscular junction that is characterized by muscle weakness and autonomic dysfunction. Electromyography testing in a patient with LEMS reveals a low compound muscle action potential. Almost 60% of those diagnosed with LEMS also have a diagnosis of SCLC detected within 2 years of the diagnosis of LEMS. In rare cases, these individuals can also develop cerebellar degeneration.[11]

Cerebrovascular Complications of Cancer

A variety of cerebrovascular disorders can be found in the cancer population which may be a direct or indirect result of the tumor. Early recognition of acute stroke within the cancer population is vital to improve the overall patient outcome.[13] Intratumoral parenchymal hemorrhage and subdural hemorrhage can be related to the tumor. Metastatic tumors are more often associated with hemorrhage than primary tumors. Predisposing factors associated with intratumoral hemorrhage include head trauma, hypertension, coagulopathy, shunting procedures, and anticoagulation.[13] Factors related to the histology are rapid tumor growth, tumor necrosis, vessel thrombosis, tumor invasion of cerebral vessels, or vessel wall degeneration.[13] These individuals may benefit from treatment with steroids and external radiation to help with cerebral edema. Surgical evacuation of the hemorrhage may be performed dependent upon individual's presentation. Subdural hemorrhages are typically associated with dural tumor metastasis. Treatment of this type of tumor is palliative and can include drainage of subdural fluid, brain radiation, and even surgical evacuation. If surgery is performed, it is important to adequately biopsy

the dural membrane, after which radiation can be performed once the diagnosis is confirmed.[13]

Medical Assessment Tools

Medical assessments that are performed specifically for persons diagnosed with brain and spinal cord tumors are important to understand how the initial diagnosis is made and subsequent follow-up assessments help determine treatment.

Magnetic Resonance Imaging/Computed Tomography Scan/Positron Emission Tomography

High-Definition Fiber Tractography

High-definition fiber tractography (HDFT) is an advanced MRI-based noninvasive imaging technique pioneered by researchers at the University of Pittsburg School of Medicine. HDFT allows direct visualization of the three-dimensional structure of the axonal fiber damage and loss of cortical projections as well as quantifies the degree damage and predicts functional deficits. HDFT provides a presurgical evaluation of the damage to the fiber tracts of the underlying white matter, that, in combination with neuroanatomical knowledge, is able to design a less invasive trajectory into a target lesion[14] (Figure 8.15).

Computed Tomography

A CT scan is a noninvasive diagnostic imaging that uses X-ray beams to produce horizontal or axial slices of the brain. Brain CTs can provide more detailed information about the brain tissue and brain structures. These can be done with or without contrast. A CT may be performed to assess brain tumors, intracranial bleeding, and structural anomalies especially when another exam may be inconclusive.[15]

Brain Perfusion Scan

A brain perfusion scan is an image that shows the amount of blood taken up in certain areas of your brain. A single photon emission computed tomography (SPECT) scan or a positron emission tomography (PET) scan uses radiotracers which emit tiny

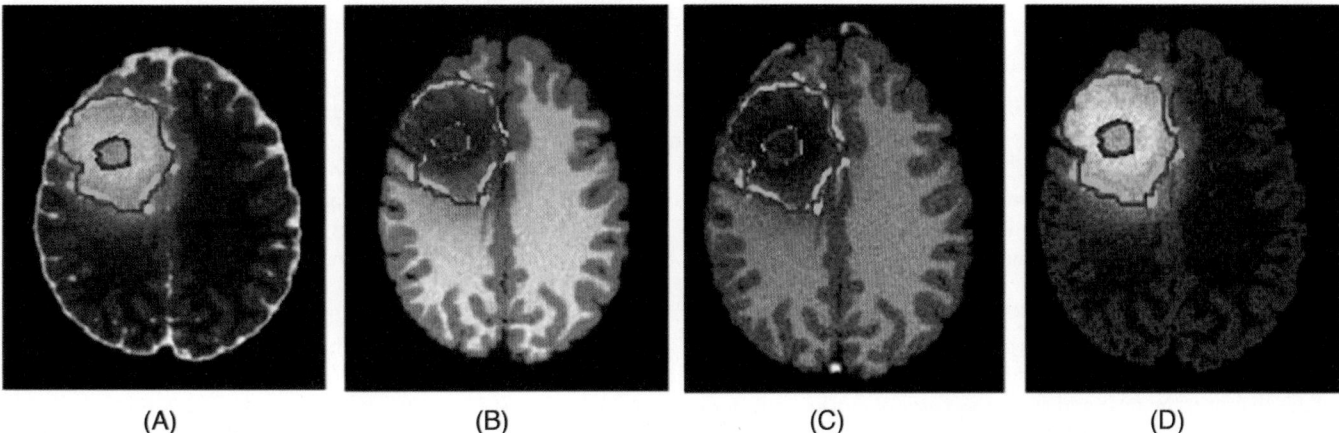

(A)   (B)   (C)   (D)

• **Fig. 8.15** Brain MRI Image. Blue curve = tumor, red curve = edema, yellow curve = tumor ground truth, green curve = edema ground truth. (A) T2 image; (B) T1 image; (C) T1C image; (D) FLAIR image. (Reprinted with permission from Njeh I, Sallemi L, Ayed IB, et al. 3D multimodal MRI brain glioma tumor and edema segmentation: a graph cut distribution matching approach. *Comput Med Imaging Graph*. 2015;40:108–119.)

particles that are radioactive. The areas of the brain that are more active show a greater blood supply as well as greater oxygen and glucose use. It is important to note areas where there is less activity as this area of the brain may be impaired.[15]

Sensory Evoked Potentials

Sensory evoked potentials are studies that measure electrical activity in the brain in response to stimulation by sight, sound, or touch. A visual evoked response test can diagnose problems with the optic nerves that affect sense. Electrodes are placed along the scalp and record signals as a checkerboard pattern is flashed across a screen for several minutes. Brainstem auditory evoked response test can diagnose hearing ability and can point to brainstem tumors or multiple sclerosis. Electrodes are placed along the scalp and earlobes, and an auditory stimulus such as a clicking noise or tone is delivered to one ear and then the other. Somatosensory evoked response can detect problems in the spinal cord that cause numbness of the arms and legs. Electrodes are placed on the wrist, back of knee, and other specific locations. An electrical stimulation is sent through the electrode which sends a signal to the electrodes placed on the scalp to determine how long the signal takes to travel along the nerves to the brain.[16]

Cerebrospinal Fluid Analysis

Lumbar puncture requires a hollow needle to be inserted into the subarachnoid space of the spinal column in the lower back. CSF a clear fluid that cushions the brain and spinal cord and contains cells, water, protein, sugars, and other substances that are essential to maintain balance in the nervous system. After a lumbar puncture, the fluid is analyzed for pathology or for other diagnostic purposes.[17] Typically a patient is advised to lay supine for several hours (usually 4 hours) after a lumbar puncture to preven the onset of a headache from the reduced CSF volume.

Medical Treatment for Primary and Metastatic Brain and Spinal Cord Tumors

This next section includes a description of medical treatment for primary and metastatic brain and spinal cord tumors that includes surgery, radiation, chemotherapy, including treatment adverse effects and considerations.

Surgery

The three most common types of brain surgeries include: (1) endoscopic endonasal approach (EEA); (2) craniotomy including expanded bifrontal craniotomy and supraorbital craniotomy; and (3) spinal tumor resection including posterolateral resection, en bloc resection and metastatic tumor surgery.

Endoscopic Endonasal Approach

EEA is a surgical technique that is used to remove brain tumors and lesions through the nose. This is the only minimally invasive procedure that uses the nose and sinuses as corridors to access tumors at the base of the skull or top of the spine. EEA can help to resect tumors that were once considered inoperable due to the extensive damage that would have been done to the face and skull. EEA is most used for sellar and parasellar lesions, such as a pituitary adenoma. A specially designed endoscope is used to provide light and

a lens for viewing the internal images, while small tools are placed in the other nostril to perform the surgical removal. The tools are diamond-encrusted to help minimize bleeding during the surgical procedure.[14]

Craniotomy

A craniotomy is a surgical removal of part of the skull to expose the brain. In oncology, a craniotomy is used to gain access to and resect a brain tumor. The section of the bone removed, called a bone flap, is replaced when the surgical procedure has been completed. This differs from a craniectomy, a procedure where the bone flap is permanently or temporarily removed. Craniectomies are often performed when there is significant brain swelling. The bone flap may be replaced during a second surgery once the cerebral edema has decreased.

Expanded bifrontal craniotomy is a traditional skull-based approach used to target difficult tumors toward the anterior portion of the brain. An incision is made in the scalp behind the hairline and the portion of the skull is removed that forms the contour of the orbits and forehead. This procedure is typically used for meningiomas, esthesioneuroblastomas, and malignant skull-based tumors that are not a candidate for EEA because of anatomy, possible pathology of the tumor, or goals of surgery.[18]

Supra-Orbital Craniotomy

Supra-orbital craniotomy is performed to remove pituitary tumors when the tumor is too large or too close to the optic nerves or vital arteries for EEA. A small incision is made within the eyebrow to access these tumors in the front of the brain.[18]

Retro-Sigmoid Craniotomy

Retro-sigmoid craniotomy is used to remove meningiomas or vestibular schwannomas/acoustic neuromas. With this procedure, an incision is made behind the ear and provides access to the cerebellum and brain stem.[18]

Patients typically remain in the hospital for 3 to 7 days after craniotomy, and depending upon their deficits, they may require inpatient rehabilitation before returning home.[18]

Spinal Tumor Resection

Surgery is not typically the first line of treatment for spinal tumors. Surgical removal of a tumor carries the additional risk of causing damage to the spinal cord or nerves.[19] Surgical resection of the tumor may be indicated when there is spinal cord compression, if the tumor is not responding to conventional radiation therapy, or there is spinal instability that a minimally invasive procedure cannot fix.

Posterolateral resection is a procedure used to remove the spinal tumor and reinforce the spine via a posterior midline incision. This allows the surgeon a direct route to the ventral canal. Typically, hardware is required to stabilize the spine where the tumor was previously located.[19]

En bloc resection is used to remove a tumor in a single piece. This is used to completely eliminate primary tumors that are located in bones of the spine or next to the spine.[19]

Metastatic spine tumor surgery can include both spinal cord decompression and spinal instrumentation decompression to relieve pressure and create space to allow for high-dose radiation without causing risk to the spinal cord. Instrumentation often includes the placement of pedicle screws and rods to redistribute stress and align the spine. This procedure is performed when there is significant spinal cord compression or a collapsed vertebra or burst fracture that cannot be repaired with a kyphoplasty.[19]

Radiation

See Chapter 5 for background and general procedures for radiation therapy. Here specific radiation for brain and spinal cord tumors will be discussed.

Whole Brain Radiation

Individuals with multiple brain metastases or an aggressive primary tumor may benefit from whole brain radiotherapy. Whole brain radiotherapy is often used to treat metastatic brain tumors and can extend survival from 1 to 2 months to 6 months, and it was found that fractionation schedules (radiation therapy lasting for several weeks) did not influence survival.[20] Fractionation is a process by which an radiation therapy dose is divided into multiple smaller (or a fraction) parts, thus requiring multiple treatments with a smaller amount of radiation therapy. This procedure aims to maximize malignant cell destruction while protecting and decreasing the damage to the healthy tissues. There are multiple long-term adverse effects of whole brain radiation therapy including but not limited to neurocognitive decline and early onset dementia.[20]

Spinal Tumors

Both internal and external radiation therapy can be part of the treatment plan for spinal tumors. Benefits of radiation therapy for these tumors include pain reduction, eliminating metastatic spine tumors, shrinking tumors for easier removal, and preventing the recurrence of spinal tumors.

Brachytherapy

Brachytherapy is a form of internal radiation therapy where high doses of radiation therapy are placed into the tumor for a short time period. Brachytherapy plaques are thin pieces of silicone that are coated with a high-dose radioactive film which are applied directly to tumor cells. For spinal tumors, this film is placed during surgery and then removed before the operation ends. Brachytherapy catheters are inserted into or near the tumor while the patient is under general anesthesia. After placement, a prescribed amount of radiation therapy is dispensed through each catheter. A patient undergoing this procedure will remain hospitalized until the catheters are removed.[19]

Common Adverse Events From Radiation

Nerve Palsies or Plexopathies

Radiation-induced polyneuropathy (RIPN) is a progressive, usually irreversible adverse effect of radiation therapy that may appear months to years after radiotherapy.[21] While the occurrence of RIPN is rare, <1% to 2% in persons receiving usual plexus total doses of <55 Gy,[21] rates are increasing due to improved long-term cancer survival. The pathophysiology is not yet understood but nerve compression by indirect extensive radiation therapy fibrosis likely plays a central role. It is thought that there is also axonal damage and demyelination as well as injury to blood vessels by ischemia following capillary network failure. Electroneuromyography is used to identify the level of plexus injury. There can be involvement proximal to the dorsal root ganglia where the sensory potentials are preserved. A proximal conduction block of the motor fibers origin may be compression by fibrosis but also direct damage of myelin by radiation therapy.[21]

The most common type of RIPN in the upper limb is radiation-induced brachial plexopathy (RIBP), a progressive injury in the axillary-supraclavicular ipsilateral node volume after radiation therapy for breast cancer.[21] Clinically, RIBP begins with a person reporting paresthesia, which progresses to anesthesia. In RIBP, the person will exhibit a positive Tinel sign when pressure in the zone of axillary and/or supraclavicular induration triggers the paresthesia. Motor weakness is progressive and often delayed by several months and associated with fasciculations and amyotrophy. The common presentation usually starts at the median nerve which will clinically present like carpal tunnel syndrome before spreading to the forearm and then upper arm.[21] Rapid neurological worsening is possible after trauma such as unusual traction on the affected limb. Arm lymphedema is strongly linked to combined extensive lymph node dissection and high dose radiation therapy and is not predictive of RIBP but may enhance upper limb nerve compression.

Lower limb RIPN is rare and was first described after testicular irradiation. Delayed, progressive radiation-induced lumbosacral radiculoplexopathy occurs after high-dose radiation therapy in a moderate area of radiation therapy and also after a moderate-dose radiation therapy in large area of radiation therapy. However, it presents earlier in high-dose radiation therapy.[21] a The usual neurological deficits are bilateral but initially they most often present as asymmetric due to unilateral damage in the radiation therapy zone. Eventually symptoms move into a bilateral presentation. Unlike RIBP, radiation-induced lumbosacral radiculoplexopathy tends to affect motor function as opposed to sensory functions, and paresthesia is typically absent or noted very late. Sudden worsening of neurological deficit with lumbar pain may indicate vertebral compression with underlying radiation-induced vertebral osteoporosis. This may occur following a fall due to walking difficulties. Intestinal and/or urinary disorders are associated after pelvic radiation therapy either by peripheral neurogenic damage or by pelvic fibrosis.[21] Electroneuromyography determines whether sensory potential is preserved. An MRI may show bony changes in the radiation therapy field including osteoporosis of the vertebral bodies which would also indicate that adjacent nerve roots also received radiation therapy. Treatment for RIPN is based on symptoms. Pain can be treated with nonopioid analgesics, benzodiazepines, tricyclic antidepressants, and anti-epileptics. Neurolysis or surgical manipulation can worsen nerve wall ischemia but mechanical separation of the fibrotic tissues from the nerves may help relieve symptoms. Often vitamins B1–B6 are used but evidence is still lacking.[21]

Oncology rehabilitation (Onc R) is recommended to maintain function and prevent joint complications which can cause pain and decrease movement. It is important to prevent any stretching of a plexus immobilized by fibrosis, including avoiding carrying heavy loads and limiting end-range movements.[21]

Chemotherapy

Platinum-Based Antineoplastics

This class of drugs includes oxaliplatin (Eloxatin), cisplatin (Platinol), and carboplatin (Paraplatin). These chemotherapeutic agents are used to treat a wide variety of solid tumors. Oxaliplatin is primarily used for treatment of advanced colorectal, esophageal, stomach, liver, and pancreatic cancers. Cisplatin and carboplatin are used for treatment of small-cell lung cancer, testicular, ovarian, brain, uterine, and bladder. This drug class can cause acute and chronic neurotoxicity which can lead to an increase in infusion time, dose reductions, and treatment delays, or cessation of treatment. A unique adverse effect of oxaliplatin is cold-induced neuropathy, which presents acutely with pharyngolaryngeal dysesthesias, jaw spasms, fasciculations, muscle cramps, and cold-related paresthesia of the hands and feet.[22] One study found that the duration of cold evoked pain reported within the first three cycles of oxaliplatin was associated with the extent of the chronic form of chemotherapy-induced polyneuropathy (CIPN) experienced 1 year later.[23] These drugs induce the activation of glial cells which leads to the activation of immune cells and the release and elevation of pro-inflammatory cytokines. This release of cytokines results in nociceptor sensitization, hyperexcitability of peripheral neurons, and damage to the blood-brain barrier, resulting in neuroinflammation.[22]

Immunomodulatory Drugs

Thalidomide (Thalomid) is a chemotherapeutic agent that is a glutamic acid derivative and immunomodulatory drug that is used in the treatment of multiple myeloma. Thalidomide-induced polyneuropathy occurs in 25% to 75% of patients with dose-dependent prevalence and severity.[22] Thalidomide can cause the classic sensory symptoms but may also induce motor impairment and GI and cardiovascular autonomic manifestations. Risk factors for thalidomide-induced polyneuropathy include advanced age or prior neuropathy caused by the myeloma itself or by drugs. The role of genetics has not been consistently studied but may be a factor.[22]

Taxanes

Common taxanes include paclitaxel (Taxol), docetaxel (Taxotere), and cabazitaxel (Jevtana). This class of chemotherapeutic agents act on microtubules which cause impairment of cancer cell division, ultimately leading to cell death. The cancers that are commonly treated with these drugs include ovarian, breast, non-small cell lung, and prostate. The incidence of CIPN ranges from 11% to 87%, with the highest rates for paclitaxel.[22] This neuropathy presents as a sensory-dominant neuropathy mostly affecting small diameter sensory fibers. Motor and autonomic symptoms develop less frequently. The symptoms are dose dependent and may start days after the first dose and tend to improve after completion of treatment. Some persons living with and beyond cancer (PLWBCs) that have been diagnosed with taxane-induced neuropathy can continue to have symptoms 1 to 3 years after completion of treatment and it can be lifelong.[22]

Epothilones

Epothilones (ixabepilone) are a new antineoplastic drug with similar mechanisms to taxanes as tubulin destabilizers and causing cell death. The prevalence for CIPN with this drug class is 67%.[22] This drug class is typically used as second line treatment; therefore, many patients have already been treated with another chemotherapeutic agent so they may have already exhibited some symptoms of CIPN. The manifestations are mild or moderate sensory-dominant neuropathy affecting small-diameter sensory fibers. Motor involvement is less frequent but possible and is typically from disuse due to the sensory impairments. Autonomic manifestations occur in less than 1% of patients treated with this drug.[22]

Vinca Alkaloids

This class of drugs includes vincristine (Oncovin, Vincasar PFS), vinblastine (Alkaban-AQ, Velban), and vinorelbine (Navelbine).

Vinca alkaloids are commonly used to treat Hodgkin and non-Hodgkin lymphoma, testicular cancer, and non-small cell lung cancer. The drugs inhibit the assembly of the microtubules which disrupts axonal transport. Acting on the cell body of the peripheral nerve, they induce sensorimotor neuropathy that is dose dependent. The onset of symptoms appears within the first 3 months of treatment and will include pain in the hand and feet, muscle weakness of the wrist extensors and dorsiflexors, and muscle cramping.[22]

Protease Inhibitors

Bortezomib (Velcade) is used to treat multiple myeloma and certain types of lymphomas. The sensory neuropathy that presents is very painful and sometimes weakness with demyelinating neuropathy may be seen. It has been found that 34% of patients treated with protease inhibitors will develop chronic, distal, and symmetrical sensory peripheral neuropathy with a neuropathic pain syndrome.[22]

Chemotherapeutic Adverse Effects on the Nervous System

Chemotherapy-Induced Polyneuropathy

The six main agents listed above can cause damage to the peripheral sensory, motor, and autonomic neurons resulting in CIPN. The most neurotoxic are the platinum-based drugs, taxanes, and epothilones and immunomodulatory drugs.[22] CIPN occurs as a result of damage to sensory and motor neurons outside the BBB. The underlying cause of CIPN is multifactorial with various sites of involvement. Physical neuronal damage contributes to functional impairment and hyperexcitability of peripheral nerves through oxidative stress, neuroinflammation, apoptosis, and electrophysiological disturbances. These chemotherapeutic agents can easily penetrate the blood-nerve barrier and bind to the dorsal root ganglion and nerve terminals. The endoneural compartment lacks the lymphatic system components to remove the neurotoxins from the distal aspects of these nerves. At a cellular level there is damage to the DNA, interruption of mitochondrial function, and damage to microtubule-based axonal transport system.[24]

CIPN is one of the most common and significant adverse effects of taxane-based chemotherapy.[25] Taxanes are an established treatment that greatly improve survival rates among persons diagnosed with breast cancer. Thirty to sixty percent of patients have persistent CIPN beyond treatment.[26] Taxane-induced polyneuropathy can affect any of the three divisions of the peripheral nervous system: motor, sensory, or autonomic. Taxane-based chemotherapy targets cancer cells by inhibiting microtubule depolymerization and causing mitotic arrest.[22]

Symptom presentation can include numbness, tingling, pain in a stocking and glove distribution, decreased positional, vibratory, and temperature perception, as well as weakness. It can be difficult to monitor these individuals due to their large variability in symptom presentation. Symptom monitoring can be done by both patient-reported outcomes (PROs) as well as quantitative sensory testing.[26]

The prevalence of CIPN is very wide, ranging from 19% to over 85%. It is primarily a sensory neuropathy.[22] CIPN symptoms usually emerge late which can be weeks or months after the completion of chemotherapy, and the severity is usually proportional to the dose of the drug. Some PLWCs will experience "coasting," a term used to describe the development of a new, or exacerbation of, an existing CIPN when treatment has been completed. This situation is challenging for oncologists as there are no signs or indications for a change in dosage.

Sensory symptoms usually develop first involving the feet and hands and commonly present in a stocking and glove pattern starting distally and moving proximally. The symptoms are often described as numbness, tingling, altered touch sensation, impaired vibration, paresthesias, and dysesthesias induced by touch and warm or cool temperatures. Motor symptoms occur less frequently than sensory symptoms and are typically distal weakness, gait and balance disturbances, and impaired movements. Autonomic symptoms that can occur based on CIPN include orthostatic hypotension, constipation, and altered sexual or urinary function.

CIPN is underappreciated especially on the impact of QOL and safety. A survivor of cancer who develops CIPN are three times more likely to fall.[22] Predisposing factors of CIPN include patient age (increased risk in older patients); the co-occurrence of neuropathy before the start of chemotherapy, a history of smoking; impaired renal function; exposure to other neurotoxic chemotherapeutic agents; paraneoplastic antibodies; and independent direct cancer-associated neuropathy.[22]

Autonomic Symptoms From CIPN

Autonomic dysfunction is not as common as sensory changes, but the system lies outside the BBB and can affect these neurons which leads to signs and symptoms of autonomic dysfunction (Figure 8.16). Symptoms may include orthostatic hypotension potentially leading to syncope. Anhidrosis (inability to sweat normally) may occur early in the course of treatment and is often distal to the trunk and progresses medially. The opposite can also occur, with excessive sweating, typically in the head and neck area.

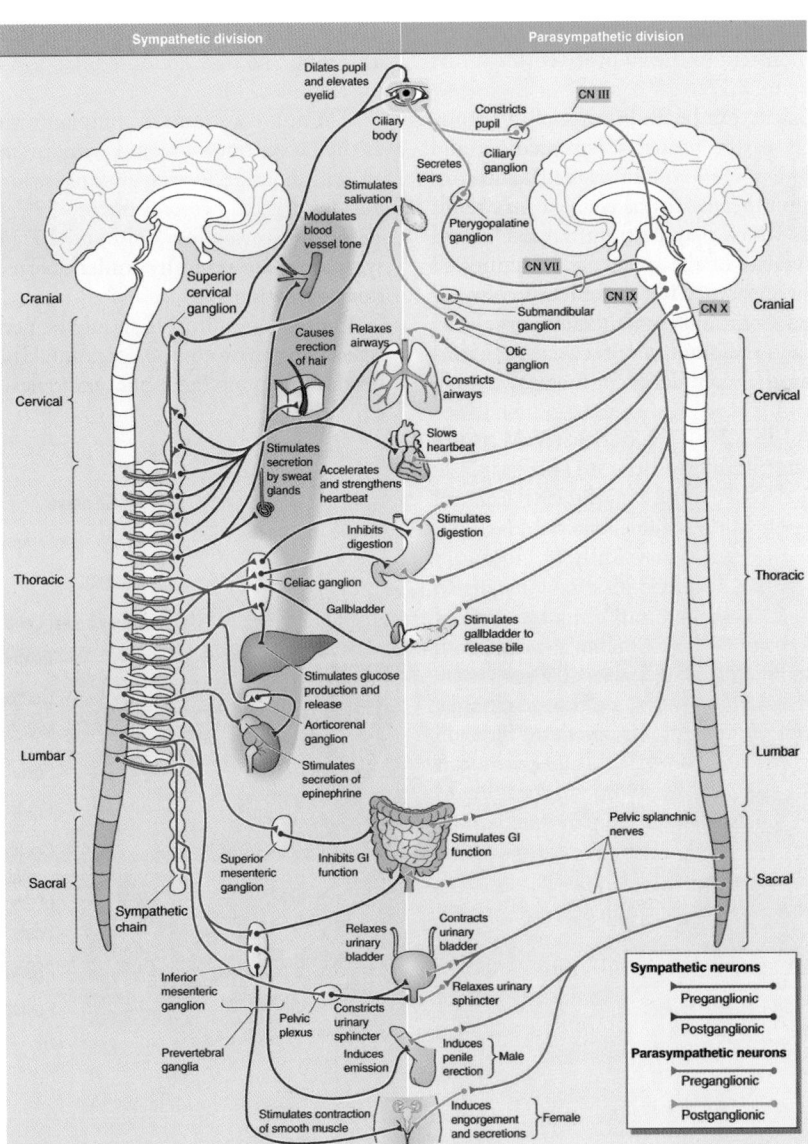

• **Fig. 8.16** Autonomic Nervous System. (Printed with permission. Created by George B Richerson, Medical Physiology. Published December 31, 2016. © 2017.)

Arrhythmias can also occur, which is why cardiovascular exercise should be assessed and prescribed as a part of a PLWC's treatment plan. Dryness of the eyes and mouth is often seen and changes in visual acuity have been reported. Gastrointestinal dysmotility often presents with alternating constipation and diarrhea. Urinary dysfunction may also occur, causing an atonic bladder and overflow incontinence. Erectile dysfunction may also present in men as an early autonomic symptom.[27]

Ototoxicity

Ototoxicity is a common adverse effect with various treatments, including cisplatin as well as radiation therapy or surgery involving the ear and auditory nerve.[28] The ear is made up of three divisions known as the external, middle, and inner ear. The external ear helps to amplify and direct sound towards the middle ear. Once the sound is in the middle ear it transmits through the ossicles and transforms the sound waves into mechanical energy. The inner ear then transmits the mechanical energy into hydraulic waves by the cochlea to stimulate the sensory hair cells. This causes the release of neurotransmitters allowing the auditory nerve to transmit a neural signal through the brainstem to the auditory cortex in the opposite temporal lobe[29] (Figure 8.17).

Radiation-induced ototoxicity can be multifactorial in nature. Persons who receive ≥30 Gy to the posterior nasopharynx and mastoid are at high risk of developing serous otitis media and conductive hearing loss. Radiation therapy to the cochlea may result in sensorineural hearing loss which may be from damage to the small vessels resulting in hypoxia of the inner ear structures or direct damage to the cochlear apparatus, but the exact mechanism is unknown. The loss caused from radiation therapy is typically permanent and progressive and the onset may occur acutely during treatment or several years after completion of therapy.[29]

Chemotherapy-related ototoxicity is typically from platinum-based chemotherapy or aminoglycoside antibiotics. Cisplatin has been found to be the most ototoxic agent with complaints of hearing loss, tinnitus, and postural imbalance. The prevalence of this toxicity is 50% to 80% in adults and 60% to 90% in children.[30] This toxicity is characterized by toxic levels of reactive oxygen species to the cochlea, which causes damage to the cochlear hair cells and damage to the stria vascularis and spiral ganglion cells. This damage is dose-dependent, bilateral, and irreversible due to cochlear sensory hair cells being unable to regenerate. Higher frequency sound is affected first, progressing into lower frequency sound loss if the chemotherapy dosage continues. This can be especially detrimental in children as a high frequency hearing loss can interfere with the process of acquiring language and communication skills.[29]

Surgical-related ototoxicity can be related to a tumor in or near the auditory structures. Surgery to resect such a tumor can affect the auditory nerve itself, or it can affect the central nervous system structures that interpret the sound.[29] The effects are bilateral high-frequency sensorineural hearing loss and tinnitus. Vestibular dysfunction can also be common, and the dizziness is described as feeling like they are on a boat and they have a sense of overall unsteadiness.[28]

Tinnitus is a common complaint with ototoxicity and is defined as the perception of sound without an external source. Individuals will describe it as a buzzing, whistling, or hissing sound. In persons treated with cisplatin, 59% experienced tinnitus only, 18% had hearing loss only, and 23% had both symptoms. These symptoms are typically underreported and underappreciated in this population.[30]

Ototoxic monitoring should be performed for any person who is receiving an ototoxic medication. This should include a full diagnostic audiogram (air, bone, and reflexes), full acoustic immittance

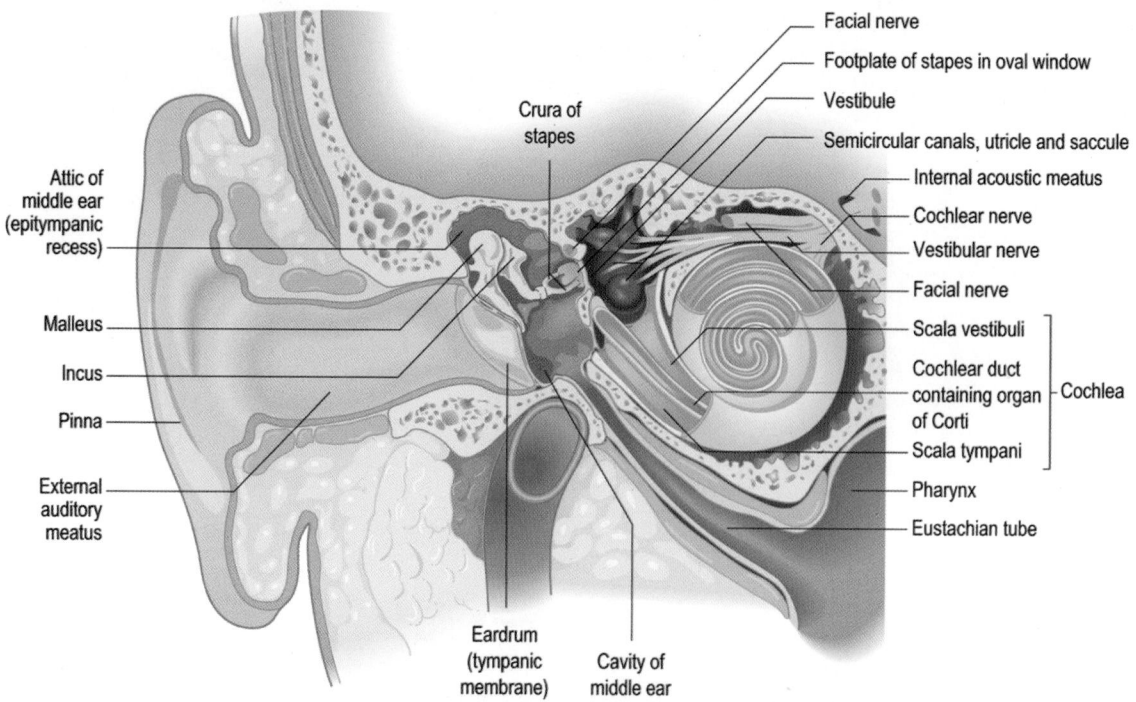

• **Fig. 8.17** Anatomy of the Ear. (Reprinted with permission. Wilson, Janet. Published December 31, 2017. © 2018.)

testing, and speech discrimination. Pure-tone audiometry is the criterion standard for hearing assessments. This involves presenting sounds across a wide range of frequencies from 500 to 8000 Hz. The frequency of testing should be performed at baseline and then at every 1 to 2 courses of the platinum-based chemotherapy (especially in children) which will allow for early detection and auditory intervention as needed. Monitoring should continue for persons who have received chemotherapy for 2 years and then as clinically indicated. If a person received radiation therapy to the head or ear, monitoring is recommended every 5 years due to the potential of a progressive loss over time.[29]

A thorough vestibular screen should be performed as well looking at vestibular-ocular reflex (VOR), balance, and oculomotor systems.[28] This will be described more in the balance/vestibular section of this chapter. Vestibular effects are less frequently documented as compared to auditory symptoms with platinum-based chemotherapy. More than 50% of patients who reported subjective dizziness had reduced efficiency at work, 27% had to change jobs, and 21% were not able to work anymore.[30] Bilateral symmetrical decline is found with platinum-based chemotherapy, and this loss correlates to disequilibrium, postural imbalance, or oscillopsia (visual perception of jumping or jittering). This loss may not be seen until the patient loses cues from vision or somatosensory inputs when walking in the dark or dimly lit places or when they develop concomitant peripheral neuropathy.[30]

Treatment of ototoxicity can include hearing aids, cochlear implants, assistive devices, and special accommodations. Hearing aids can benefit the amplification of sound and have advanced speech processing features in the newest models. Unfortunately, sometimes the quality is distorted, and it can be difficult to discriminate speech in a noisy environment. Cochlear implants can be beneficial as they offer a direct stimulation of the auditory neural pathway and can provide transmission of a sound to the brain, even though the severely damaged sensory hair cells. Ongoing audiology and speech language pathology rehabilitation programs are required. Auditory trainers, phone amplifiers, audio streamers, and the use of text messaging can help with supplementary communication especially in noisy environments. They must be compatible with the device being used and be replaced, as technology evolves. Special accommodations include specialized service at the public expense which can be helpful for children who are attending school or for adults in the work environment. These services are not always available and there needs to be appropriate application and evaluative procedures.[29]

Cancer-Related Cognitive Impairment

Cognitive function includes six domains: perception, memory, executive function, attention, decision making, and language abilities.[31] Perception is how sensory information is processed and integrated. It can be tested by identification of objects from sensory information, by the ability to recognize objects and sounds, and by the intactness of perceptual fields. Memory is most complex and multifaceted, having several subdomains. Working memory is the ability to hold information in consciousness for adaptive use. This includes memory for verbal information, spatial information, and emotional memory across multiple sensory channels. Episodic/declarative/explicit memory is what interacts with working memory to encode, maintain, and retrieve information into and out of longer-term storage. Procedural memory is for motor actions or skills. This is how we remember how to type

or ride a bike without having to re-learn every time we perform the activity.

Executive functioning, referred to as reasoning or problem solving, is a set of processes that is utilized to solve problems and plan and perform complex tasks. This domain requires flexibility in that novel tasks require new strategies or rapid rejection of failed efforts. A few patient populations have pre-existing issues with executive function which can be exacerbated with cancer treatments. These populations include persons with attention deficit hyperactivity disorder (ADHD), depression, obsessive-compulsive disorder, and schizophrenia. Attention is divided into two subdomains: selective attention and sustained attention. Selective attention is the process of attending to information that is relevant and important. Distractors can be presented in auditory or visual information. Dual task processing is also a selective attention paradigm. Sustained attention can also be termed vigilance. Tasks that measure vigilance require detection of simple stimuli within a continuous performance task. Performance of this is indexed by correct detections, missed target stimuli, and responses to nontarget stimuli. Processing speed refers to tasks that require rapid performance that range from simple to complex. It is an important cognitive ability and is correlated with impairments in everyday functioning. Language skills include receptive and productive abilities and the ability to understand language, assess semantic memory, and respond to verbal instruction with behavioral acts.[32]

Cognitive changes can impact an individual's QOL, interfere with a person's ability to work and contribute to society, and lead to poor compliance with treatment and follow-up.[17] Chemotherapy is associated with long term toxicity that includes cognitive dysfunction. The National Health and Nutrition Examination Survey notes that there is a 40% likelihood of cancer survivors reporting cognitive concerns.[33] It should be noted that there can be some persons who have not received chemotherapy that may exhibit cognitive decline due to the cancer process itself. There is increasing evidence that it can affect both subjective (patient-reported) and objective changes. Most of the effects are short-term with improvements expected farther out of treatment.

These individuals may benefit from cognitive rehab. Pharmacologic treatments have not been proven to help in the management of CRCI. There are some factors and cognitive domains that can be affected based on the time point in their cancer journey. Prior to cancer diagnosis factors that can influence this domain include age, education, diabetes, and cardiovascular comorbidity.[17]

A study of persons diagnosed with colon cancer reported showed that 37% demonstrated cognitive impairment prior to systemic treatment,[34] and among persons diagnosed with testicular cancer evaluated after surgery but prior to chemotherapy, the incidence of cognitive impairment was 46%.[35] In general, postoperative cognitive dysfunction may be due in part to the inflammatory and immune response to surgery lasting for days to months.[36] Studies continue to be done on the effects of anxiety and depression and the impact on cognitive behavior. It is important to note QOL when reporting outcome measures, as this can be correlated with self-perceived cognitive concerns.[37]

In the older adult population, recall, orientation, and executive function become more impaired as they undergo treatment for their cancer diagnosis. Impairments in these cognitive processes are associated with increased risk of falls, decreased gait speed, and impaired balance.[38] Structural MRIs have demonstrated a reduction in gray matter density in patients with breast cancer exposed to chemotherapy. These changes appear to improve over time after recovery from chemotherapy.[39] Functional MRI studies have shown that if there was a prior chemotherapy exposure there was a reduced activation of certain brain regions during a cognitive task when compared to baseline results.[40] These studies are allowing researchers to try and determine patterns based on treatment and patient presentation.

Some individuals may demonstrate a phenomenon called cognitive compensation, which is where the person has adequate cognitive reserve to overcome the effects of chemotherapy by involuntarily utilizing other parts of the brain which are affected less by the chemotherapy. This could be an explanation of discrepancies between cognitive complaints and neuropsychological testing.[41]

Subjective reports of factors affecting peoples' cognitive function include anxiety, depression, fatigue, and sleep disturbance. When establishing a treatment plan for cognitive impairment, it is important to address these areas, as well as to note any medications that may affect cognitive function.

Hormone and Biological Therapies

This section will present cognitive adverse effects from hormone and biological therapy for all cancers (see Chapter 5 for more details about these treatments).

Cognitive Changes

Multiple studies have confirmed that hormonal therapy for both men and women have an impact on cognitive function.[42] A meta-analysis of persons diagnosed with prostate cancer who were treated with androgen deprivation therapy showed that they performed worse on visuomotor tasks compared with their own baseline performance as well as healthy controls.[43] A study looking at tamoxifen and exemestane showed that PLWBCs who were taking tamoxifen (Nolvadex) for 1 year did significantly worse on verbal and executive function tests compared to healthy controls but the same was not observed for those who took exemestane (Aromasin).[44] Studies of persons diagnosed with breast cancer who were treated with only tamoxifen revealed impaired processing speed and verbal memory.[45] On the other hand, there have been studies that have noted no negative impact from the use of tamoxifen or aromatase inhibitors.[46]

Neurological Rehabilitation Assessment Measures

This section will discuss specific assessment measures that can be used during the Onc R evaluation of all individuals experiencing neurological adverse effects from either a cancer diagnosis or treatment. Studies have shown that after an average of 6 years after treatment for breast cancer 47% of women still reported symptoms of CIPN. These women had significantly worse self-reported and objectively measured function with the exception of maximal leg strength and base of support during a usual walk.[47]

Sensation

Tactile detection threshold can be determined by a set of 20 Von Frey filaments calibrated to generate a force in grams within a 5% standard deviation.[26] The testing procedure involves the person closing their eyes and then the clinician touches the dorsum of the distal interphalangeal joint of the right and left middle fingers,

and the right and left great toes with the filaments. Starting with the smallest size filament at a 90-degree angle, the filament is pressed against the testing site until the filament bends. This is repeated with subsequently larger filament sizes until the patient is able to report tactile sensation at the testing site. This is graded as normal (0.008–0.07 g); diminished light touch (0.16–0.4 g); loss of protective sensation (4–180 g); deep pressure sensation only (300 g).[26]

Vibration detection threshold can be assessed using a hand-held biothesiometer (Figure 8.18) at the dorsum of the distal interphalangeal joints of the right and left index fingers, and the right and left great toes. The person is positioned and the biothesiometer is placed on the testing site and the amplitude of the device vibration (microns) is gradually increased until the person first perceives a vibration sensation. The average of three recordings are then documented. The vibration perception for normal subjects is 0.42 microns at the index finger and 0.84 microns at the great toe. The grading for vibration threshold is mild loss of perception (index finger 0.43–4.0 microns, great toe 0.84–4.0 microns); moderate loss of perception (index finger >4 microns, great toe 4.0–11.8 microns); severe loss of perception (only observed at the great toe >11.8 microns).[26]

Reflexes

Deep tendon reflexes may be diminished by abnormalities in muscles, sensory neurons, lower motor neurons, the neuromuscular junction, acute upper motor neurons, and mechanical factors such as joint disease. Abnormally increased reflexes are associated with upper motor neuron lesions. These can also be influenced by age, metabolic factors, and the anxiety level of the patient. See Tables 8.10 and 8.11 for the main spinal nerve roots and grading

TABLE 8.10 Deep Tendon Reflexes

Reflex	Main Spinal Nerve Root Involved
Biceps	C5, C6
Brachioradialis	C6
Triceps	C7
Patellar	L4
Achilles Tendon	S1

Created by Frannie Westlake. Printed with permission.

TABLE 8.11 Grading of Deep Tendon Reflexes

0	Absent reflex
1+	Trace, or seen only with reinforcement
2+	Normal
3+	Brisk
4+	Nonsustained clonus
5+	Sustained clonus

Created by Frannie Westlake. Printed with permission.

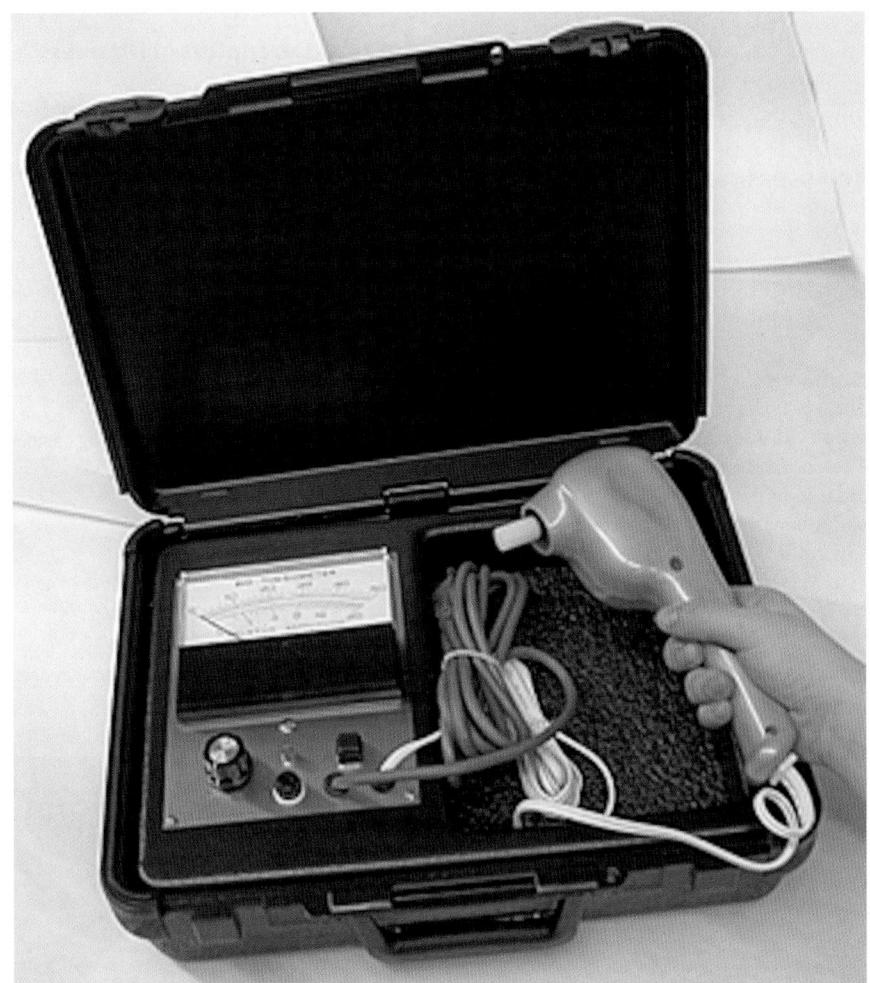

criteria.[48] See Figure 8.19 for a depiction of the mechanism of deep tendon reflexes.

Coordination

Coordination should be tested, as normal performance of motor tasks depends on the interdependence of multiple sensory and motor subsystems. These subsystems include position sense pathways, lower and upper motor neurons, basal nuclei, and the cerebellum. These subsystems can be affected by CNS tumors or adverse effects of cancer treatment. It is important to first test for normal joint position sense, strength, and reflexes. Appendicular ataxia is usually caused by lesions of the cerebellar hemispheres while truncal ataxia is often caused by damage to the midline cerebellar vermis and associated pathways.[49]

To test rapid alternating movements, have the person wipe one palm alternately with the palm and dorsum of the other hand. In testing finger to nose, have the patient alternately touch their nose and the examiner's finger as quickly as they can. The examiner should observe for dysmetria (past-pointing) or ataxia with the person unable to accurately touch the examiner's finger or their nose. Caution should be taken to not mistake weakness or a tremor for discoordination. To identify an individual's ability to

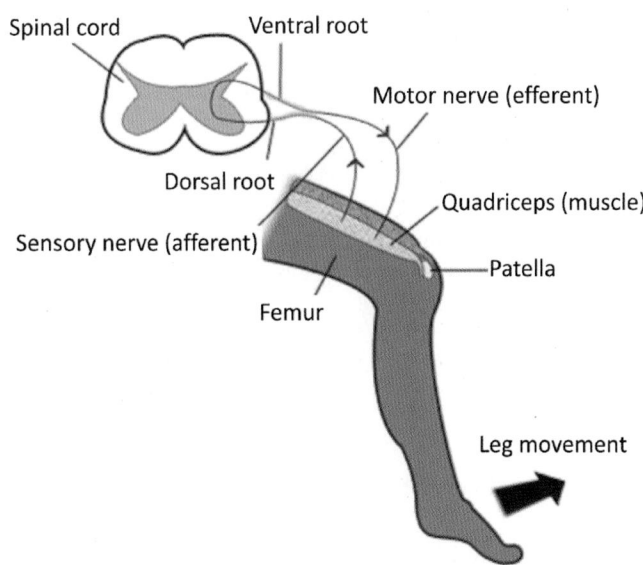

• **Fig. 8.19** Diagram of Deep Tendon Reflexes. (Open access permission under Creative Commons Attribution License from ChristinaT3 at English Wikipedia, CC BY-SA 3.0.)

touch the heel to the shin, have the patient touch the heel of one foot to the opposite knee and then drag their heel in a straight line all the way down and back up again. This test should be done in the supine position to eliminate the effect of gravity.[49]

Neuropathy Specific Assessments

Neuropathic Pain Scale

The neuropathic pain scale (NPS) is a 10-item questionnaire that quantifies specific qualities of neuropathic pain such as intense, sharp, hot, dull, cold, itchy, sensitive to describe the reaction to light touch, timing of the pain, overall unpleasantness, and the intensity of the deep and surface pain.[50] The minimally clinically important difference for this scale is 33% by the end of six weeks. If the total score is >5.53, this will indicate the patient has neuropathic pain.[51] A higher NPS score indicates more severe symptoms. This measure has been validated in patients with neuropathic pain and more specifically in patients with taxane-induced CIPN. Ratings are considered 0 to 30 mild pain, 31 to 70 moderate pain, and 71 to 100 with severe pain.[52]

Functional Assessment of Cancer Therapy-Gynecologic Oncology Group/Neurotoxicity

The Functional Assessment of Cancer Therapy-Gynecologic Oncology Group/Neurotoxicity subscale is a questionnaire that assesses sensory-, motor-, and hearing-related neurotoxic symptoms. This 11 item self-report tool describes CIPN symptoms, severity, and functional consequences. A lower score indicates more functional disability and more severe neurotoxicity with a 0 to 44 total score range. It is important to note that this questionnaire is looking at QOL versus actual functional performance.[26]

Comprehensive Assessment Scale for Chemotherapy-Induced Peripheral Neuropathy

The Comprehensive Assessment Scale for Chemotherapy-induced Peripheral Neuropathy (CAS-CIPN) is an assessment tool with high reliability and validity. This subjective assessment consists of 15 items that provides their medical team with information on their CIPN. It is divided into four subscales: threatened interference in daily life by negative feelings, impaired hand fine motor skills, confidence in the choice of treatment/management, and dysesthesia of the palms and soles.[53]

Total Neuropathy Score, Clinical Version

The Total Neuropathy Score, Clinical Version is a 7-item assessment tool that combines patient report with objective measures. It looks at subjective sensory, motor, and autonomic symptoms. The assessor then performs deep tendon reflexes, manual muscle testing of the distal muscles, pin sensibility, and semi-quantitative vibration sensibility using a graduated Rydel-Seiffer tuning fork. The grading scale is 0 to 28 points with a higher score indicating worse neuropathy.[54]

Vestibular Assessment

The vestibular system is responsible for gaze stability, orientation in space, and postural stability. See Table 8.12 for descriptors of dizziness. A scoping review of the literature of platinum-based chemotherapy adverse effects found that cochleotoxicity is well documented but vestibulotoxicity is not well established in the literature.[55] The conclusion emphasized the need for more attention

TABLE 8.12	Descriptors of Dizziness[55]
Vertigo	False sense of self-motion (rotational or linear)
Dizziness	Disturbed spatial orientation without a sense of self-motion
Oscillopsia	Gaze instability
Unsteadiness	Instability, disturbed postural control
Pulsion	Imbalance with a tendency to fall in a particular direction
Visual vertigo/dizziness	Evoked with complex or moving visual stimulus
Presyncope	Feeling of faintness

Created by Frannie Westlake. Printed with permission.

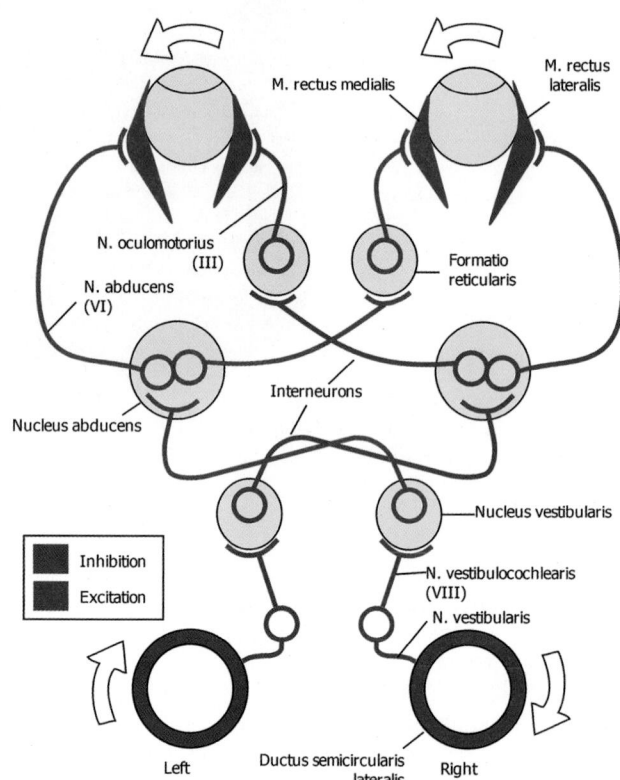

• **Fig. 8.20** Vestibulo-Ocular Reflex. (Permission under GNU Free Documentation License from Häggström M. ThreeNeuronArc.png. October 27, 2007.)

and evaluation of the vestibular system as several studies showed significant evidence of vestibular toxicities.

Vestibular-Ocular Reflex

The function of the VOR is to stabilize visual images on the retina during head movements by producing eye movement of equal velocity but in opposite direction of head movement (Figure 8.20). VOR is mediated by a three-neuron arc: primary vestibular afferent, secondary vestibular efferent, and oculomotor neurons. It is important to remember that each of the three semicircular canals

TABLE 8.13 — Oculomotor Exam[55]

Observation	Head tilt, Ocular Tilt Reaction, Ptosis, etc.
Visual Fields	Confrontation testing to determine field cuts
Pupillary Light Reflex	Optic nerve
Extraocular Movements	Range of motion of eyes—monocular and binocular
Ocular Alignment	Cover Tests; Alternate Cover Tests; Maddox Rod
Gaze Fixation/Holding	Ability to maintain stable gaze without generation of other eye movements in nine cardinal planes
Smooth Pursuit	Ability to maintain slowly moving target on fovea of retina
Saccades	Ability to make single rapid eye movement to refocus image on fovea of retina
Optokinetic Nystagmus	Reflexive jerk nystagmus occurring w/ visual flow
Vestibular/Vesitublar Ocular Reflex (VOR)	Ability to stabilize gaze while head moves; Benign paroxysmal positional vertigo
VOR Cancellation	Ability to suppress VOR response centrally
Vergence	Ability to move eyes simultaneously in opposite directions to fixate on object

ROM, Range of motion; *VOR*, Vestibular-Ocular Reflex.
Created by Frannie Westlake. Printed with permission.

TABLE 8.14 — Sensory Organization Balance Conditions[55]

Eyes	Surface	Unaltered Sensory Information
Open	Firm	Vision, somatosensation, vestibular
Closed	Firm	Somatosensation, vestibular
Open	Foam	Vision, vestibular
Closed	Foam	Vestibular

Created by Frannie Westlake. Printed with permission.

nighttime, and the cones help with color vision. It is ideal to make sure that a PLWBC has had a recent vision testing by an ophthalmologist or optometrist prior to initiating any vision retraining.[57]

Sensory receptors also provide information about motion, equilibrium, and spatial orientation. Information is obtained from the utricle, saccule, and semicircular canals which were discussed above. Any time balance is assessed with eyes closed and on an unstable surface, the primary system being used to stabilize the balance is the vestibular system.[57]

Other sensory receptors in the skin, muscles, and joints can be affected by chemotherapy and general deconditioning. Many times, after cancer treatments these receptors are slowed or diminished which impairs the body's ability to react to internal and external stimuli appropriately affecting normal function. (See Figure 8.22).[30]

Ankle strategy is one of the first balance strategies that we use. For small perturbations and also in quiet standing. Next is the hip strategy which happens when the perturbation is too large for the ankles to control. The hip joint moves in all directions and is used to defend against falling because it can correct any medium to large perturbation. The step strategy is the last line of defense for standing balance before a fall. This only kicks in when the perturbation is so large the ankle or hip cannot prevent a loss of balance. This strategy is what the body uses once we go outside our base of support and cone of stability (See Figure 8.22).[58]

The presence of CIPN is associated with impaired postural stability during eyes-closed balance conditions (Table 8.14). Medial-lateral postural instability was more pronounced in the CIPN group. This is consistent for impaired peripheral sensation.[59]

A systematic review demonstrated that lower limb kinetic exercises showed a decrease in tingling sensation, decrease in pain, and improvement in balance.[60] Working on strength and endurance training also showed positive effects for balance, lower extremity (LE) strength, function, and QOL. Interactive sensory training showed an increase in tandem stance balance with eyes open. This review helps to demonstrate the need for Onc R intervention for individuals with CIPN and that exercise can help to improve static and dynamic balance, increase lower extremity strength, and reduce CIPN symptoms such as pain and paresthesia. More research needs to be completed to show how these improvements correlate to a decrease in falls risk and improve QOL.[60]

lies in a different plane, and they are considered orthogonal to one another. Stimulation of an individual semicircular canal will produce movements of the eyes in the same plane of that canal. The ratio of eye velocity to head velocity is referred to as the gain of the VOR. VOR gain has been shown to be reduced to 25% to 50% in humans immediately following unilateral labyrinthine lesions during head movements toward the affected side. The VOR is compensatory for high frequency head movements (up to 2 cycles/second); however, the ability to compensate can be negatively affected by chemotherapy, causing patients to have dizziness with daily activities.[56]

The oculomotor system plays a major part in the balance system. A thorough assessment of the oculomotor system should be completed prior to assessing the vestibular system, see Table 8.13 for oculomotor examination that can be performed.[55] Although research is investigating the adverse effects of chemotherapy on this system, some patients subjectively report visual acuity changes during chemotherapy, although the mechanism is unknown at this time.

Balance Assessments

Balance is defined as the ability to maintain the body's center of mass over its base of support. Balance comes from three peripheral sources: visual, vestibular, and proprioceptive (See Figure 8.21). When performing balance assessments, knowing the system you are looking at will help you determine the appropriate interventions for the individual patient.[57]

Sensory receptors that can be affected by chemotherapy in the retina are called the rods and cones. The rods assist with vision at

Gait Analysis

Gait measures that should be assessed with CIPN include cadence, stride length, swing, double support, stride length variability, and swing time variability which can all increase the risk of falls. It has been shown that individuals who have received a taxane or

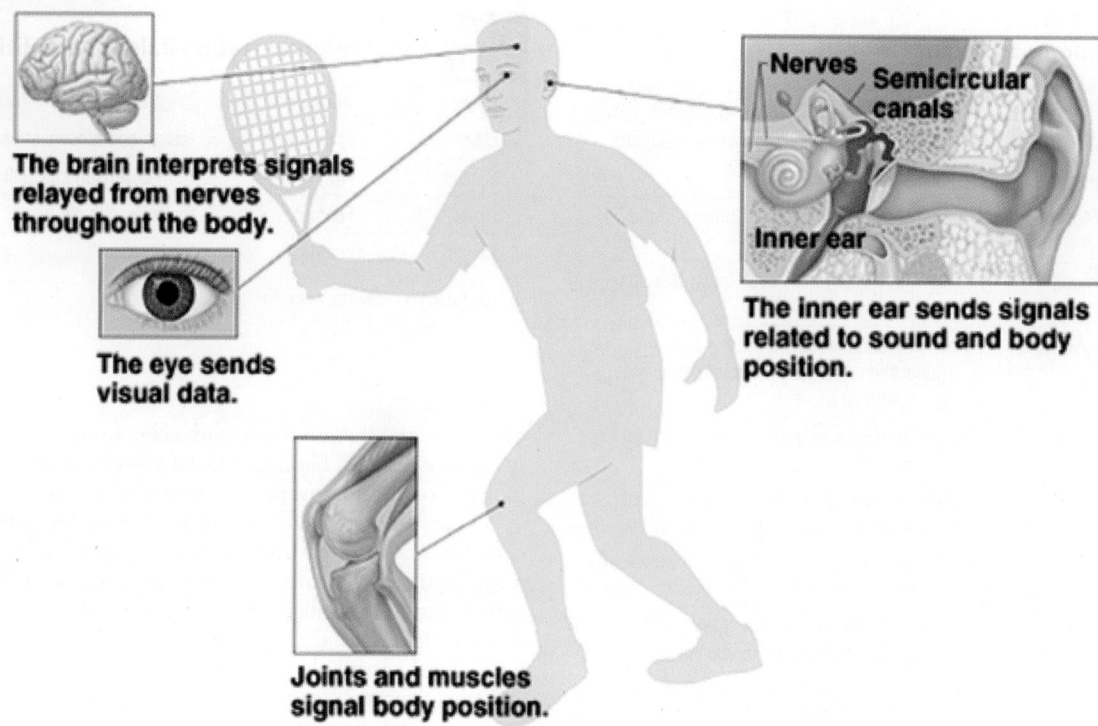

Fig. 8.21 Balance Systems. (Open access permission under Creative Commons Attribution License from Vestibular Disorders Association. 2008.)

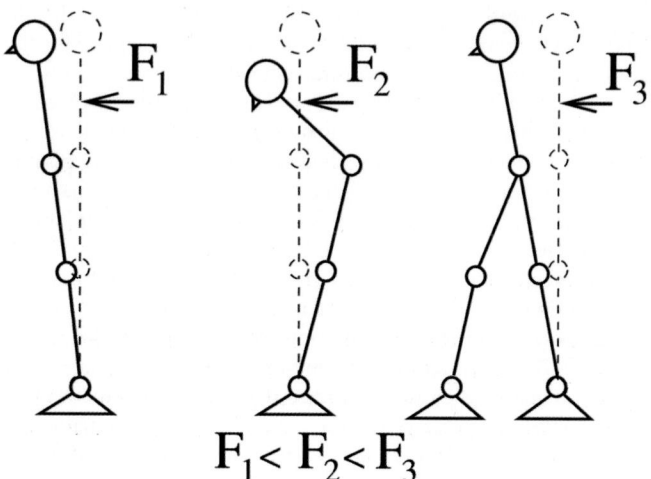

$$F_1 < F_2 < F_3$$

Fig. 8.22 Balance Strategies. (Open access under Creative Commons License from Shen K, Chemoir A, Hayashibe M. Human-like balance recovery based on numerical model predictive control strategy. *IEEE Access*. 2020;8:92050–92060.)

platinum-based chemotherapy demonstrated a slower cadence and shorter step length which may increase their risk of falls. A slower cadence has also been shown to increase energy expenditure which can also correlate to an increase in cancer related fatigue.[61] Subjective reports of decline in walking ability and balance have been correlated with a decline in the objective physical performance measures such as gait speed and balance (with eyes opened or closed). It was noted during this study that there was a decline in gait speed by 5% as they progressed through their chemotherapy regimen.[62]

Cognitive Measures

The International Cognition and Cancer Task Force recommends the following tests be used to assess cancer treatment-related cognitive dysfunction: The Hopkins Verbal Learning Test-Revised, the Trail Making Test, and the Controlled Oral Word Association of the Multilingual Aphasia Examination to measure learning and memory, processing speed, and executive function.[63] Objective neurocognitive tests may not be as sensitive as patient-perceived domains, so it is extremely important to employ standardized patient-reported measures for use in daily practice.

Common Treatments for Cognitive Therapy

Interventions should focus on cognitive training, cognitive rehabilitation, physical activities, and pharmacological interventions as recommended by their physician. Cognitive training is based on neuroplasticity and is a behavioral method of training by using cognitive exercise drills to stimulate the brain. Cognitive rehabilitation is where a patient learns new compensatory strategies to improve their everyday skills.[64] There are many web-based and in-person training methods, and it is important for a PLWC to be evaluated by a neuropsychologist, speech language pathologist, or an occupational therapist to help determine the specific interventions that would be of benefit to them. Physical activity should also be individualized for the PLWC to help mitigate the effect of cancer-related fatigue. Current recommendations are to complete 150 minutes per week of aerobic exercise, with 2 days per week of resistance exercise. See Chapter 23 for more information on exercise prescription. Exercise also positively affects QOL as well as body image.[65] Lastly, pharmacologic interventions can be prescribed as needed. The two most common medications used are methylphenidate (Ritalin) and modafinil (Alertec), both of which are stimulants and help decrease cancer-related fatigue and improve wakefulness. Studies have shown that they help with fatigue but not necessarily cognitive function; however, individuals using these medications report improved reported outcomes.[66]

Exercise has been shown to improve overall cognitive function and self-reported cognitive function; however, more research needs to be completed on which aspects of cognitive function are specifically improved. There is a paucity of studies where cognitive function is the primary outcome. Preliminary studies suggest that exercise is equally likely to result in gains in cognitive function during and/or following cancer treatments.[67] Aerobic exercise (10–60 minutes/week) has demonstrated benefits for cognitive function. The level of training should be between moderate and vigorous but specific parameters have yet to be studied.[67]

A decrease in reaction time right was observed after a bout of exercise compared to after a bout of rest demonstrating that persons were able to perform a cognitive task faster without sacrificing accuracy.[68] An improvement in the accuracy of responses on a spatial working memory task was noted immediately after aerobic exercise. More research needs to be conducted examining cognitive function as compared to rest as great potential is being found with aerobic exercise and the overall effect of cognitive function.[68]

Strategies have been identified that can be incorporated in rehabilitation treatments for the PLWBC that aims to return to work.[69,70] The first strategy is to re-organize work. Examples include dividing a large task into smaller tasks, working less hours, or switching to a less demanding position. Another strategy is to apply compensatory strategies such as taking notes, working in a less stimulating environment, using feedback from others to monitor work accuracy, and recording conversations. There have also been individual reports of the importance of being open and honest regarding their cognitive problems to the people around them. This can help with coping as well as providing a higher level of understanding by their peers. Lastly, there needs to be instruction on how to deal with fatigue from both a physical and mental perspective. Energy conservation is an essential component of patient education to provide the tools that will assist their (Table 8.15).[70]

Conclusion

The neurological system is always affected when there is a cancer diagnosis, either directly from a primary cancer of the brain or spinal cord, from metastases to the system or suffer adverse effects caused from the treatments for cancer. The damage to the neurological system determines the level of functional deficits and sometimes disabilities that a person will experience. Onc R clinicians are experts in treating all potential adverse effects, including nerve palsies, plexopathies, CIPN, ototoxicity, CRCI and more. These adverse effects can cause a short term inconvenience or a long term impairment that will negatively affect a person's physical, cognitive, emotional well-being for a lifetime. It is imperative to persons diagnosed as well as living with and beyond cancer to be referred to Onc R to mitigate and/or manage the adverse effects to the neurological system from cancer treatment to preserve QOL.

Critical Research Needs

- Diagnosis and treatment of cancer-related cognitive impairment from other causes besides chemotherapy

TABLE 8.15	Energy Conservation Techniques[70]
Technique	**Examples of Technique**
Distraction	Takes break and listen to music or meditate
	Adjust work and lifestyle balance
	Do activities that allow for fun and escape from every life
Comfort	Monitor posture with activities
	Use a chair with backrest and armrests
	Wear clothing that is easy to put on and comfortable to wear
Burden Reducing	Avoid crowded times when shopping
	Make plans regarding steps and process prior to doing a large task
	Follow regular pattern of everyday activities
	Structure activities according to energy level
Labor Saving	Monitor naps and take just enough that it does not affect nighttime sleep
	Skip or avoid activities that are not necessary
	Avoid lifting or moving heavy objects
	Sit to perform tasks (i.e., prepping food)

Modified and adapted from Sadeghi E et al. Effects of energy conservation strategies on cancer related fatigue adn health promotion lifestyle in breast cancer survivors: A randomized controlled trial. APJPC. 2016; 17 (10):4783-4790. Created by Frannie Westlake. Printed with permission.

- Incidence, assessment, and treatment of polyneuropathy from cancer surgeries and radiation therapy
- Prevalence, assessment, and treatment of autonomic nervous system changes caused from chemotherapy
- Assessment and treatment of vestibular system deficits caused form chemotherapy
- Paraneoplastic neurologic syndrome.

Case Study

A 69-year-old woman who was diagnosed with endometrial cancer grade III, stage 1A uterine serous carcinoma presented for a physical therapy evaluation with complaints of chemotherapy-induced peripheral neuropathy, lower extremity weakness, and fatigue. Her initial cancer treatments included a complete hysterectomy with lymph node removal (no positive lymph nodes per the patient report). Following surgical resection, she underwent chemotherapy and completed six rounds of carboplatin (Paraplatin) and paclitaxel (Taxol).

Her past medical history included a history of Graves disease which was currently controlled with medication and a left ankle fusion. She lived with her husband in a ranch-style house with a walk-out basement. She reported being retired and spent most of her free time going to her grandchildren's swim meets. Prior to chemotherapy she enjoyed walking a mile, biking for two miles, and lifting weights for 20 minutes. She had been unable to return to this activity since chemotherapy due to fatigue.

Her chief complaint was the neuropathy in her toes which she described as numbness that got worse as the day goes on. She had difficulty standing on one foot which made it hard for her to put her pants on and to perform stairs without holding on to a railing.

She reported one fall earlier in the year when she turned quickly and tripped due to the neuropathy in her feet.

The review of systems consisted of assessment of the cardiovascular, musculoskeletal, and neuromuscular systems. Examination revealed the following: Blood pressure: 144/85; Heart rate: 65 beats per minute. Range of motion was within functional limits for all upper and lower extremity joints, manual muscle testing was 4/5 for gross leg and arm muscle strength. She was able to complete the cardiovascular testing a few weeks after the evaluation as this was performed by another physical therapist in the clinic. She had diminished vibration sense in both ankles and great toes. She displayed normal light touch of both lower extremities (LEs) and normal proprioception in bilateral great toes. Her balance reactions were fair on a compliant surface with her eyes closed, both in single leg stance and in tandem. She was able to attain the tandem stance position without use of her upper extremities (UEs).

The initial hypothesis was that this patient was unable to return to her normal exercise routine and continued to have difficulty with her activities of daily living due to sensory and motor deficits following the development of CIPN. Due to this hypothesis the Onc R clinician administered the following tests and measures which would quantify her dynamic balance, functional mobility, subjective report, and current exercise capacity based on her cardiovascular assessment.

Test and Measure	Initial Evaluation	Reassessment 1	Reassessment 2	Reassessment 3 (After Back Pain)
FACT GOG/NTX-13	134/160	Did not answer	141/160	141/160
McGill Pain Questionnaire—SF	Sensory: 6/33 Affective: 0/12 VAS: 7/10	Sensory: 4/33 Affective: 0/12 VAS: 2.5/10	Sensory: 3/33 Affective: 0/12 VAS: 3.8/10	Sensory: 6/33 Affective: 0/12 VAS: 2/10
Five Times Sit to Stand	9.44 seconds with no UE	10.9 seconds with no use of UEs and increased fatigue	8.46 seconds with no use of UEs	9.84 with no use of UEs, recent complaints of back pain
ABC	79%	88%	88%	90%
mCTSIB	30/30/30/30, inc sway during conditions 3 and 4	30/30/30/30, no postural sway indicated	30/30/30/30, no postural sway noted	30/30/30/30, no postural sway noted
LEFS	54/80	55/80	61/80	61/80
Gait Speed	0.82 m/s	1.24 m/s	1.24 m/s	1.25 m/s
Vibration Sense	Diminished B great toe and ankles	Diminished B great toe and ankles	Diminished B great toe and ankles	Diminished in B great toes and ankle
SLS	R: 11.6 seconds L: 5.4 seconds	R: 30 seconds L: 30 seconds	R: 30 seconds L: 30 seconds	R: 30 seconds L: 30 seconds
Tandem	R: 20 seconds L: 20 seconds	EO: B feet 30 seconds EC: 7.34 seconds	EO: B feet 30 seconds EC: 14.09 seconds	EO: B feet 30 seconds EC: 20 seconds

FACT-GOG/NTX-13, Functional Assessment of Cancer Therapy-Gynecologic Oncology Group - Neurotoxicity- 13; SF, short form; mCTSIB, modified Clinical Test of Sensory Interaction in Balance; B, bilateral; VAS, visual Analog Scale. UE, upper extremity; ABC, Activities Balance Confidence Scale; EC, eyes closed; EO, eyes open; inc, increased; m/s, meters/seconds; R, right; L, Left; SLS, single leg stance; LEFS, Lower Extremity Functional Scale. Created by Frannie Westlake. Printed with permission.

Cardiovascular Assessment: She was able to complete stage 8 out of 21 (21 is the best or highest) of the University of Northern Colorado Cancer Rehabilitation Institute (UNC-CRI) treadmill test without holding onto the handrails. Her peak O_2 was predicted at 21.3 mL/kg/min, and this classified her as above aerobic capacity when compared to other cancer survivors for her age, and poor aerobic capacity when compared to the general public for her age. She was currently in phase 2 of cardiac rehab with the goal of working at 40% to 60% heart rate reserve for 20 to 30 minutes. She performed these 2-3 times per week. for a duration of three months. At the completion of 3 months, she would return for another cardiovascular assessment. Her target heart rate zone was calculated as 102 to 118 beats per minute.

In this case, the patient was functional and lived at home with her husband. She presented to physical therapy for her neuropathy symptoms and her inability to return to her exercise routine that she performed a few times a week. She also wanted some recommendations to help with the pain/discomfort she had from the CIPN.

Onc R intervention included short- and long-term goals. Short term goals were focused on LE strengthening, improved balance reactions to help decreased postural sway on a compliant surface, scheduling of a cardiovascular assessment, education on CIPN, and prescription of a home exercise program. Long term goals included: improving her gait speed, increasing her ability to go up/down a flight of stairs without a handrail, LE strengthening, and decreasing her risk of falls as evidenced by outcome measure performance.

She participated in physical therapy once a week for 12 weeks after which a reassessment was performed. As she met several of her goals, she transitioned to every other week so the therapist could continue to monitor her symptoms as she continued to increase her activity at the gym and home.

Impairment	Intervention	Prognosis (Goal of Care)
CIPN	Sensory integration, foot mobility, manual therapy to improve joint mobilization and for sensory feedback	Decrease patient report of pain, improve balance and walking on compliant surfaces
Fatigue	UNCCRI Treadmill Assessment, cardiovascular training, LE/UE strengthening	Improvement of gait speed, decreased patient report of fatigue with ADLs
Weakness	LE/UE strengthening	To improve her LE/UE strength to help with ADLs, increase muscular endurance
Impaired Balance	Balance on compliant surface, core strengthening	To help with stairs with use of railing, improve walking and balance on compliant surfaces, increase ankle strategy

CIPN, Chemotherapy-Induced Polyneuropathy; UNCCRI, University of North Carolina Cancer Research Institute; LE, lower extremity; UE, upper extremity. ADLs, activities of daily living. Created by Frannie Westlake. Printed with permission.

Review Questions

Reader can find the correct answers and rationale in the back of the book.

1. The vestibulocochlear (CN VIII) nerve is a part of which of the following systems?
   A. Central nervous system
   B. Peripheral nervous system
   C. Somatic nervous system
   D. Autonomic nervous system
2. A patient was recently diagnosed with breast cancer and they have just begun treatment which includes a platinum-based chemotherapy. They present today for an evaluation. What symptom below would most likely be their complaint since recently starting chemotherapy?
   A. Muscle cramping
   B. Tingling in toes and fingers
   C. Urinary incontinence
   D. Headache
3. What is the phenomenon called that describes chemo-induced peripheral neuropathy that worsens or develops once chemotherapy treatment is completed?
   A. Coasting
   B. Static
   C. Progressing
   D. Transmitting
4. Which of the following systemic chemotherapies have the most neurotoxic adverse effects resulting in the need for patients to be monitored during ADLs for balance impairments?
   A. Paclitaxel (Taxol)
   B. Doxorubicin (Adriamycin)
   C. Capecitabine (Xeloda)
   D. Gemcitabine (Gemzar)
5. Which of the following cognitive processes helps to determine how sensory information is processed and integrated?
   A. Perception
   B. Memory
   C. Executive function
   D. Attention
6. Which of the following outcome measures would you want to give your patient with complaints of neuropathy to assess his quality of life?
   A. Dizziness Handicap Index
   B. Activities Balance Confidence Scale
   C. McGill Pain Questionnaire—Short Form
   D. FACT-GOG NTX/13
7. Which of the following cancers is not common to have brain or spinal metastasis?
   A. Breast
   B. Lung
   C. Stomach
   D. Melanoma
8. Which of the following is a common gait kinematic change that is seen with patients who have received a neurotoxic chemotherapy?
   A. Increased step length
   B. Narrow base of support
   C. Decreased cadence
   D. Increased single support time
9. Which of the following balance strategies should be used with small perturbations and is typically the most commonly affected one for patients diagnosed with CIPN?
   A. Ankle strategy
   B. Hip strategy
   C. Stepping strategy
   D. Reaching strategy
10. The type of nerves that are most affected by chemotherapy are?
    A. Sensory nerves
    B. Motor nerves
    C. Autonomic nerves
    D. Somatic nerves

References

1. American Brain Tumor Association. Brain tumor education. American Brain Tumor Association. https://www.abta.org/about-brain-tumors/brain-tumor-education/. June 28, 2020.
2. Dangond F. What is central nervous system? Definition, function & parts. *eMedicineHealth*. https://www.emedicinehealth.com/anatomy_of_the_central_nervous_system/article_em.htm. Accessed April 15, 2020.
3. Zhou Y, Wu Y, Liu Y, et al. The cross-talk between autophagy and endoplasmic reticulum stress in blood-spinal cord barrier disruption after spinal cord injury. *Oncotarget*. 2017;8(1):1688–1702.

4. Suzuki Y, Sa Q, Ochiai E, Mullins J, Yolken R, Halonen S. Cerebral toxoplasmosis. In: *Toxoplasma Gondii*. Elsevier; 2014:755–796.

5. A Text and Atlas, LIppincott, Williams and Wilkins.

6. Carlson NR. *Physiology of Behavior*: Pearson Education (Allyn & Bacon). 2010.

7. American Association of Neurological Surgeons. Brain tumors. https://www.aans.org/en/Patients/Neurosurgical-Conditions-and-Treatments/Brain-Tumors. Accessed October 1, 2020.

8. Pace A, Dirven L, Koekkoek JA, et al. European Association of Neuro-Oncology (EANO) guidelines for palliative care in adults with glioma. *Lancet Oncol*. 2017;18(6):e330–e340.

9. Day J, Yust-Katz S, Cachia D. Interventions for the management of fatigue in adults with a primary brain tumour. *Cochrane Database Systematic Revs*. 2016;4:CD011376. doi:10.1002/14651858. CD011376.pub2.

10. American Association of Neurological Surgeons. Spinal tumors. https://www.aans.org/en/Patients/Neurosurgical-Conditions-and-Treatments/Spinal-Tumors. Accessed October 1, 2020.

11. Honnorat J, Antoine JC. Paraneoplastic neurological syndromes. *Orphanet J Rare Dis*. 2007;2(1):1–8.

12. Darnell R, Posner J. Paraneoplastic syndromes involving the nervous system. *New Eng J Med*. 2003;349:1543–1554.

13. Mehta D, El-Hunjul M, Leary M. Cerebrovascular complications of cancer. In: *Primer on Cerebrovascular Diseases*. Elsevier; 2017:573–579.

14. University of Pittsburgh School of Medicine. Endoscopic endonasal approach (EEA). https://www.upmc.com/services/neurosurgery/brain/treatments/brain-mapping/high-definition-fiber-tracking. September 23, 2020.

15. Johns Hopkins Medicine. Computed tomography (CT or CAT) scan of the brain. https://www.hopkinsmedicine.org/health/treatment-tests-and-therapies/computed-tomography-ct-or-cat-scan-of-the-brain. Accessed August 14, 2020.

16. John Hopkins Medicine. Sensory evoked potentials studies. https://www.hopkinsmedicine.org/health/treatment-tests-and-therapies/sensory-evoked-potentials-studies. Accessed November 3, 2020.

17. American Association of Neurological Surgeons. Spinal tumors. https://www.aans.org/en/Patients/Neurosurgical-Conditions-and-Treatments/Spinal-Tumors. Accessed October 1, 2020.

18. Johns Hopkins Medicine. Craniotomy. https://www.hopkinsmedicine.org/health/treatment-tests-and-therapies/craniotomy. Accessed October 18, 2020.

19. Memorial Sloan Kettering Cancer Center. Spine tumors surgery. https://www.mskcc.org/cancer-care/types/spine-tumors/treatment/surgery; 2019. Accessed May 29, 2022.

20. Suteu P, Fekete Z, Todor N, Nagy V. Survival and quality of life after whole brain radiotherapy with 3D conformal boost in the treatment of brain metastases. *Med Pharm Rep*. 2019;92(1):43–51.

21. Delanian S, Lefaix JL, Pradat PF. Radiation-induced neuropathy in cancer survivors. *Radiiother Oncol*. 2012;105(3):273–282.

22. Zajaczkowska R, Kocot-Kepska M, Leppert W, Wrzosek A, Mika J, Wordliczek J. Mechanisms of chemotherapy-induced peripheral neuropathy. *Intl J Mol Sci*. 2019;20(6):1451–1480.

23. Attal N, Cruccu G, Baron R, et al. EFNS guidelines on the pharmacological treatment of neuropathic pain: 2010 revision. *Eur J Neurol*. 2010;17(9):1113–1e88. doi:10.1111/j.1468-1331.2010.02999.x.

24. Wang XM, Lehky TJ, Brell JM, Dorsey SG. Discovering cytokines as targets for chemotherapy-induced painful peripheral neuropathy. *Cytokine*. 2012;59(1):3–9.

25. Bao T, Basal C, Seluzicki C, Li S, Seidman A, Mao J. Long-term chemotherapy-induced peripheral neuropathy among breast cancer survivors: prevalence, risk factors and fall risk. *Breast Cancer Res Treat*. 2016;159:327–333.

26. Zhi W, Chen P, Kwon A, et al. Chemotherapy-induced peripheral neuropathy (CIPN) in breast cancer survivors: a comparison of patient-reported outcomes and quantitative sensory testing. *Breast Cancer Res Treat*. 2019;178(3):587–595.

27. Izycki D, Niezgoda AA, Kazmierczak M, et al. Chemotherapy-induced peripheral neuropathy—diagnosis, evolution and treatment. *Ginekol Pol*. 2016;87(7):516–521.

28. Paken J, Govender CD, Pillay M, Sewram V. Perspectives and practices of ototoxicity monitoring. *S Afr J Commun Disord*. 2020;67(1):685.

29. Landier W. Ototoxicty and cancer therapy. *Cancer*. 2016; 122(11):1647–1659.

30. Baguley DM, Prayuenyong P. Looking beyond the audiogram in ototoxicity associated with platinum-based chemotherapy. *Cancer Chemother Pharmacol*. 2019;85:245–250.

31. Kiely KM. *Encyclopedia of Quality of Life and Well-Being Research*. Springer; 2014.

32. Harvey PD. Domains of cognition and their assessment. *Dialogues Clin Neurosci*. 2019;21(3):227–237.

33. Koppelmans V, Breteler M, Boogerd W. Neuropsychological performance in survivors of breast cancer more than 20 years after adjuvant chemotherapy. *J Clin Oncol*. 2012;30(10):1080–1086.

34. Crizado J, Lopez-Santiago S, Martinez-Marin V. Longitudinal study of cognitive dysfunctions induced by adjuvant chemotherapy in colon cancer patients. *Support Care Cancer*. 2014;22:1815–1823.

35. Wefel JS, Vidrine DJ, Veramonti TL, et al. Cognitive impairment in men with testicular cancer prior to adjuvant therapy. *Cancer*. 2011;117(1):190–196.

36. Rundshagen I. Postoperative cognitive dysfunction. *Dtsch Arztebl Int*. 2014;111(8):119–125.

37. Biglia N, Moggio G, Peano E, et al. Effects of surgical and adjuvant therapies for breast cancer on sexuality, cognitive function and body weight. *J Sexual Med*. 2010;7(5):1891–1900.

38. Blackwood J. The influence of cognitive function on balance, mobility, and falls in older cancer survivors. *Rehabil Oncol*. 2019;37(2):77–82.

39. McDonald BC, Conroy S, Ahles T. Gray Matter reduction associated with systemic chemotherapy for breast cancer: a prospective MRI study. *Breast Cancer Res Treat*. 2010;123(3):819–828.

40. McDonald BC, Conroy S, Ahles T. Alterations in brain activation during working memory processing associated with breast cancer and treatment: a prospective fMRI study. *J Clin Oncol*. 2012;30(2):2500–2508.

41. Moore H. An overview of chemotherapy-related cognitive dysfunction, or 'chemobrain'. *Cancer Network*. 2014;28(9):797–804.

42. Hardy SJ, Krull KR, Wefel JS, Janelsins M. Cognitive changes in cancer survivors. *Am Soc Clin Oncol*. 2018;38:795–806.

43. McGinty H, Phillips K, Jim H. Cognitive functioning in men receiving androgen deprivation therapy for prostate cancer: a systematic review and meta analysis. *Support Care Cancer*. 2014;22(8):2271–2280.

44. Schilder C, Seynaeve C, Beex L. Effects of tamoxifen and exemestane on cognitive functioning of postmenopausal patients with breast cancer: results from the neuropsychological side study of the tamoxifen and exemestane adjuvant multinational trial. *J Clin Oncol*. 2010;28(8):1294–1300.

45. Ahles T, Saykin A, McDonald B. Cognitive function in breast cancer patients prior to adjuvant treatment. *Breast Cancer Res Treat*. 2007;110:143–152.

46. Hermelink K, Henschel V, Untch M. Short-term effects of treatment-induced hormonal changes on cognitive function in breast cancer patients: results of a multicenter prospective, longitudinal study. *Cancer*. 2008;113(9):2431–2439.

47. Winters-Stone KM, Horak F, Jacobs PG, et al. Falls, Functioning, and disability among women with persistent symptoms of chemotherapy-induced peripheral neuropathy. *J Clin Oncol*. 2017;35(23):2604.

48. Bloomfield H. Deep Tendon Reflexes. Neuroexam.com. http://neuroexam.com/neuroexam/content31.html. Accessed October 18, 2020.

49. Bloomfield H. Appendicular Coordination. Neuroexam.com. http://neuroexam.com/neuroexam/content36.html. Accessed October 18, 2020.

50. Liberia J, Reicherter A. Neuropathic Pain Scale (NPS). APTA. https://www.apta.org/patient-care/evidence-based-practice-resources/test-measures/neuropathic-pain-scale-nps. Accessed November 11, 2020.

51. Smith EM, Cohen JA, Pett MA, Beck SL. The validity of neuropathy and neuropathic pain measures in patients with cancer receiving taxanes and platinums. *Oncol Nurs Forum.* 2011;38(2):133–142.

52. Fishbain D, Lewis J, Cutler R. Can the neuropathic pain scale discriminate between non-neuropathic and neuropathic pain? *Pain Med.* 2008;9(2):149–160.

53. Kanda K, Fujimoto K, Mochizuki R, Ishida K, Lee B. Development and validation of the comprehensive assessment scale for chemotherapy-induced peripheral neuropathy in survivors of cancer. *BMC Cancer.* 2019;19(1):1–11.

54. Cavaletti G, Frigeni B, Lanzani F, et al. Multi-center assessment of the Total Neuropathy Score for chemotherapy-induced peripheral neurotoxicity. *J Peripheral Nerv Sys.* 2006;11(2):135–141.

55. Prayuenyong P, Taylor JA, Pearson SE, et al. Vestibulotoxicity associated with platinum-based chemotherapy in survivors of cancer: a scoping review. *Front Oncol.* 2018;8:363.

56. Herdman SJ. *Vestibular Rehabilitation.* F.A. Davis Company; 2007.

57. Watson M, Black F, Crowson M. The Human Balance ANATOMY System: A Complex Coordination. Vestibular Disorders Association; 2016. https://vestibular.org/wp-content/uploads/2011/12/Human-Balance-System_36.pdf.

58. Blenkinsop GM, Pain MT, Hiley MJ. Balance control strategies during perturbed and unperturbed balance in standing and handstand. *R Soc Open Sci.* 2017;4(7):161018. doi:10.1098/rsos.161018.

59. Monfort SM, Pan X, Loprinzi CL, Lustberg MB, Chaudhari AM. Impaired postural control and altered sensory organization during quiet stance following neurotoxic chemotherapy: a preliminary study. *Integr Cancer Ther.* 2019;18:1–8.

60. Brayall P, Donlon E, Doyle L, Leiby R, Violette K. Physical therapy-based interventions improve balance, function, symptoms, and quality of life in patients with chemotherapy-induced peripheral neuropathy: a systematic review. *Rehabil Oncol.* 2018;36(3):161–166.

61. Marshall TF, Zipp GP, Battaglia F, Moss R. Chemotherapy-induced peripheral neuropathy, gait and fall risk in older adults following cancer treatment. *J Cancer Res Prac.* 2017;4(4):134–138.

62. Monfort SM, Pan X, Patrick R, et al. Gait, balance and patient-reported outcomes during taxane-based chemotherapy in early stage breast cancer patients. *Breast Cancer Res Treat.* 2017;164(1):69–77.

63. Wefel JS, Vardy J, Ahles T, Schagen S. International Cognition and Cancer Task Force recommendations to harmonise studies of cognitive function in patients with cancer. *Lancet Oncol.* 2011;12(7):703–708.

64. Bray V, Dhillon H, Bell M. Evaluation of a web-based cognitive rehabilitation program in cancer survivors reporting cognitive symptoms after chemotherapy. *J Clin Oncol.* 2017;35(2):217–225.

65. Schmitz K, Courneya K, Matthews C, et al. American College of Sports Medicine roundtable on exercise guidelines for cancer survivors. *Med Sci Sports Exer.* 2010;42(7):1409–1426.

66. Gong S, Sheng P, Jin H. Effect of methylphenidate in patients with cancer-related fatigue: a systematic review and meta-analysis. *PLoS One.* 2014;9(1):e84391. doi:10.1371/journal.pone.0084391.

67. Campbell KL, Zadravec K, Bland KA, Chesley E, Wolf F, Janelsins MC. The effect of exercise on cancer-related cognitive impairment and applications for physical therapy: systematic review of randomized controlled trials. *Phys Ther.* 2020;100(3):523–542.

68. Salerno EA, Rowland K, Kramer AF, McAuley E. Acute aerobic exercise effects on cognitive function in breast cancer survivors: a radomized crossover trial. *BMC Cancer.* 2019;19(1):1–9.

69. Klaver KM, Duijts SF, Engelhardt EG, et al. Cancer-related cognitive problems at work: experiences of survivors and professionals. *J Cancer Surviv.* 2020;14(2):168–178.

70. Sadeghi E, Gozali N, Tabrizi FM. Effects of energy conservation strategies on cancer related fatigue and health promotion lifestyle in breast cancer survivors: a randomized control trial. *Asia Pac J Cancer Prev.* 2016;17(10):4783–4790.

9

Lymphatic and Integumentary Systems

JULIA C. OSBORNE, BSC (HONS) PT, CLT-LANA, CAROLINE S. GWALTNEY, PT, DPT, CWS

CHAPTER OUTLINE

Lymphatic System

Oncology-related lymphedema is classified as a secondary lymphedema. It is an accumulation of protein-rich fluid within the interstitium that exceeds the transport capacity (TC) of the lymphatic system and its ability to transport the fluid. Lymphostasis associated with lymphedema can occur anywhere in the body, including the arms, legs, genitals, face, neck, chest wall, oral cavity, and pharyngeal cavity. The word "lymphedema" reflects more than a static, linear disease process. It represents a chronic, progressive disease process that involves a complex network of biologic processes.[1] Both its prophylaxis and treatment present a varied trajectory of surveillance, referral pathways, management, and patient experiences. An in-depth understanding of the pathophysiology of this disease process, as well as the intricacies of the functional anatomy of this incredibly vital and remarkable system in the human body is important and critical to the management of lymphedema. Broadening knowledge and understanding in both areas of study will allow for advancements in skill set to optimize the functioning of the "remaining" lymphatic system and to facilitate lymphangiogenesis in persons living with lymphedema.

Secondary Lymphedema

Secondary lymphedema occurs when a previously functioning lymphatic system becomes impaired secondary to insult, injury, or obstruction to a specific region, known as a lymphatic territory, within the lymphatic system. In developed countries, the predominant cause of lymphatic injury resulting in mechanical insufficiency relates to cancerous malignancies and their associated medical treatment interventions.[2] Secondary lymphedema is one of the most significant sequelae relating to the surgical, radiological, and chemotherapy-based management of persons treated for cancer. Breast cancer is the most common cancer associated with secondary lymphedema in developed countries.[3] Secondary lymphedema is characterized by an accumulation of protein-rich lymphatic fluid in the affected part of the body,[4] and has significant physical, functional, occupational, recreational, community-based, and economic consequences in persons living with lymphedema.

Incidence

The reported incidence of lymphedema relating to oncologic diagnosis and treatment varies widely depending on the population studied, body areas selected, measurement criteria, absence or presence of comorbidities, timing of onset, and reported length of follow up. The most current statistics indicate that one in five persons with breast cancer will develop breast cancer-related clinical lymphedema (BCRCL).[5] Within a range from 3 months post-treatment to 20 years post-treatment, there is an overall incidence rate of 16.6% of BCRCL, with a subset of people with axillary lymph node dissection (ALND) with a reported incidence of 19.9%.[6] Sentinel lymph node biopsy (SLNB) is the gold standard for lymph node preserving surgical biopsy, however, clinically, the evidence suggests that BCRCL is still of concern given that the incidence of onset ranges from 0% to 63.4% within 6 to 12 months post biopsy.[7] Additional research results show that overall, 87% to 89% of those diagnosed with BCRCL have a clinical onset within 2 to 3 years post treatment,[8] however it is well documented that the risk of onset remains for life.[9]

Evidence-based research about lymphedema incidence in other cancer disease sites shows that within the first 18 months post treatment, greater than 90% of persons living with and beyond cancer (PLWBCs) of the head and neck experience varying forms of both external and internal clinical lymphedema[10]; and within 12 months post treatment, 37% of PLWBC of the gynecological region demonstrated a measurable clinical lymphedema.[11]

The Functioning of the Lymphatic System

The primary functional role of the lymphatic system is to maintain fluid equilibrium and local physiological homeostasis within the immediate environment of every cell in all tissues of the body.[12] Homeostasis is attained by removing waste byproducts resulting from cellular activity, as well as optimizing immunity against bacteria, viruses, parasites, and other pathogens. The role of the lymphatic system therefore is to optimize immune function, and to establish homeostasis within tissue microenvironments to optimize tissue function. Illustrated in Figure 9.1, it is important to

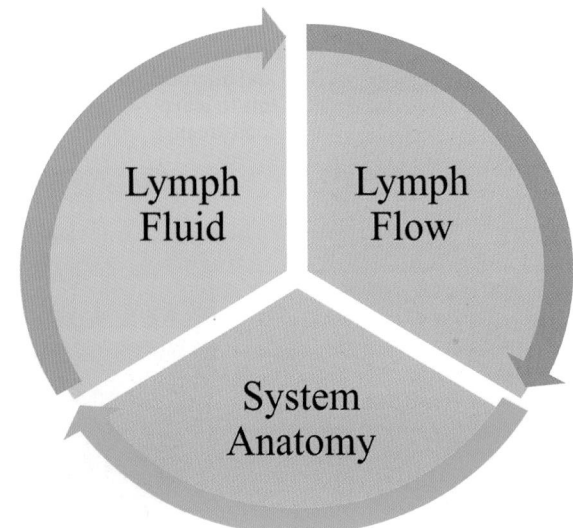

• **Fig. 9.1** The Mechanisms of Relationship of the Lymphatic System— Lymph Fluid, Lymph Flow, System Anatomy. (Created by Julia C. Osborne. Printed with permission.)

consider the trifecta of components (lymph fluid, lymph flow, system anatomy) that make up the overall mechanisms of relationship of functioning of the lymphatic system.

Lymph Fluid

Lymph fluid is made up of protein macromolecules, long chain fatty acids, and other unwanted foreign particles including bacteria, viruses, and other pathogens. Its composition is dependent on two functions: (1) the ultrafiltration of plasma proteins as well as protein macromolecules; and (2) molecules derived from the metabolic and catabolic activities of each parenchymal organ from which the lymph drains. In more recent years, studies have shown that the composition of lymph fluid will reveal both physiological and pathological activity in a local area.[13]

Lymph Flow

Lymph fluid is extracellular fluid that is collected from the periphery of the body and transported through deep, central lymphatic ducts, against hydrostatic pressure and protein concentration gradients, and ultimately drains into the venous system.[14] The formation of the extracellular fluid occurs during the process of microcirculation. To understand this effectively, it is important to look at the four main components of microcirculation function in Figure 9.2 and gain insight in the relationship between capillaries, the surrounding tissue channels, plasma proteins (macrophages), and the initial lymphatics.

Microcirculation and the formation of lymph fluid depends on the overall balance between the hydrostatic and osmotic pressure gradients in the capillary beds and the composition of the glycocalyx.[15] The glycocalyx is a micro thin gel layer that protects the inner lining of the entire blood system, including that of arterial and venous capillaries. The glycocalyx acts like a "sieve" at both arterial and venous ends of the capillary bed, responding to the physiological needs of the local tissue, as well as the local pressure gradients to filter the right balance of nutrients, proteins, and waste product through to make up the extracellular fluid.

One of the most impactful discoveries made about the glycocalyx is that while it acts like a sieve and is a vital part of fluid exchange in capillary beds, it also has a hydrophobic component to it. In this

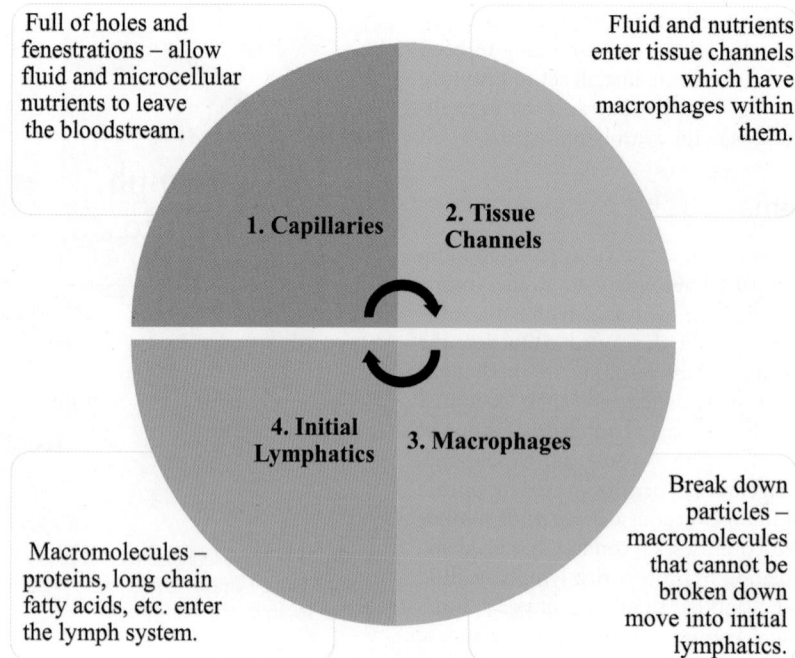

1. Capillaries — Full of holes and fenestrations – allow fluid and microcellular nutrients to leave the bloodstream.

2. Tissue Channels — Fluid and nutrients enter tissue channels which have macrophages within them.

3. Macrophages — Break down particles – macromolecules that cannot be broken down move into initial lymphatics.

4. Initial Lymphatics — Macromolecules – proteins, long chain fatty acids, etc. enter the lymph system.

• **Fig. 9.2** The Formation of the Extracellular Fluid Occurs During the Process of Microcirculation of Which There Are Four Main Components. (Created by Julia C. Osborne. Printed with permission.)

capacity it can change hydrostatic pressures and, more importantly it resists fluid exudate from the arterial capillaries from being reabsorbed from across the capillary bed into the venous capillaries. This means that almost all the lymph fluid generated within the capillary bed is absorbed by the initial lymphatics (Figure 9.3). The lymphatic system becomes the low-pressure outlet for fluid.[16]

Lymph Flow — Lymph Time Volume, Transport Capacity, Functional Reserve

The amount of lymph fluid the system can move in a unit of time is called the lymph time volume (LTV). The TC of the lymph system is the maximal amount of fluid that the lymph system can move at maximal amplitude and frequency of its vessel and node function. At rest, the LTV is only at approximately 10% of the TC. The remaining 90% of the TC is called the functional reserve (FR) as seen in Figure 9.4.

The FR allows the lymph system to adjust to increased fluid volume demands within the system. When there is increased lymph fluid production, the lymph collector vessels (see in section below) increase their frequency of contractions per minute thereby increasing the TC of the system and utilizing some of the FR. When there is loss of lymph system function, then the system's ability to maintain fluid equilibrium is compromised and the lymphatic load (LL) becomes more elevated than the available TC in the system (Figure 9.5).

Anatomy of the Lymphatic System

The lymphatic system is made up of lymphatic vessels and lymph nodes. The system runs throughout the body from superficial to deep, permeating through all body systems, moving fluid from initial lymphatic vessels, to precollector vessels, to collector vessels that feed directly into lymph node beds. Lymph fluid is filtered through lymph node beds, and ultimately cleansed filtrate is moved into the deepest vessels of the lymphatic system, namely

the lymphatic ducts. The lymphatic ducts deposit cleansed filtrate back into the venous system via the left and right subclavian veins (Figure 9.6).

The anatomy of the lymphatic system is further divided into two broad dimensions of system function. The first is the functioning of the system within territories and watersheds; and the second is the functioning of the system across superficial, deep, and visceral areas in the body.

Territories and Watersheds

The lymphatic system is divided into territories which are delineated by watershed lines (Figure 9.7). These watershed lines are formed naturally by the system itself. Their formation takes place at the subfascial level with deep, regional collector vessels feeding into associated regional lymph node basins. These regional drainage patterns allow for the formation of lymphatic territories which are divided from one another by the correlating formation of natural watershed lines (see Box 9.1).[17]

Superficial, Deep, and Visceral Drainage Regions

The lymphatic system is additionally divided into three layers of function within each territory. The "superficial lymphatics" as they are called, drain the dermal and epidermal layers of the body. The "deep lymphatics" drain the subfascial neuromusculoskeletal and myofascial tissues layers of the body. The "visceral lymphatics" drain fluid from all viscera in the body (see Figure 9.8 and Box 9.2).[18]

Rehabilitation Management of the Lymphatic System — Leveraging Its Anatomy and Relationship With Body Systems to Optimize Function

To fulfill its system-wide function, the architectural structure of lymphatic vessels and nodes is complex. Keeping in mind the

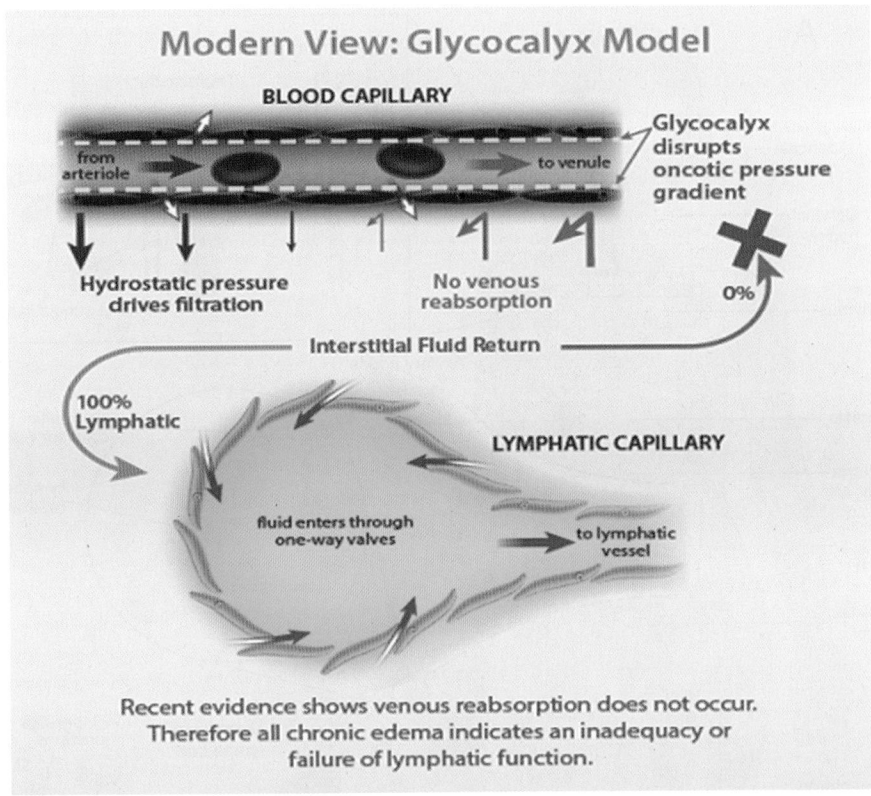

• **Fig. 9.3** Hundred Percent Fluid Absorption Into Initial Lymph Vessels.[16] (Reprinted with permission from Levick JR, Michel CC. Microvascular fluid exchange and the revised Starling principle. *Cardiovasc Res.* 2010;87(2):198–210.)

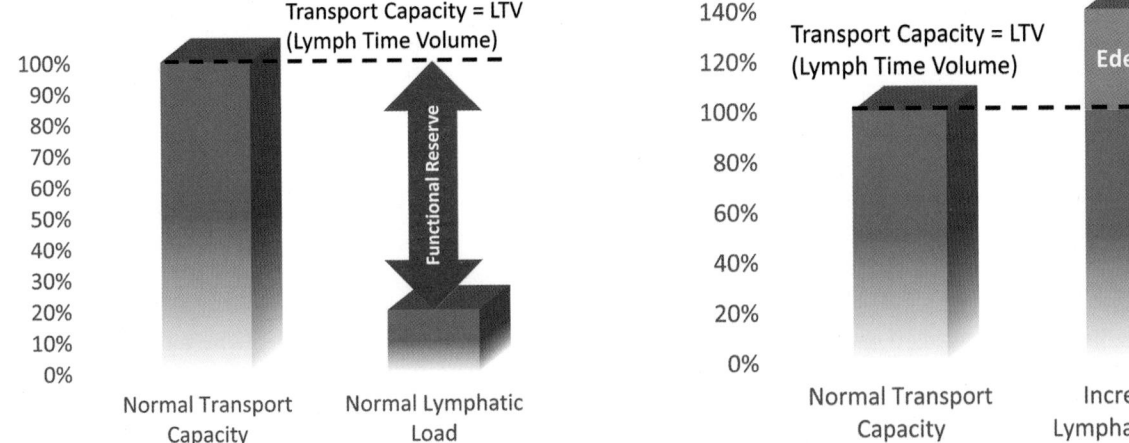

• **Fig. 9.4** Transport Capacity and Functional Reserve. (Created by Chris Wilson. Printed with permission.)

• **Fig. 9.5** Lymphatic Load Elevated Above the Transport Capacity. (Created by Chris Wilson. Printed with permission.)

overarching functions of the system as a whole and being mindful of this as an important focus in the management and treatment of the lymphatic system in persons living with lymphatic system compromise. Lymphatic vessels maintain normal tissue fluid equilibrium throughout the body by returning the capillary ultrafiltrate and extravasated plasma proteins to the central circulation via lymphatic ducts that drain into the left and right subclavian veins. The lymphatics in the abdominal region additionally have a vital role in the transport of lipids absorbed in the gastrointestinal tract. The lymphatic system also plays an integral role throughout the body in the identification of antigens and the mediation of immunological responses.[12] Loss of function in any lymphatic territory is therefore extremely impactful and has significant physiological and pathological consequences that affect all body systems and affects the overall health and wellness of persons living with lymphatic system compromise (see Box 9.3).

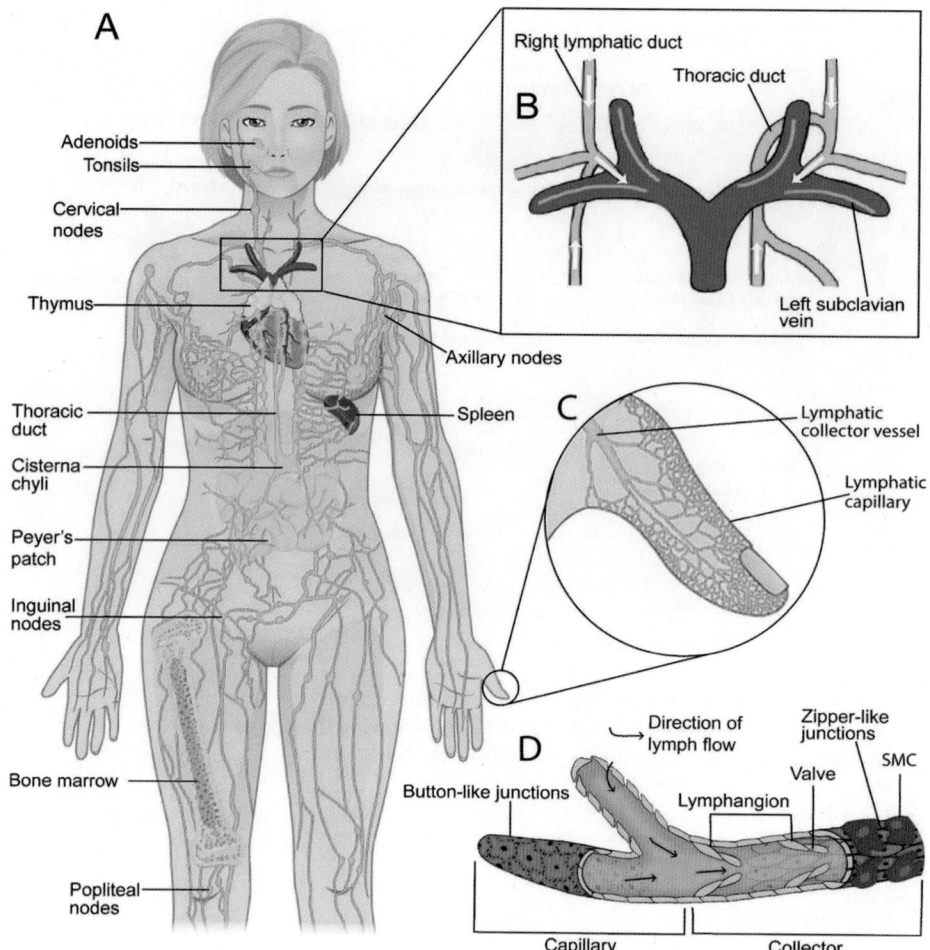

• **Fig. 9.6** SMC, smooth muscle cell. Anatomic Overview of the Lymphatic System (A) Overview of the interacting lymphatic and immune system structures, (B) Introduction of lymph into the central venous system, (C) Illustration of small lymphatic capillaries, (D) Close-up view of lymphatic capillaries to collector ducts. (This file is licensed under the Creative Commons Attribution-Share Alike 4.0 International License. Sif Nielsen and eLearning Unit members Sheetal Kavia and Dhillon Khetani from St George's, University of London (SGUL) have assisted with figure preparation. Image in (A) modified from OpenStax College under a CC BY 3.0 license. (C) Modified from OpenLearn Create under a CC BY-NC-SA 4.0 License. Reprinted with permission from commons.wikimedia.org.)

Lymphatics are organized sequentially (Figure 9.9) with open-ended initial lymphatics leading into precollector vessels, followed by prenodal collecting lymphatics feeding into lymph nodes, followed by postnodal collecting lymphatics moving cleansed filtrate into the deepest and largest lymph vessels in the body, namely the thoracic duct, and left and right lymphatic ducts. These connect to the left and right subclavian veins.

Initial Lymph Vessels

Initial lymph vessels (ILs) are in all connective tissue spaces between all cells of the body. ILs are the entry point of extracellular filtrate that needs to be absorbed by the immediate ILs in order to maintain fluid equilibrium and optimal immune function. The extracellular filtrate that moves into the immediate ILs is called the LL. See Box 9.4.

From a treatment perspective, consideration must be given as to how best to access the available ILs interspersed within body systems within an affected territory. The most remarkable feature of ILs is that, from an architectural perspective, they are the only vessel in the body designed to open wide enough to absorb large macromolecules that cannot be absorbed by other vessel systems in the body. This unique functional ability of ILs needs to be taken advantage of by oncology rehabilitation (Onc R) clinicians working to reduce lymphatic compromise, as well as working to improve overall lymphatic function. The more lymphostatic lymph fluid that can be moved from territory-based body systems into the lymphatic system, the more effective the resolution of impairment as well as the restoration of lymphatic functioning (Figure 9.10).

Epidermal/Dermal System and Initial Lymph Vessels

There are ILs throughout the dermal layer of the human body (Figure 9.11). Access to initial lymphatic vessels within this body system is one of the most important in facilitating movement of lymphostatic fluid into the regional, territory-based lymphatic

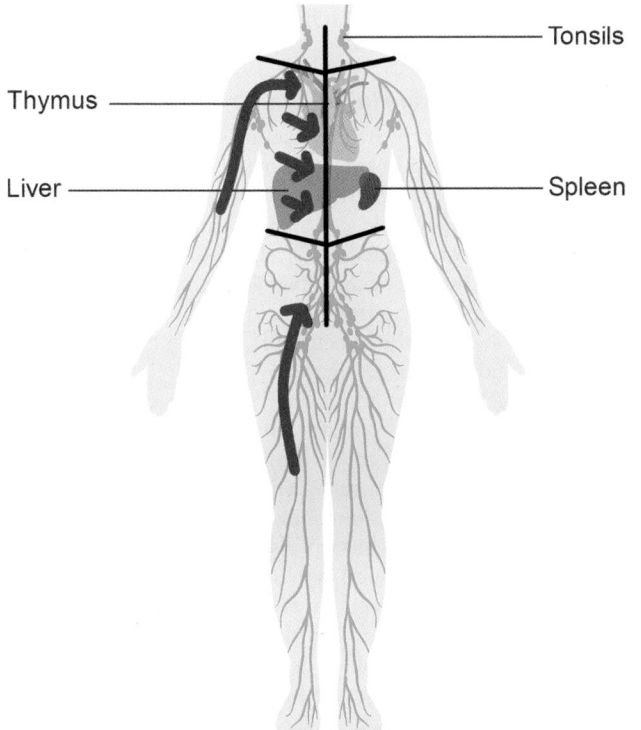

• **Fig. 9.7** Watershed Lines and Territories. (Adapted from Cancer Research UK Creative Commons Cancer Research UK. Creative Commons, CC BY-SA 4.0 https://creativecommons.org/licenses/by-sa/4.0, via Wikimedia Commons.)

The lymph system can be divided into three areas of function within territories

The Superficial Lymph System	The Deep (Subfascial) Lymph System	The Visceral Lymph System
Drains the cutis and subcutis. Superficial vessels cross watershed lines	Drains lymph from deeper structures such as the joints, synovia, nerves, and muscles	Drains via collectors which run parallel to the blood vessels of the viscera

All drain to Local Node Beds then to Ducts, then into Venous system

• **Fig. 9.8** System Function Across Superficial, Deep, and Visceral Regions. (Created by Julia C. Osborne. Printed with permission.)

• BOX 9.2   Clinical Pearl

Manual lymph drainage techniques applied to the epidermis of persons living with lymphedema is effective in draining lymphostasis from the dermal and epidermal layers of the system, across watershed lines, through superficial lymphatic vessels, from one territory to an adjacent territory to allow for "territory to territory" drainage. Manual lymph drainage aimed at draining lymphostasis from the subfascial neuromusculoskeletal and myofascial tissues layers, and visceral organs is effective when drainage techniques are focused within an affected territory, moving fluid from collector vessels to territory-based lymph node beds, to territory based lymphatic ducts thereby focusing more on "within territory" drainage.

Created by Julia C. Osborne. Printed with permission.

• BOX 9.1   Clinical Pearl

Superficial dermal and epidermal lymphatic vessels cross watershed lines, thereby allowing the movement of fluid from one territory into adjacent territories. However, deep, subfascial collector vessels do not cross watershed lines, thereby only allowing fluid movement of the deep lymphatic system to remain within the regional territory, draining into regional lymph node basins, and ultimately into either the thoracic and left lymphatic ducts, or the right lymphatic duct.

Created by Julia C. Osborne. Printed with permission.

• BOX 9.3   Clinical Pearl

Physical therapy evaluation must be inclusive of all impacted body systems and yield a set of management objectives that extend beyond the single focus of fluid volume reduction as the primary measurable outcome in managing this population.

Created by Julia C. Osborne. Printed iwth permission.

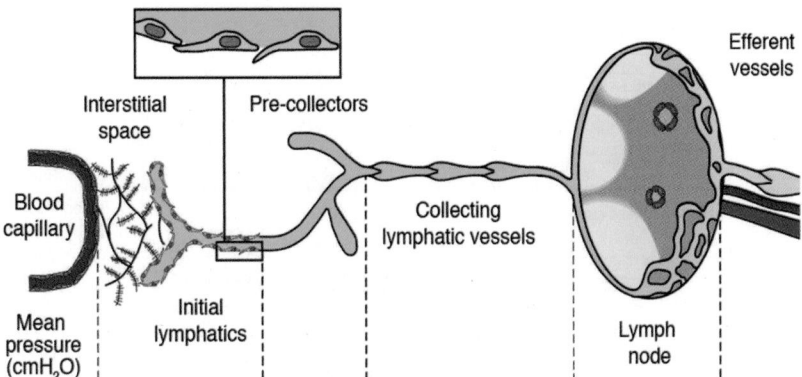

• **Fig. 9.9** Sequence of Lymphatic Vessels From Initial Lymph Vessels to Lymph Nodes. (This article is licensed under a Creative Commons Attribution 4.0 International License, https://creativecommons.org/licenses/by/4.0/. (Reprinted with permission from Jamalian S, Jafarnejad M, Zawieja SD, et al. Demonstration and analysis of the suction effect for pumping lymph from tissue beds at subatmospheric pressure. *Sci Rep.* 2017;7:12080. doi:10.1038/s41598-017-11599-x.)

When there is lymphatic territory-based impairment and henceforth local and regional lymphostasis, the clinical advantage achieved in delivering effective treatment is to assist in moving excess lymphostatic fluid into the immediate, available, initial lymph vessels. Given that these are interspersed within the connective tissue spaces between all cells of the body, clinical consideration must be given to include treatment to all body systems within, and immediately surrounding, an affected territory (Figure 9.10).

Created by Julia C. Osborne. Printed with permission.

system. This is where manual lymphatic drainage, performed by a clinician trained in the techniques, is an integral part of the treatment system for managing lymphatic impairment. Manual lymph drainage is only effective when performed optimally, and for this to happen, it is important to fully engage the biomechanical functioning of the ILs. Their biomechanical functioning is as follows: Radial tension exerted through anchoring filaments attached to the single layer of endothelial cells making up the lumen walls pulls the endothelial cells apart from each other, thereby expanding the opening of the lumen into which lymph fluid flows, as well as creating large, permeable spaces between

the cells, through which lymph fluid can also flow (Figure 9.12). See Box 9.5.

Myofascial System and Initial Lymph Vessels

In skeletal muscle both arcade arterioles and initial lymphatic vessels run side by side in the endomysial and perimysial spaces. Mechanical forces are transmitted through both vessels during muscle stretch, muscle contraction, and muscle relaxation phases of movement (Figure 9.16).[19] There is a direct relationship between the functioning of these two vessels in that arcade arterioles provide the primary pumping action required for mechanical opening and closing of the lumens of ILs during muscular stretch, contraction, and relaxation (Figure 9.17).[19]

On a more gross anatomical scale, it is also clinically important to release myofascial tension across entire muscle structures through myofascial release mechanisms. Increased myofascial tension will hold muscles in a state of increased intramuscular tension, which will reduce the functional differential needed between a contraction and a stretch but will also contribute to a widespread occlusion pressure on the local system within the muscle. The latter is substantiated by the fact that the lumens of ILs are not circular, which means that circumferential hoop stress cannot be supported by the lymphatic wall, as it can for example in arterioles. Initial lymphatics are compressed and expanded by local tissue

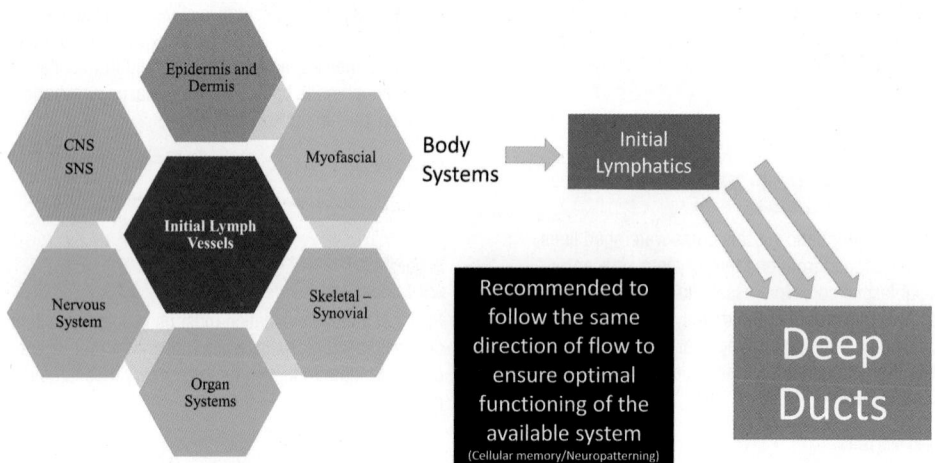

• **Fig. 9.10** The Lymphatic System Is in Relationship With All Surrounding Body Systems. (Created by Julia C. Osborne. Printed with permission.)

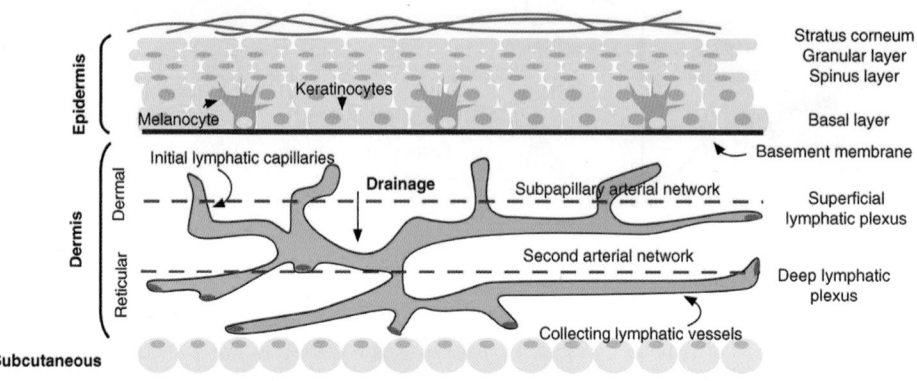

• **Fig. 9.11** Initial Lymph Vessels in the Dermis. (Reprinted with permission from Lund AW, Medler TR, Leachman SA, Coussens LM. Lymphatic vessels, inflammation, and immunity in skin cancer. *Cancer Discov.* 2016;6(1):22–35. doi:10.1158/2159-8290.CD-15-0023.)

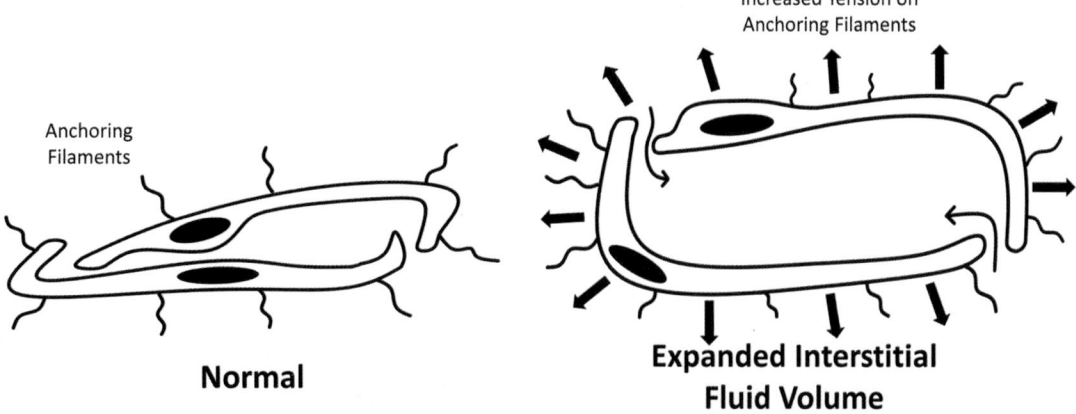

Anchoring
Filaments

Normal

Increased Tension on
Anchoring Filaments

**Expanded Interstitial
Fluid Volume**

• **Fig. 9.12** Radial Tension Through the Anchor Filaments of Initial Lymph Vessels. (Created by Julia C. Osborne. Printed with permission.)

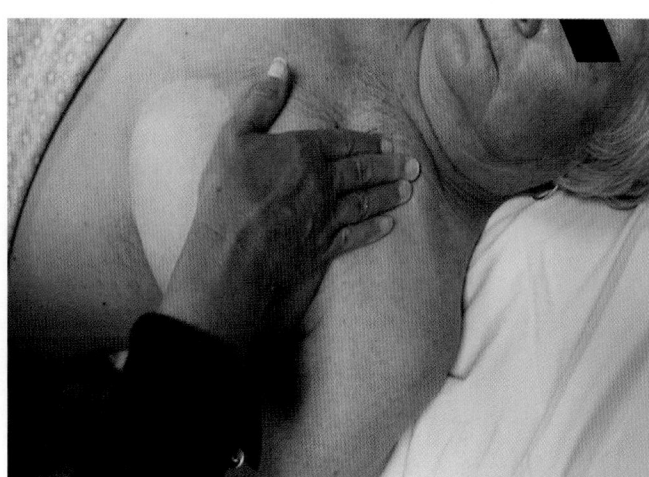

• **Fig. 9.14** Position 1: Beginning of Skin Stretch. (Photograph provided by Julia C. Osborne. Printed with permission.)

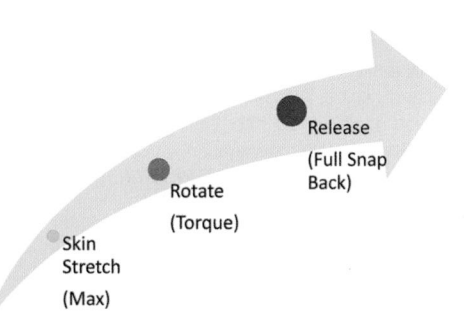

Release
(Full Snap
Back)

Rotate
(Torque)

Skin
Stretch
(Max)

• **Fig. 9.13** The Mechanics of Manual Lymph Drainage. (Created by Julia C. Osborne. Printed with permission.)

deformation and in many organs are positioned strategically in the adventitia of arterioles, bronchi, or mucosal smooth muscle, as well as other tissue structures to offer surrounding support (see Box 9.6).[20]

Skeletal System and Initial Lymph Vessels

Micromolecules in intra-articular structures are removed by synovial capillaries, however macromolecules within the synovium of joints are removed by the lymphatic system (see Box 9.7 and Figure 9.18).[21]

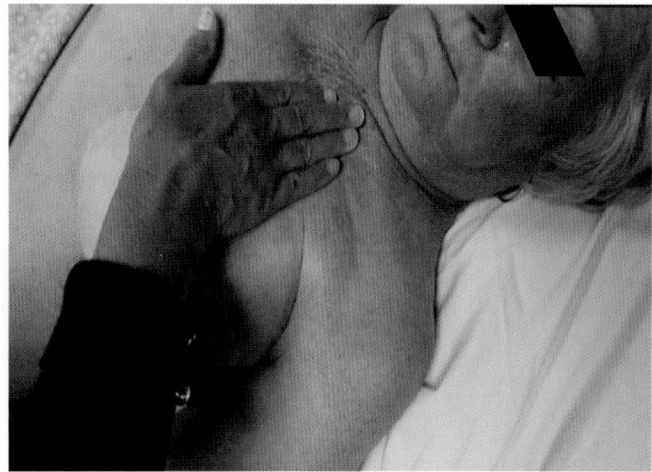

• **Fig. 9.15** Position 2: Horizontal Skin Stretch. (Photograph provided by Julia C. Osborne. Printed with permission.)

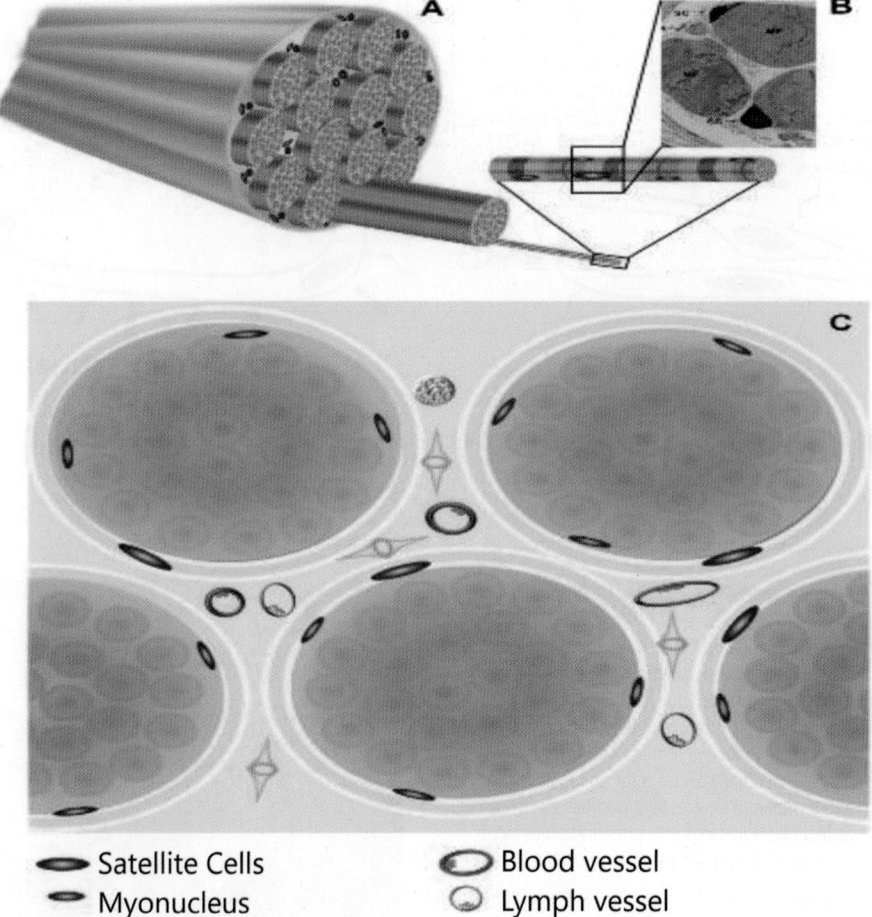

• **Fig. 9.16** Relationship Between Blood Vessels and the Initial Lymph Vessels in Skeletal Muscle. (A) The connective tissue surrounding each muscle is called epimysium, and its projections that separate muscle bundles are called perimysium. (B) The connective tissue between single muscle fibers is called endomysium and servers as the muscle satellite cells (SCs) niche. SCs are subsarcolemmal cells that can be activated to regenerate new muscle fibers. (C) Skeletal muscle tissue is not only formed by muscle fiber, but also by acellular matrix, cellular components, blood and lymphatic vessels and nerves. Altogether, these muscle niche components play a distinct role on muscle regeneration and on muscle progenitor cell regulation. (Reprinted with permission from Zouraq FA, Stölting M, Eberli D. Skeletal muscle regeneration for clinical application. In: *Regenerative Medicine and Tissue Engineering*. InTech Open; 2013. doi:10.5772/55739.)

Skeletal Muscle System

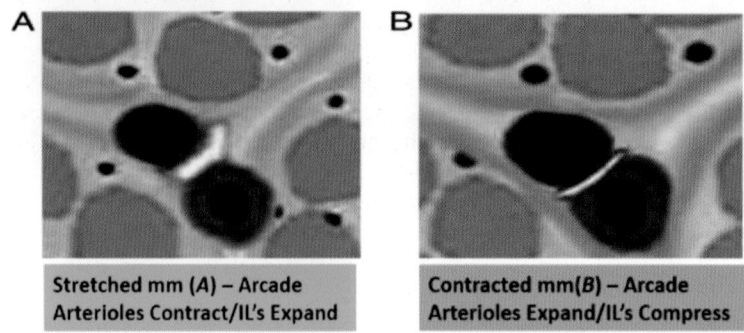

• **Fig. 9.17** Direct Relationship Between the Filling and Emptying of Arcade Arterioles and the Opening and Closing of Initial Lymph Vessels. *ILs*, Initial lymph vessels. Conceptual drawing of muscle cross-section stretched (A) and contracted (B). The arteriole and venule pairs in the perimysial space expand and compress the adjacent IL vessels during a stretch and a contraction, respectively. (Reprinted with permission from Causey L, Cowin SC, Weinbaum S. Quantitative model for predicting lymph formation and muscle compressibility in skeletal muscle during contraction and stretch. *Proc Natl Acad Sci U S A*. 2012;(23):9185–9190.)

Onc R clinicians managing and treating PLWBCs with lymphatic compromise can leverage the movement of lymph fluid into the ILs within skeletal muscle by ensuring exercise prescription that is inclusive of optimal muscle pump action. This will affect an optimal differential between a functional muscle contraction and a functional muscle stretch, facilitating the opening of IL's within the perimysial spaces. Also important for this differential to occur would be to ensure effective functional movement patterns through full range movement in all activities of daily living (ADLs) as well as reducing protective posturing which holds muscles in a shortened contracted position for prolonged periods of time, thereby further inhibiting lymph flow within the myofascial structures within an affected territory.

Created by Julia C. Osborne. Printed with permission.

Onc R clinicians managing and treating PLWBCs with lymphatic compromise can leverage the movement of lymph fluid into the ILs within joint structures by ensuring exercise prescription that is inclusive of optimal, full range joint mobility. Joints that become restricted and compressed by surrounding tightening tissue will not only create occlusion pressure on the intra-articular ILs, but also deform and distort the synovial environment thereby reducing the ability of the anchoring filaments to receive enough radial tension for optimal luminal opening. Encouraging persons living with risk of lymphatic compromise to move joints in the body through full functional range on a daily basis is important. Joint restriction results in lymphatic functional limitation.

Created by Julia C. Osborne. Printed with permission.

Lymph Precollector Vessels

Precollector vessels are next in line after lymph fluid has moved into the ILs. These vessels are made up of several layers of endothelial cells and contain valves to ensure there is no retrograde flow of lymph fluid once it enters the lymphatic system. Precollectors transport the fluid collected in the ILs to the prenodal collector vessels. These vessels are usually subfascial given that they move fluid towards the local regional lymph node beds within a territory.

Lymph Collector Vessels

Collector vessels form the primary pulsatile function of the lymphatic system in that they are lined with a layer of smooth muscle.

This facilitates their ability to be pulsatile, and to propel lymph fluid through the system towards the lymph nodes. Lymph flow through collector vessels is governed by extrinsic forces due to the movements of organs and skeletal muscles which exert external pressure on the lymphatic walls, and by the intrinsic forces due to rhythmic contractions of smooth muscle within the walls of the collector vessels (Figure 9.19).[22] Intensities of the smooth-muscle contractions are also mediated by humoral mediators such as epinephrine, serotonin, and PGE1.[22] These physiological mediators combined with the principles of mechanics, result in a very powerful system of fluid movement into lymph nodes (see Box 9.8).

Lymph Nodes

Lymph nodes are vital immunological organs, each of which has its own blood supply and nerve supply. Nodes are very complex structures at the microscopic level. Surrounded by a cortex, each node is made up of specific areas of lobules and sinuses. The lobules lie together within the sinus system and lymphocytes float within the sinus doing surveillance for antigens. Once an antigen is identified, there is active antibody secretion that occurs, as well as ongoing lymph fluid filtration.[23] It is the outer cortex

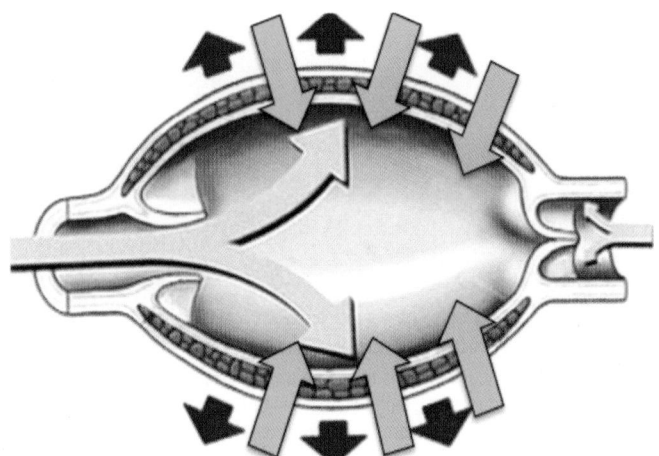

• **Fig. 9.19** Extrinsic and Intrinsic Forces Propel Fluid Through the Lymphangion of a Collector Vessel. (Reprinted with permission from Quere I. Lymphatic system: anatomy, histology, and physiology. *Presse Med.* 2010;39(12):1269–1278.)

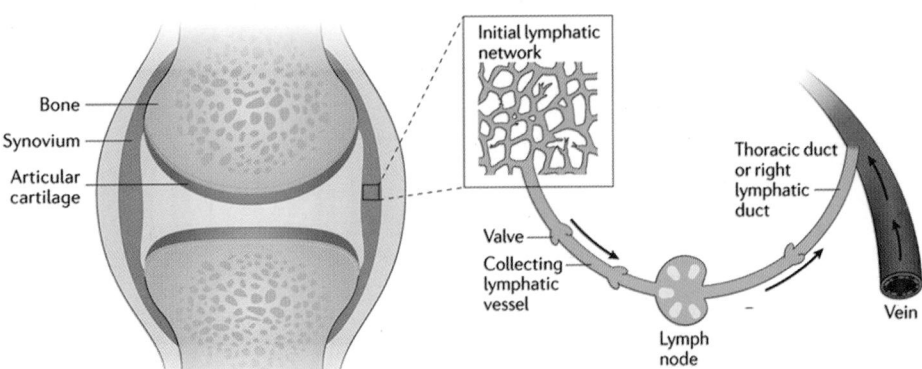

• **Fig. 9.18** Relationship of Initial Lymph Vessels in the Synovium of Joints. (Reprinted with permission from Bouta E, Bell R, Rahimi H, et al. Targeting lymphatic function as a novel therapeutic intervention for rheumatoid arthritis. *Nat Rev Rheumatol.* 2018;(14):94–106.)

The principles of mechanics affecting the contractility of the collector vessels translates into the same emphasis of the importance of practitioners ensuring functional movements within optimal range that is inclusive of the myofascial system, the skeletal system, the neural system, and the visceral system in the treatment plans of persons living with lymphatic compromise.

Created by Julia C. Osborne. Printed with permission.

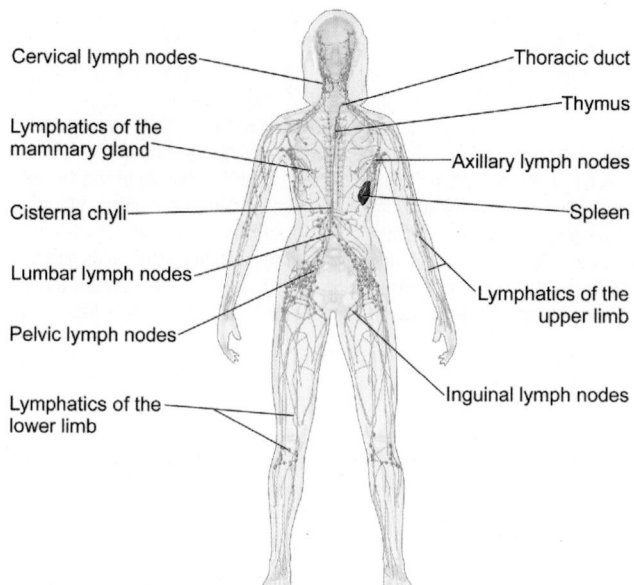

• **Fig. 9.21** Lymph Node Regions and Primary Joint Areas in the Body. (Reprinted with permission from Blausen.com staff. Medical gallery of Blausen Medical 2014. *WikiJournal Med.* 2014;1(2). doi:10.15347/wjm/2014.010. ISSN 2002-4436. Printed using CC-BY 3.0. http://creativecommons.org/licenses/by/3.0/.)

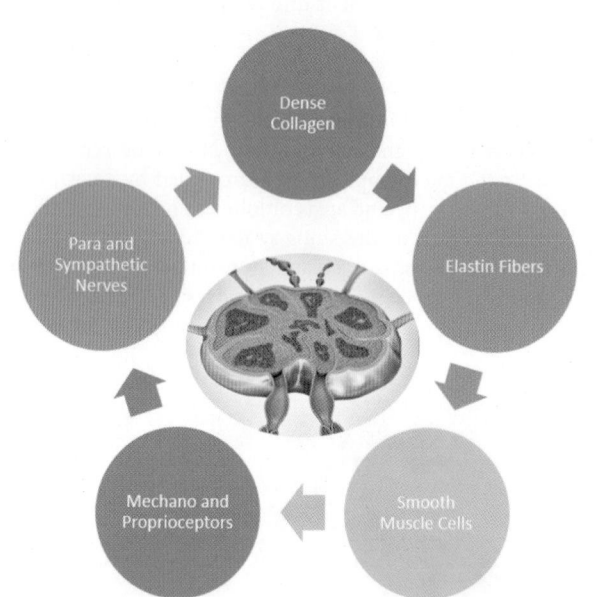

• **Fig. 9.20** The Outer Cortex of a Lymph Nodes. (Created by Julia C. Osborne. Printed with permission.)

• BOX 9.9 **Clinical Pearl**

It is important for Onc R clinicians to ensure transmission of mechanical forces onto the cortical surfaces of lymph nodes when engaging in the lymph node component of treating the system. The mechanical forces will have a function stimulating effect on elastin fibers, which are malleable, smooth muscle cells through changes in action potentials, mechanoreceptors and proprioceptors, and the sympathetic nervous system. This will assist in fluid movement within the system and help move fluid through to the lymphatic ducts and into the subclavian veins.

Created by Julia C. Osborne. Printed with permission.

(Figure 9.20) that is most important for practitioners to clinically understand and leverage in the treatment of lymphatic compromise. The outer cortex responds to mechanical forces exerted upon it, exactly in the same way as the entire lymphatic system does.

The outer cortex is made up of elastin fibers, mechanoreceptors and proprioceptors, sympathetic and parasympathetic nerves, and smooth muscle cells all enmeshed in dense collagen (see Box 9.9).

It is worth noting that the main lymph node beds are closely associated with joint structures of the skeletal system of the body (Figure 9.21). This is in part because they respond to the mechanics of joint movement. Once again this demonstrates the importance of directing mechanical input through functional movement into the system. Joints that become restricted will impact

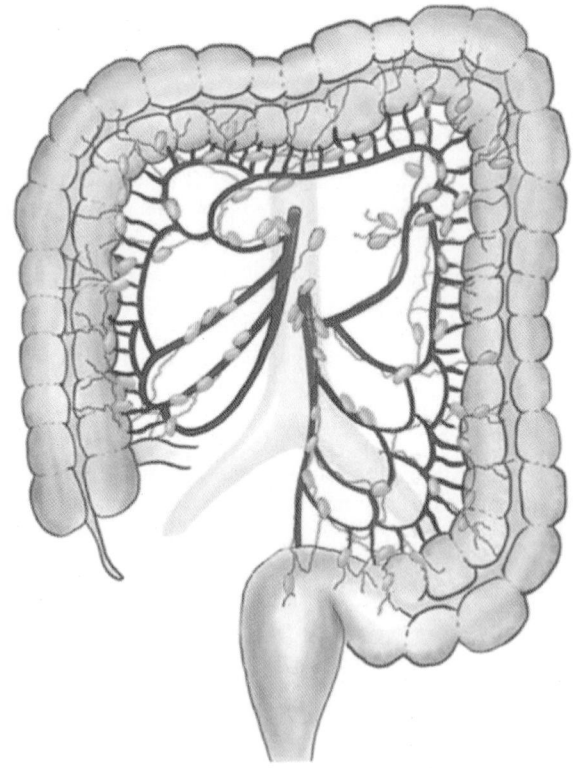

• **Fig. 9.22** Lymph Nodes Associated With the Viscera. (Reprinted with permission from *Sabiston Textbook of Surgery.* 20th ed. Elseiver: 1322.)

the transmission of mechanical forces into associated lymph node beds and this will contribute to the overall compromise of the system. The same can be applied to lymph nodes in the viscera. These are not associated with joints, but with visceral organs that also have functional movement that occurs within and around them (Figure 9.22). The functional movement of the viscera, as well as visceral mobilization techniques stimulate optimal functioning of associated lymph nodes.

Further to the discussion about the myofascial and skeletal systems, it is also worth noting that both systems play a vital role in lymph fluid movement throughout the body from the periphery to central, and into the venous system (Figure 9.23). This provides another critical reason for the importance of optimal, functional, full-range muscle contraction of all major muscle groups and optimal, full-range joint mobility of all joints in the body.

In prescribing exercises to persons living with lymphatic compromise it is important to emphasize that they are intentional about achieving this. The third driving force for lymph fluid movement in the body is the pressure difference between the thorax and the abdomen (Figure 9.24). This pressure difference is achieved functionally through effective diaphragmatic breathing. As the diaphragm alters the pressure in the thorax and the abdomen reciprocally, a pressure differential is established and lymph fluid is moved upwards, through the thoracic duct and into the left and right lymphatic ducts, and ultimately into the left and right subclavian veins.

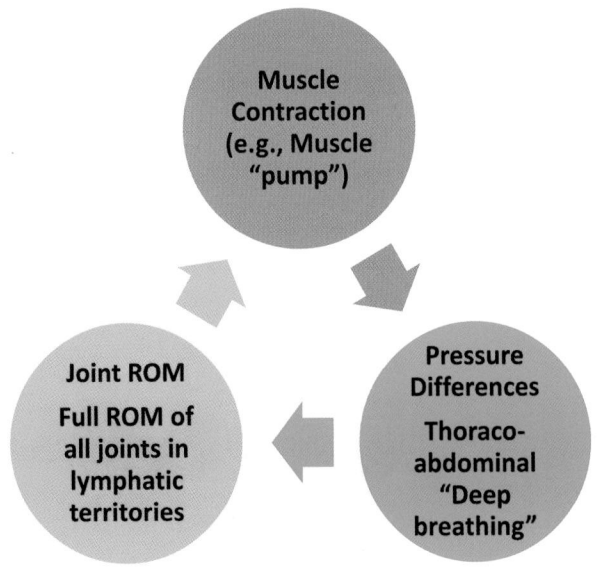

• **Fig. 9.23** The Movement of Lymph Fluid. *ROM,* Range of motion. (Created by Julia Osborne. Printed with permission.)

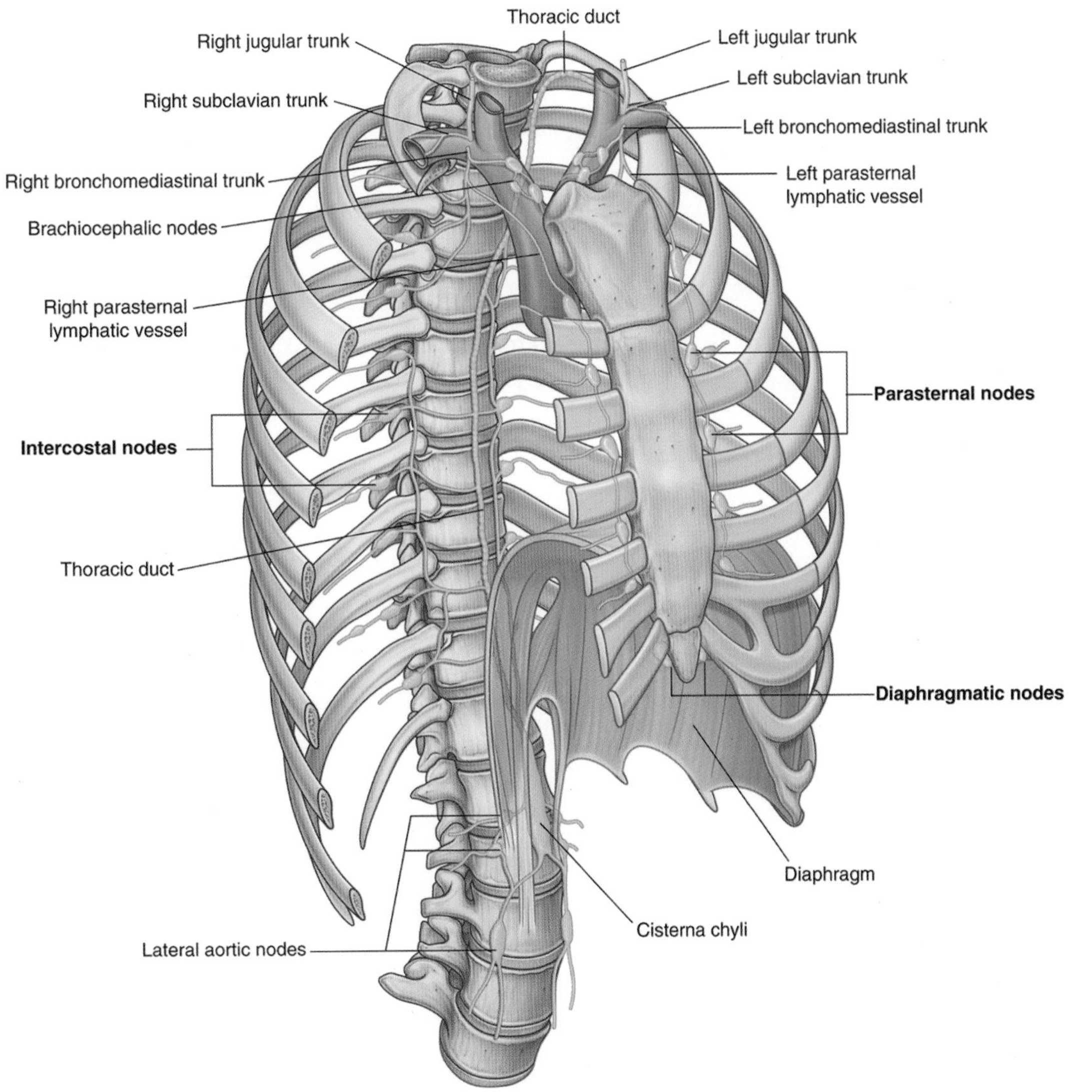

• **Fig. 9.24** Thoraco-Abdominal Pressure Difference. (Reprinted with permission from Drake RL, Vogl AW, Mitchell A. *Gray's Anatomy for Students.* Elsevier; 2020.)

Staging of Lymphedema

Clinical lymphedema is a serious medical condition. It is a chronic disease process and a progressive disease process.[1] The stages of lymphedema speak to both subclinical and clinical lymphedema and delineate the clinical presentation at the time of diagnosis of persons living with lymphatic compromise (Figure 9.25). The staging of lymphedema takes multifactorial signs and symptoms into consideration at each stage (Table 9.1).

Lymphedema Measurement

This has traditionally been performed with the use of a tape measure obtaining circumferential measurements at predetermined

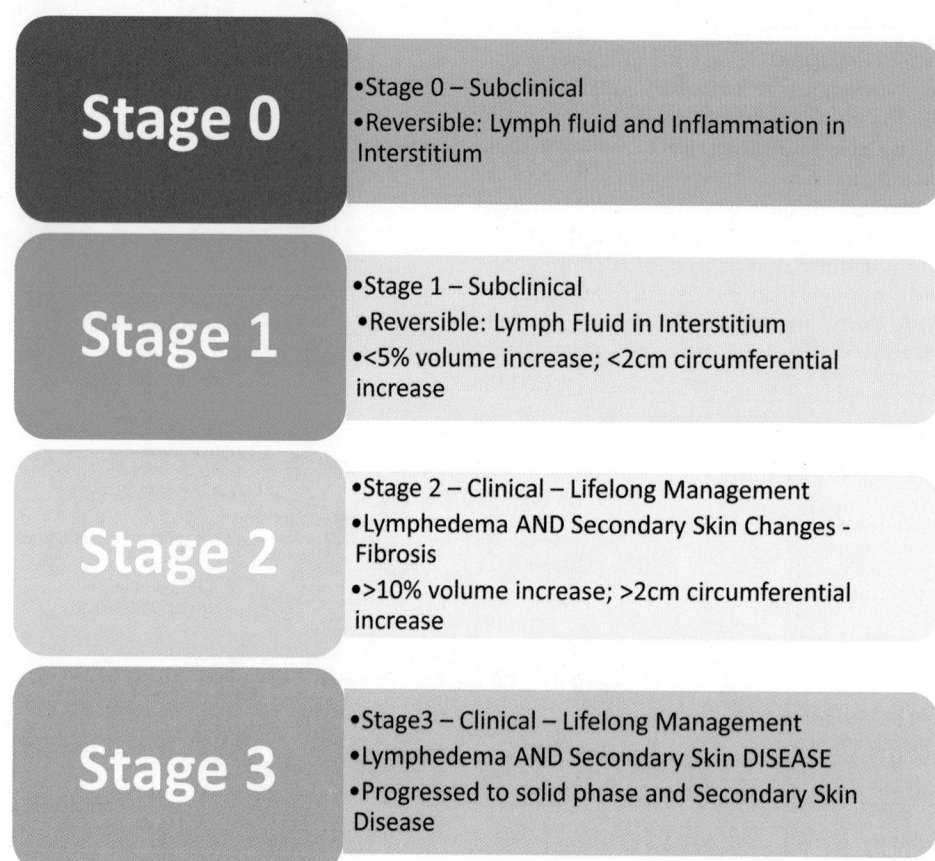

Stage 0
- Stage 0 – Subclinical
- Reversible: Lymph fluid and Inflammation in Interstitium

Stage 1
- Stage 1 – Subclinical
- Reversible: Lymph Fluid in Interstitium
- <5% volume increase; <2cm circumferential increase

Stage 2
- Stage 2 – Clinical – Lifelong Management
- Lymphedema AND Secondary Skin Changes - Fibrosis
- >10% volume increase; >2cm circumferential increase

Stage 3
- Stage3 – Clinical – Lifelong Management
- Lymphedema AND Secondary Skin DISEASE
- Progressed to solid phase and Secondary Skin Disease

• **Fig. 9.25** Stages of Subclinical and Clinical Lymphedema. (Created by Julia C. Osborne. Printed with permission.)

TABLE 9.1	The Stages of Lymphedema

Stage 0: Subclinical Lymphedema (Reversible)
- Risk of subclinical lymphedema progressing to a clinical lymphedema but does not present with outward signs of swelling
- Lymphatic transport capacity has been reduced — predisposes the patient to lymphatic overload and resultant edema

Stage 1: Subclinical Lymphedema (Reversible)
- Liquid phase of subclinical lymphedema
- Swelling at this stage is soft, pitting edema

Stage 2: Clinical Lymphedema (Irreversible)
- Secondary tissue changes — tissue fibrosis/induration and skin and tissue thickening occur as the limb volume increases
- Pitting may be present, but there is transition from liquid phase to solid phase edema

Stage 3: Lymphostatic Elephantiasis (Irreversible)
- Solid phase clinical lymphedema
- Nonpitting fibrotic lymphedema
- Secondary skin disease — dermal thickening, papillomas, increased risk of infections/cellulitis

Created by Julia C. Osborne. Printed with permission.

TABLE 9.2	Volumetric Measurements Compared to Bioimpedance Measurements	
At Risk Early-Stage Upper Extremity Lymphedema (Stage 0–1)	**Bioimpedance Spectroscopy (BIS) Analysis**	**Volumetrics Using a Tape Measure**
	BIS analysis is sensitive enough to be used to detect early, subclinical Stage 0–1 lymphedema, allowing for effective prospective assessment	Circumferential measurements are appropriate for detecting clinical Stage 2 or 3 lymphedema but are not sensitive enough to detect early-stage subclinical Stage 0–1 lymphedema
	BIS analysis yields and L-Dex Score (Lymphedema Index Score) where the inter-arm ratio ranges from a score of 10 = mean + 3standard deviation (SD) to a score of −10 = mean −3SD. The total change in score from a presurgical baseline to a postsurgical baseline must be considered (e.g., a PLWC could have a presurgical score of −4 and a postsurgical score of +7. Total change is 11 which is greater than 10 and a SD of 3)	When using circumferential measurements, total volume change should be calculated. Volume is commonly calculated using the formula representing the frustum of a cone: $V = h * (C2 + Cc + c2)/(12 * \pi)$ V = volume of a segment measured every 4 cm C and c represent the circumferential measurements in cm of each segment. h = the distance between the circumferences ($h = 4$ cm)
	Cut off point of >10 from preoperative values should be used to diagnose breast cancer-related lymphedema[24]	Calculated volume changes between affected and nonaffected limbs of >200 mL or a difference ratio of > 1.04 (affected: nonaffected) are indicative of clinical lymphedema
	Cut off point of >7 should be used to diagnose breast cancer-related lymphedema when preoperative measurements are not available[24]	Measuring and calculation methods are noninterchangeable. Calculated volume changes < 200 mL or < 1.04 do not necessarily rule out the onset of clinical lymphedema

Created by Julia C. Osborne. Printed with permission.
Volume calculation using formula representing the frustrum of a cone is courtesy of Bevilacqua JLB, Kattan MW, Changhong Y, et al. Nomograms for predicting the risk of arm lymphedema after axillary dissection in breast cancer. *Ann Surg Oncol.* 2012;19(8):2580.

points in an area of lymphedema. In addition to the use of a tape measure, in more recent years bioimpedance spectroscopy (BIS) has emerged as another clinically relevant form of measurement. BIS provides a lymphedema index measurement which is especially helpful in its accuracy in providing subclinical and early-stage clinical lymphedema measurements.[24] Table 9.2 provides an example of the measurement parameters for both tape measure measurement and BIS measurement in the upper extremity. BIS uses tissue resistance to electrical current, known as impedance, to compare the volume of fluid in the intercellular compartment to the fluid in the extracellular (interstitial fluid) compartments. The level of impedance of electrical current through these fluid compartments is inversely proportional to the volume of fluid within them. Therefore, when clinical lymphedema is present, the accumulation of excess interstitial fluid results in a decrease in tissue impedance.[25]

Prospective Surveillance Model of Care

When it is detected at its earliest onset, therapeutic management has a greater likelihood of reducing short and long-term morbidity. Evidence supports the prospective surveillance model (PSM) for early identification and treatment to prevent or mitigate many of these concerns.[26] Dr. Stout's landmark study[26] in 2012 demonstrated that using the PSM approach to asses subjective and objective signs and symptoms of lymphedema by advocating for early referral and providing surveillance throughout the trajectory of the disease process and its treatment, holds the greatest promise for earlier identification and treatment of lymphedema. The PSM allows for identification of Stage 0 to 1 lymphedema, which is reversible. This is especially important because subclinical lymphedema can exist without an increase in volume. The PSM is best initiated in a prehabilitative setting where baseline measurements including volumetrics and BIS

can be gathered. The PSM should continue for the PLWBC into Onc R treatment postsurgery and throughout cancer treatment.

Effective intervention includes the PSM to identify earliest signs of meaningful clinical change (Table 9.3). These have been developed through an international consensus of stakeholders.[26]

Risk Assessment

The impacts on the lymphatic system are multifactorial and layer into a complex management system. Risk assessment models are evolving in research. Lymphedema should not only be measured by the presence of swelling, but also by other symptoms and contributing factors.[27] To this end, early implementation of these in initial prehabilitative and rehabilitative settings assist in building appropriate plans of care for Persons Living With Breast Cancer (PLWBCs). Risk assessment and stratification models (Table 9.4) are inclusive of individualized objective and subjective data collected from PLWBCs allowing Onc R clinicians to be able to assess the potential risk of subclinical lymphedema progressing to clinical lymphedema.

Early Treatment Intervention

Early intervention provides the Onc R clinician with a window of opportunity to initiate CDT and concurrent rehabilitation using the principles of treatment delineated earlier in the chapter. This will assist in the mitigation of the onset of clinical lymphedema and to facilitate the optimal recovery and function of the local area of lymphatic injury.

Early Referral to Lymphatic Surgery Assessment

This is an area of intervention that is evolving with increasing sophistication of both technique and type of procedure. Currently

TABLE 9.3	The Prospective Surveillance Model of Care[26]

Baseline Clinical Assessment at the Time of Cancer Diagnosis

- Identify normal lifestyle behaviors
- Identify normal physical activity levels
- Screening of the affected territory
- ROM, strength, function
- Volumetrics (tape measure, Bioimpedance Spectroscopy (BIS) — L-Dex/SOZO)
- Tissue assessment (palpation, MoistureMeter)

Ongoing Model of Interval Surveillance at Determined Time Points

- Noticeable swelling (visible, palpable, experienced)
- Symptoms — Develop screening questions (heaviness, achiness, fatigue, numbness, and tingling)
- Territory-based Screening — Function, volumetrics (tape measure or bioimpedance spectroscopy), tissue assessment

Created by Julia C. Osborne. Printed with permission.

TABLE 9.4	Systemic Checklist for Risk Assessment/ Stratification

Lymph Node Biopsy/Dissection

- Extent of dissection

Surgical Intervention(s)

- Extent of surgery and reconstructive surgeries; healing issues; scar tissue necrosis
- Number of phases to complete surgical and reconstructive process
- Fluid dynamic issues — seroma formation, hematoma formation
- Infection

Radiation — Regional and Targeted

- Regional radiation with local lymph node involvement
- Targeted radiation with no nymph node involvement

Chemotherapy — Systemic, Targeted, Hormone, Immunotherapy

- Taxane-based chemotherapy — increased extracellular fluid volume (Tokumoto et al., 2020).
- Targeted therapies — soft tissue inflammation and joint arthralgia
- Hormone therapies and immunotherapies have a common side effect of joint arthralgia often resulting in joint restriction and decreased range of motion.

Infection — Cellulitis

Genetic Predisposition

- Genetic susceptibility may influence risk (Newman, 2012)

BMI >30

- Occlusion pressure on lymphatic vessels; disruption in metabolic & endocrine function

Comorbidities — Vascular, Cardiopulmonary, Renal, Autoimmune

Created by Julia C. Osborne. Printed with permission.

there are three types of lymphatic surgery, namely lympho-venous anastomosis (LVA), vascularized lymph node transfer (VLNT), and suction-assisted protein lipectomy (SAPL).

Lympho-Venous Anastomosis

This is the least invasive of the three surgical interventions and is most successfully performed with Stage 0 or Stage 1 lymphedema diagnoses. Early referral for assessment is important within the first 3 to 6 months postsurgery with Sentinel Lymph Node Biopsy (SNLB) or Axillary Lymph Node Dissection (ALND).[28] An advanced form of micro-vascular surgery, lymph vessels in the affected body region are connected to nearby veins. These connections create additional outflow pathways to drain excess lymph fluid. This surgery can be very effectively performed on PLWBCs who have a subclinical presentation of lymphedema. The research shows that the progression to clinical lymphedema is significantly reduced.[29] Research also shows that prophylactic LVA has been shown to decrease the incidence of postoperative lymphedema among individuals receiving mastectomy with ALND, and additionally, prophylactic LVA is economically preferred over mastectomy and ALND alone from a cost minimization perspective.[30] Performing a prophylactic LVA results in an average of $7646.65 (45.2%) cost saving per patient over the course of their lifetime where lifetime costs average around $13,942.26.[30] It is for these reasons that LVA should be a part of the pathway of management for PLWBCs who are at risk of clinical lymphedema.

Vascularized Lymph Node Transfer

This is also a microsurgical procedure that can improve the PLWBC's own physiologic drainage of lymphatic fluid in an affected area.[29] The surgery involves the transfer of functional lymph nodes, usually associated with tissue flaps harvested from within the axillary, inguinal, abdominal, or cervical lymph node basins, which are then connected to recipient node beds with micro-anastomoses of local vasculature to maintain their blood supply and to ensure their viability.[31] This surgery is also an early intervention and prophylactic procedure. It is often performed at the same time as reconstructive surgery, or free flap surgeries at the time of tumor removal and lymph node biopsy.

Suction-Assisted Protein Lipectomy

This surgery is most effective with solid phase advanced Stage 2 and Stage 3 clinical lymphedema diagnoses.[32] In cases where SAPL is needed, the lymphedema disease process has progressed to such an extent that adipose tissue deposition has occurred as well as the laying down of severe fibrosis and dermal thickening. With the presence of such dense tissue, improving the drainage pathways by performing an LVA or a VLNT is futile. The SAPL procedure uses a narrow-gauge cannula to remove the excess adipose and fibrotic tissue in the extremity, thereby restoring some degree of fluid drainage capability of the lymphatic system. Once some of the drainage pathways have been reestablished, the SAPL surgery can be followed by either an LVA or a VLNT to improve the system's own physiological drainage capacity.[32]

The Future of Lymphedema Care

There is still so much to be learned and understood about the lymphatic system and the disease process of lymphedema. Study of both the functioning of the system and the physiology of the disease is still today a growing science. As research increases in its sophistication and discovery, our clinical opportunity to be successful in both mitigating the onset of clinical lymphedema and reducing its disease impact will continue to evolve in its effectiveness. As Onc R clinicians, we must continue our focused study in this area of clinical management and consider the importance of treating persons living with lymphatic compromise from a body system-based functional impairment model of care that is inclusive of physical and psychological considerations in response to this disease process.

Integumentary System

The skin is the largest organ of the body, and like many other body systems, the skin is negatively impacted both directly and indirectly by cancer and its treatments. Research has highlighted the similarities between wound healing and tumor progression; therefore, an understanding of the wound healing cascade may also lead to better insight into cancer pathology and treatment.

Anatomy of the Skin

The skin is composed of three layers: epidermis, dermis, and hypodermis. Each layer contains cells and structures vital to the various functions of the skin. Skin thickness varies from 5.5 mm thick at the palms and soles to less than 1 mm thick at the eyelid.[33]

For a more thorough discussion of each skin layer and key cells/structures, please refer to the enhanced e-book. eFigure 9.1 depicts the layers of the epidermis while eFigure 9.2 highlights the various layers and structures found in the dermis. Refer to Table 9.5 for a description of important cells and structures located in the skin that are related to wound healing.

Epidermis

The epidermis, the outer-most layer of the skin, consists of four or five distinct layers, depending on location (stratum basale, stratum spinosum, stratum granulosum, stratum lucidum, and the stratum corneum) (eFigure 9.1) and is primarily composed of keratinocytes. As keratinocytes migrate toward the surface of the epidermis, they go through a process of proliferation, cell differentiation, and eventually cell death, followed by sloughing off of the outermost cell layer. The time for cell to migrate from the basal layer to slough off is up to 30 days in young people; 50 days in the elderly.[33]

The deepest layer of the epidermis, called the stratum basale or stratum germinavatum is attached to the basement membrane via hemidesmosomes. This layer is made up of metabolically active keratinocytes, called basal cells, which contain keratin. These cells actively divide and migrate toward the outer layer, where the cells begin a process called keratinization. The epidermis is avascular but receives its blood supply by osmosis from the dermis through the basement membrane.

Superficial to the basal layer is the stratum spinosum, or spiny layer, and is where production of keratin and other proteins begin.[34] The keratinocytes in this layer have a characteristic

TABLE 9.5 Key Epidermal and Dermal Wound Healing Cells and Structures

Skin Layer	Cell/Structure	Function
Epidermis	Keratinocyte	Wound re-epithelialization
	Melanocyte	Protects against ultraviolet light, gives skin/hair its color
	Langerhans cell	Initiates the immune response activates T-cell lymphocytes
Dermis	Macrophage	M1 phenotype: digests bacteria M2 phenotype: Slows inflammatory process, digests byproducts of inflammatory phase including cellular debris Promotes proliferative phase
	Fibroblast	Produces extracelluar matrix components: collagen, elastin, proteoglycans
	Myofibroblast	Contracts wound edges, produces collagen, aligns collagen fibers
	Mast cell	Produce histamine to increase capillary permeability, allowing migration of wound healing cells
	Dermal Appendages Hair follicle Sweat gland Sebaceous gland	Assist with re-epithelialization, lined with epithelium, hair follicle bulge is the source of keratinocyte stem cells

Created by Caroline S. Gwaltney. Printed with permission.

"spiny" appearance when stained, thus giving the layer its name. The keratinocytes synthesize tonofibrils that connect to desmosomes,[35] which are one of the structures that adhere the cells of the epithelium together to provide strength to the skin.

Keratinocytes in the stratum granulosum, or granular layer, become dehydrated and start to lose their cellular organelles.[36] The granules located in the keratinocytes contain lipids, enzymes, and proteins which are precursors to keratin filaments that connect the cells.[36,37] This creates a highly soluble keratin matrix that acts as a scaffold for attachment of the lipids and "cornified cell envelope."[37,38] This hydrophobic envelope prevents fluid loss from the epidermis, and also prevents invasion of allergens, toxins, and infectious bacteria and viruses.[36,37]

The stratum lucidum (found in thicker, hairless skin of the palms of the hands, and soles of the feet) consists of dead keratinocytes that have a clear characteristic under a microscope.[34] This layer adds additional protection against the shear and friction forces common to the hands and feet, as well as additional moisture barrier protection.[34]

The stratum corneum is composed of the keratinized cells surrounded and protected by the lipid corneal envelope, sometimes called corneocytes[34] or squamous cells, which provides significant protection for the skin. The cells are connected by corneodesmosomes that naturally degrade over time, thereby allowing desquamation, defined as the natural process of sloughing the outer layer of the epidermis.[39] This process is controlled through the production and tight regulation of proteases. Epidermal thickness is maintained by balancing the production of new keratinocytes at the basal layer with desquamation.[39,40]

Key Cells of the Epidermis

Although keratinocytes are the primary cells of the epidermis, there are other key epidermal cells. The keratinocytes are the key cell involved in re-epithelialization of wounds, during which a thin layer of actively dividing basal keratinocytes will migrate across the open wound in order to close it. Melanocytes, located in the basal layer and hair follicles of the skin,[34] produce varying amounts of melanin among individuals. The melanin is then absorbed by and stored in the keratinocytes. Melanin gives hair and skin its color; the more melanin produced, the darker the skin or hair color.

Langerhans cells are both native to the epidermis in the stratum spinosum and also derived from bone marrow during an inflammatory response.[41] These cells act as the skin's first line of defense against bacteria.[35] They initiate an immune response by producing antigens that attract lymphocytes and T-cells to the wounded area. Langerhans cells and T-cells are common targets in immunotherapy treatments that target cancer.[41]

Basement Membrane

The basement membrane serves as an anchor between the epidermis and the dermis, providing stability as well as a diffusion barrier.[42] It consists of Type IV collagen, at least one type of laminin, the protein nidogen, and the proteoglycan perlecan.[42] Keratin filaments in the keratinocytes are connected to hemidesmosomes, which attach the epidermis to the basement membrane. Anchoring filaments and fibrils attach to the underlying dermis. Of note, a breach in the basement membrane of the skin or vascular tissue is an indicator of the progression and invasiveness of cancer.[42]

Dermis

The dermis is much thicker than the epidermis, but less defined, with two main layers: the papillary and reticular layers.[43] The papillary dermis is directly beneath the basement membrane. The connection between the epidermis and dermis consists of a mortise-like link between epidermal pegs that project downward and dermal papillae that project upward, giving this junction a wavy appearance called rete ridges. This integration provides protection from forces of friction and shear.[34] The rete ridges flatten with age, making older individuals more susceptible to skin tears.

The papillary layer consists of loose collagen, thin elastin, fibroblasts, and blood vessels.[44] Capillary loops extend into the dermal papillae where diffusion of blood occurs through the basement membrane to support the avascular epidermis. The deeper, reticular layer is thicker than the papillary dermis and has a denser concentration of collagen and elastin.[44] The collagen and elastin in the reticular dermis run parallel to the surface of the skin, but in multiple directions, thus giving skin its ability to withstand stretch in all directions. The dermis gives skin structure, strength, and elasticity while supporting the skin appendages, sensory structures, and superficial lymphatic vessels (eFigure 9.3).

Skin Appendages

The skin appendages arise and/or pass through the dermis and epidermis and include the hair, sweat glands, sebaceous glands, and nails. The sebaceous glands and hair shaft can be further grouped into a pilosebaceous unit which also includes the hair follicle and erector pili muscle.[45] The hair follicle is continuous with the epidermis and is, therefore, lined with epithelial cells (melanocytes, keratinocytes, and stem cells).[45] Further, the bulge of the hair follicle is a source of stem cells that differentiate into keratinocytes.[46] The hair follicle is an important structure to consider regarding wound healing; if the hair follicle is not lost, this can be a source of new epithelial growth to resurface the wound.

Sebaceous glands are connected to the hair follicle and are located throughout the skin (except in the palms, soles, lips, and dorsum of the feet).[45] The lobules of these glands produce sebum, or oil, which lubricates the skin and hair. Sebum combined with sweat also provides immunity and protection against bacteria by contributing to the acidity of the skin.[34,44] Loss of the sebaceous glands in tissue injury leads to dry, fragile skin that is at increased risk for breakdown.

Two types of sweat glands exist throughout the body: eccrine and apocrine glands. Eccrine glands are located deep in the dermis and hypodermis (except the lips and external genitalia) but are most concentrated in the palms, soles, and head.[45,47] Eccrine sweat glands are controlled by the parasympathetic system and function to cool the skin for temperature regulation.[47] These glands secrete merocrine, a hypotonic saline sweat solution[47] that is odorless due to a lack of a cellular component to the sweat.[45] Conversely, the apocrine glands are under adrenergic control and become active during puberty.[47] Located primarily in the axillae, nipple, genital region, and groin, the apocrine glands produce sweat that is oilier and contains odor.[47]

Key Cells of the Dermis

The dermis gives rise to many cells that are key to wound healing. Fibroblasts produce collagen, elastin, and proteoglycans, key components of the dermis that provide strength and elasticity.[43] Wound-activated fibroblasts produce much more collagen that fibroblasts in normal tissue.[48] Fibroblasts are capable of differentiating into the myofibroblast, which is characterized by the presence of the protein α-smooth muscle actin (α-SMA).[49] As the name suggests, this protein gives the myofibroblast the ability to contract like smooth muscle, which is critical to wound contraction while healing. There are a variety of factors that control myofibroblast activation and function, but the growth factor TGF-β1 has been shown to be the most significant.[50,51] Myofibroblasts are not located in normal tissues, but are differentiated in wound healing and pathology, including cancer. These cells have been implicated in diseases involving fibrosis, which will be discussed later in the chapter.

Circulating monocytes become macrophages when they reach the dermis, and these "big eaters" of bacteria and byproducts of other inflammatory cells are key to the inflammatory phase, but they also play a role in the proliferative and remodeling phases. Mast cells of the dermis produce histamine, which is important for the immune response. Histamine allows increased permeability of the capillaries to allow leukocytes and proteins to diffuse into the wounded area where they phagocytose bacteria and debris.

Hypodermis

While not considered a true layer of the skin, the hypodermis is below the dermis and contains some of the dermal appendages and deeper lymphatic vessels.[43] The hypodermis allows free movement of the skin over the deeper muscles and bones and consists of loose connective tissue, adipose cells of varying numbers throughout the body, and blood vessels.[34] Adipose tissue stores the fat-soluble vitamins A, D, E, and K while also providing energy, insulation, and cushioning of underlying structures.[43]

Fascia, considered a part of the hypodermis, is thick, fibrous tissue that covers and separates many structures, such as muscle, tendon, and bone. Visualization of the fascia also gives the Onc R clinician an idea of the depth of tissue injury, and as a rule should not be debrided.

Functions of the Skin

The skin performs a variety of functions integral to survival, comfort, and quality of life (QOL). As the body's outer-most barrier, the skin provides protection from the outside environment in a variety of ways. The waterproof epidermal layers are the first line of defense preventing excessive fluid loss while regulating fluid absorption from outside the body. The keratinized skin cells work together with immune cells in the skin to prevent against viral and bacterial invasion.[52] Skin immunity is further strengthened by the Langerhans cells located in the epidermis. These cells are the first to recognize a foreign invader of the epidermis, inciting an immune response by activating T-lymphocytes.[34]

The skin is healthiest at an acidic pH of 4.0 to 5.5, called the acid mantle.[53] The acidity contributes to the immune function of the skin, preventing excessive growth of resident bacteria normally found on the surface while also strengthening the permeability barrier.[54] The pH is maintained by secretions from the sweat and sebaceous glands as well as proton pumps which pump hydrogen ions onto the skin's surface.[36]

Melanin, produced by the melanocytes, is absorbed by the keratinocytes of the epidermis and protects the body from ultraviolet (UV) radiation while also absorbing resulting reactive oxygen species (ROS) that results from exposure.[55] Although melanin provides protection against UV light, it has also been implicated in the development of skin cancer later in life.[56]

UV light is essential for vitamin D synthesis in the skin, a vitamin critical for bone health; however, vitamin D is also implicated in a variety of conditions, including cancer.[57] Because few foods contain vitamin D, exposure to sunlight is essential for its synthesis by the skin. Upon exposure to sunlight, vitamin D hydroxylase is secreted by keratinocytes which converts 7-dehydrocholesterol to previtamin D_3, then a temperature-dependent process converts previtamin D_3 to vitamin D_3.[34,57] Further conversion is performed in the liver, creating the active form of vitamin D.[57]

The skin is a sensory organ, and intact tactile sensation is critical to both development and survival.[58] For example, loss of pain sensation elevates the risk of skin breakdown due to mechanical forces. Several structures in the skin provide input on touch, pain, pressure, and vibrations sensations. These can be broken down into low-threshold mechanoreceptors that sense gentle touch, and nociceptors which sense more threatening inputs such as heat, pain, and chemical stimuli.[58] Merkel cells, which are light touch receptors, are found in the basal layer of the epidermis near the rete ridges in hairless skin.[58] Free nerve endings that sense temperature, pain, and touch are also found in the basal layer. The dermis contains several different structures related to sensation. Messner's corpuscles and Pascinian corpuscles sense low-frequency and high-frequency vibration, respectively while Raffini endings sense stretch.[58] The base of the hair follicle also contains Merkel cell-like structures that sense gentle touch and pressure.

The skin is critical for thermoregulation, acting first as an outer "coat." Sweat glands and superficial vasculature of the skin work together to maintain normal body temperature. As core temperature rises, the body increases sweat production to cool the body via evaporation while simultaneously sending increased blood flow to the periphery for cooling. Conversely, when core body temperature is low, the body shunts blood flow more centrally to preserve temperature. With additional cooling, the body attempts to create heat through involuntary shivering. The reflexive responses to excess heat and cold are controlled by the autonomic nervous system.[59]

Finally, the skin has a role in identity and communication. A person's unique appearance is, in part, related to skin color, freckles, skin texture, and skin appearance.[34] Wrinkles indicate age, skin color can suggest ethnicity and culture, and facial skin can imply emotion. Pheromones are released through the apocrine sweat glands after puberty, contributing to a method of social and sexual communication.[34]

Wound Healing

Wound healing is a complex, orchestrated process that occurs in an anticipated, overlapping sequence of events in healthy individuals, but can be altered, delayed, or even stalled in the presence of many disease states, infection, or improper wound care. The cells are the performers, but the great "conductor" of this orchestra is cell signaling. Cellular communication via cell signaling is essential in each phase, taking place via chemical messengers, such as growth factors, cytokines, chemokines, and interleukins released by multiple cells at various timepoints during wound healing.[60] These substances can alter the growth, movement, or differentiation of the target cell, which can be the cell itself (autocrine mechanism of action), a cell in contact with the original cell (juxtracrine), a neighboring cell (paracrine), or a cell within the circulating system (endocrine).[61] Cells are activated or suppressed in response to the chemical signal at various stages of wound healing, and the temporospatial aspects of release of signals is critical to normal healing. Various cells also alter their phenotype and role in wound healing in response to these signals.[60]

Four distinct yet overlapping phases of wound healing have been identified: hemostasis, inflammatory, proliferative, and remodeling. An understanding of the cellular activity during each phase helps Onc R clinicians recognize the similarities between wound healing and cancer. The Onc R clinician should also consider the implications of abnormal lab values as it relates to these processes, including anemia, neutropenia/leukopenia, and thrombocytopenia.

Hemostasis Phase

The hemostasis phase is initiated immediately after injury. Vasoconstriction occurs reflexively, and hemostasis is achieved by the activation of the platelets. Once a platelet plug is formed, a plasma clotting cascade is started which ultimately creates a fibrin mesh, thereby strengthening the clot.[62,63] The platelets and fibrin mesh serve as the initial matrix on which the wound healing cells migrate and begin to rebuild tissue.[51,62] The fibrin mesh also serves as a reservoir for growth factors and cytokines that are essential to wound healing.[64]

The activated platelets release alpha granules which contain several cytokines and growth factors, including platelet-derived growth factor (PDGF), epidermal growth factor (EGF), and transforming growth factor beta (TGF-β), all of which signal inflammatory cells to migrate to the area.[61] Upon injury to the epidermal layer, keratinocytes immediately release the pro-inflammatory interleukin 1 (IL-1) to recruit inflammatory cells, and later release interleukin 6 (IL-6).[61] Histamine and serotonin are released, which increase vascular permeability to allow other cells to enter the wounded area.[60]

At the time of wounding, ROS are produced at the wound site.[65] ROS are essential to the healing cascade but can also be detrimental in higher quantities. Excess ROS are implicated in poor wound healing and cancer pathology. One ROS, hydrogen peroxide (H_2O_2), is an important attractor of inflammatory cells in this phase, but also attracts fibroblasts and vascular endothelial cells later to start the proliferative phase.[66] Many ROS are produced during the wound healing process, acting as signaling molecules but also assisting with cleansing of the wound area.

Inflammatory Phase

The goal of the inflammatory phase, which begins within the first hour after wounding,[60] is to remove bacteria, debris, and cellular byproducts that occur with phagocytosis. Many signals expressed in the inflammatory phase also stimulate cellular activity that is essential to the proliferative phase of healing. Leukocytes, especially the neutrophils, are first to act.[67] Neutrophils have the ability to kill bacteria through phagocytosis and by trapping bacteria in neutrophil extracellular traps (NETs).

Neutrophils are significant producers of nitric oxide (NO), which is a potent signaling molecule involved in many processes of wound healing. NO supports neutrophil function through the formation of cytonemes. which allow the cells to bind to bacteria extracellularly and essentially trap the bacteria, thus rendering them harmless.[67] Only recently discovered, the full scope of NO action has yet to be elucidated; however, it is known to be a potent vasodilator, cell signaler, a key player in the inflammatory phase of healing, a key regulator of inflammation, and a scavenger of ROS. The effects of NO can be both positive and negative, however, as it can react with superoxide to form a cytotoxic byproduct.[67]

Neutrophils undergo apoptosis, or preprogrammed cell death, causing a release of pro-inflammatory cytokines that calls additional monocytes to the area. Monocytes differentiate into macrophages once they arrive in the tissues, while dermal macrophages also become activated. Macrophages, key cells in both the inflammatory and proliferative phases of wound healing, will take on one of two phenotypes: M1 or M2. M1 macrophages, also called wound-activated macrophages (WAMs) scavenge the wound area by phagocytosing bacteria and releasing pro-inflammatory cytokines to ensure proper wound cleaning, including IL-1 and IL-6.[68] M1 macrophages are strong players in the inflammatory phase while also mediating ROS-related tissue damage. M1 macrophages release free radicals, including NO, H_2O_2, and the superoxide radical ion (O_2^-), which decreases the pH of the wound environment and further assists with phagocytosis of bacteria, viruses, and fungi.[60,69] These cells also play a role in anti-tumor activity.[70]

A change in phenotype from M1 to the M2 macrophage is critical to wound healing. Unlike M1 cell types, the M2 macrophage is a reparative cell.[68] The M2 macrophages decrease production of ROS, NO, and transforming growth factor alpha (TGF-α), which slows the inflammatory process.[71] The M2 macrophages clean up the wound by phagocytosing dead or no longer needed neutrophils, bacteria, and debris left at the end of the inflammatory phase which prevents further damage to the tissues; however, the M2 macrophages also express anti-inflammatory mediators and are involved in the recruitment of fibroblasts, production of the extra-cellular matrix (ECM), and the process of new blood vessel growth, called angiogenesis.[68] Growth factors secreted by M2s include fibroblast growth factor (FGF), EGF, TGF-β, and vascular endothelial growth factor (VEGF).[61] Notably, tumor-associated macrophages (TAMs) are implicated in the link between cancer and inflammation,[70] but over time, TAMs take on an M2 phenotype that promotes cancer growth through immunosuppression, promotion of angiogenesis, and anti-inflammatory action.

Early angiogenesis takes place during the inflammatory phase and continues more robustly in the proliferative phase. In order to support newly formed granulation tissue and remove waste products during phagocytosis, new capillary growth must occur. Fibroblasts are activated by the TGF-β produced by platelets and macrophages.[60] Along with macrophages, the fibroblasts produce FGF and VEGF, which are key signalers to proteases that must carve a path in the basement membrane and ECM for endothelial cells to migrate to the wound area, proliferate, and form new capillary tissue.[60] Once formed, the capillaries differentiate into arterioles or venules.[60]

Clinical observations that indicate a wound is in the inflammatory phase include relatively large amounts of wound exudate, periwound redness, and the potential presence of necrotic tissue. The wound edges will not yet be migrating, and the granulation tissue growth is minimal. It is important to recognize the difference between normal inflammatory phase characteristics and infection, which will present with more profound exudate that is often purulent and odorous, more robust and extensive redness extending >2 cm beyond the wound borders,[72] peri-wound induration, warmth >3 degrees measured with an infrared skin thermometer,[73] and systemic signs, including fever, edema, pain.

Proliferative Phase

The proliferative phase is hallmarked by activity of the fibroblasts and keratinocytes to generate granulation tissue and re-epithelialize the wound, respectively. Fibroblasts, activated by PDGF, TGF-β, and FGF during the early phases of wound healing, create collagen, glycosaminoglycans (GAGs), and fibronectin, all key components of the ECM. Wound-activated fibroblasts also produce NO during wound healing,[74] which has been correlated to their increased production of collagen.[48] The provisional clot matrix formed during the hemostasis phase is replaced by a stronger ECM made of collagen.[75] Fibroblasts located in the wound bed synthesize new collagen by the 5th day of healing.[60] Early in healing, the fibroblasts create Type III collagen, which is quickly, but irregularly deposited in a matrix. During the remodeling phase, Type III will be replaced by Type I collagen, which is stronger and well-organized.

Actin and myosin bundles within the myofibroblast contract while extracellular fibrils adhere to the ECM, causing overall wound contraction.[49] This contraction aids in wound closure while making less work for the keratinocytes during re-epithelialization. The myofibroblasts are also significant producers of collagen.

Tissue production and breakdown as well as cellular migration are highly regulated processes in wound healing, tightly controlled by the balance of matrix metalloproteinases (MMPs) and tissue inhibitors of metalloproteinases (TIMPs). MMPs, secreted by nearly all wound healing cells[76] are critical to ECM formation and remodeling, as these proteinases break down ECM and basement membrane structures to pave a path for cells to reach the wounded area. In addition, MMPs disrupt cell-cell and cell-matrix adhesions in order to allow cells to migrate to the wound area, or in the case of the keratinocytes, across the wound surface. The MMPs are involved in all stages of wound healing, but left uncontrolled, tissue breakdown will exceed tissue formation, prohibiting cell migration due to a lack of ECM on which to attach. Dysregulation of MMPs has also been implicated in all phases of cancer, from development to metastasis.[77] Too few MMPs will also impede healing by not allowing a path to migrate, not allowing cells to detach from one another, or not allowing the matrix to reach the wounded area. MMPs are implicated in hypertrophic scarring and fibrosis, although it is unclear which MMPs are pro-fibrotic and which are anti-fibrotic.[78] The TIMPs act to regulate MMP activity through a variety of cellular processes during normal wound healing. At least 28 MMPs have been identified, but only four TIMPs regulate these MMPs.[79] Interestingly, while TIMPs normally reduce MMP activity, they can also increase MMP activity indirectly, making their action paradoxical and complicating the use of TIMP gene therapy in the treatment of chronic wounds and cancer.[79]

The keratinocytes begin the process of re-epithelialization within hours after wounding,[60] a process that is promoted by many cytokines and growth factors. Keratinocyte growth factor (also called FGF-7) secreted by the fibroblasts, EGF and TGF-α produced by both the platelets and macrophages, and NO produced by the macrophages all stimulate keratinocyte migration. In addition, keratinocytes produce IL-1 immediately after wounding, acting in an autocrine fashion to activate themselves.[80]

There are several theories about how keratinocyte migration across the wound bed occurs, and understanding these processes helps to understand migration and metastasis in cancer, as some of these mechanisms occur in cancer cells.[65] Basal keratinocytes flatten and elongate, develop extensions called lamellipodia, lose some of the desmosomal connections while retracting the tonofilaments, and form actin filaments to assist with migration.[80] It is thought that some of the cell-to-cell connections are not lost, and the keratinocytes can migrate as a cohesive sheet, while some researchers have found a tumbling of epidermal cells that contributes to re-epithelialization.[60,80] Cells behind this "leading edge" of migrating cells are stimulated to proliferate and continue to push the migrating keratinocytes across the wound. The keratinocytes must migrate over granulation tissue; therefore, they lose their hemidesmosomal connections to the basement membrane during re-epithelialization by altering the integrin receptors on the cell surface that allow the cell to interact with the ECM instead of the basement membrane. These integrins are not present in uninjured or noncancerous skin.[65]

Keratinocytes produce collagenases and MMPs, which allows them to migrate across the ECM.[65] Once the wound is fully covered, the contact between migrating keratinocytes is a mechanical cue to stop migrating, to begin proliferating and differentiating, and to begin the process of stratification. The single-layer basal keratinocytes return to a cuboidal shape and are no longer activated for mobility but rather for proliferation and stratification. The cells resume the process of keratinization to create the stratified epithelium with cell-to-cell connection via desmosomes. Meanwhile, the basement membrane is repaired by laminins[60] and the basal layer again becomes firmly attached through hemidesmosomes.

Wounds in which the basement membrane is not disrupted and are superficial, only involving the epidermis, heal simply by re-epithelialization only. There is no scar tissue formation since the dermis is not involved, and there is no need to replace tissue since the epidermis is constantly replenishing itself under normal circumstances. All four phases of healing are only necessary when the defect extends into the dermal layers and beyond. Further, it has been found that keloid or hypertrophic scarring is a phenomenon only seen in wounds in which the deeper reticular dermis is involved, not in superficial dermal wounds.[81]

Clinical observations of a wound in the proliferative phase include a reduction in the amount of drainage due to the decrease in phagocytosis and byproducts being flushed from the wound. The wound bed will demonstrate growth of granulation tissue with reducing or no necrotic tissue, and the wound edges will begin to demonstrate migration. This is noted by a less defined wound border, with a thin, leading edge beginning to form across the wound surface. Wound contraction may be visible at the periphery. All of these observations are reflected in decreasing wound width, length, and depth.

Maturation and Remodeling Phase

Once the wound is fully re-epithelialized, the maturation and remodeling phase begins. During the initial phase, the wound is very weak because remodeling of the epidermis and dermis takes time. The skin is not yet strong due to the lack of rete ridges; however, these will form during the last phase of wound healing which can take 1 to 2 years. Early granulation tissue is very dense with cells and vasculature; however, this matures into organized scar tissue consisting of varying amounts of collagen and elastin. Hypertrophic and keloid scar tissue has a much higher collagen content than normal skin.[82]

During the initial phase of remodeling, myofibroblasts are involved through continued contraction and facilitation of collagen alignment along the lines of stress.[60] Eventually the number of myofibroblasts and fibroblasts decrease, along with a reduction in the density of the capillaries that are no longer required to support the tissue. MMPs produced by multiple cells during the healing process remain to remodel the immature Type III collagen into the stronger and better organized Type I collagen. This increases the tensile strength of the remodeled tissue; however, tensile strength of healed tissue is only about 80% as strong as the original.[60]

Onc R clinicians have utilized appropriate range of motion (ROM) interventions to provide safe stress to healing tissues after orthopedic injuries, ligament and tendon repairs, and burns. The use of ROM for skin healing is paradoxical, however. While joint ROM must be preserved through stretching, mechanical stress can be detrimental to skin healing.[83,84] Tension on healing skin can lead to increased scar formation, causing changes at both the cellular level and the ECM. Mechanical forces can cause increased ECM stiffness and stronger cell adhesion, leading to subsequent scarring.[83] Interestingly, ECM stiffness is also implicated in cancer growth and metastasis.[83] Interventions such as pressure garments, silicone sheets, negative pressure wound therapy (NPWT), and even botulism toxin A have proven to be helpful in reducing scarring by reducing mechanical tension on the skin.[84] It must be noted that NPWT is contraindicated for use on malignant wounds due to the high risk of bleeding.

Chronic Wounds

A discussion of chronic wounds is available in the electronic version of this text. The details of cellular and acellular activity in wound healing are intricate, interrelated, and in some cases, relate to the development of cancerous cells. For example, in a prolonged inflammatory state, macrophages release excess pro-inflammatory cytokines that increase MMPs while reducing TIMPs.[64] Hypoxic conditions, common in chronic wounds, also foster the release of pro-inflammatory cytokines which are related to excessive ROS; alternatively, ROS can facilitate the release of pro-inflammatory cytokines, creating a perpetuating loop.[64,85] NO, which can regulate ROS, is decreased in hypoxic environments. Since NO is involved in the mechanism to move from the inflammatory to the proliferative phase by turning off a potent regulator of inflammation, nuclear factor kB (NF-kB), a lack of NO perpetuates the inflammatory phase.[64] As a result of all of these factors, the migration and proliferation of fibroblasts and keratinocytes are stalled, and tissue breakdown occurs at a faster rate than ECM production, thus creating a vicious cycle that keeps the wound in the inflammatory phase. Notably, chronic inflammation is also implicated in the development of most cancerous tumors.[85]

Wound healing is complex, and while there are some redundancies and alternate pathways to ensure wounds heal properly, chronic wounds remain a significant problem across the globe. It is estimated that 1% to 2% of people in developed countries will suffer from a chronic wound at some point in their lifetime.[86] A wound is considered chronic when healing is slow, delayed, or stalled.[87]

Disruptions to cell migration, differentiation, and proliferation (often caused by improper cellular communication or an ineffective balance of growth factors, cytokines, and other chemical messengers), lead to chronic wounds.[64] As mentioned, the spatiotemporal release of these messengers is critical for the proper timing of events. Wounds that are stuck often have elevated pro-inflammatory cytokines and MMPs with a reduction in TIMPs.[88] This leads to wounds that are stalled in the inflammatory phase, where continued bacterial invasion prevents the body's ability to progress to the proliferative phase of healing.

Excessive neutrophil presence is a common biological marker in chronic wounds.[89] In chronic wounds, neutrophils release MMPs that break down the ECM and elastase which degrades PDGF and TGF-β, thereby preventing progression along the wound healing cascade. Additionally, excessive ROS are released which causes additional damage to cells and tissues.[89] A balance of ROS presence in the wound is necessary to harness the positive antimicrobial effects while preventing the harmful effects ROS can have on healthy tissue. This is achieved through ROS scavengers, such as NO, Vitamins C and E, and glutathione.[90]

While it might seem tempting to intervene to eliminate inflammation in order to prevent chronic wounds, adult wounds rely on an organized inflammatory phase to transition to proliferation. Prolonged inflammation can also lead to problems in the proliferative and remodeling/maturation phases of wound healing. Chronic inflammation has been identified as a factor in fibrotic changes such as keloids and hypertrophic scars with several pro-inflammatory cytokines noted to be increased.[81] Upregulation of TGF-β, which has been the focus of research on fibrosis and scarring, can lead to excessive collagen formation by the fibroblasts and myofibroblasts, thus leading to abnormal scarring or fibrosis. TGF-β has also been shown to be upregulated in keloid scars, and fibroblasts of keloid scars produce 2 to 3 times more collagen than fibroblasts of normal skin of the same individual.[89] Finally, increased angiogenesis also plays a role in fibrosis, and a reduction in both inflammation and angiogenesis/blood flow has been found to successfully reduce keloids and hypertrophic scarring.[81]

Similarities Between Wound Healing and Cancer

Many authors have discussed the similarities between the wound healing cascade and the growth and metastasis of tumors. More specifically, tumors behave like "wounds that do not heal."[91] Many of the same concepts of tissue healing are paralleled in cancer; however, the outcomes are different. Whereas wound healing is an organized and self-limiting process, cancer development and progression is a disorganized process that is perpetuated.[65]

The tumor microenvironment, or the area surrounding tumor cells, is becoming an increasing focus of research due to its role in tumor progression,[92] and includes the stroma, blood supply, ECM, and cells communicating with the tumor.[93] Stroma (defined as the cells in an organ that are not related to its function) is found throughout the body under normal and pathological conditions. In noncancerous tissue, stroma presents

with limited numbers of fibroblasts, well-organized type I collagen, and low amounts of MMPs.[51] Conversely, tumor stroma, which is found at the periphery of tumors, more closely resembles newly formed granulation tissue at the start of the maturation phase. This stromal tissue is dense, highly cellular/vascular, and saturated with Type I and III collagen, MMPs, and fibrous proteins.[51] This increased density is one reason anti-tumor medications cannot effectively invade cancer cells in hard-to-treat tumors.[51,93] Further, the way in which the collagen and fibronectin is organized creates channels for tumor cells to migrate to other areas, increasing the risk of metastasis.[51] Cells within the tumor and the tumor microenvironment communicate, which further supports tumor growth and metastasis.[51]

It is well established that tumors cannot grow beyond 1 to 2 mm without additional blood supply,[91,94] making angiogenesis another common feature between wounds and cancer. In noncancerous wound healing, angiogenesis is driven by growth factors, primarily VEGF. Endothelial cells, in response to VEGF, become migratory and travel to the wound area, guided by cues from other growth factors and the ECM itself. Early vessel development is immature, but with time, the new vessels go through a maturation process, forming lumen, a basement membrane, and reducing permeability through pericytes and vascular smooth muscle cells.[94] In contrast, angiogenesis in cancer is poorly organized. The vessels of the tumor microenvironment are not like normal vessels. Rather, they are tortuous, disorganized, have varying endothelial wall thicknesses, and are leaky.[65,94,95] Significant perfusion differences are also noted in various aspects of the tumor due to the lack of consistency in vessel growth. Malignant wounds bleed very easily and profusely due to the irregular vascular nature of the tumor and stroma.

The abnormalities in cancer vasculature contributes to difficulties delivering cancer therapies, which fosters cancer growth and metastasis.[65,94,95] The leaky vessels do not allow medications to reach the tumor; instead, they diffuse into the interstitial tissue, where they cannot perform the required action.[94] The leaky vessels also provide a pathway for cancer cells to metastasize after entering the blood stream.

Vascular normalization is a targeted therapy being explored using anti-angiogenic treatment; while its success has been promising, the results vary by tumor type.[94] Methods currently being used or investigated include using agents that block VEGF, blocking PDGF in combination with VEGF treatments in order to reduce recruitment of pericytes, or promoting pericyte recruitment through PDGF to strengthen and thereby "fix" the leaky vessels that promote metastasis.[94] Careful use of this intervention is necessary because complete blocking of vessel growth can lead to hypoxia of the tumor microenvironment which can contribute to additional immature vessel growth and metastasis.[65,95] As with other therapies, dose and timing are crucial, and the full understanding of these parameters is still unclear.

Inflammation is critical to both wound healing and cancer. In noncancerous tissue healing, inflammation is regulated by cytokines and growth factors that move the wound to proliferation. Chronic inflammation is related to poor wound healing but has also been linked to cancer.[65] Unregulated activation of the NF-kB pathway leads to continued inflammation, which contributes to the tumor growth and metastasis.[96] Prolonged activation of inflammatory cells and cytokines causes proliferation of harmful ROS due to the overactivity of neutrophils and macrophages. These signals also attract preneoplastic cancer cells to the area.[65] As discussed, NO can mediate both of these harmful pathways, and could be an important advancement in cancer therapy.

Prolonged inflammation is also linked to the overexpression of TGF-β which can cause excessive proliferation of the fibroblasts and subsequently lead to fibrosis, which is a common problem in chronic wounds and cancer. Fibroblasts are significantly activated in tumor stroma and are differentiated into myofibroblasts by TGF-β.[65] This over-activation leads to excessive production of collagen and eventual fibrosis. The increased stiffness further inhibits anti-cancer medication access to tumors by preventing diffusion, acting as a firm barrier to medication delivery.[94,95] The fibrotic changes also reduce blood supply to the tumor area by compressing local blood vessels, thereby promoting hypoxia in the tumor microenvironment. This is problematic for several reasons. First, this inhibits cancer medication effectiveness; potent medications cannot reach the tumor. Second, many cancer treatments require oxygen to be effective.[95] Without adequate blood supply, the medications are ineffective. Finally, chronic hypoxia drives the process of angiogenesis, which again promotes cancer metastasis.

The role of TGF-β in cancer prognosis is paradoxical. High levels of TGF-β in early-stage cancer is correlated to a favorable prognosis while high levels in late stages appear to promote tumor progression.[65] Nonetheless, medications targeting TGF-β have been useful in the treatment of cancer, both to treat the cancer itself or to improve blood flow, thereby increasing the effectiveness of chemotherapy.[92,97] Other anti-fibrotic agents have shown promise in improving cancer therapies, including relaxin and the common medication losartan, which is an angiotensin II receptor blocker that reduces collagen production.[95]

Many of the same growth factors and cytokines that are implicated in tumor growth and metastasis have parallels to wound re-epithelialization. A break in the basement membrane is necessary for the "leading edge" of the cancer cells to migrate, similar to the keratinocytes in the process of re-epithelialization.[65] Cancer-activated fibroblasts (CAFs) take on a myofibroblast phenotype, and have been found to both soften the basement membrane and tunnel through matrix proteins in order to pave the way for cancer cells to metastasize.[65] Similarly, macrophages have been found to transport cancer cells to nearby blood vessels, thus contributing to metastasis.[65] Both phenotypes of macrophages are found in cancers; however, the tumor microenvironment creates a strong shift to the M2 phenotype, which are anti-inflammatory, but immunosuppressive, pro-angiogenic, and pro-tumor.[71]

Wounds and Cancer

PLWBCs can experience a wound due to a variety of reasons. The wound can be the result of an adverse effect of adjunct interventions or medications used to treat the cancer. Skin cancers are examples of primary cancers that present as wounds; chronic ulcers can also develop into malignancies over time. Additionally, wounds can occur due to metastases or at the end of life.

Wound healing in PLWBCs is complicated by a variety of factors, including the disease process itself, treatments for the disease that affect neighboring healthy cells, comorbidities, and nutritional status, among others.[98] Understanding the mechanisms by which these factors affect healing can assist the Onc R clinician in decision-making regarding prognosis and interventions.

Radiation therapy is considered an essential aspect of cancer treatment, and nearly 50% of PLWBCs will undergo this type of therapy.[99] The ionizing radiation causes direct DNA damage as well as ROS production, both of which attack cancer cells but also damage neighboring healthy cells.[100] Cells that are rapidly dividing, such as cancer cells, are most susceptible to radiation-induced cell damage; however, the cells of the basal layer in the epidermis and mucosal cells have high turnover rates, so these areas are also highly susceptible to damage.[98] Of those PLWBCs who undergo radiation treatment, 95% will develop radiation dermatitis of some form.[101]

Acute effects of radiation are seen within 90 days of treatment[99] and include erythema, hyperpigmentation, blistering, or dry or wet desquamation (peeling of the skin). Radiation dermatitis is classified into four stages, and treatment varies based on classification. Refer to Table 9.6 for a definition of each stage and treatment indicated.[102]

Chronic, long-term effects are more severe and include fibrosis, skin atrophy, telangiectasis, and chronic ulceration.[99,100] Radiation decreases tissue healing in a variety of ways. In addition to epidermal cell death, altered dermal cellular function causes fibrotic changes in the tissues (described in further detail below), and microvascular damage leads to sclerotic arteries and arterioles, creating chronic tissue hypoxia.[98,100] The DNA damage caused by radiation prevents cellular regeneration, causing problems with wound healing years after treatment. Radiation therapy also damages the hair follicle which complicates healing since hair follicle-derived stem cells have been shown to be necessary for re-epithelialization.[103]

The amount of radiation skin damage is directly related to the total radiation dose, the fraction size or dose per treatment, the volume of tissue treated, total treatment time, type of radiation used, and individual patient factors.[98,104] Advances in radiation therapy have reduced the damage to healthy cells, but science has yet to eliminate unintended damage because many of the factors targeted by the treatment are found in the skin, such as EGF receptors and VEGF.[105] In addition, many genes predispose

TABLE 9.6	National Cancer Institute Radiation Dermatitis Classification[167]	
Grade	Definition	Treatment
Grade 1	Faint erythema, dry desquamation	Moisturizers, low-dose steroids for pruritis, and irritation
Grade 2	Moderate to brisk erythema, patch desquamation confined to skin folds and creases	Hydrogel and/or hydrocolloid dressings to prevent infection
Grade 3	Moist desquamation outside of folds, pitting edema, bleeding from minor trauma	Hydrogel and/or hydrocolloid dressings to prevent infection
Grade 4	Full-thickness skin necrosis or ulceration with spontaneous bleeding	Debridement, moisture-retentive dressings; may require skin grafts or flaps

Created by Caroline S. Gwaltney. Printed with permission.

certain PLWBCs to radiation injury, especially radiation-induced fibrosis (RIF).[106]

RIF is a result of the tissue damage and inflammation caused by radiation injury, and TGF-β has been highly associated with the pathology. This association is paradoxical, however since a reduction in TGF-β leads to weak tissue healing, but an increase leads to fibrosis. Further, reduced TGF-β can perpetuate inflammation which has been linked to fibrosis.[81] Prolonged inflammation subsequently causes a release of TGF-β which stimulates fibroblasts to differentiate into myofibroblasts, which then proliferate excessively. Excess collagen and ECM components are produced with a concurrent reduction in MMPs and other enzymes that would normally balance collagen production.[106] The result is fibrosis of the tissues, a reduction in tissue extensibility (especially in areas of skin with minimal subcutaneous tissue, such as the head, neck, and upper chest), and an increased risk of future skin breakdown due to reduced vascularity of the fibrotic tissue.[106]

Management of skin injury after radiation is focused on supportive wound care, and wound dressings or creams that maintain an appropriate moist wound environment are recommended.[100] Gentle washing of radiated skin with mild soap and water is now recommended, after years of debate.[107] Harsh antiseptics and cleansers should be avoided on previously radiated skin. Onc R interventions including ROM, stretching, and functional mobility are essential to reduce the functional consequences of tissue fibrosis, as has been demonstrated in people after burn injury.[106] Many topical agents have been studied with no significant benefit, however topical corticosteroids[101,108] and silver sulfadiazine[109] have been found to reduce acute radiation dermatitis (ARD) and are currently recommended to reduce pain or itching and improve QOL for PLWBCs in the early phases of radiation therapy.[110] Long-pulsed dye laser (LPDL) has been recommended to reduce telangiectasis, and pentoxifylline with vitamin E is a promising intervention for chronic RIF.[100,101,107] Ongoing studies are exploring stem cell therapy, TGF-β modification, biologic matrix dressings, growth factors, and anti-oxidant therapies.[100]

Radiation recall is a rare, but a well-recognized condition affecting PLWBCs who undergo chemotherapy after radiation treatment. The hallmark of this acute inflammatory reaction is a rash that occurs, most often in normal-appearing skin that was previously irradiated, when a new medication is introduced. While the skin is most often affected, one-third of the reactions have occurred in previously irradiated organs such as the lungs, bowel, oral mucosa, genitourinary tract, central nervous system, neck, and head.[111,112] The pathophysiology is not well-understood, but theories include keratinocyte necrosis due to DNA damage and oxidative stress, malnutrition affecting the endogenous immune response, a lowered inflammatory response threshold, and mutations at the cellular level that cause a "remembered" response when the chemotherapy medication is introduced.[112,113] While chemotherapeutic medications have been implicated, other medications have been found to cause radiation recall, including simvastatin, tamoxifen, antibiotics, anti-tuberculosis medications, and UV light exposure.[111–113]

In order for radiation recall to be diagnosed, there must be complete resolution of dermatitis that evolved after radiation treatment.[112] Time is also a factor. Reactions to medications given within 7 days of radiation treatment are more likely due to radiosensitization, not radiation recall.[112] Radiation recall can occur after 7 days and up to several years after initiation of a new medication.

There is currently no method to predict which PLWBCs will react to which medications, making it hard to prevent radiation recall. The severity of reactions is also diverse, ranging from mild erythematous rash, dry desquamation, and/or itching to more severe pain, edema, skin eruptions, to the most severe ulceration with necrosis.[111,112] Reactions can occur immediately after the first chemotherapy treatment, but may not be evident until several infusions/oral doses. Treatment for radiation recall involves eliminating the causative medication, either for a short time or completely. Corticosteroids are often used, either topically or systemically. Antihistamines may assist with symptom management, and antibiotics are used if there are signs of cellulitis or mastitis.[111] Some PLWBCs will respond well to a different chemotherapeutic agent while others can be rechallenged with the original agent with possible use of a concurrent systemic corticosteroid.[112]

Surgical interventions remain the most effective method of treatment for most types of cancer; therefore, many PLWBCs with cancer will undergo a surgery at some point in their healing.[114] Biopsies also create tissue trauma that requires wound healing. Despite advances in surgical techniques, healing after surgery can be compromised.

Both chemotherapy and radiation can damage cells critical to wound healing, causing a delay or disruption to the normal healing process; therefore, timing of the interventions is an important consideration to allow optimal healing. The optimal time to schedule surgery after neoadjuvant chemotherapy or radiation treatment is 4 to 6 weeks.[105] Wound healing complications have been noted with neoadjuvant radiation doses above 50 gray or when radiation therapy is less than 3 weeks before surgery.[98]

When chemotherapy is given after surgery, treatment should wait 7 to 10 days, which appears to have the most limited effects on wound healing.[98] Radiation therapy is recommended to begin 6 to 8 weeks postoperatively.[98] Waiting longer is not advantageous due to the late effects of radiation damage to tissues.

Anti-angiogenesis agents (bevacizumab, aflibercept) impair angiogenesis by impeding VEGF or by inhibiting enzymes necessary for new blood vessel growth.[115] While this can assist with tumor management, the effects are not specific to tumors. Healing wounds require angiogenesis to support the growth of granulation tissue and ECM components, therefore these agents can impair wound healing. The recommendation is to avoid use of these medications within 28 to 30 days of surgery.[115]

Corticosteroids are commonly used to treat pain and inflammation related to cancer, and they are also components of chemotherapeutic regimens; however, this medication is known to alter healing by reducing the inflammatory response and thereby reducing the growth of granulation tissue. The effects are seen with both long and short-term use. Taking vitamin A with corticosteroids can offset some negative effects; however, it is best to delay prescribing corticosteroids until the wound has completed the inflammatory phase of healing, generally after 7 to 10 days.[98] The Onc R clinician should be aware of PLWBCs who have a history of long-term corticosteroid use, as the inflammatory phase can take longer in those PLWBCs.

Skin Cancer

Skin cancer is the most common type of cancer, and the majority of these are nonmelanoma basal and squamous cell carcinomas (SCC).[116] Basal cell carcinomas (BCC) are the most common, making up 80% of the diagnosed nonmelanoma cases, followed by SCC. Melanomas are found in only 2% of people, but these are the deadliest.[117] Many skin cancers can present as open wounds; therefore, it is essential for Onc R clinicians to recognize when a wound doesn't look typical or heal as expected. A differential diagnosis is imperative to ensure early medical treatment.

The primary risk factor for all types of skin cancer is chronic UV light exposure. Other common risk factors include fair skin, light eye color, and older age.[117–119] For both BCC and SCC, immunosuppression is a significant risk factor. The risk of developing a BCC or SCC is twice as high in people who are HIV positive and up to 250 times higher in people following organ transplant.[119,120] The incidence of all skin cancers is increasing worldwide, which is thought to be due to better detection, but also increased UV exposure.

Basal Cell Carcinoma

BCC are slow-growing cancers that arise in the basal layer of the epidermis. A UV-induced activation of a specific intracellular signaling pathway leads to the development of BCC tumors, and this is a potential target of treatment.[117,118,121] These cancers do not typically metastasize; however, the risk of metastasis is greater for tumors larger than 2 cm.[118]

Because of the influence of UV light in the pathogenesis, these tumors are often found on sun-exposed areas such as the nose, face, ears, neck, and the back of the hands, but BCC can occur anywhere in the skin. Earlier onset of BCC has been correlated to the use of tanning beds.[122] There are three main subtypes: nodular, superficial, and morpheaform (listed in order of most to least common). See Figure 9.26. Other less common variants are not discussed here. Nodular BCCs present as a papule or raised area of skin that can be pink or skin-colored, and is often translucent or pearly with telangiectasias.[118] Nodular BCCs are often found on the face and may have an ulcer within the papule. Superficial BCCs typically present as scaly, pink plaques that can be mistaken for eczema or psoriasis.[118] The border can be raised, with translucent papules and an atrophic center and are typically found on the trunk.[117] Morpheaform are higher risk BCCs and have a higher rate of recurrence due to invasion of the space around a nearby nerve, termed perineural invasion. This type of BCC can present as a waxy, scar-like plaque that may have induration or a depressed center. The lesion can be skin-colored or red and can also have ulceration.[117,118]

Medical treatment for BCC involves local excision, either surgically, with curettage and electrodessication, or using the Mohs micrographic surgical technique (a procedure in which the tumor is removed one layer at a time, the tissue is analyzed, and more layers are removed until no abnormal cells are found).[121] Typically, no wound care is necessary unless the surgical wound becomes infected or does not heal properly, in which case moist wound healing is recommended.[123] PLWBCs should

be assessed by a dermatologist yearly to ensure no new growth of BCC lesions.

Squamous Cell Carcinoma

Cutaneous SCC develops due to uncontrolled proliferation in the outer layer of the epidermis.[119] Lesions are typically found on areas exposed to the sun, but can occur anywhere. Other risk factors include exposure to arsenic, hydrocarbons, nitrosamines, and alkylating agents.[119] Human papillomavirus is also associated with SCC of the finger and toenails and anogenital areas.[119] Rare genetic conditions that are hallmarked by skin disorders, such as epidermolysis bullosa and albinism, predispose people to SCCs at a younger age.[119] Previous trauma, especially burns, can also lead to the development of cutaneous SCC, termed a Marjolin's ulcer[123,124] (see Box 9.10).

An SCC lesion can present as a single rough, red, scaly plaque, but can also appear as a papule or nodule.[117,119] The lesions can also present with crusted edges and may appear in multiples.[119] See Figure 9.27. Recurrence of an SCC leads to greater risk of metastasis, and perineural involvement is also linked to worse prognosis.

The treatment for SCCs is similar to BCCs, except surgical incision or Mohs surgery is preferred[119]; therefore, wounds are common after surgery. Chemotherapy and radiation treatment are used when the SCC has metastasized.[123] Radiation therapy may also be used for larger tumors or PLWBCs who cannot tolerate surgery.[117] Standard wound care is recommended, including gentle cleansing, dressings to manage drainage while maintaining a moist wound environment, infection control with antimicrobial dressings, and lymphedema management if necessary. Aseptic agents are not advised for cleaning postsurgical wounds due to cytotoxicity to healing cells.

Melanoma

Melanoma is the most aggressive form of skin cancer, arising from the melanocytes at the basal layer of the epidermis as well as melanocytes outside of the skin, such as the eye or gastrointestinal mucosa.[125] The American Cancer Society estimates that approximately 106,110 people will be diagnosed and 7,180 people will die due to melanoma in 2021.[126] Melanoma is more prevalent in older men, however in those under the age of 60 who have melanoma, more PLWBCs are women.

UV light exposure is the largest risk, causing DNA damage and mutations that lead to activation of oncogenes with concurrent inactivation of tumor suppressor genes. These changes allow uncontrolled proliferation of melanocytes which leads to melanoma. Melanomas are categorized based on depth using the Breslow Depth scale and staged based on tumor size, lymph node involvement, and metastasis using the American Joint Committee

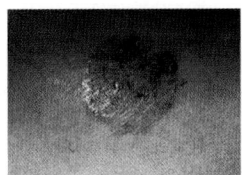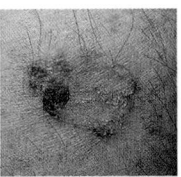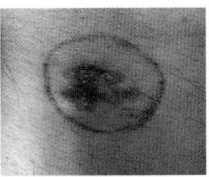

• **Fig. 9.26** A Comparison of the Three Most Common Basal Cell Carcinomas (BCC). Left to Right: Nodular BCC, Superficial BCC, and Morpheaform BCC. (Left and right photos reprinted with permission from Cockerell CJ, Tran KT, Carucci J, et al. Basal cell carcinoma. In: Rigel DS, Robinson JK, Ross M, et al. eds. *Cancer of the Skin*. 2nd ed. Elsevier; 2011:99–123. Middle photo reprinted with permission from Chapman MS. Premalignant and malignant non-melanoma skin tumors. In: Habif TP, Dinulos JGH, Chapman MS, Zug KA, eds. *Skin Disease: Diagnosis and Treatment*. 4th ed. Elsevier; 2018:454–494.)

• **BOX 9.10   Clinical Pearl**

A wound arising in previously burned, wounded, or injured scar or a change in a chronic wound should be biopsied to rule out a Marjolin's ulcer, which is a cancerous wound. While rare, these "scar-associated carcinomas" present a greater risk of metastasis, worse prognosis, and higher mortality than skin cancers.[122] Kanth[122] suggests that everted edges, irregularity at the base of the wound, and hypergranulation tissue growth beyond the borders of the ulcer should cause an Onc R clinician to suspect malignancy in a chronic wound, especially one in scar tissue.

Created by Caroline S. Gwaltney. Printed with permission.

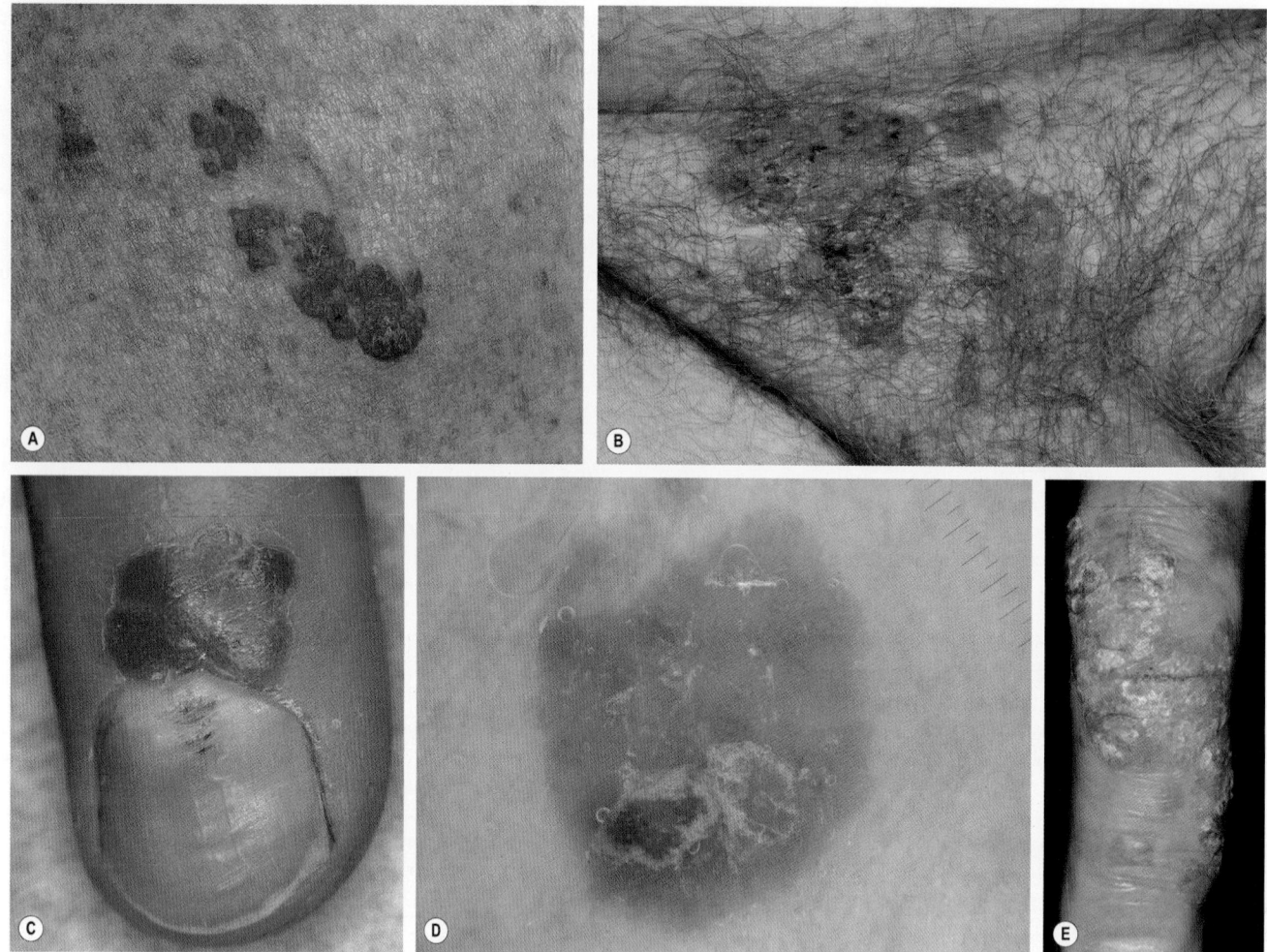

• **Fig. 9.27** Examples of Various Presentations of Squamous Cell Carcinoma. (A) Scaly red plaque on the chest with skip areas and background photodamage. (B) Larger broken-up pink plaque with scale-crust in the pubic region, a sun-protected site. This type of lesion is often misdiagnosed as dermatitis or psoriasis and treated with topical corticosteroids. (C) Bright red, well-demarcated plaque on the proximal nail fold with associated horizontal nail ridging; the possibility of HPV infection needs to be considered. (D) Dermoscopic findings of tiny dotted vessels in the upper half of the lesion combined with superficial scales. (E) Extensive involvement of the finger which was misdiagnosed clinically as an inflammatory dermatosis and treated for years with corticosteroid creams. (Reprinted with permission from Colegio OR, O'Toole EA, Pontén F, Lundeberg J, Asplund A. Actinic keratosis, basal cell carcinoma, squamous cell carcinoma. In: Bolognia JL, Schaffer JV, Ceronni L, eds. *Dermatology.* 4th ed. Elsevier; 2018:1872–1893.)

on Cancer's staging system. The tumors initially grow at the skin level, then begin to grow vertically once they invade the dermal layers.[117]

PLWBCs and Onc R clinicians are taught to look for spots that are unlike others on the body, the so-called "ugly duckling sign."[117] Lesions can be superficial or nodular, appearing as plaques, macules, papules, or flat discolored areas. Acral lentiginous lesions appear on the palms, soles, or nailbeds.[127] The acronym ABCDE is useful to identify potential malignant melanomas[127] (see Figure 9.28).

- Asymmetry of the discoloration; one side does not match the other
- Borders that are irregular, notched, blurred, or jagged
- Color that is varying or uneven shades of dark brown or black, sometimes with patches of pink, blue, red, or white
- Diameter greater than 6 millimeters, or larger than a pencil-top eraser
- Evolution of the lesion in size, shape, or color

Malignant melanomas must be biopsied, and once a diagnosis is made, medical treatment is based on staging and depth. Surgical excision is required in all cases; however, lymph node dissection is indicated in Stage III melanoma or in lower stages where lymph node biopsy indicates metastasis.[117] Chemotherapy and radiation are also indicated in more severe cases, therefore incisional wound healing may be compromised. In this case, standard wound care is indicated.

Cancerous tumors can eventually invade and break through the skin, causing a malignant wound. These wounds are often fungating wounds, characterized by significant amounts of wound drainage, malodor, pain, and itching, all of which contribute to a reduced QOL.[128] These wounds present with either raised, cauliflower-like wound beds (proliferating wounds) or with deep, cratered appearances (destructive wounds).[128,129] Both types of wounds bleed very easily and are prone to infection.[129] The vasculature is very fragile, leading to hypoxic tissues, and poor healing

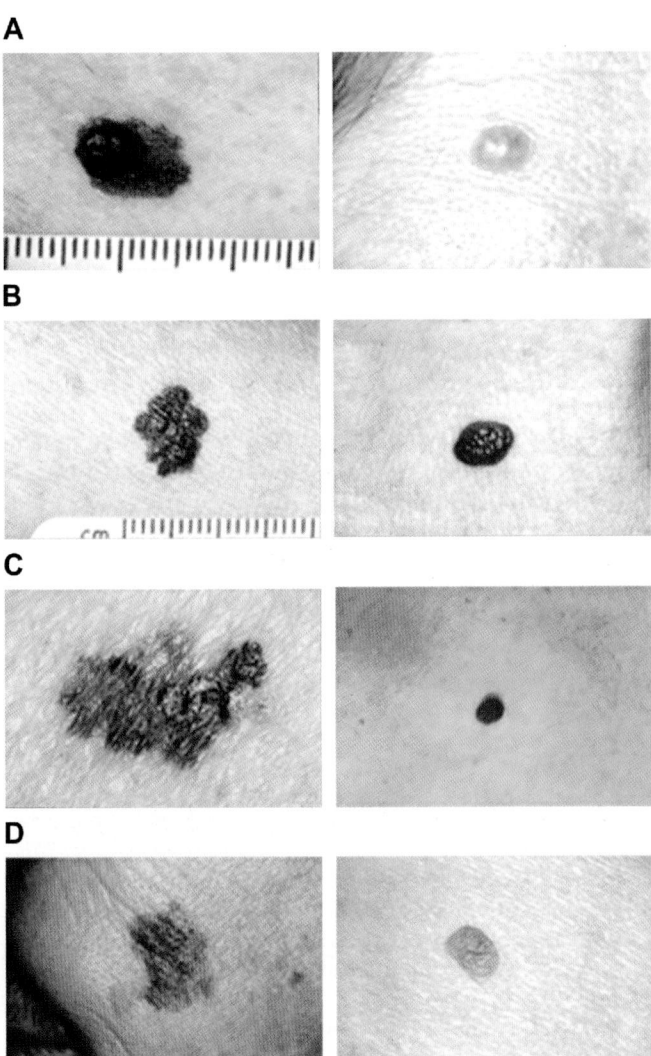

• **Fig. 9.28** The ABCDEs of Malignant Melanoma, Shown on the Left in Comparison to Non-Malignant Skin Moles on the Right. A=Asymmetry, B=irregular Borders, C=Color variation, D=Diameter larger than 6 mm. Not pictured is the characteristic of a mole Evolving in size, shape, color, or scabbing. (Reprinted with permission from Linares MA, Zakaria A, Nizran P. Skin cancer. *Prim Care*. 2015;42(4):645–659.)

outcomes.[128] It is estimated that half of PLWBCs who are diagnosed with a fungating wound will die within 6 months.[129] See Box 9.11 for information on the phenomenon known as the Kennedy Terminal Ulcer.[130]

Wound Care

Good wound care involves holistic care of the PLWBC, not just the wound itself. PLWBCs may have wounds due to the cancer itself or other factors, therefore the first step is to identify the underlying pathology of the wound as well as comorbidities that will affect healing.[88] It has been noted that PLWBCs tend to have more comorbidities,[132] and wounds caused or influenced by conditions such as diabetes, arterial insufficiency, venous insufficiency, pressure, or cancer will all require different medical management. Comorbidities such as obesity, poor nutrition, smoking, pressure,

---

• BOX 9.11   Clinical Pearl

A Kennedy Terminal Ulcer is a phenomenon in which a characteristic ulcer presents at the end of life, indicating skin organ failure.[130] This type of ulcer may be suspected when the following characteristics are noted:

- Has a pear shape (later may expand to butterfly or horseshoe-shape)
- Occurs usually on the sacrum or coccyx (has been reported elsewhere at times)
- Presents with red, yellow, or black tissue
- Has a sudden onset
- Is associated with imminent death (within 2–6 weeks)[130,131]

Created by Caroline S. Gwaltney. Printed with permission

---

or reduced mobility will also need to be addressed in order for successful wound healing to occur. All wounds that do not respond to treatment in PLWBCs should be biopsied to rule out malignancy.

Once the underlying etiology is addressed, wound care concepts are similar for any wound; however, there are unique considerations for wounds related to cancer. Fungating, malignant wounds are found in 5% to 10% of patients diagnosed with cancer at the end of life due to advanced, metastatic cancer invading the skin.[105] In these cases, the goals of wound care include odor control, pain management, prevention of infection, and management of drainage. Metronidazole gel has been found to reduce odor,[133] but application of a gel may not be indicated in highly exudating wounds. Dressings containing activated carbon are well-known to control odor, but silver, honey, and iodine also provide benefits.[133] Dakin's solution or other cytotoxic antiseptics may be used to manage odor and bacterial bioburden only when tissue healing is not expected. When wound healing is not a realistic or achievable goal, such as in the case of a Kennedy Terminal Ulcer, palliative care is recommended. Dressings that manage drainage, require less frequent changes, and minimize pain with removal are indicated as part of palliative care.

Diabetes affects wound healing in multiple ways, and all stages of healing are affected.[134] Uncontrolled blood glucose levels can cause damage at the cellular level due to glycation of proteins, or the attachment of sugar, which leads to the formation of advanced glycation end products (AGEs) that in turn cause thickening of the vessels and eventually ischemia and hypoxia.[134] Impaired glucose control can also affect NO production and the body's innate ability to scavenge harmful ROS. In contrast, too little insulin leads to protein damage and poor collagen formation, also negatively affecting wound healing.

Proper blood glucose control is essential to prevent complications of diabetes and facilitate wound healing. Though no correlation has been found between glycosylated hemoglobin (Hg A1c) levels and healing,[135] a Hg A1c level below 7.0% is recommended for people diagnosed with diabetes. Further, peripheral polyneuropathy is common in diabetes and can predispose patients to neuropathic ulcers due to a lack of protective sensation. Onc R clinicians are advised to test protective sensation using a 10 g monofilament in at least four plantar foot surfaces: distal great toe, and the first, third, and fifth metatarsal heads (the primary sites of skin breakdown in someone with diabetes).[136] Adding vibration testing using a 128-Hz tuning fork can increase the reliability of sensory testing.

People with diabetes are at risk for foot deformities due to motor neuropathy as well as glycosylation of tendons leading to stiffness.[136] Deformities such as pes cavus, hammer toes, and claw toes lead to prominent metatarsal heads that are susceptible to high pressures and tissue breakdown. Callus formation is an indication of excessive friction, and deep purple wounds an indication of shear, but a thorough biomechanical evaluation can identify PLWBCs at risk for diabetic foot ulcer formation. Onc R clinicians can intervene early for muscle and joint tightness and early weakness; however, surgical correction is often warranted. Offloading is the gold standard for any patient with diabetes, foot deformities, and evidence of excessive pressure. The total contact cast (TCC) is considered by many to be the best choice for offloading; the TCC forces compliance due to its unremovable nature. Offloading boots have demonstrated similar reductions in pressure; however, if the PLWBC can take them off, the benefit is of little value.

PLWBCs with arterial insufficiency are at risk for skin breakdown due to ischemia. Palpation of pedal pulses is not sufficient to diagnose adequate circulation; an ankle brachial index (ABI) or toe pressures are indicated. The ABI uses a doppler ultrasound to test both the dorsalis pedis and brachial arteries, then dividing the ankle by the brachial pressure. Normal perfusion status is found with an ABI of 1.0; a diagnosis of lower extremity arterial disease is made at or below 0.9. Severe ischemia is diagnosed with an ABI of 0.5, and critical limb ischemia is 0.4 or below.[137] Onc R clinicians should note that an ABI of 1.3 or greater can indicate calcification of blood vessels, commonly seen in patients with diabetes, in which case the ABI is not reliable and toe pressures would be indicated. Toe pressures less than 50 mmHg in a patient with diabetes or less than 30 mmHg without diabetes indicate critical limb ischemia. PLWBCs with an ABI of 0.9 or less who present with nonhealing ulcers after 2 to 4 weeks of treatment, patients with intermittent claudication, or patients with toe pressure less than 30 mmHG should be referred to a vascular surgeon.[137]

Chronic venous insufficiency leads to excessive edema, most often due to incompetent valves in the deep or superficial venous system. The function of the valves is to prevent blood from flowing backward in the system, however when the valves no longer fully close, retrograde blood flow occurs, causing hypertension in the venous system.[138] Over time, the pressure in the venous system causes damage to the microvasculature, allowing red blood cells (RBCs) to leak into the interstitial space. The RBCs subsequently leak hemoglobin, which is then phagocytosed by macrophages, leaving a ruddy, brown discoloration called hemosiderin staining.[138] This staining is indicative of chronic venous insufficiency. Thickening of the skin also occurs over time, called lipodermatosclerosis.

The hallmark of treatment for venous insufficiency is compression to counteract the incompetent vessels, to assist with blood return to the heart. Prior to applying compression, the clinician must assess the lower extremity vascular status, usually with an ABI to ensure adequate blood flow for wound healing. See eTable 9.1 for clinical decision-making regarding use of compression based on ABI assessment.

Compression options exist in many forms, including multilayer wrap systems, medical compression stocking ulcer kits, UNNA boots, short stretch bandaging, and compression stockings. A recent consensus paper review found similar results between multi-layer wraps and the ulcer kits; however, the multilayer wraps require more skilled application.[139] The panel recommended the ulcer kits for healing of venous leg ulcers. Compression stockings are also recommended for prevention of ulcer recurrence as well as patient comfort to reduce pain, aching, swelling, and heaviness in the legs with or without ulcers.

Pressure injuries occur due to excessive pressure, either high pressures for a short duration or low pressures for prolonged periods. The occlusion pressure at the capillary level is 32 mmHg, and tissues cannot tolerate prolonged pressure beyond this level without tissue ischemia, tissue death, and ultimately ulceration.[140] The obvious focus of treatment for PLWBCs with pressure injuries is pressure redistribution using specialized seating, mattress surfaces, turning schedules, and functional mobility training to improve the person's inherent mobility and ability to reposition with less assistance.

Other comorbid factors that affect tissue healing include obesity, smoking, vaping, and alcohol abuse. Obesity affects wound healing due to the increased risk of wound infection related to the avascularity of adipose tissue.[134] PLWBCs who are obese are also potentially protein malnourished, and since wound healing relies on protein stores, this may pose a problem for timely healing. Smoking negatively affects wound healing because the nicotine causes vasoconstriction which can cause tissue hypoxia at the wound site. The immune response is also reduced in smokers, leading to increased risk of infection and delayed healing.[134] Alcohol abuse affects many aspects of wound healing. Decreases in the inflammatory and immune responses increase the risk of infection while decreased fibroblast activity and angiogenesis are noted in the proliferative phase.[141] During the remodeling phase, MMP activity is increased while Type 1 collagen production is decreased.[141] These changes in the wound healing process lead to delayed healing and a weaker wound that is likely to recur.[141]

Nutrition and Wound Healing

Good nutritional status is of paramount importance to wound healing and is often compromised in PLWBCs due to multiple factors, including increased metabolic demand due to the disease and its treatments, stress, and lack of appetite (refer to Chapter 30). Malnutrition is common in PLWBCs, and consequences can include increased risk of infection, delayed healing, impaired QOL, poor response to cancer-related treatment, and/or increased mortality.[142] A commonly used nutritional screening, assessment, and progress-tracking tool used for PLWBCs is the Patient-Generated Subjective Global Assessment.[143] Current nutritional recommendations include at least 30 kcal/kg body weight/day and 1.2 g protein/kg body weight/day, although higher levels are recommended if the PLWBC already has a wound or if the wound is very large.[144]

Vitamin C is critical for the formation of collagen through its involvement in the hydroxylation of lysine to proline.[145] Wound tensile strength is decreased and the risk of surgical wound dehiscence is increased with inadequate vitamin C.[98] Further, vitamin C is required for adequate neutrophil function, as it is thought that vitamin C protects neutrophils from oxidative stress. Vitamin C itself is a potent antioxidant that can scavenge reactive oxidants while blocking inflammatory signaling pathways, and it can also increase NO production, thereby leading to vasodilation and reduced hypoxia.[145,146] These roles highlight the importance of vitamin C in the immune response. Since the body cannot store vitamin C, supplementation is critical. To facilitate wound healing, 1 to 2 grams of vitamin C are recommended daily.[98]

Vitamin A deficiency is also linked to decreased collagen formation as well as decreased re-epithelialization and slow wound closure.[98] Macrophage recruitment is improved with vitamin A supplementation, leading to an improved inflammatory response.[98] Vitamin A can mitigate the negative effects of corticosteroids, and topical doses may provide benefit locally without affecting systemic corticosteroid action.[98] A recommended daily supplement of vitamin A is 25,000 IU per day.

Zinc is a cofactor for DNA and RNA synthesis and is important in all phases of wound healing; however, it is important to supplement only in cases of deficiency. Excess zinc can affect collagen cross-linking and interfere with iron and copper absorption.[98,141] Recommended dosing for patients who are deficient is up to 220 mg twice per day for 10 to 14 days.[141]

The amino acid arginine is essential to protein synthesis, collagen production, and immune function.[141] Arginine added to other micronutrient supplementation has been found to improve healing in patients with pressure injuries.[147] NO is synthesized by arginine by a group of enzymes called nitric oxide synthases (NOS), and this signaling molecule plays many important roles in immune function and inflammation, vasodilation, and angiogenesis, which are all critical to wound healing. Neural functions impacted by NO include cognition, stress, and muscle and gastrointestinal tone. There is a dichotomous role of NO in cancer pathogenesis, acting to either promote or defend against cancer growth, depending on cancer type and concentration.[148] NO can also help to mitigate the harmful effects of ROS. Clearly, there is a need for arginine supplementation in PLWBCs in need of wound healing, and 4.5 mg per day has been suggested.[141,149]

Wound Bed Preparation

Wound bed preparation is critical to wound healing. The DIME approach to wound bed preparation has been established to guide Onc R clinicians and focuses on **D**ebridement, managing **I**nfection and/or persistent **I**nflammation, and **M**oisture balance, then addressing the wound **E**dge to promote re-epithelialization.[150]

The presence of necrotic tissue will prevent healing, impede cellular migration, and promote inflammation and/or infection. Removal of necrotic tissue, such as slough, eschar, debris, or biofilm is essential and can occur in a variety of ways. Excisional debridement, in the form of serial sharp debridement using scissors, scalpel, curette and/or forceps is the preferred method of selective debridement to spare healthy tissue for most PLWBCs, and the recommended frequency is weekly.[150] Selective sharp debridement of only necrotic or nonviable tissue is within the scope of Onc R practice for physical therapists in the US; however, Onc R clinicians must always consider their personal scope of practice when utilizing modes of treatment. Onc R clinicians are strongly encouraged to pursue additional training in sharp debridement prior to practice and to meet their facilities' competencies.

Some PLWBCs may require surgical debridement, performed under anesthesia for faster, more complete removal of devitalized tissue. Enzymatic debridement can selectively cleave collagen connections and break down the necrotic tissue; however, this is much slower than sharp debridement. The only available enzyme on the US market currently is a collagenase. Autolytic debridement is achieved using the body's endogenous enzymes to break down necrotic tissue, but this method is also slower compared to other methods. Biological debridement is the use of medical-grade maggots to debride the wound via phagocytosis and enzymatic mechanisms. Finally, mechanical debridement uses some mechanical force, such as irrigation with pulsed lavage with suction or syringes, abrasion with moist gauze, or removal of a dried dressing to remove nonviable tissue; however, mechanical debridement using wet to dry dressings is not selective and should be avoided when healthy granulation tissue is visible.

Wound infection is determined by the number and virulence of the microbes in the wound, coupled with the host's defense system.[150] There is a continuum of infection that progresses from contamination to systemic infection, see eFigure 9.3.[151,152] Note that classic signs of local infection may be present (erythema, warmth, swelling, purulent drainage), however it has been found that the more subtle signs are better indicators of chronic wound infection than the classic signs.[153]

Biofilms are defined by the International Wound Infection Institute as "a structured community of microbes with genetic diversity and variable gene expression (phenotype) that creates behaviors and defenses used to produce unique infections (chronic infection)."[150] Planktonic, or free-floating bacteria are weakly attached to the wound surface and are the target of many antimicrobial treatments. When attachments become stronger and irreversible, biofilm formation begins.[150] Bacteria develop a unique, 3-D polysaccharide structure that creates an environment in which groups of bacteria thrive in communities while protected from the environment, endogenous immune cells, and exogenous antibacterial treatments.[154] Biofilms exist in most chronic wounds in both superficial and deep tissues and contribute to delayed healing, inflammation, and infection.[150,155] Weekly debridement is one of the few interventions that can remove or reduce biofilm, which grows back quickly; however, the biofilm is rarely fully removed and other interventions such as ultraviolet C are needed to manage local bacteria.[150]

Making the decision to treat infection locally or systemically is made easier using the mnemonics NERDS and STONEES, depicted in eFigure 9.4.[156] The use of antimicrobial dressings is not recommended prophylactically, unless the patient is at high risk for developing infection, such as patients who are immunocompromised. Various dressing types are available to treat bacteria locally, including dressings that contain silver, honey, iodine, polyhexamethylenebiguanide (PHMB), or methylene blue/crystal violet.[156] Silver and honey also help manage inflammation.[156] These dressings should be used for 2 weeks, then the wound reassessed to determine the need for continued use. PLWBCs with systemic infections will need to be referred to their physician for systemic antibiotics. Wound perfusion and comorbidities must be taken into account when determining oral versus intravenous administration of antibiotics.

Swab cultures may be used to determine the amount and type of microbe in a wound, although the punch biopsy is considered best practice. Wound biopsies are less commonly performed due to pain, damage to the already struggling wound bed, and cost[150]; however, they are necessary in any wound that is suspected of being malignant. Biopsies should be taken at several areas of the wound since cancer cells are often not homogeneous within a wound bed. The Levine technique for swab cultures has been found to be the most reliable measure of wound bioburden.[157] In this technique, the wound is debrided and cleansed prior to taking the culture. The swab is moistened with normal saline, then firmly pressed and rotated in a 1 cm² area of clean wound tissue (not in necrotic tissue) in order to express wound fluid. The swab is returned to the culture tube and brought to the lab.[150] Point-of-care fluorescence imaging has been shown to have excellent predictive value in identifying bacterial load in a wound, allowing the clinician to make faster clinical judgments regarding anti-bacterial dressing use.[158]

Inflammation is normal during wound healing in adults; however, prolonged inflammation can lead to many problems, as described previously. Further, prolonged inflammation can weaken the body's natural immune response and allow bacteria to proliferate, thus leading to infection. Multiple biomarkers have been identified in prolonged inflammatory states, including ILs, cytokines, MMPs, NF-kB, c-reactive proteins, among others.[150] Advances in both wound care and cancer treatment are investigating interventions aimed at these biomarkers to return cell function to normal.

Dressing options to address chronic inflammation in wounds include collagen dressings that can regulate MMPs in the wound while also scavenging excessive ROS to promote healing.[90,134] MMPs, which degrade collagen and ECM proteins, prefer the easy-to-access collagen of the wound dressing, thereby sparing the ECM collagen required for the migration and proliferation of cells needed to advance wounds to the proliferative phase of healing. Stabilized collagen dressings have also been found to improve the efficiency of macrophages, then rapidly facilitate movement through the inflammatory phase, measured using the pro-inflammatory biomarkers.[159]

Wound fluid is also high in pro-inflammatory substances, including MMPs, IL-8, and NF-kB which contribute to a sustained inflammatory phase if not removed from the wound bed.[160] These inflammatory substances are harmful to the cells involved in wound healing, and if left in contact with the wound surface, healing will be delayed.[150] Exudate needs to be managed through proper wound dressings to promote proper healing, leading to the next consideration in the DIME concept.

Moisture balance is essential for normal cellular function. With too little moisture, the ECM and cells dry up and cannot migrate to the wound area. Conversely, too much moisture can macerate the skin, leading to poor re-epithelialization and potentially causing additional skin breakdown and increased risk of infection.

A proper moisture balance is achieved through the use of appropriate dressings. If a wound is dry, a dressing that will donate moisture to the area is indicated. This is best achieved through hydrogel dressings, which are water or glycerin-based (available in sheets, amorphous gels, or impregnated gauze forms). Thin film dressings, while moisture neutral,[156] can create a moister environment in a dry wound when used over a hydrogel, a combination which promotes autolytic debridement. The necrotic tissue is solubilized, and the cellular byproducts are subsequently flushed from the wound as exudate. Frequent assessment is always indicated to ensure the right dressing is used as the wound characteristics change.

If the wound is draining, a dressing that will absorb the excess drainage while leaving the right amount within the wound is required. See eTable 9.2 for a list of dressing categories in order of absorptive capability. Often, dressings are used in combination, one to fill wound space (termed primary dressing) and one to cover, protect, and absorb excessive drainage (termed secondary dressing). Alginates and hydrofiber dressings have similar absorptive qualities and uses. Alginates are made from a derivative of seaweed and are bio-degradable, meaning if a small portion of the dressing is left in the wound bed, the body does not create an inflammatory response to fight it. Foam dressings are highly absorptive and most have the ability to lock drainage into the dressing to thereby avoid perpetuating the inflammatory response while preventing skin maceration. Superabsorbent dressings are relatively new and absorb the most drainage, locking away moisture even under compression dressings. These dressings are valuable for highly-draining venous ulcers.

PLWBCs who do not demonstrate healing after 4 weeks of standard wound care can qualify for adjunctive therapies in the outpatient setting. These therapies include NPWT, bioengineered skin substitutes, human fibroblast-derived dermal substitutes, porcine extracellular matrices, amniotic tissue grafts, and acellular dermal scaffolds. Other interventions that can be initiated after 4 weeks of nonhealing include electrical stimulation and hyperbaric oxygen therapy. It should be noted that current Centers for Medicare and Medicaid guidelines do not limit advanced dressings in the inpatient setting, they are only limited in the outpatient setting at the time of this writing. Biological and cellular/tissue dressings can only be applied by a physician or by a licensed provider under the supervision of a physician.

Attempts have been made to provide growth factors to a wound exogenously. The growth factor recombinant PDGF (becaplermin) is FDA approved for use in diabetic foot ulcers, and has been shown to improve healing time by an average of 6 weeks and increase full wound closure by 43%.[161] Caution is advised in PLWBCs with known malignancy since PDGF over-signaling is associated with multiple cancers.[65,162]

The Future of Wound Healing and Cancer Treatment

The science of wound healing parallels the pathology of cancer. The cells, growth factors, cytokines, and ROS involved in wound healing are also involved in tumor growth and metastasis; therefore, researchers in both fields have come to realize what can be learned from one another. The future of interventions in both areas is focused at the cellular and molecular levels in an effort to normalize infection control cell proliferation and manage disease. Research is also focused on the role of oxygen, including ROS and their mediators, to identify methods that balance and harness the power of both in order to promote optimal tissue health. As discoveries are made in the field of wound care, the field of cancer research will benefit and vice versa. It is, indeed, an exciting time for both fields.

Conclusion

The lymphatic system and the integumentary system are nearly inseparable and the Onc R clinician rarely will be able to treat one without addressing the other. There is still much to be learned and understood about the lymphatic system and the disease process of lymphedema. Study of both the functioning of the system and the physiology of the disease is still a growing science. As research increases in its sophistication and discovery, our clinical opportunity to be successful in both mitigating the onset of clinical lymphedema and reducing its disease impact will continue to evolve in its effectiveness. As clinicians we must continue our focused study in this area of clinical management with consideration of the importance of treating persons living with lymphatic and integumentary compromise from a body system-based, functional impairment model of care that is inclusive of physical and psychological considerations in response to these disease processes. Cancers of the integumentary system most predominantly include basal cell carcinoma, squamous cell carcinoma, and melanoma, and collectively are the most frequently diagnosed cancers. Prevention education and screening are within the purview of the Onc R clinician. Further, the wound healing cascade offers insight into cancer pathology and treatment, as similarities between wound healing and tumor progression have been identified.

Critical Research Needs

- Benefits of prospective surveillance to prevent and manage lymphedema with all stages of breast cancer and gynecological cancers is vital in guiding the management needs of PLWBCs who are at risk for lymphedema. Determine the efficacy of directing early postsurgical management and treatment towards improving/optimizing the functional recovery of the impacted lymphatic system within a lymphatic territory. Determine how lymphedema manifests, behaves and responds to treatment intervention, as well as on different objective measures that measure outcomes with patients diagnosed with head and neck cancer, gynecological cancers, and genitourinary cancers.

- Determine the targeted cell therapies that are the most effective in preventing tumor growth and metastasis while minimizing damage to multiple cell types. Elucidate interventions that modulate the growth factors responsible for over-activation of fibroblasts. Identify key growth factors and cytokines that are linked to the development of each cancer type that can unlock even more specific treatments which could also prevent common integumentary system complications.
- In addition to fibrosis, tissue damage after radiation therapy is due to the formation of ROS, which are highly reactive with NO. Determine the most effective effectiveness of interventions that utilize NO to increase circulation, improve tissue healing, and/or manage ROS within postoperative or postradiated tissue. Determine the specific matrices that can alter cancer growth and metastasis in the tumor microenvironment, in vivo.

Case Studies

Lymphedema Case Study

A patient with breast cancer-related lymphedema presented with chronic Stage 3 lymphedema. Her initial onset of clinical lymphedema was Stage 2 lymphedema in early 2014 which progressed into Stage 3 lymphedema by early 2015 and was still currently present at the time of evaluation.

Patient and Tumor Identification

Patient was a 64-year-old female diagnosed in 2014 with left (L) sided Stage 2, Grade 2 invasive ductal carcinoma.

Pathology: ER+/PR+/HER 2-; Axillary lymph node dissection: 1+/15.

Genetic Testing: Patient tested negative for BRCA 1 & 2, as well as other genetic markers.

Family History: No reported family history of breast cancer or any cancers related to the BRCA genes.

Medical History: Previously healthy; no significant past medical history.

Patient presented with acute onset of clinical lymphedema in April 2014 approximately 1 month after the completion of her bilateral mastectomy with expander placement, systemic chemotherapy, and radiation therapy.

Purpose of the Study

The purpose of this case study is to describe the treatment approach for this patient. The treatment approach was inclusive of the clinical parameters of best practice management presented in the content of this chapter. Additionally, the skilled interventions described within this case study are aligned with the current standards of skilled intervention in accordance with the Chronic Disease Model of Care.

Clinical Parameters of Best Practice Management
See Figure 9.29.

Skilled Intervention and the Chronic Disease Model of Care

The definition of the Chronic Disease Model of Care is to rehabilitate functional impairments to a level where impairments are optimized and symptoms are controlled, not cured. The latter would pertain to a Curative Model of Care. Lymphedema is a chronic, progressive disease process and therefore it should be treated in alignment with the Chronic Disease Model of Care. Within this model of care, the constructs of skilled intervention are as follows:

1. Improve and optimize functional impairments.
2. Stabilize symptoms of optimized functional impairments.
3. Monitor and address safety and effectiveness of function in all activities of daily living.
4. Reduce or slow down further deterioration of the chronic health condition.
See Table 9.7.

There is emerging research that taxane-based chemotherapy results in lymphatic system toxicity (see eTable 9.2).[33] The predominant causative impact to the lymphatic system is fluid retention. This can result in adding accumulative stress to the ratio between TC and lymph obligatory load within the impacted lymphatic territory in which the ALND has been performed. See Tables 9.8 and 9.9.

Surgery and Radiation Therapy
See Table 9.10

Treatment Considerations

The clinical parameters of best practice are to ensure rehabilitative treatment addresses the lymphatic system function across all three superficial, subfascial, and deep regions, as well as addressing the surrounding body systems (Figure 9.30).

Treatment of the lymphatic system was focused within the affected lymphatic territory, addressing the remaining lymphatic system to engage its function and provide opportunity to optimize its locoregional function (Figures 9.31 and 9.32).

Treatment of surrounding body systems was focused within the affected quadrant both anteriorly, anterolaterally, and posteriorly, as well as inclusive of the ipsilateral upper extremity. The neuromuscular-skeletal systems are addressed, as well as the visceral system. Myofascial trigger point release is performed on affected myofascial structures (Figures 9.33 and 9.34), neural tension release techniques are performed with upper tension release techniques, joint mobilization is performed to all joint structures in the quadrant, and visceral mobilization if performed to visceral organs in the abdominal region.

Results of Treatment
See Figure 9.35.

Discussion

Stage 3 lymphedema remained exacerbated significantly through January 2016 and January 2017. This was attributed to patient being immunosuppressed during this time. The patient's immunosuppression was secondary to recovering from DIEP (deep inferior epigastric perforator) flap surgery, and additionally enduring repeated cellulitis infections in the ipsilateral upper extremity.

The patient consistently received treatment once a week to once every 2/3 weeks from 2016 through to the present. The Chronic Disease Model of Care has remained the primary focus

Left sided Stage 2, Grade 2, Invasive Ductal Carcinoma
Pathology: ER+/PR+/HER2-. Axillary nodes: 1 of 15+; BRCA-

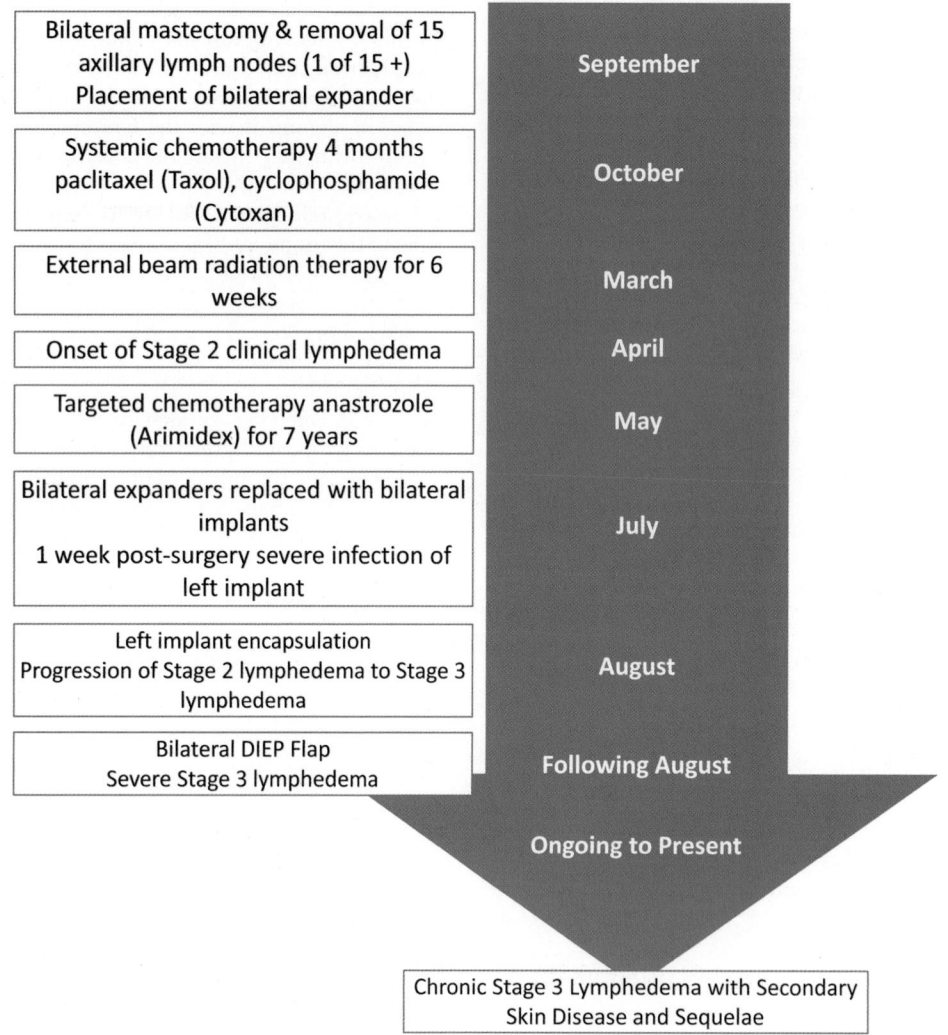

• **Fig. 9.29** Timeline of Treatment Sequence. (Created by Julia C. Osborne. Printed with permission.) *DIEP*, Deep inferior epigastric perforator.

TABLE 9.7	Systemic Chemotherapy Toxicities: Taxol and Cytoxan		
Drug	Drug Class	Delivery Method	Salient Toxicity and Clinical Pathway of Management
Cyclophosphamide (Cytoxan)	Alkylating Agent	IV every 2 or 3 weeks	General toxicity
Paclitaxel (Taxol)	Taxane	IV every 2 or 3 weeks or 12 weeks	Chemotherapy-induced neuropathy

Created by Julia C. Osborne. Printed with permission.

of patient treatment and management. Within this model of care, the constructs and the goals of skilled intervention were integrated into the treatment plan (see Figure 9.10):

Goal 1: Improve and optimize functional impairments — this was achieved from January 2018 and January 2021 by clinically addressing both the lymphatic system and the concurrent treatment of the surrounding body systems.

Goal 2: Stabilize symptoms of optimized functional impairments — this was achieved from January 2020 through January 2021 by ensuring sustainability of treatment results whilst the patient engaged in activities of daily living with minimal fluctuations of lymphedema.

Goal 3: Monitor and address safety and effectiveness of function in all activities of daily living — this was achieved by

TABLE 9.8 Body Systems Evaluation — Systemic Chemotherapy

Body System	Toxicity	Evaluation and Treatment Considerations
Cardiopulmonary	Cardiovascular tolerance	Physical therapist or exercise physiologist
Lymphatic	Extracellular fluid overload	Lymphedema risk assessment
Nervous: central	Cognitive impairment	Screen — occupational therapy or speech language pathology
Nervous: peripheral	Chemotherapy-induced polyneuropathy (CIPN)	CIPN and balance assessments
Skeletal	Osteopenia/osteoporosis	Pain, posture, weight bearing
Myofascial	Adenosine triphosphate (ATP) metabolism	Flexibility, strength, coordination
Gastrointestinal	Inflammation — colitis, constipation, decreased bowel function	Decreased nutritional and hydration status — weakness, debilitation, poor balance — fall risk
Urogenital	Bladder instability and inflammation	Urinary urgency, frequency, stress incontinence

Created by Julia C. Osborne. Printed with permission.

TABLE 9.9 Body Systems Evaluation — Targeted Chemotherapy (Anastrozole [Arimidex])

Body System	Toxicity	Evaluation and Treatment Considerations
Skeletal	Arthralgic pain, soft tissue inflammation	Arthralgic pain, posture, types of exercises
Vascular	Bleeding, delayed healing	Surgical recovery, other trauma
Dermal	Skin rash	Patient education — skin/nail care and awareness of onset of cellulitis infection
Gastrointestinal	Inflammation — colitis, constipation, decreased bowel function	Decreased nutritional and hydration status — weakness, debilitation, poor balance — fall risk

Created by Julia C. Osborne. Printed with permission.

TABLE 9.10 Body Systems Evaluation — Surgery and Radiation Therapy

Body System	Impairment	Evaluation and Treatment Considerations
Dermal	Incisional scar adhesions	Myofascial release, stretching program
Skeletal	Postural changes; joint restrictions	Joint mobilization, range-of-motion (ROM) exercises, strengthening and conditioning, postural education
Myofascial	Tissue restrictions	Manual therapy, strengthening and stretching program
Lymphatic	Acute injury to local lymphatic system	Complete decongestive therapy, trigger point release, joint mobilization, visceral mobilization, diaphragmatic breathing, stretching program
Vascular	Local vascular compromise	Heart rate range monitoring for optimal perfusion to local areas of surgical and radiation intervention
Neural	Pain, peripheral neural tension	Neural glides, spinal ROM

Created by Julia C. Osborne. Printed with permission.

closely monitoring body systems and structures for any need of additional patient education and/or for any need of assistive devices. Additionally, the safety and effectiveness were used as a function of decreasing the incidence and frequency of cellulitis infections.

Goal 4: Reduce or slow down further deterioration of the chronic health condition — this was achieved by optimizing the function of the remaining lymphatic system and effective stable results over the long term.

Integument Case

Case Description

A 76-year-old male was referred to home health physical therapy due to a nonhealing wound on his anus. His diagnosis was ulcer of the anus and rectum, suspected due to hemorrhoid. He had been treated by his primary care physician and home nursing for the last 2 to 3 months with no change in wound size. Dressings used included a topical corticosteroid, zinc oxide

Treat the LYMPHATIC SYSTEM

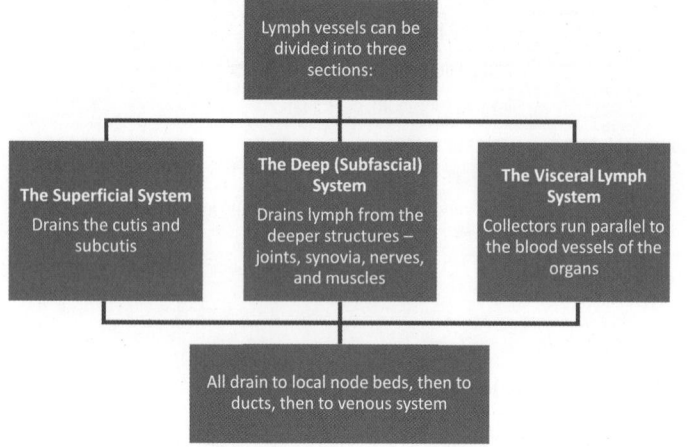

Lymph vessels can be divided into three sections:

The Superficial System
Drains the cutis and subcutis

The Deep (Subfascial) System
Drains lymph from the deeper structures – joints, synovia, nerves, and muscles

The Visceral Lymph System
Collectors run parallel to the blood vessels of the organs

All drain to local node beds, then to ducts, then to venous system

Treat the SURROUNDING BODY SYSTEMS

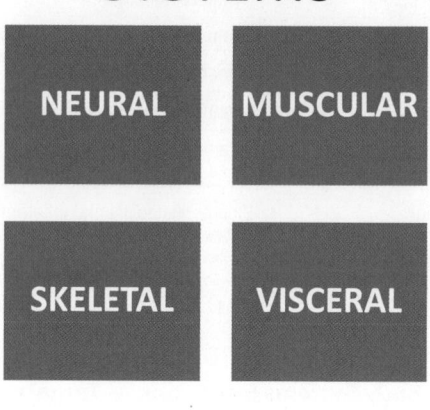

NEURAL **MUSCULAR**

SKELETAL **VISCERAL**

• **Fig. 9.30** Planning the Treatment Requirements. (Created by Julia C. Osborne. Printed with permission.)

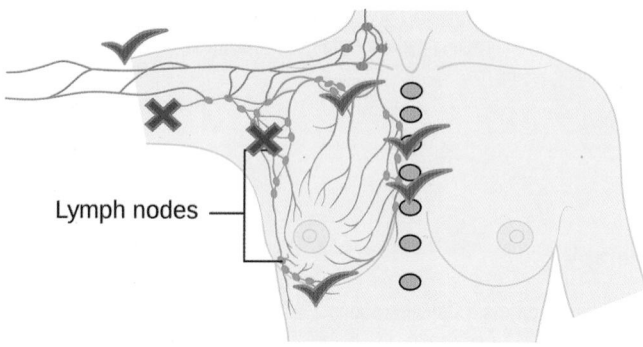

Lymph nodes

• **Fig. 9.31** Access points to the "Remaining" Lymphatic System. Anterior: Cephalic pathway, intercostal nodes, and parasternal nodes. Posterior: Paraspinal lymph nodes (not shown). (Adapted from Cancer Research UK under Creative Commons Attribution-Share Alike 4.0 International license.)

paste, bacitracin cream, and the current application of gentian violet solution applied twice daily. An ABD pad was also used to absorb drainage and bleeding and to protect his clothes from the gentian violet.

The patient's medical history was significant for hypertension, controlled with benazepril hydrochloride. He was a former smoker with a 30-pack year history; he quit smoking 5 years ago. He reported occasional constipation and used psyllium regularly, docusate sodium when constipation was more severe. More recently, he complained of loose stools and had since discontinued his daily psyllium. He also noted bleeding with bowel movements since the wound was noted.

The patient reported pain in the wound area and lower abdomen that he rated as a 4/10 on the visual analog scale. He also stated that bowel movements were "uncomfortable." His main complaint was fatigue and weakness that increased over the last 3 to 4 months. He reported difficulty walking and had recently begun to use a front-wheeled walker (FWW) to assist with

balance. He denied needing assistance from his wife for mobility. The patient also reported weight loss of approximately 15 pounds in the last 3 months.

He was previously able to ambulate without a device in the community and in the woods behind his property. His goals for therapy were to improve his mobility so he could return to walking in the woods and to heal the wound.

Clinical Impression 1

Several red flags were noted in the subjective information. A non-healing wound is always concerning and alternative etiologies should be considered. The patient's recent change in bowel habits, recent decline in function, and significant weight loss were also concerning. His smoking history was a red flag. The wound location alone was not unusual, but coupled with the other red flags, the location became a concerning factor. Malignancy was a possible concern, and a thorough wound evaluation would need to be performed. A mobility exam would also need to be performed.

Examination

Upon observation, the patient appeared thin with muscle wasting noted in the extremities and trunk. He was alert and oriented × 4. He was observed to shift his position in sitting often, taking weight from buttock to buttock without bearing weight centrally on the coccyx.

Upper and lower quarter screens were negative for any neurological involvement, but general weakness was noted. ROM of his bilateral upper and lower extremities was full throughout. A strength assessment revealed global functional weakness in his trunk and lower extremities, graded 4- to 4/5 throughout.

The patient demonstrated modified independence with sit to stand transfers from all surfaces; he needed to use his arms to assist with all transfers. He required stand-by assistance for gait with the FWW due to occasional unsteadiness with turns. Gait was limited to 300 feet (91 meters) due to fatigue. He was slow during bed mobility tasks but did not require physical assistance.

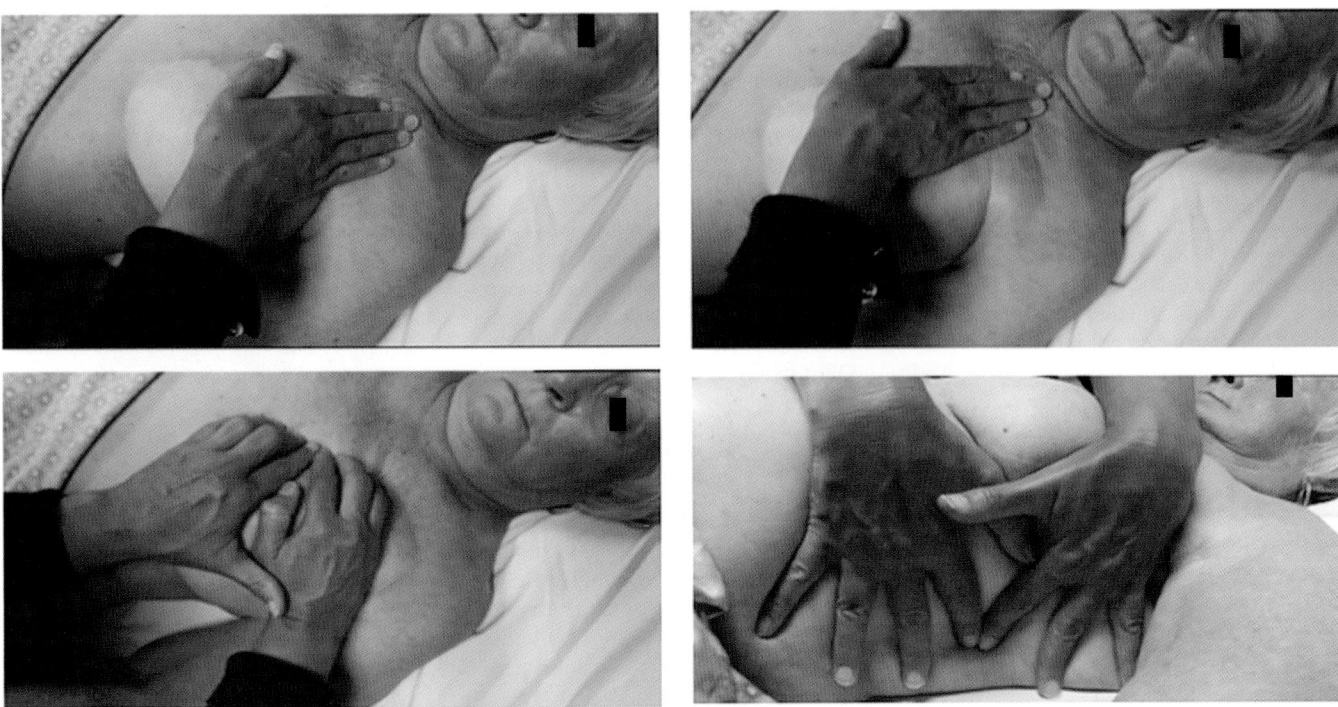

• **Fig. 9.32** Manual Lymphatic Drainage Techniques Applied Within the Ipsilateral Territory. (Created by Julia C. Osborne. Printed with permission.)

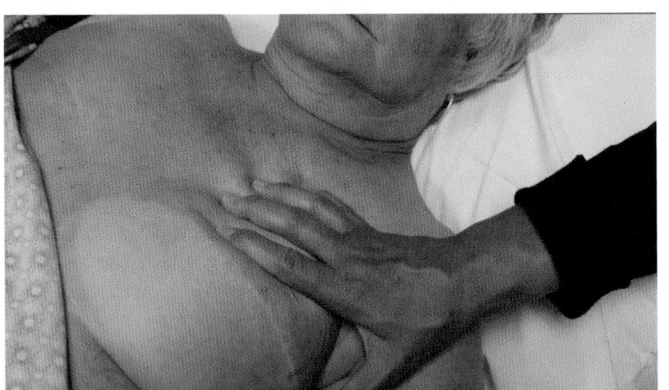

• **Fig. 9.33** Treatment of the Myofascial System — Pectoralis Major. (Created by Julia C. Osborne. Printed with permission.)

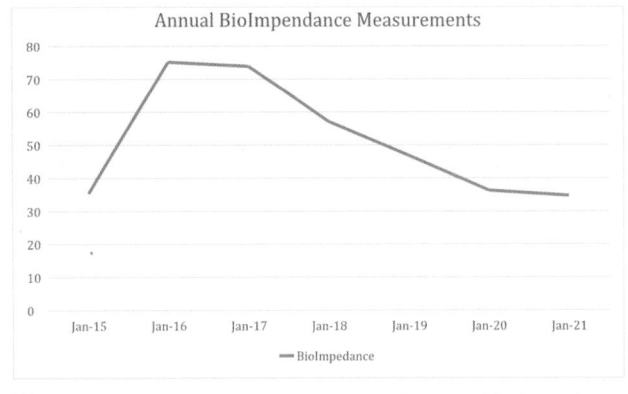

• **Fig. 9.35** Bioimpedance Measurements January 2015 to January 2021. (Created by Julia C. Osborne. Printed with permission.)

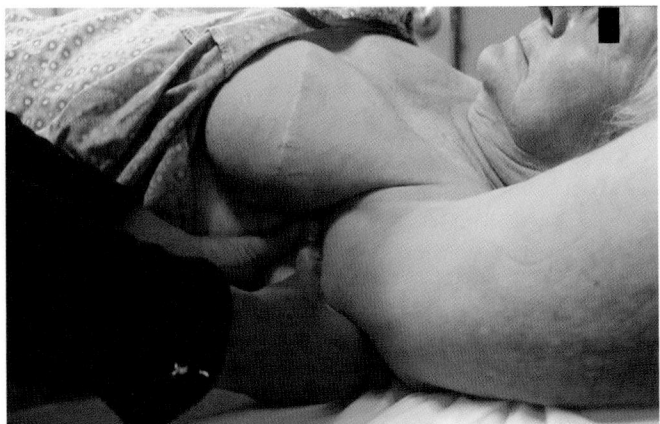

• **Fig. 9.34** Treatment of the Myofascial System — Subscapularis and Latissimus Dorsi. (Created by Julia C. Osborne. Printed with permission.)

A Tinetti Performance Oriented Mobility Assessment was performed, the patient scored 16/28, indicating a high risk of falling. He lost points during balance testing and because of his use of the FWW.

The wound was assessed with the patient in modified plantigrade standing. Gentian violet staining was noted, even after cleansing. The wound presented with a raised, cauliflower-like wound bed and demarcated edges that extended from the skin near the edge of the anus into the anal canal. The wound bed presented with a translucent quality at the surface with a red base. There was no slough or eschar noted.

All borders of the wound were visible when the gluteal tissue was stretched. The wound measured 4.5 cm in length by 2.5 cm in width. Depth was listed at 0.1 cm due to a disruption in the epithelium, but no measurable depth was noted. The wound was friable and bleeding was noted with minor cleansing. The periwound tissue was intact with mild erythema extending approximately

1.0 cm beyond the wound edge. No edema, warmth, or indura-tion was noted upon palpation of the periwound area. There was no significant odor noted. Drainage was noted on the ABD pad, assessed to be moderate drainage, tinted with gentian violet.

Clinical Impression 2

The suspicion of a malignant wound was heightened after the examination; the appearance of the wound bed was alarming. The cauliflower-like appearance along with the translucent character were not consistent with a typical wound bed presentation. This, coupled with the friable wound bed was enough to warrant a biopsy of the wound bed. Infection was not suspected based on a lack of erythema >2 cm from the wound edge, no induration, no warmth. The edges were demarcated, demonstrating no signs of re-epitheliazation after 3 months of intervention, further indicat-ing a nonhealing wound. The clinician's concerns were reported to the primary care physician and a biopsy was scheduled.

Interventions

The patient's primary care physician performed biopsies of various aspects of the wound, and a diagnosis of Stage III rectal cancer was made. The patient underwent chemotherapy and radiation treat-ments; surgery was potentially planned after reassessment upon completion of those interventions. Nursing managed the wound care as there were no debridement needs by the physical therapist. The patient was seen by physical therapy for 3 weeks at home for education in energy conservation techniques to maximize func-tion, balance training, functional strengthening, and gait training. A home exercise program was provided to allow continuation of the program after discharge.

Outcomes

The patient was discharged from home physical therapy prior to the completion of his chemotherapy and radiation treatment, demon-strating significant functional progress such that he was no longer homebound. He improved on the Tinetti assessment (24/28) but was still at mild risk of falling due to reliance on an assistive device and decreased steadiness with eyes closed. He demonstrated improved tolerance for ambulation with incorporation of energy conservation techniques. He was ambulating variable distances of up to 1500 feet (457 m) with a standard cane on level surfaces at discharge. He did not meet his goal of walking in the woods, but he chose not to pur-sue outpatient physical therapy at that time. He planned to attend outpatient physical therapy after completion of his cancer treatments. He demonstrated a good understanding of the home program and indications to request a follow-up physical therapy evaluation. He was motivated to continue with the home program.

Discussion

This case highlights an important aspect of clinical reasoning when assessing a nonhealing wound: if the wound appearance looks unusual, a biopsy is likely warranted. This nonhealing wound presented with characteristics inconsistent with a "typi-cal" wound bed. Further, the patient's history was rife with red flags that were missed by other healthcare providers. It took a "new set of eyes" to assess the entire case and recognize that there were enough flags to warrant a biopsy. Often, the Onc R clini-cian is not a key player in the management of cancerous wounds, but all Onc R clinicians must be able to recognize wounds that might be malignant.

Review Questions

Reader can find the correct answers and rationale in the back of the book.

Case 1 (for questions 1–5): A 48-year-old female presents with left sided Stage 3, HER2-, hormone negative (triple nega-tive) breast cancer. She is treated with neoadjuvant chemo-therapy which includes doxorubicin (Adriamycin), cyclophos-phamide (Cytoxan), carboplatin (Paraplatin), and paclitaxel (Taxol). This is followed with a bilateral mastectomy, removal of 3 axillary lymph nodes, and expander placement. The pathology post-neoadjuvant chemotherapy revealed a pathological com-plete response in the tumor, however residual tumor cells were noted in the three axillary lymph nodes. Four weeks post-sur-gery, the patient underwent 6 weeks of external beam radiation therapy to the left chest wall and axillary region. During this time, the patient developed an acute cellulitis infection in the tissue over her left expander and lateral chest area. She was hos-pitalized for three days and received intravenous antibiotics to treat the infection. The patient has just completed phase two of her reconstructive surgery in which her bilateral expanders were replaced with bilateral implants. Currently she is six weeks post-surgery and is mildly weakened and deconditioned secondary to her extensive treatment and recent surgery. She presents with a BMI of 36. Her volumetric measurements of her left upper extremity compared to her right upper extremity show a 6% increase on the left. Prior to diagnosis, the patient had a history of left shoulder impingement syndrome, but overall was very active, and she expresses a strong desire to get back to her prior activity levels.

1. What is the first evidence-based lymphedema risk stratifica-tion consideration encountered in this patient's treatment pathway?
   A. The HER2 biomarker
   B. The hormone biomarkers
   C. Patient's age
   D. Systemic chemotherapy

2. When is the most effective time to initiate lymphedema surveillance with this patient?
   A. At 6 weeks after phase two reconstructive surgery
   B. At prehab at the time of her initial diagnosis
   C. As she goes through her neoadjuvant chemotherapy regimen
   D. Immediately after her phase one bilateral mastectomy

3. With a 6% increase in fluid volume in the left upper extrem-ity compared to the right, we can conclude that that patient is presenting with:
   A. Subclinical lymphedema in her left upper extremity
   B. Clinical lymphedema in her left upper extremity
   C. An irreversible form of lymphatic compromise
   D. Postsurgical edema

4. Which additional comorbidity is the most likely to signifi-cantly increase her risk of developing clinical lymphedema?
   A. Her BMI status
   B. Her history of shoulder impingement syndrome
   C. Her cellulitis infection
   D. Her phase 2 reconstructive surgery

5. The patient inquires about lymphatic surgery options that could help mitigate progression to secondary lymphedema. The evidence-based research advice you provide to her is the following:
   A. It's too early in her recovery process to consider the need for lymphatic surgery
   B. The timing is just right for considering a LVA surgery
   C. The timing is just right to consider a VLNT surgery
   D. The timing is just right to consider a SAPL surgery
   Review Questions for Integumentary System, 6 to 10
   Based on the Following Case Vignette: A 53-year-old female was referred to the wound clinic with an ulcer that erupted 2 months ago on her left, lateral, lower leg. The wound has not healed, despite the use of appropriate wound dressings. She reports itching in the periwound area, but pain is minimal. Her past medical history is significant for rheumatoid arthritis (RA), osteoarthritis (OA) of both knees, and a full-thickness burn to the left leg after an automobile accident 25 years ago. Her burn wounds healed, but grafting was necessary after 4 weeks of conservative wound care. She currently takes methotrexate and prednisone for RA and ibuprofen for OA. She reports she has been walking 30 minutes each day to assist with wound healing and overall health. The wound presents with hypergranulated tissue growing above the rolled, irregular borders of the wound. There is moderate clear drainage, but no odor noted. The wound measures 4.0 cm in length by 3.0 cm in width. The periwound skin presents with scar tissue that demonstrates decreased mobility to stretch and minimal localized edema surrounding the wound area

6. Based on the wound presentation, what is the most likely etiology of this wound?
   A. Venous wound
   B. Pressure injury
   C. Marjolin's ulcer
   D. Arterial wound

7. What is the recommended initial treatment for this type of ulcer?
   A. Serial debridement and moisture-retentive dressings
   B. Biopsy followed by wound excision
   C. Electrical stimulation and moisture-retentive dressings
   D. Compression dressings

8. What dressing would be an appropriate choice for this patient's wound?
   A. Hydrogel
   B. Thin film
   C. Hydrofiber
   D. Superabsorbent

9. The methotrexate, prednisone, and ibuprofen can affect healing most in what stage?
   A. Hemostasis
   B. Inflammatory
   C. Proliferative
   D. Maturation

10. What vitamin can be given to offset the effects of the patient's current medications on wound healing?
    A. Vitamin A
    B. Vitamin B6
    C. Vitamin C
    D. Vitamin D

References

1. Rockson SG. Acquired lymphedema: abnormal fluid clearance engenders tissue remodeling. *Lymphat Res Biol.* 2014;12(1):1. doi:10.1089/lrb.2014.1211.
2. Sleigh BC, Manna B. Lymphedema., *StatPearls*: StatPearls Publishing; 2020 July 26.
3. Cormier JN, L Rourke, Crosby M, et al. The surgical treatment of lymphedema: a systematic review of the contemporary literature (2004–2010). *Ann Surg Oncol.* 2012;19:642–651.
4. Armer JM, Ostby PL, Ginex PK, et al. ONS Guidelines™ for cancer treatment-related lymphedema. *Oncol Nurs Forum.* 2020;47(5):518–538.
5. Davies C, Gilchrist L, Levenhagen K, et al. Interventions for breast cancer-related lymphedema: clinical practice guideline from the academy of oncologic physical therapy of APTA. *Phys Ther.* 2020;100(7):1163–1179.
6. Disipio TRS, Newman B, Hayes S. Incidence of unilateral arm lymphedema after breast cancer: a systematic review and meta-analysis. *Lancet Oncol.* 2013;14:500–515.
7. Gebruers N, Verbelen H, De Vrieze T, Coeck D, Tjalma W. Incidence and time path of lymphedema in sentinel node negative breast cancer patients: a systematic review. *Arch Phys Med Rehabil.* 2015;96(6):1131–1139.
8. Rupp J, Hadamitzky C, Henkenberens C, Christiansen H, Steinmann D, Bruns F. Frequency and risk factors for arm lymphedema after multimodal breast-conserving treatment of nodal positive breast cancer—a long-term observation, *Radiat Oncol.* 2019;14(1):39. doi:10.1186/s13014-019-1243-y.
9. Rockson SG, Keeley V, Kilbreath S, Szuba A, Towers A. Cancer-associated secondary lymphoedema. *Nat Rev Dis Primers.* 2019;5(1):22. doi:10.1038/s41572-019-0072-5.
10. Ridner SH, Dietrich MS, Niermann K, Cmelak A, Mannion K, Murphy B. A prospective study of the lymphedema and fibrosis continuum in patients with head and neck cancer. *Lymphat Res Biol.* 2016;14(4):198–205.
11. Hayes SC, Janda M, Ward LC, et al. Lymphedema following gynecological cancer: results from a prospective, longitudinal cohort study on prevalence, incidence and risk factors. *Gynecol. Oncol..* 2017;146(3):623–629.
12. Breslin JW, Yang Y, Scallan JP, Sweat RS, Adderley SP, Murfee WL. Lymphatic vessel network structure and physiology. *Compr Physiol.* 2018;9(1):207–299.
13. Hansen KC, D'Alessandro A, Clement CC, Santambrogio L. Lymph formation, composition and circulation: a proteomics perspective. *Int Immunol.* 2015;27(5):219–227.
14. von der Weid PY. Lymphatic vessel pumping. *Adv Exp Med Biol.* 2019;1124:357–377.
15. Santambrogio L. The lymphatic fluid. *Int Rev Cell Mol Biol.* 2018;337:111–133.
16. Levick JR, Michel CC. Microvascular fluid exchange and the revised Starling principle. *Cardiovasc Res.* 2010;87(2):198–210.
17. Suami H, Kato S. Anatomy of the lymphatic system and its structural disorders in lymphoedema. In: Lee BB, Rockson S, Bergan J, eds. *Lymphedema*: Springer; 2018. doi:10.1007/978-3-319-52423-8_5.
18. Földi M, Földi E, Kubik S. *Textbook of Lymphology for Physicians and Lymphedema Therapists*: Urban & Fischer; 2003.
19. Causey L, Cowin SC, Weinbaum S. Quantitative model for predicting lymph formation and muscle compressibility in skeletal muscle during contraction and stretch. *Proc Natl Acad Sci U S A.* 2012;109(23):9185–9190.
20. Schmid-Schönbein GW, Ikomi F. Biomechanics of lymph transport. In: Jaffrin MY, Caro CG, eds. ***Biological Flows***; 1995:353–360.

21. Evans CH, Kraus VB, Setton LA. Progress in intra-articular therapy. *Nat Rev Rheumatol.* 2014;10(1):11–22.

22. Reddy NP. Lymph circulation: physiology, pharmacology, and biomechanics. *Crit Rev Biomed Eng.* 1986;14(1):45–91.

23. CL Willard-Mack. Normal structure, function, and histology of lymph nodes. *Toxicol Pathol.* 2006;34(5):409–424.

24. Levenhagen K, Davies C, Perdomo M, Ryans K, Gilchrist L. Diagnosis of upper quadrant lymphedema secondary to cancer: clinical practice guideline from the oncology section of the American Physical Therapy Association. *Phys Ther.* 2017;97(7):729–745.

25. Forte AJ, Huayllani MT, Boczar D, et al. Use of bioimpedance spectroscopy for prospective surveillance and early diagnosis of breast cancer-related lymphedema. *Breast Dis.* 2021;40(2):85–93. doi:10.3233/BD-201008.

26. Stout NL, Binkley JM, Schmitz KH, et al. A prospective surveillance model for rehabilitation for women with breast cancer. *Cancer.* 2012;118(8 suppl):2191–2200.

27. Bundred N, Foden P, Todd C, et al. Increases in arm volume predict lymphoedema and quality of life deficits after axillary surgery: a prospective cohort study. *Br J Cancer.* 2020;123(1):17–25.

28. Kilgore LJ, Korentager SS, Hangge AN, et al. Reducing breast cancer-related lymphedema (BCRL) through prospective surveillance monitoring using bioimpedance spectroscopy (BIS) and patient directed self-interventions. *Ann Surg Oncol.* 2018;25(10):2948–2952.

29. Granzow JW. Lymphedema surgery: the current state of the art. *Clin Exp Metastasis.* 2018;35(5–6):553–558.

30. Squitieri L, Rasmussen PW, Patel KM. An economic analysis of prophylactic lymphovenous anastomosis among breast cancer patients receiving mastectomy with axillary lymph node dissection. *J Surg Oncol.* 2020;121(8):1175–1178.

31. Schaverien MV, Badash I, Patel KM, Selber JC, Cheng MH. Vascularized lymph node transfer for lymphedema. *Semin Plast Surg.* 2018;32(1):28–35.

32. Gallagher KK, Lopez M, Iles K, Kugar M. Surgical approach to lymphedema reduction. *Curr Oncol Rep.* 2020;22(10):97. doi:10.1007/s11912-020-00961-4.

33. SEER Training Modules. U.S. National Institutes of Health, National Cancer Institute. Layers of the skin. https://training.seer.cancer.gov/. Accessed October 10, 2020.

34. Hamm RL. Anatomy and physiology of the integument system. In: Hamm RL, ed. *Text and Atlas of Wound Diagnosis and Treatment,* McGraw-Hill Education; 2019:3–13.

35. Yousef H, Alhajj M, Sharma S. Anatomy, skin (integument), epidermis [July 27, 2020], *StatPearls* [Internet], StatPearls Publishing; 2020 January.

36. Agrawal R, Woodfolk JA. Skin barrier defects in atopic dermatitis. *Curr Allergy Asthma Rep.* 2014;14(5):433. doi:10.1007/s11882-014-0433-9.

37. Palmer CN, Irvine AD, Terron-Kwiatkowski A, et al. Common loss-of-function variants of the epidermal barrier protein filaggrin are a major predisposing factor for atopic dermatitis. *Nat Genet.* 2006;38(4):441–446.

38. Sandilands A, Sutherland C, Irvine AD, McLean WH. Filaggrin in the frontline: role in skin barrier function and disease. *J Cell Sci.* 2009;122(Pt 9):1285–1294.

39. Ishida-Yamamoto A, Kishibe M. Involvement of corneodesmosome degradation and lamellar granule transportation in the desquamation process. *Med Mol Morphol.* 2011;44(1):1–6.

40. Del Rosso JQ, Levin J. The clinical relevance of maintaining the functional integrity of the stratum corneum in both healthy and disease-affected skin. *J Clin Aesthet Dermatol.* 2011;4(9):22–42.

41. Rajesh A, Wise L, Hibma M. The role of Langerhans cells in pathologies of the skin. *Immunol Cell Biol.* 2019;97(8):700–713.

42. Breitkreutz D, Koxholt I, Thiemann K, Nischt R. Skin basement membrane: the foundation of epidermal integrity—BM functions and diverse roles of bridging molecules nidogen and perlecan, *Biomed Res Int.* 2013;2013:179784.

43. Myers BA. Integumentary anatomy. In: Myers BA, ed. *Wound Management: Principles and Practice,* Pearson; 2014:3–10.

44. Losquadro WD. Anatomy of the skin and the pathogenesis of nonmelanoma skin cancer. *Facial Plast Surg Clin North Am.* 2017;25(3):283–289.

45. Yousef H, Miao JH, Alhajj M, et al. Histology, skin appendages. [Updated May 7, 2020], *StatPearls* [Internet]: StatPearls Publishing; 2020. January. https://www.ncbi.nlm.nih.gov/books/NBK482237/.

46. Garcin CL, Ansell DM, Headon DJ, Paus R, Hardman MJ. Hair follicle bulge stem cells appear dispensable for the acute phase of wound re-epithelialization. *Stem Cells.* 2016;34(5):1377–1385.

47. Vary Jr JC. Selected disorders of skin appendages—acne, alopecia, hyperhidrosis, *Med Clin North Am.* 2015;99(6):1195–1211.

48. Witte MB, Thornton FJ, Efron DT, Barbul A. Enhancement of fibroblast collagen synthesis by nitric oxide. *Nitric Oxide.* 2000;4(6):572–582.

49. Yuan Q, Tan RJ, Liu Y. Myofibroblast in kidney fibrosis: origin, activation, and regulation. *Adv Exp Med Biol.* 2019;1165:253–283.

50. Myofibroblasts Hinz B. *Exp Eye Res.* 2016;142:56–70.

51. Huet E, Jaroz C, Nguyen HQ, et al. Stroma in normal and cancer wound healing. *FEBS J.* 2019;286(15):2909–2920.

52. Sherwani MA, Tufail S, Muzaffar AF, Yusuf N. The skin microbiome and immune system: potential target for chemoprevention? *Photodermatol Photoimmunol Photomed.* 2018;34(1):25–34.

53. Lynde C, Tan J, Skotnicki S, et al. Skin surface pH. *J Drugs Dermatol.* 2019;18(12):214.

54. Angelova-Fischer I, Fischer TW, Abels C, Zillikens D. Accelerated barrier recovery and enhancement of the barrier integrity and properties by topical application of a pH 4 vs. a pH 5.8 water-in-oil emulsion in aged skin. *Br J Dermatol.* 2018;179(2):471–477.

55. Moran B, Silva R, Perry AS, Gallagher WM. Epigenetics of malignant melanoma. *Semin Cancer Biol.* 2018;51:80–88.

56. Brash DE. UV-induced melanin chemiexcitation: a new mode of melanoma pathogenesis. *Toxicol Pathol.* 2016;44(4):552–554.

57. Bergqvist C, Ezzedine K. Vitamin D and the skin: what should a dermatologist know?. *G Ital Dermatol Venereol.* 2019;154(6):669–680.

58. Jenkins BA, Lumpkin EA. Developing a sense of touch. *Development.* 2017;144(22):4078–4090.

59. Charkoudian N. Human thermoregulation from the autonomic perspective. *Auton Neurosci.* 2016;196:1–2.

60. Luttrell T. Healing response in acute and chronic wounds. In: Hamm RL, ed. *Text and Atlas of Wound Diagnosis and Treatment,* McGraw-Hill Education; 2019:15–66.

61. Barrientos S, Stojadinovic O, Golinko MS, Brem H, Tomic-Canic M. Growth factors and cytokines in wound healing. *Wound Repair Regen.* 2008;16(5):585–601.

62. Golebiewska EM, Poole AW. Platelet secretion: from haemostasis to wound healing and beyond. *Blood Rev.* 2015;29(3):153–162.

63. Smith SA, Travers RJ, Morrissey JH. How it all starts: initiation of the clotting cascade. *Crit Rev Biochem Mol Biol.* 2015;50(4):326–336.

64. Zhao R, Liang H, Clarke E, Jackson C, Xue M. Inflammation in chronic wounds. *Int J Mol Sci.* 2016;17(12):2085. doi:10.3390/ijms17122085.

65. MacCarthy-Morrogh L, Martin P. The hallmarks of cancer are also the hallmarks of wound healing. *Sci Signal.* 2020;13(648):eaay8690. doi:10.1126/scisignal.aay8690.

66. Dunnill C, Patton T, Brennan J, et al. Reactive oxygen species (ROS) and wound healing: the functional role of ROS and emerging ROS-modulating technologies for augmentation of the healing process. *Int Wound J.* 2017;14(1):89–96.

67. Galkina SI, Golenkina EA, Viryasova GM, Romanova YM, Sud'ina GF. Nitric oxide in life and death of neutrophils. *Curr Med Chem.* 2019;26(31):5764–5780.

68. Sorg H, Tilkorn DJ, Hager S, Hauser J, Mirastschijski U. Skin wound healing: an update on the current knowledge and concepts. *Eur Surg Res.* 2017;58(1–2):81–94.

69. Dryden M. Reactive oxygen species: a novel antimicrobial. *Int J Antimicrob Agents.* 2018;51(3):299–303.

70. Shapouri-Moghaddam A, Mohammadian S, Vazini H, et al. Macrophage plasticity, polarization, and function in health and disease. *J Cell Physiol.* 2018;233(9):6425–6440.

71. Brown JM, Recht L, Strober S. The promise of targeting macrophages in cancer therapy. *Clin Cancer Res.* 2017;23(13):3241–3250.

72. Lavery LA, Armstrong DG, Murdoch DP, Peters EJ, Lipsky BA. Validation of the Infectious Diseases Society of America's diabetic foot infection classification system. *Clin Infect Dis.* 2007;44(4):562–565.

73. Fierheller M, Sibbald RG. A clinical investigation into the relationship between increased periwound skin temperature and local wound infection in patients with chronic leg ulcers. *Adv Skin Wound Care.* 2010;23(8):369–381.

74. Kwesiga MP, Cook E, Hannon J, et al. Investigative study on nitric oxide production in human dermal fibroblast cells under normal and high glucose conditions. *Med Sci (Basel).* 2018;6(4):99. doi:10.3390/medsci6040099.

75. Hinz B. The role of myofibroblasts in wound healing. *Curr Res Transl Med.* 2016;64(4):171–177.

76. Rohani MG, Parks WC. Matrix remodeling by MMPs during wound repair. *Matrix Biol.* 2015;44–46:113–121.

77. Mondal S, Adhikari N, Banerjee S, Amin SA, Jha T. Matrix metalloproteinase-9 (MMP-9) and its inhibitors in cancer: a mini-review. *Eur J Med Chem.* 2020;194:112260. doi:10.1016/j.ejmech.2020.112260.

78. Robert S, Gicquel T, Victoni T, et al. Involvement of matrix metalloproteinases (MMPs) and inflammasome pathway in molecular mechanisms of fibrosis. *Biosci Rep.* 2016;36(4):e00360. doi:10.1042/BSR20160107.

79. Jiang Y, Goldberg ID, Shi YE. Complex roles of tissue inhibitors of metalloproteinases in cancer. *Oncogene.* 2002;21(14):2245–2252.

80. Rousselle P, Montmasson M, Garnier C. Extracellular matrix contribution to skin wound re-epithelialization. *Matrix Biol.* 2019;75–76:12–26.

81. Ogawa R. Keloid and hypertrophic scars are the result of chronic inflammation in the reticular dermis. *Int J Mol Sci.* 2017;18(3):606. doi:10.3390/ijms18030606.

82. Ghazawi FM, Zargham R, Gilardino MS, Sasseville D, Jafarian F. Insights into the pathophysiology of hypertrophic scars and keloids: how do they differ? *Adv Skin Wound Care.* 2018;31(1):582–595.

83. Wong VW, Akaishi S, Longaker MT, Gurtner GC. Pushing back: wound mechanotransduction in repair and regeneration. *J Invest Dermatol.* 2011;131(11):2186–2196.

84. Lee HJ, Jang YJ. Recent understandings of biology, prophylaxis and treatment strategies for hypertrophic scars and keloids. *Int J Mol Sci.* 2018;19(3):711. doi:10.3390/ijms19030711.

85. Gupta SC, Kunnumakkara AB, Aggarwal S, Aggarwal BB. Inflammation, a double-edge sword for cancer and other age-related diseases. *Front Immunol.* 2018;9:2160. doi:10.3389/fimmu.2018.02160.

86. Gottrup F. A specialized wound-healing center concept: importance of a multidisciplinary department structure and surgical treatment facilities in the treatment of chronic wounds. *Am J Surg.* 2004;187(5A):38S–43S.

87. Swanson T, Angel D. Wound infection in clinical practice update. *Aust Nurs Midwifery J.* 2017;24(8):33.

88. Snyder RJ, Fife C, Moore Z. Components and quality measures of DIME (Devitalized Tissue, Infection/Inflammation, Moisture Balance, and Edge Preparation) in wound care. *Adv Skin Wound Care.* 2016;29(5):205–215.

89. Diegelmann RF, Evans MC. Wound healing: an overview of acute, fibrotic and delayed healing. *Front Biosci.* 2004;9:283–289. doi:10.2741/1184.

90. Bryan N, Ahswin H, Smart N, Bayon Y, Wohlert S, Hunt JA. Reactive oxygen species (ROS)—a family of fate deciding molecules pivotal in constructive inflammation and wound healing, *Eur Cell Mater.* 2012;24:249–265.

91. Dvorak HF. Tumors: wounds that do not heal. Similarities between tumor stroma generation and wound healing. *N Engl J Med.* 1986;315(26):1650–1659.

92. Boesch M, Baty F, Rumpold H, Sopper S, Wolf D, Brutsche MH. Fibroblasts in cancer: defining target structures for therapeutic intervention. *Biochim Biophys Acta Rev Cancer.* 2019;1872(1):111–121.

93. Henke E, Nandigama R, Ergün S. Extracellular matrix in the tumor microenvironment and its impact on cancer therapy. *Front Mol Biosci.* 2020;6:160. doi:10.3389/fmolb.2019.00160.

94. Viallard C, Larrivée B. Tumor angiogenesis and vascular normalization: alternative therapeutic targets. *Angiogenesis.* 2017;20(4):409–426.

95. Jain RK. Normalizing tumor microenvironment to treat cancer: bench to bedside to biomarkers. *J Clin Oncol.* 2013;31(17):2205–2218.

96. Whiteside TL. The tumor microenvironment and its role in promoting tumor growth. *Oncogene.* 2008;27(45):5904–5912.

97. Polydorou C, Mpekris F, Papageorgis P, Voutouri C, Stylianopoulos T. Pirfenidone normalizes the tumor microenvironment to improve chemotherapy. *Oncotarget.* 2017;8(15):24506–24517.

98. Payne WG, Naidu DK, Wheeler CK, et al. Wound healing in patients with cancer. *Eplasty.* 2008;8:e9.

99. Leventhal J, Young MR. Radiation dermatitis: recognition, prevention, and management. *Oncology (Williston Park).* 2017;31(12): 885–899.

100. Jacobson LK, Johnson MB, Dedhia RD, Niknam-Bienia S, Wong AK. Impaired wound healing after radiation therapy: a systematic review of pathogenesis and treatment. *JPRAS Open.* 2017;13:92–105.

101. Singh M, Alavi A, Wong R, Akita S. Radiodermatitis: a review of our current understanding. *Am J Clin Dermatol.* 2016;17(3):277–292.

102. Friedstat J, Brown DA, Levi B. Chemical, electrical, and radiation Injuries. *Clin Plast Surg.* 2017;44(3):657–669.

103. Liu JQ, Zhao KB, Feng ZH, Qi FZ. Hair follicle units promote re-epithelialization in chronic cutaneous wounds: a clinical case series study. *Exp Ther Med.* 2015;10(1):25–30.

104. Gosselin TK, Schneider SM, Plambeck MA, Rowe K. A prospective randomized, placebo-controlled skin care study in women diagnosed with breast cancer undergoing radiation therapy. *Oncol Nurs Forum.* 2010;37(5):619–626.

105. Deptuła M, Zieliński J, Wardowska A, Pikuła M. Wound healing complications in oncological patients: perspectives for cellular therapy. *Postepy Dermatol Alergol.* 2019;36(2):139–146.

106. Straub JM, New J, Hamilton CD, Lominska C, Shnayder Y, Thomas SM. Radiation-induced fibrosis: mechanisms and implications for therapy. *J Cancer Res Clin Oncol.* 2015;141(11):1985–1994.

107. Wong RK, Bensadoun RJ, Boers-Doets CB, et al. Clinical practice guidelines for the prevention and treatment of acute and late radiation reactions from the MASCC Skin Toxicity Study Group. *Support Care Cancer.* 2013;21(10):2933–2948.

108. Haruna F, Lipsett A, Marignol L. Topical management of acute radiation dermatitis in breast cancer patients: a systematic review and meta-analysis. *Anticancer Res.* 2017;37(10):5343–5353.

109. Hemati S, Asnaashari O, Sarvizadeh M, et al. Topical silver sulfadiazine for the prevention of acute dermatitis during irradiation for breast cancer. *Support Care Cancer.* 2012;20(8):1613–1618.

110. Bolton L. Acute radiation therapy-related dermatitis. *Wounds.* 2020;32(2):66–68.

111. Bourgeois A, Grisoli SB, Soine EJ, Rosen LB. Tamoxifen-induced radiation recall dermatitis. *Dermatol Online J.* 2017;23(2) 13030/ qt1d38c9c7.

112. Burris HA III, Hurtig J. Radiation recall with anticancer agents. *Oncologist.* 2010;15(11):1227–1237.

113. Azria D, Magné N, Zouhair A, et al. Radiation recall: a well recognized but neglected phenomenon. *Cancer Treat Rev.* 2005;31(7):555–570.

114. Wyld L, Audisio RA, Poston GJ. The evolution of cancer surgery and future perspectives. *Nat Rev Clin Oncol.* 2015;12(2):115–124.

115. Beitz JM. Pharmacologic Impact (aka "Breaking Bad") of medications on wound healing and wound development: a literature-based overview. *Ostomy Wound Manage.* 2017;63(3):18–35.

116. American Cancer Society. Skin cancer. https://www.cancer.org/cancer/skin-cancer.html. Accessed November 14, 2020.

117. Linares MA, Zakaria A, Nizran P. Skin cancer. *Prim Care.* 2015;42(4):645–659.

118. Kim DP, Kus KJB, Ruiz E. Basal cell carcinoma review. *Hematol Oncol Clin North Am.* 2019;33(1):13–24.

119. Waldman A, Schmults C. Cutaneous squamous cell carcinoma. *Hematol Oncol Clin North Am.* 2019;33(1):1–12.

120. Silverberg MJ, Leyden W, Warton EM, Quesenberry Jr CP, Engels EA, Asgari MM. HIV infection status, immunodeficiency, and the incidence of non-melanoma skin cancer. *J Natl Cancer Inst.* 2013;105(5):350–360.

121. Tanese K. Diagnosis and management of basal cell carcinoma. *Curr Treat Options Oncol.* 2019;20(2):13. doi:10.1007/s11864-019-0610-0.

122. Karagas MR, Zens MS, Li Z, et al. Early-onset basal cell carcinoma and indoor tanning: a population-based study. *Pediatrics.* 2014;134(1):e4–e12. doi:10.1542/peds.2013-3559.

123. Hamm RL, Shah JB. Atypical wounds. In: Hamm RL, ed. *Text and Atlas of Wound Diagnosis and Treatment*, McGraw-Hill Education; 2019:235–268.

124. Kanth AM, Heiman AJ, Nair L, et al. Current trends in management of Marjolin's Ulcer: a systematic review. *J Burn Care Res.* (2020), doi:10.1093/jbcr/iraa128.

125. Shannan B, Perego M, Somasundaram R, Herlyn M. Heterogeneity in melanoma. *Cancer Treat Res.* 2016;167:1–15.

126. American Cancer Society. Key statistics for melanoma skin cancer. https://www.cancer.org/cancer/melanoma-skin-cancer/about/key-statistics.html. Accessed May 27, 2021.

127. Kozovska Z, Gabrisova V, Kucerova L. Malignant melanoma: diagnosis, treatment and cancer stem cells. *Neoplasma.* 2016;63(4):510–517.

128. Adderley UJ, Holt IG. Topical agents and dressings for fungating wounds. *Cochrane Database Syst Rev.* 2014;2014(5):CD003948. doi:10.1002/14651858.CD003948.pub3.

129. Alexander S. Malignant fungating wounds: epidemiology, aetiology, presentation and assessment. *J Wound Care.* 2009;18(7):273–280.

130. Kennedy KL. The prevalence of pressure ulcers in an intermediate care facility. *Decubitus.* 1989;2(2):44–45.

131. Hanson D, Langemo DK, Olson B, et al. The prevalence and incidence of pressure ulcers in the hospice setting: analysis of two methodologies. *Am J Hosp Palliat Care.* 1991;8(5):18–22.

132. McNees P. Skin and wound assessment and care in oncology. *Semin Oncol Nurs.* 2006;22(3):130–143. doi:10.1016/j.soncn.2006.04.003.

133. Akhmetova A, Saliev T, IU Allan, Illsley MJ, Nurgozhin T, Mikhalovsky S. A Comprehensive review of topical odor-controlling treatment options for chronic wounds. *J Wound Ostomy Continence Nurs.* 2016;43(6):598–609.

134. de Leon J, Bohn GA, DiDomenico L, et al. Wound care centers: critical thinking and treatment strategies for wounds. *Wounds.* 2016;28(10):S1–S23.

135. Fesseha BK, Abularrage CJ, Hines KF, et al. Association of hemoglobin A1c and wound healing in diabetic foot ulcers. *Diabetes Care.* 2018;41(7):1478–1485. doi:10.2337/dc17-1683.

136. Rhim B, Harkless L. Prevention: can we stop problems before they arise? *Semin Vasc Surg.* 2012;25(2):122–128. doi:10.1053/j.semvascsurg.2012.05.002.

137. WOCN Clinical Practice Wound Subcommittee, 2005. Ankle brachial index: quick reference guide for clinicians. *J Wound Ostomy Continence Nurs.* 2012;39(2 suppl):S21–S29. doi:10.1097/WON.0b013e3182478dde.

138. Woelfel S, Ochoa C, Rowe VL. Vascular wounds. In: Hamm RL, ed. *Text and Atlas of Wound Diagnosis and Treatment*, McGraw-Hill Education; 2019:101–143.

139. Rabe E, Partsch H, Hafner J, et al. Indications for medical compression stockings in venous and lymphatic disorders: an evidence-based consensus statement. *Phlebology.* 2018;33(3):163–184. doi:10.1177/0268355516689631.

140. Bhattacharya S, Mishra RK. Pressure ulcers: current understanding and newer modalities of treatment. *Indian J Plast Surg.* 2015;48(1):4–16. doi:10.4103/0970-0358.155260.

141. Hamm RL, Luttrell T. Factors that impede wound healing. In: Hamm RL, ed. *Text and Atlas of Wound Diagnosis and Treatment*: Hill Education; 2019:321–346.

142. Müller-Richter U, Betz C, Hartmann S, Brands RC. Nutrition management for head and neck cancer patients improves clinical outcome and survival. *Nutr Res.* 2017;48:1–8. doi:10.1016/j.nutres.2017.08.007.

143. Jager-Wittenaar H, Ottery FD. Assessing nutritional status in cancer: role of the Patient-Generated Subjective Global Assessment. *Curr Opin Clin Nutr Metab Care.* 2017;20(5):322–329.

144. Talwar B, Donnelly R, Skelly R, Donaldson M. Nutritional management in head and neck cancer: United Kingdom National Multidisciplinary Guidelines. *J Laryngol Otol.* 2016;130(S2):S32–S40.

145. Carr AC, Maggini S. Vitamin C and immune function. *Nutrients.* 2017;9(11):1211.

146. Cavezzi A, Troiani E, Corrao S. COVID-19: hemoglobin, iron, and hypoxia beyond inflammation: a narrative review. *Clin Pract.* 2020;10(2):1271.

147. Schneider KL, Yahia N. Effectiveness of arginine supplementation on wound healing in older adults in acute and chronic settings: a systematic review. *Adv Skin Wound Care.* 2019;32(10):457–462.

148. Keshet R, Erez A. Arginine and the metabolic regulation of nitric oxide synthesis in cancer. *Dis Model Mech.* 2018;11(8):dmm033332.

149. Leigh B, Desneves K, Rafferty J, et al. The effect of different doses of an arginine-containing supplement on the healing of pressure ulcers. *J Wound Care.* 2012;21(3):150–156.

150. Gupta S, Andersen C, Black J, et al. Management of chronic wounds: diagnosis, preparation, treatment, and follow-up. *Wounds.* 2017;29(9):S19–S36.

151. Swanson T, Angel D, Sussman G, et al. International Wound Infection Institute Wound Infection in Clinical Practice: Principles of Best Practice. https://www.woundsinternational.com/resources/details/iwii-wound-infection-clinical-practice. Accessed November 3, 2020.

152. Walters E. Raising awareness for sepsis, sepsis screening, early recognition, and treatment in the emergency department. *J Emerg Nurs.* 2018;44(3):224–227.

153. Gardner SE, Frantz RA, Doebbeling BN. The validity of the clinical signs and symptoms used to identify localized chronic wound infection. *Wound Repair Regen.* 2001;9(3):178–186.

154. Solano C, Echeverz M, Lasa I. Biofilm dispersion and quorum sensing. *Curr Opin Microbiol.* 2014;18:96–104.

155. Schultz G, Bjarnsholt T, James GA, et al. Consensus guidelines for the identification and treatment of biofilms in chronic nonhealing wounds. *Wound Repair Regen.* 2017;25(5):744–757.

156. Sibbald RG, Elliott JA, Ayello EA, Somayaji R. Optimizing the moisture management tightrope with Wound Bed Preparation 2015©. *Adv Skin Wound Care.* 2015;28(10):466–478. doi:10.1097/01.ASW.0000470851.27030.98.

157. Gardner SE, Frantz RA, Saltzman CL, Hillis SL, Park H, Scherubel M. Diagnostic validity of three swab techniques for identifying chronic wound infection. *Wound Repair Regen.* 2006;14(5):548–557. doi:10.1111/j.1743-6109.2006.00162.x.

158. Rennie MY, Lindvere-Teene L, Tapang K, Linden R. Point-of-care fluorescence imaging predicts the presence of pathogenic bacteria in wounds: a clinical study. *J Wound Care.* 2017;26(8):452–460.

159. El Masry MS, Chaffee S, Das Ghatak P, et al. Stabilized collagen matrix dressing improves wound macrophage function and epithelialization. *FASEB J.* 2019;33(2):2144–2155. doi:10.1096/fj.201800352R.

160. Saleh K, Strömdahl AC, Riesbeck K, Schmidtchen A. Inflammation biomarkers and correlation to wound status after full-thickness skin grafting. *Front Med (Lausanne).* 2019;6:159.

161. Wieman TJ, Smiell JM, Su Y. Efficacy and safety of a topical gel formulation of recombinant human platelet-derived growth factor-BB (becaplermin) in patients with chronic neuropathic diabetic ulcers. A phase III randomized placebo-controlled double-blind study. *Diabetes Care.* 1998;21(5):822–827.

162. Smith and Nephew. Regranex product information page. https://www.smith-nephew.com/professional/products/all-products/regranex/. Accessed November 29, 2020.

10

Cardiovascular and Pulmonary Systems

SARA K. ARENA, PT, MS, DSCPT, MEGHAN K. HUBER, PT, DPT, CLT, ACSM CERTIFIED EXERCISE PHYSIOLOGIST

CHAPTER OUTLINE

Introduction

Diagnosis and Prevalence

Cardiac Cancers

Malignant Primary Cardiac Tumors

Primary cardiac tumors are extremely rare and account for approximately 0.001% to 0.28% of all tumors.[2] Malignancy has been reported to represent 25% of neoplasms originating in the cardiac tissues of adults.[3] Sarcomas account for two-thirds of malignant primary cardiac tumors (MPCT) with primary cardiac angiosarcoma (PCA) accounting for nearly three-fourths of all MPCT.[3,4] These aggressive neoplasms originate from the epithelial cells of the cardiac tissues, are most common in the right atrium, and have a high localized recurrence and metastasis rate.[5] PCA has an increased incidence among males in the fourth and fifth decades of life and a poor long-term prognosis with a projected 9- to 12-month survival rate of 10%.[6] Individuals with a PCA diagnosis commonly present with dyspnea, chest discomfort, shortness of breath, and/or pericardial effusion.[6] Delayed diagnosis from onset of symptoms is not uncommon given the similar clinical presentation to other more common diagnoses such as heart failure; however, this delay may contribute to the poor prognosis of PCA.[7]

Rhabdomyosarcoma is the second most common MPCT arising from striated muscle differentiation and may occur in any chamber of the heart, although seldom occurs in the left atrium.[8] While rare, this type of malignant tumor is most commonly diagnosed in children and young adults and often is accompanied by poor prognosis secondary to complexity of diagnosis and rapid growth.[4] Brain metastases have been cited to occur in 31% of people diagnosed with primary cardiac sarcomas as compared to 8% of those with noncardiac sarcomas, which further contributes to a poor prognosis.[9]

Primary cardiac lymphoma accounts for 1% of primary cardiac tumors and is described as infiltrative, intramural, and epicardial with about one-third involving the pericardium.[10] Cardiac lymphoma typically presents on the right side of the heart with an increased risk in those who are immunocompromised, including individuals with human immunodeficiency virus (HIV), acquired immunodeficiency syndrome (AIDS), and allograft transplant.[10]

Mesothelioma is an asbestos exposure-related malignant cancer that typically affects the lining of the lungs but can develop in other locations including the lining of the heart (pericardial mesothelioma).[11] A 21 to 70 year latency in the presentation of cancer has been reported after asbestos exposure contributing to its continued diagnosis today, despite being banned in the United States (US) since 1970. Deaths among those ≥85 years old likely represent exposure many years ago; however, the occurrence of mesothelioma deaths among persons aged <55 years old suggests ongoing occupational and environmental exposures to asbestos fibers and other causative factors.[12] The median survival after being diagnosed with this rare malignant cancer is approximately 1 year.[12]

Benign Primary Cardiac Tumors

Benign cardiac tumors comprise 75% of all adult primary cardiac tumors with myxoma occurring in 80% of benign cases. Myxoma is a tumor composed of primitive connective tissue that commonly originates in the left atrium.[13] These tumors are more common in women, with 10% reported as familial. Benign cardiac tumors occurring less frequently include papillary, fibroelastomas, rhabdomyomas, fibromas, hemangiomas, teratomas, lipomas, paragangliomas, and pericardial cyst types. About 83% of those diagnosed with a benign cardiac tumor will survive five years or longer.[8] Although less common, malignant tumors of the left atrium include pleomorphic sarcoma, fibrosarcoma, and leiomyosarcomas.[3]

Cardiac Metastases

Cardiac metastases are more common than primary cardiac malignancies with up to 25% of postmortem autopsies uncovering cardiac metastases as a secondary cause of death.[14] Cardiac metastases present most frequently in the pericardium, followed by epicardium and the myocardium.[2] Primary lung cancer accounts for 36 to 39% of all cardiac metastases, followed by breast cancer 10% to 12% and hematologic malignancies 10% to 21%.[15]

Pulmonary Cancers

Malignant Pulmonary Tumors

Lung and bronchus cancers comprise the second leading cancer diagnosis and are the leading cause of worldwide cancer death in both males and females.[16] Lung cancer risk increases after the fifth decade of life with a higher incidence among males than females.

All forms of smoking and smoking exposure significantly increase an individual's risk of cancer cell proliferation. Approximately 80% to 85% of all lung cancers are non-small cell lung carcinomas (NSCLC) and are further classified as adenocarcinoma, squamous cell carcinoma, or large cell carcinoma.[17] Among nonsmokers, NSCLC is the most common lung tumor diagnosis. Those with localized NSCLC have a 5-year survival rate of 61%; whereas, those with distant disease have a 6% 5-year survival rate.[18]

The remaining 10% to 15% of primary malignant lung cancer diagnoses are classified as small cell lung carcinomas (SCLC) and arise from neuroendocrine cell precursors. These cancers are most common in those with a smoking history and are more aggressive as evidenced by a more rapid cell division and growth than that of NSCLC. The 5-year survival rate for those diagnosed with local SCLC is 27%; whereas those with distant disease have a 3% 5-year survival rate.[18]

Lung Metastases

While the mortality rates of primary lung cancers are concerning, these rates are even more alarming when metastatic lung tumors are considered. Specifically, the lungs are a common, first metastatic site of other primary cancers. The most common primary cancers to metastasize to the lungs include colorectal (25.8%), head and neck (19.4%), urological (14.7%), gastrointestinal (10.9%), breast (10.7%), melanoma (6.5%), and gynecological (6.1%).[19] While lung cancers will be described in more detail in Chapter 18, it is essential for oncology rehabilitation (Onc R) clinicians to understand the prevalence of metastatic lung tumors given its potential impact on care of any person living with and beyond cancer (PLWBC).

Common Adverse Effects of Treatment

Radiation Therapy

Radiation therapy radiation therapy plays an important role in the treatment of thoracic cancer.[20] Despite several advancements over recent decades in the delivery of radiation therapy, including the mechanism by which the radiation is delivered and the use of concurrent chemotherapy, damage to both cardiovascular and pulmonary (CVP) tissues continue to occur.[21] Radiation leaves the tissues at high risk for pathology and can impact normal physiologic adaptations to physical activity. Radiation therapy delivery has seen positive advancements over the past few decades including stereotactic radiation therapy, three-dimensional conformal radiation therapy, and the intensity-modulated radiation therapy that allows radiation dose escalation with more precise target tissue delivery. Despite these advances, a reported 43% of individuals experience adverse effects impacting the surrounding tissue as a result of radiation therapy.[22]

Radiation therapy has been identified as a major contributor in the progression of coronary artery disease (CAD) among those with a cancer diagnosis. Radiation-associated CAD is most commonly experienced after mantle radiation for hematologic malignancies, especially Hodgkin lymphoma.[2] The risk increase is dose-dependent with every 1 Gray (Gy) delivered to the heart resulting in a 7.4% increased risk of myocardial infarction (MI), need for cardiac revascularization surgery, or death from ischemic heart disease.[2] With advanced technology and treatment options in combination with ventricular dose limits of 15 Gy and total heart dose limits of 30 Gy,[2] collateral damage to the heart tissues from radiation therapy has decreased.

Although rare, phrenic nerve paralysis may occur from radiation therapy, chemotherapy, or surgery for primary lung cancers or Hodgkin/non-Hodgkin lymphomas. Individuals with this impairment may present with dyspnea in supine relieved by upright positioning.[2] Other adverse effects including esophagitis, pneumonitis, lung fibrosis, toxicities, and death and have been reported as sequelae of radiation therapy. One systematic review detailed the radical radiotherapy of NSCLC and has identified predictors of radiotoxicity which include "age, gender, performance status, tumor stage, fractionation, radiotherapy technique, and molecular markers."[22] However, the most common statistically significant risk factor for radiotoxicity is concurrent chemotherapy.

Chemotherapy/Immunotherapy

Chemotherapy results in an array of adverse effects despite advancing interventions and medications designed to address chemotherapy-induced symptomatology. While each chemotherapy agent may present with different symptom sequelae, the majority have adverse effects of nausea, vomiting, fatigue, and appetite changes. Platinum-based chemotherapy remains the standard of care for advanced NSCLC treatment.[23] Cisplatin (Platinol, Platinol-AQ) and carboplatin (Paraplatin) are commonly used for the treatment of lung cancer but result in short- and long-term adverse effects. Among the 40 possible adverse effects, the dose-limiting adverse effect for cisplatin is nephrotoxicity, whereas myelosuppression is the dose-limiting adverse effect for carboplatin.[24]

Chemotherapy medications can impact the heart through a variety of systemic mechanisms, with cardiomyopathy and subsequent heart failure being most common. Many factors contribute to cancer-related cardiac dysfunction including hormonal suppression experienced in tyrosine kinase inhibitors (e.g., dasatinib [Sprycel], nilotinib [Tasigna], and ponatinib [ICLUSIG]) or hyperglycemia and hyperlipidemia, resulting in progression or development of already present atherosclerosis.[2] Given that cancer-related cardiac dysfunction has been reported in 10% of individuals receiving chemotherapy, Onc R clinicians should be alert to this adverse effect and adapt treatment appropriately.

Additional CVP adverse effects of these chemotherapy medications include anemia, low potassium, heart failure, and blood clots. These conditions can significantly limit functional capacity and exercise safety and should be monitored closely while under the care of the Onc R clinician. Medications and their role in Onc R interventions are further described in Chapter 6. An overview of immunotherapy medication categories and adverse effects most common to the CVP system are detailed in the enhanced eBook (eTable 10.1).

Cardiotoxicity

While there are many adverse effects of chemotherapy and immunotherapy, cardiotoxicity is one of the most commonly experienced adverse effects. Adverse effects may include cardiomyopathy, myocarditis, pericarditis, and acute coronary syndrome, any of which may result in cardiac pump dysfunction.[25] While each may have a different clinical presentation, common symptoms include: shortness of breath, chest pain, heart palpitations or arrhythmias, fluid retention in the legs, distention of the stomach and/or dizziness. Cardiotoxicity may result from a combination of chemotherapy-induced cardiomyopathy, radiation toxicity, cumulative effects of comorbidities including hypertension (HTN), CAD, and valvular disease. Patient-related risk factors for cancer-related cardiotoxicity include pre-existing CAD, sedentary lifestyle, smoking history, female sex, postmenopausal, HTN, and hyperlipidemia.[26] Medical therapy-induced cardiotoxicity risk factors include high dose chemotherapy in bolus form, combination of chemotherapies, prior anthracycline use, and concurrent mediastinal radiation.[26]

Irreversible chemotherapy-induced myocardial damage is most common among individuals treated for breast cancer, lymphoma, and many childhood cancers with anthracycline agents (e.g., doxorubicin [Adriamycin], daunorubicin [Cerubidine], epirubicin [Ellence], idarubicin [Idamycin]).[2] Nitric oxide involvement in anthracycline-related cardiac damage has been suggested as a contributing factor to the myocardial damage, as it has a role in producing reactive oxygen species imbalance.[27] Furthermore, a PLWBC using angiogenesis inhibitors (to suppress vascular endothelial growth factor for the ultimate purpose of thwarting tumor growth) or tyrosine kinase inhibitors (to reduce tumor cell signaling, growth, and division) should be monitored for signs and symptoms of cardiotoxicity to assure optimal clinical outcomes.[28] Cardiotoxicity is dose-dependent and most prevalent with a cumulative dose >550 mg/m^2 of doxorubicin or 900 mg/m^2 of epirubicin.[2] MI resulting in mortality has been reported at a rate of 25% in long-term survivors of Hodgkin lymphoma.[29] Cardiotoxicity may also result in dose-independent reversible myocardial injury as seen when trastuzumab (Herceptin) is used in the medical management of breast cancer.[26]

HTN is another factor contributing to cancer-related cardiotoxicity. Typically, large volumes of intravenous fluids are administered prior to treatment for individuals receiving anthracycline, platinum-based agents, or high-dose methotrexate chemotherapy, which results in an increased intravascular volume and afterload.[2] Specifically, the stress associated with an increased afterload may be the tipping point for an individual with borderline ventricular dysfunction into an overt heart failure.[2] Furthermore, the stress, anxiety, and emotional turmoil associated with a cancer diagnosis may also contribute to HTN, which can exacerbate cardiotoxic sequelae.

Pulmonary Toxicity

Pulmonary toxicity, commonly manifested as pneumonitis, is characterized by inflammation of the lung tissue. It has been observed in PLWBCs who have received radiation therapy, chemotherapies, or biologic therapies.[30] Chest X-rays and pulmonary function tests are useful in establishing a clinical diagnosis. It can result in symptoms, including shortness of breath, dry cough, fullness in chest, and/or flu-like symptoms. Additionally, fever and chest pain are associated with radiation pneumonitis, which can occur as an outcome of radiation to the chest. It most commonly develops one to three months after treatment is completed, but it can happen up to six months after treatment.[31] Chronic pneumonitis, which presents similarly to interstitial lung disease, is also possible. It is most commonly associated when high doses of radiation are administered or if radiation is administered in combination with chemotherapies known to increase the risk, such as bleomycin (Blenoxane), cyclophosphamide (Procytox), and carmustine (BiCNU, BCNU).[31]

Surgical Procedures

Surgery is the main treatment for primary heart and lung cancers with thoracic surgical entry points most common. While contemporary surgical practices reduce collateral tissue damage, approaches such as thoracotomies and median sternotomies can alter the chest wall mechanics and impact breathing patterns, thereby resulting in reduced inspiratory capacity, cough strength, and scapular/upper extremity (UE) function. Additionally, surgical intubation and sedating medications alter mucociliary function and can result in poor secretion clearance, which can increase the risk for respiratory infections.

Complex cardiac reconstruction is frequent in the treatment of primary cardiac tumors. Patients with secondary cardiac tumors are less frequently candidates for surgery given the complexity of the surgical approach and the need for highly skilled and experienced multidisciplinary teams.[32] Despite surgical interventions, long-term prognosis remains poor for those with primary cardiac tumors.[7]

Techniques such as video-assisted thoracoscopic surgery (VATS) and robotic-assisted thoracoscopic surgery (RATS) offer a less invasive approach for lung and mediastinal tumors.[33] These approaches offer the advantage of excellent access to remove lymph nodes with low morbidity and mortality, less trauma and pain, shorter chest drainage duration, decreased hospital stay, and preservation of short-term pulmonary function.[34] Disadvantages of the VATS surgical procedure include the surgeon's intraoperative loss of binocular vision and a limited maneuverability of thoracoscopic instruments, an unstable camera platform, and poor ergonomics for the surgeon; however, the RATS requires additional cost for the specialized equipment, hospital stay, and may result in an extended operation time.[33-35] Thoracotomy incisions using posterior, posterior-lateral, lateral, and anterior approaches are still utilized. This approach results in dissection of the intercostal musculature and can produce rib fractures when the rib retractors are expanded. This procedure may also increase the risk of adhesive capsulitis if shoulder range of motion is not incorporated into the postoperative care plan.

Comorbidities

Comorbidities, outside the scope of the cancer diagnosis, must be considered when conducting an examination and intervention of a PLWBC with a documented or presumed CVP diagnosis. This is especially relevant given that heart disease and chronic lower airway respiratory disease are among the leading causes of mortality in the US.[1] While a PLWBC of the heart and lungs will inevitably have short- and long-term sequelae related to the cancer and its associated treatments, Onc R clinicians should also consider how secondary comorbidities may impact the PLWBC. For example, a PLWBC with a comorbidity of diabetes mellitus (DM) may require specific attention to blood glucose levels during care to ensure safety when initiating exercise or to assure adequate postsurgical wound healing. A sedentary lifestyle before a cancer diagnosis can impact exercise dosing and prescription for the PLWBC, as well as intolerance to medical treatment. Additionally, atrial fibrillation (AFib) is frequently observed in patients being treated for cancer.[36] Given that AFib increases an individual's morbidity and mortality risk, assessment of heart rate (HR) using a manual technique or automatic unit with sensitivity for this arrhythmia should be considered. Furthermore, given that tobacco use has a strong causative effect on lung cancer, PLWBCs of the lung often experience other cardiovascular and respiratory comorbidities including HTN and chronic obstructive respiratory diseases (COPD).[37] These diagnoses in isolation or combination can alter the performance

status of a PLWBC and, in some cases, more so than the cancer diagnosis itself.[37]

Vena Cava Syndrome

Vena cava syndrome occurs when there is an obstruction, either intrinsic or extrinsic, of the vena cava. Approximately 2% to 4% of persons diagnosed with lung cancer will develop superior vena cava syndrome (SVCS).[38] Episodes of intrinsic obstructions from SVCS often originate from intrathoracic malignancies of NSCLC (50%), SCLC (25%–35%), and non-Hodgkin lymphoma (10%–15%).[38] This syndrome can also occur via extrinsic factors including thrombosis secondary to pacemaker placement, central venous catheters, endocardial defibrillator, pacemaker leads, and dialysis catheters.[39] SVCS can have a gradual or rapid onset of symptoms including chest pain, dyspnea, dysphagia, jugular distention, edema of head and neck, headaches, and/or confusion.[38,40] The focus of treatment for SVCS is to treat the cancer with radiation therapy or chemotherapy. However, associated swelling or fluid retention may be reduced with corticosteroids or diuretics. In severe cases, central airway obstruction and/or coma secondary to cerebral edema can result in a medical emergency.[38]

Hematologic Disorders

Hematologic disorders related to cancer and cancer treatment may include anemia, thrombocytopenia, leukopenia, pancytopenia, tumor lysis syndrome, thrombosis, and embolism. Iron-deficiency anemia has been reported to impact 39% of individuals with cancer at initial presentation and increases to 69% at the 6-month follow-up.[41] This disorder can have a negative impact on an individual's quality of life (QOL).[41] Malnutrition, malabsorption, systemic infection, surgery, and myelosuppression, which all reduce red blood cell formation in the bone marrow are among the most common factors leading to the development of anemia.

Venous thromboembolism (VTE) is a disorder that includes deep vein thrombosis (DVT) and pulmonary embolism (PE) which occurs in higher frequencies among PLWBCs than among the noncancer population.[42,43] As compared to healthy peers, the risk of thrombosis increases 4.1 times with a cancer diagnosis and further increases to 6.5 times following chemotherapy.[44] Furthermore, one-third of patients with advanced cancer admitted to a specialist palliative care unit were found to have a femoral DVT. Cancer treatments, specifically surgery, chemotherapy, hormonal therapy, antiangiogenic drugs, immunomodulatory agents, erythropoiesis-stimulating agents, blood transfusions, and central venous catheters are all reported to be associated with an increased risk of DVT.[42]

Deconditioning

Deconditioning is a significant symptom burden among many individuals with a cancer diagnosis. Tests, measures, and interventions aimed at assessing an individual's exercise capacity will be discussed later in this chapter as well as throughout this book. However, it is important for Onc R clinicians to recognize deconditioning as an impairment of the CVP systems and that it can bring about short- and long-term impacts to exercise capacity and function. Furthermore, those with cancer-induced cachexia and myelosuppression can experience QOL-related impairments when considering the combined impact of the conditions and will require an interdisciplinary approach to regain function and reduce further loss of ability.

Persistent physical disability due to deconditioning has also been among the most important concerns of PLWBCs during the postoperative period after receiving surgical interventions for lung cancer.[45] However, one study identified that physicians reported mortality and complications to be among their most important considerations, thereby creating a divergence in patient-physician shared goals.[45] Onc R clinicians are well-positioned to address reduced physical capacity and should be considered essential survivorship team members to assist in bridging this gap. Furthermore, addressing existing and future deconditioning can and should be addressed from the onset of diagnosis through prehabilitation programming.

An 8-week exercise program encompassing both aerobic exercise and respiratory muscle training demonstrated improvements in exercise capacity and respiratory muscle strength in individuals with NSCLC after lung resection.[46] Furthermore, exercise training may improve or avoid a decline in exercise capacity for adults with advanced stage lung cancer when conducting a review of available randomized controlled trials.[47] Short-term, high-intensity interval training also has evidence for its utility in a prehabilitation program in PLWBCs who are deconditioned.[48] However, exercise dosing aimed at achieving moderate levels of exercise intensity can be specifically useful in the cancer population while undergoing treatment, as it is both preventative to thwart deconditioning and protective against the negative sequelae associated with the increased oxidative stress levels brought about by cancer treatment, specifically chemotherapy.[49]

Edema

Edema, or fluid buildup, may occur in a variety of different body structures and for a variety of reasons. Edema may occur as a result of a cancerous tumor leading to obstruction, malignant ascites, or may occur during chemotherapy infusions during which there may be increased fluid intake. Other etiologies of edema include heart failure, cirrhosis, nephrotic syndrome, or disease localized to venous and lymphatic systems.[50]

Edema occurs when fluid moves from the vascular space into the interstitium, reducing plasma volume and tissue perfusion. In response, the kidneys retain sodium and water, which alters capillary hemodynamics causing an increase of fluid in the interstitium.[50] With an increased fluid load in the interstitium, edema formation begins. Edema becomes clinically apparent when the interstitial volume has increased by 2.5 to 3 L.[50] Presenting symptoms include pitting of the tissue upon pressure, subjective reports of extremity fullness and heaviness, as well as shiny taut skin. Less commonly, some individuals may experience difficulty breathing or heart arrhythmias.

Although onset of edema is typically slow, pulmonary edema may become life threatening and requires immediate medical attention.[50] Acute cardiogenic pulmonary edema often results from acute decompensated heart failure with elevation of left ventricular filling pressures. This results in significant dyspnea due to fluid accumulation in the interstitial and/or alveolar spaces of the lungs.[51] Flash pulmonary edema is a severe form of acute cardiogenic pulmonary edema and typically occurs from a hypertensive episode when left ventricular end diastolic pressure raises. It may also be resultant of acute ischemia as seen with MIs, tachyarrhythmia, stress induced cardiomyopathy, or obstructive valvular disease such as acute severe mitral regurgitation or aortic regurgitation.[51] Noncardiogenic pulmonary edema (i.e., not associated

with left ventricular failure and when pulmonary capillary wedge pressures are low) is due to conditions that result in increased pulmonary endothelium tissue permeability leading to diffuse fluid accumulation into the alveolar spaces.[51]

Lymphatic obstruction and vascular damage can result in the development and formation of lymphedema associated with malignancy. Lymphedema and Onc R management is discussed as a component of Chapter 9.

Phrenic Nerve Neuropathy

While chemotherapy-induced polyneuropathy has been well described in the literature, evidence for phrenic nerve neuropathy brought on by this therapy is emerging.[52,53] As the phrenic nerve innervates the diaphragm, respiratory dysfunction may occur. Case reports describe initial presentation to include dyspnea on exertion,[52] hiccups, and/or acute respiratory distress.[53] Specifically, phrenic nerve dysfunction following vincristine (Oncovin, Vincasar PFS) treatment has been reported.[53] While breath sound auscultation may be within normal limits, rapid decreases in oxygen saturation on room air have been identified among individuals with suspected phrenic nerve neuropathy.[53,54] Additionally, abnormal test and measure findings may include: (1) a restrictive pattern noted on pulmonary function testing with low maximal inspiratory and expiratory pressures; (2) evidence of diaphragmatic weakness when assessed using fluoroscopic sniff evaluation; (3) atelectasis and associated reduced lung volumes assessed with a chest computed tomography scan; and (4) phrenic nerve electromyography findings that are asymmetric or with conduction discrepancies consistent with possible fascicular phrenic neuropathy.[52-54] Additional contributions to the evidence into this rare sequelae of chemotherapy is warranted; however, phrenic nerve neuropathy in the presence of new onset exertional dyspnea should be considered in a PLWBC.[52]

Measurement Tools to Screen for Adverse Effects

Integumentary Observation

Onc R examination most commonly starts with observation of the skin. This is especially relevant among individuals who have received radiation therapy, as 85% will experience adverse effects to the skin.[55] Radiation therapy can result in significant integumentary damage and is discussed in more detail in Chapter 9. Considerations specific to the CVP systems include cyanosis and pallor of the extremities since the endothelial lining of the vasculature can be damaged during radiation therapy. Additionally, nail bed clubbing may be present when oxygen perfusion is chronically limited due to vascular damage.

Laboratory Values

The Academy of Acute Care Physical Therapy—Laboratory Values Interpretation Resource[56] provides a comprehensive source detailing with common laboratory measures, causes, presentation, and clinical implications in physical therapy practice. The document cautions there is a paucity of universal reference ranges available for laboratory measures[56] so clinicians should utilize all resources available to determine safe and effective intervention plans that encompass laboratory values. The following is a summary of the measures available within the Laboratory Values Interpretation Resource: (1) Complete blood count (CBC) (white blood cells, platelets, hemoglobin, hematocrit); (2) Electrolyte panel (sodium, potassium, calcium, chloride, phosphate, magnesium); (3) Kidney function (blood urea nitrogen, serum creatinine); (4) Endocrine testing (glucose/criteria for diagnosis of diabetes, Hgb A1C, thyroid function tests); (5) Acid–base disorders (respiratory alkalosis, respiratory acidosis, metabolic alkalosis, metabolic acidosis); (6) Liver function/hepatic panel (serum albumin/prealbumin, serum bilirubin, ammonia, model for end-stage liver disease, FK trough [Tacrolimus/Prograf Test]; (7) Lipid panel (high-density lipoprotein, low-density lipoprotein, triglycerides, total cholesterol); (8) Bleeding ratio/viscosity (international normalized ratio [INR], activated partial thromboplastin time [aPTT], prothrombin time [PT], anti-factor Xa assay, D-dimer, algorithm for mobilizing patients with known lower-extremity deep vein thrombosis); and (9) Cardiovascular-specific labs (troponin, B-Type natriuretic peptide, creatinine kinase). eTable 10.2, available in the enhanced eBook, also provides common myoglobin and inflammatory marker laboratory measures, normal ranges, as well as possible causes of elevated and decreased measurement values as these may be relevant measures for an Onc R clinician.[57–60] While the role of myoglobins in cancer propagation is not clearly understood, immunoreactivity is used in the confirmation of myogenic phenotype of tumor cells.[61] Inflammatory markers indicate the degree of inflammation in the body by detecting levels of circulating protein in the blood. The incidence of cancer increases with rising inflammatory markers in an exposure–response relationship.[62]

Additionally, it should be noted that clinical laboratories conduct sputum and tissue sample testing to assess for the presence of abnormal and malignant cells. More specifically, sputum testing uses exfoliative cytology based on spontaneous shedding of cells derived from the mucociliary lining in the lungs to detect cancer cells within these tissues. Conditions which can be identified via lab testing include but are not limited to anemia, thrombocytopenia, leukopenia, and pancytopenia. Please refer Chapter 24 for further direction and assist with clinical decision making related to new or persistent abnormal laboratory values in the oncology population.

Medication Review

A review of CVP medications as a component of both assessment and intervention is essential. Details of medications applicable to the care of PLWBCs is detailed in Chapter 6. However, it is worth mentioning in the context of this chapter that an Onc R clinician's understanding of normal and abnormal exercise responses related to medication use is essential when providing care to all individuals. Attention to the clinical presentation associated with medication use among individuals with compromised systems due to cancer, cancer treatment, or an unrelated co-morbidity must not be underestimated as it is essential for providing safe patient care.

Cardiovascular Tests and Measures

Heart and Pulse Rate

HR can be measured using electrocardiography (ECG) or by auscultation over cardiac windows with a stethoscope (i.e., apical HR). Pulse rate (PR) is a measurement obtained by manual palpation over an artery using the second and third digits. The HR

and PR measures are commonly in congruence; however, in the presence of peripheral vascular disease or compromised cardiovascular function, it is possible that the PR may be lower than the HR. Both measures are useful to establish a baseline rate and to detect irregularities or arrhythmias. These measures are also useful in establishing intensity parameters when designing an exercise program or when considering exercise prescription.

Manual assessment of HR/PR requires the Onc R clinician to use a timepiece capable of measuring seconds. While there are a variety of equations that can be used to calculate the 60 seconds HR/PR, use of the 15 seconds × 4 or 30 seconds × 2 is advantageous in that the relatively longer timeframe assists in identifying irregularities when compared to a 6 seconds × 10 calculation.

A normal HR/PR is regular and reflects the time interval between each heartbeat. It also has a strength or pulse pressure that correlates with the volume of blood being ejected from the heart with each contraction. Weak pulse pressures, scar tissue (e.g., from radial arterial lines), sensation loss in the fingers of the person obtaining the PR measure, or difficulty locating the point of maximal apical impulse for HR measures can all be barriers to obtaining an accurate measurement.

The radial artery is most commonly utilized as the palpation location as it is relatively easy to access and a comfortable touch location for most individuals. The brachial, carotid, femoral, dorsalis pedis, and posterior tibial arteries are also acceptable choices and may be warranted depending on considerations of surgical or tumor sites, chemotherapy ports, pain, or a myriad of other clinical presentations. Oxygen saturation monitors and automated blood pressure (BP) devices are also capable of measuring PR; however, measures obtained from these devices should be used with caution as accuracy of the equipment may be a limitation, especially in the presence of an arrhythmia.

While the normative values for an adult HR/PR is generally accepted as 60 to 100 beats per minute, sources have identified 50 to 95 beats per minute as a normal range.[63,64] An Onc R clinician should expect HR/PR to rise in proportion to increase in workload; however, confounding factors such as medications may blunt or exaggerate the HR response. When tachycardia (>100 beats per minute) is identified in a PLWBC, dehydration, anemia, congestive heart failure, hemorrhage, or shock should be considered as a component of the clinical presentation. In contrast, when bradycardia is observed among PLWBCs, medication use, hyperkalemia, and cardiac arrhythmia should be considered as possible contributors.

Heart Sounds

While the use of heart sounds may not always be considered as having a prominent role in the routine Onc R assessment and care of PLWBCs, the assessment is an essential component of a complete cardiac examination and can be useful for screening and differential diagnosis. There are a variety of interactive websites and resources to assist Onc R clinicians in reviewing and assuring skill in this measure.[65]

S1 and S2 are considered the normal heart sounds which result from closure of the atrioventricular and semilunar valves, respectively. These sounds can be auscultated at the onset of ventricular systole (S1) as a "LUP" (also referred to as "LUB") sound and diastole (S2) as a "DUP" (also referred to as "DUB") sound. The S3 heart sound is an abnormal heart sound that is best heard over the apex and, when present, can be auscultated early in diastole. It is commonly heard as a "LUP-DUP-*dup*" sound and is the hallmark heart sound associated with acute decompensated heart failure.

The S4 is an abnormal sound heard in late diastole or presystole, is commonly heard as a "*la*-LUP-DUP" sound, and is present with resistance to filling as would be present in HTN.[66]

Heart Rhythm and Electrocardiography

Irregularities of heart rhythms are a common complication of cancer therapies among PLWBCs. Chemotherapy has an effect on intracellular signaling pathways and may result in new onset of AFib and other supraventricular arrhythmias.[67] Furthermore, use of oncologic medications can result in QT prolongation and increase the risk of developing ventricular arrhythmias including torsades de pointes.[67] A rhythm reference guide has been included in the supplemental enhanced eBook (eFig. 10.1) to assist Onc R clinicians in identifying and making clinical decisions for some of the possible arrhythmias that may be encountered in clinical practice.

Blood Pressure

Measurement of BP is useful to Onc R clinicians in that it provides a primary prevention strategy and an opportunity for secondary prevention through early identification of HTN. Additionally, assessment of a baseline BP aids the clinician in determining if it is safe to initiate exercise. During exercise, cardiac output increases to meet the demands of exercise. Systolic BP increases steadily until peak exercise is achieved, and then an increase in HR is experienced to maintain cardiac output. For an increase in 1 metabolic equivalent of a task (MET), BP is expected to increase 8 to 12 mmHg.[61] When BP does not increase in response to increasing workload and the PLWBC becomes hypotensive, underlying pathology may include severe left ventricular dysfunction, dehydration, myocardial ischemia, or sepsis.[61]

The importance of BP assessment among PLWBCs is highlighted by one study stating, "The importance of adequately diagnosing and managing HTN in this patient population arises from the facts that HTN is well established as a risk factor for chemotherapy-induced cardiotoxicity and that poorly controlled HTN can significantly influence cancer management and even lead to the discontinuation of certain therapies."[40,62] Furthermore, the role of BP is important in Onc R. One author emphasized stating: "95% of cancers occur in adults, and of those adults, 53% are older than 70 years, one would expect HTN to be present in a large percentage of our patients simply because of their age and, in point of fact, the prevalence of HTN before chemotherapy is similar to that of the general population."[63] Furthermore, chemotherapies such as vascular signaling pathway inhibitors have been identified as causative factors to new HTN and are a common adverse effect of chemotherapy.[62] Therefore, Onc R clinicians are key players in identifying, monitoring, and communicating with other healthcare providers when abnormalities in BP are identified.

The publication entitled *Blood Pressure Screening by Outpatient Physical Therapists: A Call to Action and Clinical Recommendations* provides significant detail on the methodology of BP measurement, normal resting measures and exercise responses, clinical decision making, and referral and it suggests an ethical duty of Onc R clinicians to incorporate BP measure into practice.[68-70] The publication includes resources that may be helpful to clinicians caring for PLWBC. Additionally, the Cardiovascular and Pulmonary Section of the American Physical Therapy Association (APTA) has 12 videos freely available that overview various aspects of BP measures and methodologies as a component of its "VitalsAreVITAL" Campaign.[71] Finally, the *Rehabilitation*

TABLE 10.1 Angina Scale

Numeric Rating	Description
0	No angina
1	Light, barely noticeable
2	Moderate, bothersome
3	Severe, very uncomfortable: Possible preinfarction
4	Most angina ever experienced: Possible infarction

Created by Sara Arena and Meghan Katherine Huber Printed with permission.

Provider Blood Pressure Decision Making Algorithm is a useful reference in clinical practice and is available as eFig. 10.2 of the enhanced eBook.

Angina Scale

Utilization of the Angina Scale is appropriate when PLWBCs are participating in exercise and physical activity, especially in the presence of a known cardiovascular history or risk. The Angina Scale is a 0 to 4 point scale (with 0 being no angina pain and 4 being the most severe or intense angina pain ever experienced) utilized to measure the amount of chest discomfort a person may experience during exercise and is visualized in Table 10.1. Rate pressure product (RPP) is a measure calculated using an individual's HR and systolic BP and represents the degree of stress placed on cardiac muscle. In the presence of an imbalance between myocardial oxygen supply and demand (i.e., elevated HR or SBP common to physical activity and exercise), angina pectoris may arise. This occurrence can be exacerbated or provoked in the presence of low hemoglobin or SpO_2; therefore, monitoring for this adverse event necessitates clinician monitoring of the timing, character, and resolution of anginal symptoms.[72] If the patient experiences a 3 or a 4 out of 4 on the Angina Scale, a seated rest recovery should be provided. If chest discomfort does not subside, urgent medical attention is warranted.

Perceived Exertion

The Borg rating of perceived exertion (RPE) is a way of measuring the intensity level of physical activity. The measure is based on the individual's perception of how hard the body is working and asks the individual to incorporate physical sensations inclusive of HR, increased respiration and breathing rate, sweating, and muscle fatigue. The person is asked to rate their exertion from 6 to 20 with 6 being the lowest exertion and 20 being the highest. Although it is a subjective measure, the individual's exertion rate provides a good estimate of the HR during activity.[73] Furthermore, Borg has reported a high correlation between a person's perceived exertion rating times 10 and HR (e.g., if a 11 was verbalized, this may indicate an approximate HR of 110).[73] When dosing an exercise, a RPE value of 12 to 14 would suggest a moderate level of activity and corresponds to 60% of the HR range; whereas a value of 16 would correspond to 85% of the HR range.[63]

In addition to the 6 to 20 RPE scale, the BORG CR10, 0 to 10 category-ratio scale, and the OMNI scale (acronym for the word omnibus) have all demonstrated efficacy in clinical practice including when dosing resistance training.[74] Use of perceived exertion scales are a useful and complementary tool for PLWBCs to self-monitor the intensity of exercise in both the clinical and home

TABLE 10.2	Rate Perceived Exertion Scales: Borg 6–20 and CR10

Rating of Perceived Exertion *Description and Comparison of the 6–20 and 0–10 Scales*

Borg 6–20 Scale	Borg CR10 Scale
6 No exertion at all	0 Nothing at all
7 Extremely light	
8	0.5 Very, very light
9 Very light	1 Very light
10	
11 Light	2 Light (weak)
12	
13 Somewhat hard	3 Moderate
14	4
15 Hard (heavy)	5 Heavy (strong)
16	6
17 Very hard	7 Very heavy
18	8
19 Extremely hard	9
20 Maximal exertion	10 Very, very heavy (maximal)

Modified from Hillegass E. *Essentials of Cardiopulmonary Physical Therapy-E-Book.* 4th ed. Elsevier Health Sciences; 2016 and Borg G. *Borg's Perceived Exertion and Pain Scales.* Human Kinetics; 1998.
Created by Sara Arena and Meghan Huber. Printed with permission.

settings, and is especially important for those using beta blockers or other medications that blunt HR response. For a side by side comparison of the 6 to 20 RPE scale and the BORG CR0 10 scale, please refer to Table 10.2.

Superficial Vascular Response

As described earlier in this chapter, radiation exposure results in damage to the vasculature within the bounds of the radiation field and ultimately increases the risk of cardiovascular disease. Many PLWBCs have completed radiation therapy and thus may experience altered perfusion and diffusion capabilities of the vascular system. A plethora of research has concluded that aerobic exercise training improves the vasodilator function and reduces peripheral vascular resistance which is most evident in the endothelium versus the smooth muscle.[75] Furthermore, one benefit of exercise is improvement in generalized systemic endothelial function. In other words, engaging in lower extremity (LE) exercise training will result in adaptations of the UE endothelial function.[75] Exercise training mitigates the effects of aging on baroreflex functioning, decreases muscle sympathetic nerve activity, and improves activation of the brainstem, which modulates central sympathetic output and thus sympathetic nervous system-mediated vasoconstriction.[75] Along with sympathetic nervous system mediation, humoral vasoconstrictors are affected by exercise training and regular bouts of exercise suppress circulating concentrations of angiotensin II as well as lower the plasma concentration of endothelin 1.[75] Therefore, an aerobic exercise session decreases the vasoconstrictor tone, which ultimately leads to vasodilation. The importance of a proper cool down following aerobic exercise

cannot be overstated as abrupt cessation of exercise may cause a drop in venous return and result in hypotension and a possible exacerbation of underlying ischemia due to decreased perfusion.[76]

Exercise Participation Screening

In order to overcome barriers to exercise participation, the American College of Sports Medicine (ACSM) has developed an updated screening algorithm for individuals desiring to participate in regular exercise.[77] Given PLWBCs can experience short- and long-term cardiovascular adverse effects from treatment, it is important to screen this population appropriately. The ACSM preparticipation screening algorithm is presented in eFig. 10.3 of the enhanced eBook.

The preparticipation health screening questionnaire has three main focuses: (1) current level of physical activity; (2) current signs/symptoms of known cardiac, renal, or metabolic disease; and (3) desired exercise intensity level.[72] Physician clearance for exercise is recommended for an individual with known cardiovascular, metabolic, or renal disease who was previously sedentary. For previously active individuals, physician clearance is recommended when the individual has known cardiovascular, metabolic, or renal disease and is symptomatic. Physician clearance is also warranted for previously active individuals with a history of cardiovascular, metabolic, or renal disease who wish to participate in vigorous exercise.

The ACSM's preparticipation algorithm serves as a foundation to initiate a safe and person-focused exercise prescription for a PLWBC. Further exercise prescription principles will be reviewed in more detail in Chapter 23.

Pulmonary Tests and Measures

Oximetry

Oximetry is a measurement of the saturation of oxygen in hemoglobin. It can be measured directly using an arterial puncture and reported as the saturated hemoglobin (SaO_2) or by using pulse oximetry which is measured using a noninvasive probe (oxygen saturation [SpO_2]). Additionally, the partial pressure of oxygen and carbon dioxide in the arterial blood can be obtained through an arterial puncture and is reported as partial pressure of oxygen (PaO_2) or partial pressure of carbon dioxide ($PaCO_2$), respectively. Table 10.3 provides an overview of normal and abnormal measures of pulse oximetry and arterial blood assays.

The oxygen-hemoglobin dissociation curve plots the proportion of SaO_2 on a vertical axis to the PaO_2, or oxygen tension, on the horizontal axis. While there are several factors that can lead to shifts within this curve (e.g., fever, pH levels, temperature), it provides Onc R clinicians with a reference to relate the noninvasive SpO_2 measure of how readily hemoglobin acquires and releases oxygen before, during, and after therapeutic interventions.

It is essential for clinicians to determine both baseline and exercising levels of oxygen bound to hemoglobin to assure that there is an ample supply of oxygen for muscles and organs to function. Low amounts of oxygen can result in tissue ischemia and therefore place the patient at significant risk for an adverse event. Given the risk of anemia and low hemoglobin (Hgb) among PLWBCs, this measure may be telling of an underlying physiologic concern. The *Acute Care Handbook for Physical Therapists, 5th edition* provides additional detial and describes the relationship of both the SaO_2 and PaO_2 to the signs and symptoms of hypoxemia.[78]

Use of a pulse oximeter is not without limitations. Barriers to obtaining the measure from these devices specific to the

TABLE 10.3	Blood Gas Normal Values
Measure	Normal Values
PaO$_2$	80–100 mmHg
PaCO$_2$	35–45 mmHg
pH	7.35–7.45
SaO$_2$	97%–99% is normal Generally, >90%–92% safe to initiate exercise with close monitoring
SpO$_2$	97%–99% is normal Generally, >90%–92% safe to initiate exercise with close monitoring

PaO$_2$, partial pressure of oxygen; PaCO$_2$, partial pressure of carbon dioxide; pH, potential of hydrogen (acidic or basic); SaO$_2$, oxygen saturation of arterial blood; SpO$_2$, oxygen saturation of peripheral blood.
Created by Meghan Katherine Huber. Printed with permission.

TABLE 10.4	Common Breathing Patterns and Associated Descriptions
Breathing Pattern	Description
Eupena	Normal rate, depth, rhythm
Apnea	Absence of breathing
Bradypnea	Slow, shallow or normal depth; regular rhythm
Tachypnea	Fast rate, shallow depth, regular rhythm
Hyperpnea	Normal rate, increase depth, regular rhythm
Hypopnea	Slow or shallow breathing
Orthopnea	Difficulty breathing in positions other than upright
Cheyne-Stokes	Increase then decrease depth with periods of apnea interspersed
Biot's	Slow rate, shallow depth, apneic periods, irregular rhythm
Periodic breathing	Oscillations between hypopnea and hyperpnea; no true apnea

Created by Sara Arena. Printed with permission.

oncologic population include: nail polish and artificial nails, dark skin pigmentation, decreased circulation and perfusion to the area being measured (e.g., cold fingers), anemia, certain medications, shivering, those of advanced age, arrhythmias, and obtaining the measurement in bright artificial light. Given the devices may also provide a HR, accuracy can be checked against a manual PR measure to assure accuracy. However, Onc R clinicians should also consider investing in medical grade devices (versus widely available screening finger probes) when working with at-risk populations including those with cancer diagnoses.

Pulmonary Function Testing

Outcomes of pulmonary function testing (PFT) can be important when determining if the flow and/or volume of air in the lungs is altered. This understanding can be useful in choosing the best treatment strategy to address a given impairment. Normal PFT values have been established for individuals that take into considerations age, gender, weight, height, and racial background.

Spirometry is most commonly used to measure lung mechanics including rate of flow. The forced vital capacity (FVC) and the forced expiratory volume in 1 second (FEV1) are considered normal if they fall above 80% of the predicted value for each individual. Body plethysmography is commonly used to measure lung volumes with total lung capacity (TLC), vital capacity (VC) and residual volume (RV) most useful to rehabilitation clinicians as a guide for intervention. The normal range for TLC is 80% to 120% with levels above 120% indicative of lung hyperinflation.

It is not uncommon to have an annual decline in FVC and FEV1 at rates of 20 cc and 30 cc as individuals age. Furthermore, tobacco use can result in an additional 50 to 100 cc/year reduction. Given a strong correlation between tobacco use and lung cancer reduced airflow may be a baseline finding in a PLWBC of the lung which could be potentially compounded by surgery and other cancer-related therapies. Therefore, a thorough chart review to assess for availability of PFT measures would allow Onc R clinicians insight into a patient's baseline values and the ability to alter their rehabilitation program as warranted.

Breath Sounds and Breathing Patterns

Auscultation of breath sounds and assessment of breathing patterns to determine if a PLWBC has optimal availability of oxygen for exercise and physical activity can be helpful. Table 10.4 provides an overview of many common breathing patterns and the associated descriptions.

In addition to assessment of the breathing pattern, breath sounds can be assessed through lung auscultation to determine if there are adventitious (abnormal) sounds that might suggest pathology. Crackles (previously known as rales), high-pitched wheezes, low pitched wheezes (previously known as rhonchi), and stridor are among sounds considered abnormal. Diminished or absent breath sounds may also be indicative of an abnormality as it is suggestive of decreased air flow to an area of the lung field. A PLWBC may present with diminished breath sounds due to a variety of conditions that result in air or fluid in or around the lungs. Among these conditions, heart failure as a result of cardiotoxicity, pneumonia, or postsurgical atelectasis should be considered. Table 10.5 provides a summary of possible medical interpretations of these adventitious breath sounds.

Finally, vocal transmission during auscultation should be loudest at the trachea and the mainstem bronchi. Words should be intelligible, though softer and less clear distally. Abnormal sound transmissions may be heard through fluid filled areas, effusions, tumor, or other lung consolidation.

Dyspnea Measures

Dyspnea is a sensation of difficult or labored breathing that can occur at rest and/or with activity. It is the most prevalent symptom among individuals with cardiac and respiratory disease and can be brought on or exacerbated during the course of medical treatments for cancer. Additionally, dyspnea is an independent predictor of mortality.[79] Therefore, it is a symptom that should be at the forefront of assessment by Onc R clinicians.

Dyspnea triggers most common to PLWBCs include: pulmonary dysfunction, deconditioning, obesity, anemia, and heart failure however there are several other plausible contributors. The Total Dyspnea Scale for Cancer Patients (TDSC) has emerging evidence for its efficacy in assessing the effects on daily living activities, psychology, and on social activity among PLWBCs. Hashimoto and Kanda provide evidence for its acceptable

TABLE 10.5 Adventitious Breath Sounds and Possible Clinical Interpretations

Sound	Possible Clinical Interpretation[a]
Crackles (rales)	• Pulmonary edema • Atelectasis • Interstitial lung disease • Infection • Pneumonia • Secretions • Chronic obstructive pulmonary disease
High and low pitched wheezes (rhonchi)	• Small airway bronchoconstriction • Focal masses • Asthma • Chronic obstructive pulmonary disease
Stridor	• Extra thoracic upper-airway obstruction if auscultated on inspiration • Intrathoracic tracheobronchial lesions if auscultated on expiration • Stenosis if auscultated on both inspiration and expiration
Absent or diminished breath sounds	• Pneumothorax • Pleural effusion • Pneumonia • Increased thickness of the chest wall. • Over-inflation of a part of the lungs • Reduced airflow to part of the lungs

[a]List is not all inclusive.
Created by Sara Arena. Printed with permission.

reliability, reference-related validity, and discriminant validity. Therefore, this may be one useful tool when assessing cancer-related dyspnea.[80]

Pulmonary Outcome Measures
Table 10.6 provides details of common pulmonary-focused outcome measures, measurement domains, and general descriptions of each outcome.

Other Tests and Measures

Aerobic Capacity/Endurance

VO_2 Maximal Test
The criterion standard of assessing cardiopulmonary reserve and aerobic capacity is via a VO_2 maximal (max) test which evaluates an individual's maximal oxygen uptake during intense exercise.[2] VO_2 (also referred to as oxygen consumption) is a measure of the volume of oxygen that is used by your body to convert the energy from the food sources to energy molecules. Ultimately, an individual's maximal VO_2 provides insight into a person's cardiorespiratory fitness. Relative energy expenditure is expressed in mL/kg/min and accounts for individuals with differing body weights.[81] Absolute energy expenditure is expressed in METs and will be further described in the next section of this chapter.

Treadmill and cycle ergometry are the most common modes when administering a VO_2 max test. Chapter 23 will discuss specific protocols that have been developed to accurately assess VO_2

TABLE 10.6 Pulmonary Outcome Measures

Outcome Measure	General Description
0–10 category-ratio scale (CR10)[108]	Subjective measure/rating of exertion and/or breathlessness during exercise or exercise testing[108]
Visual Analogue Scale (VAS)[109]	Can be used to measure dyspnea during exercise using a line 100mm in length with written anchors at the extremes of dyspnea (e.g., "not breathless at all" to "extremely breathless")[109]
Modified Medical Research Council (mMRC) Dyspnea Scale for COPD[110]	Used to measure the degree of breathlessness related to activities.[a,110]
Baseline and Transition Dyspnea Index[111]	Measures change in dyspnea severity from baseline in three categories: functional impairment, magnitude of task, and magnitude of effort[111]
Chronic Respiratory Questionnaire (CRQ) Dyspnea Component[112]	Used to measure physical and emotional aspects of chronic respiratory disease[a,112]
University of California, San Diego-Shortness of Breath Questionnaire (UCSD-SOBQ) for COPD[109]	Self-report questionnaire that measures severity of shortness of breath/dyspnea during various activities of daily living in individuals with various forms of lung pathology[109]
The Medical Research Council (MRC) Breathlessness Scale[113]	It quantifies the disability associated with breathlessness by identifying that breathlessness occurs when it should not (Grades 1 and 2) or by quantifying the associated exercise limitation (Grades 3–5)[113]
St. George's Respiratory Questionnaire (SGRQ)[114]	Used to measure the impact of respiratory disease on participation in activities[a,114]
Borg RPE/RPD[108]	A way of measuring physical activity intensity level and uses an individual's self-reported perception of how hard they are working[73]
Talk Test[115]	Informal, subjective method of estimating cardiorespiratory exercise intensity. Reports support usefulness and ability to closely reflect actual HR and VO_2 levels[115]

List is not all inclusive. [a]COPD is the target population of this tool. *COPD*, Chronic obstructive pulmonary disease; *HR*, heart rate; *RPD*, rating of perceived dyspnea; *RPE*, rating of perceived exertion, VO_2, volume of oxygen consumption
Created by Sara Arena. Printed with permission.

TABLE 10.7 Quick Reference for Activity and Associated METs[84]

	Very Light/Light (<3 METs)	Moderate (3–5.9 METs)	Vigorous (>6 METs)
Walking	Walking slowly around the home	Walking at a brisk pace 3–4 mph (4.8–6.4 kph)	Walking >4.5 mph (7.2 kph), hiking with pack or elevation, jogging, running
Household and occupation	Making the bed, washing dishes, cooking	Washing windows, car, cleaning garage, sweeping, vacuuming, mowing, carrying/stacking wood	Shoveling, farming, bailing hay, digging
Leisure and sports	Playing cards, billiards, boating, darts, fishing, playing music	Badminton, shooting baskets, slow ballroom dancing, golf, table tennis, tennis doubles, noncompetitive volleyball	Bicycling, basketball game, cross-country skiing, soccer, swimming, tennis singles, competitive volleyball

MET, metabolic equivalent of task; mph, miles per hour; kph, kilometers per hour.
Created by Sara Arena and Meghan Katherine Huber. Printed with permission.

max, although each protocol is designed to increase speed, incline, or resistance every few minutes until the participant has reached volitional fatigue. Each mode and protocol presents advantages and disadvantages, thus history taking is important to select the most appropriate protocol for each individual.

Gas analysis is the best indicator in determining if a true VO_2 max was reached during the exercise test. During gas analysis, the individual wears a mask surrounding the nose and mouth. The mask is connected to laboratory equipment via a tube. Gas concentrations of both inspired and expired air are measured throughout the test with this equipment. A true VO_2 max is completed when 4/5 criteria have been achieved. These criteria include; plateau of VO_2, respiratory exchange ratio (RER) of >1.10, HR within ±10 to 12 beats per minute (bpm) of age predicted max or failure of HR to increase with increasing workload, blood lactate >8 mM, and subjective report of RPE >17 on the Borg 6 to 20 scale.[76] If an individual does not reach the previously stated variables or if local muscular fatigue limits participation in continued testing (as seen most commonly in cycle ergometer testing), VO_2 peak (highest value attained during a test) has been achieved as opposed to VO_2 max (highest value attainable by the individual).[81]

While many individuals with a prior cancer diagnosis experience CVP decline and deconditioning, the decline in VO_2 max can be attributed to compromised oxygen utilization that is a result of the cancer treatments.[2] VO_2 peak in individuals with cancer has been found to be ~30% lower than that of age and sex matched sedentary individuals who are otherwise healthy.[82] Due to deconditioning, many PLWBCs may not be able to endure the intensity of a VO_2 max test, thus VO_2 peak or submaximal testing may be more appropriate an achievable.

METs

METs quantify the absolute intensity of a particular activity and can be calculated based on an individual's VO_2 max. METs represent the intensity of a given activity or achieved workload relative to the metabolic expenditure for basal homeostasis (i.e., sleeping and resting), which is considered to be 1 MET and equivalent to approximately 3.5 mL/kg/min.[76] In other words, a five MET activity would expend five times the energy used by the body at rest. However, when using METs to guide the intensity of an activity, regard for the individual's age, sex, and fitness level must be considered. For example, the Ainsworth Compendium suggests making a bed would require approximately three MET levels of energy expenditure.[83] For a healthy, physically active, 24-year-old male triathlete with no underlying medical conditions or comorbidities,

this activity will be completed quickly without fatigue. The same activity for an 80-year-old male who is undergoing chemotherapy and radiation therapy for metastatic lung cancer and has a history coronary artery bypass graft x 4 may find this activity to be more physically demanding and fatiguing. It is feasible that the energy used to complete the tasks for the 80-year-old individual would be above the three MET level. These examples emphasize the shortcomings of using METs in isolation when determining exercise dosing as contextual factors can impact the person's response and associated outcome.

VO_2 max and MET levels are pertinent in treating PLWBCs as these measurements provide a means of consistent and objective data throughout the course of an individual's rehabilitative programming. Discharge recommendations created by Onc R clinicians in the acute care setting can be guided by an individual's ability to tolerate a certain MET level and thereby assure a safer discharge to the home environment. Specifically, it is recommended that individuals over the age of 85 demonstrate a VO_2 max of at least 15 to 18 mL/kg/min in order to be successful in an independent living environment.[2] To determine the conversion of METs to/from VO_2, utilize the following equation: 1 MET=VO_2 (mL/kg/min)/3.5 mL/kg/min. This would indicate that a MET level of 4.2 to 5.1 is the threshold for independent living. Table 10.7 provides an abbreviated reference for METs associated with common activities. For more in-depth MET equivalent activities, the Ainsworth Compendium is a valuable resource.[83]

VO_2 Submaximal Test

Submaximal VO_2 testing is utilized when a patient may not be able to tolerate a VO_2 max test or VO_2 max testing is deemed unsafe. This test is used to predict VO_2 max and may be completed using a treadmill, cycle ergometer, or step test. In order to complete the VO_2 submaximal test accurately the following methods should be employed: steady state HR is obtained at each workload, linear relationship with HR and work rate is evident, the patient has not taken any medications affecting HR response, has avoided large amounts of caffeine, is not sick, and the room is not at extreme high or low temperatures.[81]

There are many different protocols for submaximal testing, with each protocol requiring an increase in either speed or incline every 2 to 3 minutes while monitoring HR, BP, and RPE at least two times at each stage. When the HR is >110 bpm, a steady state must be reached prior to advancing to the next stage. Steady state requires the measured HR to be within 5 bpm between readings prior to advancing speed and incline. A submaximal test is terminated when the patient has reached 85% of age-adjusted HR max, the patient requests to terminate, or the patient has any adverse symptoms/reactions as described as "red flag symptoms" listed in Table 10.10. Upon termination of the test, there are equations that are utilized to best predict VO_2 max for the individual, based on the submaximal test performance. The different modes and equations will be reviewed in Chapter 23.

Field Tests

Six Minute Walk Test

Many PLWBCs demonstrate severely decreased functional and aerobic reserve and may be unable to tolerate a traditional VO_2 max exercise test. The six minute walk test (6MWT) has been validated as a field test to assess the functional capacity of cancer survivors who are unable to tolerate a VO_2 max test.[85,86] In the 6MWT the individual is instructed to cover as much distance as possible in six minutes. Assistive devices can be utilized if needed, and the person may take as many rest periods as required but the six-minute timer will not stop. The Onc R clinician is responsible for monitoring HR, BP, and SpO_2 prior to, during, and after exercise.

After two cycles of chemotherapy treatment in lung cancers, a statistically significant decline in the 6MWT distance has been demonstrated mostly in those with lower body mass index (BMI) and advanced disease.[87,88] Prior studies also established an initial distance of ≥400 m during the 6MWT prior to lung cancer treatment as a good prognostic indicator for positive outcomes, tolerance to treatment, and overall survival.[87] This 6MWT initial distance is similar to prognostic indictors among individuals with COPD, pulmonary HTN, and heart failure.

Two Minute Walk Test

The two-minute walk test may be utilized for those individuals presenting with significantly limited functional reserve and aerobic capacity. The test is administered in the same manner as the 6MWT with the exception of a shorter time, two minutes versus six minutes. It has been found that a change of 5.5 meters is a clinically meaningful difference.[89] Normative data specific to the oncology population have yet to be established.

Step Test

Step tests are utilized as submaximal exercise tests that can estimate VO_2 max. The test requires a step or platform (40 cm for males and 33 cm for females), stopwatch, metronome or cadence tape, and a body weight scale. The step test typically requires a minimum VO_2 of 25.8 to 29.5 mL/kg/min to complete, thus is not recommended for deconditioned individuals and those with debilitating medical conditions.[81] The step test may be more appropriate for individuals in the outpatient rehabilitation setting as opposed to acute care.

Peripheral Vascular Tests

Girth Measurements

Girth measurements assist in assessing and screening for lymphedema. Chapter 9 provides a more comprehensive explanation of these measurements as it relates to lymphedema.

Assessing for Deep Vein Thrombosis

As previously discussed in this chapter, VTE, which includes both DVT and PE, can result as a serious adverse effect of cancer-related therapies. Thrombosis most commonly occurs in the LE although it can dislodge and become a life-threatening PE. Contrast venography has historically been the criterion standard for diagnosis of DVT, but this procedure is invasive and requires expertise, as well as

TABLE 10.8 Wells Criteria for Deep Vein Thrombosis

Active cancer: ongoing treatment, within previous 6 months
Paralysis, paresis, recent immobilization of LE
Recently bedridden for 3 days or major surgery within 4 weeks
Localized tenderness along deep venous system distribution assessed by firm palpation in posterior calf, the popliteal space, and along the femoral vein in anterior thigh and groin
Entire LE swelling
Calf swelling >3 cm when compared with asymptomatic LE (measured 10 cm below tibial tuberosity)
Pitting edema (greater in symptomatic LE)
Collateral superficial veins (nonvariceal)
Alternative diagnosis as likely or greater than that of proximal DVT: cellulitis, calf strain, Baker's cyst, and postoperative swelling

DVT, deep vein thrombosis; *LE*, lower extremity.
Wells PS, Anderson DR, Rodger M, et al. Evaluation of D-dimer in the diagnosis of suspected deep-vein thrombosis. N Engl J Med. 2003;349(13):1227-1235. doi:10.1056/NEJMoa023153
Adapted by Meghan Huber. Printed with permission.

intravenous contrast.[90] LE venous duplex combines B-mode (grayscale) imaging and transducer compression maneuvers to produce doppler imaging and waveform analysis.[90] Ultrasound criteria for diagnosis of a LE DVT includes inability to compress the vein.[90] Doppler imaging can also distinguish between acute and chronic DVTs. Doppler ultrasound is 89% sensitive, 100% specific, and 94% accurate in diagnosis of DVT.[91] The pros of a venous duplex scan are that it is noninvasive, quick/easy, readily available, and portable. The cons of venous duplex scan are that it is less sensitive among those who are obese, have significant edema, or have physical barriers including casts, immobilizers, and bandages.

If a DVT is suspected, but no imaging has been completed, the Wells Criteria (Table 10.8) for DVT is a predictive screen that can be employed by a clinician to determine the risk of DVT presence.[92] For each symptom/criterion present in the individual being evaluated, the person is scored one point. Once all the criteria have been reviewed, the Onc R clinician tallies the total points. A total score of 0 is considered low risk, 1 to 2 equates to moderate risk, and 3 or higher establishes the person to be at a high risk of having a DVT. It is important to note that any patient with active cancer or undergoing oncologic treatment is already at a moderate risk of developing a DVT when using the Wells Criteria.

D-dimer

D-dimer, a biological marker, is a small protein segment found in the blood when fibrin is present as a result of blood clot disintegration.[93] The biomarker elevates with clot formation and is a predictor of DVT, PE, or disseminated intravascular coagulation.[93] D-dimer levels have evidence of predicting cancer progression, recurrence, and prognosis in colorectal, lung, prostate, and gastric cancers.[93] High levels of plasma D-dimer present in PLWBCs indicates a significantly increased risk of mortality, is a poor prognostic indicator for those diagnosed with terminal cancer of all types, and may be a predictor of survival time of less than one week in patients with a terminal prognosis.[93]

Vascular Assessments

The Buerger test and Ankle Brachial Index (ABI) are useful when screening for circulation deficits or ischemia to the LE. The

Buerger test is completed with the individual positioned in supine and legs elevated to 60° while observing the plantar surface of the feet.[82] The person then sits up with the feet in a dependent position while the Onc R clinician continues to observe the feet. A flush red color may appear in the feet and travel proximally.[94] A positive test is elicited when pallor is observed on the LE in an elevated position or rubor is noted in a dependent position and may indicate peripheral vascular disease.[95] A positive Buerger test indicates severe ischemia in the limb; however, a negative test does not necessarily rule out ischemia.[94] While not a test specific to the oncologic population, it may assist with differential diagnosis when new conditions and presentations arise during the course of care in PLWBCs.

A useful resource to understand the methods of performing an ABI is available at https://stanfordmedicine25.stanford.edu/the25/ankle-brachial-index.html.[96] In this assessment, the systolic BP is obtained in the bilateral brachial artery, anterior tibial (dorsalis pedis) artery, and posterior tibial artery using a sphygmomanometer and a doppler device with an 8 MHz continuous wave probe.[97] Two measurements are taken at each site. To calculate the ABI the highest measurement of dorsalis pedis or posterior tibial artery is divided by the higher reading of the brachial artery pressure. This mathematical equation will yield a value. When ABI is <0.90 there is clinical suspicion for peripheral arterial disease (PAD).[98] The severity of the PAD increases as the ABI value decreases (e.g., ABI of 0.40 indicates severe PAD). It is also important to note older adults and those with diabetes can present with an elevated ABI (values >1.3) which can also be concerning as it represents noncompressible calcified blood vessels. An abnormal ABI is considered a predictor of cancer mortality, with an increased risk in those individuals with an abnormal ABI (<0.9 and >1.3) and history of cardiovascular events.[99] Details of normal and abnormal ABI values are detailed in Table 10.9.

TABLE 10.9 Ankle Brachial Index Measures and Interpretation

Ankle Brachial Index Value	Possible Interpretation	Recommendation
Greater than 1.4	Calcification/Vessel hardening	Refer to vascular specialist
1.0–1.4	Normal	None
0.9–1.0	Acceptable	
0.8–0.9	Some arterial disease	Treat risk factors
0.5–0.8	Moderate arterial disease	Refer to vascular specialist
Less than 0.5	Severe arterial disease	Refer to vascular specialist

Modified from Medicine S. Introduction to Measuring the Ankle Brachial Index. https://stanfordmedicine25.stanford.edu/the25/ankle-brachial-index.html; 2020.
Created by Sara Arena and Meghan Huber. Printed with permission.

Contraindications and Indications to Terminate Exercise

Signs and Symptoms in Response to Increased Oxygen Demand With Exercise/Activity

Given the complex medical status of PLWBCs, Table 10.10 provides details of specific vital signs, symptoms, and observations that warrant termination of exercise or contraindication to initiating exercise.

TABLE 10.10 Contraindications for Starting Exercise or Rationale for Termination of Exercise

	Contraindications for Exercise or Physical Activity	Indications to Terminate Exercise or Physical Activity
Resting heart rate	>100 beats per minute or <50 beats per minute	Sudden drop >15 beats per minute, change from regular to irregular rhythm, or exceeds heart rate maximum
Resting systolic blood pressure	>200 mmHg or <90 mmHg	>200 mmHg, decrease to <90 mmHg, drop >20mmHg from resting or with increasing exercise
Resting diastolic blood pressure	>110 mmHg	115 mmHg
Oxygen saturation	<90%	<90%
Symptoms	Shortness of breath, angina, dizziness, severe headache, sudden onset of numbness or weakness, painful calf suggestive of deep vein thrombosis	Shortness of breath, angina, dizziness, severe headache, sudden onset of numbness or weakness
Observation	Cyanosis, diaphoresis, bilateral edema in a patient with congestive heart failure, pallor, fever, weight gain >4–6 lb/day (1.8–2.7 kg/day), abnormal change in breath sounds or heart sounds, Cheyne-Stokes breathing, jugular distention, mottling, vertebral artery compression signs (dizziness, diplopia, dysarthria, dysphagia, drop attack, nausea/vomiting, nystagmus, numbness)	Cyanosis, diaphoresis, bilateral edema in a patient with congestive heart failure, pallor, fever, weight gain >4–6 lb/day (1.8–2.7 kg/day), abnormal change in breath sounds or heart sounds, ataxia, Cheyne-Stokes breathing, jugular distention, mottling, vertebral artery compression signs (dizziness, diplopia, dysarthria, dysphagia, drop attack, nausea/vomiting, nystagmus, numbness)
Other	Fever >101°F (38.3 C), hemoglobin <8 mg/dL, neutropenia—white blood cells <10³/µL, platelets <25–50 × 10³/µL	

Modified from APTA Physical Fitness for Special Populations, Exercise & Physical Activity Guidelines Based on Best Available Evidence and the American College of Sports Medicine exercise testing guidelines.
Created by Meghan Huber. Printed with permission.

Additionally, the Joint Task Force of APTA Acute Care and the Academy of Cardiovascular & Pulmonary Physical Therapy of the American Physical Therapy Association published recommendations for the interpretation of adult vital signs in the acute care setting with specific reference to the oncologic population. Specifically, it recommends that exercise should be terminated if (1) HR and BP decrease with an increased workload; (2) there is new onset of a dysrhythmia; (3) SpO_2 is <88%; (4) respiratory rate is <5 breaths/minute or >40 breaths/minute; and (5) to avoid exercise if body temperature >38.3°C (101°F).[100] Additionally, the task force suggests the use of the Borg Breathlessness Scale, Borg, or Modified Borg RPE Scale to monitor appropriate progression of rehabilitation intervention. Elevated fall risk and associated injury among PLWBCs with the possibility of HR and BP alterations among individuals undergoing neck radiation therapy due to arterial baroreceptor disruptions are also cited within the Joint Task Force document.[100] Onc R clinicians are encouraged to actively collaborate with the medical team to determine safe exercise and recommend adaptations to exercise programs base on health status, adjuvant treatments, and anticipated disease trajectory.[100]

Common Treatments for Adverse Effects

Aerobic Exercise Modes

There are many modes of aerobic exercise that could be of benefit in PLWBCs. Continuous, interval, circuit, and cross training are all aerobic modes available for improving physical performance and function. Further discussion and review of each specific exercise prescription will be addressed in Chapter 9.

Role of Aerobic Exercise in Cancer-Related Fatigue

Among the plethora of adverse effects from cancer and cancer treatment, cancer-related fatigue (CRF) is among the most common experiences. It is estimated that overall, 48% of cancer survivors experience CRF, with a higher prevalence in among those with a pancreatic, breast, or lymphoma cancer diagnosis.[101] It is estimated that 25% to 30% will experience CRF in the five years following cancer treatment.[101] Symptoms include, but are not limited to, extreme fatigue to a point of exhaustion, significant lack of energy, memory and concentration difficulties, and loss of personal drive and interest.[102] PLWBCs have reported that CRF is more severe than other fatigue, impacts daily function and quality of life, is not relieved by rest or sleep and is not proportional to the activity performed.[103]

CRF is multifactorial with a host of underlying conditions including pulmonary edema and valvular dysfunction each of which can be brought on or exacerbated by the gamut of cancer-related medical interventions. It is important for the Onc R clinician to recognize the underlying cause of the fatigue will need to be addressed if the outward signs and symptoms are to be relieved. Despite the high prevalence of CRF in a PLWBC, fatigue levels are often underreported via the patient and often undertreated by Onc R clinicians.[101] Furthermore, while CRF has been reported as most debilitating during chemotherapy, radiation therapy, surgery, or a combination thereof it can remain and persist following treatment.[102] Those with CRF typically have higher protein oxidation and lower antioxidant capacity as compared to individuals without cancer.[104] The combination of these two physiological alterations can lead to a state of systemic oxidative stress which may contribute to the underlying mechanism of CRF.[104]

Treatment should be initiated soon after diagnosis in order to prevent CRF from becoming a chronic sequela of cancer.

Management should be multifocal and likely interdisciplinary to address the physical, psychological, and cognitive aspects of the PLWBC. Additionally, any associated chronic pain, sleep disturbances, and stress levels/management should be addressed. Referrals for nutrition assessment and medication management may also be warranted. Furthermore, nonpharmacological interventions could include cognitive behavioral therapy, energy conservation, activity modification, mindfulness-based stress reduction, and physical activity/exercise.[102]

Exercise has been found to be of benefit in managing CRF. Current recommendations include 150 minutes a week of moderate intensity or 75 minutes of vigorous intensity aerobic exercise (walking, cycling, water aerobics, stair climbing) and 2 to 3 exercise sessions a week of strengthening to each major muscle group.[72,101] A 10-week study investigating the effect of exercise on cardiorespiratory fitness, muscular strength, and plasma markers for oxidative stress, DNA oxidation, and antioxidant capacity in those who have completed chemotherapy or radiation therapy was conducted.[104] The investigators reported exercise improved antioxidant capacity and decreased protein oxidation which may impact systemic oxidative stress.[104]

While it is important to engage in exercise during cancer treatments, appropriate exercise dosing and prescription are of utmost importance. Moderate intensity dosing of exercise has been suggested as a strategy to balance the important health benefits of exercises while mediating oxidative stress production. Additionally, exercise can assist the body in adapting and preparing for the higher levels of oxidative stress that may be experienced during cancer treatment.[49] Higher levels of oxidative stress, as may be experienced with high intensity aerobic exercise sessions, may overwhelm the antioxidant defense system and cause oxidative damage in persons undergoing cancer treatments.[49]

Protective Effects of Physical Activity and Exercise

As described earlier in this chapter, cancer and cancer-related medical treatment result in damage to the CVP systems. The most efficient way to improve cardiac muscle endurance is through aerobic exercises that increase cardiac filling and cardiac output.[2] Aerobic exercise may provide protective roles in cardiac function before, during, and after cancer treatment, specifically radiation therapy.[2] Exercise has also been linked to longer disease-free cancer survival rates as well as reducing the risk of cancer recurrence.[105]

Energy Conservation Principles

Although energy conservation is most commonly referred to in the scope of pulmonary rehabilitation or among those with heart failure, the principles have application to a wide array of impairments relevant to primary and secondary cancer diagnosis and the cancer medical intervention sequelae. While aerobic conditioning is essential for optimization of function, there are situations for which an individual may need to buffer energy expenditure, either as a short- or long-term solution, in order to function safely and independently. Pursed lip breathing, prioritizing activities, advanced planning to streamline activities, reducing the speed or pace of an activity to minimize the sympathetic response and positioning of the body to optimize thoracic excursion and diaphragmatic contraction are elements of a good energy conservation program.

An example of how incorporating these principles into care may be useful is illustrated in an individual who recently started a regime of daily radiation therapy concurrent with chemotherapy every two weeks. These therapies would need to be highly *prioritized* into the PLWBC's day as they are needed to treat the cancer. The individual may need to *plan activities* (shower in the evening versus the morning, have help with transportation so they can rest in the car) to accommodate fatigue associated with the treatments and the stress of the diagnosis. *Pursed lip breathing* and *body positioning* can be incorporated as both a strategy to decrease shortness of breath and an adjunct to relaxation and stress management. Specifically, relaxation and stress management are essential to reduce the sympathetic state that can be induced with an unchecked release of catecholamines that may result from the demands of a cancer diagnosis and the associated interventions.

Airway Clearance Techniques With Consideration for Obstructive Tumors, Pulmonary Fibrosis, and Inflammation

Airway clearance techniques including interventions to optimize breathing and coughing as well as manual and mechanical techniques can be useful tools for PLWBC. Choosing the appropriate technique is unique to each individual's presentation. The measurement and screening tools previously described in this chapter and throughout this book can be helpful resources to determine which airway clearance technique may be appropriate. Some potential breathing techniques that may be useful include paced breathing, diaphragmatic breathing, pursed lip breathing, and the active cycle of breathing. Additionally, coughing techniques including huffing and self- and external-assisted cough may be useful. Manual techniques including postural drainage, chest percussion, vibration and shaking, and chest wall mobilization can be used in isolation or combination to open and drain airways. Furthermore, mechanical devices including percussion vests, inspiratory muscle trainers, and positive pressure devices may have utility to mediate complications from surgery and immobility. Finally, it is essential that Onc R clinicians utilize physical activity as a focal point in addressing airway clearance. An outstanding free resource that covers each of these techniques is publicly available (https://youtu.be/kbidrfSCgfs). The video was created as a component of the Post-Acute COVID-19 Exercise and Rehabilitation (PACER) project; however, the techniques have application to the vast array of strategies that can be used when addressing the unique needs of PLWBCs.

Conclusion

Pulmonary cancers are the second leading cause of cancer deaths. While primary malignant cardiac cancers are rare, cancer of either the pulmonary or cardiac organ systems can have a significant impact on those who are living with and beyond an initial cancer diagnosis. Of further significance, is the impact that cancer interventions can have on the CVP systems among all PLWBC. Evidence-based assessments, tools, and directed interventions are available; however, further validation for use among populations with varied cancer diagnosis is warranted. Clinicians should approach each patient/client encounter with attention to the CVP system and with attention to its impact on aerobic endurance and ultimately physical activity and function. Furthermore, the potential for adverse effects brought about by cancer treatment and any serious contraindications to activity should be in the forefront of every rehabilitation encounter among individuals with risk factors for future cancer onset, a new cancer diagnosis, or a prior cancer history.

Critical Research Needs

- Characteristics, lifestyle risk factors, or physical activity levels of individuals with a diagnosed with primary cardiac cancers
- Epigenetic factors that may be contributing to the development of primary cardiac tumors
- Cardiovascular and pulmonary related epigenetic factors in primary and secondary prevention of all cancers and recurrence
- Large scale randomized controlled trials examining exercise volumes that reduce oxidative stress and optimize aerobic capacity in cardiovascular and pulmonary cancers
- Large scale randomized controlled trials of prehabilitation on long term heart and lung function after cancer interventions
- Role of oxidative stress and inflammatory markers in cancer propogation
- Correlations between static cardiac measures (i.e., echocardiogram) versus aerobic capacity exercise testing
- Uniform use of exercise (moderate versus vigorous) and physical activity definitions and terminology across study methodology
- Studies examining validity and reliability of cardiovascular and pulmonary focused outcome measures on PLWBCs

Case Study

A 63-year-old male with non-Hodgkin lymphoma (Stage IIIb), with a peripheral T-cell lymphoma (PTCL) subtype, and thymus involvement is referred for outpatient physical therapy to address impairments of weakness and fatigue (Tables 10.11 and 10.12).

TABLE 10.11 Case Study Results of Pulmonary Function Tests

	Actual Measure	Predicted Measure	% Predicted
Spirometry—Lung Mechanics			
FVC (L)	1.90	4.00	48
FEV1 (L)	1.75	3.50	50
FEV1/FVC (%)	92.1	82.0	112
Lung Volumes			
TLC (L)	2.20	4.40	50
VC (L)	2.10	4.60	46
RV (L)	1.09	1.69	64

FVC, Forced vital capacity; *FEV1,* forced expiratory volume over 1 second; *TLC,* total lung capacity; *VC,* vital capacity; *RV,* residual volume.
Created by Sara Arena and Meghan Katherine Huber. Printed with permission.

TABLE 10.12 Results of Select Laboratory Tests

Hemoglobin (Hgb)	7.4 g/dL
Red blood cell (RBC) count	5.1 M/μL
White blood cell (WBC) count	10.0 K/μL
Platelets (PLT)	400 K/μL

Created by Sara Arena and Meghan Katherine Huber. Printed with permission.

Diagnosis-Related Medical Interventions
- External beam radiation to anterior upper thoracic region 5 times a week x 6 weeks
- Two doses of chemotherapy using a CHOP protocol (cyclophosphamide [Cytoxan], hydroxydaunorubicin [Adriamycin], vincristine [Oncovin], and prednisone)
- Rituximab (Rituxan) was used as an immunotherapy intervention

Physical Therapy Evaluation

Interview: Fatigue and generalized weakness impacting ability to be independent with activities of daily living (dressing, bathing, and vacuuming) and community independence within neutropenic precautions (walking into doctor appointment, riding in car greater than 20 minutes) and with no assistive device. The patient does have 4-wheeled walker available as needed

Lung auscultation: Diminished breath sounds throughout bilateral lung fields but no adventitious sounds present

Heart auscultation: Regular rate and rhythm (RRR)—S1, S2

Vitals: *Heart Rate:* 96 bpm, *Blood Pressure:* 106/58 mmHg, O_2 *Saturation:* 94% on room air

Pain: Denies

Fatigue: 7/10

Postural assessment: Kyphotic posture with decreased thoracic extension

Shoulder range of motion: Limited to three-fourths normal range in horizontal abduction, internal rotation and abduction bilaterally

Strength and power assessment: Decreased for expected age/sex

6MWT: 400 m with 1 standing rest

Dyspnea: 2+ With minimal exertion

Integumentary: Altered skin turgor and discoloration to skin which received radiation

Tinetti: 19/28

Functional Assessment of Chronic Illness Therapy—Fatigue (FACIT F): Total Score: 60/160, where a score of 160 is best and a score of 0 is the worst[106]

Physical Therapy Program:
1. Provide education and reinforcement of the following:
   a. Energy conservation principles
   b. Importance of adequate fluid and caloric intake
   c. Skin protection with radiation therapy
   d. Cancer-related fatigue and deconditioning
2. Establish an exercise regime that addresses the key areas of both fitness and therapeutic exercise prescription
   a. Aerobic (using energy conservation principles)
   b. Flexibility (focus UE and thoracic region)
   c. Muscular endurance
   d. Resistance training (*caution due to low platelet counts)
   e. Balance and coordination challenges
3. Breathing and relaxation exercises (e.g., pursed lip breathing, guided imagery)
4. Durable medical equipment—ambulatory assistive devices (e.g., 4 wheeled walker with seat for community ambulation and energy conservation), transport chair, shower modifications (e.g., removable shower head, tub bench)
5. Home modification—assure rails for exit and entry are secured, install grab bars in shower and other key locations
6. Referrals—consider dietician, occupational therapy, medical social worker, home health aide

Review Questions

Reader can find the correct answers and rationale in the back of the book.

Case Scenario #1

A 66-year-old female is referred for outpatient physical therapy s/p fall with resultant left hip fracture with open reduction internal fixation (ORIF) 3 weeks ago. Her medical history reveals invasive ductal carcinoma of the left breast (Stage 2b, estrogen receptor (ER)-positive, progesterone receptor (PR)-negative, human epidermal growth factor receptor 2 (HER2)-negative). She underwent a surgical resection 3 months ago and has completed radiation therapy. Additionally, she opted for chemotherapy based on her oncotype outcomes, but had a reaction to chemo during her second round of intervention, so further treatment was discontinued. Examination of her left lower extremity identifies edema through the extremity and tenderness with firm palpation in posterior calf and the popliteal space.

1. Which of the following is a common arrhythmia to observe for in this individual?
   A. Ventricular fibrillation
   B. Atrial flutter
   C. Atrial fibrillation
   D. Second degree Mobitz II heart block

2. Using the Wells Criteria this individual would be at what risk level for deep vein thrombosis?
   A. No risk
   B. Low risk
   C. Moderate risk
   D. High risk

3. This patient's laboratory values are as follows:

White Blood Cells	5.6 K/µL
Hemoglobin	8.3 g/dL
Platelets	204 K/µL
Potassium	3.5 mmol/L

If the individual experiences an elevated HR, dyspnea, and a decrease in activity/exercise tolerance, which lab value may be the MOST likely a contributor?
   A. Platelets
   B. White blood cell
   C. Hemoglobin
   D. Potassium

4. Use of METs is pertinent in the rehabilitative treatment of this individual because METs:
   A. Are a valid and reliable tool that stay constant in every patient scenario

B. Quantify the intensity of a particular activity

C. Are calculated based on an individual's HR and rate perceived exertion

D. Should be used in isolation to guide exercise intensity parameters for PLWBC

5. Three minutes into an exercise test performed at the initial evaluation visit the following is observed:

Heart rate	Changes from regular to irregular rhythm
Blood pressure	Decreases from 132/70 mmHg to 86/52 mmHg
Oxygen saturation	91%
Symptoms	Patient reports shortness of breath and dizziness

The MOST appropriate immediate action regarding the exercise test is to:

A. Stop activity and call the physician

B. Stop and have the patient come back to be retested

C. Continue with the exercise

D. Continue with the exercise and call the physician

Case Scenario #2

A 48-year-old male is referred to home healthcare s/p right atrial resection for malignant PCA 4-month ago. He has since received adjuvant therapy inclusive of chemotherapy (ifosfamide [Ifex] combined with docetaxel [Taxotere]) and radiation therapy, and targeted biologic immunotherapy. He is O_2 dependent (3L O_2 via nasal cannula) and meets homebound criteria due to an inability to leave home without significant effort and assistance. Patient self-reports intermittent chest tightness and a nonproductive cough. At the initial therapy assessment, the patient reports 1+ dyspnea at rest and 3+ dyspnea on exertion (DOE); however, SpO_2 remains within normal range (96%). His resting HR is 64 beats per minute. Additionally, impairment in lower extremity strength and balance are identified.

6. A symptom this individual is encountering that is common to both pulmonary and cardiac toxicity is:

A. Shortness of breath

B. Dry cough

C. Heart palpitations

D. Fluid retention in the legs

7. Cardiotoxicity risk would increase in this individual for each of the following cancer-related interventions EXCEPT:

A. High dose chemotherapy in bolus form

B. Combination chemotherapy delivery

C. Anthracycline use in the course of treatment

D. Nonconcurrent mediastinal radiation

8. When educating this patient in energy conservation principles, which of the following is MOST correct:

A. Perform activities quickly to allow time for rest

B. Pursed lip breathing can be a useful adjunct to reduce stress and promote relaxation

C. Position the body to increase the work of breathing

D. Plan the day to get things done promptly followed by long rest times

9. During the therapy exercise session the patient identifies he is at a 13 on the Borg 6 to 20 rating of perceived exertion scale. Which of the following MOST likely represents an associated intensity measurement for this patient?

A. Estimated HR of 180 beats per minute

B. Estimated HR of 80 beats per minute

C. Workload is at 85% of the HR range

D. Workload is at 60% of the HR range

10. Which of the following statements concerning dyspnea is MOST correct?

A. It is an independent predictor of mortality in heart disease

B. It is an objective measure of difficult, labored breathing

C. The Total Dyspnea Scale for Cancer is not recommended to measure dyspnea

D. It is uncommon in individuals with cardiac disease

References

1. Center for Disease Control and Prevention. Leading Cause of Death. https://www.cdc.gov/nchs/fastats/leading-causes-of-death.htm. Accessed September 25, 2020.

2. Bartels M, Syrkin G. Cardiac complications of cancer and their treatment. In: Stubblefield MD, ed. *Cancer Rehabilitation Principles and Practice.* 2nd ed., Springer Publishing Company; 2019:413–420.

3. Leja MJ, Shah DJ, Reardon MJ. Primary cardiac tumors. *Texas Hear Inst J.* 2011;38(3):261–262. http://doi.org/10.1097/00007611-198210000-00023.

4. Orlandi A, Ferlosio A, Roselli M, Chiariello L, Spagnoli LG. Cardiac sarcomas: an update. *J Thorac Oncol.* 2010;5(9):1483–1489. http://doi.org/10.1097/JTO.0b013e3181e59a91.

5. Nakamura-Horigome M, Koyama J, Eizawa T, et al. Successful treatment of primary cardiac angiosarcoma with docetaxel and radiotherapy. *Angiology.* 2008;59(3):368–371. http://doi.org/10.1177/0003319707308212.

6. Doherty D, Arena S, Claucherty E, Moore S. Primary cardiac angiosarcoma. *Rehabil Oncol.* 2019;37(2):64–69. http://doi.org/10.1097/01.REO.0000000000000147.

7. Patel SD, Peterson A, Bartczak A, et al. Primary cardiac angiosarcoma: a review. *Med Sci Monit.* 2014;20:103–109. http://doi.org/10.12659/MSM.889875.

8. Hoffmeier A, Sindermann JR, Scheld HH, Martens S. Herztumoren—diagnostik und chirurgische therapie, *Dtsch Arztebl Int.* 2014;111(12):205–211. http://doi.org/10.3238/arztebl.2014.0205.

9. Siontis BL, Zhao L, Leja M, et al. Primary cardiac sarcoma: a rare, aggressive malignancy with a high propensity for brain metastases. *Sarcoma.* 2019;2019:1–6. http://doi.org/10.1155/2019/1960593.

10. Jeudy J, Burke AP, Frazier AA. Cardiac lymphoma. *Radiol Clin North Am.* 2016;54(4):689–710. http://doi.org/10.1016/j.rcl.2016.03.006.

11. Scherpereel A, Wallyn F, Albelda SM, Munck C. Novel therapies for malignant pleural mesothelioma. *Lancet Oncol.* 2018;19(3):e161–e172. http://doi.org/10.1016/S1470-2045(18)30100-1.

12. Mazurek JM, Syamlal G, Wood JM, Hendricks SA, Weston A. Malignant mesothelioma mortality—United States, 1999–2015, *MMWR Morb Mortal Wkly Rep.* 2017;66(8):214–218. http://doi.org/10.15585/mmwr.mm6608a3.

13. Mankad R, Herrmann J. Cardiac tumors: echo assessment. *Echo Res Pract.* 2016;3(4):R65–R77. http://doi.org/10.1530/ERP-16-0035.

14. Reynen K, Köckeritz U, Strasser RH. Metastases to the heart. *Ann Oncol.* 2004;15(3):375–381. http://doi.org/10.1093/annonc/mdh086.

15. Goldberg AD, Blankstein R, Padera RF. Tumors metastatic to the heart. *Circulation.* 2013;128(16):1790–1794. http://doi.org/10.1161/CIRCULATIONAHA.112.000790.

16. Siegel RL, Miller KD, Jemal A. Cancer statistics, 2018. *CA Cancer J Clin.* 2018;68(1):7–30. http://doi.org/10.3322/caac.21442.

17. American Cancer Society. What is lung cancer? https://www.cancer.org/cancer/lung-cancer/about/what-is.html; 2019. Accessed September 23, 2020.

18. American Cancer Society. SEERs lung cancer survival rates; 2019. https://www.cancer.org/cancer/lung-cancer/detection-diagnosis-staging/survival-rates.html. Accessed September 23, 2020.

19. Jamil A, Kasi A. *Cancer, Metastasis to the Lung.* StatPearls Publishing; 2020. https://www.ncbi.nlm.nih.gov/books/NBK553111/.

20. Fay M, Poole CM, Pratt G. Recent advances in radiotherapy for thoracic tumours. *J Thorac Dis.* 2013(Suppl 5):S5. http://doi.org/10.3978/j.issn.2072-1439.2013.08.46.

21. Wirsdörfer F, de Leve S, Jendrossek V. Combining radiotherapy and immunotherapy in lung cancer: can we expect limitations due to altered normal tissue toxicity? *Int J Mol Sci.* 2018;20(1):24. http://doi.org/10.3390/ijms20010024.

22. Walls GM, Hanna GG, Qi F, et al. Predicting outcomes from radical radiotherapy for non-small cell lung cancer: a systematic review of the existing literature. *Front Oncol.* 2018;8:1–9. http://doi.org/10.3389/fonc.2018.00433.

23. Rossi A, Di Maio M. Platinum-based chemotherapy in advanced non-small-cell lung cancer: optimal number of treatment cycles. *Expert Rev Anticancer Ther.* 2016;16(6):653–660. http://doi.org/10.1586/14737140.2016.1170596.

24. Oun R, Moussa YE, Wheate NJ. The side effects of platinum-based chemotherapy drugs: a review for chemists. *Dalt Trans.* 2018;47(19):6645–6653. http://doi.org/10.1039/C8DT00838H.

25. National Comprehensive Cancer Network. Cardiac toxicity; 2021. https://www.nccn.org/patients/resources/life_with_cancer/managing_symptoms/cardiac_toxicity.aspx. Accessed August 1, 2021.

26. Perez IE, Taveras Alam S, Hernandez GA, Sancassani R. Cancer therapy-related cardiac dysfunction: an overview for the clinician. *Clin Med Insights Cardiol.* 2019;13. http://doi.org/10.1177/1179546819866445.

27. Fogli S, Nieri P, Cristina Breschi M. The role of nitric oxide in anthracycline toxicity and prospects for pharmacologic prevention of cardiac damage. *FASEB J.* 2004;18(6):664–675. http://doi.org/10.1096/fj.03-0724rev.

28. Touyz RM, Herrmann J. Cardiotoxicity with vascular endothelial growth factor inhibitor therapy. *NPJ Precis Oncol.* 2018;2(1):13. http://doi.org/10.1038/s41698-018-0056-z.

29. Mendes A. Cardiotoxicity of cancer therapy and current research efforts. *Br J Community Nurs.* 2020;25(6):308. http://doi.org/10.12968/bjcn.2020.25.6.308.

30. Rashdan S, Minna JD, Gerber DE. Diagnosis and management of pulmonary toxicity associated with cancer immunotherapy. *Lancet Respir Med.* 2018;6(6):472–478. http://doi.org/10.1016/S2213-2600(18)30172-3.

31. Canadian Cancer Society. Radiation Pneumonitis. https://www.cancer.ca/en/cancer-information/diagnosis-and-treatment/managing-side-effects/radiation-pneumonitis/?region=on; 2021. Accessed August 1, 2021.

32. Yanagawa B, Mazine A, Chan EY, et al. Surgery for tumors of the heart. *Semin Thorac Cardiovasc Surg.* 2018;30(4):385–397. http://doi.org/10.1053/j.semtcvs.2018.09.001.

33. Kanzaki M. Current status of robot-assisted thoracoscopic surgery for lung cancer. *Surg Today.* 2019;49(10):795–802. http://doi.org/10.1007/s00595-019-01793-x.

34. Melfi FMA, Fanucchi O, Davini F, Mussi A. VATS-based approach for robotic lobectomy. *Thorac Surg Clin.* 2014;24(2):143–149. http://doi.org/10.1016/j.thorsurg.2014.02.003.

35. Hu X, Wang M. Efficacy and safety of robot-assisted thoracic surgery (RATS) compare with video-assisted thoracoscopic Surgery (VATS) for lung lobectomy in patients with non-small cell lung cancer, *Comb Chem High Throughput Screen.* 2019;22(3):169–178. http://doi.org/10.2174/1386207322666190411113040.

36. Asnani A, Manning A, Mansour M, Ruskin J, Hochberg EP, Ptaszek LM. Management of atrial fibrillation in patients taking targeted cancer therapies. *Cardio-Oncology.* 2017;3(1):2. http://doi.org/10.1186/s40959-017-0021-y.

37. Leduc C, Antoni D, Charloux A, Falcoz PE, Quoix E. Comorbidities in the management of patients with lung cancer. *Eur Respir J.* 2017;49(3):1–12. http://doi.org/10.1183/13993003.01721-2016.

38. Straka C, Ying J, Kong FM, Willey CD, Kaminski J, Kim DWN. Review of evolving etiologies, implications and treatment strategies for the superior vena cava syndrome. *Springerplus.* 2016;5(1):1–13. http://doi.org/10.1186/s40064-016-1900-7.

39. Lepper PM, Ott SR, Hoppe H, et al. Superior vena cava syndrome in thoracic malignancies, *Respir Care.* 2011;56(5):653–666. http://doi.org/10.4187/respcare.00947.

40. Cohen R, Mena D, Carbajal-Mendoza R, Matos N, Karki N. Superior vena cava syndrome: a medical emergency?. *Int J Angiol.* 2008;17(1):43–46. http://doi.org/10.1055/s-0031-1278280.

41. Busti F, Marchi G, Ugolini S, Castagna A, Girelli D. Anemia and iron deficiency in cancer patients: role of iron replacement

therapy. *Pharmaceuticals.* 2018;11(4):1–14. http://doi.org/10.3390/ph11040094.

42. Timp JF, Braekkan SK, Versteeg HH, Cannegieter SC. Epidemiology of cancer-associated venous thrombosis. *Blood.* 2013;122(10): 1712–1723. http://doi.org/10.1182/blood-2013-04-460121.

43. White C, Noble SIR, Watson M, et al. Prevalence, symptom burden, and natural history of deep vein thrombosis in people with advanced cancer in specialist palliative care units (HIDDen): a prospective longitudinal observational study. *Lancet Haematol.* 2019;6(2):e79–e88. http://doi.org/10.1016/S2352-3026(18)30215-1.

44. Lee HH, Hwang IC, Shin J. Association between D-dimer levels and the prognosis of terminal cancer patients in the last hours of life. *Korean J Hosp Palliat Care.* 2020;23(1):11–16. http://doi.org/10.14475/kjhpc.2020.23.1.11.

45. Handy JR, Asaph JW, Skokan L, et al. What happens to patients undergoing lung cancer surgery? Outcomes and quality of life before and after surgery. *Chest.* 2002;122(1):21–30. http://doi.org/10.1378/chest.122.1.21.

46. Messaggi-Sartor M, Marco E, Martínez-Téllez E, et al. Combined aerobic exercise and high-intensity respiratory muscle training in patients surgically treated for non-small cell lung cancer: a pilot randomized clinical trial. *Eur J Phys Rehabil Med.* 2019;55(1). http://doi.org/10.23736/S1973-9087.18.05156-0.

47. Peddle-McIntyre CJ, Singh F, Thomas R, Newton RU, Galvão DA, Cavalheri V. Exercise training for advanced lung cancer. *Cochrane Database Syst Rev.* 2019;2019(2). http://doi.org/10.1002/14651858.CD012685.pub2.

48. Bhatia C, Kayser B. Preoperative high-intensity interval training is effective and safe in deconditioned patients with lung cancer: a randomized clinical trial. *J Rehabil Med.* 2019;51(9):712–718. http://doi.org/10.2340/16501977-2592.

49. Arena SK, Doherty DJ, Bellford A, Hayman G. Effects of aerobic exercise on oxidative stress in patients diagnosed with cancer: a narrative review. *Cureus.* 2019;11(8):1–12. http://doi.org/10.7759/cureus.5382.

50. Sterns RH. Adverse consequences of overly-rapid correction of hyponatremia. *Front Horm Res.* 2019;52:130–142. http://doi.org/10.1159/000493243.

51. Duane S Pinto, Garan AR. Pathophysiology of Cardiogenic Pulmonary Edema. UpToDate; 2019. https://www.uptodate.com/contents/pathophysiology-of-cardiogenic-pulmonary-edema; 2019.

52. Norton M, Alkurashi AK, Hasan Albitar HA, Almodallal Y, Iyer VN. A rare case of chemotherapy induced phrenic neuropathy. *Respir Med Case Reports.* 2020;30(May):101117. http://doi.org/10.1016/j.rmcr.2020.101117.

53. Chahin A, Riestra Guiance I, Than A, Srinivasamurthy R, Rajagopalan N. Chopping phrenic nerve—chemotherapy induced unilateral phrenic neuropathy. In: American Thoracic Society 2020 International Conference, May 15–20, 2020—Philadelphia, PA: A7491–A7491. doi: http://doi.org/10.1164/ajrccm-conference.2020.201.1_meetingabstracts.a7491.

54. Stevens WW, Sporn PHS. Bilateral diaphragm weakness after chemotherapy for lymphoma. *Am J Respir Crit Care Med.* 2014;189(7):201304. http://doi.org/10.1164/rccm.201304-0642IM.

55. Bray FN, Simmons BJ, Wolfson AH, Nouri K. Acute and chronic cutaneous reactions to ionizing radiation therapy. *Dermatol Ther (Heidelb).* 2016;6(2):185–206. http://doi.org/10.1007/s13555-016-0120-y.

56. Therapy Academy of Acute Care Physical Therapy—APTA Acute Care Task Force on Lab Values. *Laboratory values interpretation resource; 2017.* https://cdn.ymaws.com/www.aptaacutecare.org/resource/resmgr/docs/2017-Lab-Values-Resource.pdf.

57. Medline Plus. Myoglobin blood test. U.S. National Library of Medicine.

58. Medline Plus. C-Reactive protein (CRP) test. U.S. National Library of Medicine; 2020. https://medlineplus.gov/lab-tests/c-reactive-protein-crp-test/

59. Medline Plus. Erythrocyte sedimentation rate (ESR). U.S. National Library of Medicine; 2020. https://medlineplus.gov/lab-tests/erythrocytesedimentation- rate-esr/.

60. Késmárky G, Kenyeres P, Rábai M, Tóth K. Plasma viscosity: a forgotten variable. *Clin Hemorheol Microcirc.* 2008;39(1–4):243–246. http://doi.org/10.3233/CH-2008-1088.

61. Oleksiewicz U, Daskoulidou N, Liloglou T, et al. Neuroglobin and myoglobin in non-small cell lung cancer: expression, regulation and prognosis. *Lung Cancer.* 2011;74(3):411–418. http://doi.org/10.1016/j.lungcan.2011.05.001.

62. Watson J, Salisbury C, Banks J, Whiting P, Hamilton W. Predictive value of inflammatory markers for cancer diagnosis in primary care: a prospective cohort study using electronic health records. *Br J Cancer.* 2019;120(11):1045–1051. http://doi.org/10.1038/s41416-019-0458-x.

63. Hillegass E. *Essentials of Cardiopulmonary Physical Therapy-E-Book.* 4th ed.: Elsevier Health Sciences; 2016.

64. Palatini P. Need for a revision of the normal limits of resting heart rate. *Hypertension.* 1999;33(2):622–625. http://doi.org/10.1161/01.HYP.33.2.622.

65. Keroes J LD. Normal heart sounds. Medical Training and Simulation LLC; 2017. https://www.practicalclinicalskills.com/auscultationcourse- contents?courseid=22. Accessed June 27, 2020.

66. Arena S. Heart sounds, physical therapy, and home healthcare, *Home Healthc Now.* 2018;36(6):392. http://doi.org/10.1097/NHH.0000000000000742.

67. Viganego F, Singh R, Fradley MG. Arrhythmias and other electrophysiology issues in cancer patients receiving chemotherapy or radiation. *Curr Cardiol Rep.* 2016;18(6):52. http://doi.org/10.1007/s11886-016-0730-0.

68. McLaughlin AN, Policarpo G. Hypertension in cancer patients. *Community Oncol.* 2012;9(10):324–330. http://doi.org/10.1016/j.cmonc.2012.09.013.

69. Morris GS. Oh blood pressure measurements—where art thou? *Rehabil Oncol.* 2018;36(2):79–80. http://doi.org/10.1097/01.REO.0000000000000118.

70. Severin R, Sabbahi A, Albarrati A, Phillips SA, Arena S. Blood pressure screening by outpatient physical therapists: a call to action and clinical recommendations. *Phys Ther.* 2020;100(6):1008–1019. http://doi.org/10.1093/ptj/pzaa034.

71. Association C and PS of the APT Vitalarevital; 2019. https://www.cardiopt.org/vitalsarevital/. Accessed June 27, 2020.

72. Riebe D, Franklin BA, Thompson PD, et al. Updating ACSM's recommendations for exercise preparticipation health screening. *Med Sci Sports Exerc.* 2015;47(11):2473–2479. http://doi.org/10.1249/MSS.0000000000000664.

73. Borg G. *Borg's Perceived Exertion and Pain Scales.* Human Kinetics; 1998.

74. Morishita S, Tsubaki A, Nakamura M, Nashimoto S, Fu JB, Onishi H. Rating of perceived exertion on resistance training in elderly subjects. *Expert Rev Cardiovasc Ther.* 2019;17(2):135–142. http://doi.org/10.1080/14779072.2019.1561278.

75. Green DJ, Spence A, Halliwill JR, Cable NT, Thijssen DHJ. Exercise and vascular adaptation in asymptomatic humans. *Exp Physiol.* 2011;96(2):57–70. http://doi.org/10.1113/expphysiol.2009.048694.

76. Riebe D, Ehrman J, Liguori G, Magal M. Clinical exercise testing and interpretation, In: *American College of Sports Medicine,* 10th ed.: Wolters Kluwer; 2018:126.

77. Riebe M, Riebe D, Ehrman J, Liguori G, Magal M. Exercise preparticipation health screening, In: *American College of Sports Medicine,* 10th ed.: Wolters Kluwer; 2018:29.

78. Paz JC, West M. *Acute Care Handbook for Physical Therapists.* 5th ed.: Butterworth-Heinemann; 2019.

79. Pesola GR, Ahsan H. Dyspnea as an independent predictor of mortality. *Clin Respir J.* 2016;10(2):142–152. http://doi.org/10.1111/crj.12191.

80. Hashimoto H, Kanda K. Development and validation of the Total Dyspnea Scale for Cancer Patients. *Eur J Oncol Nurs.* 2019;41(May):120–125. http://doi.org/10.1016/j.ejon.2019.05.007.

81. Riebe D, Ehrman J, Liguori G, Magal M. Health related physical fitness testing and interpretation. In: *American College of Sports Medicine.* 10ᵗʰ ed.: Wolters Kluwer; 2018:81.

82. Jones LW, Liang Y, Pituskin EN, et al. Effect of exercise training on peak oxygen consumption in patients with cancer: a meta-analysis. *Oncologist.* 2011;16(1):112–120. http://doi.org/10.1634/theoncologist.2010-0197.

83. Ainsworth BE, Haskell WL, Herrmann SDet al. 2011 Compendium of physical activities. *Med Sci Sport Exerc.* 2011;43(8):1575–1581. http://doi.org/10.1249/MSS.0b013e31821ece12.

84. American College of Sports Medicine. ACSM's Guidelines for Exercise Testing and Prescription,11th ed., Lippincott Williams & Wilkins, 2022.

85. Schmidt K, Vogt L, Thiel C, Jäger E, Banzer W. Validity of the six-minute walk test in cancer patients. *Int J Sports Med.* 2013;34(7):631–636. http://doi.org/10.1055/s-0032-1323746.

86. Gilchrist S, Barac A, Ades P, et al. Cardio-oncology rehabilitation to manage cardiovascular outcomes in cancer patients and survivors: a scientific statement from the American Heart Association. *Circulation.* 2019;139:e997–e1012. http://doi.org/10.1161/CIR.0000000000000679.

87. Kasymjanova G, Correa JA, Kreisman H, et al. Prognostic value of the six-minute walk in advanced non-small cell lung cancer. *J Thorac Oncol.* 2009;4(5):602–607. http://doi.org/10.1097/JTO.0b013e31819e77e8.

88. Lee H, Kim HK, Kang D, et al. Prognostic value of 6-min walk test to predict postoperative cardiopulmonary complications in patients with non-small cell lung cancer. *Chest.* 2020;157(6):1665–1673. http://doi.org/10.1016/j.chest.2019.12.039.

89. Johnston KN, Potter AJ, Phillips AC. Minimal important difference and responsiveness of 2-minute walk test performance in people with COPD undergoing pulmonary rehabilitation. *Int J Chron Obstruct Pulmon Dis.* 2017;12:2849–2857. http://doi.org/10.2147/COPD.S143179.

90. Karande GY, Hedgire SS, Sanchez Y, et al. Advanced imaging in acute and chronic deep vein thrombosis. *Cardiovasc Diagn Ther.* 2016;6(6):493–507. http://doi.org/10.21037/cdt.2016.12.06.

91. Markel A, Weich Y, Gaitini D. Doppler ultrasound in the diagnosis of venous thrombosis. *Angiology.* 1995;46(1):65–73. http://doi.org/10.1177/000331979504600109.

92. Sartori M, Gabrielli F, Favaretto E, Filippini M, Migliaccio L, Cosmi B. Proximal and isolated distal deep vein thrombosis and Wells score accuracy in hospitalized patients. *Intern Emerg Med.* 2019;14(6):941–947. http://doi.org/10.1007/s11739-019-02066-8.

93. Hwan YJ, Shin J, Jin YJ, Lee JW. Comparison of clinical manifestations and outcomes of noncirrhotic and cirrhotic hepatocellular carcinoma patients with chronic hepatitis B. *Eur J Gastroenterol Hepatol.* 2020;32(1):66–73. http://doi.org/10.1097/MEG.0000000000001478.

94. Insall RL, Davies RJ, Prout WG. Significance of Buerger's test in the assessment of lower limb ischaemia. *J R Soc Med.* 1989;82(12):729–731. http://doi.org/10.1177/014107688908201209.

95. Wright WF, Rajachandran M. Buerger test for erythromelalgia revisited. *J Am Osteopath Assoc.* 2017;117(2):124–126. http://doi.org/10.7556/jaoa.2017.023.

96. Stanford Medicine. Introduction to Measuring the Ankle Brachial Index. https://stanfordmedicine25.stanford.edu/the25/ankle-brachial-index.html. 2020. Accessed April 11, 2022.

97. Espinola-Klein C, Rupprecht HJ, Bickel C, et al. Different calculations of ankle-brachial index and their impact on cardiovascular risk prediction. *Circulation.* 2008;118(9):961–967. http://doi.org/10.1161/CIRCULATIONAHA.107.763227.

98. Aboyans V, Criqui MH, Abraham P, et al. Measurement and interpretation of the Ankle-Brachial Index: a scientific statement from the American Heart Association. *Circulation.* 2012;126(24):2890–2909. http://doi.org/10.1161/CIR.0b013e318276fbcb.

99. Visonà A, De Paoli A, Fedeli U, et al. Abnormal ankle-brachial index (ABI) predicts primary and secondary cardiovascular risk and cancer mortality. *Eur J Intern Med.* 2020;77:79–85. http://doi.org/10.1016/j.ejim.2020.02.033.

100. APTA—Acute Care Section and Academy of Cardiovascular and Pulmonary Physical Therapy, *Adult Vital Sign Interpretation in Acute Care Guide 2021* (2021). https://www.aptacvp.org/clinical-practice-guidelines.

101. Ebede CC, Jang Y, Escalante CP. Cancer-related fatigue in cancer survivorship. *Med Clin North Am.* 2017;101(6):1085–1097. http://doi.org/10.1016/j.mcna.2017.06.007.

102. Horneber M, Fischer I, Dimeo F, Rüffer JU, Weis J. Tumor-assoziierte fatigue: epidemiologie, pathogenese, diagnostik und therapie, *Dtsch Arztebl Int.* 2012;109(9):161–172. http://doi.org/10.3238/arztebl.2012.0161.

103. Bower JE. Cancer-related fatigue—mechanisms, risk factors, and treatments. *Nat Rev Clin Oncol.* 2014;11(10):597–609. http://doi.org/10.1038/nrclinonc.2014.127.

104. Repka CP, Hayward R. Oxidative stress and fitness changes in cancer patients after exercise training. *Med Sci Sports Exerc.* 2016;48(4):607–614. http://doi.org/10.1249/MSS.0000000000000821.

105. Repka CP, Hayward R. Effects of an exercise intervention on cancer-related fatigue and its relationship to markers of oxidative stress. *Integr Cancer Ther.* 2018;17(2):503–510. http://doi.org/10.1177/1534735418766402.

106. K. Webster D, Cella, K Yost. The functional assessment of chronic illness therapy (FACIT) measurement system: properties, applications, and interpretation. *Heal Qual Life Outcomes.* 2003;1(79). http://doi.org/10.1186/1477-7525-1-79.

107. Naylor EC, Desani JK, Chung PK. Targeted therapy and immunotherapy for lung cancer. *Surg Oncol Clin N Am.* 2016;25(3):601–609. http://doi.org/10.1016/j.soc.2016.02.011.

108. Heart Online. Rating of perceived exertion: Borg scales. Heart Education Assessment Rehabilitation ToolKit; 2014. https://www.sralab.org/sites/default/files/2018-04/Rating_of_perceived_exertion_-_Borg_scale.pdf. Accessed April 11, 2022.

109. Ries AL. Minimally clinically important difference for the UCSD Shortness of Breath Questionnaire, Borg Scale, and Visual Analog Scale. *COPD J Chronic Obstr Pulm Dis.* 2005;2(1):105–110. http://doi.org/10.1081/COPD-200050655.

110. Pulmonary Rehabilitation Toolkit. Lung Foundation Australia. https://pulmonaryrehab.com.au/patient-assessment/resources/; 2016. Accessed April 11, 2022

111. Shirley Ryan Ability Lab. Baseline and transitional dyspnea index. https://www.sralab.org/rehabilitation-measures/transition-dyspnea-index. Accessed April 11, 2022.

112. Moran LA, Guyatt GH, Norman GR. Establishing the minimal number of items for a responsive, valid, health-related quality of life instrument. *J Clin Epidemiol.* 2001;54(6):571–579. http://doi.org/10.1016/S0895-4356(00)00342-5.

113. Williams N. The MRC breathlessness scale. *Occup Med (Chic Ill).* 2017;67(6):496–497. http://doi.org/10.1093/occmed/kqx086.

114. Barr JT, Schumacher GE, Freeman S, LeMoine M, Bakst AW, Jones PW. American translation, modification, and validation of the St. George's Respiratory Questionnaire. *Clin Ther.* 2000;22(9):1121–1145. http://doi.org/10.1016/S0149-2918(00)80089-2.

115. Persinger R, Foster C, Gibson M, Fater DCW, Porcari JP. Consistency of the talk test for exercise prescription. *Med Sci Sports Exerc.* 2004;36(9):1632–1636. http://www.ncbi.nlm.nih.gov/pubmed/15354048.

11

Gastrointestinal System

LORI E. BORIGHT, PT, DPT, DSCPT, EMILY COMPAGNER, PT, DPT

CHAPTER OUTLINE

Introduction

Gastrointestinal (GI) cancers are collectively among the most commonly diagnosed of all cancers worldwide. GI cancers include esophageal, stomach, pancreatic, small intestine, liver and intrahepatic bile duct, colon, rectum, and anus. The oncology rehabilitation (Onc R) management of cancers of the colon, rectum, and anus will be discussed in Chapter 17. Colon cancers account for the most significant portion, approximately one-third of all GI cancers.[1] Males are also generally more susceptible to cancers of the GI system than females (refer to Table 11.1). Significant post-treatment complications and higher rates of morbidity are also associated with cancers of the GI system due principally to the invasive nature of surgical intervention, as well as need for neoadjuvant and/or adjuvant chemotherapy and radiation.[1] As such, implications relative to potential functional compromise and diminished quality of life (QOL) secondary to neoplasm and adverse effects of treatment are of paramount importance to Onc R disciplines. The primary aim of this chapter is to highlight the most commonly encountered adverse effects of the medical management of GI cancers and provide strategies for Onc R assessment and management.

Considerations of these diagnoses are significant because many pancreatic and esophageal cancers are not diagnosed until later stages. Therefore, these diagnoses carry greater cumulative treatment and rehabilitative burden as well as significantly lower 5-year survival rates, 10% and 19.9%, respectively.[2] As with pancreatic cancers, gastric cancers tend to behave more aggressively and carry lower 5-year survival rates as well (see Table 11.2).[2]

Risk Factors

Risk factors for developing cancers of the GI system vary slightly by region and can be categorized by dietary and nondietary influences. Risks generally increase with age, consumption of any type of tobacco, and obesity. Dietary risk factors for the development of esophageal cancer include low consumption of fruits and vegetables and consumption of very high-temperature liquids.[3] Nondietary risk factors of esophageal cancer include the presence of Barrett's esophagus and GI reflux disease (GERD), human papillomavirus (HPV) infection, and occupational chemical exposure.[3] Dietary risk factors for gastric cancers include consumption of pickled foods, cured meats, and high-temperature foods. Nondietary risk factors for gastric cancer include *H. pylori* bacterial infection, family history, and occupational chemical exposure.[3] Hepatitis B infection is a risk factor for developing liver cancer.[3]

Anatomy of the Gastrointestinal System

GI cancers traditionally encompass those of the esophagus, stomach (gastric), pancreas, liver (biliary), small intestine, colon, and rectum (see Figure 11.1). In all, GI cancers are more commonly diagnosed as primary cancers, although in pancreatic, gastric, biliary, and colorectal cancers (CRC), there are few if any observable symptoms; therefore, metastatic disease spread is common at the time of diagnosis.

Physiology of the Gastrointestinal System

The collective functions of the GI tract are digestion and absorption of nutrients from ingested food. These functions are supported

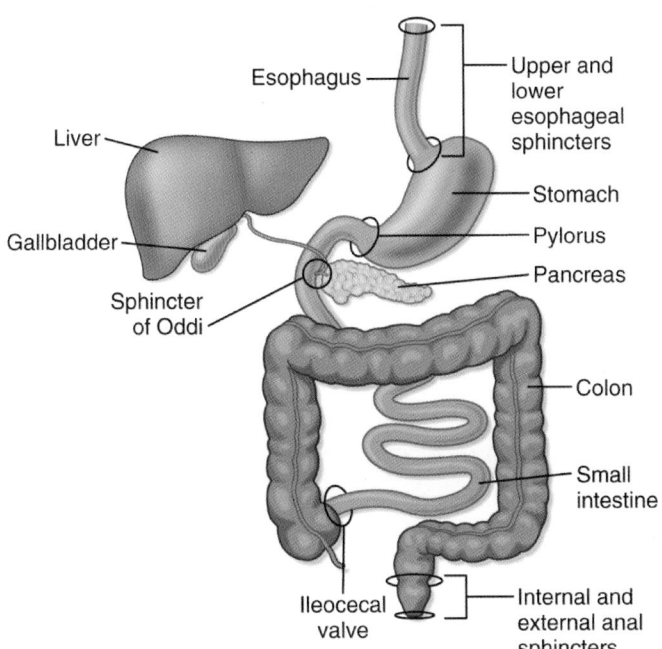

• **Fig. 11.1** Anatomy of GI System.[4] (Reprinted with permission from Koppen BM, Stanton BA. Chapter 27: Functional anatomy and general principles of regulation in the gastrointestinal tract. In: *Berne & Levy Physiology*. 7th ed. Elsevier; 2018:511–519.)

by (1) movement of food from the mouth to the rectum (esophagus, stomach, small and large intestines); (2) enzyme, electrolyte, and mucous secretions (pancreas and liver) aid in digestion (stomach and small intestine); and (3) absorption of water, electrolyte, and nutrients into the bloodstream (small and large intestines).[5]

The physiologic consequence of GI cancers has manifold impact owing to the significant supportive and vital functions of this complex system on the human body.

Primary Versus Secondary Disease

Primary cancers in the GI system are more common and more likely than secondary or metastatic cancers at advanced stages. When cancer is detected in proximal lymph nodes, there is an increased risk of metastasis in distant lymph nodes, derived from colon, biliary, and gastric cancers. However, these diagnoses still carry a smaller probability of metastatic disease.[6] Direct infiltration of cancer from a local site is more common within the GI tract than through vascular spread.[7] Cancers that commonly manifest secondary neoplasms in this region include malignant melanoma, breast cancer, and pancreatic cancer.[7]

Diagnosis/Staging Criteria

Imaging studies are useful tools for correlating cancer diagnoses of the GI system. Ultrasound (US), computed tomography (CT), and magnetic resonance imaging (MRI) are useful for detecting primary lesions, whereas positron emission tomography (PET) scanning is helpful for determining presence and extent of distant metastatic disease.[8] Refer to Table 11.3 for staging by cancer type.

Continuum of Care for Gastrointestinal Population

Evidence for prehabilitation, or pretreatment physiologic optimization, is strongest among the CRC population and is gaining traction with many other cancer diagnoses.[10] Chapter 27 is

TABLE 11.3 Cancers of the GI System Follow the Tumor, Node, Metastasis (TNM) System of Staging

Esophageal Cancer		Stomach Cancer		Pancreatic Cancer	
Primary Tumor		**Primary Tumor**		**Primary Tumor**	
Tis:	High-grade dysplasia	Tx:	Tumor cannot be assessed	Tx:	Primary tumor cannot be assessed
T1:	Invasion into lamina propria, muscularis mucosae, or submucosa	T0:	No evidence of primary tumor	T0:	No evidence of tumor
T2:	Invasion into muscularis propria	Tis:	Carcinoma in situ	Tis:	Carcinoma in situ
T3:	Invasion into adventitia	T1:	Invades the lamina propria or submucosa and ≤1 cm in size	T1:	Tumor limited to pancreas ≤2 cm in greatest dimension
T4a:	Invasion into respectable adjacent structures (i.e., pleura, pericardium, diaphragm)	T2:	Invades the muscularis propria or ≥1 cm in size	T2:	Tumor limited to pancreas, in 2–4 cm in dimension
T4b:	Invasion into unresectable adjacent structures (i.e., aorta, trachea, vertebral body)	T3:	Invades through the muscularis propria into subserosal tissue without penetration of overlying serosa	T3:	Tumor more than 4 cm in greatest dimension
Regional Lymph Nodes		T4:	Invades visceral peritoneum (serosa) or other organs or adjacent structures	T4:	Tumor involves celiac axis superior mesenteric artery and or common hepatic artery regardless of size
N0:	No regional lymph node metastasis	**Regional Lymph Nodes**		**Regional Lymph Nodes**	
N1:	Metastases in 1–2 regional lymph nodes	Nx:	Regional lymph nodes cannot be assessed	Nx:	Regional lymph nodes cannot be assessed

Continued

TABLE 11.3   Cancers of the GI System Follow the Tumor, Node, Metastasis (TNM) System of Staging Adapted From the American Joint Committee on Cancer[9]—cont'd

Esophageal Cancer		Stomach Cancer		Pancreatic Cancer	
N2:	Metastases in 3–6 regional lymph nodes	N0:	Zero regional lymph node metastasis	N0:	Zero regional lymph node metastasis
N3	7+ positive regional lymph nodes	N1:	Regional lymph node metastasis	N1:	Metastases in 1–3 regional lymph nodes
Distant Metastases		Distant Metastasis		N2:	Metastases in 4+ regional lymph nodes
M0:	No distant metastases	M0:	No distant metastasis	Distant Metastases	
M1:	Distant metastasis	M1:	Distant metastasis	M0:	No distant metastases
		M1a:	Metastasis confined to liver	M1:	Distant metastasis
		M1b:	Metastases ≥1 extrahepatic site (i.e., any site other than the liver)		
		M1c:	Both hepatic and extrahepatic metastases		

Liver Cancer		Colon Cancer	
Primary Tumor		Primary Tumor	
Tx:	Primary tumor cannot be assessed	Tx:	Primary tumor cannot be assessed
T0:	No evidence of primary tumor	T0:	No evidence of primary tumor
T1:	Tumor ≤2 cm	Tis:	Carcinoma in situ; intramucosal carcinoma (involvement of lamina propria with no extension through muscularis mucosae)
T2:	Tumor >2 cm but no more than 5 cm	T1:	Carcinoma in situ
T3:	Tumor 5–10 cm	T2:	Invades through muscularis propria into pericolorectal tissues
T4:	Tumor >10 cm in greatest dimension	T3:	Invades through inter subserosa
Regional Lymph Nodes		T4:	Directly invades or adheres to adjacent organs or structures
N0:	No regional lymph node metastasis or unknown lymph node status	Regional Lymph Nodes	
N1:	Regional lymph node metastasis	Nx:	Regional lymph nodes cannot be assessed
Distant Metastases		N0:	No regional lymph node metastasis
M0:	No distant metastasis	N1:	One to three regional nodes are positive (tumor in lymph nodes measuring 0.2 mm+ or any number of tumor deposits are present and all identifiable lymph nodes are negative)
M1:	Distant metastasis	N1a:	One regional lymph node is positive
		N1b:	Two to three regional lymph nodes are positive
		N1c:	No regional nodes are positive, but there are tumor deposits in subserosa, mesentery, or nonperitonealized pericolic or perirectal/mesorectal tissues
		N2:	Four or more regional nodes are positive
		N2a:	Four to six regional nodes are positive
		N2b:	Seven or more regional nodes are positive
		Distant Metastases	
		M0:	No distant metastasis
		M1:	Metastasis to 1+ distant sites or organs, or peritoneal metastasis is identified
		M1a:	Metastasis to one site or organ without peritoneal metastasis
		M1b:	Metastasis to two or more sites or organs without peritoneal metastasis
		M1c:	Metastasis to peritoneal surface alone or with other site or organ metastases

M, Metastasis; *N*, lymph node; *T*, tumor.
Adapted from American College of Surgeons. *AJCC Cancer Staging Manual.* 8th ed. Springer International Publishing; 2017.

dedicated to the discussion of this pivotal time for assessment and intervention along the cancer continuum of care. The opportunity to gather baseline metrics, to educate the person living with and

beyond cancer (PLWBC), and provide therapeutic interventions to address the anticipated adverse effects of surgery, radiation, and/or chemotherapy among other medical interventions is invaluable and should be exercised. Prehabilitation has been found to improve overall functional status based on outcome measures.[11] The PRE-PARE program is a multimodal oncology prehabilitation program developed by Imperial College Healthcare NHS Trust for patients with esophageal cancer. The outcomes of this program included reduced length of hospital stay and postoperative morbidity.[12]

Other prehabilitation interventions that are of paramount importance when working with this population include smoking cessation and optimization of nutritional status. Smoking is a risk factor for many GI cancers and is also a known detriment to tissue healing and overall recovery. Providing the necessary resources and strategies to eliminate tobacco use prior to the onset of treatment bears significant advantage to the PLWBC. Additionally, optimizing nutritional status prior to medical intervention bears similar advantage in that there is an anticipated postoperative weight loss/cachexia resultant of difficulty with swallowing and digestion, and therefore the potential need for nutritional supplementation in the presentation of severe cachexia or inability to maintain adequate caloric intake is a principal consideration.

Enhanced Recovery After Surgery (ERAS) is an evidence-based method of implementing early postoperative exercise for the PLWBC of the GI system to encourage faster recovery, decrease postoperative complications, and increase functional outcomes.[13] These benefits are likely due to decreased perioperative stress, which has also been suspected to cause an increase in cancer recurrence.[13] ERAS protocols have been found to enhance immune response postoperatively and are likely connected to the improved outcomes and 5-year survival rates, within the CRC population.[13] PLWBCs' compliance with ERAS programming further benefits outcomes.[13,14] Additionally, an inverse relationship has been identified with increased compliance leading to shorter length of hospital stay for ERAS participants.[14] Staff education and participant encouragement fuels compliance to the ERAS protocol, and further supports positive outcomes.[15]

The postoperative Onc R course for the PLWBC of the GI system can include admission to an inpatient rehabilitation unit for comprehensive multidisciplinary interventions that promote functional independence and facilitate a safe home discharge. Home healthcare rehabilitation provides continued care for PLWBCs of the GI system to maximize independence with functional tasks and activities of daily living (ADLs). Outpatient Onc R is often viewed as the most traditional setting to receive rehabilitation services, though it is important to recognize and advocate for Onc R throughout the continuum of care as needs arise.

Common Adverse Effects

Common adverse effects resultant of GI malignancy management bear significant consequence due to the role that nutritional status plays in optimization of recovery from medical intervention. As with other diagnoses, and discussed in detail in Chapter 14, the psychological consequences of stress and anxiety are substantial considerations with this population. The following is an overview of the most commonly observed adverse effects as they relate to the GI system.

Cachexia

Though problematically common among persons diagnosed with cancer, cachexia has historically been an underfunded area of clinical research. See Figure 11.2 for a clinical presentation of a person with cachexia. Broadly, cachexia is a multifactorial sequelae

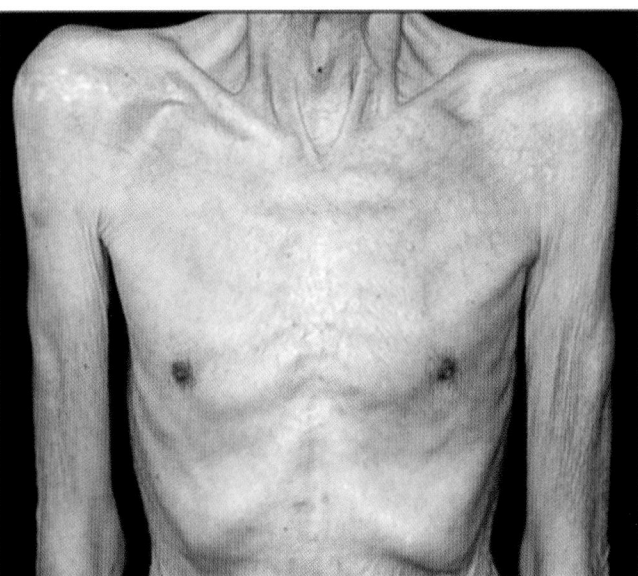

• **Fig. 11.2** Cachexia.[16] (Reprinted with permission from Muscaritoli M. Targeting cancer cachexia: we're on the way. *Lancet Oncol.* 2016;17(4): 414–415.)

resultant of malnutrition and of particular consequence to persons diagnosed with GI cancers. It is primarily characterized by anorexia, asthenia, and loss of skeletal muscle mass,[17] though recent research suggests that other tissues are adversely affected (brain, liver, heart) and contribute to muscle atrophy.[18] Further, the impact on cardiac muscle tissues, cardiac atrophy, should not be underscored and contributes to the potentially fatal consequences of cachexia.[18,19] Research is beginning to support physical exercise as a modality to attenuate cardiac atrophy resultant of cachexia.[18] Research states that nutritional therapies are ineffective at reversing the syndrome and global consequences include declines in functional status.[20] Pathophysiologically, the syndrome can be described as a negative protein and energy balance that is fueled by diminished food intake and abnormal metabolic activity.[20] A framework has been developed to stratify the diagnosis and portrays precachexia, cachexia, and refractory cachexia as a continuum. It should be noted that not all persons will advance through every stage, and some are able to reverse course based on the effectiveness of their medical interventions (see Figure 11.3).[20] Multimodal intervention during the precachexic and cachexic stages is imperative for prevention and is aimed at slowing the progression of sequelae to promote function and improve QOL.[19]

Malnutrition

Malnutrition and malabsorption are complex and manifold in etiology, though both are significant considerations in the continuum of survivorship for PLWBCs of the GI system. Consequences of malnutrition include diminished function, compromised QOL, increased length of hospital stay, and poorer prognosis.[21] Thus, nutritional support at the time of diagnosis, at regular intervals through active treatment, and into survivorship is of paramount importance to maintain or improve status before, during, and after medical treatment which increases the risk of developing malnutrition and subsequently prevents future complications. Sarcopenia, loss of skeletal muscle, is an associated factor of malnutrition, and as such contributes to the negative

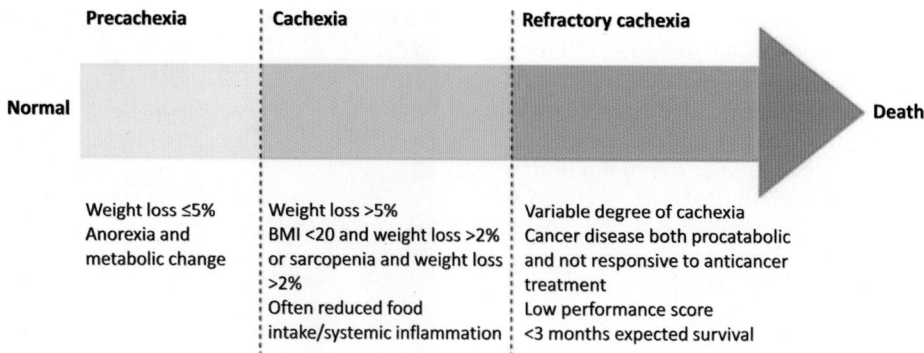

• **Fig. 11.3** Stages of Cachexia.[19,20] (Reprinted with permission from Ozorio GA, Barão K, Forones NM. Cachexia stage, patient-generated subjective global assessment, phase angle, and handgrip strength in patients with gastrointestinal cancer. *Nutr Cancer.* 2017;69(5):772–779.)

energy-protein balance (see Chapter 7 for more on sarcopenia). Medical assessment for malnutrition typically encompasses a combination of anthropometric measurements (height, weight, body mass index [BMI]) and blood samples.[22] Evidence supports the use of various malnutrition indicators such as serum albumin and c-reactive protein for prognosis of pancreatic, gastric, and CRC malignancies.[21] Referral to a registered dietitian (RD) or registered dietitian nutritionist (RDN) is warranted for all PLWBCs of the GI system though principally when risk of malnutrition is suspected. In many cancer centers, these clinicians are part of the multidisciplinary team and address needs throughout the continuum of care. See Chapter 30 for a discussion on the importance of the Onc R clinician's role in nutrition counseling.

Hernia

For the purpose of this discussion, hernia is a protrusion of the intestines through the abdominal wall and is a common consequence of GI surgery. Evidence suggests that females are more likely to develop a hernia postsurgically. Persons >65 years of age, those who have received open procedures, and have had surgical intervention in a low surgical volume institution are risk factors for developing postsurgical hernias within 3 years of surgical intervention.[23] Hernias may cause pain and intestinal obstruction and can require emergent care in cases where intestinal strangulation is present. Though less common, minimally invasive, or laparoscopic, procedures carry consequences as well if the incision/port site is greater than 10 mm with concurrent fascial defect of the same size.[24] On average, hernias present within 3 to 4 months following surgical intervention, and require additional surgical intervention to resolve. Early postoperative bowel obstruction has been correlated with hernias, with midline and umbilical port sites translating far greater incidences of this complication than other port site locations.[24] Hernia prevention consists of adherence to a prescribed diet, abdominal muscle strengthening under supervision of an Onc R clinician, use of an abdominal binder, correct body mechanics for transfers and lifting, and avoidance of straining when passing urine or stool.[25]

Ascites

Ascites is the accumulation of intra-abdominal fluid resulting from portal hypertension that can occur with malignant disease, cirrhosis, and heart failure. Medical management involves use of diuretics, serial paracentesis, or removal via indwelling catheter, though

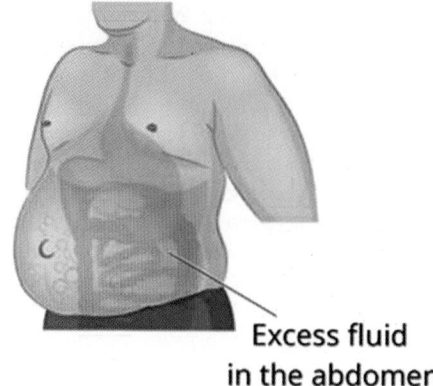

Excess fluid in the abdomen

• **Fig. 11.4** Ascites.[26] (Reprinted with permission from Elsevier. Ascites. Elsevier Patient Handouts.)

adverse events such as bacterial infection (often) and catheter malfunction (less common) can manifest.[27] A long-term abdominal drain (e.g., PleurX) generally provides more sustainable symptom palliation over paracentesis by allowing the PLWBC to drain intermittently at home versus requiring repeated serial procedures for those with persistent ascites. Prevalence of ascites in persons with malignant GI cancers is cited as high as 21% and is primarily seen in those with pancreatic, CRC, gastric, liver, and gallbladder cancers.[27] Palliative services are encouraged at the onset of ascites as short-term impairments and poor prognosis are common. One study noted the average survival after diagnosis of cancer-related ascites was 5.7 months.[28] Only 11% of persons diagnosed with ascites related to their cancer diagnosis survive longer than 6 months.[29] See Figure 11.4 for a clinical presentation of a person with ascites.

Diarrhea and Constipation

Chemotherapy-induced diarrhea (CID) and chemotherapy-induced constipation (CIC) are commonly reported adverse effects and are often a primary cause of treatment delay and reported reductions in QOL.[30] Incidence of CIC is reported at 16% where CID is cited as high as 80% depending on specific treatment protocol and medication dosages.[30] Etiology is not well understood but believed to be multifactorial and inclusive of inflammation, intestinal neuropathy, and secretory dysfunction.[30] Persistent CID and CIC contributes to alterations in treatment protocols, dose

TABLE 11.4 Criteria for Chemotherapy-Induced Diarrhea and Chemotherapy-Induced Constipation

Adverse Effect	Grade 1	Grade 2	Grade 3	Grade 4	Grade 5
	Uncomplicated		Complicated		
Diarrhea	Less than four stools over baseline/day	Four to six stools over baseline/day	Greater than seven stools over baseline/day	Life threatening, requires urgent intervention	Fatal
	Present for >4 weeks		Present for <4 weeks		
Constipation	Occasional/intermittent symptoms, occasional use of stool softeners, laxatives, enema	Persistent symptoms, regular use of laxatives or enemas, limits instrumental ADLs	Obstipation with manual evacuation, limits self-care ADLs	Life threatening, requires urgent intervention	Fatal

ADL, Activities of daily living.
Adapted from National Cancer Institute Common Terminology Criteria for Adverse Events.[31]

reductions, treatment delays, as well as treatment suspensions and, therefore, significantly impacts clinical outcomes for this population (see Table 11.4 for criteria for CID and CIC). CID is different from average diarrhea as the chemotherapy targets the rapidly dividing cells of the GI system. Improvement in diarrhea likely requires cessation or limiting of chemotherapy treatment, so cells are able to build back up in the GI system. Residual effects have also been noted to persist up to 10 years post-treatment and is a significant contributing factor in the aforementioned cachexic and malnutrition sequelae.[30] Treatment strategies are relative to classifications in Table 11.4 and include antidiarrheal medication, diet modification, and energy conservation in uncomplicated CID to more aggressive symptom management in a hospital setting with more severe cases of complicated CID. Interventions initially recommended for the management of CIC include increasing physical activity as well as fluid and fiber consumption. Medically managed measures to address CIC include various laxative options (oral and/or rectal bulk forming, emollient, osmotic/saline, and lubricant).[30]

Adverse Effects From Radiation

The adverse effects of radiation will vary depending on the field, mechanism of delivery, and patient dose response. Adverse effects related to the mucosal layer that lines the GI system can perpetuate acute effects from radiation that include radiation gastritis and radiation enteritis. These acute adverse effects manifest in persons living beyond cancer (PLBCs) as nausea, vomiting, stomach cramps, diarrhea, and or constipation.[32] Subacute adverse effects of radiation include changes in the liver, which can manifest in radiation-induced liver disease, approximately 2 to 3 months after radiation at or near the liver is complete. The subacute adverse effects are related to the mean dose delivered during the radiation cycle. Chronic or late term adverse effects of radiation therapy include fibrosis, mucosal dysfunction, stricture, intestinal dysmotility, nutritional deficits, and bile acid malabsorption.[32] The clinical manifestations of the chronic adverse effects present months to years after radiation as ulceration, dietary intolerance, vitamin deficiency, diarrhea, bloating, constipation, and secondary malignancy.

Radiation-Induced Fibrosis

Radiation-induced fibrosis (RIF) is an abnormal wound healing process following radiation therapy that can occur weeks to years

later. Along with causing DNA damage, ionized radiation results in reactive oxygen and nitrogen species that lead to acute and potentially chronic inflammation. Radiated tissue can result in tissue hardening from the increased deposition of collagen matrix causing reduced perfusion and scarring of the impacted tissue, which can have significant effects on the GI system.[33] Resultantly, this progressive fibrotic tissue sclerosis creates decreased tissue mobility and delayed or absence of wound healing. RIF is modulated by the area being radiated, the dose of radiation, and fraction size of radiation.[34] Damage to and tissue fibrosis of the mucosal layer of the GI system can cause chronic issues such as dysmotility, stenosis, and fistula formation.[32] Furthermore, PLBCs are at an increased risk of fibrosis if they have any history of smoking, poor diet, diabetes, and other inflammatory diseases.[32] These PLBCs are also at higher risk of late term effects that are additive including but not limited to transmural fibrosis, collagen deposition, and inflammatory infiltration of the mucosa.[32] After medication use for RIF, moderate exercise is recommended to facilitate return to everyday activities.[34] Participation in moderate exercise in many cases is linked to increased QOL and increased ability to manage day-to-day activities, by including range of motion (ROM), muscle strengthening, and cardiovascular interventions to promote physical efficiency and functional sustainability.[34] Onc R, and specifically the use of manual therapy, is a major part of supportive care as well as functional retraining for PLBCs post-treatment for cancer and RIF.

Radiation Gastritis

Radiation gastritis is an injury to the stomach secondary to increased gastric doses of radiation, especially dosages ≥550 cGy.[35] Radiation gastritis is a common occurrence following radiation of the esophagus, stomach, biliary duct, and pancreas due to their close proximity to the stomach during radiation treatment.[35] Radiation doses of 20 to 30 Gy can cause nausea and vomiting at 2 to 3 weeks post-treatment and is related to radiation gastritis. Mainstream medical management of radiation gastritis does not exist at the time of this publication beyond the use of antacids.[35]

Radiation Enteritis and Colitis

Radiation enteritis is a disorder that alters the function of the small bowel, commonly occurring during and after a course of radiation therapy to the abdomen, pelvis, or rectum. Signs and symptoms include diarrhea and nausea due to the altered mucosal lining of the intestinal tract. Efforts to mitigate radiation enteritis can be accomplished through altered positioning during radiation treatments to minimize exposure to unintended tissues. Chronic adverse effects of radiation enteritis can also lead to fibrosis and vasculitis of the bowel, which can manifest in chronic dysmotility, stricture formation, and malabsorption of the intestine.[32] Conversely, diarrhea may occur as well due to radiation treatments causing malnutrition and subsequent anemia. Alternate methods of providing nutrition such as total parenteral nutrition (TPN) is recommended to reduce further adverse effects of radiation treatment in those with severe malnutrition in this population. Tissue alterations in the small bowel have been found to increase surgical morbidity and necessitate surgical revision due to the changes in the mesentery and intestinal tract.[32] It is important to note that radiation enteritis is likely to occur during a course of radiation treatment, as acute adverse effects of radiation enteritis often occur at 10 Gy, well below the threshold of the curative dosage for abdominal/pelvic tumors of 50 to 75 Gy.[32]

Constipation

Constipation after radiation can be due to a variety of factors including dysmotility, narrowing of the intestinal lumen, and/or stricture formation in the large intestine. The narrowing of the intestinal lumen can result in additional stricture formation due to the dilation of the proximal portion of the bowel and the fibrosis of the mucosa, further increasing the likelihood of constipation symptoms. The amount of narrowing is related to the amount of radiation over time to a localized area of the bowel. When these dosages exceed 50 Gy or more within 5 weeks, there is increased incidence of small bowel obstruction and surgical intervention is required in 25 to 50% of cases.[36] Medications also alter the course of constipation symptoms so medication review should also be considered as an important component of rehabilitative assessment.

Radiation Considerations

Radiation can have a significant effect on the cancer treatment process, and each PLWBC should be treated individually depending on cancer type and the total treatment course received. Adverse effects of radiation treatment do present slightly differently depending on the treatment course. The following offers considerations for each PLWBC depending on when they received radiation during their cancer continuum. Radiation recall is an acute inflammatory response of previously radiated regions to certain pharmacologic agents including chemotherapies.[37] Incidence is low and pathophysiology is poorly understood, though Onc R clinicians should remain aware of this phenomenon. They should institute similar precautions as to recently radiated areas, avoiding direct contact with the skin for approximately 3 weeks after onset. Refer to Chapter 9 for additional information.

Neoadjuvant/Preoperative

Neoadjuvant radiation is used to treat local disease minimizing invasiveness of surgical resection and increasing the opportunity for complete resection. The use of radiation before surgical intervention is beneficial in many cases although the effect on the tumor depends on the field, delivery mechanism, and dose response to the area. For a person living with cancer (PLWC) in advanced stages, it has been found to not always be beneficial to incorporate neoadjuvant approaches to minimize morbidity with

surgical management and it may not change the need for further adjuvant therapies postoperatively in the lower GI cancers.[38] The use of neoadjuvant therapies increases the potential for reduced tumor size, especially in esophageal cancers, as well as proximal lymph node involvement, potentially downgrading tumor staging.[39] Preoperative radiation for CRC has been shown to decrease local recurrence and increase sphincter preservation.[40] Evidence supports decreased tissue toxicity following neoadjuvant radiation prior to surgical resection in patients with rectal cancer.[41]

Postoperative Radiation

Administration of radiation following surgical interventions requires special considerations when surgical clips or mesh have been used to secure and reconstruct tissues. Appropriate postoperative planning decreases severity of potential adverse effects by limiting the radiation field and avoiding surgically implanted devices. Surgical interventions may also aim to limit radiation to noncancerous tissues through use of clips suspending the intestines to condense the area to be radiated and limit implications to the genitourinary system from possible exposure. Similarly, these surgically implanted devices can be used to contain and protect other organs not intended to be radiated, to reduce radiation exposure to healthy tissues.[32] The use of a pelvic mesh has also shown to significantly decrease morbidity of bowel adhesions and does not significantly increase the length of the surgical procedure. This mesh is also reabsorbed by the body months after the surgical intervention, mitigating the need for a second surgery for removal.[32]

Chemotherapeutic Agents and Their Implications

The use of chemotherapeutic interventions for the management of GI cancers has expanded substantially. Increased 5-year and long-term survival rates are owed to this expanded implementation alongside early detection screening for CRC. Therefore, understanding the adverse effects of chemotherapy on the human body and the implications for QOL and physical function are of paramount importance for this population.

Fluoropyrimidines: Fluorouracil and Capecitabine

Fluorouracil (5-FU) (Adrucil) and capecitabine (Xeloda) are useful chemotherapeutic agents that integrate into the genetic material through the use of uracil to mimic natural human compounds. These chemotherapies are used to combat esophageal, gastric, hepatobiliary, and CRCs. Common adverse effects of fluoropyrimidines are myelosuppression (damage to bone marrow diminishing total blood count), mucositis, stomatitis, hand–foot syndrome (HFS), and adverse cardiac events.

Implications to therapy for the use of fluorouracil and capecitabine as a chemotherapeutic agent create physiologic changes in the digestive system in turn, altering blood lab values secondary to dehydration.[42] Cardiac toxicity is another common adverse effect that is dependent on the tolerated dose of treatment.[42] PLWBCs should be monitored for cardiac symptoms such as angina, palpitations, or malaise, especially with exercise. Cardiac toxicity may be fully reversed over two or more years after the treatment is discontinued, although the patient should still be monitored for adverse responses during therapeutic exercise.[42]

TABLE 11.5 **FDA-Approved Targeted and Chemotherapeutic Agents by GI Cancer Diagnosis[44]**

Type of Cancer	Chemotherapeutic Agents Approved for Use by the United States Food and Drug Administration
Esophageal	Pembrolizumab (Keytruda), nivolumab (Opdivo)
Gastroesophageal junction	Ramucirumab (Cyramza), trastuzumab (Herceptin), pembrolizumab (Keytruda), trifluridine and tipiracil hydrochloride (Lonsurf), docetaxel (Taxotere)
Stomach	Ramucirumab (Cyramza), fluorouracil (5-FU), doxorubicin hydrochloride, trastuzumab (Herceptin), pembrolizumab (Keytruda), trifluridine and tipiracil hydrochloride (Lonsurf), mitomycin (Mutamycin), docetaxel (Taxotere),
Gastrointestinal stromal tumors	Avapritinib (Ayvakit), imatinib mesylate (Gleevec), ripretinib (Quinlock), regorafenib (Stivarga), sunitinib malate (Sutent)
Pancreatic	Paclitaxel (Abraxane), everolimus (Afinitor), fluorouracil (5-FU), gemcitabine (Gemzar), irinotecan hydrochloride liposome (Onivyde), olaparib (Lynparza), mitomycin, sunitinib malate (Sutuent), erlotinib (Tarceva), capecitabine (Xeloda)
Liver	Bevacizumab (Avastin), cabozantinib (Cabometyx), ramucirumab (Cyramza), pembrolizumab (Keytruda), lenvatinib (Lenvima), sorafenib (Nexavar), nivolumab (Opdivo), pemigatinib (Pemazyre), regorafenib (Strivarga), atezolizumab (Tecentriq)
Colon	Bevacizumab (Avastin), irinotecan hydrochloride (Camptosar), capecitabine (Xeloda), ramucirumab (Cyramza), oxaliplatin (Eloxatin), cetuximab (Erbitux), fluorouracil (5-FU), pembrolizumab (Keytruda), folinic acid (leucovorin calcium), trifluridine and tipiracil hydrochloride (Lonsurf), bevacizumab (Mvasi), nivolumab (Optivo) regorafenib (Strivarga), panitumumab (Vectibix), ipilimumab (Yervoy), ziv-aflibercept (Zaltrap)
Rectal	Bevacizumab (Avastin), irinotecan hydrochloride (Camptosar), ramucirumab (Cyramza), oxaliplatin (Eloxatin), cetuximab (Erbitux), fluorouracil (5-FU), pembrolizumab (Keytruda), folinic acid (leucovorin calcium), trifluridine and tipiracil hydrochloride (Lonsurf), bevacizumab (Mvasi), nivolumab (Optivo), regorafenib (Strivarga), panitumumab (Vectibix), capecitabine (Xeloda), ipilimumab (Yervoy), ziv-aflibercept (Zaltrap)

Adapted from National Cancer Institute. Drugs approved for different types of cancer. https://www.cancer.gov/about-cancer/treatment/drugs/cancer-type. 2020. Accessed January 15, 2021.

Oxaliplatin

The use of platinum-based drugs, such as oxaliplatin (Eloxatin), aim to damage the DNA in tumor cells that are based on the formation of platinum-DNA.[42] Oxaliplatin is commonly used to treat esophageal, gastric, pancreatic, and CRCs. Common adverse effects of oxaliplatin exposure include disruption of hematologic values, nausea/vomiting, infusion reactions, and neurotoxicity.[42]

Oxaliplatin can be dose-limited to mitigate the intensity of adverse effects. These adverse effects also have implications to Onc R that should be addressed as appropriate throughout the treatment continuum. Specifically, PLWBCs should be screened continuously for neurotoxic effects of the oxaliplatin agents which manifest as peripheral neuropathy and may progress up to 8 weeks after the final dose.[43] Noticeable acute changes in the sensory and muscular system may occur 1 to 2 days after the first administration of oxaliplatin, and symptoms include paresthesia/dysesthesia within the upper and lower extremities, muscle hyperactivity, cramps, and muscle fasciculations.[43] Chronic adverse effects of oxaliplatin include functional changes resultant of neurotoxicity that also increase in magnitude with each dose and may manifest as muscle weakness, sensory changes, gait ataxia, vestibular deficits, and bowel and bladder dysfunction.[43]

Irinotecan

Irinotecan (Camptosar) utilizes a cascade of changes that alters cholinergic levels in the blood and causes increased amplitude of other adverse effects during treatment. Irinotecan is commonly used to treat rectal cancer and metastatic colon cancer. Common adverse effects include but are not limited to hematologic abnormalities, nausea/vomiting, mucositis/diarrhea, and alopecia.[42]

The most common and significant adverse effects of irinotecan is CID, resulting from severe mucositis. Implications to Onc R include low blood volume which necessitates increased oral (and potentially intravenous fluid) intake to combat the water volume loss.[43] Blood pressure and the timing of physical activity should be monitored to ensure safe mobilization and engagement in functional activities.

Chemotherapy During the Continuum of Cancer Treatment

Individualized treatment goals are determined by the medical oncologist with potential input from the interdisciplinary team and determine the type, frequency, and duration of each chemotherapy regimen. Additional considerations are given based on where in the continuum of care chemotherapy occurs. For example, a PLWC who undergoes chemotherapy prior (neoadjuvant) to surgical intervention is likely to have increased fatigue and weakness and potentially has increased need for therapeutic intervention following surgery. The Onc R team should have knowledge of the chemotherapeutic agents and their adverse effects when determining an individualized therapy plan of care. Adverse effects should be monitored, and referral to the treating physician is appropriate if deviation in plan of care occurs during the Onc R treatment secondary to adverse effects from chemotherapeutic agents. Close communication between the Onc R team and the medical oncologist allows for ease of dissemination of relevant information, questions, or concerns from both parties promoting patient-centered care. This allows for improved functional outcomes and expedited return to ADLs.

TABLE
11.6   **Biologic Therapies Per Cancer Diagnosis**[44]

Type of Cancer	Approved Targeted Biologic Therapies
Colorectal	Cetuximab (Erbitux), panitumumab (Vectibix), bevacizumab (Avastin), ziv-aflibercept (Zaltrap), regorafenib (Strivarga), ramucirumab (Cyramza), nivolumab (Opdivo), ipilimumab (Yervoy), encorafenib (Braftovi)
Esophageal	Trastuzumab (Herceptin), ramucirumab (Cyramza), pembrolizumab (Keytruda)
Gastrointestinal stromal	Imatinib mesylate (Gleevec), sunitinib (Sutent), regorafenib (Strivarga), avapritinib (Ayvaki)
Liver	Sorafenib (Nexavar), regorafenib (Strivarga), nivolumab (Opdivo), lenvatinib mesylate (Lenvima), pembrolizumab (Keytruda), cabozantinib (Cabometyx), ramucirumab (Cyramza), ipilimumab (Yervoy)
Pancreatic	Erlotinib (Tarceva), everolimus (Afinitor), sunitinib (Sutent), olaparib (Lynparza)
Gastric	Pembrolizumab (Keytruda), trastuzumab (Herceptin), ramucirumab (Cyramza)

Adapted from National Cancer Institute. Drugs approved for different types of cancer. https://www.cancer.gov/about-cancer/treatment/drugs/cancer-type. 2020. Accessed January 15, 2021.

Biologic Therapies

Biologic therapies for cancer management include immunotherapy that target domains of cancer cells and have seen substantial expansion in use for GI malignancy in recent years. This increase is largely due to continued advancements of successful phase II and III clinical trials. Refer to Chapter 5 for mechanisms of action, treatment delivery, and goals of intervention. What follows in this chapter is a summary of the most commonly used therapies for the GI cancer diagnoses as well as an interpretation of the Onc R implications of commonly encountered adverse effects. Refer to Tables 11.5 and 11.6 summaries of chemotherapeutic and biologic agents used in this population.

Vascular Endothelial Growth Factor Inhibition: Bevacizumab, Aflibercept, and Ramucirumab

Vascular endothelial growth factor (VEGF) inhibition is a type of biologic agent that is used in bevacizumab (Avastin), ziv-aflibercept (Zaltrap), and ramucirumab (Cyramza). These agents inhibit angiogenesis, slowing the growth of tumors through the decreased vascularization to the tumor. These targeted agents are commonly used in combination with other systemic chemotherapeutic agents as a primary line of treatment for gastric cancer and metastatic CRC.[42] Common adverse effects include but are not limited to hypertension, proteinuria, mucosal bleeding, arterial thrombosis, wound healing complications, and GI perforation.[42]

Considerations for Onc R for PLWBCs managed with VEGF inhibition are significant and include monitoring vitals during treatments to prevent large increases in blood pressure and heart rate with activity. Another Onc R consideration starting at 6 months after initiation of bevacizumab includes consideration of increased risk of GI perforation for PLWBCs who have undergone treatment for CRC.[42] Patient presentations of this adverse effect include patient reports of quick onset of severe stomach pain, fever, chills, nausea, and vomiting.[42]

Epidermal Growth Factor Receptor Inhibition: Cetuximab, Panitumumab

Epidermal growth factor receptor (EGFR) inhibition works to regulate the growth of epidermal cells and is specifically used for cancers located in the epidermis including RAS-wildtype tumors. These targeted chemotherapeutic agents have been used to manage colon cancers as well as pancreatic cancers as primary or secondary treatment. Common adverse effects associated with cetuximab (Erbitux) and panitumumab (Vectibix) include skin toxicity, hypomagnesemia, and infusion reactions.[42]

Adverse effects of EGFR inhibition include acute implications to Onc R clinicians if the patient is concurrently receiving infusions and Onc R services. EGFR inhibitors present an increased risk of dermatologic infections of the face, scalp shoulders, and upper trunk.[42] It is common for PLWCs to develop eczema and fissures. Open fissures present increased infection risk necessitating additional precautions. Long-term effects include EGFR inhibitor-induced magnesium wasting which manifests as progressive muscle dysfunction. Common symptoms of this sequelae may include tetany, weakness, ataxia, spasticity, tremor, and cramps. Cardiovascular disorders and neurocognitive changes may also present as a result of magnesium wasting.[42]

Targeted Therapies

Targeted therapies work to interface with specific proteins located on the tumor surface and work to treat/manage the disease in a variety of ways, including assisting the immune system to identify cancer cells, preventing tumor cell division, preventing angiogenesis, hormone suppression, facilitating tumor cell death, and delivering cell-killing agents to cancer cells.[45]

Targeted therapies often work best in combination with systemic chemotherapy or radiation to avoid resistance. The most common adverse effects of targeted therapies include elevated liver enzymes and diarrhea. Additional adverse effects may include issues with blood clotting, delayed wound healing, joint arthralgias, myalgias, hypertension, fatigue, mouth sores, nail changes, the loss of hair color, and skin problems (rash or dry skin).[45] Fistula formation is rare though possible and can affect the esophagus, stomach, small intestine, large bowel, rectum, or gallbladder.[45]

Many adverse effects can be managed effectively with Onc R interventions, though some circumstances may require medications prescribed by a physician. These may be used for the purpose of adverse effect prevention and others for palliation of symptoms once the adverse effects occur.[45]

Immunotherapy

Immunotherapies consist of immune checkpoint inhibitors, T-cell transfer therapy, monoclonal antibodies, treatment vaccines, and immune system modulators.[46] Adverse effects of immunotherapy include pain, swelling, redness, and itchiness at the injection site.[46]

Flu-like symptoms may also occur following treatment and include fever, chills, weakness, dizziness, nausea and/or vomiting, muscle and/or joint pain, fatigue, headache, trouble breathing, and low or high blood pressure.[46] Additional adverse effects may include swelling and weight gain resultant of fluid retention, heart palpitations, sinus congestion, diarrhea, risk of infection, and organ inflammation.[46]

Adverse effects specific to immune checkpoint inhibitors may are similar to an allergic reaction resulting from an overaction of the immune system. Adverse effects of particular relevance to the GI system include diarrhea, constipation, and nausea. Adverse effects that occur less commonly though that are of increased severity include hepatitis, colitis, and pancreatitis.[47] Specific symptomatology of hepatitis includes nausea, vomiting, dark urine, and bleeding/bruising easier than normal. In the case of colitis, diarrhea, increased frequency of bowel movements, stools that are black or tarry, sticky, and severe stomach pain are to be expected and may limit participation in Onc R.[47]

Implications for Oncology Rehabilitation

The cumulative physiologic burden of biologic therapy adverse effects specifically as they relate to the GI system is significant. Short- and long-term consequences of nausea, vomiting, and diarrhea can contribute to dehydration and malnutrition, impacting tolerance to continued medical management as well as strength and stamina to participate in Onc R programs manifesting further functional decline. Individualized exercise designed to meet current and evolving tolerance level, with careful vital sign monitoring and ongoing assessment of subjective symptoms is effective in mitigating functional decline throughout treatment, though evidence relative to medical treatment protocol completion is scant. Onc R assessments and interventions relative to the adverse effects noted will be discussed in detail later in this chapter.

Surgical Interventions and Adverse Effects

The intent of surgical interventions for GI cancers can be curative or aimed at disease management, though surgery potentially introduces significant postoperative complications for the PLWBC such as mobility and functional limitations, as well as morbidity and mortality. Oncologic surgical intervention of the GI system is invasive, possibly requiring sizable incisions, and encompasses cancer lesion resections including vascular and lymphatic pedicles as well as approximating structures such as partial or full organs, fascia, and mesentery. The PLWBC is at risk of developing visceral lymphedema if lymphatic tissue is disrupted and/or resected. Additionally, postoperative prophylactic blood thinning protocols are employed to reduce the risk of blood clot and embolism development. Major abdominal oncologic surgical procedures discussed in this section include: esophagectomy, gastrectomy, liver resection, Whipple procedure, and hyperthermic intraperitoneal chemotherapy (HIPEC).

There are several surgical options for esophagectomies: Ivor Lewis esophagectomy (incisions made in the center of the abdomen and in the back of the neck), transhiatal esophagectomy (two incisions including one in the neck and one in the abdomen, the remaining esophagus being attached to the stomach through the neck incision), McKeown esophagectomy (also known as three hole esophagectomy, three incisions in abdomen, neck, and right

upper back), and a minimally invasive procedure that entails the use of a laparoscope into the abdomen and chest through these three small incisions.[48]

Surgical options for gastrectomy include: subtotal gastrectomy (removal of cancerous part of the stomach, nearby lymph nodes, and other parts of other organs near the tumor such as the pancreas or small intestine), and total gastrectomy (removal of the entire stomach, nearby lymph nodes, and the small intestine which is then reconnected with the esophagus).[49]

Postsurgically, esophagectomy and gastrectomy patients require multiple tubes and lines which necessitates careful management on the part of the Onc R clinician with respect to all mobility activities. Clinical intervention suggestions entail: ambulating every 2 hours with assistance for line management and use of incentive spirometry and breathing exercises every 1 to 2 hours to prevent blood clot development and pneumonia. Onc R clinicians are advised to observe for any change in incision appearance which indicates a potential sign of infection. A recommendation to expedite return to function includes engagement of the surgical side during ADL performance and mobility to restore functional movement. The PLWBC is advised to avoid driving until functional ROM is restored which can take at least 4 to 6 weeks after surgery.[48,49]

A variety of surgical options exist for partial and total oncologic liver resection and the PLWBC may receive neoadjuvant chemotherapy prior to surgical intervention. Partial resection includes removal of one or more pieces of the liver while total liver resection involves removal of the entire organ and necessitates subsequent transplantation. The Onc R clinician must be mindful of postoperative bleeding risks due to proximity of major blood vessels as well as the highly vascular nature of the organ itself.[50]

The Whipple procedure is an invasive intervention that involves combination removal of the head of the pancreas, duodenum, gallbladder, the end of common bile duct, lymph nodes and occasionally part of the stomach typically via a single large incision.[51] Postoperative Onc R efforts should emphasize general mobility, elongated postures for sitting and standing tolerance, trunk strengthening, use of incentive spirometry, and coughing and breathing exercises.[51] Onc R clinicians should be advised that the acute postoperative PLWBCs will likely have multiple chest tubes. Postoperative restrictions include no lifting greater than 5 pounds and no strenuous activities for 8 weeks. Extreme precautions including use of assistive devices should be taken with early mobility to ensure safety during weight bearing postures for fall prevention.

HIPEC is a surgical technique that involves infusion of heated high-concentration chemotherapeutic agents through a surgically implanted catheter directly into the peritoneum (abdominal cavity) after tumor resection for the purpose of treating any remaining residual cancer cells within the cavity. The liquid is then evacuated from the peritoneum via a second catheter after a protocol-specified duration. Adverse effects related to chemotherapy exposure through HIPEC remain, though are reported less severely compared to systemic intravenous administration due to the reduced amount of chemotherapeutic agents systemically circulating through the bloodstream. Adverse effects related to the invasive surgical intervention conducted in tandem with HIPEC also remain and are similar to other major abdominal oncologic surgical procedures mentioned previously. The use of HIPEC for CRC and appendix cancers has gained traction in regions of the United States. Clinical trials at many nationally renowned cancer institutions are ongoing and continue to define efficacy for other GI and GYN cancers.[52]

Measurement Tools for Screening and Evaluation of Adverse Effects

Examination

Evidence for measurement tools related to the Onc R of the person diagnosed with GI cancer remains limited. What follows in this section are key recommendations to glean impactful data to enhance each PLWBC's Onc R journey. Each subsequent section reviews tests and measures that can be utilized for this population to identify Onc R needs and establish collaborative goals for treatment sessions.

Subjective History

Subjective history allows for individualized Onc R assessment and treatment and directs functional goals to encompass the PLWBC's ADLs to improve QOL. The PLWBC's subjective reports provide insights toward functional movement, cancer status, medical management, and dietary/medication concerns. Principal subjective assessments include medication review to identify potential adverse effects altering vital signs or ability to engage in exercise. Assessment of health status and home environment determines potential needs for assistive devices to support safety and/or independence with mobility, as well as the need for environmental modifications. Functional status and activity level assessments establish a baseline for comparative analysis throughout the survivorship continuum. Additionally, the PLWBC's function and activity level allows the Onc R clinician to establish patient-centered goals to increase adherence to therapy.

The Health Behavior Questionnaire (HBQ) is a useful tool[53] to assess and address potential dietary concerns and readiness for health behavior change. It is important to address dietary/

Imaging studies warrant review, due to potential impact on mobility and functional movement, especially in the presence of metastatic disease to the bone to determine appropriate weight bearing status. Comprehensive review of laboratory values is imperative to identify any concerns about blood cell counts particularly in relation to fatigue, infection, and bleeding risk.

nutrition status with this population due to the negative impact malnutrition has on functional activity tolerance. Referral to a registered dietician is appropriate especially in the absence of one on the multidisciplinary team.

Comprehensive understanding of the patient's previous medical history relating to their cancer journey is integral to create an appropriate assessment and treatment plan. The subjective interview should include questions to elicit diagnosis, stage/grade, locations of metastasis to glean perspective on the PLWBC's understanding of their diagnosis as well as direction the therapeutic approach toward rehabilitation or palliative care. Information regarding previous and current medical intervention assists in understanding and anticipating adverse effects as reported by the PLWBC or assessed by the clinician and should be addressed as appropriate (Box 11.1).

Objective Tests and Measures

Objective assessment should consist of a systematic and consistent approach of appropriate body systems that is repeatable and reliable to measure status change in the PLWBC. Table 11.7 provides considerations for inclusion in the objective assessment by body system for persons with GI cancers.

TABLE 11.7 Objective Assessment for People Living With or Beyond GI Cancer[19,54–67]

Body System	Evaluation Type/Tool	Evidence for Practice
Integumentary	Scar evaluation	Ziyu et al., 2019, examined the postsurgical outcomes of patients with surgery for gastric cancer and those who received laparoscopic surgical intervention had better postoperative safety and adjuvant chemotherapy tolerance than a patient with an open surgical intervention[54]
	Radiation burns	Hojan et al. 2014 indicated the importance of assessment of radiation fibrosis and radiation burns in patients. They stressed the importance of not mobilizing burned skins for 6 weeks and the importance of initiating treatment to maximize outcomes for radiation patients[59]
	Applied Wound Management Tool/The National Wound Assessment Form	Greatrex-White and Moxey, 2015, determined the Applied Wound Management Tool, and the National Wound Assessment Form were the most optimal tools to assess the areas of need of a specific wound. These assessment tools include evaluation of monitoring healing and guiding practice[60]
	Incision appearance integrity, skin hypersensitivity, sensitivity, radiation-induced fibrosis, other fascial restrictions	No direct evidence found regarding assessment tools but list includes other options to be considered for needs assessment
Cardiopulmonary	Aerobic assessment	Peel et al., 2009, suggesting better aerobic capacity and ability is related to improved outcomes with those diagnosed with colon, colorectal, and liver cancer especially in men[61]
	Six-Minute Walk Test	The Six-Minute Walk Test is a functional assessment of cardiorespiratory fitness that is valid and reliable in cancer populations[62]
	Two-Minute Walk Test	The Two-Minute Walk Test is a suitable alternative to the Six-Minute Walk Test[63]
Neurological	Numbness/neuropathy[a] (dermatomes, monofilament testing)	Chemotherapy-induced Peripheral Neuropathy Assessment Tool (CIPNAT) Rasch-built Overall Disability Scale for Patients with CIPN (CIPN-R-ODS)

TABLE 11.7   Objective Assessment for People Living With or Beyond GI Cancer—cont'd

Body System	Evaluation Type/Tool	Evidence for Practice
		European Organization for Research & Treatment in Cancer Quality of Life Quest—CIPN 20 Item (EORTC QLQ-CIPN 20) Patient Neurotoxicity Questionnaire (PNQ Taxanes, Cisplatin, and Carboplatin version) Modified Total Neuropathy Score (mTNS) Total Neuropathy Score, clinical version (TNSc) Five-item reduced Total Neuropathy Score (TNSr 5-item) Peripheral Neuropathy Scale (PNS) Scale for Chemotherapy-induced Neurotoxicity (SCIN)
Musculoskeletal	Strength (hand grip, thoracic, lumbar spine, core)	Liu et al., 2019, identified within cancer patients a decrease in grip strength as measured with a handheld dynamometer was associated with worse survival. The EDGE Taskforce has suggested to use hand-held dynamometry for muscle strength testing to establish changes from baseline in persons with CRC[64]
	Hand grip	Ozorio et al., 2017, established within patients with GI cancers or with cachexia secondary to cancer the patient's physical activity was correlated with handgrip strength[19,65]
	Range of motion (thoracic, lumbar spine, core)	No direct evidence found regarding assessment tools but list includes other options to be considered for needs assessment
Specific Functional Quality of Life Measures	Functional Assessment of Cancer Therapy (FACT)-Ga	Garland et al., 2011, demonstrated use of the FACT-Ga previously with patients diagnosed with gastric adenocarcinoma, it has been deemed as a useful instrument to assess QOL. The FACT-Ga can also detect significant changes in individual patients[66] The FACT-Ga identifies many things regarding the care of a person's treatment that is important to address and consider during their treatment (refer to Chapter 17 for additional Assessment Tools)
	FACT-E, FACT-HEP, FACT-C	No direct evidence found regarding assessment tools but list includes other options to be considered for needs assessment
Fatigue	Multidimensional fatigue symptom inventory short forms	The EDGE Task Force has identified multidimensional fatigue symptom inventory short forms with other cancer patients—assessment of fatigue is important and is effective through use of these assessments to identify fatigue in cancer patients[58]
	Modified Brief Fatigue Inventory (BFI), Visual Analog Scale (VAS)	No direct evidence found regarding assessment tools but list includes other options to be considered for needs assessment
Pain	Brief Pain Index (BFI)	The EDGE Task Force has identified the BFI to properly assess pain[58]
	VAS, numeric pain rating scale, McGill Pain Questionnaire (and short form)	No direct evidence found regarding assessment tools but list includes other options to be considered for needs assessment
Breathing	Use of incentive spirometry	Boden et al., 2018, concluded the use of an incentive spirometer as beneficial in the use postsurgical measurement of emergency abdominal surgical patients for tumor removal[67]
	Completion of diaphragmatic breathing, rib cage breathing	No direct evidence found regarding assessment tools but list includes other options to be considered for needs assessment
Cognitive Screen (CICI)	European Organization for Research & Treatment in Cancer Quality of Life Quest (EORTC QLQ-C30)	Baekelandt et al., 2016, demonstrated that a patient's presurgical cognitive function is a strong independent predictor of survival with pancreatic cancer[55]
	Mini-BEST, clock drawing, mini mental, trail making	No direct evidence found regarding assessment tools but list includes other options to be considered for needs assessment
Balance	Clinical Test of Sensory Integration on Balance (CTSIB)	Monfort et al., 2019, identified a need for assessment with patients who have been exposed to oxaliplatin secondary to increased risk for CIPN and used parts of CTSIB for analysis. Refer to Chapter 17 for further assessments regarding balance and colorectal cancer[56] Schmitt et al., 2017, identified that cancer survivors present with increased postural sway when compared to age-matched individuals. To assess postural sway. They used a modified CTSIB or recommend center of pressure measure to track progress of the individual to decrease fall risk[57]
	Four step, Berg Balance Test	No direct evidence found regarding assessment tools but list includes other options to be considered for needs assessment

[a]The EDGE taskforce research on CIPN in breast cancer patients recommends the following assessments to identify the impact of CIPN[58]: Oncology Group-Taxane (FACT/GOG-Taxane)
CIPN, Chemotherapy-induced polyneuropathy; CR, colorectal; CRC, colorectal cancer; E, esophageal; EDGE, Taskforce, evaluation database to guide effectiveness; FACT, functional assessment of cancer therapy; Ga, gastric; HEP, hepatic/liver; QOL, quality of life.
Created by Emily Compagner, PT, DPT.

Precautions and Contraindications for Treating Adverse Effects

Precautions

It is crucial that the Onc R clinician remain attentive to all nuances of medical management as well as the person's responses. The Onc R clinician should be prepared to alter assessments, re-assessments, and interventions as needed throughout the survivorship trajectory.[68] Special considerations for the treatment of PLBWCs who have an ostomy will be discussed in Chapter 17. Chemotherapeutic agents carry the potential for diminished blood counts (myelosuppression) and thus increased levels of fatigue, infection, and bleeding risk are present.[68] In the event of metastatic disease to bone, exercise should be carefully prescribed and monitored.[68] Chapters 7 and 20 provide further detail for these considerations. Knowledge of the PLWBC's chemotherapeutic history in relation to cardiotoxicity is important for exercise prescription, and Chapter 6 can be referenced for additional details. Rehabilitative neurotoxicity management details can be found in Chapter 8. Lifting and mobility precautions as prescribed by the referring physician must be adhered to status post abdominal surgery due to compromise of abdominal musculature and therefore core stability.[68] Refer to Chapter 17 for additional information on lifting and mobility precautions.

Red Flags

Signs and symptoms that warrant prompt attention and referral to an appropriate multidisciplinary team member are commonly referred to as red flags. A few red flags for which clinical surveillance is required will be covered in this section. Ongoing assessment of deep vein thrombosis (DVT) is critical at all times for PLWBCs and should be considered as a differential diagnosis for onset of edema. Appropriate attention to the international normalized ratio (INR) and referral to a member of the medical management team when DVT is suspected is important to minimize any risk of a pulmonary embolism.[68] Signs and symptoms of DVT include warmth, erythema, and pain in a localized area. Laboratory values require monitoring to ensure white blood cell counts are within the appropriate range to avoid compounding immunocompromise. Refer to Chapter 24 for additional information on laboratory values and monitoring in this population. Reported symptoms of fever, chills, and night sweats are indications of infection warranting referral to a physician for work up. Bladder dysesthesia, a consequence of neurotoxicity resultant of chemotherapeutic intervention for GI cancers will be discussed in detail in Chapters 12 and 16. Surgical incisions should be monitored postoperatively for signs of infection including dehiscence, redness, swelling, warmth to touch, and fever.[68]

Access the patient information handout on red flags online at http://www.expertconsult.com.

Rehabilitation Strategies for Prevention and Management of Adverse Effects

Prehabilitation

Evidence for the efficacy of health optimization before cancer treatment, termed prehabilitation, is mounting in the oncology domain. Prehabilitation for GI cancers, especially CRC, is among the most prevalent in the literature. Interventions should encompass multiple domains including physical, nutritional, and psychological. A systematic review and meta-analysis in 2018 revealed that prehabilitation significantly decreased days spent in the hospital compared with controls (weighted mean difference of length of hospital stay = 2.2 days; 95% confidence interval = 3.5–0.9).[69] Analysis of the individual studies showed multimodal prehabilitation significantly improved results of the 6-minute walk test at 4 and 8 weeks after surgery compared with standard Enhanced Recovery Pathway care and at 8 weeks compared with standard Enhanced Recovery Pathway care with added rehabilitation.[69] Additional details on prehabilitation mode, frequency, duration relative to cancer type will be explored in Chapter 27.

Patient Education

Providing education to the PLWBC and approved their support person(s) is a hallmark of comprehensive Onc R intervention. Information can be provided during treatment sessions and evolve organically based on the PLWBC's needs and inquiry. However, topics should include information on the adverse effects of surgery, chemotherapy, radiation therapy, and biologic therapies. Additionally, progressive home exercise program (HEP) instruction should be a cornerstone of educational interventions. A HEP should be provided in many forms such as verbal, visual, and written. Providing education over the course of several treatment sessions/weeks of Onc R lessens the burden of incoming information for the PLWBC. Information handouts, videos, and references on these and other topics prove to be beneficial resources to the PLWBC and their support network throughout the survivorship trajectory and minimize the need to commit to memory and/or take notes during sessions. Some handouts are available in the enhanced eBook. With the PLWBC's consent, involving the support person(s) during treatment sessions proves improved retention of educational concepts provided.

Additional information that can be considered important to include under the auspices of PLWBC education include benefits of physical activity as well as local and national support group opportunities for people with GI cancers. Information on what to expect during therapy sessions as well as a "red flags" for when to consult their physician or the Onc R clinician are also important inclusions in a comprehensive patient education model of care. Refer to the enhanced eBook for a sample educational handout.

Manual Therapy

Evidence is scant for the efficacy of many manual techniques (myofascial release, joint mobilization, soft tissue mobilization) used for the purpose of restoring proper soft tissue mobility for this population of patients diagnosed with cancer. Recommendations for manual interventions for genitourinary/gynecological and CRC populations will be formally addressed in Chapters 16 and 17.

Exercise Recommendations

The benefits of exercise/physical activity are becoming increasingly more apparent in the literature.[70–73] Meta-analyses demonstrate statistically significantly reduced risk of esophageal adenocarcinoma and gastric cancers for individuals that engage in highest versus lowest levels of activity.[72] Optimal programs begin at the point of diagnosis, to establish baseline status, provide education, and fortify physiologic reserves in advance of anticipated stressors. Refer to Chapter 23 for more on this topic.[74] There is sufficient and evolving evidence to demonstrate that exercise/physical activity provides benefits to QOL as well as muscular and aerobic status for PLWBCs before, during, and after treatment. The Canadian Society for Exercise Physiology's Canadian Physical Activity Guidelines and the American College of Sports Medicine (ACSM) support this growing evidence.[71,75] It is also principally important to note that these benefits can be realized in the absence of causing harm.[71] The ACSM guidelines specify 150 minutes of moderate intensity aerobic exercise per week over 3 to 5 days as tolerated should be completed by the PLWBC.[71,75] Resistance exercises should include all major muscle groups 2 to 3 days/week.[71,75] Refer to Chapter 23 for additional information regarding exercise prescription.

A comprehensive and patient-centered plan of care includes exercise that addresses functional, physiologic, and biomechanical deficits inclusive of breathing exercises (incentive spirometer, refer to breathing exercise video in the enhanced eBook), ROM, flexibility training, extremity and trunk strengthening, balance training, and aerobic exercise. Breathing exercises promote relaxation as well as reduction of potential respiratory complications (Video 11.1).[76]

Resistance exercise to promote strengthening should address the individual deficits of the PLWBC relative to identified extremity and especially trunk weakness in this population. Restoration of optimal posture to restore mobility, breathing, balance, and digestion is another important component of a comprehensive plan of care. Trunk and functional strengthening exercises can assist in this effort as well as patient-specific body mechanics training. Detailed interventions are provided in Chapter 17. Similarly, ROM and flexibility exercises should encompass extremities as well as spine interventions designed to address restricted areas, especially in those who have undergone surgery and radiation therapy. Aerobic exercise to address cardiopulmonary deficits and combat potential cancer-related fatigue is an additional integral component to a comprehensive plan of care.[77] Balance interventions for the purpose of fall risk mitigation, maximizing home safety, and to facilitate community integration should also be considered a cornerstone of a comprehensive plan of care. Cumulatively, supervised clinic exercise and HEP should meet the aforementioned ACSM recommendations for frequency and intensity. Postoperative mobility training, particularly log roll techniques for bed mobility, mitigates threats of incisional dehiscence and other potential postoperative compilations.[25,78]

Conclusion

Cancers of the GI system create a myriad of adverse effects resultant of medical management. Many of these adverse effects may be effectively mitigated, and in some cases prevented, with timely intervention by a skilled Onc R clinician. It is imperative to consider the implications of cachexia, metastases, chemotherapy, surgical intervention, and radiation on a PLWBC. Physical assessment and Onc R intervention can have large impacts to the QOL, strength, ROM, and functional capacity of a PLWBC in the GI cancer domain.

Critical Research Needs

- Exercise dosing for all GI cancers
- Evidence for efficacy for manual therapeutic interventions for PLWBCs in the GI cancer domain
- Outcomes assessment research is needed for validity and reliability of functional measures for PLWBCs

Case Study

By Alaina Newell, PT, DPT

Background: The patient is a 56-year-old man with Stage III pancreatic cancer. He presents 4 weeks following a Whipple procedure with a plan to resume medical treatment with capecitabine (Xeloda). He reports he had 4 weeks of neoadjuvant chemotherapy (oral Xeloda) before surgery to reduce the tumor size. At this time, he reports pain, a pulling sensation along his abdominal incision, low back pain, and fatigue. He has lost 30 pounds (18.6 kg) since his diagnosis and is having difficulty eating many foods. He is currently 180 lbs (81.6 kg), 6′4″ ft (1.93 m) tall with a BMI 21.9. His past medical history is unremarkable and had a prior right anterior cruciate ligament (ACL) knee surgery 20 years ago. He is a father of three children with two young boys at home and is employed as a software engineer. Before diagnosis he stayed active with his family and exercised 3 times/week with walking/biking.

Objective Findings:

Pain: average 4/10, best 4/10, worst 8/10 in his abdomen following meals

Abdominal Surgery Impact Scale: 56/72 72 = most difficulty

Five time Sit-to-Stand: 14 seconds with use of his arms on descent and reduced anterior pelvic tilt

Hand grip strength: average: R 25 kg L 23 kg

Gait: Normal speed 1.10 m/s with reduced arm swing, trunk rotation, hip extension, heel strike, and toe off

Spinal ROM: Flexion 60 degree, Extension -5 degree, Side bend R 15 degree L 10 degree, Rotation R 25% L 25%

Transverse abdominal incision: closed, mild erythema, mild–moderate edema superior

Posture: forward flexed with guarding in abdominal musculature, rounded shoulders, and forward head

Balance: Modified Clinical Test of Sensory Interaction in Balance (mCTSIB): conditions 1 to 3 = 30 seconds each, condition 4 = 23 seconds (best of three trials)

Assessment:

The patient is a 56-year-old man with Stage III pancreatic cancer who has undergone neoadjuvant chemotherapy, Whipple procedure and will continue to maintenance chemotherapy. He presents today with global strength deficits including focused deficits in his abdominal musculature noted from limited spinal ROM and muscle guarding present. These have led to altered posture and gait mechanics. Additionally, he has impaired balance noted by mCTSIB which elevates his fall risk in addition to his strength and posture deficits. He has had significant weight loss and is at risk for further loss secondary to pain with eating and continued treatment with a mucositic chemotherapy agent. He will benefit from Onc R to restore his ROM, abdominal strength to be consistent with his global strength to support his gait, balance, and functional tolerance for daily activity and community participation as he continues on his oncologic treatment. He will be treated twice per week for an initial 6 weeks followed by monthly surveillance.

Intervention:

Postural lengthening: progressive supine positioning with overhead can flexion, shoulder abduction, diaphragmatic breathing, knee to chest with opposite leg extension, and lower trunk rotations.

Abdominal strengthening: de-weighted positioning at countertop with weight through forearms and feet. Spinal sagittal (flexion–extension) ROM followed by neutral spine transverse abdominis activation. The progression includes weight shifting (anterior–posterior, lateral), marching, squats, and hip abduction.

Gait training: Initiate training on mechanics to include heel strike, big (long) stepping with upright trunk, ball holding with trunk rotation, and exacerbated arm swing

Transfers: Initiate at elevated surface with seated weight shifting, pelvic tilts, and foot positioning

Manual therapy: trigger point release, scar mobilization, rib mobilization, and hip distraction

Outcomes:

The following outcomes are reflected after initial 6 weeks of physical therapy. He was treated a total of 8 sessions (vs. 12 sessions) secondary to need for additional medical appointments during this time period.

Pain: average 4/10, best 2/10, worst 6/10 in his abdomen following 50% meals

Abdominal surgery impact scale: 36/72 (72 = most difficulty)

Five time sit-to-stand: 11 seconds without use of arms

Hand grip strength: average: R 27 kg L 25 kg

Gait: Normal speed 1.10 m/s with mild reduction trunk rotation, hip extension still present

Spinal ROM: Flexion 70 degrees, Extension 5 degrees, Side bend R 25 degrees L 15 degrees, Rotation R 50% L 50%

Transverse abdominal incision: closed, 0-mild edema superior

Posture: forward flexed without guarding in abdominal musculature

Balance: mCTSIB: conditions 1 to 4 = 30 seconds each (best of three trials)

Work: returned to work at 50% capacity due to new onset of HFS while on Xeloda that limited his ability to type

Activity: walking 3 times/week for 20 minutes. Reduced confidence for bike riding though is feeling limited with walking secondary to his HFS

Referrals:

Certified Dietary Nutritionist: to support caloric and protein intake with meal planning

Support group: peer support for pancreatic cancer for the PLWC and his family

Occupational therapy: for hand therapy and work adaptations

Review Questions

Reader can find the correct answers and rationale in the back of the book.

A 45-year-old male with Stage IB/grade 2 esophageal squamous cell carcinoma presents to therapy for evaluation and exercise prescription 6 weeks post-McKeown esophagectomy. He received neoadjuvant radiation to reduce the size of the tumor and reduce surgical consequences. He has a corporate office job where he sits for the majority of his workday and reports being mostly sedentary at home. Since radiation treatments and postsurgery, he is distressed by the exhaustion that does not remit with rest, has difficulty ascending a flight of stairs to access his bedroom, and comfortably walking the required distance to enter his office building.

1. What is the MOST appropriate way to objectively evaluate the multidimensional complaints of fatigue with this PLWBC?
   A. Asking the PLWBC to rate fatigue as minimal, moderate, or severe
   B. Having the PLWBC complete the Modified Brief Fatigue Inventory
   C. Having the PLWBC complete the Multidimensional Fatigue Symptom Inventory
   D. Having the PLWBC to rate fatigue on the Visual Analog Scale
2. What is the MOST appropriate functional assessment for evaluating cardiopulmonary fitness for the PLWBC?
   A. Bruce treadmill protocol
   B. YMCA Bike Test
   C. Six-minute walk test
   D. Timed Up and Go Test
3. Which of the following objective approach is MOST appropriate for comprehensive wound assessment?
   A. Visual observation
   B. Taking a digital photograph for the electronic medical record
   C. Use of the Applied Wound Management Tool and the National Wound Assessment Form
   D. There is no need to evaluate the postsurgical wound 6 weeks postsurgery

A 63-year-old female with Stage IIIA liver cancer presents to the physical therapy clinic with a report of numbness and tingling in her hands and feet, impaired balance, nausea, and fatigue. Presence of ascites that has been previously managed with paracentesis. She is currently receiving a monoclonal antibody (pembrolizumab [Keytruda]). Examination and evaluation reveals a frail habitus and signs of malnutrition, she demonstrates extremity weakness, impaired balance, and decreased endurance.

4. What is the MOST appropriate referral you can make relative to your findings of malnutrition?
   A. Provide advanced nutritional education as a physical therapist
   B. Primary care physician
   C. Registered dietitian/registered dietitian nutritionist
   D. Psychologist
5. What is the MOST appropriate course of action related to your observation of ascites?
   A. Refer to the patient back to the oncologist
   B. Consider the patient's treatment plan and implement palliative therapeutic goals
   C. Modify exercise programs to utilize more abdominal strengthening to assist in moving the fluid buildup out of the area
   D. Educate the patient on the paracentesis protocol and how it will impact their abdominal muscle activation
6. What is the LEAST appropriate strategy to address her symptoms of chemotherapy-induced polyneuropathy long-term?
   A. Implement dynamic standing balance activities
   B. Refer back to oncologist for antioxidant supplementation
   C. Provide an exercise protocol to strengthen the distal lower extremities.
   D. Provide patient education regarding CIPN including training for alternative balance strategies including vestibular and visual balance systems
7. What balance assessment is the MOST appropriate for this PLWC?
   A. Clinical Test of Sensory Integration and Balance (CTSIB)
   B. Self-perception of fall risk

C. Observe static balance

D. Record of fall history

A 62-year-old male that is 5 days status post-Whipple procedure for Stage III/grade 2 pancreatic cancer, has been transferred from the intensive care unit (ICU) to the medical–surgical floor. A referral has been placed for physical therapy and occupational therapy for progressive mobility. The electronic medical record indicates minimal functional mobility in the ICU and presently stable vital signs and lab values. Additionally the patient has received pain medication 30 minutes prior to your session.

8. Select the BEST sequence for bed mobility progression from supine to sit at the edge of the bed.

A. Apply abdominal binder by rolling left and right, carefully bend both lower extremities until feet are flat on the surface of the bed, perform a modified log roll to one side (head of bed elevated to comfort), advance lower extremities toward the edge and off of the side of the bed as upper extremities push down with same-side elbow and alternate-side hand across body, ensure both feet are flat on the floor before preparing to exit the bed.

B. Assume a long sit position, advance lower extremities to the edge of the bed, scoot hips to edge of bed to prepare to exit the bed.

C. Use the mechanics of the hospital bed to elevate the head of the bed to a comfortable height, advance lower extremities to the edge of the bed, scoot hips to edge of bed to prepare to exit the bed.

D. Apply abdominal binder by rolling left and right, use the mechanics of the hospital bed to elevate the head of the bed to a comfortable height, advance lower extremities to the edge of the bed, scoot hips to edge of bed to prepare to exit the bed.

9. Which of the following activities would contradict typical surgical precautions during his early weeks of recovery?

A. Drinking coffee while sitting at a table

B. Lifting his 4-year-old granddaughter for a hug

C. Returning to work at his desk job

D. Walking while talking in his neighborhood

10. At this time, the patient would benefit from initiation of an exercise program while in the hospital. What exercises are NOT appropriate at this time?

A. Ambulation in the hallway with assistance

B. Cough and breathing exercise

C. Repeated sit to stand transfers

D. Supine trunk strengthening program

References

1. Siegel RL, Miller KD, Fuchs HE, Jemal A. Cancer statistics, 2021. *CA Cancer J Clin.* 2021;71(1):7–33.

2. Surveillance, Epidemiology and ERP. Cancer stat facts. https://seer.cancer.gov/statfacts/. 2020. Accessed March 12, 2021.

3. Mysuru Shivanna L, Urooj A. A review on dietary and non-dietary risk factors associated with gastrointestinal cancer. *J Gastrointest Cancer.* 2016;47(3):247–254.

4. Koppen BM, Stanton BA. Chapter 27: Functional anatomy and general principles of regulation in the gastrointestinal tract. In: BM Koppen, BA. Stanton (Eds.) *Berne & Levy Physiology*, 7th ed., Elsevier, 2018, pp. 511–519.

5. Costanzo LS. Chapter 8 Gastrointestinal physiology. In: Costanzo LS. ed. *Physiology.* 6th ed. Elsevier; 2017:339–394.

6. Budczies J, von Winterfeld M, Klauschen F, et al. The landscape of metastatic progression patterns across major human cancers. *Oncotarget.* 2015;6(1):570–583.

7. Gilg MM, Gröchenig H-P, Schlemmer A, Eherer A, Högenauer C, Langner C. Secondary tumors of the GI tract: origin, histology, and endoscopic findings. *Gastrointest Endosc.* 2018;88(1):151–158.e1. https://linkinghub.elsevier.com/retrieve/pii/S0016510718301330.

8. Bentley-Hibbert S, Schwartz L. Use of imaging for GI cancers. *J Clin Oncol.* 2015;33(16):1729–1736, doi: 10.1200/JCO.2014.60.2847.

9. American College of Surgeons. *AJCC Cancer Staging Manual.* 8th ed. Springer International Publishing; 2017.

10. Boright L, Doherty DJ, Wilson CM, Arena SK, Ramirez C. Development and feasibility of a prehabilitation protocol for patients diagnosed with head and neck cancer. *Cureus.* 2020;12(8), doi: 10.7759/cureus.9898.

11. Silver JK. Cancer prehabilitation and its role in improving health outcomes and reducing health care costs. *Semin Oncol Nurs.* 2015;31(1):13–30.

12. Doganay E, Wynter-Blyth V, Halliday L, MacKinnon T, Osborn H, Moorthy K. Study of long-term follow-up of exercise levels following participation in a prehabilitation program in esophagogastric cancer. *Rehabil Oncol.* 2020;38(3):110–115.

13. Gustafsson UO, Oppelstrup H, Thorell A, Nygren J, Ljungqvist O. Adherence to the ERAS protocol is associated with 5-year survival after colorectal cancer surgery: a retrospective cohort study. *World J Surg.* 2016;40(7):1741–1747.

14. Pędziwiatr M, Kisialeuski M, Wierdak M, et al. Early implementation of enhanced recovery after surgery (ERAS®) protocol—compliance improves outcomes: a prospective cohort study. *Int J Surg.* 2015;21:75–81.

15. Kim JY, Wie GA, Cho YA, et al. Diet modification based on the enhanced recovery after surgery program (ERAS) in patients undergoing laparoscopic colorectal resection. *Clin Nutr Res.* 2018;7(4):297, doi: 10.7762/cnr.2018.7.4.297.

16. Muscaritoli M. Targeting cancer cachexia: we're on the way. *Lancet Oncol.* 2016;17(4):414–415, doi: 10.1016/S1470-2045(16)00085-1.

17. Sadeghi M, Keshavarz-Fathi M, Baracos V, Arends J, Mahmoudi M, Rezaei N. Cancer cachexia: diagnosis, assessment, and treatment. *Crit Rev Oncol Hematol.* 2018;127(2018):91–104.

18. Belloum Y, Rannou-Bekono F, Favier FB. Cancer-induced cardiac cachexia: pathogenesis and impact of physical activity. *Oncol Rep.* 2017;37(5):2543–2552, doi: 10.3892/or.2017.5542.

19. Wheelwright SJ, Hopkinson JB, Darlington A-S, et al. Development of the EORTC QLQ-CAX24, a questionnaire for cancer patients with cachexia. *J Pain Sympt Manage.* 2016;53(2):232–242.

20. Fearon K, Strasser F, Anker SD, et al. Definition and classification of cancer cachexia: an international consensus. *Lancet Oncol.* 2011;12(5):489–495.

21. Sachlova M, Majek O, Tucek S. Prognostic value of scores based on malnutrition or systemic inflammatory response in patients with metastatic or recurrent gastric cancer. *Nutr Cancer.* 2014;66(8):1362–1370.

22. Ryu SW, Kim IH. Comparison of different nutritional assessments in detecting malnutrition among gastric cancer patients. *World J Gastroenterol.* 2010;16(26):3310–3317.

23. Seo GH, Choe EK, Park KJ, Chai YJ. Incidence of clinically relevant incisional hernia after colon cancer surgery and its risk factors: a nationwide claims study. *World J Surg.* 2018;42(4):1192–1199.

24. Owens M, Barry M, Janjua AZ, Winter DC. A systematic review of laparoscopic port site hernias in gastrointestinal surgery. *Surgery*. 2011;9(4):218–224.

25. Cheifetz O, Lucy SD, Overend TJ, Crowe J. The effect of abdominal support on functional outcomes in patients following major abdominal surgery: a randomized controlled trial. *Physiother Canada*. 2010;62(3):242–253.

26. Elsevier. Ascites. Elsevier Patient Handouts. 2022;2.

27. Hicks AM, Chou J, Capanu M, Lowery MA, Yu KH, O'Reilly EM. Pancreas adenocarcinoma: ascites, clinical manifestations, and management implications. *Clin Colorectal Cancer*. 2016;15(4):360–368.

28. Ayantunde AA, Parsons SL. Pattern and prognostic factors in patients with malignant ascites: a retrospective study. *Ann Oncol*. 2007;18(5):945–949, doi: 10.1093/annonc/mdl499.

29. Nakano M, Ito M, Tanaka R, et al. PD-1+ TIM-3+ T cells in malignant ascites predict prognosis of gastrointestinal cancer. *Cancer Sci*. 2018;109(9):2986–2992, doi: 10.1111/cas.13723.

30. McQuade RM, Stojanovska V, Abalo R, Bornstein JC, Nurgali K. Chemotherapy-induced constipation and diarrhea: pathophysiology, current and emerging treatments. *Front Pharmacol*. 2016;7:1–14, doi: 10.3389/fphar.2016.00414.

31. U.S. Department of Health and Human Services. Common terminology criteria for adverse events (CTCAE) version 5.0. https://ctep. cancer.gov/protocoldevelopment/electronic_applications/docs/CT-CAE_v5_Quick_Reference_8.5x11.pdf. Published 2017. Accessed April 20, 2021.

32. Tanksley JP, Willett CG, Czito BG, Palta M. Acute and chronic gastrointestinal side effects of radiation therapy. In: Feldman M, Friedman LS, Brandt LJ, eds. *Sleisenger and Fordtran's Gastrointestinal and Liver Disease—2 Volume Set*. Elsevier; 2020:606–618.e6, doi: 10.1016/B978-0-323-60962-3.00041-2.

33. Straub JM, New J, Hamilton CD, Lominska C, Shnayder Y, Thomas SM. Radiation-induced fibrosis: mechanisms and implications for therapy. *J Cancer Res Clin Oncol*. 2015;141(11):1985–1994.

34. Purkayastha A, Sharma N, Sarin A, et al. Radiation fibrosis syndrome: the evergreen menace of radiation therapy. *Asia-Pacific J Oncol Nurs*. 2019;6(3):238, doi: 10.4103/apjon.apjon_71_18.

35. Sourati A, Ameri A, Malekzadeh M. *Acute Side Effects of Radiation Therapy A Guide to Management*, Springer, 2017.

36. Shadad AK. Gastrointestinal radiation injury: symptoms, risk factors and mechanisms. *World J Gastroenterol*. 2013;19(2):185, doi: 10.3748/wjg.v19.i2.185.

37. Burris HA, Hurtig J. Radiation recall with anticancer agents. *Oncologist*. 2010;15(11):1227–1237, doi: 10.1634/theoncologist.2009-0090.

38. Perri G, Prakash L, Malleo G, et al. The sequential radiographic effects of preoperative chemotherapy and (chemo)radiation on tumor anatomy in patients with localized pancreatic cancer. *Ann Surg Oncol*. 2020;27(10):3939–3947.

39. Zhan Q, Wang L, Song Y, et al. Esophageal carcinoma. In: Liu X, Pestka S, Shi Y, eds. *Recent Advances in Cancer Research and Therapy*. 1st ed. Elsevier; 2012:493–534.

40. Mitry E. Colorectal cancer. In: Cockerham WC, ed. *International Encyclopedia of Public Health*. 2nd ed. Elsevier; 2017:75–81.

41. Minsky BD, Rödel C, Valentini V. Rectal cancer. In: Gunderson LL, Joel ETepper JE, eds. *Clinical Radiation Oncology*. 3rd ed. Elsevier; 2012:989–1015.

42. Dicato MA, ed. *Side Effects of Medical Cancer Therapy*. London: Springer London; 2013. http://link.springer.com/10.1007/978-0-85729-787-7.

43. August D, Shah M, Chapter Huhmann MB. 139: Nutrition support. In: DeVita V, Lawrence T, Rosenberg S, eds. *DeVita, Hellman, and Rosenberg's Cancer: Principles & Practice of Oncology*. 11th ed.; 2018:3869–3880.

44. National Cancer Institute. Drugs approved for different types of cancer; 2020. https://www.cancer.gov/about-cancer/treatment/drugs/cancer-type. Accessed January 15, 2021.

45. National Cancer Institute at the National Institutes of Health. Targeted therapy to treat cancer. https://www.cancer.gov/about-cancer/treatment/types/targeted-therapies, 2020. Accessed April 20, 2021.

46. National Cancer Institute. Immunotherapy to treat cancer. https://www.cancer.gov/about-cancer/treatment/types/immunotherapy, 2019. Accessed April 20, 2021.

47. Weber JS. Cancer Research Institute. Immunotherapy side effects. https://www.cancerresearch.org/immunotherapy-side-effects. 2019. Accessed April 20, 2021.

48. Center MSKC. About your esophagectomy surgery. https://www.mskcc.org/cancer-care/patient-education/about-your-esophagectomy-surgery. 2021. Accessed January 15, 2021.

49. Memorial Sloan Kettering Cancer Center. About your gastrectomy surgery. https://www.mskcc.org/cancer-care/patient-education/about-your-gastrectomy-surgery. 2021. Accessed April 20, 2021.

50. Memorial Sloan Kettering Cancer Center. Surgery for liver cancer. https://www.mskcc.org/cancer-care/types/liver/treatment/surgery, 2021. Accessed April 20, 2021.

51. Memorial Sloan Kettering Cancer Center. The whipple procedure: a brief overview for family and friends. https://www.mskcc.org/cancer-care/patient-education/whipple-procedure-brief-overview-family-and-friends. 2021. Accessed April 20, 2021.

52. Napolitano E. Heated chemotherapy: using robust science to guide clinical decisions. https://www.mskcc.org/news/heated-chemotherapy-using-robust-science-guide-clinical-decisions. 2013. Accessed April 20, 2021.

53. Black B, Marcoux BC, Stiller C, Qu X, Gellish R. Personal health behaviors and role-modeling attitudes of physical therapists and physical therapist students: a cross-sectional study. *Phys Ther*. 2012;92(11):1419–1436.

54. Li Z, Shan F, Ying X, et al. Assessment of laparoscopic distal gastrectomy after neoadjuvant chemotherapy for locally advanced gastric cancer. *JAMA Surg*. 2019;154(12):1093, doi: 10.1001/jamasurg.2019.3473.

55. Baekelandt BMG, Hjermstad MJ, Nordby T, et al. Preoperative cognitive function predicts survival in patients with resectable pancreatic ductal adenocarcinoma. *HPB*. 2016;18(3):247–254.

56. Monfort SM, Pan X, Loprinzi CL, Lustberg MB, Chaudhari AMW. Impaired postural control and altered sensory organization during quiet stance following neurotoxic chemotherapy: a preliminary study. *Integr Cancer Ther*. 2019;18, doi: 10.1177/1534735419828823.

57. Schmitt AC, Repka CP, Heise GD, Challis JH, Smith JD. Comparison of posture and balance in cancer survivors and age-matched controls. *Clin Biomech*. 2017;50(2016):1–6.

58. Litterini A, Inscore E. APTA Oncology EDGE Task Force Report Summaries. Oncology EDGE taskforce annotated bibliography. https://oncologypt.org/wp-content/uploads/2020/03/EDGE-Annotated-Bibliography-8.19-update-1.pdf. 2019. Accessed May 18, 2021.

59. Hojan K, Milecki P. Opportunities for rehabilitation of patients with radiation fibrosis syndrome. *Rep Pract Oncol Radiother*. 2014;19(1):1–6.

60. Greatrex-White S, Moxey H. Wound assessment tools and nurses' needs: an evaluation study. *Int Wound J*. 2015;12(3):293–301.

61. Peel JB, Sui X, Matthews CE, et al. Cardiorespiratory fitness and digestive cancer mortality: findings from the aerobics center longitudinal study. *Cancer Epidemiol Biomark Prev*. 2009;18(4):1111–1117.

62. Schmidt K, Vogt L, Thiel C, Jäger E, Banzer W. Validity of the six-minute walk test in cancer patients. *Int J Sports Med*. 2013;34(07):631–636.

63. Bohannon RW. Normative reference values for the two-minute walk test derived by meta-analysis. *J Phys Ther Sci*. 2017;29(12):2224–2227.

64. Liu MA, DuMontier C, Murillo A, et al. Gait speed, grip strength, and clinical outcomes in older patients with hematologic malignancies. *Blood*. 2019;134(4):374–382, doi: 10.1182/blood.2019000758.

65. Ozorio GA, Barão K, Forones NM. Cachexia stage, patient-generated subjective global assessment, phase angle, and handgrip strength in patients with gastrointestinal cancer. *Nutr Cancer*. 2017;69(5):772–779.

66. Garland SN, Pelletier G, Lawe A, et al. Prospective evaluation of the reliability, validity, and minimally important difference of the functional assessment of cancer therapy-gastric (FACT-Ga) quality-of-life instrument. *Cancer*. 2011;117(6):1302–1312.
67. Boden I, Sullivan K, Hackett C, et al. ICEAGE (Incidence of Complications following Emergency Abdominal surgery: Get Exercising): study protocol of a pragmatic, multicentre, randomised controlled trial testing physiotherapy for the prevention of complications and improved physical recovery aft. *World J Emerg Surg*. 2018;13(1):29, doi: 0.1186/s13017-018-0189-y.
68. Cristian A, Tran A, Patel K. Patient safety in cancer rehabilitation. *Phys Med Rehabil Clin N Am*. 2012;23(2):441–456, doi: 10.1016/j.pmr.2012.02.015.
69. Gillis C, Buhler K, Bresee L, et al. Effects of nutritional prehabilitation, with and without exercise, on outcomes of patients who undergo colorectal surgery: a systematic review and meta-analysis. *Gastroenterology*. 2018;155(2):391–410.e4, doi: 10.1053/j.gastro.2018.05.012.
70. Stuecher K, Bolling C, Vogt L, et al. Exercise improves functional capacity and lean body mass in patients with gastrointestinal cancer during chemotherapy: a single-blind RCT. *Support Care Cancer*. 2019;27(6):2159–2169.
71. Segal R, Zwaal C, Green E, Tomasone JR, Loblaw A, Petrella T. Exercise for people with cancer: a clinical practice guideline. *Curr Oncol*. 2017;24(1):40–46, doi: 10.3747/co.24.3376.
72. Mctiernan A, Friedenreich CM, Katzmarzyk PT, et al. Physical activity in cancer prevention and survival: a systematic review. *Med Sci Sport Exerc*. 2019;51(6):1252–1261.
73. Rizzo A. The role of exercise and rehabilitation in the cancer care plan. *J Adv Pract Oncol*. 2016;7(3):339–342, doi: 10.6004/jadpro.2016.7.3.20.
74. Ven Fong Z, Chang D, Lillemoe K, Nipp R, Tanabe K, Qadan M. Contemporary opportunity for prehabilitation as part of an enhanced recovery after surgery pathway in colorectal surgery. *Clin Colon Rectal Surg*. 2019;32(2):095–101.
75. Campbell KL, Winters-Stone KM, Wiskemann J, et al. Exercise guidelines for cancer survivors: consensus statement from international multidisciplinary roundtable. *Med Sci Sport Exerc*. 2019;51(11):2375–2390.
76. Airway Clearance by Anne Mejia-Downs. *APTA cardiovascular & pulmonary PT*. https://www.youtube.com/watch?v=kbidrfSCgfs&t=1s. 2020. Accessed April 15, 2022.
77. Stout NL, Santa Mina D, Lyons KD, Robb K, Silver JK. A systematic review of rehabilitation and exercise recommendations in oncology guidelines. *CA Cancer J Clin*. 2021;71(2):149–175, doi: 10.3322/caac.21639.
78. Vatwani A. Caregiver guide and instructions for safe bed mobility. *Arch Phys Med Rehabil*. 2017;98(9):1907–1910, doi: 10.1016/j.apmr.2017.03.003.

12

Genitourinary and Gynecological Systems

**ALLEGRA ADAMS, PT, DPT, BOARD CERTIFIED
WOMEN'S HEALTH CLINICAL SPECIALIST**

CHAPTER OUTLINE

Introduction

Impairments in the genitourinary and gynecological (GU/GYN) systems are prevalent in the general population. 25% to 67% of women report at least one form of pelvic floor dysfunction.[1,2] 25% to 51% of women and 11% to 34% of men report some degree of urinary incontinence (UI).[3,4] Among women with suspected gynecological malignancy, 40% reported UI at baseline.[5] Risk factors for developing UI include: increasing age, increasing body mass index, diabetes, increased parity (the number of pregnancies resulting in birth), constipation or other chronic straining, chronic cough or other respiratory disease, smoking, high impact athletes, menopause, medications, and concurrent musculoskeletal, neurological, or cognitive impairments.[6,7] This chapter will explore how various cancers and cancer treatments further exacerbate many of these pre-existing risk factors. Other forms of voiding dysfunction include urinary urgency without incontinence, urinary frequency, nocturia (nighttime frequency), urinary retention (including hesitancy to initiate flow and interrupted flow), and painful urination (dysuria). A combination urgency, frequency, and/or nocturia may be referred to as "overactive bladder."

Up to 27% of women[8] and up to 15% of men[9] report chronic pelvic pain. A survey of premenopausal women in primary care offices revealed that a quarter to a half of women experience painful intercourse (dyspareunia).[10,11] In some instances, chronic pelvic pain is attributable to pathology such as endometriosis, interstitial cystitis, or prostatitis. For many people experiencing pelvic pain, however, the underlying mechanism is poorly understood. In most cases, there is a large component of abdominal and pelvic myofascial restriction or pelvic floor muscle (PFM) overactivity.[12-14] Other factors contributing to the development of pelvic pain and sexual dysfunction include recurrent genitourinary infections, irritable or inflammatory bowel conditions, poor posture, degenerative joint diseases, hernias, depression and anxiety, and trauma.[7,15] Surgery and radiation therapy especially have high rates of chronic pelvic pain as a long-term adverse effect.[16]

Menopause, and the associated vulvovaginal atrophy, is a common cause of pelvic floor dysfunction in women, in regard to both bladder control and pain. As will be described below, menopause is often a consequence of many cancer treatments. While the resultant GU/GYN adverse effects may be obvious in the case of pelvic organ cancers, they are often underdiagnosed and remain untreated in persons living with and beyond cancer (PLWBCs) of other systems.

Common Adverse Effects to the Genitourinary and Gynecological Systems

Here we define general symptoms of the GU/GYN systems that may arise after cancer treatment, regardless of cancer diagnosis or treatment protocol.

Bladder irritation
Daytime frequency
Dysuria
Fistula
Hesitancy
Neurogenic bladder conditions
Nocturia
Pelvic organ prolapse
Strictures
Urinary incontinence
Urinary retention
Urinary urgency

Advancing age
Alzheimer's disease or dementia
Arthritis or other musculoskeletal problems
Overweight/obese
Chronic cough
Chronic constipation
History of recurrent urinary tract infection
History of sexually transmitted disease
Enlarged abdomen (e.g., ascites, pregnancy, obesity, tumor)
Diabetes mellitus
Neurologic disorder
Medication
    Sedatives
    Diuretics
    Estrogens
    Anticholinergics
    Antibiotics
    Alpha-adrenergic blockers (antihistamines, decongestants)
    Calcium channel blockers
    Antipsychotics
    Antidepressants
    Antiparkinsonian drugs
    Laxatives
    Opioids
    Vincristine [Oncovin, Vincasar PFS]
    Angiotensin-converting enzyme (ACE) inhibitors
Caffeine, alcohol
Female gender (see below)
Specific to Women
Pregnancy (multiparity)
Vaginal or cesarean[a] birth
Previous bladder or pelvic surgery
Pelvic trauma or radiation
Bladder or bowel prolapse
Menopause (natural or surgically induced; estrogen deficiency)[b]
Tobacco use
Specific to Men
Enlarged prostate gland
Prostate or pelvic surgery
Radiation (acute and late complications), especially when combined with brachytherapy

[a]Although the abdominal muscles are disrupted with a cesarean section and limit how much the woman can bear down on the bladder, abdominal tone and function are essential for pelvic muscle function.

[b]Urinary incontinence in middle-aged women may be more closely associated with mechanical factors, such as childbearing, history of urinary tract infections, gynecological surgery, chronic constipation, obesity, and exertion, than with menopausal transition.

Used with permission from Goodman CC, Heick J, Lazaro RT. Screening for urogenital disease. In: *Differential Diagnosis for Physical Therapists: Screening for Referral.* 6th ed. St. Elsevier Inc.; 2018:372.

Genitourinary System

Common adverse effects of any cancer treatment on the genitourinary system are highlighted in Box 12.1. Systemic chemotherapy, local radiation therapy, and some hormonal and immunotherapy treatments can create acute bladder irritation, with or without blood in the urine (hematuria) and/or dysuria. These acute symptoms are usually limited to the time period a person with cancer (PWC) is actively receiving treatment.

Acute irritation may result in urinary urgency and daytime or nighttime urinary frequency. Urinary urgency is defined by the International Urogynecological Association and International Continence Society (IUGA/ICS)[17] as "a sudden, compelling desire to pass urine which is difficult to defer," which may or may not be accompanied by an incontinent episode. Urinary urgency is often accompanied by urinary frequency, which is voiding more frequently during waking hours than considered previously normal for that person—generally more than nine times in a 24-hour period or more than every 2 to 3 hours.[7] The person may also experience nighttime urinary frequency (nocturia) of waking to void more than once, where each void is preceded and followed by sleep.[7,17] These symptoms can resolve upon completion of treatment but may become chronic due to permanent fibrotic tissue changes of the bladder lining which reduces bladder filling capacity. Development of adjacent scar tissue or fascial restrictions placing abnormal pressures or tensions on the bladder may also cause detrusor irritability, reduced bladder storage capacity, PFM overactivity, or nerve damage.[18]

There are many forms of UI that may occur, in isolation or concurrently, and as previously noted are not all unique to the PLWBC. Box 12.2 lists all-cause risk factors for developing UI.[6]

The IUGA/ICS defines UI as the "complaint of involuntary loss of urine."[17] These organizations further subcategorize eight distinct types of UI including: stress, urgency, mixed, postural, nocturnal enuresis, coital, continuous, and insensible. Stress urinary incontinence (SUI) is the involuntary loss of urine due to an increase in abdominal pressure with effort or physical exertion. Urgency urinary incontinence (UUI) occurs in response to a sudden desire to void which is not possible to be delayed. Mixed incontinence is a combination of SUI and UUI. Postural incontinence occurs with a change in position and includes postmicturition leakage (upon standing from the toilet). Nocturnal enuresis occurs during sleep (not to be confused with nocturia which is nighttime frequency) and coital incontinence occurs during intercourse, either with penetration or at orgasm. Continuous UI is uninterrupted continual urine loss while insensible UI is leakage that occurs without

the person sensing it. Some sources also recognize "functional" UI as an involuntary loss of urine due to gross or fine motor limitations from musculoskeletal or neurological impairments (such as arthritis or a stroke) or cognitive deficits (such as dementia) rather than a defect in the genitourinary system itself.[6] Also described is "overflow" UI due to an overfull bladder which generally occurs due to outlet obstruction or neurological damage of the voiding mechanism.[6,7] Factors that may contribute to overflow UI include an acontractile, hypotonic, or over-distended detrusor muscle of the bladder from neurological damage or medications which leads to the bladder not emptying completely. Alternately, the urethra may be blocked due to a prolapse or mass, as in prostate cancer,

TABLE 12.1 **Definitions of Types of Urinary Incontinence**

Type of Urinary Incontinence (UI)	Definition
Stress urinary incontinence (SUI)	The involuntary loss of urine due to an increase in intraabdominal pressure with effort or physical exertion
Urgency urinary incontinence (UUI)	UI in response to a sudden desire to void which is not possible to be delayed
Mixed	Both SUI and UUI
Postural	UI occurs with a change in position
Nocturnal enuresis	UI occurs while asleep (i.e., bed wetting)
Continuous	Constant UI, with or without provocation
Insensible	UI occurs without awareness
Coital	UI occurs during intercourse
Functional	UI due to gross or fine motor limitations from musculoskeletal or neurological impairments or cognitive deficits rather than a defect in the genitourinary system itself
Overflow	Leakage of an overfull bladder which generally occurs due to outlet obstruction or neurological damage to the voiding mechanism

Created by Allegra Adams, PT, DPT. Printed with permission.

causing the bladder to overfill. The definitions of these various types of UI are summarized in Table 12.1.

Aside from the risk factors for developing UI previously described, there are other factors relating to the bladder or bladder outlet that may contribute to developing problems with urine containment.[19] The bladder may be directly affected by a tumor or it may be compressed by an adjacent pelvic tumor; incontinence may be neurogenic from a spinal metastasis interrupting the complex micturition reflexes; or there may be inflammation of the bladder wall due to infection, radiation cystitis, or chemotherapeutic agents. The bladder outlet/sphincter may be impaired due to local cancer invasion into the sphincter or damage to the regulating pelvic nerves due to surgery or chemotherapy treatments, such as antiestrogens or vincristine [Oncovin, Vincasar PFS]. Medications, such as diuretics, sleep aids, sedatives, muscle relaxants, anticholinergics, antibiotics, narcotics, antihistamines, antidepressants, antipsychotics, calcium channel blockers, angiotensin-converting enzyme (ACE) inhibitors, and laxatives can disrupt the voiding mechanism at various levels.[6,19] Box 12.3 outlines a full list of medications that have adverse effects on the genitourinary system.

Stool impaction, impaired core muscle function due to surgery, core muscle incoordination (dyssynergia), or pain inhibition may also contribute to bladder dysfunction. Functional incontinence is when a person has physical or functional limitations where they cannot physically get to the bathroom or bedside commode or undress in time. Functional incontinence is common in the PLWBC due to musculoskeletal and neurological adverse effects of cancer and cancer treatment, as described in Chapters 7 and 8, respectively. Surgery or radiation may result in development of a vesicovaginal or urethrovaginal fistula, an opening between the bladder and vagina and between the urethra and vagina respectively, which would result in continuous incontinence.

Conversely, a PWC may experience urinary retention, or the inability to pass urine or fully empty the bladder, despite effort.[17] Causes for retention originating from the bladder include bladder or gastrointestinal cancers, neurological regulation (spinal metastasis, spinal fractures due to osteoporotic changes), or local damage to pelvic nerves from chemotherapy-induced polyneuropathy (CIPN), surgery, or radiation therapy. Causes for retention affecting the sphincter include: localized cancer or tumor invasion,

• **BOX 12.3** **Medications That Have Adverse Effects on the Genitourinary System**

Angiotensin-converting enzyme (ACE) inhibitors
Antibiotics
Antidepressants
Antihistamines
Antipsychotics
Calcium channel blockers
Cyclophosphamide [Cytoxan]
Diuretics
Laxatives
Muscle relaxants, anticholinergics
Narcotics, opioids
Sleep aides, sedatives
Tamoxifen
Vinca-alkaloids (e.g., vincristine [Oncovin, Vincasar PFS])

• **BOX 12.4** **Potential Reversible Causes of Urinary Incontinence or Retention**

D—Delirium or other cognitive causes
I—Infection/inflammation of the urinary tract
A—Atrophic vaginitis (menopause, estrogen antagonists)
P—Pharmaceuticals, pain, psychological
E—Endocrine (diabetes mellitus)
R—Restricted mobility
S—Stool impaction

compression from pelvic tumors, or bladder prolapse (cystocele). A urethral stricture from surgery or fibrosis from infection, catheterization, or radiation may also impair the bladder outlet. Medications, pain, and dyssynergia can also cause urinary retention.[19] Box 12.4 offers a helpful mnemonic in remembering potentially reversible causes of UI or retention, not specific to the oncology population.[7,19,20]

Urinary hesitancy, or a delay in initiating urine flow, may be due to psychological or neurological causes. A weak stream may be an early sign of a bladder outlet obstruction or dysfunction. The urine stream may be intermittent, or interrupted, due to neurological causes or PFM overactivity or dyssynergia.

A cystocele may occur for many of the same reasons that UI develops including parity, obesity, and constipation.[7] A cystocele may additionally occur due to surgery affecting PFM strength or ligamentous supports, such as a hysterectomy. Similarly, abdominal surgeries, such as a cesarean section delivery, can restrict the bladder from rising out of the pelvic cavity and into the abdominal cavity while filling. Tamoxifen (a selective estrogen receptor modulator, SERM [Nolvadex]) has also been shown to contribute to the development of pelvic organ prolapse (POP) in healthy postmenopausal women.[21] Regardless of the cause, a cystocele may result in obstructed voiding and urinary retention or overflow incontinence. In some cases, a cystocele may actually mask underlying PFM weakness as the kinked urethra may provide passive (structural) continence. Surgical correction of a cystocele may therefore result in UI if the active continence mechanism (PFM strength) is lacking.

Surgical or radiation damage to the core muscles or innervating nerves, CIPN, or steroidal- or hormonal- induced muscle atrophy will impair active continence. Other passive continence mechanisms are also disrupted with cancer treatment. For example, an enlarged prostate provides passive bladder continence due to the pressure inwards on the urethra. However, during a prostatectomy, the prostate is removed which reduces pressure on the urethra, and the part of the urethra passing through the prostate (prostatic urethra) is removed thereby shortening the overall length of the urethra and reducing passive continence. For women, the health and vascularity of the pelvic tissues contributes to passive continence through coaptation of the vaginal walls providing some degree of compression and closure for the urethra. When vaginal tissue atrophy and vaginal dryness develop during and after menopause, whether natural or due to cancer related treatments, underlying PFM weakness is often revealed and UI, typically SUI, may develop.

The physiology of micturition (voiding) and maintaining continence requires a complex system of somatic and autonomic innervation including lumbar and sacral spinal reflex loops and cortical centers. Therefore, beyond damage to active continence mechanisms, upper motor neuron damage either directly due to tumor location, cancer treatment itself, or a cerebrovascular accident due to cancer treatment may result in a hyperreflexic bladder dysfunction. Even in the absence of true neurological damage, the fascia of the bladder is continuous along the deep front line fascial chain to the sphenobasilar joint and therefore dysfunction here may result in distal bladder dysfunction.[18,22,23] Conversely, lower motor neuron damage from surgery, radiation, CIPN, or spinal compression fracture due to spinal metastasis or cancer treatment-related osteoporosis can result in an areflexic or flaccid bladder. The PWC with neurogenic bladder conditions will be closely monitored and instructed in a bladder management program by their medical care team which may include: continuous or intermittent self-catheterization, fluid intake maintenance, medication, and possibly surgery to minimize infections, optimize continence, and maintain safe bladder pressures and residual volumes to maximize quality of life (QOL) and minimize burden of care.[19]

Gynecological System and Sexual Function

With everything that happens during the initial stages of cancer diagnosis and treatment, sexual function may not be a high

---

• BOX 12.5 Gynecological and Sexual Adverse Effects

Anorgasmia
Decreased arousal
Dyspareunia, sexual dysfunction
Erectile dysfunction
Genitourinary syndrome of menopause (GSM)
Infertility
Poor or absent libido
Psychosocial
  Depression, anxiety
  Body image changes or actual disfigurement
  Fear of recurrence
  Change in roles of relationship
  Socioeconomic strains

---

priority, though for younger PWC, fertility preservation may be a critical consideration (see below). Eventually, however, the PWC will likely be faced with challenges impairing their sexual health and function as a result of their cancer treatment, both acutely and in the long term. While this is frequently readily recognized for PWC of the genital or gynecological organs, less attention is paid to sexual dysfunction in PWC of other systems. However, considering that sexuality and sexual function are important factors for QOL, they should be assessed and addressed. Common gynecological and sexual adverse effects of cancer treatment are highlighted in Box 12.5.

While chemotherapy and hormonal therapy may have a direct impact on libido, one must also consider the effect of psychosocial factors on sexual interest including anxiety and depression, relational and financial stressors, and altered body image. Additionally, cancer or cancer treatment can lead to nausea, fatigue, weakness, pain, or impaired mobility which can not only limit one's libido, but also their ability to participate in sexual activity.

Neurovascular damage from chemotherapy, radiation, or surgery can all reduce genital sensitivity resulting in decreased arousal, erectile dysfunction, and anorgasmia. PFM weakness from all cause neuropathy (e.g., chemotherapy, diabetes, alcohol abuse, nerve injury locally, spinal injury, and peripheral vascular disease), surgical or radiation nerve damage, or pre-existing risk factors may also lead to sexual dysfunction.

A systematic review of worldwide literature reports that up to 64% of women living with or beyond cancer report sexual pain; this includes 45% of women with a history of breast cancer and 55% of women with a history of either gynecological or rectal cancers.[24] Dyspareunia among women is multifactorial and is impacted by PFM tone, vaginal dimensions, and lubrication. PFM hypertonicity may arise from neurovascular damage from chemotherapy, surgery, or radiation. It may more often be a reaction to fascial and joint restrictions created by surgery and radiation through abnormal tensions and pressures on the lumbopelvic muscles, ligaments, and organs. Hypertonicity of the PFM may also be a guarding response due to pain—real or anticipated—or prolonged or recurrent infection. Finally, musculoskeletal changes from treatment may change the length-tension relationship of the PFM, interrupt the core muscle synergies, or create compensatory movement patterns that result in PFM overuse. Overuse also occurs with chronic cough, dyssynergic constipation, or chronic bladder or bowel urge suppression. While PFM underactivity can contribute to decreased erection and anorgasmia, overactivity can result in dyspareunia and pain with ejaculation. Surgery and radiation can result in reduced vaginal dimensions—either due to anatomical changes from surgery or stenosis from radiation fibrosis—which can lead to dyspareunia. Men likewise report pain with intercourse, generally during ejaculation, which is most often due to PFM overactivity, myofascial restrictions of the urogenital triangle muscles at the base of the penis, or neurovascular impingement of the inguinal canal contents.

Chemotherapy, radiation therapy, surgery, and hormonal therapy may all result in premature menopause due to a decline in ovarian function and a deficiency of estrogen. The pelvic organs and support structures are dense with estrogen receptors[25] and therefore symptoms arise due to a lack of estrogen. Pelvic symptoms of this nature, collectively termed genitourinary syndrome of menopause (GSM) (which replaces the previous term vulvovaginal atrophy), are not unique to the oncology population.[26,27] 51% of postmenopausal women report at least one vulvovaginal symptom affecting urinary or sexual function.[28] Symptoms of GSM, as listed in Box 12.6, include: vaginal dryness, itching, burning, irritation, dyspareunia, vaginal bleeding or spotting with intercourse, dysuria, urinary urgency and frequency, UI, recurrent urinary tract and yeast infections, decreased genital sensation, and decreased arousal or orgasm.[26,27]

Infertility is an adverse effect of all systemic cancer treatment modalities (chemotherapy, hormonal therapy, and stem cell transplant). It may be reversible for males, however, without intentional efforts to preserve fertility, will be permanent for women.

Infertility is also probable with any localized surgery or radiation therapy in the low back, abdomen, and/or pelvis due to organ resection or fibrosis. Fertility preservation options will be discussed later in the chapter.

Genitourinary and Gynecological Adverse Effects of Cancer Treatments

Treatments for non-GU/GYN cancers can still have lasting impacts on the pelvic viscera, pelvic nerves, and PFM that influence bladder and sexual function. Table 12.2 provides an overview of GU/GYN adverse effects from each form of cancer treatment.

• BOX 12.6   Genitourinary Syndrome of Menopause

Decreased genital sensation
Dyspareunia
Dysuria
Recurrent urinary tract and yeast infections
Urinary urgency, frequency, incontinence
Vaginal bleeding or spotting with intercourse
Vaginal burning, itching, irritation
Vaginal dryness

TABLE 12.2 Genitourinary and Gynecological Adverse Effects of Cancer Treatments

Surgery	Radiation	Chemotherapy	Hormonal/ Biological	Stem Cell Transplant	Immunotherapy
Chronic pelvic pain	Acute bladder irritation	Acute bladder irritation	Infertility	Infertility	Acute bladder irritation
Damage to pelvic nerves	Bladder fibrosis	Acute change in urine	Menopause	Kidney damage	Hematuria
Direct organ damage	Damage to pelvic nerves	Damage to pelvic nerves	Muscle atrophy	Menopause	Kidney damage
Menopause	Decreased vascularity	Infertility	POP	UTI/yeast infections	Urinary frequency
Fistula formation	Direct organ damage	Kidney/bladder damage	Sexual dysfunction		
Impaired core muscle function	Fistula formation	Menopause	UI		
Infertility	Infertility	PFM weakness			
Lymphedema	Menopause	POP			
Myofascial/scar/ visceral restrictions	Myofascial/visceral restrictions	Sexual dysfunction			
PFM overactivity, trigger points	PFM fibrosis	UI			
POP	Pelvic radiation disease				
Sexual dysfunction	Second cancer				
UI	Sexual dysfunction				
Urinary retention	Urinary urgency/ frequency				
Urinary urgency/ frequency	UTI/yeast infections				
	UI				
	Vaginal stenosis				

PFM, Pelvic floor muscle; *POP,* pelvic organ prolapse; *UI,* urinary incontinence; *UTI,* urinary tract infection.
Created by Allegra ADams, PT, DPT. Printed with permission.

From Surgery

Surgery is a mainstay treatment for many solid tumor types, from biopsy to resection. Often, the impact is viewed as localized to the incised muscles and adjacent joints. Evolving laparoscopic approaches to replace open procedures create even less visible evidence of systemic disruption. Nonetheless, surgery can have deleterious physical effects on not only the musculoskeletal system but also neurological controls, hormonal regulation, blood and lymphatic circulation, and abnormal strains on the organs and even distal tissues. Physical adverse effects in the pelvic region such as bladder, bowel, or sexual dysfunction, pain, and disfigurement can have deeper psychological effects including isolation, depression, embarrassment, inability to return to vocation, and relational strains.

All surgeries carry with them the expectation of postoperative pain. However, genetic predispositions to scar formation, other influencers of tissue healing (e.g., co-morbid conditions, infection, nutritional status and habits, age, stress, smoking), incision location and dimensions, and lack of early scar mobilization can all contribute to the development of chronic abdominal, back, and pelvic pain through joint restrictions and malalignment, impaired muscle function, development of compensatory postures or movement patterns, neurovascular impingement, and/or ischemia. Pain may also be accompanied by muscle overactivity in an effort to splint or guard the healing area or pain inhibition of a muscle's function. If the body's main goal is to preserve vital organ, nerve, or vascular function, it will contort to reduce strain on that structure which may result in recurrent alignment asymmetries and muscle imbalances.[29] Take, for instance, the uterus in a patient who has had a hysterectomy. There may remain surgical restrictions to the uterosacral ligament which will result in a recurrent sacral torsion and all of the joint strain, change in muscle length-tension relationship, and nerve impingement that may follow.[18]

Surgeries above or below the diaphragm can affect breathing mechanics. Movement of the diaphragm has a stimulatory effect on the vagus nerve for parasympathetic innervation of the viscera (e.g., voiding, sexual arousal), stimulates gastrointestinal motility, acts as a muscle pump for venous and lymphatic drainage, and performs a "piston pump" synergy with the PFM.[30,31] Therefore, restricted ability of the diaphragm to descend can contribute to PFM tension or overactivity as well as weaken the PFM ability to generate strength and stability.

Open surgeries of the abdominal cavity clearly disrupt the synergy of the PFM with the transversus abdominus.[32] They may also result in surgical hernias or leave a diastasis rectus abdominus (DRA) when the incision is through the linea alba. However, even laparoscopic surgeries can disrupt the abdominal muscles' force generating capacity. All open and laparoscopic incisions disrupt the parietal peritoneum which is the layer deep to the transversus abdominus and can thereby impact abdominal muscle function.[33] Many laparoscopic approaches go through the umbilicus which can have inadvertent effects on the bladder via the urachus, which is the suspensory ligament of the bladder.[18] Umbilical incisions are also often a common site for postoperative pain.

Restricted peritoneal mobility can also place abnormal pressures downward on the infraperitoneal pelvic viscera and musculature resulting in impaired detrusor muscle function of the bladder (overactivity or retention), restricted bladder storage capacity, POP and a functionally shortened vaginal vault, and PFM overactivity which can result in pain, urinary urgency, retention, and/or incontinence.[18]

The lymphatic system is commonly interrupted due to surgery, whether from lymph node biopsy or dissection, or as a result of constriction of deep drainage pathways, notably the iliac and lumbar nodes, the cisterna chyli, the thoracic duct, and even the greater omentum, which is often damaged or removed during abdominal surgeries. For the purposes of this chapter, this disruption to the lymphatic system can result in genital edema and pelvic congestion; Chapter 9 discusses adverse effects to the lymphatic system in more detail.

Bladder and urinary dysfunction are more directly related to surgery in the pelvic region. Surgical scar restrictions can place abnormal tensions on the bladder resulting in detrusor overactivity and thereby contribute to urinary urgency, frequency, incontinence, or pain. Conversely, surgeries can result in ineffective detrusor contraction, again due to abnormal tensions or neurovascular damage, resulting in urinary retention and increased risk of urinary tract infections. Damage or removal of support structures could result in cystocele which may cause outlet obstruction and retention. Outlet obstruction could also occur from strictures secondary to surgery. Beyond the immediate urological organs and ligaments, surgery can damage the complex neurological network responsible for continence and micturition, including somatic and parasympathetic innervation from sacral nerves 2 to 4 and sympathetic innervation from the hypogastric nerve (T11-L2).[34] Figures 12.1 and 12.2 provide an in-depth view of the multiple levels of somatic and autonomic innervation for the pelvic viscera. Surgical resection of a tumor in the brain or spinal cord could also cause mobility impairments that may result in functional incontinence. Direct injury of an organ could occur during surgery, including the kidneys, ureters, bladder, prostate, or urethra, depending on the surgical site. Rarely, a vesicovaginal or urethrovaginal fistula can form, resulting in continuous incontinence.

Damage to or resection of the uterus, ovaries, fallopian tubes, or testicles can all cause pain, sexual dysfunction, infertility, and for women, premature menopause and the associated GSM, previously discussed. A hysterectomy, with or without unilateral or bilateral salpingo-oophorectomy, can cause chronic pelvic pain or pain with deep vaginal penetration and is often accompanied by a structural shortening of the vaginal vault depth. Dyspareunia can also be a result of myofascial restrictions, PFM overactivity, or vaginal atrophy or dryness due to reduced estrogen.

For males, erectile dysfunction following surgery for the treatment of cancer is mostly a result of neurological damage. Specifically, disruption of the superior hypogastric plexus (sympathetic, T10-L2) and sacral nerves 2 to 4 (parasympathetic pelvic plexus and somatosensory pudendal nerve) will adversely affect erectile function.[35] PFM weakness, specifically of the urogenital triangle which is innervated by the pudendal nerve, can also impair occlusion of penile vasculature to maintain erection.[35] It then follows that vascular damage from surgery can also contribute to erectile dysfunction.

From Radiation

Radiation therapy is ever evolving to minimize the scatter and damage to unintended tissues. Therefore, most adverse effects to the GU/GYN systems are from direct radiation to the region. In fact, more people with pelvic tumors are treated with radiation therapy than any other anatomical site of cancer.[36] It follows then that PWCs of pelvic organs treated with radiation therapy have a high likelihood of developing pelvic radiation disease (PRD).

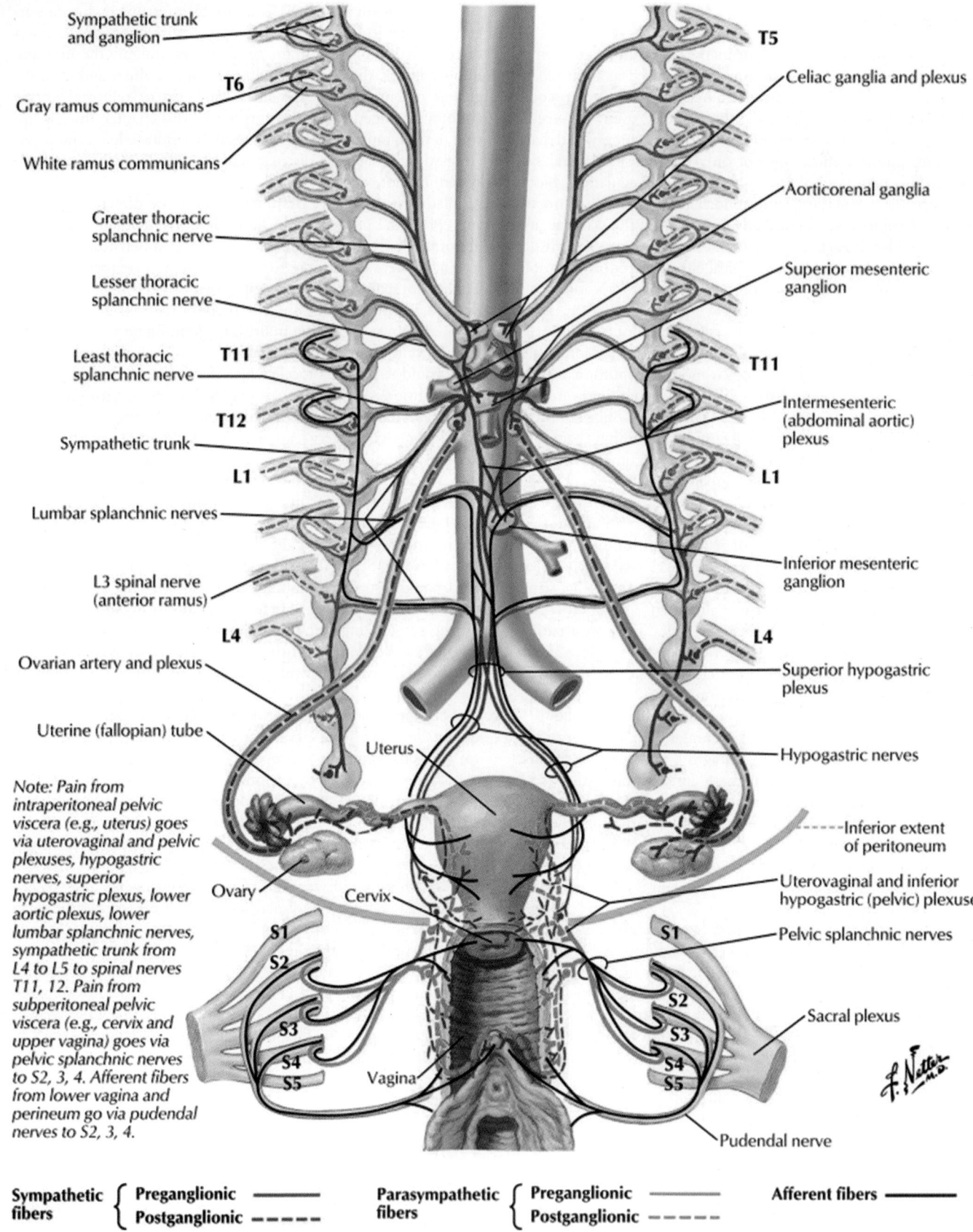

Sympathetic trunk and ganglion

Gray ramus communicans

White ramus communicans

Greater thoracic splanchnic nerve

Lesser thoracic splanchnic nerve

Least thoracic splanchnic nerve

Sympathetic trunk

Lumbar splanchnic nerves

L3 spinal nerve (anterior ramus)

Ovarian artery and plexus

Uterine (fallopian) tube

Note: Pain from intraperitoneal pelvic viscera (e.g., uterus) goes via uterovaginal and pelvic plexuses, hypogastric nerves, superior hypogastric plexus, lower aortic plexus, lower lumbar splanchnic nerves, sympathetic trunk from L4 to L5 to spinal nerves T11, 12. Pain from subperitoneal pelvic viscera (e.g., cervix and upper vagina) goes via pelvic splanchnic nerves to S2, 3, 4. Afferent fibers from lower vagina and perineum go via pudendal nerves to S2, 3, 4.

T6

T11

T12

L1

L4

Uterus

Ovary

Cervix

S1

S2

S3

S4

S5

Vagina

T5

Celiac ganglia and plexus

Aorticorenal ganglia

Superior mesenteric ganglion

Intermesenteric (abdominal aortic) plexus

Inferior mesenteric ganglion

Superior hypogastric plexus

Hypogastric nerves

Inferior extent of peritoneum

Uterovaginal and inferior hypogastric (pelvic) plexuses

Pelvic splanchnic nerves

Sacral plexus

Pudendal nerve

T11

L1

L4

S1

S2

S3

S4

S5

Sympathetic fibers { Preganglionic ——— Postganglionic ─ ─ ─ ─ ─

Parasympathetic fibers { Preganglionic ——— Postganglionic ─ ─ ─ ─ ─

Afferent fibers ———

• **Fig. 12.1** Somatic and Autonomic Innervation of the pelvic floor muscle (PFM) and Viscera, Female. Note that the pudendal nerve also supplies efferent innervation to the pelvic floor muscles. (Reprinted with permission from Netter FH. Chapter 6: Pelvis and perineum. In: Netter FH, ed. *Atlas of Human Anatomy.* 7th ed. Elsevier; 2019:367–441, Plate 397.)

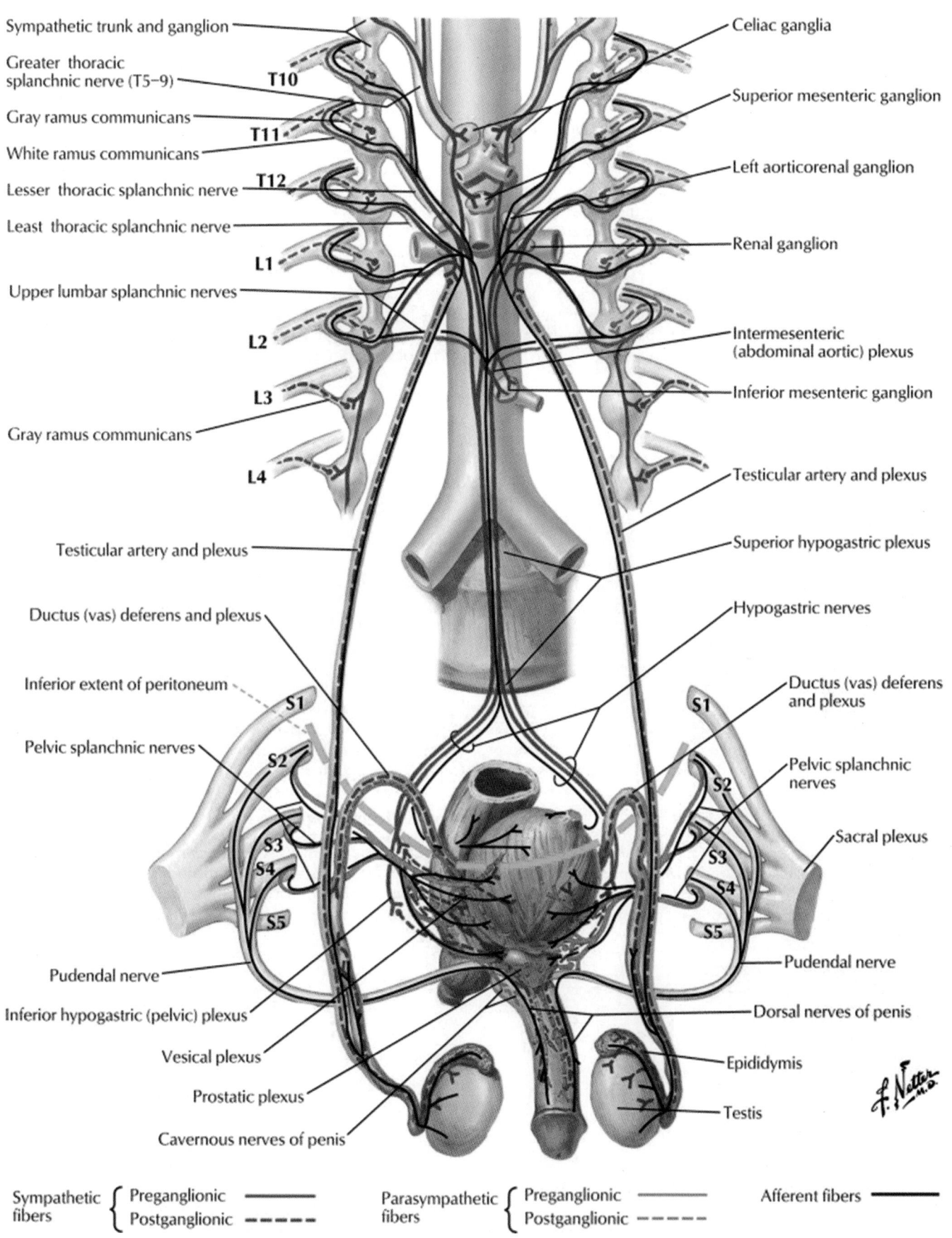

Sympathetic trunk and ganglion

Greater thoracic splanchnic nerve (T5–9)

Gray ramus communicans

White ramus communicans

Lesser thoracic splanchnic nerve

Least thoracic splanchnic nerve

Upper lumbar splanchnic nerves

Gray ramus communicans

Testicular artery and plexus

Ductus (vas) deferens and plexus

Inferior extent of peritoneum

Pelvic splanchnic nerves

Pudendal nerve

Inferior hypogastric (pelvic) plexus

Vesical plexus

Prostatic plexus

Cavernous nerves of penis

Celiac ganglia

Superior mesenteric ganglion

Left aorticorenal ganglion

Renal ganglion

Intermesenteric (abdominal aortic) plexus

Inferior mesenteric ganglion

Testicular artery and plexus

Superior hypogastric plexus

Hypogastric nerves

Ductus (vas) deferens and plexus

Pelvic splanchnic nerves

Sacral plexus

Pudendal nerve

Dorsal nerves of penis

Epididymis

Testis

T10
T11
T12
L1
L2
L3
L4

S1
S2
S3
S4
S5

S1
S2
S3
S4
S5

| Sympathetic fibers | Preganglionic ——— Postganglionic ----- | Parasympathetic fibers | Preganglionic ——— Postganglionic ----- | Afferent fibers ——— |

• **Fig. 12.2** Somatic and Autonomic Innervation of the pelvic floor muscle (PFM) and Viscera, Male Note that the pudendal nerve also supplies efferent innervation to the pelvic floor muscles. (Reprinted with permission from Netter FH. Chapter 6: Pelvis and perineum. In: Netter FH, ed. *Atlas of Human Anatomy*. 7th ed. Elsevier; 2019:367–441, Plate 398.)

It is common to experience some acute irritation of the bladder or vaginal mucosa during radiation treatment, though this is typically transient and may be mitigated by using L-argenine.[37] Corticosteroids and anti-inflammatories may be protective in the acute prefibrotic stages but are not effective in chronic stages.[38] The more debilitating adverse effects of radiation therapy are often long- or late-term onset, as the radiation never truly leaves the tissues and has a cumulative and progressive damaging effect as time goes on.[19,36]

Radiation fibrosis results from DNA damage by ionization followed by an inflammatory response with the abnormal deposition of collagen, accumulation of fibrin, and progressive ischemia resulting in fibrosis.[19,36] In addition to fibrosis, tissue atrophy due to loss of neurovascular innervation can occur. Pain, sensory loss, neuropathy, weakness, muscle spasm, loss of joint range of motion or contracture, bone pathology (osteopenia, osteoporosis, or osteonecrosis), and lymphedema are common long-term consequences of radiation therapy, which can collectively be referred to as radiation fibrosis syndrome (RFS).[19,36,39,40]

When RFS occurs in the pelvic structures, it is more commonly referred to as pelvic radiation disease (PRD). PRD is characterized by radiation enteritis, proctitis, and cystitis, ulceration, and vaginal stenosis.[36,38,41,42] Radiation therapy directly affects the PFM structure (dimensions, morphology, and composition) and function (resting and squeeze pressures, decreased contractile response to stimulation).[43] A PWC may develop myotomal muscle weakness, focal myopathy, or muscle spasm resulting in functional weakness of the contractile unit and/or pain. A PWC's risk of developing PRD is proportional to the total dose of radiation, total volume of tissue treated, tissue type, prolongation of therapy, and concurrent use of chemotherapy and/or surgery. Risk is also increased with concurrent comorbidities or lifestyle factors including: pre-existing connective tissues disease, genetic predisposition, hypertension, arterial disease, inflammatory bowel disease, tobacco use, previous pelvic or abdominal surgery, a body mass index less than 30, or diabetes mellitus. In fact, a diagnosis of diabetes doubles the risk of developing PRD within 5 years of radiation therapy.[36] Risk factors for developing PRD are summarized in Box 12.7.

Radiation therapy can have significant effects on the pelvic organs, causing fibrosis of the bladder which will result in reduced storage capacity, urinary urgency and frequency, and, in some instances, UI. Vaginal stenosis secondary to pelvic radiation can lead to dyspareunia. Restricted joint range of motion from muscle contracture due to radiation fibrosis of ligaments or joint capsules

---

• BOX 12.7   Risk Factors for Developing Pelvic Radiation Disease

Body mass index less than 30
Concurrent use of chemotherapy, surgery
pre-existing connective tissues disease
Diabetes
Genetic predisposition
Hypertension, arterial disease
Inflammatory bowel disease
Previous pelvic or abdominal surgery
Prolongation of therapy
Tissue type
Tobacco use
Total dose of radiation
Total volume of tissue treated

---

can pose positioning limitations during intimacy. Radiation can also damage the ovaries or testes resulting in infertility, and in women, the onset of premature menopause. Early menopause brings with it a plethora of genitourinary symptoms, as previously described, including UI, overactive bladder, and dyspareunia. The bowel is the most negatively affected site from radiation therapy, with 9 out of 10 PWC reporting chronic changes in bowel habits after receiving radiation to the pelvic region.[36] Refer to Chapter 17 for a complete discussion on bowel-related effects from radiation therapy.

Beyond direct fibrotic damage to the urogynecological organs and PFM, radiation therapy can also damage the surrounding nerves and blood vessels. Damage to the pudendal nerve (sacral nerve roots 2–4) can result in impaired somatic function for muscle contraction (incontinence) and sensory input (lack of awareness of bladder filling, insensate incontinence, reduced genital sensitivity, anorgasmia). Radiation damage to the autonomic nerve plexuses can result in abnormal smooth muscle contractility (overactive bladder, erectile dysfunction).[36] Nerve damage from radiation therapy within or outside the pelvis can contribute to functional incontinence by way of joint and muscle contractures, limited mobility, or impaired fine motor ability to get to the toilet and undress in time. Damage to blood vessels can contribute to decreased vascularity in the vaginal canal, UI, urinary tract and yeast infections, dyspareunia, and erectile dysfunction.

Vertebral compression fractures can occur due to osteopenia and osteoporosis secondary to radiation therapy. Nerve root compression can create pain or pelvic organ, muscle, or sensory dysfunction as previously described. Partial or complete spinal cord injury (SCI) could also result from radiation therapy. A full review of urological and sexual dysfunction from SCI is outside the scope of this text but is covered extensively by Stubblefield.[19] Osteonecrosis should be considered as a differential diagnosis for hip and pelvic pain.

As always, radiation therapy exposure also carries the risk of inducing a second cancer in the area. Since radiation therapy is widely used for pelvic organ cancers, this may mean a second pelvic organ cancer later on in life.[19]

From Chemotherapy

Chemotherapy is a mainstay treatment for hematological cancer types and is an adjuvant treatment to most other higher-grade cancers. Given its systemic nature, many acute adverse effects are obvious, including nausea and vomiting, fatigue, and chemotherapy-induced cognitive impairment (CICI). In the pelvic organs, acute changes in urine color or smell and bladder irritation may occur as the chemicals pass out of the body. However, chemotherapy may have the largest "silent" long- and late-term effects on the pelvic organs and muscles from seemingly unrelated cancers.

Kidney and bladder, in addition to liver, toxicity or damage is common from metabolizing and excreting these toxic chemicals and their byproducts. The toxic nature of chemotherapy can also damage the ovaries and testes, or perhaps more importantly the germ cells, leading to infertility and, in women, early onset of menopause. Women are born with their lifetime supply of oocytes (eggs), and therefore, these may be permanently damaged. Conversely, spermatozoa are continually regenerating and therefore men may be cleared for reproduction as early as 6 months after completing chemotherapy treatment.[44]

CIPN is well known for parethesias in the extremities. What is less often discussed is the effect of CIPN on the sacral nerves (somatic innervations of PFM) and the autonomic nervous system (ANS) which can contribute to GU/GYN symptoms. Chemotherapeutic agents commonly associated with the development of CIPN include: vinca-alkaloids (vinblastine [Alkaban-AQ, Velban], vincristine [Oncovin, Vincasar PFS]), and vinorelbine [Navelbine]), taxanes (paclitaxel [Taxol, Onxal], docetaxel [Taxotere], cabazitaxel [Jevtana]), podophyllotoxins (etoposide [Toposar, VePesid]), epothilones, thalidomide, bortezomib, and interferon which can cause symptoms after first dose. Platinum compounds (cisplatin [Platinol, Platinol AQ], carboplatin [Paraplatin], oxaliplatin [Eloxatin]) may not have effects until several weeks or months after the last dose. Risk factors that increase the chance of developing CIPN include: pre-existing neuropathy from alcoholism, diabetes, malnutrition, increased age, HIV, smoking, and vitamin B12 deficiency.[45–48] For a full discussion on CIPN, the reader is referred to Chapters 6 and 8.

Chemotherapy can cause myopathic PFM weakness contributing to UI and anorgasmia. Chemotherapy can also reduce sensations of bladder filling, result in overflow and/or insensate incontinence, and reduce genital sensation for sexual stimulation. Damage to the ANS includes overactive bladder symptoms, reduced detrusor contractility and urinary retention, and erectile dysfunction. Given the large range of musculoskeletal and neurological adverse effects from chemotherapy (discussed in detail in Chapters 7 and 8), there are any number of reasons that a PLWBC may also experience functional incontinence.

Chemotherapy may reduce a PLWBC's libido or impair their body image. Chemically-induced menopause resulting in vaginal thinning and dryness may lead to chafing, bleeding, and dyspareunia. Sexual dysfunction among PWCs receiving chemotherapy can also stem from a lack of interest due to other adverse effects, such as nausea, diarrhea, fatigue, or weakness. Psychosocial effects from the overall cancer diagnosis may also weigh heavy on the PWC and intimate partner relations.

From Hormonal and Biological Therapies

Hormonal therapies are primarily used for the treatment of breast, prostate, uterine, and ovarian cancers. They carry with them all the effects of reducing or blocking the sex-specific hormones. For men, reduced testosterone levels can result in erectile dysfunction and impotence, decreased sexual desire and reduced libido, and muscle atrophy. Men undergoing androgen deprivation therapy (ADT) are at an increased risk of falls, osteoporosis, and fractures. One in five men receiving ADT will experience a fracture within 5 to 6 years of ADT.[49]

For women, estrogen deprivation forces them into menopause and its associated GSM, including infertility, decreased sexual desire and reduced libido, dyspareunia, and UI. The bladder, urethra, and vagina and the pelvic support ligaments are rich in estrogen receptors[25] SERMs (such as tamoxifen [Nolvadex]) have an antiestrogen effect on the pelvic tissues. Tamoxifen, as used in treatment for some breast cancers, has been shown to increase the risk of developing POP. In a study of healthy postmenopausal women given tamoxifen for 20 weeks, 60% demonstrated an increase in POP measurements.[21]

From Stem Cell Transplant

The GU/GYN adverse effects experienced by the PWC receiving stem cell transplant are mostly due to adjuvant chemotherapy and radiation therapy. The most significant consequence affecting the urinary system is chronic kidney damage from graft versus host disease (GVHD).[50] Also, due to immunosuppressants, the PWC is at increased risk of recurrent urinary tract or yeast infections. Early menopause and infertility are also possible.

From Immunotherapy

Immunotherapy is frontline treatment for bladder cancer using Intravesical Bacillus Calmette-Guerin (BCG), which is a derivative of tuberculosis.[19] Acute bladder irritation, urinary frequency, and hematuria are common adverse effects. Chronic kidney damage is among long- or late-term effects of immunotherapy for all cancer types.

From Cancers of the GU/GYN System

The reader is referred to Chapter 16 for a full description of cancers of the GU/GYN systems including: risk factors, screening and diagnosis, staging, treatment pathways, and treatment specific adverse effects.

Measurement Tools to Screen for and Evaluate Adverse Effects

Referrals to pelvic floor physical therapy (PFPT) for bladder or sexual dysfunction rarely come from the oncology team itself. The PLWBC will likely be referred back to their primary care physician with such complaints who will then refer the person to either a urologist or gynecologist. Once at the specialists' office, the practice generally has their own screening questions for bladder or sexual dysfunction with several available medical self-report questionnaires. These are not the same as the self-report patient outcome measures utilized by the PFPT which will be discussed in Chapter 16. A urologist or urogynecologist may ask the person to complete a 24- to 72-hour bladder diary or, rarely, quantify volume of leakage with a pad test (pad weighed before and after a set period of time or after incontinence-provoking activity). Often the first, and sometimes only, test ordered by a physician for a person presenting with urological complaints is a urine culture to rule out infection, although some may initially treat irritative bladder symptoms (urgency, frequency, dysuria) with antibiotics without a urine culture.[7]

Additional imaging to quantify or categorize voiding dysfunction may be performed. A measure of postvoid residual (PVR), or the amount of urine left in the bladder after volitionally emptying, may be measured either with a bladder scanner or through catheterization. A PVR volume of 50 mL or less is normal; however, up to 100 mL is generally acceptable. While this is a measure of bladder emptying, it does not specify the type of voiding dysfunction. However, this is a simple test that can be performed in the physician's office. Less commonly used are a variety of urodynamic studies (UDS), ranging in complexity of equipment that may or may not be readily available in office—from simple cystoscopy to cystourethrography. UDS objectively measure bladder characteristics including: sensation, detrusor stability and contractility, urethral reaction during filling or emptying, bladder capacity, urethral pressure, and flow rate.[19]

Medical tests are rarely ordered for sexual dysfunction but may include imaging studies of the pelvic cavity or organs (ultrasound or magnetic resonance imaging), imaging of genital or pelvic circulation, pudendal nerve conduction/latency, or electromyography of the pelvic floor musculature.

Common Treatments for Each Adverse Effect

This chapter will discuss possible medical management interventions that PWC may receive to prevent adverse effects during treatment and interventions PLWBC may try to mitigate long- or late-term adverse effects. Physical therapy primary, secondary, and tertiary prevention methods for these adverse effects are presented in Chapter 16.

A person undergoing radiation therapy may benefit from taking anti-inflammatories, corticosteroids, antibiotics, or antioxidants to offset the development of PRD, though once fibrosis starts to develop, these treatment options are no longer viable.[38] Alternatively, as ischemia is a major contributing factor in the development of fibrosis or necrosis, hyperbaric oxygen therapy can temporarily increase the amount of oxygen carried to the tissues in the blood to stimulate healing and fighting infections.[38,51,52] If bladder capacity is reduced by radiation cystitis, the PLWBC may receive some relief of bladder pain, urinary urgency or frequency through bladder instillations or a hydrodistension. Bladder instillations are an intravesical therapy to repair the mucosal lining of the bladder using either heparin or hyaluronic acid and chondroitin sulfate.[53] A hydrodistension is an outpatient procedure performed under anesthesia in which the bladder is filled with water through a catheter in the urethra to a pressure to stretch the bladder walls which is held for several minutes. A hydrodistension will transiently increase bladder capacity but usually needs to be repeated every 6 months for maintenance; instillations may be received up to weekly in between distensions.

There is a plethora of medications that can be used to treat bladder storage dysfunction. Overactive bladder (UUI) is more successfully treated pharmacologically than SUI and may be helped with anticholinergics (oxybutynin [Ditropan], tolterodine [Detrol]), muscarinic antagonists (Solifenacin [Vesicare]), or beta-3 adrenergic agonists (mirabegron [Mirbetriq]) to relax the detrusor. Alpha-adrenergic agonists (e.g., ephedrine, phenylpropanolene), beta-adrenoceptor agonists (clenbuterol), beta-adrenoceptor antagonists (propranolol), tricyclic antidepressants (imipramine), and serotonin and norepinephrine reuptake inhibitors (duloxetine [Cymbalta]) increase the urethral sphincter tone for SUI whereas alpha-adrenergic blocking agents (e.g., baclofen, diazepam, dantrolene) improve bladder emptying in patients with outlet obstruction. Bethanechol chloride ([Urecholine]) can be used to treat urinary retention due to a hypocontractive bladder.[7,19] Azo or pyridium may be used to treat painful urination.

Surgery may be performed to treat persistent and bothersome SUI including bladder or urethral slings (success rate of 76%–79% and 61%–69%, respectively), injection of periurethral bulking agents (success rate of 38%), or an artificial urinary sphincter (15%–87% success).[54,55]

The use of hormone replacement therapy (HRT) for urinary and sexual dysfunction in women due to GSM, though effective, remains controversial. Current evidence demonstrates no excess risk of recurrence of gynecological cancers for patients taking HRT, though there are safety concerns about the use of systemic and local HRT in women with current or past history of estrogen-dependent breast cancer.[56,57] HRT has been shown to be protective against cardiovascular and skeletal morbidity (e.g., osteoporosis). For epithelial ovarian cancer, HRT even improved overall survival, in addition to QOL.[58] In terms of GSM, local HRT helps vaginal revascularization and thickening of vaginal epithelium, increasing lubrication and elasticity and decreasing vaginal pH, thereby preventing recurrent urinary tract infections and overactive bladder symptoms.[56-59]

For erectile dysfunction, men will be instructed in penile rehabilitation which includes oral vasodilators (sildenafil [Viagra], tadalafil [Cialis], or vardenafil [Levitra]), optional penile suppository (Alprostadil) or intracavernosal injection of vasodilators, a vacuum erection device or a penile exercise device, and self-stimulation (masturbation). Rarely, men may opt for an implanted penile prosthesis.[19]

Chronic pelvic pain is poorly understood in the general population and therefore is generally not well managed. Medical treatments are often trial and error and involve a variety of pain medications, muscle relaxants, selective serotonin reuptake inhibitors (SSRIs), corticosteroid injections, Botox injections to the PFM for spasticity, or pudendal nerve blocks.

For the PWC in their reproductive and childbearing years, fertility preservation will likely be a concern. There are several options, depending on cancer type, stage, and anticipated course of treatment. For males, some cancers, like Hodgkin lymphoma or testicular cancer, may be the cause of impaired sperm production. Surgery for testicular or prostate cancer will disrupt ejaculation. In cases of testicular cancer, the tumor typically presents unilaterally, and fertility may be preserved in the remaining testicle. "The primary threat for fertility in men is compromised sperm production, quality and mobility, and DNA damage secondary to chemotherapy and/or radiotherapy exposure."[44] However, this is usually transient and spermatogenesis and sperm health may be restored by 2 years after completion of treatment, provided appropriate shielding was used during radiation therapy. There is no documented increase in birth defects after this time. Nonetheless, the best option for males is cryopreservation of sperm. Harvesting takes an average of 5 days and long-term follow up shows that the sperm can be conserved up to 28 years.[44]

Fertility preservation options for females are less advanced; most are experimental with variable levels of success. Females are born with a finite number of oocytes and "most anticancer treatments can induce … immediate, definitive infertility, premature menopause, (or) compromised ability to carry a pregnancy due to uterine damage."[44] The standard method of preservation is in vitro fertilization and embryo banking; unfertilized oocyte cryopreservation is also promising. Nonetheless, it takes 2 to 6 weeks for harvesting which will delay the initiation of treatment, sometimes up to 2 months. This also requires ovarian hyperstimulation which may cause progression in hormone-sensitive cancers. Research is still being conducted regarding the viability of harvesting immature oocytes or cryopreservation of ovarian tissue to later be transplanted back to the woman. This latter option carries the risk of reintroducing latent cancer cells. Hormonal suppression of ovulation prior to and during chemotherapy may reduce the risk of premature ovarian failure, particularly for women being treated for breast cancer. Other options include: ovarian transposition (oophoropexy) by laparoscopy moving the ovaries as far as possible from the radiation field, gonadal shielding during radiation therapy, or conservative gynecologic surgery in early-stage cervical, ovarian, or endometrial cancers. Regardless, it is generally recommended that women wait an average of 2 to 5 years after completing cancer treatment prior to attempting to achieve spontaneous or medically assisted pregnancy. However, there is no evidence that a cancer history, cancer treatment, or fertility preservation measures increase the risk of birth defects or cancer in these children, though there is a slightly increased risk of miscarriage or preterm birth.[44]

Conclusion

Adverse effects to the GU/GYN systems are not unique to cancers of these systems and may arise from cancer treatment anywhere in the body, through direct or indirect mechanisms. Primary prevention of these effects is lacking as QOL is not always taken into account in the urgency to deliver lifesaving cancer care. Therefore, improved secondary prevention of increased awareness, enhanced screening, and early referral to a qualified oncology rehabilitation (Onc R) provider needs to be developed.

Critical Research Needs

- Urological and sexual function among PLWBC not of the GU/GYN systems
- Primary prevention of adverse effects before or during cancer treatment; secondary prevention through enhanced awareness, screening, and follow-up

Case Study

A 52-year-old woman presents to PFPT with complaints of UI, diminished sensation of bladder filling, and anorgasmia. Four years ago, she was diagnosed with left-sided Stage IIA multi-focal invasive ductal breast carcinoma, triple negative (estrogen receptor negative [ER-], progesterone receptor negative [PR-], HER2 negative). She received neoadjuvant chemotherapy with AC-T (doxorubicin [Adriamycin], cyclophosphamide [Cytoxan], paclitaxel [Taxol, Onxal]), lumpectomy and sentinel lymph node biopsy, followed by adjuvant radiation to the breast. Medical history is significant for hypothyroidism for which she takes levothyroxine. Her current BMI is 29. She was premenopausal at the time of diagnosis but now has not had a menstrual period in 3 years. She had three pregnancies, one miscarriage, and two cesarean deliveries. She notes onset of symptoms 2 years ago with progressive worsening of UI.

She is a nurse on a general orthopedics floor. She notes UI with sneezing and assisting patients with bed mobility. She would like to increase her exercise for weight loss but this also causes leakage. She finally mentioned her symptoms to her gynecologist who provided the referral to PFPT. Her PVR on bladder scan was 115 mL.

Discussion

This case illustrates how a PWC likely already has several risk factors for developing pelvic floor dysfunction, whether or not they are already symptomatic. Parity of three, two cesarean deliveries, and being overweight all increase a person's risk of developing UI. Even a cesarean delivery increases the risk of incontinence as the woman still carried the fetus for 9 months putting strain on the PFM. Many women go through labor and pushing for several hours prior to being converted to a cesarean which can damage the PFM. Moreover, the cesarean scar tissue can restrict bladder filling and impairs abdominal muscle function which creates a key synergy with the PFM (refer to Chapter 16). A symptom of hypothyroidism is constipation and therefore chronic straining may predispose someone to pelvic floor dysfunction. Her treatment course for breast cancer included cyclophosphamide and doxorubicin which are known to cause medical menopause, in addition to her age where she may have experienced menopause naturally. Many women with history of pelvic floor injury are still asymptomatic until they go through menopause when the drop in estrogen thins the vaginal tissues which were providing a structural means of bladder control revealing underlying pelvic muscle weakness. Cyclophosphamide can also cause adverse effects of the bladder through damage of the bladder walls. Finally, taxanes like paclitaxel are significantly linked to CIPN which can reduce afferent, efferent, and autonomic nerve function contributing to her loss of bladder sensation, decreased sensation with intercourse, and PFM weakness contributing to SUI and anorgasmia. Her self-image following cancer treatment as well as breast sensitivity as an erotic zone may also affect her libido contributing to sexual dysfunction. Urinary retention may occur due to decreased contractility of the detrusor muscle during voiding or she may have some degree of bladder prolapse which impairs bladder emptying. A bladder that never fully empties also increases the likelihood of incontinence with increases in intraabdominal pressure.

Treatment

The general course of treatment for this PLWBC will include assessment of breathing mechanics and chest wall mobility due to surgery and radiation. Abdominal wall integrity (DRA), abdominal scar mobility, and abdominal muscle strength for synergy with the PFM will also need to be addressed. General assessment and retraining of posture, bony alignment asymmetries, and lumbopelvic muscle length-strength imbalances will need to be normalized. PFM tone will be assessed and trigger points resolved prior to functional progression of strengthening for both power and endurance. PFM strength will help with both voluntary bladder control and sexual function. Functional progression of core (diaphragm, abdominal, and PFM) strengthening and integration into daily activities is required in addition to training proper body mechanics for home and work-related responsibilities. The woman may require sacral or intravaginal electrical stimulation to improve PFM strength, bladder and/or vaginal sensation. It is possible that she will require a pessary for prolapse support or urethral closure either worn continuously, only at work, or during exercise. Exercise safety to prevent progression of pelvic floor dysfunction and instruction in an exercise protocol appropriate for her level of training will conclude her PT treatment.

Review Questions

Reader can find the correct answers and rationale in the back of the book.

1. Which of the following is an example of an active continence mechanism that is interrupted by cancer treatment?
   A. Prostatectomy
   B. PFM atrophy as a result of androgen-deprivation therapy
   C. Vaginal atrophy as a result of surgically induced menopause
   D. Tamoxifen (Soltamox) treatment exacerbating bladder prolapse

2. A PLWBC is likely to develop functional UI as a result of:
   A. Cerebrovascular accident due to thrombus formation
   B. Fibrotic changes of the bladder due to radiation therapy for colorectal cancer
   C. PFM weakness due to CIPN from cisplatin (Platinol, Platinol AQ) for small cell lung cancer
   D. Bladder wall irritation due to cyclophosphamide (Cytoxan) for breast cancer
3. Which of the following is NOT a cause of urinary retention?
   A. Spinal metastasis resulting in lower motor neuron injury and an areflexic bladder
   B. Urethral stricture from radiation fibrosis
   C. Antiemetic medications to treat chemotherapy-induced nausea and vomiting
   D. Constipation from abdominal surgery for tumor resection
4. Urinary tract or yeast infections may become recurrent in a PLWBC for all of the following reasons except:
   A. Chemotherapy-induced myelosuppression
   B. Treatment-induced menopause and associated changes in vaginal pH
   C. Radiation cystitis from treatment for endometrial cancer
   D. Immunosuppression for stem cell transplant
5. Which of the following is LEAST LIKELY to be true regarding fertility during/after cancer treatment?
   A. A woman who requires pelvic radiation may be able to have the ovaries surgically moved out of the radiation field to preserve fertility
   B. A man who has received chemotherapy will not be able to father a child of his own unless he banks his sperm prior to treatment
   C. It takes an average of 6 weeks to harvest oocytes which may result in a worse prognosis by delaying the initiation of care
   D. A man can still father children after testicular cancer treatment
6. A prepubescent female underwent treatment for acute lymphoblastic leukemia over the course of 2.5 years. Her treatment included methotrexate (Trexall), prednisone (Deltasone), and vincristine (Oncovin, Vincasar PFS). She is now 25 years old, nulliparous, and is a competitive dancer. She has complaints of SUI. Her incontinence is likely due to all of the following EXCEPT:
   A. Recurrent urinary tract infections and kidney stones due to methotrexate resulting in PFM overactivity
   B. Proximal muscle wasting due to prolonged corticosteroid use
   C. CIPN due to vincristine
   D. Engaging in a high-impact sport

7. A 72-year-old male presents with complaints of urinary retention. His medical history is significant for Stage II non-small cell lung cancer of the right lung treated with lobectomy and regional lymph node dissection, cisplatin (Platinol, Platinol AQ), and docetaxel (Taxotere). Which of the following is NOT a contributing factor to his bladder dysfunction?
   A. ANS dysfunction due to CIPN
   B. Impaired breathing mechanics due to lobectomy
   C. PFM weakness due to chronic cough
   D. Opioids for postoperative pain
8. A 65-year-old African American man presents to his primary care physician with complaints of erectile dysfunction. His cancer history is significant for Stage III melanoma on his left torso treated with wide local excision of the melanoma and regional lymph node dissection followed by adjuvant treatment with an immune check point inhibitor. His other medical history includes obesity, hypertension, type 2 diabetes mellitus, and a right total hip replacement. His erectile dysfunction is likely due to:
   A. Scar tissue from the local excision restricting chest wall expansion and breathing mechanics
   B. Subclinical lymphedema from lymph node dissection
   C. Use of immune check point inhibitors
   D. He has other risk factors and his cancer history is likely not relevant to his erectile dysfunction
9. A 56-year-old woman is referred to PFPT with complaints of dyspareunia following treatment for rectal cancer. Her treatment included fluorouracil (Adrucil), oxaliplatin (Eloxatin), leucovorin (Wellcovorin), external beam radiation, and proctectomy with colo-anal anastomosis. Which of the following is NOT likely to contribute to her complaints?
   A. Vaginal fibrosis/stenosis due to external beam radiation
   B. Vaginal dryness due to chemoradiation
   C. CIPN from oxaliplatin
   D. Pelvic muscle overactivity due to surgical scar restriction and/or change in bowel habits
10. A 17-year-old male was treated for high-grade osteosarcoma in the distal femur with neoadjuvant and adjuvant methotrexate (Trexall), doxorubicin (Adriamycin), and cisplatin (Platinol, Platinol AQ) in addition to surgical resection. He is referred to physical therapy with complaints of ipsilateral testicular and groin pain. Which of the following is the likely cause of this pain?
   A. Altered gait mechanics from surgery resulting in pelvic asymmetry and altered lumbopelvic muscle length-tension relationships
   B. Impaired spermatogenesis from chemotherapy
   C. He likely has an inguinal hernia from straining
   D. He likely has a second unrelated cancer of the testicle

References

1. Wu JM, Vaughan CP, Goode PS, et al. Prevalence and trends of symptomatic pelvic floor disorders in U.S. women. *Obstet Gynecol*. 2014;123(1):141–148. http://doi.org/10.1097/AOG.0000000000000057.
2. Kepenekci I, Keskinkilic B, Akinsu F, et al. Prevalence of pelvic floor disorders in the female population and the impact of age, mode of delivery, and parity. *Dis Colon Rectum*. 2011;54(1):85–94. http://doi.org/10.1007/DCR.0b013e3181fd2356.
3. Buckley BS, Lapitan MCM. Prevalence of urinary incontinence in men, women, and children-current evidence: findings of the fourth international consultation on incontinence. *Urology*. 2010;76(2):265–270. http://doi.org/10.1016/j.urology.2009.11.078.
4. Markland AD, Richter HE, Fwu CW, Eggers P, Kusek JW. Prevalence and trends of urinary incontinence in adults in the United States, 2001 to 2008. *J Urol*. 2011;186(2):589–593. http://doi.org/10.1016/j.juro.2011.03.114.
5. Bretschneider CE, Doll KM, Bensen JT, Gehrig PA, Wu JM, Geller EJ. Prevalence of pelvic floor disorders in women with suspected

gynecological malignancy: a survey-based study. *Int Urogynecol J.* 2016;27(9):1409–1414. http://doi.org/10.1007/s00192-016-2962-3.

6. Goodman CC, Heick J, Lazaro RT. *Differential Diagnosis for Physical Therapists: Screening for Referral.* 6th ed. Elsevier Inc.; 2018.

7. Irion JM, Irion G. *Women's Health in Physical Therapy.* Wolters Kluwer Health/Lippincott Williams & Wilkins; 2010.

8. Ahangari A. Prevalence of chronic pelvic pain among women: an updated review. *Pain Physician.* 2014;17(2):E141–E147.

9. Tran CN, Shoskes DA. Sexual dysfunction in chronic prostatitis/chronic pelvic pain syndrome. *World J Urol.* 2013;31(4):741–746. http://doi.org/10.1007/s00345-013-1076-5.

10. Tennfjord MK, Hilde G, Stær-Jensen J, Ellström Engh M, Bø K. Dyspareunia and pelvic floor muscle function before and during pregnancy and after childbirth. *Int Urogynecol J.* 2014;25(9):1227–1235. http://doi.org/10.1007/s00192-014-2373-2.

11. Jamieson DJ, Steege JF. The prevalence of dysmenorrhea, dyspareunia, pelvic pain, and irritable bowel syndrome in primary care practices. *Obstet Gynecol.* 1996;87(1):55–58. http://doi.org/10.1016/0029-7844(95)00360-6.

12. Hoffman D. Understanding multisymptom presentations in chronic pelvic pain: the inter-relationships between the viscera and myofascial pelvic floor dysfunction, *Curr Pain Headache Rep.* 2011;15(5):343–346. http://doi.org/10.1007/s11916-011-0215-1.

13. Spitznagle TM, McCurdy Robinson C. Myofascial pelvic pain. *Obstet Gynecol Clin North Am.* 2014;41(3):409–432. http://doi.org/10.1016/j.ogc.2014.04.003.

14. Bonder JH, Chi M, Rispoli L. Myofascial pelvic pain and related disorders. *Phys Med Rehabil Clin N Am.* 2017;28(3):501–515. http://doi.org/10.1016/j.pmr.2017.03.005.

15. Moore J, Kennedy S. Causes of chronic pelvic pain. *Bailliere's Best Pract Res Clin Obstet Gynaecol.* 2000;14(3):389–402. http://doi.org/10.1053/beog.1999.0082.

16. Hwang S, Clark M. Cancer-related pelvic pain. In: Gulati A, Puttanniah V, Bruel BM, Rosenberg WS, Hung JC, eds. *Essentials of Interventional Cancer Pain Management.* Springer Nature; 2018:385–393.

17. Haylen BT, De Ridder D, Freeman RM, et al. An International Urogynecological Association (IUGA)/International Continence Society (ICS) joint report on the terminology for female pelvic floor dysfunction. *Int Urogynecol J.* 2010;21(1):5–26. http://doi.org/10.1007/s00192-009-0976-9.

18. Barral J-P. *Urogenital Manipulation.* 2nd ed. (Anderson S, Bensky D, eds.). Eastland Press; 2006.

19. Stubblefield MD, ed. *Cancer Rehabilitation: Principles and Practice.* 2nd ed. Springer Publishing Company; 2019.

20. Resnick NM. Geriatric incontinence. *Urol Clin North Am.* 1996;23(1):55–74. http://doi.org/10.1016/S0094-0143(05)70293-7.

21. Vardy MD, Lindsay R, Scotti RJ, et al. Short-term urogenital effects of raloxifene, tamoxifen, and estrogen. *Am J Obstet Gynecol.* 2003;189(1):81–88. http://doi.org/10.1067/mob.2003.374.

22. Myers TW. *Anatomy Trains: Myofascial Meridians for Manual Therapists and Movement Professionals.* 4th ed. Churchill Livingston/Elsevier; 2020.

23. Upledger JE. *Craniosacral Therapy II: Beyond the Dura.* Eastland Press; 1987.

24. Coady D, Kennedy V. Sexual health in women affected by cancer: focus on sexual pain. *Obstet Gynecol.* 2016;128(4):775–791. http://doi.org/10.1097/AOG.0000000000001621.

25. Lang JH, Zhu L, Sun ZJ, Chen J. Estrogen levels and estrogen receptors in patients with stress urinary incontinence and pelvic organ prolapse. *Int J Gynecol Obstet.* 2003;80(1):35–39. http://doi.org/10.1016/S0020-7292(02)00232-1.

26. Portman DJ, Gass MLS. Genitourinary syndrome of menopause: new terminology for vulvovaginal atrophy from the International Society for the Study of Women's Sexual Health and the North American Menopause Society. *Maturitas.* 2014;79(3):349–354. http://doi.org/10.1016/j.maturitas.2014.07.013.

27. Kim H-K, Kang S-Y, Chung Y-J, Kim J-H, Kim M-R. The recent review of the genitourinary syndrome of menopause. *J Menopausal Med.* 2015;21(2):65. http://doi.org/10.6118/jmm.2015.21.2.65.

28. Fried TR, Erekson EA, Li F-Y, Martin DK. Vulvovaginal symptoms prevalence in postmenopausal women and relationship to other menopausal symptoms and pelvic floor disorders. *Menopause.* 2016;23(4):368–375. http://doi.org/10.1097/GME.0000000000000549.

29. Barral J-P, Merier P. *Visceral Manipulation,* Revised Edition. Eastland Press; 2005.

30. Talasz H, Kremser C, Kofler M, Kalchschmid E, Lechleitner M, Rudisch A. Phase-locked parallel movement of diaphragm and pelvic floor during breathing and coughing-a dynamic MRI investigation in healthy females. *Int Urogynecol J.* 2011;22(1):61–68. http://doi.org/10.1007/s00192-010-1240-z.

31. Bordoni B, Zanier E. Anatomic connections of the diaphragm: Influence of respiration on the body system. *J Multidiscip Healthc.* 2013;6:281–291. http://doi.org/10.2147/JMDH.S45443.

32. Sapsford RR, Hodges PW, Richardson CA, Cooper DH, Markwell SJ, Jull GA. Co-activation of the abdominal and pelvic floor muscles during voluntary exercises. *Neurourol Urodyn.* 2001;20(1):31–42. http://doi.org/10.1002/1520-6777(2001)20:1<31::AID-NAU5>3.0.CO;2-P.

33. Barral J-P, Mercier P. *Visceral Manipulation II, Revised Edition.* Eastland Press; 2007.

34. Fowler CJ, Griffiths D, De Groat WC. The neural control of micturition. *Nat Rev Neurosci.* 2008;9(6):453–466. http://doi.org/10.1038/nrn2401.

35. Dean RC, Lue TF. Physiology of penile erection and pathophysiology of erectile dysfunction. *Urol Clin North Am.* 2005;32(4):379–395. http://doi.org/10.1016/j.ucl.2005.08.007.

36. Morris K AL, Haboubi NY. Pelvic radiation therapy: between delight and disaster. *World J Gastrointest Surg.* 2015;7(11):279–288. http://doi.org/10.4240/wjgs.v7.i11.279.

37. Costa WS, Ribeiro MN, Cardoso LEM, et al. Nutritional supplementation with l-arginine prevents pelvic radiation-induced changes in morphology, density, and regulating factors of blood vessels in the wall of rat bladder. *World J Urol.* 2013;31(3):653–658. http://doi.org/10.1007/s00345-012-0938-6.

38. Frazzoni L, La Marca M, Guido A, Morganti AG, Bazzoli F, Fuccio L. Pelvic radiation disease: updates on treatment options. *World J Clin Oncol.* 2015;6(6):272–280. http://doi.org/10.5306/wjco.v6.i6.272.

39. Hojan K, Milecki P. Opportunities for rehabilitation of patients with radiation fibrosis syndrome. *Reports Pract Oncol Radiother.* 2014;19(1):1–6. http://doi.org/10.1016/j.rpor.2013.07.007.

40. Delanian S, Lefaix JL. Current management for late normal tissue injury: radiation-induced fibrosis and necrosis. *Semin Radiat Oncol.* 2007;17(2):99–107. http://doi.org/10.1016/j.semradonc.2006.11.006.

41. Andreyev HJN, Wotherspoon A, Denham JW, Hauer-Jensen M. "Pelvic radiation disease": new understanding and new solutions for a new disease in the era of cancer survivorship, *Scand J Gastroenterol.* 2011;46(4):389–397. http://doi.org/10.3109/00365521.2010.545832.

42. Andreyev HJN, Wotherspoon A, Denham JW, Hauer-Jensen M. Defining pelvic-radiation disease for the survivorship era. *Lancet Oncol.* 2010;11(4):310–312. http://doi.org/10.1016/S1470-2045(10)70026-7.

43. Bernard S, Ouellet MP, Moffet H, Roy JS, Dumoulin C. Effects of radiation therapy on the structure and function of the pelvic floor muscles of patients with cancer in the pelvic area: a systematic review. *J Cancer Surviv.* 2016;10(2):351–362. http://doi.org/10.1007/s11764-015-0481-8.

44. Caroline D, Ries F. Preservation of fertility in the cancer patient. In: Dicato MA, VanCutsem E, eds. *Side Effects of Medical Cancer Therapy: Prevention and Treatment.* 2nd ed. Springer International Publishing AG; 2018:355–366. http://doi.org/10.1007/978-0-85729-787-7.

45. Society. American Cancer, What is Peripheral, Neuropathy? (2019). https://www.cancer.org/treatment/treatments-and-side-effects/

physical-side-effects/peripheral-neuropathy/what-is-peripherial-neuropathy.html.

46. Argyriou AA, Kyritsis AP, Makatsoris T, Kalofonos HP. Chemotherapy-induced peripheral neuropathy in adults: a comprehensive update of the literature. *Cancer Manag Res.* 2014;6(1):135–147. http://doi.org/10.2147/CMAR.S44261.

47. Seretny M, Currie GL, Sena ES, et al. Incidence, prevalence, and predictors of chemotherapy-induced peripheral neuropathy: a systematic review and meta-analysis. *Pain.* 2014;155(12):2461–2470. http://doi.org/10.1016/j.pain.2014.09.020.

48. Addington J, Freimer M. Chemotherapy-induced peripheral neuropathy: an update on the current understanding [version 1; referees: 2 approved], *F1000Research.* 2016;5(F1000 Faculty Rev):1466. http://doi.org/10.12688/f1000research.8053.1.

49. Shahinian VB, Kuo Y-F, Freeman JL, Goodwin JS. Risk of fracture after androgen deprivation for prostate cancer. *N Engl J Med.* 2005;352(2):154–164. http://doi.org/10.1097/S0022-5347(01)68451-9.

50. Sawinski D. The kidney effects of hematopoietic stem cell transplantation. *Adv Chronic Kidney Dis.* 2014;21(1):96–105. http://doi.org/10.1053/j.ackd.2013.08.007.

51. Oscarsson N. *Hyperbaric Oxygen Treatment in Radiation-Induced Injuries: From a Multicenter Randomized Controlled Trial to an Experimental Cell Model [Doctoral thesis].* University of Gothenburg; 2020.

52. Craighead P, Shea-Budgell MA, Nation J, et al. Hyperbaric oxygen therapy for late radiation tissue injury in gynecologic malignancies. *Curr Oncol.* 2011;18(5):220–227. http://doi.org/10.3747/co.v18i5.767.

53. Giannitsas K, Athanasopoulos A. Intravesical therapies for radiation cystitis. *Curr Urol.* 2014;8(4):169–174. http://doi.org/10.1159/000365711.

54. Nikolopoulos KI, Betschart C, Doumouchtsis SK. The surgical management of recurrent stress urinary incontinence: a systematic review. *Acta Obstet Gynecol Scand.* 2015;94(6):568–576. http://doi.org/10.1111/aogs.12625.

55. Linder BJ, Rangel LJ, Elliott DS. Evaluating success rates after artificial urinary sphincter placement: a comparison of clinical definitions. *Urology.* 2018;113:220–224. http://doi.org/10.1016/j.urology.2017.10.033.

56. The North American Menopause Society. The 2017 hormone therapy position statement of The North American Menopause Society. *Menopause J North Am Menopause Soc.* 2017;24(7):728–753. https://www.menopause.org/docs/default-source/2017/nams-2017-hormone-therapy-position-statement.pdf.

57. Pinkerton JV, Changing the conversation about hormone therapy. *Climacteric.* 2017;20(4):293–295. http://doi.org/10.1080/13697137.2017.1346380.

58. Eeles RA, Morden JP, Gore M, et al. Adjuvant hormone therapy may improve survival in epithelial ovarian cancer: results of the AHT randomized trial. *J Clin Oncol.* 2015;33(35):4138–4144. http://doi.org/10.1200/JCO.2015.60.9719.

59. Chambers LM, Herrmann A, Michener CM, Ferrando CA, Ricci S. Vaginal estrogen use for genitourinary symptoms in women with a history of uterine, cervical, or ovarian carcinoma. *Int J Gynecol Cancer.* 2020;30(4):515–524. http://doi.org/10.1136/ijgc-2019-001034.

13

Immune System

SOPHIA ANDREWS, PT, DPT, CLAIRE CHILD, PT, DPT, MPH

CHAPTER OUTLINE

Introduction

A rehabilitation professional is trained to be an expert in movement science, assessing for impairments in various body structures and functions that contribute to changes in movement quality. To be highly effective movement specialists working in ever-more specialized areas of oncology rehabilitation (Onc R) across the care continuum, a more advanced understanding of the immune system and its various components and functions is essential. Most persons living with and beyond cancer (PLWBCs) will experience changes in the normal function of the immune system at some point during their cancer treatment course. Certain changes in immune function (e.g., aging, autoimmune conditions) may increase the risk of malignant transformation of cells. Other changes occur as part of the primary pathophysiology of a specific type of cancer. Alterations in immune function are some of the most common adverse effects

of current cancer treatment regimens. The skilled clinician working with persons diagnosed with cancer (PDWC) must be able to recognize changes in the immune system and interpret implications for movement, safety, and exercise capacity.

Onc R clinicians must be knowledgeable about the normal function of innate and adaptive immunity (including cellular and humoral responses) and considerations for genetic variation. Pathological trends during malignancy that impact the immune system are highlighted here, building upon other chapters. Many medical treatments for solid and hematologic malignancies are associated with adverse effects on the homeostasis of the immune and hematologic systems, which can have specific implications for Onc R clinicians working with PLWBCs.

Humans live within a complex environment of microorganisms and have developed systems of host defense to protect against potentially dangerous microbial infections. Elements of host

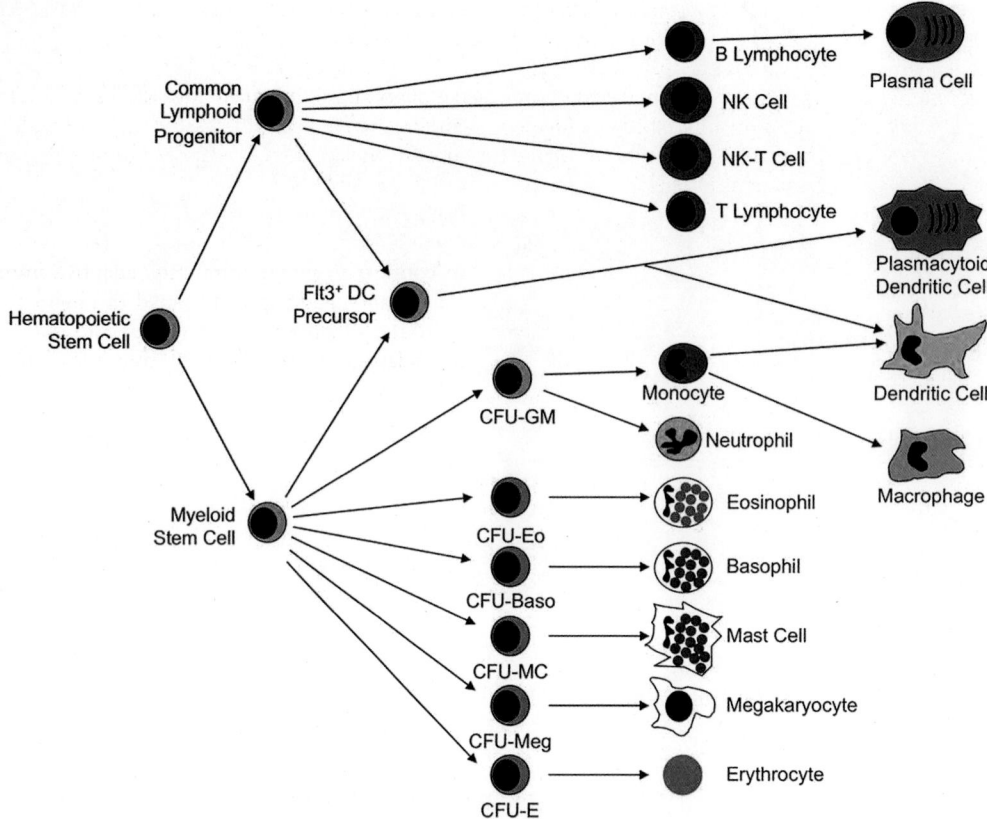

• **Fig. 13.1** Hematopoietic Stem Cell-Derived Cell Lineages. Pluripotent hematopoietic stem cells differentiate in bone marrow into common lymphoid or common myeloid progenitor cells. Lymphoid stem cells give rise to B cell, T cell, and NK cell lineages. Myeloid stem cells give rise to a second level of lineage specific colony form unit (CFU) cells that go on to produce neutrophils, monocytes, eosinophils, basophils, mast cells, megakaryocytes, and erythrocytes. Monocytes differentiate further into macrophages in peripheral tissue compartments. Dendritic cells (DC) appear to develop primarily from a DC precursor that is distinguished by its expression of the Flt3 receptor. This precursor can derive from either lymphoid or myeloid stem cells and gives rise to both classical DC and plasmacytoid DC. Classical DC can also derive from differentiation of monocytoid precursor cells. *NK,* Natural killer. (Reprinted with permission from Chaplin DD. Overview of the immune response. *J Allergy Clin Immunol.* 2010;125(2 suppl 2):S3–S23. doi:10.1016/j.jaci.2009.12.980.)

defense systems are phylogenetically ancient and shared in some form with all living organisms, including insects and plants.[1,2] Key components and normal functions of human immune defense systems are presented below, including descriptions of the innate and adaptive cellular and humoral immune systems.

Innate Immunity

Innate immunity refers to immune system responses that are present from birth, genetically inherited from parents, and are not learned, adapted, or permanently heightened as a result of exposure to microbes or vaccines. Genetic variation accounts for some differences between parents and offspring and within a population. Many cellular components of innate immunity are derived from hematopoietic stem cells including, but not limited to lymphocytes, monocytes, and neutrophils (Figure 13.1). Each derived cell type has a different role within the immune system.[3]

The innate immune system protects the host during the time between pathogen exposure and adaptive responses. The generation time of most bacteria is about 20 to 30 minutes, whereas the development of a specific adaptive immune response with antibody and T cells takes days to weeks[4] in healthy individuals. Innate immune system receptors are able to recognize specific

patterns on foreign microbial pathogens and trigger nonspecific reactionary mechanisms to minimize infectious damage.

Some cells produce cytokines and chemokines that participate in essential processes of phagocytosis, inflammation, and the synthesis of acute phase proteins. The cardinal signs of inflammation (tumor, rubor, calor, and dolor) are products of the protective action of innate immunity. To limit damage to the host, these responses must also be terminated when no longer needed. There are many different etiologies of inflammation (Table 13.1). For persons living with cancer (PLWC), acute inflammatory responses can become life-threatening, such as a high-grade fever that triggers an increase in respiratory rate. Subsequent hyperventilation can lead to changes in the partial pressure of carbon dioxide in the blood and abnormal blood pH levels. In most malignancies, proinflammatory pathways along the inflammation-immune axis become chronically overactive.

Host physical barriers, structural components of cells, and the host microbiome may also be considered ancillary components of the innate immune system, as they function as barriers to infection. Table 13.2 lists some of the critical functions and host components of the innate immune system.

Multiple innate immune mechanisms are known to trigger endogenous T cell-mediated responses to tumor-specific antigens (TSAs).[5]

Innate pathways involved in the recognition of tumors continue to be explored by researchers and characterized as promising avenues for the design of new therapeutic strategies for cancer immunotherapy treatments. The innate immune system also activates and primes the adaptive immune system to interact with a microbe or other antigen. The recognition of conserved features of microbial pathogens by the innate immune system is mediated by pattern-recognition receptors (PRRs), which detect danger by recognizing conserved pathogen-associated molecular patterns (PAMPs),[6] including bacterial and fungal cell-wall components and viral nucleic acids. Toll-like receptors (TLRs) are one of these PRRs expressed by a variety of immune cells.[7] The detection of PAMPs by PRRs triggers inflammatory responses and other innate host defenses. Dendritic cells and other antigen-presenting cells can sense microbes with PRRs and tailor the subsequent activation of adaptive immune responses.[8]

Adaptive Immunity

In contrast to innate immunity, adaptive immune responses are continually changing and refined throughout the lifetime of the host. The adaptive immune system consists of two principal arms that adapt to defend the body from infections and malignancy—T lymphocytes (also referred to as T cells) and B lymphocytes (also referred to as B cells). The main functions of T lymphocytes are described as adaptive cellular response, and the main functions of B lymphocytes, including antibody development, are described as adaptive humoral response.

Over several decades of research and practice, our contemporary understanding of the duality of adaptive immunity has been refined. Immature B and T cells originate in the bone marrow and then migrate either to peripheral lymphoid tissues (immature B cells) or the thymus (immature T cells) to mature.[9] After cell-mediated "education" and specialized adaptations, they then leave to seed peripheral tissues.[10] Basic science laboratory investigation has elucidated much about the anatomic origins and development of two separate lineages of adaptive immunity—how T and B cells collaborate for effective immune responses within different peripheral tissues, how they contribute to host defense, how they

---

TABLE 13.1 Etiology of Inflammation

Noninfectious Factors	Infectious Factors
Physical: burn, frostbite, physical injury, foreign bodies, trauma, ionizing radiation	Bacteria, viruses, fungi, other microorganisms
Chemical: glucose, fatty acids, toxins, alcohol, chemical irritants (including fluoride, nickel, and other trace elements)	
Biological: damaged cells	
Psychological: excitement, emotional stress	

Adapted from Chen L, Deng H, Cui H, et al. Inflammatory responses and inflammation-associated diseases in organs. *Oncotarget*. 2017;9(6):7204–7218. doi:10.18632/oncotarget.23208.

TABLE 13.2 Critical Functions and Host Components of Innate Immunity

Critical Functions of Innate Immunity	Description and Examples
Detection of micro-organisms and first-line defense	Microbial detection through pattern recognition and complement cascade
Regulation of inflammation	To limit damage to the host, acute inflammatory responses must also be terminated when no longer needed.
Maintenance of immunologic homeostasis	Microbe-induced activation of the innate immune system is tightly linked to the concurrent induction of down-regulatory mechanisms to regain immune homeostasis.
Activation and instruction of the adaptive immune responses	Pattern recognition receptors (PRRs) on innate immune cells recognize microbes and activate dendritic cells, macrophages, and other facilitators of an adaptive immune response.
Host Components	**Description and Examples**
Physical barriers	Tight junctions in the skin, epithelial and mucous membrane surfaces, mucus itself, and vascular endothelial cells that prevent pathogen penetration of the intestines
Antimicrobial enzymes	Found in epithelial and phagocytic cells (e.g., lysozyme)
Inflammation-related serum proteins	(e.g., complement components, C-reactive protein [CRP], and lectins [carbohydrate-binding proteins])
Toll-like receptors (TLRs)	Cell receptors that sense micro-organisms and signal a defensive response
Macrophages, mast cells, natural killer (NK) cells, innate lymphoid cells (ILCs)	Cells that release cytokines and other inflammatory mediators
Phagocytes	Neutrophils, monocytes, macrophages
The inflammasome	A central signaling system that regulates the innate inflammatory response
The microbiome	The collection of bacteria, fungi, and viruses that live in and on the body, may also be considered a component of the innate immune system, as it profoundly impacts mechanisms of host defense.

Created by Claire Child and Sophia Andrews. Printed with permission.

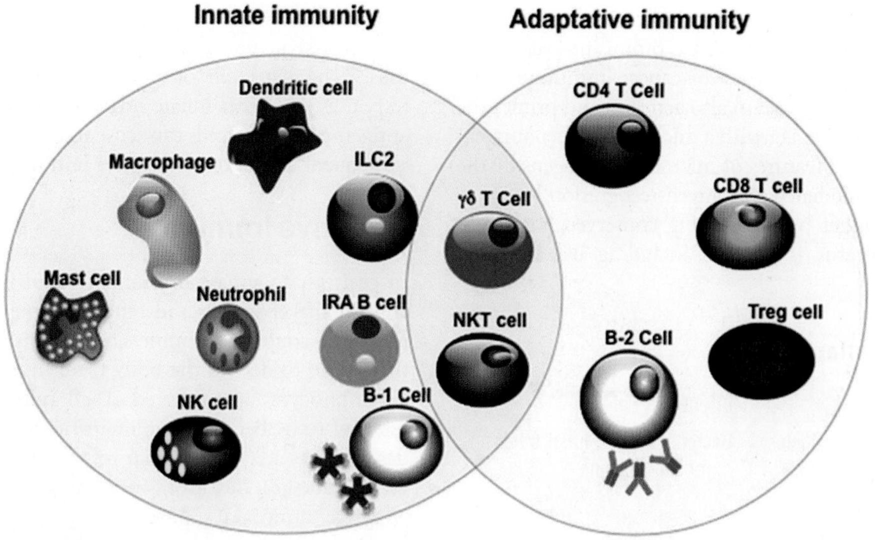

• **Fig. 13.2** Innate and Adaptive Cellular Response. Innate immune cells are characterized by a rapid but poorly specific responses, whereas adaptive responses are more delayed but specifically recognize epitopes. Strong interactions between innate and adaptive systems have been highlighted during the past decade with several cell subsets positioned at the interface between both systems. *ILC2*, Type 2 innate lymphoid cells; *IRA B cell*, innate response activator B cell; *NK*, natural killer; *Treg*, regulatory T cells. (Reprinted with permission from Ait-Oufella H, Sage AP, Mallat Z, Tedgui A. Adaptive (T and B cells) immunity and control by dendritic cells in atherosclerosis. *Circ Res.* 2014;114(10):1640–1660.)

communicate in initiating and regulating immune responses, and how defects in their development give rise to specific forms of immunodeficiency and cancers.[11]

Cellular Immunity

Cellular immunity describes a set of cell-mediated immune responses that are diverse and dynamic in nature (Figure 13.2).[12] T cell-mediated mechanisms involve elaborate effector functions, such as the production of cytokines and chemokines. Naïve T cells are cells that have not yet encountered a specific antigen. A specific co-receptor (cluster of differentiation 8 or 4 [CD8 or CD4]) helps differentiate a naïve T cell into one of the major types of effector T-cells. A naïve T cell with co-receptors for CD8 will become a cytotoxic T cell, which functions to kill target cells by releasing cytotoxic granules into an infected cell. A naïve T-cell with co-receptors for CD4 will become a T helper cell, which has a wide range of effector functions and the ability to further differentiate into subtypes that help activate other immune cells, release cytokines, and facilitate B cell antibody production.

Cell-mediated immunity plays a principal role in controlling viral infections. These immune responses are not only effective during the acute phase of an infection, but can also establish long-lived memory via the perpetuation of memory T cells.[13] Memory T cells can be rapidly re-activated when they encounter the same or similar antigens on infected cells in the future.

Although many pathogens are effectively cleared from the host as a result of cell-mediated immunity, certain viruses can remain in the host indefinitely following infection, which is called lysogeny. Lysogeny is common with all types of herpesviridae and some retroviruses. Eight herpes viruses routinely infect humans. Of the eight strains, herpes simplex virus types 1 and 2, varicella-zoster virus, cytomegalovirus, Epstein-Barr virus (EBV), and Kaposi's sarcoma virus (or human herpesvirus 8) are commonly activated in immunocompromised persons, including PLWCs, and can result in increased morbidity and mortality. Retroviruses, such as the human immunodeficiency virus (HIV), have an RNA genome

and can utilize reverse transcriptase to reactivate an infectious cycle in the setting of immunosuppression. In these instances, T cell responses can bring the same level of containment of the infection and operate to control the infection at a steady state level over time.[14] Persons living with HIV are regularly monitored for adequate CD4+ counts as a measure of critical levels of cell-mediated immunity. Occasionally, cell-mediated responses during viral infection cause damage to host tissues,[15,16] which can manifest as immunopathology and/or an autoimmune condition.

In healthy individuals, there are multiple mechanisms that regulate the normal function of cellular immunity. In contrast, in PLWBCs, the normal function of T-cells is often disrupted by primary malignancy and/or treatment effects, resulting in an immunocompromised state. Cellular immunity requires a delicate harmony of finely tuned processes and immune system components, thus complicating the clinical management of cellular immunodeficiencies.

Clinical Pearl

HIV and other lentiviruses are highly effective at integrating their viral genome into the genome of a host cell, thereby infecting nondividing cells, as well as rapidly dividing cells. Inactivated lentiviruses are commonly used as vectors for gene therapies and adoptive T-cell therapies because they can become endogenous, integrating artificially designed genetic material into the host genome so that the therapeutic DNA is inherited by host descendants.

Humoral Immunity

Humoral immunity refers to antibody-mediated immune responses and all of the accessory processes that accompany them. Most B cells are dependent upon T helper cells to recognize the presence of an antigen. With assistance from T helper cells, B cells will differentiate into plasma B cells that can produce specific antibodies against an antigen. In contrast to T-cells, which mediate cellular immune responses by binding to antigens on the surfaces of infected cells, immunoglobulin G (IgG) antibodies bind primarily

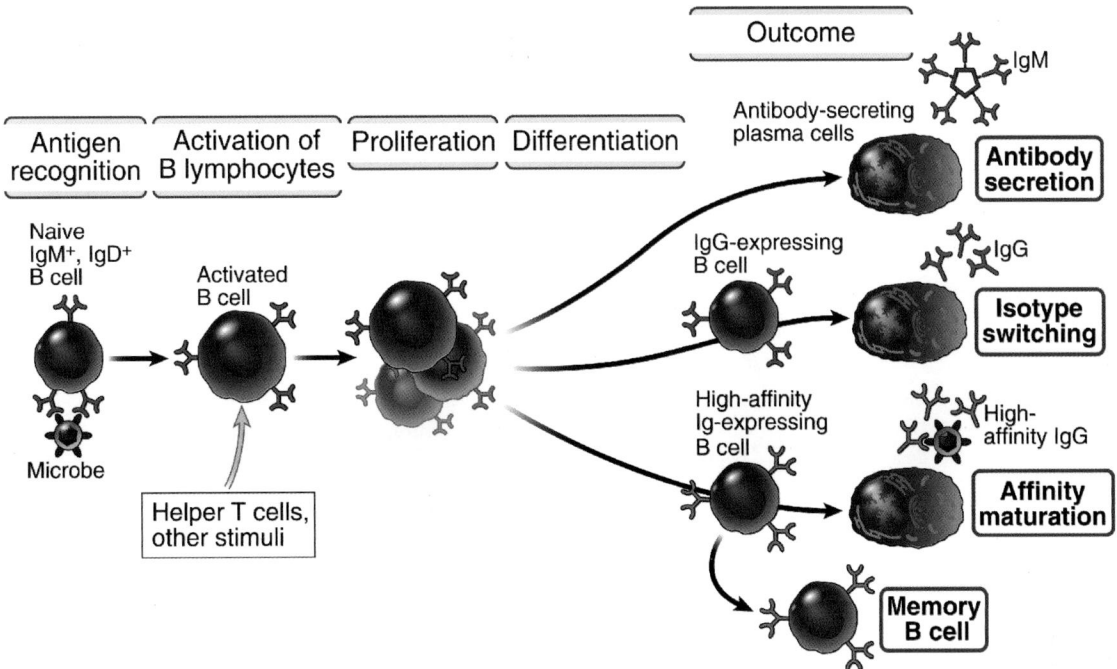

• **Fig. 13.3** Naïve B lymphocytes recognize antigens, and under the influence of helper T cells and other stimuli (not shown), the B cells are activated to proliferate, giving rise to clonal expansion, and to differentiate into antibody-secreting plasma cells. Some of the activated B cells undergo heavy-chain isotype switching and affinity maturation, and some become long-lived memory cells. (Reprinted with permission from Abbas AK, Lichtman AH, Pillai S. Humoral Immune Responses: Activation of B Lymphocytes and Production of Antibodies. In: *Basic Immunology: Functions and Disorders of the Immune System.* Elsevier; 2020: 137–157.)

with pathogenic antigens that are freely circulating in the blood or extracellular fluid. Other antibodies directly target cell surface antigens within a plasma membrane. These cell-specific molecules often have key functional roles in immunity and may be targeted for diagnostic testing or drug targets.

Antibodies are produced by plasma B cells and protect the host from infection in three main ways: (1) by binding to pathogens to inhibit their toxic effects or infectivity (neutralization); (2) by coating pathogens and facilitating their uptake and killing by phagocytes (opsonization); and (3) by activating the complement cascade.[17]

Naïve B cells are able to recognize and bind to a single, randomly determined antigen. Binding to that specific target activates the B cell and recruits Helper T cells to facilitate proliferation and differentiation into antibody-secreting plasma cells or B cells with different roles. Some B cells with a high affinity for a specific antigen will become perpetuating memory B cells to provide long-lived immunity against the specific antigen. The phases of the humoral immune response are summarized in Figure 13.3.

The Pathophysiology of Malignancy and Coagulopathies

Cancer immunosurveillance refers to the immune system's ability to identify molecular signatures of a neoplasm, including TSAs and stress ligands on transformed cells that have escaped cell-intrinsic tumor suppressor mechanisms, and eliminate them before they can establish malignancy.[18] While antitumor immune responses recognize and eliminate the vast majority of nascent neoplasms over the course of an individual's life, occasionally the transformed cells are able to escape immune system control.

Tumor growth and dissemination or metastasis to local and distant sites may follow.

Coagulopathies

Bleeding related to coagulopathies is a common problem for persons with cancer (PWCs). Bleeding may occur as a result of tumor invasion of capillaries and other blood vessels, tumor-related angiogenesis, or anti-cancer treatments. Once bleeding has started, it can be exacerbated by the use of nonsteroidal anti-inflammatory drugs (NSAIDs) and anticoagulants. Clinically, bleeding may present as abnormal bruising, petechial rashes, epistaxis (bleeding from the nose), hemoptysis (coughing up blood), hematemesis (vomiting blood), hematochezia (bleeding from the rectum), melena (blood in the stool), hematuria (blood in the urine), or excessive vaginal bleeding.[19]

Medical interventions to stop or slow bleeding may include systemic agents or transfusion of blood products, including platelets. More conservative, noninvasive treatment options include applying pressure to localized sources of bleeding, pressure dressings, packing, and radiation therapy. More invasive options may be considered in circumstances of severe bleeding, including surgical embolization and endoscopic procedures.[19]

Certain types of cancer and the systemic effects of cancer can place a patient in a hypercoagulable state with an increased risk for venous thromboembolism (VTE). The use of the Two-level Wells Criteria Score for deep vein thrombosis (DVT) (Table 13.3)[20] may be helpful to screen for the likelihood of hypercoagulopathy and to make evidence-based clinical decisions. In addition to assessing for abnormal signs and symptoms, the Onc R clinician should determine the Wells Criteria Score prior to contacting the referring provider to make a recommendation for further testing backed by an evidence-based screening tool.

TABLE 13.3	Two-Level Deep Vein Thrombosis (DVT) Wells Criteria Score	
Clinical Feature		**Points**
Active cancer (treatment ongoing, within 6 months, or palliative)		1
Paralysis, paresis, or recent plaster immobilization of the lower extremities		1
Recently bedridden for 3 days or longer or major surgery within 12 weeks requiring general or regional anesthesia		1
Localized tenderness along the distribution of the deep venous system		1
Entire leg swollen		1
Calf swelling at least 3 cm larger than asymptomatic side		1
Pitting edema confined to the symptomatic leg		1
Collateral superficial veins (nonvaricose)		1
Previously documented DVT		1
Alternative diagnosis at least as likely as DVT		−2
Clinical Probability Simplified Score		
DVT likely		2 points or more
DVT unlikely		Less than 2 points

Adapted from Wells PS, Anderson DR, Rodger M, et al. Evaluation of D-dimer in the diagnosis of suspected deep-vein thrombosis. *N Engl J Med.* 2003;349:1227–1235.

Lab values (including D-dimer testing), duplex venous ultrasound, clinical decision rules for pulmonary embolism, and other forms of diagnostic imaging are used to more definitively diagnose a VTE prior to the initiation of more aggressive medical treatment.[20, 21] The first line of pharmacologic treatment for a hypercoagulable state is the initiation of an anticoagulant and careful monitoring of the patient's blood coagulation profile. Mobilization should be encouraged for prevention of further coagulopathies.

Onc R clinicians can play an important role in the prevention, screening, and treatment of VTE in PLWBCs. A clinical practice guideline titled the "Role of Physical Therapists in the Management of Individuals at Risk for or Diagnosed with Venous Thromboembolism: Evidence-Based Clinical Practice Guideline" was developed and published in 2016 by the American Physical Therapy Association (APTA), in conjunction with the Academies of Acute Care and Cardiovascular and Pulmonary Physical Therapy.[21] See Table 13.4 for a summary of each Key Action Statement. Collectively, the key action statements are valuable guidelines to inform best practices for the PWC that is at risk for, is currently diagnosed with, or has previously been diagnosed with VTE or post-thrombotic syndrome.

In PLWBCs, consider the patient's goals of care when formulating therapeutic interventions for bleeding and clotting coagulopathies. Treatments should be guided by patient-centered goals and quality of life (QOL). Certain medications and therapies should be adjusted or discontinued, including the reversal of anticoagulation, if they are interfering with palliative care.

Clinical Pearl

When a PLWBC presents with new clinical signs and symptoms concerning for possible VTE, it can be difficult to isolate the primary etiology without further medical diagnostic testing, such as a duplex ultrasound to rule out DVT. Extremity pain and edema are common adverse effects of many types of cancer therapy and are also associated with peripheral neuropathy, fluid overload, organ dysfunction, and lymphedema. Be sure to rule out VTE prior to considering other interventions. When VTE is ruled out, the patient is therapeutically anticoagulated, and there are no other contraindications, the application of mechanical compression to involved extremities may also help with symptom management of pain and edema resulting from other etiologies.

Hematologic Malignancies Versus Solid Malignancies

Disease pathologies and treatments considerations for solid malignancies and hematologic malignancies can be generally categorized, as described in previous chapters in this text. Table 13.5 outlines key differences in the types of immune system compromise in solid tumor versus hematologic malignancies, looking specifically at lung cancer and leukemia as examples.

Autoimmune Diseases

An autoimmune disease occurs when the immune system aberrantly attacks the body's own cells. The immune system can normally differentiate between native and foreign cells. In autoimmune disorders, the immune system recognizes host antigens as foreign. Based on where the autoantigen is expressed, autoimmune sequelae can be limited to a specific organ or can be systemic in nature. Many pathological mechanisms for the development of autoimmune conditions have been identified. Genetics and chronic inflammation (related to diet, infection, or chemical exposure) likely play a role, as do other environmental factors. An antinuclear antibody (ANA) panel is a common blood test used to screen for certain autoimmune diseases, but is not highly specific to one type of disease. Treatment of an autoimmune disease usually involves suppressing the autoimmune cellular response with immunosuppressive medications. Figure 13.4 presents common associations between autoimmunity, chronic inflammatory diseases, and risks for the development of cancer.[22]

Some autoimmune diseases are associated with chronic inflammation and the development of specific cancer types (Table 13.6). During a patient intake, note any current or prior autoimmune conditions. The presence of an autoimmune condition may guide one's monitoring for related physical impairments.

Prior to a cancer diagnosis, persons living with an autoimmune disorder may have received long-term, systemic immunosuppressive treatments, such as glucocorticoids. This not only has implications for the function of their immune system, but can also affect their functional status. Be sure to monitor for steroid-related adverse effects, including myopathies, osteoporosis, and changes in blood pressure, triglycerides, cholesterol, and glucose levels.

Hypersensitivity Reactions

Hypersensitivity reactions occur as an overreaction to an irritant, such as from a microbial infection or allergen. They can be idiopathic in nature or have a known allergic trigger. There are four types (I–IV) of immune hypersensitivity reactions, as classified by Gell and Combs.[23] Access the specifics of each type of immune hypersensitivity online at http://www.expertconsult.com. See Table 13.7 for abbreviated information about each type of hypersensitivity reaction.

	TABLE 13.4	**Key Action Statements**	

Number	Statement	Key Phrase
1	Advocate for a culture of mobility and physical activity unless medical contraindications for mobility exist. (Evidence Quality: I; Recommendation Strength: A-Strong)	Advocate for a culture of mobility and physical activity
2	Screen for risk of VTE during the initial patient interview and physical examination. (Evidence Quality: I; Recommendation Strength: A-Strong)	Screen for risk of VTE
3	Provide preventive measures for patients who are identified as high risk for LE DVT. These measures should include education regarding signs and symptoms of LE DVT, activity, hydration, mechanical compression, and referral for medication. (Evidence Quality: I; Recommendation Strength: A-Strong)	Provide preventive measures for LE DVT
4	Recommend mechanical compression (e.g., IPC, GCS) when individuals are at high risk for LE DVT. (Evidence Quality: I; Recommendation Strength: A-Strong)	Recommend mechanical compression as a preventive measure for LE DVT
5	Establish the likelihood of an LE DVT when the patient has pain, tenderness, swelling, warmth, or discoloration in the lower extremity. (Evidence Quality: II; Recommendation Strength: B-Moderate)	Identify the likelihood of LE DVT when signs and symptoms are present
6	Recommend further medical testing after the completion of the Wells criteria for LE DVT prior to mobilization. (Evidence Quality: I; Recommendation Strength: A-Strong)	Communicate the likelihood of LE DVT and recommend further medical testing
7	When a patient has a recently diagnosed LE DVT, (clinicians) should verify whether the patient is taking an anticoagulant medication, what type of anticoagulant medication, and when the anticoagulant medication was initiated. (Evidence Quality: V; Recommendation Strength: D-Theoretical/Foundational)	Verify the patient is taking an anticoagulant
8	When a patient has a recently diagnosed LE DVT, initiate mobilization when therapeutic threshold levels of anticoagulants have been reached. (Evidence Quality: I; Recommendation Strength: A-Strong)	Mobilize patients who are at a therapeutic level of anticoagulation
9	Recommend mechanical compression (e.g., IPC, GCS) when a patient has an LE DVT. (Evidence Quality: II; Recommendation Strength: B-Moderate)	Recommend mechanical compression for patients with LE DVT
10	Recommend that patients be mobilized, once hemodynamically stable, following IVC filter placement. (Evidence Quality: V; Recommendation Strength: P-Best Practice)	Mobilize patients after IVC filter placement once hemodynamically stable
11	When a patient with a documented LE DVT below the knee is not treated with anticoagulation and does not have an IVC filter and is prescribed out of bed mobility by the physician, the (clinician) should consult with the medical team regarding mobilizing versus keeping the patient on bed rest. (Evidence Quality: V; Recommendation Strength: P-Best Practice)	Consult with the medical team when a patient is not anticoagulated and without an IVC filter
12	Screen for fall risk whenever a patient is taking an anticoagulant medication. (Evidence Quality: III; Recommendation Strength: C-Weak)	Screen for fall risk
13	Recommend mechanical compression (e.g., IPC, GCS) when a patient has signs and symptoms suggestive of PTS. (Evidence Quality: I; Recommendation Strength: A-Strong)	Recommend mechanical compression when signs and symptoms of PTS are present
14	Monitor patients who may develop long-term consequences of LE DVT (e.g., PTS severity) and provide management strategies that prevent them from occurring to improve the human experience and increase quality of life. (Evidence Quality: V; Recommendation Strength: P-Best Practice)	Implement management strategies to prevent future VTE

GCS, Graduated compression stockings; *IPC*, intermittent pneumatic compression; *IVC*, inferior vena cava; *LE DVT*, lower extremity deep vein thrombosis; *PTS*, post-thrombotic syndrome; *VTE*, venous thromboembolism.

Adapted from Hillegass E, Puthoff M, Frese EM, et al. Role of physical therapists in the management of individuals at risk for or diagnosed with venous thromboembolism: evidence-based clinical practice guideline. *Phys Ther.* 2016;96(2):143–166. doi:10.2522/ptj.20150264.

Type I and IV hypersensitivity reactions are caused by medications more often than Type II and III reactions. Type II reactions present based on cell types affected, such as hemolytic anemia, thrombocytopenia, or neutropenia. Medication-related hemolytic anemia is typically triggered by cephalosporins, penicillin, and NSAIDs. It presents with clinical symptoms of fatigue, pallor, jaundice, dark urine, and splenomegaly. Drug-induced thrombocytopenia manifests as bleeding in the skin and buccal mucosa and can be caused by heparin, abciximab, quinine, quinidine, sulfonamides, vancomycin, gold compounds, beta-lactam antibiotics, carbamazepine, and NSAIDs. Of note, heparin-induced thrombocytopenia (HIT) increases clotting due to the activation of platelets from auto-antibody reactions. Drug-induced neutropenia often presents with clinical symptoms of infection,

TABLE 13.5   Types of Immune System Compromise Differentiated by Major Classifications of Malignancies

Type of Malignancy	Medical Treatment	Type of Immune System Compromise
Solid Malignancy (Example: Lung Cancer)[69]	Surgery	Infection and inflammation
	Radiation	Inflammation
	Chemotherapy	Increased infection from neutropenia, thrombocytopenia, anemia
	Targeted Drug Therapy	Neutropenia, increased infections
	Immunotherapy[70]	Infusion reaction and autoimmune response
Hematologic Malignancy: (Example: Chronic Myeloid Leukemia)	Immunotherapy Bone Marrow Transplant	Infusion reaction and autoimmune response, increased risk for infection
	Chemotherapy	Increased infection from neutropenia, thrombocytopenia, anemia, neutropenic fevers, disseminated intravascular congestion, neutropenic enterocolitis

Adapted from Carbone DP, Gandara DR, Antonia SJ, Zielinski C, Paz-Ares L. Non-small-cell lung cancer: role of the immune system and potential for immunotherapy. *J Thorac Oncol.* 2015;10(7):974–984. doi:10.1097/JTO.0000000000000551; Midthun DE. Overview of the initial treatment and prognosis of lung cancer. In: Post T, ed. *UpToDate.* UpToDate; 2020. www.uptodate.com. Accessed July 22, 2020; and Schiffer CA, Atallah E. Overview of the treatment of chronic myeloid leukemia. In: Post T, ed. *UpToDate.* UpToDate; 2020. www.uptodate.com. Accessed July 22, 2020.

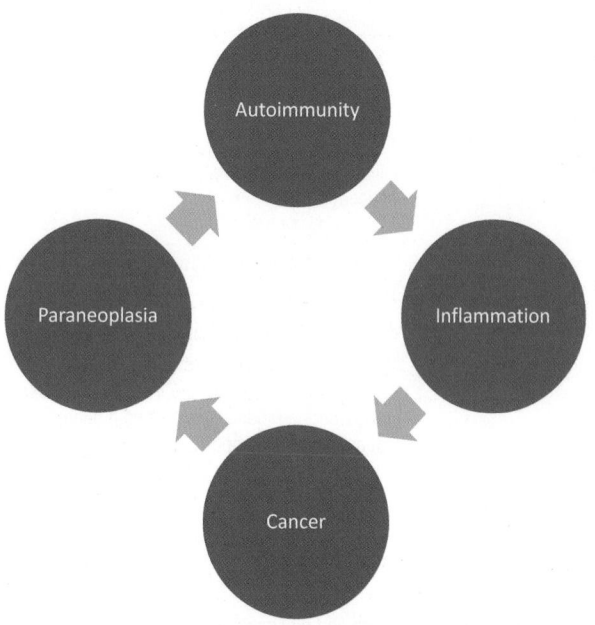

• **Fig. 13.4** Associations Between Autoimmunity and Cancer. Persons with non-Hodgkin lymphoma have an increased rate of developing autoimmune diseases. Persons with breast, GI, lung, ovarian, and lymphoproliferative cancers can develop a rheumatoid arthritis-like clinical picture. Chronic inflammation leads to an increased risk of developing lymphoproliferative malignancies. GI, Gastrointestinal. (Adapted from Franks AL, Slansky JE. Multiple associations between a broad spectrum of autoimmune diseases, chronic inflammatory diseases and cancer. *Anticancer Res.* 2012;32(4):1119–1136.)

TABLE 13.6   Common Autoimmune Diseases, Chronic Inflammation, and Associations in Cancer Types

Common Autoimmune Diseases	Cancer Type
Scleroderma	Lung
Multiple Sclerosis	Nervous system, breast
Myasthenia Gravis	Thymoma tumors, lung
Rheumatoid Arthritis	Lung cancer, lymphoma
Thyroid Disease	Thyroid
Inflammatory Bowel Disease	Gastric cancer
Lupus	Lung, breast, cervical, lymphoma
Diabetes Mellitus Type 1	Stomach, liver, pancreas, endometrium, ovary, and kidney
Vasculitis	Bladder cancer

Adapted from Franks AL, Slansky JE. Multiple associations between a broad spectrum of autoimmune diseases, chronic inflammatory diseases and cancer. *Anticancer Res.* 2012;32(4):1119–1136.

including systemic inflammatory response syndrome (SIRS) and sepsis.[23] Propylthiouracil, amodiaquine, and flecainide are most commonly associated with drug-induced neutropenic reactions.

Type III reactions usually manifest with symptoms of serum sickness, vasculitis, or fever. These reactions are uncommon and are typically only seen after prolonged drug administration. Serum sickness presents with fever, urticarial rash, arthralgias, or acute glomerulonephritis. Serum sickness is different from a serum sickness-like reaction, which presents almost identically, but does not create immune complexes. The most common medications that cause serum sickness include penicillins, cephalosporins, sulfamides, bupropion, fluoxetine, and thiouracil.[24] Vasculitis symptoms include purpura, petechiae, fever, urticaria, arthralgias, lymphadenopathy, and elevated erythrocyte sedimentation rate (ESR), and can be caused by penicillins, cephalosporins, sulfonamides, phenytoin, and allopurinol. An Arthus reaction is a Type III hypersensitivity reaction that can cause local swelling, redness, and tissue necrosis of the skin due to the deposition of antibody-antigen complexes in the walls of small blood cells. The Arthus phenomenon typically follows a skin injection of an antigen or vaccine into a previously immunized individual by a series of similar injections.[24]

Type IV reactions usually have a long latency period, as seen classically with Stevens-Johnson syndrome and drug-induced hypersensitivity reactions. These reactions occur much later after a seemingly uncomplicated treatment course. The immune

TABLE 13.7 **Types of Hypersensitivity Reactions**

	Type I	Type II	Type III	Type IV
Common Allergens	Pollen, food, allergens, drugs, eczema/atopic dermatitis	Infectious agents or autoimmune reactions (immune thrombocytopenia, autoimmune hemolytic anemia, and autoimmune neutropenia)	Inhaled molds, infused foreign proteins (serum sickness), tetanus, vaccine (Arthus reaction) Rheumatoid arthritis	Contact allergens
Onset	Seconds to minutes (immediate)	Several minutes to hours	3–12 hours	12 hours to 2 days
Immune reactant	IgE, mast cells, and/or basophils	IgG or IgM	IgG or IgM	T cells
Mechanism	Antibodies from allergens (IgE) bind to mast cells and basophils which release histamine and cause inflammation	Antibody binds to an antigen on a host cell that the immune system labels as "foreign." IgG & IgM damage "foreign" cells by phagocytosis	Antibody binds to a soluble antigen creating an immune complex with IgG. These complexes can activate complement in tissues, such as blood vessels, leading to an inflammatory response	T effector cells are stimulated by an antigen cell. Antigen appears again and memory T cells activate macrophages and create an inflammatory reaction
Clinical Signs	Urticaria, hypotension, conjunctivitis, rhinitis, bronchial asthma, vomiting, diarrhea, anaphylaxis	Secondary symptoms according to cells affected (example: purpura in thrombocytopenia)	Cutaneous vasculitis, allergic alveolitis, serum sickness, Arthus reaction	Allergic contact eczema, Stevens-Johnson syndrome, drug-induced hypersensitivity reaction

IgG (immunoglobulin G) IgE (immunoglobulin E); IgM (immunoglobulin M) all antibodies.
Adapted from Justiz Vaillant AA, Vashisht R, Zito PM. Immediate hypersensitivity reactions. [Updated June 15, 2020]. In: *StatPearls* [Internet]. StatPearls Publishing; 2020 January. https://www.ncbi.nlm.nih.gov/books/NBK513315/.

symptoms of Stevens-Johnson syndrome tend to present suddenly on the skin and mucous membranes and can become severe and life-threatening if not immediately recognized and treated. Stevens-Johnson syndrome is a known adverse effect of allopurinol, carbamazepine, lamotrigine, phenobarbital, phenytoin, sulfa antibiotics, sertraline, and nevirapine. Symptoms most often begin with flu-like symptoms, and then a diffuse red/purple rash develops and begins to form blisters.[25]

To maintain the safety of the PLWBC during Onc R, the clinician should understand common triggers of hypersensitivity reactions and recognize concerning symptoms quickly. Hypersensitivity reactions can become very serious if not quickly identified and medically managed. PWC receiving new induction chemotherapy or follow-up cycles of treatment may develop a hypersensitivity reaction(s). Sometimes PWCs are hospitalized for pharmacological desensitization and close monitoring prior to and during the initiation of a new therapeutic agent that is highly associated with the development of hypersensitivity reactions.

Clinical Pearl

Hypersensitivity reactions are important to monitor in persons with a new diagnosis of cancer that are receiving treatment for the first time. A PWC may end up needing transition to the intensive care unit (ICU) for severe allergic reactions and subsequently require intensive Onc R related to critical illness and ICU-acquired weakness.

Tumor Lysis Syndrome

In persons living with hematologic cancers, tumor lysis syndrome (TLS) is one of the most common emergency situations that can develop. TLS is usually caused by chemotherapy or another aggressive cancer treatment, but it can also be unprompted. TLS is most commonly encountered with acute leukemia or non-Hodgkin lymphoma (NHL) after a massive release of tumor cell contents into the bloodstream. When tumor cells lyse or die, they release their intracellular components into the bloodstream, including potassium, phosphorus, and nucleic acids, which are then metabolized by many processes into uric acid.[26] The rapid increase in uric acid can cause an acute kidney injury and cytokine release, potentially resulting in systemic inflammatory response and multiple organ failure. A massive shift in electrolyte levels disrupts normal homeostasis, leading to metabolic changes that can produce renal insufficiency, cardiac arrhythmias, seizures, and potentially death. The most common TLS-related electrolyte derangements seen on laboratory testing are hyperuricemia (uric acid >8.0 mg/dL), hyperkalemia (potassium >6.0 mmol/L), hyperphosphatemia (phosphorus >4.5 mg/dL in adults and >6.5 mg/dL in children), and hypocalcemia (calcium <7.0 mg/dL).[26]

There are two broad classifications of TLS: laboratory and clinical. Laboratory TLS is defined as two or more metabolic abnormalities present in the first 3 days prior to or within 7 days after the start of therapy. These metabolic changes must occur within the same 24-hour period and demonstrate a 25% change from baseline. Clinical TLS is defined as the development of overt signs and symptoms in the presence or absence of laboratory abnormalities, including increased creatinine (>0.3 mg/dL), seizures, cardiac arrhythmias, oliguria, or death.[27]

Many risk factors have been identified for the development of TLS during or after treatment. First, prior underlying conditions that limit the ability to excrete blood waste products, such as renal insufficiency, nephropathy, dehydration, oliguria, hypotension, and acidic urine output, increase the likelihood for TLS to occur with treatment. Therefore, oncology teams will attempt to correct any modifiable abnormalities prior to the initiation of therapy in order to prevent further renal malfunction. In addition, the magnitude of the tumor burden is taken into consideration; the larger the neoplasm, the higher the number of cellular contents that might be released into the bloodstream after tumor lysis. TLS is commonly seen in high-grade lymphomas, leukemias, and other cancers that have infiltrated the bone marrow, liver, spleen, or kidney.[27] The lysis potential of tumors is weighed carefully by the oncologist when making decisions about treatment protocols. Tumors with increased cellular proliferation or high sensitivity to treatment place the PLWBC at a greater risk of developing TLS.

TLS can quickly become critical, and the best way to treat it is with prevention. The medical treatment of TLS depends on the severity, and the goal is usually to preserve renal function. The first line of defense is the administration of intravenous fluids to assist with renal perfusion and minimize acidosis. In addition, rigorous monitoring of blood lab values and continuous cardiac monitoring can help guide interdisciplinary efforts to halt TLS progression. Depending on the extent of TLS and associated renal injury, hemodialysis may be initiated to assist with filtration.[28] Medications can also be administered. Diuretics are commonly used to promote excretion of uric acid. Rabricase is an enzyme that acts as a uricolytic agent, and allopurinol reduces uric acid level.[29] Both of these medications have demonstrated efficacy in reducing the severity of TLS. For persons with B-cell NHL or Burkitt lymphoma, conditioning with vincristine and prednisone prior to intensive chemotherapy has demonstrated efficacy in slowing the lytic process.

Clinical Pearl

TLS is considered a medical emergency. At most cancer centers, the signs of symptoms of tumor lysis syndrome call for immediate termination of exercise and notification of the medical team. Many new leukemia diagnoses are automatically admitted to the ICU for critical monitoring due to a high risk for TLS during treatment initiation.

Infections and Sepsis

Having cancer and undergoing certain treatments, including chemotherapy, can make the body unable to fight off infections in the manner that it normally would. PLWBCs are at an increased risk for infection, SIRS, and sepsis. Sepsis is a life-threatening complication caused by the body's overwhelming response to infection. For PWCs, a microbial infection at any location of the body can rapidly progress to sepsis.

Sepsis is a life-threatening situation that requires immediate medical intervention. Care providers often look for early signs of systemic inflammation using the SIRS criteria (Table 13.8) before

a pathogen is identified. In 2016, a shortened Sequential Organ Failure Assessment score (SOFA score), known as the quick SOFA score (qSOFA) (Table 13.9), was created to supplement the SIRS system of screening and diagnosis.[30] qSOFA criteria for sepsis include the presence of at least two of the following three: increased respiratory rate, change in the level of consciousness, and low blood pressure.

Other clinical indicators of sepsis include confusion, decreased alertness, changes in white blood cell (WBC) count, and symptoms related to a specific source infection such as a cough and shortness of breath secondary to pneumonia.[31] Severe sepsis is defined as reduced blood flow to vital organs, resulting in at least one organ failing to function properly.

Episodes of infection and sepsis are common in PLWCs. Onc R clinicians must know the signs and symptoms of possible sepsis and be able to decide when to modify or terminate treatment. Onc R clinicians should know when to seek urgent medical referral and/or emergency services. Sepsis and septic shock are leading causes of death worldwide, and one of the leading causes of death for PLWBC. Targeted campaigns seek to expedite the response time to sepsis in order to optimize outcomes, such as the *It's About Time* campaign by the Sepsis Alliance (Figure 13.5).[32]

Clinical Pearl

The SIRS and qSOFA criteria include data points obtained via resting vitals and lab values. Onc R clinicians may observe other signs and symptoms during exertion that are concerning for SIRS/sepsis, including orthostatic hypotension, exercise-induced hypotension, diaphoresis, dizziness/lightheadedness, or excessive fatigue with exertion. Consider SIRS/sepsis as a possible etiology if a PLWBC exhibits an inappropriate response to exercise.

Neutropenia and Sepsis

Neutropenic sepsis is a complication of multiple forms of cancer treatment and can become more serious in the presence of a presumed microbial infection. The risk of a life-threatening infection is estimated by the degree of immunosuppression, commonly assessed by the absolute neutrophil count (ANC) on a complete blood count (CBC) with differential in the laboratory.[33] Patients with a low neutrophil count may be placed on "neutropenic precautions" for protective isolation.

The neutrophil-mediated immune response is muted when patients are neutropenic. Sometimes a neutropenic fever is the only early indication of SIRS/sepsis. When patients are neutropenic, conditions of bacteremia and sepsis can progress very quickly to become life-threatening. In a neutropenic patient, high fevers

TABLE 13.8 Systemic Inflammatory Response Syndrome (SIRS) Criteria

Meet Two or More of the Following:	
Temperature (<36°C or >38°C)	1
Increased heart rate (>90 beats/min)	1
Increased respiratory rate (≥22 breaths/min)	1
White blood cell count <4000 cells/mm³ or >12,000 cells/mm³, or >10% immature (band) forms	1

TABLE 13.9 Quick Sequential Organ Failure Assessment (qSOFA) Criteria

Meet Two or More of the Following:	
Low blood pressure (SBP ≤100 mmHg)	1
Increased respiratory rate (≥22 breaths/min)	1
Altered mentation (Glasgow Coma Scale ≤14)	1

SBP, systolic blood pressure.
Tables 13.8 and 13.9 adapted from Singer M, Deutschman CS, Seymour CW, et al. The third international consensus definitions for sepsis and septic shock (Sepsis-3). *JAMA.* 2016;315(8):801–810. doi:10.1001/jama.2016.0287.

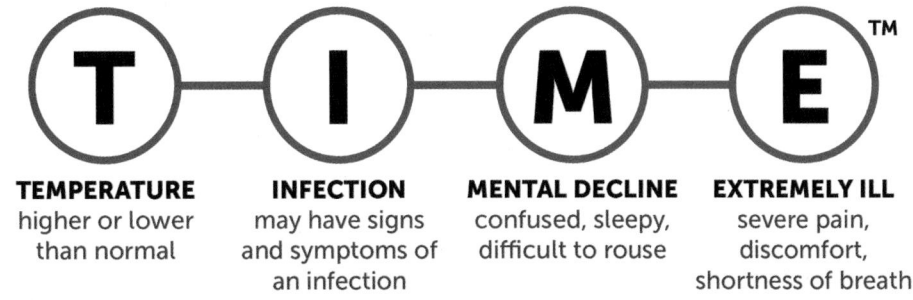

When it comes to sepsis, remember
IT'S ABOUT TIME™. Watch for:

TEMPERATURE higher or lower than normal

INFECTION may have signs and symptoms of an infection

MENTAL DECLINE confused, sleepy, difficult to rouse

EXTREMELY ILL severe pain, discomfort, shortness of breath

If you experience a combination of these symptoms: seek urgent medical care, call 911, or go to the hospital with an advocate. Ask: **"Could it be sepsis?"**

©2020 Sepsis Alliance   sepsis.org

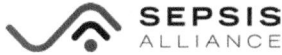

• **Fig. 13.5** Sepsis: It's About Time™. (Reprinted with permission from Sepsis Alliance. What Is Sepsis? https://www.sepsis.org/sepsis-basics/what-is-sepsis/. Accessed March 1, 2021.)

(body temperature >39°C) may start in response to an infection and can be difficult to autoregulate. However, microbial infections can also trigger sepsis in the *absence* of a fever.[34]

Neutropenic sepsis is associated with unique clinical and biological characteristics, with emerging data showing distinct differences in the pathophysiology of neutropenic fever/sepsis and non-neutropenic fever/sepsis. PWCs who have neutropenic sepsis demonstrate a higher risk for acute kidney injury and higher concentrations of the inflammatory mediators interleukin (IL) 6 and IL 8, and granulocyte-colony stimulating factors, relative to non-neutropenic persons experiencing sepsis.[35]

For persons receiving treatment for cancer, clinicians should have a very low threshold to suspect neutropenic sepsis anytime the patient appears generally unwell. Other signs and symptoms associated with neutropenic sepsis include mucositis, chills, clinical signs of infection, and altered mental status. Because of the high prevalence of neutropenic sepsis in persons receiving chemotherapy and other cancer treatments, the Onc R clinician should always be monitoring for concerning signs and symptoms.

PWCs that develop neutropenic sepsis have a high risk for morbidity and mortality, often requiring hospitalization and care escalation to the ICU empiric antibiotics are often initiated. In PW. Rapid initiation of an appropriate antimicrobial therapy is key to mitigating the infectious and immune system sequelae and decreasing the risk of mortality. If a pathogen cannot be quickly identified, empiric antibiotics are often initiated. In PWCs, infections are most frequently caused by gram-positive organisms, but the mortality rate is higher for gram-negative infections.[36] Increasing challenges with multiple drug resistant organisms (MDROs) have significant implications for the successful treatment of neutropenic sepsis for PWCs.

Cytokine Release Syndrome

Cytokine release syndrome is a form of SIRS that can be triggered by a variety of etiologies, including infection, sepsis, and certain drugs. Specific to PLWCs, monoclonal antibody therapies and adoptive T-cell therapies are known to have adverse effects of cytokine release

syndrome. Sometimes referred to in lay terms as a "cytokine storm," this life-threatening complication occurs when a large number of WBCs tivated and release inflammatory cytokines are activated and release inflammatory cytokines into the bloodstream. Cytokines can trigger a positive feedback loop, activating even more WBCs and culminating in massive systemic hyperinflammation, hypotensive shock, and organ failure if not urgently treated and reversed.

Post-Transplant Lymphoproliferative Disease

Post-transplant lymphoproliferative disease (PTLD) is the most common type of malignancy after an allogeneic transplant. PTLD is an abnormal proliferation of lymphoid cells that can occur after solid organ transplant or allogeneic stem cell transplant and can progress to lymphoma.[37] Risk factors for PTLD include infection, degree of immunosuppression, age, race, genetics, and type of allograft. In addition, a history of pretransplant malignancy (in solid tumor transplant) and lower levels of human leukocyte antigen (HLA)-matching are associated with increased risks for the development of PTLD. Notably, the risk for PTLD is highest in the first few months after transplant due to large doses of immunosuppressive medications.[38] Chronic graft-versus-host disease is another risk factor for late onset PTLD.

EBV, commonly known as the virus that causes infectious mononucleosis, has a strong association with many PTLD cases. As is the case with many lysogenic viruses during transplant, infection with EBV can occur from the host or the donor. In a normal infection, EBV antigens expressed by infected B cells cause a T-cell response that eliminates most of the virus-infected cells. However, a small amount of host B cells harbor a latent infection and remain in circulation until T cell depletion occurs with immunosuppression. A latent EBV infection may become activated and contribute to the development of PTLD.[38]

The World Health Organization classifies four categories of PTLD: plasmacytic hyperplasia and infectious mononucleosis-like PTLD, florid follicular hyperplasia, polymorphic PTLD (usually containing EBV), and classic Hodgkin lymphoma-like PTLD. Monomorphic PTLD is further classified based upon the type of lymphoma, such as diffuse large B cell lymphoma, Burkitt lymphoma, plasma cell neoplasm, and peripheral T cell lymphoma. Most tumors associated with a diagnosis of PTLD are B cell lymphomas.[39]

Diagnosis is suspected in patients that have had a solid organ or allogenic transplant with adenopathy, fever, weight loss, night sweats, unexplained hematologic abnormalities, or signs of infiltration of extra lymphatic tissue. Individuals may experience symptoms similar to those of organ or tissue rejection. A positron emission tomography (PET) scan with the presence of a mass and elevated serum markers is suggestive of PTLD. Patients may also present with an increasing EBV viral load.[28] Transplant centers have incorporated EBV monitoring into treatment and maintenance protocols for persons that are considered high risk for the development of PTLD.

The treatment of PTLD aims to preserve the function of the transplanted graft, but also stop the spread of malignancy. There is no standardized treatment approach. Reduction in immunosuppressive medications and chemotherapy with use of rituximab (Rituxan) in combination with cyclophosphamide (Cytoxan), hydroxydanorubicin hydrochloride, vincristine (Oncovin), and prednisone (R-CHOP) has been shown to be effective. R-CHOP will be further discussed in the Monoclonal Antibodies (mAbs) section of this chapter. Radiation may be used for local malignancies. Antiviral medications can be used prophylactically and for treatment of EBV-related PTLD.

This can be a challenging patient population to work with during Onc R. Persons with PTLD have often received multiple advanced medical and/or surgical therapies over a span of many years and have multiple comorbidities. They may have limited remaining treatment options available. Exercise may help persons with PTLD to minimize adverse symptoms and maximize QOL.

Challenges in Cancer Immunology: Antimicrobial Resistance and Stewardship, Novel Pathogens, and COVID-19

One of the ever-present challenges for PLWBCs who experience immsses, which can negatively impact prognosis and overalntivirals, and other antimicrobial agents. Many of the infectious diseases that develop in PWCs are opportunistic in nature, and the culpable microbes are evolving rapidly to become increasingly drug resistant. Global antibiotic resistance is of particular concern because antibiotics are so essential to the treatment of bacterial sepsis. Providers are increasingly being held to standards for antimicrobial stewardship. Quality improvement initiatives driven by regulatory agencies, health systems, insurance companies, and professional organizations are evaluating adherence to evidence-based recommendations and strategies to better implement best prescribing practices.

Microbes and viruses have persisted through the epochs of time by evolving and proliferating, while still maintaining key pathogenic phenotypes.[40] In recent years, a number of novel pathogens have jumped from animal species into humans, resulting in significant global morbidity and mortality. Each novel pathogen presents new challenges to public health, immunology, and infectious disease professionals as they work to rapidly study the pathogen, design tests, optimize clinical management, and develop and distribute treatment regimens and vaccines as quickly as possible.

Coronavirus disease 2019 (COVID-19) is caused by the novel coronavirus severe acute respiratory syndrome coronavirus 2 (SARS-CoV-2), which became virulent in humans starting at the end of December 2019. This novel pathogen created a pandemic with unprecedented health and economic tolls. It is a unique virus in that it is highly contagious and also causes variable disease severity among different populations and demographics. PLWBCs are at an increased risk for severe illness during COVID-19 infection due to the effects of the cancer itself, cancer treatments, and other secondary health problems that are not related to cancer. The risk for severe COVID-19-related illness also goes up for PLWCs that have other comorbid risk factors, including advanced age, hypertension, and/or diabetes. Certain races/ethnicities and socioeconomic levels are also at an increased risk for severe illness. During a pandemic, PLWBCs may have less access to outpatient infusion centers, rehabilitation therapy sessions, and exercise and wellness classes, which can negatively impact prognosis and overall QOL.

Common Adverse Effects of Treatments

Most of the contemporary treatment approaches for cancer impact the immune system at some point during the treatment course. Effects can include suppressing host immunological function, initiating the inflammatory cascade, increasing the risk for infection, and delaying healing time and return to homeostasis. Some medical treatments work by recruiting, upregulating, and engineering components of the immune system to target specific malignant markers and antigens. PWCs that choose to receive medical and surgical treatments will usually have a specialized multidisciplinary care team that includes an oncologist with advanced training and experience in the recognition and mitigation of negative effects on the immune system. The Onc R clinician working in this multidisciplinary team needs to recognize common adverse effects on the immune system as part of the primary disease sequelae and secondary to treatments received. Onc R clinicians need to advocate for the role of exercise and mobility in boosting immune system function in PLWCs. Specific implications for the immune system of each major oncology treatment for PLWBCs are summarized below.

Surgery

The immune system participates in the early postsurgical phase by initiating and facilitating the inflammatory cascade in response to tissue damage during and after the surgical procedure. PWCs that choose to undergo surgical treatment may be given intravenous antibiotics prior to and during surgery to prevent secondary infections. However, the risk of infection after surgery is still elevated due to the compromise of physical protective barriers and potential loss of blood and other bodily fluids that normally enable proper immune system function. Providers should closely monitor clinical presentations and lab values after surgery for the detection of possible signs of infection.

Surgical interventions for cancer are most successful in the earlier stages, before extensive local invasion or metastasis has occurred. Many advanced tumors will be surgically excised, even if only for palliative purposes. Cancer surgery may follow a precise, evidence-based protocol when excising smaller tissues and organs, such as the prostate, skin lesions, or localized involvement of the lung, or when operating in complex areas such as the face. Surgery may also be more exploratory in nature, requiring the surgeon to take a careful approach using advanced technologies to remove all malignant tissue. Surgeons may work closely with a surgical pathologist to make sure that all margins are clear of malignancy.

The blood contains key components for normal immune and coagulation function, including red blood cells, WBCs, platelets, clotting factors, and other plasma components. Loss of blood volume due to malignancy, during and after surgery, or as a complication of other therapies may result in a decrease in immune function. Immunosuppression may persist until key components of the blood are restored by allogeneic transfusions of blood products and/or autogenic regeneration.

The amount of blood loss is often greater during exploratory surgeries for tumor debulking or for removal of metastatic lesions, compared to surgeries for low grade malignancy or using precise protocols.[41] Bleeding complications can prolong the duration of critical care needs and hospital length of stay.[42] Further emergent interventions may be needed for complications of bleeding, including surgical embolization, revascularization, management of compartment syndrome, or critical management of hemorrhagic shock.

Surgery may involve the removal of lymph nodes if there are concerns for lymphatic malignancy and/or metastatic spread through the lymphatic system. This can also negatively affect normal immune system function, which relies heavily on the lymphatic network of vessels and nodes for transport and function. The lymphatic system transports and filters lymph fluid, which contains antibodies and lymphocytes, as well as inactivated microbial components. See Chapter 9 for more information about the effects of cancer and therapies on the lymphatic system.

Radiation

Another pillar in the management of cancer is radiation therapy, which may impact the immune system in a variety of ways. This type of cancer therapy is used at some point during the course of care for curative, adjuvant, or palliative purposes in a majority of treatment regimens for solid malignancies. The primary goal of radiation therapy is to kill cancer cells or slow their growth by damaging their DNA. Once a cancer cell is damaged beyond repair, it will stop dividing and die. Damaged cells then either undergo apoptosis or are broken down and removed by various cellular components of the host immune system.

The effects of ionizing radiation are seen not only in the tumor cells, but also in the tumor microenvironment, and can upregulate or downregulate the cancer immunoediting functionality of the host immune system. Radiation can stimulate the immune system to participate in immunogenic cell death, regulate inflammatory, necrotic, and apoptotic pathways after nonimmunogenic cell death, or cause immunosuppression. Radiation therapy is more likely to cause immunosuppression if it is directed at the bones, especially the bones of the pelvis, femur, and other large bones that contain bone marrow, host to hematopoietic stem cells.

Ionizing radiation can also damage healthy cells and immune system function, although the radiation oncology team minimizes this whenever possible. Developments in technologies for radiotherapy delivery have led to higher precision and better sparing of normal tissue,[43] thereby optimizing the desired local action and minimizing unwanted systemic effects.

Radiation is commonly used in combination with surgery and/or chemotherapy to target residual malignant cells after removal of localized tumors and chemotherapy treatment. Increasingly, radiation therapy is being used in combination with immunotherapy to promote an effective antitumor immune response. Cell death induced by radiation therapy is thought to be immunogenic in nature. It is thought that this immunogenic reaction results in increased lymphocyte effector function in the tumor microenvironment, thus increasing the effectiveness of adjuvant immunotherapies.[44]

A systemic immune response can also be elicited through combined therapies to upregulate lymphocyte effector function and other immunogenic antitumor effects outside of the irradiation field. This systemic effect is called an abscopal effect and is a relatively rare phenomenon.[45] The abscopal effect occurs when radiation treatment or another type of local therapy shrinks the targeted tumor and also leads to the shrinkage of other untreated tumors elsewhere in the body. The precise biological mechanisms that cause this effect are still being investigated, but is it logical that the immune system plays a key role.

Some of the conceptualized mechanisms by which combined radiation therapy and immunotherapy are thought to complement each other and upregulate antitumor immune system function are presented in Figure 13.6. Ideal combination therapy protocols are still being studied, with multiple clinical trials ongoing.

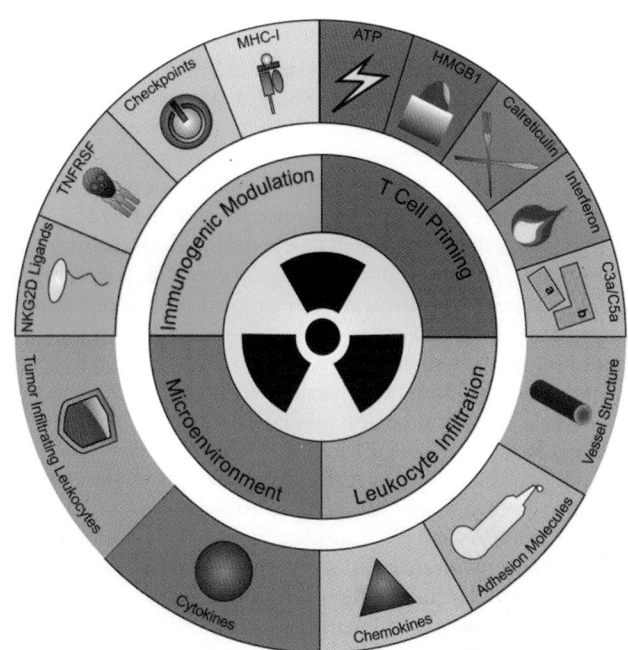

• **Fig. 13.6** Principles of the Radiation-Induced Immune Response. The effects of RT on the immune system are conceptualized in four major organizing principles (inner circle): (a) the priming of TA-specific T cells; (b) leukocyte infiltration into the tumor tissue; (c) changes in the immunosuppressive TME; and (d) immunogenic modulation of the tumor cell phenotype, leading to increased sensitivity of irradiated tumor cells to lymphocyte-mediated lysis. The mechanisms involved in each of these organizing principles are displayed in the outer circle. (A) RT primes tumor antigen-specific T cells by inducing antigen uptake and maturation of dendritic cells. Five signals triggered by RT have been implicated in this process: the secretion of ATP and the alarmin HMGB1, the cell surface exposure of the eat-me signal calreticulin, radiation-induced interferons and activated complement fragments C5a/C3a. (B) RT drives leukocyte infiltration into the tumor tissue by three different mechanisms: changes in vessel structure, increased adhesion molecule expression on endothelium and the induction of chemokines. (C) RT also shapes the TME by triggering secretion of a plethora of cytokines and changing the presence and function of immunosuppressive leukocytes in the TME. (D) RT also modulates the immunophenotype of cancer cells by inducing the expression of MHC-I, ligands for the NKG2D receptor, ligands for immune checkpoint molecules and TNFRSF member Fas. These surface molecules increase or lower susceptibility of cancer cells to T and natural killer cell-mediated lysis. The different organizing principles are highly interconnected and influence each other's occurrence and effect on tumor growth. *ATP*, Adenosine triphosphate; *HMGB1*, high mobility group box; *MHC-I*, major histocompatibility complex I; *NKG2D*, natural killer cell lectin-like-receptor K1; *RT*, radiotherapy; *TA*, tumor antigen; *TME*, tumor microenvironment; *TNFRSF*, tumor necrosis factor superfamily. (Reprinted with permission from Walle T, Martinez Monge R, Cerwenka A, Ajona D, Melero I, Lecanda F. Radiation effects on antitumor immune responses: current perspectives and challenges. *Ther Adv Med Oncol*. 2018;10:1758834017742575. doi:10.1177/1758834017742575.)

The disruption of the integrity of skin, organs, and other localized tissues by radiation triggers an inflammatory response, which is regulated by the immune system to promote tissue healing. In some individuals, the acute inflammatory state persists and can cause secondary complications. The presence of chronic inflammation may lead to fibrotic changes in vital tissues and organs, including the vascular and lymphatic systems that promote normal immunocellular transport and function. See Chapter 9 for more information about the effects of radiation therapy on the lymphatic system and the Onc R management of lymphedema.

Chemotherapy

Immune system changes during and after chemotherapy regimens directly or indirectly contribute to the burden of disease experienced by PWCs. A PWC is likely to experience more severe adverse effects associated with immunosuppression at the start of new chemotherapy regimens during the induction phase.

Cytotoxic chemotherapeutic agents are administered in doses close to the maximum-tolerated dose, which is determined in part by anticipated immunosuppressive adverse effects including myelo- and lymphopenia.[46] Patients may be prophylactically admitted to the hospital during the induction phase of chemotherapy for closer monitoring of their clinical status, lab values, and immune system function. Specific immune cells can be used as biomarkers for the effectiveness of chemotherapy on clinical goals for disease management. Refer to eTable 13.1 in the enhanced eBook for more information. High-dose, intensive chemotherapy is also used as a preliminary step in many advanced treatment protocols (e.g., conditioning prior to stem cell transplantation (SCT) or adoptive cell therapy), with the overt goals of inducing rapid myelo- and lymphodepletion and achieving desired immunocellular outcomes.

Most chemotherapy regimens target rapidly dividing cancerous cells with poor repair mechanisms. Conventional chemotherapeutics exhibit a wide range of effects on malignant lesions and the host immunosurveillance. For more information regarding the specific immunological effects of the most conventional chemotherapy drugs, refer to eTable 13.2 in the enhanced eBook.

Novel combination therapies and chemotherapy approaches are continually being designed and studied in clinical trials at cancer centers throughout the world. The Onc R clinician working at a comprehensive cancer center will inevitably treat a PWC that has received or is currently receiving a novel drug regimen that is part of a clinical trial. They are encouraged to discuss each new clinical trial regimen with the prescribing oncologist prior to initiating an evaluation and designing a rehabilitation plan of care for the recipient. They must be vigilantly aware of any clinical presentation that is indicative of an adverse drug event and be able to communicate this efficiently with the medical provider.

Chemotherapy also destroys other rapidly dividing cells, including normal immune and hematological cells in the blood, lymph, bone marrow, mouth, intestinal tract, nose, nails, and hair. Once the chemotherapy treatment terminates and toxic effects subside, healthy cells can typically repair cell and tissue damage, including immune system modulator cells. However, if treatment regimens or malignancies have damaged the bone marrow, then the marrow may have a decreased ability to produce sufficient red blood cells, WBCs, and platelets. This may be partially mitigated in some diagnoses by allogeneic plasma infusions from healthy donors.[47] Table 13.10 summarizes common adverse effects, signs, and symptoms associated with chemotherapy. Adverse effects that are caused primarily by immunosuppression

TABLE 13.10	Common Negative Adverse Effects of Chemotherapy Associated With Immunosuppression
Immunosuppression	Multiple Contributing Mechanisms (Including Immunosuppression)
• Microbial infections • Neutropenia • Neutropenic sepsis • Easy bruising and bleeding • Anemia (low red blood cell counts) • Delayed healing	• Fatigue • Nausea/vomiting • Appetite changes • Constipation • Diarrhea • Weight changes • Mouth, tongue, and throat sores and pain with swallowing • Bladder and kidney problems • Insomnia • Impaired cognition, difficulty focusing • Mood changes • Changes in libido and sexual function • Fertility problems

Other Mechanisms

- Hair loss
- Peripheral neuropathy
- Skin and nail changes

Created by Sophia Andrews. Printed with permission.

are grouped together in order to differentiate from other pathological mechanisms.

Immunosuppression during and after chemotherapy regimens is a prevalent challenge for PLWBCs, as it places them at an increased risk for infections. All interprofessional members of the comprehensive cancer care team must perform evidence-based infection control practices when working with PLWBCs. Figure 13.7 below summarizes key personnel and environmental considerations that are important to protect PLWBCs from opportunistic infections.[48] The Onc R clinician should refer to their institution's guidelines for infection control practices.

Hormonal and Biological Therapies

A stronger association is well-established between the female sex and a more robust immune response to pathogens compared to the male sex. Females are also more susceptible to the development of autoimmune disorders than males. This phenomenon is sometimes referred to as biological sex-related "immune tone" at baseline, prior to the development of malignancy, and is presumably related to the mechanisms of sex hormones.

Hormone therapy is a type of treatment used to slow or stop the growth of cancerous cells that rely on hormones to grow.[49] It can treat the cancer or assist in reducing the symptoms of cancer in those that cannot receive other forms of treatment. There are two main types of hormone therapy: those that impair the hormone's function and those that reduce the production of the hormones. Hormone therapy is a conventional therapy for prostate and breast cancers. It can be administered as a neoadjuvant therapy to reduce tumor burden prior to the initiation of another therapy. It is also used as an adjuvant therapy to reduce the

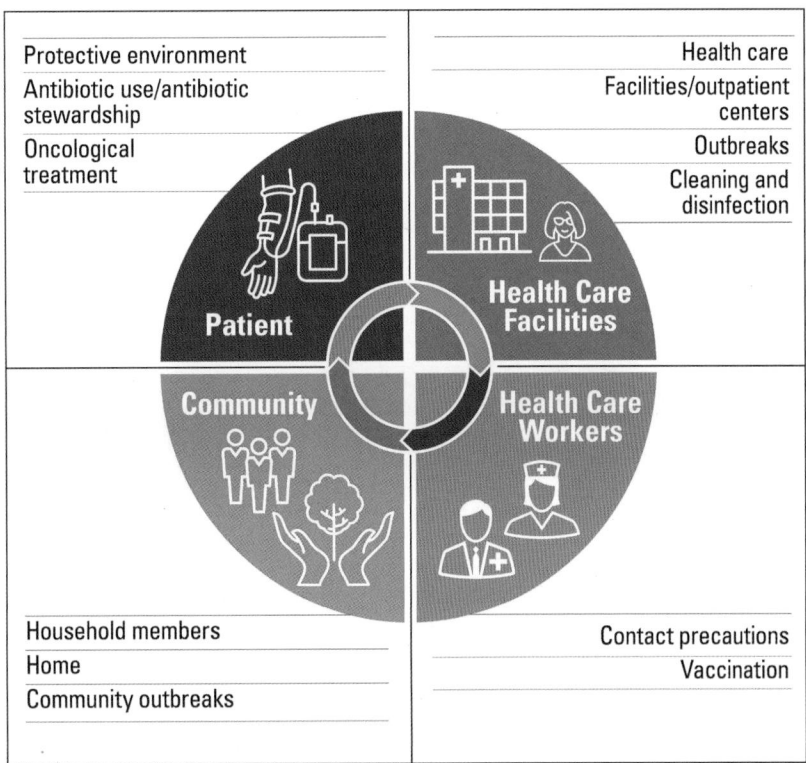

• **Fig. 13.7** Important Aspects of Infection Control and Prevention in Patients Living With Cancer. (Reprinted with permission from Ariza-Heredia EJ, Chemaly RF. Update on infection control practices in cancer hospitals. *CA Cancer J Clin.* 2018;68(5):340–355. doi:10.3322/caac.21462.)

risk for cancer recurrence. Adverse effects of hormone therapy depend upon the type of hormone administered. They include hot flashes, fatigue, nausea, and mood changes. Hormone therapy can be administered orally, by injection, or surgically.[49] Surgery may involve the removal of hormone-producing endocrine organs, such as the ovaries in women and the testicles in men.

Two thirds of breast cancers have hormone receptors that have been identified. Estrogen receptors (ERs) (subtypes alpha and beta) manage the effects of estrogen. Tamoxifen (Nolvadex) is a commonly prescribed hormonal therapy and estrogen modulator (ER alpha receptor antagonist) used to treat ER alpha positive breast cancer.[49] Hormone therapy for breast cancer is frequently administered in combination with other chemotherapy and/or checkpoint inhibitors. There is minimal literature demonstrating direct adverse effects of estrogen-based hormone therapy alone on the immune system, but other therapeutic agents used in combination with hormones may alter immune function. Estrogen-based hormone therapy is associated with an increased risk for hypercoagulopathy and VTE,[21] which the Onc R clinician should monitor for.

Androgen deprivation therapy is commonly used in the treatment of prostate cancers that are responsive to the activation or deactivation of androgens.[50,51] This type of therapy often causes immunosuppression as a result of suppression of T cell and B cell maturation, decreased antibody production, and increased cytokine production. Figure 13.8 summarizes the effects of androgens on cancer and cellular immunity.

Biologic (or biological) therapy is a class of therapeutics defined by the derivation of agents from living organisms. Donor organisms commonly used for biologic therapies include animal models in laboratory settings and human subjects. Immunotherapies, including immune checkpoint inhibitors and monoclonal antibodies (mAbs), are considered biological therapies and will be discussed later in the chapter.

Stem Cell Transplant

Bone marrow transplant (BMT), or hematopoietic SCT, is a potentially curative treatment for many neoplastic disorders. It is most commonly used for hematologic malignancies. There are three main platforms for the medical prescription of SCT—to rescue, replace, or promote immunologic function. Rescue involves destroying the malignant cells, in addition to the stem cells. Replacement refers to the exchange of diseased stem cells with healthy new ones.[52] Use of a SCT as an immunologic platform may be used to prime the recipient and create an environment that is optimized for further immunologic therapy. The essential components of the BMT process are (1) conditioning, (2) infusion, and (3) engraftment. A conditioning chemotherapy regimen immediately prior to hematopoietic cell infusion is essential to deplete the recipient's underlying disease, minimize the risk for transplant rejection, and maximize engraftment.

There are two main classifications of stem cells used in transplant: autologous and allogeneic. Autologous transplantation involves the collection and infusion of the patient's own cells, whereas allogeneic transplantation uses cells from an HLA-matched or partially matched donor. The preference is always to use a fully matched-related donor (MRD) that is HLA-identical to the person receiving the transplant, but this is not always available.[52] HLA typing is a screening process that uses markers on cells (antigens) to identify similarities between donors and recipients in order to decrease the risk and severity of an immunological response by the recipient. Donors can be matched-unrelated

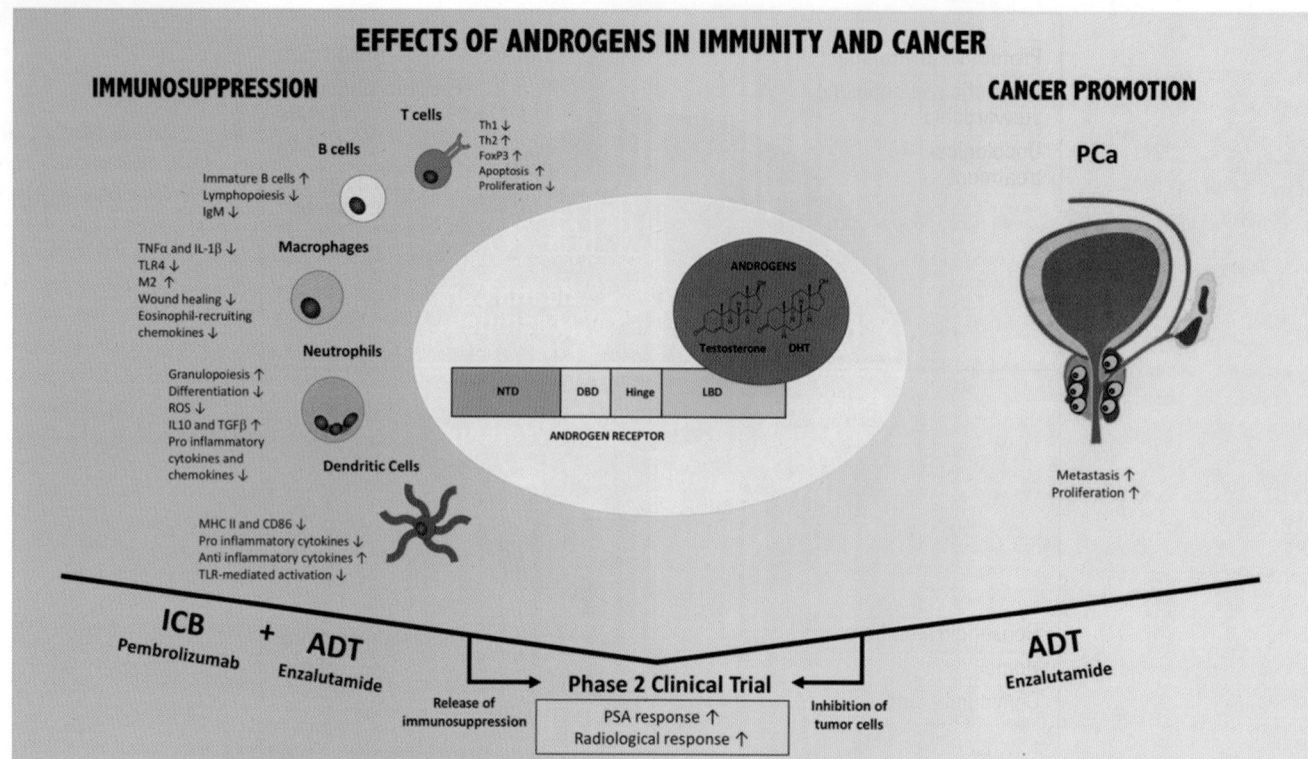

• **Fig. 13.8** The Effects of Androgens in Immunity and Cancer. AR/androgens can influence different immune cell subsets, including T cells, B cells, macrophages, neutrophils, and dendritic cells (Left part of the figure). Overall, their effect is immunosuppressive. In addition, AR/androgens directly and indirectly promote prostate cancer (PCa) via different mechanisms (Right part of the figure). Thus, the combination of ADT with immune checkpoint blockade could foster anti-tumor immune responses (ICB+ADT) while ADT additionally inhibits PCa directly. This combination strategy has resulted in improved patient responses compared to either monotherapy in Phase 2 clinical trials. Confirmatory Phase 3 trials are warranted and ongoing. *ADT*, Androgen deprivation therapy; *DBD*, DNA binding domain; *DHT*, dihydrotestosterone; FoxP3, forkhead box P3; *ICB*, immune checkpoint blockade; *IgM*, immunoglobulin M; *LBD*, ligand binding domain; *MHC II*, major histocompatibility complex II; *NTD*, N-terminal domain; *PCa*, prostate cancer; *PSA*, prostate specific antigen; *TLR4*, toll-like receptor 4; *TNF-α*, tumor necrosis factor α. (Reprinted with permission from Ben-Batalla I, Vargas-Delgado ME, Amsberg GV, Janning M, Loges S. Influence of androgens on immunity to self and foreign: effects on immunity and cancer. *Front Immunol.* 2020;11:1184. doi:10.3389/fimmu.2020.01184.)

donors (MUDs), MRDs, haploidentical donors, or otherwise partially HLA-matched donors. Recently, innovative protocols for transplantation, such as haploidentical matching, require less HLA matching and less intensive conditioning chemotherapy, thereby increasing the availability of potential donors.

Preferred sources of hematopoietic cell grafts include bone marrow from the iliac crest, peripheral blood stem cells, and umbilical cord blood. Increased pre-transplant comorbidities in the recipient are correlated with a higher post-transplant morbidity and mortality. The health status of the donor and recipient are carefully considered when determining candidacy for SCT.

Engraftment is the process by which the transplanted stem cells enter the recipient's bone marrow, start to function, and proliferate. Successful engraftment is clinically defined by the sustained production of healthy red blood cells, WBCs, and platelets. Diagnostic criteria for engraftment include 3 consecutive days with a peripheral neutrophil count of >500 × 10⁶/L and independence from platelet transfusion with a platelet count of >20 × 10⁹/L for 7 consecutive days.[53] Choices of graft sources and conditioning regimens strongly correlate to the success rates of engraftment.

Engraftment syndrome (ES) describes the development of a fever and other symptoms of vascular leakage that may occur during engraftment. Some refer to ES as "early graft-versus-host disease." These symptoms usually occur at the timepoint of neutrophil recovery and are managed with corticosteroids if symptoms persist for greater than 1 week.

Graft failure is a major complication of SCT that occurs after insufficient stem cell engraftment and greatly increases morbidity and mortality. Clinical factors that can increase the risk of graft failure include HLA disparity, ABO mismatching (conflicting blood types), reduced-intensity conditioning, underlying primary diagnosis, cell dosage, graft source, and viral status. Primary graft failure is defined as no engraftment or donor cell recovery in the first 30 days after transplant with no evidence of disease relapse. Secondary graft failure refers to the destruction of the graft that was previously functioning. Graft rejection occurs when the recipient's immune system response to the graft is the leading cause of graft failure.

A second allogeneic transplant may be considered for patients with graft failure and rejection. Patients with poor graft function, but without evidence of graft rejection, may be candidates to receive a T cell infusion from the donor to try to improve the graft function.[53] There are many other complications that can occur after SCT. These include, but are not limited to neutropenia, anemia, thrombocytopenia, mucositis, diarrhea, liver dysfunction, renal complications, pulmonary complications, and graft versus host disease (GVHD).[54]

Mucositis is defined as the inflammation of the mucosal epithelial cells in response to the cytotoxic effects of chemotherapy and radiation. It is also one of the most common adverse effects of bone marrow transplantation protocols that include intensive conditioning chemotherapy. The onset of mucositis typically occurs within the first 100 days after transplantation and affects the mucosal-lined surface all the way from the mouth to the rectum.[54] Clinical manifestations start with erythema and cracking of the mucosa and can progress to bleeding and ulceration. Pain is the most common symptom. Treatment options include pain medication, topical agents, and good oral care. Mucositis can interfere with speaking and swallowing, impair nutritional intake, and increase the risk for mucosal infections. Transplant recipients that experience mucositis also report lower levels of energy and decreased sleep quality, which may impact participation in post-transplant Onc R and overall QOL.[54] See a grading scale for mucositis in the enhanced eBook on eTable 13.3.

The potential adverse effects and complications of SCT can affect multiple systems along the inflammation-immune axis. In the musculoskeletal system, steroid myopathy is the most common adverse effect resulting from the extended use of corticosteroids. Myopathies occur as a result of type II muscle fiber atrophy and phagocytosis replacing the original fibrous muscle tissue with adipose tissue.[55] The symptoms of steroid myopathy may include hip girdle weakness or proximal muscle weakness, especially shown through difficulty with sit to stand transfers.[56] Strength improvements during Onc R tend to occur slowly. Strengthening exercises should focus on proximal muscles with low resistance to prevent further muscle breakdown.

Cytotoxic chemotherapies administered for cancer treatment prior to and during transplant conditioning frequently result in the development of peripheral neuropathies. Central neuropathy and metabolic encephalopathy are also common adverse effects of chemotherapy and SCT. Typically, changes in mental status that are related to metabolic changes can be reversed by addressing the cause.

Cancer-related fatigue (CRF) is commonly experienced by persons that have or are receiving SCT. Many factors can contribute to CRF, including metabolic abnormalities, anemia, infection, decreased nutritional status, pain, deconditioning/inactivity, depression, insomnia, other alterations in sleep/wake cycle, and medications such as opioids, antihistamines, antidepressants, and immunosuppressants. The best interventions for fatigue are correcting the associated medical causes, altering contributing medications, exercise, energy conservation, and assisting with coping.[55]

Clinical Pearl

Health care providers may want persons undergoing SCT to receive "prehabilitation" (see Chapter 27) prior to transplant in order to increase their overall fitness for candidacy. These treatment regimens can have positive effects on the strength and functional exercise capacity of persons living with advanced cancer. However, gains may be quickly lost due to detraining and illness during the acute post-transplant phase while engraftment is occurring. Onc R clinicians may be able to minimize detraining effects post-transplant by facilitating regular participation in functional mobility and aerobic exercise.

Graft Versus Host Disease

GVHD is a common complication of allogeneic hematopoietic stem cell transplants. In GVHD, an immune reaction occurs between the transplanted (graft) immune cells and the recipient (host) tissues. The grafted immune cells recognize the recipient cells as "foreign." Body systems most commonly involved are the skin, liver, and gastrointestinal (GI) system.

There are two main classifications of GVHD: acute and chronic. Symptoms of acute GVHD (aGVHD) include a classic maculopapular rash or lichenoid, nausea/vomiting, abdominal cramps, diarrhea, and an increase in serum bilirubin.[57] These occur around the same time as WBC engraftment. Chronic GVHD (cGVHD) symptoms include sclerodermatous skin involvement, dry oral mucosa, mucosal ulceration, GI tract sclerosis, and an increase in serum bilirubin.[57] A diagnosis is typically made on clinical evaluation alone, but in some complex cases, biomarker testing and tissue biopsies are used for more definitive diagnoses.

GVHD-associated skin lesions may involve the dermal and epidermal layers, manifesting as a maculopapular rash or a sclerotic plaque. These skin lesions can be quite painful and commonly involve the neck, ears, shoulders, soles of feet, and hands. In severe cases, bullous lesions can form.

GI involvement usually includes both the upper and lower tract. Clinical symptoms may include diarrhea, nausea, vomiting, anorexia, and abdominal pain. Upper GI symptoms (anorexia, food intolerance, nausea, and vomiting) tend to respond better to immunosuppressive therapy. It is very rare to have manifestations of liver GVHD without concurrent involvement of the skin and GI systems. A liver biopsy is required to diagnose liver involvement. Clinical symptoms of liver involvement include abnormal liver function tests, including a rise in serum bilirubin. Hepatomegaly, dark urine, pale stool, fluid retention, and pruritus may also be seen.[57]

The Glucksberg Grading System for the Severity of GVHD (Table 13.11) is the most commonly used grading system. A single, succinct grade can be given after staging the involvement of each of the three most commonly involved tissues or organs (skin, liver, and GI tract). Primary organ involvement of GVHD involves the skin, liver, and GI tract, however other organ involvement can occur as well. These include involvement of the lungs, kidneys, eyes, and bone marrow.[58] Hematopoietic involvement is normally seen through thymic atrophy and cytopenia. The effects of GVHD on the ocular system include photophobia, hemorrhagic conjunctivitis, and lagophthalmos. See Table 13.12 for distinctive characteristics of GVHD by system or tissue affected.

There are many risk factors for the development of aGVHD. These include the degree of HLA disparity, biological sex disparity between donor and recipient, intensity of transplant conditioning treatment, type of GVHD prophylaxis used, source of the graft (blood or bone marrow more so than umbilical cord), age, and cytomegalovirus status of donor.[57] In addition, the severity of post-transplant GVHD is associated with the number of pre-transplant comorbidities. The initiation of a prophylaxis regimen is imperative to lower the risk of peri-transplant GVHD.

Prophylaxis focuses on immunosuppression of the donor cells either with medication or with T cell depletion. The uses of antithymocyte globulin (ATG) in the pre-transplant period and rituximab in the post-transplant period have been found to be beneficial in preventing cGVHD.[57] Logically, the severity of cGVHD is strongly associated with the use of prophylaxis for aGVHD in the pre- and post-transplant phases.

After a diagnosis of GVHD is made, the choice of treatment depends on which organs are involved and the severity of involvement. There is no consensus approach to treating GVHD; the use of corticosteroids is a common initial strategy in the acute phase.

TABLE 13.11   Grading the Severity of Graft-Versus-Host Disease

Organ	Stage	Description
Skin	1	Maculopapular rash <25% of body area
	2	Maculopapular rash 25%–50% of body area
	3	Generalized erythroderma
	4	Generalized erythroderma with bulbous formation
Liver (bilirubin)	1	2.0–3.0 mg/dL
	2	3.1–6.0 mg/dL
	3	6.1–15.0 mg/dL
	4	>15.0 mg/dL
Gut (diarrhea)	1	>30 mL/kg or >500 mL/day
	2	>60 mL/kg or >1000 mL/day
	3	>90 mL/kg or >1500 mL/day
	4	>120 mL/kg or >2000 mL/day or severe abdominal pain

Glucksberg Grade	
I	Stage 1 or 2 skin involvement; no liver or gut involvement
II	Stage 1–3 skin involvement; Grade 1 liver or gut involvement
III	Stage 2 or 3 skin, liver, or gut involvement
IV	Stage 1–4 skin involvement; Stage 2–4 liver or gut involvement

Adapted from Chao NJ. Clinical manifestations, diagnosis, and grading of acute graft-versus-host disease. In: Post T, ed. *UpToDate*. UpToDate; 2019. www.uptodate.com. Accessed August 7, 2020.

Glucocorticoids are administered to those with Grade II or higher.[58] Topical steroids can be used with skin involvement and supplemental nutrition will also be needed with GI involvement.

The treatment for GVHD involves dampening the immune reaction, which is typically achieved through the use of corticosteroids. Table 13.13 lists some common components of cGVHD in addition to potential interventions. The most common musculoskeletal impairments seen in those with GVHD include soft tissue contractures and fasciitis from skin involvement and steroid-induced myopathy (as discussed earlier). Cutaneous involvement is the most common symptom in cGVHD affecting 90% of people.[57] It presents as a combination of dermal and fascial involvement. Sclerodermoid GVHD mimics scleroderma and results in skin tightening and joint contractures which affect functional mobility.[56] Distal joints are affected first. The clinical presentation is almost always symmetric. Treatment options are limited but stretching and splinting have shown mild benefits in the literature. Treating pain and soft tissue impairments may benefit from use of transcutaneous electrical nerve stimulation (TENS) or therapeutic ultrasound to assist with tissue healing. Myofascial release can assist with inflammation. In addition, edema can sometimes result from GVHD leading to range-of-motion (ROM) restrictions and mobility.[56] The goal of therapy is to safely reduce the edema and improve function. This can be done through fluid restriction, diuretic medications, and compression therapy.

Avascular necrosis and osteoporosis may result from long-term corticosteroid use. Avascular necrosis presents with pain and limited ROM and is when the blood supply to the joints, most commonly the femoral head, is disrupted. It can be managed conservatively with medication and physical therapy or with more invasive surgical intervention. Nonoperative intervention involves decreasing the compressing and shear forces around the joint. This can be done through assistive devices, increasing joint mobility, and strengthening muscles around the joint. In addition, due to nutritional status and decreased vitamin D, there is a higher risk for osteoporosis secondary to use of glucocorticoids due to increased

TABLE 13.12   Diagnostic and Distinctive Clinical Manifestations of GVHD

Organ	Distinctive Characteristics
Skin	Depigmentation, fibrosis, maculopapular rash, sclerodermoid GVHD
Nails	Dystrophy, longitudinal ridging, splitting, or brittle, nail loss, onycholysis, pterygium unguis
Scalp and Body Hair	New onset of scarring or nonscarring scalp alopecia (after recovery from chemoradiotherapy)
Mouth	Xerostomia, mucocele, mucosal atrophy, pseudomembranes, ulcers, restriction of mouth opening from sclerosis
Eyes	New-onset dry, gritty, or painful eyes, cicatricial conjunctivitis, keratoconjunctivitis sicca, confluent of punctuate keratopathy, photophobia, hemorrhagic conjunctivitis, lagophthalmos
Genitalia	Erosions, fissures, ulcers, vaginal scarring, or stenosis
Gastrointestinal Tract	Diarrhea, nausea, vomiting, anorexia, abdominal pain
Hepatic	Increase in serum bilirubin, hepatomegaly, dark urine, pale stool, fluid retention, pruritus
Cardiopulmonary	Increased resting heart rate, decreased stroke volume, decreased VO_2 max, lower extremity edema, increased cardiac afterload, bronchiolitis obliterans, and obstructive pulmonary disorders
Hematopoietic	Thymic atrophy and cytopenia
Neurological	Nerve entrapment, mononeuropathies, peripheral neuropathy, inflammatory neuropathy
Musculoskeletal	Soft tissue contractures, fasciitis, steroid myopathy, avascular necrosis, osteoporosis, decreased muscle mass

GVHD, Graft versus host disease Vo_2 max, Maximal volume of oxygen consumed..
Adapted from Chao NJ. Clinical manifestations, diagnosis, and grading of acute graft-versus-host disease. In: Post T, ed. *UpToDate*. UpToDate; 2019. www.uptodate.com. Accessed August 7, 2020.

TABLE 13.13	Common Impairments Seen and Potential Interventions in Persons With Chronic GVHD (cGVHD)	
COMMON REHABILITATION ISSUES IN cGVHD		
Organ	Problem	Intervention
Skin/Fascia	Sclerodermatous contractures	ROM and strengthening, splinting, iontophoresis. Surgery likely ineffective and may have negative outcomes.
Muscle	Myopathy	Fall prevention and strengthening. Bracing for weak muscles. Adaptive equipment (canes, walkers) as indicated.
Bone	Osteoporosis	Core stabilization, bracing for pain or stability
Peripheral Nervous System	Peripheral neuropathy	Bracing for motor weakness, nerve stabilizing agents for pain, wound prevention (proper footwear, frequent skin checks)
Cardiopulmonary	Physical deconditioning	Exercise program, consider pulmonary or cardiac rehab for specific issues in these organ systems

ROM, Range of motion.
Adapted from Smith S, Haig A, Couriel D. Musculoskeletal, neurologic, and cardiopulmonary aspects of physical rehabilitation in patients with chronic graft-versus-host disease. *Biol Blood Marrow Transplant.* 2015;21(5):799–808. Used with Permission.

bone turnover. Please see Chapter 7 for more information about the management of musculoskeletal impairments.

Significant loss of muscle mass is also commonly seen in persons with GVHD. This can result from deconditioning and/or adverse effects of immunosuppressive medication such as corticosteroids. With high levels of inactivity and bed rest, the weight bearing lower extremities and back extensor muscles are more affected than upper extremities. This can make transfers and ambulation challenging. Muscle repair is also altered due to increased catabolism from the glucocorticoids in the bloodstream. In addition, poor nutritional status is seen with GVHD due to GI involvement. Poor nutritional status can affect muscle mass and energy level and it is imperative that this is addressed in order to progress a strengthening program. Initiating a strength and resistance program and early Onc R can assist with prevention of muscle atrophy. Relative precautions should be taken for those with severe thrombocytopenia (<20,000), as increased intracranial pressure during a Valsalva maneuver with resistance exercises may increase the risk of subarachnoid hemorrhages and retinopathy.[56] Multiple factors must be taken into consideration for developing a treatment plan to address musculoskeletal impairments in those with GVHD.

cGVHD is also associated with neurologic impairments such as mononeuropathies, peripheral neuropathy, and inflammatory neuropathy. Additionally, steroid-induced peripheral neuropathy may develop after extended corticosteroid use. cGVHD is known to cause inflammatory demyelinating polyneuropathy due to T cell infiltration of nerves.[56] Nerve entrapment is a potential cause of mononeuropathies in GVHD. Compression from fascial inflammation can occur in nerves with little surrounding protective tissue. Treatment for most neuropathies includes medications such as gabapentin and physical therapy to restore function.

Finally, cardiopulmonary compromise frequently occurs in individuals with GVHD as a result of increased sedentary behaviors. Aerobic deconditioning can result in an increased resting heart rate, decreased stroke volume, and decreased VO_2 max.[56] Those with liver involvement from GVHD may develop lower extremity edema, leading to congestion and increasing cardiac afterload. Rehabilitation strategies include increasing activity through a structured Onc R program. Loss of function and independence may occur for individuals with GVHD. Comprehensive, multidisciplinary Onc R interventions may help to improve musculoskeletal function and cardiopulmonary endurance.

Clinical Pearl

Persons with GVHD may have decreased energy reserves and activity tolerance, especially with involvement of the liver and GI system. They may have decreased oral intake and frequent diarrhea, leading to nutritional deficits and electrolyte abnormalities. Consider coordinating Onc R therapies after meals and discussing a nutritional plan with dieticians in order to optimize rehabilitation potential.

Checkpoint Inhibitor Immunotherapy

Checkpoints are cellular molecules along the immune response cascade that are either activated or inactivated to facilitate an immune response. Checkpoint inhibitor immunotherapy does not work directly on the tumor, but instead slows or speeds up the immune response to the cancer. Checkpoint inhibitors are mostly used to treat solid tumors. Programmed cell death protien-1 (PD-1) and cytotoxic T-lymphocyte-associated protein 4 (CTLA-4) are two commonly targeted checkpoint proteins found on T cells. Checkpoint inhibitors help promote antitumor immunity while minimizing immunosuppression.[59] They are increasingly used in combination with hormone therapy for the treatment of prostate and breast cancers, with results demonstrating safety and efficacy in promoting antitumor T cell activation and NK cell depletion.[60]

Monoclonal Antibodies

MAbs are biologic proteins that are created in a laboratory setting. They help the host immune system to recognize antigens on pathological cells, such as viruses and cancer cells, and brand them for termination. MAbs are used to treat a variety of cancers. Since the first therapeutic monoclonal antibody came to market in 1975, there has been an explosion in the number of therapeutic mAbs successfully developed and applied to different diagnoses (Figure 13.9).[61] Adverse effects of mAbs include flu-like symptoms, allergic reactions, cytokine release syndrome, and capillary leak syndrome.[62]

MAbs are also used to treat autoimmune disorders such as rheumatoid arthritis (RA) and allograft rejection. Rituximab is commonly used to treat RA and NHL, in combination with chemotherapy. Persons living with NHL usually receive combination therapy in cycles of R-CHOP as a first line therapy.[62]

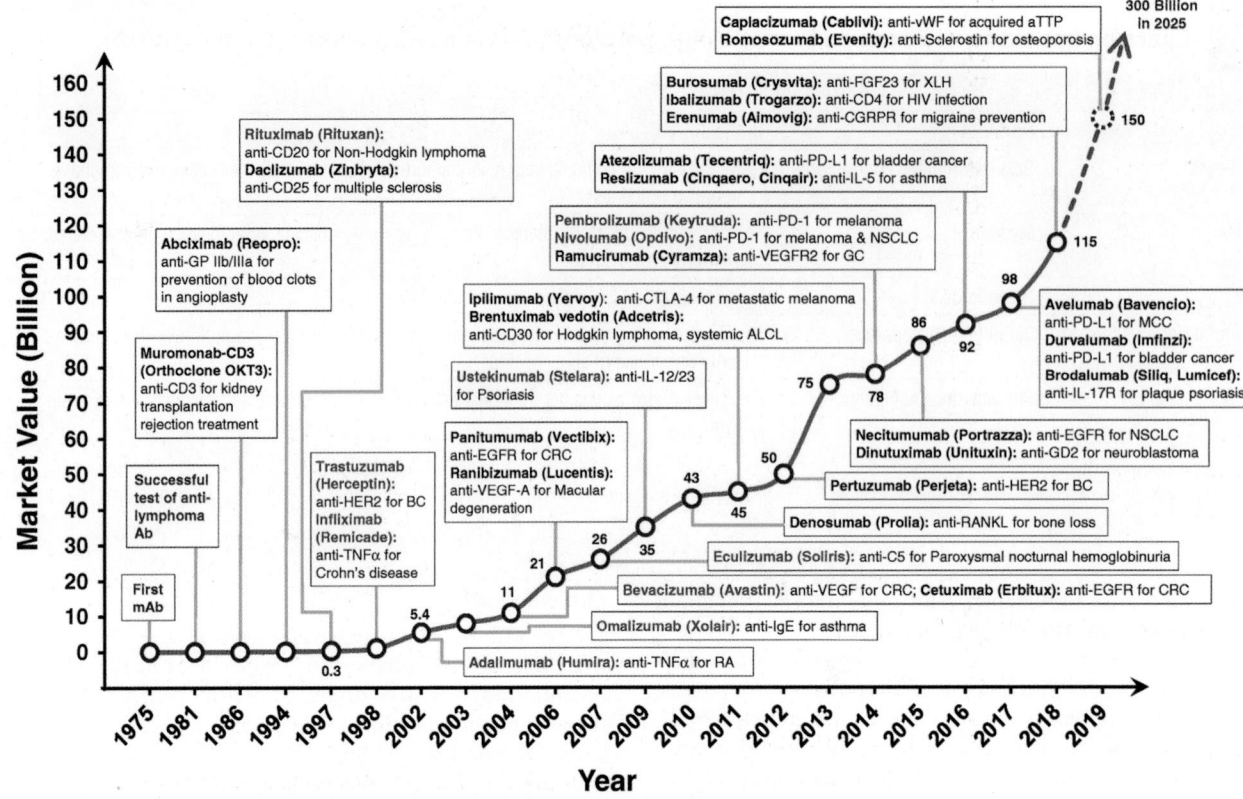

• **Fig. 13.9** Timeline From 1975 Showing the Successful Development of Therapeutic Antibodies and Their Applications. Many biotech companies that promised antibodies as anticancer "magic bullets" were launched from 1981 to 1986. The height of the line and numerical annotations represent the estimated market value of mAb therapeutics in each indicated year (shown as billions of US dollars). Antibodies colored in red represent the top 10 best-selling antibody drugs in 2018. *Ab*, Antibody; *ALCL*, systematic anaplastic large-cell lymphoma; *aTTP*, acquired thrombotic thrombocytopenic purpura; *BC*, breast cancer; *CD*, cluster of differentiation; *CGRP*, calcitonin gene-related peptide; *CGRPR*, calcitonin gene-related peptide receptor; *CRC*, colorectal cancer; *CTLA-4*, cytotoxic T-lymphocyte-associated protein 4; *EGFR*, epidermal growth factor receptor; *FGF*, fibroblast growth factor; *GC*, gastric cancer; *GD2*, disialoganglioside GD2; *HER2*, human epidermal growth factor receptor 2; *IgE*, immunoglobulin E; *IL*, interleukin; *IL-17R*, interleukin-17 receptor; *mAb*, monoclonal antibody; *MCC*, merkel-cell carcinoma; *NSCLC*, nonsmall cell lung cancer; *PD-1*, programmed cell death protein 1; *PD-L1*, programmed death-ligand 1; *RA*, rheumatoid arthritis; *RANKL*, receptor activator of nuclear factor kappa-B ligand; *TNFα*, tumor necrosis factor *α*; *VEGF-A*, vascular endothelial growth factor A; *VEGFR2*, vascular endothelial growth factor receptor 2; *vWF*, von Willebrand factor; *XLH*, X-linked hypophosphatemia. (Reprinted with permission from Lu RM, Hwang YC, Liu IJ, et al. Development of therapeutic antibodies for the treatment of diseases. *J Biomed Sci.* 2020;27:1. doi:10.1186/s12929-019-0592-z.)

This combination therapy can be quite taxing on the immune system and sometimes requires hospitalization for close monitoring.

Clinical Pearl

There are many exciting immunotherapies recently FDA approved and currently in clinical trials. Limited evidence is available to inform effective Onc R protocols after immunotherapies. More research is needed to guide best practices and establish Onc R guidelines.

Adoptive Cell Therapies

An innovative new class of cancer therapeutics has been developed through a series of translational science breakthroughs in the fields of genetics, engineering, and cellular immunology. Adoptive cell therapy, also referred to as cellular immunotherapy, refers to

therapeutic approaches that utilize autogenic or allogenic immune effector cells to treat certain types of cancer. Autogenic strategies include taking T cells from a person's own blood or tumor tissue, replicating them to reach large numbers, and then reinfusing them back into the patient's blood to help fight malignancies. Other approaches involve the use of gene therapy to selectively engineer TSAs and other cellular components on the T cells to target malignant biomarkers.

Current adoptive cell therapy treatment strategies[63] are summarized in Table 13.14 and Figure 13.10. This area of oncological research and clinical medicine is rapidly developing and evolving, with a large number of available clinical trials evaluating immunocellular therapies alone and in combination with other treatment approaches, such as with chemotherapy and radiation.[64] There is evidence of positive outcomes after immunotherapy for certain types of pediatric and adult cancer, including a high percentage of partial and complete responses. FDA approval has been granted

TABLE 13.14	Overview of Treatment Modalities of Adoptive Cell Therapy		
	TIL	**TCR**	**CAR**
First evidence of clinical benefit	1994	2006	2013
Production method	Isolation of T cells from tumors and expansion ex vivo	Isolation of peripheral T cells via apheresis and ex vivo transduction with a TCR against tumor antigen	Isolation of peripheral T cells via apheresis and ex vivo transduction with a CAR against tumor antigen
Target	MHC-peptide complex	MHC-peptide complex	Non-MHC cell surface proteins
Lymphodepleting preparative regimen	Yes	Yes	Yes
Supportive IL-2	Yes	Varying	No
Specificity	Polyclonal	Monoclonal	Monoclonal
Main toxicity	Lymphodepleting regimen IL-2 mediated (chills, fever, edema) Seldom autoimmune	Lymphodepleting regimen "On-target, off-tumor" CRS	Lymphodepleting regimen "On-target, off-tumor" CRS Neurological
Restrictions	Complex Heterogeneous infusion product	MHC-restricted Currently not yet tumor-specific Toxicity	Currently only effective for treatment of hematological malignancies Toxicity

CAR, Chimeric antigen receptor; *CRS*, cytokine release syndrome; *IL-2*, interleukin-2; *MHC*, major histocompatibility complex; *TCR*, T cell receptor; *TIL*, tumor-infiltrating lymphocytes.
Adapted from Rohaan MW, Wilgenhof S, Haanen JBAG. Adoptive cellular therapies: the current landscape. *Virchows Arch.* 2019;474:449–461. doi:10.1007/s00428-018-2484-0.

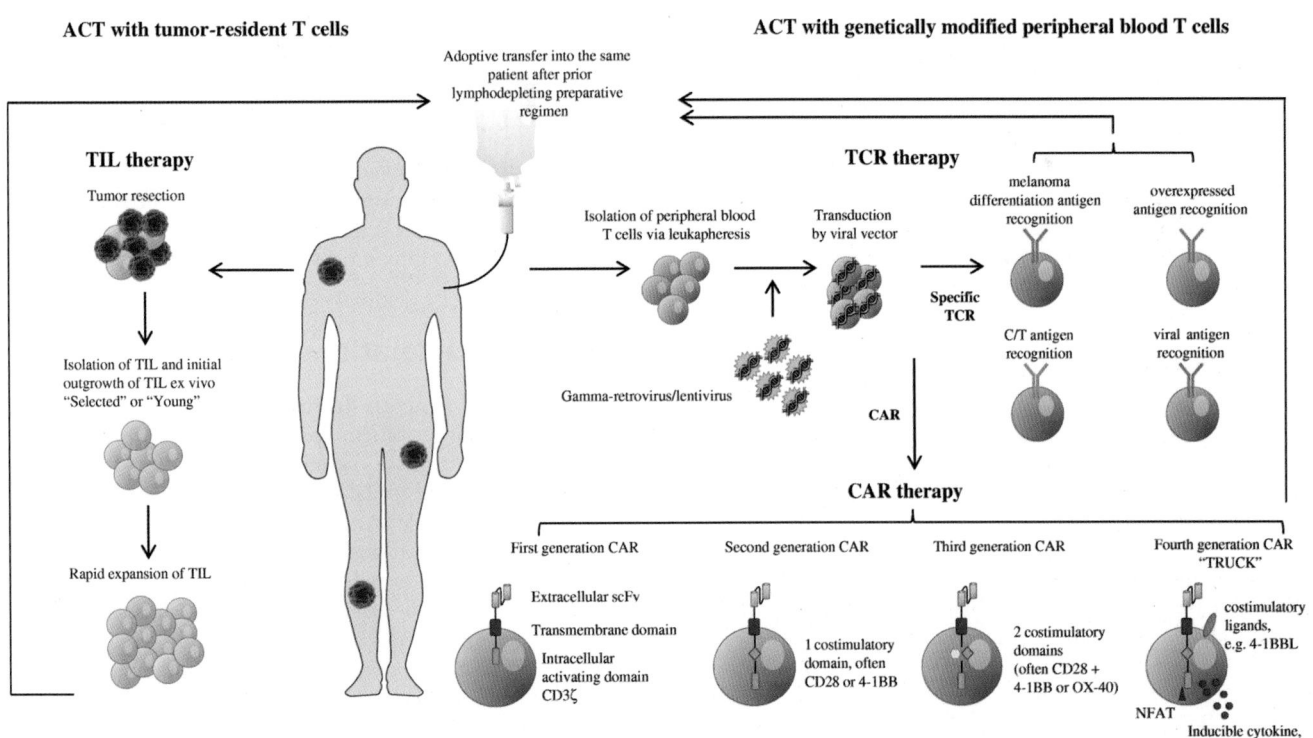

• **Fig. 13.10** Schematic Overview of the Processes for Adoptive Cell Therapy. Adoptive cell therapy (ACT) of tumor-infiltrating lymphocytes (TIL), ACT with T cell receptor (TCR) gene therapy and ACT with chimeric antigen receptor (CAR)-modified T cells. In ACT with TIL, tumor-resident T cells are isolated and expanded ex vivo after surgical resection of the tumor. Thereafter, the TILs are further expanded in a rapid expansion protocol (REP). Before intravenous adoptive transfer into the patient, the patient is treated with a lymphodepleting conditioning regimen. In ACT with genetically modified peripheral blood T cells, TCR gene therapy and CAR gene therapy can be distinguished. For both treatment modalities, peripheral blood T cells are isolated via leukapheresis. These T cells are then transduced by viral vectors to either express a specific TCR or CAR, respectively. (Reprinted with permission from Rohaan MW, Wilgenhof S, Haanen JBAG. Adoptive cellular therapies: the current landscape. *Virchows Arch.* 2019;474:449–461. doi:10.1007/s00428-018-2484-0.)

for the use of Chimeric antigen receptor T cell (CAR-T) immunocellular therapies to treat certain forms of leukemia and lymphoma. See Chapter 5 for more on CAR-T.

Current protocols for clinical management after adoptive cell therapy are also focused on strategies to mitigate the serious potential adverse effects that have been documented during and after immunocellular therapy infusions. Serious adverse effects can become life-threatening, resulting in hemodynamic and neurological changes that can negatively affect a patient's activity tolerance. Onc R clinicians, in collaboration with other members of the health care team, should be able to recognize and appropriately respond to the signs and symptoms of cytokine release syndrome and neurotoxicity in the acute phase during and after infusion therapy.[65] The patient, family, and caregivers are also educated to regularly monitor for signs and symptoms related to known potential adverse effects. The early detection of adverse effects[66] is important to limit progression to more critical stages, to minimize damage to body structures and functions, and to determine patient eligibility for pharmacological therapies and other clinical management.

Clinical Pearl

Some individuals that receive CAR-T cell immunotherapies can experience persistent adverse effects of immune effector cell-associated neurotoxicity syndrome that last beyond the acute phase, resulting in more long-term impairments in physical and neurocognitive function. Research efforts are ongoing to understand the complex mechanisms of injury and treatment approaches for severe central neurotoxicity. Individuals that experience severe adverse effects of neurotoxicity are more likely to need extensive Onc R to promote return to function and maximize QOL.

Cancer Vaccines

A vaccine works by enhancing the body's immune system in order to defend against a virus. The same works with cancer vaccines. The vaccine works to defend the body against cancer by reinforcing the body's own immune system. Prevention-oriented vaccines target known mechanisms for the malignant transformation of cells. Treatment vaccines are focused on attacking already malignant cancer cells.[67]

Treatment vaccines are comprised of TSAs that are not found in normal, healthy cells. Vaccines train the host immune system to selectively react to TSAs on cancerous cells. They can be made precisely using the PWC's own cells, from the dendritic cells of the PWC, or from TSAs commonly expressed on a type of malignant cell. Adverse effects of a treatment vaccine include fever, chills, weakness, dizziness, muscle and joint pain, fatigue, or severe allergic reactions.[67] Currently, there is only one FDA-approved dendritic vaccine that is used for the treatment of prostate cancer if persons have not responded to hormone therapy (Sipuleucel-T [Provenge]).

Measurement Tools to Screen for and/or Evaluate Each Adverse Effect

The careful monitoring of pertinent lab values and signs and symptoms is essential during all phases of Onc R for the PLWC. Clinical changes in the immune system and hematologic function may be regularly monitored via lab values on a CBC with differential and other clinical pathology assays. The 2017 Lab Values Interpretation Resource and Point-Of-Care Document (updated 2019) from the APTA Academy of Acute Care Physical Therapy

are helpful resources to use during the acute management of hospitalized patients with oncological diagnoses, but also for the management of PLWCs across the care continuum. Refer to Chapter 24 on the acute care management of PLWCs and Chapter 21 about leukemia/lymphoma for more thorough discussions of possible changes in lab values in the acute care setting and associated clinical decision-making.

PLWCs can experience changes in immune system and hematologic function as a result of malignancy and cancer therapeutics. Because many cancer therapies are delivered in the home and outpatient settings, outpatient lab reports can also provide important measurements of immune system and hematologic function. It is essential for the Onc R clinician to review the most recent lab values prior to starting any session. Lab values are useful to inform safety precautions for exercise and rehabilitation.

Clinical Pearl

There is limited evidence available to validate thresholds and cutoff scores for risks related to lab values. The Onc R clinician should ask their respective institution for specific guidelines for exercise precautions related to WBC, hemoglobin, and platelets. These guidelines vary by institution and cancer center. For individuals that are not candidates to receive transfusions of blood products and other therapeutic approaches for correction of lab values, the Onc R clinician is advised to take an individualized approach to each patient. This includes considering the risks versus benefits of exercise compared to rest, using clinical judgment to tailor an activity program, and consulting with experienced members of the care team.

There are a variety of clinically useful measurement tools and outcomes available to quantify and qualify the activity and participation limitations and QOL associated with immunosuppression and other immunological adverse effects of cancer therapies. Measurement tools are commonly validated for specific types of cancer therapies and diagnoses. Please refer to other pertinent chapters in this textbook for more information about appropriate outcome measures to use.

General Considerations for Onc R

Emerging research supports the role of exercise and physical activity as an adjuvant treatment for boosting the immune system during all types of cancer therapies for PLWBCs. In 2016, one study proposed a conceptual framework to discern the potential role of exercise in regulating inflammation-immune axis function in cancer initiation and progress. This framework presents multiple mechanisms by which long-term exercise (as opposed to acute, single bouts of exercise) may modulate specific interactions between normal cells within the immune system, and steps at which the immune response fails to eliminate malignantly transformed cells (Figure 13.11).[68] Refer to Chapter 23 for more information regarding the positive systemic effects of exercise for PLWC. Exercise immunology is a promising area of research that aims to elucidate the biomedical mechanisms by which the functions of the immune system are enhanced by exercise and physical activity in healthy individuals, as well as in PWC.

Conclusion

Onc R clinicians that choose to specialize in the area of Onc R will serve an integral role on any cancer care team, contributing positively to the management of immune system pathologies for PWC. This chapter summarizes the major components of the immune system and the deleterious effects of malignancy and cancer treatments

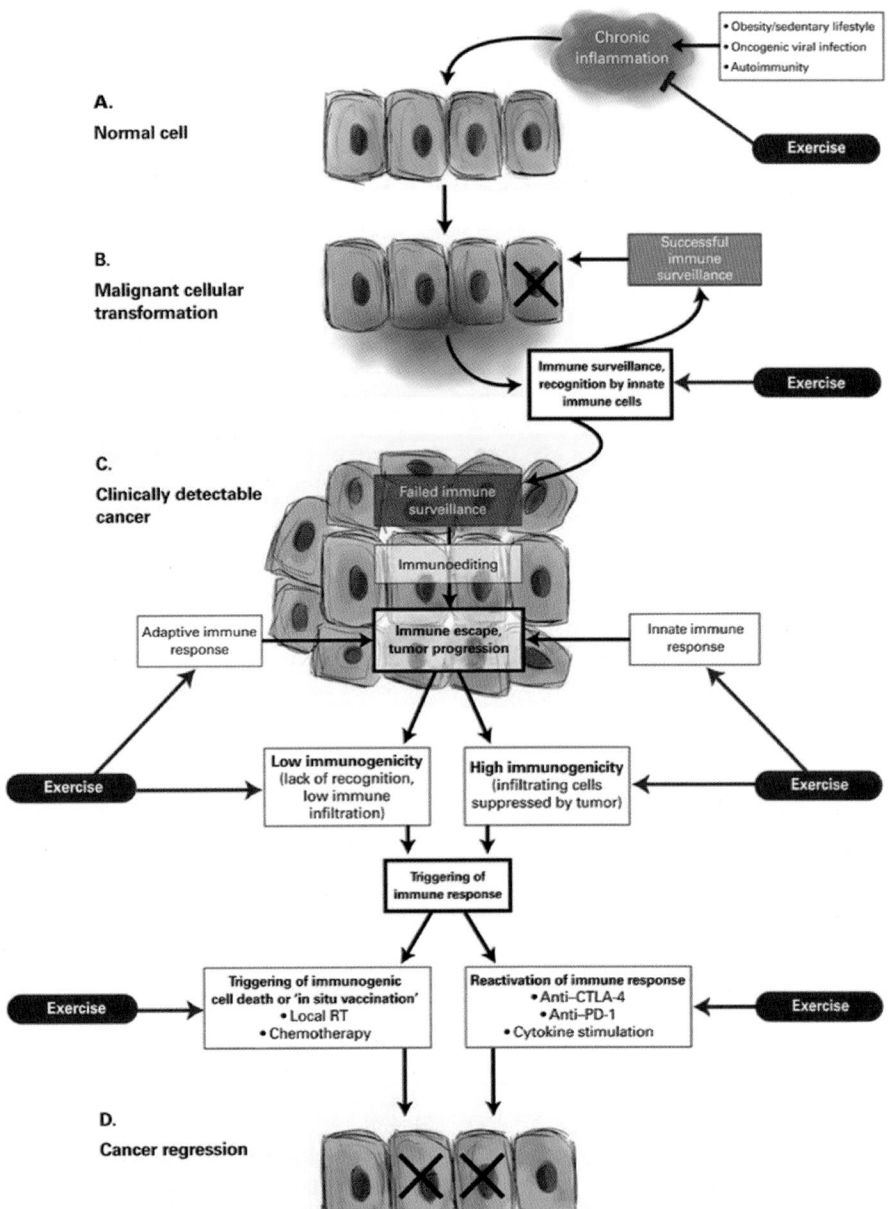

• **Fig. 13.11** A Conceptual Framework to Discern the Potential Role of Exercise in Regulating Inflammation-Immune Axis Function in Cancer Initiation and Progression. (A) Chronic inflammation can be initiated and maintained in patients suffering from a variety of conditions, including autoimmune reactions, persistent viral infections, and obesity (due to pro-inflammatory adipokine secretion). Sustained secretion of pro-inflammatory cytokines can result in transformation of cells that can ultimately lead to cancer. There is emerging evidence that exercise can reduce a variety of markers of inflammation. (B) Most premalignant cells are eliminated by innate immune cells in a process of immune surveillance, particularly by NK cells that are specialized in eliminating cells infected by viruses or undergoing cellular transformation. It has been reported that exercise leads to increased numbers of circulating NK cells, as well as to potentiated NK cell cytotoxic function, although the evidence is inconclusive. (C) In cases where transformed cells are able to avoid elimination, they are instead kept in equilibrium with surrounding immune cells. Over long periods of time and sustained immunologic pressure, a Darwinistic microselection process takes place in which tumor cells that acquire additional mutations become resistant to killing by immune cells, surviving and making the emerging tumor decreasingly immunogenic. Ultimately, the tumor is able to escape from immune control, the growth rate accelerates, and the cancer becomes clinically detectable. Although minimal evidence exists, exercise may positively influence innate and adaptive immune responses following immune escape and subsequent tumor growth. (D) The occurrence and strength of spontaneous tumor-specific immune responses varies significantly depending on the tumor type and the affected individual. In tumors that have evidence of a pre-existing adaptive immune response (high immunogenicity), the infiltrating tumor-specific T cells can be reactivated by the use of immune checkpoint inhibitors (anti-CTLA-4, anti-PD-1), thus triggering a direct antitumor effect. In tumors that have low immunogenicity, there is a lack of recognition of tumor antigens, which renders the tumor invisible to T-cell attack. In order to generate an adaptive immune response in such tumors, a de novo antitumor immune response must be initiated. Localized tumor irradiation has been shown to trigger immunogenic cell death of tumor cells, resulting in release of tumor antigens and concomitant danger-associated molecular patterns (DAMPs) that allow tumor-resident dendritic cells to become activated, engulf the exposed tumor antigens, and subsequently present the antigens to naïve T cells to trigger tumor-specific immune responses. Minimal evidence suggests that dendritic cell number may increase with exercise; currently, no evidence exists for the role of exercise in triggering immunogenic cell death or reactivation of the immune system. *CTLA-4*, Cytotoxic T-lymphocyte-associated antigen 4; *NK cell*, natural killer cell; *PD-1*, programmed death 1; *RT*, radiation therapy. (Reprinted with permission Koelwyn GJ, Wennerberg E, Demaria S, Jones LW. Exercise in regulation of inflammation-immune axis function in cancer initiation and progression. *Oncology (Williston Park)*. 2015;29(12):908–922.)

on normal immune system function. As new therapeutics emerge that use the immune system to help combat cancer, Onc R specialists will be called on to use evidence-based clinical reasoning, skills, and advanced knowledge to manage the changing rehabilitation needs of PLWBCs. Specialists are encouraged to review the literature often in order to stay contemporary. Opportunities may arise for specialists to participate in research and quality improvement initiatives to improve the trajectories for functional recovery for PLWBC across the continuum of care.

Critical Research Needs

- Risk stratification for adverse events during exercise or physical activity at different platelet, hemoglobin, and WBC counts
- Randomized controlled trails demonstrating the effectiveness of specific parameters of standardized pre- and post-BMT rehabilitation protocols
- Rehabilitation implications for cytokine release syndrome, neurotoxicity, and other adverse effects of novel immunotherapies and adoptive cell therapies
- Mechanisms of physical rehabilitation-facilitated repair of damaged body functions and structures related to acute and cGVHD
- Mechanisms of exercise immunology in cancer, and clarification of the risks versus protective effects of exercise while receiving different types of cancer treatment

Case Studies

Case Study #1—Outpatient

A 56-year-old female presents to outpatient therapy who has a history of acute myeloid leukemia and had an allogeneic stem cell transplant 4 months ago. She had complications post-transplant including neutropenic sepsis requiring a stay in the intensive care unit for 3 days due to shock and hypotension. The order from the physician is to evaluate and treat the "decreased ROM and balance." The patient had lab values drawn at a clinic visit 1 day ago, which read as follows:

Hemoglobin: 8.6 g/dL
Hematocrit: 32.1%
WBC Count: 1.1×10^9/L
Platelets: 148,000/microliter

The patient's chief complaint is a "tightness" in her upper extremities (right >left) limiting her from performing activities of daily living. The ROM in the right shoulder is limited and is noted below:

Shoulder Flexion: 100 degrees
Shoulder Abduction: 110 degrees
Shoulder Internal Rotation: 80 degrees
Shoulder External Rotation: 40 degrees

The patient removed her garments and a red, raised rash appears over both extremities in what appears to be a distal to proximal pattern. She also reported two falls in the past month due to "loss of balance." Muscle strength in lower extremities was within normal limits. There was diminished sensation in the bilateral feet from neuropathy due to chemotherapy conditioning treatment involving vincristine prior to transplant, of which the patient is taking gabapentin to assist with.

Guiding Questions:
1) Would you refer the patient to anyone?
   It is concerning that this person is possibly developing signs and symptoms of chronic skin GVHD. The Onc R clinician

should ask the person if they had any skin reactions similar to this during the initial post-transplant period in order to determine type and extent of GVHD. Then, a call to the referring physician is warranted as this person may need an adjustment in immunosuppressive medications or further testing.

2) What is your immediate treatment plan?
   The initial goal of treatment is to assist the person with performing their activities of daily living. As mentioned previously in the chapter, stretching and myofascial release can assist in preventing joint contracture that can occur with GVHD of the skin. In addition, gentle Grade I or II joint mobilizations can assist with mobility at the shoulder joint.

   Consider endurance and light resistance training for this type of patient. It is likely that this person is deconditioned from extensive treatment and hospitalization in addition to the long-term corticosteroid use post-transplant to prevent deconditioning. This weakness and limited endurance could be a contributing factor to the falls.

   Neuropathy is a common adverse effect from intensive treatment especially in this population. In addition, vincristine is well known for its neurotoxic adverse effects. It is important to educate the person with neuropathy regarding self-care. Daily skin assessment especially for the bottom of the feet and areas not easily visible can assist in catching infections early on.

   While focusing more on the falls, this person might need a rolling walker or any other type of durable medical equipment to assist with balance and mobility. A full balance and mobility assessment is warranted. Conducting balance measures, such as gait speed or the Berg Balance Scale can assist with insurance approval and justify need.

Case Study #2—Inpatient

A 54-year-old female currently enrolled in a clinical trial for new combination therapy (chemotherapy + hormone therapy) for metastatic breast cancer was admitted to the hospital yesterday directly from the outpatient infusion clinic with hypotension and tachycardia. Although she is neutropenic, she is currently afebrile and reports feeling a little better after receiving fluids and blood products. Her oncologist would like to prescribe filgrastim (Neupogen) to boost her neutrophil counts, but she is still awaiting insurance authorization to pay for this drug, which may take a few days. A consult is placed for physical therapy and occupational therapy to evaluate and treat for discharge planning, with possible discharge to home planned for tomorrow morning.

Pertinent lab values (CBC with differential drawn at 8:00 am):
Hemoglobin: 9.1 g/dL
Hematocrit: 28.3%
WBC Count: 2.4×10^9/L
Neutrophils (Absolute Neutrophil Count/ANC): 953/mL
Platelets: 118,000/mL

Upon entering the room and beginning the examination, the therapist noticed that the patient was increasingly lethargic as the session progresses, especially in upright positions. She was also having difficulty answering questions and following commands. Another set of vitals was promptly taken in standing to assess for orthostatic hypotension. The patient's blood pressure did drop, but not enough to classify as orthostasis. Her supine resting vitals and vitals in standing were as follows. The therapist decided to return the patient to supine and call in the nurse.

Vitals:

Supine (rest):	HR 110	BP 101/59	SpO$_2$ 96% on room air	RR 20
Standing (1 min):	HR 126	BP 89/51	SpO$_2$ 97% on room air	RR 24
Supine (2 min recovery):	HR 124	BP 90/56	SpO$_2$ 94% on room air	RR 25

Guiding Questions:

1) What is concerning about this patient's clinical presentation during the therapy session? How would you summarize key findings to the bedside nurse and/or the provider?

The patient is demonstrating multiple signs of possible SIRS or sepsis, including tachycardia, increased respiratory rate, low WBC count, hypotension, and altered mental status. It is not the Onc R therapist's role to diagnose the presence of SIRS/sepsis, but instead to notify the nurse and/or on-call provider of signs and symptoms that are concerning for impending sepsis. A useful tool to communicate these important findings promptly and appropriately to the rest of the team is the SBAR format, which stands for Situation, Background, Assessment, Recommendation.

2) The patient is known to be neutropenic. How is this important to the current clinical picture?

This clinical picture is concerning for possible neutropenic sepsis in the absence of a fever. When an individual is neutropenic, the magnitude of the neutrophil-mediated immune response to infection is muted and conditions of bacteremia and sepsis can progress very quickly to become life-threatening. The medical team should be notified immediately by the therapist, the nurse, or another care team member in order to (1) closely monitor the patient's status, (2) consider further infectious workup, and (3) make decisions regarding the possible need for care escalation.

3) During the therapy session, the patient required supervision for all bed mobility and transfers, but was unable to safely ambulate. She will have consistent supervision and assistance available from her husband at discharge. Is this patient ready for discharge to home? Why or why not?

The patient is not currently medically appropriate for discharge from the hospital. She will likely undergo further tests to determine the etiology of the change in her clinical presentation. The therapist is advised to objectively document the events of the session, including the patient's observed functional level during task performance. This data can be used to inform discharge planning for when the patient is more medically stable.

Review Questions

Reader can find the correct answers and rationale in the back of the book.

1. You are treating a person with a new diagnosis of leukemia in the intensive care unit. The person is being monitored for TLS. Which of these scenarios are indicative of the person having TLS?
   A. Inflammatory response of the skin 24 hours after treatment demonstrated by a raised and red symmetrical rash
   B. Elevated creatinine the day of treatment
   C. Hypocalcemia and hyperphosphatemia both occurring on the second day following treatment
   D. Nausea and vomiting prior to initiation of treatment leading to poor oral intake

2. Which cells of the immune system do hormone therapy for both androgen and breast cancers affect?
   A. T cells
   B. Cytokines and B cells
   C. Antibodies
   D. Dendritic cells

3. You are treating a person with a history of myelodysplastic syndrome (MDS) and an uncomplicated allogeneic stem cell transplant who was admitted to the hospital for fever, lymph node swelling, and recent sudden weight loss. A positron emission tomography (PET) scan was completed upon admission shows a new mass in the left groin not seen on previous scans. What most likely is the medical diagnosis for this person's admission?
   A. Progression of MDS
   B. TLS
   C. Septicemia infection
   D. PTLD

4. An autoimmune disorder, such as RA, can increase a person's risk of developing cancer due to what reason?

   A. Increased risk of infection due to high-dose steroids
   B. Chronic inflammation increases a person's lymphoproliferative malignancy risk
   C. Development of post-transplant lymphoproliferative disorder
   D. Innate immunity

5. Stevens-Johnson syndrome is what type of hypersensitivity reaction characterized by a long latency period?
   A. Type I
   B. Type II
   C. Type III
   D. Type IV

6. You are treating a person status post 9 days after allogeneic stem cell transplant complicated by mucositis and skin and liver graft-versus-host disease. Which of the following treatments is most appropriate for your rehabilitation treatment session?
   A. Light aerobic exercise with focus on sit to/from transfers in order to assist with proximal muscle strengthening
   B. Higher level balance exercises on foam with reaching activity to address neuropathy
   C. Stretching and gentle joint mobilizations (Grade I or II) of the proximal muscle joints
   D. Resistance training for shoulder girdle

7. Select the correct representation of the hematopoietic stem cell-derived cell lineage of the T lymphocyte:
   A. Hematopoietic stem cell – myeloid stem cell – CFU-GM – T lymphocyte
   B. Hematopoietic stem cell – myeloid stem cell – CFU-Baso – T lymphocyte
   C. Hematopoietic stem cell – common lymphoid progenitor – T lymphocyte
   D. Hematopoietic stem cell – common lymphoid progenitor – plasma cell – T lymphocyte

8. Which of the following cancer therapeutics is most likely to cause systemic immunosuppression?
   A. Intrathecal chemotherapy administered via lumbar puncture for CNS lymphoma
   B. Chemotherapy administered through a central line for hematologic malignancy
   C. Localized ionizing radiation therapy for solid malignancy
   D. Surgical tumor debulking for solid malignancy

9. Which if the following is NOT one of the clinical criteria for SIRS/sepsis, as measured by the SIRS criteria or the qSOFA score?
   A. Increased heart rate
   B. Altered mental status
   C. Abnormal WBC count
   D. Palpable lymph node

10. Choose the statement that best describes the relationship between the innate and adaptive immune systems.
    A. The adaptive immune system protects the host during the time between microbial exposure and individualized innate immune system responses to microbes.
    B. The innate immune system utilizes two principal arms to adapt and defend the body from infections and malignancy—T lymphocytes and B lymphocytes.
    C. The adaptive immune system serves critical functions of first line defense, regulation of inflammation, and activation and instruction of the innate immune system responses.
    D. The innate immune system serves critical functions of first line defense, regulation of inflammation, and activation and instruction of the adaptive immune system responses.

References

1. Travis J. On the origin of the immune system. *Science.* 2009;324(5927):580–582.
2. Medzhitov R, Janeway CA Jr. Innate immunity: the virtues of a nonclonal system of recognition. *Cell.* 1997;91(3):295–298.
3. Chaplin DD. Overview of the immune response. *J Allergy Clin Immunol.* 2010;125(2 suppl 2):S3–S23.
4. Medzhitov R, Janeway CA Jr. Innate immunity: the virtues of a nonclonal system of recognition. *Cell.* 1997;91(3):295–298.
5. Medzhitov R. Pattern recognition theory and the launch of modern innate immunity. *J Immunol.* 2013;191(9):4473–4474.
6. Iwasaki A, Medzhitov R. Control of adaptive immunity by the innate immune system. *Nat Immunol.* 2015;16(4):343–353.
7. Vijay K. Toll-like receptors in immunity and inflammatory diseases: past, present, and future. *Int Immunopharmacol.* 2018;59:391–412.
8. Iwasaki A, Medzhitov R. Regulation of adaptive immunity by the innate immune system. *Science.* 2010;327(5963):291–295.
9. Cooper MD, Miller JFAP. Discovery of 2 distinctive lineages of lymphocytes, T cells and B cells, as the basis of the adaptive immune system and immunologic function: 2019 Albert Lasker Basic Medical Research Award. *JAMA.* 2019;322(13):1247–1248.
10. Miller JF, Mitchell GF. The thymus and the precursors of antigen reactive cells. *Nature.* 1967;216:659–663.
11. Garcia K. Dual arms of adaptive immunity: division of labor and collaboration between B and T cells. *Cell.* 2019;179(1):3–7.
12. Ait-Oufella H, Sage AP, Mallat Z, Tedgui A. Adaptive (T and B cells) immunity and control by dendritic cells in atherosclerosis. *Circ Res.* 2014;114(10):1640–1660.
13. Sasson SC, Gordon CL, Christo SN, et al. Local heroes or villains: tissue-resident memory T cells in human health and disease. *Cell Mol Immunol.* 2020;17:113–122.
14. Zajac AJ, Harrington LE. Immune response to viruses: cell-mediated immunity. *Reference Module in Biomedical Sciences:* Elsevier; 2014. ISBN 9780128012383, https://doi.org/10.1016/B978-0-12-801238-3.02604-0. (https://www.sciencedirect.com/science/article/pii/B9780128012383026040).
15. Teijaro JR. Too much of a good thing: sustained type 1 interferon signaling limits humoral responses to secondary viral infection. *Eur J Immunol.* 2016;46(2):300–302.
16. Honke N, Shaabani N, Merches K, et al. Immunoactivation induced by chronic viral infection inhibits viral replication and drives immunosuppression through sustained IFN-I responses. *Eur J Immunol.* 2016;46(2):372–380.
17. Shishido SN, Varahan S, Yuan K, Li X, Fleming SD. Humoral innate immune response and disease. *Clin Immunol.* 2012;144(2):142–158.
18. Schreiber RD, Old LJ, Smyth MJ. Cancer immunoediting: integrating immunity's roles in cancer suppression and promotion. *Science.* 2011;331:1565–1570.
19. Johnstone C, Rich SE. Bleeding in cancer patients and its treatment: a review. *Ann Palliat Med.* 2018;7(2):265–273.
20. Wells PS, Anderson DR, Rodger M, et al. Evaluation of D-dimer in the diagnosis of suspected deep-vein thrombosis. *N Engl J Med.* 2003;349:1227–1235.
21. Hillegass E, Puthoff M, Frese EM, et al. Role of physical therapists in the management of individuals at risk for or diagnosed with venous thromboembolism: evidence-based clinical practice guideline. *Phys Ther.* 2016;96(2):143–166.
22. Franks AL, Slansky JE. Multiple associations between a broad spectrum of autoimmune diseases, chronic inflammatory diseases and cancer. *Anticancer Res.* 2012;32(4):1119–1136.
23. Justiz Vaillant AA, Vashisht R, Zito PM. Immediate hypersensitivity reactions. [Updated June 15, 2020]. In: *StatPearls [Internet]:* StatPearls Publishing; 2020. January. https://www.ncbi.nlm.nih.gov/books/NBK513315/.
24. Rixe N, Tavarez MM. Serum sickness. [Updated September 3, 2020]. *StatPearls [Internet]:* StatPearls Publishing; 2021. January. https://www.ncbi.nlm.nih.gov/books/NBK538312/.
25. Pichler WJ. Drug hypersensitivity: classification and clinical features. In: Post T, ed. *UpToDate:* UpToDate; 2018. www.uptodate.com. Accessed July 7, 2019.
26. Gupta A, Moore JA. Tumor lysis syndrome. *JAMA Oncol.* 2018;4(6):895.
27. Firwana BM, Hasan R, Hasan N, et al. Tumor lysis syndrome: a systematic review of case series and case reports. *Postgrad Med.* 2012;124(2):92–101.
28. Findakly D, Luther RD, Wang J. Tumor lysis syndrome in solid tumors: a comprehensive literature review, new insights, and novel strategies to improve outcomes. *Cureus.* 2020;12(5):e8355. doi:10.7759/cureus.8355.
29. Lopez-Olivo MA, Pratt G, Palla SL, Salahudeen A. Rasburicase in tumor lysis syndrome of the adult: a systematic review and meta-analysis. *Am J Kidney Dis.* 2013;62(3):481–492.
30. Singer M, Deutschman CS, Seymour CW, et al. The third international consensus definitions for sepsis and septic shock (Sepsis-3). *JAMA.* 2016;315(8):801–810.
31. Rhodes A, Evans LE, Alhazzani W, et al. Surviving sepsis campaign: international guidelines for management of sepsis and septic shock: 2016. *Intensive Care Med.* 2017;43:304–377.
32. Sepsis Alliance. What is sepsis? https://www.sepsis.org/sepsis-basics/what-is-sepsis/. Accessed March 1, 2021.
33. National Collaborating Centre for Cancer. *Neutropenic sepsis: prevention and management of neutropenic sepsis in cancer patients.*

National Institute for Health and Clinical Excellence (UK); 2012. Sep. (NICE Clinical Guidelines, No. 151.) 2, Diagnosis of neutropenic sepsis. https://www.ncbi.nlm.nih.gov/books/NBK373673/.

34. Hakim H, Flynn PM, Srivastava DK, et al. Risk prediction in pediatric cancer patients with fever and neutropenia. *Pediatr Infect Dis J*. 2010;29(1):53–59.

35. Reilly JP, Anderson BJ, Hudock KM, et al. Neutropenic sepsis is associated with distinct clinical and biological characteristics: a cohort study of severe sepsis. *Crit Care*. 2016;20(1):222.

36. Stephens RS. Neutropenic fever in the intensive care unit. *Oncologic Critical Care*. 2019:1297–1311.

37. Singavi AK, Harrington AM, Fenske TS. Post-transplant lymphoproliferative disorders. *Cancer Treat Res*. 2015;165:305–327.

38. Al-Mansour Z, Nelson BP, Evens AM. Post-transplant lymphoproliferative disease (PTLD): risk factors, diagnosis, and current treatment strategies. *Curr Hematol Malig Rep*. 2013;8(3):173–183.

39. Negrin RS, Brennan DC. Epidemiology, clinical manifestations, and diagnosis of post-transplant lymphoproliferative disorders. In: Post T, ed. *UpToDate*: UpToDate; 2018. www.uptodate.com. Accessed July 7, 2020.

40. Held T, Klemmer D, Lässig M. Survival of the simplest in microbial evolution. *Nat Commun*. 2019;10:2472. https://doi.org/10.1038/s41467-019-10413-8.

41. Curnow J, Pasalic L, Favaloro EJ. Why do patients bleed? *Surg J (N Y)*. 2016;2(1):e29–e43.

42. Al-Attar N, Johnston S, Jamous N, et al. Impact of bleeding complications on length of stay and critical care utilization in cardiac surgery patients in England. *J Cardiothorac Surg*. 2019;14(1):64. doi:10.1186/s13019-019-0881-3.

43. Carvalho HA, Villar RC. Radiotherapy and immune response: the systemic effects of a local treatment. *Clinics (Sao Paulo)*. 2018;73(suppl 1):e557s. doi:10.6061/clinics/2018/e557s.

44. Walle T, Martinez Monge R, Cerwenka A, Ajona D, Melero I, Lecanda F. Radiation effects on antitumor immune responses: current perspectives and challenges. *Ther Adv Med Oncol*. 2018;10:1758834017742575. doi:10.1177/1758834017742575.

45. Nobler MP. The abscopal effect in malignant lymphoma and its relationship to lymphocyte circulation. *Radiology*. 1969;93(2):410–412.

46. Galluzzi L, Buqué A, Kepp O, Zitvogel L, Kroemer G. Immunological effects of conventional chemotherapy and targeted anticancer agents. *Cancer Cell*. 2015;28(6):690–714.

47. Azzariti A, Iacobazzi RM, Di Fonte R, et al. Plasma-activated medium triggers cell death and the presentation of immune activating danger signals in melanoma and pancreatic cancer cells. *Sci Rep*. 2019;9(1):4099.

48. Ariza-Heredia EJ, Chemaly RF. Update on infection control practices in cancer hospitals. *CA Cancer J Clin*. 2018;68(5):340–355.

49. Ben-Batalla I, Vargas-Delgado ME, Amsberg GV, Janning M, Loges S. Influence of androgens on immunity to self and foreign: effects on immunity and cancer. *Front Immunol*. 2020;11:1184. doi:10.3389/fimmu.2020.01184.

50. Silvestri I, Cattarino S, Giantulli S, Nazzari C, Collalti G, Sciarra A. A perspective of immunotherapy for prostate cancer. *Cancers*. 2016;8(7):64.

51. Pu Y, Xu M, Liang Y, et al. Androgen receptor antagonists compromise T cell response against prostate cancer leading to early tumor relapse. *Sci Transl Med*. 2016;8(333):333ra47. doi:10.1126/scitranslmed.aad5659.

52. Nikiforow S, Spitzer TR. Overview of clinical bone marrow transplantation. In: Chabner BA, Longo DL, eds. *Harrison's Manual of Oncology, 2e*: McGraw-Hill. https://hemonc.mhmedical.com/content.aspx?bookid=1799&sectionid=124753048. Accessed August 19, 2020.

53. Hutt D. Engraftment, graft failure, and rejection. In: Babic A, Kenyon M, eds. *The European Blood and Marrow Transplantation Textbook for Nurses*: Springer; 2017:259–270.

54. Jo KS, Kim NC. Incidence and factors influencing oral mucositis in patients with hematopoietic stem cell transplantation. *J Korean Acad Nurs*. 2014;44(5):542.

55. Mohammed J, Savani BN, El-Jawahri A, Vanderklish J, Cheville AL, Hashmi SK. Is there any role for physical therapy in chronic GvHD? *Bone Marrow Transplant*. 2017;53(1):22–28.

56. Smith S, Haig A, Couriel D. Musculoskeletal, neurologic, and cardiopulmonary aspects of physical rehabilitation in patients with chronic graft-versus-host disease. *Biol Blood Marrow Transplant*. 2015;21(5):799–808.

57. Chao NJ. Clinical manifestations, diagnosis, and grading of chronic graft-versus-host disease. In: Post T, ed. *UpToDate*: UpToDate; 2019. www.uptodate.com. Accessed October 20, 2020.

58. Chao NJ. Treatment of acute graft versus host disease. In: Post T, ed. *UpToDate*: UpToDate; 2020. www.uptodate.com. Accessed August 7, 2020.

59. Shoushtari AN, Hellman M. Principles of cancer immunotherapy. In: Post T, ed. *UptoDate*: UptoDate; 2020. www.uptodate.com. Accessed September 16, 2020.

60. Richards JO, Albers AJ, Smith TS, Tjoe JA. NK cell-mediated antibody-dependent cellular cytotoxicity is enhanced by tamoxifen in HER2/neu non-amplified, but not HER2/neu-amplified, breast cancer cells. *Cancer Immunol Immunother*. 2016;65(11):1325–1335.

61. Lu RM, Hwang YC, Liu IJ, et al. Development of therapeutic antibodies for the treatment of diseases. *J Biomed Sci*. 2020;27(1). https://doi.org/10.1186/s12929-019-0592-z.

62. Manis JP. Overview of therapeutic monoclonal antibodies. In: Post T, ed. *UpToDate*: UpToDate; 2020. www.uptodate.com. Accessed September 16, 2020.

63. Rohaan MW, Wilgenhof S, Haanen JBAG. Adoptive cellular therapies: the current landscape. *Virchows Arch*. 2019;474:449–461.

64. Magalhaes I, Carvalho-Queiroz C, Hartana CA, et al. Facing the future: challenges and opportunities in adoptive T cell therapy in cancer. *Expert Opin Biol Ther*. 2019;19(8):811–827. doi:10.1080/14712598.2019.1608179.

65. Lee DW, Santomasso BD, Locke FL, et al. ASTCT consensus grading for cytokine release syndrome and neurologic toxicity associated with immune effector cells. *Biol Blood Marrow Transplant*. 2019;25(4):625–638.

66. Lee DW, Santomasso BD, Locke FL, et al. ASTCT Consensus grading for cytokine release syndrome and neurologic toxicity associated with immune effector cells. *Biol Blood Marrow Transplant*. 2019;25(4):625–638.

67. Chabner BA, Longo DL. *Harrisons Manual of Oncology*. 2nd ed. McGraw-Hill Professional; 2014.

68. Koelwyn GJ, Wennerberg E, Demaria S, Jones LW. Exercise in regulation of inflammation-immune axis function in cancer initiation and progression. *Oncology (Williston Park)*. 2015;29(12):908–922.

69. Carbone DP, Gandara DR, Antonia SJ, Zielinski C, Paz-Ares L. Non-small-cell lung cancer: role of the immune system and potential for immunotherapy. *J Thorac Oncol*. 2015;10(7):974–984.

70. American Cancer Society. Lung cancer immunotherapy: immune checkpoint inhibitors. https://www.cancer.org/cancer/lung-cancer/treating-non-small-cell/immunotherapy.html. Accessed July 17, 2020.

14

Psychosocial Considerations

LAURA MUNGER, LMSW, DEBORAH J. DOHERTY, PT, PhD

CHAPTER OUTLINE

Introduction

As an oncology rehabilitation (Onc R) clinician considers the adverse effects of cancer and its treatments, it is critical to have a deep understanding of the psychosocial issues that can arise throughout the cancer care voyage. The National Cancer Institute (NCI) defines psychosocial as "In medicine, having to do with the mental, emotional, social, and spiritual effects of a disease, such as cancer. Some of the psychosocial effects of cancer are changes in how a patient thinks, their feelings, moods, beliefs, ways of coping, and relationships with family, friends, and co-workers."[1] The American Cancer Society concurs that cancer impacts the person diagnosed with cancer (PDWC) and their loved ones, affecting the physical, social, emotional, and spiritual parts of life. Examples include trouble coping with being diagnosed and treated for cancer, feeling apart from family and friends, changes in how a family gets along and works together, problems with making a decision, concern about not being able to do enjoyable activities, problems working or going back to work, worries about money, stress from making choices about care, problems talking about one's feelings, changes in body image and sexual self, fear of cancer recurrence, and fear of death and dying.[2]

As an Onc R clinician, it is important to be very cognizant of when, where, and how these issues manifest themselves during different phases of the cancer treatment trajectory. It is also crucial to understand that every person living with and beyond cancer (PLWBC) will experience psychosocial issues differently. It is therefore the responsibility of each Onc R clinician to be very alert, observant, and attentive to the ways in which psychosocial issues present and be prepared to intervene through screening, culturally appropriate intervention, and referral to other healthcare professionals of the cancer care team as needed.

When evaluating the psychosocial impact on a PLWBC, it is important to assess the following three domains: *emotional, social, and financial Cognitive considerations will also be discussed later in the chapter.* The authors believe that categorizing the psychosocial issues into these three domains will help Onc R clinicians more accurately identify the main source of psychosocial stress. This, in turn, will guide the Onc R clinician in determining the most appropriate treatment and/or referral. Table 14.1 provides a list of common psychosocial issues and how they present. This is not an exhaustive list but a helpful tool to recognize issues that are witnessed or that a person talks about that could be a red flag identifying a need for some psychosocial intervention.

TABLE 14.1 Common Cancer-Related Psychosocial Issues

- Anxiety
- Anger
- Body image issues
- Crying spells
- Confusion
- Decline in physical or emotional intimacy
- Diminished self-esteem
- Fear/worry
- Fear of recurrence
- Guilt over change in role/abilities
- Guilt of comparison (others have it worse)
- Problems with primary relationships
- Heightened vulnerability
- Isolation
- Loss of control
- Loss of sexual and/or reproductive capacity
- Loss of interest and/or motivation
- Mood swings
- Sadness
- Somatic complaints (stomach, headache, muscle tension, loss of appetite, heart rate)

Created by Laura Munger. Printed with permission.

Psychosocial adverse effects from cancer and its treatments present in various ways throughout the changing phases of cancer care and present differently for each individual. Psychosocial concerns such as fear and loss of control begin soon after diagnosis. Onc R clinicians need to advocate for psychosocial assessment and referrals upon diagnosis and at various points throughout the cancer journey. It is important for a PDWC to learn effective coping strategies very early on in the cancer trajectory to facilitate the treatment and healing process. Common psychosocial considerations for Onc R clinicians will be reviewed during the different phases of care including when newly diagnosed as well as during and after surgery, chemotherapy, and radiation. The concerns of most PLWBCs can be categorized into three major categories: emotional, social and financial. Cognitive considerations are also important and will addressed later in the chapter. Preliminary and common concerns will be summarized followed by more in-depth discussions of each category. This chapter will bring awareness to the Onc R clinician about the importance of providing the PDWCs and the PLWBCs with the opportunity and a safe space in which to share psychosocial concerns. Onc R clinicians need to ask the pertinent questions, provide valid measurement tools, and learn how to respond to psychosocial issues that could impact an individual's success in rehabilitation and their quality of life (QOL). The clinician also needs to know when and where to refer a person that has psychosocial needs beyond the scope of practice of the Onc R clinician. Mitigating and managing psychosocial issues will create the opportunity for the individual to be successful in the recovery from cancer.

Newly Diagnosed With Cancer

Emotional

When a person is diagnosed with cancer, the psychosocial whirlwind begins. The severity of the cancer can matter tremendously but does not necessarily coincide with severity of the individual's reaction. Once the word "cancer" is spoken, many people associate this diagnosis with dying and the fear can be very real. Many questions begin to swirl in one's mind related to how they will manage work, children, parents, partner, and so much more. Examples of questions that a newly diagnosed patient may be contemplating include: What type of treatment will I receive? Will I lose my hair? Am I going to have surgery or chemo or radiation? How much pain will I be in? How long am I going to live? Can I still work? How am I going to tell my husband, children, family? The list of potential questions can be extensive.

Social

There are two major areas to consider here—issues about how a person identifies within their social setting as well as what type of social support system they have. Issues related to race, ethnicity, religion, and sexual orientation are all critical components to be considered when delivering medical information of this magnitude. Culturally appropriate explanations, education, and communication are essential when delivering information as well as working through the diagnosis and its implications. The person's support system is also a large component of a person's coping abilities. Family, friends, neighbors, loved ones, work, and religious families can help or hinder a person's successful navigation of the cancer journey. Questions to consider include: Do they have transportation to and from treatments? Will someone to be able to attend their appointments with them to serve as another set of eyes and ears? Do they have help for household chores, grocery shopping, meal preparation, childcare or elder care (if needed)? Are there any cultural or religious considerations that need to be understood or learned before beginning treatment? For example, Orthodox Jewish men are generally not comfortable or allowed to be touched by a female clinician. Some Muslim women are not allowed to be treated by a male clinician nor take their head covering off unless in a private room with a female clinician. Families from some cultures do not want the patient to know they have been diagnosed with cancer. Every Onc R clinician should ask what cultural, religious, race, and pronoun considerations are important to the PLWBC to provide for a more culturally appropriate, respectful and affirming treatment.

Financial

Financial toxicity encompasses the adverse effects of excess financial strain. The first concern is whether treatment for cancer will impact the PDWC's ability to work. If so, are they the only source of income to the household? Does the person have reliable transportation? Is gas money going to be a problem? Do they have insurance? If so, what are the deductibles, copayments, coinsurance, and out-of-pocket costs? Individuals may be concerned about continuing sports and music lessons for their children, special food, or interventions for a child or parent with special needs. What about a breakdown in a major appliance, like a refrigerator, washing machine, microwave, or furnace? How will it be replaced? Financial toxicity may also be referred to as financial stress, hardship or burden, or economic burden. The cancer diagnosis can also greatly impact these questions. Is the cancer easily treated, curable or is it at an advanced stage? Is this a recurrence of cancer? Is there more than one diagnosis of cancer? Does the PDWC also have another chronic disease like diabetes, heart disease or an autoimmune disease along with the cancer? See Chapter 33 for more information on financial toxicity.

Surgery

Emotional

There is a wide variety of potential challenges to be considered when evaluating the emotional impact of surgery. There is always anxiety around most types of surgery, and this is certainly the case in oncologic surgery. For some, there are fears of what will be found once a surgeon performs surgery and because some will lose a body part, organ, or be disfigured as a result of the surgery. The fear around not knowing what things will be like when they wake up is terrifying. However, when there is a loss of a sexual organ (breast, penis, scrotum, uterus, ovary, etc.) the emotional impact can be even more significant as our sexual beings are a part of our identity. Furthermore, if someone already struggles with body image issues or is having problems in their sexual relationship with a partner, losing a body part may magnify the stress. The same is true of many head and neck surgeries causing facial disfigurement which can further complicate emotions. In some cases, a person may choose not to have a surgery due to the potential adverse effects, such as erectile dysfunction from prostate removal. Losing sexual ability can potentially be too devastating to justify the treatment.

Another consideration is whether or not this is the person's first surgery along the course of their cancer journey. If they have had other surgeries for their cancer, the emotional toll can also be magnified. Although surgery is most often the first step in treatment for cancer, it can also occur after chemotherapy. If chemotherapy has been utilized to shrink a tumor prior to surgery, by the time the person's surgery is scheduled, emotional reactions may have already formed. Treatment weariness is a factor for the Onc R clinician to have heightened awareness of, and be prepared to manage.

Surgery can also cause incontinence issues. This is one of the most emotionally debilitating issues that a PLWBC can experience. If the person was continent before the cancer diagnosis and treatment, this change can cause tremendous stress, body image issues, and a loss of dignity. This has the potential to cause problems with sexuality and sexual relationships especially if a person's caregiver is also their sexual partner and helps with physically caring for the person. A loss of feeling attractive is common. Isolation, embarrassment, lack of confidence, fear of bladder, and anal leakage are all potential problems. Incontinence may cause a person to stay home due to fear of not finding a bathroom when needed or lack of financial stability preventing the purchase of proper supplies needed. There are some people who will refuse treatment if there is a chance of incontinence. It is important as an Onc R clinician to not only be sensitive to potential emotional challenges but also to provide a safe space for a person to share their concerns so help can be provided through appropriate referral.

Social

A support system is very important for any PLWBC. Who brings the PLWC to surgery? Who will help after surgery? Who will manage needs at work and at home? Those with young children will have a lot of anxiety around who is taking care of their children. Their children's anxiety may also focus on who is taking care of them. Teenagers frequently struggle with talking about their parent's cancer diagnosis with anyone. Teenagers may begin acting out or not studying due to the fear of not knowing what is happening with their parent and whether they may die. Peer support is crucial. Sometimes children will have behavioral, somatic, or academic symptoms that need to be looked out for. Interfacing with the school to develop a plan for if/when this occurs is very important.

Older adults may be alone or may not be physically or mentally able to take care of themselves when returning home from the hospital. They could also be a caregiver for their spouse. It is important to explore if they have support at home and if their support at home is adequate. It may be necessary to formally obtain permission to talk to a friend or family member about the person or make referrals for supportive service if their support is limited.

It is also critical to consider the social needs of patients in terms of cultural norms, family, and religious or spirituality beliefs, as well as those persons in the LGBTQIA+ community. It is important for the Onc R clinician to not make assumptions about the social needs of their patients. Not all people are traumatized with the loss of a sexual organ that they do not identify with. Others may have cultural rituals that are essential to deal with such severe changes in their body. As a clinician, the social, cultural, and spiritual needs of each PDWC is essential for patient-centered and whole person care. It is important to show respect to each PDWC by taking the time at the first visit to ask questions about their cultural, social, and spiritual needs and concerns. The Onc R clinician should strive to show true interest and convey the desire for Onc R to be a very valuable experience physically, psychosocially and psychoemotionally.

Financial

The financial stress of surgery will depend mostly on insurance and employment. Surgery is very expensive. If someone is uninsured or underinsured that is an obvious challenge. However, with current high deductibles and out of pocket maximums, a costly surgery could mean a significant financial burden even for someone who is well insured. If the person is employed with no paid time off, they will likely require unpaid time or reduced pay, if they have short-term disability insurance through their employer. Even if they have paid time off, the length of recovery time could exhaust their paid time off. If a person has financial stress due to surgery, or any other aspect of treatment, they will often feel a sense of anxiety and/or depression over the feelings of putting themselves and possibly their family in financial distress. They will often have substantial concerns about the security of their job and may experience guilt for putting managers and co-workers in a compromised position. They may also request fewer Onc R visits and ask to be taught what things they can do on their own. With the significant increase in telerehabilitation services, this provides the Onc R clinician with another option for providing logistical ease in continuing Onc R if time off work cannot be obtained.

For those already retired and on a fixed income, financial concerns are even greater. Inability to manage the cost of the surgery can cause tremendous amounts of stress. Onc R clinicians should ask every PLWBC if they would like to be referred to a financial counselor or automatically provide a list of resources for them to consider.

Chemotherapy and Immunotherapy

Emotional

The emotional stress of chemotherapy/immunotherapy is focused on the adverse effects caused from these treatments. A primary concern is the emotional impact of needing the treatment of chemotherapy/immunotherapy to stay alive; a secondary concern is the potential depression and anxiety that often occurs when people experience the adverse effects of treatment. Examples of adverse effects include cancer-related cognitive impairment, polyneuropathy, nausea, cancer-related fatigue, cardiotoxicity, muscle loss and weakness, loss of hearing, difficulty with balance, hair loss, fingernails and toenails become thin and peel, loss of function in taste buds, and decreased work efficiency, just to name a few.

Loss of hair, when applicable, is one of the most traumatic adverse effects. Many people feel ashamed of the fact that this is so devastating to them. They feel embarrassed that they are upset about losing their hair. As clinicians, it is important to make an effort to normalize the fact that it is valid for the experience of losing one's hair to be a traumatic event. A useful phrase is "most patients that have walked in your shoes feel exactly the same way you do."

The physical symptoms of nausea, vomiting, and extreme fatigue are also very difficult to deal with because of the profound impact these symptoms have on a person's ability to engage in their normal activities and maintain their QOL. If a person is suffering from these adverse effects, their anxiety goes up prior to their next infusion once they have knowledge of what the week ahead will look like. For most, infusion can mean the loss of 3 days to a week of feeling good which is not to be minimized. They learn to have to schedule their lives based on when their next infusion is. This keeps them constantly connected to the painful reminder that they have cancer which has a major impact on their emotional health. Even in the event of oral chemotherapy, taking that pill every day is still that painful reminder. This is not the case with all PLWCs, however, as many are relieved that they do not have to go to the hospital or clinic to get an infusion; the adverse effects can still limit their lifestyle.

Another issue to consider is that for many people, living a clean lifestyle void of chemicals and impurities is critical to their life philosophy. Chemotherapy goes against everything they believe in yet not having chemotherapy is terrifying to them. This inner conflict is important to be aware of. Naturopaths and integrative medicine practitioners can be a critical member of the existing oncology team and work in conjunction with and as partners with the oncology team to assist people in the healing process. Remember that one of the most critical adverse effects on mental health for PDWCs and PLWBCs is loss of control. Consider stating to a PLWBC: "We are in the business of creating healthy cells so everything you can do to contribute to creating healthy cells will help you feel in control. Every healthy cell that you create in your body matters, every healthy muscle cell matters, every flexible muscle matters, every healthy bite of food, drink of water, and good night's sleep matters."

Dignity issues discussed earlier apply here as well due to the potential incontinence that can also be caused by chemotherapy. Onc R clinicians need to be comfortable with asking the right questions to know when referral is appropriate. There are many QOL survey tools that can and should be used on a regular basis (please refer to Chapter 16).

Social

A person's support system is vital. For those getting infusions (vs. oral chemotherapy), infusion day can often be a very long day. Having a support person with them while they are being infused can be as important as having support people that are able to take care of the unexpected at home. However, other persons may want to complete their infusions without a support person due to the need for solitude, prayer, or wanting to participate in activities to take their mind off the chemotherapy like reading, working or other sedentary hobbies. Even for those using oral chemotherapy medication at home, there is a ritual that must be developed to make sure the medication is taken on the schedule prescribed. This has its own set of stressors due to the concerns of scheduling work, other obligations, and activities around the schedule.

Chemotherapy involves blood work that can sometimes lead to a cancellation of treatment, blood transfusions, or even hospitalizations. This change in treatment may cause an increase in stress and a feeling of losing control. It is important to have dependable family and friends to assist with these schedule changes. It is also important to recognize that not all persons with cancer (PWC) have a support system they can rely on so involving a navigator or case manager, if available, will be helpful to with these challenges.

Alcohol and drug use or abuse is an important factor due to its contraindication for chemotherapy. Even those who are in recovery may relapse due to the stress and inability to cope with the adverse effects. If an Onc R clinician has any concerns about a person's potential substance use disorder, due to their behavior or what they may have shared during a treatment, should contact the primary care physician or oncologist.

A public health crisis, such as the COVID-19 pandemic, can also be devastating to the person receiving the infusion as they are worried about their support person who wants to be with them but has to wait outside of the infusion clinic or possibly the hospital. This adds another level of stress to both the patient and their caregiver. Clinicians need to be aware of social concerns, provide verbal support, and refer to a mental health practitioner for assistance as needed.

Financial

The cost of chemotherapy/immunotherapy is compounded by the cost of medications to prevent nausea, treat the pain and dysfunction of polyneuropathy, cancer-related fatigue, cardiotoxicity, and more. There are many financial assistance programs and strategies to help with the expenses. If the expenses of the treatment are too high, a person may choose to omit rehabilitation due to the cost. It is important to inquire about financial stress and refer to social workers or financial counselors in the organization or the local community to assist with this process.

Radiation

Emotional

It is imperative that PDWCs are educated on what the radiation treatments will encompass in terms of logistics as well as the potential for adverse effects. Treatment appointments are commonly scheduled 5 days/week for several weeks but each session only lasts a short duration of time. This can allow some people to still work and receive treatments before or after work as well as on their lunch break. Because these appointments tend to be quicker, the stressors are different. For some, the stress of scheduling daily transportation can be difficult and as a result treatment can be missed, affecting the overall efficacy of the radiation therapy.

Claustrophobia can also cause increased stress. Some are affected by the machine itself while others struggle if they have to wear a mesh mask holding the head and neck in place to avoid movement during radiation. Physical adverse effects such as skin changes including discoloration, burning, and scarring may cause additional stress. The changes in the skin can be physically painful but the disfiguration that may also appear may affect body self-image. Cancer-related fatigue is the most commonly reported adverse effect during and after radiation that can change a person's lifestyle. These stressors, like all the other parts of treatment, can add to one's anxiety and depression.

Social

One of the most critical aspects of this portion of the person's journey is the frequency of treatments and not missing appointments to assure the efficacy of the treatment. For a person scheduled for radiation treatments 5 times per week for 6 to 12 weeks, this is a substantial commitment; it will be important to have a conversation about reliable transportation as well as the importance of attending all appointments. Some people will travel long distances for treatment, therefore lodging during the course of this treatment may also be needed. Some may not have reliable transportation and may need assistance with getting to their appointments.

Financial

In addition to previously mentioned financial stressors, if lodging is necessary, that is another expense unless the cancer center where they are being treated has resources to provide this amenity.

Hormonal Therapies

Emotional

Some hormonal therapies cause women to experience temporary or permanent menopause. This drastic change causes new symptoms and adverse effects that can have a profound effect on emotions. The hormones themselves can exacerbate emotions. Some women will struggle with the concept of experiencing menopause younger than anticipated. Often women will experience weight gain and in the context of already losing a body part (e.g., their breast), body image dilemmas can be exacerbated. Some women choose to "put their ovaries to sleep" or have their ovaries removed prophylactically to prevent cancer. Either way, it changes their hormonal status and makes it challenging to manage emotional symptoms. It is difficult to determine where the hormonal impact ends and mental health impact begins.

Men receiving hormonal therapies, for example androgen deprivation therapy, can experience erectile dysfunction, obesity, anemia, loss of bone mineral density, muscle atrophy, gynecomastia, fatigue, decreased sexual desire as well as mood changes such as irritability, depression, and cognitive changes. Onc R clinicians need to be prepared to inquire about these issues as some PWCs do not think it is important in a rehabilitation setting, while others will not want to discuss these issues. Onc R clinicians need to assure every PWC that their whole person is important in this recovery, not just one body part and even though each clinician works within their scope of practice, they can easily refer to other professionals that can provide support and help as needed.

Hormonal therapies for males and females are often prescribed to be taken daily for 5 to 10 years. This can become tiresome for some, while others may forget to take their medications, which can affect the efficacy of the treatment. There is an emotional exhaustion associated with the thought of treating the cancer for many years and in some cases an individual will simply refuse to continue. Furthermore, the adverse effects from the medications can also be so overwhelming that a person decides not to continue taking the medication. They can struggle with the guilt of not taking the medications but are also overwhelmed with the physical and emotional toll on their body. If a person shares these concerns with the Onc R clinician, it is important to refer the person to the oncologist and a mental health practitioner to discuss the options and make an informed decision.

Social

An emotional roller coaster can easily occur with hormonal therapy treatment. As a result, some PWCs will have difficulty maintaining a social circle. Friends may not know what to say or how to deal with the emotional ups and downs, thereby reducing time spent with the person going through the treatments. For the PWC receiving the treatments, the emotional insecurity prevents them from wanting to spend time with friends. If a woman still wanted to have children but chemical perimenopause or menopause was induced, she may find it too stressful to spend time with friends who are having children. Relationships can be strained. Some adverse effects may significantly affect sexual intimacy causing strain on marital or partner relationships. Spousal/partner support is greatly needed if available. In that case, it is important to refer the person to a social worker to help work through the emotional stressors.

Financial

Financial toxicity can be an issue if insurance does not pay for the hormonal treatment. There is greater risk of noncompliance if finances to afford the treatment are not available. This can affect the efficacy of the treatment.

Long Treatment Course

Emotional

Treatment weariness is a critical consideration. A long treatment course takes a major toll on one's emotions and QOL. Those with chronic, incurable cancers have a long journey of fighting for time and some QOL. There can be restlessness, mood swings, and being emotionally unsettled. Patients have voiced sentiments that some days "it is all worth fighting for" and other days there is a feeling of giving up due to the fatigue of the fight. It is important to continue to provide that safe space to let the PWC share these emotions and then refer as needed.

Social

Support systems are often strained over time. Caregivers (often termed carers) may have needed to take time off from work, juggle their schedules, and cancel attendance at usual church functions or other pleasurable scheduled outings. They often bear the strain of being a confidant and cheerleader, all the while worrying silently while attempting to be strong for their loved one. Most PLWBCs are keenly aware of this and feel tremendous guilt. Sometimes PWCs stop asking for help and will often verbalize sentiments that reflect that they are more worried for their support people than they are for themselves. Considering the aforementioned, it is not unusual to see a PLWBC's support people withdraw after a period of time, leaving the PLWBC feeling alone and isolated.

Financial

The longer the course of cancer treatment, the more likely that out-of-pocket expenses will build up. In some cases, the financial strain will be so great that some people will decide to stop treatment. Although often perceived as an inspirational act of kindness, fund raisers or Go Fund Me webpages are likely a temporary solution and PWCs often find that the money runs out, but the financial burden has not and treatment is still continuing. People can feel shame and embarrassment and very humbled when money is received that was gathered for them. An additional stressor may include the occasional donor who starts to question how the PWC used the money. Although fundraisers seem ubiquitous, it is important to note that many PWCs do not have support systems that can assist with fundraisers or gathering of funds so they are left to deal with this burden alone.

Post-Treatment Survivorship

Emotional

When treatment concludes, a person is given the "cancer free" trophy and routine follow-up appointments are scheduled every 4, 6, or 12 months. Shouldn't this be a time to celebrate? This is not always the situation. Often, this is the time when the support system cheers and goes back to their "normal" lives. This is frequently one of the more anxiety producing times in a PLWBC's journey when the support system withdraws and the highly qualified team of caregivers are no longer encountered on a daily basis. Weekly or monthly blood draws and imaging studies for status updates can also lead to scan anxiety. "Scanxiety," as it is often referred to, is when someone goes in for post-treatment follow up scans for routine monitoring yet they have anxiety around whether or not they will get a clear scan. Scanxiety may also occur in persons in active cancer treatment to determine if a current regimen is effective.

In addition to the rallying support of their social network, a PLWBC also grows to feel secure and supported by their clinical team. When this highly structured series of appointments and visits is taken away, it can leave the person feeling very fearful and very alone in that fear. An Onc R clinician interfacing with a person during this phase of their cancer experience can play an important role in providing them with support and working with them to improve their functioning, self-confidence, and QOL. Regaining these things can play an integral part in helping them begin to assemble a level of normalcy—even a new normal—and help them to reduce fear as they begin to take control of their wellness again.

Social

Relationships can be strained if those in one's support system are ready to move on and do not understand the lingering or new treatment adverse effects and/or the fear of recurrence that often exists in the background of a person's mind after completing cancer treatment. The PLWBC is often still feeling fatigued and anything but normal; they may feel that they are unable to talk to their support system anymore either because they do not understand or because they feel that they have exhausted them and feel guilty to still be "burdening" them.

Financial

If someone is feeling the effects of the financial strains of cancer treatment, they may return to work too soon, return to full-time when part-time may be more appropriate, or feel pressured to get a job if they were not previously employed. They may also be feeling guilty for any additional pressure put on a partner or parent due to this treatment course or feel guilty about inconveniencing their coworkers who may have taken over some of their responsibilities during their absence and therefore feel reluctant to put any more burdens on their work colleagues.

Cognition

Cognitive status cuts across all phases and stages of the cancer journey. It is very important to understand a person's premorbid status, if possible, either from the PWC themselves or their caregiver. Premorbid cognitive function can have a major effect on self-esteem issues when cognition is challenged secondary to the cancer or its treatments. Did the PWC have a learning disability or were they diagnosed with a traumatic brain injury (TBI) prior to their cancer diagnosis? If there was baseline cognitive impairment, this will affect how the PWC presents information, it may change the way they interpret what they hear, and it may impact their emotional capacity to respond. Sometimes a TBI can cause a person to over-emote or conversely under-emote as a result of this underlying pathology. Although a prior cognitive impairment may affect the PWC's motivation to participate in Onc R, motivation can also be affected in a person without a diagnosed pathology. As a result, the person with a flat affect may not be able to explain what is really wrong with them in terms of their rehabilitation or psychosocial needs; this may impact the Onc R clinician's ability to provide the most optimal goals or treatment intervention. If a person over-emotes either due to cognitive challenges or cultural norms, the Onc R treatment may be reduced in intensity and thus becomes less effective. The premorbid personality is also important to determine. For example, if a PWC cries easily and always has, and the Onc R clinician is someone who does not cry easily, the clinician may overreact to the tears instead of helping the person continue to participate in Onc R.

Persons who over-emote in terms of increased episodes of crying or emotion can also be a sign of deeply embedded emotions from past traumas brought to light or revisited due to the cancer journey. For example, if a patient was assaulted as a child and now is facing a pelvic or abdominal cancer, additional challenges can be experienced as this new bodily invasion can bring buried emotions to the surface. Situations such as these require professional clinicians who are trained to work through these issues and referrals should be made immediately. Clinicians may note a withdrawn, flat affect which may be indicative of an undiagnosed depressive episode, especially if this new affect is different from that of their "normal" or baseline status. If a person commonly exhibited negative behaviors or outlook prior their cancer, these defeatist remarks may be more pronounced; however, if this is new, it could be a sign of hopelessness and a referral would be warranted.

Another challenging cognitive issue for Onc R clinicians include those who exhibit catastrophic thought processes, in which the person thinks the worst in every situation. This is also referred to as cognitive distortion. This is important to understand as well while working through the rehabilitation process. As a result of all these considerations, it is important to understand that one's personality, cognitive challenges, or cultural norms can cause over- or under-emoting, can cause a person to have flat affect or be guarded and thus have a difficult time expressing himself or herself. In addition, some individuals process new information at different rates which requires the Onc R clinician to adapt their communication style to the needs of the person. The Onc R clinician should take into consideration these precancer baselines in order to help assess if someone is in distress, if this is a reaction to the cancer disease process or is there another underlying factor which warrants referral.

The Onc R clinician should consider asking questions like— "What kinds of things helped you before in stressful situations?", "What kinds of things made you feel better in other situations?", "How do you handle other stressful situations?" The goal with questions like these is to help the person remember if they already had successful strategies that have worked for them in the past that they could use again.

Words of comfort from the Onc R clinician could include some gentle acknowledgements like—"this is hard" and "this is tough." Give the person space to acknowledge their feelings and then ask for them to continue to work with the next rehabilitation intervention. Clinicians are advised against using phrasing such as "*I know* this is hard" especially when the Onc R clinician has not experienced cancer or its treatments themselves. A PWC may subsequently point out the fact that the clinician does not "*know*." More beneficial phrasing may include, "We will work through this together," or " I will help you learn strategies to get stronger," or "…to decrease pain," or that the clinician will help them achieve new tasks with the Onc R interventions. Some clinicians have difficulty navigating the situation where a person is crying. Some patients will apologize for crying, and the Onc R clinician is advised to always assure them and provide comfort with phrasing such as, "never apologize for crying, it is important to work through this emotionally as well as physically." A useful follow up question may be, "Is crying a normal way for you to cope or is this new for you?" This also helps to understand their premorbid personality. Other useful lines of inquiry include asking, "When you had huge challenges or hit hard times before, what helped you get through?" This may also provide some openings to conversations about their own strategies for coping. Perhaps they liked to watch a movie, read a book, take a walk outside, take a drive, etc. to try and get through the struggle. Even momentary breaks from the cancer world help with decreasing stress.

If an emotional crisis is preventing the Onc R sessions, or causing them to be stalled or nonproductive, it is important to refer the person to a mental health practitioner—social worker, psychologist or spiritual counselor. It is important to share that the Onc R clinician is providing a referral. This may involve a statement such as, "Here is someone that can help you in great detail but what can we do right now to help?" Perhaps they will consider the referral to be a relief and will be able to work through the remainder of the Onc R session.

A person's overall belief system can also greatly impact the cancer journey. This conversation may be started by a question such as "How do you look at the world?" Some people may exhibit negative self-talk and the Onc R clinician can help to refocus or reframe this conversation. For example: If someone says they are never going to get better, the Onc R clinician can suggest that it might be helpful for the PWC to instead state "I'm frustrated but I know this will get easier." A key question posed to the patient is, "What statements or thoughts serve you and what statements do not?"

Cognition after diagnosis and during or after treatment can also be a challenge due to the actual physical changes in the brain secondary to cancer treatment as well as the emotional changes. Cancer-related cognitive impairment can be caused from chemotherapy or other metabolic adverse effects (see Chapter 8 for more details). These cognitive changes can be difficult to acknowledge or admit. It is frustrating and embarrassing to have difficulty with remembering dates and names, have word finding difficulty, or forget to reply to emails, answer calls or texts or inadvertently miss appointments or other obligations. This can affect household chores, family obligations, or the workplace. Multitasking may be very stressful when it was easy prior to the cancer treatments. All of these issues can result in a state of increased distress. Exercise has been shown to improve cognition (see Chapter 23 for evidence for practice), however, referrals may be needed to a speech language pathologist for compensatory strategies or a neuropsychologist for further evaluation.

For those that have had chemotherapy, re-entering normal activities can leave them feeling inadequate if they are feeling the effects of the cognitive impairments that come with chemotherapy. Returning to work where expectations of their precancer performance run high can leave a person feeling fearful that they will lose their job if mistakes are made or they have difficulty keeping up with their workload. Often, these PLWBCs may attempt to hide their cognitive challenges which further amplify the pressure and their anxiety. Hiding cognitive challenges can also lead to mistakes on the job resulting in disciplinary action. It is important for individuals to ask for accommodations up front instead of waiting until there is disciplinary action which could result in the loss of their job. PLWBCs with cognitive impairments should be encouraged to pursue information regarding options offered by the Americans with Disabilities Act[3] as in many instances they can request accommodations. Learn more at Americans With Disabilities Act: Information for People Facing Cancer.[3]

Psychosocial Challenges—A Deeper Dive

This section will provide an in-depth examination into the common categories of psychosocial challenges, including emotional, social, and financial. Some PWCs may experience little to no distress. Others will experience severe distress in one or more categories. The remainder fall somewhere in between.

Emotional

When someone is told that they have cancer, the mental swirl begins. There can be a wide range of emotional responses that vary in type, intensity, and duration. The most common are depression, anxiety, post-traumatic stress disorder (PTSD), and grief and loss.

Depression

According to the National Institute of Mental Health (NIMH)[4], there are specific signs and symptoms that may indicate if a person is suffering from depression (see Table 14.2). It is important

TABLE 14.2	Signs and Symptoms of Depression

- Persistent sad, anxious, or empty mood
- Feelings of hopelessness
- Irritability
- Feels of guilt, worthlessness, and/or helplessness
- Loss of interest or pleasure in things that used to be enjoyable
- Decreased energy; fatigue
- Moving or talking slowly
- Restlessness
- Difficulty concentrating, remembering, or making decisions
- Irregular sleep: problems falling or staying asleep or sleeping too much
- Appetite disturbances with or without weight changes
- Thought of suicide or death
- Somatic complaints such as headaches, digestive issues, without a clear medical basis

Created by Laura Munger. Printed with permission.

to note if the symptoms persist for most of the day and for the majority of days over a 2-week period. A person does not have to have all of these symptoms but if a few to multiple symptoms are encountered, it likely indicates a clinical depressive episode. This may be difficult to identify in a PDWC as some of the symptoms of depression may mimic some of the adverse effects of cancer treatment. Examples of this could be fatigue, irregular sleep, and appetite disturbances. Frequency, severity, and persistence over 2 weeks become important information to consider. When a person is experiencing cancer, it is not difficult to see how the stress of treatment, fear, guilt for pressure on their support system, and feelings of loss of control can contribute to a depressive episode.

In one study, the prevalence of depression varied between 3% and 49% depending on the cancer diagnosis and treatment setting. Depression prevalence was found to be between 5% and 16% in outpatients, 4% to 14% in inpatients, 4% to 11% in mixed outpatient and inpatient samples, and 7% to 49% in palliative care.[5] The specific point in time in the person's cancer journey impacts the prevalence of depression with the highest prevalence occurring during treatment (14%), the first year after diagnosis (9%), and one year or more after treatment (8%).[5] The prevalence of depression also differs with diagnosis as the prevalence in lung cancer was only 3%, but in cancer of the digestive tract, it was 31%.[5] Depression in ovarian and prostate cancer was found to be highest pretreatment at 25% and 17% respectively decreasing to 23% and 1% during treatment, however, while prevalence post-treatment dropped to 13% in the ovarian cancer population, it increased to 18% for men in the prostate cancer population, above pretreatment status.[5] Overall 15% to 25% of PWC will suffer from depression and 75% of those patients will receive little or no psychological support.[6] In a sample of 57 PWCs with a variety of diagnoses (breast, uterine, lung, rectal, stomach, and hematological) anxiety and depression rates varied from mild (19%–30%) to moderate (5%–7%) and severe (5%). However, the average prevalence of depression in the cancer population ranges between 15% and 30% depending on the specific screening tool and diagnosis criteria chosen.[7]

Anxiety

One of the most common forms of anxiety is generalized anxiety disorder (GAD). NIMH defines GAD as "excessive anxiety and worry about a variety of events or activities that occurs more days

TABLE 14.3	Signs and Symptoms of Generalized Anxiety Disorder

- Feeling restless or on edge
- Easily fatigued
- Difficulty with concentration
- Irritability
- Muscle tension
- Heightened worry
- Difficulty falling or staying asleep
- Somatic complaints such as digestive issues, heart palpitations, or rapid breathing

Created by Laura Munger. Printed with permission.

than not, for at least six months. People with GAD find it difficult to control their worry, which may cause impairment in social, occupational, or other areas of functioning." Signs and symptoms of GAD are listed in Table 14.3.

There is some overlap in symptoms with anxiety from a cancer diagnosis which is why it is important that a person experiencing cancer that exhibits any of these symptoms of distress be evaluated by a mental health professional. Additionally, it is very important to note that there are many forms that anxiety can take. Often, they can branch into things such as phobias, panic disorders, social anxiety, or PTSD.

Onc R clinicians need to be diligent with screening and referral for depression and anxiety due to its potential effect on cancer recurrence, all-cause mortality, and cancer-specific mortality. A systematic review and meta-analysis of breast cancer survivors found that the presence of depression/anxiety was associated with a 24%/17% higher risk of cancer recurrence, 30%/13% increase risk of all-cause mortality, and 29%/0% increase risk of breast cancer-specific mortality.[8] These authors described depression as indicated by depressive mood, slow thinking, and loss of interest, more prone to committing suicide while they defined anxiety as being characterized by worry, tension and feelings of apprehension. Both depression and anxiety can cause insomnia. In addition, overall depression and anxiety were found to have a significant association with increased risk of cancer incidence for lung, oral cavity, prostate, and skin cancers.[9] It is also associated with cancer-specific mortality in lung, bladder, colorectal, hematopoietic, kidney, and prostate and all-cause mortality in patients diagnosed with lung cancer.[9]

Post-Traumatic Stress Disorder/Post-Traumatic Stress Symptoms

Cancer is a traumatic event but is only rarely viewed as such and, therefore, PTSD presentation can be underreported and underdiagnosed. NIMH defines PTSD as "a disorder that develops in some people who have experienced a shocking, scary, or dangerous event."[10] This definition provides a clear understanding as to how a cancer experience would result in PTSD. The "fight or flight" response is very characteristic of PTSD and often happens when a person is not in immediate danger. Often, PWCs can have this reaction simply by entering the cancer center or any medical facility, smelling certain things, or experiencing other external stimuli, such as seeing someone with no hair. PTSD has been reported to range from 4% to 55% in PDWCs.[11] Another study found PTSD rates ranging from 6.4% to 13.8% for clinically diagnosed PTSD while another 10% to 20% experienced subclinical PTSD

which is also associated with impaired QOL.[12] Childhood cancer survivors are also susceptible to PTSD with prevalence ranging from 0% to 12.5%.[12] Authors reported that PTSD often does not disappear when cancer treatments are completed.[11] These authors report that while some survivors have a decrease in PTSD symptoms with time, others have the opposite trajectory and may have full blown PTSD at four years post-treatment and can also last for years. Common behaviors of PTSD in a PLWBC include missing appointments, failing to finish cancer treatments, withdrawing from friends, or avoiding speaking to anyone about cancer. They may also suffer from a preoccupation of the fear of trauma preventing them from returning to their previous precancer work, relationships, and hobbies. Risk factors for PTSD include stage of diagnosis, socioeconomic and environmental factors, such as educational level, income, minority racial and ethnic groups, younger women, prior life stress, and the fear of recurrence. It is noteworthy that a link has been found in women diagnosed with breast cancer, between chronic stress, inflammation, and PTSD.[13] Chronic stress increases endogenous glucocorticoid release which promotes cancer and depresses the immune system by increasing and maintaining a proinflammatory state in the body. Inflammation is prevalent in both cancer and PTSD and is considered a means by which one can exacerbate the other.

Grief and Loss

Often people consider grief and loss as occurring through the death of a loved one, but grief and loss can be experienced with any loss. Cancer can result in loss of a body part, loss of normal life, loss of functioning, loss of health, loss of work, loss of relationships, and more. The Kubler-Ross Model describes the five stages of grief that a person can experience including: denial, anger, bargaining, depression, and acceptance.[14] These stages are not experienced in a linear timeline nor do people go through these stages one at a time. Similarly, movement through the stages should not be viewed as once they pass a stage they have mastered it. A person will cycle back and forth through some or all stages in random order, often numerous times. Please see Figure 14.1. Furthermore, when a person is going through the cancer experience,

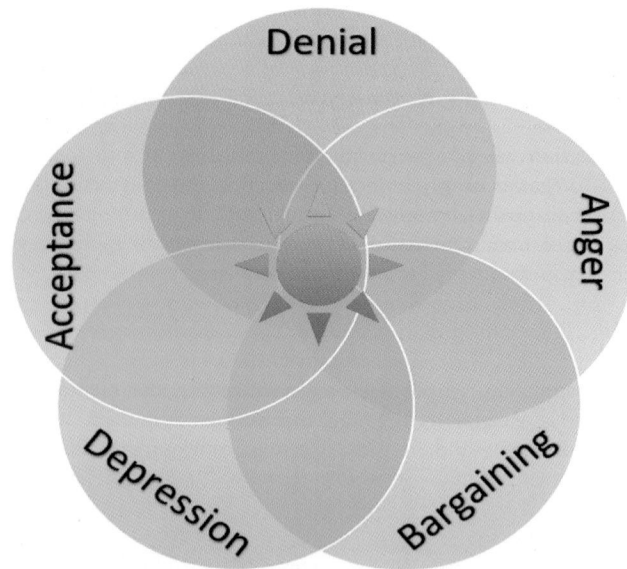

• **Fig. 14.1** Stages of Grief. (Created by Laura Munger. Printed with permission.)

this can be very episodic in nature. They may experience all of these stages with a new diagnosis, then again when there is a change in treatment, surgery, cancer recurrence, return to work, or changes in relationships.

For example, the decision to have one's breast removed (mastectomy) as a result of breast cancer causes a lot of distress dealing with the loss of a body part that significantly changes one's self-identity, and negatively impairs one's perception of womanhood and femininity. In a meta-analysis of the impact of breast cancer, women have reported that the loss of a breast causes negative feelings of disfigurement, due to scarring and the feeling of never being a "normal person" again.[15] Other consequences included a loss of security in relationships and sexuality which can lead to sexual abstinence and a loss of identification as a woman, a wife, or a mother.[15]

Social

Support System

Whether someone has a support system or not is vital to their treatment outcomes. The most optimal situation is that every person has a caregiver to accompany them on all of their appointments and treatments to provide another set of eyes and ears to ask important questions, listen to the clinician's answers, help provide clarity, and even write down information to allow the PWC to be able to read and think about the information later. Often, the PWC is overwhelmed by the experience and information overload can occur quickly.

There are many ways to provide support to a PWC. In addition to having someone attend appointments, it is also helpful to have someone to drive to appointments, be an emotional support to process events, help with tasks at work or home, and to be available to do routine activities with, like grocery shopping or going to church. Some even find it helpful to have a support person that manages the array of information sharing that happens after appointments via social media rather than the PWC having to contact everyone separately with individual updates. Every person's support needs are different, and questions need to be asked to determine help needs to prevent a PWC from missing appointments or developing more anxiety from not being able to physically and emotionally handle the new schedule.

Support can also come in the form of emotional support. Local cancer support groups can provide wonderful support to both the PLWBC and their caregivers. There are numerous organizations that provide various forms of support, for example, "Reach for Recovery" provided by the American Cancer Society,[16] and Cancer Survivors Network[17] which provides virtual chat rooms and discussion boards. Additional, virtual communities through Cancer Support Community[18] and Cancer Hope Network[19] will match a cancer survivor with someone that has experienced the same challenges.

Some survivors needing assistance with activities of daily living (ADLs) may not have the social support necessary to provide this assistance. It is important to identify these PWCs and to connect them with a case manager, navigator, or mental health practitioner so that are able to meet their needs for food, cleanliness, and assistance for other daily tasks.

Premorbid Stressors

There are two major considerations to be aware of: (1) a stressful support system or no support system; and (2) history of or current mental illness. Cancer is hard enough to manage when things are going well in one's life and a rich support team is present. The

difficulty is compounded when there is no support system available or when the support system is toxic. It can be very common for a support person, like a partner, to be someone who the PWC has a tumultuous relationship with and now they are the primary caregiver. This adds increased strain to already strained relationships and can be a big contributing factor to anxiety and depression. Having a support person who is negative can actually detract from the experience and cause more stress. For example: Consider the spouse of the PWC who is verbally or emotionally abusive and tries to control the appointment by answering all the questions and interrupting the PWC. This can cause excessive levels of anxiety for the PWC. In this case, it is imperative to intervene and come to agreement that another friend or family member be designated to bring the PWC to the appointments.

Mental illness can be a substantial confounding factor during cancer treatment that must be monitored and addressed. Working closely with a person's mental health provider (if they already have a provider and have granted permission to contact) is very important as some cancer treatments can exacerbate a pre-existing mental health diagnosis.

The issue of substance abuse with the potential for substance use disorder must also be considered. Cancer is considered not only life threatening but also psychotraumatic.[20] Investigators report that substance abuse carries with it significant psychological, social, and economic consequences, but it also is linked to cancer development and reducing treatment compliance (e.g., unreliability with appointment attendance or maintaining a treatment regimen) which will significantly decrease the efficacy of the cancer and Onc R treatment plan.[20] Substance abuse can also negatively affect cancer prognosis and QOL. It is important to be aware of this history if it is documented in medical records. Furthermore, if the Onc R clinician is the first person to identify substance abuse, it is important to notify the cancer care team to initiate appropriate referrals to support the person through these challenges.

Religion/Spirituality

Spiritual well-being has been defined as "one's perception regarding seeking congruent, intrinsic, meaningful purpose of life and self-confidence to overcome challenges and achieve life goals."[21] In a study of 150 elderly Taiwanese participants aged 65 to 84, higher levels of spiritual well-being were associated with a higher health-related QOL and lower levels of depression. Evidence is growing rapidly demonstrating that a person's spiritual well-being is essential to health-related QOL and is integral in truly providing patient-centered care. Spiritual/religious belief systems of PWCs need to be embraced and integrated into clinical practice during cancer diagnosis, treatment, and survivorship. Research has shown that those that particpate in some kind of spiritual practice have better outcomes.[22] High levels of spiritual well-being have been specifically studied in PDWC and found to directly affect health outcomes, including QOL, lower levels of depression, distress, and anxiety. Spirituality is a source of hope and strength in coping with their cancer diagnosis, treatment, and subsequent adverse effects. It is found to help individuals find meaning in their lives and find meaning in their cancer journey.

Among Black breast cancer survivors, spirituality/religion played an integral role in providing strength to cope with their diagnosis and treatment. Overall, most studies found that spirituality/religion was quite variable as it related to participant demographics, methodology, and where they were at along the cancer trajectory. However, it is clear that the incorporation of spirituality/religion impacts QOL and decisions related to cancer care. As Onc R clinicians, it is important to make sure that awareness of and respect for the spirituality/religious beliefs and needs of each PLWBC is essential to provide culturally appropriate holistic care.[23]

Race/Cultural Issues

Cultural bias for underserved and marginalized groups can come in the form of lack of access to healthcare services. It can also be hindered by language barriers. Having access to translators is a vital resource. Some cultures also have challenges with talking to healthcare providers regarding physical and emotional issues that they consider to be private but also some cultures view illness as shaming. One author of this chapter once worked with a family of Middle Eastern descent that did not want the social workers to tell the woman with cancer that she had breast cancer as this was seen as making her less desirable for a partner. The ethical issues that arose from this were significant since our American laws did not match up with the cultural beliefs of these individuals.

LGBTQIA+

By Morgan Shaw-Andrade

Sexual and romantic identity pertains to whom an individual is sexually or romantically attracted to, respectively. Whereas gender identity pertains to how an individual identifies their gender. These entities are separate. For example, a transgender woman is an individual who was assigned a male sex at birth and identifies as female. Nonbinary individuals may fall in between the dichotomy of male and female gender, potentially utilizing pronouns such as "they/them/theirs." Since gender identity is a spectrum, some individuals may fall more toward the side of masculine and others toward the side of feminine. To account for nonbinary individuals that may undergo feminizing or masculinizing medical interventions, it may be more applicable to utilize the terms "transfeminine individual" and "transmasculine individual" in place of transgender woman or transgender man.

In cancers such as penile, prostate, breast, uterine, cervical, and ovarian, conversations about sexual identity, gender identity, and self-image are essential. It is vital to not make assumptions and to be highly sensitive to how someone identifies and to ask questions rather than make statements. Small, but highly impactful gestures such as asking the PLWBC for their pronouns help to build a sound patient–clinician relationship. Ultimately, our patients are the experts of their own life experience, and it is crucial that they are treated as such experts. When working with the transgender and nonbinary community, neutral terms such as "reproductive organs" can be utilized until it can be established what the individual prefers their reproductive organs to be called. It is equally vital to recognize that as all people are unique, all transgender PLWBCs are unique. Transgender individuals may undergo various medical interventions, including but not limited to hormone replacement therapy, "top surgery" (mastectomy or breast augmentation), "bottom surgery" (phalloplasty or vaginoplasty), and more. Despite the numerous medical interventions available to the transgender PLWBC, transgender individuals may opt out of various interventions for their own personal reasoning. It is not the Onc R clinicians' place to inquire about the personal choices of a transgender PLWBC unless medically relevant. It is, however, the Onc R clinicians' place to recognize that gender identity is a spectrum, and all transition processes are unique. This means transgender PLWBCs may have various emotional reactions to procedures that require removing sexual reproductive organs or sexual accessory organs, all of which are valid. In addition, when working with PLWBCs within and outside of the LGBTQIA+

community, it should not be assumed whether or not an individual wishes to bear children. People of all sexual and gender identities may or may not wish to bear children, making conversations about germ cell preservation applicable to all individuals that still have their original reproductive organs. Finally, when the Onc R clinician is concerned if a question may be interpreted as invasive when it is in fact medically relevant, the Onc R clinician should explain their inquiries prior to asking. This shows the Onc R clinician is well intentioned and helps build patient confidence with all patient populations. The health and QOL of PLWBCs are of utmost importance to the Onc R clinician and questions pertaining to ensuring the PLWBC's well-being are appropriate.

Financial

The NCI defines financial toxicity as: "problems a patient has related to the cost of medical care."[24] A lack of health insurance and excessive costs of medical interventions can cause devastating financial problems, and may lead to debt and possibly bankruptcy. This stress can affect access to medical care and affect a patient's QOL. Any financial stresses could increase the likelihood of a person experiencing or having an episode of depression and/or anxiety and/or grief.

Burden

Missed work, loss of paid time off, missed work by loved ones, and added daycare expenses are just a few examples of how treatment can burden one's financial picture. This added burden will also have an impact on someone's emotional well-being due to the stress and may also impact their social situation as relationships can potentially become strained.

Insurance Status

There are a few considerations regarding insurance. Some people are insured but in order to keep their premiums down have opted into plans where the deductible and/or copays are very high. Even "covered services" with the concurrent out-of-pocket costs can financially devastate a person/family. Sometimes the PWC retains health insurance through their employer. In these instances, the balance between treatment and work can be complicated as they risk losing their insurance if they do not work. Other situations where someone may be uninsured also exist. Some cancer treatment programs are equipped to help to support these individuals. Lastly, there are also situations where someone is uninsured but whose cancer has progressed to a level where they are eligible for social security disability (SSD). Once approved for SSD, it may take up to two years to obtain Medicare for their health insurance coverage. Although this will eventually be beneficial in the long run, the 2-year waiting period can be a strain. Finally, PLWCs may be eligible for Medicaid in some states if there is an established financial need but this varies widely by the state that the PLWC lives in.

Service Needs

One of the biggest areas of need for PLWCs is financially affording medications or even items such as compression sleeves for lymphedema. There are a variety of programs that exist to assist PLWBCs with these strains. Many pharmaceutical companies have coupons or financial assistance programs to help to reduce or alleviate the cost of very expensive medications. Often the cancer center where someone is treated will have readily available resources to assist with this process. There are also websites such as Needy Meds (needymeds.org) that can be an avenue for a person to access these programs.

Employment

Those that are employed will often fear losing their jobs. Employers with less than 50 people are not held to the protection of the Family Leave Act[25] so they will not have the protection of this act to hold their job for 12 weeks while they are undergoing treatment. Other individuals may not have paid time off so using sick or vacation time for cancer treatments is not an option. Going weeks without pay is devastating. It is common to see people forcing themselves to still work when they are physically struggling due to these circumstances. A final note is in regards to the Americans with Disabilities Act.[3] There are specific guidelines that an employer must follow. For example, it would be illegal to fire someone because they have cancer. The act is very extensive and has a specific section to address cancer, and Onc R clinician are encouraged to familiarize themselves with it or at least direct a PLWBC to look through this if they feel their employer is treating them unfairly. If necessary, an advocate or legal representation may be beneficial to assure that employers are following these laws.

Measurement Tools for Screening or Evaluation

There are numerous valid measurement tools for screening and evaluation of psychosocial issues. Six tools are described here including: NCCN Distress Thermometer, PROMIS, FACT-G, The National Cancer Center Psychological Symptom Inventory (NCC-PSI), Patient Health Questionnaire (PHQ-9) and (PHQ-2), and Center for Epidemiological Studies Depression Scale (CES-D).

NCCN Distress Thermometer

Distress is considered the 6th vital sign in oncology care.[26] Evidence is clear that with increased distress, PLWBCs will often not complete treatment plans, are dissatisfied with their cancer care, have a lower QOL, and even have lower survival rates.[26] The prevalence of distress is reported as ranging from 41% to 60%.[27] Due to this high prevalence of distress, it is important to identify persons at high risk for distress and provide interventions to prevent and manage distress early in the cancer trajectory. The NCCN has established the distress thermometer (DT) and problem list to quantify distress and distressing problems. The DT has well established validity for this population, is available in multiple languages, is brief to fill out, and is easy for clinicians to interpret. The DT uses a 0 (no distress) to 10 (severe distress) scale to rate distress over the past week. The ease of use of this tool makes it ideal for use multiple times throughout the course of cancer care. A cutoff score of "3" on the DT is recommended which indicate clinically elevated levels of distress.[28] Further, they found that PDWC 1 to 4 weeks prior to the assessment noted the highest levels of distress. This tool can be obtained through the National Comprehensive Cancer Network (NCCN) at https://www.nccn.org/patients/resources/life_with_cancer/distress.aspx

Patient-Reported Outcomes Measurement Information System

PROMIS is the Patient-Reported Outcomes Measurement Information System that measures physical function, fatigue, pain interference and intensity, depression, and anxiety. A systematic review found that the PROMIS was increasingly popular with the cancer population due to the various short forms and the ability to administer electronically through the web or a smart phone.[29] The systematic review examined studies with patients with a variety of cancer diagnoses and gathered data at pre-, during, or post-treatment. The most common measurement tool used was the PROMIS Global Health Short Form while the PROMIS-29 was the second most popular form. The responsiveness of eight PROMIS measures was studied in 2968 patients diagnosed with a variety of cancers. All measures studied were found to be sensitive to patient-perceived changes in their clinical experiences, whether worsening or improving.[30] The PROMIS tools can be obtained via Health Measures at https://www.healthmeasures.net/explore-measurement-systems/promis/obtain-administer-measures.

Functional Assessment of Cancer Therapy Tools

The functional assessment of cancer therapy–General (FACT-G) questionnaire contains four health related QOL domains—physical, social, emotional, and functional well-being. This questionnaire has 27-items with a 5-point Likert-type response scale, can be delivered via paper or electronic mode, and only requires 5 to 10 minutes to complete. It was created and validated in 1993[31] and was updated in 2019 with a bifactor analysis completed to confirm the factorial structure. It is available in over 70 languages. The FACT-G is one of over 100 different questionnaires for various cancer diagnosis and adverse effects caused from the treatments for cancer available through www.facit.org. The four domains provide comprehensive and identified areas of distress. It is recommended to be provided to a PLWBC upon diagnosis and frequently throughout cancer care due to the changes in health-related QOL with each treatment and throughout survivorship.[32]

The National Cancer Center Psychological Symptom Inventory

The NCC-PSI screening tool measures insomnia, depression, and anxiety. This tool uses a 1 to 10 rating scale for six questions and a check mark on the 7th question regarding what symptoms the person desires help with. The cut off score severity for insomnia was 5, while depression and anxiety were 4/5. This tool is fairly new, but the evidence demonstrates that its performance is comparable to the NCCN Distress Thermometer.[33]

Patient Health Questionnaire With 9 and 2 Questions

The Patient Health Questionnaire with 9 questions (PHQ-9) is a self-administered tool to assess depression. It includes the DSM-IV depression criteria as well as other common symptoms and is a useful tool for screening, diagnosing, and monitoring treatment outcomes. It is available in over 30 languages. The nine questions have four potential answers (0–3). 0 is not at all, 1 is several days, 2 is more than half of the days, and 3 is nearly every day, resulting in a sum score range of 0 to 27. The degree of depression is mild (>5), moderate (>10), and severe (>15). In 2016, it was confirmed that the PHQ-9 was applicable for assessing for depression in PDWC.[34] The PHQ-2 includes two questions from the PHQ-9. This tool is screening for a depressed mood and anhedonia over the past 2 weeks. This is scored from 0 to 6 and a score of 2 or more is considered meeting the criteria for depression. This is often used first and if it is positive for depression, the PHQ-9 is then administered. The PHQ-2 was studied in persons diagnosed with cancer receiving treatment in community-based radiation oncology practices and it demonstrated good psychometric properties.[35] The authors concluded that screening for mood disorders with the PHQ-2 was equivalent to the PHQ-9 and superior to the NCCN-DT.[35]

Center for Epidemiological Studies Depression Scale

The CES-D is used to measure depressive symptoms in PWCs.[36] The CES-D has been found to be valid and reliable with PWCs.[37] The CES-D measures 20 items associated with depression within 1 week. A 0 to 3 Likert scale is used where 0 = rarely or never; 1 = occasionally or 1 to 2 days; 2 = occasionally or 3 to 4 days; and 3 = most of the time or 5 to 7 days. The total scores range from 0 to 60 with higher scores indicating more depressive symptoms. This tool can be obtained from: https://www.apa.org/pi/about/publications/caregivers/practice-settings/assessment/tools/depression-scale.

When Is a Person in Distress?

Distress is a common adverse effect of cancer and its treatments. Although incidents of distress can be chronic, it is also common for distress to be episodic in nature especially throughout the journey of cancer. For example, it is important for an Onc R clinician to be prepared for and observe for changes in a PLWBC as they go through treatment transitions. When a PWC is having a change in their treatment (e.g., surgery scheduled or completed, the start of chemotherapy, radiation now being recommended when it was not previously), changes in the levels of distress are common and should be expected and addressed. While some people react with distress during the treatment phase, others will not experience distress until the treatments are completed and the adverse effects are affecting their QOL. It also may begin as survivorship evolves and changes in lifestyle and abilities become a reality. If a person cannot return to the same level of function as they had prior to the cancer diagnosis, depression can occur. Finding the appropriate measurement tool is important to provide at every appointment, especially as treatment changes.

What Should the Onc R Clinician Ask and When?

Onc R clinicians are very familiar with the process of assessing a person's premorbid functioning and, subsequently reassessing current function and how it changes ADL performance and function. This same tact should be taken with mental health. It is important to ask questions that will establish a baseline mental health, cognitive, and emotional status as well as coping levels to proactively identify for any distress and promptly address it. Some Onc R clinicians may have concerns that they are not experts in mental health and may be reluctant to assess for these issues, but it should be remembered that the main goal in this line of questioning is to establish if support is needed. This may be as simple as asking the PLWC if what they are currently feeling is normal for them or if what they are experiencing is something new.

For example, a PLWBC comes to their Onc R appointment visibly upset. They may be withdrawn or weepy. The Onc R clinician asks them how they are doing, and they begin to tear up and cry then say, "I am having a hard time." The Onc R clinician could follow up with a familiar question such as, "Are you still experiencing pain?" If the person responds with, "Yeah, but I mean I am struggling in general." This might be a good point to ask them, "Are these feelings normal for you or do you feel like it's bigger than that?" The PLWBC might immediately say, "Oh yeah, totally normal. I am just having a bad week." At this point, it may be appropriate to proceed with treatment with the plan to discuss coping strategies at a future time and ongoing monitoring for these symptoms. If these symptoms do not improve over subsequent weeks or begin to worsen, it would be time to inquire further and refer the patient back to their physician for further support and resources.

Conversely, upon inquiry, the person may also say, "I don't know.", or "No, this feels awful. I am normally such an 'up' person." In either case, an appropriate follow up question is recommend such as, "Do you feel like you are having a hard time engaging in normal daily life?" As an Onc R clinician, a useful transition may be to inquire about ADL performance such as, "Are you showering daily?", "Are you getting up and getting dressed?", "Are you doing things that you normally enjoyed?" If it appears as though they are not functioning at a level that would be normal for them, then this would be the time to utilize any of the aforementioned distress measurement tools that will help the Onc R clinician and the PLWBC to identify if more intervention is needed. Please refer to video with 5 steps for OncR clinicians to empower PLWBC (acknowledge, get curious, reflect back, shift from feeling out of control to in control, and look for opportunities to empower and to encourage) (Video 14.1).

Treatment Interventions

Psychosocial Prehabilitation

Just as prehabilitation is recommended for all the potential physical and functional adverse effects that can result from treatment for cancer, it is also recommended for the potential psychosocial and psychoemotional adverse effects that may occur (see Chapter 27).

A psychosocial prehabilitation program should include "Coping 101." People preparing for cancer treatment need to know what to expect in terms of potential emotional and social challenges, areas of stress, and financial considerations. It is always much easier to hear and comprehend these issues when in a calmer state. Teaching coping strategies is not only a valuable educational intervention but also provides the PLWBC with basic strategies to deal with the emotional, social, and financial stressors along the entire cancer journey and in life. This may include, but is not limited to, the importance of including communication with the medical team, communication with family/friends, importance of support system and how best to utilize them (or how to access support if no support system is available), teaching key points to helping a person "stay who they are," understanding how not to let cancer define them, and coping strategies such as meditation or art therapy.

Mindfulness Based Stress Reduction

Mindfulness Based Stress Reduction (MBSR) theory was developed by Jon Kabat-Zinn in the 1970s.[38] This treatment method incorporates the elements of mindfulness and meditation. Mindfulness "is an awareness that arises through paying attention, on purpose in the present moment, nonjudgmentally."[38] Mindful approaches work to have the person not focus on thoughts that may draw them to the past or future, rather keep their focus upon the present moment. Meditation practices are often used as a strategy to pursue mindfulness. As can be imagined, when someone is told they have cancer, the mental swirl begins. Fear about what lies ahead for them or anger about what they did in the past that may have caused this can leave people in a mental space that results in fear, sadness, and anxiety. Keeping someone as present as possible can go a long way in helping them to cope. MBSR is a structured 8-week program that combines mindfulness meditation, yoga, and other stress reduction techniques to improve overall well-being and QOL.[39] MBSR has been shown to improve mood disorders, reduce fear of recurrence and stress, and improve physical functioning thereby reducing stress and anxiety in women diagnosed with breast cancer.[39] It is important to note that MBSR also positively alters cortisol release and immune functioning.[39]

Clinician Tools

An Onc R clinician, while not a mental health provider, can use many of these techniques to help a person reduce their stress while providing Onc R services. If a person begins to talk about their fears for the future, the PLWBC can be redirected to the present moment in a nonjudgmental way. Useful phrasing may include, "I know this can be scary but tell me about something in the present moment that makes you feel encouraged." Mindfulness-based breathing techniques can be employed—5 counts in, 1 second hold, 5 counts out. If they are in pain during an exercise, this breathing technique can be used and accompanied by key verbiage and visual imagery such as, "breathe in good, healing oxygen to the place that hurts and blow out the pain or tension." Onc R clinicians should also listen to the words that their patients are using to assist them in cognitively reframing a situation. For example, if a PLWBC uses phrases like "this is my bad side," the Onc R clinician should redirect them away from judgmental words like "bad" and instead suggest something like, "This is the side I need to work on." It may also be useful to instruct the PLWBC to focus on to the clinician's voice while the clinician counts out their exercise reps in a quiet, calm voice. Finally, it may be effective to have some calming music to listen to while participating in Onc R. These may seem like small things, but lessons will empower and equip a PLWBC to face future issues which will be crucial to their overall coping.

Cognitive Behavioral Therapy

"Cognitive behavioral therapy (*CBT*) is based on the idea that how we think (cognition), how we feel (emotion) and how we act (behavior) all interact together. Specifically, our thoughts determine our feelings and our behavior. When a person suffers with psychological distress, the way in which they interpret situations becomes skewed, which in turn has a negative impact on the actions they take. CBT helps to develop alternative ways of thinking and behaving which aims to reduce psychological distress."[40] CBT has core principles that psychological problems are based on unhelpful ways of thinking or learned patterns of unhelpful behavior that can be positively affected through learned coping strategies.[41]

Clinician Tools

As discussed above with MBSR, an Onc R clinician can actively listen for phrases that a person uses that reflects a defeatist, fearful, negative, and out of control mindset. If a person says, "I can't do it.", have them change it to "I can't do it YET." or "I will do it eventually." If they say, "I am never going to be the same.", help them reframe their words to something like "I may be different, but I am going to work as hard as I can to be the best that I can in this moment." One of the most common statements that a PLWBC may voice if they begin to cry is, "I'm so sorry." or "How embarrassing?", or "Why can't I cope better?" To reframe these statements away from the judgment and stigma of crying

	TABLE 14.4 Clinical Tools for Reframing Negative Self-Talk to Positive Self-Talk
Negative or Defeating Self-Talk	**Positive/Empowering Reframe**
"I just can't do this."	"This is really hard but I will get there."
"Why do I always cry? I'm so stupid."	"Crying is normal and vulnerability is courageous! These are healing waters! It's healthy to get this out."
"I hate coming here. All you do is hurt me."	"I am proud of myself for doing something hard."
"This was bound to happen to me because my mother and father both have had cancer."	"Even with genetics, there is a lot you have control of."
"Bad things always happen to me."	"Hardship happens to the best of people."

Created by Laura Munger. Printed with permission.

into something positive, useful phrases may include, "Those are healing waters!", or "Crying is healthy!" Statements such as these often help to put someone at ease. Refer to Table 14.4.

Mindfulness Based Cognitive Therapy

Dr. Zindel Segal took the concept of MBSR and combined it with CBT to help "individuals better understand and manage their thoughts and emotions in order to achieve relief from feelings of distress."[42]

Clinician Tools

Many of the tools in the previous section are applicable in mindfulness based cognitive therapy (MBCT) as well. It is important to reiterate the following points: (1) Keep the individual feeling in *control*. When they talk about things that are out of their control (e.g., multiple physician appointments, recurrence, financial issues), remind them of what they do have control of, like their exercise program, sleep habits, nutrition, attending appointments, etc.; (2) The astute clinician should listen for sentences that start with "what if." (e.g., "what if I had a bad scan?", "what if I never get better?", "what if these exercises don't help?"). If a patient is participating in negative self-talk, the Onc R clinician should actively help them refocus (see Table 14.4). For example, "If you think that you are not going to get better, then you aren't."; and (3) Another useful intervention is to redirect the person to keep them in the *present*. When the person's thoughts are swirling about things that have already happened or things that are going to happen, the Onc R clinician should bring them back to the here and now. Consider these motivational sayings to share with a PLWBC:

Thoughts are the first critical step in our ability to manifest our outcomes.

Laura Munger

It all starts in your mind, what you give power to has power over you!

Leon Brown

Don't go with the flow, be the flow!

Shams Tabrizi

Motivational Interviewing

"Motivational interviewing (MI) is a counseling method that helps people resolve ambivalent feelings and insecurities to find the internal motivation they need to change their behavior. It is a practical, empathetic, and short-term process that takes into consideration how difficult it is to make life changes."[43] A meta-analysis was conducted including 15 studies that used MI with PWCs. MI was used to address behaviors of diet, exercise, smoking cessation, cancer-related stress, and fatigue management. The authors concluded that there was evidence that demonstrated the efficacy of MI to deal with psychosocial and lifestyle behaviors in PDWC.[44] Motivational interviewing is discussed in greater detail in Chapter 30.

Clinician Tools

Onc R clinicians routinely work with patients or clients who have limited motivation or are not invested in the rehabilitative process. PLWBCs are often feeling futile, treatment-weary, and fatigued. In order to gain buy-in and actively promote the process, the Onc R clinician can use the following strategy. First the person should be encouraged to identify what they would like to work on, and then have them set their own short- and long-term goals. Questions to initiate this conversation and consideration of their future may include: "What would you like to gain out of this process?", "What things are difficult to do that you would like to gain some independence with?", or "What has you feeling discouraged that you would like to feel encouraged by?"

Integrative Therapies/Integrative Oncology

Integrative therapies are utilized along with conventional treatments and can enhance outcomes and reduce symptom burden. In some cases, PWCs and PLWBCs may actively seek these therapies out. Onc R clinicians would benefit from understanding the evidence for and against these therapies. These may include, but are not limited to acupuncture/acupressure, massage, art therapy, and music therapy. An Onc R clinician should actively inquire within their organization and community to be become familiar with what is available in the area. The Society for Integrative Oncology (https://integrativeonc.org/about-us) defines *Integrative Oncology* as "a patient-centered, evidence-informed field of cancer care that utilizes mind and body practices, natural products, and/or lifestyle modifications from different traditions alongside conventional cancer treatments. Integrative oncology aims to optimize health, QOL, and clinical outcomes across the cancer care continuum and to empower people to prevent cancer and become active participants before, during, and beyond cancer treatment."[45] They define specific modalities of Integrative Oncology to include diet, physical activity, dietary supplements, mind-body modalities, acupuncture, and massage therapy.[45] The National Center for Complementary and Integrative Health (www.nccih.nih.gov/) developed a five-domain concept: (1) manipulative and body-based methods; (2) mind-body medicine; (3) alternative medical systems; (4) energy therapies; and (5) biologically-based therapies.[46] Due to its increasing popularity and acceptance, more organizations related to this realm of practice are being established and increased research and evidence-based practice guidelines are being undertaken. This will provide integrative therapeutic providers with more tools to treat the adverse effects from cancer treatment in collaboration with the medical team to improve QOL. Although a comprehensive discussion of these topics and their respective evidence bases is beyond the scope of this textbook, evidence is growing rapidly in the following interventions:

Oncology Massage

Oncology massage is used to decrease stress, pain, anxiety, depression, nausea, and fatigue. The Society for Oncology Massage (www.s4om.org/oncology-massage-overview) provides very helpful information regarding the training and benefits of oncology massage.

Art Therapy

Art therapy is used to express emotions in a creative, nonverbal way using visual art. Art therapy can decrease anxiety and depression, increase QOL, and has shown to have positive effects on personal growth, coping with the disease, developing a new form of self-expression, and increasing social interaction.[47] The authors of this chapter have observed that art therapy anecdotally improves coping skills, emotional wellbeing, and QOL. One author personally attended cancer center-based art gallery events and it was evident in talking to the artists that it profoundly impacted their emotions and coping by giving them a beautiful and creative process to express and tell their story.

Music Therapy

Music therapy can assist in providing distraction from adverse effects, promoting relaxation, reducing anxiety, and increasing feelings of well-being. Music often results in a connection with an individual providing a more comfortable environment to express their feelings.[48]

Meditation and Mindfulness

Meditation and mindfulness are effective ways to help anyone become more present in their existence as opposed to ruminating in the past or worrying about/fearing the future. When working with a PLWBC, an Onc R clinician may hear elements of regretting past choices (e.g., where a person feels they might have done something that caused their cancer). They also may be worrying about upcoming scans or recurrence. In addition to helping someone focus on the present, which is the only time frame that they have control over, meditation may assist in actually reprogramming the brain to be more calm and less reactive. Mindfulness meditation is described as focusing attention on the full and nonjudgmental experience of creating a positive outcome for wellbeing through curiosity, openness, and acceptance. It can promote relaxation and decreased stress.[49] As it relates to the theme of feeling in control versus out of control, relaxation can facilitate improved feelings of control, while distress can further exacerbate an out-of-control feeling. Please refer to three meditations (Audio 14.1, Audio 14.2, Audio 14.3).

Deep Breathing

Deep breathing is one of the simplest skills to teach and learn. It can have a profound impact the vagus nerve (VN) which subsequently lowers blood pressure, heart rate, and respirations.[50] This is thought to be the result of the modulation of respiration where the VN activity is suppressed during inhalation and facilitated during exhalation.[50] The VN also influences physical health by suppressing inflammation.[50] Not only does the VN control heart rate and slow deep breathing, slow respiration rates with extended exhalation could also activate the PNS by VN afferent function in the airways.[50] This is a form of respiratory biofeedback. Slow, deep breathing with long exhalation increases relaxation via the VN which then is on a feedback loop, resulting in more VN activity and further relaxation.[50] This is associated with better mental, emotional, and physical health as well as improved cognition.[50] Diaphragmatic breathing promotes parasympathetic responding which is the higher executive functioning needed for coping and problem-solving versus they sympathetic/fight-or-flight response. All of this can be achieved in just 10 minutes of deep breathing. Several breathing techniques are available in the enhanced eBook in Chapter 11.

Spiritual Practices

Spiritual practices are very individualized and have been shown to improve outcomes for PWCs. Spiritual practices provide inner peace, hope, acceptance of reality, opportunity to seek meaning and purpose in life, and seek forgiveness. Spiritual needs of PWCs need to be considered and respected and encouraged at any point during their cancer journey.[51]

Peer Support and Support Groups

Even with the employment of strategic and well-intentioned psychosocial and emotional interventions, many people going through the cancer experience find irreplaceable relief by speaking with other people that have lived through the same or similar experience. It is important to match people up as closely as possible to an individual person and/or group/organization that best matches them. For example, there are many groups such as Livestrong and Cancer Sucks that aim for those who are young people (under the age of 40) dealing with cancer and have unique needs (dating, childbearing, jobs, school, etc.). Other groups may focus on type of cancer, stage of cancer, or racial demographics, to name a few.

Support for Families and Children of PWCs

Children and families are often under supported when they are living with a loved one going through the cancer experience. For children, parents act with the best of intentions to try and do what they feel is protecting their children from knowing too much. They feel that the more they know, the more anxiety they cause. In some ways, the opposite can be true. Children are very aware and very smart. No matter what age, they know when things are not normal, routines are different, and energies/emotions in their parents are off. Denying children age-appropriate information actually increases their anxiety and depression. The PWC should be encouraged to let their children know what to anticipate in terms of appointments, changes in routine, hair loss, or other symptoms or life changes. The PWC should strive to be calming and encouraging but should not lie.

Children in distress will also exhibit identifiable behavior changes. These may include appetite changes, sleep disturbances, and/or problems in school. Especially for older children and teenagers, they are likely to use the internet in an attempt to find health information; it is critically important to be proactive and honest with information as internet-based health information without context can increase anxiety as opposed to lessen it. The PWC should be coached to pursue resources or support groups in their community that are aimed at supporting these children and their unique needs. In addition, older children should be encouraged to speak to their friends about their concerns and issues as peer support is critical. It is recommended to assure that the family has an open dialog to facilitate questions, concerns, and discussing fears. It is natural to not want to make this disease process the center of all family interactions but discussing it should not be taboo either. Facilitating this conversation can help all involved to cope together, come to mutual understanding, and strengthen the bonds of the PWC's support network at a time when it is needed most.

Coordination of Care

Making a Referral

As an Onc R clinician, it is important to be aware of the psychosocial issues that a PWC has. Utilization of measurement tools should be common practice. Every interaction with a PWC offers the opportunity for observation and discussions that may identify concerns and possible need for referral. It is the responsibility of Onc R clinicians to ask the right questions, provide the right measurement tools, and refer to a mental health practitioner in a timely manner.

If the Onc R clinician practices within a health system with an established cancer center, this process should be a simple one. Most cancer centers have social work departments, psychoncology clinics, and/or patient and family support services that can be readily referred to. Even if the Onc R provider is not a part of that health system's cancer center, it is the responsibility of the Onc R clinician to locate services in the community that patients can be referred to. Many cancer centers have charitable endeavors and may provide some support services to patients who do not receive any cancer services at that health system, but this varies widely.

Building relationships with mental health practitioners is essential for patient-centered and whole person care. Another useful resource is the website Psychology Today which provides lists of therapists and their specialty information in the PWC's in geographic area that specialize in working with patients diagnosed with cancer (https://www.psychologytoday.com/us). The Association of Oncology Social Workers also has a directory that is easily accessible (https://aosw.org/).

If someone is in financial distress, useful resources can be accessed at the local cancer center which should include assistance in working with pharmaceutical companies or charitable organizations that provide medication discount coupons or have assistance programs to help with the costs of treatments. Some resources include: Needymeds (https://www.needymeds.org/), the American Cancer Society (https://www.cancer.org/), Cancer.net (https://www.cancer.net/navigating-cancer-care/financial-considerations/financial-resources), or Cancer Financial Assistance Coalition (https://www.cancerfac.org/). If transportation is a concern, the local American Cancer Society office may be able to provide volunteer drivers.

What If Psychiatric Medications Are Needed?

Working With the Mental Health Professional

There will be times where the PLWBC's distress is unrelated to the Onc R. It may be financial issues or relationship issues, for example. However, if someone is experiencing depression and anxiety related to their treatment it might be helpful to converse with the mental health practitioner. This exchange of ideas can help with treatment outcomes, as well as offering the PLWBC an opportunity for a more comprehensive approach that will help their mental health goals. To meet the tenets of patient confidentiality, the PLWBC would have to sign releases both with the Onc R clinician's office and with the mental health practitioner's office before conversations occur regarding specifics of the patient's case.

Compassion Fatigue in the Clinician

Compassion fatigue (CF), also called Secondary Traumatic Stress (STS) or vicarious traumatization has been defined as the "natural consequent behaviors and emotions resulting from knowing about a traumatizing event experienced by a significant other—the stress resulting from helping, or wanting to help, a traumatized or suffering person."[52] It is also described as the "combined effects of the caregiver's continuous visualizing of clients' traumatic images added to the effects of burnout can create a condition progressively debilitating the caregiver."[53] It is an extreme state of excessive concern for the suffering of those being helped. CF stress results in a state of physical and mental exhaustion caused by a depleted ability to cope with one's everyday environment. It is important to note that both clinicians and caregivers

to the PLWBC are at increased risk for CF. Evidence shows that 25% of healthcare professionals working in cancer care are at risk for CF.[54] They found a positive correlation between personal distress and CF that may impact negatively on professional QOL. The authors state that this research implies a need for identifying which healthcare providers are at risk for CF. See Box 14.1 for common symptoms of CF.

Who Is at Risk for Compassion Fatigue?

Medical professionals, law enforcement officers, first responders, genetic counselors and caregivers, and anyone who is taught at an early age to put the needs of others before themselves are at risk of CF. It is common to find a history of CF in those that grew up in homes where there was a chronic illness, substance use/abuse,

---

• BOX 14.1 Symptoms of Compassion Fatigue

Symptoms of Compassion Fatigue		
Emotional	**Behavioral**	**Cognitive**
• Powerlessness	• Impatient	• Perfectionism
• Anxiety	• Withdrawn	• Spacing out
• Guilt	• Irritable	• Loss of meaning
• Anger/rage	• Sleep disturbances	• Self-doubt
• Hypersensitivity	• Hypervigilance	• Minimization
• Overwhelmed	• Accident prone	• Distractibility
• Detachment from emotion	• Losing things	• Memory issues
• Depression	• Crying spells	• Losing things
• Emotional roller coaster	• Self-destructive decision making (drugs, alcohol, food, etc.)	• Negative or defeating self-talk
		• Preoccupation with trauma
Physical	**Personal Relationships**	**Spiritual**
• Shock	• Withdrawal	• Loss of purpose
• Rapid heartbeat	• Mistrust	• Questioning the meaning of life
• Dizziness and disorientation	• Loneliness	
• Depleted energy	• Isolation	• Lack of self-satisfaction

Created by Laura Munger. Printed with permission.

Life Balance Worksheet

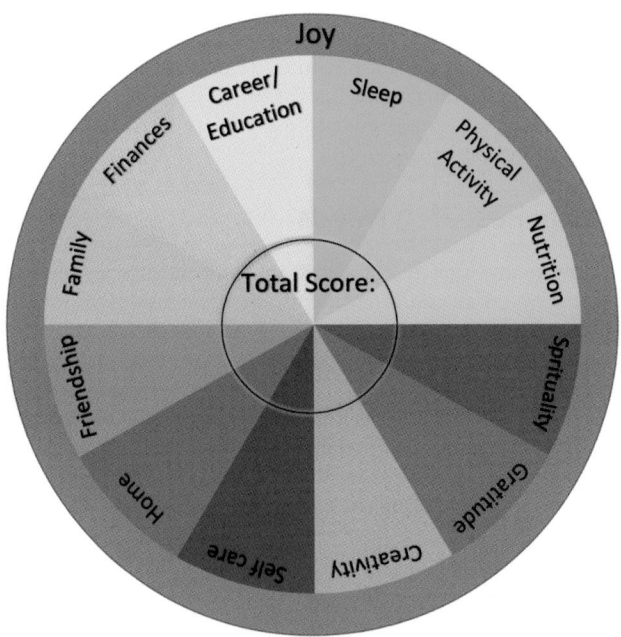

physical/emotional abuse, or simply homes where this was modeled in some way.

How to Treat Compassion Fatigue

Munger Theory

Created by Laura Munger, LMSW, this worksheet was designed to determine the current perceived level of life balance. The worksheet should be completed by both a PLWBC and an Onc R clinician regarding their respective situations. There should be concern for CF if either the clinician or PLWBC has a low score. This lack of emotional acuity from both parties has the potential to cause a huge challenge as the Onc R clinician is working from a less capable place and their best self is reduced. It is important to keep the life balance strong in clinicians to prevent CF and be emotionally available for their patients. See Figure 14.2—Life Balance Worksheet. Instructions: In each slice of the Life Balance Pie, the person should rate how satisfied/happy that they are with this area of our life. Ratings are as follows: 1—Not satisfied at all; 2—Dissatisfied but working on it; 3—Neither satisfied nor dissatisfied; 4—Fairly satisfied but need to devote more time to it; 5—Completely satisfied. Total: Add the numbers together for a total life balance score.

Other Interventions for Compassion Fatigue

Self-Care

Self-care is essential for each Onc R clinician to keep their physical, mental, emotional, and social wellness at the highest function level possible. Self-care practices may include a healthy plant-based nutritional program, regular physical activity including aerobic, resistive and flexibility exercises, yoga, Tai chi, Qigong,

• **BOX 14.2**   **Prevention Through Gratitude**

Prevention Through Gratitude
Grateful
Release what isn't mine
Awareness within me (symptoms)
Trust
I am statements
Tools
Unapologetically me and it's enough
Define where my responsibility begins and ends
Enjoy my life

walking out in nature, massage, mental health therapy, counseling, meditative practices (singing bowls, guided meditations/imagery, pranayama, or breathing practices). It is important to find what self-care intervention works for each Onc R clinician to assist in providing balance to life.

Prevention Through Gratitude

Below is an acronym created by Laura Munger, LMSW, used for PLWBCs and Onc R clinicians. This serves as a quick reference, can be easily remembered, and is convenient to carry in a wallet or purse or keep a picture on one's phone to assist with reducing consuming thoughts and the corresponding depression and anxiety. See Box 14.2 Prevention Through Gratitude for an in-depth description of what the process is with each letter of the acronym.

G/Grateful: Utilizing the power of gratitude to help us develop a mindset that promotes positive thinking and effective coping. When we are going through difficult times, it is easy to become focused on all of the negative and traumatic events that are going on in our lives. However, when you have daily rituals to practice gratitude via meditation, prayer, or journaling, evidence shows that we re-train our minds to look for these elements more often versus focusing on the distressing events.

R/Release What Isn't Mine: Another source of stress for many people is worry, stress, or taking responsibility for things or people that are not their responsibility. For example, as a clinician you may find yourself agonizing over different ways to get through to a client that is resistant, yet the responsibility to buy into the therapy process also lies heavily with the PLWBC. It is important to set boundaries on what we can each do within our scope of practice. We can provide resources to PLWBC and their caregivers and then release the responsibility to the PLWBC.

A/Awareness Within Me (symptoms): For many of us, this is a very critical step. That is, we must develop the awareness around what it feels like in our bodies to be stressed, anxious, overwhelmed, or depressed. Many people are not in tune with this. In meditation, this is a key skill that is developed: the art of knowing when and how emotions show up in our bodies. How does that feel to us? Although the "A" is third in the acronym, it is often the first step in knowing when we need to sit quietly to engage in any relaxation technique. Awareness is also about being aware of our thoughts and emotions. Many people are so used to "pushing through" or "pushing past" instead of hitting the pause button to fully connect to what is going on with them so that they can work through it.

T/Trust: If you are going to release what is not your responsibility that means that you have to entrust someone else in whatever it is. Who do you trust—the medical team?, the follow through of the PLWBC?, your spiritual higher power (if this is something that you believe in)? It is important to trust that what you are doing will have a positive outcome.

I/I Am Statements: Dr. Wayne Dyer speaks of the power of the "I am…" statement. It is considered that we manifest whatever comes after the "I am." For example, statements like "I am so tired.", "I am afraid.", "I am so sick of this." are said to actually attract more of these things in our life. In the theory such as the Law of Attraction, we are like human magnets. So, with these statements, the theory is that we are attracting more reasons to be tired, afraid, and frustrated. However, if you change those statements to "I am excited to get more rest.", "I am confident in the steps that I am taking to help the PLWBC.", "I am proud of myself. I am a good clinician.", "I am looking forward to better days ahead.", "I am healthy.", and "I am faithful." These types of statements also manifest attraction, only now we have changed our "magnet" to attract the things we want to attract.

T/Tools: Once we learn coping skills, it is important that we use them! Utilizing coping tools only when in a therapy session will not provide positive outcomes. Just as it is important to complete physical exercises and follow instructions for good posture prescribed by clinicians, it is also important to complete coping exercises and follow instructions for stress relief. It is the dedication to using the tools learned on a regular basis that will provide the strategies for success.

U/Unapologetically Me and It's Enough: There is nothing more important than developing a strong sense of self. In the book, *The Gifts of Imperfection* by Brene Brown, she discusses the difference between fitting in and belonging. When we try to fit in, she says, we end up hustling for our worth. However, when learn to be authentic, we naturally belong. We are *enough* as is. Be confident in all that you are doing, be confident in who you are and be unapologetic about it. It's enough.

D/Define Where Your Responsibility Begins and Ends: This is simply for emphasis, and you can refer to R/Release What Isn't Mine. This is a tough habit to break and needs lots of repetition.

E/Enjoy Your Life: The whole reason that Laura Munger developed this acronym is because when we are weighted down by the things that cause us distress, it can often prevent us from experiencing joy. The goal is to feel joy. You work so hard caring for others. When the workday is over, it is time for you. Enjoy your life. You deserve it and have earned it.

Conclusion

The psychosocial elements of persons diagnosed with, treated for, and living with or beyond cancer are multifaceted and deep. This multitude of emotional, social, financial, and cognitive influences can truly shape one's life each and every day. As Onc R clinicians,

it is imperative to have a thorough understanding of the potential impact that psychosocial and psychoemotional issues have on healing and QOL of each individual. It is also necessary to know when to refer to a mental health practitioner or other professional to assist the individual in building strategies to cope with the issues. With all that Onc R clinicians provide for patients and others, Onc R clinicians are at risk for CF. Prevention through gratitude and self-care needs to be a priority in the daily lives of Onc R clinicians.

Critical Research Needs

- How many Onc R clinicians are screening for psychosocial issues and what tools they are using?
- What is the referral pattern from Onc R clinicians to social work, psychology, and counseling after screening for psychosocial issues?
- What is the most prevalent psychosocial issue for cancer survivors—emotional, social, or financial?
- What is the greatest barrier to evaluation and treatment of psychosocial issues during the cancer journey?

Case Study

A 38-year-old female was recently diagnosed with Stage 3 estrogen receptor (ER)+/progesterone receptor (PR)+/and human epidermal growth factor receptor 2 (HER2-) breast cancer. She is referred to outpatient physical therapy. The medical record reflects that she had been scheduled for lumpectomy, chemotherapy, and radiation and her surgery was scheduled for one week after the initial physical therapy evaluation. The patient entered the physical therapy treatment room to meet the physical therapist (PT) for the first time. She appeared extremely angry and after introductions, the PT began the subjective portion of the examination. After only asking a few initial questions regarding when the cancer was diagnosed, the patient burst out in anger. She very loudly described how she had spent her life doing "everything right," including running 5 days/week, eating healthy food all the time, never smoking, and never drinking. She did not cry but was enraged that this could ever happen to her as she had "taken perfect care of herself." The PT tried to divert the conversation to describing what she could do now to prepare for her procedures, what red flags to look for, and which medical professional to contact if there were signs of any of the potential adverse effects. The patient sat with her arms crossed and did not answer, respond, or in any way participate in the conversation. The PT completed her physical examination, but the patient refused a treadmill test to determine baseline cardiorespiratory function. The patient never returned for follow-up visits nor answered any phone calls from the PT. The PT was also devastated by this encounter. She felt great guilt in not being able to connect with the patient and never knowing how she managed her treatments.

How could the PT have handled this situation differently?

This is where the Onc R clinician needs to allow a patient some safe space and time to talk before pushing too fast into evaluation and treatment. Using refocusing techniques may also help, such as, "How about considering saying to yourself—'I have always taken good care of myself and I will continue to. I am a healthy individual and working through this will make me even stronger.'" Of course, referral to a mental health practitioner is absolutely necessary.

What can the PT do to help him/her mentally and emotionally move past this encounter?

Onc R clinicians should also allow themselves time to talk about challenges with patients. Finding a kind ear to listen and keeping confidentiality of the person involved, can assist the clinician in mentally and emotionally working through the challenge.

Making an appointment with a mental health professional can help a clinician as well. Finding a meditation, mindfulness, or yoga practice can decrease the stress of the day. It is important to take the Life Balance screening to also identify areas that need work. We are all a work in progress.

Review Questions

Reader can find the correct answers and rationale in the back of the book.

1. The four areas of most importance in the psychosocial realm include all of the following except:
    A. Emotional
    B. Social
    C. Cognitive
    D. Spiritual

2. A patient exhibits muscle irritability, is easily fatigued, has heightened worry and somatic complaints such as digestive issues. You are concerned that they are suffering from:
    A. Depression
    B. Anxiety
    C. PTSD
    D. Grief and loss

3. A patient reports feelings of hopelessness, sadness, restlessness, and feelings of guilt and worthlessness. You are concerned that they may be suffering from:
    A. Depression
    B. Anxiety
    C. PTSD
    D. Grief and loss

4. Evidence shows that _____% of healthcare professionals working in cancer care are at risk for CF.
    A. 15%
    B. 20%
    C. 25%
    D. 30%

5. The 6th vital sign is:
    A. Distress
    B. Anxiety
    C. Depression
    D. PTSD

6. When a child exhibits behavior changes such as appetite changes, sleep disturbances, and/or problems in school, they may be suffering from _____.
    A. Social awkwardness
    B. Distress
    C. Sore throat
    D. Sadness

7. During chemotherapy, patients sometimes dwell on the future and their fears of "what may happen" and "what could happen" with significant focus only on the future. Onc R clinicians should:
    A. Redirect to the present moment by saying: I know this can be scary but tell me what you'll do if this treatment doesn't work
    B. Redirect to the present moment by saying: I know this can be scary but tell me something that makes you feel encouraged today
    C. Reframing the situation: Let's talk about your nutrition intake
    D. Reframing the situation: Let's do some deep breathing exercises

8. The presence of depression in breast cancer survivors is associated with a _____ higher risk of cancer recurrence.
    A. 4%
    B. 14%
    C. 24%
    D. 34%

9. A patient displays negative self-talk during physical therapy treatment. The most effective intervention is to reframe the self-talk to positive and empowering words. If a person states: "I just can't do this," the MOST EFFECTIVE reframe is:
    A. I am proud of myself for doing something hard
    B. Crying is normal and vulnerability is courageous.
    C. This is really hard but I will get there
    D. Even with genetics, there is a lot that I can control.

10. One form of Compassion fatigue can be described as:
    A. natural consequent behaviors and emotions resulting from thinking about a traumatizing event experienced in one's youth
    B. combined effects of the caregiver's continuous visualizing of client's traumatic images added to the effects of burnout causing caregiver debilitation
    C. extreme state of excessive concern for the suffering of oneself during an illness
    D. State of physical and mental exhaustion caused by one's own cancer diagnosis and treatment

References

1. National Cancer Institute. Dictionary of cancer terms—psychosocial. https://www.cancer.gov/publications/dictionaries/cancer-terms/def/psychosocial. Accessed January 20, 2021.
2. American Cancer Society. Psychosocial support options for people with cancer. https://www.cancer.org/treatment/survivorship-during-and-after-treatment/coping/understanding-psychosocial-support-services.html. Accessed April 25, 2021.
3. American Cancer Society. Americans with disabilities act: information for people facing cancer. https://www.cancer.org/treatment/finding-and-paying-for-treatment/understanding-health-insurance/health-insurance-laws/americans-with-disabilities-act.html. May 13, 2019. Accessed January 21, 2021.

4. National Institute of Mental Health. National Institute of Health. Depression. https://www.nimh.nih.gov/health/topics/depression/?ftag=MSF0951a18. February 2018. Accessed February 21, 2021.

5. Niedzwidez CL, Knifton L, Robb KA, Katikireddi SV, Smith DJ. Depression and anxiety among people living with and beyond cancer: a growing clinical and research priority. *BMC Cancer.* 2019;19:943. doi:10.1186/s12885-019-6181-4.

6. Milligan F, Martinez F, Aal SHMA, et al. Assessing anxiety and depression in cancer patients. *Br J Nurs.* 2018;27(10):S18–S23. doi:10.12968/bjon.2018.27.10.S18.

7. Bortolato B, Hyphantis TN, Valpione SV, et al. Depression in cancer: the many biobehavioral pathways driving tumor progression. *Cancer Treat Rev.* 2017;52:58–70.

8. Wang X, Wang N, Zhong L, et al. Prognostic value of depression and anxiety on breast cancer recurrence and mortality: a systematic review and meta-analysis of 282,203 patients. *Mol Psychiatry.* 2020;25:3186–3197.

9. Wang YH, Li JQ, Shi JF, et al. Depression and anxiety in relationship to cancer incidence and mortality: a systematic review and metaanalysis of cohort studies. *Mol Psychiatry.* 2020;25:1487–1499.

10. National Institute of Mental Health. National Institute of Health. Post-traumatic stress disorder. https://www.nimh.nih.gov/health/publications/post-traumatic-stress-disorder-ptsd/. 2020. Accessed February 21, 2021.

11. Leano A, Korman MB, Goldberg L, Ellis J. Are we missing PTSD in our patients with cancer? Part I *Canadian Oncol Nurs J.* 2019;9(2):141–146.

12. Cordova MJ, Riba MB, Speigel D. Post-traumatic stress disorder and cancer. *Lancet Psychiatry.* 2017;4(4):330–338. doi:10.1016/S2215-0366(17)30014-7.

13. Brown LC, Murphy AR, Lalonde CS, et al. Posttraumatic stress disorder and breast cancer: risk factors and the role of inflammation and endocrine function. *Cancer.* 2020;126(14):3181–3191.

14. Psycom. The 5 stages of grief. https://www.psycom.net/depression.central.grief.html. May 4, 2021. Accessed May 15, 2021.

15. Sun L, Ang E, Ang WHD, Lopez V. Losing the breast: a metasynthesis of the impact in women breast cancer survivors. *Psycho-Oncology.* 2017;27(2):376–385.

16. American Cancer Society. Sources of support. https://www.cancer.org/treatment/Carers/listen-with-your-heart/sources-of-support.html. July 12, 2019. Accessed March 27, 2021.

17. Cancer Survivors Network. American Cancer Society. https://csn.cancer.org/. Accessed March 27, 2021.

18. Cancer Support Community. American Cancer Society. https://www.cancersupportcommunity.org/virtual-programs. Accessed on March 27, 2021.

19. Cancer Hope Network. American Cancer Society. https://www.cancerhopenetwork.org/get-support/support/. Accessed March 27, 2021.

20. Moussas GI, Papadopoulou AG. Substance abuse and cancer. *Psychiatriki.* 2017;28:234–241.

21. Lee YH, Salman A. The mediating effect of spiritual well-being on depressive symptoms and health related quality of life among elders. *Arch Psychiatr Nurs.* 2018;32:418–424.

22. Lee YH. Spiritual care for cancer patients. *Asia Pac J Oncol Nurs.* 2019;6(2):101–103. doi:10.4103/apjon.apjon_65_18.

23. Kelly EP, Paredes AZ, Tsilimigras DI, Hyer JM, Pawlik TM. The role of religion and spirituality in cancer care: an umbrella review of the literature. *Surg Oncol.* 2020. doi:10.1016/j.suronc.2020.05.004.

24. National Cancer Institute. Definition: financial toxicity. https://www.cancer.gov/search/results?swKeyword=financial+toxicity. Accessed February 21, 2021.

25. Family and Medical Leave Act. https://www.dol.gov/agencies/whd/fmla. Accessed May 15, 2021.

26. Ownby KK. Use of the distress thermometer in clinical practice. *J Adv Pract Oncol.* 2019;10(2):175–179.

27. Cormio C, Caporale F, Spatuzzi R, et al. Psychosocial distress in oncology: using the distress thermometer for assessing risk classes. *Support Care Cancer.* 2019;27:4115–4121.

28. Cutillo A, O'Hea E, Person S, et al. NCCN distress thermometer: cut off points and clinical utility. *Oncol Nurs Forum.* 2017;44(3):329–336.

29. Tran TXM, Park J, Lee J, Junt YS, Chang Y, Cho H. Utility of the patient-reported Outcomes Measurement Information System (PROMIS) to measure primary health of cancer patients: a systematic review. *Support Care Cancer.* 2021;29:1723–1739.

30. Jensen RE, Moinpour CM, Potosky AL, et al. Responsiveness of 8 PROMIS measures in a large, community-based cancer study cohort. *Cancer.* 2017;123(2):327–335.

31. Cella DF, Tulsky DS, Gray G, et al. The Functional Assessment of Cancer Therapy (FACT) scale: development and validation of the general measure. *J Clin Oncol.* 1993;11(3):570–579.

32. Pelpert JD, Cella D. Bifactor analysis confirmation of the factorial structure of the Functional Assessment of Cancer Therapy-General (FACT-G). *Psychooncology.* 2019;28:1149–1152.

33. Shim EJ, Hahm BJ, Yu ES, et al. Development and validation of the National Cancer Center Psychological Symptom Inventory. *Psychooncology.* 2017;26(7):1036–1043.

34. Hinz A, Mehnert A, Kocalevent RD, et al. Assessment of depression severity with PHQ-9 in cancer patients and in the general population. *BMC Psychiatry.* 2016;16:22. doi:10.1186/s12888-016-0728-6.

35. Wagner LI, Phgh SL, Small W Jr, et al. Screening for depression in cancer patients receiving radiotherapy: feasibility and identification of effective tools on NRG Oncology RTOG 0841. *Cancer.* 2017;123(3):485–493.

36. American Psychological Association. Center for epidemiological studies, depression. https://www.apa.org/pi/about/publications/caregivers/practice-settings/assessment/tools/depression-scale. 2011. Accessed February 21, 2021.

37. Hann D, Winter K, Jacobsen P. Measurement of depressive symptoms in cancer patients: evaluation of the Center for Epidemiological Studies Depression Scale (CES-D). *J Psychosom Res.* 1999;46(5):437–443.

38. Mindfulness Based Stress Reduction. https://mbsrtraining.com/jon-kabat-zinn/. Accessed February 21, 2021.

39. Sarenmalm EK, Martensson LB, Anderson BA, Karlsson P, Bergh I. Mindfulness and its efficacy for psychological and biological responses in women with breast cancer. *Cancer Med.* 2017;6(5):1108–1122.

40. Simply Psychology. Cognitive behavioral therapy. https://www.simply-psychology.org/cognitive-therapy.html. Accessed February 21, 2021.

41. American Psychological Association. What is cognitive behavioral therapy? https://www.apa.org/ptsd-guideline/patients-and-families/cognitive-behavioral. Accessed April 25, 2021.

42. Mindfulness Based Cognitive Therapy. https://www.mbct.com/. Accessed April 25, 2021.

43. Psychology Today. Motivational interviewing. https://www.psychologytoday.com/us/thrapy-types/motivational-interviewing. Accessed April 25, 2021.

44. Spencer JC, Wheeler SB. A systematic review of motivational interviewing interventions in cancer patients and survivors, *Patient Educ Couns.* 2016;99(7):1099–1105.

45. Society for Integrative Oncology. What is integrative oncology. https://integrativeonc.org/knowledge-center/what-is-integrative-oncology. Accessed April 25, 2021.

46. Viscuss PV, Price K, Millstine D, et al. Integrative medicine in cancer survivors. *Curr Opin Oncol.* 2017;29(4):235–242.

47. Geue L, Goetze J, Buttstaedt M, et al. An overview of art therapy interventions for cancer patients and the results of research. *Comp Ther Med.* 2010;18(3–4):160–170.

48. Breastcancer.org. Music therapy. https://www.breastcancer.org/treatment/comp_med/types/music; September 19, 2018. Accessed April 25, 2021.

49. American Institute for Cancer Research. How mindfulness meditation can help cancer survivors cope with stress. https://www.aicr.org/news/how-mindfulness-meditation-can-help-cancer-survivors-cope-with-stress/. Accessed April 25, 2021.

50. Gerritsen RJS, Band GPH. Breath of life: the respiratory vagal stimulation model of contemplative activity. *Front Hum Neurosci.* 2018;12:397. doi:10.3389/fnhum.2018.00397.

51. Hatamipour K, Rassouli M, Yaghmaie F, Zendedel K, Majd HA. Spiritual needs of cancer patients: a qualitative study. *Indian J Palliat Care.* 2015;21(1):61–67.

52. Sabo B. Reflecting on the concept of compassion fatigue. *Online J Issues Nurs.* 2011;16(1):1. doi:10.3912/OJIN.Vol16No01Man01.

53. Gentry JE. Compassion fatigue: a crucible of transformation. *J Trauma Pract.* 2002;1(3–4):37–61. doi:10.1300/J189v01n03_03.

54. Hunt P, Denieffe S, Gooney M. Running on empathy: relationship of empathy to compassion satisfaction and compassion fatigue in cancer healthcare professionals. *Eur J Cancer Care.* 2019;28:e13124.

UNIT III

Management of Common Oncologic Diagnoses

15

Breast Cancer

JILL BINKLEY, PT, MSc, CLT, PAAOMPT, DEBORAH DOHERTY, PT, PhD

CHAPTER OUTLINE

Introduction

Currently, breast cancer (BC) is the most diagnosed cancer worldwide with 2.26 million cases in 2020 and the fifth leading cause of cancer death (after lung, colorectal, liver, stomach).[1] Incidence rates vary across the globe. Belgium has the highest rate of BC in women (113.2 per 100,000), Luxembourg is the second highest (109.3 per 100,000) and the United States (US) is 22nd (84.9 per 100,000).[2]

Statistics

In 2021, it is estimated that 281,550 (up from 276,480 in 2020) new cases of BC were diagnosed in women in the US[3] and 2650 in men.[4] BC represents 14.8% of all new cancer cases in the US in women[3] and less than 1% in men. Globally, BC is the fifth most common cause of death from cancer in women and represents about 25% of all cancers in women. Within the US, BC is the third leading cause of cancer-related deaths in women (after lung and colorectal) with an estimated 43,600 (up from 42,170 in 2020) deaths occurring estimated for 2021[3] and 530 deaths in men.[4] BC accounts for 7.2% of all cancer deaths in the US.[3] Approximately 12.9% of women, or one in eight, will be diagnosed with BC in their lifetime.[3] Today there are approximately 3.8 million women living with BC in the US.[4] and the 5-year relative survival rate (from 2011 to 2017 data) is 90.3% for females of all races. This includes 99% with localized stage BC, 86.8% with regional stage, and 29.0% with distant stage.[3]

Female BC incidence rates are highest among non-Hispanic (NH) White women at 130.8 per 100,000, followed closely by NH Black women (126.7 per 100,000). However, the BC death rate is highest among NH Black women at 28.4 deaths per 100,000 which is estimated at greater than double that in Asian/Pacific Islander women (11.5 per 100,000) where the lowest incidence and death rates are found.[5] The lifetime risk for men is 1 in 833.[4] NH Black men had the highest incidence of BC at 1.89 cases per 100,000 standard population and death rates at 0.53 deaths per 100,000 standard population compared to men in other racial and ethnic groups.[6]

Risk Factors

Established[7–9] and emerging[9] risk factors for BC in females are noted in Tables 15.1 and 15.2. The most common risk factors for BC in males are noted in Table 15.3. These risk factors are essential information for oncology rehabilitation (Onc R) clinicians to provide education at all levels of prevention (see Chapter 2 for the five levels of prevention).

Family history of BC is associated with a higher risk of the disease: women with one first-degree relative with BC have almost twice the risk of women without a family history. If two first-degree relatives have a history of BC then the risk is five times higher than a woman without a family history.[10] Some inherited mutations, particularly BRCA1, BRCA2 and p53, result in a very high risk of BC. While the incidence of BC in the general population is 13%, the incidence of BC in an individual who inherits the BRCA1 variant is 55% to 72% and the BRCA2 variant is 45% to 69%.[10–11] Germline mutations in these genes are infrequent and account for only 2% to 5% of cases. During the carcinogenic process, mutations and epigenetic modifications in oncogenes and tumor suppressor genes may be acquired by cancer cells (see Chapter 4 for more details).

Pathogenesis

Breast tissue varies at different stages of life in response to host hormonal status and other environmental influences. As such, some risk factors may have different effects at different ages. Hormones play an important role in BC because they modulate the structure and growth of epithelial tumor cells.[8] Different cancers vary in hormone sensitivity. The immunohistochemical profile of a BC tumor is analyzed for hormone involvement. This assists in determining the diagnosis of the BC and guides subsequent treatment. BCs are classified by the extent to which they are responsive to progesterone and estrogen related to growth. BC cells that have estrogen receptors are referred to as estrogen-positive (ER+) and cells that have progesterone receptors are called progesterone-positive (PR+) cancers. If they do not have these receptors, they are in turn referred to as estrogen-negative (ER-) and progesterone-negative (PR-). ER+ is expressed in approximately 80% of

TABLE 15.1 Established Risk Factors for Breast Cancer in Women

1. Being a woman
2. Age
3. Family history of cancer
4. Genetics/genetic mutations
5. Personal history of breast cancer
6. Radiation to chest or face before age 30
7. Certain breast changes, such as atypical hyperplasia
8. Race/ethnicity, higher risk in White women, more aggressive triple negative breast cancer in Black women
9. Being overweight or obese
10. Pregnancy/reproductive history
11. Breastfeeding history, breastfeeding reduces risk due to decreased number of menstrual cycles
12. Early menarche and/or late menopause, period of time between onset and cessation of menstrual cycling strongly correlates with increased breast cancer risk in women
13. Use of hormone replacement therapy
14. Alcohol consumption
15. Dense breasts
16. Sedentary lifestyle, lack of physical activity
17. Smoking
18. History of taking the drug diethylstilbestrol (DES) to prevent miscarriage, have a higher risk or women whose mothers took DES.
19. Breast implants

Created by Deborah J. Doherty. Printed with permission.

TABLE 15.2 Emerging and Proposed Risk Factors for Breast Cancer in Women

1. Low vitamin D levels
2. Light exposure at night/shift work
3. Nutritional contributors
4. Exposure to chemicals in cosmetics, food, lawn and garden treatments, plastic, sunscreen, water, and grilled foods

Created by Deborah J. Doherty. Printed with permission.

TABLE 15.3 Established Risk Factors for Male Breast Cancer

1. Age
2. Family history of breast cancer
3. Genetic mutations (such as BRCA1/BRCA2)
4. Radiation therapy to chest
5. Increased estrogen levels
   a. Hormone therapy treatments that contain estrogen
   b. Overweight or obese, which increases production of estrogen
   c. Exposure to environmental estrogens (hormone fed beef cattle or chemical products of pesticide DDT that mimic effects of estrogen in body)
   d. Liver disease (including heavy use of alcohol)—cirrhosis lowers androgen levels and raises estrogen
6. Klinefelter's syndrome results in lower levels of androgens and higher levels of estrogen and can increase risk of BC along with radiation exposure to chest, if being treated for lymphoma
7. Conditions that affect the testicles such as injury, swelling, or removal

Created by Deborah J. Doherty. Printed with permission.

term utilized is HER2 positive (HER2+).[12] Of these, at least 50% are co-expressed with hormone receptors.[12,13] As a result, it plays an important role in the tumor cell proliferation and survival pathways. There are also subtypes of HER2 with the most common subtype called HER2-enriched or HER2-E. About 50% of HER2+ tumors are HER2-E.[12]

The androgen receptor (AR) is another protein marker that is immunoexpressed in 60% to 80% of BCs.[12,13] It appears to have conflicting roles in BCs. Interestingly this is also expressed in prostate tumors and most often expressed with HER2+ and triple negative (ER-, PR-, HER2-) breast tumors.[13] This represents challenges that are being investigated but also opportunities as AR appears to either stimulate or inhibit cellular proliferation and promote metastases in ER+ BC cells. The role of AR is conflicting as it appears that the tumor microenvironment and circulating levels of estrogens and androgens play a role in its function. While AR is usually considered to be associated with positive prognosis in ER+ BC, there are now findings that suggest if the levels of AR are too high, it can contribute to the cells becoming resistant to therapies. AR is also known to stimulate cellular proliferation in the BCs that are classified as triple negative.[13] This will be discussed later. AR represents a new target for therapeutic interventions.

Other biomarkers include the epidermal growth factor receptor (EGFR), p53, c-myc, and proliferation markers such as Ki-67.[12] Hormone sensitivity, biomarkers and gene expression will determine treatment and subsequent potential adverse effects from those treatments. Onc R clinicians can utilize this information to strategize a treatment plan for preventing and managing the potential adverse effects.

Diagnosis, Staging, and Classification of BC

Classification of BC involves a multitude of factors that require extensive study to understand the details. More common classifications will be addressed here. Clinical staging of BC begins with the TNM System. This staging system categorizes the cancer in terms of tumor (T) size, regional lymph node (N) involvement

BCs and PR+ in about 65%.[12] They co-express in the majority of BCs. When co-expressed, they are referred to as hormone-receptor-positive (HR+) cancers. This is the most common subtype of BC (60%–90%). They have a relatively better prognosis than hormone-receptor-negative (HR-) cancers, which are likely to be of higher pathological grade and can be more difficult to treat. Many BCs also produce hormones, such as growth factors, that act locally, and these can both stimulate and inhibit the tumor's growth.

The human epidermal growth factor receptor 2 (HER2) is a protein biomarker that is present in about 15% to 20% of BC.[12] HER2 is a protein on the outside of all breast cells that promotes growth. When this biomarker is overexpressed or amplified, the and absence or presence of metastases (M). BC can also be categorized using a 5-stage system: Stage 0 describes noninvasive ductal carcinoma in situ (DCIS) and Stages I through IV indicate invasive BC. Within each of these stages are many subcategories and variables. Numerous online resources are available to discover the details of all of the categories. When considering the tumor size, the acronym TX refers to a tumor that cannot be evaluated. T0 means there is no evidence of cancer, Ts refers to carcinoma exclusively in the ducts. The T with a number (1–4) and letter (a–d) following determines the size of the tumor. For example, T2 represents a tumor between 20 and 50 mm. Lymph nodes are also analyzed and designated as an N. Regional lymph nodes include those located in the axilla, above or below the clavicle, and those under the sternum. If there is a designation of NX, then nodes were not evaluated, and N0 indicates no cancer was found in nodes or areas of cancer are smaller than 0.2 mm. N followed by a number (1–3) denotes the range of number of nodes where the cancer has spread. For example, N2 means there is spread of cancer to either 10 or more axillary lymph nodes or to clavicular nodes. Lastly, the M designation refers to whether there is spread of cancer to other areas of the body. MX means spread cannot be evaluated. M0 refers to no evidence of distant metastases, M0(i+) means no clinical evidence of metastases but there is evidence of tumor cells in the blood, bone marrow, or other nodes, while M1 indicates that there is evidence of metastasis to other body parts. In this case, the tumor size and node involvement are not relevant. Each staging category provides the oncologist with more information that is used to determine medical treatment. Refer to Cancer. Net at https://www.cancer.net/cancer-types/breast-cancer/stages and American Cancer Society at https://www.cancer.org/cancer/breast-cancer/understanding-a-breast-cancer-diagnosis/stages-of-breast-cancer.html for a detailed list of all TNM staging categories. Please refer to Chapters 1 and 4 for further explanation.

BC is classified as noninvasive (preinvasive) or invasive with numerous subtypes. If there are no special features to determine a special subtype, then it may also be called not otherwise specified (NOS) or no special type (NST). Noninvasive BC refers to BC that is localized in either the milk duct (ductal carcinoma in-situ [DCIS]) or lobules of the breast (lobular carcinoma in-situ [LCIS]). Noninvasive cancers not found can become invasive.[14]

DCIS, also called intraductal carcinoma, is considered Stage 0 BC. DCIS is a proliferation of neoplastic luminal cells confined to the ductolobular system.[14] This type of cancer cell is found within the milk ducts, but with no evidence of spread to nearby tissue or beyond. DCIS represents about 20% to 25% of all BC in the US, or over 60,000 new diagnoses annually. In the UK and the Netherlands there are over 7000 and 2500 annual DCIS diagnoses, respectively.[14] LCIS and atypical lobular hyperplasia (ALH) are both considered a lobular neoplasia. Lobular refers to abnormal cell growth starting in the lobules, which are glands responsible for milk production at the end of a breast duct. In LCIS and ALH, there is no spread to surrounding tissues. LCIS represents 5.3% of all in situ cancers and is thought to have a low risk for transforming into an invasive lobular BC. Further categorization occurs in both DCIS and LCIS and will be discussed below.

The majority of BC in women and men is invasive. Invasive BC is the type of cancer that occurs when abnormal cell growth extends out of the lobules or milk ducts and moves into nearby breast tissue or lymph nodes. Invasive ductal carcinoma or infiltrating ductal carcinoma (IDC) is the most common form of invasive BC with a rate of occurrence at 70% to 75% of all BCs, followed by invasive lobular carcinoma (ILC) at 5% to 15% of cases.

Figure 15.1 demonstrates the normal breast and where the ducts are located. Figure 15.2 demonstrates the microscopic level of the normal breast duct and the changes to hyperplasia, to DCIS, and finally to IDC.

Mixed invasive ductal and lobular carcinoma (IDLC) represents 5% of the cases.[15] IDC are abnormal cells originating in lining of the breast milk duct that have invaded surrounding tissue.

The remainder and less common IDCs are classified into many special types often named for the microscopic description, including adenoid cystic carcinoma, low-grade adenosquamous carcinoma or metaplastic carcinoma, medullary carcinoma, mucinous or colloid carcinoma, and papillary carcinoma. Another example is invasive cribriform carcinoma (ICC) that invades stroma or connective tissues of the breast in nest-like formations between ducts and lobules. There are distinctive holes between the cancer cells. ICC constitutes only 0.3% to 6% of invasive BC, and some DCIS is also cribriform. It is reported to occur predominantly in women who exhibit a lower tumor grade. ICC can be diagnosed independently but can also be accompanied by other cancers such as tubular carcinoma (TC) upon which it would be classified as a mixed type. TC is also another subcategory of IDC. This low-grade cancer grows slowly and can occur in about 1% to 2% of all BCs.[16,17]

Invasive or infiltrating lobular carcinoma (ILC) starts in breast lobules that produce milk. It is the second most common form of invasive BC with a 5% to 15% occurrence rate.[18] ILC can also be classified into six histological subtypes, including solid, alveolar, tubulolobular, pleomorphic, classical, and mixed.

Triple negative BC (TNBC) accounts for 10% to 15% of all BCs. This BC is characterized by the absence of expression of ER, PR, and HER2 receptors, thus the designation of ER-, PR-, HER2-.[19] This BC has the poorest prognosis of all the BC subtypes because it is more aggressive and there are fewer treatment options.[20] There are six basic subtypes of TNBC including basal-like 1 (BL1), basal-like 2 (BL2), mesenchymal (M), mesenchymal stem-like (MSL) immunomodulatory (IM), and luminal androgen receptor (LAR) as well as an unspecified group (UNS). Additional newly discovered genomic alterations are further stratifying BC into at least 10 subtypes.[21] Seventy-five percent of the TNBCs are the basal-like subtype and are associated with an elevated DNA damage response and high Ki67 levels.

With consideration of the receptor or protein status of the BC cells, four main molecular subtypes have been identified for easy classification. The female BC subtypes and the percent prevalence of each are listed in Table 15.4. The most common BC subtype is luminal A or hormone positive (HR+) and HER2 negative (HER2-).[22,23]

Inflammatory BC (IBC) is a rare and aggressive form of BC. It is diagnosed in approximately 1% to 6% of BCs in the US but is responsible for 10% of BC deaths. However, IBC is diagnosed in 5% to 11% of women in Northern Africa.[24] IBC is further classified into two categories: primary IBC and secondary IBC, based on whether there is a sudden onset of skin changes or after a long history of non-inflammatory changes in the breast.[24] According to one study, there is no definitive molecular diagnosis criteria for IBC, although there are several molecular findings that have been identified in numerous studies including dermal lymphatic emboli, ductal or lobular, luminal, triple negative, and HER+.[24] The majority of women have had a recent breast abscess or non-inflammatory locally advanced BC.[25] The diagnosis is based on clinical findings including erythema, edema, and peau d'orange texture of the skin. Peau d'orange means "skin of an orange" describing the dimpled, thickened skin textured and may exhibit a red or darkened color.

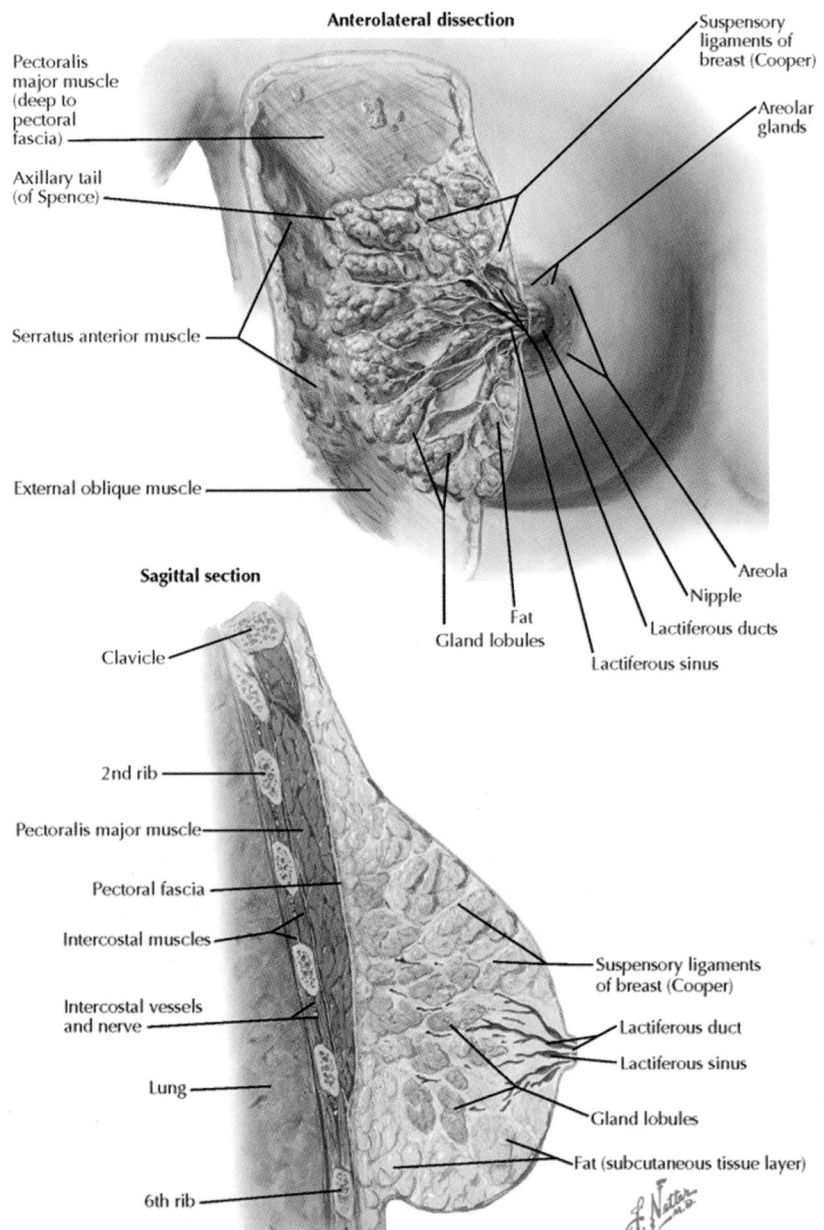

Anterolateral dissection

Suspensory ligaments of breast (Cooper)

Pectoralis major muscle (deep to pectoral fascia)

Areolar glands

Axillary tail (of Spence)

Serratus anterior muscle

External oblique muscle

Areola
Nipple
Lactiferous ducts
Lactiferous sinus
Fat
Gland lobules

Sagittal section

Clavicle

2nd rib

Pectoralis major muscle

Pectoral fascia

Intercostal muscles

Intercostal vessels and nerve

Lung

6th rib

Suspensory ligaments of breast (Cooper)
Lactiferous duct
Lactiferous sinus
Gland lobules
Fat (subcutaneous tissue layer)

• **Fig. 15.1** Normal Breast. (Reprinted with permission from Smith RP, Turek PJ. *Netter Collection of Medical Illustrations: Reproductive System*. Elsevier; 2011: Plate 13-1.)

Some risk factors have been identified, including women who experience menarche at an early age as well as the birth of their first child occuring after the age of 35. Breastfeeding that may exceed 24 months increases the risk as does obesity in premenopausal women. Although there are still a lot of unknowns and misdiagnoses, researchers are working globally to standardize the diagnosis and treatment for IBC. See Figure 15.3 for an example of the skin changes in IBC.

Paget disease, also referred to as Paget disease of the nipple or mammary Paget disease, is a rare cancer that is designated by cancer cells (called Paget cells) collecting in the epidermis of the skin around the nipple including the areola.[26] The nipple and areola become scaly, red, itchy, and/or irritated. The skin can become crusty or thickened and the nipple may flatten. Yellow or bloody nipple discharge can occur. Paget disease represents 1% to 4% of all BCs. In 80% to 90% of cases, there will also be either DCIS or another form of IDC.[26]

There are several rare BCs, two are noted here. Signet ring cells (SRCs) are found in IDC, ILC, and mucinous carcinoma.[27] They are categorized as a high (greater than 31%) or low (less than 30%) SRC tumor. SRCs are types of epithelial cells that contain intracytoplasmic mucins that can push the nucleus to one side. The cells appear like signet rings. Phyllodes tumors are a rare tumor (less than 1%) of the breast and most of them are benign.[28] A malignant phyllode tumor requires immediate intervention as they grow quickly but rarely spread outside the breast. These tumors invade the connective or stromal tissue of the breast. They resemble a leaf, thus the name phyllode which means leaf. Surgery is the main treatment as there is no evidence for the use of chemotherapy or

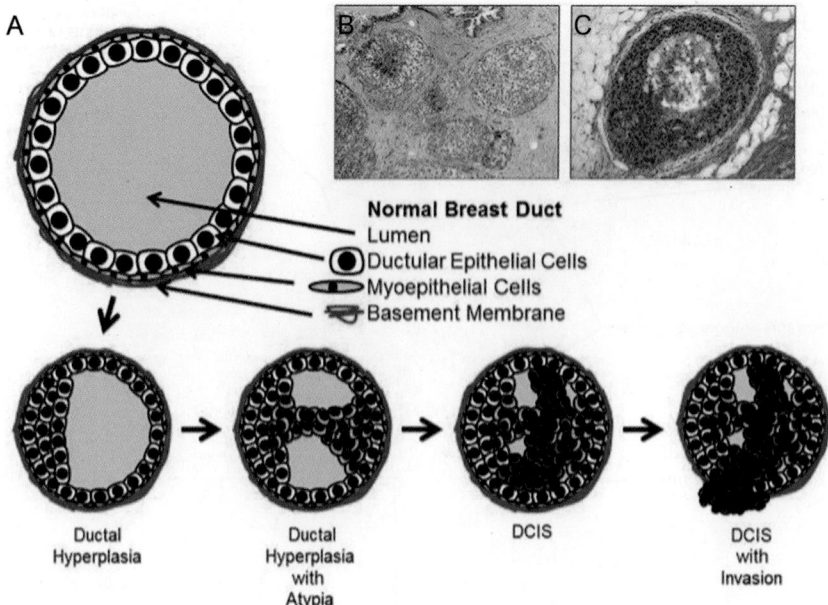

• **Fig. 15.2** Breast Duct Changes From Normal to Invasive Breast Cance. *DCIS,* Ductal carcinoma in situ. A Schematic normal to invasive DCIS; B and C Microscopic example of DCIS. (Reprinted with permission from Coleman WB. Breast ductal carcinoma in situ precursor to invasive breast cancer. *Am J Pathol.* 2019;189(5):942–945.)

TABLE 15.4	**Female Breast Cancer Subtypes**		
BC Subtype		Protein Status	Prevalence
Luminal A/normal-like		HR+/HER2–	68%
Luminal B		HR+/HER2+	10%
Triple negative		HR-/HER2–	10%
HER2-enriched or over-expressed		HR-/HER2+	4%
Unknown			7%

Created by Deborah J. Doherty. Printed with permission.

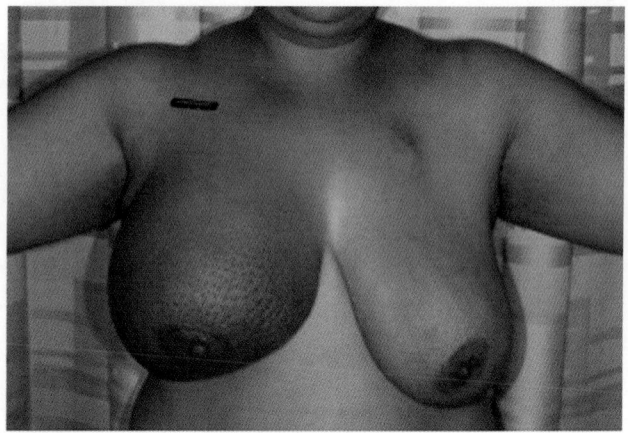

• **Fig. 15.3** Inflammatory Breast Cancer. (Reprinted with permission from TurningPoint Breast Cancer Rehabilitation.)

radiation. There can be recurrence as well as metastases which would occur in the lung, mediastinum, and skeleton.

Researchers are continually learning more about the molecular variation and histopathology of the many types and subtypes of BC. As such, it is imperative that an Onc R clinician be diligent in investigating the pathology of the BC diagnosis unique to each person with cancer (PWC). As details are gleaned about each diagnosis, medical management may be altered, impacting the timing and types of adverse effects encountered by the Onc R clinician.

Other Pathological Findings

Tumor Grade

The American Joint Committee on Cancer recommends the Modified Nottingham (Scarff-Bloom Richardson or SBR) tumor grade.[29] Nottingham grade is a multiparameter grading system where a grade is determined by totaling the score of three characteristics: (1) tubule formation: extent to which the tumor tissue

has normal breast (milk) duct structures; (2) nuclear pleomorphism grade: an evaluation of the size and shape of the nucleus in the tumor cells; and (3) mitotic count (how many dividing cells are present) which is a measure of how fast the tumor cells are growing and dividing the nuclear pleomorphism. The grade scoring is from GX to G3 and is determined by the following: each of the characteristics above gets a score between 1 and 3; a "1" means the cells and tumor tissue look the most like normal cells; "3" means the cells and tissue look the most abnormal. The scores for the three categories are added for a total score of 3 to 9. Total score = GX means the grade cannot be assessed.
• G1: Score is between 3 and 5 (Low combined histological grade or well differentiated).
• G2: Score is between 6 and 7 (Intermediate combined histologic grade or moderately differentiated).
• G3: Score is between 8 and 9 (High combined histologic grade).

The absence or presence of residual tumor after surgical treatment of BC is determined and categorized as follows: R0 = No residual tumor (or negative margins); R1 = Microscopic residual tumor (or micro + margin where tumor is not identified grossly at the margin but present microscopically at the margin); R2 = Macroscopic residual tumor (or macro + margin where tumor is identified grossly at the margin); RX = Presence of residual tumor cannot be assessed.[30] This is important to understand. A lack of clean margins may indicate that an additional surgery or a change in cancer treatment is likely.

Rate of Cell Growth

Rate of cell growth is important to determine how aggressive the BC is. Two common measurement tools for determining rate of cell growth are Synthesis Phase fraction (S Phase) and Ki-67.[31] S Phase fraction reports the percentage of cells in the sample that are in the process of copying their genetic information or DNA. The S-phase is low if it is <6%, intermediate if it is between 6% and 10%, and high if it is >10%. *Ki-67* is a cancer antigen (protein) in cells that functions in both interphase and mitotic cells. It sits on the surface of a cell and stimulates the production of an antibody. This protein increases as the cells prepare to divide into new cells. The more positive (+) cells there are, the more quickly they are dividing and forming new cells. Low protein count is 10%, moderate is 10% to 20%, and high is >20%.

Genomic Assays

Genomic assays (multigene signatures) have been developed commercially to assist in the prediction of clinical outcomes for persons diagnosed with BC.[32] Currently there are several types that are approved by the US Food and Drug Administration, including but not limited to: MammaPrint (70 gene signature), Veridex (76 gene signature), Genomic grade index (e.g., MapQuant Dx [97 gene signature], MapQuant Dx simplified (8 gene signature), Oncotype DX (21 gene recurrence score), Pro Signa test (50 gene signature), IHC4 assay, EndoPredict test (11 gene signature), and Theros (2 gene ratio molecular grade index). These assays are helpful in determining prognosis, including rate of recurrence, distant metastasis, and predicted response to therapy. The assay is selected based on hormone receptor status, histologic grade, *Ki*67 expression, HER2 status, and tissue type to determine which assay to use.

As Onc R clinicians, it is important to understand the value of these tests and how they assist the oncologist and PWC to determine the most effective treatment regimen. Increasing specificity of genetic profiling for BC will continue to promote individualized, person-centered, targeted medical managment.

Breast Cancer Surgeries

Surgical options for the treatment of BC include mastectomy (removal of the breast) with or without reconstruction and breast-conserving surgery (BCoS) (removal of only the tissue with cancer and just enough surrounding tissue to ensure clean margins).[33,34] In 2019–2020, 34% of women in the US with Stage I and II BC had mastectomies, 61% had BCoS, and 5% did not have surgery.[35] For individuals with Stage III BC, 68% had mastectomy, 20% had BCoS, and 12% did not have surgery. For PWC diagnosed with Stage IV metastatic BC (MeBC), 12% had mastectomies, 5% had BCoS, and 82% did not have surgery.[35] In women under age 40 with Stage I invasive BC examined between

2004 and 2014, 57.2% underwent mastectomy and 42.8% preferred BCoS.[35] During that same time, the rate of mastectomy increased from 43.6% to 62.5%.[35] Bilateral mastectomy was also significantly higher in 2014 at 73% compared to 31.5% in 2004. This increase in contralateral prophylactic mastectomy has interestingly demonstrated a significant increase in 10-year survival rate as compared to unilateral mastectomy. However, BCoS showed a significant increase in 10-year survival when compared to bilateral mastectomy. One study analyzed the trends of mastectomy and BCoS in a cohort in Saudi Arabia between 2009 and 2017 and found that 62.4% of females diagnosed with BC chose a mastectomy while 37.6% had BCoS. Approximately 60% to 70% (mastectomy-BCoS) of these women were over 40 years of age and another 20% to 30% (BCoS-mastectomy) were over 60 years.[36]

Mastectomy[33,34]

Mastectomy is the surgical removal of the whole breast. There are six common mastectomy procedures:

1. Simple (total)—removal of the entire breast including the nipple, areola, and skin; lymph nodes may be removed (Figure 15.4)
2. Skin sparing—most of the skin over the breast is left intact while breast tissue, nipple, and areola are removed
3. Nipple sparing (subcutaneous)—skin and nipple are left in place while the breast tissue is removed
4. Modified radical—removal of the breast (simple mastectomy) and removal of the axillary lymph nodes
5. Radical—removal of the entire breast, axillary lymph nodes, and pectoral muscles
6. Double or bilateral mastectomy—both breasts are removed often as a risk-reducing surgery or as a choice to provide symmetry for bilateral reconstruction

Breast-Conserving Surgery[34]

BCoS is the removal of the cancer with a small amount of normal breast tissue surrounding the cancer to obtain clean margins. This may include some lymph nodes for biopsy or chest wall lining if cancer is near it. This surgery may also be called: lumpectomy, re-excision quadrantectomy, wedge resection, partial mastectomy, breast-conserving or breast preservation surgery, or segmental mastectomy. Figure 15.5 is an example of a BCoS, or lumpectomy. Note the mild erythema and swelling related to radiation.

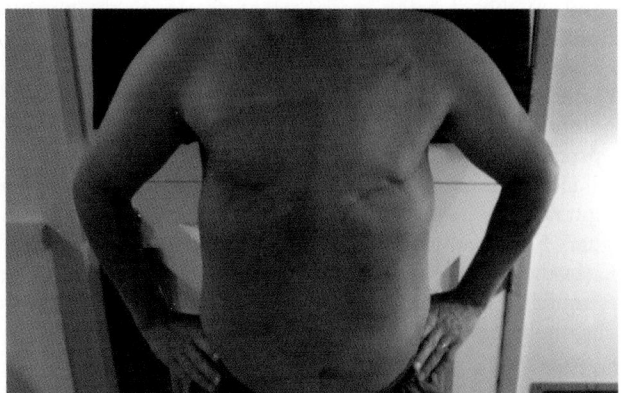

• **Fig. 15.4** Bilateral Mastectomies With Radiation Tanning of Right Chest Wall. (Reprinted with permission from TurningPoint Breast Cancer Rehabilitation.)

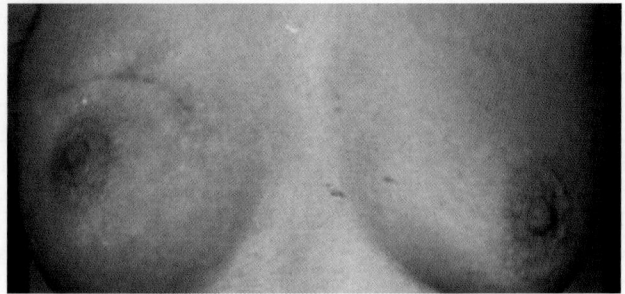

• **Fig. 15.5** Breast Conserving Surgery (Lumpectomy) on Right. (Reprinted with permission from Dixon JM, Macaskill FJ. *Breast Surgery*. Elsevier; 2019:86–104.)

Lymph Node Dissection

A varying number of lymph nodes are removed and biopsied to determine the spread of the BC. They can be removed during a biopsy, during breast surgery, or at some point after breast surgery. There are three levels of lymph nodes in the axilla with level I located at the bottom or lower edge of the pectoralis minor muscle; level II lies underneath the pectoralis minor muscle and level III is above the pectoralis minor muscle. Lymph node dissection can be completed via sentinel lymph node dissection (SLND) or through axillary lymph node dissection (ALND).

Sentinel Lymph Node Biopsy[37]

The lymphatic vessels in the breast area first drain on a path merging into one or only a few nodes before moving into nodes further away from the breast. These are called the "guarding, or sentinel, lymph node(s). The sentinel nodes are identified through a mapping procedure. See Figure 15.6 demonstrating how the radioactive substance is injected. Due to the small size of cancer cells, it is difficult to trace their path from the primary tumor so a tracking substance is injected into the lymphatic channels that are near the cancer to identify the potential path that cancer cells might take as well as the sentinel node(s) where the cancer cells may collect first. Most commonly used tracking substances are usually a radioactive tracer (isotope) called technetium 99 and a blue dye called isosulfan blue. Because the dyes follow the same route as cancer cells, they locate the sentinel node(s). Sentinel lymph node biopsy (SLNB) provides the PWC with more individualized care. A fewer number of lymph nodes are removed as a result of this objective measurement decreasing the potential adverse effects of lymph node dissection including the development of lymphedema.

Axillary Lymph Node Dissection[38]

Depending on the results of the SNB, further investigation of levels I and II lymph nodes may be carried out by removing 5 to 30 lymph nodes. Figure 15.7 is a schematic diagram of an ALND and Figure 15.8 demonstrates the ALND performed on a person with BC. In the case of a mastectomy, this is often completed through the same incision or may be a separate 2 to 3 inch incision in the axilla. In the case of BCoS, there is almost always a separate axillary incision.

Historically, the goal of ALND was to remove all lymph nodes that contained cancer cells to increase survival rates. However, the outcomes of ALND often were life altering due to significant adverse effects, including high risk of lymphedema, reduced

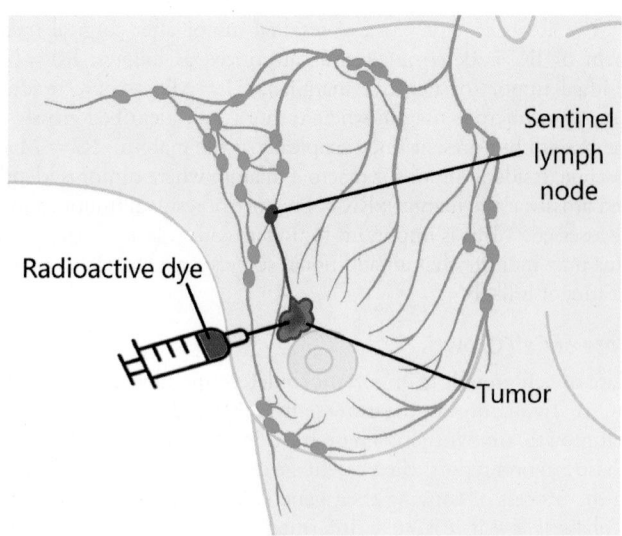

• **Fig. 15.6** Sentinel Lymph Node Biopsy. (Created by Chris Wilson. Adapted from Cancer Research UK under creative commons license CC BY-SA 4.0.)

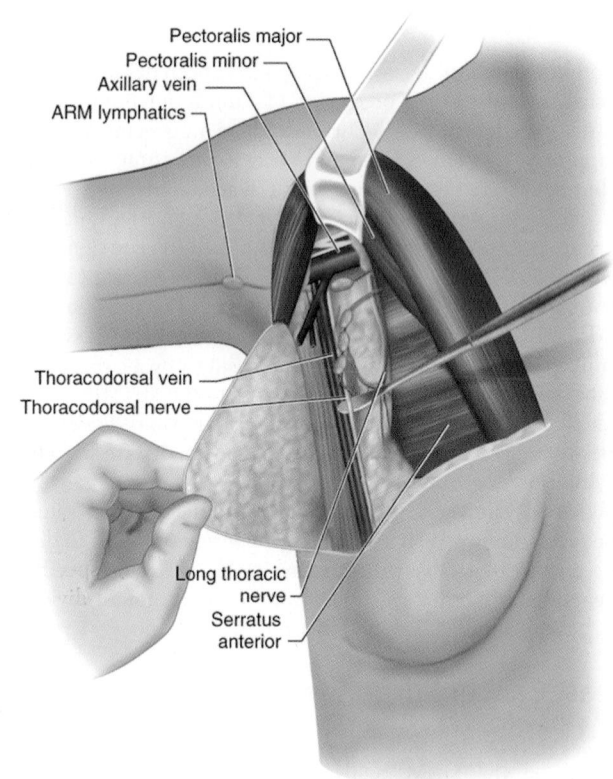

• **Fig. 15.7** Schematic Diagram of Axillary Lymph Node Dissection. (Reprinted with permission from Klimberg VS, Coffman DR, Cochran J. Axillary lymph node dissection: procedure video. Elsevier; 2021.)

mobility, and limited function. Researchers are working to determine which BC diagnoses requires SLND versus ALND in order to balance risk and benefit. A 10-year study found that SLND was

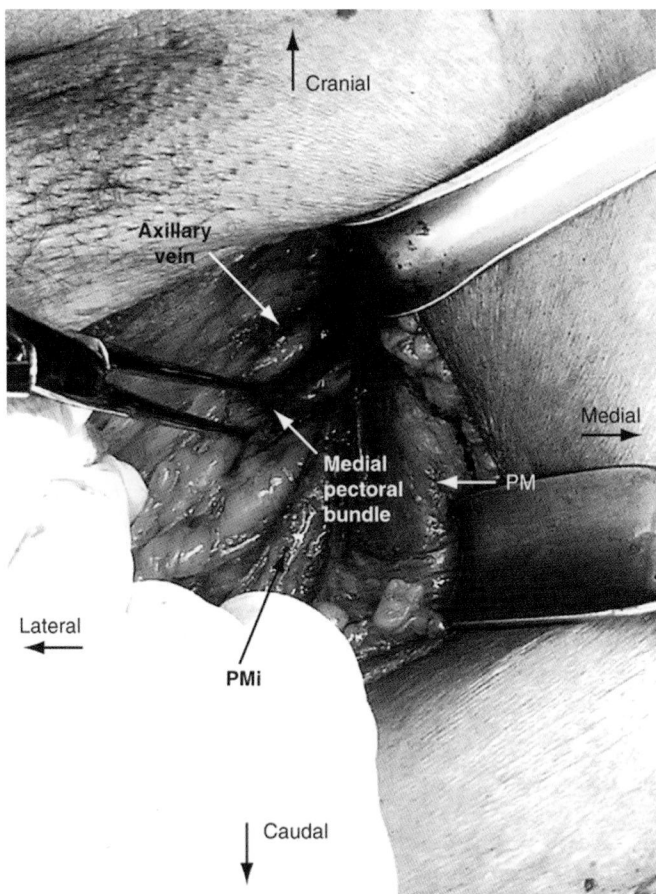

• **Fig. 15.8** Axillary Lymph Node Dissection. (Reprinted with permission from Klimberg VS, Coffman DR, Cochran J. Axillary lymph node dissection: procedure video. Elsevier; 2021.)
PM - pectoralis major; *PMi* - pectoralis minor.

superior to ALND in women with T1 or T2 invasive primary BC. The 10-year overall survival was 86.3% in the SLND alone group and 83.6% in the ALND group.[39] When neoadjuvant chemotherapy is provided, thereby converting some nodes from clinically positive to negative, researchers found that both the ALND group and the SLNB group had similar rates of recurrence concluding that SLNB is the most optimal strategy for outcomes and fewer adverse effects.[40] It has also been concluded by other researchers that removal of more than 10 lymph nodes does not provide any significant survival benefit regardless of how high risk the BC is.[41] More research is warranted.

Reconstruction After Mastectomy

The breast reconstruction rate after mastectomy is reported to be approximately 42% with 25% of women beginning reconstruction at the time of surgery for mastectomy and 17% delaying reconstruction.[42] Women who choose autologous reconstruction may have higher satisfaction than those who had a mastectomy alone, as measured by the Breast Q survey.[42] More women are opting for contralateral prophylactic mastectomy, bilateral reconstruction, and implants instead of autologous tissue breast reconstruction.[43] Data suggests that the reasons for this may be improvement in surgical techniques such as nipple sparing procedures, using fat grafting around implants, and a decreased postoperative recovery period, all of which have improved satisfaction

in persons with BC. Autologous fat grafting has evolved significantly over the last two decades and can be used during and as follow up to implant placement. Fat grafting may result in improved cosmetic results, and chest wall healing and may reverse damage to soft tissue by stabilizing the soft tissue during the process of tissue expansion.[44]

Racial disparities exist in the ability to secure breast reconstruction after a mastectomy. Compared with White women with BC, Black women are more likely to undergo autologous-based reconstruction and be underinsured. It is unclear to what extent this disparity stems from socioeconomic issues or individual preference.[45] One study found that in the US, demographics for those women most likely to undergo breast reconstruction included women who are White, young, have a higher income and education level, are covered by private insurance, and are treated at academic or private hospitals. Women whose demographics include minority race or ethnicity, lower socioeconomic level, or public or no insurance are less likely to undergo reconstruction. Women in low- and middle-income countries are less likely to undergo breast reconstruction as it is not often available.[46]

Implant Reconstruction

During the process of implant reconstruction, tissue expanders are placed behind the pectoralis major muscle to stretch the muscle allowing for increased space to insert an implant (Figure 15.9).[47] Note that there are a variety of shapes, sizes, and types of tissue expanders. Expanders and implants may be used alone or as part of a flap procedure such as the latissimus flap. Figure 15.10 depicts a person 1-week post mastectomy with expander and drain in place. Figure 15.11 demonstrates a silicone implant. Figure 15.12 helps to visualize how the implant is usually positioned under the pectoralis major muscle. Bioprosthetic material is used to cover the inferior pole of the breast.

In the case of a skin-sparing mastectomy, it may be possible to pursue implant reconstruction without the need for expanders. The choices for implants include:
1. Saline
2. Silicone—There are two types, including gel implants and cohesive gel implants (also called gummy bear implants which form stable implants). Cohesive gel implants are made with thicker saline that decreases their risk for rupture.

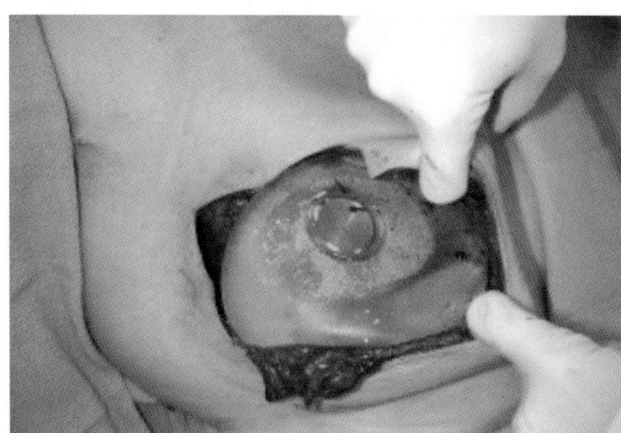

• **Fig. 15.9** Tissue Expander in Place in Mastectomy Incision. (Reprinted with permission from Hammond DC. Latissimus dorsi flap breast reconstruction. *Clin Plast Surg.* 2007;34(1):75–82.)

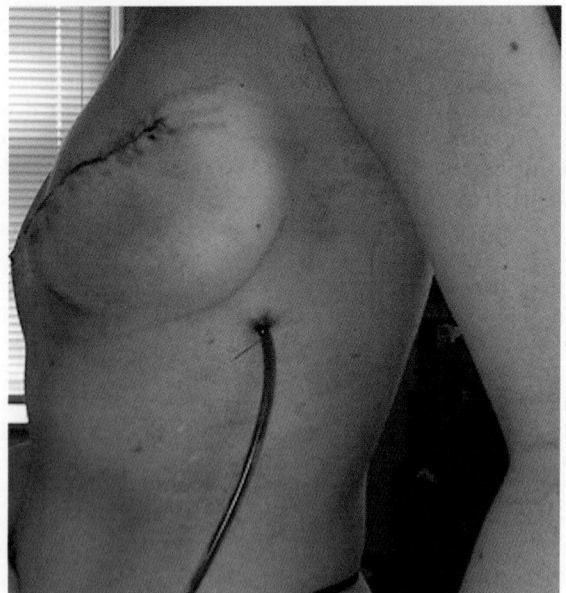

• **Fig. 15.10** One Week Post Mastectomy With Expander, Drain in Place. (Reprinted with permission from TurningPoint Breast Cancer Rehabilitation.)

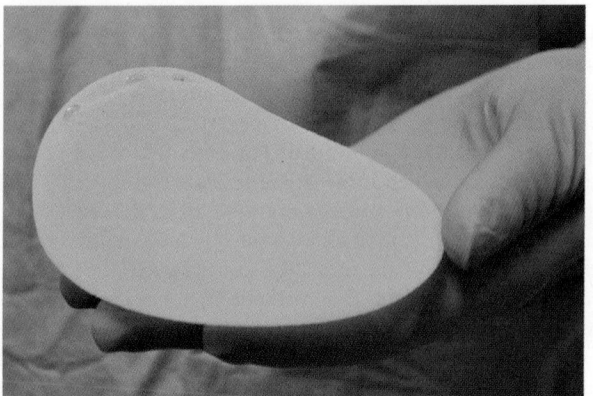

• **Fig. 15.11** Silicone Implant. (Reprinted with permission from "Breast Implant" by Dr. Spitalier is licensed under CC BY-SA 2.0. https://creativecommons.org/licenses/by-sa/2.0/.)

Tissue support or scaffolding is sometimes needed for greater soft tissue coverage and implant support. Acellular dermal matrix (ADM) is a soft connective tissue graft made from human-, bovine-, or porcine-derived tissue generated by a decellularization process. See Figure 15.13 to demonstrate the results of implants.

Autologous Breast Reconstruction[48]

With autologous (sometimes referred to as autogenous or flap) reconstruction, a new breast-like shape is created from a flap of muscle, fat and/or skin taken from the abdomen, buttocks, back, or inner thigh. In a "free flap," tissue is separated from its original blood vessels, moved to the breast area and vessels are reattached through microvascular surgery. In a "pedicled flap," tissue remains attached to its original blood vessels and moved under the skin to the chest wall. See Table 15.5 for a list of autologous reconstruction options. See Figure 15.14 for an example of a transverse rectus abdominis muscle (TRAM) flap procedure. Figures 15.15 and 15.16 provide examples of a schematic diagram of latissimus flap reconstruction as well as latissimus flap reconstruction on the right side with radiation tanning.

There are two common procedures to create nipples, if desired. A skin flap from another area of the body can be used, often from the donor site of flap reconstruction. Nipple tattooing can be used to create an areola with or without a nipple graft. 3D tattooing can be used to create the shape of a nipple as well as the color of the areola. See Figures 15.17 and 15.18.

Delayed breast reconstruction may be the appropriate choice in the case where a person has health problems that prevent immediate reconstruction, is not able to cope with another cancer treatment at the same time, or needs radiation therapy that could negatively affect the implant or prevent healing. The reconstruction timeline is an important decision that needs thoughtful consideration and consultation with the oncologic surgeon, medical oncologist, caregiver, and patient in a shared decision-making forum.

It is important as an Onc R clinician to be sensitive and neutral in the discussion with an individual making this very personal decision. Often a person recently diagnosed is unsure of their options and decisions and may ask for the clinician's opinion. It is important to provide resources and an understanding of the expected

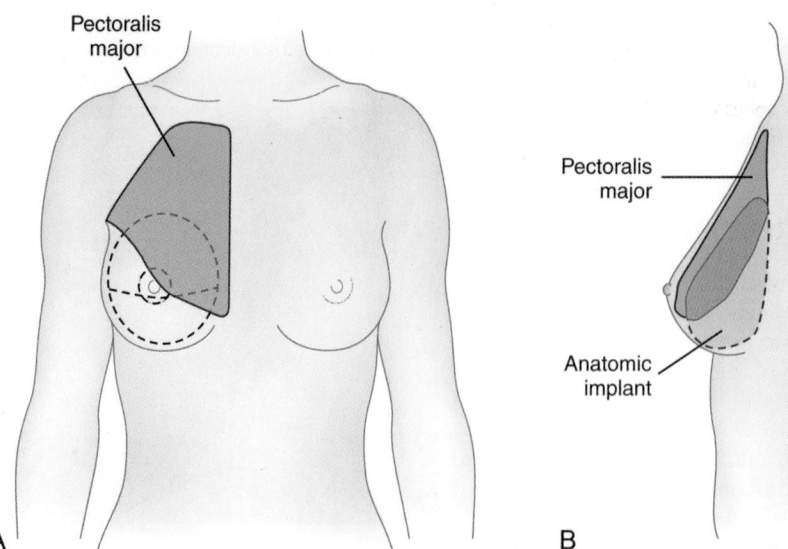

• **Fig. 15.12** Schematic Representation of Implant Position Under Pectoralis Major. (Reprinted with permission from Breuing KH, Warren SM. Immediate bilateral breast reconstruction with implants and inferolateral AlloDerm slings. *Ann Plast Surg.* 2005;55:232–239.)

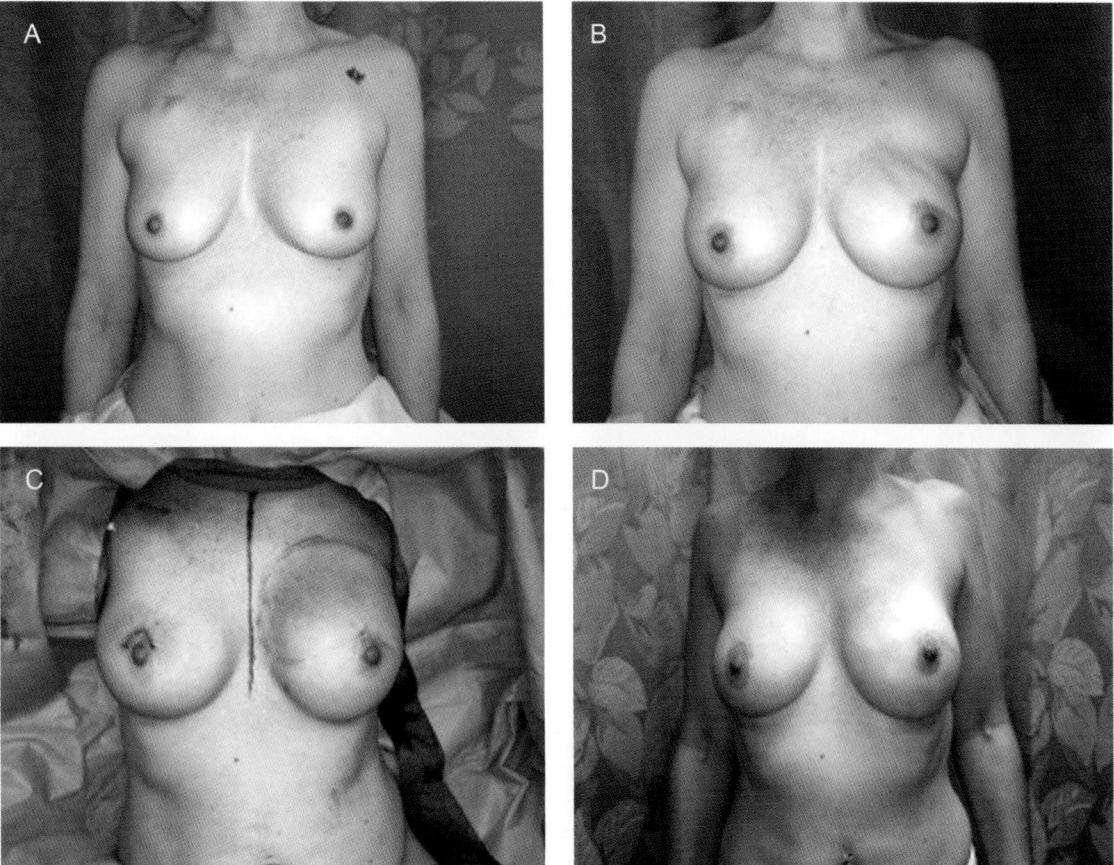

• **Fig. 15.13** Implant Outcomes. (A) Preoperative, (B) post left skin and nipple-sparing mastectomy and immediate prepectoral implant reconstruction (no expander phase) and right breast augmentation for symmetry, (C) immediate fat grafting to correct hollowing and rippling in superior and medial pole of breast, (D) 6 months following surgery. (Reprinted with permission from Gabriel A, Patrick Maxwell G. *The Evolution of Breast Implants.* Vol. 42. Elsevier; 2015: 399–404.)

recovery experience and functional change, but not bias the discussion. Having a network of persons living with and beyond cancer (PLWBCs) that can share their experiences and the pros and cons of each procedure can be helpful to assist patients in decision-making and decrease the overall psychosocial burden of a PLWBC.

There is some ambiguity regarding the optimal time for post-mastectomy radiation therapy (PMRT). In a systematic review,[49] evidence was clear that the incidence of infection was statistically higher when PMRT was performed prior to implant exchange in a 2-stage expander-implant reconstruction versus post implant.[49] PMRT following prosthetic reconstruction posed greater risks of reconstruction failure and capsular contractures at a rate of over 9% versus 0.5% for those who received implants without radiation. The failure rate is not only with radiation on the implant but there is also a substantially high failure rate (40%) when radiation is provided over the expander. Capsular contractures are more common when PMRT is performed on tissue expanders. There is no consensus on proper timing of radiation due to the multifactorial considerations involved in this decision including both the person receiving the radiation and the parameters of the radiation secondary to the diagnosis.[49] It is important for individuals to have a detailed discussion with their radiation oncologist and plastic surgeon to determine the best treatment for positive outcomes.

Medical Treatment Modalities for Breast Cancer

There are four major medical treatment modalities for BC:

1. Chemotherapy
2. Endocrine therapy
3. Targeted agents
4. Bone-modifying agents

Chemotherapy

Chemotherapy may be utilized prior to or following surgery. Neo-adjuvant chemotherapy is given prior to surgery with the goal to shrink tumors before removal, minimizing the invasiveness of the anticipated surgical procedure. The purpose of adjuvant chemotherapy, given following surgery, is to eradicate micro-metastatic disease or those BC cells that have moved out of the breast tissue and into the lymph nodes or beyond. For early-stage cancers, the purpose of chemotherapy is to eliminate cancer cells left behind after surgery to reduce risk of recurrence. In more advanced stages, the purpose of chemotherapy is to destroy or at least damage cancer cells and slow down the growth to prevent more metastasis or growth outside the breast tissue. To date, there is no cure for MeBC, although in many cases individuals with MeBC are living for many years with advancements in treatment. Chemotherapy

TABLE 15.5   **Autologous Reconstruction Options**

Autologous abdominally-based flap reconstruction	a) TRAM flap—(transverse rectus abdominis muscle)—skin, fat, and all or part of the TRAM are used to reconstruct the breast. Can be free flap or pedicled flap. b) DIEP flap—(deep inferior epigastric perforator)—fat, skin, and blood vessels are moved from the wall of the lower abdomen to the chest to rebuild the breast with muscle sparing. Requires incision in rectus abdominis muscle fascia. Free flap (tissue is separated from its original blood vessels, moved to the breast area and vessels are reattached through microvascular surgery.) c) APEX flap^CM (abdominal perforator engineered vascular exchange flap)—fat, skin, and blood vessels from wall of lower abdomen are moved to the chest to rebuild the breast (similar to DIEP flap but an option for women who have small abdominal blood vessels or vessels that are not in the correct location for easy access). d) SIEA flap—(superficial inferior epigastric artery or epigastric perforator)—engineering of the blood vessel skin and fat anatomy with no disturbance to the muscle thus called muscle sparing. Similar to DIEP flap but with blood vessels from different area of abdomen. No incision in rectus abdominis fascia is required. Free flap.
Latissimus-based flap reconstruction (see Figures 15.15 and 15.16)	Latissimus dorsi flap (lat flap)—skin, fat, muscle, and blood vessels are used from the latissimus dorsi muscle to reconstruct the breast. Blood vessels of the flap are left attached to their original blood supply in the back; pedicled. An implant is typically utilized to form the breast mound under the skin and muscle flap.
Gluteal-based flap reconstruction	a) SGAP flap/hip flap—(superior gluteal artery perforator or gluteal perforator hip flap)—skin, fat from upper buttocks/hip (love handles), with muscle sparing. Free flap. b) IGAP flap—(inferior gluteal artery perforator)—skin, fat, and blood vessel from the lower buttocks near the crease with muscle sparing. Free flap.
Thigh-based flap reconstruction	a) TUG flap—(transverse upper gracilis muscle)—skin, fat, muscle, and blood vessels from the upper thigh including the gracilis muscle. b) PAP flap—(profunda perforator)—skin, fat from the back of the upper thigh along with the blood vessel with muscle sparing.
Multi-component "hybrid" flap reconstruction (tissue from abdomen/hips)	a) Stacked DIEP flap—using flaps from both sides of the lower abdomen and stacking or folding them for women who do not have enough tissue on one side or if reconstructing both breasts. b) Body lift perforator flap—combination of DIEP flap with SGAP/hip flap—lift results from both the "tummy tuck" from the lower abdomen tissue used and "butt lift" from the butt flaps for increased body contour. c) Stacked/"hybrid" GAP flap—using flaps from both sides of the upper buttock and stacking or folding them for women who do not have enough tissue on one side or if reconstructing both breasts.
Autologous breast reconstruction using fat tissue removed from the abdomen, buttocks, and/or thighs by liposuction	Fat grafting—also called lipofilling

Created by Deborah J. Doherty. Printed with permission.

is used to extend the survival time by slowing the progress of the disease and provide symptom relief.

Classes of Chemotherapy Drugs for Breast Cancer and General Toxicities[50]

1. Anti-microtubule agents (taxanes, ixabepilone [Ixempra], eribulin [Halaven], and vinca alkaloids). Anti-microtubule agents interfere with cell division and share the toxicities of chemotherapy-induced polyneuropathy (CIPN), myelosuppression, and loss of hair. Paclitaxel (Taxol), docetaxel (Taxotere), and paclitaxel protein-bound (Abraxane) are examples of taxanes commonly used in BC.
2. Anthracyclines (doxorubicin [Adriamycin, Rubex], epirubicin [Ellence], daunorubicin [Cerubidine], mitoxantrone [Novantrone], liposomal doxorubicin [Doxil], and non-pegylated liposomal doxorubicin [Myocet]). Anthracyclines are chemically similar to an antibiotic. Anthracyclines damage the genetic material of cancer cells, which makes the cells die.
   Anthracyclines have many adverse effects at the molecular level, with negative effects on the cell membrane as one

example. These agents cause the toxicities of cardiac damage, myelosuppression, and emesis.
3. Antimetabolites (5-fluorouracil [Adrucil], methotrexate [Otrexup, Rasuvo, Rheumatrex, Trexall], capecitabine [Xeloda], and gemcitabine [Gemzar]). Three classes exist: nucleoside analogues, thymidylate synthase inhibitors, and dihydrofolate reductase inhibitors. The toxicities from these agents include mucositis, diarrhea, and myelosuppression.
4. Alkylating agents (cyclophosphamide [Cytoxan, Neosar], cisplatin [Platinol], and carboplatin [Paraplatin]). This class of agents create similar toxicities, including myelosuppression, gonadal dysfunction, and rarely pulmonary fibrosis. They are also responsible for causing secondary neoplasms, particularly leukemia.

Dose-Dense Chemotherapy: Dose-dense refers to the administration of drugs with a shortened interval between treatment cycles. Dose-dense anthracycline- and taxane-based chemotherapy is a common adjuvant regimen for BC. Over and above the toxicities of the standard dose, these agents cause a higher risk of anemia, thrombocytopenia, and mucositis.

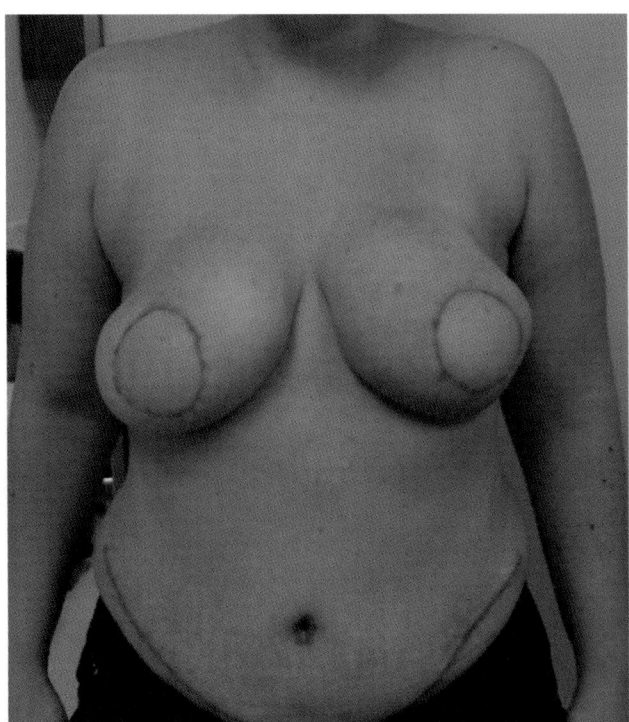

• **Fig. 15.14** Free Tram Flap Reconstruction Demonstrating Skin Graft Islands and Abdominal Donor Site Incision. (Reprinted with permission from Nahabedian MY. *Plastic Surgery*. Elsevier; 2018: 350–372.e2.)

Common Chemotherapy Drugs Used in the Management of Breast Cancer[51]

See Table 15.6 for common chemotherapy drugs used in the management of BC.

Combinations of two or three drugs are commonly a treatment of choice, however, while combination therapies are considered to have a higher efficacy in comparison to single-agent therapy, the risk of increased toxicity is also higher. The combinations of drugs depend on many variables, including the stage, grade, risk of recurrence, metastasis, co-morbidities of the person receiving the medication and more. It is important to communicate with the medical oncologist to understand the planned treatment regimen for the PWC. Examples of common drugs used in combination include[51]: (1) AT: Adriamycin and Taxotere; (2) AC ± T: Adriamycin and Cytoxan, with or without Taxol or Taxotere; (3) CMF: Cytoxan, Methotrexate, and Fluorouracil; (4) CEF: Cytoxan, Ellence, and Fluorouracil; (5) FAC: Fluorouracil, Adriamycin, and Cytoxan; (6) CAF: Cytoxan, Adriamycin, and Fluorouracil; (7) The FAC and CAF regimens use the same medicines but use different doses and frequencies; (8) TAC: Taxotere, Adriamycin, and Cytoxan; and (9) GET: Gemzar, Ellence, and Taxol.

Endocrine Therapy[50,52–54]

Endocrine therapy is a targeted therapy specifically deployed to create an antitumor reaction for persons diagnosed with breast tumors that are expressing estrogen receptors (ER+) and/or progesterone receptors (PR+).[53,54] For BC at early or advanced stages there are three classes of endocrine agents (SERMs, AIs, and SERDs) used based on the mechanism of action[53,54] (see Chapter 5 for additional information).

Selective Estrogen Receptor Modulators[53,54]

Selective estrogen receptor modulators (SERMs) occupy the estrogen receptor, preventing estrogen from attaching or sitting in the receptor and thus will interfere with its transcriptional activity in breast cells but because it is selective will not occupy the estrogen receptors in other cells, like bone, liver or uterine.[53] Examples are tamoxifen (Nolvadex, Evista, Raloxifene) and toremifene (Fareston). Common adverse events in women are risk of blood clots in the lungs and legs, stroke, cataracts, endometrial cancer and uterine sarcoma, bone loss, hot flashes, vaginal dryness or discharge, arthralgias, osteoporosis, increased risk for uterine cancer, headaches, mild nausea and mood changes. In men, the common adverse effects are headaches, nausea, vomiting, skin rash, impotence and sexual problems, fatigue, hot flashes, increased weight, and mood changes.

Aromatase Inhibitors[53,54]

In postmenopausal women, the largest source of estrogen is through the aromatization of fat cells. Aromatase inhibitors (AIs) block or inhibit the enzyme aromatase and profoundly reduce estrogen levels in postmenopausal women so there is less stimulation of HR+ BC cells. Examples of AIs are anastrozole (Arimidex), exemestane (Aromasin), and letrozole (Femara). Common adverse events include risk of heart attack, angina, heart failure, hypercholesterolemia, bone loss, joint and muscle pain, mood swings, and depression.

Selective Estrogen Receptor Down Regulator

Selective estrogen receptor down regulators (SERDs) do not mimic estrogen but bind to the ER and target its destruction.[53,54] One example is fulvestrant (Faslodex). Common adverse events are gastrointestinal symptoms, including nausea, vomiting, constipation, weakness, fatigue, joint pain, headaches, hot flashes, breathing problems, and loss of appetite.

Luteinizing Hormone-Releasing Hormone

Ovarian suppression drugs are used to block the production of estrogen from the ovaries in premenopausal women.[55] Examples are leuprolide (Lupron) and goserelin (Zoladex). Common adverse events are bone loss, mood swings, depression, and loss of libido.

Targeted Agents[50]

In BC, there is targeted therapy specifically for the overproduction of the HER2 protein. Targeted agents have toxicity profiles different from traditional cytotoxic chemotherapy and are class specific and agent specific. Monoclonal antibodies may generate immediate infusion reactions. Small molecule inhibitors cause diarrhea and skin rash; all HER2 agents potentially cause left ventricular myocardial dysfunction; bevacizumab (Avastin) causes hypertension, bleeding, thrombosis, impaired wound healing, and myocardial dysfunction. Examples of drugs used include: (1) trastuzumab (Herceptin) monoclonal IgG1 class humanized murine antibody that binds the extracellular portion of the HER2 transmembrane receptor; (2) pertuzumab (Perjeta); (3) ado-trastuzumab emtansine (T-DM1, Kadcyla); (4) neratnib (Nerlynx); (5) bevacizumab (Avastin); (6) everolimus (Afinitor); (7) palbociclib (Ibrance); and (8) margetuximab-cmkb (Margenza).

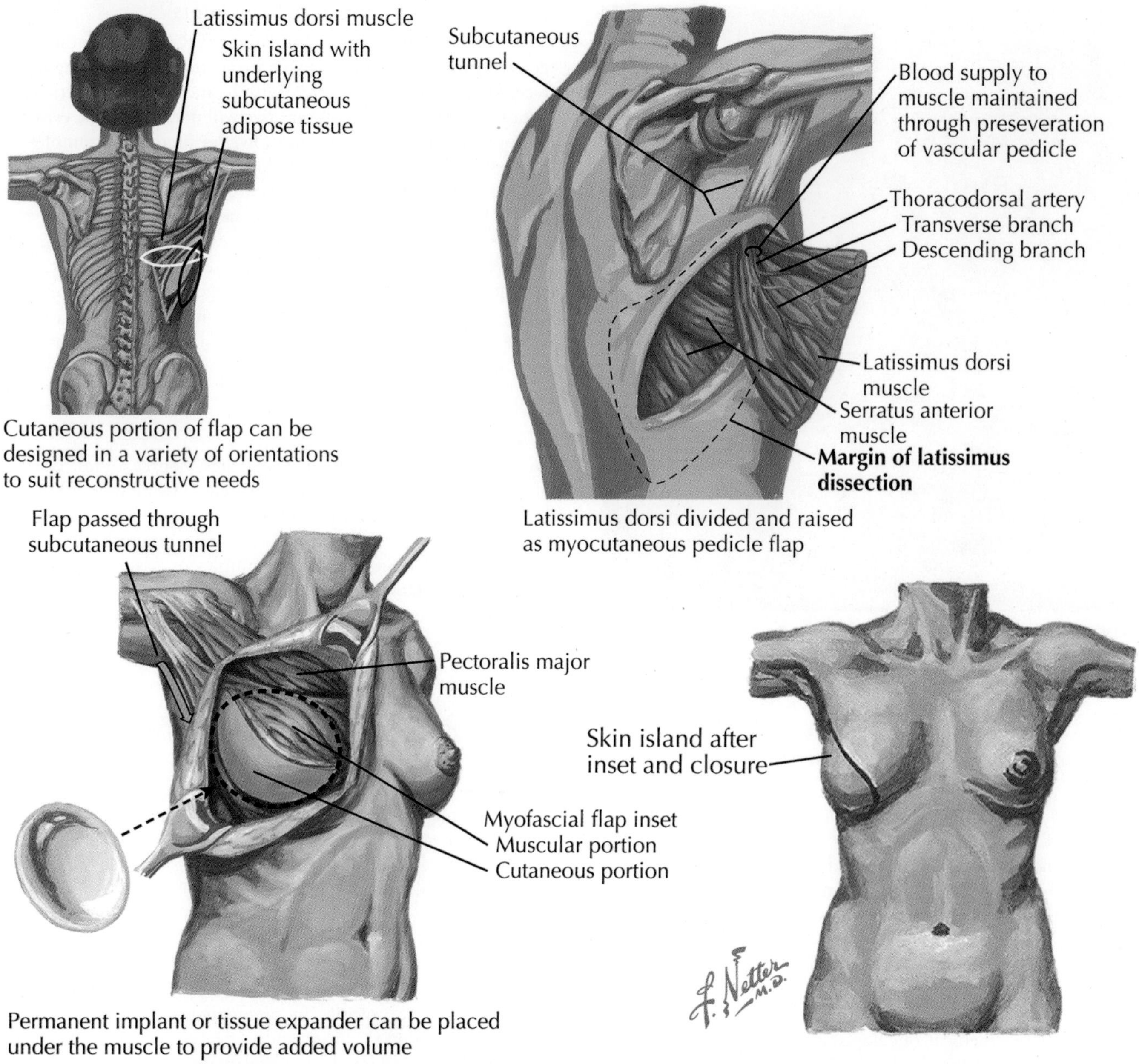

Latissimus dorsi muscle

Skin island with underlying subcutaneous adipose tissue

Cutaneous portion of flap can be designed in a variety of orientations to suit reconstructive needs

Subcutaneous tunnel

Blood supply to muscle maintained through preseveration of vascular pedicle

Thoracodorsal artery
Transverse branch
Descending branch

Latissimus dorsi muscle

Serratus anterior muscle

Margin of latissimus dissection

Latissimus dorsi divided and raised as myocutaneous pedicle flap

Flap passed through subcutaneous tunnel

Pectoralis major muscle

Myofascial flap inset
Muscular portion
Cutaneous portion

Skin island after inset and closure

Permanent implant or tissue expander can be placed under the muscle to provide added volume

• **Fig. 15.15** Schematic Diagram of Latissimus Flap Reconstruction. (Reprinted with permission from Craig JA. Breast cancer surgery: breast reconstruction with latissimus dorsi myocutaneous flap and implant. Netterimages.com. https://www.netterimages.com/breast-cancer-surgery-breast-reconstruction-with-latissimus-dorsi-myocutaneous-flap-and-implant-unlabeled-surgery-john-a-craig-29301.html.)

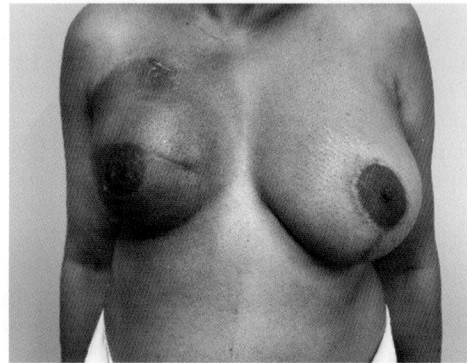

• **Fig. 15.16** Latissimus Flap Reconstruction On Right Side With Radiation Tanning, Breast Lift for Symmetry on Left Side. (Reprinted with permission from TurningPoint Breast Cancer Rehabilitation.)

Bone Modifying Agents[50]

Bone mineral density (BMD) loss is common with anticancer treatments. Whether cancer is localized or metastatic, bone complications are a major risk. Studies report that 70% of persons diagnosed with and treated for MeBC will suffer from osseous degradation and decreased integrity of the bone matrix.[56] Bisphosphonates prevent skeletal related events (SREs) and reduce the risk of BC recurrence. Examples of bone modifying agents include: (1) denosumab (receptor activator of nuclear factor kappa-B ligand or RANKL [Prolia, Xgeva]) and (2) zoledronic acid (bisphosphonate [Reclast]). They both modulate osteoclastic activity decreasing

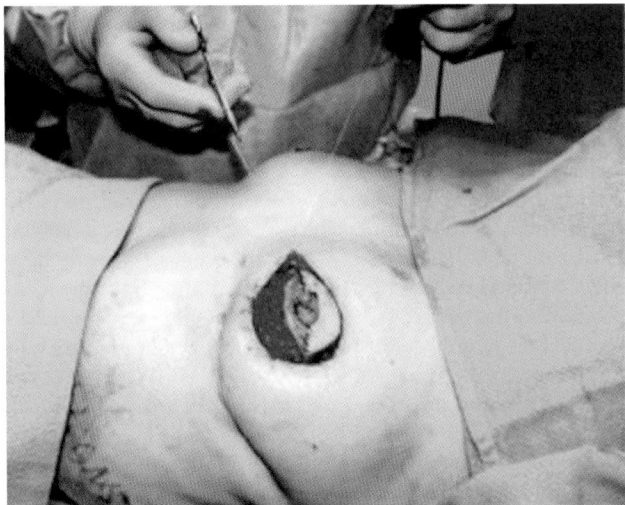

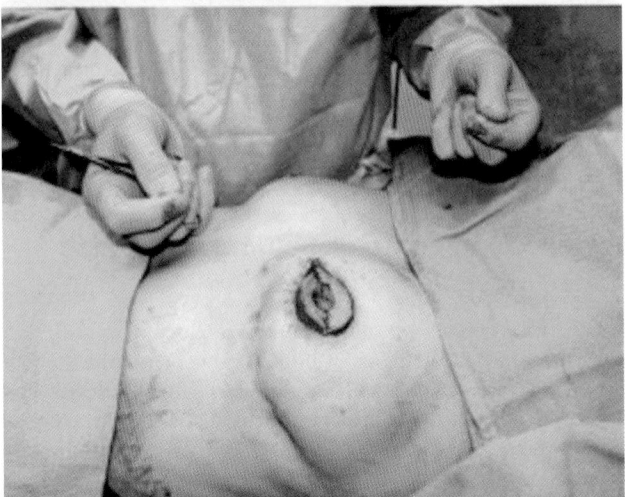

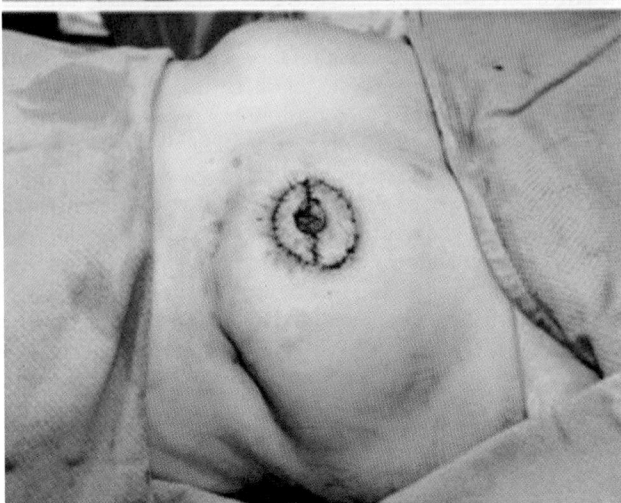

• **Fig. 15.17** Nipple Grafting From Donor Skin Site to Create a Nipple, Subsequent Intradermal Tattoo Will Provide Color and Disguise Incisions. (Reprinted with permission from Davidson EH, Ergo FM, Shestak KC. Reconstruction of the nipple areolar complex. In: Nahabedian MY, Neligan PC, Liu DZ, eds. Plastic Surgery: Volume 5: Breast. 4th ed. 2018; 501-508.e2.)

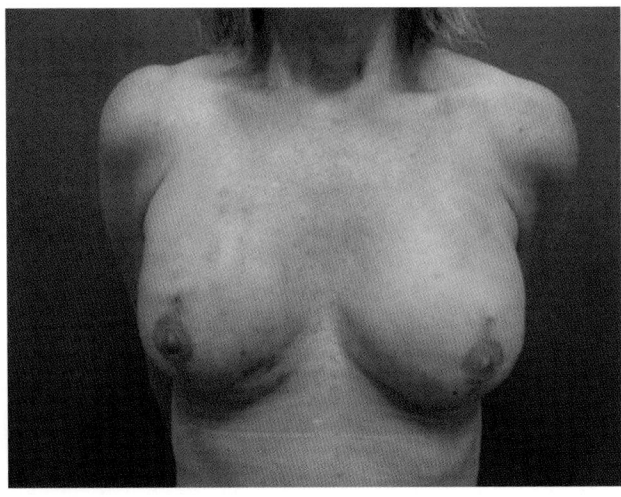

• **Fig. 15.18** 3D Tattooing Creates Color of the Areola and the Illusion of Projection of the Nipple Following Bilateral Implant Reconstruction. (Reprinted with permission from TurningPoint Breast Cancer Rehabilitation.)

TABLE 15.6	Common Chemotherapy Drugs Used in the Management of Breast Cancer
i.	Abraxane (chemical name: albumin-bound or nab-paclitaxel)
ii.	Adriamycin (chemical name: doxorubicin)
iiii.	Carboplatin (brand name: Paraplatin)
iv.	Cytoxan (chemical name: cyclophosphamide)
v.	Daunorubicin (brand names: Cerubidine, DaunoXome)
vi.	Doxil (chemical name: doxorubicin)
vii.	Ellence (chemical name: epirubicin)
viii.	Fluorouracil (also called 5-fluorouracil or 5-FU; brand name: Adrucil)
ix.	Gemzar (chemical name: gemcitabine)
x.	Halaven (chemical name: eribulin)
xi.	Ixempra (chemical name: ixabepilone)
xii.	Methotrexate (brand names: Amethopterin, Mexate, Folex)
xiii.	Mitomycin (chemical name: mutamycin)
xiv.	Mitoxantrone (brand name: Novantrone)
xv.	Navelbine (chemical name: vinorelbine)
xvi.	Taxol (chemical name: paclitaxel)
xvii.	Taxotere (chemical name: docetaxel)
xviii.	Thiotepa (brand name: Thioplex)
xix.	Vincristine (brand names: Oncovin, Vincasar PES, Vincrex)
xx.	Xeloda (chemical name: capecitabine)

Created by Deborah J. Doherty. Printed with permission.

Radiation Therapy

Radiation is utilized to destroy cancer cells via high-energy X-rays or other particles.[57] There are several different types of radiation therapy for BC: (1) External-beam radiation therapy: Most common type of radiation treatment given to the whole or partial breast from a machine outside the body. Also, accelerated

bone loss and destabilizing the environment to decrease tumor cell growth. Onc R clinicians need to be very aware of the potential bone loss both in skeletal bone and the potential for osteonecrosis of the jaw.

radiation is an option for some PWCs and is completed in a few days instead of a few weeks. This can be achieved through intensity-modulated radiation therapy (IMRT), which is more targeted to the breast tissue with reduced radiation dose and decreased immediate adverse effects and damage to nearby organs. Proton therapy, that utilizes protons rather than X-rays, is also a more targeted approach that reduces the radiation dose; (2) Intra-operative radiation therapy: Radiation treatment is given in an operating room with the use of a probe placed into the tumor; and (3) Brachytherapy: Radiation therapy provided through the use of radioactive sources that are placed into the tumor. A radiation therapy regimen, or schedule, usually consists of a specific number of treatments given over a set period. The goal of radiation therapy is to lower the risk of recurrence in remaining breast tissue. In fact, with modern surgery and radiation therapy, recurrence rates in the breast are now less than 5% in the 10 years after treatment, and survival is the same with lumpectomy or mastectomy. If there is cancer in the axillary lymph nodes, radiation therapy may also be given to the same side of the neck or underarm near the breast or chest wall. Adjuvant radiation therapy is given after surgery. Most commonly, it is given after a lumpectomy, and sometimes after chemotherapy. Individuals who have a mastectomy may not need radiation therapy, depending on the features of the tumor and the number of positive lymph nodes. Radiation therapy may be recommended after mastectomy in patients with larger tumors, positive lymph nodes, cancer cells outside of the capsule of the lymph node, or cancer that has grown into the skin or chest wall, as well as for other reasons. Radiation can also be given before surgery. This is called neoadjuvant radiation and is sometimes used to shrink a large tumor to make it easier to surgically resect.

Common Findings and Evaluation

Research suggests that women are often unaware of the adverse-effects of treatment for BC and express surprise that pain, fatigue, and impaired upper extremity (UE) movement do not always disappear after treatment but remain part of their lives, even years later.[58] Women report shock at the impact that pain, limitations in range of motion (ROM), and fatigue have on daily life.[58] As PLWBCs begin the process of moving on after treatment, they often experience lingering physical symptoms that are ongoing reminders of their BC that may increase fear of recurrence. Restrictions in activities of daily living (ADL) are compounded by lack of preparation and a sense of being misunderstood. Particularly distressing limitations are those that impact usual roles, such as work or childcare involving lifting, carrying, or bathing a child.[58–60] Lymphedema and the risk of lymphedema impose limitations on their lives as well. Some PLWBCs report more distress related to the threat of lymphedema than with BC itself. Finally, research suggests that many PLWBCs withhold concerns because they believe disabling adverse effects are a normal part of BC treatment. Others are concerned with bothering their doctors and loved ones with unreasonable complaints.[58–60]

Most individuals have a general understanding that they will have pain, stiffness, swelling, numbness after common orthopedic surgeries and have a general understanding of the role of rehabilitation in their return to usual function. Most persons diagnosed and treated for BC, however, are unprepared for the impact of the BC treatment on impairment and function and do not have a clear understanding of the role of rehabilitation. At the same time, the Onc R clinician is often the first person with whom the PWC shares their intimate story and often one of the few people who has seen their surgical site(s). For these reasons, Onc R clinicians must be prepared to allow persons with BC time and space to tell their story, share their fears, and ask questions. They must meet the PWC where they are in their life and BC journeys. The assessment phase of Onc R care is necessarily carried out with compassion and the clinician should be attentive to truly developing an understanding of a person's needs and concerns. It may be important to pause the history-taking to allay fears related to issues such as lymphedema or to ensure the person that they will be able to return to usual ADL.

There are common adverse effects from the treatments for BC including mastectomy, BCoS, ALND, flap reconstruction, reconstruction with implants, chemotherapy, endocrine therapy, targeted agents and radiation. See Table 15.7 of the common adverse effects by treatment type. Figure 15.19 demonstrates radiation tanning, keloid scarring, and soft tissue tightness and adhesions following left mastectomy, ALND, latissimus flap reconstruction and radiation.

Human Movement Issues in Breast Cancer

Incidence and Common Findings Related to Human Movement and Function

Figure 15.21 depicts the multi-dimensional impact of BC and its treatment on all domains of human movement and function. This includes the cardiovascular, pulmonary, integumentary, musculoskeletal, endocrine, and nervous systems. The most common adverse effects are then delineated from each system. In some instances, there is more than one system whose dysfunction or challenges contribute to an adverse effect. For example, the common cardiovascular adverse effects from treatment for BC are cardiotoxicity and decreased endurance. However, the two colors (green and yellow) demonstrate that both the cardiovascular and the pulmonary systems can contribute to decreased endurance. Cancer-related fatigue (CRF) is surrounding all systems as it is a condition that is multifactorial, and all systems can contribute to CRF as well as help prevent or manage it. Psychosocial issues are listed in the blue circle surrounding the systems. These issues are equally important and require proper screening, referral and treatment as needed. This figure was created to provide an overview and reminder to Onc R clinicians to include screening and treatment for all the biopsychosocial/emotional components of the PLWBC for true individually based whole-person centered care. In the next sections, the impact on each of the key dimensions of human movement will be addressed. Functional limitations as well as impairments such as pain, numbness, limitation of shoulder ROM, and weakness are common and well documented following surgery for BC.[61–66]

Measurement of Human Movement and Function

The following are self-reported measures particularly applicable in BC populations. Further detail on the evaluation of function, including performance-based functional tests are described in Chapter 7.

Patient-Specific Functional Scale

The patient-Specific Functional Scale (PSFS) allows patients to state activity limitations that are unique, important, and meaningful to them. The measurement properties of the PSFS have been reported for individuals with orthopedic conditions and in BC.[67–70] The PSFS has been shown to be reliable, valid, sensitive to change and is superior to relevant condition-specific or generic health status measures. The scale takes approximately

4 minutes to complete with the PWC. They are asked to identify up to three functional items that they are unable to do or have difficulty with related to the issue they are seeking care for, in this case BC-related issues such as shoulder dysfunction. The PWC is encouraged to consider functional activities, such as "lifting my baby" or "combing my hair" rather than impairment such as "shoulder stiffness." They are then asked to rate their limitation on an 11-point scale, from "0" (severely

TABLE 15.7	Common Adverse Effects by Treatment Type
Mastectomy	• Pain • Tenderness at surgical site • Neuropathic—hypersensitivity, burning or shooting pain in chest wall, axilla • Postmastectomy pain syndrome (PMPS) • Edema • Hematoma • Seroma • Limited range of motion of the shoulder joint complex, cervical spine, thoracic spine, rib joints • Numbness or deceased sensation—chest wall and/or upper extremity • Scar adherence to underlying tissue
Breast conserving surgery	• Pain • Painful, tight scar tissue region of surgery and/or SNB/ALNB incision • Breast edema or lymphedema
Lymph node dissection (SNB or ALND)	• Lymphedema • Loss or decreased sensation, tingling or numbness in the upper extremity or axilla which can be temporary or permanent • Stiffness of the upper extremity • Weakness • Inflammation of arm veins passing through axilla • Winged scapula • Axillary web syndrome (cording)

Flap reconstruction	• Necrosis of tissue
	• Fat necrosis—hardened areas in the reconstructed breast caused from scar tissue replacing the fat related to poor blood supply
	• Hernia at donor site
	• Pain, tissue tightness and seroma in donor site or reconstruction site
	• Pain secondary to tissue and/or muscle removal (latissimus dorsi, transverse abdominis)
	• Asymmetry and poor cosmesis of donor and/or or reconstruction site
	• Fat transfer reabsorption
	• Latissimus flap reconstruction
	  • Donor site seroma
	  • Muscle contraction of breast mound during activity if latissimus muscle innervated
	  • Lateral chest wall pain and tightness

Reconstruction with implant(s)	• Pectoral and peri-implant pain and tightness • Capsular contraction of implant resulting in pain and/or poor cosmesis • Incision failure during expander or implant phase, particularly related to radiation changes • Implant leakage, rupture, or displacement • Breast implant-associated anaplastic large cell lymphoma (BIA-ALCL)—may occur 8–10 years after implant was placed. It can appear as a collection of fluid near the implant, a lump, pain, swelling or asymmetry (https://www.plasticsurgery.org/patient-safety/breast-implant-safety/bia-alcl-summary)
Chemotherapy	• Cancer-related fatigue • Febrile neutropenia • Chemotherapy-induced emesis • Chemotherapy-induced polyneuropathy • Cardiotoxicity • Gastrointestinal adverse effects: mucositis, diarrhea, and constipation • Chemotherapy-related cognitive impairment (CRCI) • Infertility • Altered body image and sexual dysfunction • Secondary malignancies • Acute myeloid leukemia (AML) with or without preleukemic myelodysplastic syndrome (MDS)

Continued

TABLE 15.7	Common Adverse Effects by Treatment Type—cont'd
Endocrine therapy: tamoxifen and aromatase inhibitors	• Hot flashes due to estrogen deprivation, greater with tamoxifen, incidence is 35%–40%; if premenopausal undergoing ovarian suppression combined with tamoxifen, incidence is 90% • Gynecological adverse effects, including, estrogen effects on uterus, endometrial cancer risk, benign hyperplasia, benign uterine polyps • Vision and eye issues: increased rate of cataracts, retinopathy and ocular toxicity, retinal opacities (tamoxifen) • Abnormal vaginal bleeding, discharge, or spotting • Vaginal dryness and loss of libido • Thromboembolic disease (aromatase inhibitors) • Osteoporosis and osteopenia, increased fracture • Arthralgia and other joint pain • Weight gain • Cancer-related cognitive impairment • Cardiovascular events—myocardial ischemia and stroke, angina, cardiac failure significantly higher in aromatase inhibitors compared to tamoxifen
Targeted agents	• Cardiovascular toxicity—left ventricular dysfunction, left ventricular systolic dysfunction, rare arterial and venous thromboembolic events • Hypertension—causing neurological symptoms like headache, impaired vision, and rare leukoencephalopathy syndrome • Infusion reactions—mild to moderate fever, chills, headache, nausea, bronchospasm, cardiac arrest which are immune mediated, cytokine release and type I hypersensitivity reaction • Hepatotoxicity—liver toxicity • Gastrointestinal perforation, wound healing complications and bleeding • Diarrhea • Skin rash • Interstitial pneumonitis • Hematological toxicity
Radiation	• Lymphedema of upper extremity • Cancer-related fatigue • Discoloration, redness, hyperpigmentation of skin (see Figure 15.19) • Epilation • Radiodermatitis; red, dry tender or itchy skin (see Figure 15.20) • Skin peeling; desquamation with weeping of serous fluid • Breast heaviness • Skin irritation • Pain • Breast edema or lymphedema • Fat necrosis • Hair loss, nausea, rib fracture • Cardiotoxicity • Radiation pneumonitis • Brachial plexopathy • Scarring in lungs from radiation • Risk of secondary cancer

Created by Jill Binkley. Printed with permission.

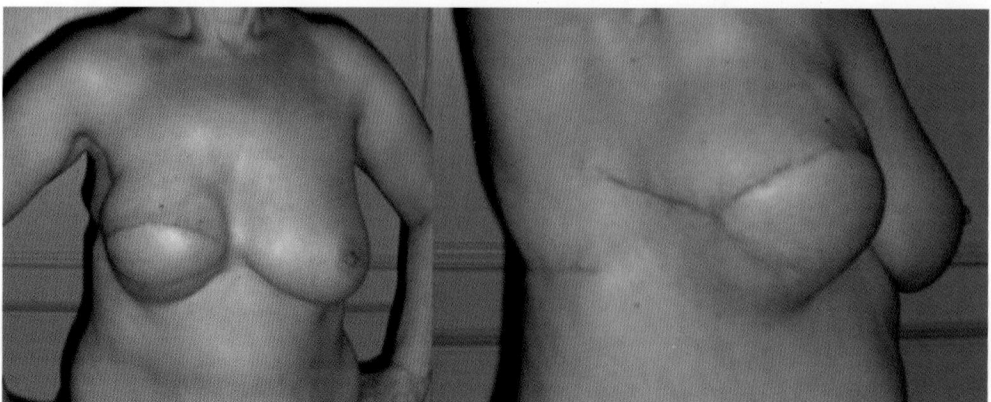

• **Fig. 15.19** Right Latissimus Flap Reconstruction. (Reprinted with permission from TurningPoint Breast Cancer Rehabilitation.)

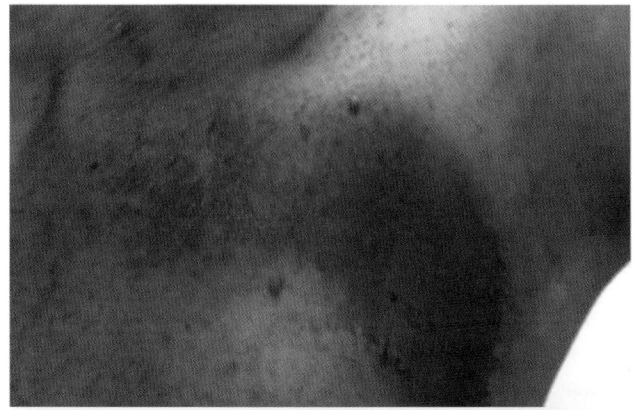

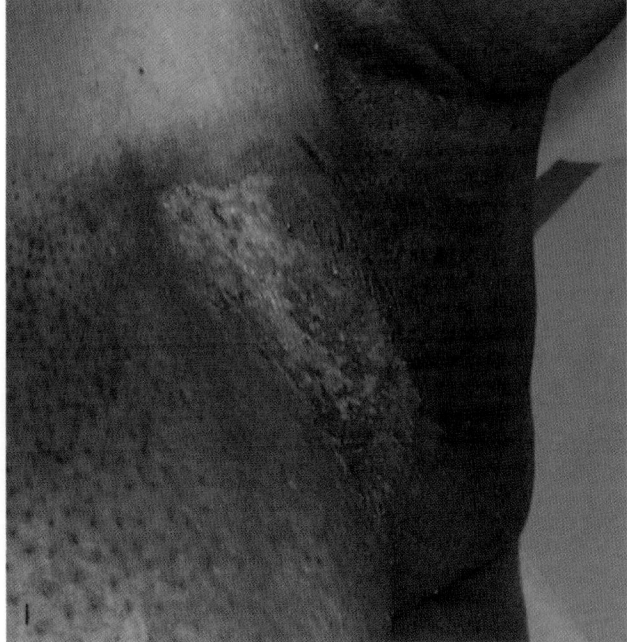

• **Fig. 15.20** Moderate (Top) and Severe (Bottom) Radiation Dermatitis, With Wet Desquamation on Bottom. (Reprinted with permission from TurningPoint Breast Cancer Rehabilitation.)

limited) to "10" (no limitation). Individual items and/or the scale average can be used to set goals and measure change in function.

Measures of Upper Extremity Function

Considering the incidence of UE issues in persons with BC, the assessment of UE function is critical. The Academy of Oncology Physical Therapy Task Force (AOPTTF) of the American Physical Therapy Association (APTA) on Breast Cancer Outcomes reviewed 21 self-reported measures of UE function.[71] The Disabilities of the Shoulder, Arm and Hand scale (DASH) and QuickDASH were recommended by the Task Force and in a systematic review based on psychometric properties reported in a BC population.[71,72] The QuickDASH, a shortened version of the DASH, is a self-report UE measure that assesses function as well as pain and abnormal sensations.[73] It consists of 11 items that inquire about physical function (8-items) and symptoms (3-items asking about pain or abnormal sensations) of

musculoskeletal disorders of the UE. The items are scored on a 5-point Likert scale with 1 indicating no limitation and 5 indicating extreme limitation. Raw scores are transformed to yield a total score out of 100 with lower scores indicating higher levels of function. The measurement properties of the QuickDASH are well documented in orthopedic populations and one study has reported acceptable reliability and validity in the context of PLWBC.[74]

The Upper Extremity Functional Index (UEFI) is a self-reported measure of UE functional status.[75] The UEFI consists of 20 activities or participatory items. Each item is scored from 0 to 4 to determine difficulty with each activity. Extreme difficulty is rated as a 0 and no difficulty is rated as a 4. Total scores range from 0 to 80 with higher scores representing greater levels of functional status. The minimal clinically important difference (MCID) is 9 scale points. All items address function and do not inquire about pain, abnormal sensations, or impairments. The UEFI was developed to be a clinically efficient, homogenous measure of function for UE musculoskeletal issues. It is a single page consisting of 20 items and it can be administered, scored, and interpreted in 3 to 5 minutes without computation aids. The reliability, validity, and sensitivity to change of the UEFI has been documented in the context of persons with orthopedic conditions and BC.[75-78]

From a clinical point of view, impairments and functional limitations seen in persons with BC commonly involve the entire UE. An example of this is axillary cording that may impact shoulder, elbow, wrist, and hand function. In the BC population, it makes sense to select a measure that addresses UE function globally, rather than shoulder function specifically. The UEFI, DASH, QuickDASH meet this criterion. Onc R clinicians should be aware that the DASH and QuickDASH, include questions related to impairments such as pain, weakness, and stiffness. When measuring change in function of an individual, it is generally recommended that pain, physical function, motion, swelling, and function not be combined into a single score. The inclusion of impairments in a scale designed to measure function may attenuate the ability of the scale to assess true function and change in function.[79] Different concepts, such as swelling versus UE function, may change at different rates and may require different clinical interventions.[80] If the goal is to measure functional status and change in function related to Onc R interventions, a unidimensional measure of function, such as the UEFI, is a reasonable choice.

Physical and Psychosocial Function in Breast Cancer: FACT-B+4 Scale

The Functional Assessment of Cancer Therapy—Breast (FACT-B) is a widely used questionnaire that measures physical, social, functional, emotional, and BC-specific domains during and after treatment for BC.[81-83] In the FACT-B+4 version of the scale, four items were added that assess UE function and impairment for patients with lymphedema. The items are: (1) Movement of my arm on this side is painful; (2) I have a poor range of arm movements on this side; (3) My arm on this side feels numb; and (4) I have stiffness of my arm on this side. Each item is scored on a Likert scale from 0 to 4. Total domain scores can vary from 0 to 16 with higher scores representing greater levels of disability or abnormal sensation. This questionnaire has been shown to be reliable and valid in persons with BC, is available in 57 languages and can be attained through Facit.org.

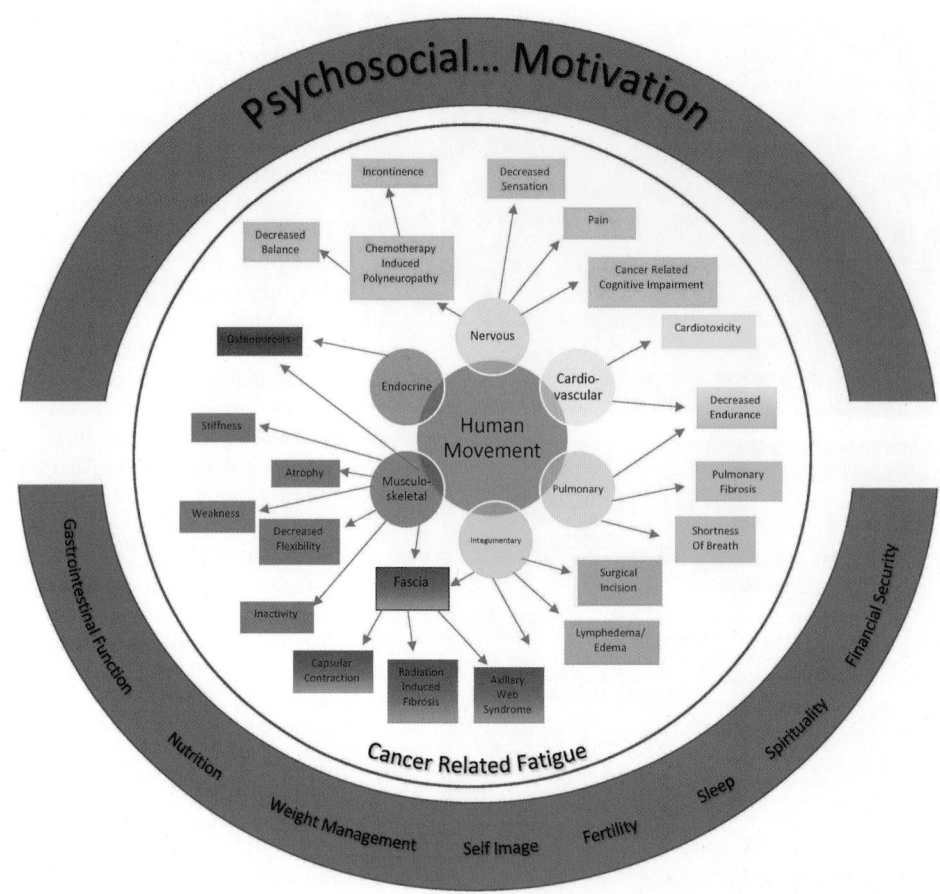

• **Fig. 15.21** Impact of Breast Cancer on Human Movement Domains. (Modified and reprinted with permission from The American Physical Therapy Association.)

Nervous System Issues

Chemotherapy-Induced Polyneuropathy and Balance

CIPN is a common, painful, and debilitating adverse effect of many standard BC chemotherapy regimens. Taxanes, platinum agents, vinca alkaloids, and proteasome inhibitors are known to be associated with CIPN. It may develop within weeks or months after the initiation of chemotherapy and may last from months to years after chemotherapy completion. PLWBCs report paresthesia, tingling, numbness, pain, muscle weakness, shortness of breath, incontinence, and balance impairments. The most reported areas of polyneuropathy are in the hands and feet; however, other peripheral nerves are also commonly involved, including the vestibulocochlear nerve, rectal nerve, and phrenic nerve. The neuropathy can be serious enough to limit or delay the dose of administered chemotherapy and may cause a discontinuation of treatment. Long-term CIPN has been associated with functional decline and diminished quality of life (QOL).[84,85] The course of CIPN is unpredictable and symptoms may improve in time, others may persist or worsen and can interfere with key aspects of QOL, including physical, social, and emotional well-being. Further detail on the assessment and management of CIPN can be found in Chapter 8.

Pain

Incidence and Common Findings

Postoperative pain is experienced by the majority of persons after a BC surgery in the following areas: chest wall, breast, primary and donor incision regions, drain sites, as well as the axilla

and upper extremity. Pain related to axillary cording is also common. Chronic postmastectomy pain syndrome (PMPS) has been reported in up to 30% of people with BC and appears to be related to younger age, tumor staging, history of chronic pain, and ALND. It is related to negative body image, sexual enjoyment, and QOL.[86]

Measurement

Pain assessment includes pain location, behavior, and intensity. The AOPTTF of the APTA on clinical measures of pain identified and evaluated 22 outcome measures used to assess pain in adults with a diagnosis of cancer.[72] On the basis of the psychometric properties, clinical utility, and relevance to adults with a diagnosis of cancer, the following three measures were highly recommended: McGill Pain Questionnaire–Short Form, Numeric Rating Scale (NPS), and Visual Analog Scale. The 11-point NPS, from 0 (no pain) to 10 (worst imaginable pain), is the most commonly used form of the NPS, easy to use in the clinic, and the value can be utilized to set goals and evaluate progress. Minimal detectable change (MDC) and MCID have been reported for orthopedic populations: MDC: 3 points and MCID: 3 points.[87–89]

Further detail on the assessment and management of cancer-related pain can be found in Chapter 22.

Musculoskeletal System

Posture and Breathing Patterns

In the postoperative period, it is common for PWCs to develop a protective posture and more shallow and rapid breathing. Many

PWCs have significant postural changes due to muscle and joint tightness, guarding, fibrosis, expanders, and implants, as well as pain. Forward head posture, protracted shoulders, and abnormal scapular position are all common. Reconstruction donor sites may also impact posture, such as tightness in an abdominal incision related to an abdominally-based reconstruction procedure (Figure 15.22).

Evaluation of the Mobility of the Shoulder Complex

Incidence and Common Findings

Reduced ROM of the shoulder complex is common and often continues several years after the conclusion of cancer treatment.[90–92] Evaluation of the shoulder complex in persons diagnosed with BC is similar to an orthopedic evaluation of the shoulder complex but key aspects are highlighted here. Active functional ROM is evaluated with the person in a standing position, when possible.[92] Following BC surgery, active and passive flexion and abduction are the most common ROM limitations and abduction is often the motion that elicits the symptoms of pain and restriction related to axillary cording and radiation fibrosis syndrome. Abduction is also where cording may be the most visible. Glenohumeral rotation should be assessed but is often not significantly restricted except where a PLWBC has a restriction of rotation related to frozen shoulder, significant pectoral tightness, or pre-existing pathology.

Evaluation of Shoulder Complex Motion

There is reasonable reliability for utilization of the goniometer to measure active shoulder ROM.[93] Passive ROM testing of the shoulder complex in supine with and without the scapula stabilized provides information regarding the relative contribution of articular restriction, muscle and soft tissue tightness and weakness to the functional limitation. The evaluation of shoulder motion through passive testing has been "highly recommended" by the AOPTTF on Breast Cancer Outcomes: Shoulder and Glenohumeral Outcome Measures based on psychometric properties but has not been evaluated in persons with BC.[93] Further work is needed related to establish adequate intra-rater and inter-rater reliability of active and passive goniometric shoulder measurements in a BC population. When active ROM is limited, passive joint accessory motion is evaluated to determine the extent to which each component of shoulder complex motion contributes to the restriction. Joints that should be assessed include glenohumeral, acromio-clavicular, sterno-clavicular, and scapulothoracic (Table 15.8). The reliability of determining glenohumeral stiffness in subjects without pathology and in persons with adhesive capsulitis is acceptable.[94] Good reliability was reported for the

assessment of anterior-to-posterior stiffness and posterior-to-anterior stiffness and the utilization of glenohumeral accessory motion testing was recommended for use by the AOPTTF based on good psychometric properties.[93] The reliability and validity of accessory motion testing of the other joints of the shoulder complex has not been reported.

Restriction and abnormal mechanics related to the scapulothoracic joint is common in people during and after treatment for BC (Table 15.9). There is good reliability reported for position assessment of the scapula, such as noting anterior/posterior tilt of the scapula in standing, but positional assessment is not necessarily predictive of pathology or motion abnormality since there are normal variations within and between people with and without pathology.[95] The scapulothoracic joint may be restricted, with tightness of soft tissues and limited motion on the chest wall. The scapula may be held in a protracted and laterally rotated position due to tightness of the anterior structures of the shoulder complex, such as pectoralis minor. The passive mobility of the scapula can be evaluated in side-lying. There are no studies to date that document the reliability of scapular mobility testing. Abnormal scapular mechanics, or scapular dyskinesia, have been reported in persons diagnosed and treated for BC[96] and are common clinically (Figure 15.23). The Dynamic Movement Assessment test has been shown to have reasonable reliability and validity, but has not

TABLE 15.8	Clinical Summary: Key Passive Motion Testing of Shoulder Complex (Supine)
Passive flexion, abduction, ER, IR with and without scapula stabilized	
G-H joint	
Inferior glide in abduction and flexion	
Posterior-anterior movement (P-A) in elevation	
A-C joint	
Posterior rotation of lateral clavicle in shoulder neutral position, abduction and supported elevation (restriction may contribute to limited shoulder elevation)	
S-C joint	
Inferior glide (restriction may contribute to limited shoulder elevation)	
Posterior glide (restriction may contribute to limited shoulder retraction)	

A-C, Acromioclavicular; *ER*, external rotation; *G-H*, glenohumeral; *IR*, internal rotation; *S-C*, sternoclavicular.
Created by Jill Binkley. Printed with permission.

TABLE 15.9	Clinical Summary: Scapular Mobility Assessment

Assess at rest and during motion:
- Muscle atrophy in scapular region
- Resting scapular position
- Prominence of the inferior and medial scapular border
- Elevation and anterior displacement of superior border
- Winging
- Note if dyskinesia is "present/absent"

Created by Jill Binkley. Printed with permission.

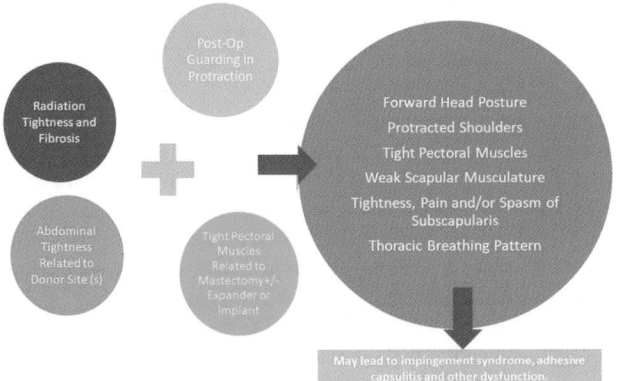

• **Fig. 15.22** Postural Relationships and Challenges During and After Treatment for Breast Cancer. (Created by Jill Binkley, printed with permission.)

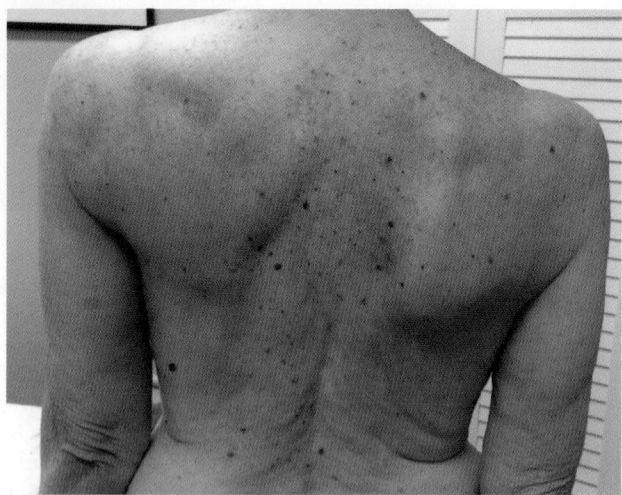

• **Fig. 15.23** Scapular Position Abnormality, Muscle Imbalance and Trunk and Shoulder Mobility Issues Following Bilateral Mastectomies With Implant Reconstruction and Radiation on Left. (Reprinted with permission from TurningPoint Breast Cancer Rehabilitation.)

been examined in a BC population.[97] Agreement between raters is increased when the original 4 point rating scale is collapsed to yes/no options with respect to the presence of scapular dyskinesia.[95,98]

Muscle Length Assessment

Muscles that commonly contribute to shoulder complex dysfunction in persons diagnosed and treated for BC through tightness or weakness include pectoralis minor, pectoralis major, subscapularis, latissimus dorsi, serratus anterior and sternocleidomastoid (Figure 15.24).

Other muscles may be involved as well and should be assessed based on clinical judgment. Tests for muscle length lack supporting evidence with respect to reliability and validity.[93,99] As such, the information gained from muscle length testing should be corroborated with other clinical findings, such as ROM testing, and should not be utilized as measures of outcome. The exceptions to this are several tests for pectoralis minor tightness that have been examined with respect to reliability. The Scapular Index

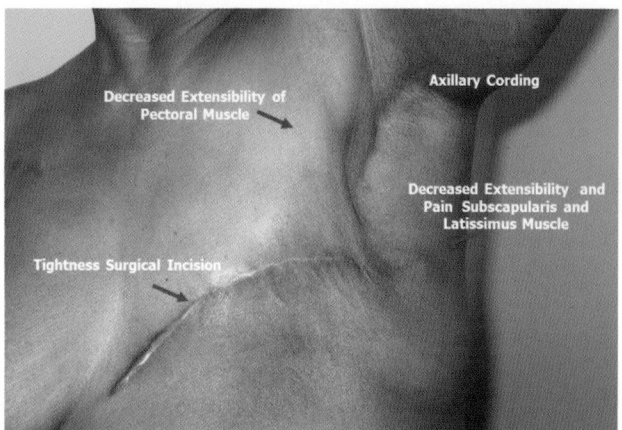

• **Fig. 15.24** Tightness and Decreased Extensibility of Surgical Incision, Subscapularis, and Latissimus Muscles With Axillary Cording Following Left Mastectomy and Radiation. (Reprinted with permission from Turning-Point Breast Cancer Rehabilitation.)

TABLE 15.10	**Clinical Note**

While assessing muscles of the shoulder complex, consider:
- Length-tension
- Tenderness
- Hypertrophy
- Spasm
- Atrophy

Created by Jill Binkley. Printed with permission.

measures—the distance between the sternal notch and the coracoid process anteriorly and the distance between the posterolateral angle of the scapula to the thoracic spine posteriorly—is measured with a tape measure.[100] It is recommended by the AOPTTF on Scapular Assessment, but further studies are needed to determine the validity and reliability, particularly in a BC population.[93] Please see Table 15.10 Clinical Note for overall considerations when assessing muscles of the shoulder complex. The mobility of the cervical and thoracic spine as well as ribcage should be assessed depending on postural and mobility findings.

Strength

Incidence of Weakness and Common Findings

Persons with BC have weakness and related functional loss compared to healthy women.[61,62] Scapular dyskinesia, shoulder joint position sense, and UE strength imbalances are also prevalent after BC surgery.[101] A meta-analysis that examined aerobic capacity and UE strength in women diagnosed with BC found generally these to be reduced compared to population norms.[102] Overall, persons living beyond BC have lower force production for shoulder muscle groups compared with controls and there is some indication that generalized weakness, including shoulder and knee extensors, is greater for individuals on tamoxifen.[103]

A literature review that included 13 studies concluded that latissimus dorsi reconstruction leads to measurable reductions in shoulder joint stability, strength, ROM, and general functioning.[104] These authors suggest that these deficiencies resolve in the majority of women within 6 to 12 months, but many of the studies reviewed did not have data on long-term follow-up.

There is impact on abdominal strength in individuals undergoing abdominal-based breast reconstruction. Strength deficits are greater in persons undergoing non muscle-sparing free TRAM flap surgery compared with DIEP flap surgery at early and late follow-up.[105] A systematic review examined abdominal strength deficits in persons with pedicled TRAM, free TRAM, and DIEP reconstruction, as measured by rectus abdominus and abdominal oblique muscle function, overall flexion and extension strength and ability to carry out ADL.[106] The review concluded that, with the exception of those who had bi-pedicled TRAM or bilateral free TRAM (which had significant impact on abdominal strength and function), most persons reported return to their preoperative function without a decrease in their ability to perform ADL.[106] A more recent study that included long-term follow up on function and QOL showed that there was no significant long-term impact of abdominally-based autologous breast reconstruction related to function and QOL.[107] The exception was in obese women, but it is not clear that this is related to the type of surgery.

Upper Extremity and Core Strength Assessment

Manual muscle testing is a common approach to assessment of strength in the clinic, but the grading system of 0 through 5 may not be useful when differentiating minor weakness. One approach to assessing UE strength is to assess grip strength as proxy measure for overall strength. However, there appears to be minimal correlation between grip strength and 1-repetition maximum (RM) bench press in individuals with BC.[108]

In early postoperative weeks, core strength can be evaluated by observing the individual moving from supine to sitting and standing. Clinical assessment of core strength is described in Chapter 7.

Integumentary System

Common Findings Related to Skin, Fascia, and Surgical Incisions

The person's chest wall, breast area, axilla, and abdominal wall should be examined and palpated, as applicable, considering:

- Skin condition
  - Erythema, rash, dryness, shiny appearance, necrosis
  - Secondary to radiation, particularly note erythema, tightness, skin changes
  - Rash and peau d'orange—note that these can be a sign of BC recurrence or IBC
- Skin hypersensitivity and numbness
  - Numbness of the skin of the breast, proximal UE, and/or axilla following mastectomy or BCoS
  - Hypersensitivity to light touch in the chest wall, especially the first several weeks postoperatively
- Seroma (accumulation of serous fluid) in area of surgical incisions, most common in mastectomy without reconstruction, donor latissimus site and lumpectomy incisions
- Bruising or hematoma
- Surgical incisions—location, healing status and condition, including drain, donor, port and SLNB/ALND sites, if applicable. See Figures 15.24–15.28
- Reconstruction-specific assessment
  - TRAM or DIEP reconstructions—tightness of abdominal wall and incision site

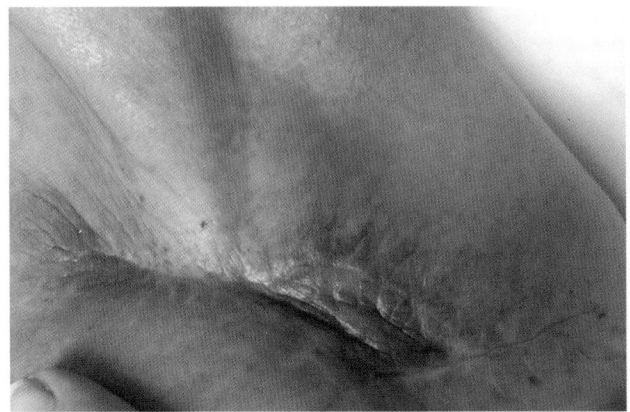

• **Fig. 15.26** Tightness and Reduced Mobility of Axillary Lymph Node Dissection (ALND) Incision Following Radiation. (Reprinted with permission from TurningPoint Breast Cancer Rehabilitation.)

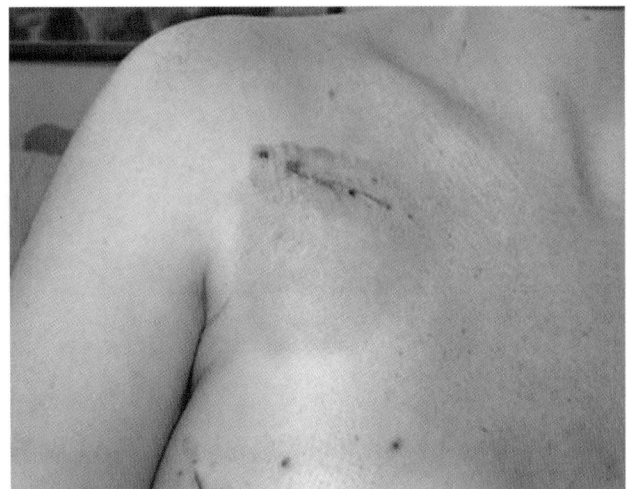

• **Fig. 15.27** Chemotherapy Port Site. (Reprinted with permission from TurningPoint Breast Cancer Rehabilitation.)

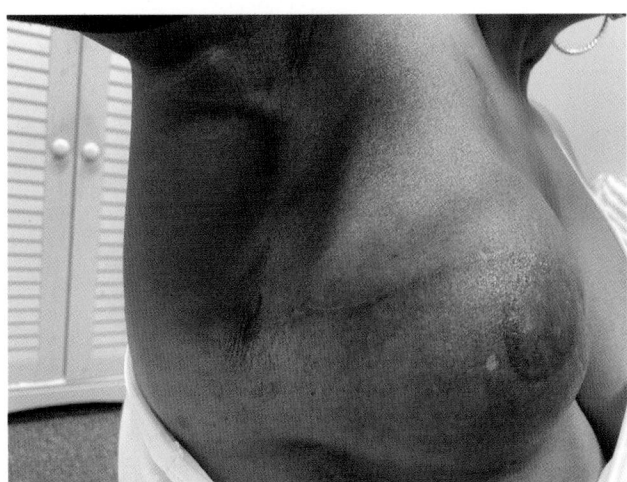

• **Fig. 15.25** Skin and Fascial Tightness of Lateral Chest Wall, Axilla and Breast Incision, Particularly Lateral End Where it is Bound Down. (Reprinted with permission from TurningPoint Breast Cancer Rehabilitation.)

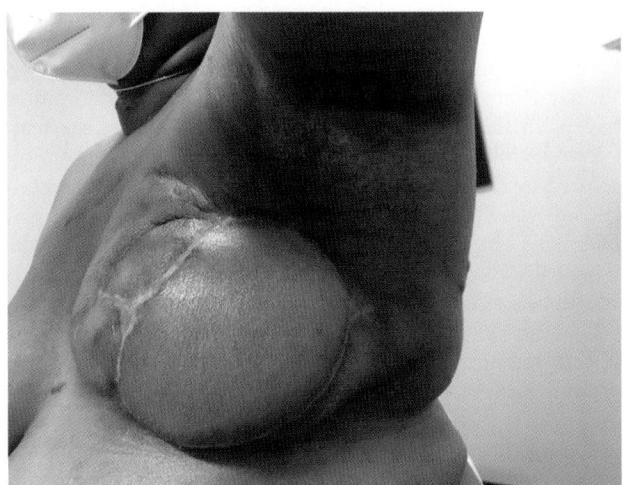

• **Fig. 15.28** Significant Tightness and Keloid Scarring Incisions, Lateral Chest Wall and Pectoralis Following Left Mastectomy With Latissimus Flap and Implant Reconstruction and Radiation. (Reprinted with permission from TurningPoint Breast Cancer Rehabilitation.)

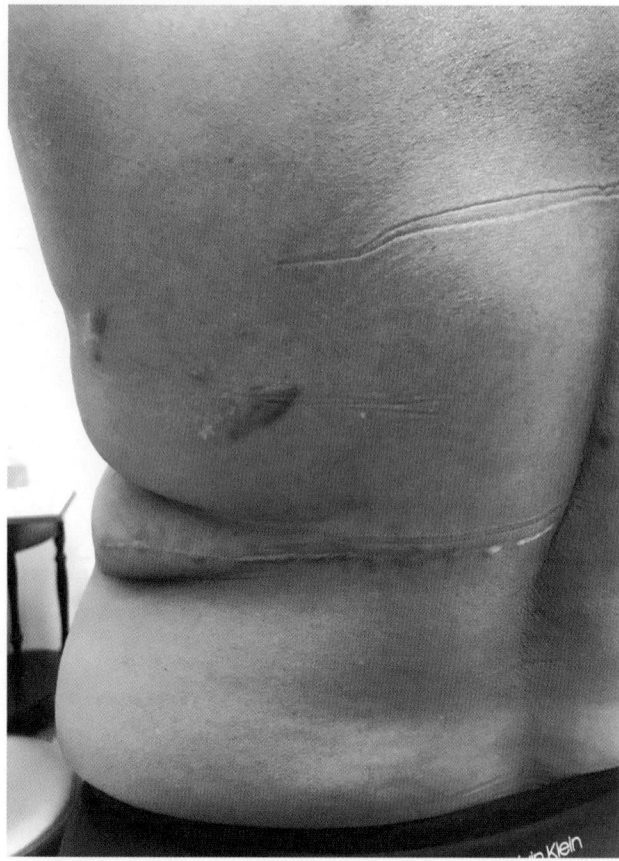

• **Fig. 15.29** Latissimus Flap Donor Site Incision, Skin and Fascial Tightness. (Reprinted with permission from TurningPoint Breast Cancer Rehabilitation.)

- Latissimus flap—tightness of soft tissue and skin mobility at incision site, lateral chest wall. See Figure 15.29
- Swelling of the mons pubis region

Further detail of integumentary issues can be found in Chapter 9.

Axillary Cording/Axillary Web Syndrome

The incidence of axillary cording, also known as axillary web syndrome, has been reported to range from 30%[109] to over 80%.[110] One study reported that cording occurs in approximately 50% of women following BC surgery, can persist for 18 months or longer and may recur months or years after resolution.[111] It commonly develops in the early postoperative stage, typically in the first 2 to 4 weeks following surgery. In a prospective study, most cords appeared by the seventh day (66.1%), and the total incidence of the cords was 90.9% at 6 months.[112] The location of cording was in the axilla for 80% of persons with BC and over 70% of cording was palpable. Flexion and abduction of the shoulder was reduced, and pain was associated with cording in about 40% of the persons in this study. Women with a body mass index (BMI) of less than 30, undergoing chemotherapy,[113] and those with hypertension are more likely to develop cording, while those with diabetes had lower risk.[112] There is conflicting evidence related to the relationship between age and the risk of developing cording. Individuals with cording in the first postoperative month have up to three times greater risk of developing lymphedema within the first postoperative year.[109,113] The pathogenesis of cording is not clear, some studies have associated it with lympho-venous injury, hypercoagulability due to superficial venous stasis, lymphatic disruption, and tissue injury after axillary lymph node removal.[114,115]

Axillary cording can often be visualized during active ROM assessment, particularly shoulder abduction. It can be more specifically evaluated by palpation assessed in supine, with the arm supported in abduction and the effect of positioning of the shoulder, elbow, and wrist can be assessed. Cording may be present in the axilla only or may extend in a common pattern into the medial upper arm, anterior elbow, forearm, and/or to the lateral wrist at the base of the thumb (Figures 15.30–15.33).

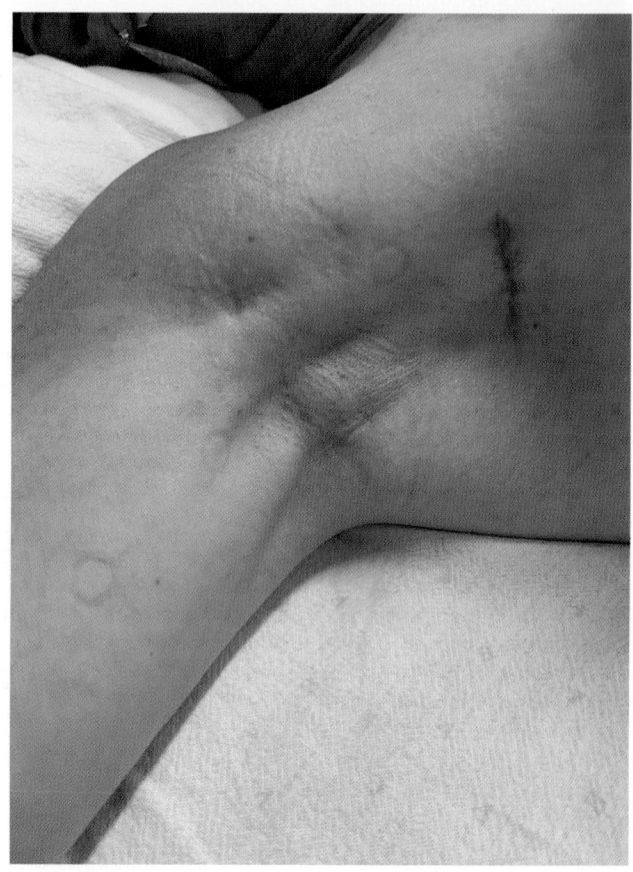

• **Fig. 15.30** Axillary Cording (Supine in Abduction). (Reprinted with permission from TurningPoint Breast Cancer Rehabilitation.)

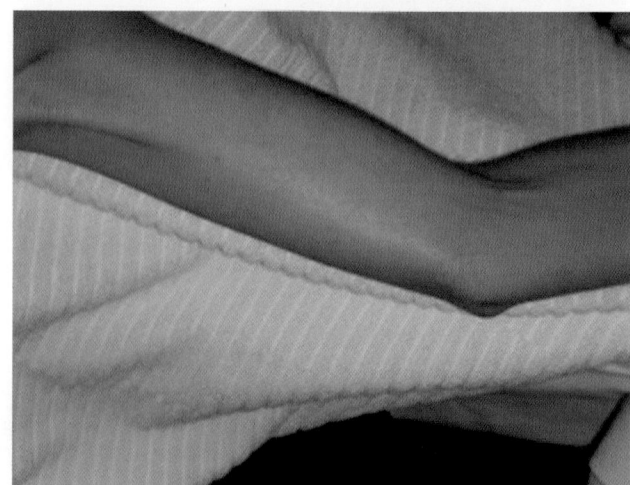

• **Fig. 15.31** Axillary Cording Extending From Axilla to Cubital Fossa, Increasing Stretch and Pain With Elbow Extension. (Reprinted with permission from TurningPoint Breast Cancer Rehabilitation.)

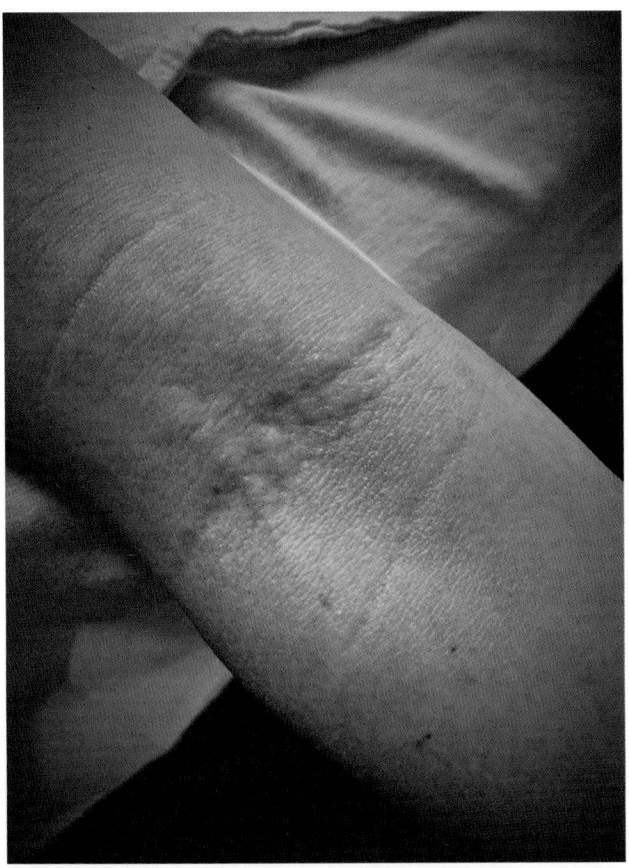

Fig. 15.32 Axillary Cording at Cubital Fossa. (Reprinted with permission from TurningPoint Breast Cancer Rehabilitation.)

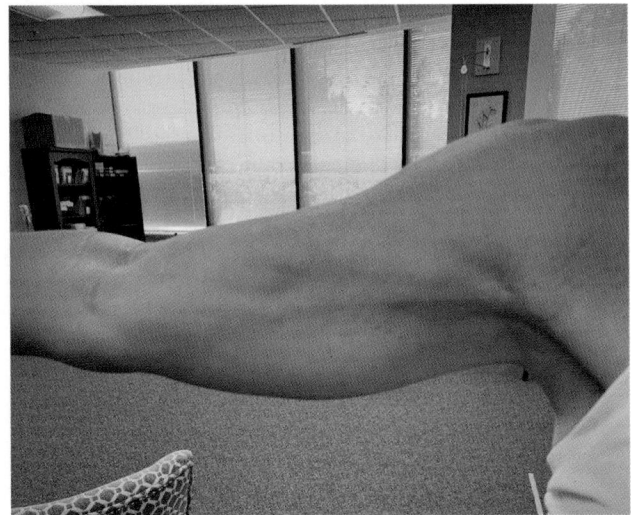

Fig. 15.33 Axillary Cording Extending From Axilla to Forearm in Standing Abduction. (Reprinted with permission from TurningPoint Breast Cancer Rehabilitation.)

Pain and tightness are often exacerbated with elbow and wrist extension. Pain level, motion restriction, and tightness and quality (e.g., thickness, extensibility, number) of cords are considered when evaluating axillary cording. Although most persons report cording in the axilla or arm, cording in the inframammary region is a common etiology of pain after BC surgery (Figure 15.34).[113]

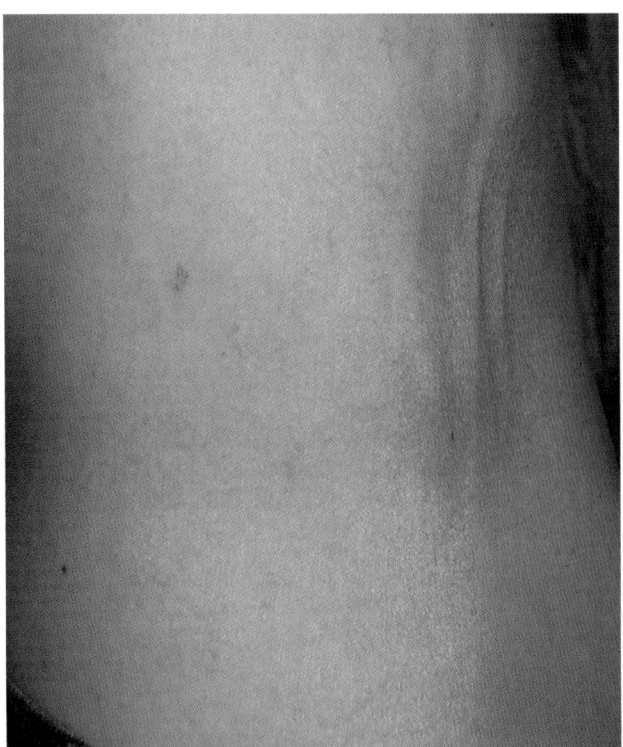

Fig. 15.34 Inframammary Cording (Standing). (Reprinted with permission from TurningPoint Breast Cancer Rehabilitation.)

Lymphedema

Incidence, Common Findings, and Evaluation

BC survivors are at risk for BC-related lymphedema (BCRL) for an average of 3 years following treatment for BC.[116] The reported incidence of BCRL ranges from 5% to 40%, with higher risk of lymphedema for persons who underwent axillary radiation, have a BMI in the obese range, who have developed a seroma, underwent chemotherapy infusion in the affected limb, and are diagnosed with advanced disease.[117,118] Taxane chemotherapy has been associated with increased lymphedema risk[119] while other studies suggest that taxane drugs do not present an increased risk.[120]

Infection or inflammation of the hand or arm, such as following a cut, can overload the lymph system and be a trigger for lymphedema. As such, education for individuals at risk should include simple precautions such as gloves while gardening, monitoring, and managing cuts for infection, and sun protection. Air travel, needlesticks, and blood pressure assessments have been discussed as potential triggers of BCRL. In a large prospective study, however, no evidence was found that these activities were risk factors for lymphedema.[121] In PLWBC at risk for lymphedema, it is suggested that, when feasible, the unaffected UE be utilized for blood pressure and needlesticks—but they do not need to feel anxiety related to these issues nor air travel. In the authors' experience, those at risk who are travelling longer distances should take fitted compression sleeves and, if appropriate, hand garments to allow early management should swelling occur while away. With respect to intravenous fluids administration, it is recommended that patients avoid these due to more prolonged tissue trauma and introduction of fluid to the limb.

Differences in defining and measuring lymphedema, time since diagnosis, and accurate risk stratification contribute to the wide variation in estimates of lifetime incidence of BCRL. There is, however, broad consensus that the lifetime incidence of lymphedema in persons with BC is approximately 20%.[90,91,116,122] BCRL is one of the most feared adverse effects of BC treatment and can lead to reduced health-related QOL, activity and participation restrictions, cosmetic concerns and economic hardship.[58,59,123] Early detection and management of lymphedema through prospective surveillance appears to reduce the progression of BCRL. This reduces both the impact to the person as well as cost to the healthcare system.[123–125]

There are challenges related to the accurate and efficient identification and measurement of UE lymphedema. While clinical examination is critical in the diagnosis of lymphedema, common approaches to detecting and quantifying lymphedema in a clinical setting include bioimpedance analysis and calculation of arm volume.[126] Bioimpedance analysis to detect early lymphedema has been shown to have good diagnostic accuracy for the detection of early lymphedema, when volume changes may not be detectable.[126–129] However, a more recent study investigated the diagnostic accuracy of bioimpedance analysis by comparing it to the reference test of iodocyanine green lymphography. The study found a high rate of false negative results for bioimpedance, suggesting that it may not be a valid method of detecting early lymphedema.[130] Additionally, in moderate to severe lymphedema, connective tissue changes such as fibrosis may make bioimpedance less accurate for assessing lymphedema.[126]

There is no gold standard for limb volume calculation. Methods of calculating limb volume include water displacement methods, limb circumferences converted mathematically to volume, and infrared three-dimensional sensor imaging devices.[126] Each of these methods demonstrate clinically sufficient reliability and validity.[131–134] Water displacement, often considered a reference standard, lacks feasibility in a clinical setting.[126] The perometer is the most commonly used infrared imaging device to quantify limb volume and has been shown to be efficient to use, reliable and valid when compared to water displacement (Figure 15.35).[126–131]

LymphaTech is a software application that utilizes custom software to capture three-dimensional depth data on an iOS mobile device. It has been shown to be reliable and valid and is portable.[135] The standard error of measurement and minimal

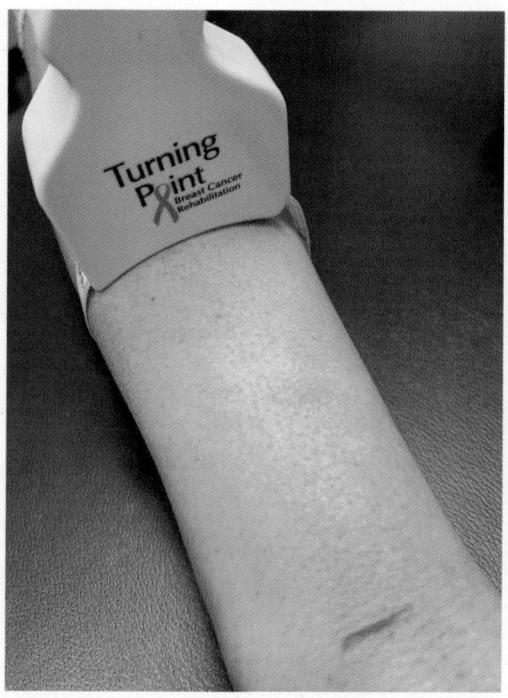

• **Fig. 15.36** Caliper Tape Measure Circumference Measures for In-clinic, Telerehabilitation and Home Self-Monitoring Usage. (Reprinted with permission from TurningPoint Breast Cancer Rehabilitation.)

detectable difference for the perometer and the LymphaTech is similar, both are able to detect change in limb volume between affected and unaffected by about 5%.[135,136] The perometer is expensive, large, and not easily available for purchase or to service in the US.[126] Serial circumference measures converted to volume are cost-efficient but can be time-consuming in a clinical setting, depending on the number of circumference measures required. A recent study demonstrated the reliability and validity of self-measure of arm circumference utilizing an inexpensive caliper tape measure[60,137] (Figure 15.36). Circumferences are obtained at five points, 10 cm apart, starting distally at the wrist. The circumference measures can be converted to volume. The method is efficient, useful in clinic settings as well as in telerehabilitaiotn applications and allows home self-monitoring.[138]

In early and mild lymphedema, persons may report the following signs and symptoms:
• Mild visible swelling in wrist or hand, particularly visible around tendons or bony prominences (Figures 15.37 and 15.38)
• Sensation of heaviness, fullness, or tingling in arm
• Clothing and/or jewelry feeling tight
• Increased swelling through the day that resolves overnight
• Lymphedema without other accompanying conditions, such as cording, and not typically painful

In moderate to severe lymphedema, swelling is more significant (Figure 15.39). It must be differentiated from a vascular issue such as a blood clot or disease recurrence in the axilla based on history and diagnostic testing, if applicable.

Detection of Early, Sub-Clinical Lymphedema: A Diagnostic Challenge

Sub-clinical lymphedema is defined as lymphedema that is developing but not yet visible. Research suggests that if identified and treated in this early phase, outcomes are improved with respect to limiting progression of the condition.[90,139] Accurate detection

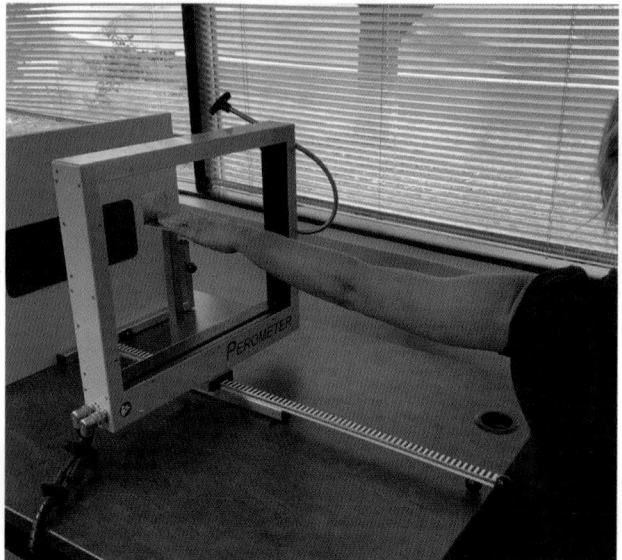

• **Fig. 15.35** Perometer Measure of Comparative Arm Volume. (Reprinted with permission from TurningPoint Breast Cancer Rehabilitation.)

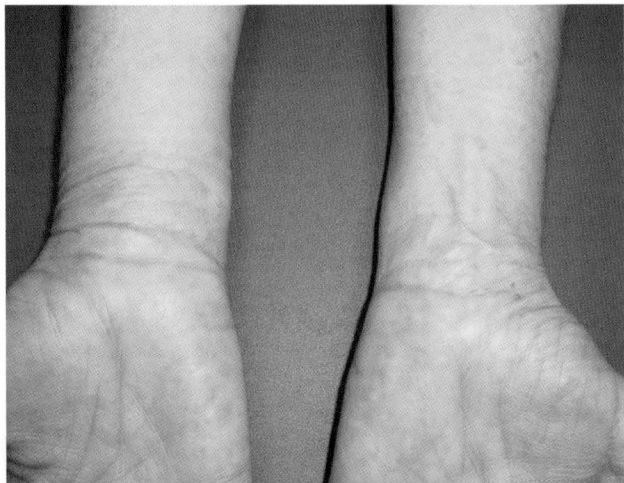

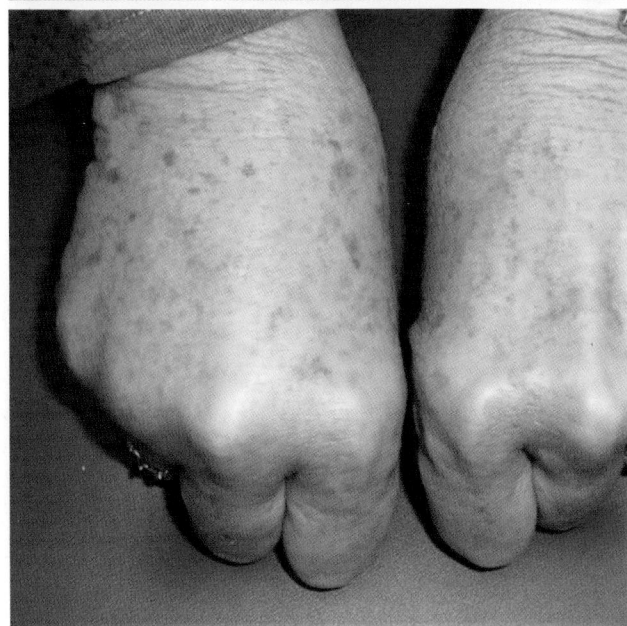

• **Fig. 15.37** Mild Lymphedema of the Right Upper Extremity Showing Filling in of Anterior Wrist Tendons and Skin Folds (Top) With Visible Swelling Over Radial Styloid and Filling of the Space Between the MCP Joints "Knuckle Check" (Bottom). (Reprinted with permission from TurningPoint Breast Cancer Rehabilitation.)

of early lymphedema—especially prior to a measurable volume change—is a diagnostic challenge for clinicians. Diagnostic accuracy, or the ability of a measurement system to accurately identify the presence or absence of lymphedema, is of critical importance when the goal is to detect early lymphedema.

Measurement and Staging of Visible Lymphedema

When nonpainful visible swelling is present in the affected upper limb or hand in a person with known risk factors for lymphedema and other causes of swelling can be ruled out, a clinical diagnosis of lymphedema can be made. At this stage, the goal is to have a measure of swelling that is as accurate as possible. While current measures of volume may lack the diagnostic accuracy to detect sub-clinical lymphedema, limb volume measures obtained by a perometer or sequential circumferences converted to volume are recommended for the assessment of lymphedema.[126] Obtaining these measures preoperatively, or at least early postoperatively, prior to any signs or symptoms of swelling can assist the clinician in determining the existence of swelling

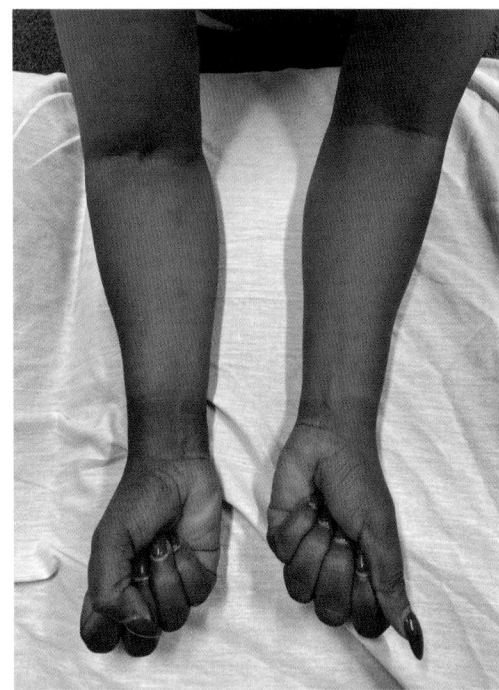

• **Fig. 15.38** Mild Lymphedema of Right Forearm. (Reprinted with permission from TurningPoint Breast Cancer Rehabilitation.)

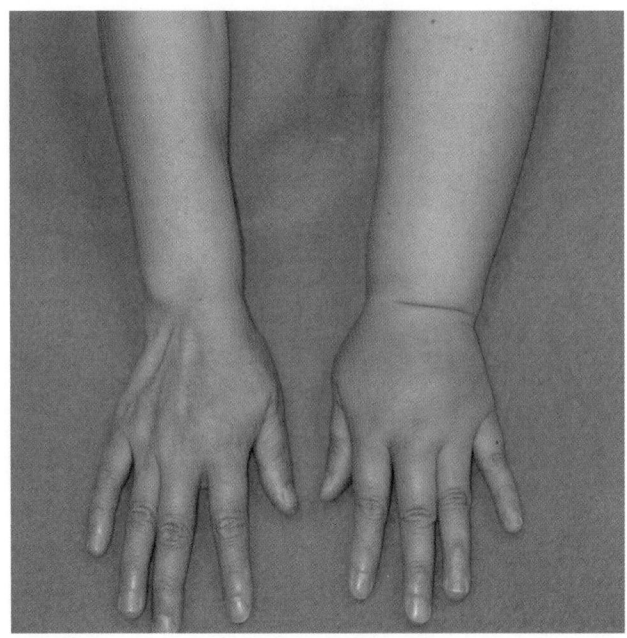

• **Fig. 15.39** Severe Lymphedema of Left Upper Extremity with Visible Swelling of Left Forearm, Wrist and Thenar Eminence. Left Upper Extremity is 28% Larger then Right. (Reprinted iwth permission from TurningPoint Breast Cancer Rehabiliation.)

by allowing a comparison to baseline. Weight gain and other causes of swelling, such as chemotherapy, can make interpretation of volume changes difficult even when a baseline is available. In addition, most persons have normal volume differences between dominant and nondominant arms. For these reasons, Onc R clinicians should consider changes from the baseline difference for both the affected and unaffected UEs to determine the volume and severity of lymphedema (affected to unaffected volume ratio). See Table 15.11 for an evidence-based approach to lymphedema management.

TABLE
15.11   Evidence-Based Approach to Lymphedema Management

	Transient Lymphostasis	Sub-Clinical Lymphedema	Mild Lymphedema (Stage I)	Moderate Lymphedema (Stage II)	Severe Lymphedema (Stage III)
Signs and Symptoms	Swelling of arm that occurs soon after surgery (either initial surgery or reconstruction) that resolves with or without treatment. Swelling easily reversible—usually diminishes at night. Note: Typically, transient lymphostasis is only identified when there is full resolution of swelling and no recurrence. Therefore, transient lymphedema is treated as per sub-clinical or mild lymphedema, depending on volume.	Heaviness, fullness, tingling sensations in affected arm. Affected to Unaffected Volume Ratio increased by 3%–5% compared to baseline. No obvious visible swelling, but there may be palpable soft tissue evidence of swelling.	Mild visible swelling in hand and/or arm. Swelling easily reversible—usually diminishes at night. Affected to Unaffected Volume Ratio increased by 3%–10% compared to baseline.	Nonreversible. Could be reversible with mild tissue changes Affected to Unaffected Volume Ratio increased by 8%–15% compared to baseline. Decreased visibility of veins. Visible swelling with fullness of the elbow, forearm, or wrist contours. Increases skin thickness with or without hand swelling.	Nonreversible. Affected to Unaffected Volume Ratio increased by greater than 15% compared to baseline. Skin changes with adhesions and fibrosis, skin may be indurated and dry.
Short-term management approach	Education: Skin and injury precautions—avoid infection and strain/sprain Signs & symptoms of lymphedema progression Nutrition and hydration issues Weight management Intervention: Exercise, compression, and intervention for upper extremity range of motion and/or strength per sub-clinical.	Education: See Transient. Intervention: *Compression*: Class I compression sleeve (Ready-made or custom as needed) for 2–3 weeks during waking hours until reduced, then as needed if swelling recurs; glove or gauntlet per judgment. *MLD*: Use with discretion ensuing that addition of MLD procedures measurable change. *Exercise*: Aerobic and progressive upper body resisted exercise. Assess and treat limitation in upper extremity range of motion and strength.	See Sub-Clinical.	Education: See Transient. Intervention: *Compression*: Course of lymphedema bandaging 23 hours/day for 2–4 weeks until volume reduced and plateaued. *MLD*: Use with discretion ensuring that addition of MLD produces measurable change. *Exercise*: Aerobic and progressive upper body resisted exercise. Assess and treat limitation in upper extremity ROM and strength.	Education: See Transient. Intervention: *Compression*: Course of lymphedema bandaging 23 hours/day for 2–4 weeks until volume reduced and plateaued. *Manual lyimphatic drainage*: Not indicated. Soft tissue techniques: Focus on areas of tissue changes to address fibrosis and adhesions. *Exercise*: Aerobic and progressive upper body resisted exercise. Assess and treat limitation in upper extremity ROM and strength. Trial of pump if indicated by lack of progression with above approaches.

TABLE 15.11	Evidence-Based Approach to Lymphedema Management—cont'd				
	Transient Lymphostasis	Sub-Clinical Lymphedema	Mild Lymphedema (Stage I)	Moderate Lymphedema (Stage II)	Severe Lymphedema (Stage III)
Long-term management approach	Surveillance to determine lymphostasis versus lymphedema.	Ongoing education and weight management *Compression*: Sleeve as needed or measurable swelling. Sleeve as determined for athletics or travel. *Exercise*: Aerobic and progressive upper body resisted exercise. Surveillance and adjustment of management plan as needed.	See Sub Clinical.	Ongoing education and weight management *Compression*: As needed to maintain lymphedema at goal volume. This may be a combination of compression sleeve and/or intermittent bandaging. Sleeve as determined by clinician for athletics or travel. *Exercise*: Aerobic and progressive upper body resisted exercise. Surveillance and adjustment of management plan as needed.	Ongoing education and weight management *Compression*: As needed to maintain lymphedema at goal volume. May be a combination of compression sleeve and/or intermittent bandaging. Local treatment with compression for areas of fibrosis. *Exercise*: Aerobic and progressive upper body resisted exercise. Surveillance and adjustment of management plan as needed.

Created by Jill Binkley. Printed with permission.

Cardiovascular and Pulmonary Issues

Reduction in Aerobic Capacity

Aerobic capacity has been shown to be reduced in persons diagnosed with BC during and after treatment compared to population norms.[102,140] Decreased aerobic capacity has been shown to be associated with lower QOL in persons diagnosed with and treated for BC.[141] Reduced aerobic capacity may be caused by cancer-related reductions in skeletal muscle mass and lower oxidative capacity may contribute to cardiovascular disease risk in this population by limiting the ability to engage in aerobic exercise.[140] Aerobic capacity is addressed in more detail in Chapter 23.

Fatigue

Incidence and Common Findings

Cancer-related fatigue is a significant issue that impacts QOL during and after treatment for BC and about 25% of individuals have severe fatigue.[142] Risk factors for severe fatigue are higher disease stages, chemotherapy, and receiving the combination of surgery, radiotherapy, and chemotherapy.[143] Hormone therapy does not appear to be a significant risk factor for severe fatigue. Having a partner, receiving only surgery, or surgery and radiation without chemotherapy decreased severe fatigue risk in individuals with BC.[143] Psychological factors, including depression, childhood trauma and factors such as younger age, obesity, physical inactivity, sleep problems, hot flashes, and lack of social support appear to be risk factors for more significant fatigue related to chemotherapy and radiation in BC.[144,145]

Measures of Fatigue

Inquiry should be made during the assessment related to fatigue and the impact of fatigue on usual activities and roles. While there are numerous fatigue scales, for clinical use the AOPTTF on Measures of Cancer-Related Fatigue suggest that the 11-point numeric pain rating scale for fatigue is appropriate as a screening tool.[146,147] The suggested format is to ask the person to rate their fatigue on a scale of 0–10 with 0 being "no fatigue" and 10 being the "worst possible fatigue." The scale has good test-retest reliability.[95] Further detail on CRF, including measures and management is found in Chapter 8.

Cancer-Related Cognitive Impairment

Chemotherapy and hormonal therapy for BC can have adverse effects on cognition during and after treatment, particularly in the domains of verbal and visuospatial ability, termed cancer-related cognitive impairment (CRCI).[148] These cognitive deficits and have been shown to persist in as long as 20 years post-treatment and may be related to persistent elevated inflammatory markers.[149] See Chapter 8 for further detail on cognitive changes, evaluation, and management of cognitive issues relevant to Onc R.

Pelvic Floor Issues and Urinary Incontinence Issues

A metanalysis found that women with BC had a higher prevalence of urinary incontinence (38%) compared to women without BC (21%).[150] Urinary incontinence is highly prevalent at BC diagnosis and appears to be worse following adjuvant therapy.[151] Endocrine therapy for BC can exacerbate menopausal symptoms, but to date, there does not appear to be an association between urinary incontinence and hormone therapy use, nor does there appear to be a difference between tamoxifen and AI use compared to no use.[152] Please refer to Chapter 12 for more information about pelvic floor issues.

Onc R Management Approach

International Classification of Functioning, Disability, and Health (ICF) Model Application to Breast Cancer Rehabilitation

The ICF system addresses human functioning, providing a standard language and framework that describes how people with a health condition function in their daily lives, rather than focusing on a labeled diagnosis or the presence or absence of disease. Cancer is truly a multisystem disease process. Careful attention needs to be placed on assessment of all body systems as designed in the movement system figure (see Movement System Figure 15.21). Whether treating specifically or referring to another discipline or specialty, the comprehensive management of PLWBCs is essential for truly individualized care. Each clinician has the autonomy to determine what model of care works best for their discipline and practice. Regardless of the model of care, shared decision making is essential (see Chapter 2). Due to the potentially overwhelming nature of adverse effects and needs of some, it is imperative to develop a strategic plan of short- and long-term goals in collaboration with the PWC and, when applicable, the caregiver.

Prospective Surveillance

The prospective surveillance model of rehabilitation was developed by an expert panel based on evidence supporting improved outcomes with early detection and management of impairment and functional issues (Figure 15.40).[125] The model includes early baseline assessment of impairment and function, ideally preoperatively with ongoing intermittent follow-up assessment postoperatively and throughout the trajectory of care. As issues are identified, rehabilitation can be initiated early for optimum outcomes. Education and exercise is woven throughout the model. Implementation of the model has been shown to be an effective approach to identifying the need for rehabilitation as well as reducing and even preventing the impact of adverse effects.[123,153,154]

Telerehabilitation

Telerehabilitation, online education, and virtual support groups for individuals during and after BC treatment provided a safe alternative for rehabilitation during the COVID-19 pandemic (Figure 15.41).[155] Several advantages were realized, including increased flexibility for PLWBCs related to scheduling and the potential for improved caregiver involvement in their family member's care.

Using telerehabilitation, observing a person in their home provides additional benefits when Onc R clinicians were able

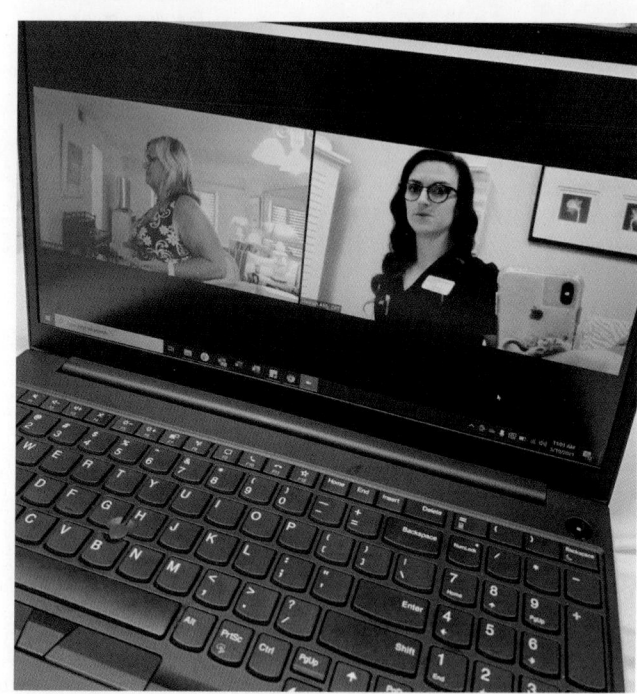

• **Fig. 15.41** Instruction in Resistance Exercise via Telerehabilitation. (Reprinted with permission from TurningPoint Breast Cancer Rehabilitation.)

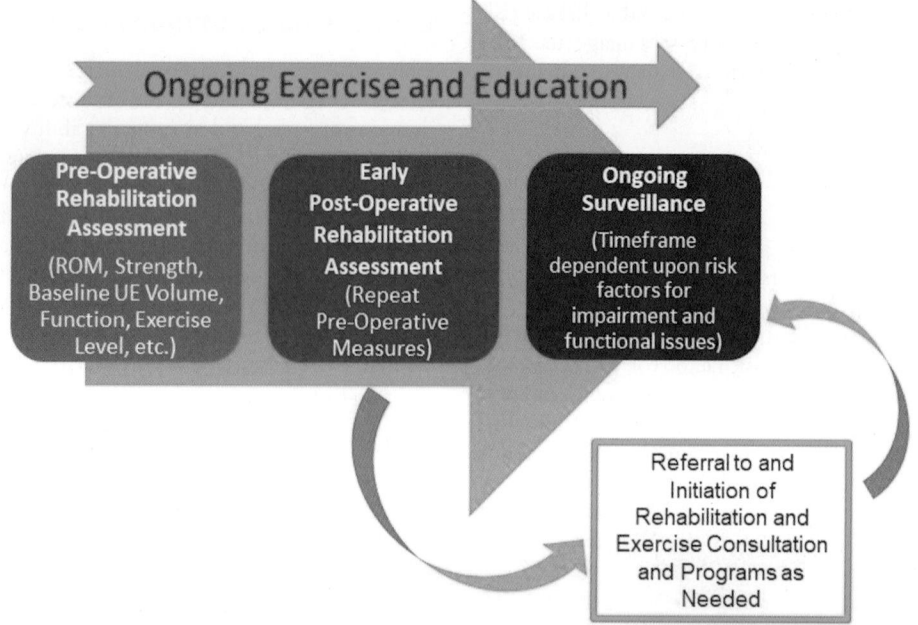

• **Fig. 15.40** Schematic Diagram of the Prospective Surveillance Model of Breast Cancer Rehabilitation. (Created by Jill Binkley. Printed with Permission.)

to observe an exercise program in the PWC's, usual environment. Onc R clinicians can evaluate and advise related to issues such as home office space ergonomics and sleep position via this method. Reported success of a live interactive web-based format for education, group exercise, and support groups demonstrate an opportunity for clinicians to lead broad community cancer survivorship education and exercise initiatives. Implementation of telerehabilitation, virtual education, and support programs offered by Onc R clinicians has opened frontiers in caring for PLWBC that will continue to expand and can be offered stand alone or in combination with in-person care.[155] These care options may reduce barriers to the prospective model of care for preoperative and long-term surveillance by increasing access to care remotely. This model can be applied to other cancer populations.

Education

Research is clear that rehabilitation, including exercise, improves QOL, and reduces or prevents treatment-related issues, but it is estimated that less than 20% of cancer survivors are referred for care.[60] PLWBCs voice a need for information and education related to the incidence and management of BC survivorship issues. The following topics should be included in a comprehensive oncology education program that focuses on empowering each person with knowledge and promoting self-efficacy:

- Early postoperative expectations, including activity level, sleep positions, functional expectations, cording and ROM exercise
- Understanding individual risk, incidence, risk reduction strategies, early detection and basic management related to lymphedema
- Importance of physical activity during and after treatment for BC and home exercise program that includes components of stretching, resistive, and aerobic exercise depending on phase of surgical and medical treatment
- Understanding and managing fatigue
- Effects of radiation, radiation recall and fibrosis, if applicable
- Knowledge of red flags during and following treatment (Table 15.12)
- Emotional, psychosocial, nutritional, and financial impact of BC and awareness and referral to other resources, including counseling, massage therapy, nutrition, financial counseling

TABLE 15.12	When to Call The Onc R Clinician

Call your Onc R clinician if you experience:

New swelling of your hand or arm

Decreased mobility and function

Increased tightness, restriction, or skin issues following radiation

Change in ability to carry out your usual functional activities or exercise program

Increased fatigue

Significant increase in usual pain over 2–3 days

<u>It is important to call your physician immediately</u> if you experience symptoms such as fever, redness, or drainage from surgical sites or new areas of pain

Created by Jill Binkley. Printed with permission.

Manual Therapy

Evidence and Experience

A systematic review identified five randomized clinical trials for inclusion in a meta-analysis on manual therapy as a treatment for chronic musculoskeletal pain in PLWBCs.[156] Manual therapy techniques included myofascial release, massage, and/or trigger point release. The metanalysis demonstrated a significant effect of manual therapy on pain compared to controlled conditions. A significant improvement in ROM was reported in one high quality study.[157] There was no significant difference in QOL reported in three studies and no change in shoulder function reported in one study.[156]

In the authors' experience, manual techniques are important components of the management of soft tissue and joint restriction related to surgery, both in the region of the surgery and reconstruction as well as soft tissue adhesions in the areas of donor, drain, and port sites. Manual therapy is useful in the management of radiation-induced tissue tightness and fibrosis with the caveat that the actual radiation site should be avoided during radiation and until the acute inflammatory reaction settles. Manual therapy techniques are also useful in the management of cording, dealt with later in this section.

Joint Mobilization

Shoulder and trunk mobility limitation seen early postoperatively is typically a result of soft tissue, incision pain and tightness, as well as cording, rather than shoulder and trunk joint restriction. The exception is if the limitation was pre-existing. In more chronic mobility limitations, mobilization of the glenohumeral, sternoclavicular, and acromioclavicular joints as well as the ribs and spine are useful in the treatment of more specific joint restriction (Figure 15.42). Delay in postoperative rehabilitation, radiation changes, and chronic pain may contribute to specific articular restriction.

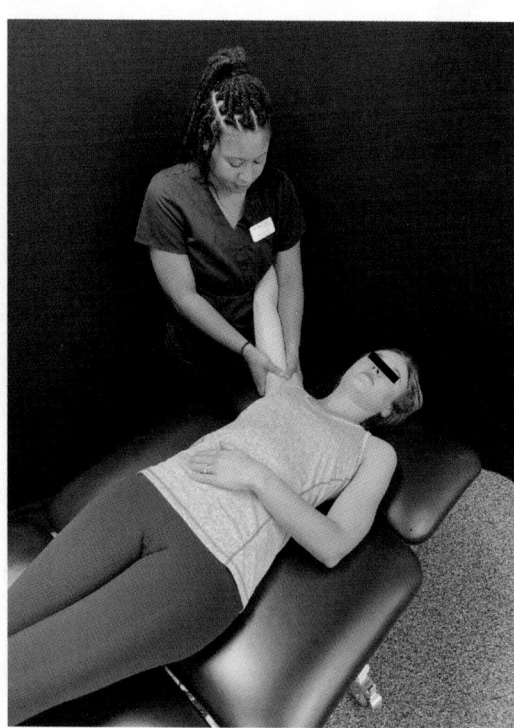

• **Fig. 15.42** Glenohumeral Joint Mobilization for Articular Restriction. (Reprinted with permission from TurningPoint Breast Cancer Rehabilitation.)

Soft Tissue Mobilization

Pectoralis major and minor are commonly restricted postoperatively but are most significant in persons who have had reconstruction with expanders and/or implants. Manual techniques that incorporate supported muscle stretch, gentle contract/relax, and myofascial work are useful to facilitate stretch of the pectoral muscles. Subscapularis is commonly tight and painful in PLWBCs, contributing to lateral chest wall pain and tightness. Manual techniques combined with gentle stretch are useful to reduce this tightness as well as restriction in the scapulothoracic joint (Figures 15.43 and 15.44).

Management of Cording

A systematic review of the management of axillary cording identified two randomized trials that manual therapy, including stretching and manual lymph drainage are beneficial in the management of cording.[158] In another systematic review, myofascial release, scar massage, stretching, and manual lymph drainage appeared to be effective components of cording management.[110] Several studies have shown the benefit of Onc R intervention for cording that included manual techniques in addition to therapeutic exercise.[159–162]

Another systematic review of axillary cording concluded that there is good quality evidence to support therapeutic exercise and a possible role of nonsteroidal anti-inflammatory agents (NSAIDs) for the management of cording.[110] In the authors'

experience, NSAIDs may be most useful during the acutely painful and inflammatory phase of treatment in combination with specific stretching, therapeutic exercise, and manual techniques.

While research supports manual therapy in general in the management of cording, the authors' experience suggests that some specific techniques are valuable in the management of cording, including segmental stretch, soft tissue massage, and self-massage of cording in progressive stretch positions (Figures 15.45–15.47). The stretch of the cording may be produced through shoulder abduction, elevation, and elbow extension, alone or in combination. In the initial and very painful postoperative phase of cording, very gentle supported stretch and manual techniques are most effective in reducing pain and increasing extensibility of cording and ROM. As pain decreases and healing phase allows, the stretch and manual techniques can be slightly more forceful. Gentle release, or popping, can sometimes be felt during stretch and manual techniques. While it is not a goal to "pop" inflamed cords, this phenomenon is considered harmless, often resulting in subjective relief of pain and tightness and may be due to release of scar tissue around the cord.

Exercise

Early postoperative shoulder ROM exercise has been shown to increase ROM and function initially and in the long-term.[163] A systematic review of exercise related to upper limb morbidity

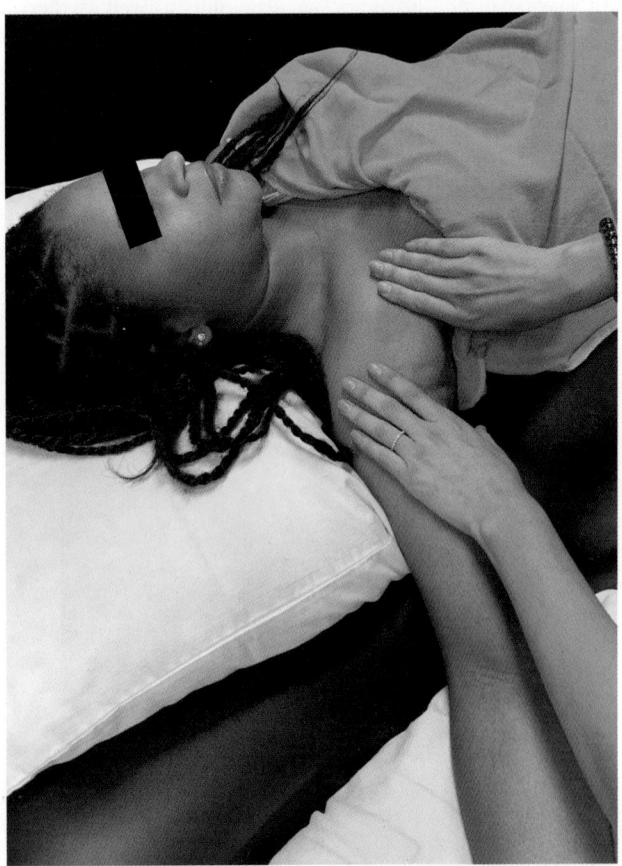

• **Fig. 15.43** Manual Therapy Techniques for Pectoral Tightness in Supported Abduction. (Reprinted with permission from TurningPoint Breast Cancer Rehabilitation.)

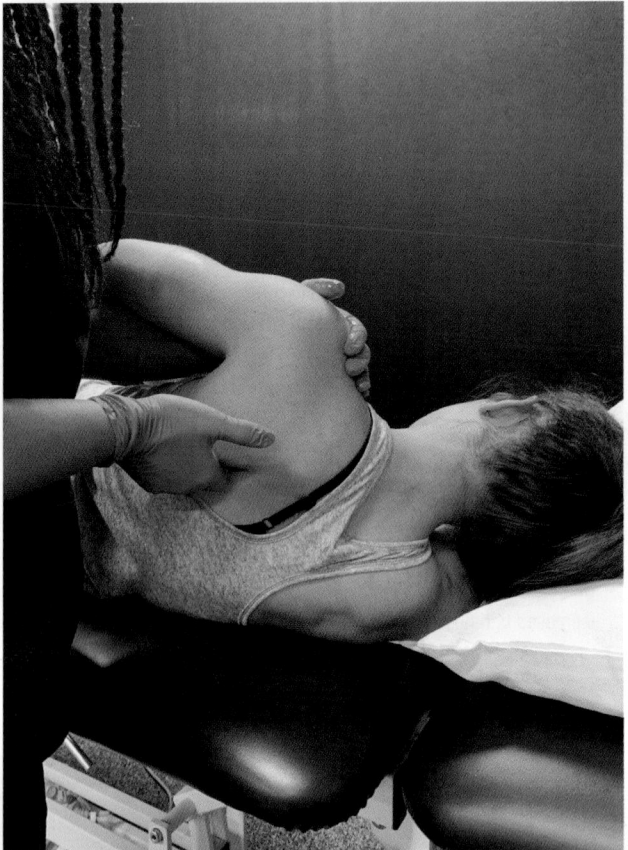

• **Fig. 15.44** Scapular Mobility in Side-Lying. (Reprinted with permission from TurningPoint Breast Cancer Rehabilitation.)

was no indication that upper-limb exercise was associated with increased lymphedema risk.[164]

PLWBCs have increased risk for UE strength imbalance. An 8-week resistance training program was shown to improve strength.[101] Shoulder retractor weakness and protective protraction is common in even the early postoperative phase and active and isometric shoulder retraction can be initiated in this early phase.

There is strong evidence to support aerobic and resistance exercise alone and combined in improving QOL, physical fitness, and fatigue during and after treatment for BC.[169] Persons diagnosed and treated for BC may benefit from exercise during adjuvant cancer treatment through improved cognitive function and improved cancer site-specific QOL. Aerobic and resistance exercise has been shown to be effective for the management of AI-induced arthralgia. Exercise appears to lower the risk of lymphedema and is important in the management of lymphedema.[165–168] Importantly, exercise reduces the risk of recurrence of BC.[165,169–171]

Key Exercises for Shoulder and Trunk Mobility

In the first 2 weeks postoperatively, posture, breathing, shoulder retraction and posterior shoulder rolls, sleep positions, and gentle ROM below 90 degrees of shoulder elevation are emphasized (Figures 15.48 and 15.49).

In weeks 2 to 4, gentle ROM exercises are emphasized and several key exercises are shown in Figures 15.50–15.52.

In later stages of recovery, weeks 4 to 6 and beyond, stretching is progressed based on tissue healing, pain, tolerance, and other individual factors such as ongoing fills of tissue expanders. Some examples of progressing stretches for the upper quadrant and trunk are in eFigures 15.1–15.3. A series of stretching and strengthening exercises are available in the Breast Cancer Recovery Exercise series in the Enhanced e-Book.

Resistance Exercise

UE resistance exercise can be initiated for nonsurgical region muscle groups, such as hand squeeze, biceps, triceps, core engagement at 2 to 3 weeks postoperatively. When there is no delayed healing or persistent seroma, resistance exercises can be added 6 weeks postoperatively and gradually progressed. Resistance exercise is individualized and should include the major muscle groups of the UE, lower extremity and core.[163]

Aerobic Exercise

Light aerobic exercise, typically walking, should be encouraged within a few days postoperatively. PLWBCs should be encouraged to build up to 150 minutes of moderate intensity per week or 5 times per week for 30 minutes.[163] In individuals without postoperative complications, aerobic exercise can gradually be increased at 6 weeks following surgery.

Aerobic exercise should be encouraged during chemotherapy and radiation to reduce fatigue and improve QOL.[163] For individuals with fatigue, encouraging light aerobic exercise such as walking or cycling for as much as can be tolerated, even 10 minutes, should be encouraged.

Overall resistance training or resistance training in combination with cardiovascular endurance training provides the best results, especially on physical performance and perceived fatigue.[172] It appears that resisted exercise modulates proinflammatory cytokine levels elevated by chemotherapy and radiation. Aerobic and resistance exercise benefits can be gained from many

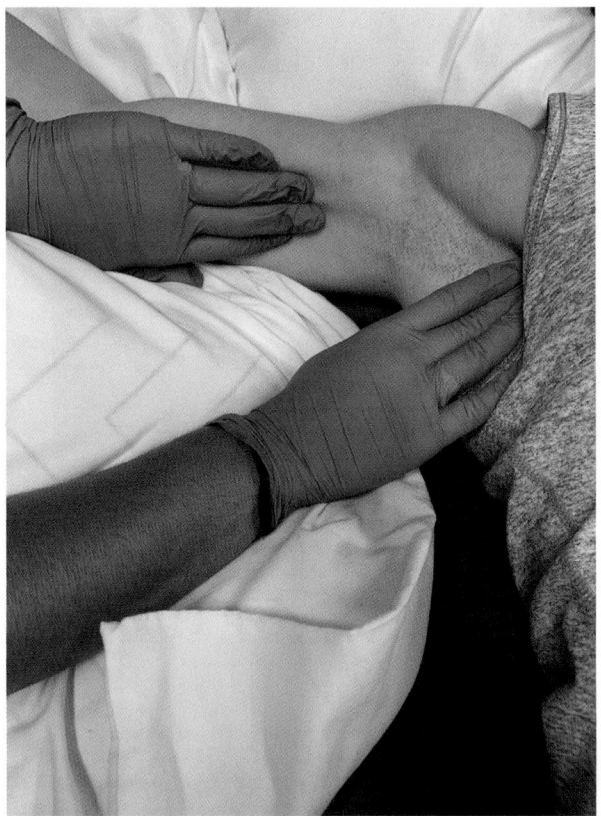

• **Fig. 15.45** Gentle Segmental Stretching of Cording in Supported Abduction. (Reprinted with permission from TurningPoint Breast Cancer Rehabilitation.)

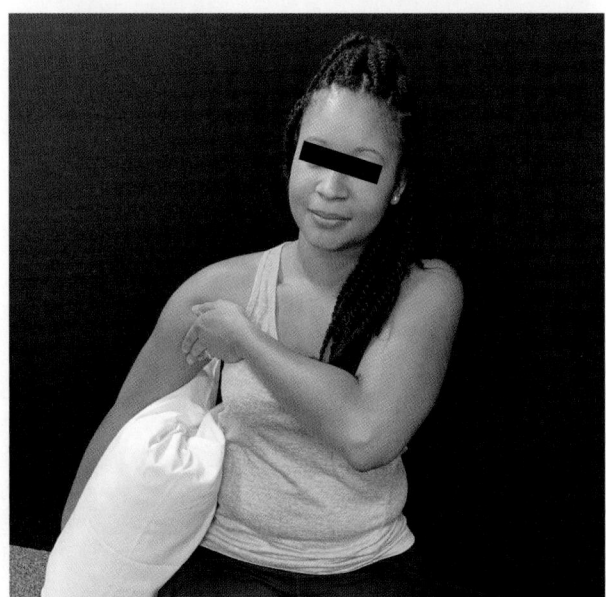

• **Fig. 15.46** Gentle Self-Massage of Acute Cording in Early Phase of Treatment. (Reprinted with permission from TurningPoint Breast Cancer Rehabilitation.)

found that shoulder ROM and stretching is helpful in recovering upper-limb movement following surgery for BC.[164] Starting exercise early after surgery may result in more wound drainage and require the drains to be in place longer than if exercise is delayed by about 1 week. This review showed that more structured exercise programs, such as Onc R, delivered in the early weeks following surgery are beneficial to regain movement and function. There

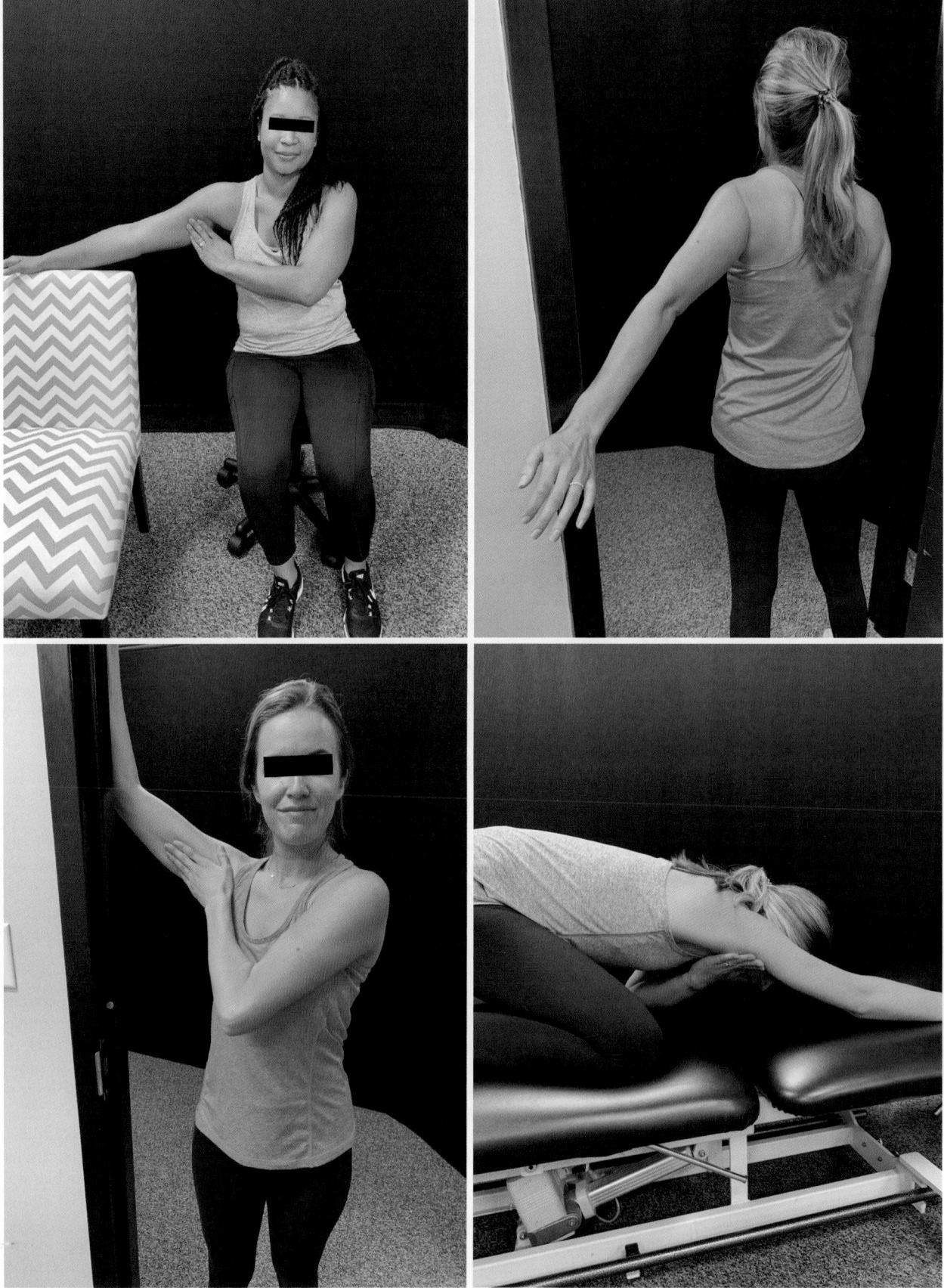

• **Fig. 15.47** Progressing Stretch and Self-Massage for Axillary Cording: Outstretched Over Chair or Table, Can Add Wrist Extension and Rotation Away for Increased Stretch as Tolerated (Top Left); Single Arm Doorway Stretch "Flossing" with Gentle Wrist Flexion and Extension During Stretch, Can Progress to Increased Elevation as Tolerated (Top Right); Doorway Stretch in Elevation (Bottom Left); Child's Pose Position (Bottom Right). (Reprinted with permission from TurningPoint Breast Cancer Rehabilitation.)

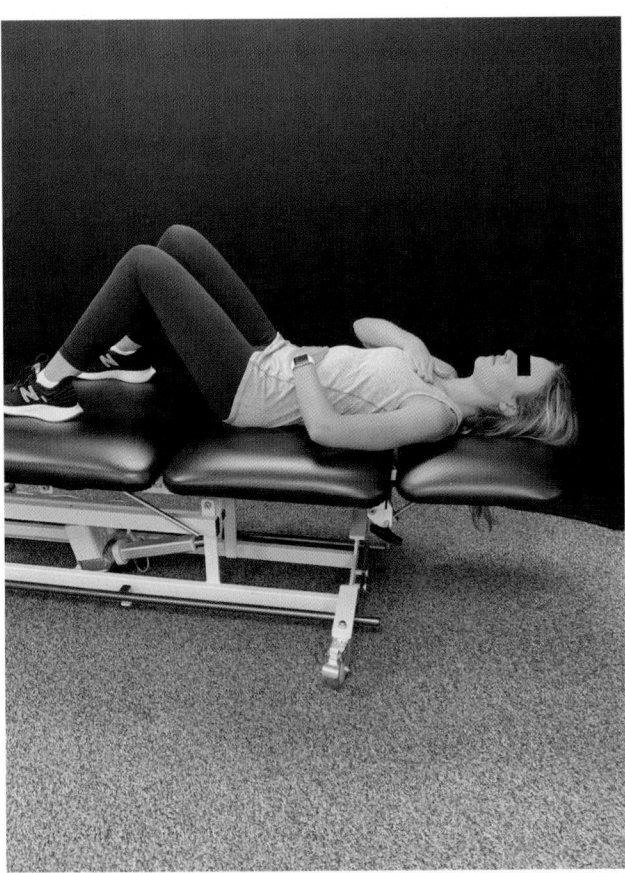

• **Fig. 15.48** Diaphragmatic Breathing Exercise. (Reprinted with permission from TurningPoint Breast Cancer Rehabilitation.)

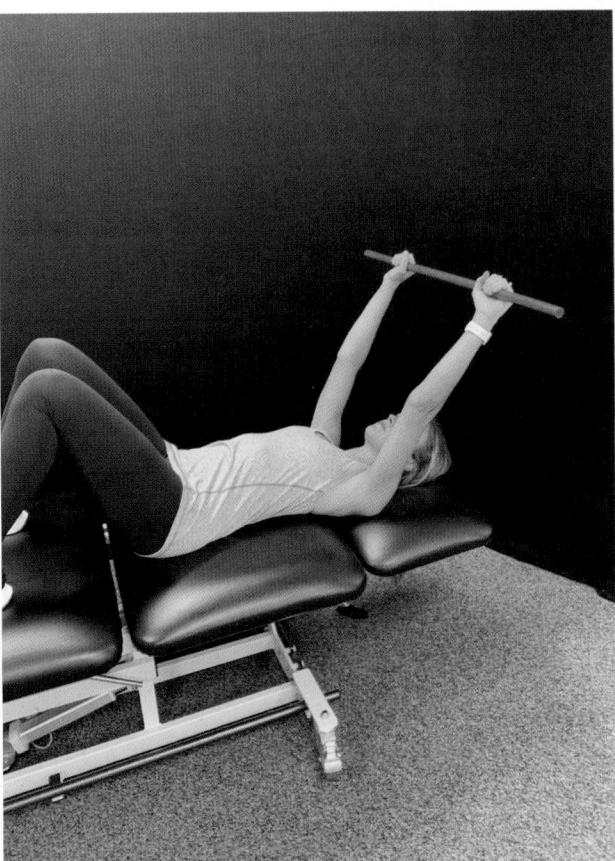

• **Fig. 15.50** Overhead Stretch With Stick. (Reprinted with permission from TurningPoint Breast Cancer Rehabilitation.)

different types of exercise programs during adjuvant therapy. It is important to identify the exercise that works for the PLWBC that can be sustained throughout treatment and beyond.

The Onc R clinician is instrumental in providing guidance related to balancing activity and fatigue during this time. A daily log of activity and fatigue level can be helpful to encourage activity while acknowledging, tracking, and reporting fatigue. Refer to Chapter 23 for more information on resistance training.

Special Exercise Approaches: Yoga, Pilates, and Water Aerobics

There is evidence to support the safety and benefits of yoga[173–176] and water aerobics[177–179] for BC survivors. Specialized programs led by instructors familiar with BC surgery and medical treatment may be of particular benefit. Group exercise classes led by Onc R clinicians have been shown to be of particular value during and after BC treatment and for persons diagnosed with MeBC.[180–182]

Lymphedema Management

Evidence and Experience (see also Chapter 9)

There is significant evidence to guide the management of BCRL. Managing lymphedema in the earliest phase is most effective in reducing progression. This is facilitated by obtaining baseline volume measures for comparison during prospective surveillance and education related to early signs and symptoms of lymphedema.[124,125] In general, the goal is to detect mild visible swelling and/or small volume increases of about 5% compared to baseline on the same

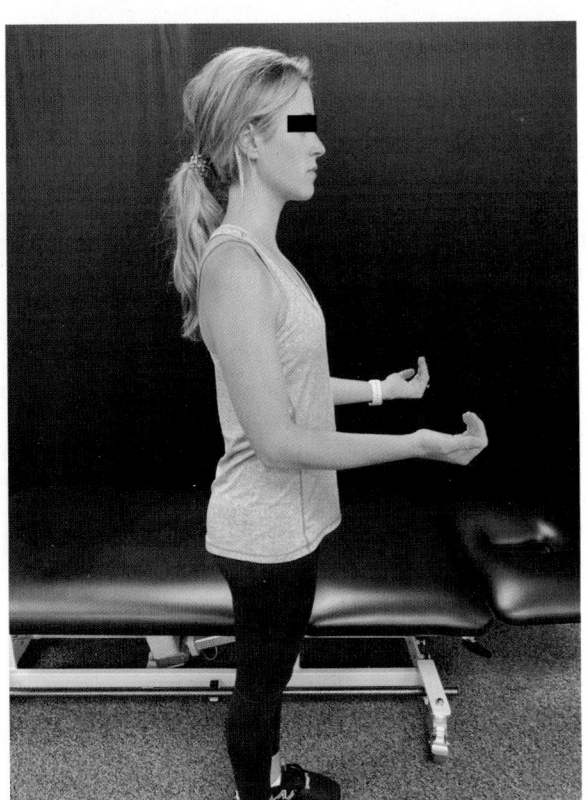

• **Fig. 15.49** Shoulder Retraction and Posterior Shoulder Rolls. (Reprinted with permission from TurningPoint Breast Cancer Rehabilitation.)

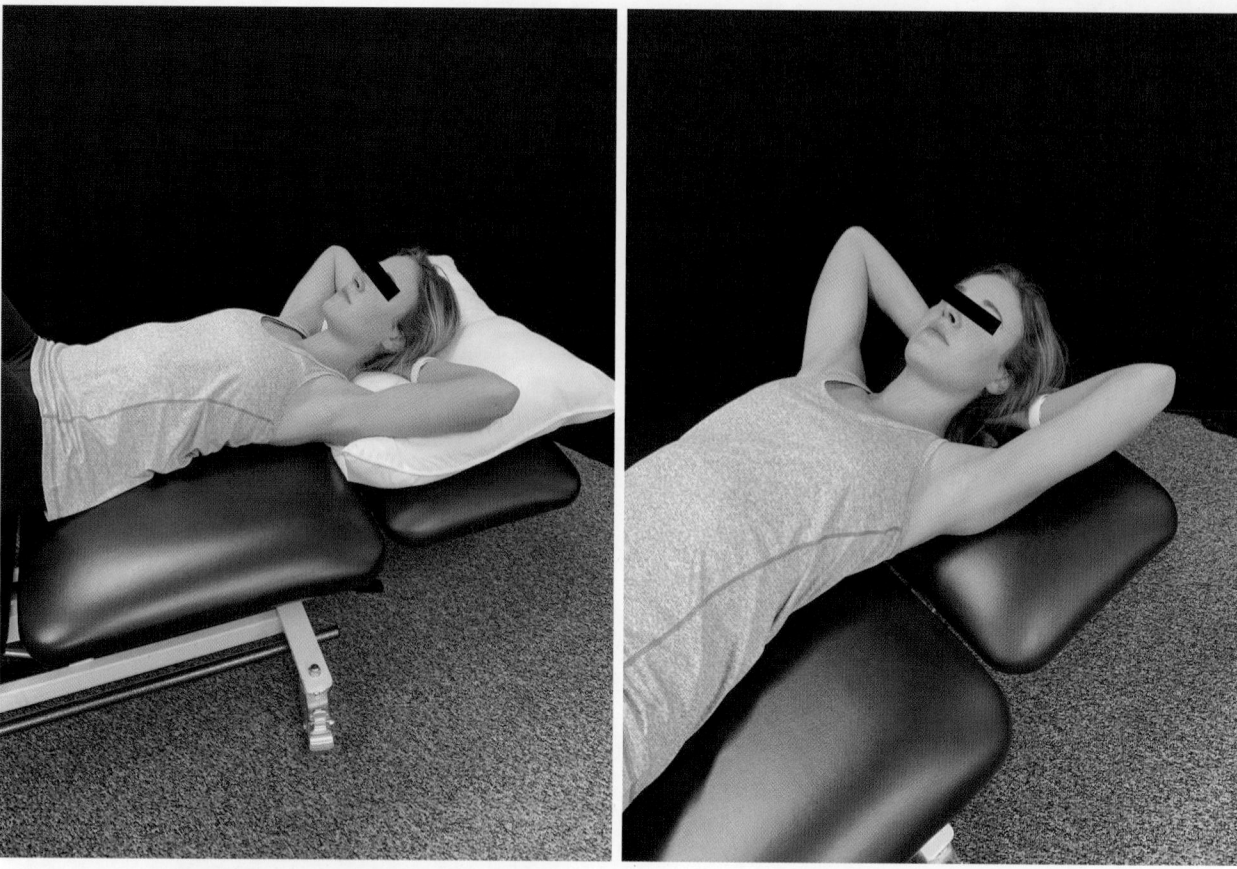

• **Fig. 15.51** Butterfly Stretch With Pillow, Progressing to Flat as Able. (Reprinted with permission from Turning-Point Breast Cancer Rehabilitation.)

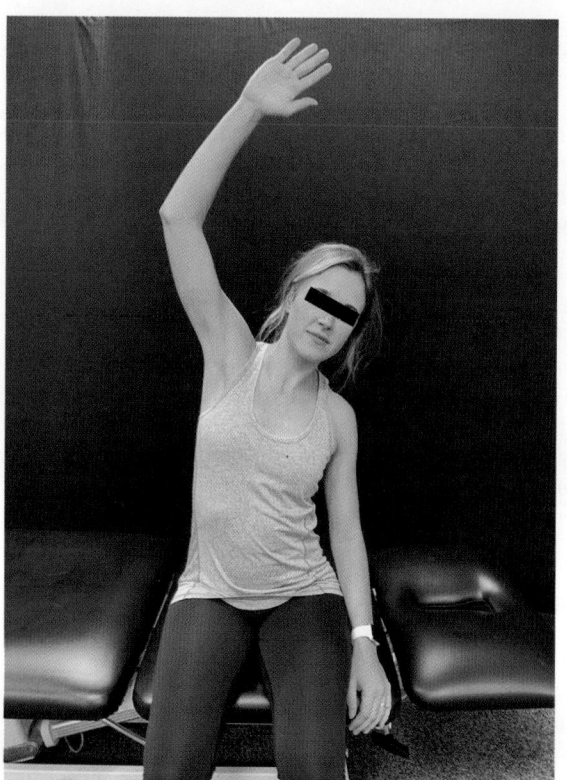

• **Fig. 15.52** Teapot Stretch, Can be Progressed With Hand Under Thigh and by Adding Trunk Rotation Toward and Away From Elevated Arm. (Reprinted with permission from TurningPoint Breast Cancer Rehabilitation.)

side.[124,138] At this early, mild-stage lymphedema, a compression sleeve, active and resisted exercise with or without manual lymph drainage, may be enough to reduce or control lymphedema (Figure 15.53)[124] (see Table 15.11 on management for stages of lymphedema).

In lymphedema greater than 5%, the AOPT clinical practice guidelines (Figure 15.54) support a similar management approach with good evidence that includes compression, aerobic and resistance exercise, and education.[182] For lymphedema that is more significant, compression may include bandaging and increased level of compression (Figure 15.55).

Breast and Chest Wall Lymphedema and Swelling

Breast lymphedema and painful incision sites are not uncommon in women following breast conserving surgery. Management with soft tissue massage, manual lymph drainage, compression bras, or camisoles with foam inserts for local treatment can all be effective. Trunk swelling is also common following surgery, particularly related to flap procedures, and a similar approach can be effective. Aerobic and resisted exercise, when appropriate, are important components in the management of breast and trunk swelling.

Precautions and Contraindications

Prior to initiating treatment for significant lymphedema, cardiac issues such as congestive heart failure should be ruled out. Axillary spread of cancer can be a cause of UE lymphedema. In this case, axillary pain and palpable lymph nodes may be present and symptoms may be unresponsive to initial attempts to treatment. Management of UE swelling in the presence of active axillary disease must be carried out in close communication with the PLWBC's

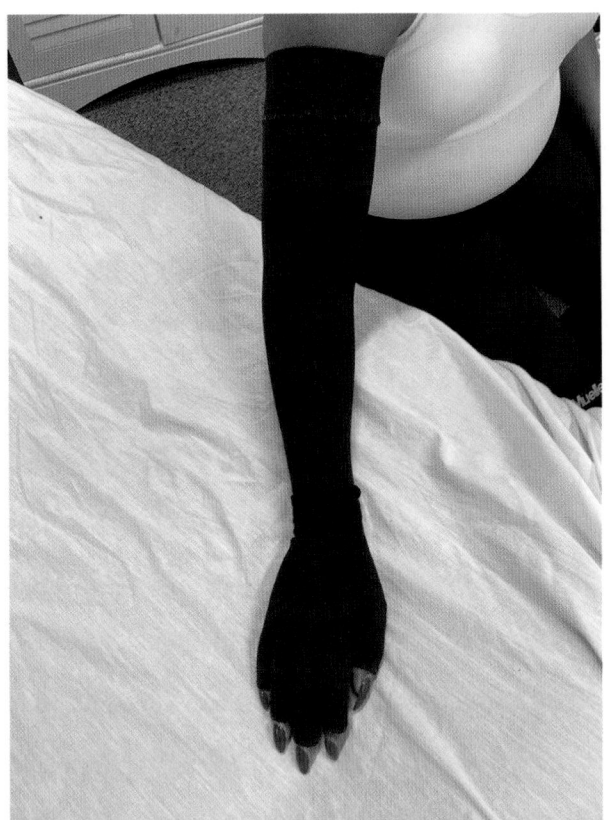

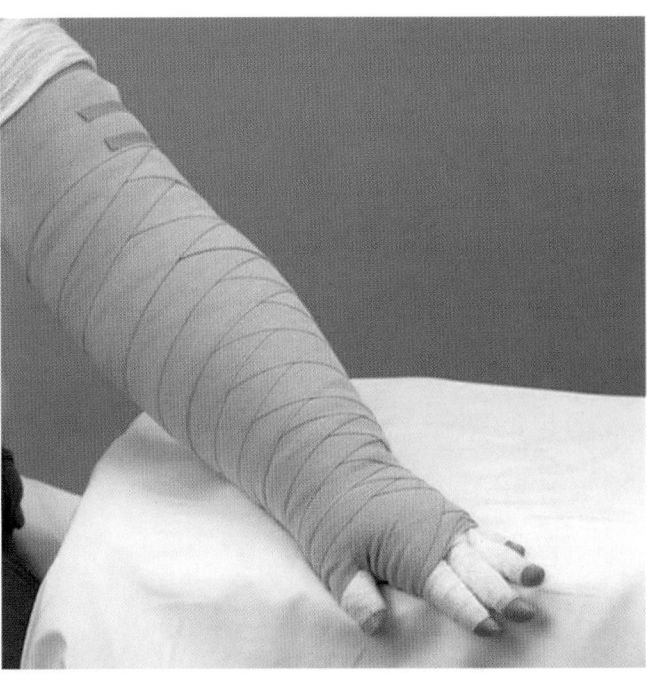

• **Fig. 15.55** Bandaging (Wrapping) for Upper Extremity Lymphedema. (Reprinted with permission from TurningPoint Breast Cancer Rehabilitation.)

• **Fig. 15.53** Compression Sleeve and Glove for Mild to Moderate Lymphedema. (Reprinted with permission from TurningPoint Breast Cancer Rehabilitation.)

oncologist but may provide important comfort and improved function.

Persons with lymphedema are at risk for developing cellulitis in the UE or breast. Common indicators of cellulitis are a mottled pink or red rash that may be warm to touch. The skin may also be sensitive to touch, painful, and/or reports of a burning sensation. Often a fever may accompany more severe cases. In this case, the PLWBC should be referred to their physician immediately for

management of potential infection and lymphedema intervention should be held until the infection is under control and symptoms have subsided (Figure 15.56).

Modalities/Biophysical Agents

The utilization of modalities/biophysical agents to treat PLWBCs is controversial. The debate exists in part due to the lack of research to determine the safety and efficacy of each agent. It is of growing interest and an emerging field of study in Onc R Regarding specific use of modalities/biophysical agents for PLWBCs, there is some recent evidence to provide guidance to Onc R clinicians who want to include this intervention in their treatment protocol. Limited evidence is available for the use of transcutaneous electrical nerve stimulation (TENS), low level laser treatment (LLLT) (also known

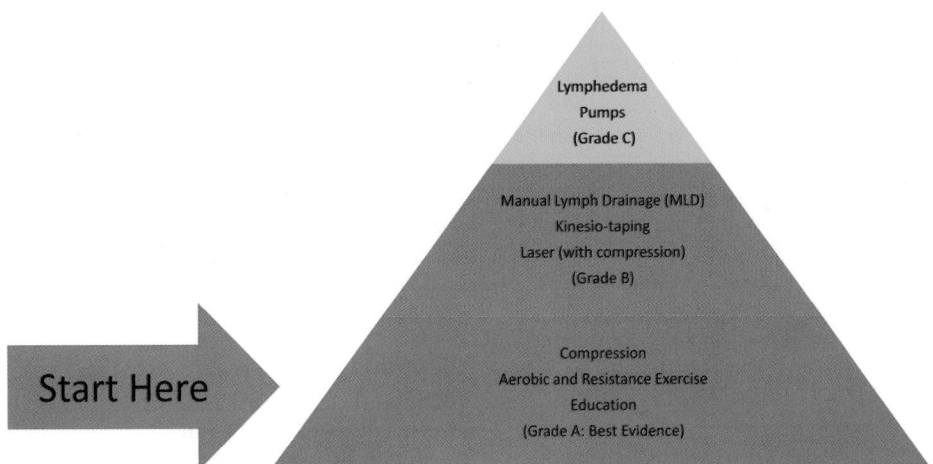

• **Fig. 15.54** Summary of American Physical Therapy Association Academy of Oncologic Physical Therapy Clinical Practice Guidelines for the Management of Lymphedema.[182] (Created by Jill Binkley. Printed with Permission.)

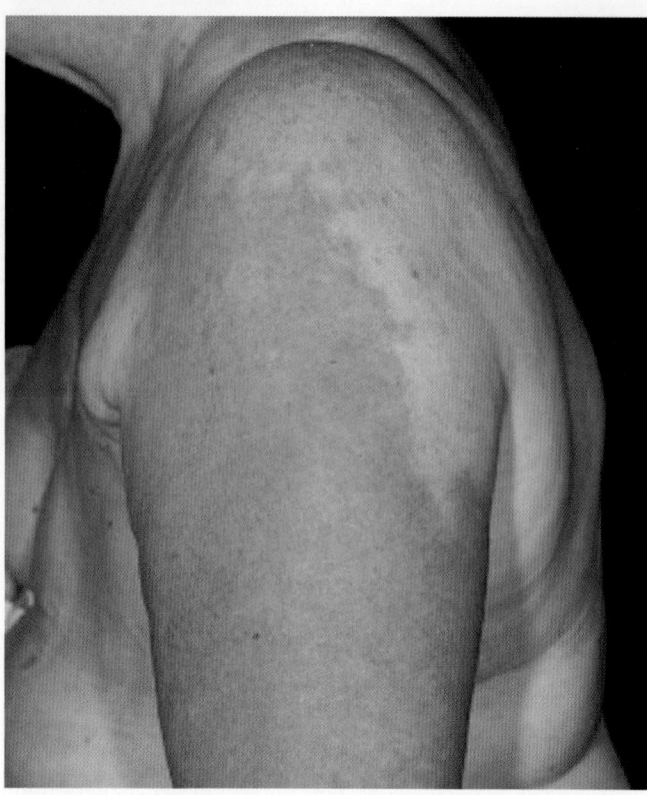

• **Fig. 15.56** Severe Cellulitis of the Upper Extremity. (Reprinted with permission from TurningPoint Breast Cancer Rehabilitation.)

as photobiomodulation therapy [PBMT)], neuromuscular electrical stimulation (NMES), vibration, cryotherapy, and dry needling for persons diagnosed specifically with BC.

Transcutaneous Electrical Nerve Stimulation

TENS assisted in decreasing vertebral bone pain in women diagnosed with Stage IV BC.[183] This study utilized both high and low frequency TENS to achieve the reduced reports of refractory pain due to thoracic and/or lumbar vertebral bone metastasis.[183] In another study, women who underwent BC surgery including an axilectomy of all three levels of lymph nodes and reported changes in cutaneous sensibility after 3 months, were treated with TENS.[184] The area of greatest concern, the intercostobrachial nerve (ICBN) related dermatome, demonstrated significant decreases in dysesthesia intensity after only 20 treatments of TENS. Interestingly insomnia, dyspnea, and fatigue were also improved.[184] Lastly, TENS was utilized to treat CIPN on 15 participants (58% female and 90% Caucasian) who had completed treatment with neurotoxic chemotherapy agents for 3 months. These participants had unsuccessfully been prescribed gabapentin, duloxetine, or opioids previously to treat their CIPN symptoms. After 6 weeks of TENS treatments, improvements were found in pain and neuropathy in the questionnaires and decreases in pain, tingling, numbness, and cramping were noted in their daily diaries. Eighty-one percent of participants reported improvement from baseline of at least one symptom (pain, numbness, tingling, cramping).[185]

Low Level Laser Treatment (LLLT)/Photobiomodulation (PBMT)

This intervention is reported to have potential to treat radiodermatitis, lymphedema, CIPN, oral mucositis, and osteonecrosis of the jaw in PLWBCs. PBMT has been suggested to increase "cellular migration, proliferation and metabolism, induce collagen synthesis and growth

factor secretion while decreasing the production of pro-inflammatory cytokines and cell apoptosis."[186] This review article provided evidence for the use of PBMT in reducing pain and swelling from lymphedema, decreasing chemotherapy induced oral mucositis, decreasing the severity of radiodermatitis, reducing CIPN, as well as reducing pain, infection and edema while increasing function from medication related osteonecrosis of the jaw. Although treatment protocols differed for each diagnosis, successful outcomes were gained.[186]

A systematic review noted that the majority of the studies on PBMT therapy observed no negative adverse effects from treatment when utilizing PBMT for the management of cancer related toxicities. At the same time, this study provided evidence that PBMT is effective in the prevention and treatment of BCRL, oral mucositis, radiodermatitis, and peripheral neuropathy.[186] There is also evidence of statistically significant improvements in emotional distress in individuals with BCRL treated just two times per week along with their complete decongestive therapy.[187] Finally, eleven clinical trials and seven randomized controlled trials (RCTs) were analyzed.[188] Authors found strong evidence showing LLLT (PBMT) was more effective than sham treatment for limb circumference/volume reduction at a short-term follow-up and moderate evidence indicating that LLLT (PBMT) was more effective than sham laser for short-term pain relief. This study concludes that LLLT was not effective for decreasing actual limb swelling for women with BCRL.[188]

Electrical Stimulation or Neuromuscular Electrical Stimulation

Investigators evaluated whether NMES could be used in place of exercise to improve skeletal muscle fiber size or function in persons diagnosed with cancer and currently receiving treatment. They found the beneficial effects to be encouraging in utilizing NMES to promote muscle fiber hypertrophy and fiber type transitions that are similar to resistance exercise. Functional benefits of NMES have historically been considered related to the intensity of muscle contraction, while this study suggests that the benefits of electrical stimulation are primarily related to contractile stress/strain. The nine studies included in this analysis demonstrated statistically significant improvement in health-related QOL. However, there is need for greater standardization.[189]

An interesting study treated women diagnosed with chronic postmastectomy pain, including postlumpectomy pain.[190] Scrambler therapy (ST) was delivered as treatment to three patients. This is a noninvasive electrical neurocutaneous stimulation. In this study, treatment consisted of 45 minutes daily for several consecutive days until pain relief was achieved. The ST device used synthesizes 16 different waveforms, delivered to the surface receptors of the c-fibers. This sends "nonpain" information along the damaged pathways to reduce central sensitization. The results were positive with all three participants achieving 75% reduction of allodynia, hyperalgesia, and pain as well as increase in QOL and normal function. One person was able to stop chronic opioid use.[190] This treatment deserves more research as no adverse effects were observed.

Vibration

Vibration therapy may have the potential to improve some of the adverse effects of BC treatment. In one study 14 persons diagnosed with BC were treated with vibration therapy treatment for ten 15-minute sessions on their affected upper limb. Participants were evaluated before and after treatment, and 3 months later. Vibration therapy attenuated pain symptoms, improved shoulder movements (extension, abduction, and adduction movements of the horizontal shoulder), activated muscle contraction mechanism, and increased shoulder strength.[191]

Cryotherapy

Cryotherapy appears to have promise in providing a simple, safe, and effective strategy for the prevention of CIPN caused from the use of paclitaxel for the treatment of BC. In one study, 119 subjects received cryotherapy when CIPN symptoms appeared in 2016 and in 2017 another 96 women received prophylactic cryotherapy.[192] The goal was to complete nine cycles of paclitaxel. Only 64% of participants completed the planned 720 mg/m^2 in the 2016 group compared to 77% completion with the 2017 cohort. This study suggests that prophylactic cryotherapy has the potential to assist in increasing the proportion of persons completing the planned dose of paclitaxel without delays from CIPN in adjuvant treatment of early-stage BC.[192] In another study, 36 women diagnosed with BC were treated weekly with paclitaxel (80 mg/m^2 for 1 hour). They all wore frozen gloves and socks on their dominant side for the entire duration of the drug infusion (90 minutes) and no participants needed to drop out secondary to cold intolerance.[193] Objective and subjective CIPN signs were clinically and statistically lower on the intervention side than on the control side as measured with tactile sensitivity of hands and feet, warm sense, peripheral neuropathy questionnaire, (PNQ), and manipulative dexterity.[194]

Dry Needling

Dry needling is receiving significant attention in the rehabilitation field. State Boards of Physical Therapy in the US have specific position statements that designate the legal standing of this intervention and should be referred to. In a 2014 literature review on dry needling, an overview of the physiological changes that may occur from dry needling as well as the legal considerations and clinical implications are discussed. More research is needed in the cancer population to determine the benefits and efficacy.[194] Ultrasound-guided dry needling (USGDN) has been found to not only reduce pain and disability but to decrease opioid use in post mastectomy pain syndrome (PMPS) by addressing myofascial pain.[195] This suggests a myofascial contribution to pain and disability in PMPS.

Important Considerations, Timelines, and Contraindications for Manual Therapy, Exercise, and Modalities

Onc R intervention, including manual therapy, active and resisted exercise and modalities must consider surgery type, phase of BC treatment, stages of healing, insult to the lymphatic system as well as the potential for adverse consequences, such as seromas.

In the first 2 weeks postoperatively (mastectomy, BCoS, with or without ALND), manual lymph drainage, breathing exercises, and gentle ROM can be utilized to address swelling, as well as reducing pain and postural compensations. Daily walking should be encouraged. During this time, gentle shoulder ROM is recommended but typically is restricted to approximately 90 degrees of elevation to allow healing to occur and reduce the risk of seroma development. After the first 2 weeks postsurgery, ROM can be progressed. Resisted exercise that includes the muscles and joints in the surgical sites, including donor sites, should not be initiated until 6 weeks postoperatively and then only if healing is progressing as expected.

Two weeks after surgery, manual therapy to gently stretch the surrounding soft tissue and axillary cording can be initiated but tension should be avoided on healing incisions. Soft tissue and joints around expanders or implants are commonly tight and can be gently and safely stretched. Expanders, however, should not be mobilized or moved as they are sutured in place to create expansion only in the desired location. Implants, conversely, are intended to be mobile and gentle soft tissue procedures are appropriate to maintain this mobility. Radiation is not a contraindication for manual therapy, but direct contact with the radiation site(s) must be avoided as soft tissue inflammation develops, typically in weeks three to four of radiation. During this time, gentle stretching of soft tissue and joints surrounding the radiation site can continue.

The potential of metastatic disease needs to be considered. It is not unusual for the Onc R clinician treating a PLWBC to notice concerning signs and symptoms, such as skin rash indicating local recurrence or persistent joint pain in the spine suggesting bone metastases. For PWCs with known metastatic disease, caution should be taken in the region(s) of metastases, and mobilization and end-range stretches should be avoided. However, metastatic disease alone is not a contraindication to treatment and many PLWBCs with MeBC have impairments that are amenable to Onc R.[196] In addition, exercise is a critically important aspect for QOL in these PWCs.[177,179,181,197,198]

Special Topics

Breast Cancer in Males

BC in males is rare and only 1% of all BCs diagnosed are in males. However, there are more recent epidemiologic studies showing the incidence is rising to 15% although due to a dearth of research in this area, the cause is not yet determined.[199] There are two classifications of male BC—male complex subtype (similar to female luminal BC) and male simplex subtype (not a classification in female BC).[200] It is most commonly diagnosed in men 60 to 70 years of age. The most common types of male breast cancer (MBC) include IDC, DCIS, inflammatory, Paget disease of the nipple. Male breast duct cells are less developed than females and they normally have lower levels of female hormones that affect the growth of breast cells. The most common causes of BC in men overall include increased estrogen from hormone imbalance, medication, radiation exposure, obesity, and Klinefelter's syndrome (which affects the balance of androgen/estrogen). Predisposing factors also include aging, genetic mutations, radiation exposure, alcohol abuse, liver disease, and testicular conditions. MBCs are most often hormone receptor positive (+) (including the AR [Klinefelter's syndrome]), have the BRCA2 mutations, and are often dependent on family history.[201] Males are also at higher risk of recurrence and metastasis. MBCs are treated with the same interventions as females with additional consideration for orchiectomy (removal of testicles). Treatment of ER+/PR+ BC in men is commonly treated with endocrine agents, most commonly tamoxifen. AIs, although used, have been found to be less optimal since the hormonal status of men is more closely related to the premenopausal status of women.[202]

There is psychological and societal stigma of men suffering from what is sometimes considered a "woman's disease" and men are striving to reconstrue their masculinity and personal strength to manage their illness.[203] Stigmatization is particularly evident in the management phase of BC treatment.[204] As a result, there tends to be limited resources for psychosocial support, delayed diagnosis due to lack of understanding, education, and a paucity of research regarding unmet psychosocial needs of this population; all of which result in poorer outcomes. In a recent study regarding unmet needs of men with BC, there are numerous issues related to lack of information and education about acute and late adverse effects and sexual adverse effects.[205,206] Limited educational information was available for healthcare professionals to provide to these men. As this has been identified as an issue, there are many resources available now for men diagnosed with BC (eTable 15.1).

Triple-Negative Breast Cancer

Triple-negative breat cancer (TNBC) accounts for about 10% to 15% of all BCs.[19] The term *triple-negative BC* refers to the fact that the cancer cells have fewer estrogen and progesterone receptors so they are considered hormone receptor negative (HR-). In addition, they demonstrate a very low expression of HER2. Thus, all three tests are negative. TNBC is considered more aggressive with poorer prognosis due to fewer targeted medications. It is more often diagnosed as a higher grade (Grade 3) and 70% to 90% of TNBC contains the "basal like" cell type.[207] Basal-like cancers are more aggressive and have a higher grade.[208] These cancers tend to be more common in women younger than age 50, who are Black or Hispanic, or who have a BRCA1 mutation. Twenty-five percent of TNBC tumors express the AR. This is a growing area of research to determine if targeting this receptor can provide better outcomes. Compared with the other major types of BC, TNBC is characterized by higher rates of recurrence, increased occurrence of metastasis, and shorter overall survival.[209] The racial disparities are very evident. Not only are socioeconomic factors contributing to poorer outcomes and survival rates, but also genetic risk factors and aberrant activation of oncogenic pathways have been identified in several studies.[210] There is also evidence of the connection between obesity and the TNBC molecular circuitry that drives the aggressive progression of this disease. This is known as the obesity-TNBC axis and demonstrates the need for a multidisciplinary approach to treatment (eTable 15.2).

Metastatic Breast Cancer

MeBC is diagnosed as a Stage IV BC. This refers to cancer that has spread to other parts of the body through the bloodstream, lymphatic system, or growth to local tissue. MeBC consists of recurrence of BC as well as de novo BC. De novo (meaning *from the beginning*) BC is when metastatic cancer is the first diagnosis and the cancer was not detected until it had already moved to other parts of the body. While 6% of all MeBC diagnoses are de novo, 20% to 30% of early stage BC will recur at a distant site thus becoming metastatic.[211] While the overall 5-year relative survival rate for women diagnosed with metastatic BC is 28% and 22% for men, a recent study demonstrated a distinct increase in the survival rate for women diagnosed with de novo MeBC between 15 and 49 years of age to 36% and 29.7% for women diagnosed between 50 and 64 years of age. Hundred percent of deaths from BC are from MeBC.[212] 16% of the deaths for BC occur in women under 50 years of age.[212] The most common sites for metastasis from BC include the bone, lung, brain, liver.[213] Common symptoms associated with these areas of metastasis are listed below in Table 15.13. Onc R clinicians should be aware of these symptoms to facilitate a referral back to the appropriate physician for follow up.

TABLE 15.13 **Common Sites and Symptoms of Metastasis**

- Bone—Severe, persistent, and/or progressive pain, swelling, bone fractures
- Brain—Persistent headaches that worsens, problems with vision, seizures, nausea or vomiting, behavioral or personality changes
- Liver—Jaundice, itchy skin or rash, elevated liver enzymes, abdominal pain, loss of appetite, nausea and vomiting
- Lungs—Chronic cough, difficulty with deep breathing, abnormal chest radiograph, chest pain, fatigue, weight loss, poor appetite

Created by Deborah J. Doherty. Printed with permission.

MeBC can also be identified as poly-metastatic or oligometastatic. While the majority of metastatic disease is classified as poly-, 1% to 3% of MeBC is oligo. Oligometastatic BC (OMBC) is limited metastatic disease and can be defined as five or fewer metastases that were identified through imaging and is amenable to curative therapy.[211,214] Recent studies are considering OMBC as a genetically distinct diagnosis of metastatic cancer instead of a transitional stage. More research is needed in relation to new medical treatments. These new therapies could increase the potential for better outcomes for those diagnosed with MeBC. This will provide more opportunities for Onc R and improving QOL. More information can be obtained from http://wwwcases.mbcn.org/.

Young Cancer Survivors

BC is the most diagnosed cancer in Adolescent and Young Adults (AYAs) (ages 15–39) resulting in 30% of all cancers among AYA women. Approximately 12,000+ BCs are diagnosed in AYA women each year. During that same time, more than 1,000 women under 40 will die from BC. One in every 3,000 pregnant women will be diagnosed with BC[215] and more than 30% of BC in young women will be diagnosed in a few short years after having a baby. 20% of women who are age 25–29 at the time of BC diagnosis have completed a pregnancy within the past 12 months.[216] There are approximately 250,000 women living in the US today that were diagnosed with BC under the age of 40. Due to dense breast tissue, routine mammograms are not useful for screening. In these women, cancers may be more aggressive and pose a higher risk of metastasis. Women under the age of 30 are often found to have a gene mutation of BRCA1, BRCA2, or TP53.[217] While AYA persons with BC accounts for less than 2% of all BC cases, they have been found to have a higher percentage of TNBC, HER2+ BC, and have more advanced disease resulting in higher rates of mastectomy and use of chemotherapy than adult women with BC.[218]

Young women diagnosed with BC face unique challenges including a potential loss of fertility, difficulty in raising children while going through treatment, early menopause and sexual dysfunction, early ovarian decline, body image and intimacy issues, decreased sex drive, financial instability due to potential inability to work full-time while going through treatment, and higher prevalence of anxiety and depression. They are also under-represented in research studies due to the smaller population size. See Table 15.14 or more AYA resources. Please see Chapter 26 for more information about AYA cancers.

TABLE 15.14 **Adolescent and Young Adult Resources**

- Young Survival—https://www.youngsurvival.org
- Fertile Hope—http://www.fertilehope.org/.
- Living Beyond Breast Cancer —http://www.lbbc.org/Audiences/ Young-Women/FAQs-about-Breast-Cancer-in-Young-Women.

Created by Deborah J. Doherty. Printed with permission.

Health Disparities in Breast Cancer

Racial disparities are multifactorial and can be divided into two categories including biologic (genetics and molecular changes) and nonbiologic (sociodemographic issues and lifestyle behaviors) factors. The incidence of BC in Black and White women in the US is similar in diagnosis at 135 cases per 1,000,000 women annually; however, the descrepancy in mortality rate continues to increase with a 42% higher rate of death in Black women. The 5-year BC-specific survival rate is 78.9% in Black women and 88.6% in NH White women.[219] While access to care has been shown to be a major factor in survival, recent data has emerged regarding inherent biological tumor differences that could also contribute to health disparities. There are higher frequencies of TNBC in Black women. This includes Black women in the US, women in sub-Saharan Africa, the Caribbean, and South Africa.[210] This diagnosis itself is more difficult to treat due to reasons explained earlier. Racial differences have been found to be significant in somatic mutation analysis and gene expression. In other studies, racial differences such as enhanced p53, BRCA1, Aurora A, Aurora B, and polo-like signaling networks as well as intratumor genetic heterogeneity have been shown to be greater in tumors from Black PLWBCs as compared to tumors from women of European descent. These molecular differences also contribute to the aggressiveness of TNBC.[220]

Significant molecular differences have been identified between invasive BC in Black versus White women diagnosed with BC. Gene expression, protein, DNA copy number, DNA methylation are genomic features that differ between the two groups. Black women have a higher risk of recurrence in comparison to White women. Research has concluded that 40% of the variations in BC subtypes can be attributed to inherited germline variants. This suggests that racial differences in the frequency of BC subtypes are resultant of genetic factors.[220]

Nonbiologic issues are now being recognized and documented. Disparities resultant of socioeconomic issues, including access to care, income, and treatment delays and specific social determinants of health. One study noted that the social determinants of TNBC in Black women include socioeconomic status, younger age, more advanced stage of disease, larger tumors, being unmarried, living in lower socioeconomic neighborhoods, lack of health insurance and financial hardships caused by cancer care, taking time off work, problems with travel, and not receiving standard of care.[221]

There is also evidence of a strong correlation between the socioeconomic factors, obesity, and diet. The prevalence of obesity is higher among Black women than NH White women at 58.6% versus 33.4%, respectively. Since evidence demonstrates that obesity predicts poor survival, it is hypothesized that obesity may contribute to aggressive TNBC in Black women. The most likely explanation is that obesity is an inflammatory disease and promotes elevation of numerous inflammatory cytokines that activate pathways that predict poor prognosis in women with TNBC. Disparities in access to healthy food, like fresh fruits and vegetables, unsafe neighborhoods, and lack of physical activity can promote obesity and poor metabolic health in Black women and more aggressive TNBC.[219] Prediagnostic breastfeeding and BMI were studied in Hispanic and NH White women diagnosed with BC. Longer duration of breastfeeding was associated with a lower risk of mortality and a reduced risk of BC specific and overall mortality in women with a BMI less than 25 kg/m^2 but did not provide protection if the BMI was greater than 25 kg/m^2.[222] Onc R clinicians are well positioned and possess the knowledge and resources to provide education regarding lifestyle behaviors that can help to decrease inflammatory processes and related obesity. Advocacy for policy change to impact the socioeconomic and sociodemographic factors that can lead to racial disparities is an expectation of all healthcare practitioners.

LGBTQIA+ Disparities

Specific considerations are needed to improve the care of persons within the LGBTQIA+ population. LGBTQIA+ persons fear stigmatization and as a result more often remain silent regarding health issues. Other barriers to healthcare include structural barriers like cost as well as a lack of trust in the physician-patient relationship in terms of confidentiality and lack of standard care. There is also a lack of knowledge about LGBTQIA+ specific issues and unmet needs by many healthcare professionals with some evidence of negative attitudes towards them.[223] Compared to cisgender men, there is an increased risk of BC in transfeminine individuals; however, the risk is lower in transmasculine individuals when compared to cisgender women. Hormone treatment can increase the risk of BC in transfeminine individuals undergoing hormone replacement therapy although studies show that this resembles a more female presentation. Annual BC screening is essential for transgender people using hormone treatment. BC in transmasculine individuals is very rare after mastectomy and gender affirmation surgery.[223] However, there is a chance that continuously receiving testosterone could increase risk of BC.[224] There is a dearth of research on transgender people with BC. It is challenging to recruit this population due to financial hardships, social biases against them, mental struggles, and internal self-rejection that prevent them from taking surveys or participating. Studies describing BC in gay and bisexual men do not exist currently. There is one study identifying 13 male to female and 12 female to male transgender persons with BC, of which 10 were veterans, but details were not available. A study specific to California Health identified prevalence for BC in lesbians is 17.8%, bisexual women is 13.3% and heterosexual women, in comparison, is 20.6%. Lesbian and bisexual women receive less routine healthcare according to some studies. Reasons include fear of discrimination, lack of health insurance, and negative experiences with healthcare providers.[225] Recommendations for screening are the same as with cisgender women.

Risk factors include smoking, excess alcohol use, parity after age 30 or nulliparity, unhealthy weight/obesity, avoidance or delay of health screenings and medical care secondary to fear of discrimination or past negative experiences with doctors. Lesbian women have a greater disease-specific mortality compared to heterosexual women.

Conclusion

The management of individuals diagnosed with BC presents an incredible opportunity for Onc R clinicians. It is important for Onc R clinicians to understand the common classifications of BC, the most common treatments, potential adverse effects of all treatments, keep informed about new therapies and become familiar with their adverse effects. As the regimen for the chemotherapy agents is rapidly changing in not only the drugs used but the amount used, the toxicities are ever changing. It is extremely important to understand the PLWBC's treatment protocol, medications from their co-morbidities and their state of health overall to help determine the Onc R plan of care. Onc R clinicians are well positioned to develop, not only rehabilitation strategies to mitigate potential adverse effects, but greatly improve the QOL of each PLWBC.

Critical Research Needs

Effectiveness of telerehabilitation in different treatment phases and populations:

- Group therapy (patient education and intervention)—determine effective strategies to create a standard of care that includes Onc R for all PLWBCs. Most valid clinical tool to measure CIPN report it and measure change
- Pathophysiology of cording and most effective treatments
- Effectiveness of laser treatment on lymphedema, cording, and radiation fibrosis
- Prevention or reduction of recurrence of BC with a multimodal approach to treatment, including nutrition, exercise, emotional wellness, massage therapy, education on sleep, physical activity, lifestyle behavior and recurrence reduction
- Disparity in BC survivorship and access to specialized BC rehabilitation and exercise

Case Studies

Case 1

History and Current Complaints

A 38-year-old black woman was diagnosed with Stage III left invasive ductal carcinoma (LIDC) 18 months prior to being seen by the physical therapist. Her tumor was classified as triple negative. She had 8 rounds of neoadjuvant chemotherapy (Adriamycin, Cytoxin, and Taxotere) followed by mastectomy and ALND (13 nodes removed, 2 positive) with DIEP reconstruction and breast reduction on the right. She then received 28 radiation treatments to left chest wall and axilla. No other significant medical issues.

Social History

The PWC reported she was married with two children, ages 4 and 6 years. She worked full-time in insurance sales. She reported working about 60% of her usual hours due to COVID-19 and BC treatment. She usually exercised regularly, including spin classes, yoga, and strength training with resistance bands. She had not exercised regularly since her surgery. She expressed frustration about not feeling listened to, deep concern about the aggressiveness of her TNBC, caring for her children, and financial concerns.

She presented to Onc R clinicians with onset of swelling of her left forearm and thenar eminence and ongoing pain and restriction of her left shoulder and chest wall.

Key Impairment and Functional Outcomes

Pain: 3/10 (left axilla and upper arm)
  PSFS:
1. Reaching high kitchen cabinets 5/10
2. Throwing ball with her children 4/10
3. Working >1 hour on computer for work 3/10
  Average: 3/10
  UEFI: 58/80
  Active ROM:

Shoulder ROM	Left	Right
Flexion	134° with pain and tightness in pectoral region at end range	165°
Abduction	123° with pain and tightness lateral chest wall	165°
Hand behind back motion	To iliac crest	To L1
External rotation (elbow 90° flexion, arm at side)	20°	45°

Visual Inspection: Forward head posture, protracted shoulders. Mild swelling of thenar eminence and between the MCPs as well as in the region of her anterior wrist and forearm. Skin hyperpigmentation in area of radiation field.

Palpation: Very tight left pectoral musculature, subscapularis, and lateral chest wall soft tissue. Decreased mobility of left glenohumeral and acromioclavicular motion. No evidence of cording.

Volume: Perometer measure indicated that left affected nondominant UE is 7% larger than right.

Key Rehabilitation Issues

The PWC was a young black woman who had received little support related to treatment adverse effects over 18 months since her diagnosis. She reported feeling unheard by her healthcare providers. She was at high risk for lymphedema based on number of nodes removed, radiation and her race and in fact, has early, mild swelling. She had not received education related to lymphedema or symptom management. Racial disparity and financial toxicity are impacting her.

The PWC had a longstanding painful limitation in shoulder mobility and potentially early adhesive capsulitis. She exhibited mild lymphedema and was not exercising regularly.

Domains of Human Movement and Function Impacted: Integumentary, musculoskeletal, cardiovascular, pulmonary, nervous, plus financial security, self-image.

Rehabilitation Approach

The short-term rehabilitation approach included manual therapy and exercise to increase shoulder ROM. Manual therapy focused on soft tissue techniques for pectoral and subscapular tightness and glenohumeral and acromioclavicular mobilization. Posture education and upper body stretching was initiated. She was provided with a class 1 compression sleeve and glove to wear during all waking hours. Education related to lymphedema was provided. She was referred to counseling for emotional support.

At week 3, her shoulder flexion and abduction increased to 158 degrees and 155 degrees, respectively. There was minimal visible swelling, and volume decreased to 3%. Pain reduced to 1/10 at end range only. Core strengthening was added as well as upper body resistance exercise was added for strengthening and for lymphedema management.

At week 5, there was no visible swelling, no pain, and full range of shoulder motion. Her sleeve and glove wearing schedule gradually was weaned off over a 3-week period while her arm volume was monitored at home and in the clinic.

At week 8, active treatment is discontinued. She returned to her usual exercise program that included upper body and core stretching and strengthening. She was scheduled to return for prospective surveillance for lymphedema and other adverse treatment adverse effects every 3 months. She was instructed to use the sleeve as needed for occasional visible swelling.

Summary

Onc R clinicians must be aware of their own unconscious bias to address and not perpetuate racial disparity and bias that hinders building a therapeutic relationship. It is not unusual for a PWC to present with complex, multi-dimensional issues that need to be addressed simultaneously. Management of the lymphedema in the early phases and through prospective surveillance may reduce lymphedema to a point where it can be managed with the least impact to PLWBC's QOL. Onc R clinicians need to be aware of when to refer to other professionals, such as counseling and nutrition, is needed.

Case 2

History and Current Complaints

A 65-year-old Caucasian woman was diagnosed with Stage II ER/PR+, HER2neu+ BC 8 years ago. She was well known to her Onc R clinician and had participated in long-term surveillance and management program for lymphedema. At her most recent check-in visit, she presented with recurrence of BC, including metastatic disease at T6 and iliac crest as well as her liver. She received targeted radiation for her bone metastases, followed by ongoing Gemzar chemotherapy.

She was teary during the evaluation and expressed fear and anxiety over her diagnosis of MeBC and fear of death. She stated that she has significant fatigue and pain in her back as well as difficulty sleeping due to discomfort. She was not currently exercising due to fatigue and expressed concern about picking up and playing with her young grandchildren considering her MeBC.

Social History

The PWC was retired, and her husband died 3 years ago of heart disease. She reported having three adult children, one of whom lived close by and three grandchildren, ages 6 months, 2 and 5 years. She volunteered once weekly at her church's food pantry, but had not been doing that since her recent diagnosis.

Key Impairment and Functional Outcomes

Pain: 5/10 (thoracic, mid scapular, and upper trapezius region)
    PSFS:
1. Lifting her 6-month-old grandchild 0/10
2. Sleeping 2/10
3. Exercising due to fatigue 3/10
    Average: 1.7/10
    UEFI: 52/80
    Fatigue Scale: 7/10
    UE and Trunk Evaluation: Exhibited protracted shoulders, forward head posture. Shoulder ROM was full. Tender and tight on palpation of upper trapezius and mid-scapular musculature.

Key Rehabilitation Issues

This PWC had significant anxiety, fatigue, sleep issues, pain related to bone metastases, soft tissue and postural issues and ongoing lymphedema risk. She lived alone and felt isolated, particularly considering her diagnosis of MeBC.

Domains of Human Movement and Function Impacted: Musculoskeletal, cardiovascular, pulmonary, integumentary, nervous, plus sleep and spirituality.

Rehabilitation Approach

Multi-faceted Onc R support including guided exercise coaching and activity modification to address fatigue was provided. Education included approaches to maximizing QOL and activity level with MeBC, posture, sleep positions and body mechanics for safe lifting. Gentle soft tissue massage and stretching program were provided for upper trapezius and mid scapular soft tissue tightness and pain while avoiding end range rotation motions. Other Onc R support included counseling, nutrition, and massage therapy. The PWC joined a support group for persons with MeBC.

In the long term, ongoing surveillance, and support for lymphedema as well as new and increasing adverse side effects of treatment protocols would continue.

Summary

The Onc R clinician must be prepared to address the multitude of physical, emotional, and psychosocial aspects of caring for PLWBC. In persons with MeBC, issues that are amenable to Onc R intervention are often not addressed, and it is assumed that reduced activity and QOL is inevitable with a trajectory that cannot be altered. There is an important role for the Onc R in understanding the myriad of medical treatment for MeBC and providing ongoing support throughout the journey (see Chapter 29). In addition, the Onc R clinician can provide other professional resources and education that are crucial to the well-being of persons with MeBC. Finally, the Onc R clinician must be aware of the impact of difficult emotional situations on their own mental health as a caregiver, and seek out support from other clinicians, counseling, and self-care strategies.

Case 3

History and Current Complaints

A 45-year-old White man was diagnosed with Stage II BC on the left, BRCA 2+, ER+. He underwent 8 rounds of neoadjuvant chemotherapy (Cytoxan, Taxotere) and is now 2 weeks post left mastectomy with ALND (8 nodes removed, 3 positive). The drain remains in situ lateral to his mastectomy incision, and had drained approximately 50 cc in 24 hours. The goal is that drainage would be reduced to less than 20 cc in 24 hours for removal of drain. He also had radiation planned.

Social History

The PWC was married and had two children, ages 13 and 15. He reported working in sales and was currently off work postoperatively. He has a strong family history of BC, including his aunt, sister, and mother. He expressed anxiety regarding lack of understanding about BC in men by society in general, and his family and friends particularly. He expressed fears about his family history related to his children, as well as concerns regarding cosmesis and body image. He reported playing recreational tennis regularly. His BMI was 27.4 and he had diet-controlled diabetes and hypertension. He reported being on Lisinopril.

Key Impairment and Functional Outcomes

Pain: 5/10 (axilla, medial upper arm, cubital fossa with stretch into elevation).

PSFS:
1. Reaching overhead trunk door 3/10
2. Driving 2/10
3. Tennis 0/10
   Average: 1.7/10
   UEFI: 55/80
   Active ROM:

Shoulder ROM	Left	Right
Flexion	145° with pain and tightness in axilla and pectoral region at end range	172°
Abduction	98° with pain and tightness lateral chest wall; visible axillary cording extending to cubital fossa	170°
Hand behind back motion	To L2	To L2
External rotation (elbow in 90° flexion, arm at side)	80°	78°

Visual Inspection: Forward head posture, protracted shoulders. Incision is healing well, with no open areas, mild swelling, and erythema surrounding incision. Visible cording on abduction. No visible swelling in left UE or hand.

Palpation: Palpable seroma with fluid wave beneath mastectomy incision. Palpable and painful cording in left axilla with shoulder positioned in supported abduction; cording extended into upper arm, cubital fossa, and anterior wrist at base of thumb; pain increased with elbow and wrist extension.

Volume: Perometer measure indicated that left affected dominant UE is 3% larger than right.

Review Questions

Reader can find the correct answers and rationale in the back of the book.

1. A person is at a higher risk for breast cancer related lymphedema if they have all of the following except:
   A. Underwent axillary radiation
   B. Were taking tamoxifen (Soltamox)
   C. Developed a seroma
   D. Diagnosed with advanced disease

2. The most common sites for breast cancer to metastasize to are all of the following except:
   A. Bone
   B. Brain
   C. Liver
   D. Pancreas

3. Triple negative breast cancer is diagnosed as:
   A. ER+ PR- HER2-
   B. ER- PR- HER2-
   C. ER- PR+ HER2-
   D. ER+ PR+ HER2+

Key Rehabilitation Issues

There was significant pain, loss of mobility and function related to surgery and axillary cording. He was at fairly high risk for lymphedema based on the number of nodes removed, planned radiation, presence of seroma and cording, as well as BMI. As expected, there was no evidence of lymphedema this early postoperatively, but baseline measures were acquired to facilitate prospective surveillance and early detection should it occur. He had significant anxiety related to his strong family history of BC and shame related to being diagnosed with BC as a man.

Domains of Human Movement and Function Impacted: Musculoskeletal, integumentary, nervous, plus self-image.

Rehabilitation Approach

Manual therapy and targeted therapeutic stretching were utilized to address cording and shoulder ROM. Education was provided regarding lymphedema risk and risk reduction, as well as prospective surveillance and early detection. Expectations regarding radiation-related skin changes and fatigue were provided. He was gradually encouraged to begin a walking program that was increased as tolerated to 30 minutes daily.

At weeks 6 postoperatively and with 1 week of radiation complete, his abduction ROM increased to 155°, pain decreased to 2/10, and cording was much less prominent and painful. He was followed through radiation and monitored for loss of motion, lymphedema, fatigue, and to progress his home stretching and exercise program.

Summary

Loss of shoulder ROM, axillary cording, and seroma are common postoperative adverse effects in people going through BC. The Onc R clinician's role is to follow a PLWBC throughout the trajectory of their treatment and beyond through prospective surveillance as this is critical for early detection of new adverse treatment effects. As with women, mastectomy in a man can be disfiguring and can result in body image issues. Sensitivity on the part of the Onc R clinician is critical when caring for a man going through BC.

4. When should a patient contact their Onc R clinician?
   A. Increased fatigue
   B. Drainage from surgical site
   C. Redness
   D. New area of pain

5. When assess muscles of the shoulder complex, the most important considerations include all of the following except:
   A. Length-tension
   B. Tenderness or pain
   C. Hypertrophy or atrophy
   D. Strength at a 4/5

6. Scapular mobility assessment should always include all of the following except:
   A. Muscle atrophy in scapular region
   B. Prominence of lateral and superior borders
   C. Winging
   D. Resting scapular position

7. Cancer related fatigue, lymphedema, breast heaviness, brachial plexopathy, and risk of secondary cancer are possible results from:
   A. Taxanes
   B. Radiation
   C. Axillary lymph node dissection
   D. Breast reconstruction
8. Using flaps from both sides of the lower abdomen and stacking or folding them for women who do not have enough tissue on one side or if reconstructing both breasts describes:
   A. Stacked DIEP flap surgery
   B. Body lift perforator flap
   C. IGAP flap
   D. SCAP flap
9. The most common female breast cancer subtype is:
   A. HER2-enriched
   B. Triple negative
   C. Luminal B
   D. Luminal A
10. The risk factors for male breast cancer include all of the following except:
    A. BRCA1 genetic mutation
    B. Overweight or obese
    C. Decreased estrogen levels
    D. Liver disease

References

1. World Health Organization. Cancer, the problem. https://www.who.int/news-room/fact-sheets/detail/cancer. Accessed May 23, 2021.
2. World Cancer Research Fund. Breast cancer statistics. https://www.wcrf.org/dietandcancer/breast-cancer-statistics/; October 2018. Accessed February 21, 2021.
3. National Cancer Institute. Cancer stat facts: female breast cancer. https://seer.cancer.gov/statfacts/html/breast.html. Accessed May 23, 2021.
4. American Cancer Society. Key statistics for breast cancer in men. https://www.cancer.org/cancer/breast-cancer-in-men/about/key-statistics.html. Accessed May 23, 2021.
5. American Cancer Society. Breast at a glance; 2020. https://cancerstatisticscenter.cancer.org/#!/cancer-site/Breast. Accessed May 23, 2021.
6. Center for Disease Control. Male breast cancer incidence and mortality, United States: 2013–2017. https://www.cdc.gov/cancer/uscs/pdf/USCS-DataBrief-No19-October2020-h.pdf#:~:text=Male%20Breast%20Cancer%20incidence%20and%20Mortality%2C%20United%20States,2017%2; October 1, 2020. Accessed May 23, 2021.
7. Centers for Disease Control and Prevention. Breast cancer: what are the risk factors? https://www.cdc.gov/cancer/breast/basic_info/risk_factors.htm. September 14, 2020. Accessed December 1, 2020.
8. World Cancer Research Fund. Breast cancer. https://www.wcrf.org/dietandcancer/breast-cancer/. Accessed December 1, 2020.
9. Breastcancer.org. Breast cancer risk factors. https://owl.purdue.edu/owl/research_and_citation/ama_style/electronic_sources.html; April 21, 2021. Accessed April 23, 2021
10. Breastcancer.org. Breast cancer risk factors—family history. https://www.breastcancer.org/risk/factors/family_history. April 21, 2021. Accessed May 23, 2021.
11. National Cancer Institute. BRCA gene mutations: cancer risk and genetic testing. https://www.cancer.gov/about-cancer/causes-prevention/genetics/brca-fact-sheet#how-much-does-an-inherited-harmful-variant-in-brca1. November 19, 2020. Accessed December 20, 2020.
12. Godoy-Ortiz A, Sanchez-Munoz A, Parrado MRC, et al. Deciphering HER2 breast cancer disease: biological and clinical implications. *Front Oncol.* 2019;9:1124. doi:10.3389/fonc.2019.01124.
13. Loibl S, Gianni L. HER2-positive breast cancer. *Lancet.* 2017;389:2415–2429.
14. Giovannelli P, Di Donato M, Galasso G, DiZazzo E, Bilancio A, Migliaccio A. The androgen receptor in breast cancer. *Front Endocrin.* 2018;9:492. doi:10.3389/fendo.2018.00492.
15. van Seijen M, Lips EH, Thompson AM, et al. Ductal carcinoma in situ: to treat or not to treat, that is the question. *BJC.* 2019;121:285–292.
16. Duraker N, Hot S, Akan A, Nayir PO. A comparison of the clinicopathological features, metastasis sites and survival outcomes of invasive lobular, invasive ductal and mixes invasive ductal and lobular breast carcinoma. *Eur J Breast Health.* 2020;16(1):22–31.
17. Limaiem F, Mlika M. *Tubular Breast Carcinoma.* Stat Pearls Publishing; 2020. https://www.ncbi.nlm.nih.gov/books/NBK542223/.
18. Adachi Y, Ishiguro J, Kotani H, et al. Comparison of clinical outcomes between luminal invasive ductal carcinoma and luminal invasive lobular carcinoma. *BMC Cancer.* 2016;16:248. doi:10.1186/s12885-016-2275-4.
19. American Cancer Society. Triple-negative breast cancer. https://www.cancer.org/cancer/breast-cancer/about/types-of-breast-cancer/triple-negative.html. Accessed December 20, 2020.
20. Mehanna J, Haddad FGH, Eid R, Lambertini M, Kourie HR. Triple negative breast cancer: current perspective on the evolving therapeutic landscape. *Int J Women's Health.* 2019;11:431–437.
21. Wang DY, Jiang Z, Ben-David Y, Woodgett JR, Zacksenhaus E. Molecular stratification within triple-negative breast cancer subtypes. *Sci Rep.* 2019;9:19107. doi:10.1038/s41598-019-55710-w.
22. Dai X, Li T, Bai Z, et al. Breast cancer intrinsic subtype classification, clinical use and future trends. *Am J Cancer Res.* 2015;5(10):2929–2943.
23. National Cancer Institute. Cancer stat facts: female breast cancer subtypes. Surveillance, epidemiology and end results program. https://seer.cancer.gov/statfacts/html/breast-subtypes.html. Accessed December 20, 2020.
24. Mamouch F, Berrada N, Aoullay Z, Khanoussi B, Errihani H. Inflammatory breast cancer: a literature review. *World J Oncol.* 2018;9(5–6):129–135.
25. Barlartalo S, Joglekar-Javadekar M, Bradfieldd P, Murphy T, Dickson-Witmer D, van Golen KL. Inflammatory breast cancer: a panoramic overview. *J Rare Dis Res Treat.* 2018;3(2):37–43.
26. National Cancer Institute. Paget disease of the breast. https://www.cancer.gov/types/breast/paget-breast-fact-sheet. April 10, 12. Accessed December 20, 2020.
27. Ohashi R, Hayama A, Yanagihara K, et al. Prognostic significance of mucin expression profiles in breast carcinoma with signet ring cells: a clinicopathological study. *Diag Pathol.* 2016;11:131.
28. National Center for Advancing Translational Sciences. Phyllodes tumor of the breast. Genetic and rare disease information center. https://rarediseases.info.nih.gov/diseases/9514/phyllodes-tumor-of-the-breast. July 5, 2016. Accessed December 20, 2020.
29. National Cancer Institute, SEER Registrar Staging Assistant. Nottingham or Bloom-Richardson (BR) Score/Grade. https://staging.seer.cancer.gov/cs/input/02.05.50/breast/ssf7/?breadcrumbs=(~view_schema~,~breast~). Accessed May 23, 2021.
30. Gress DM, Edge SB, Greene FL, et al., http://www.cancerstaging.org/references-tools/deskreferences/Documents/Principles%20of%20Cancer%20Staging.pdf.

31. Breastcancer.org. Rate of Cell Growth. https://www.breastcancer.org/symptoms/diagnosis/rate_grade. September 21, 2020. Accessed December 20, 2020.

32. Győrffy B, Hatzis C, Sanft T, Hofstatter E, Aktas B, Pusztai L. Multigene prognostic tests in breast cancer: past, present, future. *Breast Cancer Res.* 2015;17:11. doi:10.1186/s13058-015-0514-2.

33. Breastcancer.org. Surgery. https://www.breastcancer.org/treatment/surgery/. December 14, 2020. Accessed December 20, 2020.

34. American Cancer Society. Surgery for breast cancer. https://www.cancer.org/cancer/breast-cancer/treatment/surgery-for-breast-cancer.html. September 18, 2019. Accessed December 20, 2020.

35. Lazow SP, Riba L Alapati A, James TA. Comparison of breast-conserving therapy vs mastectomy in women under age 40: national trends and potential survival implications. *Breast J.* 2019;25(4):578–584.

36. Al-Gaithy ZK, Yaghmoor BE, Koumu M, Alshehn KA, Saqah AA. Alshehn H. Trends of mastectomy and breast-conserving surgery and related factors in female breast cancer patients treated at King Abdulaziz University Hospital, Jeddah, Saudi Arabia, 2009–2017: a retrospective cohort study. *Ann Med Surg (Lond).* 2019;41:47–52.

37. Heerdt AS. Lymphatic mapping and sentinel lymph node biopsy for breast cancer. *JAMA Oncol.* 2018;4(3):431. https://jamanetwork.com/journals/jamaoncology/fullarticle/2663957.

38. Breastcancer.org. Axillary lymph node dissection. https://www.breastcancer.org/treatment/surgery/lymph_node_removal/axillary_dissection. September 19, 2018. Accessed December 20, 2020.

39. Giuliano AE, Ball KV, Beitsch P. Effect of axillary dissection vs no axillary dissection on 10-year overall survival among women with invasive breast cancer and sentinel node metastasis: the ACOSOG Z0011 (Alliance) randomized clinical trial. *JAMA.* 2017;318(10):918. doi:10.1001/jama.2017.11470.

40. Kang YJ, Han W, Park S, You JY, Yi HW, Park S, et al. Outcome following sentinel lymph node biopsy-guided decisions in breast cancer patients with conversion from positive to negative axillary lymph nodes after neoadjuvant chemotherapy. *Breast Cancer Res Treat.* 2017;166:473–480.

41. Ebner F, Wockel A, Schwentner L, et al. Does the number of removed axillary lymphnodes in high risk breast cancer patients influence the survival? *BMJ.* 2019;19:90. doi:10.1186/s12885-019-5292-2.

42. Munday LR, Homa K, Klassen AF, Pusic AL, Kerrigan CL. Breast cancer and reconstruction: normative data for interpreting the Breast Q. *Plast Reconstr Surg.* 2017;139(5):1046e–1055e.

43. Panchal H, Matros E. Current trends in post-mastectomy breast reconstruction. *Plast Reconst Surg.* 2017;140(5):7S–13S.

44. Turner A, Abu-Ghname A, Davis MJ. Fat grafting in breast reconstruction. *Surg Semin Plast.* 2020;34:17–23.

45. Sharma K, David G, Parikh R, Myckatyn T. Race and breast cancer reconstruction: is there a health care disparity? *Plastic Reconstr Surg.* 2016;138(2) 3554–3361.

46. Hart SE, Momoh AO. Breast reconstruction disparities in the United States and internationally. *Curr Breast Cancer Rep.* 2020;12:132–139.

47. American Cancer Society. Breast reconstruction using implants. https://www.cancer.org/cancer/breast-cancer/reconstruction-surgery/breast-reconstruction-options/breast-reconstruction-using-implants.html. September 18, 2019. Accessed February 21, 2021.

48. Breastcancer.org. Autologous or "flap" reconstruction. https://www.breastcancer.org/treatment/surgery/reconstruction/types/autologous. March 9, 2019. Accessed February 21, 2021.

49. Oliver JD, Boczar D, Huayllani MT, et al. Postmastectomy radiation therapy before and after 2-stage expander-implant breast reconstruction: a systematic review. *Medicina.* 2019;55(6):226. doi:10.3390/medicina55060226.

50. Lambertini M, Afrimos P, Gombos A, Awada A, Piccart M. in: MA Dicato, EV Cutsen (Eds.), Breast Cancer, 2nd ed., Springer International Publishing, 2018.

51. Breastcancer.org. Chemotherapy medicines. https://www.breastcancer.org/treatment/chemotherapy/medicines. October 29, 2020. Accessed January 20, 2021.

52. Denk F, Ramer LM, Erskine ELKS, et al. Tamoxifen induces cellular stress in the nervous system by inhibiting cholesterol synthesis. *Acta Neuropathol Commun.* 2015;3:74. doi:10.1186/s40478-015-0255-6.

53. Breastcancer.org. Hormonal therapy. https://www.breastcancer.org/treatment/hormonal. March 28, 2020. Accessed January 20, 2021.

54. National Cancer Institute. Hormone therapy for breast cancer. https://www.cancer.gov/types/breast/breast-hormone-therapy-fact-sheet. March 4, 2021. Accessed April 20, 2021.

55. American Cancer Society. Hormone therapy for breast cancer. https://www.cancer.org/cancer/breast-cancer/treatment/hormone-therapy-for-breast-cancer.html. Accessed January 20, 2021.

56. Heeke A, Nunes MR, Lynce F. Bone-modifying agents in early-stage and advanced breast cancer. *Curr Breast Cancer Rep.* 2018;10(4):241–250.

57. Cancer.net. Breast Cancer: types of treatment. https://www.cancer.net/cancer-types/breast-cancer/types-treatment. Accessed February 20, 2021.

58. Binkley JM, Harris SR, Levangie PK, et al. Patient perspectives on breast cancer treatment side effects and the prospective surveillance model for physical rehabilitation for women with breast cancer. *Cancer.* 2012;118(8 suppl):2207–2216.

59. Rosedale M, Fu MR. Confronting the unexpected: temporal, situational, and attributive dimensions of distressing symptom experience for breast cancer survivors. *Oncol Nurs Forum.* 2010;37(1):E28–E33.

60. Rafn BS, Singh CA, Midtgaard J, Camp PG, McNeely ML, Campbell KL. Self-managed surveillance for breast cancer-related upper body issues: a feasibility and reliability study. *Phys Ther.* 2020;100(3):468–476.

61. Harrington S, Padua D, Battaglini C, Michener LA. Upper extremity strength and range of motion and their relationship to function in breast cancer survivors. *Physiother Theory Pract.* 2013;29(7):513–520.

62. Harrington S, Padua D, Battaglini C, et al. Comparison of shoulder flexibility, strength, and function between breast cancer survivors and healthy participants. *J Cancer Surviv.* 2011;5(2):167–174.

63. Levangie PK, Drouin J. Magnitude of late effects of breast cancer treatments on shoulder function: a systematic review. *Breast Cancer Res Treat.* 2009;116(1):1–15.

64. Levy EW, Pfalzer LA, Danoff J, et al. Predictors of functional shoulder recovery at 1 and 12 months after breast cancer surgery. *Breast Cancer Res Treat.* 2012;134(1):315–324.

65. McNeely ML, Binkley JM, Pusic AL, et al. A prospective model of care for breast cancer rehabilitation: postoperative and postreconstructive issues. *Cancer.* 2012;118(8 suppl):2226–2236.

66. Zabit F, Iyigun G. A comparison of physical characteristics, functions and quality of life between breast cancer survivor women who had a mastectomy and healthy women. *J Back Musculoskelet Rehabil.* 2019;32(6):937–945.

67. Chatman AB, Hyams SP, Neel JM, et al. The Patient-Specific Functional Scale: measurement properties in patients with knee dysfunction. *Phys Ther.* 1997;77(8):820–829.

68. Davies C, Lengerich A, Bugajski A, Brockopp D. Detecting change in activity using the patient-specific functional scale with breast cancer survivors. *Rehabil Oncol.* 2018;36(2):117–122.

69. Horn KK, Jennings S, Richardson G, et al. The patient-specific functional scale: psychometrics, clinimetrics, and application as a clinical outcome measure. *J Orthop Sports Phys Ther.* 2012;42(1):30–42.

70. Westaway MD, Stratford PW, Binkley JM. The patient-specific functional scale: validation of its use in persons with neck dysfunction. *J Orthop Sports Phys Ther.* 1998;27(5):331–338.

71. Miale S, Harrington S, Kendig T. Oncology section task force on breast cancer outcomes: clinical measures of upper extremity function. *Rehabil Oncol.* 2013;30(4):27–34.

72. Harrington S, Gilchrist L, Sander A. Breast Cancer EDGE Task Force outcomes: clinical measures of pain. *Rehabil Oncol.* 2014;2(1):13–21.

73. Kennedy CA, Beaton DE, Smith P, et al. Measurement properties of the QuickDASH (disabilities of the arm, shoulder and hand) outcome measure and cross-cultural adaptations of the Quick-DASH: a systematic review. *Qual Life Res.* 2013;22(9):2509–2547.

74. LeBlanc M, Stineman M, DeMichele A, Stricker C, Mao JJ. Validation of QuickDASH outcome measure in breast cancer survivors for upper extremity disability. *Arch Phys Med Rehabil.* 2014;95(3):493–498.

75. Stratford PW, Binkley JM, Stratford DM. Development and initial validation of the upper extremity functional index. *Physiother Can.* 2001;53:259–267.

76. Binkley JM, Stratford P, Kirkpatrick S, et al. Estimating the reliability and validity of the upper extremity functional index in women after breast cancer surgery. *Clin Breast Cancer.* 2018;18(6):e1261–e1267.

77. Lehman LA, Sindhu BS, Shechtman O, Romero S, Velozo CA. A comparison of the ability of two upper extremity assessments to measure change in function. *J Hand Ther.* 2010;23(1):31–39.

78. Razmjou H, Bean A, van Osnabrugge V, MacDermid JC, Holtby R. Cross-sectional and longitudinal construct validity of two rotator cuff disease-specific outcome measures. *BMC Musculoskelet Disord.* 2006;7:26. doi:10.1186/1471-2474-7-26.

79. Bellamy N, Kirwan J, Boers M, et al. Recommendations for a core set of outcome measures for future phase III clinical trials in knee, hip, and hand osteoarthritis. Consensus development at OMER-ACT III. *J Rheumatol.* 1997;24(4):799–802.

80. Duncan PW. Stroke disability. *Phys Ther.* 1994;74(5):399–407.

81. Andrade Ortega JA, Millán Gómez AP, Ribeiro González M, et al. Validation of the FACT-B+4-UL questionnaire and exploration of its predictive value in women submitted to surgery for breast cancer. *Med Clin (Barc).* 2017;148(12):555–558.

82. Brady MJ, Cella DF, Mo F, et al. Reliability and validity of the functional assessment of cancer therapy-breast quality-of-life instrument. *J Clin Oncol.* 1997;15(3):974–986.

83. Nguyen J, Popovic M, Chow E, et al. EORTC QLQ-BR23 and FACT-B for the assessment of quality of life in patients with breast cancer: a literature review. *J Comp Eff Res.* 2015;4(2):15–166.

84. Pachman DR, Barton DL, Swetz KM, Loprinzi CL. Troublesome symptoms in cancer survivors: fatigue, insomnia, neuropathy, and pain. *J Clin Oncol.* 2012;30(30):3687–3696.

85. Pachman DR, Barton DL, Watson JC, Loprinzi CL. Chemotherapy-induced peripheral neuropathy: prevention and treatment. *Clin Pharmacol Ther.* 2011;90(3):377–387.

86. Gong Y, Tan Q, Qin Q, Wei C. Prevalence of postmastectomy pain syndrome and associated risk factors: a large single-institution cohort study. *Medicine (Baltimore).* 2020;99(20):e19834. doi:10.1097/MD.0000000000019834.

87. Childs JD, Piva SR, Fritz JM. Responsiveness of the numeric pain rating scale in patients with low back pain. *Spine.* 2005;30(11):1331–1334.

88. Farrar JT, Young JP, LaMoreaux L, Werth JL, Poole RM. Clinical importance of changes in chronic pain intensity measured on an 11-point numerical pain rating scale. *Pain.* 2001;94(2):149–158.

89. Spadoni GF, Stratford PW, Solomon PE, Wishart LR. The evaluation of change in pain intensity: a comparison of the P4 and single-item numeric pain rating scales. *J Orthop Sports Phys Ther.* 2004;34(4):187–193.

90. Hayes SC, Johansson K, Stout NL, et al. Upper-body morbidity after breast cancer: incidence and evidence for evaluation, prevention, and management within a prospective surveillance model of care. *Cancer.* 2012;118(8 suppl):2237–2249.

91. Hayes SC, Rye S, Battistutta D, Newman B. Prevalence of upper-body symptoms following breast cancer and its relationship with upper-body function and lymphedema. *Lymphology.* 2010;43(4):178–187.

92. Muir SW, Corea CL, Beaupre L. Evaluating change in clinical status: reliability and measures of agreement for the assessment of glenohumeral range of motion. *N Am J Sports Phys Ther.* 2010;5(3):98–110.

93. Perdomo M, Sebelski C, Davies C. Oncology Section Task Force on breast cancer outcomes: shoulder and glenohumeral outcome measures. *Rehabil Oncol.* 2013;30(4):19–26.

94. Lin HT, Hsu AT, An KN, et al. Reliability of stiffness measured in glenohumeral joint and its application to assess the effect of end-range mobilization in subjects with adhesive capsulitis. *Man Ther.* 2008;13(4):307–316.

95. Fisher M, Levangie P. Oncology Section Task Force on breast cancer outcomes: scapular assessment. *Rehabil Oncol.* 2013;30(4):11–18.

96. Rietman JS, Dijkstra PU, Hoekstra HJ, et al. Late morbidity after treatment of breast cancer in relation to daily activities and quality of life: a systematic review. *Eur J Surg Oncol.* 2003;29(3):229–238.

97. Kibler WB, Uhl TL, Maddux JW, et al. Qualitative clinical evaluation of scapular dysfunction: a reliability study. *J Shoulder Elbow Surg.* 2002;11(6):550–556.

98. Uhl TL, Kibler WB, Gecewich B, Tripp BL. Evaluation of clinical assessment methods for scapular dyskinesis. *Arthroscopy.* 2009;25(11):1240–1248.

99. Lewis JS, Valentine RE. The pectoralis minor length test: a study of the intra-rater reliability and diagnostic accuracy in subjects with and without shoulder symptoms. *BMC Musculoskelet Disord.* 2007;8:64. doi:10.1186/1471-2474-8-64.

100. Borstad JD. Measurement of pectoralis minor muscle length: validation and clinical application. *J Orthop Sports Phys Ther.* 2008;38(4):169–174.

101. Benton MJ, Schlairet MC. Upper extremity strength imbalance after mastectomy and the effect of resistance training. *Sports Med Int Open.* 2017;1(5):E160–E165.

102. Neil-Sztramko SE, Kirkham AA, Hung SH, et al. Aerobic capacity and upper limb strength are reduced in women diagnosed with breast cancer: a systematic review. *J Physiother.* 2014;60(4):189–200.

103. Bertoli J, de Souza Bezerra E, Dias Reis A, et al. Long-term side effects of breast cancer on force production parameters. *J Strength Cond Res.* 2020. doi:10.1519/JSC.0000000000003631.

104. Smith SL. Functional morbidity following latissimus dorsi flap breast reconstruction. *J Adv Pract Oncol.* 2014;5(3):181–187.

105. Selber JC, Nelson J, Fosnot J, et al. A prospective study comparing the functional impact of SIEA, DIEP, and muscle-sparing free TRAM flaps on the abdominal wall: part I. unilateral reconstruction. *Plast Reconstr Surg.* 2010;126(4):1142–1153.

106. Atisha D, Alderman AK. A systematic review of abdominal wall function following abdominal flaps for postmastectomy breast reconstruction. *Ann Plast Surg.* 2009;63(2):222–230.

107. Nelson JA, Tecci MG, Lanni MA, et al. Function and strength after free abdominally based breast reconstruction: a 10-year follow-up. *Plast Reconstr Surg.* 2019;143(1):22e–31e.

108. Rogers BH, Brown JC, Gater DR, Schmitz KH. Association between maximal bench press strength and isometric handgrip strength among breast cancer survivors. *Arch Phys Med Rehabil.* 2017;98(2):264–269.

109. Ryans K, Davies CC, Gaw G, et al. Incidence and predictors of axillary web syndrome and its association with lymphedema in women following breast cancer treatment: a retrospective study. *Support Care Cancer.* 2020;28(12):5881–5888.

110. Yeung WM, McPhail SM, Kuys SS. A systematic review of axillary web syndrome (AWS). *J Cancer Surviv.* 2015;9(4):576–598.

111. Koehler LA, Blaes AH, Haddad TC, et al. Movement, function, pain, and postoperative edema in axillary web syndrome. *Phys Ther.* 2015;95(10):1345–1353. doi:10.2522/ptj.20140377.

112. Figueira PVG, Haddad CAS, de Almeida Rizzi SKL, Facina G, Nazario ACP. Diagnosis of axillary web syndrome in patients after breast cancer surgery: epidemiology, risk factors, and clinical aspects: a prospective study. *Am J Clin Oncol.* 2018;41(10):992–996.

113. Brunelle C L, Roberts SA, Shui AM, et al. Patients who report cording after breast cancer surgery are at higher risk of lymphedema: results from a large prospective screening cohort. *J Surg Oncol.* 2020;122(2):155–163.

114. Leidenius M, Leppanen E, Krogerus L, von Smitten K. Motion restriction and axillary web syndrome after sentinel node biopsy and axillary clearance in breast cancer. *Am J Surg.* 2003;185(2):127–130.

115. Moskovitz AH, Anderson B O, Yeung RS, et al. axillary web syndrome after axillary dissection. *Am J Surg.* 2001;181(5):434–439.

116. Hayes SC, Janda M, Cornish B, Battistutta D, Newman B. Lymphedema after breast cancer: incidence, risk factors, and effect on upper body function. *J Clin Oncol.* 2008;26(21):3536–3542.

117. Nguyen TT, Hoskin TL, Habermann EB, Cheville AL, Boughey JC. Breast cancer-related lymphedema risk is related to multidisciplinary treatment and not surgery alone: results from a large cohort study. *Ann Surg Oncol.* 2017;24(10):2972–2980.

118. Ribeiro Pereira ACP, Koifman RJ, Bergmann A. Incidence and risk factors of lymphedema after breast cancer treatment: 10 years of follow-up. *Breast.* 2017;36:67–73.

119. Kilbreath SL, Refshauge KM, Beith JM, et al. Risk factors for lymphoedema in women with breast cancer: a large prospective cohort. *Breast.* 2016;28:29–36. doi:10.1016/j.breast.2016.04.011.

120. Swaroop MN, Ferguson CM, Horick NK, et al. Impact of adjuvant taxane-based chemotherapy on development of breast cancer-related lymphedema: results from a large prospective cohort. *Breast Cancer Res Treat.* 2015;151(2):393–403.

121. Ferguson CM, Swaroop MN, Horick N, et al. Impact of ipsilateral blood draws, injections, blood pressure measurements, and air travel on the risk of lymphedema for patients treated for breast cancer. *J Clin Oncol.* 2016;34(7):691–698.

122. Norman SA, Localio AR, Potashnik SL, et al. Lymphedema in breast cancer survivors: incidence, degree, time course, treatment, and symptoms. *J Clin Oncol.* 2009;27(3):390–397.

123. Chance-Hetzler J, Armer J, Van Loo M, et al. Prospective lymphedema surveillance in a clinic setting. *J Pers Med.* 2015;5(3):311–325.

124. Stout Gergich NL, Pfalzer LA, McGarvey C, et al. Preoperative assessment enables the early diagnosis and successful treatment of lymphedema. *Cancer.* 2008;112(12):2809–2819.

125. Stout NL, Binkley JM, Schmitz KH, et al. A prospective surveillance model for rehabilitation for women with breast cancer. *Cancer.* 2012;118(8 suppl):2191–2200.

126. Levenhagen K, Davies C, Perdomo M, Ryans K, Gilchrist L. Diagnosis of upper quadrant lymphedema secondary to cancer: clinical practice guideline from the Oncology Section of the American Physical Therapy Association. *Phys Ther.* 2017;97(7):729–745.

127. Bundred NJ, Stockton C, Keeley V, et al. Comparison of multifrequency bioimpedance with perometry for the early detection and intervention of lymphoedema after axillary node clearance for breast cancer. *Breast Cancer Res Treat.* 2015;151(1):121–129.

128. Fu M R, Cleland C M, Guth AA, et al. L-dex ratio in detecting breast cancer-related lymphedema: reliability, sensitivity, and specificity. *Lymphology.* 2013;46(2):85–96.

129. Smoot BJ, Wong JF, Dodd MJ. Comparison of diagnostic accuracy of clinical measures of breast cancer-related lymphedema: area under the curve. *Arch Phys Med Rehabil.* 2011;92(4):603–610.

130. Qin ES, Bowen MJ, Chen WF. Diagnostic accuracy of bioimpedance spectroscopy in patients with lymphedema: a retrospective cohort analysis. *J Plast Reconstr Aesthet Surg.* 2018;1(7):1041–1050.

131. Deltombe T, Jamart J, Recloux S, et al. Reliability and limits of agreement of circumferential, water displacement, and optoelec-

132. Sander AP, Hajer NM, Hemenway K, Miller AC. Upper-extremity volume measurements in women with lymphedema: a comparison of measurements obtained via water displacement with geometrically determined volume. *Phys Ther.* 2002;82(12):1201–1212.

133. Sharkey AR, King SW, Kuo RY, et al. Measuring limb volume: accuracy and reliability of tape measurement versus perometer measurement. *Lymphat Res Biol.* 2018;6(2):182–186.

134. Stanton AW, Northfield JW, Holroyd B, Mortimer PS. Levick JR Validation of an optoelectronic limb volumeter (Perometer). *Lymphology.* 1997;30(2):77–97.

135. Binkley J, Weiler M, Frank N, et al. Reliability and convergent validity of the lymphatech system to assess arm volume in patients during and after treatment for breast cancer. *Phys Ther.*100(3):457–467.

136. Hidding JT, Viehoff PB, Beurskens CH, et al. Measurement properties of instruments for measuring of lymphedema: systematic review. *Phys Ther.* 2016;96(12):1965–1981.

137. Rafn BS, McNeely ML, Camp PG, Midtgaard J, Campbell KL. Self-measured arm circumference in women with breast cancer is reliable and valid. *Phys Ther.* 2019;99(2):240–253.

138. Binkley J, Mark M, Finley J, Brazelton A, Pink M. Meeting the rehabilitation and support needs of breast cancer patients during Covid-19: opening new frontiers in models of care delivery. *Rehabil Oncol.* 2020;38(4):159–168.

139. Springer BA, Levy E, McGarvey C, et al. Pre-operative assessment enables early diagnosis and recovery of shoulder function in patients with breast cancer. *Breast Cancer Res Treat.* 2010;120(1):135–147.

140. Zieff GH, Wagoner CW, Paterson CL, Lassalle PP, Lee JT. Cardiovascular consequences of skeletal muscle impairments in breast cancer. *Sports (Basel).* 2020;8(6):80.

141. Kim DY, Kim JH, Park SW. Aerobic capacity correlates with health-related quality of life after breast cancer surgery. *Eur J Cancer Care (Engl).* 2019;28(4):e13050. doi:10.1111/ecc.13050.

142. Abrahams HJG, Gielissen MFM, Verhagen C, Knoop H. The relationship of fatigue in breast cancer survivors with quality of life and factors to address in psychological interventions: a systematic review. *Clin Psychol Rev.* 2018;63:1–11.

143. Abrahams HJG, Gielissen MFM, Schmits IC, et al. Risk factors, prevalence, and course of severe fatigue after breast cancer treatment: a meta-analysis involving 12,327 breast cancer survivors. *Ann Oncol.* 2016;27(6):965–974.

144. Han TJ, Felger JC, Lee A, et al. Association of childhood trauma with fatigue, depression, stress, and inflammation in breast cancer patients undergoing radiotherapy. *Psychooncology.* 2016;25(2):187–193.

145. Kishan AU, Wang PC, Sharif J, et al. Clinical indicators of psychosocial distress predict for acute radiation-induced fatigue in patients receiving adjuvant radiation therapy for breast cancer: an analysis of patient-reported outcomes. *Int J Radiat Oncol Biol Phys.* 2016;95(3):946–955.

146. Fisher MI, Davies C, Lacy H, Doherty D. Oncology section EDGE task force on cancer: measures of cancer-related fatigue: a systematic review. *Rehabil Oncol.* 2018;36:93–105.

147. Temel JS, Pirl WF, Recklitis CJ, Cashavelly B, Lynch TJ. Feasibility and validity of a one-item fatigue screen in a thoracic oncology clinic. *J Thorac Oncol.* 2006;1(5):454–459.

148. Jim HS, Phillips KM, Chait S, et al. Meta-analysis of cognitive functioning in breast cancer survivors previously treated with standard-dose chemotherapy. *J Clin Oncol.* 2012;30(29):3578–3587.

149. van der Willik KD, Koppelmans V, Hauptmann M, et al. Inflammation markers and cognitive performance in breast cancer survivors 20 years after completion of chemotherapy: a cohort study. *Breast Cancer Res.* 2018;20(1):135. doi:10.1186/s13058-018-1062-3.

150. Colombage UN, Lin KY, Soh SE, Frawley HC. Prevalence and impact of bladder and bowel disorders in women with breast cancer: a systematic review with meta-analysis. *Neurourol Urodyn.* 2021;40:15–27.

151. Chung CP, Behrendt C, Wong L, Flores S, Mortimer JE. Serial assessment of urinary incontinence in breast cancer survivors undergoing (neo)adjuvant therapy. *J Natl Compr Canc Netw.* 2020;18(6):712–716.

152. Landi SN, Doll KM, Bensen JT, et al. Endocrine therapy and urogenital outcomes among women with a breast cancer diagnosis. *Cancer Causes Control.* 2016;27(11):1325–1332.

153. Lai L, Binkley J, Jones V, et al. Implementing the Prospective Surveillance Model (PSM) of rehabilitation for breast cancer patients with 1-year postoperative follow-up, a prospective, observational study. *Ann Surg Oncol.* 2016;23(10):3379–3384.

154. Gerber LH, Stout NL, Schmitz KH, Stricker CT. Integrating a prospective surveillance model for rehabilitation into breast cancer survivorship care. *Cancer.* 2012;118(8 suppl):2201–2206.

155. F Pinheiro da Silva, Moreira GM, Zomkowski K, M Amaral de Noronha, Flores Sperandio F. Manual therapy as treatment for chronic musculoskeletal pain in female breast cancer survivors: a systematic review and meta-analysis. *J Manipulative Physiol Ther.* 2019;42(7):503–513.

156. De Groef A, Van Kampen M, Dieltjens E, et al. Effectiveness of postoperative physical therapy for upper-limb impairments after breast cancer treatment: a systematic review. *Arch Phys Med Rehabil.* 2015;96(6):1140–1153.

157. Luz CMD, Deitos J, Siqueira TC, Palu M, Heck APF. Management of axillary web syndrome after breast cancer: evidence-based practice. *Rev Bras Ginecol Obstet.* 2017;39(11):632–639.

158. Cho Y, Do J, Jung S, Kwon O, Jeon JY. Effects of a physical therapy program combined with manual lymphatic drainage on shoulder function, quality of life, lymphedema incidence, and pain in breast cancer patients with axillary web syndrome following axillary dissection. *Support Care Cancer.* 2016;24(5):2047–2057.

159. Lauridsen MC, Christiansen P, Hessov I. The effect of physiotherapy on shoulder function in patients surgically treated for breast cancer: a randomized study. *Acta Oncol.* 2005;44(5):449–457.

160. Torres Lacomba M, Mayoral Del Moral O, Coperias Zazo JL, et al. Axillary web syndrome after axillary dissection in breast cancer: a prospective study. *Breast Cancer Res Treat.* 2009;117(3):625–630.

161. Torres Lacomba M, Yuste Sánchez MJ, Zapico Goñi A, et al. Effectiveness of early physiotherapy to prevent lymphoedema after surgery for breast cancer: randomised, single blinded, clinical trial. *BMJ.* 2010;340:b5396.

162. Campbell KL, Winters-Stone KM, Wiskemann J, et al. Exercise guidelines for cancer survivors: consensus statement from international multidisciplinary roundtable. *Med Sci Sports Exerc.* 2019;51(11):2375–2390.

163. McNeely ML, Campbell KL, Rowe BH, et al. Effects of exercise on breast cancer patients and survivors: a systematic review and meta-analysis. *CMAJ.* 2006;175(1):34–41.

164. Furmaniak AC, Menig M, Markes MH. Exercise for women receiving adjuvant therapy for breast cancer. *Cochrane Database Syst Rev.* 2016;9:CD005001. doi:10.1002/14651858.cd005001.pub3.

165. Hasenoehrl T, Palma S, Ramazanova D, et al. Resistance exercise and breast cancer-related lymphedema-a systematic review update and meta-analysis. *Support Care Cancer.* 2020;28(8):3593–3603.

166. Schmitz KH, Ahmed RL, Troxel A, et al. Weight lifting in women with breast-cancer-related lymphedema. *N Engl J Med.* 2009;361(7):664–673.

167. Schmitz KH, Ahmed RL, Troxel AB, et al. Weight lifting for women at risk for breast cancer-related lymphedema: a randomized trial. *JAMA.* 2010;304(24):2699–2705.

168. Friedenreich CM, Gregory J, Kopciuk KA, et al. Prospective cohort study of lifetime physical activity and breast cancer survival. *Int J Cancer.* 2009;124(8):1954–1962.

169. Harris SR, Schmitz KH, Campbell KL, McNeely ML. Clinical practice guidelines for breast cancer rehabilitation: syntheses of guideline recommendations and qualitative appraisals. *Cancer.* 2012;118(8 suppl):2312–2324.

170. Holmes MD, Chen WY, Feskanich D, Kroenke CH, Colditz GA. Physical activity and survival after breast cancer diagnosis. *JAMA.* 2005;293(20):2479–2486.

171. Gebruers N, Camberlin M, Theunissen F, et al. The effect of training interventions on physical performance, quality of life, and fatigue in patients receiving breast cancer treatment: a systematic review. *Support Care Cancer.* 2019;27(1):109–122.

172. Cramer H, Lange S, Klose P, Paul A, Dobos G. Yoga for breast cancer patients and survivors: a systematic review and meta-analysis. *BMC Cancer.* 2012;12:412. doi:10.1186/1471-2407-12-412.

173. Cramer H, Lauche R, Klose P, et al. Yoga for improving health-related quality of life, mental health and cancer-related symptoms in women diagnosed with breast cancer. *Cochrane Database Syst Rev.* 2017;1:CD010802. doi:10.1002/14651858.CD010802.pub2.

174. Cramer H, Rabsilber S, Lauche R, Kummel S, Dobos G. Yoga and meditation for menopausal symptoms in breast cancer survivors: a randomized controlled trial. *Cancer.* 2015;121(13):2175–2184.

175. Pinto-Carral A, Molina AJ, de Pedro A, Ayan C. Pilates for women with breast cancer: a systematic review and meta-analysis. *Complement Ther Med.* 2018;41:130–140.

176. Cantarero-Villanueva I, Fernandez-Lao C, Cuesta-Vargas AI, et al. The effectiveness of a deep water aquatic exercise program in cancer-related fatigue in breast cancer survivors: a randomized controlled trial. *Arch Phys Med Rehabil.* 2013;94(2):221–230.

177. Cantarero-Villanueva I, Fernandez-Lao C, Fernandez-de-Las-Penas C, et al. Effectiveness of water physical therapy on pain, pressure pain sensitivity, and myofascial trigger points in breast cancer survivors: a randomized, controlled clinical trial. *Pain Med.* 2012;13(11):1509–1519.

178. Fernandez-Lao C, Cantarero-Villanueva I, Ariza-Garcia A, et al. Water versus land-based multimodal exercise program effects on body composition in breast cancer survivors: a controlled clinical trial. *Support Care Cancer.* 2013;21(2):521–530.

179. Delrieu L, Pialoux V, Perol O, et al. Feasibility and health benefits of an individualized physical activity intervention in women with metastatic breast cancer: intervention study. *JMIR mHealth uHealth.* 2020;8(1):e12306. doi:10.2196/12306.

180. Ligibel JA, Giobbie-Hurder A, Shockro L, et al. Randomized trial of a physical activity intervention in women with metastatic breast cancer. *Cancer.* 2016;122(8):1169–1177.

181. Yee J, Davis GM, Beith JM, et al. Physical activity and fitness in women with metastatic breast cancer. *J Cancer Surviv.* 2014;8(4):647–656.

182. Davies C, Levenhagen K, Ryans K, Perdomo M, Gilchrist L. Interventions for breast cancer-related lymphedema: clinical practice guideline from the academy of oncologic physical therapy of APTA. *Phys Ther.* 2020;100(7):1163–1179.

183. Sampaio LR, deResende MA, Pereira LSM. Cutaneous electrical nerve stimulation on vertebral metastatic bone pain of breast cancer patients: single case experimental study review. *Dor Sao Paulo.* 2016;17(2):81–87.

184. Mendonca ACR, Rett MT, Garcez PA, et al. TENS effects on dysesthesia and quality of life after breast cancer surgery with axilectomy: randomized controlled trial. *Fisioter Mov.* 2017;30(suppl 1):S285–S295.

185. Gewandter JS, Chaudrari J, Ibegbu C, et al. Wireless transcutaneous electrical nerve stimulation device for chemotherapy-induced peripheral neuropathy: an open-label feasibility study. *Support Care Cancer.* 2019;27(5):1765–1774.

186. Paglioni MdP, Araujo ALD, Arboleda LPA, et al. Side effects of photobiomodulation therapy used for prevention and management of cancer treatment toxicityies. A systematic review. *Oral Oncol.* 2019;93:21–28.

187. Kilmartin L, Denham T, Fu MR, et al. Complementary low-level laser therapy for breast cancer-related lymphedema: a pilot, double-blind, randomized, placebo-controlled study. *Lasers Med Sci.* 2020;35:95–105.

188. Baxter GD, Liu L, Petrich S, Gisselman AS, Chapple C, Anders JJ, Tumilty S. Low level laser therapy (Photobiomodulation therapy) for breast cancer-related lymphedema: a systematic review. *BMC Cancer.* 2017;17:83.

189. O'Connor D, Caulfield B, Lennon O. The efficacy and prescription of neuromuscular electrical stimulation (NMES) in adult cancer survivors: a systematic review and meta-analysis. *Supportive Care in Cancer.* 2018;26(12):3985–4000.

190. Smith T, Cheville AL, Loprinzi CL. Schoberlein DL. Scrambler therapy for the treatment of chronic post-mastectomy pain (cPMP). *Cureus.* 2017;9(6):e1378. doi:10.7759/cureus.1378.

191. Mendes IdS, Lima FPS, de Freitas STT, et al. Effects of vibration therapy in the musculoskeletal system in post-surgical breast cancer women: longitudinal controlled clinical study. *Res Biomed Eng.* 2016;32(3). doi:10.1590/2446-4740.00915.

192. Rosenbaek F, Holm HS, Hjelmborg B, Ewertz M, Jensen JD. Effect of cryotherapy on dose of adjuvant paclitaxel in early stage breast cancer. *Supportive Care Cancer.* 2020;28:3763–3769.

193. Hani A, Ishiguro H, Sozu T, et al. Effects of cryotherapy on objective and subjective symptoms of paclitaxel-induced neuropathy: prospective self-controlled trial. *JNCI.* 2018;110(2):djx178. doi:10.1093/jnci/djxt178.

194. Dunning J, Butts R, Mourad F, Young I, Flannagan S, Perreault T. Dry needling: a literature review with implications for clinical practice guidelines. *Phys Ther Rev.* 2014;19(4):252–265.

195. Vas L, Pai R. Ultrasound-guided dry needling as a treatment for postmastectomy pain syndrome—a case series of twenty patients. *Indian J Palliat Care.* 2019;25(1):93–102.

196. Cheville AL, Troxel AB, Basford JR, Kornblith AB. Prevalence and treatment patterns of physical impairments in patients with metastatic breast cancer. *J Clin Oncol.* 2008;26(16):2621–2629.

197. Ahmed RL, Thomas W, Yee D, Schmitz KH. Randomized controlled trial of weight training and lymphedema in breast cancer survivors. *J Clin Oncol.* 2006;24(18):2765–2772.

198. Ten Tusscher MR, Groen WG, Geleijn E, et al. Physical problems, functional limitations, and preferences for physical therapist-guided exercise programs among Dutch patients with metastatic breast cancer: a mixed methods study. *Support Care Cancer.* 2019;27(8):3061–3070.

199. Yousef AJA. Male breast cancer: epidemiology and risk factors. *Semin Oncol.* 2017;44(4):267–272.

200. Gucalp A, Traina TA, Eisner JR, et al. Male breast cancer: a disease distinct from female breast cancer. *Breast Cancer Res Treat.* 2019;173:37–48.

201. Ferzoco RM, Ruddy KJ. The epidemiology of male breast cancer. *Curr Oncol Rep.* 2016;18:1. doi:10.1007/s11912-015-0487-4.

202. Massarweh SA, Choi GL. Special considerations in the evaluation and management of breast cancer in men. *Curr Probl Cancer.* 2016;40:163–171.

203. Midding E, Halbach SM, Kowalski C, et al. Men with a "woman's disease": stigmatization of male breast cancer patients—a mixed methods analysis. *Am J Men's Health.* 2018;12(6):2194–2207.

204. Younas A, Sundus A, Inayat S. Transitional experience of men with breast cancer from diagnosis to survivorship: an integrative review. *Eur J Onc Nurs.* 2019;42:141–152.

205. Bootsma TI, Duijveman P, Pijpe A, et al. Unmet information needs of men with breast cancer and health professionals. *Psycho-Oncology.* 2020;29:851–860.

206. Silva TD. Male breast cancer: medical and psychological management in comparison to female breast cancer: a review. *Cancer Treat Commun.* 2016;7:23–34. doi:10.1016/J.CTRC.2016.03.004.

207. Triple Negative Breast Cancer Foundation. Understanding TNBC. tnbcfoundation.org\what-is-tnbc. Accessed April 25, 2021.

208. Breastcancer.org. Triple negative breast cancer. breastcancer.org/symptoms/types/triple-negative. April 9, 2021. Accessed April 25, 2021.

209. Garrido-Castro AC, Lin NU, Polyak K. Insights into molecular classifications of triple-negative breast cancer: improving patient selection for treatment. 2019;9(2):176–198. doi:10.1158/2159-8290.CD-18-1177.

210. Siddhartha S, Sharma D. Racial disparity and triple-negative breast cancer in African-American women: a multifaceted affair between obesity, biology, and socioeconomic determinants. *Cancers.* 2018;10(12):514. doi:10.3390/cancers10120514.

211. Maklin I, Fox K. Oligometastatic breast cancer. *Curr Oncol Rep.* 2020;22(2):15. doi:10.1007/s11912-020-0867-2.

212. Metastatic Breast Cancer Network. http://mbcn.org/death-mortality-rates/. Accessed April 25, 2021.

213. National Breast Cancer.org. Metastatic breast cancer. https://www.nationalbreastcancer.org/metastatic-breast-cancer. Accessed April 25, 2021.

214. Kanedan H, Saito Y. Oligometastases: defined by prognosis & evaluated by cure. *Cancer Treat Commun.* 2015;3:1–6. s.

215. John Hopkins Medicine. Pregnancy related breast cancer. https://www.hopkinsmedicine.org/kimmel_cancer_center/cancers_we_treat/breast_cancer_program/treatment_and_services/rare_breast_tumors/pregnancy_related_breast_cancer.html#:~:text=Pregnancyrelated%20breast%20cancer%20is,3000%20pregnant%20women%20are%20diagnosed. Accessed April 25, 2021.

216. Cathcart-Rake EJ, Ruddy KJ, Bleyer A, Johnson RH. Breast cancer in adolescent and young adult women under the age of 40 years. *JCO Oncol Prac.* 2021;17(6):305–313. doi: 10.1200/OP.20.00793.

217. Young Survival.org. Breast cancer risk factors. https://www.young-survival.org/learn/about-breast-cancer/breast-cancer-risk-factors-/. Accessed April 25, 2021.

218. Murphy BL, Day CN, Hoskin TL, Habermann EB, Boughey JC. Adolescents and young adults with breast cancer have more aggressive disease and treatment than patients in their forties. *Ann Surg Oncol.* 2019;26(12):3920–3930.

219. Prakash O, Hossain F, Danos D, Lassak A, Scribner R, Miele L. Racial disparities in triple negative breast cancer: a review of the role of biologic and non-biologic factors. *Front Public Health.* 2020;8:576964. doi:10.3389/fpubh.2020.576964.

220. Keenan T, Moy B, Mroz EA, et al. Comparison of the genomic landscape between primary breast cancer in African American versus white women and the association of racial differences with tumor recurrence. *J Clin Oncol.* 2015;33(31):3621–3627.

221. Huo D, Hu H, Rhie SK, et al. Comparison of breast cancer molecular features and survival by African and European ancestry in The Cancer Genome Atlas. *JAMA Oncol.* 2017;3(12):1654–1662. doi:10.1001/jamaoncol.2017.0595.

222. Connor AE, Visvanathan K, Baumgartner KB, et al. Pre-diagnostic breastfeeding, adiposity and mortality among parous Hispanic and non-Hispanic white women with invasive breast cancer: the breast cancer health disparities study. *Breast Cancer Res Treat.* 2017;161(2):321–331.

223. Quinn GP, Sanchez JA, Suttun SK, et al. Cancer and lesbian, gay, bisexual, bisexual, transgender/transsexual, and queer/questioning populations (LGBTQ). *CA Cancer J Clin.* 2015;65(5):384–400.

224. de Blok CJ, Wiepjes CM, Nota NM, et al. Breast cancer risk in transgender people receiving hormone treatment: Nationwide cohort study in the Netherlands. *BMJ.* 2019;365:l1652. doi:10.1136/bmj.l1652:10.1136/bmj.l1652.

225. American Cancer Society. Breaking down barriers for LGBT community. https://www.cancer.org/latest-news/breaking-down-health-care-barriers-for-lgbt-community.html. June 5, 2018. Accessed April 25, 2021.

16

Genitourinary and Gynecological Cancers

ALLEGRA ANN ADAMS, PT, DPT, BOARD CERTIFIED WOMEN'S HEALTH CLINICAL SPECIALIST

CHAPTER OUTLINE

Introduction

Prostate cancer is the most commonly diagnosed cancer in men and accounts for 21% of new cancer cases. It is the second leading cause of cancer-related death in men at 10%. Cancer of the urinary bladder is the fourth most common cancer in men and accounts for 7% of cancer-related deaths. In women, uterine cancer is the most common gynecological cancer and fourth most common cancer overall, at 7% of new cases. However, ovarian cancer has the highest mortality rate for gynecological cancers and accounts for 5% of cancer-related deaths.[1]

The direct effect of genitourinary and gynecological (GU/GYN) cancers and their treatments on urinary and sexual function is often quite apparent and well researched and therefore may result in earlier referral to rehabilitation directly from the surgeon, medical oncologist, or radiation oncologist rather than the person living with and beyond cancer (PLWBC) having to either "accept a new normal" or navigate through referrals to multiple specialists prior to referral to rehabilitation. Moreover, the oncology care team may start interventions related to behavior modification, bladder retraining, and dilator therapy prior to the referral to rehabilitation and occasionally as prehabilitation.

Cancers of the Genitourinary and Gynecological Systems

The following sections describe risk factors, signs and symptoms, screening and diagnosis, staging, treatment, and urinary and sexual adverse effects of treatment for bladder, prostate, testicular, endometrial, ovarian, and cervical cancer. A summaritive table is provided for each cancer type for quick reference.

Bladder Cancer

Bladder cancer is two to three times more common in men than in women. New cases have been slightly declining in both sexes, though the mortality rate in men has remained unchanged. Half of the new cases of bladder cancer are found in situ, with a 96% survival rate. Overall, the survival rate is 77% for all stages combined.[2] The following information is summarized in Table 16.1.

Risk Factors

The risk of developing bladder cancer increases with age, with most cases occurring in persons over the age of 55 years old and the average age at diagnosis of 73. It is more common in Caucasians, though African Americans are more likely to be diagnosed with more advanced disease. A personal or family history of bladder cancer also increases risk. Current or a history of tobacco use is present in one third of cases and occupational exposure to carcinogens contributes to 20% of cases. Risk increases with prolonged use of an indwelling catheter, parasitic infections, or cystitis. Treatment for other cancers is also a risk factor, including systemic use of cyclophosphamide or arsenic or radiation therapy for pelvic cancers.[2–4]

Signs and Symptoms

Bladder cancer is almost always symptomatic, with a relatively short time between the occurrence of disease and the onset of symptoms. Symptoms include blood in the urine, pain with urination (dysuria), urinary urgency (with or without frequency), and difficulty voiding. The location of the mass may compromise the integrity of the bladder lining, impair contraction of the detrusor muscle, or obstruct the outlet, thereby contributing to voiding dysfunction and symptoms.[2–4]

TABLE 16.1 Bladder Cancer

Risk Factors	Signs and Symptoms	Screening And Diagnosis	Treatment	Adverse Effects
Increased age, >55 yo Caucasian race Personal or family history Tobacco use Occupational exposure to carcinogens Prolonged use of indwelling catheter Parasitic infections, cystitis Systemic use of cyclophosphamide or arsenic Pelvic radiation therapy	Dysuria Urinary urgency, frequency Straining to void Hematuria Urinary retention	Urinalysis, urine culture, urine cytology Cystoscopy, cystourethroscopy Tumor biopsy (TURBT) Intravenous pyelogram or urogram (IVP or IVU) Ultrasound CT scan, MRI, bone scan, chest X-ray Urine marker tests	Surgery • TURBT • Partial or radical cystectomy • Ileal conduit and urostomy • Continent stoma • Neobladder Immunotherapy • Intravesical Bacillus Calmette-Guerin (BCG) • Immune checkpoint inhibitors • Monoclonal antibodies Chemotherapy • Mitomycin • Methotrexate • Vinblastine • Doxorubicin • Cisplatin • Gemcitabine • Paclitaxel External beam radiation Targeted therapy	Acute bladder irritation Systemic flu-like symptoms Bladder scarring, decreased bladder volume Urinary urgency/frequency Bladder, abdominal, pelvic pain Cancer recurrence Stoma problems (infection, tissue breakdown, leakage, incontinence) Intestinal reservoir problems (pouch stones, blockages due to stricture or mucous from intestinal lining, intestinal malabsorption, metabolic imbalances) Erectile dysfunction, dry ejaculation Dyspareunia, anorgasmia, decreased arousal

CT, computed tomography; *MRI*, magnetic resonance imaging.
Created by Allegra Adams. Printed with permission.

0— The tumor has only invaded the surface of the inner lining of the bladder, carcinoma in situ (CIS)
I— Tumor has invaded deeper into the lining of the bladder
II— The cancer has invaded through to the detrusor muscle
III— Tumor growth reaches adjacent organs including: prostate, uterus, vagina
IV— Invasion of the pelvic or abdominal wall or at least one lymph node or metastasis

Created by Allegra Adams. Printed with permission.

Diagnosis and Staging

Urothelial, or transitional cell, carcinoma is by far the most common form of bladder cancer, accounting for roughly 95% of cases. Other types of bladder cancer include: squamous cell carcinoma (1%–2%), adenocarcinoma (1%), small cell carcinoma (<1%), and sarcoma (<1%).[2] Bladder cancer diagnosis includes urinalysis to check for blood, urine culture to rule out infection as a differential diagnosis, urine cytology to check for precancerous and cancerous cell types, and cystoscopy or cystourethroscopy with tumor biopsy through Transurethral Resection of Bladder Tumor (TURBT). Imaging studies will also likely be performed to check for metastasis, including: intravenous pyelogram or urogram (IVP or IVU) which is a radiograph of the urological tract with contrast; ultrasound of the bladder, abdomen, or pelvis with or without additional needle biopsy; computed tomography (CT) or magnetic resonance imaging (MRI) scan of the pelvis, abdomen, and/or chest; bone scan; and chest radiograph. There are also several new urine marker tests available of variable utility.[2,4] Bladder cancer staging is summarized in Box 16.1.

Medical Treatment

Surgery is the main treatment intervention for bladder cancer. A TURBT may be sufficient for early stages of cancer though, with more advanced stages, a partial or a radical cystectomy or removal of the bladder may be necessary. A radical cystectomy will be followed by creation of an ileal conduit and urostomy (incontinent diversion to pass urine through the abdominal wall), a continent stoma requiring intermittent catheterization, or a neobladder for cases where the urethra can be preserved. These diversions are shown in eFigure 16.1. All diversions require harvesting a segment of intestines as a reservoir.[2,4]

Intravesical therapy, with immunotherapy or chemotherapy, is typically performed immediately after a TURBT and is generally used for Stage II or less. Intravesical Bacillus Calmette-Guerin (BCG) is a relative of the tuberculosis bacteria and is used in early-stage cancers to prevent recurrence through stimulating an immune response. Intravesical chemotherapy is used when local immune therapy does not work to kill actively growing cancer cells. Mitomycin is the most commonly used agent.[2,4]

Systemic chemotherapy may be used as neoadjuvant treatment to shrink a tumor before surgery or as adjuvant treatment during radiation, after surgery, or for metastatic disease. Common agents include: mitomycin (Mutamycin), methotrexate (Otrexup, Rasuvo, Rheumatrex, Trexall), vinblastine (Alkaban-AQ, Velban), doxorubicin (Adriamycin), cisplatin (Platinol), gemcitabine (Gemzar), or paclitaxel (Taxol).[2]

External beam radiation may be used in combination with surgery and chemotherapy or for a person with cancer (PWC) who cannot tolerate surgery or chemotherapy.[2]

Other forms of immunotherapy include immune checkpoint inhibitors to allow the immune system to recognize and target cancer cells or monoclonal antibodies that target specific cancer cell types. Targeted therapy to inhibit the Fibroblast Growth Factor Receptor (FGFR) is also under development.[2,4]

Genitourinary and Gynecological Adverse Effects of Bladder Cancer and Its Treatment

In cases of early-stage bladder cancer treated only with TURBT, there is a high rate of recurrence of up to 70%. Following a TURBT with intravesical BCG can reduce the risk of recurrence 30% to 40%.[4] Often, cancer recurrences are treated similarly, which can result in bladder scarring and decreased bladder volume, urgency and/or frequency, and pain. Even 10% of patients who undergo cystectomy will later develop urethral cancer distal to the perineal membrane. Intravesical therapies, and some systemic approaches, often result in acute bladder irritation. Intravesical BCG can cause systemic flu-like symptoms. Resections are accompanied by the usual effects of surgery (anesthesia reactions, bleeding, blood clots, infection, damage to adjacent organs, and pain) but also problems related to the stoma including infection, tissue breakdown, and leakage. Complications may also be related to the intestinal reservoir such as pouch stones, blockages due to stricture or mucous from the intestinal lining, and intestinal malabsorption or metabolic imbalances as the intestinal segments are permeable to urine.[2] Even with formation of an orthotopic neobladder, urinary incontinence (UI) rates for women are up to 43% during the day and 67% at night.[5] Hypercontinence (inability to void or urinary retention), vaginal prolapse, and neobladder-vaginal fistula are also common, at 69%, 6%, and 3% to 10% respectively.[5] For men, surgical resections can cause nerve damage resulting in erectile dysfunction. In a radical cystectomy, the prostate and seminal vesicles are removed resulting in a dry ejaculation with no semen. For women, surgical damage or tissue restriction results in dyspareunia (painful intercourse), anorgasmia, and decreased arousal. Psychosocial factors associated with a stoma also factor into sexuality in PLWBCs of the bladder.[2] The reader is referred to Chapter 12 for a full discussion of adverse effects of chemotherapy and radiation therapy on bladder and sexual function.

Prostate Cancer

Prostate cancer is the most commonly diagnosed cancer in men in the United States (US) (after skin cancer), with a one in eight lifetime risk, and the second leading cause of cancer-related death in men.[6] Globally, prostate cancer is the second most frequent cancer diagnosis made in men and the fifth leading cause of death.[7] An estimated 1.3 million cases of prostate cancer were diagnosed worldwide in 2018.[7] Localized and regional cancers have a nearly 100% 5-year relative survival rate and a combined 98% survival rate. That equates to 3.1 million men living in the US with a history of prostate cancer potentially dealing with treatment-related sequelae.[6] The following information is summarized in Table 16.2.

Risk Factors

The risk of developing prostate cancer increases with age, with the majority of cases occurring in men over 65 years of age and an average age at diagnosis of 66 years. A family history of prostate cancer, genetic factors (e.g., *BRCA* 2 mutations), and African American race are other nonmodifiable risk factors for developing prostate cancer. Extensive research has been done regarding

TABLE 16.2	Prostate Cancer			
Risk Factors	**Signs and Symptoms**	**Screening And Diagnosis**	**Treatment**	**Adverse Effects**
Increased age, >65 yo Family history *BRCA* 1 and 2 mutations African American race Obesity Diet high in animal fat or meat Low levels of vitamins or selenium Multiple sex partners Viruses Occupational exposure to chemicals/metals	Asymptomatic Obstruction of LUT • Urinary hesitancy • Weak stream • Small voiding volumes • Urinary frequency, nocturia • Post-void drip • Palpable bladder above the pubic symphysis • Urinary retention • Lower abdominal, suprapubic discomfort with urge to void Low back, pelvic, hip, or upper thigh pain or stiffness Difficulty having erection Blood in semen Hematuria Bone pain CBC changes Signs of spinal cord compression Weight loss Lymphedema of LE, scrotum	Age 50, or 45 with known risk factors Digital rectal exam (DRE) Prostate-specific antigen (PSA) Transrectal ultrasound-guided biopsy CT/PET scan, chest X-ray, bone scan	Watchful waiting/active surveillance Surgery • Prostatectomy • Transurethral resection of prostate (TURP) Radiation therapy • External beam • Brachytherapy Hormonal therapy • Androgen deprivation therapy (ADT) • Luteinizing hormone-releasing hormone (LHRH) agonists or antagonists • Androgen receptor antagonists, antiandrogens • Bilateral orchiectomy • Adrenal suppression Chemotherapy • Docetaxel, taxanes • Prednisone Cryotherapy Immunotherapy Targeted therapy • PARP (poly (ADP)-ribose polymerase) inhibitors	Acute bladder irritation, bleeding, dysuria Urinary incontinence Urinary retention Radiation cystitis, fibrosis Urinary urgency, frequency, nocturia Chronic pelvic pain Impaired core muscle function Low back pain Pain with ejaculation Erectile dysfunction Decreased sexual desire Infertility Genital, lower extremity lymphedema Inguinal or umbilical hernia Decreased muscle mass Osteoporosis Falls, fractures Menopausal symptoms

CBC, complete blood count; *CT*, computed tomography; *LE*, lower extremity; *LUT*, lower urinary tract; *PET*, positron emission tomography.
Created by Allegra Adams. Printed with permission.

potential modifiable risk factors in the prevention of prostate cancer including: obesity, a diet high in animal fat or meats, other dietary or nutrient levels (i.e., selenium), smoking and alcohol consumption, hormone levels, multiple sex partners, viruses, and environmental or occupational exposure to certain chemicals (including Agent Orange) or metals. Unfortunately, to date there is limited evidence of efficacy.[3,4,6,8]

Signs and Symptoms

Prostate cancer is a typically slow-growing cancer type; cell changes may be present 10 or more years prior to the onset of symptoms. Therefore, early stages of prostate cancer may be asymptomatic. Early signs of prostate pathology correspond with obstruction of the lower urinary tract, including: urinary hesitancy, weak stream, small voiding volumes, urinary frequency especially nocturia (nighttime frequency), postvoid drip, a palpable bladder above the pubic symphysis indicating urinary retention, or lower abdominal or suprapubic discomfort with an urge to void. It is therefore possible that treatment for prostate cancer may actually improve more genitourinary symptoms than it causes. It is worth noting that many of these symptoms may occur with benign prostatic hyperplasia (BPH), which is decidedly not cancerous.[3,6] eFigure 16.2A shows the bladder-prostate anatomy demonstrating how prostatic enlargement will impinge on the urethra, as the prostate typically grows inward.

Other signs of prostate cancer may include low back, pelvic, hip, or upper thigh pain or stiffness; erectile dysfunction; or blood in the urine or semen. *Low back pain with sciatica is a red flag in men with a history of prostate cancer.* Prostate cancer most commonly metastasizes to the bone and therefore may present as bone pain, anemia or other blood count changes, or neurological changes associated with spinal cord compression. Weight loss or lymphedema of the lower extremities and scrotum may also suggest metastatic disease.[3,6]

Diagnosis and Staging

Prostate cancer is most commonly adenocarcinoma. 90% of cases are detected pre-metastasis.[4] The US Preventative Services Task Force and the American Urological Association (AUA) recommend screening for prostate cancer to begin at age 50, or age 45 with known risk factors.[6,9] Screening typically includes a digital rectal exam (DRE) to assess for size, texture, and pain, and testing of prostate-specific antigen (PSA) through a blood draw. eFigure 16.2B shows the anatomical relationship of the rectum to the prostate for how a DRE would allow for access to the posterior aspect of the prostate. Recently, there has been significant controversy regarding over-diagnosis and over-treatment of prostate cancer as PSA is prostate, but not cancer, specific. For example, PSA increases as prostate size increases, such as with age or BPH, or with recent ejaculation. Additionally, African Americans tend to have higher levels of PSA and some medications can lower PSA. Poorly differentiated prostate carcinomas produce minimal or no PSA. There is a small benefit of testing PSA levels in men between the ages of 55 to 69 years old, but no net benefit of testing over age 70 and therefore this is not recommended. There is no normative value that definitively indicates cancer, though higher values and rapidly increasing values may signal the need for further testing. PSA levels have more utility as a measure of recurrence of prostate cancer.[4,6] A urine test is currently under development which has been shown in clinical trials to accurately discriminate cases of elevated PSA levels associated with clinically significant prostate cancer (grade group two or above) with the hope to avoid

• BOX 16.2 Prostate Cancer Staging

I— Tumor not palpable during rectal exam; found during surgery for another reason (i.e., BPH); Gleason score ≤6; PSA <10

II— Tumor palpable during rectal exam or with biopsy; no evidence of metastasis; Gleason score 6–7; PSA 10–20

III— Metastasis to nearby tissues (i.e., seminal vesicles, rectum, bladder, pelvic walls); Gleason score 8–9; PSA 20+

IV— Metastasis to lymph nodes or other parts of body; any Gleason score/ PSA

BPH, Benign prostatic hyperplasia; *PSA*, prostate specific antigen.
Created by Allegra Adams. Printed with permission.

unnecessary invasive and costly testing (e.g., biopsy and MRI) in persons with PSA levels elevated for other reasons.[10]

If symptomology and screening suggest, a transrectal ultrasound-guided biopsy will be performed to collect tissue samples to detect the presence of cancer. At least two core needle specimens will be collected and the primary and secondary glandular patterns will be graded from 1 to 5 (histologically similar to undifferentiated) and summed to give a Gleason score between 2 and 10. Cell differentiation for the Gleason scores is depicted in eFigure 16.3.

A low grade (less than or equal to 6) indicates a well-differentiated, less aggressive cancer with a better prognosis.[4,6] Gleason grade groups indicating risk level are defined in eTable 16.1. The Gleason score is not the same as the stage of prostate cancer, defined in Box 16.2.[6] If metastasis is suspected, a CT or positron emission tomography (PET) scan of the pelvis, abdomen, and/or chest, a chest radiograph, or a bone scan may also be performed.[4,6]

Medical Treatment

Treatment for prostate cancer is dependent on the age and overall health of the PWC, symptom burden, Gleason score, and stage of cancer. Older persons with comorbidities, a lower Gleason score (less than or equal to six), and a lower stage (Stage I) of cancer may be offered observation ("watchful waiting") or active surveillance, with continued screening but no immediate intervention or treatment.[4,6]

Surgical excision of the prostate and seminal vesicles, or a radical prostatectomy, is the most common treatment for localized prostate cancer. Surgery can either be open, with a single long incision from umbilicus to pubis, or laparoscopic. It may be done directly by the surgeon or robotic assisted. Overall, outcomes seem to be more related to the skill of the surgeon and extent of cancer rather than the surgical approach.[6] eFigure 16.2D shows the postprostatectomy anatomy. The indwelling catheter remains in place for 7 to 10 days to allow for healing. For metastatic disease, a transurethral resection of prostate (TURP) may be performed as a debulking procedure to lessen obstructive symptoms rather than have a curative intent. Radical prostatectomy will not be performed for metastatic disease due to the burden of adverse effects for a noncurative procedure.[4,6]

Radiation therapy may be used for local prostate cancer with similar cure rates as a prostatectomy. Radiation will also be used for metastatic or recurrent disease in conjunction with hormonal therapy. Radiation may be external beam or brachytherapy (internal radiation). Brachytherapy may be permanent via placement of radioactive seeds into the prostate or temporary and may be used in combination with external beam radiation. The adverse effects

from radiation therapy, namely UI and erectile dysfunction, are similar to those of surgery, however, symptoms arise immediately after surgery and improve over time whereas symptoms are minimal postradiation and increase over several years.[4,6]

Hormonal therapy is used for prostate cancer to shrink the tumor to lessen symptom burden in persons who cannot receive surgery or radiation, or prior to radiation to improve outcomes. It may also be used in combination with radiation or surgery to prevent or treat recurrence. Hormonal therapy aims to lower testosterone levels to reduce the growth of prostate cancer, however, it is not curative. Treatment is targeted at testosterone production centers in either the testes or adrenals and includes: androgen deprivation therapy (ADT) (luteinizing hormone-releasing hormone [LHRH] agonists or antagonists, androgen receptor antagonists also called antiandrogens; medical castration), bilateral orchiectomy (surgical castration), or adrenal suppression. Due to the risk of blood clots, estrogen is rarely used.[4,6]

Chemotherapy is not a mainline treatment for prostate cancer and is typically used for metastatic disease after hormone therapy proves ineffective; it is not a curative treatment for prostate cancer.[6] The primary chemotherapeutic agent used is docetaxel (Taxotere) in combination with prednisone, followed by trials of other taxanes. Platinum-based drugs are under investigation.

Cryotherapy may be used for recurrent disease but is rarely a first line treatment. Immunotherapy, in which an individualized vaccine is created from the person's white blood cells and then injected back into circulation, is another noncurative option to extend life expectancy for a PLWBC for whom hormonal therapy is no longer effective. Targeted therapy with PARP (poly(ADP)-ribose polymerase) inhibitors can be used after hormonal therapy and chemotherapy has failed in persons with a *BRCA* mutation.[6]

Genitourinary Adverse Effects of Prostate Cancer and Its Treatment

Given the proximity of the prostate to the bladder and the associated neurovascular bundles (eFigure 16.2C), urological adverse effects are almost inevitable with either surgery or radiation therapy. UI—either stress, urgency, mixed, or continuous (refer to Chapter 12 for definitions)—is the most common.[6] UI postoperatively generally improves spontaneously within the first year with 68% of men reporting continence by two months and 75% to 92% by one year.[11] Bladder control improves first at night, then in the early morning, and finally in the evening. Conversely, but less common, surgical strictures or radiation fibrosis may result in urinary retention. Radiation therapy may result in radiation cystitis, progressing to fibrosis of the bladder, acutely causing irritation, bleeding, and/or dysuria and chronically causing urinary urgency, frequency, and/or nocturia due to reduced bladder capacity. UI may also occur with chemotherapy, though the pathophysiology is more likely neuropathy of the pelvic nerves for bladder and pelvic muscle innervation.[6]

Also due to proximity, radiation can cause proctitis and fibrosis with associated bowel symptoms including: diarrhea, constipation, bowel urgency and frequency, anal irritation and bleeding, and anal incontinence (leakage of gas, stool, or mucus). Chemotherapy is also notorious for its gastrointestinal adverse effects (see Chapter 11).[6]

Surgical incisions, scar restriction, or radiation fibrosis may cause pain at the site (abdominal, perineal) as well as pain with urination, defecation, or ejaculation. Chronic pelvic pain with activities such as sitting, walking, or other exercise can also develop. This author has found that incisions, radiation, and chemotherapy may also impair core muscle function including strength or coordination for bladder or bowel control and evacuation and for dynamic lumbopelvic stability contributing to low back pain. Midline incisions often result in a diastasis rectus abdominus.

Neurovascular damage from surgery or radiation or neuropathy from chemotherapy may all result in erectile dysfunction, which is expected to last up to 2 years postoperatively, if it is recovered at all. Rates of erectile dysfunction are reported to be as high as 87% 2 to 5 years postoperatively, with only 4% to 16% of men reporting return to baseline erectile function by 2 years.[12] Conversely, erectile function declines for the two years following radiation therapy.[13] Altered body image from these procedures or use of hormonal therapy impacting hormone levels contribute to decreased sexual desire. Though prostate cancer is more common in older men, most treatments do result in infertility as the vas deferens from the testes is cut with surgery, radiation and chemotherapy damage the spermatozoa, and hormonal therapy suppresses testosterone.[6]

Due to lymph node removal during surgery or damage with radiation therapy, genital and lower extremity lymphedema is possible. Surgery also increases the risk of developing an inguinal hernia, or depending on the surgical approach, an umbilical hernia. Metastatic disease itself, radiation therapy, hormonal therapy, and chemotherapy all decrease muscle mass and increase the risk of developing osteoporosis resulting in higher levels of fragility, falls, and fractures.[6] In fact, one in five men receiving ADT will fracture within 5 to 6 years.[14]

Hormonal therapy also creates menopausal symptoms in men, including hot flashes and gynecomastia (breast enlargement).[6]

Testicular Cancer

The following information is summarized in Table 16.3.

Risk Factors

Testicular cancer is most common in Caucasian males between the ages of 20 and 34 years. Risk is increased in males with a history of an undescended testicle (cryptorchidism), HIV infection, or genetic factors including a family history of testicular cancer or Klinefelter's syndrome. Carcinoma in situ of the testicle may develop into cancer and there is a 3% to 4% chance of developing a second cancer on the other side for males with a personal history of testicular cancer.[3,4,15,16]

Signs and Symptoms

In most cases, testicular cancer is asymptomatic. Particularly carcinoma in situ or early stage cancer may be found incidentally during routine medical examination or work up for infertility. Postpubescent males are encouraged to perform regular testicular exams and report any enlargement, swelling, or hardness of the testicle or a finding of a hard, painless lump in the testicle the size of a pea.[3,4,15]

Pain or discomfort in the testicle or scrotum is uncommon with testicular cancer but men may experience a dull ache or feeling of heaviness in the scrotum, groin, or lower abdomen. Metastatic disease may also cause low back pain, unexplained fatigue, or malaise. Some germ cell tumors produce human chorionic gonadotropin (HCG) which may enlarge the breasts or make them tender.[3,4,15,16]

Diagnosis and Staging

An ultrasound of the testicle is the first test performed to rule out a hydrocele, a varicocele, or simply inflammation of the testis or epididymis. A blood test will also be performed to measure HCG, alpha-fetoprotein (AFP), and the enzyme lactate dehydrogenase (LDH) which may all be produced by the tumor.[4,15]

A testicular biopsy may increase the risk of metastasis so often the testicle will be surgically removed (orchiectomy) and then biopsied or the biopsy will be performed during surgery prior to resection, if warranted.[15]

If testicular cancer is confirmed, other imaging tests will be performed to rule out metastasis including: a chest radiograph, CT scan, MRI, PET scan, or bone scan.[15]

Testicular cancer is staged according to the International Germ Cell Cancer Collaborative Group, as described in Box 16.3. Ninety percent of testicular cancers arise from the germ cells, or

---

• BOX 16.3   Testicular Cancer Staging

0— Germ cell neoplasia in situ (GCNIS)
I— Cancer confined to testicle or adjacent structures
II— Cancer spread to inguinal or retroperitoneal lymph nodes
III— Cancer spread beyond local lymph nodes to remote sites (lungs, brain, liver), tumor marker levels are high

Created by Allegra Adams. Printed with permission.

TABLE 16.3   Testicular Cancer

Risk Factors	Signs and Symptoms	Screening And Diagnosis	Treatment	Adverse Effects
20–34 yo Caucasian race Tall height Cryptorchidism HIV infection Personal or family history Klinefelter's syndrome	Infertility Enlargement, swelling, or hardness of the testicle Hard, painless lump in the testicle the size of a pea Pain or discomfort in the testicle or scrotum Dull ache or feeling of heaviness in the scrotum, groin, or lower abdomen Low back pain Unexplained fatigue, malaise Gynecomastia	Ultrasound Blood test • Human chorionic gonadotropin (HCG) • Alpha-fetoprotein (AFP) • Lactate dehydrogenase (LDH) Orchiectomy with biopsy CT/PET scan, MRI, chest X-ray, bone scan	Surgery • Orchiectomy, unilateral or bilateral • Spermatic cord • Retroperitoneal Lymph Node Dissection (RPLND) External beam radiation Chemotherapy • Bleomycin • Etoposide • Cisplatin Autologous stem cell transplantation	Infertility Retrograde ejaculation Decreased sex drive, erectile dysfunction, fatigue, hot flashes, loss of muscle mass Bowel dysfunction Second cancer Kidney damage

CT, computed tomography; *HIV,* human immunodeficiency virus; *MRI,* magnetic resonance imaging.
Created by Allegra Adams. Printed with permission.

the cells that make sperm, and are either seminomas, nonseminomas, or mixed.[15]

Medical Treatment

Testicular cancer has a 99% 5-year relative survival rate for localized disease and a 95% combined survival rate.[15] Surgery is performed in nearly all cases of testicular cancer to remove the testicle, spermatic cord, and, if indicated, the associated lymph nodes. Regardless of the stage of cancer, the testicle is removed through a small suprapubic incision in a radical inguinal orchiectomy. Cancer that may have spread in the lymph nodes will be removed in an open or laparoscopic Retroperitoneal Lymph Node Dissection (RPLND).[4,15]

External beam radiation may be used instead of or in combination with a RPLND or for metastatic disease at the site of the metastasis. Chemotherapy is often used to cure metastatic testicular cancer or to prevent recurrence. Agents are generally used in combination, with the current most common being: bleomycin (Blenoxane), etoposide (Toposar, VePesid), and/or cisplatin (Platinol). For recurrent testicular cancer, the PWC is treated with high-dose chemotherapy followed by autologous stem cell transplantation that was collected and frozen prior to chemotherapy to restore bone marrow function.[4,15]

Genitourinary Adverse Effects of Testicular Cancer and Its Treatment

Since testicular cancer is most common in younger men around the age of trying to start a family, fertility is often a concern. It may be complaints of infertility that uncovered the cancer to begin with. In general, a unilateral orchiectomy should not impair erections or fertility. Men should wait 2 years after chemotherapy prior to attempting to conceive a child in order to reduce the risk of birth defects from DNA damage due to chemotherapy.[17] Rarely, the nerves involved in ejaculation are affected resulting in retrograde ejaculation (ejaculation into the bladder) but this can be prevented through a nerve-sparing approach. A bilateral orchiectomy will result in infertility as well as decreased sex drive, erectile dysfunction, fatigue, hot flashes, and loss of muscle mass due to the decrease in testosterone levels. Men will likely need to be on some form of hormone replacement therapy (HRT) for the extent of their life. In men requiring a bilateral orchiectomy who desire to have biological children in the future, sperm may be collected and banked, though the cancer may make sperm counts low. For cosmetic purposes, men may opt to have an egg-shaped saline prosthesis implanted in the scrotum.[15,17]

Other adverse effects of surgery and radiation include bowel dysfunction including constipation, diarrhea, malabsorption, or obstruction. Radiation may cause a second cancer in the remaining testicle, though advances in dosing and shielding have reduced this risk. Radiation may also cause a second unrelated cancer in the adjacent tissues when treating metastatic disease. There is a 1% chance of developing a second cancer after chemotherapy treatment for testicular cancer.[15] Cisplatin (Platinol) is also known to cause kidney damage.[4,15]

Uterine (Endometrial) Cancer

Endometrial cancer arises from the inner lining of the uterus, the endometrium. It is the most common cancer of the female reproductive tract, representing 65% of gynecological cancers.[18]

It is estimated that there are 600,000 PLWBCs of the endometrium and its sequelae in the US.[18] Rarely, cancer arises in the muscular layer of the uterus (myometrium) forming a uterine sarcoma; this represents less than 10% of uterine cancers.[18] Uterine sarcoma is not discussed in this chapter, though the adverse effects of its treatment are similar. Reproductive system anatomy for the three gynecological cancers discussed in this chapter is depicted in eFigure 16.4. The following information is summarized in Table 16.4.

Risk Factors

Endometrial cancer is most common in postmenopausal women between the ages of 50 and 70 years. Risk increases with increased exposure to estrogen, therefore nulliparous or low parity women (women who have had no or few children, respectively), women receiving prolonged unopposed estrogen therapy (as in hormone replacement therapy without progesterone), women who had early menarche (first menses) or late menopause, and women with anovulation or infertility are all at greater risk of developing endometrial cancer. Adipose tissue also produces estrogen and therefore obesity is a risk factor as well. Polycystic ovarian syndrome (PCOS) results in increased estrogen levels and is often accompanied by infertility and obesity. Contraceptives that decrease the exposure to estrogen, including oral progesterone or an intrauterine device (IUD), may be protective.[3,4,18] Recently, there has been some concern regarding the role of dietary soy consumption and its relation to estrogen-dependent cancers due to its structural similarity to endogenous estrogen. Despite its phytoestrogen properties, soy intake has been shown to be inversely related to endometrial cancer risk.[19]

Endometrial cancer shares many risk factors with breast and ovarian cancers and therefore a PLWBC may experience more than one of these female cancers over her lifespan. Moreover, tamoxifen used in treating and preventing breast cancer recurrence acts as an anti-estrogen in the breasts but has an estrogenic effect in the uterus and can therefore increase the risk of endometrial cancer in a PLWBC of the breast. Pelvic radiation therapy, for ovarian or other pelvic cancer, also increases the risk of developing endometrial cancer.[3,4,18]

Endometrial cancer is more common in Caucasian women than women of other races and is twice as common in women with type 2 diabetes. Risk increases with a history of endometrial hyperplasia, family history of endometrial cancer, or genetic predisposition due to Lynch syndrome (previously hereditary nonpolyposis colon cancer [HNPCC]). Women with Lynch syndrome have a 70% chance of developing endometrial cancer.[3,4,18]

Signs and Symptoms

The most common sign of endometrial cancer is abnormal uterine bleeding, including change in menstrual cycle, intermenstrual bleeding, or postmenopausal bleeding. Abnormal uterine bleeding is present in 90% of cases of endometrial cancer[18] and is especially telling as most cases of endometrial cancer are postmenopausal. Any abnormal vaginal discharge in general, even without visible traces of blood, should be evaluated by a physician.[3,4,18]

More advanced cancer may present with fatigue, weight loss, pelvic or abdominal pain or mass, bladder pain, or dyspareunia.[3,4,18]

TABLE 16.4	Endometrial (Uterine) Cancer			
Risk Factors	**Signs and Symptoms**	**Screening And Diagnosis**	**Treatment**	**Adverse Effects**
Postmenopausal, 50–70 yo Caucasian race Increased exposure to estrogen • Nulliparity, low parity • Prolonged unopposed estrogen therapy (HRT) • Early menarche, late menopause • Anovulation, infertility • Obesity • Polycystic ovarian syndrome (PCOS) Type 2 diabetes History of breast, ovarian cancer, endometrial hyperplasia Tamoxifen Pelvic radiation therapy Family history Lynch syndrome Protective: Contraceptives • Oral progesterone • Intrauterine device (IUD) Dietary soy consumption	Abnormal uterine bleeding (AUB) • Change in menstrual cycle • Intermenstrual bleeding • Postmenopausal bleeding Fatigue Weight loss Pelvic, abdominal pain, mass Bladder pain Dyspareunia	No screening tests Education of postmenopausal women of the risk factors and signs and symptoms Lynch syndrome: • Annual endometrial biopsy >35 yo • Prophylactic hysterectomy after childbearing Ultrasound Hysteroscopy Biopsy Dilation and curettage (D&C) CT/PET scan, MRI, chest X-ray Cystoscopy, proctoscopy Blood tests • CBC • CA-125	Surgery • Hysterectomy • Parametrium • Uterosacral ligament • Proximal portion of the vagina • Bilateral salpingo-oophorectomy (BSO) • Omenectomy • Parietal peritoneum • RPLND Radiation therapy • External beam • Brachytherapy Chemotherapy • Carboplatin, paclitaxel • Cisplatin, doxorubicin Hormone therapy • Progestins • Tamoxifen • LHRH agonists • Aromatase inhibitors (Als)	Kidney damage Bladder irritation Infertility Menopause • GSM • Osteoporosis • Heart disease Vaginal, bladder, rectal fibrosis Urinary urgency/frequency Vaginal shortening, fibrosis Dyspareunia Decreased libido, decreased genital sensitivity, anorgasmia Genital, lower extremity lymphedema

CBC, complete blood count; *CT*, computed tomography; *GSM*, genitourinary syndrome of menopause; *LHRH*, luteinizing hormone-releasing hormone; *MRI*, magnetic resonance imaging; *PET*, positron emission tomography; *RPLND*, retroperitoneal lymph node dissection; *yo*, years old.
Created by Allegra Adams. Printed with permission.

Diagnosis and Staging

There is no standard screening test for endometrial cancer, except for those with confirmed or suspected Lynch syndrome, based on family history of endometrial or colon cancer. For these women, the American College of Obstetrics and Gynecology (ACOG) recommends annual endometrial biopsy after the age of 35. A prophylactic hysterectomy once childbearing is completed may also be recommended.[20] Otherwise, the American Cancer Society (ACS) recommends that women be advised of the risk factors and signs and symptoms of endometrial cancer at menopause.[4,18]

A woman presenting to her gynecologist with reports of signs or symptoms of endometrial cancer and a history of any risk factors, will first undergo an ultrasound of the reproductive tract to assess for endometrial thickening, polyps, or masses in the endometrium or myometrium (uterine sarcoma). If the ultrasound results are unclear, the gynecologist may perform a hysteroscopy with a scope inside the uterus. During the ultrasound or hysteroscopy, the gynecologist will likely take a tissue biopsy. If the biopsy is inconclusive, the woman may require a dilation and curettage (D&C) under anesthesia where the cervix is artificially dilated and the endometrial lining is scraped to obtain a tissue sample.[4,18]

When endometrial cancer is detected, the woman will also receive a chest radiograph, a CT scan, MRI, and/or a PET scan to look for metastasis. A cystoscopy or proctoscopy may also be performed to look for metastasis to the bladder or rectum, respectively, if symptoms suggest. Some blood tests may also

be performed. A complete blood count will check for anemia due to abnormal uterine bleeding. CA-125, a protein released by endometrial and ovarian cancer, can also be measured in the blood indicating metastasis and as a measure to assess response to treatment.[4,18]

Endometrial cancer is most commonly endometrioid adenocarcinoma (70%–80%).[4] Staging of endometrial cancer is based on the International Federation of Gynecology and Obstetrics (FIGO) Surgical Staging, and is described in Box 16.4.[18] Per this guidance, a stage may only be assigned after all tissue samples from surgery have been assessed, as compared to clinical staging which relies only on physical exam, imaging, and biopsy.

Medical Treatment

Endometrial cancer has a 95% 5-year relative survival rate for localized cancer and a combined survival rate of 81%.[18]

• BOX 16.4   Endometrial Cancer Staging

I— Tumor limited to endometrium, cervix, and myometrium
II— Tumor invades supportive connective tissue of the cervix (cervical stroma)
III— Tumor invades serosa or adnexa (tubes, ovaries); vaginal or parametrial metastases; metastases to pelvic/para-aortic lymph nodes
IV— Tumor invades bladder/bowel; distant metastases

Created by Allegra Adams. Printed with permission.

For those medically able to tolerate it, endometrial cancer is primarily treated with surgical removal of the uterus and cervix (total hysterectomy). A hysterectomy can be performed abdominally (total abdominal hysterectomy, TAH) or vaginally. A radical hysterectomy also removes the parametrium, uterosacral ligament, and proximal portion of the vagina. A hysterectomy is most often combined with removal of both fallopian tubes and ovaries (bilateral salpingo-oophorectomy, BSO). Rarely, the ovaries may be preserved if the woman is premenopausal. Occasionally, cancer has spread to the greater omentum and an omenectomy may be required. The parietal peritoneum may also be biopsied. Retroperitoneal pelvic and para-aortic lymph nodes are also removed for staging purposes. Another method of staging includes a peritoneal lavage where the pelvic and abdominal cavities are flooded with saline and the fluid recollected and tested for cancer cells. For advanced cancer, surgical debulking may be required in the abdominal cavity to improve the efficacy of adjuvant chemotherapy or radiation therapy.[4,18]

Depending on the stage of endometrial cancer, adjuvant radiation therapy may be required 4 to 6 weeks after surgery. Occasionally, radiation may be performed prior to surgery to shrink the tumor or as the main treatment for women who are not medically able to tolerate surgery. Radiation therapy may be provided by external beam, brachytherapy, or a combination. External beam radiation may include the vaginal vault, whole pelvis, or whole abdomen. Vaginal brachytherapy is performed to treat the proximal end of the vagina after the uterus and cervix have been removed.[4,18]

Chemotherapy is used to treat metastatic or recurrent endometrial cancer. The most common chemotherapy combination regimens are carboplatin (Paraplatin) with paclitaxel (Taxol) or cisplatin (Platinol) with doxorubicin (Adriamycin). Chemotherapy may be administered before and after radiation (sandwich therapy) or in combination with radiation (chemoradiation). Chemoradiation is more effective in treating the cancer but has greater adverse effects.[4,18]

Hormone therapy is often used in conjunction with chemotherapy for metastatic or recurrent cancer. Hormone therapy may include: progestins, tamoxifen (Nolvadex), LHRH agonists, and aromatase inhibitors (AIs). Progestins are the main hormone used in slowing the growth of endometrial cancer, particularly for women who wish to preserve fertility. Some women with endometrial hyperplasia or early endometrial cancers can be treated with an IUD that contains a progestin. Progesterone is often better tolerated when alternated with tamoxifen, an anti-estrogen. LHRH agonists, given as an injection every one to three months, block the ovaries from producing estrogen in premenopausal women in whom the ovaries have been preserved. AIs work to block estrogen production from adipose tissue.[4,18]

Targeted therapies for endometrial cancer are emerging. They exist as clinical trials or for high-risk, advanced, or recurrent cases. They are likely combined with chemotherapy after a failed trial of another drug regimen. Targeted therapies aim to block angiogenesis or mitosis.[18]

Immunotherapy options are also being developed for metastatic or recurrent cancer, particularly for cancer cells with specific genetic mutations.[18]

Genitourinary and Gynecological Adverse Effects of Endometrial Cancer and Its Treatment

According to a systematic review, prevalence of UI after treatment for uterine cancer is 2% to 44% and dyspareunia is 7% to 39%.[21]

Surgery and radiation therapy can cause direct tissue damage to adjacent organs or temporary or permanent nerve and blood vessel injury to the pelvic organs and muscles. Following a radical hysterectomy, a catheter will be in place until the bladder and nerve supply heal. Chemotherapy can also cause neuropathy and resultant somatic or autonomic dysfunction of the pelvic muscles and organs, respectively.[4] Chemotherapy, targeted therapy, and immunotherapy can all potentially cause permanent kidney damage, though mostly transient bladder irritation is experienced.[4,18]

Simple or radical hysterectomy will obviously result in inability to become pregnant. If the uterus and ovaries are not removed, they may be permanently damaged from radiation therapy or hormonal therapy may induce temporary, potentially reversible, infertility by blocking estrogen and the ovaries.[18] Surgical removal of the ovaries, radiation or chemotherapy damage to the ovaries, and hormonal therapy will all result in medically-induced menopause in premenopausal women accompanied by Genitourinary Syndrome of Menopause (GSM, discussed in Chapter 12), along with osteoporosis and an increased risk of heart disease that accompanies menopause.[18] Radiation therapy creates permanent fibrosis to the vagina, bladder, and rectum resulting in discomfort, bleeding, and urinary or rectal urgency and frequency.[22] See Chapter 12 for a full discussion of pelvic radiation disease. Vaginal shortening from surgery, fibrosis from radiation, and dryness from any cause of menopause may all contribute to dyspareunia. Chemotherapy, radiation, or hormonal therapy may all decrease libido, sensitivity, or the ability to reach orgasm.[18] Surgery to remove lymph nodes and radiation therapy that damages lymph nodes increases the risk of developing genital or lower limb lymphedema (LLL).[18] The incidence of LLL for PLWBCs of the endometrium can be up to 47%.[23] The adverse effects of surgery are compounded by radiation and the adverse effects of radiation are worsened with concurrent chemotherapy.[18]

Ovarian Cancer

Ovarian cancer is the second most common form of gynecological cancer in women but the leading cause of death from gynecological cancers due to it generally being asymptomatic until more advanced stages. It is the fifth leading cause of death from cancer among women. Epithelial ovarian cancer is the most common, representing 85% to 90% of malignant ovarian cancers,[24] and the information provided below is primarily in regards to this form. Emerging evidence suggests, however, that some ovarian cancers actually originate in the distal fallopian tubes.[24] The following information is summarized in Table 16.5.

Risk Factors

Ovarian cancer mostly occurs in postmenopausal women between the ages of 50 and 75 years, however, several forms may arise in young girls or young adults. It is more common in Caucasian women. Similar to endometrial cancer, lifetime estrogen exposure plays an important role and women who are nulliparous or low parity (less than two), had their first child after the age of 35 years old, had infertility or required assisted reproductive technologies, had early menarche or late menopause, or had prolonged (more than 10 years) postmenopausal estrogen HRT are at a greater risk. Obesity is also a risk due to estrogen production by adipose tissue. Personal or family history of endometriosis or breast, endometrial, or colorectal cancer increases a woman's risk of developing ovarian cancer. Family history of ovarian cancer increases a woman's risk

TABLE 16.5   Ovarian Cancer

Risk Factors	Signs and Symptoms	Screening And Diagnosis	Treatment	Adverse Effects
Postmenopausal, 50–75 yo Caucasian race Increased exposure to estrogen • Nulliparity, parity <2 • First child after 35 yo • Infertility, assisted reproductive technologies • Early menarche, late menopause • Postmenopausal estrogen therapy (HRT) >10 years • Obesity Personal or family history of endometriosis or breast, endometrial, or colorectal cancer Family history of ovarian cancer *BRCA* 1 or 2 gene Environmental exposure to cosmetic talc, asbestos Protective: Pregnancy, breastfeeding Birth control • Oral hormonal contraception • IUD • Tubal ligation • Hysterectomy	Bloating, indigestion, early satiety Pelvic or abdominal pain Urinary urgency, frequency AUB Dyspareunia Changes in bowel habits Back pain Pain referred to area of kidneys Abdominal distension combined with weight loss Paraneoplastic syndrome • Polyarthritis • Carpal tunnel • Myopathy • Plantar, palmar fasciitis	No screening tests Genetic predisposition • Annual pelvic exams • Transvaginal ultrasound (TVUS) • Blood test for CA-125 • Prophylactic oophorectomy TVUS Laparoscopic biopsy CT/PET scan, MRI, chest X-ray Barium enema X-ray, colonoscopy Blood tests • CBC • CA-125 • HCG • AFP • LDH	Surgery • Hysterectomy • BSO • Omenectomy • Pelvic and para-aortic lymph node sampling Chemotherapy • Platinum compound + taxane Hormonal therapy • LHRH agonists • Tamoxifen • AIs	See Endometrial cancer

AFP, alpha-fetoprotein; *AIs*, aromatase inhibitors; *AUB*, abnormal uterine bleeding; *BSO*, bilateral salpingo-oophorectomy; *CBC*, complete blood count; *CT*, computed tomography; *HCG*, human chorionic gonadotropin; *IUD*, intrauterine device; *LDH*, lactate dehydrogenase; *LHRH*, luteinizing hormone-releasing hormone; *PET*, positron emission tomography; *MRI*, magnetic resonance imaging; *yo*, years old. Created by Allegra Adams. Printed with permission.

by three to fivefold. Women who are carriers of the *BRCA* 1 or 2 gene(s) comprise 8% to 13% of cases. Environmental exposure to cosmetic talc or asbestos is also a risk factor.[3,4,24]

Factors that reduce the risk of developing ovarian cancer include pregnancy and breastfeeding, particularly before the age of 26; birth control including use of oral hormonal contraception, IUD, or tubal ligation; and hysterectomy, even without removal of the ovaries.[3,4,24]

Signs and Symptoms

The symptoms of epithelial ovarian cancer are often nondescript and not specific to the ovaries themselves. In a study by Goff et al., 72% of women reported having symptoms for 3 months before detection and 35% reported symptoms for more than 6 months.[25,26] Bloating, indigestion, pelvic or abdominal pain, early satiety, and urinary urgency or frequency are some of the early signs of ovarian cancer. Similar to endometrial cancer, abnormal uterine bleeding (between menstrual cycles, menstrual irregularity, or postmenopausal bleeding) or dyspareunia may also indicate ovarian cancer. More advanced disease may present with changes in bowel habits, particularly constipation, as well as back pain, pain referred to the area of the kidneys, or abdominal distension combined with weight loss (indicative of ascites).[3,4,24–26]

Rarely, reproductive carcinomas present with paraneoplastic syndrome with symptoms of polyarthritis, carpal tunnel, myopathy, plantar fasciitis, and/or palmar fasciitis. These cancers may therefore be misdiagnosed as complex regional pain syndrome, Dupuytren's contracture, or as a rheumatologic disorder.[3] Paraneoplastic syndrome is when a cluster of symptoms arises in response to substances produced by the tumor itself or by the body in response to the tumor being present. These symptoms may present as autoimmune, endocrine, electrolyte imbalance, or neurological (paraneoplastic neurological syndrome is discussed in Chapter 8).[3,4]

Less common cancers, including primary peritoneal carcinoma (PPC) and fallopian tube cancer, have a similar presentation to ovarian cancer and look similar during surgery and under the microscope. PPC may occur in women who have prophylactically had their ovaries removed. Both are treated similarly; PPC has similar outcomes to ovarian cancer while fallopian tube cancer has a slightly better prognosis.[3,24]

Diagnosis and Staging

There are no standard screening tests for ovarian cancer and it is often hard to detect in the early stages. Women with a genetic predisposition may be offered active surveillance which can include annual pelvic exams, transvaginal ultrasound (TVUS), and a

---

• BOX 16.5   Ovarian Cancer Staging

I— Tumor limited to ovaries or fallopian tubes
II— Tumor involving one or both ovaries with pelvic extension of disease
III— Tumor involving one or both ovaries with peritoneal implants outside the pelvis and/or positive retroperitoneal or inguinal nodes; superficial liver metastases
IV— Tumor involving one or both ovaries with distant metastases

Created by Allegra Adams. Printed with permission.

---

blood test for the CA-125 protein. However, there is no evidence to support that these tests improve outcomes.[24,26] A prophylactic oophorectomy may be recommended, depending on risk factors. Women who are diagnosed with ovarian cancer, even without family history, may be referred for genetic counseling to check for other mutations.[4,24,26]

For any history or symptoms indicating ovarian pathology, a TVUS will be performed first. This test detects cysts and masses, including those which are benign. A CT scan is not good at visualizing localized disease but can show larger masses and assess for metastasis. A barium enema radiograph or colonoscopy can detect metastasis to the colon or rectum. An MRI may be useful in detecting metastasis to the central nervous system. A chest radiograph will detect metastasis to the lungs. A PET scan may also be used to look for metastasis. A laparoscopy can be used to obtain a biopsy for those who may not medically be able to withstand surgery or to plan for a more complex surgery. Similar to endometrial cancer, blood tests including complete blood count, CA-125, HCG, AFP, and LDH may be completed.[4,24]

Staging of ovarian cancer is also based on the FIGO Surgical Staging, as described in Box 16.5.[24]

Medical Treatment

The 5-year relative survival rate for localized epithelial ovarian cancer is 92% with a combined 5-year survival rate of 47%.[24] Surgery is the standard treatment for ovarian cancer. Surgery is performed both for curative purposes and to stage the cancer to determine need for further treatment. Surgery includes hysterectomy and BSO, omenectomy, peritoneal washings, and bilateral pelvic and para-aortic lymph node sampling. The goal is to remove any visible tumor in the pelvic or abdominal cavity greater than one centimeter, which may include the peritoneum or any other affected organ. Young, low-risk patients wishing to preserve fertility may be able to have a unilateral salpingo-oophorectomy with uterine preservation to later be removed after childbearing, though this may not always be possible and carries high risk of disease progression.[4,24]

Chemotherapy for ovarian cancer may be systemic or intraperitoneal. It is usually a combination of a platinum compound and a taxane. Intraperitoneal chemotherapy is more concentrated and has more severe adverse effects. Chemotherapy is used more for higher stage, metastatic epithelial ovarian tumors than for stromal or germ cell tumors. Targeted therapy may be given in combination with or after chemotherapy to block angiogenesis and slow tumor growth or to block DNA repair within the tumor. Targeted therapy is mostly used in women with a *BRCA* mutation.[4,24]

Hormonal therapy is rarely used to treat epithelial ovarian tumors and more commonly used in ovarian stromal tumors. It includes LHRH agonists to turn off estrogen production by the ovaries, tamoxifen which acts as an anti-estrogen in the tissues, and AIs to lower estrogen levels in women after menopause.[24]

Radiation therapy is rarely used for ovarian cancers.[24]

Genitourinary and Gynecological Adverse Effects of Ovarian Cancer and Its Treatment

The adverse effects of surgery, chemotherapy, and hormonal therapy for ovarian cancer are mainly the same as those for endometrial cancer.[24] The prevalence of stress UI is 32% to 42%, urgency UI 15% to 39%, prolapse 17%, and sexual dysfunction 62% to 75%.[21] Given the greater peritoneal and omentum involvement, and the usual higher stage at which cancer is detected, the risk of lymphedema and gastrointestinal effects are higher with ovarian cancer treatment. The incidence of LLL reported following treatment for ovarian cancer is up to 41%.[23]

Cervical Cancer

Cervical cancer develops in the cervix, which is the distal part of the uterus connecting to the proximal vagina. It is perhaps one of the most screened for cancers, detected most often in the precancerous stages, and preventable by vaccine. Previously, however, cervical cancer was the leading cause of cancer-related death among women in the US and remains the leading cause of death from gynecological cancer worldwide.[27] The following information is summarized in Table 16.6.

Risk Factors

Cervical cancer is almost always caused by the human papilloma virus (HPV). Therefore, certain sexual behaviors and history that increase exposure to HPV are the primary risk factors for developing cervical cancer. Women who had an early age of first sexual intercourse (including childhood sexual abuse), multiple sex partners, unprotected sexual intercourse, and intimate partner abuse increases a woman's risk of developing cervical cancer. Specifically, a history of abuse is associated with greater risk of exposure to any sexually transmitted infection (STI) and often these women avoid or are prevented from routine gynecological care. Other correlates with cervical cancer, though not necessarily causative, include early age at first pregnancy, multiparity (greater number of pregnancies), history of any STI, and long-term oral contraceptive use. Multiparity suggests a greater number of sexual encounters increasing exposure to HPV. Hormonal changes and/or immunosuppression as a natural part of pregnancy may also increase a woman's susceptibility to HPV infection. Some studies suggest that chlamydia may promote HPV growth on the cervix. All-cause immunosuppression, including tobacco use and second-hand smoke, reduces the body's natural ability to fight precancerous changes as a result of HPV exposure allowing the infection to progress to cervical cancer. The carcinogens from smoking may also directly cause changes in the DNA of cervical tissues. Cervical cancer is more common in Hispanic women and those of low socioeconomic status with less access to routine gynecological screening. There is also a slightly greater risk among women whose mothers used the drug diethylstilbestrol (DES) during early pregnancy to prevent miscarriage (between 1938 and 1971).[3,4,27]

The HPV vaccine, either Cervarix or Gardasil, is preventative against developing cervical cancer. There is also emerging evidence to suggest that an IUD for contraception may be protective.[27]

TABLE 16.6 Cervical Cancer

Risk Factors	Signs and Symptoms	Screening And Diagnosis	Treatment	Adverse Effects
Human papilloma virus (HPV) Risky sexual behaviors • Early age of first sexual intercourse • Multiple sex partners • Childhood sexual abuse • Intimate partner abuse • Early age at first pregnancy • Multi-parity • History of any STI • Long-term oral contraception use Tobacco use, second hand smoke Hispanic ethnicity Low socioeconomic status Women whose mothers used the drug diethylstilbestrol (DES) (1938–1971) Protective: • HPV vaccine Cervarix, Gardasil • IUD	Dyspareunia General pelvic pain AUB Postcoital bleeding Unusual, foul smelling vaginal discharge that may be blood tinged Lower extremity edema Bladder, bowel changes Hematuria	Screening 25–65 yo • HPV test alone or with Papanicolaou (Pap) test every 5 years • OR Pap smear alone every 3 years Colposcopy Endocervical curettage Cone biopsy (conization) • Loop electrosurgical excision procedure (LEEP) • Cold knife cone biopsy Cystoscopy, proctoscopy, chest X-ray, CT/PET scan, MRI, IVP	Surgery • Biopsy • Cryosurgery • Laser surgery • Conization • Hysterectomy • Trachelectomy • Pelvic and para-aortic lymph node sampling • Pelvic exenteration with neobladder, abdominal stoma, colostomy or J-pouch, and neovagina Radiation therapy • External beam • Brachytherapy Chemotherapy • Cisplatin • Carboplatin • Paclitaxel • Topotecan Targeted therapy	Surgical pain Dyspareunia Vaginal shortening Pelvic radiation disease Bladder, bowel dysfunction Pelvic muscle over-activity Infertility Menopause, GSM Neuropathy Nephrotoxicity

AUB, abnormal uterine bleeding; *CT*, computed tomography; *GSM*, genitourinary syndrome of menopause; *HPV*, human papilloma virus; *IVP*, intravenous pyelogram; *IUD*, intrauterine device; *MRI*, magnetic resonance imaging; *PET*, positron emission tomography; *STI*, sexually-transmitted infection.
Created by Allegra Adams. Printed with permission.

Signs and Symptoms

Precancerous cervical dysplasia and early cervical cancer are often asymptomatic. As the cancer spreads to adjacent tissues, a woman may experience dyspareunia or general pelvic pain; abnormal vaginal bleeding including during or after intercourse or between menstrual cycles, postmenopausal bleeding, or heavier menstrual bleeding; and/or unusual and foul smelling vaginal discharge that may be blood tinged.[3,4,27] More advanced disease may present with lower extremity edema, bladder and bowel changes, or blood in the urine.[3,4,27]

Diagnosis and Staging

There are two screening tests for cervical cancer, the Papanicolaou (Pap) smear and the HPV test, which can be performed simultaneously. The ACS recommends that screening begin at age 25. The HPV test should be performed alone or with a Pap test every 5 years or the Pap test alone every 3 years until age 65. Screening should continue even in women who have had a supra-cervical hysterectomy, as the cervix is still present. Screening tests increase the odds that disease can be discovered in the precancerous or early stages of cancer and improve the prognosis.[4,27]

The screening tests look for abnormal cellular changes that warrant advanced testing and are not diagnostic. The next level of testing after screening is a colposcopy to directly look at the cervix and is usually accompanied by a biopsy. Occasionally a biopsy is able to remove all abnormal tissue and is the only treatment needed.[4,27]

If abnormal cells cannot be seen or biopsied during a colposcopy, endocervical curettage, or scraping, will be performed to sample cells closer to the uterus as compared to the superficial cells near the vagina.[27]

A cone biopsy (conization) may be required to obtain both superficial and deep cells of the cervix. This procedure may be enough to remove abnormal precancerous or early cancerous cells. Different approaches to conization include a loop electrosurgical excision procedure (LEEP) or cold knife cone biopsy.[4,27]

For confirmed and advanced cancers, additional testing is required to determine metastasis including: cystoscopy, proctoscopy, chest radiograph, CT scan, MRI, PET scan, and/or IVP.[4,27]

Ninety percent of cervical cancer is squamous cell carcinoma. Staging of cervical cancer is also based on the FIGO Surgical Staging, as described in Box 16.6.[27]

Medical Treatment

The 5-year relative survival rate for localized cervical cancer, as of 2015, was 92% with a combined survival rate of 66%.[27] The ACS anticipates that the current survival rate is much higher.[27]

• BOX 16.6   Cervical Cancer Staging

0— Precancerous, carcinoma in situ (CIS)
I— Tumor confined to the cervix
II— Tumor extends beyond the cervix and uterus but not onto the pelvic side wall
III— Tumor extends onto the pelvic side wall, lower third of vagina, blocks ureters causing hydronephrosis
IV— Tumor involves the mucosa of the bladder or rectum, metastasis to lung or bone

Created by Allegra Adams. Printed with permission.

Precancerous lesions may be resolved through ablation with cryosurgery or laser surgery or removed with conization. For more advanced cervical cancer, a simple or radical hysterectomy may be performed, though the ovaries are usually not removed. In some cases, a trachelectomy may be possible in which the cervix and proximal vagina are removed but the uterus remains intact to maintain fertility. Pelvic and/or para-aortic lymph nodes are also sampled during surgery. In rare cases of recurrent cervical cancer, pelvic exenteration surgery is required, removing all involved pelvic organs and replacing them with a neobladder from the intestines with an abdominal stoma, a colostomy or J-pouch (see Chapter 17 for more details regarding colostomy), and creation of a neovagina from graft tissue.[4,27]

Radiation therapy may be the primary treatment for some cases of cervical cancer, or it may be performed following surgery. Radiation will generally be external beam but may be followed by brachytherapy. If external beam radiation is the primary treatment, it is most commonly combined with the chemotherapeutic agent cisplatin (Platinol). Other forms of chemotherapy used for metastatic or recurrent cervical cancer are carboplatin (Paraplatin), paclitaxel (Taxol), and topotecan (Hycamtin). Targeted therapy with an angiogenesis inhibitor may be used with chemotherapy; if effective, the chemotherapy may be discontinued and the PWC will continue only with the targeted therapy. Immune checkpoint inhibitors are being developed for use in women diagnosed with cervical cancer and may be used after chemotherapy for metastatic or recurrent disease.[4,27]

Genitourinary and Gynecological Adverse Effects of Cervical Cancer and Its Treatment

The adverse effects from surgery, radiation, and chemotherapy for cervical cancer are mostly the same as those for other gynecological cancers including: surgical pain, dyspareunia, vaginal shortening, pelvic radiation disease, bladder and bowel dysfunction, pelvic muscle overactivity, infertility, menopause and GSM, and neuropathy.[22,27–29] Rates of stress UI are as high as 76% post treatment; urge UI up to 59%; urinary retention up to 39%; dyspareunia up to 58%; and vaginal dryness up to 47%.[21] LLL is reported in up to 56% of PLWBCs of the cervix.[23] Cisplatin (Platinol) may also cause nephrotoxicity. Smoking exacerbates the adverse effects of radiation and can make treatment less effective. The adverse effects of radiation are also made worse by concurrent chemotherapy.[27]

Other Genitourinary and Gynecological Cancers

Some less common cancers of the GU/GYN systems include: renal, urethral, penile, vulvar, vaginal, and fallopian tube.

Psychosocial Issues in Genitourinary and Gynecological Cancers

In addition to the usual psychosocial issues PLWBCs experience, people with cancer of the genital and gynecological organs face unique challenges. Treatments for cancers of these systems often involve removing the most fundamental part of a person's sense of self. In addition to the fear of death, treatment, and recurrence, compounded with financial strains, depression, and anxiety, a person may be left questioning their very identity. The sexual dysfunction and infertility pose a sometimes insurmountable trial to personal relationships. The bladder and bowel dysfunction is perhaps more embarrassing and isolating than any other cancer-related adverse effect. One study found that of women up to 8 years post-gynecological cancer, 10% had diagnostically-indicated definite or probable depression, 20% post-traumatic stress disorder, and 29% anxiety.[30]

Sexual dysfunction after endometrial cancer is reported in up to 90% of PLWBCs and postprostatectomy is 85%.[12,31] Sexual dysfunction is close to 60% among PLWBCs of the anorectum and 45% for PLWBCs of the breast.[32,33] Sexual dysfunction is multidimensional. Anatomical and physiological changes to the genitalia are evident, however, psychological and social factors are also at play including: decreased libido, alterations in body image, anxiety related to sexual performance, difficulty maintaining previous sexual roles, emotional distancing from the partner, and perceived change in the partner's level of sexual interest.[34] It is worth noting that bladder and bowel dysfunction may be a significant contributing factor in the avoidance of sexual activity.

The LGBTQIA+ Experience With Cancer

The lesbian, gay, bisexual, transgender, transitioning, queer, questioning, intersex, asexual, agender (LGBTQIA+) community has many barriers to health care coverage and accessibility in general, and can face discrimination within the healthcare system leading 30% of LGBTQIA+ adults to not seek regular healthcare services. This is particularly problematic considering that the LGBTQIA+ community is disproportionately affected by anal, breast, cervical, colorectal, endometrial, lung, and prostate cancers.[35] Non-GU/GYN cancers will be addressed in their respective chapters.

Heterosexual women have significantly lower rates of cervical cancer than lesbian or bisexual women. This is primarily due to higher rates of HPV transmission and lower rates of HPV vaccination among lesbian and bisexual women.[35] Lesbian women report both more overall sexual partners and higher rates of sexual intercourse before the age of 18. An average of 77% of lesbian women have had sex with men in the past.[36] Lesbian and bisexual women also have higher use rates of tobacco and alcohol, nulliparity, lower use of hormonal contraceptives, obesity, and high-fat diet consumption.[37] Nonetheless, the risk of cervical cancer among lesbian women is under-recognized by both the women themselves and providers due to a perceived lack of exposure to HPV. Lesbian women are screened 5% to 18% less than heterosexual women for cervical cancer.[36] In a study of oncology providers by Tamargo et al., just over half of respondents knew that HPV-related cervical dysplasia could be found among women who have only ever exclusively had sex with women.[38]

Considering the transgender community, a male (sex assigned at birth) whose gender identity is female may not acknowledge, and may not be screened for, prostate cancer. Even with gender affirmation surgery, including orchiectomy and penile-inversion neovagina formation, the prostate is not removed and the woman remains at risk of developing prostate cancer. Though female-to-male affirmation surgery is less common, the man remains at risk for breast, cervical, endometrial, and ovarian cancers and will require proper screening according to the standard screening recommendations and differential diagnosis.[37]

For PLWBCs within the LGBTQIA+ community, the usual psychosocial adverse effects of cancer and its treatment are often magnified due to preexisting higher rates of anxiety, depression, suicidal ideation and attempts; history of stressful life circumstances and events; history of being a target of harassment, violence, and discrimination; likely estrangement from family; and they are less likely to have adult children to care for them.[39] This in addition to the aforementioned likelihood that persons in the LGBTQIA+ community have lower use of healthcare services due to access and real or perceived system discrimination often resulting in a cancer diagnosis at more advanced stages; therefore, an overall worse prognosis with use of more invasive or extensive cancer treatments and a greater chance of developing adverse physical effects exists.[39] Many members of the LGBTQIA+ population note poorer cancer outcomes and decreased satisfaction with care, particularly in regards to GU/GYN cancers.[38]

Six themes have been developed that represent the responses from the LGBTQIA+ community regarding their experiences with their overall cancer care including: issues related to disclosure, homophobia, healthcare provider behavior, heterocentric care, support groups, and unmet needs.[39] Several studies have gauged the knowledge and attitudes of oncologists regarding the specific care needs of the LGBTQIA+ community which have revealed severe knowledge gaps but an overall positivity toward both treating this population and receiving specialized education and training specific to the health issues of this population.[38,40] Seventy-two percent of providers admit that they assume a person seeking cancer care is heterosexual upon first encounter. Additionally, only 40% to 58% of providers thought that it was necessary to know the person's sexual orientation and only 28% to 66% of providers felt that that gender identity was relevant. The most common provider response was that they treat all patients equally and therefore did not see that knowledge of the person's gender identity or sexual orientation would impact their decision making model,[38,40] despite the inequities and greater risk factors this minority population faces.

Patient Management Model

For many of the GU/GYN adverse effects of cancer treatment, pelvic floor physical therapy (PFPT) can reduce or resolve their impact.[41–45] For cancers of the GU/GYN systems, the medical care team is more aware of the consequences these cancers and their treatments may have on urological and sexual function. Some providers may include pretreatment education, employ more preventative measures during care, or initiate rehabilitation in office or a PFPT referral sooner, thereby optimizing outcomes in all cases. Unfortunately, for non-GU/GYN cancers, the effects on urinary and sexual function are often overlooked or attributed to other factors unrelated to the cancer and its treatment. These PLWBCs often go years without adequately addressing these complaints. If or when they are recognized, their care is directed by a general urologist, gynecologist, or physiatrist rather than their oncology team or even primary care physician.

Examination

The PFPT examination includes many elements of a traditional rehabilitation examination including history, systems review, and orthopedic screening with the addition of a pelvic examination. Figure 16.1 summarizes the adverse effects of GU/GYN cancers and their treatments to keep in mind while proceeding through the examination process.

History

The subjective history needs to establish what the PLWBC's baseline urological and sexual function was, including any preexisting dysfunction. Other preexisting medical conditions or surgical procedures—especially those in the pelvis, abdomen, or spine—will help guide treatment planning and influence prognosis. Next, it is important to understand the diagnostic and cancer treatment course including biopsies, surgical approach, excisions, and margins; radiation type, field, and dosage; specific chemotherapeutic agents received; targeted or immunotherapies; and any hormonal treatments received or currently taking.

The pain screening will generally focus on the areas of the abdomen, suprapubic or "bladder," "ovaries," groin, upper thighs, mid to low back, sacrum, coccyx, sacroiliac or buttock, and pelvis (including perineum, vulva, vagina, anus, rectum, testicles/scrotum, and penis). In addition to the typical questions regarding intensity, range, descriptors, and aggravating and alleviating factors, specific attention is given to pain with bladder filling or emptying (voiding) and defecation. For females, assess for any pain with external sexual stimulation, initial entry at the vaginal opening (introitus), and full penetration (including finger, speculum, menstrual products, or penis). For males, assess for any pain with external sexual stimulation, anal penetration, erection, and ejaculation. Questioning should also include arousal levels or libido, genital sensation, ability to reach orgasm, and erectile tissue function. Box 16.7 outlines questions to evaluate urological function. Imaging tests, like a bladder scan or others described in Chapter 12, are important to review.

• BOX 16.7   Evaluating Urological Function

- How often or how many times do you empty your bladder during the daytime?
- How many times do you empty your bladder at night (followed by return to sleep)?
- How much and what kinds of fluids do you consume each day?
- Are you taking any medications for bladder function or that may influence bladder function (e.g., diuretics)?
- Do you experience any involuntary leakage of urine, with or without your awareness?
- What causes you to leak urine (increases in abdominal pressure, activities, urgency)?
- Does anything cause you to have a sudden urge to empty your bladder that is hard to delay (e.g., "key-in-door")?
- Do you wear pads to contain urine leakage or have to change your clothes due to leakage?
- How heavy of a pad do you use? How many pads do you go through per day? Per night? When you change the pad, how saturated is it?
- When you have to empty your bladder, can you make it to the bathroom in time without leaking on the way?
- Do you have difficulty starting the flow of urine? How strong is your stream? Is it continuous or interrupted?
- Do you feel that you empty your bladder completely?

Created by Allegra Adams. Printed with permission.

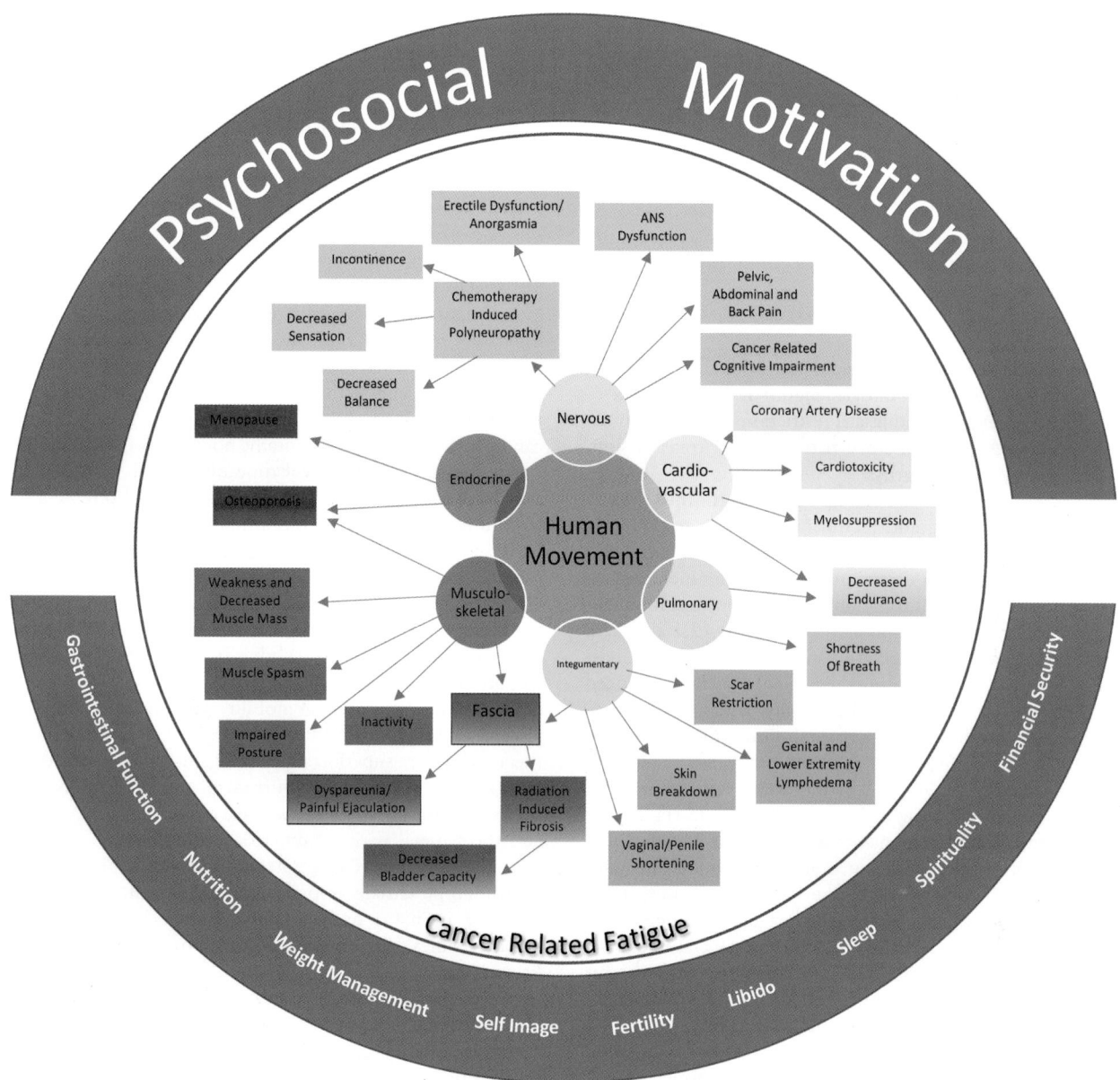

• **Fig. 16.1** Human Movement Model. (Modified and reprinted with permission from the American Physical Therapy Association. Created by Allegra Adams.)

Systems Review

While the gross and pelvic examinations will more specifically measure deficits in the integumentary, musculoskeletal, neuromuscular, and sensory systems, it is good practice to screen for any cardiopulmonary impairments including preexisting conditions, risk factors, and chemotherapeutic or hormonal therapies that influence the heart and lungs. The lungs are also a common site of metastasis and any changes at rest or with exertion should be monitored. Surgery and radiation for breast or lung cancer may also cause fibrotic and restrictive changes in the thorax as will surgeries in the upper abdomen under the diaphragm. Diaphragmatic function is essential for pelvic floor muscle (PFM) function and will need to be assessed. Refer to Chapter 10 for a full discussion on cardiopulmonary adverse effects of cancer treatment. It is also important to be cognizant of the possibility of myelosuppression from chemotherapy and radiation taking into account anemia, clotting, and risk of infection. Chemotherapy, radiation

therapy, and hormonal therapy may also place the PLWBC at risk for osteoporosis, thus be aware of any bone mineral density tests that have been performed.

A person's cognitive level of function, education, behavioral responses, learning style, and ability to communicate to provide a history, give feedback, or to follow instructions, including likelihood to be compliant with a home exercise program, are important considerations for developing a plan of care and setting the prognosis. These factors all have the potential to be influenced by adverse reactions to cancer treatment, such as chemotherapy-induced cognitive impairment (CICI) or a stroke.

Including questions regarding the PLWBC's living situation and home environment will provide insight into social support or potential barriers such as transportation or care for dependents that could impact compliance. It may also help to define goals, for instance if the PLWBC experiences leakage or pain while negotiating stairs or caring for their children. Understanding the PLWBC's vocational, educational, or recreation and leisure expectations and limitations due to symptoms will also help to direct the plan of care and establish goals.

Gross Examination

The physical examination for PFPT starts much the same as an orthopedic physical therapy examination. What makes the pelvis so unique is both that it is the interchange of all the forces below from the lower extremities during locomotion and above from the torso in addition to the multitude of roles it must play simultaneously. The PFMs are responsible for the "4 S's": visceral *Support*, lumbopelvic *Stability*, bladder and bowel *Storage* (or *sphincteric*), and *Sexual* function.

Neuromuscular assessments of gait, transitional movements, and balance give indicators of muscle length-strength imbalances, core muscle weakness, scar and fascial restrictions, deficits in muscle firing sequences, compensatory patterns, load transmission, and overall neurological integrity.

Similarly, a person's posture can also give insight into muscle imbalances as PFM firing and recruitment vary in response to posture. As the PFM attach to the innominates, sacrum, and coccyx, it is important to assess and correct alignment asymmetries. Spinal alignment throughout is also important for autonomic neurological function and pain (see Figures 12.1 and 12.2 to review spinal levels of innervation relevant to the pelvic viscera and musculature). Posture and alignment may be influenced by lower extremity and axial muscle flexibility which in turn may be influenced by surgical, fascial, visceral, dural tube, neural, or vascular restrictions.

When considering the fascia, it is important to keep in mind the continuous nature throughout the body. The fascia can be described as five chains, per the work of Thomas Myers.[46] The core musculature of the diaphragm, transversus abdominus, and PFM are on the deep front line (Figure 16.2), which traces from the sphenobasilar joint in the skull to the first and fifth metatarsals and navicular in the foot. It also includes the visceral and parietal peritoneum and the pleura, thereby involving all of the body's organs. A head injury, for instance, can cause bladder dysfunction as could ankle pronation, and vice versa. It is not uncommon for persons with pelvic dysfunction to simultaneously suffer from temporomandibular joint dysfunction, bruxism, as well as headaches, migraines, or sinus complaints as these muscles and joints are all along the deep front line.[46]

Lower extremity strength may be assessed by individual muscles, joint movements, or myotomes, as indicated. Assessment of dermatomes and deep tendon reflexes may also be indicated. The pudendal nerve, providing the primary innervation to the pelvic floor muscles, is both a sensory and motor nerve, and is made up from branches of sacral nerves S2-4. If neuropathic changes are affecting the nerves to the lower extremities, it may be an indicator that these more distal segments are also impaired.

Much of the work in treating pelvic floor dysfunction is driven by the abdominal structures. Of the abdominal muscle layers, strength testing of the transversus abdominus is most important as its fibers interdigitate with the PFM and create a synergistic relationship. Abdominal muscle strength influences PFM strength; the abdominals may be used to initiate a PFM contraction using the overflow principle.[47]

Abdominal muscle integrity, considering diastasis rectus abdominus (DRA) or widening of the linea alba, influences intraabdominal force generation for evacuation and dynamic lumbopelvic stability. A DRA may be residual from pregnancy, due to

obesity or diabetes (in both women and men), surgical, or due to visceral restriction of the parietal peritoneum and small intestines.[48,49] There is a fair amount of research that indicates that UI, pelvic organ prolapse, and low back pain are correlated with presence of a DRA[49,50] and that surgical repair improves trunk stability, UI, and quality of life.[51] However, there is conflicting evidence to this correlation.[52-54]

A DRA is easily screened by having the person in hooklying. The therapist palpates at the umbilicus as the person performs a curl up lifting their head and shoulders off the surface. This is repeated at 4 cm above and below the umbilicus. A separation greater than 2 cm (2 finger widths) is clinically significant.[55] Other indicators to consider are the end-feel (tension generated in the linea alba) and whether the gap closes or if bulging of the abdominal contents occurs with exertion. Clinically, the gap between the rectus muscles is measured by the number of fingers the clinician can fit into the space horizontally, however, for research purposes, a tape measure, calipers, real time ultrasound, CT scan, or MRI may be used.[56-58] Figure 16.3 illustrates the anatomy of a DRA.

Scar restrictions, even as seemingly insignificant as laparoscopic incisions including those through the umbilicus, impair core muscle function and place abnormal pressures down on the pelvic viscera and PFM contributing to many pelvic floor dysfunctions including detrusor or PFM overactivity, prolapse, incontinence, and pain.[59,60] Therefore, the abdominal assessment should include palpation for tenderness, measures of strength and DRA, consideration of scar integrity and mobility, and evaluation of fascial and visceral mobility, if the clinician is trained to do so. For instance, the urachus, or superior support ligament of the bladder, runs from the superior-anterior surface of the bladder, between the transverse fascia on the deep surface of the transversus abdominus and the parietal peritoneum, to the umbilicus.[60] Therefore, any midline, horizontal (e.g., cesarean), or laparoscopic umbilical incision could potentially impair bladder function.

There are many reasons a person may have impaired breathing mechanics, not limited to cancer treatment. Breathing may become impaired due to pregnancy, a self-conscious body image response, pain, overuse of accessory muscles in providing dynamic lumbopelvic stability, or scarring or fibrotic changes in the thorax or upper abdomen. Nonetheless, the diaphragm also forms a synergy, or "piston pump," with the PFM and therefore its proper mobility and function are essential to address in treating pelvic floor dysfunction.[61] During inhalation, the diaphragm contracts and descends, the abdominal cavity expands, and the PFM also descend. This is important in treating pelvic pain including fibrosis and scarring, muscle overactivity, and muscle shortening. During exhalation, the diaphragm resumes its domed shape, the abdomen reduces, and the PFM elevate to neutral. This is the natural sequencing to initiate retraining of core muscle firing and PFM recruitment.

Pelvic Examination

It is outside the scope of this text to provide a full training in PFPT. Interested readers are directed to the American Physical Therapy Association Academy of Pelvic Health (aptapelvichealth.org) or Herman and Wallace (hermanwallace.com) for continuing education options for training and certification in general PFPT and oncology rehabilitation (OncR) specific coursework. For the current PFPT, the pelvic examination is likely no different for a PLWBC than would otherwise be performed with the exception of including an assessment for radiation fibrosis. For readers who are not PFPT trained, the following provides an overview of the

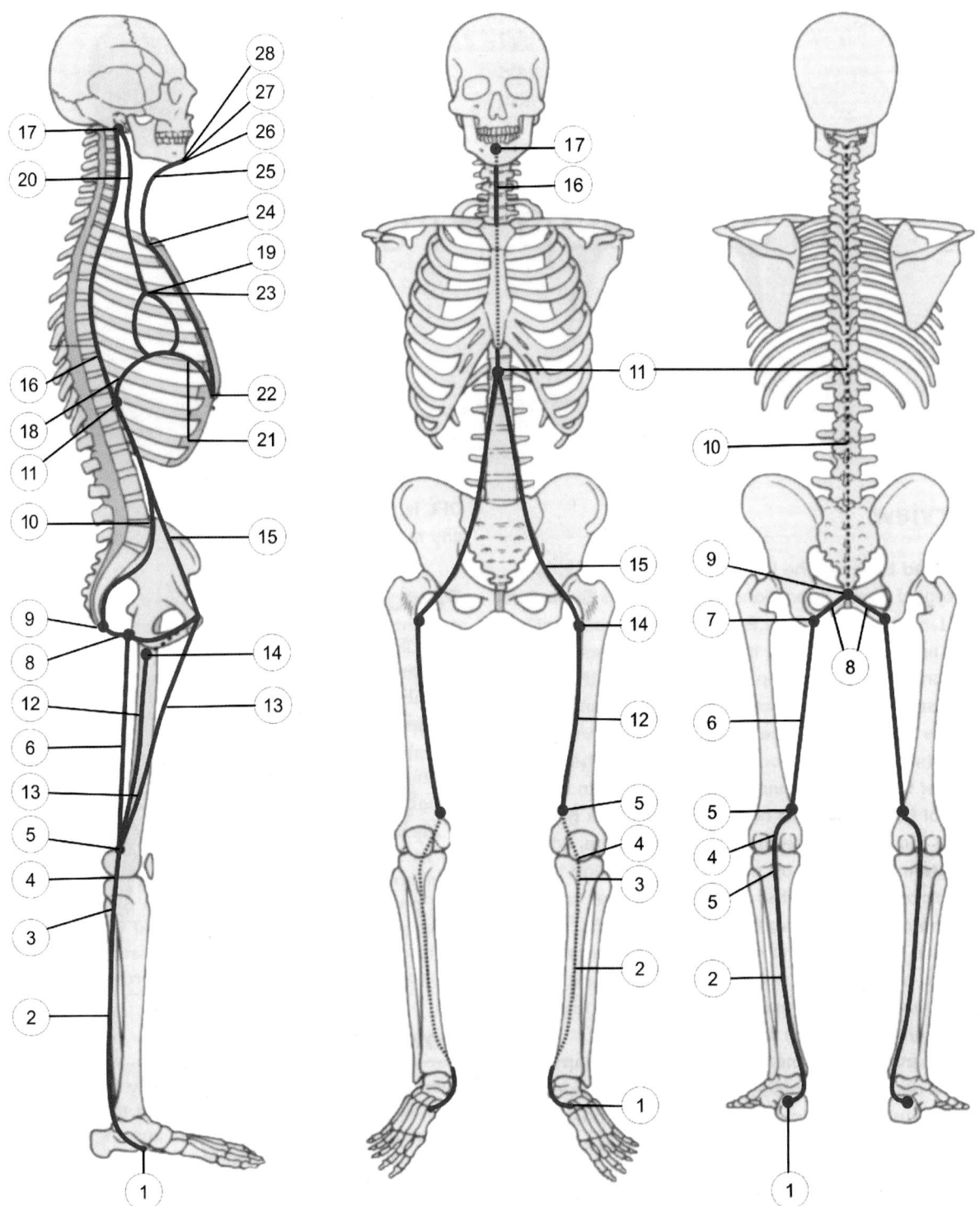

• **Fig. 16.2** Deep Front Fascial Line. (1) Plantar tarsal bones, plantar surface of toes. (2) Tibialis posterior, long toe flexors. (3) Superior/posterior tibia/fibula. (4) Fascia of popliteus, knee capsule. (5) Medial femoral epicondyle. (6) Posterior intermuscular septum, adductor magnus and minimus. (7) Ischial ramus. (8) Pelvic floor muscle and visceral fascia, levator ani, ovbturator internus fascia. (9) Coccyx. (10) Anterior sacral fascia, anterior longitudinal ligament. (11) Lumbar vertebral bodies. (12) Linea aspera of femur. (13) Medial intermuscular septum, adductor brevis/longus. (14) Lesser trochanter of femur. (15) Iliopsoas, pectineus, femoral triangle. (16) Anterior longitudinal ligament, longus coli and capitis. (17) Basilar portion of occiput. (18) Posterior diaphragm, crura of diaphragm, central tendon. (19) Pericardium, mediastinum, parietal pleura. (20) Fascia prevertebralis, pharyngeal raphe, scalene muscles and fascia. (21) Anterior diaphragm. (22) Posterior surface of subcostal, cartilages, xiphoid processes. (23) Fascia endothoracica, transversus thoracis. (24) Posterior manubrium. (25) Infrahyoid muscles, fascia pretrachialis. (26) Hyoid bone. (27) Suprahyoid muscles. (28) Mandible. (Reprinted with permission from Myers TW. *Anatomy Trains: Myofascial Meridians for Manual Therapists and Movement Professionals*. 4th ed. Churchill Livingston/Elsevier; 2020.)

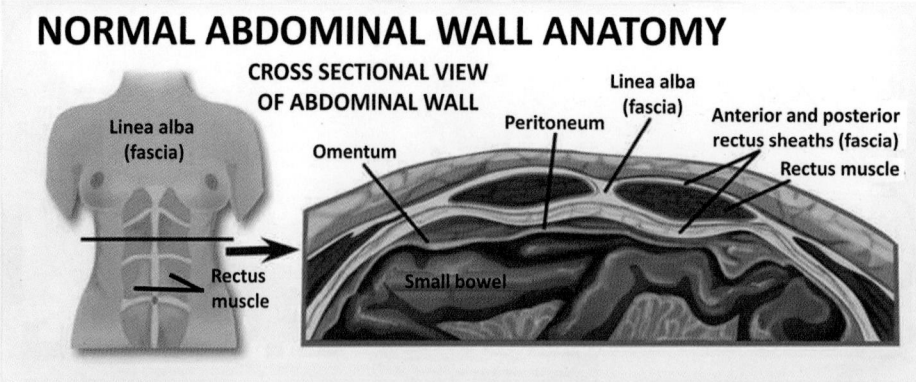

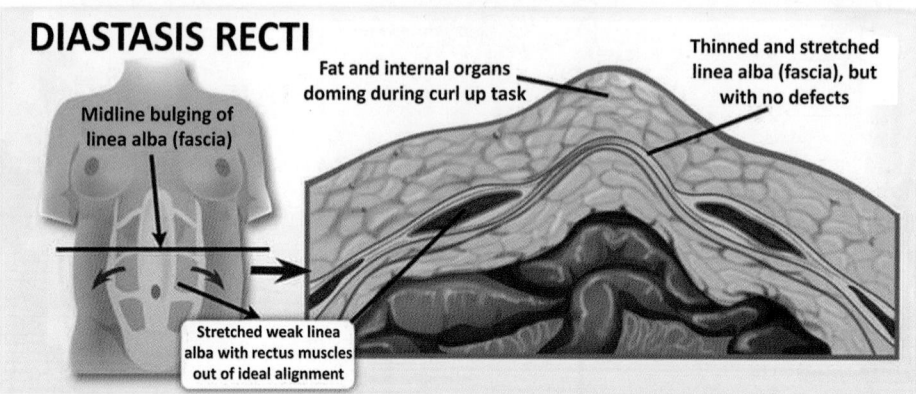

• **Fig. 16.3** Diastasus Rectus Abdominus. (Reprinted with permission from https://www.burrelleducation. com/total-core-re-hab-chichester/diastasis-recti-copyright/.)

pelvic examination in order to gauge persons who may benefit from a referral.

The PFM are divided into three layers.[62,63] The most superficial layer (Figure 16.4) includes both the urogenital and the anorectal triangles. The urogenital triangle consists of the ischiocavernosus, bulbocavernosus (female) or bulbospongiosus (male), and the superficial transverse perineal. These muscles follow the ischiopubic ramus to ischial tuberosities and then horizontally between the tuberosities connecting at the perineal body, or central tendon, the fleshy space between the vagina or base of the penis and the anus. For females, these superficial muscles in the urogenital triangle control clitoral erection and constriction of the introitus during orgasm. For males, they control erection, ejaculation, and emptying the spongy urethra (the distal portion of the urethra within the shaft of the penis). The anorectal triangle consists of the external anal sphincter and the anococcygeal ligament which stabilizes the external anal sphincter between the coccyx and the perineal body.

The intermediate layer is termed the perineal membrane, formerly the urogenital diaphragm, and consists of the deep transverse perineal, compressor urethra, sphincter urethrovaginalis, and the external urethral sphincter, with the latter three lending their function to urinary continence. The deepest, and most familiar, layer of the pelvic diaphragm (Figure 16.5) is the levator ani and ischiococcygeus (coccygeus). The levator ani is formed by: puborectalis, pubococcygeus, and iliococcygeus. The levator ani forms a sling from the pubis and the tendinous arch of the levator ani (along the medial surface of obturator internus) to coccyx. The levator ani contracts in an anterior cranial direction, flexing the coccyx, and providing closure of the pelvic outlet. Together, the piriformis, just superior to coccygeus, and the obturator internus make up the posterior and lateral muscular walls of the pelvis.

Again, visceral anatomy is important to know. For instance, the lateral vesical ligament of the bladder blends with the arcus tendoneus—the junction between the levator ani and the obturator internus—following the same pathway as the pudendal nerve, and then blending with the transverse acetabular ligament.[60] Therefore, intraarticular hip pathology or joint replacement is going to have significant impact on PFM and bladder function.

The pelvic examination begins with a visualization of the perineum, the urogenital, and anorectal triangles. Skin integrity, rashes, erythema, scars, signs of incontinence, and discharge are observed. Involuntary motor and sensory reflex contractions are observed. The external anal sphincter should contract and the perineal body elevate when the person coughs (motor, "cough reflex") and when lightly stimulated around the anus (sensory, usually with the end of a cotton swab, "anal wink").[64,65] For females presenting with the complaints of vulvodynia, mapping of sensitive areas around the introitus with a cotton swab ("Q-tip test") may also be documented as points on a clock, envisioning 12 o'clock at the clitoris and 6 o'clock at the perineal body. Perineal mobility in response to a voluntary concentric contraction (Kegel), voluntary relaxation (release), and bearing down (eccentric elongation, involuntary relaxation) may also be observed showing the PFM excursion range as an indication of muscle tone, strength, and coordination.

Palpation of muscle tone begins externally with the urogenital and anorectal triangles, levator ani, and obturator internus. For females with urinary or sexual complaints, the exam proceeds to palpation of the urogenital triangle layer at the introitus, including any perineal scars, and then finally an internal palpation of levator ani, coccygeus, obturator internus, arcus tendoneus, perineal membrane, and urethra. An intrarectal examination is indicated for males and anyone experiencing coccyx, rectal, or pudendal

A **Male**

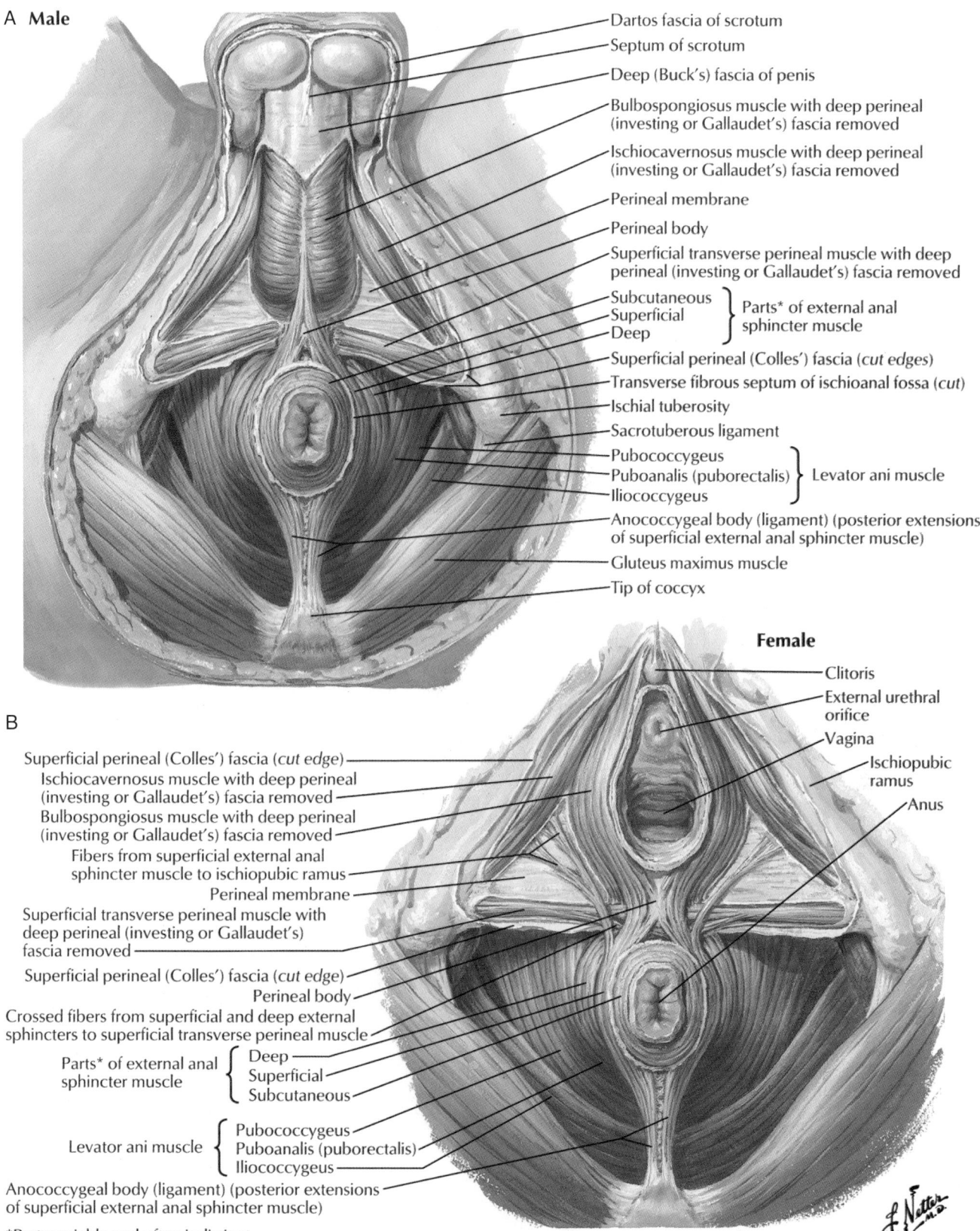

- Dartos fascia of scrotum
- Septum of scrotum
- Deep (Buck's) fascia of penis
- Bulbospongiosus muscle with deep perineal (investing or Gallaudet's) fascia removed
- Ischiocavernosus muscle with deep perineal (investing or Gallaudet's) fascia removed
- Perineal membrane
- Perineal body
- Superficial transverse perineal muscle with deep perineal (investing or Gallaudet's) fascia removed
- Subcutaneous
- Superficial   Parts* of external anal
- Deep   sphincter muscle
- Superficial perineal (Colles') fascia (*cut edges*)
- Transverse fibrous septum of ischioanal fossa (*cut*)
- Ischial tuberosity
- Sacrotuberous ligament
- Pubococcygeus
- Puboanalis (puborectalis)   Levator ani muscle
- Iliococcygeus
- Anococcygeal body (ligament) (posterior extensions of superficial external anal sphincter muscle)
- Gluteus maximus muscle
- Tip of coccyx

B

Female
- Clitoris
- External urethral orifice
- Vagina
- Ischiopubic ramus
- Anus

Superficial perineal (Colles') fascia (*cut edge*)
Ischiocavernosus muscle with deep perineal (investing or Gallaudet's) fascia removed
Bulbospongiosus muscle with deep perineal (investing or Gallaudet's) fascia removed
Fibers from superficial external anal sphincter muscle to ischiopubic ramus
Perineal membrane
Superficial transverse perineal muscle with deep perineal (investing or Gallaudet's) fascia removed
Superficial perineal (Colles') fascia (*cut edge*)
Perineal body
Crossed fibers from superficial and deep external sphincters to superficial transverse perineal muscle

Parts* of external anal sphincter muscle { Deep, Superficial, Subcutaneous

Levator ani muscle { Pubococcygeus, Puboanalis (puborectalis), Iliococcygeus

Anococcygeal body (ligament) (posterior extensions of superficial external anal sphincter muscle)

*Parts variable and often indistinct

• **Fig. 16.4** Superficial Layer of Pelvic Floor Musculature. Urogenital and Anorectal Triangle. (A) Male; (B) Female. (Reprinted with permission from Netter, FH. Chapter 6: Pelvis and perineum. In: Netter FH, ed. *Atlas of Human Anatomy.* 7th ed. Elsevier; 2019:367–441, Plate 377.)

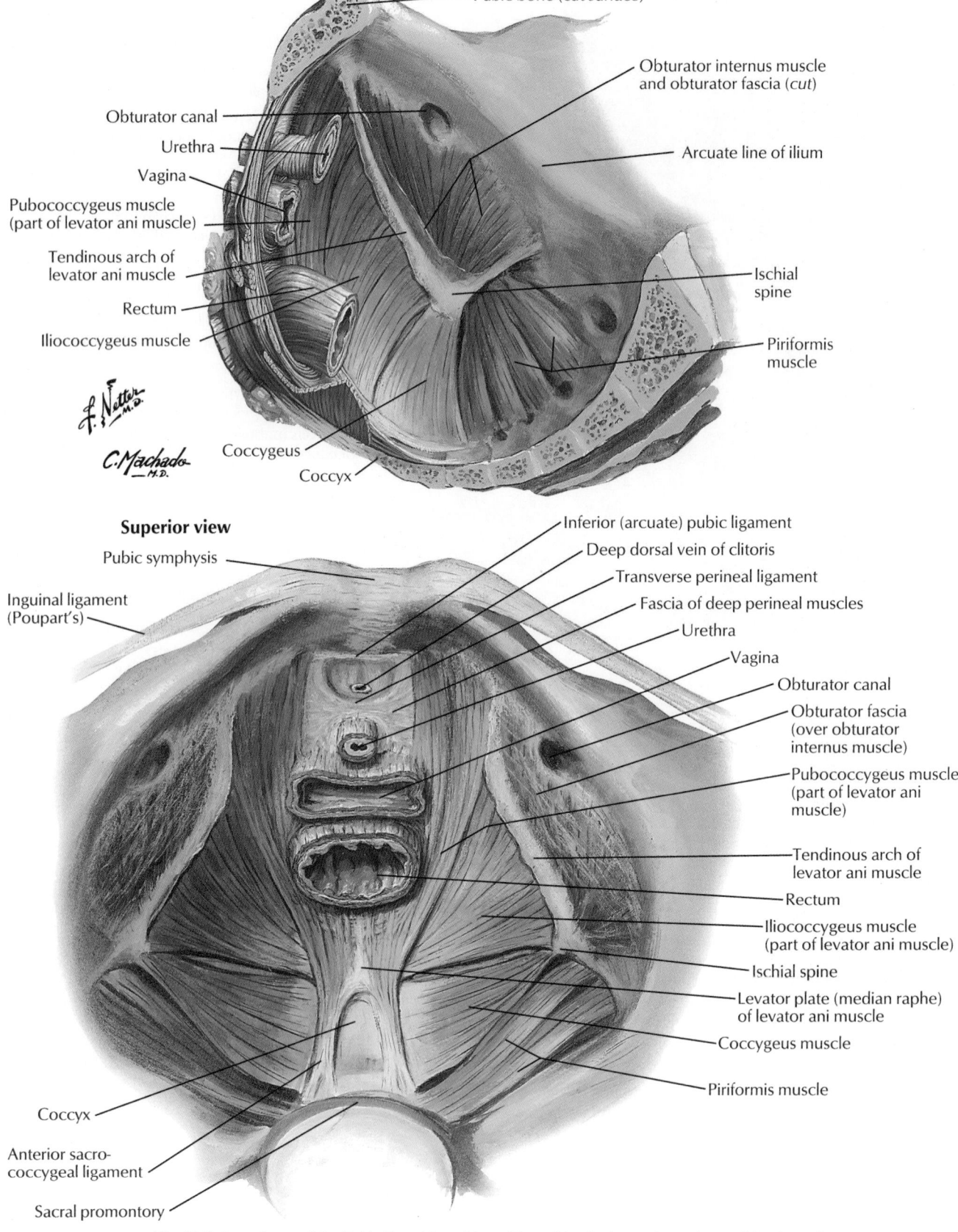

Medial view

Pubic bone (*cut surface*)

Obturator canal

Urethra

Vagina

Pubococcygeus muscle
(part of levator ani muscle)

Tendinous arch of
levator ani muscle

Rectum

Iliococcygeus muscle

Obturator internus muscle
and obturator fascia (*cut*)

Arcuate line of ilium

Ischial
spine

Piriformis
muscle

Coccygeus

Coccyx

Superior view

Pubic symphysis

Inguinal ligament
(Poupart's)

Inferior (arcuate) pubic ligament

Deep dorsal vein of clitoris

Transverse perineal ligament

Fascia of deep perineal muscles

Urethra

Vagina

Obturator canal

Obturator fascia
(over obturator
internus muscle)

Pubococcygeus muscle
(part of levator ani
muscle)

Tendinous arch of
levator ani muscle

Rectum

Iliococcygeus muscle
(part of levator ani muscle)

Ischial spine

Levator plate (median raphe)
of levator ani muscle

Coccygeus muscle

Piriformis muscle

Coccyx

Anterior sacro-
coccygeal ligament

Sacral promontory

• **Fig. 16.5** Deep Layer of the Pelvic Floor Musculature. The pelvic diaphragm is made up of: levator ani (pubococcygeus, iliococcygeus), obturator internus, coccygeus, and piriformis. (Reprinted with permission from Netter FH. Chapter 6: Pelvis and perineum. In: Netter FH, ed. *Atlas of Human Anatomy.* 7th ed. Elsevier; 2019:367–441, Plate 340.)

TABLE 16.7 Laycock PERFECT Scale

PERFECT	Measure	Description
P	Power	Grade 0- to 5-point manual muscle test
E	Endurance	Up to 10 seconds
R	Repetitions	Number of contractions at ≥50% Power and measured endurance, up to 10 repetitions
F	Fast contractions	Number of squeeze-relax contractions completed in 10 seconds
E	Elevation of perineum	Power of ≥3/5
C	Cough reflex	Present/absent
T	Transversus abdominus	Synergistic contraction with PFM

With author's modifications.
Created by Allegra Adams. Printed with permission.

BOX 16.8 Red Flags

- Pain with urination, blood in the urine, change in bladder function (e.g., more or less frequent urination, intermittent stream, hesitancy, retention)
- Vaginal or rectal spotting or bleeding in excess of small streaks of pink, red, or brown on gloved finger, pad, or bed covering
- Anyone with back, pelvic, groin, hip pain accompanied by abdominal complaints or palpable mass
- Any man with pelvic, groin, sacroiliac, or low back pain accompanied by sciatica and past history of prostate cancer
- Shoulder, back, hip, pelvic, sacral pain accompanied by change in bladder or bowel characteristics

Created by Allegra Adams. Printed with permission.

BOX 16.9 ICD-10 Diagnosis Codes for Genitourinary and Gynecological Impairments

M62.81	Muscle Weakness
M62.838	Muscle Spasm
M69.8	Disorder of Muscle, Ligament, Fascia
M79.1	Myalgia
R27.8	Other lack of coordination (dyssynergy)

Created by Allegra Adams. Printed with permission.

nerve complaints. Intrarectal palpation includes: levator ani, obturator internus, arcus tendoneus, coccygeus, coccyx, sacrospinous ligament, Alcock's canal, and prostate or urethral anastomosis, if indicated.

In the absence of PFM overactivity, muscle strength may be graded according to the Laycock PERFECT system.[66–68] **P**ower is graded on a standard 0- to 5-point manual muscle test scale. **E**ndurance is measured up to 10 seconds. The number of **R**epetitions at that power and for that endurance is counted, up to 10 repetitions. **F**ast contractions are counted for the number completed in 10 seconds. **ECT** then stands for "**E**very **C**ontraction **T**imed." This author, however, prefers to use the latter half of the mnemonic as a reminder of several other PFM functional indicators. Perineal **E**levation indicating a power of 3/5 or greater. Presence of the **C**ough reflex and synergistic contraction of the **T**ransversus Abdominus. This modified scale is represented in Table 16.7. Of note, the PFM are two-thirds tonic, slow-twitch muscle fibers and one-third fast-twitch.

Evaluation

Within PFPT, even more so for the PLWBC, it is best practice to maintain close communication with the oncology or medical care team, even in jurisdictions allowing for direct consumer access to rehabilitation services without a prescription or referral, given the visceral nature of many of the presenting complaints. Thorough imaging and lab work to rule out pathological causes of complaints is highly recommended prior to PFPT examination. Box 16.8 highlights several Red Flags that may warrant communication with or referral back to the physician, if not already ruled out.[3,4]

If the examination reveals that the presenting complaint is likely caused or contributed to by neuromusculoskeletal factors that are within the practitioner's training and scope of practice to address, care may proceed. It is not unusual for PFPT clinics to have waitlists of several months, and therefore, there are many interventions within the scope of the general orthopedic physical therapist that may be initiated to mitigate symptoms, even if PFPT is ultimately indicated.

Diagnosis and Prognosis

While a PLWBC may be referred to rehabilitation with medical diagnoses that state the person's exact complaint, such as UI, pelvic pain, anorgasmia, or erectile dysfunction, these are not reimbursable physical therapy diagnoses. Based on the results of the examination, the clinician must determine which structures and impairments will be addressed in the plan of care. Muscle weakness may be the root cause of UI whereas muscle spasm may be the cause of pelvic pain. Refer to Box 16.9 for a list of reimbursable ICD-10 codes.

The objective findings from the examination should be combined with the results of the history and systems review when developing a plan of care and determining a prognosis. Baseline function, comorbidities, cancer stage, cancer treatment, number of systems involved, chronicity, cognition, social support, financial resources including insurance coverage, transportation, and other demands on the person's time including dependents or vocation must all be considered when determining the prognosis.

It is also important to understand the PLWBC's goals for treatment. The complex, neurologically-involved person may simply wish to reduce toileting accidents to prevent skin breakdown whereas someone without preexisting dysfunction may wish to reduce incontinence or frequency for return to work or leisure or reduce pain with intercourse for eventual conception.

Intervention

The following is intended for the non-PFPT as a starting point to address GU/GYN dysfunction without specific pelvic floor training, followed by a brief overview of the types of interventions a PFPT would be able to offer.

Prehabilitation and Early Intervention

The referral rates for PWC to PFPT prehabilitation are low, however there is emerging evidence of the benefits of prehabilitation to address baseline deficits or to educate the PWC on how to prevent adverse effects throughout cancer treatment and in the early days post-treatment.[69–73] Similar to fertility preservation (see Chapter 12), there is often not enough time between diagnosis and necessity to initiate treatment to allow for a course of prehabilitation. Doing so may cost valuable time in delaying cancer treatment. Nonetheless, simple education regarding what impairments to anticipate, mitigation strategies, behavior modification, and general instruction in pelvic floor strengthening may be feasible.[69] It may be enough to simply acknowledge the known GU/GYN adverse effects and offer reassurance that these too can be treated, when the person is ready.[74]

Likewise, PLWBCs are rarely referred for Onc R during treatment for pelvic-related complaints as there are often more pressing medical issues or initiating PFPT is not indicated for some time after treatment has completed. During and immediately after radiation therapy, the initial exercise may include active and active assisted range of motion to prevent contracture, gentle strengthening to prevent deconditioning, and functional mobility. Heavy resistance with the affected areas should be minimized initially after radiation and the weight-bearing status for bones in the irradiation field should be considered before starting exercise.[4] Direct mobilizations and manipulations are contraindicated.[4] Be mindful of skin changes that are red, tender, blistered, or open secondary to radiation changes, as these tissues should not be excessively stressed to allow for healing.[4] For the PLWBC receiving brachytherapy, the radioactive status remains for as long as the radiotherapy is in place, depending on the type of cancer and the approach (e.g., implanted seeds versus intravaginal applicator). During chemotherapy, the agent remains in circulation for 48 to 72 hours after treatments, so the Onc R clinician should avoid direct contact during that time.[75] Again, Onc R clinicians must remain mindful of cardiopulmonary adverse effects, osteoporosis, and myelosuppression from the various forms of cancer treatment, discussed elsewhere in this text.[4]

Most PLWBCs are seen in rehabilitation after completion of cancer treatment, though usually no earlier than 4 to 6 weeks. A PLWBC referred to Onc R early after surgery may be monitored for appropriate wound healing timeline and early signs of complication or infection. Until the wounds are healed, stitches or staples are dissolved or removed, and in general at least 6 to 8 weeks postoperatively, no direct scar mobilization may be performed or biophysical agents/modalities used at the site (see below for a full discussion on biophysical agent use in PLWBCs). Interventions may focus on education, behavior modification, and general conditioning.

Education

Persons treated at any point along the cancer continuum will benefit from education regarding pelvic anatomy, normal physiology, and pathophysiological changes due to the cancer or its treatment. While it is outside the scope of this text to educate the reader regarding normal micturition controls and sexual response models, several normative values are presented.

For persons under 65 years old or premenopausal, normal urinary frequency is every 3 to 4 hours during the day, or five to seven times, and none at night. After 65 years old or postmenopause (including cancer treatment induced), normal urinary frequency is every two to three hours, or up to nine times per day, and once at night.[76,77] The normal bladder capacity is 400 to 500 mL. When full, the urine stream should last for at least a strong eight seconds.[76,78] A person with outlet obstruction, as in prostate cancer,

may have a much greater capacity whereas a person after radiation may have a much smaller capacity.

Education may also include topics regarding adequate hydration and dietary irritants. Hydration recommendations vary, however, it is generally accepted that the number of ounces of water a person consumes per day should be equal to half of their weight in pounds (i.e., a person who is 150 pounds should drink 75 ounces of water per day). Food or drink containing alcohol, caffeine, carbonation, acidity, certain spices, or high in sugar or artificial sweeteners may irritate the bladder, especially if it is predisposed due to radiation, chemotherapy, or immunotherapy. Bladder irritants can contribute to urinary frequency and urge UI.[79] Conversely, limiting fluid intake to reduce UI concentrates the urine making it more acidic and therefore also becomes a bladder irritant. However, if nighttime urination is a concern, it is recommended to restrict fluid intake 2 hours before bedtime.[78]

Bladder training helps to control urinary urgency and reduce frequency. PFM contractions and distraction techniques may be used to suppress an urge to void by reflexively inhibiting detrusor contractions and extending the voiding interval to approach normal limits. This technique can also be used to break classical conditioning of specific triggers of urgency such as doing the dishes or arriving home ("key-in-door" syndrome).[78]

Conversely, someone struggling with urinary retention, areflexive bladder, or increased bladder volume, may be encouraged to use timed voiding, according to normative recommendations. All persons, and especially those with difficulty voiding, should also be encouraged to sit fully on the toilet seat, with feet planted on the floor or a stool that keeps the knees at or above hip height, and not stand or hover over the toilet. Hinging forward at the hips, with or without direct pressure on the bladder (in the suprapubic area) may help to empty completely ("Crede maneuver"), though this should be used only in specific cases, as PFM dysfunction can result with long-term use.[4,78,80] For someone who has a bladder prolapse (cystocele), two fingers or a small spatula may be placed on the front wall of the vagina to empty urine that may have pooled in this pouch. A person may also practice "double voiding" by weight shifting while on the toilet, wiping, getting up and sitting back down to empty more. Occasionally, performing PFM contractions after emptying may allow more urine to be emptied. *Performing PFM contractions while actively voiding, meaning intentionally attempting to stop the flow of urine, should be discouraged.* Urine flow may also be initiated by tapping on the bladder (in the suprapubic area) or stroking the skin over the sacrum. Constipation and straining should be avoided, though pushing the abdomen out to increase intraabdominal pressure as if having a bowel movement can help to relax the pelvic floor. Contracting the abdominals during toileting should be avoided, as this can activate the PFM and contribute to incomplete emptying.[66,78]

As a special note regarding neobladder retraining after bladder cancer, these persons lack the normal desire to void in the absence of a natural feedback loop. Voiding with a neobladder occurs with PFM relaxation, slight abdominal contraction, slight hand-pressure inwards at the lower abdomen, and forward bending. Persons with a neobladder will likely continue to use intermittent self-catheterization on a regular basis to ensure emptying and utilize saline lavage to prevent mucous plugging. In contrast to prostate cancer, daytime urinary continence can be anticipated first by approximately 3 months, with nighttime continence taking up to 9 months. A timed voiding schedule is used every 2 hours during the day and 3 hours at night, using urge suppression techniques to stretch to every 4 hours around the clock, progressing to a 500-mL capacity. Given the intestinal origin of creating the neobladder, there is a risk of mucous plugging and urinary retention. Absorption is also altered, increasing the risk of metabolic acidosis, presenting with fatigue, weakness, lethargy, anorexia, nausea, vomiting, epigastric burning, and heartburn. Body weight monitoring, electrolyte and vitamin B12 monitoring, and fluid intake of 2 to 3 liters per day are recommended.[4]

A pessary is a silicone device that is fitted generally in a gynecology or urogynecology office that offers support to a pelvic organ prolapse to improve bladder emptying, reduce pelvic floor pressure or chaffing, and/or provide some urethral compression to reduce UI. For men, a penile clamp may be used transiently (less than 2 hours at a time) to prevent incontinence during activities such as giving a presentation, athletics, or swimming.

Vulvovaginal irritation from GSM or radiation can be compounded by dietary irritants (oxalates), UI or other moisture (e.g., sweating, wet swimsuit), soaps and detergents (dyes, fragrances), clothing (tightness, material, dyes), douching, vaginal deodorizers, moisturizers, and sexual lubricants. Soaps and detergents that are fragrance free and pH neutral are recommended, but the vaginal region should not be directly cleaned. The soap from washing elsewhere on the body should simply wash over the area from the shower water, followed by external rinsing of water; baths are discouraged. To decrease discomfort and irritation in the vulvar region, the area should be rinsed with warm water after voiding and patted dry rather than wiping; wet wipes should be avoided. Loose fitting, cotton undergarments and pants may help reduce moisture, compression, and risk of infection. Douching, vaginal deodorizers, and other vaginal cleaning that is not otherwise recommended by the oncology team is discouraged.[78] Vaginal moisturizers and lubricants that include glycols or have a high osmolality can also cause irritation and infections.[81]

Functional Mobility, Balance, and General Conditioning

Though direct PFM training may not be within the scope of most Onc R clinician's practice, generalized lumbopelvic strengthening, functional mobility, balance, postural retraining, and correcting spinal alignment are within the scope of a generalist and each can positively influence the PFM function. In fact, in a review of 225 persons with urgency UI, 48% received a concurrent hip or spine movement impairment diagnosis.[82]

Given the extent of musculoskeletal and neurological adverse effects of cancer treatment, outlined in Chapters 7 and 8, a significant portion of UI after cancer treatment may be functional incontinence—that the PLWBC simply cannot physically get to the bathroom or bedside commode or undress in time. There is a fair amount of evidence to support the correlation between urgency UI and rate of falls.[83–87] There is also some evidence showing that women with stress UI likewise have decreased balance ability compared to continent women.[88,89] In fact, it has been shown that the postural activity of the PFM is delayed in women with stress UI.[90]

As the PFM are part of the anticipatory postural control activity,[91] global postural retraining and trunk stabilization has been shown to increase the strength of the PFM and reduce stress UI more than isolated PFM strengthening alone, with better treatment adherence.[92,93] Similarly, coordinated retraining of diaphragmatic, deep abdominal, and PFM function resulted in decreased episodes of stress or mixed UI and increased quality of life as compared to PFM training alone.[94] It is also well established that the PFM may be activated through recruitment of the hip adductors or gluteals.[64]

In the same way, delayed activation of the transversus abdominus has been found to be present in chronic groin pain.[95] Haugstad et al. reported "a specific pattern of pain, posture, movement, muscle pathology, and reduced awareness of one's own body was found in women with chronic pelvic pain" suggesting that treatments aimed at addressing these deficits should be incorporated to reduce chronic pelvic pain.[96] Numerous researchers support this link between musculoskeletal dysfunction and chronic pelvic pain.[97–101]

In summary, strengthening of muscles involved in the lumbopelvic slings (Figure 16.6) can enhance PFM functioning and reduce UI, pelvic pain, and sexual dysfunction through use of muscle synergies and the overflow principle. This can be incorporated through exercises such as bridging with added hip abduction or adduction, trunk proprioceptive neuromuscular facilitation patterns, and dynamic balance retraining.

Alignment, Flexibility, Postural Retraining

All of the muscles of the pelvic floor, as well as the muscles of the abovementioned lumbopelvic slings, attach to the innominates, sacrum, and coccyx. Therefore, alignment asymmetries will influence the length-tension relationships of the PFM contributing to weakness or overactivity. An overstretched muscle and an overactive muscle can both be considered functionally weak and contribute to UI, predominately stress incontinence. PFM overactivity is implicated for urgency UI and also in pelvic pain conditions. Thoracic and lumbar spinal alignment is equally important due to the somatic and autonomic functions these spinal levels play in motor, sensory, and visceral innervations for the pelvic region; refer to Figures 12.1 and 12.2. The reader is referred to the work of Greenman for muscle energy techniques as a method of correcting alignment asymmetries.[102]

Standing and sitting posture can also influence PFM activation. There is greater PFM activity in all standing postures as compared with sitting, with the greatest activity measured in a hypo-lordotic position.[103] In this position, the abdominal-gluteal force couple creates a synergy with the PFM which is likely compensatory for PFM weakness. A neutral standing position provides the optimal pelvic floor length-tension relationship. In sitting, there is greater PFM activity in more upright and unsupported sitting postures as compared to slump sitting.[104,105] An upright, unsupported sitting posture recruits overall more core musculature for synergistic activity of the PFM.

Recalling the fascia of the deep front line, postural supports such as a heel lift or orthotics can reduce incontinence through corrected spinal alignment, improved PFM activity, and/or reduced strain on the bladder.

Manual Therapies

Alignment and posture can be driven or perpetuated by lumbopelvic muscle imbalances in flexibility or weakness and thereby addressed by stretching or strengthening as indicated by the examination. Of note, the wide deep squat or "Happy Baby" yoga pose is an optimal stretch position for the PFM.[78] Positional releases (Kerry J. D'Ambrogio[106]), ischemic (Travell, Simons, and Simons[107]), or strain-counterstrain (Lawrence H. Jones[108]) trigger point releases may also be utilized for focal areas of muscle overactivity. Stretching may also require mobilizations of the spine or hip capsule utilizing Kaltenborn,[109] McKenzie,[110] or Maitland[111] techniques, as trained, in addition to stretching of the sacrotuberous, sacrospinous, and sacrococcygeal ligaments. The reader is cautioned to keep in mind the fibrotic effects of radiation therapy on muscles and ligaments as well as the osteoporotic effects

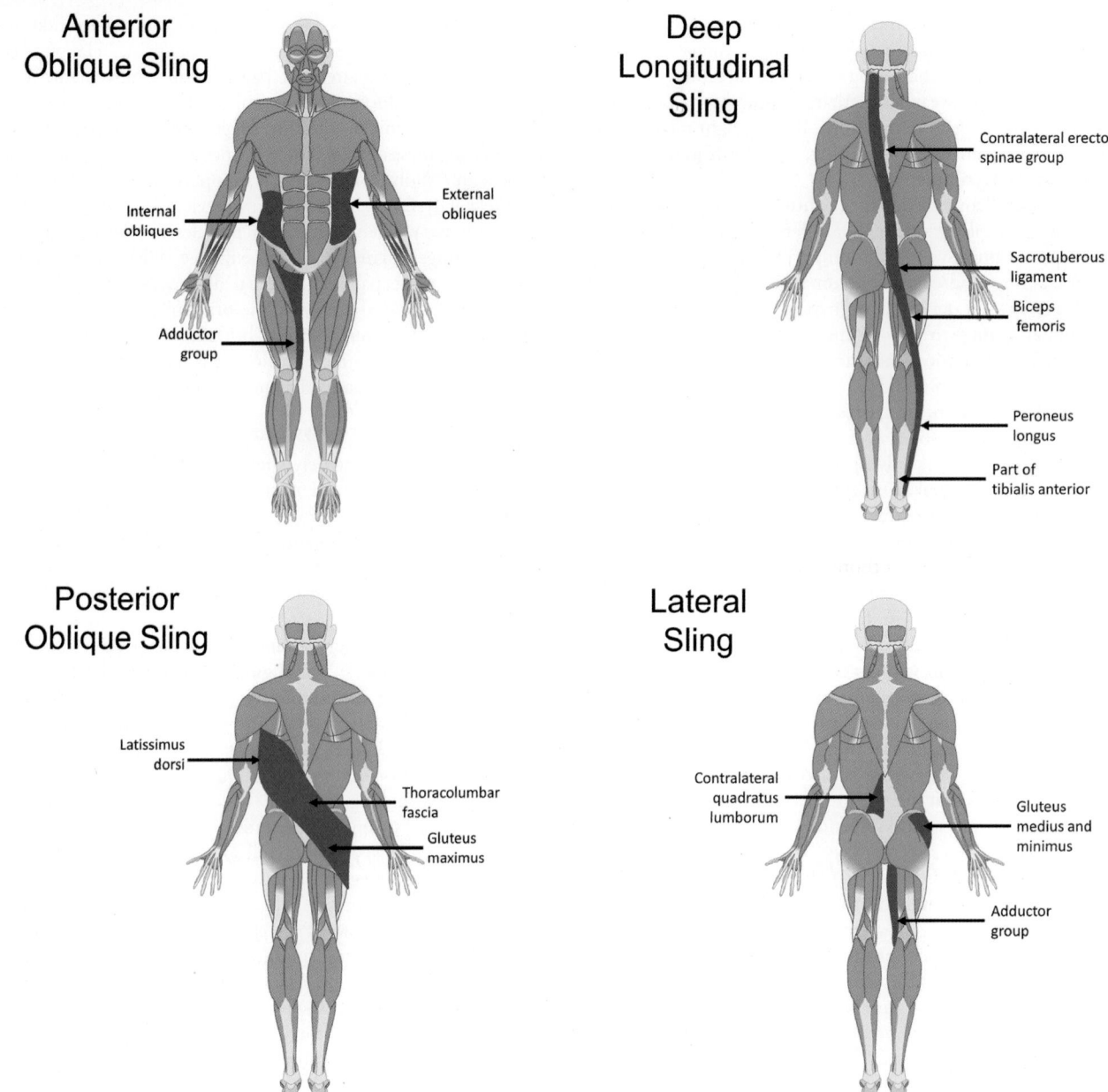

• **Fig. 16.6** Lumbopelvic Sling. (Created by Chris Wilson.) (Printed with permission.)

of treatments on bone, described in Chapter 7, when selecting interventions.

Myofascial restrictions due to antalgic postures and movement patterns, inflammation or infection, or radiation therapy, and surgical scar restrictions also contribute to alignment and postural asymmetries, restricted joint mobility, and reinforce impaired movement patterns. Myofascial release, massage, scar mobilizations, cupping, dry needling, or other soft tissue mobilizations may be useful in restoring necessary soft tissue balance.

Alignment and postural impairments may also be driven by organ, vascular, neural, or dural restrictions. For instance, during a hysterectomy for any of the gynecological cancers, the supporting ligaments are often not removed, or if they are, scar tissue develops in their place. Radiation, chemotherapy, and hormonal therapies may also cause organ restrictions, over and above those from past pathology, pregnancy, or menopause. Therefore, restriction of the uterosacral ligament may result in a sacral torsion and restriction of the broad ligament (to the innominates) or any restriction around the ovaries can result in an innominate dysfunction. Through the fascial chains previously discussed, the ligaments of the bladder can be traced to the sphenoid and occasionally manipulation of the sphenobasilar joint may be necessary to treat over-active bladder. The reader is referred to the work of Jean-Pierre Barral,[60] John E. Upledger,[112] or William G. Sutherland[113] for training in these techniques.

Ultimately, PFM dysfunction is often a consequence of a more global systemic imbalance that is well within the training of a general Onc R clinician to address. However, with direct pelvic surgeries or radiation treatment, as is the case for the GU/GYN cancers, direct pelvic floor interventions are required. A PFPT is trained to perform intravaginal or intrarectal interventions to address soft tissue impairments, often with the support of vaginal dilators or wands.

Pelvic Floor Muscle Strengthening

PFM strengthening, through performing "Kegels," is well established as a successful treatment for UI.[41,114–116] It can also be used for treatment of erectile dysfunction[117] and to some extent for anorgasmia.[118–121] There is less consensus regarding treatment parameters, which vary significantly in the literature. It is the best practice to perform the Laycock PERFECT scale previously described and then utilize traditional strength training principles of overload and specificity to set an intensity level that will encourage strength gains without resulting in compensations, overactivity, or fatigue; the muscles must remain functional for their usual functions for the remainder of the day. Moreover, the literature shows that roughly a quarter of research participants do not correctly perform a PFM contraction, which indicates the importance of a referral to PFPT.[122] Shy of an internal PFM examination, a general recommendation for someone without PFM overactivity is to perform 8 to 12 PFM contractions, holding for 10 seconds each, as well as ten fast contractions without holds, for two to three sets per day.[78,123] During radiation therapy, and for the first 4 to 6 weeks after surgery or radiation, it is this author's practice to recommend that the PLWBC perform Kegels at 50% intensity.

In addition to performing a thorough pelvic examination and providing specific PFM strengthening guidelines, a PFPT will also have access to surface EMG biofeedback to improve brain-body awareness of the PFM or, when not contraindicated (see Biophysical Agents/Modalities section below), may perform perianal, intravaginal, or intrarectal neuromuscular electrical stimulation to facilitate PFM contractions. Internal electrical stimulation may, in some cases, also be used for women who have received brachytherapy and are now lacking intravaginal sensation.

Perhaps the most important consideration regarding PFM strengthening is that Kegels are not the panacea for all pelvic floor dysfunction. In fact, stress UI and to a lesser extent erectile dysfunction and pelvic organ prolapse, are the primary diagnoses that Kegels can help. Urgency UI and the majority of pain diagnoses are generally the result of PFM overactivity and prescribing strengthening for an already shortened and functionally weak muscle may serve to compound the dysfunction. It is therefore the author's recommendation that the reader take advantage of the aforementioned muscle synergies and overflow properties rather than make blanket suggestions to the persons in their care regarding Kegels.

Biophysical Agents/Modalities

The use of biophysical agents (colloquially known as modalities) for persons seeking Onc R treatment with a past history of cancer is generally discouraged in entry level education, with the exception of palliative care. Nonetheless, the conditions with which the PLWBC are presenting are often the exact complaints which would most benefit from the use of biophysical agents. The concern is based on several principles of biophysical agent physiology:

- Physical agents and electrotherapeutic agents have the potential to break down cell membrane barriers or change transmembrane potentials thus stimulating growth of abnormal tissues.
- Increased blood flow to tissue may enhance tumor growth by supplying the tumor with necessary nutrients and encouraging development of metastatic spread via tumor angiogenesis.
- Enhanced radiation treatment effect or increased blood flow and delivery of chemotherapy to tissue.

Therefore, it is best practice to observe absolute contraindications for biophysical agent use in PLWBC and for 6 to 12 months

> ### • BOX 16.10 Absolute Contraindications for Biophysical Agent Use
>
> - Superficial and deep heat (including ultrasound) should never be applied directly over an area of active tumor due to enhanced circulation
> - Do not use heat or cold packs on areas recently treated with radiation
> - Mechanical and electrotherapeutic agents (traction, ultrasound, transcutaneous electrical nerve stimulation) should be avoided in areas of malignancy due to risk of structural instability and resultant fracture
> - Electrotherapeutic agents may result in uncontrolled growth of tumor
> - Not to be used in area:
>   - Of active infection, acute DVT, untreated cardiac edema, arterial insufficiency
>   - Of dysvascular tissue due to risk of tissue injury
>   - At risk for bleeding or hemorrhage (bone marrow suppression, long-term corticosteroids, anticoagulation therapy)
>   - Of damaged or regenerating nerves
>   - With sensory impairments, as in chemotherapy-induced polyneuropathy (risk of burns, tissue injury)
>   - Over an implanted device (pacemakers, defibrillators, joint prosthetics, plastic or cement components for orthopedic reconstruction, tissue expanders or breast implants, morphine pump)
>
> Created by Allegra Adams. Printed with permission.

following treatment, presented in Box 16.10.[4,124–126] However, "when the patient has been deemed by the medical oncologist to be free of signs or symptoms of cancer and/or has had recent negative scans, general modality guidelines can be used."[4] Nonetheless, it may be better practice for the Onc R clinician to consult the PLWBC's oncology team individually for each request to involve a biophysical agent in the plan of care.

If appropriate clearance is received to incorporate biophysical agents into the plan of care, there are several ways in which they may be used to treat GU/GYN symptoms.

Ultrasound or low level laser therapy (LLLT, cold laser) may be used to break down scar tissue from surgical incisions or radiation fibrosis prior to manual soft tissue manipulations.[127] LymphaTouch (LymphaTouch Inc., Helsinki, Finland)[128] or the 6D Action Massage Device (Mettler Electronics Corp., Anaheim, CA) may also be used as noncompressive techniques for myofascial or scar mobilization or for lymphatic drainage.[129]

Electrical stimulation may be helpful for pain modulation; improving pelvic sensation, such as the awareness of bladder filling, through application over the sacral nerves; reducing overactive bladder through application on the sacral nerves, bladder, and/or distal tibial nerve posterior to the medial malleolus; and for neuromuscular reeducation of PFM strengthening, perianally, intravaginally, or intrarectally.[78,127,130–132]

There are no contraindications for the use of surface EMG biofeedback in PLWBCs, though the practitioner is reminded not to place electrodes over recently irradiated skin or open areas.

Devices

There is a plethora of devices on the market claiming to cure GU/GYN dysfunction, with or without evidence to support them, to which a PLWBC may fall prey and occasionally cause more damage. Several of the more common one are reviewed below.

The evidence to support vaginal and rectal weights for treating UI or improving sexual function, is limited.[133] Additionally, there is significant variability in design and corresponding protocols that are delivered with the weights. Moreover, there is potential that the person's PFM are in fact already overactive, or conversely too weak to support such resistance. It is unlikely that the person intending to use the weight will in fact correctly isolate only the PFM without compensations and it is very easy to overuse the weight as some protocols recommend inserting the weight and then to walk around with a sustained contraction of up to 10 minutes.

Intravaginal pressure sensors, or perineometers, seem to come with more reasonable parameters. Caution is still necessary to be sure that the consumer is ready to initiate strengthening and that the PFM are not already overactive. Considering the above discussion of contraindications to biophysical agents, PLWBCs should be advised to discuss any over-the-counter intravaginal stimulation device for incontinence or sexual function with their oncology care team.

Vaginal dilators have been shown in the literature to be effective and safe for the treatment of dyspareunia and pelvic pain.[134–139] Vaginal dilators are available in hollow plastic, solid plastic, or silicone, and are typically available as graduated sets that increase in diameter and sometimes height. These can be used for desensitizing the vaginal tissues and stretching the vaginal opening and vaginal depth in the case of a woman who has undergone a hysterectomy and now has apical pain or vaginal vault shortening. Women with a history of cervical or endometrial cancer may have already been provided with, and/or instructed in use of, dilators by their oncology care team early post-treatment, as this is well established practice in the literature and increasingly the standard of care.[140] Another type of vaginal dilator is longer, more narrow, and either S- or C-curved for self-intravaginal trigger point release. While a person is unlikely to cause harm by using vaginal dilators, they are often intimidating and uncomfortable both to discuss and to use initially.

The International Clinical Guideline Group outlines the recommendations for vaginal dilation after pelvic radiotherapy in Box 16.11.[135,141,142] However, given the progressive nature of pelvic radiation disease, early vaginal dilation did not seem to improve vaginal dimensions[143] and therefore use may need to be extended beyond a year postradiation to be most effective.[144]

The Internation Clinical Guideline Group goals of vaginal dilation after pelvic radiotherapy are as follows:[141]

- Facilitate resumption of sexual relations after radiotherapy.
- Prevent adhesions progression to fibrosis and stenosis of the vagina, especially during the first year after completion of radiation therapy (if no intercourse is resumed and the patient is motivated to maintain vaginal patency).
- Allow the medical team to examine and assess the vaginal vault or cervix as part of on-going medical follow up.
- Reduce potential sexual difficulties (dyspareunia).
- Offer the opportunity to discuss sexual fears/myths associated with pelvic radiotherapy.
- Reduce tissue damage.
- Improve psychological well-being.

Outcomes Assessment

As always, having an objective outcome measure to compare baseline functional status and rehabilitation treatment response is desirable for reimbursement purposes as well as to intermittently take assessment of the treatment plan and to make revisions as indicated. In addition to objective examination measures, many patient-reported outcome measures are available. The American Physical Therapy Association (APTA) Academy of Oncologic Physical Therapy Evaluation Database to Guide Effectiveness (EDGE) Task Force has evaluated many of the existing measures for incontinence and sexual dysfunction.

• BOX 16.11   International Guidelines on Vaginal Dilation After Pelvic Radiotherapy

- Dilation therapy may include the use of dilators, vibrators, fingers, or similar shaped devices. It may not be necessary if vaginal intercourse is resumed weekly (or more) following treatment
- Dilation therapy should be gentle
- Dilation therapy may be commenced at approximately 2–8 weeks post radiotherapy, when the acute inflammatory response has settled
  - North American practice guidance does not recommend dilation during radiation therapy and also advises patients not to have intercourse during radiation therapy
  - Routine dilation during or too soon after cancer treatment may be harmful
  - There is limited reliable evidence to show that routine regular vaginal dilation during or after radiotherapy prevents the late effects of radiotherapy or improves QOL
- A reasonable duration and frequency of dilation may range from 3 minutes 2x/week up to 10 minutes 2x/day
- Women may be offered a range of sizes according to their anatomy. It is usual to start with the smallest and progress to whatever size is comfortable.
  - Dilator shape should be determined by the tumor site treated (pointed end for anal, low rectal/ vaginal cancer and flat end for endometrial/ cervix cancer)
- A small amount of bleeding or "spotting" after dilator use is normal; if there is a lot of bleeding or pain, a clinician should be contacted
- Review the need for dilation therapy on a regular basis, consider discontinuation of dilation therapy when no longer required (when sexually active or experiencing no discomfort during vaginal examinations at follow up 1–2 years post treatment)
  - Some women develop negative emotions regarding long-term dilator use

Created by the International Clinical Guideline Group.

For UI, the EDGE Task Force highly recommends[145]:
- American Urological Association Symptom Index
- Pelvic Floor Distress Inventory—Short Form (PFDI-20)
- Pelvic Floor Impact Questionnaire—Short Form

The Incontinence Quality of Life Questionnaire and the International Consultation Incontinence Questionnaire—Short Form are also recommended but have not been evaluated in the cancer population. Other patient-reported measures that are available include: the Urinary Distress Inventory (UDI-6), the Incontinence Impact Questionnaire (IIQ-7), and the NIH-Chronic Prostatitis Symptom Index. A bladder diary may also be useful to assist in answering many of the questions posed in the History section (Box 16.3). A "pad test" also offers an objective measure of leakage. The pad is weighed and then the person is asked to either perform specific activities (e.g., jumping, running) for a set period of time or to wear the pad for 24-hours and then is reweighed as an indication of the volume of urine leaked.[78]

For sexual dysfunction, the EDGE Task Force highly recommends[146]:
- Sexual Function—Vaginal Changes Questionnaire
- International Index of Erectile Function
- Erection Hardness Score
- Sexual Health Inventory for Men (International Index of Erectile Function-5)

The Sexual Interest and Desire Inventory is recommended but has not been evaluated in the cancer population. Other patient-report measures that are available include: the Vulvar Questionnaire (VQ), the Female Sexual Function Index (FSFI), and the NIH Chronic Prostatitis Symptom Index (NIH-CPSI). Research published in the Journal of Gynecological Oncology concluded that the FSFI "remains the most robust sexual morbidity outcome measure, for research or clinical use, in sexually active women treated for cervical or endometrial cancer."[147]

Conclusion

Cancers of the GU/GYN and their treatment can have devastating adverse effects on urological and sexual function. Fortunately, oncologists are starting to recognize these effects and incorporate a small amount of primary prevention as part of the standard of care for treatment of these cancers. Additionally, much can be done by an OncR clinician, with or without advanced PFPT training, for tertiary prevention of these long-term effects to improve the quality of life for PLWBCs of any type.

Critical Research Needs

- Pelvic floor physical therapy (PFPT) interventions for urinary and sexual adverse of effects of treatments for GU/GYN cancers
- PFPT interventions regarding GU/GYN cancers in the LGBTQIA+ populations.
- The sequelae of cancer treatment and rehabilitation interventions in the LGBTQIA+ populations.

Case Study

History: A 63-year-old man is referred to pelvic floor rehabilitation following da Vinci robotic laparoscopic prostatectomy for T3bN0M0, Gleason score 4+5 = 9, prostate cancer 6 weeks ago. He had an indwelling catheter for 10 days and noted onset of UI upon removal. He currently reports urinary frequency of every hour during the day to prevent leakage and four times per night. He does not have a strong urge to void and his stream is not very strong. He wears four heavy pads per day that are soaked when changed and one adult diaper at night that is wet in the morning. He notes UI with changes in position including sit to stand and bed mobility, as well as coughing, sneezing, lifting, bending, and yard work. He also reports back pain that interferes with sleep, bed mobility, standing longer than 20 minutes, and yard work. He is a university professor and is concerned about frequency and leakage during lecturing. He would also like to return to golfing. He reports erectile dysfunction and has not yet started penile rehabilitation.

Examination:

Outcome Measure: American Urological Association Symptom Index: 25/35 (severe)

Posture: forward head, increased thoracic kyphosis, bilateral scapular elevation and protraction L>R, slightly forward flexed at hips

Spinal Active Range of Motion: Lumbar: 50% flexion, 10% extension, 75% sidebending

Alignment: anterior rotation left innominate; sacral, lumbar within normal limits (WNL)

Standing flexion: positive on left; Stork test: positive on left; Seated flexion: Negative

Lower Extremity: Passive Range of Motion and Flexibility: moderate tightness bilateral hamstrings, iliopsoas, severe tightness piriformis, quadriceps

Joint Mobility: right hip capsule within normal limits (WNL), left hip grade 2 hypomobility (anterior and lateral glide)

Manual Muscle Tests (MMT): Transverse abdominals: dyssynergic; Bilateral lower extremities: WNL except left hip abduction 4/5

Abdominal Palpation: no tenderness to palpation

Breathing pattern: chest biased with minimal lateral rib expansion or abdominal movement

Diastasis recti abdominis: 3 cm supraumbilical with bulging during transitional movements

Scar tissue integrity/mobility: laparoscopic incisions healing appropriately (no signs of infection; scabs intact), moderate restriction with mild subdermal thickening except severe restriction and subdermal thickening of supraumbilical incision (NOTE: incisions are located at supraumbilical midline, 2 inches in vertical length, 2 inches in each lower abdominal quadrant measuring 0.5 inch horizontally)

Fascial mobility: restricted pelvic and respiratory fascial diaphragms

Visceral mobility: restricted urethral anastomosis, left lateral vesical ligament

External Pelvic Floor Palpation: minimal to moderate fascial restriction L>R urogenital triangle, minimal to moderate overactivity L>R levator ani, obturator internus

Perineum inspection/skin integrity: normal

Cough Reflex: intact

Anal Wink: intact

Perineal Mobility: diminished

Intrarectal Exam:

Anal sphincter tone: normal

Anal sphincter manual muscle test: 2/5

PFM tone: minimally to moderately increased tone L>R levator ani, obturator internus, coccygeus

PFM MMT: 2/5

Hold time: 10 seconds Repetitions: 5

Quick flicks: not assessed due to incomplete relaxation

Ability to recruit PFM: fair

Ability to release PFM: poor

Eccentric elongation: incomplete relaxation

Treatment: 6 visits, 1 hour, 1×/week for 3 visits, every other week ×2 visits, 1-month follow-up

Visit 1 (initial evaluation): Education regarding normal bladder habits, normal recovery of function, dietary irritants, and urge suppression techniques. Muscle energy techniques for innominate asymmetry. Myofascial releases. Visceral manipulation of bladder ligaments and parietal peritoneum abdominally and anastomosis intrarectally. Instruction in proper breathing mechanics and self-scar mobilizations (cross friction, skin rolling).

Visit 2: Hip capsule mobilizations, standard and with visceral fascia. Stretching for lower extremity flexibility. DRA reduction exercise. Transversus abduminus recruitment/localization. External and intrarectal fascial and ischemic trigger point releases.

Visit 3: Postural retraining including proper postures for seated worker, upper cervical flexion, lower trapezius retraining. Functional progression of transversus abduminus retraining. PFM releases and initiation of strengthening. Bridging with Theraband-resisted hip abduction and Kegel.

Visit 4–6: Functional progression of PFM strengthening from gravity eliminated to gravity resisted positions, muscle lengthened positions, with functional activities. Dynamic balance retraining (core muscle synergistic recruitment with upper or lower extremity perturbations).

Visit 1 (initial evaluation)	Education • Normal bladder habits • Normal recovery of function timeline • Dietary bladder irritants • Urge suppression techniques Muscle energy techniques for innominate asymmetry Myofascial releases Visceral manipulations • Bladder ligaments (abdominally and anastomosis intrarectally) • Parietal peritoneum Home exercise program (HEP) • Proper breathing mechanics • Self-scar mobilizations (cross friction, skin rolling)
Visit 2	Hip capsule mobilizations • Kaltenborn • With visceral fascia Neuromuscular reeducation of transversus abdominus recruitment/localization External and intrarectal fascial and ischemic trigger point releases HEP • Lower extremity stretching • DRA reduction exercise
Visit 3	PFM releases and initiation of strengthening Postural retraining • Proper postures for seated worker • Upper cervical flexion • Lower trapezius retraining HEP • Functional progression of transversus abdominus retraining • Bridging with theraband resisted hip abduction and Kegel

Visit 4–6	Functional progression of PFM strengthening • Gravity eliminated to gravity resisted positions (supine to standing) • Muscle lengthened positions (stride) • With functional activities Dynamic balance retraining (core muscle synergistic recruitment with upper or lower extremity perturbations)

Outcomes:

Subjective: Urinary frequency reduced to every 3 to 5 hours and 0 to 1x at night. Normalized urge to void and stream strength. Mild stress UI with golfing and yard work. Wears a thin shield with lecturing and golf, for peace of mind. Resolution of back pain. Participating in penile rehabilitation and meeting with sexual therapist.

Outcome Measure: American Urological Association Symptom Index: 2/35 (mild)

Objectives met:

- Reducing kyphotic posture resolved standing hip flexion
- Normalized spinal range of motion and pelvic alignment
- Flexibility improved
- Hip capsule mobility and hip abductor strength normalized
- Diastasis reduced to 1 cm, bulging reduced
- Breathing mechanics and abdominal recruitment normalized
- Abdominal strength 3/5
- Laparoscopic incision mobility normal except mild restriction/thickening at midline
- Fascial and visceral mobility normalized.
- Pelvic floor muscle tone and coordination normalized.
- PFM strength 4/5, 10 second hold, 8 repetitions, 5 fast contractions in 10 seconds.

Review Questions

Reader can find the correct answers and rationale in the back of the book.

1. Which of the following is MOST likely to be considered a red flag when working with a PLWBC in rehabilitation?
   A. Low back pain with sciatica in a man with a history of prostate cancer
   B. Low back pain in a woman with a history of TAH-BSO for endometrial cancer
   C. Hip pain in a man with a history of cystectomy for bladder cancer
   D. Dyspareunia in a woman with a history of brachytherapy for cervical cancer

2. You are working with a 48-year-old woman with a history of right breast cancer, HER-2 positive, treated with lumpectomy and sentinel lymph node dissection, chemotherapy (docetaxel [Taxotere], carboplatin [Paraplatin], trastuzumab [Herceptin]), and radiation therapy currently on tamoxifen (Nolvadex) for the last 3 years. You are seeing her for shoulder mobility when she mentions that sex is becoming painful and she is experiencing some spotting afterward. Which of the following is the MOST appropriate course of action?
   A. Reassure her that her experience is a normal part of being postmenopausal
   B. Recommend vaginal dilators to help with the pain

   C. Encourage her to follow up with her oncologist as soon as possible as tamoxifen is a risk factor for endometrial cancer and she is reporting red flags
   D. Discontinue the session and send her to the emergency room

3. You are working with a tall, Caucasian, 32-year-old male with groin pain. After a few sessions, he mentions that he and his wife have been having difficulty starting a family. Which of the following is the MOST appropriate course of action?
   A. Show empathy and reassure him that they are young and it might just take some time
   B. Recommend that they look into fertility testing and assisted reproduction
   C. Contact the referring physician to discuss concern for testicular cancer screening
   D. Refer him to a sex therapist and change the topic

4. You are a PFPT working with a 46-year-old woman for complaints of urinary urgency and chronic pelvic pain. She is on Medicaid and has six kids with several different men. You see in her chart that she has been referred to psychology for a history of abuse, though she has not gone, and that she will not let the gynecologist do a pelvic exam due to pain. After a few sessions, she agrees to start external pelvic floor work. You notice a strong odor and some blood in her underwear.

Which of the following is MOST likely to be considered a red flag for cervical cancer?

A. Overactive bladder and pelvic pain

B. Low socioeconomic status, lack of previous pelvic exam

C. Higher number of sexual partners, history of abuse, multi-parity

D. Vaginal discharge or bleeding with foul odor

5. Which of the following does NOT contribute to quality of life outcomes in a PLWBC in the LGBTQIA+ community?

A. Lower risk of developing cancer

B. Lack of routine healthcare due to actual or perceived discrimination

C. Lack of routine cancer screening due to providers' lack of awareness of risk factors leading to cancer detection at a higher stage requiring more pervasive and aggressive treatments

D. Preexisting higher rates of anxiety, depression, suicidal ideation and attempts; history of stressful life circumstances and events; history of being a target of harassment, violence, and discrimination; and likely estrangement from family and less likely to have adult children to care for them

6. You are working with a 75-year-old man who recently had a posterior hip replacement. His history is also significant for prostate cancer treated with external beam radiation. He wears adult diapers to his therapy sessions due to UI. Which exercise is MOST likely to exacerbate PFM shortening on top of radiation fibrosis?

A. Bridging with hip adductor ball squeeze

B. Sit to stand with Theraband resistance of hip abduction/external rotation

C. Forward and lateral step ups onto an exercise step

D. Dynamic balance activities

7. An 82-year-old man undergoing treatment for lung cancer complains of stress UI with coughing. Which of the following treatments would be LEAST APPROPRIATE?

A. Instruct him to contract his transversus abdominus and PFM prior to coughing/increases in intraabdominal pressure

B. Chest wall fascial/scar, thoracic, and rib cage mobilization to optimize posture and neuromuscular reeducation of diaphragmatic breathing for core muscle synergy

C. PFM stretching and trigger point releases to address overactivity due to cough reflex

D. A home exercise program of 10 PFM contractions held for 10 seconds performed three times a day

8. Which of the following is LEAST likely to be true regarding use of biophysical agents in a PLWBC?

A. Cancer history is an absolute contraindication for biophysical agent use

B. Someone with UI during cancer treatment or immediately after may benefit from use of surface EMG biofeedback to improve brain-body connection for PFM localization, recruitment, and strength

C. Ultrasound may reasonably be used on the elbow of a man choosing active surveillance of prostate cancer, providing that recent imaging is clear for metastasis

D. Intravaginal electrical stimulation may be used for urgency UI or lack of vaginal sensation in a PLWBC of the cervix after 5 years, with recent clear imaging ruling out recurrence/second cancer

9. Which of the following is MOST likely to be true regarding vaginal dilation therapy after pelvic brachytherapy?

A. Dilation should start during radiation treatment to prevent long-term adverse effects

B. Dilation should be gentle, progressive, and discontinued if bleeding greater than spotting occurs

C. Women who have had vaginal brachytherapy will have to use dilators lifelong to maintain vaginal patency

D. Vaginal dilation is not necessary if the PLWBC has no desire for penetrative intimacy

10. Which of the following is false regarding prescription of PFM strengthening?

A. All persons should perform Kegels daily to prevent or correct pelvic floor dysfunction

B. PFM strength can improve bladder control, erectile function, and orgasm

C. The same principles of exercise prescription for strengthening other muscle groups apply to the PFM (overload, specificity)

D. The PFM work in synergy with the abdominals and diaphragm and receive overflow from adjacent hip musculature

References

1. American Cancer Society. Cancer Facts & Figures 2020. Atlanta, GA; 2020. https://www.cancer.org/content/dam/cancer-org/research/cancer-facts-and-statistics/annual-cancer-facts-and-figures/2020/cancer-facts-and-figures-2020.pdf.

2. American Cancer Society. Bladder cancer; 2019. https://www.cancer.org/cancer/bladder-cancer.html. Accessed July 28, 2020.

3. Goodman CC, Heick J, Lazaro RT. *Differential Diagnosis for Physical Therapists: Screening for Referral.* 6th ed. Elsevier Inc.; 2018.

4. Stubblefield MD. *Cancer Rehabilitation: Principles and Practice.* 2nd ed. Springer Publishing Company; 2019.

5. Littlejohn N, Cohn JA, Kowalik CG, Kaufman MR, Dmochowski RR, Reynolds WS. Treatment of pelvic floor disorders following neobladder. *Curr Urol Rep.* 2017;18(1):5–10. doi:10.1007/s11934-017-0652-4.

6. American Cancer Society. Prostate cancer; 2019. https://www.cancer.org/cancer/prostate-cancer.html. Accessed August 11, 2020.

7. Rawla P. Epidemiology of prostate cancer. *World J Oncol.* 2019;10(2):63–89. doi:10.14740/wjon1191.

8. Sartor AO. Risk factors for prostate cancer. UpToDate; 2021.

9. Hoffman RM, Volk RJ, Wolf AMD. Making the grade: the newest US Preventive Services Task Force prostate cancer screening recommendation. *Cancer.* 2017;123(20):3875–3878. doi:10.1002/cncr.30941.

10. Tosoian JJ, Trock BJ, Morgan TM, et al. Use of the MyProstateScore test to rule out clinically significant cancer: validation of a straightforward clinical testing approach. *J Urol.* 2021;205(3):732–739. doi:10.1097/ju.0000000000001430.

11. Trofimenko V, Myers JB, Brant WO. Post-prostatectomy incontinence: how common and bothersome is it really? *Sex Med Rev.* 2017;5(4):536–543. doi:10.1016/j.sxmr.2017.05.001.

12. Emanu JC, Avildsen IK, Nelson CJ. Erectile dysfunction after radical prostatectomy: prevalence, medical treatments, and psychosocial interventions. *Curr Opin Support Palliat Care.* 2016;10(1):102–107. doi:10.1097/SPC.0000000000000195.

13. Katz A, Dizon DS. Sexuality after cancer: a model for male survivors. *J Sex Med.* 2016;13(1):70–78. doi:10.1016/j.jsxm.2015.11.006.

14. Shahinian VB, Kuo Y-F, Freeman JL, Goodwin JS. Risk of fracture after androgen deprivation for prostate cancer. *N Engl J Med.* 2005;352(2):154–164. doi:10.1097/S0022-5347(01)68451-9.

15. American Cancer Society. Testicular cancer; 2018. https://www.cancer.org/cancer/testicular-cancer.html. Accessed August 18, 2020.

16. Michaelson MD, Oh WK. Epidemiology of and risk factors for testicular germ cell tumors. UpToDate; 2021.

17. Caroline D, Ries F. Preservation of fertility in the cancer patient. In: Dicato MA, Van Cutsem E, eds. *Side Effects of Medical Cancer Therapy: Prevention and Treatment*. 2nd ed. Springer International Publishing AG; 2018:355–366. doi:10.1007/978-0-85729-787-7.

18. American Cancer Society. Endometrial cancer; 2019. https://www.cancer.org/cancer/endometrial-cancer.html. Accessed August 18, 2020.

19. Zhang GQ, Chen JL, Liu Q, Zhang Y, Zeng H, Zhao Y. Soy intake is associated with lower endometrial cancer risk: a systematic review and meta-analysis of observational studies. *Med (United States)*. 2015;94(50):1–10. doi:10.1097/MD.0000000000002281.

20. ACOG Practice Bulletin No. 147: Lynch syndrome. *Obstet Gynecol*. 2017;124(5):1042–1054.

21. Ramaseshan AS, Felton J, Roque D, Rao G, Shipper AG, Sanses TVD. Pelvic floor disorders in women with gynecologic malignancies: a systematic review. *Int Urogynecol J*. 2018;29(4):459–476. doi:10.1007/s00192-017-3467-4.

22. Morris K AL, Haboubi NY. Pelvic radiation therapy: between delight and disaster. *World J Gastrointest Surg*. 2015;7(11):279–288. doi:10.4240/wjgs.v7.i11.279.

23. Mendivil AA, Rettenmaier MA, Abaid LN, et al. Lower-extremity lymphedema following management for endometrial and cervical cancer. *Surg Oncol*. 2016;25(3):200–204. doi:10.1016/j.suronc.2016.05.015.

24. American Cancer Society. Ovarian cancer; 2018. https://www.cancer.org/cancer/ovarian-cancer.html. Accessed August 25, 2020.

25. Goff BA, Mandel LS, Melancon CH, Muntz HG. Frequency of symptoms of ovarian cancer in women presenting to primary care clinics. *J Am Med Assoc*. 2004;291(22):2705–2712. doi:10.1001/jama.291.22.2705.

26. Smith LH, Morris CR, Yasmeen S, Parikh-Patel A, Cress RD, Romano PS. Ovarian cancer: can we make the clinical diagnosis earlier? *Cancer*. 2005;104(7):1398–1407. doi:10.1002/cncr.21310.

27. American Cancer Society. Cervical cancer; 2020. https://www.cancer.org/cancer/cervical-cancer.html. Accessed August 25, 2020.

28. Jackson KS, Naik R. Pelvic floor dysfunction and radical hysterectomy. *Int J Gynecol Cancer*. 2006;16(1):354–363. doi:10.1111/j.1525-1438.2006.00347.x.

29. Hazewinkel MH, Sprangers MAG, van der Velden J, et al. Long-term cervical cancer survivors suffer from pelvic floor symptoms: a cross-sectional matched cohort study. *Gynecol Oncol*. 2010;117(2):281–286. doi:10.1016/j.ygyno.2010.01.034.

30. Hodgkinson K, Butow P, Fuchs A, et al. Long-term survival from gynecologic cancer: psychosocial outcomes, supportive care needs and positive outcomes. *Gynecol Oncol*. 2007;104(2):381–389. doi:10.1016/j.ygyno.2006.08.036.

31. Onujiogu N, Johnson T, Seo S, et al. Survivors of endometrial cancer: who is at risk for sexual dysfunction? *Gynecol Oncol*. 2011;123(2):356–359. doi:10.1016/j.ygyno.2011.07.035.

32. Lange MM, Van De Velde CJH. Urinary and sexual dysfunction after rectal cancer treatment. *Nat Rev Urol*. 2011;8(1):51–57. doi:10.1038/nrurol.2010.206.

33. Coady D, Kennedy V. Sexual health in women affected by cancer: focus on sexual pain. *Obstet Gynecol*. 2016;128(4):775–791. doi:10.1097/AOG.0000000000001621.

34. Abbott-Anderson K, Kwekkeboom KL. A systematic review of sexual concerns reported by gynecological cancer survivors. *Gynecol Oncol*. 2012;124(3):477–489. doi:10.1016/j.ygyno.2011.11.030.

35. Quinn GP, Sanchez JA, Sutton SK, et al. Cancer and lesbian, gay, bisexual, transgender/transsexual, and queer/questioning (LGBTQ) populations. *CA Cancer J Clin*. 2015;65(5):384–400. doi:10.3322/caac.21288.

36. Waterman BL, Voss JHPV. cervical cancer risks, and barriers to care for lesbian women. *Nurse Pract*. 2015;40(1):46–53.

37. Ceres M, Quinn GP, Loscalzo M, Rice D. Cancer screening considerations and cancer screening uptake for lesbian, gay, bisexual, and transgender persons. *Semin Oncol Nurs*. 2018;34(1):37–51. doi:10.1016/j.soncn.2017.12.001.

38. Tamargo CL, Quinn GP, Sanchez JA, Schabath MB. Cancer and the LGBTQ population: quantitative and qualitative results from an oncology providers' survey on knowledge, attitudes, and practice behaviors. *J Clin Med*. 2017;6(10):93. doi:10.3390/jcm6100093.

39. Lisy K, Peters MDJ, Schofield P, Jefford M. Experiences and unmet needs of lesbian, gay, and bisexual people with cancer care: a systematic review and meta-synthesis. *Psychooncology*. 2018;27(6):1480–1489. doi:10.1002/pon.4674.

40. Schabath MB, Blackburn CA, Sutter ME, et al. National survey of oncologists at National Cancer Institute–designated comprehensive cancer centers: attitudes, knowledge, and practice behaviors about LGBTQ patients with cancer. *J Clin Oncol*. 2019;37(7):547–558. doi:10.1200/JCO.18.00551.

41. Yang EJ, Lim JY, Rah UW, Kim YB. Effect of a pelvic floor muscle training program on gynecologic cancer survivors with pelvic floor dysfunction: a randomized controlled trial. *Gynecol Oncol*. 2012;125(3):705–711. doi:10.1016/j.ygyno.2012.03.045.

42. Zhang AY, Bodner DR, Fu AZ, et al. Effects of patient centered interventions on persistent urinary incontinence after prostate cancer treatment: a randomized, controlled trial. *J Urol*. 2015;194(6):1675–1681. doi:10.1016/j.juro.2015.07.090.

43. Dorey G, Speakman M, Feneley R, Swinkels A, Dunn C, Ewings P. Randomised controlled trial of pelvic floor muscle exercises and manometric biofeedback for erectile dysfunction. *Br J Gen Pract*. 2004;54(508):819–825.

44. Rutledge TL, Rogers R, Lee SJ, Muller CY. A pilot randomized control trial to evaluate pelvic floor muscle training for urinary incontinence among gynecologic cancer survivors. *Gynecol Oncol*. 2014;132(1):154–158. doi:10.1016/j.ygyno.2013.10.024.

45. Huffman LB, Hartenbach EM, Carter J, Rash JK, Kushner DM. Maintaining sexual health throughout gynecologic cancer survivorship: a comprehensive review and clinical guide. *Gynecol Oncol*. 2016;140(2):359–368. doi:10.1016/j.ygyno.2015.11.010.

46. Myers TW. *Anatomy Trains: Myofascial Meridians for Manual Therapists and Movement Professionals*. 4th ed. Churchill Livingston/Elsevier; 2020.

47. Sapsford RR, Hodges PW, Richardson CA, Cooper DH, Markwell SJ, Jull GA. Co-activation of the abdominal and pelvic floor muscles during voluntary exercises. *Neurourol Urodyn*. 2001;20(1):31–42. doi:10.1002/1520-6777 (2001)20:1<31::AID-NAU5>3.0.CO;2-P.

48. Kirk B, Elliott-Burke T. The effect of visceral manipulation on Diastasis Recti Abdominis (DRA): a case series. *J Bodyw Mov Ther*. 2021;26:471–480. doi:10.1016/j.jbmt.2020.06.007.

49. Wu L, Gu Y, Gu Y, et al. Diastasis recti abdominis in adult women based on abdominal computed tomography imaging: prevalence, risk factors and its impact on life. *J Clin Nurs*. 2021;30(3–4):518–527. doi:10.1111/jocn.15568.

50. Spitznagle TM, Leong FC, Van Dillen LR. Prevalence of diastasis recti abdominis in a urogynecological patient population. *Int Urogynecol J*. 2007;18(3):321–328. doi:10.1007/s00192-006-0143-5.

51. Olsson A, Kiwanuka O, Wilhelmsson S, Sandblom G, Stackelberg O. Cohort study of the effect of surgical repair of symptomatic diastasis recti abdominis on abdominal trunk function and quality of life. *BJS Open*. 2019;3(6):750–758. doi:10.1002/bjs5.50213.

52. Benjamin DR, Frawley HC, Shields N, van de Water ATM, Taylor NF. Relationship between diastasis of the rectus abdominis muscle (DRAM) and musculoskeletal dysfunctions, pain and quality of life: a systematic review. *Physiother (United Kingdom)*. 2019;105(1):24–34. doi:10.1016/j.physio.2018.07.002.

53. Wang Q, Yu X, Chen G, Sun X, Wang J. Does diastasis recti abdominis weaken pelvic floor function? A cross-sectional study. *Int Urogynecol J*. 2020;31(2):277–283. doi:10.1007/s00192-019-04005-9.

54. Bo K, Hilde G, Tennfjord MK, Sperstad JB, Engh ME. Pelvic floor muscle function, pelvic floor dysfunction, and diastasis recti abdominis: prospective cohort study. *Neurourol Urodyn.* 2017;36:716–721. doi:10.1002/nau.

55. Boissonnault JS, Blaschak MJ. Incidence of diastasis recti abdominis during the childbearing year. *Phys Ther.* 1988;68(7):1082–1086. doi:10.1093/ptj/68.7.1082.

56. Mota P, Pascoal AG, Sancho F, Carita AI, Bø K. Reliability of the inter-rectus distance measured by palpation: comparison of palpation and ultrasound measurements. *Man Ther.* 2013;18(4):294–298. doi:10.1016/j.math.2012.10.013.

57. Beamish N, Green N, Nieuwold E, McLean L. Differences in linea alba stiffness and linea alba distortion between women with and without diastasis recti abdominis: the impact of measurement site and task. *J Orthop Sports Phys Ther.* 2019;49(9):656–665. doi:10.2519/jospt.2019.8543.

58. van de Water ATM, Benjamin DR. Measurement methods to assess diastasis of the rectus abdominis muscle (DRAM): a systematic review of their measurement properties and meta-analytic reliability generalisation. *Man Ther.* 2016;21:41–53. doi:10.1016/j.math.2015.09.013.

59. Barral J-P, Mercier P. *Visceral Manipulation II (Revised Edition).* Eastland Press; 2007.

60. Barral J-P. In: Anderson S, Bensky D, eds. *Urogenital Manipulation.* 2nd ed. Eastland Press; 2006.

61. Talasz H, Kremser C, Kofler M, Kalchschmid E, Lechleitner M, Rudisch A. Phase-locked parallel movement of diaphragm and pelvic floor during breathing and coughing-a dynamic MRI investigation in healthy females. *Int Urogynecol J.* 2011;22(1):61–68. doi:10.1007/s00192-010-1240-z.

62. Perucchini D, DeLancey JO. Functional anatomy of the pelvic floor and lower urinary tract. In: Baessler K, Schussler B, Burgio KL, Moore KH, Norton PA, Stanton SL, eds. *Pelvic Floor Re-Education: Principles and Practice.* 2nd ed. Springer-Verlag; 2010:3–21. https://doi.org/10.1007/978-1-84628-505-9_1.

63. Herschorn S. Female pelvic floor anatomy: the pelvic floor, supporting structures, and pelvic organs. *Rev Urol.* 2004;6(5):S2–S10. doi:10.1097/MOU.0b013e3282f10a2b.

64. Bø K, Stien R. Needle EMG registration of striated urethral wall and pelvic floor muscle activity patterns during cough, valsalva, abdominal, hip adductor, and gluteal muscle contractions in nulliparous healthy females. *Neurourol Urodyn.* 1994;13(1):35–41. doi:10.1002/nau.1930130106.

65. Chan CLH, Ponsford S, Swash M. The anal reflex elicited by cough and sniff: validation of a neglected clinical sign. *J Neurol Neurosurg Psychiatry.* 2004;75(10):1449–1451. doi:10.1136/jnnp.2003.032110.

66. Laycock J, Haslam J. *Therapeutic Managment of Incontinence and Pelvic Pain: Pelvic Organ Disorders.* 2nd ed. Springer-Verlag; 2008. https://doi.org/10.1007/978-1-84628-756-5.

67. Newman D, J L. Clinical evaluation of the pelvic floor muscles. In: Baessler K, Schussler B, Burgio KL, Moore KH, Norton PA, Stanton SL, eds. *Pelvic Floor Re-Education: Principles and Practice.* 2nd ed. Springer-Verlag; 2010:91–104. https://doi.org/10.1007/978-1-84628-505-9_9.

68. Laycock J, Jerwood D. Pelvic floor muscle assessment: the PERFECT scheme. *Physiotherapy.* 2001;87(12):631–642. doi:10.1016/S0031-9406(05)61108-X.

69. Schneider S, Armbrust R, Spies C, du Bois A, Sehouli J. Prehabilitation programs and ERAS protocols in gynecological oncology: a comprehensive review. *Arch Gynecol Obstet.* 2020;301(2):315–326. doi:10.1007/s00404-019-05321-7.

70. Lukez A, Baima J. The role and scope of prehabilitation in cancer care. *Semin Oncol Nurs.* 2020;36(1):150976. doi:10.1016/j.soncn.2019.150976.

71. Van Rooijen S, Carli F, Dalton S, et al. Multimodal prehabilitation in colorectal cancer patients to improve functional capacity and reduce postoperative complications: the first international randomized controlled trial for multimodal prehabilitation. *BMC Cancer.* 2019;19(1):1–11. doi:10.1186/s12885-018-5232-6.

72. Treanor C, Kyaw T, Donnelly M. An international review and meta-analysis of prehabilitation compared to usual care for cancer patients. *J Cancer Surviv.* 2018;12(1):64–73. doi:10.1007/s11764-017-0645-9.

73. Sacomori C, Araya-Castro P, Diaz-Guerrero P, Ferrada IA, Martínez-Varas AC, Zomkowski K. Pre-rehabilitation of the pelvic floor before radiation therapy for cervical cancer: a pilot study. *Int Urogynecol J.* 2020;31(11):2411–2418. doi:10.1007/s00192-020-04391-5.

74. Falk SJ, Dizon DS. Sexual dysfunction in women with cancer. *Fertil Steril.* 2013;100(4):916–921. doi:10.1016/j.fertnstert.2013.08.018.

75. American Cancer Society. Chemotherapy safety; 2019. https://www.cancer.org/treatment/treatments-and-side-effects/treatment-types/chemotherapy/chemotherapy-safety.html. Accessed March 5, 2021.

76. FitzGerald MP, Stablein U, Brubaker L. Urinary habits among asymptomatic women. *Am J Obstet Gynecol.* 2002;187(5):1384–1388. doi:10.1067/mob.2002.126865.

77. Lukacz ES, Sampselle C, Gray M, et al. A healthy bladder: a consensus statement. *Int J Clin Pract.* 2011;65(10):1026–1036. doi:10.1111/j.1742-1241.2011.02763.x.

78. Irion JM, Irion G. *Women's Health in Physical Therapy*: Wolters Kluwer Health/Lippincott Williams & Wilkins; 2010.

79. Burgio KL, Newman DK, Rosenberg MT, Sampselle C. Impact of behaviour and lifestyle on bladder health. *Int J Clin Pract.* 2013;67(6):495–504. doi:10.1111/ijcp.12143.

80. Chang SM, Hou CL, Dong DQ, Zhang H. Urologic status of 74 spinal cord injury patients from the 1976 Tangshan earthquake, and managed for over 20 years using the Crede maneuver. *Spinal Cord.* 2000;38(9):552–554. doi:10.1038/sj.sc.3101060.

81. Ayehunie S, Wang YY, Landry T, Bogojevic S, Cone RA. Hyperosmolal vaginal lubricants markedly reduce epithelial barrier properties in a three-dimensional vaginal epithelium model. *Toxicol Rep.* 2017;5:134–140. doi:10.1016/j.toxrep.2017.12.011.

82. Wente KR, Spitznagle TM. Movement-related urinary urgency. *J Women's Heal Phys Ther.* 2017;41(2):83–90. doi:10.1097/jwh.0000000000000075.

83. Tinetti ME, Inouye SK, Gill TM, Doucette JT. Shared risk factors for falls, incontinence, and functional dependence: unifying the approach to geriatric syndromes. *JAMA.* 1995;273(17):1348–1353. doi:10.1001/jama.1995.03520410042024.

84. Brown JS, Vittinghoff E, Wyman JF, et al. Urinary incontinence: does it increase risk for falls and fractures? Study of Osteoporotic Fractures Research Group. *J Am Geriatr Soc.* 2000;48(7):721–725. http://www.ncbi.nlm.nih.gov/pubmed/10894308.

85. Morris V, Wagg A. Lower urinary tract symptoms, incontinence and falls in elderly people: time for an intervention study. *Int J Clin Pract.* 2007;61(2):320–323. doi:10.1111/j.1742-1241.2006.01174.x.

86. Chiarelli PE, Mackenzie LA, Osmotherly PG. Urinary incontinence is associated with an increase in falls: a systematic review. *Aust J Physiother.* 2009;55(2):89–95. doi:10.1016/S0004-9514(09)70038-8.

87. Lee C-Y, Chen L-K, Lo Y-K, et al. Urinary incontinence: an underrecognized risk factor for falls among elderly dementia patients. *Neurourol Urodyn.* 2011;30:1286–1290. doi:10.1002/nau.

88. Takazawa K, Arisawa K. Relationship between the type of urinary incontinence and falls among frail elderly women in Japan. *J Med Investig.* 2005;52(3–4):165–171. doi:10.2152/jmi.52.165.

89. Smith MD, Coppieters MW, Hodges PW. Is balance different in women with and without stress urinary incontinence? *Neurourol Urodyn.* 2008;27:71–78. doi:10.1002/nau.

90. Smith MD, Coppieters MW, Hodges PW. Postural activity of the pelvic floor muscles is delayed during rapid arm movements in women with stress urinary incontinence. *Int Urogynecol J.* 2007;18(8):901–911. doi:10.1007/s00192-006-0259-7.

91. Hodges P, Sapsford R, Pengel L. Postural and respiratory functions of the pelvic floor muscles. *Neurourol Urodyn*. 2007;26:362–371. doi:10.1002/nau.20232.

92. Sapsford R. Rehabilitation of pelvic floor muscles utilizing trunk stabilization. *Man Ther*. 2004;9(1):3–12. doi:10.1016/S1356-689X(03)00131-0.

93. Fozzatti C, Herrmann V, Palma T, Riccetto CLZ, Palma PCR. Global postural re-education: an alternative approach for stress urinary incontinence? *Eur J Obstet Gynecol Reprod Biol*. 2010;152(2):218–224. doi:10.1016/j.ejogrb.2010.06.002.

94. Hung HC, Hsiao SM, Chih SY, Lin HH, Tsauo JY. An alternative intervention for urinary incontinence: retraining diaphragmatic, deep abdominal and pelvic floor muscle coordinated function. *Man Ther*. 2010;15(3):273–279. doi:10.1016/j.math.2010.01.008.

95. Cowan SM, Schache AG, Brukner P, et al. Delayed onset of transversus abdominus in long-standing groin pain. *Med Sci Sports Exerc*. 2004;36(12):2040–2045. doi:10.1249/01.MSS.0000147587.81762.44.

96. Haugstad GK, Haugstad TS, Kirste UM, et al. Posture, movement patterns, and body awareness in women with chronic pelvic pain. *J Psychosom Res*. 2006;61(5):637–644. doi:10.1016/j.jpsychores.2006.05.003.

97. Hoffman D. Understanding multisymptom presentations in chronic pelvic pain: the inter-relationships between the viscera and myofascial pelvic floor dysfunction. *Curr Pain Headache Rep*. 2011;15(5):343–346. doi:10.1007/s11916-011-0215-1.

98. Lamvu G, Carrillo J, Witzeman K, Alappattu M. Musculoskeletal considerations in female patients with chronic pelvic pain. *Semin Reprod Med*. 2018;36(2):107–115. doi:10.1055/s-0038-1676085.

99. Mieritz RM, Thorhauge K, Forman A, Mieritz HB, Hartvigsen J, Christensen HW. Musculoskeletal dysfunctions in patients with chronic pelvic pain: a preliminary descriptive survey. *J Manipulative Physiol Ther*. 2016;39(9):616–622. doi:10.1016/j.jmpt.2016.09.003.

100. Prendergast SA. Screening for musculoskeletal causes of pelvic pain. *Clin Obstet Gynecol*. 2003;46(4):773–782.

101. Moore J, Kennedy S. Causes of chronic pelvic pain. *Bailliere's Best Pract Res Clin Obstet Gynaecol*. 2000;14(3):389–402. doi:10.1053/beog.1999.0082.

102. DeStefano LA. *Greenman's Principles of Manual Medicine*. 5th ed. Wolters Kluwer Health/Lippincott Williams & Wilkins; 2017.

103. Capson AC, Nashed J, Mclean L. The role of lumbopelvic posture in pelvic floor muscle activation in continent women. *J Electromyogr Kinesiol*. 2011;21(1):166–177. doi:10.1016/j.jelekin.2010.07.017.

104. Sapsford RR, Richardson CA, Stanton WR. Sitting posture affects pelvic floor muscle activity in parous women: an observational study. *Aust J Physiother*. 2006;52(3):219–222. doi:10.1016/S0004-9514(06)70031-9.

105. Sapsford RR, Richardson CA, Maher CF, Hodges PW. Pelvic floor muscle activity in different sitting postures in continent and incontinent women. *Arch Phys Med Rehabil*. 2008;89(9):1741–1747. doi:10.1016/j.apmr.2008.01.029.

106. D'Ambrogio KJ, Roth GB. *Positional Release Therapy: Assessment & Treatment of Musculoskeletal Dysfunction*. Mosby; 1997.

107. Donnelly JM, Fernandez-de-Las-Penas C, Finnegan M, Freeman JL. *Travell, Simons & Simons' Myofascial Pain and Dysfunction: The Trigger Point Manual*. 3rd ed. Wolters Kluwer Health/Lippincott Williams & Wilkins; 2018.

108. Jones LH, Kusunose RS, Goering EK. *Strain-Counterstrain*. Jones Strain Counterstrain Incorporated; 1995.

109. Kaltenborn F. *Manual Mobilization of the Joints, Volume II: The Spine*. 7th ed. Orthopedic Physical Therapy Products; 2018.

110. McKenzie RA, May S. *The Lumbar Spine: Mechanical Diagnosis & Therapy, Volume I and II*. 2nd ed. Spinal Publications; 2003.

111. Hengeveld E, Banks K, eds. *Maitland's Vertebral Manipulation: Management of Neuromusculoskeletal Disorders, Volume 1*. 8th ed. Churchill Livingston Elsevier.

112. Upledger JE. *Craniosacral Therapy II: Beyond the Dura*. Eastland Press; 1987.

113. Sutherland WG. *Teachings in the Science of Osteopathy*. Sutherland Cranial Teaching Foundation; 2003.

114. Bø K. Physiotherapy management of urinary incontinence in females. *J Physiother*. 2020;66(3):147–154. doi:10.1016/j.jphys.2020.06.011.

115. Price N, Dawood R, Jackson SR. Pelvic floor exercise for urinary incontinence: a systematic literature review. *Maturitas*. 2010;67(4):309–315. doi:10.1016/j.maturitas.2010.08.004.

116. Davis AM. Nonsurgical management of urinary incontinence in women. *JAMA*. 2017;317(1):79–80. doi:10.1001/jama.2016.18433.

117. Myers C, Smith M. Pelvic floor muscle training improves erectile dysfunction and premature ejaculation: a systematic review. *Physiother (United Kingdom)*. 2019;105(2):235–243. doi:10.1016/j.physio.2019.01.002.

118. de Freitas CS, HMF Pivetta, Vey APZ, Sperandio FF, Braz MM, Mazo GZ. Relationship between pelvic floor muscle and sexual function in physically active older women. *Fisioter em Mov*. 2020;33:1–9. doi:10.1590/1980-5918.033.ao23.

119. Nazarpour S, Simbar M, Majd HA, Tehrani FR. Beneficial effects of pelvic floor muscle exercises on sexual function among postmenopausal women: a randomised clinical trial. *Sex Health*. 2018;15(5):396–402. doi:10.1071/SH17203.

120. Stein A, Sauder SK, Reale J. The role of physical therapy in sexual health in men and women: evaluation and treatment. *Sex Med Rev*. 2019;7(1):46–56. doi:10.1016/j.sxmr.2018.09.003.

121. de Menezes Franco M, Driusso P, Bø K, et al. Relationship between pelvic floor muscle strength and sexual dysfunction in postmenopausal women: a cross-sectional study. *Int Urogynecol J*. 2017;28(6):931–936. doi:10.1007/s00192-016-3211-5.

122. Kandadai P, O'Dell K, Saini J. Correct performance of pelvic muscle exercises in women reporting prior knowledge. *Female Pelvic Med Reconstr Surg*. 2015;21(3):135–140. doi:10.1097/SPV.0000000000000145.

123. Kisner C, Colby L. *Therapeutic Exercise: Foundations and Techniques*. 5th ed. F.A. Davis Company; 2007.

124. Pfalzer LA. Physical agents/modalities for survivors of cancer. *Rehabil Oncol*. 2001;19(2):12–24.

125. Wilson A, Ensign G, Flyte K, Moore M, Ratliff K. Physical agents for cancer survivors: an updated literature review. *Rehabil Oncol*. 2017;36(2):1–9. doi:10.1097/01.REO.0000000000000081.

126. Cheville AL, Basford JR. Role of rehabilitation medicine and physical agents in the treatment of cancer-associated pain. *J Clin Oncol*. 2014;32(16):1691–1702. doi:10.1200/JCO.2013.53.6680.

127. Prentice WE. *Therapeutic Modalities in Rehabilitation*. 4th ed. McGraw-Hill Education; 2011.

128. LymphaTouch. *Clinical Proof Book*; 2021. https://www.lymphatouch.com/clinical-studies. Accessed June 16, 2022.

129. Gott FH, Ly K, Piller N, Mangio A. Negative pressure therapy in the management of lymphoedema. *J Lymphoedema*. 2018;13(1):43–48.

130. Stewart F, Berghmans B, Bo K, Glazener C. Electrical stimulation with non-implanted devices for stress urinary incontinence in women (Review). *Cochrane Database Syst Rev*. 2017;(12). doi:10.1002/14651858.CD012390.pub2. CD012390.

131. Stewart F, Gameiro L, El Dib R, Gameiro M, Kapoor A, Amaro J. Electrical stimulation with non-implanted electrodes for overactive bladder in adults (review). *Cochrane Database Syst Rev*. 2016;(12). doi:10.1002/14651858.CD010098.pub4. CD010098.

132. Schreiner L, dos Santos TG, de Souza ABA, Nygaard CC, da Silva Filho IG. Electrical stimulation for urinary incontinence in women: a systematic review. *Int Braz J Urol*. 2013;39(4):454–464. doi:10.1590/S1677-5538.IBJU.2013.04.02.

133. Herbison G, Dean N. Weighted vaginal cones for urinary incontinence. *Cochrane Database Syst Rev*. 2013;(7). doi:10.1002/14651858.CD002114.pub2. CD002114.

134. Liu M, Juravic M, Mazza G, Krychman ML. Vaginal dilators: issues and answers. *Sex Med Rev.* 2021;9(2):212–220. doi:10.1016/j.sxmr.2019.11.005.

135. Miles T, Johnson N. Vaginal dilator therapy for women receiving pelvic radiotherapy. *Cochrane Database Syst Rev.* 2014;2014(9):CD007291. doi:10.1002/14651858.CD007291.pub3.

136. Miles T, Johnson N. Vaginal dilator therapy for women receiving pelvic radiotherapy (Review). *Cochrane Database Syst Rev.* 2018(9). doi:10.1002/14651858.CD007291.pub3. CD007291.

137. Aslan M, Yavuzkır Ş, Baykara S. Is "Dilator use" more effective than "finger use" in exposure therapy in vaginismus treatment? *J Sex Marital Ther.* 2020;46(4):354–360. doi:10.1080/0092623X.2020.1716907.

138. Melnik T, Hawton K, McGuire H. Interventions for vaginismus. *Cochrane Database Syst Rev.* 2012;12(2):CD001760. doi:10.1002/14651858.cd001760.pub2.

139. Pacik PT. Understanding and treating vaginismus: a multimodal approach. *Int Urogynecol J Pelvic Floor Dysfunct.* 2014;25(12):1613–1620. doi:10.1007/s00192-014-2421-y.

140. Damast S, Jeffery DD, Son CH, et al. Literature review of vaginal stenosis and dilator use in radiation oncology. *Pract Radiat Oncol.* 2019;9(6). doi:10.1016/j.prro.2019.07.001.

141. Miles T. International guidelines on vaginal dilation after pelvic radiotherapy. *Int Clin Guidel Gr.* 2012. https://owenmumford.com/us/wp-content/uploads/sites/3/2014/11/Dilator-Best-Practice-Guidelines.pdf.

142. De Lima Matos SR, Cunha MLR, Podgaec S, Weltman E, Centrone AFY, Mafra ACCN. Consensus for vaginal stenosis prevention in patients submitted to pelvic radiotherapy. *PLoS One.* 2019;14(8):2–3. doi:10.1371/journal.pone.0221054.

143. Cerentini TM, Schlöttgen J, Viana da Rosa P, et al. Clinical and psychological outcomes of the use of vaginal dilators after gynaecological brachytherapy: a randomized clinical trial. *Adv Ther.* 2019;36(8):1936–1949. doi:10.1007/s12325-019-01006-4.

144. Stahl JM, Qian JM, Tien CJ, et al. Extended duration of dilator use beyond 1 year may reduce vaginal stenosis after intravaginal high-dose-rate brachytherapy. *Support Care Cancer.* 2019;27(4):1425–1433. doi:10.1007/s00520-018-4441-5.

145. Jeffrey A, Harrington SE, Hill A, Roscow A, Alappattu M. Oncology section EDGE Task Force on urogenital cancer: a systematic review of clinical measures for incontinence. *Rehabil Oncol.* 2017;35(3):130–136. doi:10.1097/01.REO.0000000000000068.

146. Alappattu M, Harrington SE, Hill A, Roscow A, Jeffrey A. Oncology section EDGE Task Force on cancer: a systematic review of patient-reported measures for sexual dysfunction. *Rehabil Oncol.* 2017;35(3):137–143. doi:10.1097/01.reo.0000000000000071.

147. White ID, Sangha A, Lucas G, Wiseman T. Assessment of sexual difficulties associated with multi-modal treatment for cervical or endometrial cancer: a systematic review of measurement instruments. *Gynecol Oncol.* 2016;143(3):664–673. doi:10.1016/j.ygyno.2016.08.332.

17

Colorectal Cancer

ALAINA M. NEWELL, PT, DPT, BOARD-CERTIFIED CLINICAL SPECIALIST IN WOMEN'S
HEALTH PHYSICAL THERAPY, BOARD-CERTIFIED CLINICAL SPECIALIST IN ONCOLOGIC
PHYSICAL THERAPY, LANA-CERTIFIED LYMPHEDEMA THERAPIST

CHAPTER OUTLINE

Anatomy and Physiology of the Colon

As one looks to provide oncology rehabilitation (Onc R) care for individuals with colorectal cancer (CRC), understanding the anatomy and physiology of the large intestine as well as the development of lesions, medical oncology treatment options, and the adverse effect presentation is critical to perform a comprehensive evaluation and construct a holistic plan of care for this population. First, the gastrointestinal (GI) tract, digestive tract, or alimentary canal encompasses many organs, which can be subdivided into the upper and lower GI tracts. The lower GI tract includes both the small intestine and large intestine. The small intestine consists of the duodenum, jejunum, and ileum and has the primary function of absorbing products from digestion (including carbohydrates, proteins, lipids, and vitamins) into the bloodstream. The large intestine, often referred to as the colon, also consists of the cecum, appendix, rectum, and anal canal (Figure 17.1). The colon is divided into the following sections, each with a different function and anatomical location: cecum, appendix, ascending colon, transverse colon, descending colon, sigmoid colon, rectum, and anus. The overall function of the large intestine is water absorption from digested food (chyme) and the formation of feces to perform

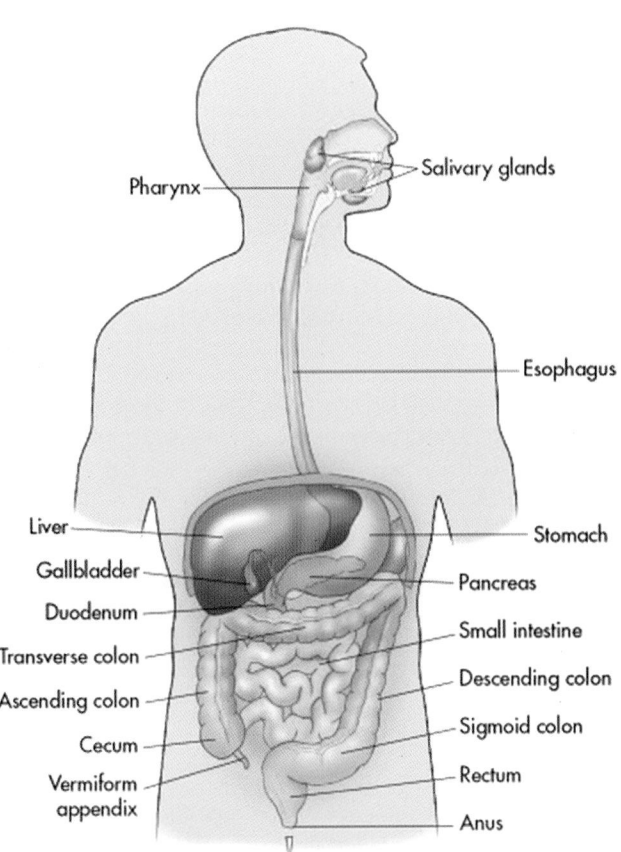

• **Fig. 17.1** The Complete Gastrointestinal System Pictured and Labeled. Colorectal Cancers are Those Present From the Cecum Through Rectum. (Reprinted with permission from Hagen-Ansert SL. *Textbook of Diagnostic Sonography*. Elsevier; 2018:64–80.)

waste removal from the body effectively. This chapter discusses the Onc R needs of persons living with and beyond cancers (PLWBCs) in the cecum through the rectum, collectively known as CRCs.

Colorectal cancer genetic markers, prognostic factors, and treatment options are partially based on the tumor location. Understanding human embryonic development aids in supporting an Onc R clinician's understanding of these factors. The gut is an endoderm-derived structure; it forms from the most inner layer of the three primary germ layers of the very early embryo. This inner layer consists of a single row of flattened cells that form the epithelial lining of multiple body systems, including the GI tract, respiratory tract, endocrine glands and organs, auditory system, and urinary system.[1] Both the GI and respiratory tracts are tubes within the body that allow the body to interact with the environment to gain vital resources necessary to continue life, including food, water, and air. As the fetus develops, the primitive gut is divided into three segments: foregut, midgut, and hindgut. The foregut consists of the esophagus to the first two sections of the duodenum. The midgut runs from the lower duodenum to the first two-thirds of the transverse colon, and the hindgut is the last third of the transverse colon to the upper part of the anal canal. These primitive gut segments are delineated by the arterial, venous, and lymphatic supply to the GI tract and are implicated in the metastatic spread of CRC.

The hollow tubular structure of the GI tract is composed of four functional layers from deep to superficial: mucosa, submucosa, muscular layer, and adventitia or serosa. The mucosa in the

innermost layer surrounds the lumen (open space within the tube) and directly interacts with the chyme. The submucosal layer is a dense irregular layer of connective tissue that includes vascular, lymphatic vessels, and nerves that serve the mucosa and muscular layer. The muscular layer performs peristalsis to propel digestive contents through the digestive system and is regulated internally as well as by the autonomic nervous system. Lastly, the external most layer of connective tissue is dependent on the location: intraperitoneal or retroperitoneal. Serosa covers the intraperitoneal to differentiate the gut and surrounding tissues and is connected to the mesentery. Adventitia covers the retroperitoneal portions (i.e., ascending and descending colon), which blend with the surrounding tissue and are fixed in place. In evaluating an individual's viscera and while performing colon massage, it is essential to recognize this anatomical location and the implications that connective tissue manipulation will have on these structures. Understanding the anatomy and base physiology of the large intestine will aid in a deeper appreciation of the changes that occur within the system during surgery, chemotherapy, and radiation and understanding medical oncology treatment options available for individuals with CRC.

Demographics, Prevalence, and Prognosis

Prevalence

CRC is often considered the most preventable yet least prevented cancer, with approximately 150,000 new cases each year.[2,3] In the United States (US), CRC is the fourth leading new cancer diagnosis and the second cause of death with around 53,200 (higher than either breast or prostate cancer). Worldwide, CRC is the third highest diagnosed cancer with 1.88 million and second highest deaths (916,000) in 2020.[4] CRC is more prevalent, with a higher mortality rate in males and Blacks, American Indians, and Alaska Natives.[3] More than 75% of persons are diagnosed between 45 and 85 years of age, with a mean age of 67. With a rise in regular screenings, the demographics of people with CRC have been a changing landscape. From 2011 to 2016 there was a 3% drop in cases among people over the age of 65 and an increase in those younger with a 1% and 2.2% increase in individuals between 50 and 64 and less than 50 years old, respectively. There has also been a shift in the mortality rate with a decline of 3% in people over 65, a decline of 0.6% in people 50 to 64 but an increase by 1.3% in those younger than 50 years old. While the population under 50 years old makes up only about 12% of all CRC cases, these cases tend to be more aggressive, diagnosed at later stages, and have higher mortality rates.[5] In the young adult population, persons aged 15 to 39 years old, CRC is now the fourth most common cancer-causing death.[3]

Risk Factors

Many lifestyle/modifiable factors have been linked to CRC, including obesity, sedentary lifestyle, tobacco use, alcohol consumption, and certain types of diets. Diets high in red and processed meats create an increased CRC risk. Additional nonmodifiable risk factors include a personal history of colorectal polyps, CRC, inflammatory bowel disease, Crohn's disease, abdominal radiation, a familial history of CRC or adenomatous polyps, having an inherited syndrome, and having Type 2 diabetes, irrespective of common characteristics such as obesity and low physical activity. While most persons with CRC do not have a family history, a third will have family members with CRC.[6] At this time, only about 5% of people who develop CRC have a known inherited genetic mutation linked to their cancer diagnosis.[6,7] While it is unclear why the rise in younger adults is occurring, investigations into dietary factors are being considered.

Prognosis

Similar to many cancers, the stage strongly influences the prognosis of CRC at diagnosis. In the CRC population, 38% are confined to the primary site (localized), 35% have a regional spread, 22% have distant or metastatic disease, and 4% have unknown staging in the US.[6] The more localized the disease, the less intervention that is typically required and with a better prognosis. Persons with localized, regional, and distant disease have a 90.2%, 71.8%, and 14.3% 5-year survival rate, respectively.[3] As Onc R clinicians, it is important to remember that many patients actively undergo treatment through their final years, and 5-year survival rates do not equate to 5 "treatment-free" years, and will have continued rehabilitation needs during this period and potentially beyond.

Investigations in the last few decades have revolved around tumor sidedness in relation to prognosis, genetic mutation presentation, and treatment efficacy. Tumor sidedness has many differential characteristics, and there is a slight majority (52.3%) of right-sided colon cancers (RCC).[8] People with these tumors have worsened survival and higher recurrence rate than left-sided colon cancers (LCC).[9] Of all CRC diagnoses, about a third are diagnosed as rectal cancer, though the rate of survival is stage-dependent. As an overall population, colon and rectal cancers have a similar prognosis.[10]

While the overall prevalence of cases and deaths has been on the decline over the last 20 years, CRC remains highly preventable as the disease has a precancerous phase, the adenomatous polyp. Adenomatous polyps originate in the epithelial lining of the mucosa and are typically slow-growing and are usually readily detectable by structural examination. The most common visual screening tools utilized are colonoscopy, sigmoidoscopy, and computed tomography colonography. To address some of the barriers to visual examination-based screening tools, stool-based screening tools have been developed to evaluate the fecal immunochemistry or detect colorectal neoplasia-associated DNA markers and the presence of occult hemoglobin. The 2018 American Cancer Society (ACS) guidelines recommend (1) screening to begin at age 45 for individuals in good health with the life expectancy of more than 10 years and continue screening through age 75; (2) clinicians individualize CRC screening for people between 76 and 85 years based on life expectancy, health status and prior screen history; and (3) clinicians should discourage individuals over 85 years old from continuing CRC screening. Options for CRC screening include fecal immunochemical test yearly; high-sensitivity, guaiac-based fecal occult blood test yearly; multitarget stool DNA test every three years; computed tomography colonography every five years; flexible sigmoidoscopy every five years; and colonoscopy every 10 years.[11] Utilization of population screening not only prevents neoplasms by precancerous polyp removal, but it also detects cancers at earlier stages. This early detection is critical to have a population shift in the overall survival rate. Unfortunately, about a third of Americans who should be screened for CRC have never been screened.[11] As healthcare professionals, Onc R clinicians have a role in patient education and advocacy for screening and early detection.

Medical Diagnosis

Screening evaluations are of principal importance because most CRCs are diagnosed as adenocarcinoma, and often symptoms do not present until later stages of the disease. When symptoms do appear, the most common include a change in bowel habits such as new diarrhea, constipation, narrowing of the stool that lasts for more than a few days, fecal urgency in the absence of stool, rectal bleeding, dark or bloody stools, abdominal cramping or pain, weakness, fatigue, and unintended weight loss. If a person presents with such symptoms, CRC should be ruled out through diagnostic colonoscopy, polypectomy, and biopsy. Multiple biopsies will be performed during a diagnostic colonoscopy to determine the immunohistochemistry and evaluation of the genetic profile and microsatellite instability (MSI). Additional imaging utilized to confirm the diagnosis includes computed tomography (CT) scan, chest X-ray, positron emission tomography (PET) scan, and endorectal magnetic resonance imaging (MRI) scan. While blood tests cannot determine CRC, they may be performed to monitor the person's overall health, including liver and kidney function, and monitoring carcinoembryonic antigen (CEA) to determine response to treatment. Based on the tumor location, histology, and metastatic spread, a diagnostic stage and grade will be determined.

Staging and Grading

After tumor identification, a stage and grade will be assigned that will influence the medical treatment. The American Joint Committee on Cancer (AJCC) classification and staging system has established a naming convention to describe the location of the primary tumor (T), invasion to regional lymph nodes (N), and presence of metastatic disease (M), known as TNM collectively, as well as the aggressive nature of the disease based on the histological presentation of the cancer cells compared to healthy cells by the grading (G) scale (Table 17.1).[12] While the stage assigned at the time of diagnosis will remain with the PLWBC through their continuum of life, healthcare providers may reassign the TNM designation to demonstrate the change in disease process over time or response to treatment (Table 17.2).

Right-Sided Versus Left-Sided Colon Cancer

Along with the stage and grade, the sidedness of colon cancer will be described with the diagnostic profile as it has implications of metastatic disease presentation, medical management, and prognosis, as previously stated. Colon cancer sidedness is based on the embryonic development division of midgut (RCC) and hindgut (LCC). The RCC involves the cecum, appendix, ascending colon, and two-thirds of the transverse colon and has neural-lymph-vascularly supplied by the superior mesenteric plexus, lymph nodes, and vessels, respectively. The LCC initiates at the distal third of the transverse colon, descending colon, and sigmoid colon and supplied by the inferior mesenteric plexus, lymph nodes, and vessels. Many differences are present between RCC and LCC, as shown in Table 17.3.[13] The therapeutic approach is enhanced through the clinician's knowledge of tumor physiology and presentation and awareness of the metastatic disease during differential diagnosis of an individual's impairments.

Genetics

The final tumor characteristics that can influence medical management are based on the person's genetic profile and the tumor.

| TABLE 17.1 | American Joint Committee on Cancer (AJCC) TNM Staging Criteria for Colorectal Cancer Along With Grading System to Describe Cancer Presentation[12] |

Tumor (T) Describes Depth of Lesion Into Bowel Lining		Node (N) Invasion of Regional Lymph Nodes		Metastasis (M) Distal Spread of Disease		Grade (G) Morphology of Cancer Cells	
TX	Primary tumor cannot be evaluated	NX	LNs cannot be evaluated	MX	Unable to evaluate	GX	Unable to evaluate
Tis	Tumor in situ	N0	No spread to LNs	M0	No distal spread	G1	Well-differentiated
T0	No evidence colorectum	N1a	Cells in 1 LN	M1a	Spread to 1 other location	G2	Moderately differentiated
T1	Tumor in submucosa	N1b	Cells in 2–3 LNs	M1b	Spread to >1 location	G3	Poorly differentiated
T2	Tumor in muscularis propria	N1c	Nodule structures near colon that do not appear to be LNs	M1c	Spread to peritoneal surface	G4	Undifferentiated, aplastic
T3	Tumor in subserosa	N2a	Cells in 4–6 LNs				
T4a	Tumor through all colon layers	N2b	Cells in 7+ LNs				
T4b	Tumor grown into or attached to other organs/structures						

LN, Lymph nodes.
Created by Alaina Marie Newell. Printed with permission.

| TABLE 17.2 | Cancer Staging Based on Combination of TNM Classifications[12] |

Stage	TNM	Description
0	Tis, N0, M0	In situ, cancer cells limited to mucosa
I	T1 or T2, N0, M0	Cancer has grown through mucosa and invaded the muscular layer
IIA	T3, N0, M0	Cancer has grown through the wall of the colon or rectum but has not spread to lymph nodes
IIB	T4a, N0, M0	Cancer has grown through the muscle to the visceral peritoneum
IIC	T4b, N0, M0	Cancer has grown through the colon or rectum and into nearby structures but not into lymph nodes
IIIA	T1 or T2, N1, or N1c, M0 T1, N2a, M0	Cancer has grown through mucosa or into muscle layer and spread to 1–3 lymph nodes or nodules near the colorectum
IIIB	T3–T4a, N1–N1c, M0 T2–T3, N2a, M0 T1–T2, N2b, M0	Cancer has grown through bowel wall or to surrounding organs and into 1–3 lymph nodes or nodules near the colorectum
IIIC	T4a, N2a, M0 T3–T4a, N2b, M0 T4b, N1–N2, M0	Regardless the depth of the tumor has spread to 4 or more lymph nodes
IVA	T1–T4b, N0–N2b, M1a	Cancer has spread to a single distant part of the body
IVB	T1–T4b, N0–N2b, M1b	Cancer has spread to more than one distant part of the body
IVC	T1–T4b, N0–N2b, M1c	Cancer has spread to the peritoneum

TNM, Location of the primary tumor (T), invasion to regional lymph nodes (N), and presence of metastatic disease (M).
Created by Alaina Marie Newell. Printed with permission.

Like many solid tissue tumors, CRC is a heterogeneous disease of subtypes based on molecular features. Approximately 85% of CRC exhibit sporadic chromosomal instability (CIN), resulting in a change in the chromosomal number or structure. The RAS family of genes is strongly linked to CRC, which presents as wild-type *KRAS* or *NRAS*. These result in overexpression of proteins, supporting cancerous growth. Some chemotherapies are ineffective if RAS wild-type is present. Another common mutation, occurring in 5% to 9% of CRC, is a *BRAF* mutation that results in rapid malignant growth and is susceptible to *BRAF* inhibitors for metastatic disease.[14] The remaining sporadic cases (~15%) have high-frequency microsatellite instability (MSI). These genetic presentations are also seen in two common inherited genetic mutations: familial adenomatous polyposis (FAP) and hereditary nonpolyposis colorectal cancer (HNPCC), also known as Lynch syndrome, respectively.[15] HNPCC is the most common hereditary CRC syndrome and accounts for 2% to 4% of all CRC.

TABLE 17.3 **Difference Between Right- and Left-Sided Colon Tumors**[13,19,34]

Right-Sided Colon Cancers	Left-Sided Colon Cancers
Mucinous adenocarcinomas, sessile serrated adenomas	Tubular, villous adenocarcinomas
Flat like morphology	Polypoid like morphology
MSI-high and MMR tumors	CIN-high tumors
Highly immunogenic, high T cell infiltration	Low immunogenic
Metastases in peritoneal region	Liver and lung metastases
Occur in older ages	Occur in younger ages
Predominately occur in female	Predominately occur in male
Better prognosis at early stages (Stage I and II)	Better prognosis at late stages (Stage III and IV)
Respond well to immunotherapy	Respond well to adjuvant chemotherapies (system and targeted)
Derive from the midgut	Derive from the hindgut

CIN, Chromosomal instability; *MMR*, mismatch repair; *MSI*, microsatellite instability.
Created by Alaina Marie Newell. Printed with permission.

In most cases, the syndrome is caused by a mutation in either the *MLH1, MSH2, MSH6,* or *PMS2* gene used to repair damaged or mismatched DNA and leads to MSI.[15] Most people diagnosed with CRC receive their diagnosis at younger ages, and the lifetime risk of developing CRC is 50%.[15] Many other cancers are linked to Lynch syndrome, including endometrial, ovarian, gastric, small intestine, pancreatic, kidney, prostate, breast, ureter, and bile duct cancers. These individuals should be placed on a higher screening protocol for those cancers.[6] The second most prevalent inherited condition, FAP, makes up 1% of all CRC. People with FAP develop hundreds or thousands of polyps due to a mutated copy of the adenomatous polyposis (APC) gene. These individuals begin developing polyps around 10 to 12 years of age, and typically, one or more become cancerous by the age of 40, in the absence of prophylactic colon removal. These individuals are also at a higher risk for cancer within other GI tract organs such as the stomach, small intestine, pancreas, and liver.[6] The genetic mutations, either sporadic or inherited, lead to variations in treatment options, specifically concerning the effectiveness of chemotherapy agents, including immunotherapy.

Surgical Management for Colon Cancer

The determination of appropriate medical management requires consideration of the multiple factors discussed above and the person's age, general health status, and potential improvement of quality of life (QOL). Surgical management is utilized for CRC of all stages, though treatment goals vary based on the stage and grade. As outlined in the National Cancer Coalition Network's (NCCN) clinical practice guidelines, local resection of Stage 0 in situ adenocarcinomas is routinely performed during diagnostic colonoscopies and is known as a polypectomy. The majority of Stage I tumors will only require surgical resection of the tumor and lymph node removal. In Stage II and III disease, surgery is recommended as the primary intervention unless the tumor is staged T4b (spread to nearby sites) or it is predetermined that the tumor cannot be removed. In these cases, neoadjuvant chemotherapy is advised before surgical removal. In the presence of metastatic disease, Stage IV cancer, the lesion(s) location and size will determine the best intervention plan. Resection of the primary tumor and

metastases may be performed, or the person may undergo neoadjuvant chemotherapy. Treatment pathways are determined by the treating medical professionals, consulting clinicians, and the person with cancer to meet their goals and QOL desires.[14]

A colectomy is the primary surgery to remove CRC lesions and remove the diseased portion of the colon and reattachment/reconnection of the healthy tissues. Concurrently, a lymphadenectomy is performed to remove the lymphatic tree, including the lymph nodes that serve the section of the colon. This allows for surveillance of regional metastatic spread. The lymph nodes are known as visceral lymph nodes, serving the organs and are not directly involved in the parietal lymphatic tree that serves the lower body. This surgery does not increase the person's risk for lower body lymphedema, but they should be evaluated for lymphedema of the remaining bowel, known as visceral lymphedema.[16] If the lesion is large, obstructing the bowel, or suspected to require additional healing time, a diversion of the colon to the abdominal wall, resulting in a stoma, may be required. For many PLWBCs, this procedure is a temporary ostomy and will be reversed later. The stoma location depends on tumor or bowel obstruction location and is placed more proximal to the obstruction in the digestive tract. Ideally, the stoma will be distal as possible to allow for as much natural digestion to occur before evacuation through the stoma.

Surgical Management for Rectal Cancer

Conceptually, surgical management of rectal cancer is similar to colon cancer except it occurs in the rectum. In Stage 0, a polypectomy will be performed with follow-up surveillance colonoscopy. The risk of recurrence will determine the plan of care for Stage I disease. Smaller (T1) and low-risk cancers will be treated with transanal local resection or transabdominal resection and follow-up surveillance. If the cancer is staged T1 and considered high-risk or T2, radiation and chemotherapy are recommended as primary interventions. Surgical and additional chemotherapeutic intervention may be considered based on the initial effectiveness of the primary treatment. For Stage II–IV rectal cancer, chemoradiation is the primary treatment recommendation. The surgical protocol is determined by the location and size of the lesion upon the conclusion of the primary treatment.[17]

TABLE 17.4 Definition of Rectal Cancer Surgical Resections

Surgery	Definition
Transanal local resection	Removal of small distal rectal tumors near the anus, fat in the region via the anal canal
Transabdominal surgery	Surgical approach through the abdominal wall
Total mesorectal excision	Removal of rectum, fat, lymph nodes, and membrane. Nerve sparing technique
Lower anterior resection	Total mesorectal excision (TME) + removal of sigmoid colon
Abdominoperineal resection	Removal of rectum, anus, levator ani musculature with diversion of colon to ostomy
Ostomy	Relocation of intestine to through the abdominal wall (formation) of a stoma

Created by Alaina Marie Newell. Printed with permission.

Transanal local resection consists of tumor resection near the anus, leaving the anal musculature intact and therefore preserving continence. Transabdominal surgery can include one of three options: total mesorectal excision (TME) + anastomosis, lower anterior resection (LAR) + anastomosis, abdominoperineal resection (APR) + permanent colostomy (Table 17.4). TME is the standard surgery for rectal cancer and involves removing the rectum, nearby fat, and lymph structures. A LAR is performed in the middle to upper rectal cancers, which includes a TME and sigmoid colon removal. Following these procedures, colon anastomosis is performed to connect the bowel together. For lower rectal cancers, an APR removes the tumor along with the anus and pelvic floor musculature (levator ani). In this case, a permanent colectomy is performed as the individual will not have bowel control following the APR.

Oncology Rehabilitation Evaluation of Persons Managed by Surgical Intervention

A comprehensive Onc R evaluation includes examining and evaluating all body systems to elucidate the severity of movement-related impact resultant of the CRC and its associated medical management (Figure 17.2). This section outlines significant impacts based on the body system of each intervention to guide Onc R clinicians through clinical pathways toward efficient and effective treatment. Onc R clinicians should recognize each PLWBC will have a unique presentation based on past medical history, medical oncology treatment, physical and social environment, and prior life experiences. More than half of people with CRC have regional or distal metastatic disease and require medical management beyond surgical resection. This is relevant because Onc R needs are derived from adverse effect presentation, resulting from surgical management and chemotherapy and radiation interventions. The predominant feature for PLWBCs who undergo surgical resections for CRC is the presence or absence of an ostomy diversion. For all PLWBCs, three major body systems are impacted: musculoskeletal, integumentary, and GI.

Gastrointestinal System Evaluation

To allow for stool evacuation, a stoma is placed in the skin to allow the bowel contents to exit the body. Proper fitting of an ostomy pouch is critical to reduce the impact on and maintain the integumentary system's integrity. A healthcare team member educates the PLWBC postoperatively on measuring, fitting, and applying an ostomy appliance. Onc R clinicians screen for signs of infection or skin irritation, especially if a PLWBC is immunocompromised from chemotherapy management. During Onc R evaluation, the skills of the PLWBC should be screened to ensure they can obtain effective appliance fit, have an emptying schedule to allow for sufficient sleep, chose clothing to avoid direct pressure, understand the impact on abdominal muscle activation, and demonstrate positioning to avoid direct pressure with activities of daily living (ADLs), work, and recreation. PLWBCs in the early postoperative phase may benefit from additional wound care follow-up or referral to a registered dietitian nutritionist (RDN) to adjust to the ostomy and support QOL with an incomplete digestive system. The ostomy location will determine the impact on digestion and nutritional status. The more distal the ostomy location, the greater the amount of digestion and water reabsorption that occurs. Screening for frequency of evacuations (>3 times/day, 1×/night), amount of hydration, and maintenance of body weight (maintain within 10% of preostomy weight) assist in determining the impact of the ostomy on the GI system as well as the PLWBC's nutritional status. Sufficient sleep is critical for healing, though it is often challenging for PLWBCs who have an ostomy. If the individual is waking >1×/night to empty their appliance, altered timing of food intake and consultation with durable medical equipment (DME) providers for larger-sized bags is suggested.

Integumentary and Lymphatic System Evaluation

Scar mobility assessment is another essential component of the PLWBC's integumentary system. Scar restrictions or adhesions can result in increased pain and inhibition of abdominal musculature. Evaluation should include mobilization in a single plane and multi-plane directions, including rotation to support the movement necessary for ADLs, work, and recreation.[18]

Regardless of the type of resection the PLWBC undergoes, the lymphatic system (in coordination with the GI), should be evaluated and managed to reduce the incidence of visceral lymphedema or bowel inflammation following lymphadenectomy. As discussed in Chapter 9, understanding the functional healing of the tissue in the presence of delayed fluid management is critical to support long-term GI function. Evaluation should include palpation of the abdomen, both intraperitoneal and extraperitoneal, to assess the presence of edema within the integumentary system, myofascial, and GI system. Extraperitoneal edema or lymphedema is an uncommon adverse effect of surgical management as visceral, not parietal lymph nodes are removed. Palpation of the colon, abdominal distention, and bowel function are utilized to determine if visceral lymphedema is present. If this is the case, follow-up care should be performed.

Musculoskeletal System Evaluation

Movement specialists understand the impact the ostomy has on the musculoskeletal system, which is critical for effective strength

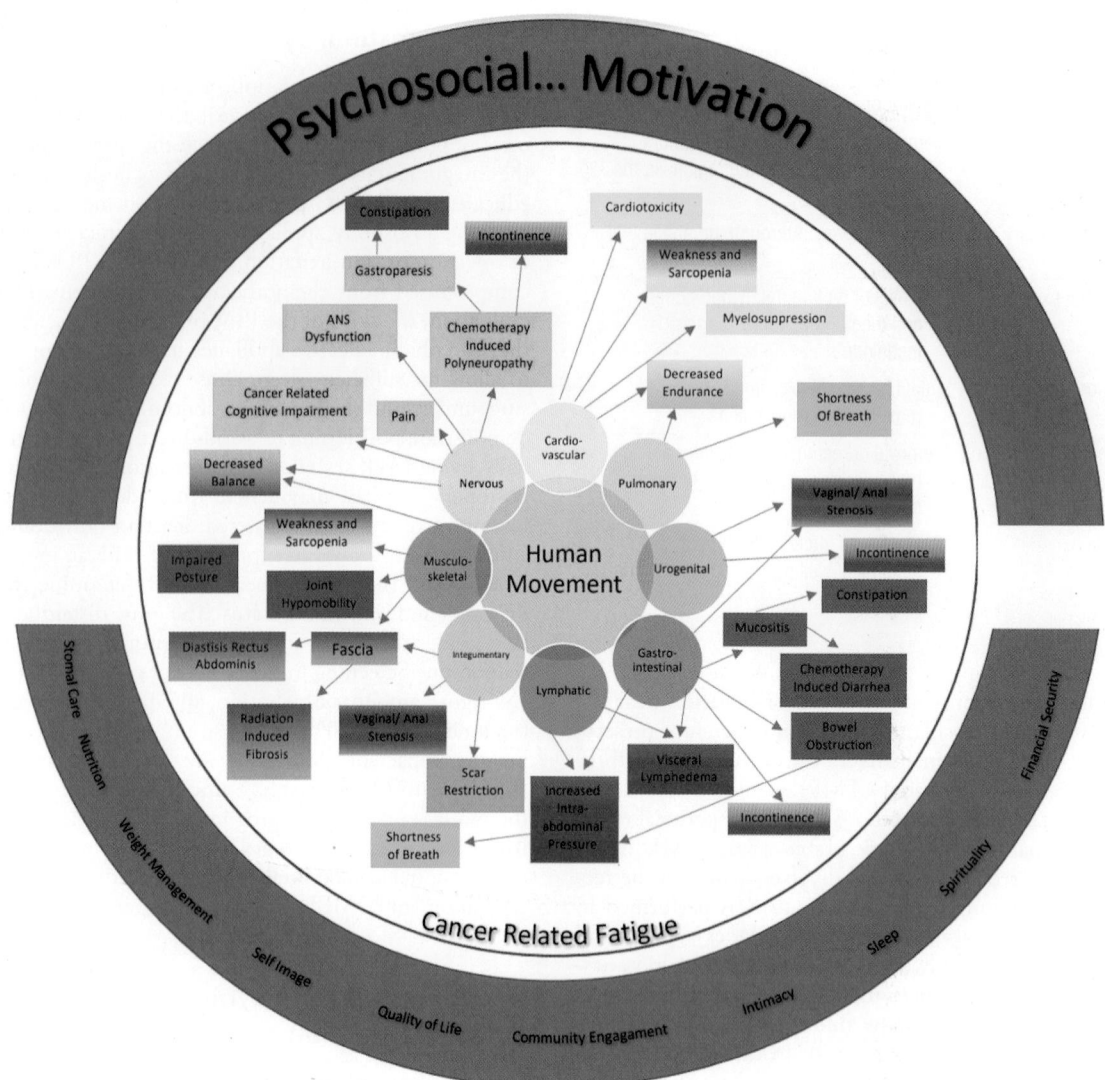

• **Fig. 17.2** The Complexity of Adverse Effects Based on Human Movement and Body Systems That Cancer Rehabilitation Providers Address are Diagramed Within the Figure. (Image was modified and reprinted with permission of the American Physical Therapy Association. © 2020 American Physical Therapy Association. All rights reserved.)

training following surgery. When a stoma is present, there is a disruption to the abdominal musculature reducing support of the trunk and spine, as evidenced with PLWBCs with complications such as abdominal hernia.[19] Patient education is essential related to the change in abdominal musculature, positional impacts (avoiding prone lying and direct pressure to the stoma), and assuring a PLWBC that they are able to return to exercise and sport with a stoma. These will help to support the return to physical activity and reduce the development of sarcopenia following surgery.[20–22] When performing functional strength assessment and exercise training, vertical positions, such as sitting and standing, are preferred to supine to reduce the tensile force applied to the fascia around the stoma (Figures 17.3 and 17.4)

For a PLWBC who is functioning at a lower level, evaluation can be performed in standing posture, as demonstrated in Figures 17.5 and 17.6. A PLWBC postcolectomy with anastomosis or following ostomy reversal should be evaluated for the presence of an abdominal hernia. Incidence of hernia following colorectal surgery ranges from 10% to 52%.[20] Hernias often form in the first few months postoperatively. They are more prevalent

in a PLWBC with the following characteristics: higher body mass index (BMI), advanced age, chronic cough, hypertension, wound healing complications, presence of a parastomal hernia, and presence of stoma prolapse.[23–25] Hernia evaluation is performed in an upright posture by observation for an outward bulge during a sit-to-stand transfer or a squat with arms overhead (Figure 17.7). Hernias often present in the abdomen near an incision and result from a greater amount of intra-abdominal pressure (IAP) than the tensile strength of the myofascial tissues can withstand. Onc R education should include hernia prevention, including proper body mechanics with lifting, squatting, carrying, toileting, and transfers as the functional strength of the abdomen is most reduced in the early phases of the postoperative period. An abdominal binder is recommended to support this musculature in early recovery as high IAP often occurs throughout daily life activities, including bed and chair transfers. Binders can be utilized in individuals with ostomies, though space should be cut out of the binder around where the ostomy site is located. While imperfect, a modified binder can help reduce hernia incidence (35%) and sequela, including low back pain in patients with ostomies.[19,26] A

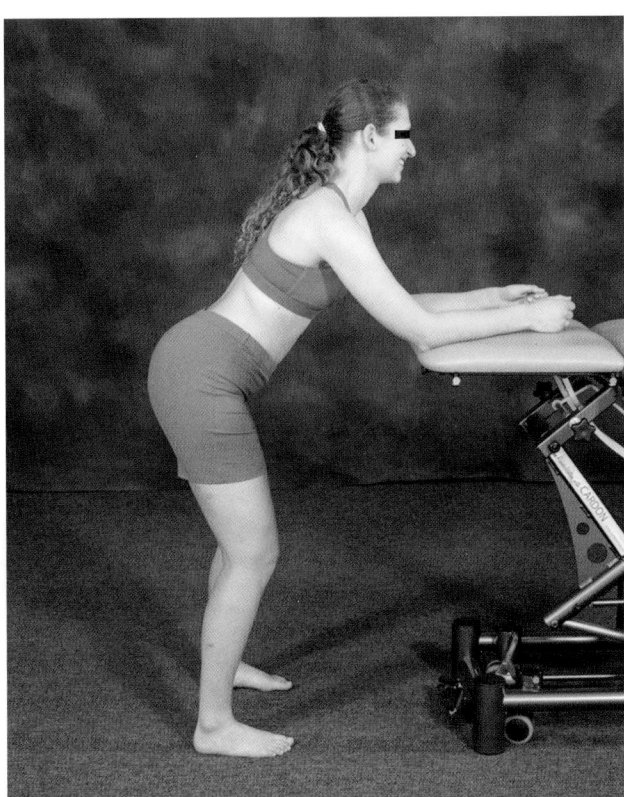

• **Fig. 17.3** Functional Strengthening Position at a Counter Allowing for Reduced Weight Bearing, Closed Kinetic Chain, and Reduced Stoma Tension for Abdominal Muscle Strengthening. (Printed with permission from John Krauss, PT, PhD, OMPT, OCS.)

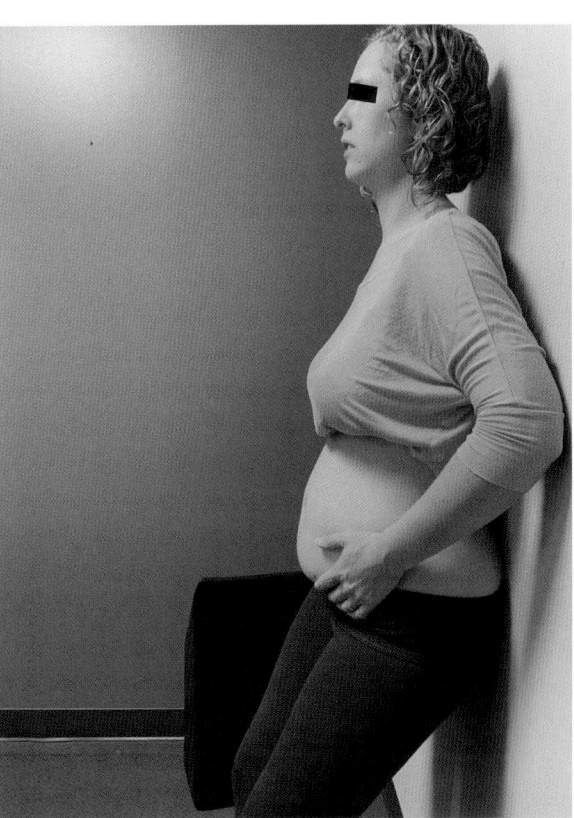

• **Fig. 17.5** Alternative Vertical Position Is Demonstrated With Use of a Wall Support. This Position Allows for Self-Palpation of Abdominal Musculature During Strengthening Exercise. (Printed with permission from Melissa Buss.)

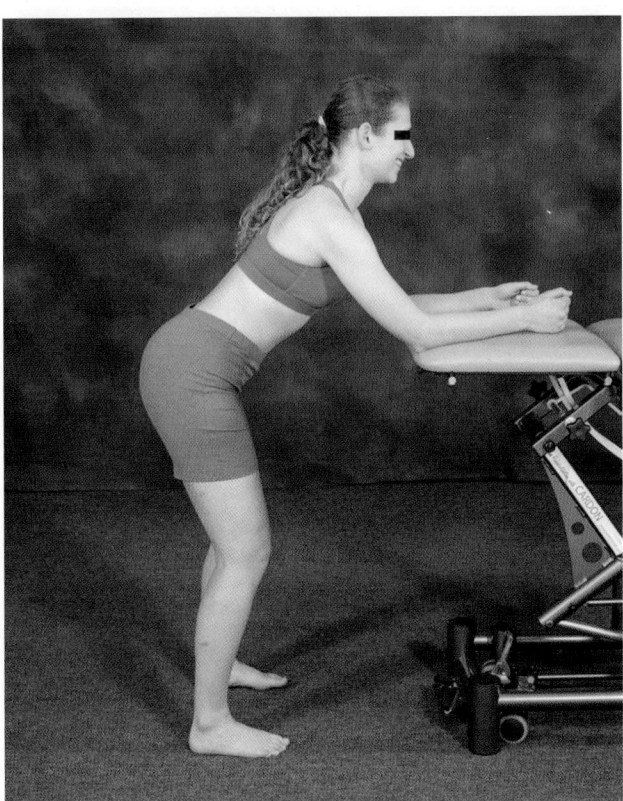

• **Fig. 17.4** Transverse Abdominal Muscle Activation is Demonstrated in a Functional Vertical Position with Counter Support. (Printed with permission from John Krauss, PT, PhD, OMPT, OCS.)

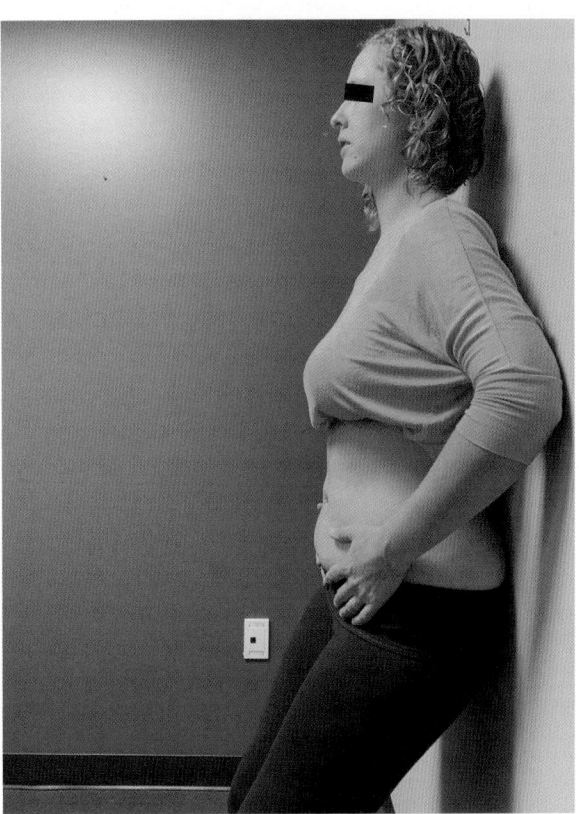

• **Fig. 17.6** Transverse Abdominal Muscle Activation Is Demonstrated in a Functional Vertical Position With Wall Support. (Printed with permission from Melissa Buss.)

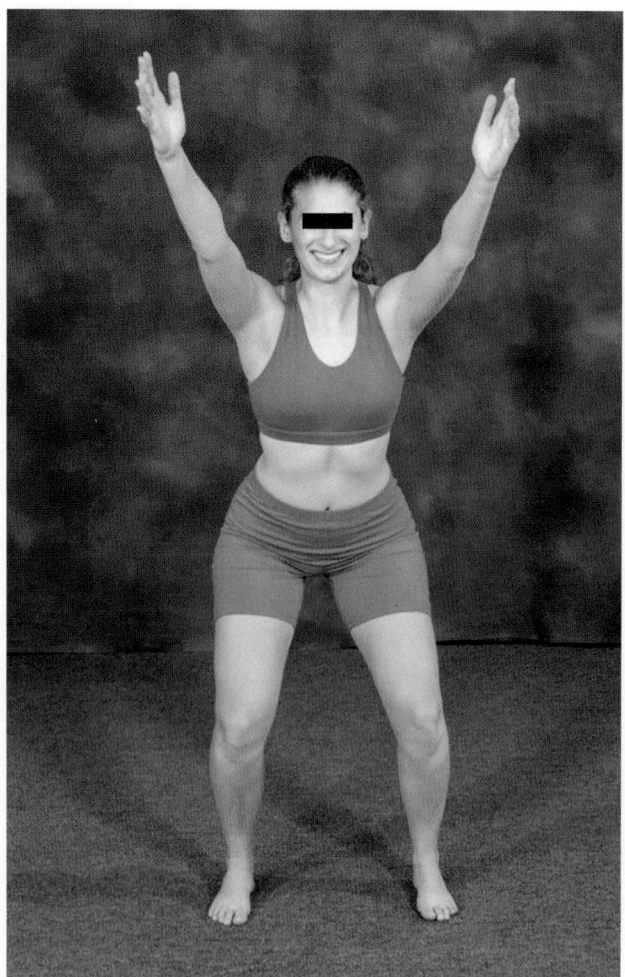

• **Fig. 17.7** Hernia Evaluation Is Completed During an Overhead Squat for Observation of an Outward Bulge. (Printed with permission from John Krauss, PT, PhD, OMPT, OCS.)

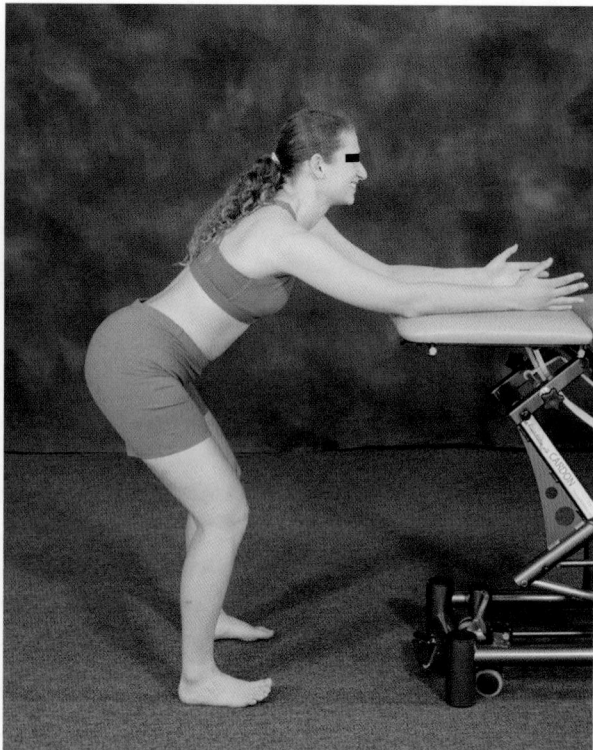

• **Fig. 17.8** Low Level Trunk Strength Assessment in De-Weighted Posture Utilizing a Counter for Support. The Person Living With and Beyond Cancer (PLWBC) Performs Abdominal Activation Throughout a Full Range Squat. (Printed with permission from John Krauss, PT, PhD, OMPT, OCS.)

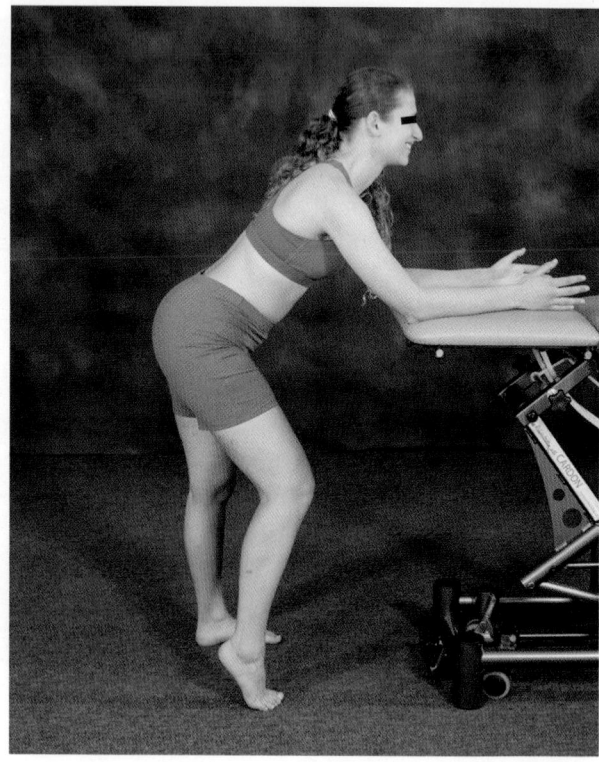

• **Fig. 17.9** Low Level Trunk Strength Assessment in a De-Weighted Posture Utilizing a Counter for Support. The Person Living With and Beyond Cancer (PLWBC) Performs Abdominal Activation and Maintains Alignment with Partial Weight Bearing Heel Raise. (Printed with permission from John Krauss, PT, PhD, OMPT, OCS.)

PLWBC's trunk strength and balance should be evaluated as there is often a reduced strength of the unilateral transverse abdominis with an ostomy present.[19] This bilateral strength differential can lead to an imbalance of forces on the spine, hip, and pelvis. Trunk strength assessment should be performed in bilateral (i.e., squat) and unilateral (i.e., single-leg standing march) tests. These can be performed in both a full standing and de-weighted posture (Figures 17.8, 17.9, 17.10, and 17.11) based on the patient's overall strength and acuity postoperatively.

Therapy Diagnostic Coding

Select diagnosis codes are applicable based on a PLWBC's presentation. Standard codes and the associated body systems involved are presented in Box 17.1.

Interventions From Surgical Adverse Effects

As discussed in Chapter 27, substantial evidence supports preoperative Onc R care to support PLWBCs' functional tolerance of medical oncological treatment. Fifty percent of people with CRC treated surgically will fail to return to preoperative physical activity levels 6-months post-treatment, and poor referral rates to physical therapy persist.[27] Advocacy for early Onc R in the acute care setting

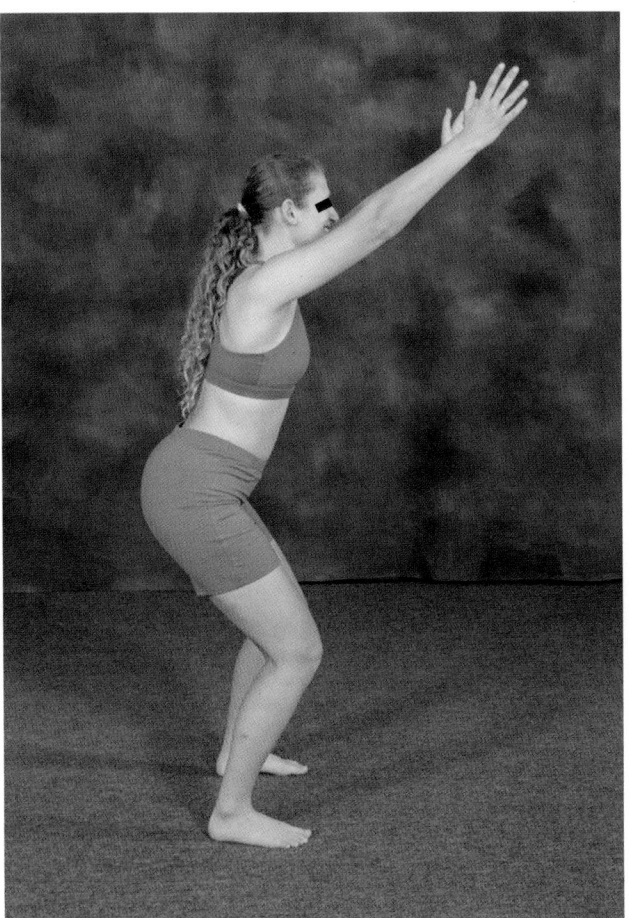

• **Fig. 17.10** Moderate Level Trunk Strength Assessment in Standing Posture. The Person Living With and Beyond Cancer (PLWBC) Performs Abdominal Activation Throughout a Full Range Squat With Arms Overhead. (Printed with permission from John Krauss, PT, PhD, OMPT, OCS.)

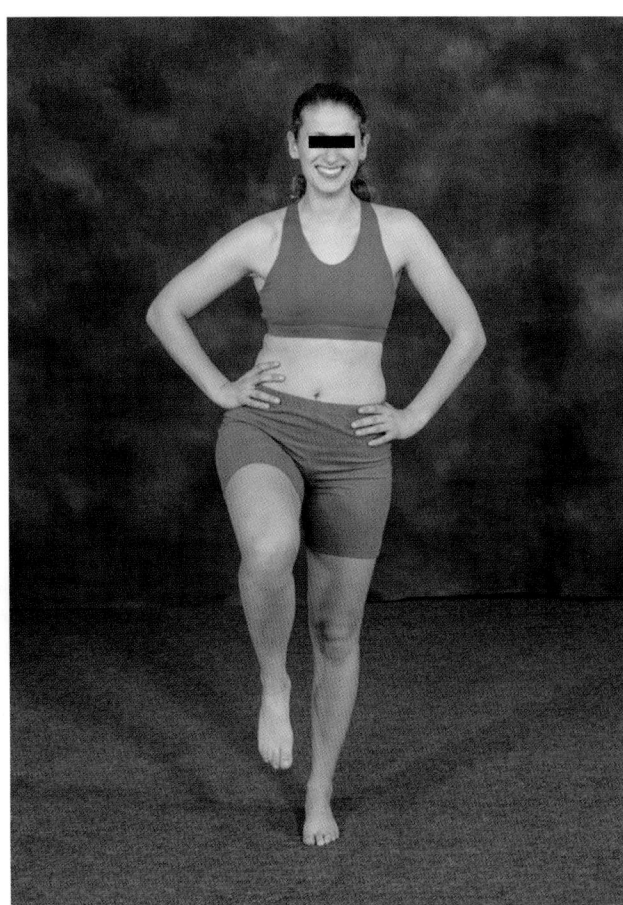

• **Fig. 17.11** Moderate Level Trunk Strength Assessment in Standing Posture. The Person Living With and Beyond Cancer (PLWBC) Performs Abdominal Activation and Maintains Alignment Throughout a Full Range March. (Printed with permission from John Krauss, PT, PhD, OMPT, OCS.)

assists with early mobilization goals as well as provides education on body mechanics for log-roll supine-to-sit transfers, postural supports including trunk strengthening for ADLs, toileting, and ambulation, and provides orthosis and assistive device recommendations including abdominal binders, walkers, and canes.[20] Additionally, prioritizing diaphragmatic breathing enhances Onc R outcomes in the CRC population. To promote tissue healing, positions and postures should be considered to avoid excessive muscle substitution and compression through the abdomen. A PLWBC should be encouraged to utilize supported, resting positions during the day when they demonstrate weakness or limited cardiovascular endurance. These supported positions allow for spinal elongation to reduce the compression of the thorax on the abdomen. Examples of these postures include supported standing, de-weighted standing, reclined sitting, or lying (refer to EBOOK: Video 2). These positions allow for full rib expansion during a breath and allow surgical sites to heal without excessive scarring into flexed postures. As the person's strength and endurance improve, advancement in strength training progression should utilize less supportive postures, involve both unilateral and bilateral weight-bearing positions, open and closed chain exercise, varying balance requirements, and progression towards patient-specific functional goals.

Some PLWBCs' strength will improve with exercise alone, but many have scarring present both superficial to and deep in the

• **BOX 17.1   Therapy Diagnosis—Surgery**

• L90.5 Scar conditions and fibrosis of skin—*Integumentary*
• K43.0 Incisional hernia—*Integumentary and Musculoskeletal*
• M62.81 Muscle weakness (generalized)—*Musculoskeletal*
• R27.8 Other lack of coordination—*Musculoskeletal*
• R15.2 Fecal urgency—*Gastrointestinal*
• I89.0 Lymphedema, not elsewhere classified—*Lymphatic*

peritoneal cavity. Addressing scar restrictions to ease tension on fascia will reduce pain and improve function.[18] Onc R clinicians can support a person's bowel function and reduce the risk of forming a bowel obstruction by implementing myofascial release, visceral mobilization, or soft tissue mobilization as scar adhesions are the primary cause of obstructions after the acute, inflammatory phase of healing, approximately 3 weeks for most individuals.[28] Onc R clinicians should avoid liberal use of instrument-assisted mobilization and high-velocity mobilization to address scar tissue in the abdomen. This concern is due to the absence of a hard (bony) end-block and the high likelihood of adverse effects if visceral tissue is lysed during mobilization. PLWBCs should be educated in self-mobilization of superficial scar tissue and exercise that will support desired movement, including diaphragmatic breathing and spinal ROM, in all directions, including rotational exercise.

Chemotherapy Interventions for Colorectal Cancer

Pharmaceutical interventions are utilized in four main ways in the CRC population: neoadjuvant, adjuvant, metastatic, and chemoradiation to treat either regional or advanced disease as seen in Stage II–IV cancers. Systemic regimens that include an anti-metabolite (and an alkylating agent) are utilized in first-line treatment (Table 17.5). Targeted and immunotherapy agents (Table 17.6) are utilized for second-line or third-line treatments. The oncogenetics of the tumor determine the appropriateness of targeted and immunotherapies, as well as the relative risk of cancer recurrence.

Chemotherapy for Colon Cancer

For colon cancer, neoadjuvant chemotherapy is most commonly utilized for T4b tumors and those that cannot be removed with surgery. The NCCN preferred regimens include leucovorin calcium (folinic acid), fluorouracil, oxaliplatin (FOLFOX), or capecitabine and oxaliplatin (CAPEOX) through a combination of chemotherapy (fluorouracil [5-FU], capecitabine or fluorouracil, leucovorin [5-FU/LV]) with radiation can be used to reduce the tumor size before surgery.[14] Commonly prescribed adjuvant chemotherapy options include FOLFOX and CAPEOX; though leucovorin calcium (folinic acid), fluorouracil, irinotecan (FOLFIRI), capecitabine, and 5-FU/LV are additional options. Targeted therapy or immunotherapy agents may be recommended in cases involving persistent metastatic disease.[14]

Chemotherapy for Rectal Cancer

Unlike colon cancer, chemotherapy or chemoradiotherapy is the first line treatment for rectal cancer.[17] Capecitabine and 5-FU are the preferred treatments, although bolus 5-FU/LV can be utilized. Following this initial cycle, surgical resection may occur, or the person will continue with an additional chemotherapy regimen described in the previous section. Similar to colon cancer, targeted therapy and immunotherapy can be utilized as second-line or third-line treatments if the initial, first-line intervention was not effective for metastatic disease.

TABLE 17.6 Targeted Chemotherapy and Immunotherapy Drugs Including Drug Class Utilized in Colorectal Cancers[14,17]

Name (Brand Name)	Drug Class
Bevacizumab (Avastin)	Anti-angiogenesis
Ramucirumab (Cyramza)	VEGFR2 Inhibitor
Ziv-aflibercept (Zaltrap)	VEGF Inhibitor
Cetuximab (Erbitux)	EGFR Inhibitor
Panitumumab (Vectibix)	EGFR Inhibitor
Regorafenib (Stivarga)	Tyrosine Kinase Inhibitor
Vemurafenib (Zelboraf)	BRAF Kinase Inhibitor
Ipilimumab (Yervoy)	PD-1 Inhibitor
Nivolumab (Opdivo)	PD-1 Inhibitor
Pembrolizumab (Keytruda)	PD-1 Inhibitor

VEGFR2, Vascular endothelial growth factor receptor 2; *VEGF*, vascular endothelial growth factor; *EGFR*, epidermal growth factor receptor; *BRAF*, B-Raf proto-oncogene serine/threonine kinase gene.
Created by Alaina Marie Newell. Printed with permission.

Oncology Rehabilitation Evaluation for PLWBCs Managed With Chemotherapy

A PLWBC of the colon or rectum will often be referred to Onc R and potentially prehabilitation based on the chemotherapy agents' anticipated adverse effects. In a prehabilitation application, Onc R clinicians would focus on building a person's functional tolerance, emphasizing exercise, nutrition, and anxiety coping strategies.[29] Patient education on common adverse effects of chemotherapy and the benefits of exercise, before, during, and after acute oncology treatment assists with anxiety coping strategies. The provision of an individualized plan of care enhances rapport and the building of the therapeutic relationship.

TABLE 17.5 Systematic Chemotherapy Regimens Including Drugs Included, Drug Class Utilized in Colorectal Cancers[12]

Regimen Name	Drug Names (Brand Names) in Regimen	Drug Classes
5-FU[a]	Fluorouracil (Adrucil)	Anti-metabolite
5-FU/LV	Fluorouracil, leucovorin	Anti-metabolite, chemo-enhancer
Capecitabine[a]	Capecitabine (Xeloda)	Anti-metabolite
Irinotecan	Irinotecan (Camptosar)	Topoisomerase I inhibitor
CAPEOX[b]	Capecitabine, oxaliplatin (Eloxatin)	Anti-metabolite, platinum/alkylating agent
FOLFIRI	Leucovorin, fluorouracil, irinotecan	Chemo-enhancer, anti-metabolite, topoisomerase I inhibitor
FOLFOX[b]	Leucovorin, fluorouracil, oxaliplatin	Chemo-enhancer, anti-metabolite, platinum/alkylating agent
FOLFOXIRI	Leucovorin, fluorouracil, oxaliplatin, irinotecan	Chemo-enhancer, anti-metabolite, platinum/alkylating agent, topoisomerase I inhibitor
Trifluridine+tipiracil	Trifluridine+tipiracil (Lonsurf)	Anti-metabolite/thymidine phosphorylase inhibitor

[a]Preferred chemotherapy for chemoradiation.

[b]Preferred chemotherapy as first-line treatment.

Created by Alaina Marie Newell. Printed with permission.

Chemotherapy is an ever-changing domain within medical oncology management, creating challenges for Onc R clinicians and textbooks to stay current with inclusive content to address impairments potentially seen during Onc R evaluations. Understanding the adverse effect impact of all systemic drugs related to the physiology of the body's systems simplifies the Onc R clinician's evaluation approach. Affording the building of clinical pathways based on impairments commonly seen based on drug classifications instead of specific drugs. Potential adverse effects of all systemic agents include myelosuppression, cancer-related fatigue, sarcopenia, weakness and debilitation, and cancer-related cognitive impairment (CRCI). For evaluation and interventions related to these adverse effects, refer to Chapters 8 and 10. Historically, CRC has been treated with three classes of systemic agents: anti-metabolites, alkylating agents, and topoisomerase inhibitors. Collectively these three classes impact four additional body systems, including the GI, integumentary, neurological, and pulmonary systems (Table 17.7). Detailed descriptions of the adverse effects of the neurological (chemotherapy-induced polyneuropathy, CRCI, vestibular toxicity, generalized pain, headaches) and pulmonary (dyspnea, cough) can be found in previously mentioned chapters.

Integumentary System Evaluation

Relative to the integumentary system, it is crucial to educate the PLWBC on the potential infection risk of compromised tissue, including incisions or dry, frail, or indurated dermis. Hand-foot syndrome (palmar-plantar erythrodysesthesia) is another adverse effect that impacts the integumentary system after exposure to anti-metabolite agents. Symptoms of this syndrome include redness, tenderness, peeling of palms and soles and are resultant of leakage of the chemotherapy agent through capillaries into the interstitial tissue beneath the skin. Factors that exacerbate hand-foot

syndrome include high chemotherapy dosage, friction, and heat exposure. Providing patient education to reduce heat exposure and maintain skin moisture can reduce symptom severity. Modifying the PLWBC's exercise program to minimize long periods of standing, walking, or jogging will reduce plantar irritation.

As mentioned in the surgical intervention section, the GI systems of PLWBCs of the colon and rectum are impacted by many factors. Chemotherapy causes an inflammatory reaction of the mucosal membranes of the entire body. Typical GI adverse effects include nausea, vomiting, diarrhea or constipation, mouth sores, low appetite, and heartburn. The severity and functional impact vary by individual and chemotherapy class but are dominant effects for anti-metabolites and topoisomerase inhibitors. See section *Gastrointestinal System Oncology Rehabilitation* below to most effectively evaluate and treat the GI system.

Therapy Diagnostic Coding

Select diagnosis codes are applicable based on the PLWBC's presentation. Common codes and associated body systems involved are presented in Box 17.2.

Radiation Therapy for Colorectal Cancer

As previously discussed, radiation therapy is primarily utilized in conjunction with chemotherapy for rectal cancer and not used as frequently for colon cancer. Chemotherapy agents, 5-FU and capecitabine, are utilized to increase the tumor's sensitivity to the radiation. While this increases the effectiveness of the radiation treatment, it does not spare healthy tissue within the radiation field and can have adverse effects both acutely and long-term. Prehabilitation before radiation therapy can support the person's movement, skincare, dietary modifications, and awareness of upcoming radiation therapy impact on all body systems. Providing surveillance and therapeutic treatment throughout radiation can ease the adverse effects in both the short and long term. The most common adverse effects include skin irritation, fatigue, weakness, bowel and bladder dysfunction, neuropathy, vaginal and rectal stenosis, and lymphedema.

Oncology Rehabilitation Evaluation for Persons Managed With Radiation Therapy

Similar to the evaluations for a PLWBC managed with surgery or chemotherapy, all body systems should be considered in the context of the phase of tissue healing. Radiation therapy creates an inflammatory-cytokine cascade in the pelvis, which precipitates

TABLE 17.7	Drug Classifications and Common Adverse Effects Based on Body Systems Involved and Ordered in Dominance of Symptoms[14,17]	
Drug Classification	Body System	Adverse Effect
Anti-metabolites	Gastrointestinal	Mucositis: nausea, vomiting, diarrhea, mouth sores, low appetite
	Integumentary	Skin and nail changes, hand-foot syndrome
Alkylating agents	Nervous	CIPN, CRCI, vestibular toxicity, generalized pain, headaches
	Gastrointestinal	Mucositis: nausea, vomiting, diarrhea, constipation, mouth sores, low appetite
Topoisomerase I inhibitor	Gastrointestinal	Mucositis: CID, nausea, vomiting, constipation, mouth sores, low appetite, heartburn
	Integumentary	Hair loss, skin and nail changes
	Pulmonary	Dyspnea, cough

CID, Chemotherapy-induced diarrhea; *CIPN*, chemotherapy-induced polyneuropathy; *CRCI*, cancer-related cognitive impairment.
Created by Alaina Marie Newell. Printed with permission.

BOX 17.2 Therapy Diagnosis—Chemotherapy

- R53.0 Cancer-related fatigue—*All Body Systems*
- M62.81 Muscle weakness (generalized)—*Musculoskeletal*
- R29.3 Abnormal posture—*Nervous and Musculoskeletal*
- G62.9 Polyneuropathy, unspecified—*Nervous*
- R26.81 Unsteadiness on feet—*Nervous*
- R06.00 Dyspnea, unspecified—*Pulmonary*
- R19.7 Diarrhea—*Gastrointestinal*
- K59.01 Slow transit constipation—*Gastrointestinal*
- N39.46 Mixed incontinence—*Urogenital*
- R39.43 Functional urinary incontinence—*Urogenital*

many short and long-term consequences. The presence of prolonged or persistent inflammation can delay healing; for example, wounds or burns may take weeks versus days to heal. Additionally, these sequelae can place the PLWBC at high risk for infection and potentially delay future surgery. As discussed in Chapter 9, prolonged inflammation impairs fluid dynamics resulting in further fibroblastic activity, decreasing the elasticity of the extracellular matrix. A downstream cascade effect of these impacts may result in lymphedema, vaginal and anal stenosis, muscle shortening, impaired postures, neuropathy including sacral nerve roots, diminished bladder capacity (urinary urgency, frequency, nocturia), diarrhea and constipation, and osteoporosis. Some of these adverse effects are considered acute or short-term, while others are late or long-term impacts and potentially not experienced until months to years post-treatment. This sequelae is collectively diagnosed as pelvic radiation disease (PRD).[30] The impact of PRD on the genitourinary (GU) system and integumentary system, including bladder dysfunction, vaginal and rectal stenosis, and sexual dysfunction, are discussed in Chapter 12 and Chapter 16. These adverse effects are commonly seen in the CRC population and should be considered part of Onc R.

As discussed above in surgical management, radiation therapy reduces the functional capacity of the lymphatic system for the local pelvic viscera and potentially for the internal and common iliac lymph nodes of the parietal tree. While not as common, individuals should be screened for lower body lymphedema as discussed in Chapter 16 due to this risk for reduced functional capacity of the deep lymphatic system.

Radiation-induced neuropathy (RIN) is not as prevalent as chemotherapy-induced polyneuropathy (CIPN), and incidence rates have improved with advancements in radiation therapy delivery.[31] Individuals with RIN should be assessed acutely and over time, as RIN is often a late-onset adverse effect after radiation-induced fibrosis and vascular stenosis have occurred. Patients exhibit similar symptoms to CIPN with sensory changes in their lower body periphery and locally around the sacral and coccygeal nerve roots, which can disrupt bowel and bladder function. Urinary or fecal incontinence without awareness is the hallmark symptom of this impairment and requires evaluation through a neuropathic clinical pathway instead of a GI/GU clinical pathway. Increased neural tension around the sacral and coccygeal nerve roots as well as the femoral and sciatic nerve distributions are additional neurological adverse effects that are observed in the initial inflammatory phase of soft tissue healing. A PLWBC presents with motor and sensory changes, including radiating pains and muscle spasms into their lower extremities, pelvis, or back. Subjective report and objective neural tissue tension evaluations performed via Slump Test, Straight Leg Raise Test, and Femoral Nerve Stretch Test can confirm the presence of increased neural tension.

It is critical to evaluate the tissues within the radiation field and regions superior and inferior to it. Many muscles are impacted by radiation-induced fibrosis, leading to sarcopenia, weakness, vaginal and anal stenosis, and joint hypomobility. These impairments impact all aspects of daily life, including ADLs, work, and recreational activities through impaired postures, abnormal gait, and sexual dysfunction. Hip flexors (iliacus, psoas, pectineus), hip adductors (adductor brevis, longus, magnus, gracilis), and hip external/lateral rotators (piriformis, gemellus superior and inferior, obturator internus and externus, and quadratus femoris) have the potential to become weak, shortened, and potentially contracted as a result of radiation exposure. Many of the external rotators of the hip become shortened and fibrotic resulting in hypomobility

- R53.0 Cancer-related fatigue—*All body systems*
- M81.8 Other osteoporosis without current pathological fracture—*Musculoskeletal*
- R29.3 Abnormal posture—*Nervous and Musculoskeletal*
- G62.9 Polyneuropathy, unspecified—*Nervous*
- R10.2 Pelvic and perineal pain—*Nervous*
- L90.5 Scar conditions and fibrosis of skin—*Integumentary*
- I89.0 Lymphedema, not elsewhere classified—*Lymphatic*
- R19.7 Diarrhea—*Gastrointestinal*
- K59.01 Slow transit constipation—*Gastrointestinal*
- N39.46 Mixed incontinence—*Urogenital*
- R39.43 Functional urinary incontinence—*Urogenital*
- N94.1 Dyspareunia—*Urogenital*
- R39.15 Urgency of urination—*Urogenital*

of the hip joint. The resting posture includes the femur being anteriorly translated and externally rotated, disrupting the hip's biomechanics and altering the pelvic position into a posterior tilt, like saddle sitting. Evaluation of the PLWBC should include hip, pelvic, and spinal range of motion (ROM), and intervention should include a flexibility program to reduce the severity of these musculoskeletal changes. An emphasis should be placed on hip internal rotation, extension and adduction, and spinal ROM.

Therapy Diagnostic Coding

Select diagnosis codes are applicable based on the presentation of the PLWBC. Common codes and associated body systems involved are presented in Box 17.3.

Interventions for Adverse Effects of Radiation

A combined manual therapy and exercise prescription approach is advised to address the neurological and musculoskeletal adverse effects evaluated above to support tissue healing by reducing inflammation, promoting angiogenesis, and mobilizing fibrous myofascial tissues. Multiple manual therapy techniques can be considered with a recommendation to avoid or minimize aggressive mobilization resulting in a significant inflammatory event. Treatment should include tissue release throughout the neurological and lymphatic territories of the impacted region and mobilization superior to the radiation field based on muscular attachments to superior structures such as the lumbar and thoracic spine and the ribcage. Moderate grade joint mobilization should be applied to the bilateral hip joints with an emphasis on posterior translation of the femur and distraction from the acetabulum. When determining the therapeutic exercise strategy for persons undergoing radiation therapy (and throughout their lifetime), a focus on tissue flexibility should be emphasized, though progression should include strength (power and endurance), balance, and cardiovascular endurance. A focused stretching program should be initiated during radiation, if not prior, and should focus on hip and spinal ROM. The most common direction of hip ROM restriction is hip internal rotation, and therefore, exercises that promote this direction of ROM should be prescribed to all PLWBCs. Additionally, flexibility exercise should target hip extension, hip abduction, and spinal (including sacrum) flexion and extension. These exercises will address musculoskeletal tissue fibrosis and inflammation and address the potential neural tension present. After the person completes radiation therapy, the PLWBC should receive a comprehensive pelvic assessment to determine the need for internal manual therapy or dilator therapy as discussed in Chapter 16.

Gastrointestinal System Oncology Rehabilitation

The aforementioned Onc R evaluation and interventions focused on common medical treatments and their impact on body systems with the exception of the GI system. This section will now provide a focused discussion on the complexity of Onc R needs around the GI system. As outlined in Figure 17.12, types of changes can be characterized in structural abnormalities, stool characteristics, or functional abnormalities. Structural changes occur from surgical resections and anastomosis. Evaluation of structural changes should include inspection of ostomy, mobility of scar restrictions, including myofascial and visceral. Subjective intake should include details (frequency, urgency, continence, stool shape and size, toileting positioning, the temporality of evacuation, and if pain present with defecation) of bowel movements and screen for changes in sexual function and bladder function. The person's response may warrant an internal (either vaginal, rectal, or both) pelvic exam to understand the severity of internal scar tissue, muscle tone, strength deficits, and pelvic floor function. Onc R clinicians should possess advanced training in pelvic floor evaluation and treatment or refer to a qualified colleague if the person is experiencing any of the above symptoms. Normal bowel function is 3×/day to 3×/week with stools that are formed and soft (Type 3–4 on Bristol Stool Scale). Evacuation should occur in less than five minutes, without excessive strain or urgency. If bowel movements take longer than this, pelvic floor Onc R should focus on normalizing pelvic floor muscle tone and scar tissue mobility as well as restoring normal defecation mechanics. If the person

has undergone a LAR, they do not have sufficient rectal capacity to store larger quantities of stool and though they will be continent, they may experience more frequent bowel movements (up to 5×/day) in addition to increased urgency. The following symptoms are consistent with lower anterior resection syndrome (LARS): fecal frequency, urgency, clustering, incontinence, gas, and abdominal pain following LAR, which significantly impacts QOL. All patients should be provided with education to address these symptoms and toileting postures and breathe with bowel movement to support effective evacuation without strain on the surgical tissue.

Changes in stool characteristics are acutely and persistently seen in individuals following radiation termed pelvic radiation disease (PRD). PRD related to the digestive system depends on the location but generally, patients acutely experience fecal urgency, frequency, and diarrhea secondary to increased mucosal permeability. Simple, bland diets reduce symptoms but rarely eliminate symptoms acutely. Frequency and urgency symptoms should decline as the person recovers from radiation exposure, and if radiation induced fibrosis becomes severe, it can result in constipation, outlet dysfunction, or bowel obstruction. The phase of healing often pairs with the function of the GI system insofar as diarrhea is seen during the inflammatory (acute or chronic) phase and constipation is more prevalent during the remodeling phase.

Changes in stool characteristics can be seen during chemotherapy alone or when combined with radiation. Primary adverse effects of chemotherapy result from either mucositis as chemotherapy induced diarrhea (CID) or neuritis as CIPN. Individuals experiencing CID, most often seen with irinotecan (Liposomal), have severe diarrhea (bowel movements >10x/day) that causes dehydration, electrolyte imbalance, weight loss, and can also be life-threatening. If a person is experiencing CID with an ostomy present, dehydration is more prevalent, and additional medical support

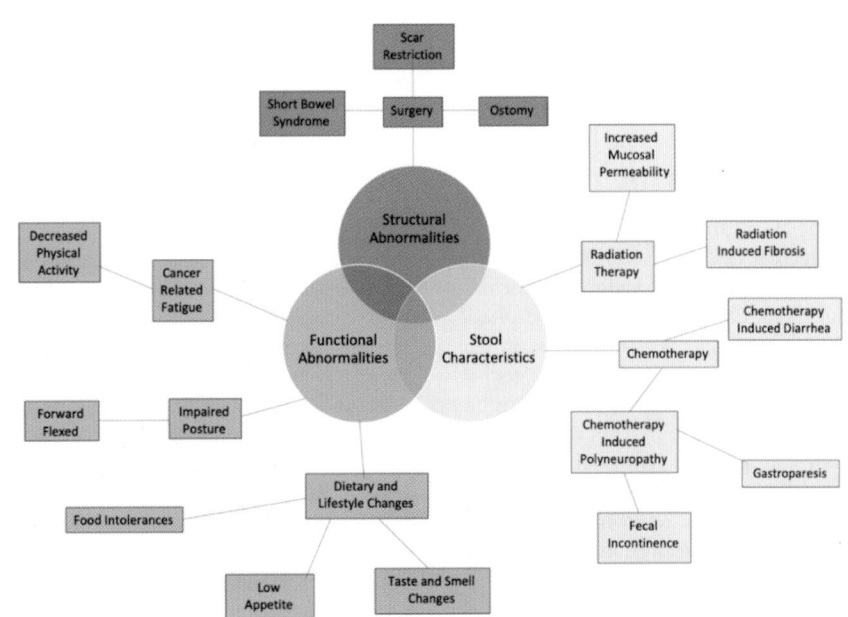

• **Fig. 17.12** Impacts to the Gastrointestinal System From Cancer and Its Treatment can be Described Through Structural Abnormalities, Functional Abnormalities, and Stool Characteristic. (Created by Alaina Newell and Carly Pawlitz. Printed with permission.)

may be required. Exercise and physical activity need to be closely monitored to avoid injury to the cardiovascular system from electrolyte imbalance. Like all peripheral nerves, patients with CIPN of the cranial nerve 10 (vagus nerve) will exhibit symptoms of gastroparesis (lack of bowel motility) with secondary constipation. Additionally, CIPN can manifest in the pudendal nerves and often result in fecal incontinence that the PLWBC is unaware of. This can vary from poor detection of stool versus gas to complete bowel emptying without awareness until after evacuation. PLWBCs with this type of incontinence should be evaluated via the CIPN clinical pathway instead of mucositis/GI clinical pathway. Assessment and intervention can include the use of rectal balloon sensory training to increase sensory awareness and continence by increasing detection of pressure changes within the rectum.

Changes in structural and stool characteristics are compounded by functional abnormalities seen in the CRC and the greater oncology population. The presence of cancer-related fatigue (CRF) often results in reduced physical activity (necessary for regular bowel motility), impaired posture from weakness, and sarcopenia, resulting in forward flexed posturing. Additionally, dietary and lifestyle changes such as low appetite and changes in taste and smell impact all patients. Clinicians need to physically evaluate or inquire about the person's prediagnosis bowel function, physical activity, posture, and diet to understand the impact of potential changes across the continuum of care. These factors are considered modifiable and should be addressed with all PLWBCs.

Therapeutic Intervention for Gastrointestinal Dysfunction

After addressing functional, modifiable factors, PLWBCs can be characterized into clinical groups, irrespective of medical treatment protocol: excessive GI motility or diminished GI motility with the goal of moderation of either extreme. Signs and symptoms of excessive motility include diarrhea, weight loss, malnourishment, dehydration, postural laxity, inflammation, fecal urgency, frequency, and incontinence. Signs and symptoms of diminished motility (constipation) include rigid or forward flexed posture, weight gain, low appetite, bowel straining, and outlet dysfunction. Both clinical pictures can result from or cause intra-abdominal pressure and are considerations for Onc R management. Manual therapy interventions to reduce intra-abdominal pressure (IAP) and support of fluid dynamics of the vascular and lymphatic systems are a priority. Manual therapy techniques focus on reducing extraperitoneal myofascial imbalances via soft-tissue mobilization, myofascial release, and superficial scar mobilization. Interventions for the musculoskeletal system reduce the tension on the peritoneum and can change the pressure dynamics to allow for normalized digestion and breathing. Secondarily, visceral and lymphatic mobilization should be performed to aid in clearing the abdominal lymph, adjust the bowel's temporal rhythm, and further reduce abdominal pressure. Patient education and exercise should emphasize diaphragmatic breathing and spinal mobilization to reduce the tension on the cisternal chyli and allow for lymphatic pumping through the abdomen to normalize the IAP.[32,33] Additional manual therapy can support joint mobility, tissue tension, and postural corrections that will further improve the pressure in the abdomen.

Exercise With Stoma Considerations

A comprehensive exercise program incorporating strength, flexibility, and balance training will be critical to maintain postural lengthening

and support bowel function long-term (refer to EBOOK: Video 3). Rotational exercises should be incorporated to provide unilateral strength training of the abdominal musculature which are necessary for activities of daily living, including walking (Figures 17.13 and 17.14 [refer to EBOOK: Video 4]). Special considerations are required for persons with an ostomy to support engagement in physical activity. No specific activity is "off-limits" for persons with ostomies, including swimming, running, endurance events, sexual intercourse, and weightlifting after the initial six postoperative weeks. A PLWBC should consult their durable medical equipment supplier for specific appliances recommended for some activities, including swimming and contact sports, to ensure the device remains adequately adhered to the stoma. All activities should begin at low intensity and be slowly progressed. A PLWBC should be educated on emptying the appliance before activity, increasing fluid intake to avoid dehydration, minimizing food intake for the hour before and during activity, and avoiding direct contact with their stoma during activity. Advancing the person's physical activity should be patient-specific and focus on individual goals while encouraging active lifestyles to improve outcomes and QOL.

Metastatic Disease

Nearly a quarter of people with CRC are diagnosed in advanced stages, and about 50% of PLWBCs will recur in the first 3 years after surgery.[34] Onc R clinician awareness of the common metastatic sites and understanding the symptomology can support timely referral to the medical oncologist if symptoms are

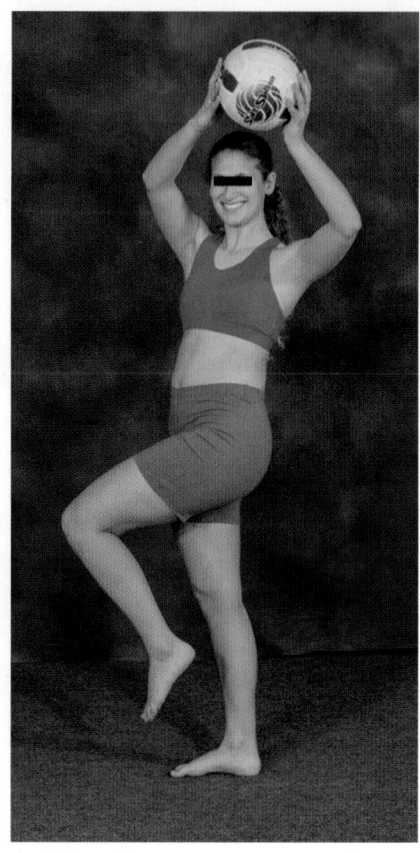

• **Fig. 17.13** High Level, Multiple Plane Exercise That Incorporates Trunk Rotation With March. Holding an Object, Such a Ball, Helps Maintain Upright Posture During Rotation. (Printed with permission John Krauss, PT, PhD, OMPT, OCS.)

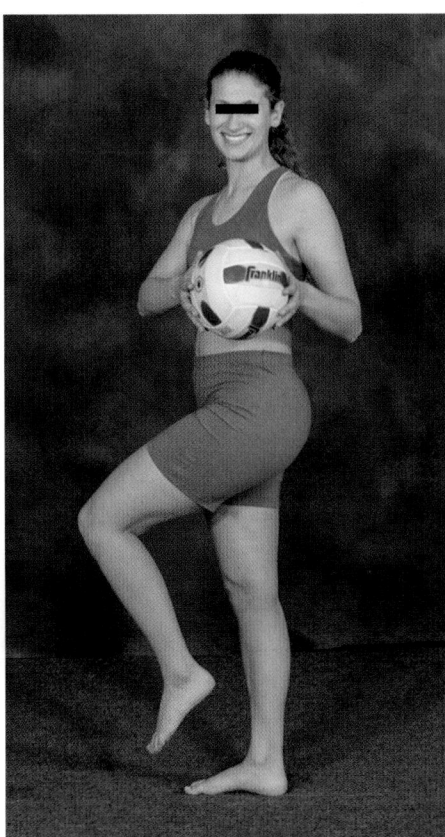

• **Fig. 17.14** High Level, Multiple Plane Exercise That Incorporates Trunk Rotation With March. Holding an Object, Such a Ball, Overhead Increases the Complexity Requiring the Person Living With and Beyond Cancers (PLWBC) to Elongate With Rotation. (Printed with permission John Krauss, PT, PhD, OMPT, OCS.)

suspected. New research shows CRC tends to spread via early seeding through the vascular and lymphatic systems that are not detectable with current diagnostic technology.[35] The liver is the most common metastatic location in patients initially diagnosed (71% colon, 60% rectal) with metastatic disease and those who develop metastasis after diagnosis.[36] The second most common site for colon cancer is the peritoneum, and the second most common site for rectal cancer is the lungs. Additional sites, though less common, are distal lymph nodes, bone, brain, spinal cord, and other rare sites.[36]

Liver Metastasis

Given the predominance of liver metastasis in CRC, understanding the signs and symptoms is critical for all Onc R clinicians working with this population (Box 17.4). Liver metastasis will typically be detected on imaging, as symptoms often do not present unless the tumor is obstructing the hepatic or portal vein, or if there is a large number of lesions or a large lesion.

In the presence of ascites and ankle swelling, Onc R clinicians should address positioning to avoid the occurrence of inferior vena cava syndrome. Ascites is an abnormal accumulation of intraperitoneal fluid that results in high intra-abdominal pressure (IAP). When a person with high IAP lays in supine, the excess fluid can occlude the posterior venous and lymphatic structures resulting in increased lower body edema, tachycardia, and dyspnea. The person should be advised to sleep in reclined positions or left side-lying to support effective oxygenation during sleep. Additionally, Onc R clinicians should provide palliative care through visceral

mobilization, diaphragmatic breathing, spinal range of motion, and cardiovascular exercise to support fluid dynamics through the inferior vena cava and thoracic duct.[32]

Nutritional Management

Effective nutritional surveillance and management are critical in the oncology population, especially those with GI system cancers, such as CRC. Malnourishment is reported in 40% to 80% of PLWBCs who have advanced disease, and has a significant impact on the person's QOL.[37] Effective referral to an RDN will support the person's nutritional needs before, during, and following active treatment. Protein-rich food intake can be provided to reduce the risk and impact of sarcopenia and weakness, thereby improving QOL. Additional resources regarding Wellness, Health Promotion, and Prevention can be found in Chapter 30.

Plan of Care

Therapeutic Goals

Regardless of surgical, chemotherapeutic, or radiation intervention, the determination of therapeutic goals should align to consider all body systems and the person's functional impairments. For many PLWBCs with CRC, their GI system will be forever changed. It is recommended that at least one goal should be framed around supporting active life in their community while living with GI changes to emphasize the importance of QOL.

Therapy Prognosis

When determining a person's prognosis for Onc R, many factors should be considered beyond the patient's medical management, as discussed in previous chapters. The therapeutic prognosis will be driven by three primary domains: functional movement, bowel and bladder function, and CIPN impact, along with the presence of metastatic disease. The number of systems involved and severity of impact should collectively be considered in prognosis development.

Outcome Measures

The selection of valid and reliable outcome measures is a pivotal component in a comprehensive evaluation and the development of an individualized plan of care. The body of evidence specific to the oncology population remains limited, and Onc R clinicians should consider utilizing theoretical application when a lack of evidence is present. The outcomes described below have evidence in the CRC population, oncology population, or GI surgical population

TABLE 17.8	Functionally Based Outcome Measures Utilized in Management of Colorectal Cancer Population	
Outcome Measure	**Assessment**
Quality of life	FACT-C, EORTC QLQ-CR38/QLQ-CR29[39,40]
Surgical impact	ASIS[41,42]
Bowel and bladder function	PFIQ-7, PFDI-20[43]
Strength	Hand-held dynamometry[38]

ASIS, Abdominal Surgery Impact Scale; *EORTC QLQ-CR*, European Organization for Research and Treatment of Cancer Quality of Life Questionnaire-Colorectal; *FACT-C*, Functional Assessment of Cancer Therapy-Colorectal; *PFDI-20*, Pelvic Floor Distress Inventory-20; *PFIQ-7*, Pelvic Floor Impact Questionnaire-7.
Created by Alaina Marie Newell. Printed with permission.

to emphasize the functional implications of the Onc R assessment (Table 17.8). Additional outcomes can be considered symptom-specific such as the outcomes discussed in previous chapters related to CRF, balance, gait, and cardiovascular endurance. Only one systematic review in the CRC population has been performed pertaining to strength and muscular endurance. The American Physical Therapy Association Oncology Evaluation Database to Guide Effectiveness Task Force (APTA Oncology EDGE Task Force) reported that no measures were highly recommended though hand grip strength using dynamometry is recommended for clinical use.[38] There is insufficient evidence to make a recommendation on an outcome measure for muscle endurance.[38] Utilization of all possible outcome measures is an inefficient use of time and resources and Onc R clinicians should consider a measure of strength, an impairment-based outcome, and a QOL measure as sufficient monitoring for a PLWBC.

Conclusion

For many PLWBCs of the colon and rectum, rehabilitation services can make a substantial impact on their QOL through generalized conditioning in the prehabilitation setting as well as therapeutic intervention addressing impacts on the musculoskeletal, integumentary, neurological, and gastrointestinal systems that occur from cancer and cancer treatments. Specific attention should be provided following surgery to restore functional movement patterns, trunk and abdominal strengthening, pulmonary hygiene, and digestive motility to allow for participation in the community. Common chemotherapeutic agents utilized in CRC have substantial neurotoxicity impacting balance, ambulation, and dexterity and increase the risk of falls as well as mucositis disrupting the full

gastrointestinal tract. These changes are areas that rehabilitation can assist to support return to work and social settings. The impact of radiation on people with CRC include acute, late, and long-lasting adverse effects that rehabilitation services can support. While the overall incidence of colorectal cancer is slowly declining, the improvement in early detection and survival is increasing, elevating the need for rehabilitation of PLWBCs of the colon and rectum.

Critical Research Needs

- Incidence of pelvic floor dysfunction in CRC including bladder and bowel urgency, frequency, and incontinence.
- Effectiveness techniques to manage adverse effects of radiation fibrosis in rectal cancer.
- Effective trunk strengthening for persons with a stoma.
- Effectiveness of manual therapy, including visceral mobilization to modulate bowel function including bowel obstruction, constipation, diarrhea.
- Benefits and risks of performing manual therapy on a person with a stoma.
- Benefits and risks of performing manual therapy on a person following abdominal or rectal radiation.

Case Study

This case details a 30-year-old female with Stage IV right-sided colon cancer with metastasis to her liver. She presents to Onc R after completing 6 cycles of FOLFOX chemotherapy and radioablation to her liver. She is scheduled for surgery (colectomy with anastomosis) in 2 weeks and is concerned as she remains symptomatic following chemotherapy. She reports symptoms of fatigue, numbness/tingling in her feet, difficulty with walking/hiking outdoors or crowded environments, and has fallen twice in the last month. Additionally, she has a low appetite and reports constipation (bowel movements once every 3 days) with need for laxatives most days.

She currently requires 10 hours of sleep at night as well as a 2-hour nap most days. Her supportive husband cooks most meals and is doing the housework. She is walking about a mile 3 to 5 days/week but must have her husband go with her due to her balance concerns. She has been on short-term disability since her second round of chemotherapy and is worried about potentially having an ostomy as her job requires public speaking and business attire. Her goal is to return to work after recovering for surgery.

Examination focused on evaluating her chemotoxicities for gait, balance, strength, and falls-safety education. Her objective measures are as follows:

Measure	Score	Assessment
Transfers: supine-to-sit, sit-to-stand	Independent	Use of arms for transfers and dizziness with supine-to-sit-to-stand
Five time sit-to-stand	13.3 seconds	Abnormal for age norms
Hand grip strength	R 54 lb (24.5 kg), L 56 lb (25.4 kg)	R-handed
Gait	Speed: 1.05 m/s	Uneven step lengths, poor toe off, reduced hip extension and low arm swing
mCTSIB	Firm Romberg EO: 30 seconds	Condition 3: increase postural sway
	Firm Romberg EC: 30 seconds	Condition 4: posterior loss of balance
	Foam Romberg EO: 30 seconds	
	Foam Romberg EC: 8.6 seconds	
Vibration sense	Diminished bilateral great toe	128 Hz tuning fork

EC, Eyes closed; *EO*, eyes open; *L*, left; *mCTSIB*, modified Clinical Test of Sensory Interaction in Balance; *R*, right.

The patient demonstrated muscle weakness (five time sit-to-stand and hand grip strength), sensory deficits (8.6 seconds on condition 4 of modified Clinical Test of Sensory Interaction in Balance [mCTSIB] and diminished vibration sense), reported fatigue of 8/10 severity and functional mobility difficulties with transfers and gait speed and pattern.

Since the patient will be going into surgery in 2 weeks, the focus of her interventions and goals will include a combination of preventative and restorative approaches. She will be seen for an additional two visits prior to surgery with the focus on building functional strength, safety with transfers and mobility, and preparation for early Onc R following surgery. The patient will be educated on techniques such as taking time with transfers and pausing between positions and leading with her eyes for transitions and turns during ambulation. Her exercise program will include use of a stationary bike to build her cardiovascular endurance, squat, mini-lunges, heel raises, standing marching for strength training, and complex balance positions including tandem stance and balancing on uneven surfaces. Additionally, to support pain and reduce herniation risk following surgery, she will be educated on log rolling during bed mobility, diaphragmatic breathing, transverse abdominis activations, and utilization of an abdominal binder for ADLs and mobility early after surgery.

Review Questions

Reader can find the correct answers and rationale in the back of the book.

1. A 67-year-old female with a history of Stage III rectal cancer presents to outpatient physical therapy with the following symptoms: urinary urgency, fecal incontinence, and vaginal stenosis. What condition are these symptoms collectively known as?
   A. Lymphedema
   B. Pelvic radiation disease
   C. Chemotoxicity
   D. Transabdominal resection

2. A 44-year-old female with Stage IV rectal cancer had undergone chemotherapy (5-FU) with radiation therapy. Based on the chemotherapy agent drug type, anticipated adverse effects will follow which clinical pathway?
   A. Cardiotoxicity pathway
   B. Chemotherapy-induced polyneuropathy pathway
   C. Myelosuppression pathway
   D. Mucositis pathway

3. A 60-year-old male diagnosed with Stage III right-sided colon cancer is seen 2 days postoperative in acute care for early mobility and strength training. Initial exercises to increase activation of his abdominal musculature should include all the following except:
   A. Abdominal crunches
   B. De-weighted transverse abdominis activation
   C. Diaphragmatic breathing
   D. Sit-to-stand transfers

4. A 52-year-old patient is looking to return to gym 4 months following abdominoperineal resection (APR) + permanent colostomy. He has progressed well in oncology rehab and the clinician is ready to discharge to a community-based exercise program. Which of the following exercises should the patient be instructed to avoid?
   A. Box jumps
   B. Prone press ups
   C. Swimming
   D. Wall push ups

5. A 32-year-old patient with Stage IV colon cancer with metastatic disease reports her metastatic disease has advanced. The patient reports she is having abdominal pain, darker urine, and wondering if her ankles are swollen. Where is the MOST LIKELY location of her metastases given this description?
   A. Liver
   B. Lung
   C. Lymph nodes
   D. Peritoneum

6. CRC is the second leading cause of death following which cancer?
   A. Breast cancer
   B. Cervical cancer
   C. Lung cancer
   D. Prostate cancer

7. Which of the following is a characteristic of right-sided colon cancer?
   A. Metastasizes to the peritoneum
   B. Occur in younger adults
   C. Predominately occur in males
   D. Responds to treatment in later stages

8. Which of the following muscles is NOT subjectively to radiation for CRC, and potentially become weak, shorted, and potentially contracted?
   A. Adductor brevis
   B. Gluteus medius
   C. Obturator internus
   D. Psoas

9. When evaluating a person who was surgically managed for CRC, which of the following body systems does NOT require a focused evaluation?
   A. Gastrointestinal system
   B. Integumentary system
   C. Musculoskeletal system
   D. Neurological system

10. What is the dominant adverse effect seen in people who undergo FOLFOX chemotherapy for CRC?
   A. Chemotherapy-induced constipation
   B. Chemotherapy-induced peripheral neuropathy
   C. Hand-foot syndrome
   D. Malnourishment

References

1. Sadler TW, Langman J. *Langman's Medical Embryology.* 11th ed.: Lippincott, Williams & Wilkins; 2010.
2. Itzkowitz SH. Incremental advances in excremental cancer detection tests. *J Natl Cancer Inst.* 2009;101(18):1225–1227. doi:10.1093/jnci/djp273.
3. Cancer of the Colon, National Cancer Institute:SEER (2019). https://seer.cancer.gov/statfacts/html/colorect.html.
4. Sung H, Ferlay J, Siegel RL, et al. Global cancer statistics 2020: GLOBOCAN estimates of incidence and mortality worldwide for 36 cancers in 185 countries. *CA Cancer J Clin.* 2020;70(4):313.
5. Simon S. *Colorectal Cancer Rates Rise in Younger Adults.* American Cancer Society, March 2020. https://www.cancer.org/latest-news/colorectal-cancer-rates-rise-in-younger-adults.html.
6. American Cancer Society. Colorectal Cancer Causes, Risk Factors, and Prevention; 2020. cancer.org.
7. Thanikachalam K, Khan G. Colorectal cancer and nutrition. *Nutrients.* 2019;11(1):164. doi:10.3390/nu11010164.
8. Ulanja MB, Rishi M, Beutler BD, et al. Colon cancer sidedness, presentation, and survival at different stages. *J Oncol.* 2019;2019:4315032. doi:10.1155/2019/4315032.
9. Lee JM, Han YD, Cho MS, et al. Impact of tumor sidedness on survival and recurrence patterns in colon cancer patients. *Ann Surg Treat Res.* 2019;96(6):296–304. doi:10.4174/astr.2019.96.6.296.
10. Lee YC, Lee YL, Chuang JP, Lee JC. Differences in survival between colon and rectal cancer from SEER data. *PLoS One.* 2013;8(11):e78709. doi:10.1371/journal.pone.0078709.
11. Wolf AMD, Fontham ETH, Church TR, et al. Colorectal cancer screening for average-risk adults: 2018 guideline update from the American Cancer Society. *CA Cancer J Clin.* 2018;68(4):250–281. doi:10.3322/caac.21457.
12. Amin MB, American College of Surgeons. *AJCC Cancer Staging Manual.* 8th ed.: Springer International Publishing; 2017.
13. Baran B, Mert Ozupek N, Yerli Tetik N, Acar E, Bekcioglu O, Baskin Y. Difference Between left-sided and right-sided colorectal cancer: a focused review of literature. *Gastroenterol Res.* 2018;11(4):264–273. doi:10.14740/gr1062w.
14. Shead D, Hanisch L, Vidic E, Clarke R, Corrigan A. *Colon Cancer, NCCN Guidelines for Patients (2018),* 2018. https://www.nccn.org/patientresources/patient-resources/guidelines-for-patients/guidelines-for-patients-details?patientGuidelineId=8.
15. Nguyen HT, Duong HQ. The molecular characteristics of colorectal cancer: implications for diagnosis and therapy (review), *Oncol Lett.* 2018;16(1):9–18. doi:10.3892/ol.2018.8679.
16. Reichert FL, Mathes ME. Experimental lymphedema of the intestinal tract and its relation to regional cicatrizing enteritis. *Ann Surg.* 1936;104(4):601–616. doi:10.1097/00000658-193610440-00013.
17. Shead D, Hanisch L, Vidic E, Clarke R, Corrigan A. *Rectal Cancer, NCCN Guidelines for Patients* (2018). https://www.nccn.org/patientresources/patient-resources/guidelines-for-patients/guidelines-for-patients-details?patientGuidelineId=36.
18. Wong YY, Smith RW, Koppenhaver S. Soft tissue mobilization to resolve chronic pain and dysfunction associated with postoperative abdominal and pelvic adhesions: a case report. *J Orthop Sports Phys Ther.* 2015;45(12):1006–1016. doi:10.2519/jospt.2015.5766.
19. Wilson IM, Lennon S, McCrum-Gardner E, Kerr DP. Factors that influence low back pain in people with a stoma. *Disabil Rehabil.* 2012;34(6):522–530. doi:10.3109/09638288.2011.613515.
20. North J. Early intervention, parastomal hernia and quality of life: a research study. *Br J Cancer.* 2014;23(5):14–19.
21. Russell S. Physical activity and exercise after stoma surgery: overcoming the barriers. *Br J Nurs.* 2017;26(5):S20–S26.
22. Mlecnik B, Bindea G, Angell HK, et al. Integrative analyses of colorectal cancer show immunoscore is a stronger predictor of patient survival than microsatellite instability. *Immunity.* 2016;44(3):698–711. doi:10.1016/j.immuni.2016.02.025.
23. *Optimizing treatment for obstructive colon cancer.* Univesity of Twente (2018) 11–23.
24. Donahue TF, Bochner BH, Sfakianos JP, et al. Risk factors for the development of parastomal hernia after radical cystectomy. *J Urol.* 2014;191(6):1708–1713. doi:10.1016/j.juro.2013.12.041.
25. Söderbäck H, Gunnarsson U, Hellman P, Sandblom G. Incisional hernia after surgery for colorectal cancer: a population-based register study. *Int J Colorectal Dis.* 2018;33(10):1411–1417. doi:10.1007/s00384-018-3124-5.
26. Bhangu A, Nepogodiev D, Futaba K. Systematic review and meta-analysis of the incidence of incisional hernia at the site of stoma closure. *World J Surg.* 2012;36(5):973–983. doi:10.1007/s00268-012-1474-7.
27. van Zutphen M, Winkels RM, van Duijnhoven FJB, et al. An increase in physical activity after colorectal cancer surgery is associated with improved recovery of physical functioning: a prospective cohort study. *BMC Cancer.* 2017;17(1):74. doi:10.1186/s12885-017-3066-2.
28. Bove GM, Chapelle SL. Visceral mobilization can lyse and prevent peritoneal adhesions in a rat model. *J Bodyw Mov Ther.* 2012;16(1):76–82. doi:10.1016/j.jbmt.2011.02.004.
29. Minnella EM, Bousquet-Dion G, Awasthi R, Scheede-Bergdahl C, Carli F. Multimodal prehabilitation improves functional capacity before and after colorectal surgery for cancer: a five-year research experience. *Acta Oncol (Madr).* 2017;56(2):295–300. doi:10.1080/0284186X.2016.1268268.
30. Huffman LB, Hartenbach EM, Carter J, Rash JK, Kushner DM, Author GO. Maintaining sexual health throughout gynecologic cancer survivorship: a comprehensive review and clinical guide. *Gynecol Oncol.* 2016;140(2):359–368. doi:10.1016/j.ygyno.2015.11.010.
31. Delanian S, Lefaix J, Pradat P. Radiation-induced neuropathy in cancer survivors. *Radiother Oncol.* 2012;105(3):273–282. doi:10.1016/j.radonc.2012.10.012.
32. Knott EM, Tune JD, Stoll ST, Downey HF. Increased lymphatic flow in the thoracic duct during manipulative intervention. *J Am Osteopath Assoc.* 2005;105(10):447–456. doi:10.7556/jaoa.2005.105.10.447.
33. Hunt L, Frost SA, Hillman K, Newton PJ, Davidson PM. Management of intra-abdominal hypertension and abdominal compartment syndrome: a review. *J Trauma Manag Outcomes.* 2014;8(2):1–8.
34. Aghili M, Izadi S, Madani H, Mortazavi H. Clinical and pathological evaluation of patients with early and late recurrence of colorectal cancer. *Asia Pac J Clin Oncol.* 2010;6(1):35–41. doi:10.1111/j.1743-7563.2010.01275.x.
35. Hu Z, Ding J, Ma Z, et al. Quantitative evidence for early metastatic seeding in colorectal cancer. *Physiol Behav.* 2019;51(7):1113–1120. doi:10.1038/s41588-019-0423-x.
36. Holch JW, Demmer M, Lamersdorf C, et al. Pattern and dynamics of distant metastases in metastatic colorectal cancer. *Visc Med.* 2017;33(1):70–75. doi:10.1159/000454687.
37. Gupta D, Lis CG, Granick J, Grutsch JF, Vashi PG, Lammersfeld CA. Malnutrition was associated with poor quality of life in colorectal cancer: a retrospective analysis. *J Clin Epidemiol.* 2006;59(7):704–709. doi:10.1016/j.jclinepi.2005.08.020.
38. Burgess F, Galambos L, Howland A, Yalamanchili M, Pfalzer LA. Oncology EDGE task force on colorectal cancer outcomes: a systematic review of clinical measures of strength and muscular endurance. *Rehabil Oncol.* 2016;34(1):36–47. doi:10.1097/01.REO.0000000000000002.
39. Ganesh V, Agarwal A, Popovic M, et al. Comparison of the FACT-C, EORTC QLQ-CR38, and QLQ-CR29 quality of life questionnaires for patients with colorectal cancer: a literature review. *Support Care Cancer.* 2016;24(8):3661–3668. doi:10.1007/s00520-016-3270-7.

40. Ward WL, Hahn EA, Mo F, Hernandez L, Tulsky DS, Cella D. Reliability and validity of the Functional Assessment of Cancer Therapy-Colorectal (FACT-C) quality of life instrument. *Qual Life Res*. 1999;8(3):181–195. doi:10.1023/a:1008821826499.

41. Urbach DR, Harnish JL, McIlroy JH, Streiner DL. A measure of quality of life after abdominal surgery. *Qual Life Res*. 2006;15(6):1053–1061.

42. Datta I, O'Connor B, Victor JC, Urbach DR. Abdominal Surgery Impact Scale (ASIS) is responsive in assessing outcome following IPAA. *J Gastrointest Surg*. 2009;13(4):687–694. doi:10.1007/s11605-008-0793-3.

43. Jeffrey A, Harrington SE, Hill A, Roscow A, Alappattu M. Oncology section EDGE task force on urogenital cancer: a systematic review of clinical measures for incontinence. *Rehabil Oncol*. 2017;35(3):130–136. doi:10.1097/01.REO.0000000000000068.

18

Lung Cancer

ANNE K. SWISHER, PT, PhD, FAPTA[a], MEGAN BURKART, PT, DPT, CLT[b]

CHAPTER OUTLINE

Overview

Demographics and Risk Factors

Lung cancer is a cancer that forms in the parenchyma or bronchi of the lung, usually due to prolonged or repeated exposure to carcinogens that leads to dysplasia and genetic mutations. The most common carcinogen is cigarette smoke which is the cause of 90% of lung cancer diagnoses.[1] There are two common broad divisions of lung cancer, including non-small cell lung cancer (NSCLC) and small cell lung cancer (SCLC), which have very different prognoses and disease progressions (Table 18.1).

The person with lung cancer may present quite differently than persons diagnosed with many other cancers including: being diagnosed often at very late stage disease, the person is often older, a chronic smoker, and will exhibit early cachexia and have multiple comorbid physical and psychological issues. In addition, there is a stigma associated with lung cancer that can make a person living with and beyond cancer (PLWBC) feel that they "deserve" the cancer and "did it to themselves" to a greater degree than many

---

[a]Board-Certified Clinical Specialist in Cardiovascular and Pulmonary Physical Therapy

[b]Board-Certified Clinical Specialist in Oncologic Physical Therapy

TABLE 18.1	Types of Lung Cancer	
Type	**Behavior**	**Subtypes**
Non-Small Cell Lung Cancer (NSCLC)	• Most common • Accounting for 85%–90% of lung cancers • Slower growing with periods of stable disease	**Adenocarcinoma** • More likely to be in the periphery of the lung and be associated with fibrous scarring **Squamous Cell Carcinoma** • Tend to be centrally located near the bronchus, cavitates, and more likely to occur with hypercalcemia **Large Cell Carcinoma** • Occurs in any part of the lung and progresses faster than adenocarcinoma or large cell
Small Cell Lung Cancer (SCLC)	• Accounts for approximately 10%–15% of all lung cancers • Often occurs centrally near the bronchus • Tends to metastasize early in the course of disease • Most commonly associated with smoking	**Oat Cell** • Named for morphology **Intermediate cell** **Combined Cell** • SCLC and NSCLC component, squamous, or adenocarcinoma

Created by Anne Swisher and Megan Burkart. Printed with permission.

other types of cancer. Alternatively, nonsmokers or never-smokers who are diagnosed with lung cancer may feel they are the undeserved target of judgment from outsiders. All these factors can make it very difficult to get a PLWBC to engage with rehabilitation or other potentially very helpful services. The clinician may need to be quite assertive in explaining the benefits of oncology rehabilitation (Onc R).

Even with advances in the medical treatment, lung cancer remains the leading cause of cancer death in men and women in the United States (US) and globally.[2] The 5-year survival rate in the US ranges from 7% to 25% for all stages combined.[3] Lung cancer rates are rising in the developing world, especially where cigarette smoking is common.[1] Commercially produced cigarettes have been shown to have at least 70 known carcinogens[4] and non-commercially produced and unregulated inhaled substances (e.g., homemade cigarettes, e-cigarettes or vaping, marijuana preparations) may have other potentially cancer-causing chemicals present in them.

Lung cancer, that was until recently exclusively impacting older men, has shifted demographics. As rates of smoking increased, starting in the post-World War II "women's liberation" movement, rates of lung cancer in women have risen.[1] For the same body size, women have smaller lungs, smaller airways, and generally poorer outcomes from smoking-related lung diseases, including lung cancer.[3] Due to lack of awareness, much like with women and heart disease, many women may not seek medical care for their symptoms (cough, progressive dyspnea, hemoptysis) as they might be dismissed as not possible to come from lung cancer. Black men are more likely than white men to develop lung cancer, but white women are more likely than black women to develop it.[3] Currently, most people diagnosed with lung cancer are over the age of 65.[2]

A small percentage, approximately 10% to 15% of all lung cancers, arise in nonsmokers that likely occur due to genetic factors.[5] These individuals can be exposed to the same stigmatizing reactions from friends, community and even healthcare providers, due to a general lack of knowledge about lung cancer in nonsmokers. It is important that Onc R clinicians recognize any internal biases and avoid blaming a PLWBC who can benefit from services, no matter the cause of the illness.

The Onc R clinician may therefore encounter a PLWBC at any point along the cancer journey—from recognizing early symptoms, to recovery from cancer-related treatment, to end-of-life care. The goal of this chapter is to illustrate effects of lung cancer and its common treatments superimposed on an individual's movement system and participation in important life roles. Each person is unique; thus the Onc R clinician needs to be aware of the complex biopsychosocial considerations that influence movement.

Effects of Lung Cancer Treatment on Movement

Surgery

Surgery is standard treatment for persons diagnosed with lung cancer as it is the most effective intervention for improving survival, especially in NSCLC. Unfortunately, some cases of lung cancer are deemed nonoperable due to comorbidities or extensive disease at diagnosis. There are a variety of surgical approaches available based on the extent of disease and amount of lung tissue that needs to be removed. Each of these has its own implications for pain, muscles involved, and need for chest tubes. Thus, it is important for the clinician to know these differences in order to develop an individualized assessment and intervention plan.

The traditional approach is an open thoracotomy, where the surgeon makes a large incision between the ribs, through layers of muscle, into the plural space. Typically, segments of ribs are also removed to allow necessary access to the lung tissue. This surgical approach leaves the patient with a large incision, which may involve direct or indirect trauma to the latissimus dorsi, serratus anterior and rhomboid muscles (depending on if the approach is anterio-lateral or posterio-lateral) as well as trauma to the intercostal muscles and nerves from placement of chest tubes (Figure 18.1).

The trauma to the muscles will contribute to changes in posture and resting position and significantly increase pain with mobility and functional activities, such as pushing up on the affected arm to transition from lying to sitting, or pushing up from a chair to a standing position. In addition, the incised muscles will also cause pain with coughing or chest wall expansion. This discomfort will affect the individual's typical positioning as well, as they usually lie on the nonoperative side. Sitting and standing posture is also impacted, as a person usually sidebends toward the operative side and hold the ipsilateral arm tightly against the chest in a protective position (Table 18.2 and Figure 18.2). In addition to posture and movement limitations due to pain, there may be specific postoperative precautions related to the specific surgery.

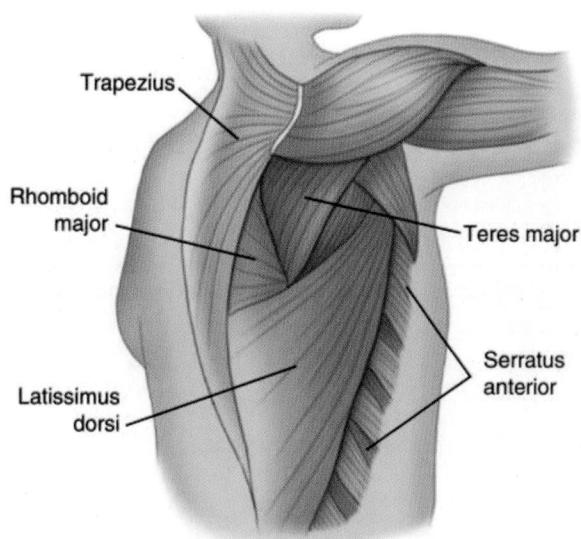

• **Fig. 18.1** Muscles Commonly Involved With a Thoracotomy. (Reprinted with permission from Hillegass E. *Essentials of Cardiopulmonary Physical Therapy.* 4th ed. Saunders; 2016. ISBN: 9780323430548.)

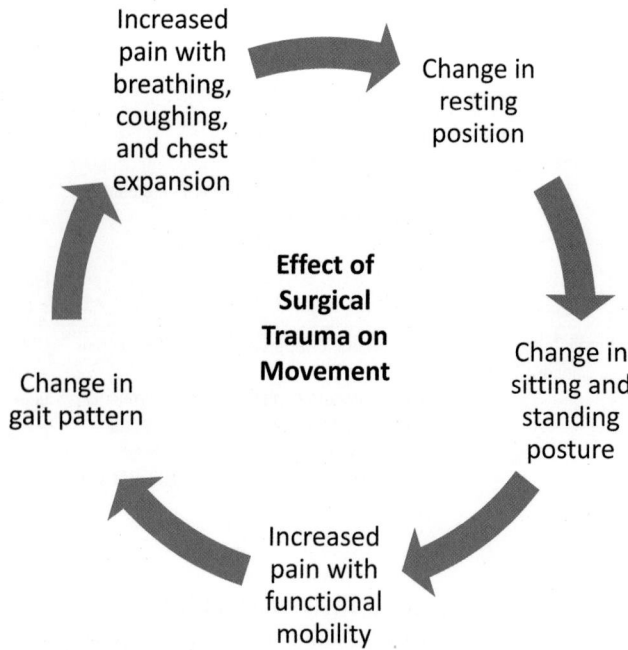

• **Fig. 18.2** Effect of Surgical Trauma on Movement. Created by Anne Swisher and Megan Burkhart. Printed with permission.

More modern surgical approaches avoid the trauma caused by large incisions and the amount of muscle affected is decreased by using smaller "minimally invasive" techniques (i.e., three 3–5 cm long access sites for instruments [Figure 18.3A] vs. a 20 cm continuous incision [see Figure 18.3B]). Individuals report a significant decrease in pain postoperatively which allows for increased ease and motivation to participate in early mobilization with robotic or video-assisted thoracic surgeries (VATS).

Less pain with movement, deep breathing, and coughing means that PLWBCs are more willing to ambulate and perform deep breathing exercises which have been shown to decrease the length of time the chest-tube is needed, postoperative complications, and length of stay. They may also require less pain medication and have fewer post-surgical movement precautions, making them more alert and active.

Both types of approaches invade the pleural space in order to remove the cancerous lung tissue, so all individuals will require chest tubes to evacuate the space for a period of a few days until the incision(s) heal. Therefore chest tube precautions must be observed. Despite some concerns, however, it is safe to lie on a chest tube and to perform manual airway clearance techniques (e.g., percussion and vibration) in this area, as long as it is not performed directly over the tube site. Certainly, it is preferable if

a person can perform active breathing techniques and progressive mobilization to clear their lungs and reverse any atelectasis.

Following the acute recovery from surgery, individuals often complain of long-standing chest wall pain.[6–8] They tend to state that the chest tube site is much more painful than any incision. The Onc R clinician should be aware that techniques to release scar tissue, normalize rib mobility, and restore active expansion of the chest wall with breathing can be very effective in pain management.

The amount of lung tissue removed surgically will certainly affect lung capacity and breathing mechanics. The clinician should expect minimal impact from a wedge resection, but significant impairment with a pneumonectomy. Principles of pulmonary rehabilitation, such as improving peripheral muscle function, energy conservation, and breathing exercises can help manage dyspnea experienced during activity.

Chemotherapy

It is important for the Onc R clinician to understand the specific chemotherapy regimens that a person might receive to treat lung cancer. As discussed in earlier chapters, this may vary by stage (limited vs. extensive), type of tumor (e.g., SCLC vs. NSCLC), and biology (e.g., tumor markers). The clinician should be aware of the potential

TABLE 18.2	Anticipated Postural and Movement Patterns Following Lung Cancer Surgery	
Possible Patient Adaptation	**Altered Postural or Movement Pattern**
Change in Resting Position	Patient will self-select to remain in bed laying on the nonoperative side
Change in Sitting and Standing Posture	Common for patients to side bend toward the operative side and hold the ipsilateral arm tightly against the chest in a protective position
Increased Pain With Functional Mobility	Difficulty performing supine to sitting and sitting to standing transfers
Change in Gait	Guarded gait pattern with decreased stride length, gait velocity, and limited to absent arm swing on the surgical side
Increased Pain With Chest Expansion	Patients will self-limit chest expansion resulting in short shallow upper chest breathing and coughing

Created by Anne Swisher and Megan Burkart. Printed with permission.

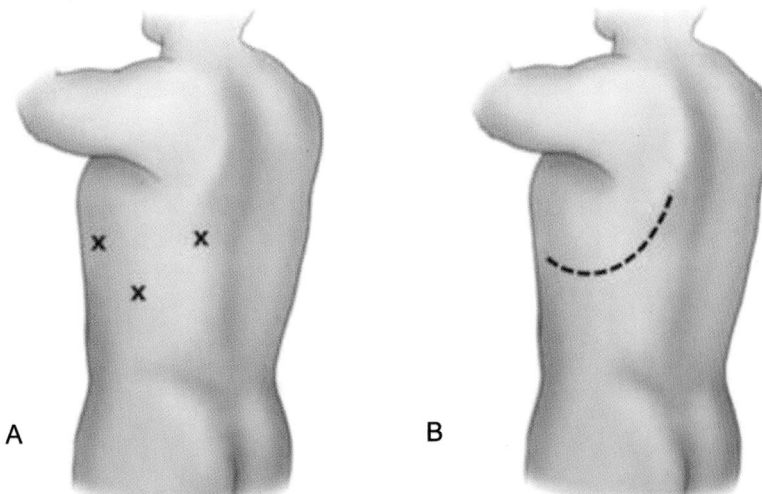

• **Fig. 18.3** Video-Assisted Thoracic Surgical Approaches (A). versus Thoracotomy (B). (Reprinted with permission from Hillegass E. *Essentials of Cardiopulmonary Physical Therapy.* 4th ed. Saunders; 2016. ISBN: 9780323430548.)

of the specific chemotherapy treatment to induce polyneuropathy and possible balance impairment, cardiotoxicity impacting exercise capacity and/or cardiac arrhythmia, and inflammation affecting lung tissue (e.g., pneumonitis). The Onc R clinician may be the first provider to recognize these issues in early stages or mild presentation, as other disciplines do not induce an exercise challenge.

Radiation Therapy

Radiation in the treatment of lung cancer can be a primary treatment or used in conjunction with surgery and chemotherapy. Early (Stage 1) cancer in persons not suitable for surgical resection or those that have limited spread of their cancer to areas like the brain or adrenals may be treated with short duration stereotactic body radiation therapy (SBRT), also known as stereotactic ablative radiotherapy (SABR), to a very focused area. Most individuals with Stage 2 (or higher) lung cancer will undergo longer duration external beam radiation to a larger area to maximize local disease control. It is important for the Onc R clinician to know the location and intensity of the radiation received in order to predict effects on tissues in the radiation field. Skin will receive the highest dose and have the greatest amount of change, from acute redness and sloughing to long-standing fibrosis and loss of tissue extensibility (Box 18.1). Radiated skin is fragile and at risk of injury from excessive forces (including so-called "instrument-assisted" manual therapy). It is also vulnerable to damage from heat modalities, sun exposure, and trauma from various types of tape (including athletic and stretchable tapes).

• BOX 18.1 Radiation-Induced Changes in the Chest

- Deeper tissues may also become fibrotic, including intercostal muscles, fascia, local nerves, local blood and lymphatic vessels, pleura, and lung parenchyma.
- This equates to a loss in tissue extensibility and tissue nutrition/healing.
- Therefore the person will have a permanent deficit in normal lung and chest wall movement.
- If the radiation field also includes the heart and pericardium, the person may also be at risk for cardiac dysfunction such as decreased ejection fraction or arrhythmias.

Fatigue is the most common complaint of a PLWBC of any diagnosis, with the effects lasting months to years after completion of treatment, and can have a significant impact on a person's ability to be physically active. This impact may be more dramatic in persons diagnosed with lung cancer as they likely led a sedentary lifestyle prior to diagnosis and dyspnea already limited their functional independence and quality of life (QOL).[6] As discussed in Chapter 23, appropriately prescribed physical activity and exercise can dramatically improve fatigue.

Late-onset complications of radiation to the lungs are common, with survivors complaining of pain, cough, and progressive stiffness in the radiation field. It is important that a PLWBC is educated on the signs and symptoms of late-onset complications, because lung cancer has a very high rate of recurrence[3] and it is difficult to distinguish these complications from tumor recurrence. A PLWBC will experience a further decrease in lung capacity due to radiation fibrosis, beyond what they already experience from surgical removal of lung tissue.

Interventions provided after completion of treatment should focus on improving chest expansion, soft tissue mobility, with a focus on methods to decrease breathlessness, especially with functional activities. Onc R clinicians should be aware that pain and other symptoms that do not improve as anticipated with mobilization of the chest wall tissues will require referral back to their medical oncologist to rule out recurrent disease.

Immunotherapy

New pharmacologic agents for treatment of lung cancer include immunotherapy. These drugs are most commonly used for a person with late-stage disease and have promise to extend life. However, these medications can cause significant adverse events that impact movement, such as pneumonitis, peripheral nerve pain or dysfunction, and cardiac arrhythmias. In addition, severe diarrhea is common and can limit the ability to participate in an exercise program and cause issues with electrolyte balance.[9] Onc R clinicians should assess balance, oxygen saturation, and heart rhythm (such as an irregular pulse) as these factors impact movement. Any impairments should be reported to the oncologist and the recommended home exercise program should be provided with options on strategies to modify the program during periods of increased adverse effects.

Movement System Implications of Lung Cancer and Treatments

The American Physical Therapy Association (APTA) has proposed a graphical way to describe the area of expertise of rehabilitation clinicians such as physical therapists—the Movement System (Figure 18.4).

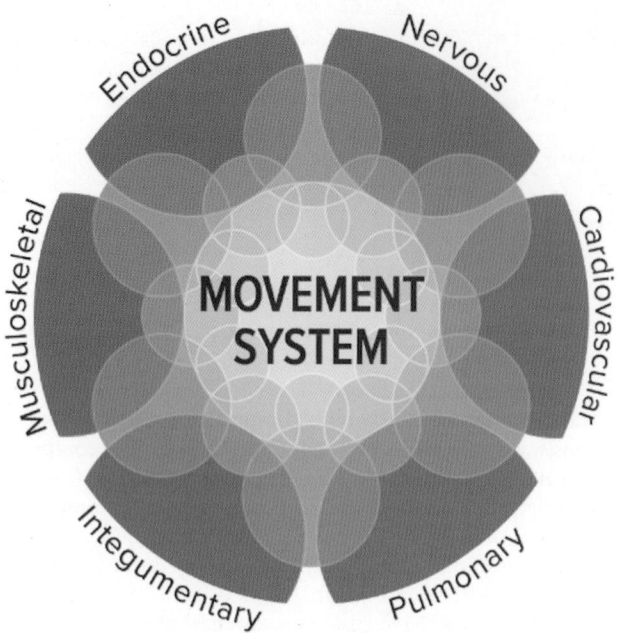

• **Fig. 18.4** American Physical Therapy Association (APTA) Movement System. (Reprinted with permission from the American Physical Therapy Association. © 2020 American Physical Therapy Association. All rights reserved.)

This model illustrates the interrelation between body systems as they are involved in movement. Thus, the Onc R clinician must be able to identify the impact of lung cancer and its treatment on not only each individual system, but also in the complex interactions required for movement. For example, surgical removal of a portion of a lung will certainly lead to deficits in the pulmonary system, but the degree of movement deficit experienced by a PLWBC is also very dependent on the function of the musculoskeletal system, cardiovascular system, endocrine system and others. Thus, the same degree of lung removal can cause little to no functional impact to a person whose other systems are optimized, but severe functional impairment for another person who has poor capacity of the other systems.

An additional level of understanding is needed to allow the Onc R clinician to determine which aspect(s) of movement are causing overall movement impairment in a PLWBC. Thus, the movement system model has been modified to add five key components of accomplishing a movement task (Figure 18.5). Common manifestations of lung cancer and their impact on components of the movement system include diminished: endurance, strength, balance/agility, flexibility, and motivation. In this figure, common issues related to lung cancer are also linked to the component of movement.

This model helps the Onc R clinician to design appropriate intervention plans intended to remediate deficits. For example, if the clinician determines that impaired endurance best explains the reason that a person cannot perform their life tasks, they can focus on a treatment plan that trains breathing and peripheral muscles to optimize the ability to perform low-intensity muscular activity for prolonged periods of time. If a person is unable to walk safely in their home due to impaired balance and fear of falling, then the clinician would focus on training muscles for quick activation to maintain dynamic balance. If a person limits their activities due

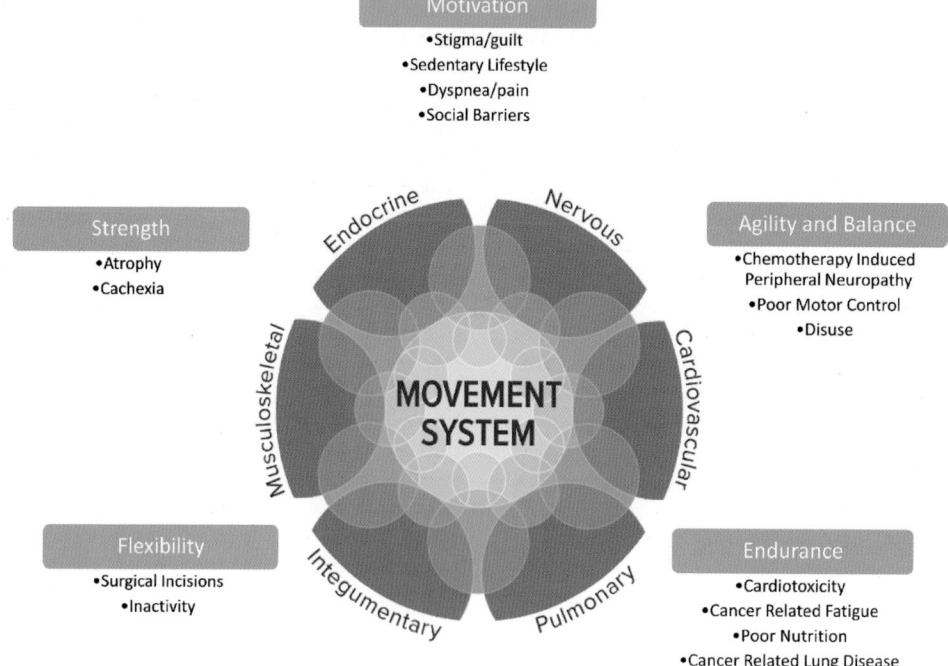

• **Fig. 18.5** Common Manifestations of Lung Cancer and Their Impact on Components of the Movement System. *CIPN*, Chemotherapy-induced polyneuropathy. Modified from the American Physical Therapy Association. (2020 American Phsical Therapy Association. All rights reserved). Movement System by Anne Swisher. Printed with permission.

to a negative memory of experiencing dyspnea during stair climbing, the clinician can include training of peripheral muscles for efficiency as well as cognitive-behavioral approaches to decrease anxiety and panic about movement.

Endurance

Limited endurance is a major symptom reported by most persons undergoing treatment for lung cancer and is associated with poor QOL.[7,8,10] In fact, fatigue and shortness of breath (dyspnea) are nearly universal issues limiting the ability to perform activities of any duration.[11] Poor endurance is multifactorial and the Onc R clinician must consider contributions of the pulmonary system, especially if there is underlying chronic lung disease. Since smoking is the primary cause of lung cancer,[1] it is very common that there is some degree of chronic obstructive pulmonary disease (COPD) present in anyone with a significant smoking history. Therefore the effects of cancer and its treatment are compounded by impaired oxygen and carbon dioxide exchange, hyperinflation, secretions, bronchoconstriction, and chest wall remodeling (e.g., barrel chest). These issues can be worsened with any exertion, leading to dyspnea. Also, physical activity levels are known to be very low in smokers, so those who develop lung cancer often already have poor aerobic capacity from a sedentary lifestyle.

In addition, the desire to avoid dyspnea leads to a downward spiral of muscular deconditioning. The fear of dyspnea results in progressively increasing kinesiophobia in which the person will self-limit all physical activity and elect to remain sedentary for symptom management. Without intervention, this spiral continues with progressive global deconditioning and increased energy demand with even low-level activities. The spiral will continue until the person is limited with basic daily activities and becomes progressively disabled. This has been called a "deconditioning storm," referring to the constellation of factors all causing poor activity tolerance.[12]

Treatment adverse events such as cardiac dysfunction from chemotherapy, impaired blood supply to peripheral muscles for oxidative metabolism, nutritional deficiencies, or fibrosis from radiation therapy can further impair endurance capacity, as the person's aerobic metabolism depends on lungs, heart, vasculature and muscle factors.

Strength

Weakness is a very common symptom of persons diagnosed with lung cancer. It can result from a variety of factors, including muscle atrophy from cachexia, impaired motor unit function and recruitment due to chemotherapy toxicity to nerves, and low baseline physical activity levels prior to their cancer diagnosis. Physical activities and tasks that require moderate-to-maximal force output from muscles are also those that are often associated with dyspnea (such as standing up from a low surface or climbing stairs). Thus, a person diagnosed with lung cancer may have a psychological aversion to performing vigorous activity and that will further compound muscle atrophy.

Onc R clinicians need to recognize the interactions between brain, motor unit, and muscle fibers that are essential for adequate strength and may need to intervene in a variety of ways to improve strength. Maximizing peripheral muscle size and force output directly improves ability to comfortably perform low-level activity, as the ceiling for strength is raised. Thus, a focus on muscle strengthening will reliably lead to improvements in endurance and daily function. Since performing isolated resistance training for a relatively few repetitions cause less dyspnea than trying to perform whole-body endurance activities, it can be a good place to start a training program that is well tolerated and acceptable by the person. Even very weak individuals can benefit from the feeling of accomplishment that comes from performing bicep curls or leg presses. The positive feelings of mastery may help to overcome fear avoidance behavior related to dyspnea.

Balance/Agility

Agility refers to the ability to perform rapid changes in direction or speed of movements. Thus, the ability to achieve and maintain balance, especially during bodily movement, is a type of agility. Falls in PLWBC is a common problem, with 25% of individuals reporting a fall within the last 12 months and 45% reporting difficulty with balance/walking[13] and therefore must be considered. Balance can be impaired by many reasons including muscle weakness, impaired ability to recruit muscles at the right time and sequence (motor control), impaired sensation and proprioception as a result of chemotherapy or comorbid polyneuropathy, and poor motor control from lack of practice, particularly in sedentary persons. The phrase, "use it or lose it" applies to balance reactions as well as muscle tissue, so persons who do not move much do not keep these complex reactions sharp.

Onc R clinicians need to consider these multiple reasons for impaired balance and determine not only which systems are involved, but also the reversibility of the impairments. Permanent changes in balance may need a compensatory approach, such as prescribing an assistive device or adaptive equipment to minimize risk of falls. Teaching how to fall safely and recover from falling can be invaluable skills for PLWBCs and can help decrease fear and increase confidence in physical activity.

Flexibility

Flexibility concerns secondary to treatment for lung cancer focus on both the chest wall and the influence of immobility. For the chest wall, surgery and radiation therapy can decrease extensibility of the rib cage, intercostal muscles, and surrounding tissues. Adopting a protective posture (e.g., side bending toward the operated side and holding the ipsilateral arm in a protective posture) can lead to having the incision heal in a shortened position resulting in loss of range of motion of the shoulder, scapula, and ribs. This can also predispose the person to developing adhesive capsulitis.

While chest wall mobility is most impacted by thoracotomy scars, chest tube scars, or radiation, the clinician should also anticipate impaired rib mobility due to altered, often long-standing upper chest-dominant breathing patterns. In addition, classic barrel-chest deformity, common with COPD, leads to adaptive shortening of neck extensors, pectoralis muscles, and thoracic spine extensors.

Many persons who develop lung cancer have long-standing postural and adaptive shortening due to a sedentary lifestyle. Therefore Onc R clinicians can expect to find tight hip flexors, knee flexors, and dorsiflexors as well as hip external rotator muscle groups. In the upper body, the person may also have scapulothoracic muscle imbalances with scapular dyskinesia, a snapping scapula, or scapular winging. A full-body assessment and flexibility interventions should be part of the clinician's plan.

Motivation

This aspect of the human movement model is the most difficult to define but may be the most important determinant of a person's movement. Even if all the physiological systems are functioning, a PLWBC may choose not to perform movement or physical activity due to fear, negative past experiences, or lack of social support.[14] Most people diagnosed with lung cancer have a history of tobacco misuse and this addictive behavior cannot be ignored.[15] Often, persons recovering from addiction need to develop new skills such as healthy ways of coping with anxiety and self-blame. Being anxious can lead to a negative association with physical manifestations of exercise, such as sweating or racing heart rate and increased respiratory rates. The clinician should consider that many of these individuals have been very sedentary and have little to no experience with exercise. Thus, they will need motivational skills, support, and encouragement with initial attempts. A PLWBC may need to exercise under supervision for longer periods of time in order to adopt the new thought processes and perspectives on physical activity.

Motivation to be physically active is also influenced greatly by the person's peer group. If all of their friends and support network smoke and are not physically active, it will be more challenging for the person to change their lifestyle behaviors. Fears of the high rate of cancer recurrence or metastasis and anticipation of having a very limited lifespan may lead to a fatalistic attitude in which the effort of becoming physically active seems overwhelming. In addition, complications of cancer treatment, such as loss of lung capacity and incisional or neuropathic pain can be barriers to physical activity which may further compound the person's motivation to be physically activity and exercise. Current smokers are significantly more likely to have higher reported pain levels and may demonstrate maladaptive behaviors with opioid use including need for higher opioid dosage and frequency of use.[15] The patient, caregiver, or provider's desire to avoid distressing symptoms such as dyspnea and pain may be more prevalent in persons being treated for lung cancer given the poor QOL and rapid decline that seem inevitable. Pain education and a medication plan developed with the person's oncologist or supportive care physician can help to avoid overmedication and potential opioid addiction. Motivational interviewing techniques can also help the Onc R clinician and a PLWBC to determine important goals and direct therapy to achieve the highest level of function and QOL, even in persons with late-stage disease.

Engaging the support of a comprehensive pulmonary rehabilitation program, where these psychological barriers are addressed, may be an optimal adjunct to a therapy plan for maximizing flexibility, strength, agility, and endurance. If such a program is not readily available to the person, the clinician should seek to engage a behavioral health professional for these services. Within an Onc R program, use of motivational interviewing and psychologically informed principles are vital to engaging the person in lifestyle changes.

History and Patient Assessment

History

It is important for the Onc R clinician to obtain a thorough history of any person at any stage of the lung cancer journey. Eliciting information about both current and prior movement impairments is necessary, as the impact of lung cancer treatment is often superimposed on poor physical health, aging, and comorbid conditions. It is important to determine any internal contextual factors (such as pre-existing medical conditions) as well as external contextual factors such as home set-up and availability of caregivers or helpers as needed.

The emphasis on each component of the history will differ by care setting. For example, the clinician working in an acute care

setting needs to focus more on ability to perform basic activities of daily living (ADLs) and safety in the home, as well as obtaining any durable medical equipment or referrals (such as home health or inpatient rehabilitation) that are deemed appropriate.

The clinician working in the home or community should delve further into chronic medical conditions and ongoing treatments that may impact function as chemotherapy and radiation therapy predominantly happen in the outpatient setting. Knowing that a person has pre-existing diabetic peripheral neuropathy, for example, helps the clinician recognize and intervene more quickly for the potential impact of chemotherapy on worsening balance.

Assessment by System

Airways/Breathing

Breathing patterns of each person, relative to use of ventilatory muscles to expand the thorax in three dimensions, should be assessed visually and by palpation (Figure 18.6).

There should be use of the diaphragm and lower costal muscles symmetrically to cause abdominal rise with inspiration (Figure 18.7).

The mid-chest should expand symmetrically in the lateral direction and there should be superior and anterior expansion of the upper chest, shoulders and sternum as well.

A PLWBC with pre-existing COPD will often lack ability to utilize the diaphragm effectively, due to hyperinflation of the lung and flattening of the dome of the diaphragm. The presence of incisions or chest tubes will lead to less lateral expansion on the affected side. A habitually- or pain-induced flexed posture will lead to decreased upper chest expansion. All of these alterations typically lead to an elevated respiratory rate and impaired inspiratory volumes.

Persons treated for lung cancer are at high risk for atelectasis in the early postoperative period and the clinician should examine any chest imaging as well as auscultate for abnormal lung sounds. Auscultation will also reveal any retained secretions from surgery or pre-existing lung disease (most smokers have a chronic productive cough). Airway clearance interventions may be indicated in addition to deep breathing exercises to normalize chest wall excursion.

The extent of lung tissue removal will impact lung volumes as well as breathing patterns. Thus, it is important for the Onc R clinician in any setting to know the extent and location of any lung surgery, as well as the location of chest tubes, as they can lead to long term alterations in breathing patterns.

Cardiovascular

The main population of persons diagnosed with lung cancer is older adults and chronic smokers.[2] These factors mean that the Onc R clinician can anticipate low physical activity and fitness levels, even before the lung cancer diagnosis. The sequalae of lung cancer treatment can be anticipated to lead to further deconditioning.[6]

The 6-minute walk test, developed in persons diagnosed with cardiovascular disease, is the most widely used functional test of endurance. It is important to follow standard protocols for performing the test and especially important to monitor oxygen saturation levels. If the Onc R clinician obtains an order for supplemental oxygen that states that the flow rate can be titrated to maintain a specific minimal SpO_2 (typically >90%), then flow rate (and possibly delivery system, such as facemask instead of nasal cannula) can be adjusted.[16]

Rest   Inspiration

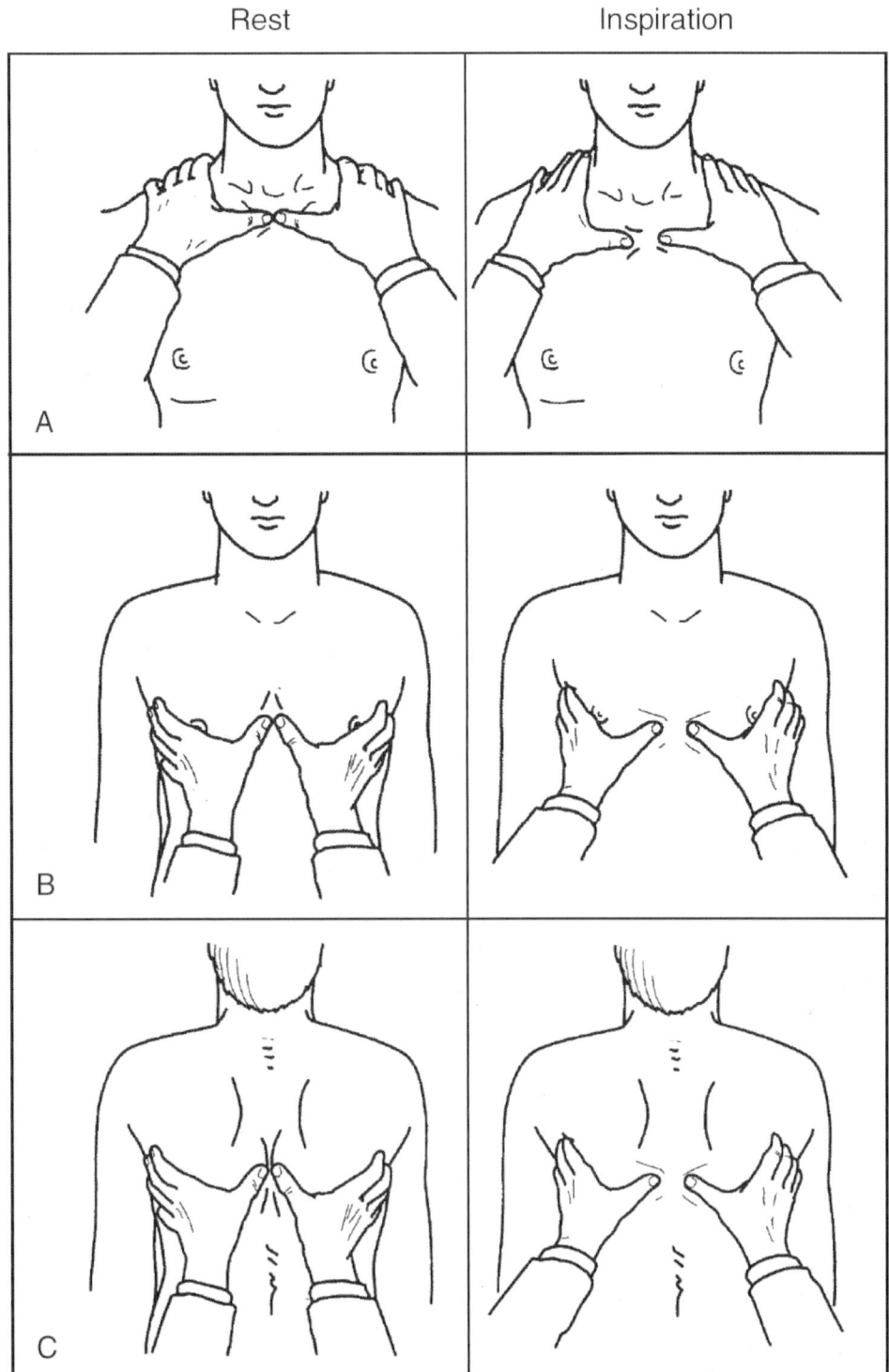

• **Fig. 18.6** Palpation of Thoracic Movement. (Reprinted with permission from Hillegass E. *Essentials of Cardiopulmonary Physical Therapy.* 4th ed. Saunders; 2016:525, Fig. 16.19. ISBN: 9780323430548.)

Pulse should also be assessed for rate and rhythm, particularly if the person has received any cardiotoxic chemotherapy or has concomitant heart disease. Edema in dependent extremities as well as cyanosis should be assessed. Oxygen saturation should be monitored to assess changes from rest to differing levels of activity. Individuals can be taught to use a dyspnea or perceived exertion rating scale as part of dyspnea management and home physical activity progression.

Musculoskeletal

Mobility of the entire chest wall can be impaired at any stage of lung cancer and treatment. Muscular flexibility of the anterior and posterior chest wall should be assessed. Typical flexed and forward-head posture will lead to tightness in pectoral muscles and neck extensors, while the scapular retractors and neck flexors are typically excessively lengthened. Intercostal muscles should be assessed, as well as muscles that connect thorax to pelvis, such as the quadratus lumborum.

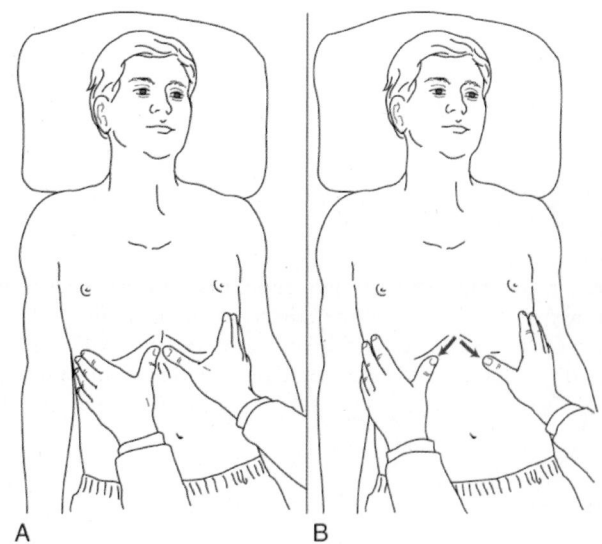

• **Fig. 18.7** Assessing Diaphragm Movement. (Reprinted with permission from Hillegass E. *Essentials of Cardiopulmonary Physical Therapy.* 4th ed. Saunders; 2016:527, Fig. 16.23. ISBN: 9780323430548.)

Overuse of the neck musculature is common in persons using an upper chest breathing pattern. Length, tone, and activation of all muscles of the trunk are important to assess, as all contribute to breathing in some way.

Mobility of bony segments should also be evaluated. It is common to find limited thoracic spinal segment extension mobility and impaired mobility of individual ribs. Shoulder complex mobility should be examined, including scapulohumeral rhythm. Limitation in overhead reaching can occur from limited mobility in many segments and each should be assessed. Limitation in trunk rotation is also common, resulting from sedentary lifestyle as well as surgical incisions or radiation fibrosis.

Neuromotor

Balance is a complex interaction of many systems that can be impacted by lung cancer and its treatments. Onc R clinicians should examine for sensory, motor, or proprioceptive impairments in the foot and ankle which can result from chemotherapy or pre-existing neuropathy. Any treatment of comorbid conditions that impacts vestibular function can also lead to imbalance.

Many different standard tests of balance can be assessed so clinicians should consider the patient's functional level, activity tolerance, and specific balance challenges to choose the most appropriate test. Assessment of strength of the major muscle groups is important to determine if weakness limits self-care, daily activity, or exercise participation. Objective and functional testing is generally preferred to manual muscle testing for improved sensitivity and carryover to daily life, especially in persons with known or suspected bone metastasis. Isometric handgrip strength is a good tool to objectively measure a key component of upper body strength and function.

A standardized assessment of the ability to perform ADLs can be done either with a patient self-report or a performance test. The Karnofsky Performance Scale (KPS) or Eastern Cooperative Oncology Group (ECOG) score (Table 18.3) are commonly used by oncologists, however tools such as the Barthel Index, Functional Independence Measure (FIM), or Physical Performance Test can give a more comprehensive picture for goal setting and intervention planning.

Nutrition

Most individuals diagnosed with lung cancer have already experienced undesired weight loss by the time the cancer is discovered. Cachexia is very common and even individuals with a normal body mass index (BMI) may have selective loss of muscle mass. Elevated work of breathing also causes an increased demand for calories, even at rest. This contributes to persons experiencing dyspnea at rest and significant anxiety-provoking shortness of breath with minimal activity. Dyspnea also impairs the ability to take in

TABLE 18.3 Functional Rating Scales Commonly Used by Oncologists

Karnofsky and Eastern Cooperative Group Performance Scales			
Percentage (%)	Karnofsky Performance Scale	Score	ECOG Performance Scale
100	Normal, no complaints, no evidence of disease	0	Normal activity; asymptomatic
90	Able to carry on normal activity; minor signs or symptoms of disease	1	Symptomatic; fully ambulatory
80	Normal activity with effort; some signs or symptoms of disease		
70	Cares for self, unable to carry on normal activity or to do active work	2	Symptomatic; in bed <50% of time
60	Requires occasional assistance, but is able to care for most of his/her needs		
50	Requires considerable, assistance and frequent medical care	3	Symptomatic; in bed 50% of time; not bedridden
40	Disabled, requires special care and assistance		
30	Severely disabled, hospitalization indicated; death not imminent		100% bedridden
20	Very sick, hospitalization indicated; death not imminent	4	
10	Moribund, fatal processes, progressing rapidly		
0	Dead	5	Dead

(Reprinted with permission from Mariano J, Min, LC. Management of Cancer in the Older Patient. Elsevier; January 2, 2012.)

nutrition, as it is difficult to breathe while eating and a full stomach impairs function of the diaphragm. Depression, anxiety, and altered appetite or taste resulting from cancer treatment will tend to decrease caloric intake.

Onc R clinicians should assess the patient's BMI but also note any comments about clothing getting loose or difficulty eating which may suggest loss of muscle mass. Working closely with a dietitian who is familiar both with chronic lung disease and with cancer treatment can be extremely helpful. It is important to ensure adequate caloric intake to be able to perform exercise.

Integumentary

Skin should be inspected for healing/nonhealing of any surgical incisions, radiation effects such as burns or fibrosis, as well as overall skin health. Edema in the dependent body parts can indicate cardiac failure or malnutrition. Cyanosis of nail beds or the perioral area can indicate hypoxemia.

Psychosocial

While psychosocial issues may not be a primary focus in the rehabilitation realm, due to the nature of practice, these issues may become evident during the assessment and examination. Mental health issues such as depression or anxiety are common in a PLWBC.[7,8,15] Issues with eating or self-care may be present, which would indicate referral to a registered dietitian and/or occupational therapist. Pain and dyspnea management may be improved with involvement of a palliative or supportive care specialist. Financial, occupational, and insurance concerns, which can lead to significant "financial toxicity" during acute treatment, would indicate consultation with a social worker and/or case manager. A multidisciplinary team dedicated to optimizing health of persons diagnosed with lung cancer has been shown to be effective in decreasing these issues.[7]

It is important to note that PLWBC may not tell their oncologist when they are having physical or emotional issues during treatment, for fear that their chemotherapy or radiation treatments might be stopped. Since they see these treatments as life-saving, they can be reluctant to report issues. The Onc R clinician should ask about physical and cognitive changes during or after treatment and seek to involve appropriate healthcare team members to address issues outside of the scope of rehabilitation. Standardized questionnaires such as the Sickness Impact Profile (SIP), DASS-21, Brief Pain Inventory (BPI), and the Distress Thermometer can be administered quickly by the clinician and guide referrals to and participation in oncologic rehabilitation.

Goals of Therapy for Different Phases of Lung Cancer

Prevention

Prevention of lung cancer is impacted primarily through prevention of or decreased amount of cigarette smoking. In fact, all other causes of lung cancer are extremely rare (e.g., radon exposure, use of open cooking fires). Therefore the primary way to decrease incidence of lung cancer is to promote tobacco/smoking avoidance. This begins in childhood/adolescence by teaching youth how to not start smoking. Nearly 90% of adult smokers first tried smoking by age 18 and 20% of high schoolers in 2020 who were tobacco users reported smoking electronic cigarettes.[17] Clinicians who work with youth in any capacity can

help promote messages of healthy lifestyle, including tobacco avoidance. Harm limiting strategies (e.g., decreasing number of cigarettes smoked) or assisting in quitting is well within the scope of Onc R clinicians. Brief counseling and motivational interviewing have been found to be acceptable and effective in assisting patients to quit.[18]

Asking all persons about their tobacco use history should be standard practice for all clinicians. Identifying persons with high risk features (e.g., age 55–74, smoking at least 30 pack-years, or quitting <15 years ago) should be routine practice to identify persons who meet the criteria for radiographic screening to identify lung cancer in its early and limited stages.[19] According to the US Center for Disease Control and Prevention,[20] low dose computed tomography (LDCT) is currently the only recommended screening measurement for lung cancer and is available from most healthcare systems in the US and many other countries. There are also mobile units available in some communities. These scans are covered by major insurers and clinicians should refer appropriate patients to this screening wherever available.

Promoting an overall healthy lifestyle, including good nutrition and regular physical activity, should be part of health promotion for persons at risk for, or diagnosed with, any stage of lung cancer. Identifying PLWBCs with psychosocial issues and referring them to appropriate services can also help persons quit smoking and address other health risks for cancer in general.

Diagnosis (System Screening and Recognition of Early Signs/Symptoms)

Onc R clinicians working with any population should recognize the early signs of lung cancer, including chronic cough (especially any hemoptysis) and dyspnea, and refer these persons for further medical evaluation. These early signs are very difficult to distinguish from smoking-related symptoms and account for much of the reason that most lung cancers are still quite advanced when diagnosed. Systematic screening of exercise tolerance, including monitoring oxygen saturation, should be part of the assessment for every PLWBC.

For persons recently diagnosed with lung cancer, the principles of prehabilitation apply (see Chapter 27). The focus should be on maximizing aerobic capacity, breathing strategies (including ventilatory muscle training and airway clearance techniques), and improving muscular strength. The more physically and mentally fit the individual becomes prior to surgery, radiation, or chemotherapy treatment, the less debility will be realized.

Preoperative exercise training, as brief as seven days, has been shown to enhance surgical recovery, decrease complications, shorten hospital length of stay, and decrease functional exercise decline.[21–23] Comprehensive training, including breathing exercises and ventilatory muscle training have been shown to be safe, acceptable, and effective in this population.[21–23]

Active Cancer Treatment

During medical treatment, functional assessment should be completed at key points in care to identify mobility complications early. Prospective surveillance models (PSM) are also appropriate for persons diagnosed with lung cancer (see Chapter 2). It is much easier to remediate or recommend adaptations for mild issues during treatment than to remediate severe issues at the conclusion of active treatment.

Recovery and Survivorship

Following active medical treatment, a person diagnosed with lung cancer should be assessed for new or worsening mobility issues. However, a person's overall ability to recover can also be significantly impacted by family, financial, or occupational issues. A multidisciplinary assessment of each person is recommended at these key time points and evidence found that 100% of persons diagnosed and treated for lung cancer reported at least one unmet physical, social, or psychological need at conclusion of the active treatment phase.[7] Early identification of issues and referral to appropriate services is key.

Palliative Care/Hospice

The clinician's role in end-of-life care for all types of cancer diagnoses are discussed in Chapter 29, but issues of dyspnea, chest pain, depression, and frailty are extremely pertinent to a person diagnosed with lung cancer. Onc R clinicians can provide strategies to decrease breathlessness, minimize energy expenditure, and manage pain that can greatly reduce the fear and discomfort for the person dying from lung cancer.

Interventions to Improve Function

Breathlessness/Endurance/Secretion Management

Any person who has decreased lung function will have challenges with breathlessness. In addition, anxiety can greatly exacerbate breathlessness. Therefore the clinician can incorporate breathing strategies, including paced breathing with activity, to help maintain the ability to function. For persons with underlying COPD especially, secretion management strategies can decrease the coughing "fits" that are so exhausting. Active cycle breathing, oscillatory positive expiratory pressure devices, and huff coughing can greatly reduce the energy required to clear secretions.

Pain Education/Management

Pain and breathlessness are the most common symptoms reported by persons diagnosed with lung cancer. Pain can be localized to surgical incisions or chest tube locations or more widespread in the chest. Tumors that invade the pleura can refer pain to the shoulder region as well. Physicians may be reluctant to prescribe pain medication, particularly opioids, as they are respiratory depressants and impair cognitive function. Nonpharmacologic approaches to pain management, including relaxation, physical activity and pain education should be integrated to help people manage pain; refer to Chapter 22 for additional information. Pain may also be due to poor posture or impaired mobility of the thorax, which can respond very well to manual therapy and muscular training.

Trunk/Chest Wall Mobility

Many people diagnosed and treated for lung cancer may have preexisting or treatment-related tightness or stiffness throughout the chest wall and thorax. A combination of manual therapy, neuromuscular re-education, and muscle strengthening can improve pain, breathlessness, and activity intolerance, but research specific to the lung cancer population is needed. Bone density and skin/soft tissue resilience can be adversely affected by radiation therapy and Onc R clinicians should be aware of these issues when considering manual therapy/joint manipulation or vigorous soft-tissue interventions.

Balance Training

Balance can be impaired by muscle atrophy, polyneuropathy, and other causes. Functional balance training should be incorporated, as well as fall recovery education, for any person with any objective signs of impaired balance or fear of falls. Practicing transfers to and from the floor and discussing home modifications to decrease fall risk can give the person confidence in daily activities and decrease unwarranted sedentary behavior.

Strengthening

Muscular weakness is also common especially those who have cachexia. Progressive resistance training, focusing on large muscle groups, has been shown to be effective and improve QOL and function in this population.[24] Performing daily activities, for persons recovering from surgery, or those with very low strength, can be important in improving daily activities. Onc R clinicians working in acute hospital or home health settings should focus strengthening exercises toward increasing independence in ADLs such as transferring from low surfaces or climbing stairs. Once the individual is independent in their home mobility, more focused muscle training can be very beneficial.

Pulmonary Rehabilitation

Pulmonary rehabilitation is an interdisciplinary, patient-centered approach to maximizing the health and function of persons diagnosed and treated for lung disease and is very appropriate for persons diagnosed with lung cancer. The goals of a program, including improving nutritional status, exercise capacity, dyspnea management, and medication adherence/education, fit very well for this population. However, disease self-management skills may be different for the person who does not fit the typical COPD profile.

Persons recovering from lung surgery will benefit from structured exercise instruction, breathing exercises, and airway clearance skills, ideally individualized and beginning immediately after surgery in the inpatient setting. Transitioning from an individualized program to a group setting is recommended, but fewer than 25% of eligible patients are referred.[25]

People with adverse events from chemotherapy that affect balance may have limitations in choices of exercise modalities. Persons with late-stage or progressive lung cancer will also present a challenge to pulmonary rehabilitation programs, as these are group classes focusing on primary lung disease. Additionally, some studies have found that elderly individuals or those at high risk for functional impairments may especially benefit from individualized and home-based programs versus group, clinic-based pulmonary rehabilitation.[26,27] The person with underlying smoking-related lung issues will more likely fit the target population for most pulmonary rehabilitation programs, but others may need more individualized programs. An Onc R clinician can, and should, incorporate the principles of pulmonary rehabilitation into any plan of care for a person diagnosed with lung cancer.

Energy Conservation and Activity Modification

Breathlessness and fatigue are major symptoms reported by this population, at least at some point in their care. Teaching energy conservation and activity modification are key elements of self-management for these individuals. Strategies include pacing breathing with activity, taking frequent rest breaks, and scheduling tasks related to their energy demands, with the most fatiguing tasks performed early in the day. Task modifications include sitting instead of standing for showering or food preparation and placing commonly used items within easy reach. Consultation with an occupational therapist and/or a pulmonary rehabilitation program can provide the clinician and the PLWBC with individualized skills to manage these most distressing symptoms.

Special Considerations Related to Lung Cancer

Stigma and Self-Blame

Cigarette smoking is by far the leading cause of lung cancer and leads to stigma and negative stereotyping that is not common in other types of cancer.[28] Many individuals feel that they are being punished for making the choice to smoke and thus, blame themselves for developing cancer. This blame can come from external sources as well, such as family members or community members. Therefore people diagnosed and treated for lung cancer may find themselves without important support for cancer or treatment-related physical, emotional, and psychological issues.

A PLWBC may also feel subtle or not-so-subtle blame from healthcare professionals, and this can be a barrier to seeking care. It is important for the Onc R clinician to provide compassionate and comprehensive care while being sensitive to the person's experiences or shame. Accepting people in their unique situation is vital to establish a therapeutic relationship. It is also important that the clinician recognize emotional issues that are beyond their scope and refer to appropriate services. Support groups may be especially helpful, as PLWBCs can share their experiences of negative stigma and find ways to overcome it.

Multiple Comorbidities and Underlying Chronic Lung Disease

Smokers who develop lung cancer typically have varying degrees of another smoking-induced lung dysfunction. Early symptoms of lung cancer closely mimic those that are common in chronic smokers, especially in those with moderate or severe COPD. The presence of a productive cough (sometimes bloody), dyspnea on exertion, weight loss, and limited activity tolerance are very familiar to people with COPD and can be dismissed as being caused by COPD. This issue accounts to a significant extent for the relatively late-stage diagnosis of most smoking-related lung cancer. Late-stage lung cancer has the poorest 5-year survival rate (≤10%).[3] Lung cancer also exacerbates the symptoms of COPD, which may be very debilitating, even at diagnosis.

Lung cancer in people who smoke is also commonly diagnosed later in life, so issues of aging must be considered. In addition, a person diagnosed with lung cancer may have other chronic diseases, such as arthritis, heart disease, and diabetes that impact physical capacity. These comorbid conditions may take a back seat during acute cancer treatment and may not be well managed. The clinician should be aware of all the person's conditions, being especially alert for signs and symptoms of poor tolerance to physical activity during the rehabilitation phase of cancer treatment (e.g., weight gain from worsening heart failure, blood glucose abnormalities, diabetic nerve issues, and heart damage).

Unusual Cases

While the stereotypical person with lung cancer is an older, male, chronic smoker, it is important to recognize that lung cancer affects other demographics. The good news is that survival is generally better for younger persons and nonsmokers, but treatment can be delayed by lack of early diagnosis. Onc R clinicians can help educate their communities about these unusual cases, especially to help younger persons and nonsmokers get early screening for symptoms, such as cough, shortness of breath, or unintended weight loss.

An emerging issue to watch closely is the possible link between inhaled substances ("vaping" or "e-cigarettes") and lung cancer development. As these devices are used by young teenagers or as a perceived safe alternative to cigarettes, they are not recognized by users as harming the lungs.[29] It stands to reason that inhalation of any substance could be an irritant to the respiratory epithelium and lead to lung damage. It may be shown in the future that this initial exposure predisposes individuals to development of precancerous and cancerous lesions later in life. Onc R clinicians can help educate their community about the dangers of these devices, especially as there is little regulation of the industry and little known about many of the substances that are "vaped."

Complex Psychosocial Situations

Chronic cigarette smoking often accompanies complicated social and psychological conditions. Persons with alcohol or other substance use disorders often also smoke.[15] Thus, some people who smoke are dependent on cigarettes for more than just the nicotine addiction. Smoking also is associated with habitual behaviors and social rituals. It can be very difficult to stop smoking if it is a person's social outlet and if all their friends also smoke. It is also very difficult to quit smoking, even if one has lung cancer, especially if family members in the same household still smoke. Thus, smoking cessation, a key component of lung cancer prevention and treatment, requires a multifaceted approach (see Pignataro et al.[18] for strategies specific to the Onc R clinician). If the patient being treated for lung cancer uses smoking as a stress management strategy or feels that their cancer is too advanced to be helped by quitting, they may feel that the short-term satisfaction of smoking outweighs the additional discomforts of trying to quit. In fact, it is not uncommon to see a person who had a laryngectomy for lung cancer smoke through their tracheostomy. Some individuals may smoke immediately before and after their chemotherapy or radiation treatment sessions as well.

Cigarette smoking is much higher in economically disadvantaged communities, minority populations, unemployed or underemployed persons, and people with mental health conditions, including homeless persons. All of these populations have poor access to cancer diagnosis and treatment and may partially account for the poor long-term prognosis at present. In addition, these populations may have challenges with poor health literacy, limited transportation and resources for medical expenses, and lack of strong social support systems.[7,8] Lack of attendance at scheduled appointments and loss to follow-up are quite common in this population.

Onc R clinicians need to recognize that this population of persons diagnosed and treated for lung cancer may have needs that are far beyond the physical issues and require much greater involvement of social services. Providing simple home exercises that require little or no equipment or cost and focusing intervention on ensuring the person can perform activities correctly and safely should predominate the program. Expecting persons to come to a clinic several times a week for passive techniques may be unrealistic.

Poor Overall Prognosis

While there is emerging hope for survival after lung cancer, due to earlier diagnosis and advanced medical treatment, the current status of survival for persons with late-stage lung cancer remains bleak. Dying from lung cancer typically includes progressive dyspnea, wasting away, and chest discomfort. Involving hospice services and supportive care specialists early after diagnosis (especially for more advanced stages) can help a PLWBC and their family to manage symptoms and plan for a "good death" (see Chapter 29).

Recent studies have documented needs of persons with inoperable lung cancer that are amenable to Onc R interventions,[30,31] as well as improved QOL and overall functional capacity from even brief home-based or virtual interventions.[32,33] The clinician can help explain the benefits of hospice care and inform the person that it is not admitting failure. Specific roles in hospice include advising on assistive and adaptive equipment and education of caregivers with the goal of maintaining functional activities that are important to the patient (see Chapter 29 for more details). Hospice care also involves psychological services that are vital to avoiding depression and despair that may begin with the initial diagnosis.

Future of Lung Cancer

Lung cancer is a huge global issue affecting persons from all walks of life. Although prognosis is currently poor, there are emerging signs of hope. Rates of cigarette smoking in the developed world have decreased over the lifetime of many current patients.[2,3] No longer is smoking seen as a socially acceptable habit in many communities and more public facilities around the world are becoming smoke-free. Legislative efforts to regulate and tax cigarettes can help discourage people from taking up smoking . Greater access to nicotine replacements and smoking cessation programs can help more people quit smoking. Screening for lung cancer is now considered a standard of care for persons with age, family history, and smoking history risk factors. No doubt, diagnosing lung cancer at earlier stages will lead to improved survival rates, less intensive treatment needs, and less treatment-related complications. New medical treatments, such as immune modulators and targeted radiation therapy are not only improving survival but also decreasing treatment adverse events that impact function and mobility. Early involvement of Onc R clinicians, especially for prevention and minimizing movement impairments is becoming standard practice. Lung cancer is represented by a "clear" or white ribbon, indicating its invisible nature. In the future, the hope is that lung cancer is something that is recognized early, not stigmatized, and managed by an interprofessional healthcare team to maximize the health and participation of the survivor.

Conclusion

Onc R clinicians are seated in a very unique and strong position to make major contributions to health of the lungs of each and every person. These clinicians can work in the realm of primordial or primary prevention leading the charge to prevent lung cancer through education of lifestyle behaviors. They are also well-situated to provide interventions to prevent, mitigate, and manage cancer treatment related adverse effects, therefore Onc R clinicians hold an advantageous status in the cancer care team to provide effective interventions at the secondary and tertiary prevention stages. Advocating for Onc R involvement across the lifespan can foster and cultivate true QOL.

Critical Research Needs

- What are the differences in mobility trajectory in newer lung cancer populations due to early screening? (Younger, more women, nonsmokers).
- What is the role of physical therapy for chest wall pain that is common in patients getting lung surgery?
- Which components of pulmonary rehabilitation need to modified for people with cancer and treatment-related issues versus those with other lung disease?
- Which patients do better with home-based versus facility-based pulmonary rehab after lung cancer?
- What are the mobility impacts of immunotherapy for lung cancer?

Case Studies

Case Study #1: Assessment

Given medical treatment and system assessment results, how do you determine movement diagnosis, prognosis, and goals?

Mary is a 72-year-old female with Stage 1 NSCLC T1N0M0 status post robotic-assisted left lower lobectomy who comes to see a physical therapist complaining of left chest wall and shoulder pain. She had an uncomplicated postoperative course, required no additional treatment, and had initiated pulmonary rehab with initial success. She reports she has a progressive increase in pain in her lateral chest wall, ribs, and shoulder with prolonged or overhead movement and deep breathing. This is limiting her ability to perform bathing and dressing due to need for additional time to complete tasks. She states she is unable to fall asleep and stay asleep for more than 2 hours due to discomfort. She reports needing assistance to perform moderate-to-heavy housework that includes carrying moderate weighted objects, pushing, or pulling. She is limiting her participation in the church choir due to breathlessness when singing and difficulty projecting well enough to be heard. She also has avoided gardening due to her daughter pushing Mary to leave her home and relocate to live with her. Mary's goal is to be able to independently do her own laundry, including carrying the basket across the house, so her daughter sees that she can remain safely in her own home. She is very anxious about her pain, as she is afraid her cancer is back and "it is a death sentence." She feels her daughter is forcing her to move out of her house.

Physical Assessment

Each assessment performed on a patient with cancer is an opportunity to identify unmet needs, both rehab-related and otherwise. These patients require a comprehensive evaluation that screens for physical impairments as well as the more common unmet needs for survivors to truly improve their QOL. Questionnaires that patients can take home and bring back to their next visit will keep the initial evaluation simpler and may help identify needs for referral to services like mental health professionals, occupational therapy, speech language pathology, pain management, nutrition/ dietician, or social work. It is also important to keep in mind that with patients diagnosed and treated for cancer we are seeking to improve and restore functional movement and participation instead of the goal being optimal movement.

Assessment/Screening Tools

1. Psychosocial screening: (Can be given at end of session for her to bring back to next session)
   Mental health: Distress Scale or Depression Anxiety and Depression Scale
   Interpersonal relations/support: Reintegration to Normal Living.
2. Cardiopulmonary: Endurance: 6-Minute Walk Test (6MWT), vitals at rest and with movement, Borg Scale of Perceived Exertion, Brief Fatigue Inventory.
3. Musculoskeletal: Strength: 5 Times Sit to Stand Test, grip strength; range of motion: goniometery (shoulder, thoracolumbar, cervical), thoracic girth measurements with respiration, joint and rib mobility.
4. Integumentary: Scar mobility assessment (incisions and drains/ chest tube sites).
5. Neuromuscular: Sensory testing (Modified Total Neuropathy Score if she reports numbness or tingling or has changes in light touch), pain pressure thresholds, Timed Up and Go or balance assessment of choice, cranial nerve and deep tendon reflexes (DTR), Comprehensive Pain (Defense and Veterans Pain Rating scale or Brief Pain Inventory).
6. Functional mobility: 10-Meter Walk Test (10MWT), Berg Balance Scale, Short Physical Performance Battery.

For this case study, the International Classification of Functional, Disability and Health (ICF) Framework is utilized (Figure 18.8) (see Chapter 2 for more information on the ICF).

Discussion: This case demonstrates how a patient with early stage lung cancer that receives curative treatment with surgery only can have a long list of impairments and unmet needs that may seem overwhelming. The selection of assessment and screening tools for the initial visit is driven by the patient's chief complaint. Once the clinician determines what is impaired then layering in the cancer-specific knowledge guides the decision. Mary's chief complaint is pain in her chest wall and her goal is to be able do her laundry. It is anticipated based on diagnosis that she will have a decrease in lean muscle mass and physical activity levels. Her goal is a functional activity so assessing strength with manual muscle testing may not give as much information as the "5 Times Sit to Stand Test" about how the strength in her legs is impacting her functional movement. As she is experiencing an acute onset of pain, the clinician would consider how the surgery could contribute to that pain and therefore aim to asses her scars, but also rib mobility and chest expansion.

Consider the movement system, ICF framework, and the patient's goals to select the optimal assessment tools. First priority for intervention is always to consider what has to be done to make the patient safe. Next, consider what impairments are leading to the patient's most distressing functional limitation. It is also important to keep in mind that people with cancer are generally seeking to improve and restore functional movement and participation instead of obtaining perfect movement. Most of the common long-lasting impairments like pain, fatigue, and shortness of breath all respond very well to increased physical activity, but especially in lung cancer, many patients are not likely to have ever been physically active or know how to begin.

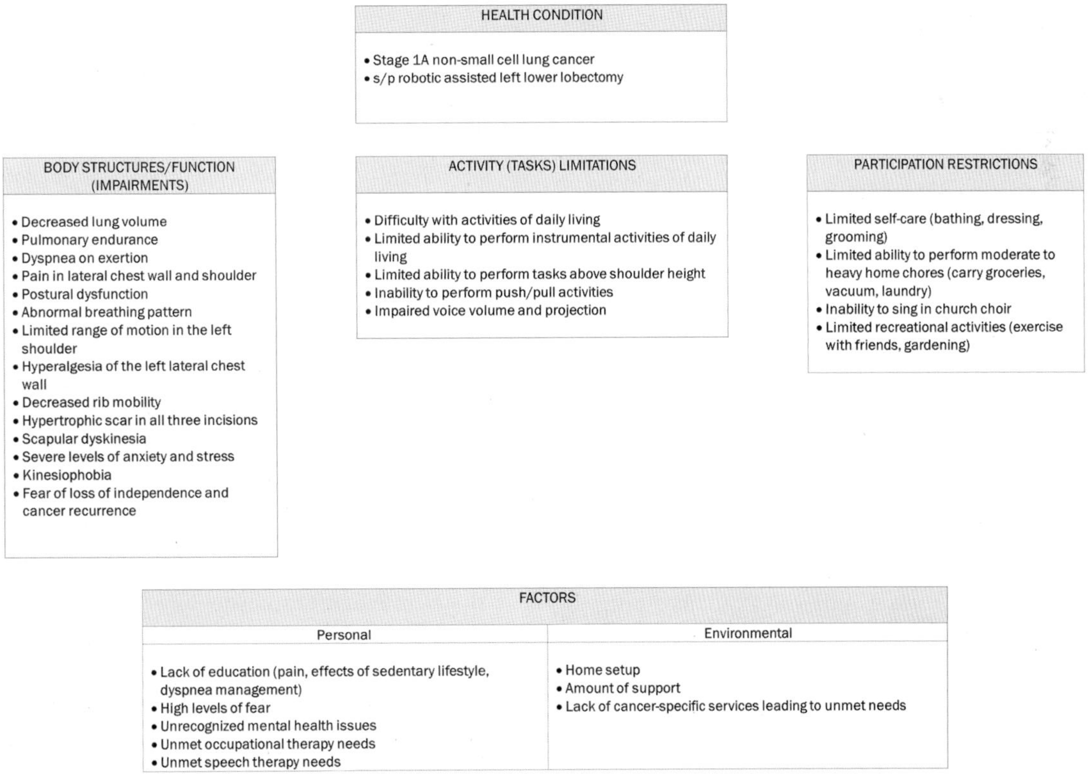

HEALTH CONDITION
- Stage 1A non-small cell lung cancer
- s/p robotic assisted left lower lobectomy

BODY STRUCTURES/FUNCTION (IMPAIRMENTS)
- Decreased lung volume
- Pulmonary endurance
- Dyspnea on exertion
- Pain in lateral chest wall and shoulder
- Postural dysfunction
- Abnormal breathing pattern
- Limited range of motion in the left shoulder
- Hyperalgesia of the left lateral chest wall
- Decreased rib mobility
- Hypertrophic scar in all three incisions
- Scapular dyskinesia
- Severe levels of anxiety and stress
- Kinesiophobia
- Fear of loss of independence and cancer recurrence

ACTIVITY (TASKS) LIMITATIONS
- Difficulty with activities of daily living
- Limited ability to perform instrumental activities of daily living
- Limited ability to perform tasks above shoulder height
- Inability to perform push/pull activities
- Impaired voice volume and projection

PARTICIPATION RESTRICTIONS
- Limited self-care (bathing, dressing, grooming)
- Limited ability to perform moderate to heavy home chores (carry groceries, vacuum, laundry)
- Inability to sing in church choir
- Limited recreational activities (exercise with friends, gardening)

FACTORS

Personal	Environmental
• Lack of education (pain, effects of sedentary lifestyle, dyspnea management) • High levels of fear • Unrecognized mental health issues • Unmet occupational therapy needs • Unmet speech therapy needs	• Home setup • Amount of support • Lack of cancer-specific services leading to unmet needs

• **Fig. 18.8** International Classification of Functional, Disability and Health (ICF) Framework for Case Study 1. *ADLs*, Activities of daily living; *NSCLC*, non-small cell lung cancer.

Pulmonary rehab is an excellent approach, but patients with lung cancer often will require modifications and an individual approach to address fears and allow them to exercise in ways that do not increase pain.

Case Study #2: Intervention

Illustrating progression of therapy interventions as patient moves from active treatment to long-term survivorship:

Bob is a 70-year-old male retired coal miner that you have worked with over the course of his initial treatment for NSCLC due to chemotherapy-induced peripheral neuropathy causing balance impairments, decreased functional mobility, and frequent falls. His initial treatment course was carboplatin (Paraplatin) and paclitaxel (Taxol) every 2 weeks for six cycles with SBRT to the isolated lesion in his right upper lobe. He was not a surgical candidate due to the severity of his COPD, type II diabetes, and hypertension. He developed chemotherapy-induced polyneuropathy (CIPN) after his first dose of chemotherapy. Over 6 weeks of intense physical rehabilitation for two to three times a week, he made significant improvements in his balance and mobility, so he was discharged to a community senior exercise program. He returns to the clinic for a 3 month follow-up with a complaint of generalized weakness and acute flare of his chronic low back pain. He was excited to report that he "rang the bell" at his last chemo treatment 2 months ago and his PET-CT last week reported negative for disease reoccurrence or any changes in baseline lung changes associated with his COPD. He denies any falls, states that his feet are a little better but still are not normal. He tried the community exercise classes but felt out of place because he was the only man attending. He has been walking his dog for 10 to 20 minutes a day and performs his balance exercises most days of the week, but otherwise he says he is not doing much due to not having any energy. He reports that he just does not feel as strong as he did after completing rehabilitation for his balance and now his back hurts too. He has experienced intermittent low back pain for 18 years that does not radiate into his legs and usually will self-resolve. He says this time his back pain is not getting worse, but it is not getting any better.

Initial Rehabilitation Care Plan

Assessment tools: 30 Second Sit to Stand Test, Dynamic Gait Index, Modified Total Neuropathy Score, 6MWT, 10MWT.

Impairments: decreased endurance, dyspnea on exertion, fear of dyspnea, static and dynamic balance impairments that were most significant in single leg stance (SLS) or with decreased visual input, and impaired sensory integrity with dull, vibration, and protective sensation.

Interventions provided: progressive aerobic exercise with a walking program, sensorimotor training, closed kinetic chain functional exercises, core strengthening, gait training on variable surfaces and over obstacles.

Re-Assessment Findings

Assessments: 30 Second Sit to Stand (moderate decrease), Dynamic Gait Index (mild decrease), Modified Total Neuropathy Score (no change), 6MWT (mild decrease), 10MWT (mild decrease), lower quarter screen and lumbopelvic evaluation (indicates mechanical low back pain).

Discussion

The focus on Bob's initial course of treatment was centered around decreasing his falls and improving his functional mobility and postural control with combined interventions to address endurance, strength, and sensorimotor training. As he continued through chemotherapy, it would be anticipated that he would experience fatigue and generalized loss of strength. Both are likely leading to the minor decrease in his balance testing scores despite his report of his balance being the same. He continued to perform exercises that improve his endurance and postural control but did not continue strength training. His new reports of fatigue and weakness are common for lung cancer survivors. The report of constant low back pain would normally raise a red flag for possible metastasis to the spine, but with negative imagining, no change in his neurological exam, and no additional concerns found on the orthopedic evaluation, he is likely experiencing mechanical low back pain that is not improving because of the weakness that is also occurring in his core musculature and spinal stabilizers.

This case demonstrates the need for continued assessments across the continuum of care and well into survivorship. Patients with lung cancer, especially those that were never physically active, will often need continued guidance in how to choose, modify, and execute their exercise prescription either through maintenance visits every 3 to 4 weeks or with planned follow-up visits at select time periods to catch small declines that can be addressed easily within a few visits.

Review Questions

Reader can find the correct answers and rationale in the back of the book.

1. A 52-year-old woman with COPD, peripheral arterial disease, and Stage I NSCLC s/p robotic-assisted left lower lobe wedge resection presents with a complaint of difficulty walking and negotiating stairs in her home. Her 5 Times Sit to Stand Test was 26.4 seconds, Timed Up and Go was 10.1 seconds, and her 6MWT was 324 m with a Modified Borg Dyspnea Scale rating of 3 (moderate). These results were likely MOST impacted by:
   A. Balance impairments due to chemotherapy induced peripheral neuropathy
   B. Radiation related fatigue
   C. Fear of cancer reoccurrence
   D. Decreased cardiopulmonary endurance

2. A patient with Stage IIB NSCLC presents mid-way through radiation for evaluation of his balance after multiple falls. He was not a surgical candidate and was treated with chemoradiation including paclitaxel (Taxol) and carboplatin (Paraplatin). What is an EARLY adverse effect of radiation that should be screened for in this patient?
   A. Fatigue
   B. Decreased soft tissue mobility
   C. Skin changes (radiation burn)
   D. Limited chest expansion

3. What postural change is COMMON in patient with a chest tube?
   A. Side bending away from the chest tube
   B. Holding bilateral upper extremities tightly across the chest in a protective position

C. Side bending toward the operative side

D. Thoracic rotation away from the operative side

4. Which of the following is NOT a cause of weakness in people with advanced lung cancer?

A. Immunotherapy-induced anemia

B. Impaired motor unit function and recruitment due to CIPN

C. Cachexia

D. Sedentary lifestyle prior to diagnosis

5. Which intervention is the LEAST appropriate for a rehabilitation oncology clinician to perform with a patient with advanced lung cancer and metastasis to the brain as they approach end of life?

A. Maximizing functional mobility and independence with task specific training

B. Passive range of motion to improve pain

C. Family training on guarding, transfers, and patient positioning

D. Educating patients and caregivers on need for transition to hospice and the services provided

6. A 61-year-old male s/p VATS right upper lobectomy wedge resection that was performed to treat his Stage II non-small cell adenocarcinoma is referred to pulmonary rehabilitation. Which of the following is MOST likely to be the goal of this program?

A. Initiate treatment 6 months after surgery to allow for complete healing

B. Provide group exercise with generalized progression

C. Medication prescription and adherence

D. Improving nutritional status and exercise capacity

Bob is a 54-year-old male electrician that presented to his primary care physician complaining of sharp, shooting low back pain with radiation into his right leg. He states that the pain initially occurred when he was working, but over time it has become constant and is worse at night. He says that the pain is keeping him from both falling asleep and staying asleep. The lack of sleep is causing him to not be able to perform his normal work tasks without resting, and he is skipping lunch to nap in his car. He has a 30 pack-year history of smoking, but recently switched to vaping after being diagnosed with emphysema. He states that he "should have kept smoking," because he is coughing more now than he did as a smoker. Observation reveals a slender man with

mildly forward flexed posture and increased respiratory rate with an abnormal breathing pattern.

7. Which of the following factors is MOST likely to qualify Bob to get a yearly low-dose CT scan to actively screen for lung cancer?

A. Age between 60 and 80 years old

B. Smoking at least 30 pack years

C. Quitting less than 5 years ago

D. Having private medical insurance coverage

8. Which of the following is MOST likely to be a component of the abnormal breathing pattern that would be expected in someone with COPD?

A. Paradoxical breathing

B. Inhibition of ventilatory muscles during expiration

C. Adaptive shortening of neck extensors and pectoralis major

D. Symmetrical use of lower costal muscles to cause abdominal rise with expiration

9. What exercise recommendations would be MOST appropriate for Bob?

A. High-intensity short-duration isolated resistance training

B. Low-intensity long-duration functional mobility training

C. Low-to-moderate intensity short duration functional exercises against body weight resistance

D. High-intensity long-duration whole body endurance exercises

10. If Bob presented to your outpatient physical therapy clinic via direct access, which of the following is the most APPROPRIATE clinical decision concerning treatment?

A. No red flags—initiate treatment for mechanical low back pain

B. Yellow flag: night pain but no cancer history—initiate treatment for mechanical low back pain and reassess in 1 month for possible need for referral to PCP if not improving

C. Red flags: night pain, constant pain, cough, age greater than 50 years, smoking history—refer to PCP due to concern for metastatic lung cancer and hold treatment until after workup

D. Red flags: night pain, constant pain, cough, age greater than 50 years, smoking history—refer to PCP due to concern for metastatic lung cancer and initiate treatment with gentle exercise and pain modulation

References

1. Siddiqui F, Siddiqui AH. Lung cancer. In: *StatPearls* [Internet]. StatPearls Publishing; 2021. https://www.ncbi.nlm.nih.gov/books/NBK482357/. Accessed February 20, 2021.

2. World Health Organization. Cancer. https://www.who.int/news-room/fact-sheets/detail/cancer. Accessed February 24, 2021.

3. American Cancer Society. Lung cancer statistics. https://www.cancer.org/cancer/lung-cancer/about/key-statistics.html. Accessed November 17, 2020.

4. American Cancer Society. Harmful chemicals in tobacco products. https://www.cancer.org/cancer/cancer-causes/tobacco-and-cancer/carcinogens-found-in-tobacco-products.html. Accessed November 17, 2020.

5. Samet JM, Avila-Tang E, Boffetta P, et al. Lung cancer in never smokers: clinical epidemiology and environmental risk factors. *Clin Cancer Res.* 2009;15(18):5626–5645.

6. Granger CL. Physiotherapy management of lung cancer. *J Physiother.* 2016;62:60–67.

7. Swisher AK, Kennedy-Rea S, Starkey A, et al. Bridging the gap: identifying and meeting the needs of lung cancer survivors. *J Public Health (Berl.).* 2020. doi:10.1007/s10389-020-01332-w.

8. Vijayvergia N, Shah PC, Denlinger CS. Survivorship in non-small cell lung cancer: challenges faced and steps forward. *J Natl Compr Canc Netw.* 2015;13(9):1151–1161.

9. Merck. Side effects of KEYTRUDA(R). https://www.keytruda.com/side-effects/. Accessed November 17, 2020.

10. Ha D, Reis AL, Mazzone PJ, Lippman SM, Fuster MM. Exercise capacity and cancer-specific quality of life following curative intent treatment of stage I–IIIA lung cancer, *Support Care Cancer.* 2018;26:2459–2469.

11. Yoo JS, Yang HC, Lee JM, et al. The association of physical functioning and quality of life on physical activity for non-small cell lung cancer. *Support Care Cancer.* 2020;28:4847–4856.

12. Messaggi-Sartor M, Marco E, Martinez-Tellez E, et al. Combined aerobic exercise and high-intensity respiratory muscle training in

patients surgically treated for non-small cell lung cancer: a pilot randomized clinical trial, *Eur J Phys Rehabil Med.* 2019;55(1): 113–122.

13. Huang MH, Blackwood J, Godoshian M, Pfalzer L. Factors associated with self-reported falls, balance or walking difficulty in older survivors of breast, colorectal, lung, or prostate cancer: results from Surveillance, Epidemiology, and End Results–Medicare Health Outcomes Survey linkage, *PLoS ONE.* 2018;13(12):e0208573.

14. Granger CL, Connolly B, Denehy L, et al. Understanding factors influencing physical activity and exercise in lung cancer: a systematic review. *Support Care Cancer.* 2017;25:983–999.

15. Dev R, Kim YJ, Reddy A, et al. Association between tobacco use, pain expression, and coping strategies among patients with advanced cancer. *Cancer.* 2019;125:153–160.

16. Hillegass E, Fick A, Pawlik A, et al. Supplemental oxygen utilization during physical therapy interventions. *Cardiopulm Phys Ther J.* 2014;25(2):38–49.

17. Centers for Disease Control and Prevention. Youth and tobacco use. https://www.cdc.gov/tobacco/data_statistics/fact_sheets/youth_data/tobacco_use/index.htm. Accessed February 24, 2021.

18. Pignataro R, Ohtake PJ, Swisher A, Dino G. The role of physical therapists in smoking cessation: opportunities for improving treatment outcomes, *Phys Ther.* 2012;92(5):757–766.

19. Smith SR, Khanna A, Wisotzky EM. An evolving role for cancer rehabilitation in the era of low-dose lung computed tomography screening. *Phys Med Rehabil.* 2017(9S2):S407–S414.

20. Centers for Disease Control and Prevention. Who should be screened for lung cancer? https://www.cdc.gov/cancer/lung/basic_info/screening.htm. Accessed February 24, 2021.

21. Lai Y, Su J, Qui P, et al. Systematic short-term pulmonary rehabilitation before lung cancer lobectomy: a randomized trial. *Interact Cardiovasc Thorac Surg.* 2017;25:476–483.

22. Li X, Li S, Yan S, et al. Impact of preoperative exercise therapy on surgical outcomes in lung cancer patients with or without COPD: a systematic review and meta-analysis. *Cancer Manage Res.* 2019;11:1765–1777.

23. Ni H-J, Pudasaini B, Yuan X-T, et al. Exercise training for patients pre- and postsurgically treated for non-small cell lung cancer: a systematic review and meta-analysis. *Integr Cancer Ther.* 2017;16(1):63–73.

24. Henshall CL, Allin L, Aveyard H. A systematic review and narrative synthesis to explore the effectiveness of exercise-based interventions in improving fatigue, dyspnea, and depression in lung cancer survivors. *Cancer Nurs.* 2019;42(4):295–306.

25. Sommer MS, Staerkind MEB, Christensen J, et al. Effect of postsurgical rehabilitation programmes in patients operated for lung cancer: a systematic review and meta-analysis. *J Rehabil Med.* 2018;50: 236–245.

26. Driessen EJ, Peeters ME, Bongers BC, et al. Effects of prehabilitation and rehabilitation including a home-based component on physical fitness, adherence, treatment tolerance, and recovery in patients with non-small cell lung cancer: a systematic review. *Critical Rev Oncol/Hematol.* 2017;114:63–76.

27. Lafaro KJ, Raz DJ, Kim JY, et al. Pilot study of a telehealth perioperative physical activity intervention for older adults with cancer and their caregivers. *Support Care Cancer.* 2020;28(8):3867–3876. doi:10.1007/s00520-019-05230-0.

28. Kornhauser C, Quinlan S, Hu N, et al. Lung cancers and stigma: perception or reality? *Oncol Nurs.* 2015;8(1). http://www.theoncologynurse.com/lung-cancer/16305-lung-cancers-and-stigma-perception-or-reality. Accessed February 24, 2021.

29. Olfert IM, DeVallance E, Hoskinson H, et al. Chronic exposure to electronic cigarettes results in impaired cardiovascular function in mice. *J Appl Physiol.* 2018;124(3):573–582.

30. Cheville AL, Rhudy L, Basford JR, Griffin JM, Flores AM. How receptive are patients with late stage cancer to rehabilitation services and what are the sources of their resistance? *Arch Phys Med Rehabil.* 2017;98(2):203–210.

31. Bayly JL, Lloyd-Williams M. Identifying functional impairment and rehabilitation needs in patients newly diagnosed with inoperable lung cancer: a structured literature review. *Support Care Cancer.* 2016;24(5):2359–2379.

32. Edbrooke L, Denehy L, Granger CL, Kapp S, Aranda S. Home-based rehabilitation in inoperable non-small cell lung cancer: the patient experience. *Support Care Cancer.* 2020;28(1):99–112.

33. Edbrooke L, Aranda S, Granger CL, et al. Multidisciplinary home-based rehabilitation in inoperable lung cancer: a randomised controlled trial. *Thorax.* 2019;74(8):787–796.

19

Head and Neck Cancers

BRYAN A. SPINELLI, PT, PHD, CYNTHIA TAN, PT, MPT, CLT-LANA

CHAPTER OUTLINE

Introduction

Approximately 4% of all cancers diagnosed in the United States (US) are head and neck cancers (HNCs).[1] This equates to approximately 65,000 people (48,000 men and 17,000 women) being diagnosed with HNC each year in the US.[1] Of the 15 million cancer survivors residing in the US, over 430,000 survivors have a history of HNC.[2]

HNC typically affects older adults who have a history of heavy tobacco and alcohol use. However, there has been an increase in HNC among younger people associated with the human papilloma virus (HPV). Although HNC is not the most common cancer, people diagnosed and treated for HNC demonstrate a high frequency, severity, and complexity of problems. HNC and its associated adverse effects can negatively impact quality of life (QOL) and can have a significant financial impact on patients and their caregivers.[3–6] Additionally, people diagnosed with HPV-positive HNC have a better prognosis meaning younger people diagnosed with HPV-positive cancer will likely have to deal with long-term negative consequences of HNC and its treatment.

Head and Neck Anatomy

The majority of HNCs begin in the squamous cells that line the mucosal surfaces of the oral cavity, nasal cavity, paranasal sinuses, pharynx, and larynx (see Figure 19.1). The oral cavity boundaries are the lips anteriorly and the tonsillar pillars posteriorly.[7] The oral cavity is separated from the nasal cavity by the hard palate.[7] Located in the oral cavity are the mandible, the hard palate, teeth, the anterior two-thirds of the tongue, and the retromolar trigone.[7]

The pharynx is located posteriorly to the nasal and oral cavities.[8] The pharynx is divided into three parts: nasopharynx, oropharynx, and hypopharynx.[8] The nasopharynx lies behind the nasal cavity and continues from the skull base to the level of the junction of the soft palates.[9] The lateral boarders include medial pterygoid plates, superior pharyngeal constrictor muscles, and the openings of the eustachian tubes.[9] The posterior border is the pharyngeal wall and continues with the oropharynx.[9] The soft palate's inferior surface forms the oropharynx's superior wall.[10] The anterior wall is formed by the base of the tongue, the vallecula, and the glossoepiglottic folds, and the lateral wall is made up of the tonsil, tonsillar fossae, and tonsillar pillars.[11] The hypopharynx is inferior to oropharynx and posterior to larynx, and ends at the pharyngoesophageal junction.[8] It comprises three subsites: the paired pyriform sinuses, the posterior pharyngeal wall, and the postcricoid area.[8]

The larynx is divided into three regions: supraglottic, glottic, and subglottic.[12] The supraglottic region consists of the epiglottis, false vocal cords, ventricles, aryepiglottic folds, and arytenoids.[12] The glottic region includes the vocal cords and the anterior and posterior commissures.[12] The subglottic larynx extends below the true cords to 5 mm below to the cricoid cartilage's inferior border.[12]

HNC can also begin in the salivary glands; however, there are numerous types of salivary gland cancers because the salivary glands consist of many different types of cells. There are three major salivary glands: sublingual, submandibular, parotid glands, and numerous minor salivary glands.[13] The sublingual glands lie underneath the mucosa of the mouth's anterior floor.[14] The submandibular glands lie in the upper neck between the mandible and the myohyoid muscle's insertion.[14] The parotid glands lie in the subcutaneous tissue of the face, overlying the mandibular ramus, and anterior-inferior to the external ear.[14]

Cancers of the head and neck can metastasize to the lymph nodes located in the neck. The sides of the neck are divided into two large triangles: anterior and posterior.[15] These triangles are divided by the sternocleidomastoid (SCM) muscle, which runs diagonally from the sternum and clavicle to the mastoid process and occipital bone. The anterior triangle is further divided into smaller triangles: the muscular, carotid, submandibular, and submental.[15] The muscular, or inferior carotid triangle, is bounded in front by the median line of the neck from the hyoid bone to the sternum and is bounded from behind by the anterior margin of the SCM and above by the superior belly of the omohyoid muscle.[15] The carotid triangle is also called the superior carotid triangle. It is bounded by the SCM's anterior border on the posterior side, by the omohyoid muscle's superior belly on the anterior-inferior border.[15] The posterior belly of the digastric muscle makes the superior border.[15] The submandibular triangle also called the submaxillary or digastric triangle, is bounded superiorly by the mandible body's lower border and a line drawn from its angle to the mastoid process.[15] The posterior border is made up of the digastric muscle's posterior belly.[15] The submental triangle, also called the suprahyoid triangle, is formed by the anterior belly of the digastric muscle laterally.[16] The medial border is formed by the midline of the neck between the mandible and the hyoid bone. The body of the hyoid bone forms the inferior border.[16]

The posterior triangle consists of two smaller triangles, the occipital and the subclavian triangles.[15] The occipital triangle is the largest division of the posterior triangle and is bound anteriorly by the SCM and posteriorly by the trapezius muscle, and inferiorly by the omohyoid muscle.[15] The subclavian triangle is also called the supraclavicular triangle.[15] It is formed superiorly by the omohyoid muscle's belly, inferiorly by the clavicle, and posteriorly by the SCM.[15]

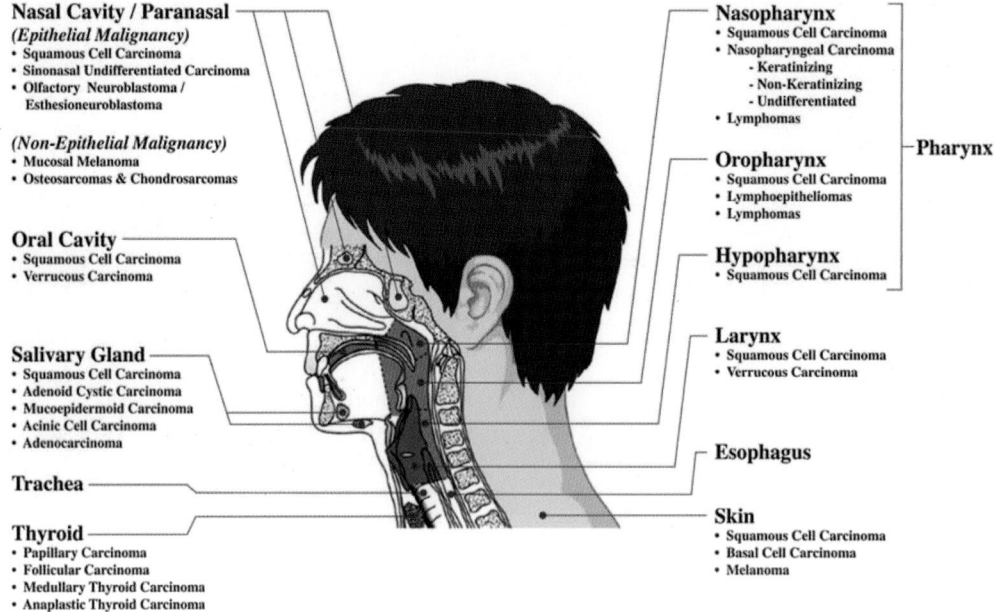

• **Fig. 19.1** *Variety of Head and Neck Cancers by Source.* (Reprinted with permission from Stadler ME, Patel MR, Couch ME, Hayes DN. Molecular biology of head and neck cancer: risks and pathways. *Hematol Oncol Clin North Am*. 2008;22(6):1099–1124, vii. doi:10.1016/j.hoc.2008.08.007.)

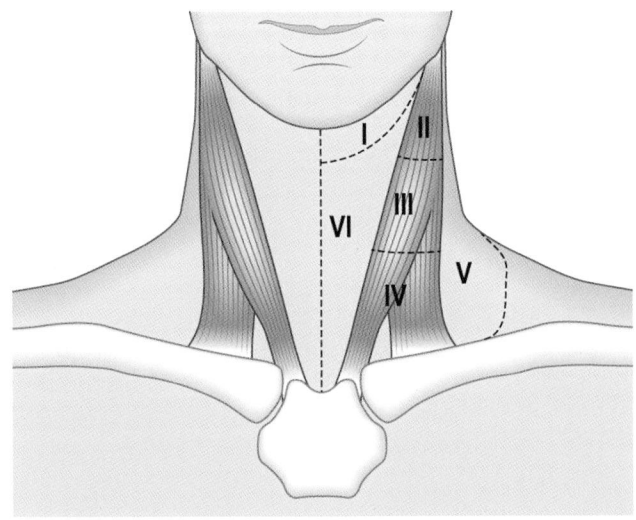

I   Submental and submandibular nodes
II   Upper third sternocleidomastoid (SCM) muscle
III Middle third SCM (between hyoid and cricoid)
IV   Lower third SCM (between cricoid and clavicle)
V   Posterior to SCM (posterior triangle)
VI   Midline from hyoid to manubrium

• **Fig. 19.2** Cervical Lymph Node Levels. (Reprinted with permission from Hathorn I. The ear, nose and throat. In: Innes JA, Dover AR, Fairhurst K, eds. *Macleod's Clinical Examination*. 14th ed. Elsevier; 2018.)

Cervical lymph nodes are divided into six levels that are useful to predict the lymph node groups that are most likely to be involved in metastatic disease for different locations of primary tumors and neck dissections (see Figure 19.2). Level I lymph nodes are related to the lymph nodes in the submandibular and submental nodes.[17] Level II, III, and IV correspond to the upper, middle, and lower jugular nodes, respectively.[17] Level V lymph nodes correspond to the posterior triangle nodes.[17] The level VI lymph nodes correspond with the neck's anterior or central compartment, located between the carotid arteries of the two sides.[17]

Medical Management of Head and Neck Cancer

Medical management of HNC will be dependent on several factors, including the type of cancer, stage of cancer, and the person's health status. Persons diagnosed with HNC may be treated with surgery or radiation alone or with a combination of surgery, radiation, and chemotherapy. Other approaches such as immunotherapy or targeted therapy may be used in the presence of metastatic or advanced recurrent disease. The following sections will provide an overview of standard medical treatment approaches for persons living with and beyond cancer (PLWBCs) of the head and neck.

Surgery

Surgical procedures may be used to resect cancerous tissue at the primary site and manage the neck and mandible structure and function. Primary tumor resection may be performed using open surgery or minimally invasive approaches. Historically, open surgery using a transcervical approach with or without

mandibulectomy had to be performed for cancers of the pharynx.[18] Although continuing to have a role in managing HNC, open surgery has largely been replaced with minimally invasive approaches for certain types and HNC stages due to the associated morbidity. Transoral robotic surgery (TORS) and transoral laser microsurgery (TLM) are two minimally invasive approaches used to resect cancers located in the oral cavity, larynx, and pharynx. TORS involves using surgical instruments and a camera attached to robotic arms inserted through the oral cavity. The surgeon performs the surgery by controlling the robotic arms from a remote console. TLM is an endoscopic surgical approach where the surgeon uses a carbon dioxide laser to remove the cancerous tissue. Another example of a minimally invasive procedure is an endoscopic nasopharyngectomy used in the management of nasopharyngeal cancer.

Neck dissection may be performed to manage the regional lymph nodes surgically.[19] Neck dissection refers to removing lymph nodes and surrounding fatty tissue. The amount of lymph node removal is dependent on the location of the primary tumor, the size of the tumor, and the extent of nodal disease based on clinical examination and imaging.[19] The terms radical neck dissection (RND) and modified radical neck dissection (MRND) were traditionally used to describe types of neck dissection. RND refers to removing cervical lymph node levels I through V and removing the SCM muscle spinal accessory nerve (SAN), and internal jugular vein (see Figure 19.3). A MRND refers to removing cervical lymph node levels I through V, but one of the following structures is preserved: SCM muscle, SAN, or internal jugular vein. Other neck dissection terms include comprehensive neck dissection, extended neck dissection, and selective neck dissection.[20,21] Comprehensive neck dissection refers to removal of the same lymph node levels as RND and MRND and possibly other structures besides lymph nodes (SCM muscle, SAN, and internal jugular vein) as well.[19] An extended neck dissection refers to removing additional lymph node groups or other nonlymphatic structures not included in a RND.[22] Selective neck dissection removes fewer than the five lymph node levels removed during a MRND or RND.[19] Selective neck dissections remove specific lymph node levels dependent on site and stage of cancer and are based on the common pattern of HNC spread to regional nodes.[20] For example, a selective neck dissection of cervical lymph node levels II through IV may be performed to remove lymph nodes where metastasis is commonly found in PLWBCs of the larynx.[20] However, due to the pattern of metastasis, selective neck dissection of cervical lymph node levels I through III may be performed in persons with cancer of the oral cavity.[20]

Depending on the extent of tissue removal, reconstructive procedures may be performed. Reconstructive procedures may involve myocutaneuous tissue or bone from other areas of the body.[23] Goals for reconstruction include restoring the head and neck areas' function and appearance. Free flap reconstruction is a type of reconstruction that involves transferring vascularized tissue from another part of the body to the area in need of tissue reconstruction.[24] Free flaps are also crucial in wound closure and protecting the head and neck area's internal structures.

An example of a bony reconstruction is a fibula flap used for mandibular reconstruction. This technique uses the middle one-third of the fibula, the donor site, to recreate the mandible (see Figure 19.4). Another example is to use a portion of the scapula to recreate the hard palate of the roof of the mouth. The iliac or radius can be used in bony reconstruction procedures as

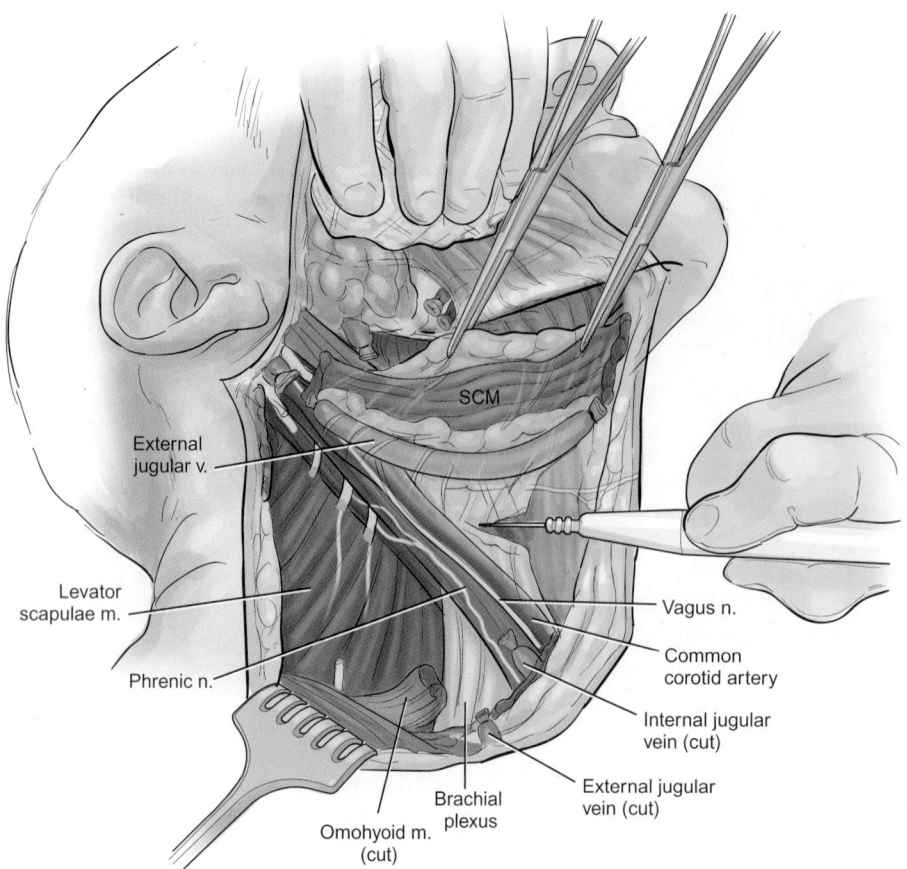

External
jugular v.

Levator
scapulae m.

Phrenic n.

Omohyoid m.
(cut)

Brachial
plexus

SCM

Vagus n.

Common
corotid artery

Internal jugular
vein (cut)

External jugular
vein (cut)

• **Fig. 19.3** Radical Neck Dissection. (Reprinted with permission from Medina JE. Radical Neck Dissection. In: Khatri VP, ed. *Atlas of Advanced Operative Surgery*. Elsevier; 2013.)

well. Soft tissue free flap procedures can be used to reconstruct the tongue, throat, neck, or lips. For example, a radial forearm flap (RFF) can be used to reconstruct the tongue and intraoral defects,[25,26] which can assist in the postsurgical recovery of speech and swallowing. However, there is a risk for donor site morbidity (limited wrist range of motion [ROM], decreased hand strength, and impaired sensation) and skin grafts are often required for closure at the donor site.[25,27] Another example of a soft tissue reconstruction is the use of the ear's cartilage to reconstruct a nose. An additional example of a soft tissue reconstruction uses a pectoralis major pedicle flap. This flap can be used as primary reconstructive procedure to address defects of neck soft tissue or pharynx, or it can be used as salvage or emergency procedure to protect the carotid artery as well as for wound closure secondary to free flap failure or refractory fistula.[28] There are many positive aspects of using the pectoralis flap for the head and neck, including that it offers a large amount of soft tissue, conforms well to various head and neck areas and minimizes operating time.[28] Some negatives of using a pectoralis flap include chest wall deformity and impaired shoulder ROM and strength (which limits function).[28] Another soft tissue flap used for HNCs is the anterolateral thigh flap (ALT). ALT is an advantageous type of flap because multiple types of tissue, skin, and subcutaneous fat tissue can be transferred, and the thickness can be varied relative to the needs of the area being covered. It also has a vascular pedicle with a relatively large diameter vessel and low donor site morbidity.[29]

General head and neck surgery complications include dysarthria, dysphagia, wound infection, delayed wound healing, wound dehiscence, hemorrhage, fistula, and venous thromboembolism.[30]

PLWBCs who undergo neck dissection may be at risk for carotid artery dissection. Risk factors for carotid artery dissection in PLWBCs of the head and neck include low body mass index, tumor located at hypopharynx or oropharynx, open wound in the neck requiring wet dressing, RND, and total radiation dose to the neck >70 Gy.[31] Other complications include facial nerve palsy if the surgery involves parotid gland or flap failure in PLWBCs who undergo reconstruction. Possible complications to the donor site need to be observed, such as seromas, hematomas, infection, dehiscence, congestion, and skin graft loss.[29] Oncology rehabilitation (Onc R) clinicians may be involved with identifying donor site morbidity. For example, a fibular flap may require physical therapy and occupational therapy to address gait, balance, strengthening, and ROM issues. The forearm flap donor site may need one or both disciplines to increase wrist and forearm ROM and grip strength.

Radiation and Chemotherapy

Radiation therapy may be recommended depending on the stage of HNC. Various techniques are used for treating a PLWBC of the head/neck. Three types of radiation therapy used in the management of HNC include intensity-modulated radiation therapy (IMRT), proton therapy, and brachytherapy. IMRT uses photon beams to deliver the radiation more precisely to the tumor and less radiation to the surrounding tissues.[32] PLWBCs that receive radiation therapy are usually treated 5 days a week for 7 weeks. A more contemporary type of radiation therapy is proton therapy which delivers proton beams to the tumor. A significant advantage of

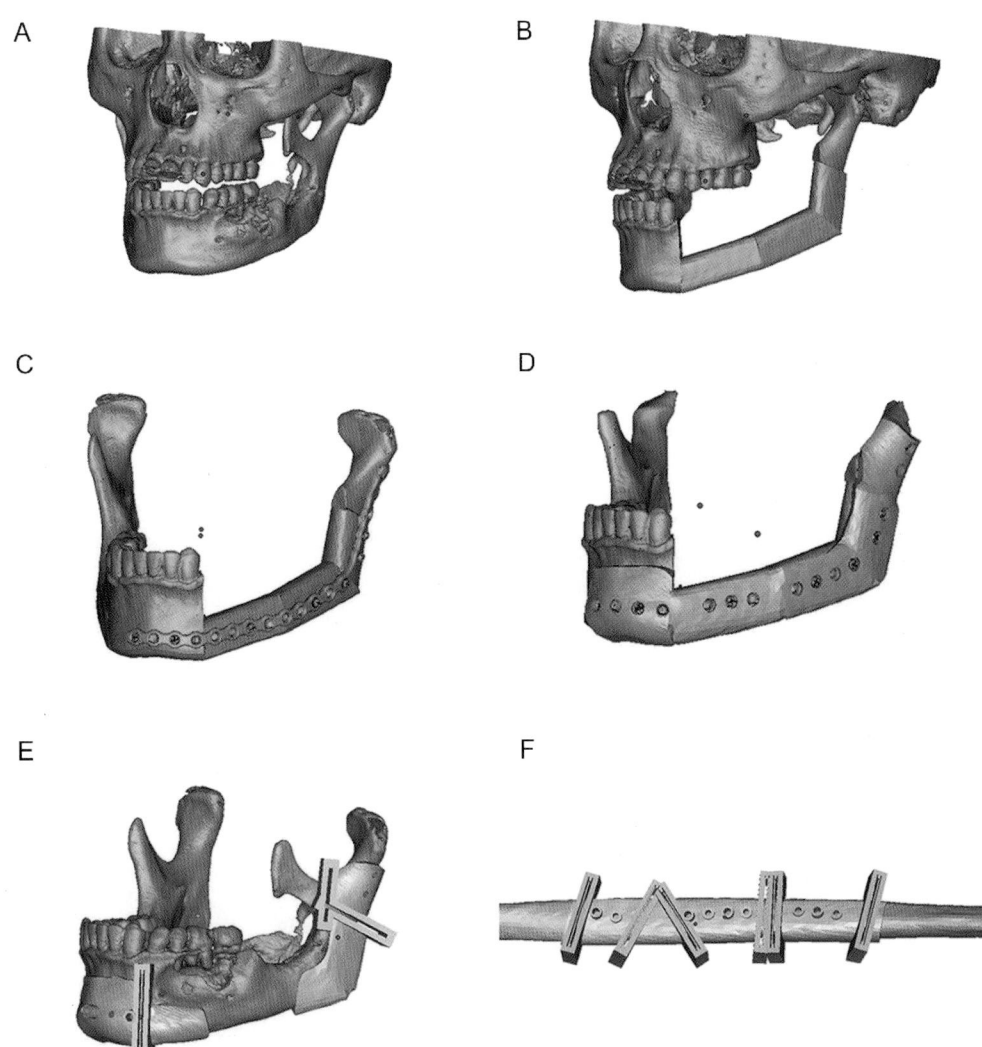

• **Fig. 19.4** Computerized Simulation of Fibular Flap Reconstruction of the Mandible. (A) Preoperative three-dimensional (3D) virtual model of a left mandibular ameloblastoma. (B) Virtual mandibular osteotomy and fibula inset. (C) A 3D model of the reconstructed mandible fixed with the pre-bent plate. (D) Design of the shaping guide with the pre-bent plate embedded. (E) Mandibular cutting guide with drill holes for fixing screws in the residual mandible. (F) Fibula cutting guide with drill holes. (Reprinted with permission from Bao T, He J, Yu C, et al. Utilization of a prebent plate-positioning surgical guide system in precise mandibular reconstruction with a free fibula flap. *Oral Oncol.* 2017;75:133–139.)

this type of radiation therapy is that there is no exit beam (dose of radiation beyond the target).[33] Thus, normal tissues are less likely to be damaged and proton therapy may cause less toxicity than photon therapy.[33] Proton therapy is the standard of care for base of skull cancer and has been used for HNCs at other locations as well.[33] Brachytherapy is used for limited tumors of the oral cavity, the oropharynx and nasopharynx, previously irradiated areas, and recurrent HNCs.[34–36]

Early or acute adverse effects of radiation therapy for this population include skin breakdown, hair loss, periodontal disease, taste changes, mucositis, xerostomia, difficulty swallowing, nausea, fatigue, and lymphedema.[2,37,38] Other adverse effects that are possible include nasal dryness and congestion, tinnitus, candidiasis, and trismus.[2,37,38] Adverse effects usually begin approximately 2 to 3 weeks after treatment has commenced, and symptoms begin to lessen 3 to 4 weeks after treatment has concluded. Other adverse effects such as ototoxicity and vision issues affect the PLWBC and

are outside of the Onc R clinician's scope of practice.[2,39] However, clinicians must be aware of these issues to refer and communicate effectively with other healthcare team members. Some adverse effects, such as taste changes, mucositis, xerostomia, and candidiasis, typically dissipate a few weeks to months after radiation has ended; however, they may persist in some PLWBCs. Other adverse effects such as fatigue and weakness may take longer to rehabilitate, though may be minimized if the PLWBC exercises throughout radiation treatment.[40] For those who have never exercised before, walking is an excellent way to begin a program, with the addition of strengthening exercises as tolerated.[41] Some late adverse effects from radiation therapy include head and neck lymphedema, carotid stenosis, osteonecrosis, fibrosis, and possible secondary cancers.[2]

For some types or stages of HNC, radiation therapy with concurrent chemotherapy is recommended. Some chemotherapy medications increase the effectiveness of radiation therapy when delivered concurrently.[42] Cisplatin (Platinol) is usually the medication of choice, and can be given weekly in lower dosages or every 3 weeks of radiation in greater amounts.[42] Adverse effects of concurrent chemoradiation with cisplatin include mucositis, xerostomia, skin toxicity, ototoxicity, kidney toxicity, neurotoxicity, low blood counts, weight loss, as well as nausea and vomiting.[42] Another type of systemic therapy for HNC is induction therapy for example, combining the medications docetaxel (Taxotere), cisplatin, and 5-FU (Adrucil)[43] or the combination of gemcitabine (Gemzar) and cisplatin.[44] Another pharmacologic approach is using immunotherapy to manage advanced or recurrent cancers. Currently, immunotherapy drugs approved by the Food and Drug Administration for cancer of the head or neck include cetuximab (Erbitux), pembrolizumab (Keytruda), and nivolumab (Opdivo); however, other treatments are being developed and investigated for persons with HNC.[45]

Multi-Disciplinary Teams

The team of physicians and nurses work closely with an ancillary team consisting of registered dietician nutritionists (RDN), speech-language pathologists (SLP), physical therapists (PT), and occupational therapists (OT). The RDN's role is to manage the PLWBCs weight while undergoing treatment, especially during radiation therapy. PLWBCs often experience decreased food intake, precipitating weight loss because of the adverse effects of radiation that causes skin damage, internal and external swelling, difficulty swallowing, as well as changes in taste. Significant weight loss may precipitate the need to stop treatment. Many PLWBCs of the head and neck undergo percutaneous endoscopic gastrostomy (PEG) tube placement to directly allow nutrition, fluids, or medications into the stomach and mitigate the weight loss/malnutrition issue if swallowing is compromised. RDNs also assist PLWBCs in the maintenance of the PEG tube. One important role of the SLP is to assess swallowing and provide treatment to address deficits and reduce risk of aspiration and malnutrition. In addition, the SLP has a critical role of rehabilitating any speech or oral motor issues that may arise after cancer treatment.

Patient Client Management

Review of Systems and Systems Review

Head and Neck Recurrence

Onc R clinicians should be aware of the signs and symptoms of HNC recurrence and refer patients to a HNC specialist if signs and symptoms are present.[2] Signs and symptoms of HNC recurrence include swelling in the head and neck region, lumps or masses, a sore that does not heal, a red or white patch in the mouth, sinus pain, persistent nasal congestion, unusual nasal discharge, nose bleeds, difficulty breathing, change in voice, change in vision, unpleasant breath odor even with consistent oral hygiene, numbness/weakness, new-onset or worsening of ear or jaw pain, persistent sore throat, difficulty swallowing, difficulty chewing or moving the jaw or tongue, blood in saliva, loosening of teeth and unexplained weight loss, and unusual fatigue.[2]

Screening for Adverse Effects of Head and Neck and Its Treatment

Due to the nature of HNC and its treatment, PLWBCs may experience problems affecting multiple body systems that may warrant referral to other health providers. Clinicians should screen for

dysphagia, speech or voice problems, hearing loss, vertigo, sleep disturbance, distress/depression/anxiety, body and self-image concerns, osteonecrosis, oral infections/candidiasis, oral hygiene, onset or worsening of gastrointestinal reflux disorder (GERD), signs or symptoms of hypothyroidism, inadequate or lack of nutrition, and dehydration.[2]

Evaluation and Diagnosis

The following sections will cover the evaluation and management of common reasons for referral to Onc R: shoulder pain and dysfunction, neck pain and dysfunction, trismus, and lymphedema.

Shoulder Pain and Dysfunction

Background and Risk Factors

Shoulder pain and dysfunction experienced by PLWBCs of the head and neck are most often associated with SAN injury. The SAN is a cranial nerve that innervates the SCM and trapezius muscle. Extracranially the SAN travels through cervical lymph node level II, where the nerve enters the SCM muscle. Typically, a single branch of the SAN exits the SCM's posterior border and travels through cervical lymph node level V to the trapezius muscle.[46] During neck dissection, the SAN may be intentionally sacrificed depending on the disease's location and extent in the neck region. However, even if the SAN is preserved, an injury may occur due to traction or trauma to the nerve, along with possible devascularization due to ligation of blood vessels during surgery.[46] Therefore, persons diagnosed with HNC who undergo neck dissection have a greater risk of experiencing shoulder pain than those who do not undergo neck dissection.[47] Wide prevalence rates of shoulder pain following neck dissection have been reported with higher rates after RND (10%–100%) and MRND (10%–100%) compared to SLND (9%–25%).[47] This highlights the risk of experiencing shoulder pain after neck dissection related to surgery's type and/or extent. Persons who undergo a RND, MRND, SND involving levels II to IV, or any neck dissection involving level V are more likely to experience shoulder pain postoperatively.[47]

Other Sources of Shoulder Pain and Dysfunction

Individuals who have their cervical nerve root branches removed may be at greater risk for shoulder pain than individuals whose cervical nerve roots are preserved.[48] The branch of the SAN innervating the trapezius communicates with cervical nerve roots 2 through 4.[46] Intraoperative stimulation of these cervical nerve roots has been shown to elicit a motor response of the trapezius muscle in 32% of individuals, so preservation of these nerves may minimize shoulder dysfunction.[46] Onc R clinicians should be aware that the cervical plexus provides sensation to the superior shoulder region via the supraclavicular nerves, so sacrificing these nerves may be a source of neuropathic pain in this region.

Individuals who undergo head and neck reconstructive procedures involving the shoulder region's anatomical structures may experience shoulder pain and dysfunction. Individuals who undergo pectoralis major pedicle flap reconstruction and neck dissection have been reported to demonstrate shoulder morbidity more frequently than individuals who undergo neck dissection only.[49] However, researchers have concluded that PLWBCs who undergo pectoralis major pedicle flap reconstruction experience minimal shoulder morbidity in addition to morbidity caused by neck dissection.[50] Another type of head and neck reconstruction that may contribute to shoulder morbidity is scapular free flap reconstruction. PLWBCs who have undergone unilateral scapular free flap reconstruction have been shown to demonstrate impaired shoulder active range of motion (AROM) (decreased shoulder abduction, flexion, and external rotation but not extension) and strength (decreased shoulder abduction, flexion, and external rotation) compared to contralateral side[51]; however, it should be noted that most PLWBCs have neck dissection surgery on the same side, so it is not clear whether the dysfunction is due to the scapular free flap or the neck dissection. In summary, PLWBCs who undergo reconstructive procedures involving anatomical structures of the shoulder girdle may experience shoulder dysfunction; however, it is likely both the reconstructive procedure and neck dissection that contributes to shoulder dysfunction in many PLWBCs.

Clinical Presentation of Spinal Accessory Nerve Palsy

Patients with spinal accessory nerve palsy (SANP) will present with decreased shoulder ROM, altered resting alignment of the shoulder girdle, scapular dyskinesis, trapezius muscle atrophy and weakness, SCM muscle atrophy and weakness, a positive scapular flip sign, and pain.[52]

The typical pattern for impaired shoulder ROM associated with SANP is decreased shoulder abduction and flexion AROM compared to passive range of motion (PROM) and other shoulder motions. On average, patients with SANP will present with less than 90 degrees of shoulder abduction AROM and 110 to 120 degrees of shoulder flexion AROM.[52,53] PLWBCs will typically present with full or near full shoulder abduction and flexion PROM.[52] There generally are no deficits found for shoulder external rotation measured at 0 degrees abduction and hand behind back internal rotation AROM or PROM.[53]

Patients with SANP can present with an altered resting position of the shoulder due to impaired trapezius muscle performance. PLWBCs may present with a depressed and forward shoulder girdle that has been commonly referred to as "shoulder droop" in the literature (see Figure 19.5).[47] The scapula's normal position on the thorax has been described as the inferior angle of the scapular aligning around the spinous process of the 8th thoracic vertebra and scapula being around 8 cm away from the thoracic spine.[54,55] Normally, the clavicle is elevated about 10 to 15 degrees at rest.[56] From a posterior view, the scapula will appear depressed (inferiorly displaced) and abducted (further away from midline) compared to the unaffected side. The clavicle may appear horizontal or depressed from an anterior view compared to the unaffected side. From a lateral view, the acromion process may appear more anterior relative to the center of the thoracic compared to the unaffected side.

Scapular dyskinesis refers to abnormal scapular motion during arm movements. During arm elevation (abduction and flexion), PLWBCs with SANP will present with altered scapular motion due to impaired trapezius muscle performance. Scapular dyskinesis is not specific for SANP, meaning altered scapular motion may be seen in other conditions such as long thoracic nerve palsy (LTNP) due to impaired serratus anterior muscle performance. However, Onc R clinicians can differentiate SANP from LTNP through visual assessment of scapular motion during shoulder flexion and abduction. During shoulder flexion and abduction, there is typically minimal scapular motion during the initial 30 to 60 degrees of arm elevation; then, the scapula should continuously upwardly rotate and elevate while it stays relatively flat against the thorax (no winging should be present).[57] Upward rotation of the scapula is produced and controlled by contraction of the trapezius and serratus anterior muscles. Therefore, decreased scapular upward rotation will be found in both SANP and LTNP.[53] Both the trapezius and serratus anterior

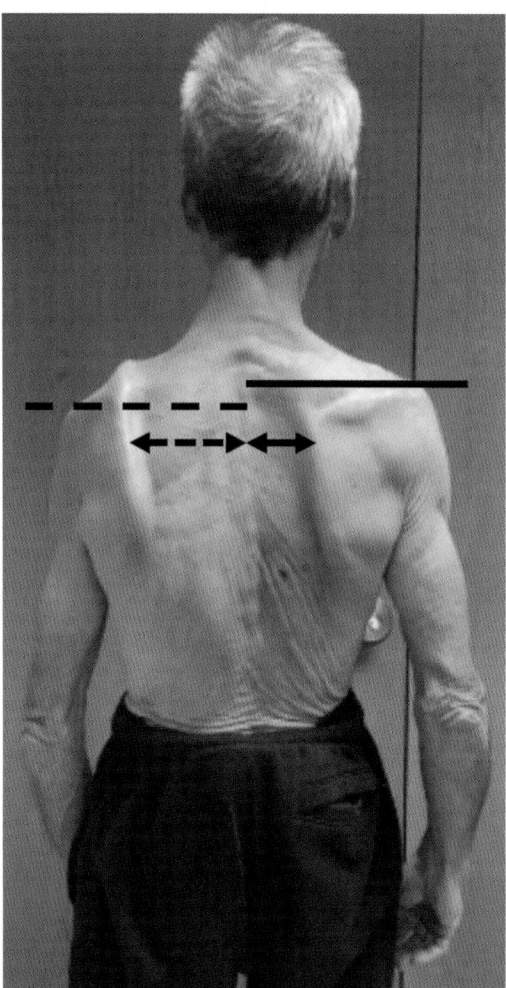

• **Fig. 19.5** Posterior View of PLWBC With Spinal Accessory Nerve Palsy. The left shoulder is depressed (*dashed line*) compared to right shoulder (*solid line*). The left scapula is more laterally displaced or abducted (*dashed arrow*) compared to the right scapular (*solid arrow*). (Photograph courtesy of Cynthia Tan. Printed with permission.)

muscles play a role in stabilizing the scapula against the thorax, so scapular winging will be seen in both conditions. However, scapular winging evident by the scapula's prominent medial border is typically more severe, especially during shoulder flexion in patients with LTNP.[52] An Onc R clinician can differentiate SANP and LTNP by noting the amount of scapular protraction (abduction or lateral displacement of scapula relative to the thorax) and elevation (superior displacement of the scapula relative to the thorax) during arm elevation. Due to the trapezius' anatomical orientation, the upper fibers contribute to scapular elevation while the middle and lower fibers contribute to scapular retraction (adduction or medial displacement of the scapula on the thorax). Therefore, patients with SANP will demonstrate decreased scapular elevation and excessive scapular protraction during arm elevation.[52,53] Excessive scapular protraction is seen due to the serratus anterior muscle's line of force causing the scapula to displace laterally and anteriorly relative to the thorax. In summary, visual assessment of scapular motion will reveal decreased scapular upward rotation, decreased scapular elevation, and excessive scapular protraction during arm elevation in patients with SANP due to trapezius weakness.

As discussed, trapezius muscle weakness and atrophy are signs of SANP. Upper trapezius muscle strength can be assessed by simultaneously resisting ipsilateral craniocervical extension-and-lateral flexion and elevation of the scapula.[58] Middle trapezius muscle strength can be evaluated by resisting horizontal abduction of the humerus or adduction of the scapula while the PLWBC is positioned prone with the shoulder externally rotated and abducted to 90 degrees.[58] Presence of a prominent medial border of the scapula or inability to adduct the scapula would indicate middle trapezius weakness. Lower trapezius muscle strength can be assessed with the PLWBC positioned in prone and the shoulder externally rotated (thumb pointed toward the ceiling) and abducted to approximately 120 to 135 degrees of abduction.[58] The Onc R clinician would then apply a downward force on the PLWBC's arm or resists adduction and depression of the scapula. A prominent medial border or inferior angle of the scapular or inability to adduct and depress the scapula would indicate lower trapezius weakness. SCM weakness and atrophy may be found as well. The SCM muscle can be assessed by positioning the PLWBC supine with the head rotated away for the muscle being tested and applying a posteromedial directed force at the temporal region as the PLWBC lifts their head off the table. Whether SCM dysfunction occurs as a result of denervation will be dependent on the location of nerve injury. SCM dysfunction is discussed further in the section on neck dysfunction.

The Scapular Flip Sign is a special test to identify if abnormal motion is due to SANP.[52] The Scapular Flip Sign is performed by the clinician resisting shoulder external rotation while the arm is by the side and visualizing the scapula's position and motion. A positive test is posterior displacement of the scapula's medial border or visualizing the scapula "flip" off the thoracic wall during resisted shoulder external rotation.[52] The medial border becomes more prominent during the test in SANP due to the middle and lower trapezius not being able to stabilize the scapula against the thorax and counteract the pull of the infraspinatus and teres minor muscles (see Figure 19.6).[52]

Pain associated with SANP may be related to upper trapezius tension, levator scapulae/rhomboid overuse or tension, thoracic outlet syndrome, or subacromial pain syndrome. The depressed and forward shoulder girdle posture associated with SANP may place excessive strain on the upper trapezius, levator scapulae, and rhomboid muscles. Additionally, the levator scapulae and rhomboids are scapulothoracic muscles that contribute to scapular elevation and retraction during arm elevation. These muscles may become overworked in the presence of SANP due to a greater responsibility needed to produce scapular motion because of trapezius muscle paralysis.[52] Pain may also occur from compression of neurovascular structures passing through the costoclavicular space to the depressed shoulder girdle. Finally, pain may arise from the irritation of structures within the subacromial space. As previously mentioned, SANP will cause abnormal scapular motion. Insufficient scapular upward rotation found in patients with SANP may reduce the size of the subacromial space, causing excessive compression of subacromial structures leading to shoulder pain.[59] Distinguishing features for sources of pain associated with SANP can be found in Table 19.1.

Differential Diagnosis

Shoulder pain and muscle power deficits[60] (e.g., rotator cuff tendinopathy) and shoulder pain and mobility deficits[60] (e.g., adhesive capsulitis) are the most likely diagnosis/classifications to consider in PLWBCs of the head and neck who present with shoulder pain and impaired shoulder mobility. Risk factors for rotator cuff tendinopathy include age and diabetes, while adhesive capsulitis risk factors include age, diabetes, thyroid disease, and surgery/prolonged immobilization.[60,61] It would not be surprising for a PLWBC of the head and neck to present with adhesive capsulitis or rotator cuff tendinopathy because (1) HNC is more

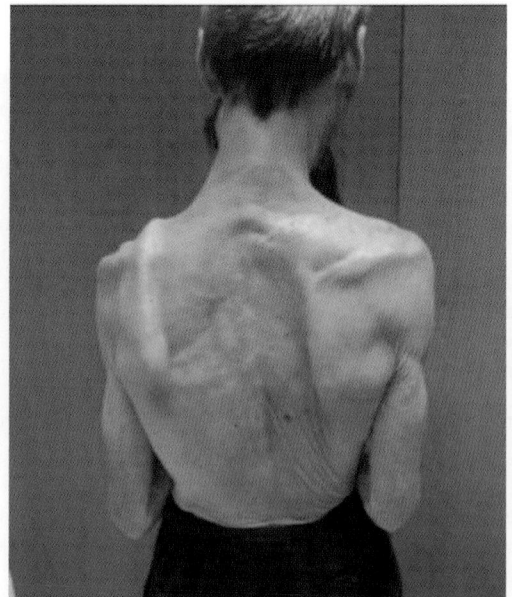
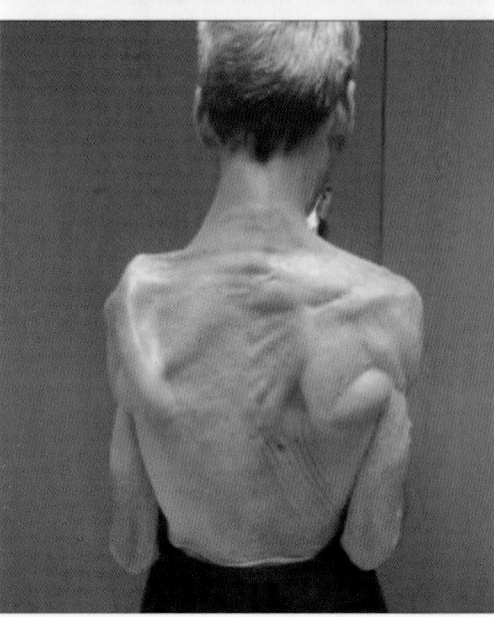

• **Fig. 19.6** Scapular Flip Sign. To perform the Scapular Flip Sign, the PLWBC's arm is positioned by side with elbow flexed to 90 degrees (top image). Next, clinician resists isometric shoulder external rotation and visualizes the scapula's position and motion. A positive test is posterior displacement of the scapula's medial border during resisted shoulder external (bottom image). (Photograph courtesy of Cynthia Tan. Printed with permission.)

common in older adults[62]; (2) diabetes may be associated with the development of HNC[63]; (3) hypothyroidism is an adverse effect of radiation therapy[2]; and (4) SANP secondary to neck dissection may cause prolonged immobilization if not educated on a home exercise program. Key findings to differentiate shoulder pain and muscle power deficits[60] (e.g., rotator cuff tendinopathy), shoulder pain and mobility deficits[60] (e.g., adhesive capsulitis), and SANP can be found in Table 19.2. Additional conditions to rule out include LTNP, as previously discussed, along with cervical myelopathy and brachial plexopathy.[52] These conditions may cause PLWBCs to experience neck/scapular pain, altered resting shoulder girdle alignment, limited active shoulder motion, and

TABLE 19.1 Key Findings for Myofascial Pain Syndrome, Thoracic Outlet Syndrome, and Subacromial Pain Syndrome

	Upper Trapezius/Levator Scapulae/ Rhomboid Myofascial Pain	Thoracic Outlet Syndrome	Subacromial Pain Syndrome
Pain	• Pain in region of upper trapezius, levator scapulae, or rhomboid muscles	• Shoulder, arm, forearm, hand pain	• Anterior or anterolateral shoulder pain
Key findings	• Reproduction of pain with palpation of upper trapezius/levator scapulae/ rhomboids • Reproduction of pain with movements that apply physical stress (stretching or resisted motions) to upper trapezius/levator scapulae/rhomboids	• Neurogenic signs: UE numbness, paresthesia, and/or weakness in the arm or hand • Positive ULNT • Vascular signs: upper limb swelling, cyanosis • Diminished pulses with positional tests • Positive Roos or elevated arm stress test • Symptoms alleviated if depressed shoulder girdle corrected	• Impingement signs (Neer, Hawkins, Jobe, Painful arc) • Pain with isometric resistance (i.e., shoulder external rotation, flexion) • Rotator cuff weakness • Positive scapular assistance test and scapular repositioning test

UE, Upper extremity; *ULNT*, Upper limb neural tension. Adapted by Bryan Spinelli and Cynthia Tan[102]

TABLE 19.2 Key Findings for Spinal Accessory Nerve Palsy, Adhesive Capsulitis, and Rotator Cuff Tear

	Spinal Accessory Nerve Palsy	Adhesive Capsulitis	Rotator Cuff Tear
Key findings to rule in	• ↓ AROM > PROM • Trapezius muscle weakness atrophy • Significant depressed and forward shoulder • Scapular dyskinesis (excessive protraction and decreased elevation) • Positive scapular flip sign	• AROM = PROM • Gradual onset and progressive worsening of pain and stiffness • ↓ Glenohumeral PROM in multiple directions (ER most limited) • Firm end feel • Joint glides/accessory motions are restricted in all directions • Scapular dyskinesis (excessive elevation)	• ↓ AROM > PROM • Recent trauma or history of shoulder pain • Catching sensation/painful arc during AROM • Rotator cuff weakness • Positive lift off or internal rotation lag sign or belly press • Positive external rotation lag sign • Supraspinatus or infraspinatus atrophy • Scapular dyskinesis (excessive elevation)
Key findings to rule out	• Significant loss of PROM • Normal scapular motion	• Normal PROM	• Significant loss of PROM • Normal rotator cuff strength

AROM, Active range of motion; *PROM*, passive range of motion; *ER*, external rotation.
Adapted by Bryan Spinelli and Cynthia Tan.[60,102]

scapular dyskinesis as well; however, these conditions do not cause isolated trapezius muscle weakness or paralysis.[52]

Interventions for Spinal Accessory Nerve Palsy

The extent of nerve injury and stage may influence the prescription of interventions. Three degrees of nerve injury have been described: (1) neurapraxia (transient disruption in nerve conduction without axon damage); (2) axonotmesis (loss of axonal integrity with no or partial damage to surrounding connective tissue layers); and (3) neurotmesis (complete disruption of entire nerve; transection).[64] With neurapraxia, muscle function will be dependent on the severity of demyelination and the extent of the conduction block.[65] With axonotmesis and neurotmesis, the nerve has no electrophysiologic function causing paralysis.[66] The following discussion on interventions for SANP will be based on expected impairments during acute and late phases of recovery.

The main goals during the acute phase are: (1) reduce the risk of developing other shoulder-related problems such as adhesive capsulitis, rotator cuff tendinopathy, thoracic outlet syndrome, myofascial pain syndrome, sternoclavicular joint instability; (2) reduce risk of shoulder passive mobility deficits; (3) maximize

muscle performance of scapulothoracic muscles (levator scapulae, rhomboids, serratus anterior) with similar function as trapezius muscle; and (4) modulate pain as needed.

PLWBCs should be educated on proper shoulder girdle posture and methods to support the shoulder girdle to: (1) reduce risk of upper trapezius/levator scapulae/rhomboid muscle pain from prolonged or excessive tension secondary to depressed shoulder posture; (2) reduce risk of thoracic outlet syndrome secondary to neurovascular compression from depressed shoulder posture; and (3) reduce risk of anterior chest wall soft tissue tightness due to a forward shoulder posture. A method to support the shoulder girdle includes instructing PLWBCs to sit with their arm supported on a pillow or armrest of a chair. PLWBCs may support the arm when standing by putting their hand in their pocket or hooking thumb on their belt. PLWBCs with severe malalignment and high pain irritability may benefit from scapular taping. Scapular taping could be performed with rigid tape or elastic kinesiology tape. A scapular elevation kinesiology taping technique slightly improved scapular depression in a single case study.[67] While not yet investigated in patients with SANP, scapular kinesiology taping techniques to facilitate middle and lower trapezius muscles and facilitation of rhomboids, middle trapezius, and lower trapezius have been found to reduce scapular winging (decreased scapular internal rotation) in children with brachial birth palsy; however, no differences were found for upward rotation.[68] Scapular taping may not be the best long-term solution to address scapular malalignment due to concern for adverse skin reaction with repeated application and need for assistance to apply taping techniques. Orthoses such as clavicle straps may effectively address forward shoulder posture[69]; however, in the authors' experience it is less effective for correcting shoulder depression. The Akman-Sari orthosis was developed to correct scapular malalignment in patients after RND (see Figure 19.7).[70] This orthosis consists of a rectangular pad and two nonelastic bands. The rectangular pad is placed on the lateral thorax covering the scapula's lateral border and inferior angle. One strap is wrapped horizontally around the PLWBC's torso. The second strap travels across the PLWBC's back and over the superior aspect of the uninvolved shoulder then is secured anteriorly to strap around the torso. Arm slings are not recommended for prolonged use due to the adverse effects of complete immobilization and limited functional use of the arm.

Exercise is an essential component for the management of SANP. ROM or stretching exercise can be prescribed to reduce the risk of developing limited passive shoulder mobility and anterior chest wall tightness. Shoulder active-assisted range of motion (AAROM)/PROM shoulder exercises may include supine forward elevation with the opposite hand; sliding the arm forward on a table to create shoulder forward elevation; supine or standing shoulder external rotation with the arm at the side using a dowel; supine hand behind head external rotation; standing shoulder extension with a dowel; and standing hand behind back shoulder internal rotation using the opposite hand, dowel, or a strap. AAROM/PROM exercises should be performed 8 to 12 times at least once per day. Stretching exercises should be prescribed to maintain the pectoralis major and minor length. It is suggested that standing pectoralis minor and major stretching exercises be performed at lower angles of humeral elevation if scapular dyskinesis is present. Examples of pectoralis muscle stretches can be found in Table 19.3. Lack of consensus exists relative to the duration of stretching that leads to the most remarkable improvement in muscle flexibility. Stretching duration may range from 5 seconds to 30 minutes, depending on the type of stretch and mode of application. Static stretches are commonly performed for 10 to 30 seconds. Cumulative total end range time or total stretching time per week is an essential factor for Onc R clinicians to consider since similar improvements have been found with different durations of stretches if the total duration of stretching was equal.[71,72]

Neuromuscular control and resistance exercise have been shown to reduce shoulder pain and disability in patients with SANP.[73,74] Neuromuscular control exercises include: (1) educating patients on the function of the scapulothoracic muscles and proper scapular alignment; and (2) providing verbal cues with or without tactile cues to facilitate desired muscle contraction and movement during exercises.[74,75] For example, Onc R clinicians may provide verbal cues for the patient to retract and elevate the scapula while providing manual contact to facilitate the motion during a shoulder shrug exercise. Manual contact could be provided to maintain proper scapular alignment and stability (no winging) during biceps curls, triceps extension, and shoulder external rotation with the arm at the side (Table 19.4).

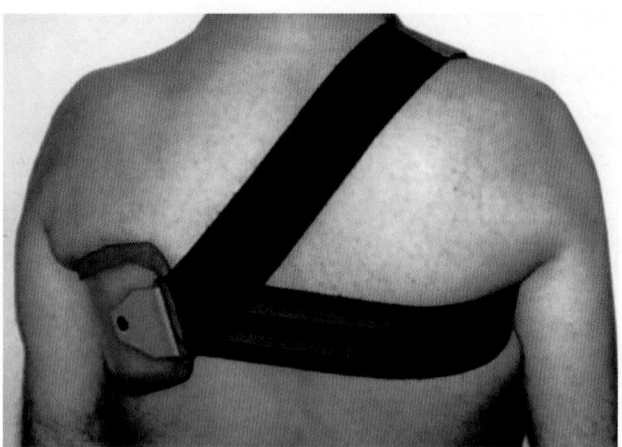

• **Fig. 19.7** Akman-Sari Orthosis. (Reprinted with permission from Kizilay A, Kalcioglu MT, Saydam L, Ersoy Y. A new shoulder orthosis for paralysis of the trapezius muscle after radical neck dissection: a preliminary report. *Eur Arch Otorhinolaryngol.* 2006;263(5):477–480. doi:10.1007/s00405-005-1017-z.)

TABLE 19.3	**Neck and Shoulder Stretching Exercises**
Exercise	**Description**
Doorway Pectoralis Stretch	While standing in a doorway and arms by side, the patient places hands on the door frame and steps forward until a stretch is felt along the front of the chest and/or shoulder.
Foam Roller Pectoralis Stretch	While supine lying on a foam roller placed longitudinally along the length of spine, the patient horizontally abducts arms until a stretch is felt along the front of the chest and/or shoulder.
Scalene/Sternocleidomastoid Stretch	While sitting and holding onto the side of a chair, the patient positions head in slight extension then laterally flexes away and rotates toward the side being stretched.
Anterior Soft Tissue Stretch	Patient places hands over skin in front of the chest and sternoclavicular joint then tilts head upwards and away from the side being stretched.
Upper Trapezius Stretch	While sitting and holding onto the side of a chair, the patient laterally flexes away from the side being stretched.
Levator Scapulae Stretch	While sitting and holding onto the side of a chair, the patient laterally flexes and rotates away from the side being stretched as if looking towards the axilla.
Rhomboid/Middle Trapezius Stretch	Patient interlocks fingers then protracts both scapula and rounds back by reaching forward with arms positioned at about 45–60° of flexion.

Created by Bryan Spinelli and Cynthia Tan. Printed with permission

TABLE 19.4 Neuromuscular Control Exercises

Exercise	Exercise Description
Elbow Flexion	With arm by side and elbow extended holding an elastic resistance band secured under the patient's foot, the patient flexes the elbow.
Elbow Extension	With arm by side and elbow flexed holding an elastic resistance band secured overhead, the patient extends the elbow.
Shoulder External Rotation	With arm by side and elbow flexed to 90°, the patient performs external rotation of the shoulder

- Verbal cues are provided to the patient to maintain proper scapular alignment during exercise.
- Manual contact is provided to assist with scapular stability and prevent winging.

Created by Bryan Spinelli and Cynthia Tan. Printed with permission.

During the acute phase, shoulder resistance exercise selection should focus on strengthening muscles with a similar function as the trapezius. Description of exercises to strengthen the levator scapulae, the rhomboids, and the serratus anterior can be found in Table 19.5. Resistance exercise programs for patients with SANP described in the literature consist of exercises performed for 2 to 3 sets of 8 to 15 repetitions progressing to intensities of 60 to 70% of 1-repetition maximum, for 8 to 12 repetitions, or RPE ranging from 11 to 15 out of 20.[76–80] Exercises can be progressed by increasing weight or resistance level by 1 to 5 pounds or next elastic resistance level once the patient can perform the desired number of sets and repetitions with proper form.[78,79]

During the late phase and if trapezius muscle recovery is evident, Onc R clinicians may prescribe exercises targeting the trapezius muscle or exercises involving a greater amount of humeral elevation. Exercises that selectively target the trapezius muscle can be found in Table 19.6. As a general guide, Onc R clinicians should ensure patients maintain proper posture and scapular stability (no scapular winging) during exercise performance.[79]

TABLE 19.5 Recommended Scapulothoracic Exercises During Acute Phase

Exercise	Muscles Targeted	Exercise Description
Shoulder shrug (scapular elevation)	Levator scapulae Upper trapezius	With arm by side and elbow extended, the patient elevates the scapula to maximum height.
Scapular elevation + retraction	Levator scapulae Rhomboids Upper trapezius Middle trapezius	With arm by side and elbow extended, the patient elevates and retracts the scapula.
Low row	Rhomboids Middle trapezius	With arm by side, the patient retracts the scapula.
Scapula protraction in supine	Serratus anterior	While supine with the shoulder flexed to 90° and elbow extended, the patient protracts the scapula.

Adapted by Bryan Spinelli and Cynthia Tan[77,78,79]

TABLE 19.6 Trapezius-Specific Exercises

Exercise	Muscles Targeted	Exercise Description
Overhead shrug	Upper trapezius	With arms in overhead position against the wall, the patient elevates the scapula to maximum height.
Overhead press	Upper trapezius	In sitting or standing with shoulders abducted to 90° and elbows flexed to 90°, the patient extends their elbows moving hands towards the ceiling.
Overhead retraction	Middle trapezius	With arms in overhead position against the wall, the patient retracts the scapula.
Elevation with external rotation	Upper trapezius Middle trapezius Lower trapezius	Holding an elastic band with arms by side and elbows flexed to 90°, the patient externally rotates about 30°, and elevates both arms to 90° in the scapular plane while maintaining tension in the band.
Prone I, T, Y	Middle trapezius Lower trapezius	Prone I In prone with arm at 90° of shoulder flexion, the patient retracts the scapula and extends the arm to neutral. Prone T In prone with arm at 90° of shoulder flexion, the patient retracts the scapula and horizontally abducts the arm while maintaining glenohumeral external rotation. Prone Y In prone with arm at 90° of shoulder flexion, the patient retracts and depresses the scapula and elevates the arm to 120°.

Adapted by Bryan Spinelli and Cynthia Tan.[58]

Prognosis/Expected Outcome

Timeframe and expected recovery level will depend on the degree of nerve injury. The timeframe for recovery after neurapraxia injury varies and may range from hours, days, weeks to months. Timeframe for recovery with axonotmesis is longer. Generally, axons regenerate at a rate of 1 mm/day or 1 inch per month; however, the nerve's proximal portion may regenerate faster than the distal portion.[65] One study found decreased trapezius muscle activity in 45% of individuals who underwent MNRD at 6 months postoperative.[81] Another study found that individuals after neck dissection (not including RND) showed signs of reinnervation 3 to 9 months after surgery; however, no individuals demonstrated electromyography activity equal to preoperative assessment.[82] Collectively, these studies suggest that recovery of SANP may take longer than 6 to 9 months in some individuals following neck dissection. In neurotmesis, nerve healing or axonal regeneration will not occur unless the nerve is surgically reattached or repaired. Hence, the reason why individuals who undergo RND demonstrate worse shoulder pain and dysfunction than those who undergo MRND or SND.[47]

Neck Dysfunction

Neck dysfunction has been shown to negatively impact QOL in PLWBCs of the head and neck.[83] Individuals are at risk of experiencing neck-related problems such as pain, limited mobility, weakness, and sensory deficits resulting from HNC and its treatment.

Neck Pain

The prevalence of neck pain in PLWBCs of the head and neck has been reported to be as high as 45% in mixed cohorts.[47] Neck pain may occur directly related to HNC secondary to nerve compression or tissue damage if the tumor invades soft tissue. Neck pain may occur as a result of HNC treatment as well. Neck pain after HNC treatment may be related to soft tissue damage and inflammation along with nerve damage. Therefore, neck pain may be nociceptive or neuropathic in nature.

Not surprisingly, most individuals who undergo RND and MRND experience neck pain immediately after surgery, with the incidence reported being as high as 70% one day after surgery.[47] Nociceptive pain after surgery may occur from surgical incisions through skin and fascia or muscle injury. Surgeons may retract the SCM to expose cervical lymph nodes during neck dissection surgery, causing trauma leading to pain and muscle hypertonicity (spasm). Also, the SCM may be sacrificed and may be a source of nociceptive pain following RND surgery. Although postsurgical pain tends to improve over time,[47] pain continues to be a significant problem for some PLWBCs. As previously mentioned, PLWBCs who undergo neck dissection may be at risk for SANP. SANP may lead to levator scapulae or rhomboid muscle injury due to overuse since the trapezius muscle is not available to assist with scapular upward rotation or elevation when reaching overhead. SANP and associated depressed and forward shoulder girdle may also contribute to nociceptive pain due to excessive tension being placed on the upper trapezius, levator scapulae, and rhomboid muscles.[52] PLWBCs with upper trapezius, levator scapulae, and rhomboid myofascial pain may present with: (1) reproduction of pain with palpation; (2) taut band of muscle or trigger point; (3) reproduction of pain with movements that apply physical stress (stretching or resisted motions) to muscles; and (4) restricted ROM.

About 1 in 4 (23%) of PLWBCs following neck dissection have been shown to demonstrate signs and symptoms of neuropathic pain.[84] Neuropathic pain after neck dissection may be due to damage or sacrifice of cervical nerve root branches.[47] Neuropathic pain is often described as burning or hot, shooting, electric shocks, pricking, pins and needles, tingling, or numbness.[85] Other findings of neuropathic pain include allodynia and hyperalgesia. Allodynia refers to pain provoked by stimuli that usually are not painful (pain exacerbated by light touch), while hyperalgesia refers to increased pain from stimuli that typically provokes pain. The presence of neuropathic pain is associated with worse neck function.[84]

Risk factors for persistent neck pain after HNC diagnosis and treatment have not been extensively researched. However, a higher incidence of neck pain has been found in PLWBCs who have had cervical nerve root branches sacrificed compared to preserved (73% vs. 37%).[47] Undergoing neck dissection and being diagnosed with hypopharyngeal cancer increases risk of developing myofascial pain.[47,86]

Differential Diagnosis for Neck Pain

Carotid Artery Dissection. Symptoms of carotid artery dissection include headache or neck pain.[87] Other clinical findings of carotid artery dissection include Horner's syndrome (constriction of the pupil, sunken eye, drooping of the upper eyelid, absence of facial sweating), pulsatile tinnitus, and cranial nerve palsies.[87] These signs and symptoms can precede cerebral ischemia (transient ischemic attack, stroke, retinal infarction).[87] Carotid artery involvement usually occurs with cancer recurrence or persistence.[88]

Limited Neck Mobility

PLWBCs of the head and neck may demonstrate restricted cervical ROM.[89] On average, PLWBCs of the head and neck demonstrate cervical ROM values less than reported normative values (flexion <50 degrees, extension <60 degrees, lateral flexion <45, rotation <80degrees).[89] However, it is important to note that the amount of cervical ROM decreases to a certain extent as a function of the aging process.[90] Decreases in lateral flexion towards the operated side, rotation towards the operated side, and flexion are associated with age in PLWBCs who underwent neck dissection. In contrast, a decrease in lateral flexion away from the operated side was associated with age and treatment factors such as the number of lymph nodes dissected and receiving radiation therapy.[90] Decreased cervical extension, and rotation to the operated and nonoperated sides have been found in PLWBCs who have undergone neck dissection compared to healthy individuals without a history of HNC.[91] PLWBCs who undergo unilateral neck dissection may present with greater difficulty rotating towards the nonoperated side compared to rotating towards the operated side as well.[47] Deficits in cervical extension and greater deficits in lateral flexion and rotation towards the nonoperated side are not surprising since these movements require soft tissue extensibility within surgical and radiation fields. Radiation therapy may lead to fibrosis and thickening of the skin.[92,93] Scars and fibrosis associated with surgery and radiation therapy may decrease tissue elasticity contributing to impaired cervical ROM.[94] Cervical muscle dystonia is another possible cause of restricted cervical ROM in PLWBCs who undergo neck dissection or receive radiation therapy.[95] Abnormal activity of nerves innervating the SCM, scalenes, and trapezius muscles may lead to involuntary contraction or spasms of these neck muscles contributing to restricted cervical ROM.[96] Finally, head and neck lymphedema can contribute to impaired cervical range of motion, likely due to lymphedema-related fibrosis involving the soft tissues of the neck.[97] Severity of external head and neck lymphedema is associated with decreased rotation ROM.[98]

Neck Weakness

Neck muscle weakness may occur as a result of HNC treatment. PLWBCs who undergo neck dissection have been shown to demonstrate decreased cervical flexor muscle strength compared to healthy controls.[91] Neck dissection may lead to weakness of the cervical flexors due to: (1) sacrifice of the SCM muscle during RND; (2) damage or sacrifice of the SAN innervating the SCM; (3) dissection of the fascia covering the SCM and retraction of muscle causing muscle trauma; and (4) devascularization of muscle from cauterizing vessels entering the SCM.[91]

Weakness of the cervical extensors may occur in PLWBCs who receive radiation therapy, likely due to a combination of damage to the spinal cord, nerves, and muscle.[95,96] Neck weakness may be worse later in the day due to poor muscle endurance and fatigue.[95,96] Weakness of the cervical extensors may compromise the ability to maintain a normal head posture.[95,96] This has been referred to as dropped head syndrome (DHS). See Chapter 7 for more information and images on DHS. PLWBCs with DHS present with a flexed and forward head posture due to an inability to extend their neck.[95,96,99] Development of cervical extensor muscle weakness in DHS may be associated with the dosage of radiation to neck extensor muscles.[100] DHS and associated neck extensor muscle weakness may be a source of neck pain and disability. Pain may occur due to prolonged tension being placed on the cervical extensors with a flexed and forward head posture or overload because of the muscle demands required during daily activities.[96] PLWBCs may report difficulty with tasks that require neck extension or stability of the head, such as overhead work, reading, or watching TV.[95,96] PLWBCs may also present with difficulty breathing and impaired swallowing.

Sensory Deficits

Loss of sensation at the neck is common for PLWBCs who undergo neck dissection, with higher prevalence rates in patients undergoing RND than MRND and SND.[47] The cervical nerve root branches are responsible for providing sensation to the anterior neck and clavicle as well as the shoulder, ear, and posterior scalp regions. These cervical nerve root branches affect sensation because they are either located within the surgical field or potentially sacrificed during neck dissection. PLWBCs may demonstrate a gradual recovery of sensation if cervical nerve root branches are preserved; however, persistent sensory deficits are to be expected if nerve root branches are sacrificed.[47]

Sensory loss is frequently observed in the anterolateral neck region, the lower part of the ear, and the posterior neck behind the border of the SCM.[90] The location of sensory deficits will be dependent on the specific cervical nerve roots affected. Cervical nerve root branches give rise to sensory nerves that emerge from the posterior aspect of the SCM. The greater auricular nerve is formed by branches from the C2 and C3 nerve roots and provides sensation to the skin over the parotid gland to the mastoid process, including the lower part of the ear.[101] The transverse cervical nerve is also formed from C2 and C3 and travels anteriorly to provide sensation to the anterior neck.[101] The lesser occipital nerve arises from the second cervical nerve root branch and provides sensation to the lateral scalp behind the ear and the upper part of the ear.[101] The supraclavicular nerve is formed by branches from C3 and C4 and travels inferiorly and laterally to provide sensation over the clavicle and superior shoulder regions.[101]

Interventions for Neck Dysfunction

The selection of interventions for neck dysfunction should be based on the identified impairments. For example, resistance exercise may be selected to address impaired muscle performance, while ROM or stretching may be selected to address passive mobility deficits. While the selection of interventions is based on impairments, the intensity of interventions should be guided by tissue irritability.[60,102] Tissue irritability refers to the tissue's ability to handle physical stress and is thought to be associated with the degree of inflammation or tissue healing.[60,102] Tissue irritability can be classified as high, moderate, or low.[60,102] Factors such as pain severity and ease of aggravation/persistence, self-report of disability, and the relationship between pain and motion are used to determine the level of tissue irritability.[60,102] Severe pain (~7/10), constant pain at rest, symptoms that are easily aggravated, if pain persists for an extended period after aggravation, and high disability are findings consistent with high irritability.[60,102] Findings consistent with moderate irritability include moderate pain (4–6/10), intermittent pain at rest, symptoms aggravated by lower demand activities, pain that returns to baseline relatively quickly after aggravation, and moderate disability.[60,102] Low irritability is characterized by low pain (≤3/10), absent pain at rest, pain aggravated when performing higher demand activities, pain that returns to baseline almost immediately after aggravation, and low disability.[60,102] Pain patterns during ROM testing can provide information on the level of tissue irritability. Aggravation of pain before the end of the available ROM and guarding suggest high irritability.[60] Moderate irritability is characterized by pain at the end of the available ROM when tissues encounter resistance, while low irritability is characterized by pain that occurs with overpressure into end ranges of motion.[60]

Range of Motion/Stretching Exercise

Cervical ROM and stretching exercises should be prescribed to address neck pain and passive mobility deficits. PLWBCs should no feel resistance or "stretching" when performing ROM. Stretching can be defined as applying a force at the end of the available ROM to elongate tissue or improve flexibility. With stretching, PLWBCs should feel a gentle "pulling" sensation towards the end of available range motion but not pain. The selection (ROM vs. stretching) and dosage of exercise should be determined by the PLWBC's level of tissue irritability. PLWBCs with high tissue irritability may respond more favorably to ROM due to the reduced level of physical stress associated with ROM exercise as compared to stretching. PLWBCs with moderate irritability may tolerate gentle shorter-duration stretching, while PLWBCs with low irritability may tolerate longer-duration stretching or a more substantial number of repetitions. Cervical ROM and stretching exercise programs commonly include cervical extension, rotation, and lateral flexion since these movements are typically restricted after HNC treatment. Exercise may be progressed by having the PLWBC perform combined movements of cervical extension and rotation and lateral flexion away from the side being elongated or stretched. Upper trapezius, levator scapulae, scalenes/SCM, and rhomboids/middle trapezius stretches may be prescribed for PLWBCs with impaired flexibility or myofascial pain. However, caution should be taken when prescribing stretches if excessive tension or elongation of muscles contributes to pain and dysfunction.

Manual Therapy and Pain Modulation Techniques

Onc R clinicians should consider the inclusion of manual therapy techniques for pain modulation. Manual therapy such as friction massage and pressure release techniques may effectively manage pain associated with trigger points.[103,104] Pressure release (Figure 19.8) involves a clinician applying gradually increasing pressure over a trigger point until increased tissue resistance

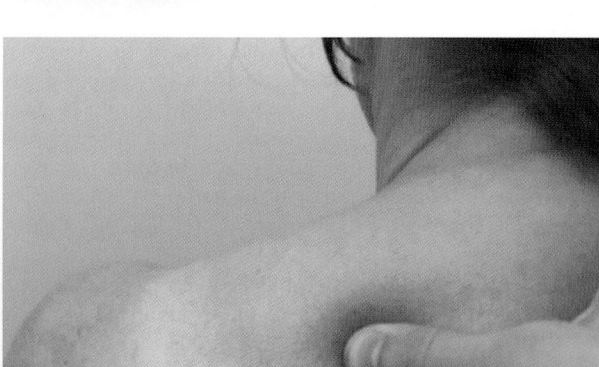
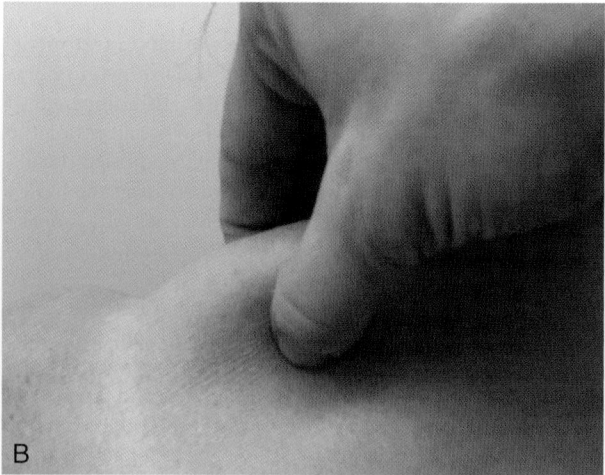

• **Fig. 19.8** Pressure Release Techniques. (A) Specific Compression technique to the levator scapula. (B) Muscle Squeezing technique for the upper trapezius. Pressure is progressively increased until tissue resistance (barrier) is perceived by the clinician. Pressure is maintained until the clinician senses a relief of the taut band. At that time, the pressure is increased again until the clinician feels the next increase in tissue resistance. (Photograph courtesy of Bryan A. Spinelli, PT, PhD. Printed with permission.)

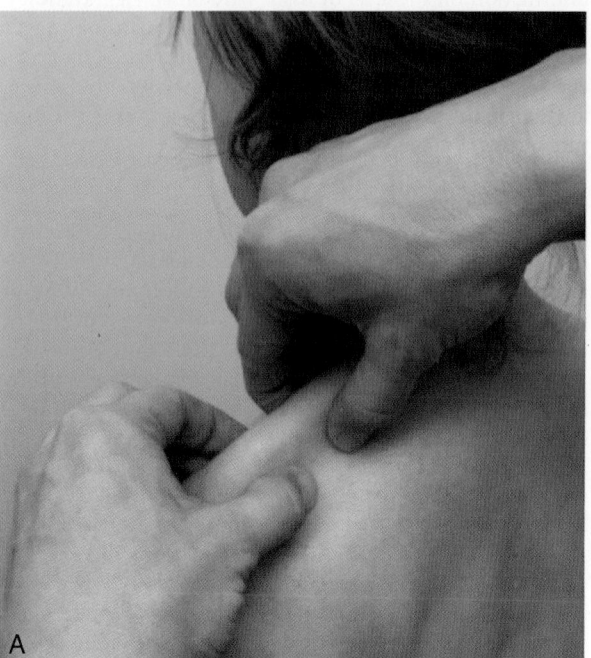
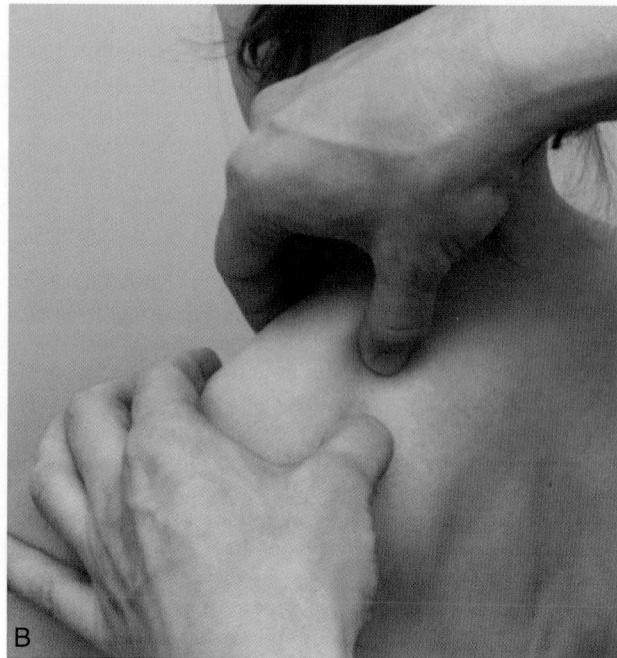

• **Fig. 19.9** Manual Stretching of Taut Bands. (A) Both thumbs of the clinician are placed over the trigger point above and below. (B) The clinician applies moderate, slow pressure over trigger point, sliding the thumbs in opposite directions. (Photograph courtesy of Bryan A. Spinelli, PT, PhD. Printed with permission.)

is felt.[103] Pressure is maintained until the muscle feels less taut, then pressure is increased again until a new barrier of tissue resistance is felt.[103] Another manual therapy technique involves manually stretching taut muscle fibers (Figure 19.9) by placing both thumbs over the taut muscle area, applying pressure, and sliding the thumbs in opposite directions.[103] Taping has been used to address musculoskeletal pain and cancer-related pain.[105,106] Kinesiology taping has been found to decrease pain pressure threshold in patients with active trapezius trigger points and trapezius myalgia.[104,107] It should be noted that a synthesis of research studies on kinesiology taping for managing different shoulder pain disorders revealed that kinesiology taping resulted in significant improvement in shoulder pain and disability when combined with exercise but was no better than placebo.[108]

Neck Strengthening and Endurance Exercises

Neck strengthening or endurance exercise and deep craniocervical flexor training have been found to improve strength and reduce pain and disability in patients with neck pain,[109,110] however, there is a lack of evidence related explicitly to PLWBCs of the head and neck. Neck strengthening or endurance exercise may include neck isometric exercise or dynamic motions. Neck isometric exercise can be performed seated with the patient resisting cervical flexion, extension, lateral flexion, and rotation motions at the forehead with one hand. If a patient has difficulty maintaining proper posture in a seated position, neck isometric exercise can be initiated supine. The following exercise dosage for seated neck isometric exercise has been found to reduce neck pain and disability and improve muscle endurance when combined with neck stretching exercises in patients with chronic nonspecific neck pain: duration of contraction: 10 seconds, repetitions: 10 to 15, rest interval: 15 seconds, intensity: initiated at submaximal progressing to maximal, frequency: 3 times/week.[111] Cervical stabilization exercises may be prescribed as well; for example, the PLWBC is positioned in standing against a wall with a ball behind their head, shoulder movements such flexion or abduction are then performed while maintaining enough pressure on the ball so that it does not fall. Additionally, semispinalis cervicis muscle training has been shown to reduce neck pain and disability and improve muscle strength and forward head posture in patients with chronic mechanical neck pain.[109] Semispinalis cervicis training involves a PLWBC maintaining neutral head and neck posture in sitting while the clinician provides manual resistance at the second cervical vertebra attempting to push their head into flexion.[109,112] Manual resistance applied at the second cervical vertebra has been shown to activate the semispinalis cervicis selectively as evidenced by an increased ratio of semispinalis cervicis and splenius capitis muscle activity as compared to the activity elicited by resistance applied at the occiput.[112]

Neck strengthening or endurance exercise can include dynamic exercises such as supine neck flexion and prone neck extension through the entire ROM. A reclined position with the head and upper body elevated from horizontal can be used if supine neck flexion is too challenging in supine. Neck extension can be modified by having the PLWBC perform the exercise in standing while in front of a table or countertop supporting the upper body on hands.

Deep craniocervical flexor (longus capitus and colli) training involves patients being instructed to perform cranial-cervical flexion by gently nodding the head as though saying "yes" while positioned supine.[113] The goal is for the patient to perform cranial-cervical flexion, causing flattening of cervical lordosis without using the large, superficial cervical muscles (SCM and scalenes).[113] Contraction of these superficial muscles can be monitored by the clinician via palpation. Deep craniocervical flexor training could be performed with or without a biofeedback device. Some Onc R clinicians will use a manual sphygmomanometer blood pressure cuff to provide feedback as to the amount of pressure the patient is providing. When using a biofeedback device, the device is inflated to 20 mmHg; then the patient performs cranial-cervical flexion attempting to reach five sequential pressure targets in 2 mmHg increments (22 mmHg, 24 mmHg, 26 mmHg, 28 mmHg, and 30 mmHg).[114] The clinician identifies the target level that the patient can hold steadily for 5 seconds without (1) extending or retracting the neck; (2) dominant use of the superficial neck flexor muscles; and (3) quick, jerky movement.[114] At the identified target level, the PLWBC can perform 10 repetitions with 3- to 5-second rest intervals and progress the contraction duration to 10 seconds.[114] Once able to perform for 10 repetitions with 10-second contraction, the PLWBC can progress to the next 2 mmHg increment.[114]

Aerobic Exercise

The addition of aerobic exercise to neck-specific exercise may lead to a more significant reduction in neck pain and disability.[115] Persons with neck pain instructed to perform 30 minutes of walking or cycling at a moderate intensity for at least 3 days/week have demonstrated a more significant reduction in pain at 3 and 6-months compared to those instructed to perform neck-specific exercises alone.[115] Interestingly, 30 minutes of moderate-intensity aerobic exercise for at least 3 days a week has been shown to lead to a similar reduction in neck pain as neck-specific

exercises in individuals with cervical radiculopathy.[116] Collectively, research suggests that aerobic exercise may have a role in addressing nociceptive and neuropathic neck pain. Exercise may reduce nociceptor activity through various mechanisms and altering cell function.[117] Regular aerobic exercise has been shown to promote nerve healing and analgesia in animal models of neuropathic pain and nerve fibers' growth in participants with diabetic neuropathy.[117] It should be noted that this is the area in need of further research for PLWBCs of the head and neck, as there is a dearth of evidence relative to the effects of aerobic exercise on neck pain for this population.

Orthotics

Cervical orthosis such as Headmaster Collar has been suggested as an intervention for PLWBCs with DHS (see Chapter 7 for an image of a DHS collar).[96,118] A cervical orthotic provides anterior support for individuals who have difficulty maintaining normal head posture due to severe neck extensor weakness. The orthotic is typically worn intermittently throughout the day to improve functional activity tolerance by providing pain relief and reducing the risk of muscle overload and fatigue.[96] PLWBCs may wear a cervical orthosis during activities such as using the computer, watching TV, traveling on an airplane, performing household chores, and walking for exercise.[96] However, it should be noted that the majority of PLWBCs with DHS who are prescribed a Headmaster Collar discontinue its use due to reasons such as discomfort, aesthetics, device being too rigid or confining, or inadequate support.[118] PLWBCs should be instructed not to wear the orthosis continuously due to risk for neck stiffness and limited passive mobility. The Headmaster Collar can also provide a low load prolonged stretch to the anterior soft tissues of the neck since the device is adjustable.

Trismus

Background and Risk Factors

Trismus can be defined as any restriction to mouth opening due to intra-articular or extra-articular temporomandibular joint (TMJ) problems.[119] The etiology of trismus in PLWBCs of the head and neck is multifactorial. Trismus may result from (1) tumor infiltrating muscles of mastication causing the reflexive spasm; (2) destruction of TMJ surfaces due to tumor infiltration; (3) damage to the trigeminal nerve causing abnormal activity and spasm; (4) scarring after surgical approaches; (5) jaw pain and the adaptive protective mechanisms; and (6) radiation-induced dystonia or fibrosis.[17]

The percentage of PLWBCs who experience trismus increases in the 6 months following HNC treatment.[120] However, the reported prevalence of trismus in PLWBC of the head and neck has varied and is dependent on tumor size, tumor location, and cancer treatment received.[17,119] Risk factors for developing trismus have been reported to include older age; smaller pretreatment amount of mouth opening; tumors located near the oral cavity, oropharynx, nasopharynx, nasal cavity, maxillary sinus, and salivary glands; reconstruction; greater radiation dosage to muscles of mastication and TMJ; receiving chemotherapy; and presence of mucositis.[120–124]

Trismus may contribute to speech deficits and negatively impact nutritional intake due to a PLWBC having difficulty putting food in their mouth, chewing, and biting. Swallowing of food may be more difficult in PLWBCs with trismus due to inadequate bolus formation and potentially cause aspiration.[119] PLWBCs may not perform adequate oral hygiene or use dentures due to the restriction in mouth opening due to trismus.

Clinical Presentation

A cut-point of 35 mm or less of mouth opening has been recommended to diagnose trismus in PLWBCs of the head and neck.[125] However, different criteria have been proposed depending on dental status (dentulous = 35 mm, endentulous = 40 mm).[125] PLWBCs with trismus associated with HNC may present with restricted lateral deviation of the mandible as well. Since trismus in PLWBCs of the head and neck is a hypomobility deficit, there is typically minimal to no difference between active and passive jaw ROM.

PLWBCs may complain of jaw aches or pain, jaw stiffness, jaw fatigue, pain when moving the jaw, and pain or soreness of jaw muscles.[126] PLWBCs may also present with involuntary contractions in the masseter muscle or hypertonicity.[127] Masseter trigger points are more common in PLWBCs of the head and neck when compared to healthy controls.[128] PLWBCs of the head and neck have also been found to have a lower pain pressure threshold at masseter muscle than healthy controls.[128] An inverse relationship between severity of jaw pain and pain pressure threshold at masseter muscle has been found in PLWBC of the head and neck.[128]

Differential Diagnosis

First Bite Syndrome

First bite syndrome is an adverse effect of surgical treatments for HNC caused by nerve damage or the tumor itself.[129] The syndrome is triggered by salivation, thinking about a meal, or by simple contact with various foods even in the absence of chewing or taking the first few bites of food during a meal, which causes pain in the mouth.[129] It is characterized by severe cramping or spasm with the first few bites but diminishes with time.[129] Another sign of first bite syndrome is a sudden onset of intense head and neck pain in the parotid region.[129] It may occur months rather than days after the surgery, and the pain can also occur in the mandibular region or oral cavity and radiate to the ear.[129]

Osteonecrosis of the Jaw

Osteonecrosis of the jaw is a condition where the bone of the lower or upper jaw becomes exposed and does not heal properly. In cases of HNCs, osteonecrosis can occur after radiation therapy, called osteoradionecrosis. It is believed that radiation therapy to the mandible disrupts fibroblast activity, and therefore may cause a decrease in blood supply to the bone, thus increasing the risk of osteonecrosis.[130] The use of concomitant chemotherapy also increases the risk of osteonecrosis, especially with the use of cisplatin.[130] There is a wide range of options to treat this condition, from close observation to radical surgical resection.[130] In addition to jaw pain and the area of exposed bone, other signs and symptoms of osteonecrosis of the jaw include mucosal swelling, erythema, and increased tooth mobility.

Interventions for Trismus

Interventions for the management of trismus typically include therapeutic exercise and manual therapy. Exercise programs may begin with jaw active ROM (opening, lateral deviation, rotations) as a warm-up followed by active or passive stretching of the jaw. The reported dosage of exercise for trismus management has significantly varied in the literature (number of sessions per day: 2–10 sessions, number of repetitions per session: 3–15, duration

of a stretch: 6 seconds to 60 minutes).[131,132] Jaw-stretching devices such as TheraBite Jaw Motion Rehabilitation System, EZBite, or Jaw Dynasplint System may be prescribed to improve jaw opening ROM in patients with trismus. The average improvement in jaw opening after using TheraBite or EZBite for 3 months has been reported to be 6.0 mm or greater.[132] The mean in improvement in jaw opening using Dynasplint is 5 to 13.6 mm, with more significant improvement noted in patients who adhered to treatment recommendations as compared to those who did not.[131,133] A static passive stretching protocol with devices such as TheraBite or EZBite include 5 repetitions—30-second hold—5 times per day. The protocol for the Dynasplint involves patients using the device for 30 minutes, 3 times/day.[134-136] Jaw-stretching devices should be prescribed with caution due to mandibular fracture risk.[137] Also, stretching devices may not be appropriate for all PLWBCs due to issues with the fit of the devices or pain during exercise.[138] Use of tongue depressors is another option to improve jaw mobility in PLWBCs with trismus.[135,136] PLWBCs may be instructed to place a maximum number of tongue depressors between their teeth to provide a gentle stretch. Tongue depressors can apply a static passive stretch for 30-second duration repeated 5 times or low load prolonged stretch up to 15 minutes.[139]

Manual therapy may help relieve pain and increase movement in patients with trismus. Manual therapy may include soft tissue mobilization to muscles of mastication. Other soft-tissue techniques may include pressure release, manual stretching of taut-band muscle fibers, and pin and stretch. Joint mobilization techniques such as inferior, inferior-lateral, inferior-medial, or inferior-anterior TMJ mobilizations may relieve pain and improve mobility in patients with trismus.

Lymphedema

Background and Risk Factors

Up to 75% of PLWBCs of the head and neck have been reported to develop HNC-related lymphedema (HNL).[140] Lymphedema associated with HNC can be external (i.e., swelling underneath the skin in the head and neck region) or internal swelling (i.e., swelling of the pharyngeal wall or epiglottis), or both.[140] Of PLWBCs who develop lymphedema, about 10% demonstrate external lymphedema only while about 40% demonstrate internal lymphedema only and about 50% demonstrate combined internal and external lymphedema.[140] Lymphedema commonly occurs 2 to 6 months after treatment; however, it may occur at any time after treatment.[141] Risk factors for HNL include (1) tumors located in pharynx associated with external and combined lymphedema; (2) number of HNC treatments associated with all types of lymphedema; (3) total dosage of radiation and number of days of radiation associated with combined lymphedema; and (4) surgery with postoperative radiation and surgery in an irradiated field associated with internal lymphedema.[141]

Clinical Presentation

PLWBCs with HNL may report sensations of discomfort, tenderness, throbbing, pressure, heaviness, numbness, warmth, tightness, and firmness.[142-144] Many of these symptoms may be due to other problems besides lymphedema. However, one study found that only one participant without HNL reported heaviness, and no participants without HNL reported warmth suggesting these symptoms might be able to differentiate between patients with and without HNL.[142]

PLWBCs with HNL may complain of difficulty with speech, eating, swallowing, breathing, mouth opening, and moving the head and neck.[141,144] PLWBCs may also report that swelling is worse when flying in an airplane.[142]

HNL is diagnosed based on history and physical examination. HNL is characterized by slow onset of swelling during or after radiation therapy or persistent swelling after HNC surgery. HNL is typically worse in the morning if the PLWBC sleeps lying down and may improve throughout the day. Physical examination findings include (1) visible swelling evident by the change in anatomical contours (i.e., increased convexity at submental region) or loss of anatomical architecture (i.e., unable to visualize jawline); (2) change in tissue texture (spongy or firm); and (3) pitting. External HNL is most frequently located at the neck and submental areas, although HNL may be present in other regions of the head.[140,143]

Moderate to severe internal lymphedema is most commonly seen at the arytenoid space, aryepiglottic folds, epiglottis, arytenoids, and base of tongue.[145] Internal lymphedema is diagnosed by fiberoptic endoscopic examination and may be graded using the Paterson scale. Endoscopic examination is beyond the scope of some Onc R clinicians. However, a clinician may suspect internal HNL if PLWBC reports difficulty breathing, voice problems, and trouble swallowing.[98,142,145]

Differential Diagnosis of Lymphedema

Superior Vena Cava Syndrome

Superior vena cava syndrome (SVCS) occurs when a person's superior vena cava is partially blocked or compressed. Usually, the leading cause is malignancy. SVCS may also occur in persons with central venous catheters, pacemakers, or other devices due to mechanical irritation and foreign body reaction, causing inflammation, fibrosis, thrombus formation, and stenosis.[146] Other causes of SVCS include radiation fibrosis, infection, mediastinal hematoma, and benign tumors.[146] Signs and symptoms of superior vena cava syndrome include swelling of face, neck, upper extremities, distended or collateral veins, dyspnea, cough, hoarseness, stridor, and possible neurologic symptoms (headache, blurry vision, loss of consciousness).[146] Symptoms of SVCS may be exacerbated when bending forward or lying down.[146]

Infection/Cellulitis

Another issue that may cause head and neck swelling is cellulitis (skin infection). Signs and symptoms of cellulitis include acute onset, redness, swelling, warmth, and flu-like symptoms. PLWBCs with an infection will require topical, oral, or intravenous antibiotics, depending on infection severity.

Interventions for Head and Neck Lymphedema

The standard of care for HNL is complete decongestive therapy (CDT). CDT is a multimodal treatment that consists of skin care, manual lymphatic drainage (MLD), compression, exercise, and instruction on self-care. Detailed discussion on the principles of CDT can be found in Chapter 9.

Head and Neck Compression

Head and neck compression options include elastic compression garments, compression bandage straps, and inelastic compression garments. The recommended type and style of compression will be dependent on several factors such as location and severity of the swelling, soft tissue texture, neck and face anatomic irregularities, presence of a tracheostomy, financial constraints, and PLWBC preference. PLWBCs who experience HNL can be measured and fitted for off-the-shelf (one size or small, medium, large) or custom (made based on individual measurements) compression garments. Both off-the-shelf and custom compression garments are offered in various styles to address lymphedema at different head and neck regions. Compression chinstraps can address edema located at the submental and mandibular region but will not address edema located at the neck or face. There are compression chin and neck straps that provide compression to the submental and mandibular region and the neck. If PLWBC presents with facial lymphedema, full face compression garments are necessary. Multi-layer short stretch bandage compression straps can be fabricated by sewing and securing Velcro to short-stretch bandages. Foam padding can be used with both compression garments and multi-layer short stretch bandage compression straps to improve pressure distribution and soften fibrotic tissue.[147] Foam padding may be purchased or fabricated using different types of foam. There are two categories of foam padding: flat pads and chip pads (bags).[147] Flat pads help re-distribute fluid to better functioning regions, re-shape edematous regions, and prevent re-accumulation of lymphedema.[147] Chip bags or Schneid packs are considered softening pads and are designed to address soft tissue firmness and fibrosis.[147] Inelastic options made of fabric and foam padding are available and include products such as the TributeNight™ Mandibular Unit and Sigvaris™ Neck and Mandible Pad. Head and neck compression is not appropriate for all PLWBCs who experience HNL. Onc R clinicians should be aware of contraindications to head and neck compression, including patients with acute infection, blockage of the carotid artery, or other vascular abnormalities such as tumor infiltrating a major blood vessel.[147] Caution should be taken if patients have a history of cardiovascular disease or a compromised airway.[147]

Decongestive Exercises

Decongestive exercises are performed while the PLWBC wears head and neck compression and is designed to increase venous and lymphatic flow. Decongestive exercises involve active, nonresistive movements. Movements should be performed slowly with a rest period between each movement that lasts at least as long as the time spent moving.[147]

Decongestive Home Exercise Program for Head and Neck Lymphedema. The exercises below should be performed in the sequence described while wearing compression.

Start by sitting with good posture. Knees should be bent and feet flat on the floor.

Abdominal Breathing (3 repetitions)
1. Place both hands over your navel area. Take a deep breath in. As you breathe in, your hands and the navel area should rise out. As you breathe out, your hands and the navel area should go in.

Shoulder Exercises (5 repetitions each)
2. Pinch shoulder blades together, then relax.
3. Raise shoulders up, then relax.
4. Perform a shoulder roll forward.
5. Perform a shoulder roll backward.

Neck Exercises (5 repetitions each)
6. Bend neck backward as if you were looking at the ceiling, then return to the starting position.
7. Rotate head to the left as if you were looking over your shoulder, then return to the starting position. Repeat to the right.
8. Tilt head to the left as if you were trying to bring your ear towards your shoulder then return to starting position. Repeat to the right.

9. Bend neck forward as if you were looking down, then return to starting position.
   Facial Exercises (5 repetitions each)
10. Frown or stick your lower lip out. You should feel the muscles contract at the front of your neck.
11. Move your lips side to side.
12. Smile
13. Close then open your eyes.

Manual Lymphatic Drainage for Head and Neck Lymphedema

Manual lymphatic drainage involves slow (one per second) and repetitive (at least 7 repetitions) hand movements that stretch the skin in a specific direction. MLD can be clinician- or caregiver-administered, or PLWBCs can be instructed on self-MLD. MLD sequences for HNL attempt to direct fluid to the bilateral axillae. Anterior and posterior sequences have been described, and the selection of sequence will be dependent on the presence of scarring that prevents fluid from being mobilized through the scarred area.[147]

Example of Self-MLD Anterior Sequence for Head and Neck Lymphedema. Self-lymphatic drainage is a gentle technique designed to help reduce edema which involves stretching the skin in a specific direction. The person should use enough pressure so that their hand does not slide across their skin, but not too much pressure. The person should not experience any pain or redness of their skin. If pain or redness is experienced, the person should be coached to stop performing this and discuss with their certified lymphedema therapist.

The patient should be educated to perform sequence below:
1. Place both hands over your naval area. Take a deep breath in. As you breathe in, your hands and the navel area should rise out. As you breathe out, your hands and the navel area should go in. Repeat 3 to 5 times.
2. Place your hand in the hollow area above your collarbone. Perform 10 stationary circles.
3. Place your hand in your armpit. Perform 10 stationary circles.
4. Place your hand on the side of your chest in line with nipple. Perform 10 stationary circles.
5. Place your hand on the front of your chest just above the nipple. Perform stationary circles stretching skin towards the armpit. Repeat 10 times.
6. Place your hand on the front of your chest just below the collarbone. Perform stationary circles stretching the skin out towards the armpit. Repeat 10 times.
7. Place your hand over your collarbone. Stretch skin out and downward towards the armpit. Repeat 10 times.
8. Place your hand on top of shoulder, reaching towards the back. Stretch skin out towards the arm. Repeat 10 times.
9. Repeat steps 2 to 8 on the opposite side.
10. Place your hand on the back of your neck. Perform 10 stationary circles stretching the skin downward and towards the front of the neck.
11. Place your hand on the side of your neck (knuckles under ears). Perform 10 stationary circles stretching the skin back and downward towards the base of the neck.
12. Place your hand on the side of your neck (knuckles under the jaw). Perform 10 stationary circles stretching the skin back and downward towards the base of the neck.
13. Place your hand on the front of your neck (knuckles under chin). Perform 10 stationary circles stretching the skin back and downward towards the base of the neck.
14. Place two fingers in front of the ear and two fingers behind the ear. Perform 10 stationary circles stretching the skin back and downward.
15. Place hand over the jaw. Perform 10 stationary circles stretching the skin back and downward.
16. Place a hand under chin. Perform 10 stationary circles stretching the skin back and downward.
17. Place hand over the cheek. Perform 10 stationary circles stretching skin back and downward.
18. Repeat steps 10 to 17 on the opposite side.
19. Repeat step 1.

Conclusion

PLWBCs of the head and neck may experience acute or long-term adverse effects that can negatively impact health-related QOL. Onc R clinicians play an instrumental role by addressing and screening for a number of these adverse effects. Common reasons for referral to Onc R include shoulder, neck, and jaw problems, as well as HNL. SANP is a shoulder problem experienced by PLWBCs of the head and neck that can cause neck and shoulder pain, impaired shoulder movement, muscle weakness, and postural deficits. Neck problems include neck pain, restricted ROM, muscle weakness, and sensory deficits. Trismus is a common jaw problem experienced by PLWBCs of the head and neck that is characterized by limited ability to open the mouth. HNL is a debilitating adverse effect of HNC and its treatment that can occur externally or internally. External HNL results in swelling underneath the skin, stiffness, tightness, difficulty moving the head or neck, and body image issues while internal lymphedema may contribute to swallowing and speech difficulties.[142,148] Problems that will require Onc R or referral to another health care provider include dysphagia; speech or voice problems, hearing loss, vertigo, sleep disturbance, distress/depression/anxiety; body and self-image concerns; osteonecrosis; oral infections/candidiasis, oral hygiene, onset or worsening of GERD, signs or symptoms of hypothyroidism, inadequate or lack of nutrition, and dehydration.[2]

Critical Research Needs

- Psychometric properties of head and neck lymphedema measures. Inter-rater reliability of tape measurements and tissue dielectric constant has been investigated but not test-retest reliability or measurement error.[149,150] More research is also needed investigating sensitivity to change.[151]
- Development and psychometric properties of patient-reported outcome measures assessing head and neck lymphedema. The authors are aware of only one patient-reported outcome specific to HNC lymphedema.[143,152]
- Randomized controlled trials investigating the effectiveness of CDT.[153]
- Clinical research investigating the following:
  - Individual contribution of manual lymphatic drainage, compression, and exercise for reducing head and neck lymphedema.
  - Comparison of advanced pneumatic compression and CDT for reducing head and neck lymphedema.
  - Effectiveness of manual therapy for addressing HNC-related trismus.
  - Effectiveness of physical therapy for managing head and neck-cancer neck pain and mobility deficits.

- The development and validity of movement system diagnoses or rehabilitation classifications specific to HNC.
- Value of matched care for patients with HNC-related neck, shoulder, and temporomandibular disorders.

Case Study

A 68-year-old male was referred to outpatient physical therapy for evaluation and treatment.

Chief complaints: pain; difficulty reaching overhead

History of present illness: The patient was diagnosed with p16-negative T3 N2 M0 squamous cell carcinoma of the oropharynx. The patient underwent TORS and left neck dissection 8 weeks ago. He reported experiencing left neck and shoulder pain and difficulty reaching overhead since surgery for HNC. His pain was reported to be worse at the end of the day. His pain was aggravated with arm motion, lifting, and driving, but is alleviated with rest. His pain at worst was rated as 5/10 (see Figure 19.10) and rated 0/10 at best. He reported seeing a speech and language pathologist for swallowing difficulty.

History of tobacco use: yes

History of alcohol use: yes

Medications: Lisinopril

Medical history: hypertension

Surgical history: TORS (10 weeks ago), left neck dissection (10 weeks ago)

Social history: lives with wife in two-story home; retired school teacher; played golf 3 times per week prior to cancer treatment

Family history: no family history of cancer; father died of myocardial infarction at 72 years of age

Fall risk assessment: history of falls in past 6 months—no; loss of balance—no; afraid of falling—no

Fatigue screen 0 to 10 scale (0 = no fatigue; 10 = worst fatigue you can imagine): 5

Insurance: Medicare

Patient goals: return to golf

Review of Systems:

- [ ] Fever, chills, sweating
- [ ] Fatigue, unusual tiredness
- [ ] Unexplained weight loss
- [ ] Nausea, vomiting, loss of appetite
- [ ] Change in vision
- [ ] Hearing loss or ringing in ears
- [ ] Nosebleeds or nasal congestion
- [ ] Hoarseness or change in voice
- [X] Trouble speaking or swallowing
- [ ] Chest pain or pressure
- [ ] Burning or cramping in legs
- [ ] Heart palpitations

- [ ] Blood in stool or urine
- [ ] Change in bowel or bladder
- [ ] Constipation or diarrhea
- [ ] Abdominal pain or bloating
- [ ] Depressed or anxious
- [ ] Memory loss
- [ ] Difficulty sleeping
- [ ] Swelling or lumps anywhere
- [ ] Skin rash or other changes
- [ ] Easy bruising
- [ ] Change in hair or nails
- [ ] Itching
- [ ] Heat or cold intolerance

- [ ] Frequent cough
- [ ] Wheezing
- [ ] Shortness of breath
- [X] Numbness or tingling
- [X] Paralysis or weakness
- [ ] Tremor
- [ ] Involuntary movements
- [ ] Headaches
- [ ] Loss of balance or falls
- [ ] Loss of consciousness or fainting
- [ ] Dizziness or lightheaded
- [X] Joint pain or stiffness
- [ ] Increased thirst

Systems Review
Musculoskeletal

ROM: impaired cervical AROM; impaired left (L) active shoulder flexion (~110 degrees) and abduction (~90 degrees); bilateral (B) elbow/wrist/hand AROM—within functional limits (WFL)

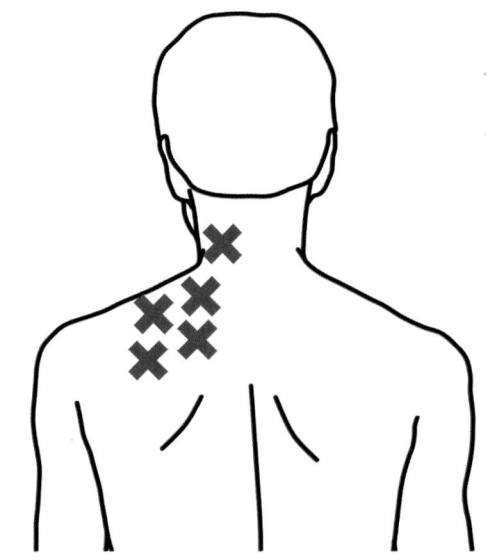

- **Fig. 19.10** Pain Body Diagram. (Created by Chris Wilson.)

Strength: weak and painful (L neck-shoulder region) resisted L shoulder abduction; strong and painless resisted elbow flexion, elbow extension, wrist extension, wrist flexion, thumb extension, finger abduction

Anthropometrics: height 5′6″ (167 cm), weight 155 pounds (70.3 kg)

Neuromuscular:

Sensation: impaired light touch left anterolateral neck; intact to light touch B upper and lower extremities grossly

Gait: ambulates without assistive device; no deviation from straight path noted

Cardiovascular/pulmonary:

Heart rate: 92 beats per minute (BPM)

Blood pressure: 129/78 mmHg

SpO_2: 95%

Respiratory rate: 14 breaths per minute

Integumentary:

Incision: left neck—clean/dry/intact

Pitting assessment: no pitting edema

Tissue texture assessment: normal tissue texture

Color: normal

Temporomandibular AROM

Opening	42 mm
Lateral deviation—Left	8 mm
Lateral deviation—Right	9 mm
Protrusion	4 mm

Comment: dentulous

Cervical AROM

Flexion	Within normal limits
Extension	Moderate restriction
Rotation-Left	Minimal restriction
Rotation-Right	Moderate restriction
Sidebend-Left	Minimal restriction
Sidebend-Right	Moderate° restriction

Shoulder ROM

	Right		Left	
	Active	Passive	Active	Passive
Forward elevation	155°	160°	110°	165°
Abduction	160°	165°	85°	160°
External rotation at 0° of shoulder abduction	60°	60°	61°	61°
Hand behind back internal rotation (Thoracic spinal level reached by hand)	T7	T7	T8	T8

Comments: 3/10 right neck-shoulder pain during left shoulder active shoulder forward elevation and abduction; pain resolved within 1 minute

Shoulder Manual Muscle Testing

	Right	Left
External rotation at 0°	5/5	5/5
Internal rotation at 0°	5/5	5/5
Rhomboids	5/5	5/5
Middle trapezius	5/5	0/5
Lower trapezius	5/5	0/5
Serratus anterior	5/5	5/5

Comments: 3/10 right neck-shoulder pain during left rhomboids, middle trapezius, and lower trapezius manual muscle testing pain resolved immediately

Palpation: tender to palpate and taut left levator scapulae and left SCM

Cervical special tests: (–) upper limb neural tension

Shoulder special tests: (–) Neer, (–) Hawkins, (–) cross body adduction, (–) external rotation lag sign, (–) belly press

Scapular special tests: (+) scapular flip sign, (–) plus sign

Posture: Flexed and forward head; left shoulder is depressed and forward compared to right

Visual assessment of shoulder motion: excessive scapular abduction (protraction), decreased scapular upward rotation, decreased clavicular elevation on left during active shoulder flexion and abduction

Assessment and plan: Patient presents with clinical findings consistent with left SANP contributing to neck-shoulder pain associated with myofascial pain due to levator scapulae overuse. Interventions may include manual techniques to address pain and levator scapulae muscle tautness and left shoulder PROM exercises to maintain shoulder passive mobility. The patient would benefit from instruction on activity modification since his symptoms were worse with overhead activities and lifting. Since the patient does not present with high pain irritability, resistance exercise may be prescribed targeting muscles with similar function as the trapezius muscle. He also presented with neck mobility deficits likely due to levator scapulae muscle tautness, SCM tautness, and a healing neck dissection scar. Interventions would include patient instruction on proper head posture and neck AROM/stretching exercises. He did not present with trismus since he was dentulous and had greater than 35 mm of mandibular opening; however, it would be reasonable to prescribe jaw ROM/stretching exercise since he presented with jaw ROM near the lower limit of normal. He did not present with any clinical signs of head and neck lymphedema.

Outcomes: Outcome for left SANP and neck-shoulder pain would be dependent on the extent of SAN injury and level of recovery. If the SAN was not sacrificed or transected, shoulder function is usually restored by 6 to 12 months after surgery. With respect to his neck mobility deficits, it would be expected that he would regain cervical range to near age-matched normative values.

Review Questions

Reader can find the correct answers and rationale in the back of the book.

1. A 58-year-old male diagnosed with HNC is currently receiving definitive radiation therapy. Patient was seen for a physical therapy evaluation with chief complaints of fatigue and neck stiffness. Resting vital signs were as follows: heart rate of 88 BPM, blood pressure of 119/68 mmHg. Musculoskeletal systems review was not remarkable except for impaired cervical AROM. Patient presented with 30 degrees of cervical extension AROM, 55 degrees of cervical rotation AROM to each direction, and 30 degrees of cervical lateral flexion to each direction. Visual inspection of the skin revealed the following: erythema and moist desquamation at anterior neck. Six Minute Walk Test distance was 78% of healthy individuals of similar sex and age. Peak heart rate during Six Minute Walk Test was 105 BPM and RPE was 13/20. Patient denied chest pain, dizziness, and extreme shortness of breath during Six Minute Walk Test. Which of the following interventions would be contraindicated at this time?

   A. Anterior neck soft tissue mobilization

   B. Cervical lateral flexion AROM exercise

   C. Upper body resistance exercise

   D. Patient instruction on walking program

2. A physical therapist evaluated a 56-year-old female who had a right modified RND 12 weeks ago. Patient presented with 75 degrees of right shoulder abduction AROM and pain located at right levator scapulae region during motion. Which of the following additional findings would be consistent with patient experiencing SANP?

   A. Similar limitation in right shoulder abduction PROM

   B. Excessive scapular abduction during active shoulder abduction ROM

   C. Deltoid muscle atrophy

   D. Resisted right shoulder external rotation weakness

3. A 53-year-old male with history of history of right mandibulectomy, fibular free flap reconstruction, and right neck dissection was seen in an outpatient physical therapy setting with chief complaint of right jaw pain. Which of the following findings would be consistent with a diagnosis of first bite syndrome?

   A. Mandibular opening ROM equal to 30 mm

   B. Area of exposed bone; tooth mobility

   C. Normal physical examination, pain in jaw that is worse taking first few bites of food

   D. Mandibular protrusion ROM equal to 10 mm

4. Which of the following is a typical finding associated with HNC-associated trismus?
   A. S-curve deviation
   B. Impaired sensation at TMJ region
   C. Masseter hypertonicity
   D. Mandibular opening between 40 mm and 60 mm

5. A 47-year-old male diagnosed with T3N2M0 squamous cell carcinoma of the oropharynx was seen for physical therapy evaluation for chief complaint of left shoulder pain. Past surgical history included TORS, anterolateral thigh free flap reconstruction, and left neck dissection (levels I–V). Patient presented with the following examination findings: left shoulder pain rated as 5/10, 90 degree of left shoulder abduction AROM and PROM, 15 degrees of shoulder external rotation AROM and PROM, strong and painless resisted shoulder abduction at 45 degrees and shoulder external rotation at 0 degree abduction, excessive scapular elevation during left shoulder abduction AROM, and right shoulder slightly depressed compared to left. Based on the clinical findings, which of the following is most likely diagnosis?
   A. Adhesive capsulitis
   B. Axillary nerve palsy
   C. Rotator cuff disease
   D. SANP

6. A 53-year-old male diagnosed with base-of-tongue squamous cell carcinoma underwent a tumor resection and right neck dissection (levels II–V). He presents with the following clinical findings: 0–3/10 right shoulder pain, 88 degrees of right shoulder abduction AROM, 0/5 right middle and lower trapezius muscle strength, positive scapular dyskinesis during shoulder abduction AROM, and positive right scapular flip sign. Which of the following exercises would be most appropriate to address shoulder pain and dysfunction at this time?
   A. Standing shoulder abduction AROM
   B. Overhead press resistance exercise
   C. Prone shoulder horizontal abduction while maintaining glenohumeral external rotation resistance exercise
   D. Standing biceps curls resistance exercise with manual assistance as needed to stabilize scapula

7. A 50-year-old female diagnosed with nasopharyngeal cancer received concurrent chemoradiation 1 year ago and was referred to physical therapy with the chief complaint of difficulty turning her head while driving. The patient reported experiencing 0/10 neck pain at rest and 3/10 neck pain described as tightness when looking over shoulder while driving. She presented with forward head posture while seated, 58 degrees of cervical flexion A/PROM, 25 degrees of cervical extension A/PROM, 45 degrees of left cervical rotation A/PROM, and 50 degrees of right cervical rotation A/PROM. Anterolateral soft tissues of the neck were firm to touch. Which of the following plans of care would likely be most effective to address patient's chief complaint?
   A. Cervical AROM: hold 5 seconds, 10 repetitions, 3 times/day
   B. Cervical dynamic stretching: hold 5 seconds, 8 repetitions, 3 times/day
   C. Cervical static active stretching: hold 30 seconds, 3 repetitions, 3 times/day
   D. Upper cervical flexion AROM: hold 10 seconds, 10 repetitions, 1 time/day

8. A 61-year-old female was seen for physical therapy evaluation with chief complaints of neck pain and difficulty working overhead. Her past medical history included T2N0M0 cancer of the larynx treated with partial laryngectomy, selective neck dissection (levels II–IV) and radiation therapy completed 4 months ago. The patient presented with the following clinical findings: flexed and forward head posture, 50 degrees of cervical flexion AROM, -5 degrees of cervical extension AROM, 50 degrees of cervical flexion PROM, and 35 degrees of cervical extension PROM. Which of the following is the most likely cause of patient's findings?
   A. Radiation-associated neck extensor muscle weakness
   B. Anterior neck soft tissue radiation fibrosis
   C. SANP
   D. Lhermitte's syndrome

9. A 67-year-old male with history of hypopharyngeal cancer treated with definitive radiation was referred for evaluation and treatment of head and neck lymphedema. Past medical history was significant for hypertension. He presented with pitting edema and firm tissue texture at submental region and anterior neck. Skin inspection revealed no redness, warmth to touch, or dilated collateral veins at bilateral upper quadrants grossly. Based on findings, patient may still present with which of the following contraindications for head and neck compression as an intervention for head and neck lymphedema?
   A. Carotid artery disease
   B. Subclavian vein deep vein thrombosis
   C. Radiation-related soft tissue fibrosis
   D. Cellulitis

10. A 63-year-old male diagnosed with head and neck lymphedema was referred for evaluation and treatment. Past medical history was significant for oropharyngeal cancer treated with TORS, bilateral neck dissection, and radiation therapy. Which of the following may indicate patient has internal head and neck lymphedema?
    A. Feeling of heaviness and warmth
    B. Difficulty breathing and swallowing
    C. Persistent cough and hemoptysis
    D. Anterior neck firmness and stiffness

References

1. Siegel RL, Miller KD, Jemal A. Cancer statistics, 2020. *CA Cancer J Clin.* 2020;70(1):7–30.
2. Cohen EE, LaMonte SJ, Erb NL, et al. American Cancer Society Head and Neck Cancer Survivorship Care Guideline. *CA Cancer J Clin.* 2016;66(3):203–239.
3. Balfe M, Butow P, O'Sullivan E, Gooberman-Hill R, Timmons A, Sharp L. The financial impact of head and neck cancer caregiving: a qualitative study. *Psychooncology.* 2016;25(12):1441–1447.
4. Hoxbroe Michaelsen S, Gronhoj C, Hoxbroe Michaelsen J, Friborg J, von Buchwald C. Quality of life in survivors of oropharyngeal cancer: a systematic review and meta-analysis of 1366 patients. *Eur J Cancer.* 2017;78:91–102.
5. Liao LJ, Hsu WL, Lo WC, Cheng PW, Shueng PW, Hsieh CH. Health-related quality of life and utility in head and neck cancer survivors. *BMC Cancer.* 2019;19(1):425. doi:10.1186/s12885-019-5614-4.
6. Wissinger E, Griebsch I, Lungershausen J, Foster T, Pashos CL. The economic burden of head and neck cancer: a systematic literature review. *Pharmacoeconomics.* 2014;32(9):865–882.
7. Montero PH, Patel SG. Cancer of the oral cavity. *Surg Oncol Clin N Am.* 2015;24(3):491–508.
8. Bruss D, Anatomy Sajjad H. Head and neck, laryngopharynx [Updated February 14, 2021]*StatPearls [Internet]*: StatPearls Publishing; 2021. January. https://www.ncbi.nlm.nih.gov/books/NBK549913/.
9. Mankowski N, Bordoni B. Anatomy, head and neck, nasopharynx [Updated February 7, 2021]*StatPearls [Internet]*: StatPearls Publishing; 2021. January. https://www.ncbi.nlm.nih.gov/books/NBK557635/.
10. Kato MG, Baek CH, Chaturvedi P, et al. Update on oral and oropharyngeal cancer staging—international perspectives. *World J Otorhinolaryngol Head Neck Surg.* 2020;6(1):66–75.
11. Cohan DM, Popat S, Kaplan SE, Rigual N, Loree T, Hicks Jr WL. Oropharyngeal cancer: current understanding and management. *Curr Opin Otolaryngol Head Neck Surg.* 2009;17(2):88–94.
12. Koroulakis A, Agarwal M. Laryngeal cancer [Updated August 10, 2020]*StatPearls [Internet].*: StatPearls Publishing; 2021. January. https://www.ncbi.nlm.nih.gov/books/NBK526076/.
13. Lin HH, Limesand KH, Ann DK. Current state of knowledge on salivary gland cancers. *Crit Rev Oncog.* 2018;23(3–4):139–151.
14. Kessler AT, Bhatt AA. Review of the major and minor salivary glands, part 1: anatomy, infectious, and inflammatory processes. *J Clin Imaging Sci.* 2018;8:47. doi:10.4103/jcis.JCIS_45_18.
15. Kikuta S, Iwanaga J, Kusukawa J, Tubbs RS. Triangles of the neck: a review with clinical/surgical applications. *Anat Cell Biol.* 2019;52(2):120–127.
16. Al-Missri M, Al Khalili Y. Anatomy, head and neck, submental triangle [Updated July 27, 2020]*StatPearls [Internet]*: StatPearls Publishing; 2021. January. https://www.ncbi.nlm.nih.gov/books/NBK545296/.
17. Abboud WA, Hassin-Baer S, Alon EE, et al. Restricted mouth opening in head and neck cancer: etiology, prevention, and treatment. *JCO Oncol Pract.* 2020;16(10):643–653.
18. Poon H, Li C, Gao W, Ren H, Lim CM. Evolution of robotic systems for transoral head and neck surgery. *Oral Oncol.* 2018;87:82–88.
19. Miller MC, Goldenberg D. Education Committee of the American Head and Neck Society (AHNS). AHNS series: do you know your guidelines? Principles of surgery for head and neck cancer: a review of the National Comprehensive Cancer Network guidelines. *Head Neck* 2017;39(4):791–796.
20. Deschler DG, Moore MG, Smith RV, eds. *Quick Reference Guide to TNM Staging of Head and Neck Cancer and Neck Dissection Classification.* 4th ed, American Academy of Otolaryngology–Head and Neck Surgery Foundation; 2014.
21. Robbins KT, Shaha AR, Medina JE, et al. Consensus statement on the classification and terminology of neck dissection. *Arch Otolaryngol Head Neck Surg.* 2008;134(5):536–538.
22. Robbins KT, Clayman G, Levine PA, et al. Neck dissection classification update: revisions proposed by the American Head and Neck Society and the American Academy of Otolaryngology–Head and Neck Surgery. *Arch Otolaryngol Head Neck Surg.* 2002;128(7):751–758.
23. Chim H, Salgado CJ, Seselgyte R, Wei FC, Mardini S. Principles of head and neck reconstruction: an algorithm to guide flap selection. *Semin Plast Surg.* 2010;24(2):148–154.
24. Kini E. Free flap procedures for reconstruction after head and neck cancer. *AORN J.* 2015;102(6) 644.e1–e6.
25. Pabst AM, Werkmeister R, Steegmann J, Holzle F, Bartella A. Is there an ideal way to close the donor site of radial forearm free flaps? *Br J Oral Maxillofac Surg.* 2018;56(6):444–452.
26. Ragbir M, Brown JS, Mehanna H. Reconstructive considerations in head and neck surgical oncology: United Kingdom National Multidisciplinary Guidelines. *J Laryngol Otol.* 2016;130(S2):S191–S197.
27. Orlik JR, Horwich P, Bartlett C, Trites J, Hart R, Taylor SM. Long-term functional donor site morbidity of the free radial forearm flap in head and neck cancer survivors. *J Otolaryngol Head Neck Surg.* 2014;43:1. doi:10.1186/1916-0216-43-1.
28. Liu M, Liu W, Yang X, Guo H, Peng H. Pectoralis major myocutaneous flap for head and neck defects in the era of free flaps: harvesting technique and indications. *Sci Rep.* 2017;7:46256. doi:10.1038/srep46256.
29. Oranges CM, Ling B, Tremp M, Wettstein R, Kalbermatten DF, Schaefer DJ. Comparison of anterolateral thigh and radial forearm free flaps in head and neck reconstruction. *In Vivo.* 2018;32(4):893–897.
30. Baehring E, McCorkle R. Postoperative complications in head and neck cancer. *Clin J Oncol Nurs.* 2012;16(6):E203–E209.
31. Chen YJ, Wang CP, Wang CC, Jiang RS, Lin JC, Liu SA. Carotid blowout in patients with head and neck cancer: associated factors and treatment outcomes. *Head Neck.* 2015;37(2):265–272.
32. Sharma A, Bahl A. Intensity-modulated radiation therapy in head-and-neck carcinomas: potential beyond sparing the parotid glands. *J Cancer Res Ther.* 2020;16(3):425–433.
33. Blanchard P, Gunn GB, Lin A, Foote RL, Lee NY, Frank SJ. Proton therapy for head and neck cancers. *Semin Radiat Oncol.* 2018;28(1):53–63.
34. Bhalavat R, Budrukkar A, Laskar SG, et al. Brachytherapy in head and neck malignancies: Indian Brachytherapy Society (IBS) recommendations and guidelines. *J Contemp Brachytherapy.* 2020;12(5):501–511.
35. Lloyd S, Alektiar KM, Nag S, et al. Intraoperative high-dose-rate brachytherapy: an American Brachytherapy Society consensus report. *Brachytherapy.* 2017;16(3):446–465.
36. Takacsi-Nagy Z, Martinez-Mongue R, Mazeron JJ, Anker CJ, Harrison LB. American Brachytherapy Society Task Group Report: combined external beam irradiation and interstitial brachytherapy for base of tongue tumors and other head and neck sites in the era of new technologies. *Brachytherapy.* 2017;16(1):44–58.
37. Tolentino Ede S, Centurion BS, Ferreira LH, Souza AP, Damante JH, Rubira-Bullen IR. Oral adverse effects of head and neck radiotherapy: literature review and suggestion of a clinical oral care guideline for irradiated patients. *J Appl Oral Sci.* 2011;19(5):448–454.
38. Sroussi HY, Epstein JB, Bensadoun RJ, et al. Common oral complications of head and neck cancer radiation therapy: mucositis, infections, saliva change, fibrosis, sensory dysfunctions, dental caries, periodontal disease, and osteoradionecrosis. *Cancer Med.* 2017;6(12):2918–2931.
39. Ganesan P, Schmiedge J, Manchaiah V, Swapna S, Dhandayutham S, Kothandaraman PP. Ototoxicity: a challenge in diagnosis and treatment. *J Audiol Otol.* 2018;22(2):59–68.
40. Lemanne D, Cassileth B, Gubili J. The role of physical activity in cancer prevention, treatment, recovery, and survivorship. *Oncology (Williston Park).* 2013;27(6):580–585.

41. Ballard-Barbash R, George SM, Alfano CM, Schmitz K. Physical activity across the cancer continuum. *Oncology (Williston Park)*. 2013;27(6):589–592.

42. Szturz P, Wouters K, Kiyota N, et al. Weekly low-dose versus three-weekly high-dose cisplatin for concurrent chemoradiation in locoregionally advanced non-nasopharyngeal head and neck cancer: a systematic review and meta-analysis of aggregate data. *Oncologist*. 2017;22(9):1056–1066.

43. Gau M, Karabajakian A, Reverdy T, Neidhardt EM, Fayette J. Induction chemotherapy in head and neck cancers: results and controversies. *Oral Oncol*. 2019;95:164–169.

44. Zhang Y, Chen L, Hu GQ, et al. Gemcitabine and cisplatin induction chemotherapy in nasopharyngeal carcinoma. *N Engl J Med*. 2019;381(12):1124–1135.

45. Sim F, Leidner R, Bell RB. Immunotherapy for head and neck cancer. *Hematol Oncol Clin North Am*. 2019;33(2):301–321.

46. Lanisnik B. Different branching patterns of the spinal accessory nerve: impact on neck dissection technique and postoperative shoulder function. *Curr Opin Otolaryngol Head Neck Surg*. 2017;25(2):113–118.

47. Gane EM, Michaleff ZA, Cottrell MA, et al. Prevalence, incidence, and risk factors for shoulder and neck dysfunction after neck dissection: a systematic review. *Eur J Surg Oncol*. 2017;43(7):1199–1218.

48. Garzaro M, Riva G, Raimondo L, Aghemo L, Giordano C, Pecorari G. A study of neck and shoulder morbidity following neck dissection: the benefits of cervical plexus preservation. *Ear Nose Throat J*. 2015;94(8):330–344.

49. Refos JW, Witte BI, de Goede CJ, de Bree R. Shoulder morbidity after pectoralis major flap reconstruction. *Head Neck*. 2016;38(8):1221–1228.

50. Merve A, Mitra I, Swindell R, Homer JJ. Shoulder morbidity after pectoralis major flap reconstruction for head and neck cancer. *Head Neck*. 2009;31(11):1470–1476.

51. Patel KB, Low TH, Partridge A, et al. Assessment of shoulder function following scapular free flap. *Head Neck*. 2020;42(2):224–229.

52. Kelley MJ, Kane TE, Leggin BG. Spinal accessory nerve palsy: associated signs and symptoms. *J Orthop Sports Phys Ther*. 2008;38(2):78–86.

53. Roren A, Fayad F, Poiraudeau S, et al. Specific scapular kinematic patterns to differentiate two forms of dynamic scapular winging. *Clin Biomech (Bristol, Avon)* 2013;28(8):941–947.

54. Cooperstein R, Haneline M, Young M. The location of the inferior angle of the scapula in relation to the spine in the upright position: a systematic review of the literature and meta-analysis. *Chiropr Man Therap*. 2015;23:7. doi:10.1186/s12998-014-0050-7.

55. da Costa BR, Armijo-Olivo S, Gadotti I, Warren S, Reid DC, Magee DJ. Reliability of scapular positioning measurement procedure using the palpation meter (PALM). *Physiotherapy*. 2010;96(1):59–67.

56. Ludewig PM, Phadke V, Braman JP, Hassett DR, Cieminski CJ, LaPrade RF. Motion of the shoulder complex during multiplanar humeral elevation. *J Bone Joint Surg Am*. 2009;91(2):378–389.

57. McClure P, Tate AR, Kareha S, Irwin D, Zlupko E. A clinical method for identifying scapular dyskinesis, part 1: reliability. *J Athl Train*. 2009;44(2):160–164.

58. Camargo PR, Neumann DA. Kinesiologic considerations for targeting activation of scapulothoracic muscles—part 2: trapezius. *Braz J Phys Ther*. 2019;23(6):467–475.

59. Lawrence RL, Braman JP, Ludewig PM. Shoulder kinematics impact subacromial proximities: a review of the literature. *Braz J Phys Ther*. 2020;24(3):219–230.

60. Kelley MJ, Shaffer MA, Kuhn JE, et al. Shoulder pain and mobility deficits: adhesive capsulitis. *J Orthop Sports Phys Ther*. 2013;43(5):A1–A31.

61. Leong HT, Fu SC, He X, Oh JH, Yamamoto N, Hang S. Risk factors for rotator cuff tendinopathy: a systematic review and meta-analysis. *J Rehabil Med*. 2019;51(9):627–637.

62. Chow LQM. Head and Neck Cancer. *N Engl J Med*. 2020;382(1):60–72.

63. Wang X, Wang H, Zhang T, Cai L, Dai E, He J. Diabetes and its potential impact on head and neck oncogenesis. *J Cancer*. 2020;11(3):583–591.

64. Althagafi A, Nadi M. Acute nerve injury *StatPearls [Internet]*: StatPearls Publishing; 2020 https://www.ncbi.nlm.nih.gov/books/NBK557635/

65. Menorca R, Fussell T, Elfar J. Peripheral nerve trauma: mechanisms of injury and recovery. *Hand Clin*. 2013;29(3):317–330.

66. Robinson LR. Traumatic injury to peripheral nerves. *Muscle Nerve*. 2000;23(6):863–873.

67. Lee JH, Yoo WG. Effect of scapular elevation taping on scapular depression syndrome: a case report. *J Back Musculoskelet Rehabil*. 2012;25(3):187–191.

68. Russo SA, Zlotolow DA, Chafetz RS, et al. Efficacy of 3 therapeutic taping configurations for children with brachial plexus birth palsy. *J Hand Ther*. 2018;31(3):357–370.

69. Bodack MP, Tunkel RS, Marini SG, Nagler W. Spinal accessory nerve palsy as a cause of pain after whiplash injury: case report. *J Pain Symptom Manage*. 1998;15(5):321–328.

70. Kizilay A, Kalcioglu MT, Saydam L, Ersoy Y. A new shoulder orthosis for paralysis of the trapezius muscle after radical neck dissection: a preliminary report. *Eur Arch Otorhinolaryngol*. 2006;263(5):477–480.

71. Cipriani D, Abel B, Pirrwitz D. A comparison of two stretching protocols on hip range of motion: implications for total daily stretch duration. *J Strength Cond Res*. 2003;17(2):274–278.

72. Thomas E, Bianco A, Paoli A, Palma A. The relation between stretching typology and stretching duration: the effects on range of motion. *Int J Sports Med*. 2018;39(4):243–254.

73. Almeida KAM, Rocha AP, Carvas N, Pinto A. Rehabilitation interventions for shoulder dysfunction in patients with head and neck cancer: systematic review and meta-analysis. *Phys Ther*. 2020;100(11):1997–2008.

74. Chen YH, Lin CR, Liang WA, Huang CY. Motor control integrated into muscle strengthening exercises has more effects on scapular muscle activities and joint range of motion before initiation of radiotherapy in oral cancer survivors with neck dissection: a randomized controlled trial. *PLoS One*. 2020;15(8):e0237133.

75. Staker JL, Evans AJ, Jacobs LE, et al. The effect of tactile and verbal guidance during scapulothoracic exercises: an EMG and kinematic investigation. *J Electromyogr Kinesiol*. 2019:102334. doi:10.1016/j.jelekin.2019.07.004.

76. Do JH, Yoon IJ, Cho YK, Ahn JS, Kim JK, Jeon J. Comparison of hospital based and home based exercise on quality of life, and neck and shoulder function in patients with spinal accessary nerve injury after head and neck cancer surgery. *Oral Oncol*. 2018;86:100–104.

77. McGarvey AC, Hoffman GR, Osmotherly PG, Chiarelli PE. Maximizing shoulder function after accessory nerve injury and neck dissection surgery: a multicenter randomized controlled trial. *Head Neck*. 2015;37(7):1022–1031.

78. McNeely ML, Parliament M, Courneya KS, et al. A pilot study of a randomized controlled trial to evaluate the effects of progressive resistance exercise training on shoulder dysfunction caused by spinal accessory neurapraxia/neurectomy in head and neck cancer survivors. *Head Neck*. 2004;26(6):518–530.

79. McNeely ML, Parliament MB, Seikaly H, et al. Effect of exercise on upper extremity pain and dysfunction in head and neck cancer survivors: a randomized controlled trial. *Cancer*. 2008;113(1):214–222.

80. McNeely ML, Parliament MB, Seikaly H, et al. Sustainability of outcomes after a randomized crossover trial of resistance exercise for shoulder dysfunction in survivors of head and neck cancer. *Physiother Can*. 2015;67(1):85–93.

81. Lanisnik B, Zitnik L, Levart P, Zargi M, Rodi Z. The impact on postoperative shoulder function of intraoperative nerve monitoring of

cranial nerve XI during modified radical neck dissection. *Eur Arch Otorhinolaryngol.* 2016;273(12):4445–4451.

82. Orhan KS, Demirel T, Baslo B, et al. Spinal accessory nerve function after neck dissections. *J Laryngol Otol.* 2007;121(1):44–48.

83. Nilsen ML, Lyu L, Belsky MA, et al. Impact of neck disability on health-related quality of life among head and neck cancer survivors. *Otolaryngol Head Neck Surg.* 2020;162(1):64–72.

84. Gane EM, O'Leary SP, Hatton AL, Panizza BJ, McPhail SM. Neck and upper Limb dysfunction in patients following neck dissection: looking beyond the shoulder. *Otolaryngol Head Neck Surg.* 2017;157(4):631–640.

85. Finnerup NB, Haroutounian S, Kamerman P, et al. Neuropathic pain: an updated grading system for research and clinical practice. *Pain.* 2016;157(8):1599–1606.

86. Cardoso LR, Rizzo CC, de Oliveira CZ, dos Santos CR, Carvalho AL. Myofascial pain syndrome after head and neck cancer treatment: prevalence, risk factors, and influence on quality of life. *Head Neck.* 2015;37(12):1733–1737.

87. Kerry R, Taylor AJ. Cervical arterial dysfunction: knowledge and reasoning for manual physical therapists. *J Orthop Sports Phys Ther.* 2009;39(5):378–387.

88. Manzoor NF, Russell JO, Bricker A, et al. Impact of surgical resection on survival in patients with advanced head and neck cancer involving the carotid artery. *JAMA Otolaryngol Head Neck Surg.* 2013;139(11):1219–1225.

89. Ghiam MK, Mannion K, Dietrich MS, Stevens KL, Gilbert J, Murphy BA. Assessment of musculoskeletal impairment in head and neck cancer patients. *Support Care Cancer.* 2017;25(7):2085–2092.

90. van Wilgen CP, Dijkstra PU, van der Laan BF, Plukker JT, Roodenburg JL. Morbidity of the neck after head and neck cancer therapy. *Head Neck.* 2004;26(9):785–791.

91. Gane EM, McPhail SM, Hatton AL, Panizza BJ, O'Leary SP. Neck and shoulder motor function following neck dissection: a comparison with healthy control subjects. *Otolaryngol Head Neck Surg.* 2019;160(6):1009–1018.

92. Baldoman D, Vandenbrink R. Physical therapy challenges in head and neck cancer. *Cancer Treat Res.* 2018;174:209–223.

93. Riekki R, Parikka M, Jukkola A, Salo T, Risteli J, Oikarinen A. Increased expression of collagen types I and III in human skin as a consequence of radiotherapy. *Arch Dermatol Res.* 2002;294(4):178–184.

94. Chin CJ, Franklin JH, Turner B, et al. A novel tool for the objective measurement of neck fibrosis: validation in clinical practice. *J Otolaryngol Head Neck Surg.* 2012;41(5):320–326.

95. DiFrancesco T, Khanna A, Stubblefield MD. Clinical evaluation and management of cancer survivors with radiation fibrosis syndrome. *Semin Oncol Nurs.* 2020;36(1):150982. doi:10.1016/j.soncn.2019.150982.

96. Stubblefield MD. Radiation fibrosis syndrome: neuromuscular and musculoskeletal complications in cancer survivors. *PM R.* 2011;3(11):1041–1054.

97. Deng J, Wulff-Burchfield EM, Murphy BA. Late Soft tissue complications of head and neck cancer therapy: lymphedema and fibrosis. *J Natl Cancer Inst Monogr.* 2019;2019(53). doi:10.1093/jncimonographs/lgz005.

98. Deng J, Murphy BA, Dietrich MS, et al. Impact of secondary lymphedema after head and neck cancer treatment on symptoms, functional status, and quality of life. *Head Neck.* 2013;35(7):1026–1035.

99. Seidel C, Kuhnt T, Kortmann RD, Hering K. Radiation-induced camptocormia and dropped head syndrome: review and case report of radiation-induced movement disorders. *Strahlenther Onkol.* 2015;191(10):765–770.

100. Inaba K, Nakamura S, Okamoto H, et al. Early-onset dropped head syndrome after radiotherapy for head and neck cancer: dose constraints for neck extensor muscles. *J Radiat Res.* 2016;57(2):169–173.

101. Waxenbaum JA, Reddy V, Bordoni B. Anatomy, head and neck, cervical nerves [Updated February 7, 2021]*StatPearls [Internet]:*

StatPearls Publishing; 2021. January. https://www.ncbi.nlm.nih.gov/books/NBK538136/.

102. McClure PW, Michener LA. Staged approach for rehabilitation classification: shoulder disorders (STAR-Shoulder). *Phys Ther.* 2015;95(5):791–800.

103. Llamas-Ramos R, Pecos-Martin D, Gallego-Izquierdo T, et al. Comparison of the short-term outcomes between trigger point dry needling and trigger point manual therapy for the management of chronic mechanical neck pain: a randomized clinical trial. *J Orthop Sports Phys Ther.* 2014;44(11):852–861.

104. Mohamadi M, Piroozi S, Rashidi I, Hosseinifard S. Friction massage versus kinesiotaping for short-term management of latent trigger points in the upper trapezius: a randomized controlled trial. *Chiropr Man Therap.* 2017;25:25. doi:10.1186/s12998-017-0156-9.

105. Banerjee G, Rebanks J, Briggs M, Johnson MI. Kinesiology taping as an adjunct for pain management in cancer? *BMJ Case Rep.* 2016;2016. doi:10.1136/bcr-2016-216439 bcr2016216439.

106. Lim EC, Tay MG. Kinesio taping in musculoskeletal pain and disability that lasts for more than 4 weeks: is it time to peel off the tape and throw it out with the sweat? A systematic review with meta-analysis focused on pain and also methods of tape application. *Br J Sports Med.* 2015;49(24):1558–1566.

107. Dones III VC, Regino JM, Esplana NTS, Rivera IRV, Tomas MKR. The effectiveness of biomechanical taping and Kinesiotaping on shoulder pain, active range of motion and function of participants with Trapezius Myalgia: a randomized controlled trial. *J Bodyw Mov Ther.* 2020;24(3):273–281.

108. Ghozy S, Dung NM, Morra ME, et al. Efficacy of kinesio taping in treatment of shoulder pain and disability: a systematic review and meta-analysis of randomised controlled trials. *Physiotherapy.* 2020;107:176–188.

109. Suvarnnato T, Puntumetakul R, Uthaikhup S, Boucaut R. Effect of specific deep cervical muscle exercises on functional disability, pain intensity, craniovertebral angle, and neck-muscle strength in chronic mechanical neck pain: a randomized controlled trial. *J Pain Res.* 2019;12:915–925.

110. Tsiringakis G, Dimitriadis Z, Triantafylloy E, McLean S. Motor control training of deep neck flexors with pressure biofeedback improves pain and disability in patients with neck pain: a systematic review and meta-analysis. *Musculoskelet Sci Pract.* 2020;50:102220. doi:10.1016/j.msksp.2020.102220.

111. Chung S, Jeong YG. Effects of the craniocervical flexion and isometric neck exercise compared in patients with chronic neck pain: a randomized controlled trial. *Physiother Theory Pract.* 2018;34(12):916–925.

112. Schomacher J, Petzke F, Falla D. Localised resistance selectively activates the semispinalis cervicis muscle in patients with neck pain. *Man Ther.* 2012;17(6):544–548.

113. Blanpied PR, Gross AR, Elliott JM, et al. Neck pain: revision 2017. *J Orthop Sports Phys Ther.* 2017;47(7):A1–A83.

114. Jull GA, Falla D, Vicenzino B, Hodges PW. The effect of therapeutic exercise on activation of the deep cervical flexor muscles in people with chronic neck pain. *Man Ther.* 2009;14(6):696–701.

115. Daher A, Carel RS, Tzipi K, Esther H, Dar G. The effectiveness of an aerobic exercise training on patients with neck pain during a short- and long-term follow-up: a prospective double-blind randomized controlled trial. *Clin Rehabil.* 2020;34(5):617–629.

116. Dedering A, Peolsson A, Cleland JA, Halvorsen M, Svensson MA, Kierkegaard M. The effects of neck-specific training versus prescribed physical activity on pain and disability in patients with cervical radiculopathy: a randomized controlled trial. *Arch Phys Med Rehabil.* 2018;99(12):2447–2456.

117. Chimenti RL, Frey-Law LA, Sluka KA. A mechanism-based approach to physical therapist management of pain. *Phys Ther.* 2018;98(5):302–314.

118. Kim A, Stubblefield MD. The role of the headmaster collar (cervical) for dropped head syndrome in Hodgkin lymphoma survivors. *PM R.* 2019;11(9):939–943.

119. Rapidis AD, Dijkstra PU, Roodenburg JL, et al. Trismus in patients with head and neck cancer: etiopathogenesis, diagnosis and management. *Clin Otolaryngol.* 2015;40(6):516–526.

120. van der Geer SJ, van Rijn PV, Roodenburg JLN, Dijkstra PU. Prognostic factors associated with a restricted mouth opening (trismus) in patients with head and neck cancer: systematic review. *Head Neck.* 2020;42(9):2696–2721.

121. Kraaijenga SA, Hamming-Vrieze O, Verheijen S, et al. Radiation dose to the masseter and medial pterygoid muscle in relation to trismus after chemoradiotherapy for advanced head and neck cancer. *Head Neck.* 2019;41(5):1387–1394.

122. Morimoto M, Bijl HP, VDS A, et al. Development of normal tissue complication probability model for trismus in head and neck cancer patients treated with radiotherapy: the role of dosimetric and clinical factors. *Anticancer Res.* 2019;39(12):6787–6798.

123. van der Geer SJ, Kamstra JI, Roodenburg JL, et al. Predictors for trismus in patients receiving radiotherapy. *Acta Oncol.* 2016;55(11):1318–1323.

124. van der Geer SJ, van Rijn PV, Kamstra JI, et al. Prevalence and prediction of trismus in patients with head and neck cancer: a cross-sectional study. *Head Neck.* 2019;41(1):64–71.

125. van der Geer SJ, van Rijn PV, Kamstra JI, Roodenburg JLN, Dijkstra PU. Criterion for trismus in head and neck cancer patients: a verification study. *Support Care Cancer.* 2019;27(3):1129–1137.

126. Thor M, Olsson CE, Oh JH, et al. Temporal patterns of patient-reported trismus and associated mouth-opening distances in radiotherapy for head and neck cancer: a prospective cohort study. *Clin Otolaryngol.* 2018;43(1):22–30.

127. Hartl DM, Cohen M, Julieron M, Marandas P, Janot F, Bourhis J. Botulinum toxin for radiation-induced facial pain and trismus. *Otolaryngol Head Neck Surg.* 2008;138(4):459–463.

128. Ortiz-Comino L, Fernandez-Lao C, Castro-Martin E, et al. Myofascial pain, widespread pressure hypersensitivity, and hyperalgesia in the face, neck, and shoulder regions, in survivors of head and neck cancer. *Support Care Cancer.* 2020;28(6):2891–2898.

129. Laccourreye O, Werner A, Garcia D, Malinvaud D, Tran Ba Huy P, Bonfils P. First bite syndrome. *Eur Ann Otorhinolaryngol Head Neck Dis.* 2013;130(5):269–273.

130. Kuhnt T, Stang A, Wienke A, Vordermark D, Schweyen R, Hey J. Potential risk factors for jaw osteoradionecrosis after radiotherapy for head and neck cancer. *Radiat Oncol.* 2016;11:101.

131. Kamstra JI, van Leeuwen M, Roodenburg JL, Dijkstra PU. Exercise therapy for trismus secondary to head and neck cancer: a systematic review. *Head Neck.* 2017;39(1):160–169.

132. Shao CH, Chiang CC, Huang TW. Exercise therapy for cancer treatment-induced trismus in patients with head and neck cancer: a systematic review and meta-analysis of randomized controlled trials. *Radiother Oncol.* 2020;151:249–255.

133. Stubblefield MD, Manfield L, Riedel ER. A preliminary report on the efficacy of a dynamic jaw opening device (dynasplint trismus system) as part of the multimodal treatment of trismus in patients with head and neck cancer. *Arch Phys Med Rehabil.* 2010;91(8):1278–1282.

134. Kamstra JI, Reintsema H, Roodenburg JL, Dijkstra PU. Dynasplint Trismus System exercises for trismus secondary to head and neck cancer: a prospective explorative study. *Support Care Cancer.* 2016;24(8):3315–3323.

135. Lee R, Molassiotis A, Rogers SN, Edwards RT, Ryder D, Slevin N. Protocol for the trismus trial-therabite versus wooden spatula in the amelioration of trismus in patients with head and neck cancer: randomised pilot study. *BMJ Open.* 2018;8(3):e021938. doi:10.1136/bmjopen-2018-021938.

136. Lee R, Yeo ST, Rogers SN, et al. Randomised feasibility study to compare the use of Therabite with wooden spatulas to relieve and prevent trismus in patients with cancer of the head and neck. *Br J Oral Maxillofac Surg.* 2018;56(4):283–291.

137. Marunick MT, Garcia-Gazaui S, Hildebrand JM. Mandibular pathological fracture during treatment with a dynamic mouth opening device: a clinical report. *J Prosthet Dent.* 2016;116(4):488–491.

138. van der Geer SJ, Reintsema H, Kamstra JI, Roodenburg JLN, Dijkstra PU. The use of stretching devices for treatment of trismus in head and neck cancer patients: a randomized controlled trial. *Support Care Cancer.* 2020;28(1):9–11.

139. Wang TJ, Su JH, Leung KW, Liang SY, Wu SF, Wang HM. Effects of a mouth-opening intervention with remote support on adherence, the maximum interincisal opening, and mandibular function of postoperative oral cancer patients: a randomized clinical trial. *Eur J Oncol Nurs.* 2019;40:111–119.

140. Deng J, Ridner SH, Dietrich MS, et al. Prevalence of secondary lymphedema in patients with head and neck cancer. *J Pain Symptom Manage.* 2012;43(2):244–252.

141. Deng J, Ridner SH, Dietrich MS, et al. Factors associated with external and internal lymphedema in patients with head-and-neck cancer. *Int J Radiat Oncol Biol Phys.* 2012;84(3):e319–e328.

142. Deng J, Murphy BA, Dietrich MS, Sinard RJ, Mannion K, Ridner SH. Differences of symptoms in head and neck cancer patients with and without lymphedema. *Support Care Cancer.* 2016;24(3):1305–1316.

143. Deng J, Ridner SH, Murphy BA, Dietrich MS. Preliminary development of a lymphedema symptom assessment scale for patients with head and neck cancer. *Support Care Cancer.* 2012;20(8):1911–1918.

144. Deng J, Ridner S, Rothman R, et al. Perceived symptom experience in head and neck cancer patients with lymphedema. *J Palliat Med.* 2016;19(12):1267–1274.

145. Jackson LK, Ridner SH, Deng J, et al. Internal lymphedema correlates with subjective and objective measures of dysphagia in head and neck cancer patients. *J Palliat Med.* 2016;19(9):949–956.

146. Azizi AH, Shafi I, Shah N, et al. Superior vena cava syndrome. *JACC Cardiovasc Interv.* 2020;13(24):2896–2910.

147. Zuther JE, Norton S. *Lymphedema Management: The Comprehensive Guide for Practioners.* Thieme Medical Publishers; 2013.

148. Doersam JK, Dietrich MS, Adair MA, Rhoten B, Deng J, Ridner SH. A comparison of symptoms among patients with head and neck or truncal lymphedema and normal controls. *Lymphat Res Biol.* 2019;17(6):661–670.

149. Chotipanich A, Kongpit N. Precision and reliability of tape measurements in the assessment of head and neck lymphedema. *PLoS One.* 2020;15(5):e0233395. doi:10.1371/journal.pone.0233395.

150. Purcell A, Nixon J, Fleming J, McCann A, Porceddu S. Measuring head and neck lymphedema: the "ALOHA" trial. *Head Neck.* 2016;38(1):79–84.

151. Pigott A, Nixon J, Fleming J, Porceddu S. Head and neck lymphedema management: evaluation of a therapy program. *Head Neck.* 2018;40(6):1131–1137.

152. Deng J, Dietrich MS, Niermann KJ, et al. Refinement and validation of the head and neck lymphedema and fibrosis symptom inventory. *Int J Radiat Oncol Biol Phys.* 2021;109(3):747–755.

153. Tyker A, Franco J, Massa ST, Desai SC, Walen SG. Treatment for lymphedema following head and neck cancer therapy: a systematic review. *Am J Otolaryngol.* 2019;40(5):761–769.

20

Bone and Soft Tissue Sarcomas

TAIRE M. THIE, PT, DPT

CHAPTER OUTLINE

Introduction

Sarcomas are relatively rare cancers that form in the body's connective tissue. Sarcomas typically occur in mesenchymal cells that create the muscles, bones, ligaments, tendons, fascia, adipose tissue, nerve sheaths, as well as blood and lymphatic vessels. Sarcomas can originate in the tissues or develop as an adverse effect from previous chemotherapy or radiation therapy treatments (e.g., second primary cancers).[1–4] Tables 20.1 and 20.2 summarize the most prevalent types of sarcoma by patient population and locations in the body.

TABLE 20.1	Most Common Types of Sarcoma by Age[5]	
Age	**Most Common Types of Sarcoma**	
Pediatrics	Osteosarcoma, rhabdomyosarcoma	
Adolescents/young adults	Ewing sarcoma, malignant peripheral sheath tumor (MPST), osteosarcoma, synovial sarcoma, undifferentiated round cell sarcoma	
Adults	Leiomyosarcoma, liposarcoma, undifferentiated high-grade sarcoma, Kaposi's sarcoma	
Geriatric adults	Chondrosarcoma, liposarcoma, myxofibrosarcoma	

Created by Taire M. Thie, DPT. Printed with permission.

TABLE 20.2	Most Common Types of Sarcoma by Location/Region in the Body[6]	
Region	**Most Common Types of Sarcoma**	
Head, neck, and throat	Angiosarcoma, fibrosarcoma, malignant peripheral sheath tumor (MPST), liposarcoma, osteosarcoma, rhabdomyosarcoma, and undifferentiated pleomorphic sarcoma (also called malignant fibrous histiocytoma)[7,8]	
Cardiac tumors	Angiosarcoma, fibrosarcoma, leiomyosarcoma, liposarcoma, myxosarcoma, neurofibrosarcoma, osteosarcoma, synovial sarcoma, rhabdomyosarcoma, and undifferentiated pleomorphic sarcoma[9]	
Chest wall and thorax	Angiosarcoma, chondrosarcoma, Ewing sarcoma, fibrosarcoma, osteosarcoma, synovial sarcoma, and undifferentiated sarcoma[10]	
Abdomen and pelvis	Gastrointestinal stromal tumor (GIST), leiomyosarcoma, liposarcoma (well-differentiated and de-differentiated)[11,12]	
Extremities	Fibrosarcoma, leiomyosarcoma, liposarcoma, osteosarcoma, rhabdomyosarcoma, and synovial sarcoma[13]	

Created by Taire M. Thie, DPT. Printed with permission.

Epidemiology

Sarcomas are divided into two main types: bony sarcomas and soft tissue sarcomas.[1–4] In 2020, the National Cancer Institute Surveillance, Epidemiology, and End Results (NCI SEER) studies estimated 13,120 new cases of soft tissue sarcomas and 3600 new cases of bony sarcomas in the United States.[1,14–17] In Europe, NCI SEER estimated 23,574 individuals are diagnosed annually with sarcomas.[18] Over 16 years from 2000 to 2016, they estimated that 80,269 people of all ages were diagnosed with sarcomas.[18]

Bony and Soft Tissue Sarcomas

Bony sarcomas can develop anywhere within the layers of bone, joints, or cartilage. The most common types are osteosarcoma, Ewing sarcoma, and chondrosarcoma. Soft tissue sarcomas can occur anywhere in the body, including in the muscles, tendons, ligaments, organs, blood vessels, nerves, and lymphatic pathways. There are over 50 different subtypes of soft tissue sarcomas, and not all are covered in this chapter.[5,7,15,19,20] These tumors can impair blood flow, affect nerve conduction rates, and cause blockages of the lymphatic pathways. They can also metabolize and cause erosion of muscles, tendons, and ligaments, resulting in permanent damage and dysfunction. Most soft tissue sarcomas grow locally; however, they frequently spread to the lungs, liver, bones, central nervous system, subcutaneous tissue, and lymph nodes if metastasized.[21] Distant metastases occur in approximately 25% to 30% of persons living with and beyond cancer (PLWBCs) at diagnosis or during follow-up. Certain sarcomas in the head and neck, such as angiosarcoma, clear-cell sarcoma, rhabdomyosarcoma, epithelioid sarcoma, and synovial sarcoma, are most likely to metastasize to the lymph nodes.[7] Because of this, PLWBCs require yearly chest imaging for their entire lifespan to monitor any future recurrence.[7]

Signs and Symptoms of Bony Sarcomas

Bone sarcomas may present with unusual pain or swelling in the PLWBC's extremities, chest, back, or pelvis.[22–27] The PLWBC could develop a fever with an unknown origin, experience a broken bone not related to trauma, or report feeling an unrelenting, constant pain that does not ease with changes in position.[22–27] Some PLWBCs report difficulty sleeping due to the pain, deep and heavy fatigue, and joint pain that is mistaken for osteoarthritis. Chondrosarcomas can cause bowel and bladder issues if found in the pelvis, or they can imitate rotator cuff syndrome if found in the shoulder region.[28] Lower extremity bone sarcomas may cause the PLWBC to experience difficulty with walking, balance, weakness, and muscle atrophy.[28,30–33] These symptoms can cause many different functional deficits and compensation patterns. Table 20.3 provides a summary of the most common bony sarcomas.

Osteosarcomas

Osteosarcomas are usually diagnosed in children and young adults, generally affect the metaphyseal joints in the body's long bones, and are more common in males. In primary osteosarcomas, the osteoblasts are affected, resulting in poor reconstruction or mineralization of the bones—this can lead to brittle bones, loss of structural integrity, pain, necrosis, or fractures.[25,29–31] The 5-year survival rate from birth to age 14 is 69%, and from ages 15 to 19 is 67%.[14] PLWBCs will most likely undergo surgery for bone resection, limb-sparing, possible amputation, or rotationplasty. Surgery is usually followed by chemotherapy and sometimes radiation. The most common chemotherapy infusions prescribed for the treatment of osteosarcomas are doxorubicin (Adriamycin), cisplatin (Platinol, Platinol-AQ), methotrexate (Otrexup, Rasuvo, Rheumatrex, Trexall), and ifosfamide (Ifex).[32,33]

Ewing Sarcoma

Ewing sarcoma is the second most common type of bone cancer and primarily occurs in pediatric and adolescent populations. It is a highly aggressive form of cancer that metastasizes quickly. Ewing sarcoma usually develops in the pelvis, tibia, femur, and ribs, and it may have a soft tissue component affecting the thorax, pleural spaces, gluteal muscles, and cervical muscles. Gene mutations alter the DNA of the bone cells and change

TABLE 20.3   Most Common Types of Bony Sarcomas

Sarcoma	Presentation	Medical Interventions and Prognosis
Osteosarcoma	• Primary osteosarcomas affect osteoblasts, resulting in poor reconstruction or mineralization of the bones—this can lead to brittle bones, loss of structural integrity, pain, necrosis, or fractures.[25,29–31] • Usually diagnosed in children and young adults. • Typically affect the metaphyseal joints in the long bones of the body. • More common in males.	• Surgery including bone resection, limb-sparing, possible amputation, or rotationplasty. • Chemotherapy infusions of doxorubicin, cisplatin, methotrexate, and ifosfamide.[32,33] Five-year survival rate: • Ages birth to 14: 69%.[14] • Ages 15–19: 67%.[14]
Ewing's Sarcoma	• Usually develops in the pelvis, tibia, femur, and ribs and may have a soft tissue component affecting the thorax, pleural spaces, gluteal muscles, and cervical muscles. • Gene mutations alter the DNA of the bone cells and change the structural blueprint of the bone.[29,34,35] • It is the second most common type of bone cancer and primarily occurs in pediatric and adolescent populations. • It is highly aggressive/can metastasize quickly.	• A combination of chemotherapy, surgery, and radiation.[36,24] • Chemotherapy infusions of doxorubicin, vincristine, dactinomycin, cyclophosphamide, ifosfamide, and etoposide.[32,33] Five-year survival rate: • Ages birth to 14: 76%.[14] • Ages 15–19: 58%.[14] • If evidence of metastasis or relapse exists, then the rate decreases to 30%.[30]
Chondrosarcoma	• Caused by cell mutations of the connective tissue that makes up cartilage. • Mainly occur in the metaphyses of the long bones or deep in the bone in the medullary cavities. • Typically occurs in the femur, tibia, humerus, scapula, pelvis, and rib cage. • May show endosteal scalloping and lead to osteolysis.[28] • Most commonly occurs in older men ages 60–80 years.	• Very resistant to radiation and chemotherapy, but surgical amputation with chemotherapy is the most common treatment option at this time. • Immunotherapy, gene therapy, and adjuvant treatment options are newer treatment options. Five-year survival rate: • 75.2% as long as it is a primary tumor, low grade, below 10 cm in size, and surgically resected.[37]

Created by Taire M. Thie, DPT. Printed with permission.

the structural blueprint of the bone.[29,34,35] In 2020, the 5-year survival rate for ages birth to 14 was 76% and from ages 15 to 19 was 58%.[14] If there is evidence of metastasis or relapse, then the 5-year survival rate decreases to 30%.[36] Ewing sarcoma must be treated with a combination of chemotherapy, surgery, and radiation.[36,24] The most common chemotherapy infusions prescribed for the treatment of Ewing sarcoma are doxorubicin, vincristine (Oncovin, Vincasar PFS), dactinomycin (Cosmegen), cyclophosphamide (Cytoxan), ifosfamide, and etoposide (Toposar, VePesid).[32,33]

Chondrosarcoma

Chondrosarcomas develop in the cartilage. There is some indication that gene mutations may cause them, but this is not conclusive. Chondrosarcomas can develop anywhere cartilage is present in the body but mainly occur in the metaphyses of the long bones or deep in the bone in the medullary cavities. This type of sarcoma typically occurs in the femur, tibia, humerus, scapula, pelvis, and rib cage. Endosteal scalloping may be present and can lead to osteolysis.[28] They most commonly occur in older men ages 60 to 80 years. Chondrosarcomas are very resistant to radiation and chemotherapy; however, surgical amputation with chemotherapy is the most common treatment option at the time of this publication. Advances in immunotherapy, gene therapy, and adjuvant treatment options show promise in the treatment of chondrosarcomas and will be discussed later in this chapter. The 5-year survival prognosis is 75.2% as long as it is a primary tumor, low grade, below 10 cm in size, and surgically resected.[37]

Soft Tissue Sarcomas

There are over 50 different subtypes of soft tissue sarcomas, and not all are covered in this chapter.[5,7,15,19,20] The most frequently discussed and researched sarcomas will be covered in this section.

Signs and Symptoms of Soft Tissue Sarcomas

Soft tissue sarcomas may present as uncomfortable lumps under the skin which grow larger but are not moveable.[22–27] PLWBCs may also report joint pain, muscle spasms, or weakness.[22–27] Symptoms of a sarcoma around the heart may include signs of intracardiac obstruction, systemic embolization, or malaise. More severe complications, including stroke, myocardial infarction, and even sudden death from arrhythmia, could also be the first signs of a soft tissue sarcoma involving the heart.[9] Signs of retroperitoneal, gastrointestinal (GI), mesenteric, or pelvic organ sarcoma may include constipation, feelings of fullness, decreased appetite, anemia, abdominal pain, nausea, difficulty swallowing, or vomiting.[27] Soft tissue sarcomas can also cause edema in the abdomen, chest, and extremities. The signs and symptoms of rhabdomyosarcoma vary greatly based on the location of the tumor. If the tumor is in the head or neck region, then the PLWBC might experience headaches, nose bleeds, or bulging eyes. Tumors present in the bladder or pelvis may cause incontinence, constipation, or blood in the urine. Rhabdomyosarcomas in the extremities may cause a painful bump under the skin. With any of these cancers, PLWBCs may experience heaviness in their pelvis, significant bleeding, nausea, sudden weight loss, prolapse, incontinence, a palpable mass, and abdominal pain.[38–41] Table 20.4 summarizes the most common soft tissue sarcomas.

TABLE 20.4   More Common Types of Soft Tissue Sarcomas

Sarcoma	Presentation	Medical Interventions and Prognosis
Angiosarcoma (Note: additional information on angiosarcomas is available in Chapter 10 Cardiovascular and Pulmonary Systems)	• One of the most common cancers found in the chest. • Aggressive sarcoma that develops and grows in the lymph or blood vessels, most often in the skin, breasts, heart, liver, and spleen.[42,43] • Reduces available space in the thorax, cause breathing restrictions and pain under or behind the ribs. • PLWBC often report a bruise that will not heal, a lesion that grows over time, edema, or an open wound that will not heal if it is bumped or scratched.[42,43] • It can present at any age but most often occurs in PLWBCs around age 70.	• Difficult to treat because of the extensive vascular, lymphatic, and nervous tissue involvement. • Surgery • Chemotherapy • Radiation can be administered before surgery to help reduce the size of the tumor margins and allow more of the tumor to be resected. • Immunotherapy Five-year survival rate: • Highly dependent on the stage and location of the angiosarcoma.[42,43] • PLWBCs diagnosed with a grade I angiosarcoma in distal blood or lymphatic vessels typically have a very good prognosis—unfortunately, most angiosarcomas are not found until after they have metastasized at a level III and IV.
Fibrosarcoma: adults and pediatrics	• Caused by chromosomal and structural mutations of fibroblasts. • Develop deep in the bone, fascia, muscles, and organs.[44] • Can be very aggressive.[44] • One of the most common forms of sarcoma, according to the SEER statistics.[44] • Frequently develops in the thighs and back of the knees but can occur in the head and neck. • Typically diagnosed in children from birth up to age four or in middle-aged adults between ages 35 and 50. • Slightly more common in men.	• Surgery and reconstruction for structural defects • Radiation • Resistant to most of the normal chemotherapy agents used to treat sarcomas. • Chemotherapy infusions that include doxorubicin, actinomycin D, mesna, ifosfamide, and dacarbazine may provide some benefit.[44] • Children receive several cycles of doxorubicin and ifosfamide to destroy cancer cells.[45] • Ongoing investigations for treatments to inhibit the growth of fibroblasts and mutations by injecting tissue inhibitors of metalloproteinases (TIMP-1-GPI) directly into the tumor.[44] Five-year survival rate: For children[45,46]: • 50% if there is bone involvement. • 80% if the tumor is limited to the soft tissues. For adults: • 55%–65% if the lesion has bone involvement, is in a common location, and is a primary cancer. • 60% if the tumor does not meet any of those three criteria.[46]
Gastrointestinal Stromal Tumor (GIST): adults and pediatrics	• A solid tumor that grows from the smooth muscle of the gastrointestinal tract.[12,18,47–50] • More common in adolescents and older females ages 50–70.[47,50] • Caused by a number of gene mutations.[48] • A mix of epithelial and mesenchymal abnormalities.[48] • PLWBCs might report feelings of nausea, lack of appetite, pain, symptoms of gastroesophageal reflux, or weight loss.[48] • PLWBCs may have evidence of an upper or lower GI bleed, bowel blockages, or anemia due to intestinal bleeding. • Can grow anywhere along the length of the digestive tract but are more common in the stomach and small intestine. • Can metastasize to the prostate, liver, and other areas of the abdomen. • Most GIST sarcomas have KIT gene mutations (the KIT gene is in charge of protein-coding for a receptor called the tyrosine kinase protein, which stimulates stem cells to grow). • GIST KIT gene mutations produce an enzyme that causes the cancer cells to grow and metastasize quickly.[48]	• Treatment options and prognosis vary due to the variety of locations along the digestive tract where the tumor can present. • Surgery must be performed very carefully since this type of tumor can rupture, which can cause spread and growth of new tumors throughout the peritoneum. • PLWBCs are prescribed 3 years of imatinib to inhibit the extracellular growth due to the high risk of relapse.[48] • Radiation is used intermittently depending on the location of the tumor.[49] Five-year survival rate: • 90% with proper management.[47]

(Continued)

TABLE
20.4 **More Common Types of Soft Tissue Sarcomas—cont'd**

Sarcoma	Presentation	Medical Interventions and Prognosis
Liposarcoma	• There are four subtypes of liposarcoma: well-differentiated; de-differentiated; pleomorphic; and myxoid.[46] • Develop in adipose tissue. • Most commonly presents in the thighs, back of the knees, and abdomen. • Usually occurs in middle-aged and older adults ages 50–65.[51–53] • De-differentiated and pleomorphic both have a poor prognosis and usually metastasize. • Myxoid are more common in children. • Myxoid appear most of the time in the mediastinum, retroperitoneum, and bone marrow.[53]	• Surgery • Pre- and/or postoperative radiation therapy. • Chemotherapy infusions of anthracyclines, specifically doxorubicin and gemcitabine. • Brachytherapy with internal radiation can be used to help decrease the size of the tumor or to prevent it from reoccurring.[51,53] Five-year survival rate: • 100% for well-differentiated.[53] • 57.2% for de-differentiated.[53] • 55%–65% for pleomorphic and myxoid.[53]
Malignant Peripheral Nerve Sheath Tumor and Neuro-fibrosarcoma	• High-grade aggressive tumor that grows from Schwann cells, from neurofibromas in the peripheral nervous system, or along the fibers of the nerve sheaths. • Evidence exists that it is related to genetic mutations that also cause neurofibromatosis type 1.[5,54] • Most commonly found in the retroperitoneum, pelvis, head, neck, and extremities.[49] • Metastasizes to the lungs, liver, adrenal glands, brain, lymph, and bone. • Typically occurs in young adults ages 20–35.[49] • Neurological symptoms may present along with the dermatomal/myotomal nerve distribution.	• Surgery • Radiation and chemotherapy can be used both pre- and postoperatively to try to shrink or eliminate the tumor.[49] Five-year survival rate: • 23%–69% depending on the tumor's size and location and on what surrounding structures are involved when it is found and removed.[49]
Rhabdomyosarcoma	• Four sub-types exist: embryonal; alveolar (loose connective tissue); pleomorphic; and spindle cell-sclerosing.[11,55] • The most common soft tissue sarcoma is seen in children. • In adults, usually diagnosed around the age of 50.[11,55,56] • Embryonal can be found in the paratesticular soft tissues, perineum, and retroperitoneal space. • Alveolar, pleomorphic, and spindle cell are typically found in the extremities, head, neck, external genitalia, and posterior abdomen.[11,55] • Spindle cell is the most aggressive form.	• Surgery • Chemotherapy • Radiation • Immunotherapy • Targeted therapy Five-year survival rate: • Ages birth to 14: 71%.[56] • Ages 15–19: 45%.[56]
Uterine Sarcoma	• Most common sub-types: uterine adenosarcoma, endometrial stromal sarcoma, uterine leiomyosarcoma, and undifferentiated uterine sarcoma. • Uterine adenosarcomas grow in the uterine wall and are not usually aggressive. • Endometrial stromal sarcomas grow rapidly and sporadically in the endometrial lining of the uterus. • Uterine leiomyosarcomas grow in the smooth muscle of the uterus and are usually undifferentiated and highly aggressive.[40] • Uterine leiomyosarcomas are most commonly diagnosed around age 40. • Uterine leiomyosarcoma is one of the known adverse effects of taking tamoxifen for breast cancer for extended periods of time.[5] • Undifferentiated uterine sarcomas mutate and grow into the endo- or myometrium, and they are very aggressive, unorganized, and prolific with cellular mutations.	• Surgery • Radiation • Uterine adenosarcoma: chemotherapy including gemcitabine, docetaxel, ifosfamide, cisplatin, and epirubicin.[38] • Endometrial stromal sarcoma: usually requires a hysterectomy and removal of the tumor, followed by hormone therapy or targeted chemotherapy and radiation.[41] • Uterine leiomyosarcoma: chemotherapy including anthracyclines. • Targeted therapy: tyrosine kinase inhibitors with pazopanib and sunitinib. • If a PLWBC is of childbearing age, surgeons and oncologists may select to surgically remove the tumor and follow up with only imaging to ensure no reoccurrence.[40,41] • Undifferentiated uterine sarcomas: surgery, radiation, and targeted chemotherapy may be used, but prognosis remains poor because of its rapid growth.[41] Five-year survival rate: • PLWBCs with endometrial stromal sarcomas have a positive prognosis if tumor is found early; otherwise, it can be very difficult to treat if it is not diagnosed until the later stages. • Uterine leiomyosarcoma: 30%.[40]

Angiosarcoma

Angiosarcoma is one of the most common soft tissue sarcomas found in the chest. It is an aggressive sarcoma that develops and grows in the lymph or blood vessels, most often in the skin, breasts, heart, liver, and spleen.[42,43] This type of tumor reduces available space in the thorax and can cause breathing restrictions and pain under or behind the ribs. The PLWBC will often report having a bruise that will not heal, a lesion that grows over time, edema, or an open wound that will not heal if it is bumped or scratched.[42,43] Angiosarcomas can present at any age but most often occur in patients around age 70. Angiosarcomas are best treated with surgery, chemotherapy, radiation, and immunotherapy. Tumors around the heart or liver are challenging to treat because of the extensive vascular, lymphatic, and nervous tissue. Radiation can be administered before surgery to help reduce the size of the tumor margins and allow more of the tumor to be resected. The 5-year survival rate is highly dependent on the stage and location of the angiosarcoma.[42,43] A person diagnosed with a grade I angiosarcoma in a distal blood or lymphatic vessel typically has an excellent prognosis. Unfortunately, most angiosarcomas are not found until after they have metastasized and are at a grade III and IV. Additional information on angiosarcomas is available in Chapter 10, Cardiovascular and Pulmonary Systems.

Fibrosarcoma: Adults and Pediatrics

Fibrosarcomas are chromosomal and structural mutations of fibroblasts. Fibroblasts are connective tissue cells that create fibers that help support the bones, muscles, and organs. Fibrosarcomas develop deep in the bone, fascia, and soft tissue and can be very aggressive.[44] It is one of the most common forms of sarcoma.[44] It frequently develops in the thighs and back of the knees, but it can also occur in the head and neck. Fibrosarcomas are typically diagnosed in children from birth up to age four or in middle-aged adults between ages 35 and 50 and are slightly more common in men. For children diagnosed with fibrosarcomas, the 5-year survival rate is 50% if there is bone involvement and 80% if the tumor is limited to the soft tissues.[45,46] If the lesion has bone involvement, is in a common location, and is a primary cancer, the adult's 5-year survival rate is 55% to 65%. If the tumor does not meet any of these three criteria, the 5-year survival rate is 40% to 60%.[46] Standard interventions include surgery, chemotherapy, and radiation. Reconstruction may be involved if cancer has caused structural defects to the bone. Fibrosarcomas are resistant to most of the standard chemotherapy agents used to treat sarcomas, but infusions include doxorubicin, dactinomycin (Cosmegen), mesna (Mesnex), ifosfamide, and dacarbazine (DTIC-Dome) may provide some benefit.[44] Children are usually administered several cycles of doxorubicin and ifosfamide to destroy the cancer cells.[45] Genetic engineers are working on medications that inhibit the growth of fibroblasts and mutations by injecting tissue inhibitors of metalloproteinases (TIMP-1-GPI) into the tumor itself.[44] The TIMP-1-GPI injections inhibit local matrix metalloproteinase (MMP) activity, thereby preventing the tumor from growing and making it vulnerable to the chemotherapy.[44]

Gastrointestinal Stromal Tumor: Adults and Pediatrics

Gastrointestinal stromal tumor (GIST) in adults is a solid tumor that grows from the smooth muscle of the gastrointestinal tract.[12,18,47–50] It is more common in adolescents and older female

PLWBCs ages 50 to 70.[47,50] It is caused by some gene mutations and is a mix of epithelial and mesenchymal abnormalities.[48] PLWBCs might report feelings of nausea, lack of appetite, pain, symptoms of gastroesophageal reflux, or weight loss, or may have evidence of an upper or lower GI bleed bowel blockages or anemia due to intestinal bleeding. This type of tumor can grow anywhere along the length of the digestive tract but is more common in the stomach and small intestine. It can metastasize to the prostate, the liver, and other areas of the abdomen outside of the intestines. Treatment options and prognosis vary due to the variety of locations along the digestive tract where the tumor can present. Most GIST sarcomas have KIT gene mutations. The KIT gene is a proto-oncogene that is in charge of protein coding for a tyrosine kinase protein receptor. Tyrosine kinase proteins stimulate stem cells to grow. GIST KIT gene mutations produce an enzyme that causes the cancer cells to grow and metastasize quickly.[48] Surgery must be performed very carefully since this type of tumor can rupture, which can cause the spread and growth of new tumors throughout the peritoneum. PLWBCs are prescribed 3 years of imatinib (Gleevec) to inhibit the extracellular growth due to the high risk of relapse.[48] Radiation is used intermittently depending on the location of the tumor.[49] The 5-year prognosis is 90% with proper management.[47]

Liposarcoma[51–53]

Liposarcoma tumors develop in adipose tissue and can grow anywhere in the body. It is most commonly seen in the thighs, back of the knees, and abdomen. It usually occurs in middle-aged and older adults ages 50 to 65.[51–53] There are several different subtypes of liposarcoma, including well-differentiated, de-differentiated, pleomorphic, and myxoid.[52] Well-differentiated liposarcomas stay local and do generally not metastasize. De-differentiated and pleomorphic liposarcomas both have a poor prognosis and usually metastasize. Myxoid liposarcomas are more common in children and appear most of the time in the mediastinum, retroperitoneum, and bone marrow.[53] The 5-year survival rates for liposarcomas are 100% for well-differentiated, 57.2% for de-differentiated, and 55% to 65% for pleomorphic and myxoid.[53] Surgery is the most common treatment for liposarcomas along with pre- or postoperative radiation therapy and anthracycline-based chemotherapy, specifically doxorubicin and gemcitabine (Gemzar). Evidence suggests that brachytherapy with internal radiation can also help decrease the size of the tumor or prevent it from reoccurring.[51,53]

Malignant Peripheral Nerve Sheath Tumor/Neurofibrosarcoma

Malignant peripheral nerve sheath tumor/neurofibrosarcoma is considered a high-grade aggressive tumor that grows from Schwann cells, from neurofibromas in the peripheral nervous system, or along the fibers of the nerve sheaths. There is evidence that it is related to genetic mutations that also cause neurofibromatosis type 1.[5,54] It can appear anywhere, but it is more common in the retroperitoneum, pelvis, head, neck, and extremities.[49] It metastasizes to the lungs, liver, adrenal glands, brain, lymph, and bone. It typically occurs in young adults ages 20 to 35.[49] There may be neurological symptoms present along with the dermatomal/myotomal nerve distribution. It is treated with surgical resection. The 5-year survival rate is 23% to 69% depending on the tumor's size and location and on what surrounding structures are involved when it is found and removed.[49] Radiation and chemotherapy can be used both pre- and postoperatively to shrink or eliminate the tumor.[49]

Retroperitoneal Sarcoma

The retroperitoneal space is unique because it is behind the posterior parietal peritoneum and the mesenteries. The adrenal glands, kidneys, ureters, abdominal aorta, inferior vena cava, lumbar nerve plexus, sympathetic trunk, sympathetic nerve ganglions, hypogastric nerves, ascending and descending colon, and lymphatic cistern chyli exist in this space.[51] Cancerous tumors in these areas can grow very large before becoming symptomatic. Most of these sarcomas are leiomyosarcomas or liposarcomas but may also be fibrosarcomas or undifferentiated pleomorphic sarcomas.[51] Cancers in this space can be very aggressive because of their location and visceral involvement and can be complicated to surgically remove. PLWBCs may report pain in their back that is not relieved by position changes, fatigue, evidence of a GI bleed (blood in stool), nausea, and vomiting.[51] They may also report symptoms related to compression of visceral organs and the vascular, lymphatic, and nerve systems.[51] It is very important that as much of the tumor as possible is surgically removed because these tumors can be very aggressive and hard to manage medically, as noted under the previous sections on leiomyosarcomas and liposarcomas.

Rhabdomyosarcoma

Rhabdomyosarcoma is the most common soft tissue sarcoma observed in children. In adults, rhabdomyosarcomas are usually diagnosed around the age of 50.[11,55,56] There are four types of rhabdomyosarcomas: embryonal, alveolar (loose connective tissue), pleomorphic, and spindle cell/sclerosing.[11,55] The embryonal rhabdomyosarcoma can be found in the paratesticular soft tissues, perineum, and retroperitoneal space. The alveolar, pleomorphic, and spindle cell rhabdosarcomas are typically found in the extremities, head, neck, external genitalia, and posterior abdomen.[11,55] Spindle cell is the most aggressive form. The signs and symptoms of rhabdomyosarcoma vary greatly based on the tumor's location. If the tumor is in the head or neck region, then the PLWBC might experience headaches, nose bleeds, or bulging eyes. Tumors present in the bladder or pelvis may cause incontinence, constipation, or blood in the urine. Rhabdomyosarcomas in the extremities may cause a painful bump under the skin. The 5-year survival rate for ages birth to 14 is 71% and for ages 15 to 19 is 45%.[56] Treatment options include surgery, chemotherapy, radiation, immunotherapy, and targeted therapy.

Uterine Sarcoma[38–41]

There are several different types of uterine sarcomas. The most common ones are uterine adenosarcoma, endometrial stromal sarcoma, uterine leiomyosarcoma, and undifferentiated uterine sarcoma. PLWBCs might experience heaviness in their pelvis, significant bleeding, nausea, sudden weight loss, prolapse, incontinence, a palpable mass, and abdominal pain with any of these cancers.

Uterine adenosarcomas grow within the uterine wall and are not usually aggressive. Uterine adenosarcomas can be treated with surgery and chemotherapy medications such as gemcitabine (Gemzar), docetaxel (Taxotere), ifosfamide, cisplatin, and epirubicin (Ellence).[38]

Uterine leiomyosarcomas grow within the smooth muscle of the uterus and are usually undifferentiated and highly aggressive.[40] Uterine leiomyosarcomas can occur at any age, but they are most commonly diagnosed around age 40. Uterine leiomyosarcoma patients have a 5-year survival rate of just 30%.[40] This type of sarcoma is one of the

known adverse effects of taking tamoxifen (Nolvadex) for breast cancer for extended periods.[5] The prognosis is dependent on the size and grade of the tumor when it is found and removed. Surgery is the most important intervention, followed by tyrosine kinase inhibitors and pazopanib (Votrient) and sunitinib (Sutent) for targeted therapy. Treatment may also include chemotherapy anthracycline infusions. If the PLWBC is diagnosed with any uterine sarcoma and of childbearing age, in an effort to save fertility, surgeons and oncologists may select to surgically remove the tumor and follow up with only imaging to ensure no reoccurrence.[40,41]

Undifferentiated uterine sarcomas mutate and grow into the endo- or myometrium. This is a very aggressive, unorganized, and very prolific subtype with cellular mutations. Surgery, radiation, and targeted chemotherapy may be used, but prognosis remains poor because of its rapid growth.[41] Endometrial stromal sarcomas grow rapidly and sporadically in the endometrial lining of the uterus. PLWBCs have a positive prognosis if the tumor is found early; otherwise, it can be very difficult to treat if it is not diagnosed until the later stages. A hysterectomy and removal of the tumor is essential, followed by hormone therapy or targeted chemotherapy and radiation.[41]

Etiology and Risk Factors of Soft Tissue and Bony Sarcomas

Each type of sarcoma is unique. Table 20.5 summarizes how the risk factors affect prognosis. Sarcomas can be idiopathic in nature, but in some cases, there are risk factors that are linked to certain types of sarcoma. General risk factors include diagnosis and treatment of other types of cancer; previous exposure to chemotherapy or radiation therapy; a previous history of sarcomas; or lymphedema or chronic lymphatic congestion leading to toxic build-up of lymph fluid.[2,26,57–59] In the case of osteosarcomas, Ewing sarcoma, angiosarcomas, and GIST sarcomas, gene mutations present a specific risk factor.[25,36,43] Exposure to toxins and heavy metals such as arsenic, thorium dioxide, and vinyl chloride are linked specifically to hepatic angiosarcomas.[7,43] Exposure to herbicides containing chlorophenol and phenoxy acids may increase the risk of soft tissue sarcomas.[60] Viral infections associated with the Epstein-Barr virus or HIV have been linked to leiomyosarcomas and Kaposi's sarcomas.[45] Use of tamoxifen has been linked to the development of uterine sarcomas.[5]

TABLE 20.5	**Prognosis Based on Risk Factors**	
Factors for Prognosis[15,22]	Better Prognosis	Worse Prognosis
Age of the patient	Less than 60 years of age	Over 60 years of age
Size of the tumor	Less than 5 cm in diameter	Greater than 5 cm in diameter
Grade of the tumor	Low grades	High grades
Margins after resection	Clear margins	Unclear margins
Gene changes	No changes present	Changes present
Lactase dehydrogenase detected	Not detected or low	High

Created by Taire M. Thie, DPT. Printed with permission.

Clinical Presentation

Diagnostic Imaging

Diagnostic testing begins with comprehensive imaging in the form of X-rays, bone scans, computed tomography (CT) scans, positron emission tomography (PET) scans, and magnetic resonance imaging (MRI), which allows oncologists and surgeons to determine the size, location, depth of the sarcoma and identifies metastases.[22,45,55] Biopsies of the bone marrow, bone, and soft tissue help determine the type, grade, and stage of the tumor. Blood tests such as complete blood count and blood chemistry panel can help identify a lactate dehydrogenase chemical, which further determines the grade and level of sarcoma.[22,45,55] Echocardiograms and angiograms are considered to be essential diagnostic tools for diagnosing cardiac sarcomas.[9] Routine pelvic floor lab testing and pelvic floor ultrasounds can assist in detecting uterine sarcomas.[61]

Staging, Grading, and Prognosis

Cancer staging and grading determine prognosis, treatment options, and course of therapy that the PLWBC will need. Grading and staging can be different depending on where the sarcoma is located. Several different staging systems take into consideration the tumor's location, size, depth (based on location), histological grade, and metastasis.[62,63] See Table 20.6 for staging based on tumor size. For more information, please refer to Chapter 5 regarding medical management.

Histological grading is the science of determining the aggressive nature of the tumor. Low-grade sarcoma cells resemble the cells of the tissue they derive from. These sarcomas are often less invasive, grow slower, and are easier to resect surgically. High-grade

sarcomas are considered to have numerous cell mutations, metastasize faster, and are deemed more aggressive.[64] Tumor cells that present in an orderly and structured manner are considered to be well-differentiated; conversely, tumor cells that appear chaotic and malformed are considered to be undifferentiated. There are four levels of grading based on order and structure: grade I is well-differentiated and defined; grade II is moderately differentiated; grade III is poorly differentiated, and grade IV is undifferentiated. Grades III and IV are considered to be high levels.[64]

Epidemiology studies have concluded that undifferentiated pleomorphic sarcomas, osteosarcomas, rhabdomyosarcomas, angiosarcomas, synovial sarcomas, and Ewing sarcomas are all considered high-grade tumors. The grade of chondrosarcomas, fibrosarcomas, liposarcomas, leiomyosarcomas, and neurogenic sarcomas depends on the tumor's location, size, and metastases.[7]

Medical Management for Sarcomas

Chemotherapy

Chemotherapy is used to stop reproduction and protein synthesis of the sarcoma, alert the immune system, and get toxins to penetrate into the cancerous cell without harming surrounding healthy cells.[45,65] Neoadjuvant chemotherapy for sarcomas can be used to help shrink tumors in the extremities before surgical resection, with the goal of avoiding amputations.[32] The possible adverse effects of chemotherapies used for the treatment of sarcomas can be found in Table 20.7. Chapters 5 and 6 provide in-depth discussions of the different chemotherapy and radiation therapy types available.

Radiation Therapy for Sarcomas

Preoperative and postoperative radiation can be used to treat sarcomas with different goals. Preoperative radiation helps shrink the tumor, minimize tissue resection, and spare unaffected tissues of the muscles, limbs, bones, nerves, and vascular and lymphatic structures.[4,66,67] Unfortunately, radiation exposure can negatively impact the surgical wound's ability to heal. Postoperative radiation can be used to treat and burn remaining tumors and prevent the sarcoma from reoccurring. Brachytherapy is a type of internal radiation that can be surgically implanted into the tumor to help radiate and destroy it from the inside out.[67,68] The adverse effects in Table 20.8 are crucial to be aware of and must be considered and listed as a precaution for manual therapy techniques and exercise.

TABLE 20.6 Staging and Size of Sarcoma[62,63]

Stages	Size
Stage I	Less than 5 cm
Stage II	5–10 cm
Stage III	10–15 cm
Stage IV	15+ cm

Created by Taire M. Thie, DPT. Printed with permission.

TABLE 20.7 Long-Term Adverse Effects of Chemotherapy[33]

Adverse Effects	Description
Cardiotoxicity/cardiomyopathy	Infusions can impair the heart musculature, specifically of the left ventricle, which is the primary pump for circulation to eject the blood from the heart to the systemic circulatory system. This can lead to heart failure, embolisms, cerebrovascular accidents, congestive heart failure, and myocardial infarction.
Second primary cancers	Chemotherapy agents can cause second primary sarcomas in the spine, breasts, lungs, and abdomen.
Neuropathies	Infusions can cause nerve damage, leading to tingling, numbness, and decreased proprioceptive awareness.
Infertility	Infusions can cause damage to the reproductive cells and make it hard to conceive and carry a child to term.
Cancer related cognitive impairment (CRCI)	Long-term use of chemotherapy agents can result in difficulty with memory, multi-tasking, and motor sequencing.

Created by Taire M. Thie, DPT. Printed with permission.

TABLE
20.8 **Treatment Considerations and Adverse Effects With Radiation[33]**

Nausea	Pain	Skin irritations/burns	Altered breathing mechanics
Neuropathy	Joint stiffness	Discoloration	Second primary cancers/sarcomas
Scar adhesions	Cardiotoxicity	Depth and area of treatment	Neuropathy
Brachial plexopathy	Lymphedema	Radiation pneumonitis	Radiation fibrosis
Altered joint mechanics due to radiation burns/restrictions	Difficulty with wound healing	Positional impairments that occurred while in radiation, not related to the radiation but rather due to the position the patient was in for prolonged periods during radiation therapy	

Created by Taire M. Thie, DPT. Printed with permission.

Adjuvant Treatment Options for Sarcomas

New developments are being made for alternative treatment interventions that can help the patient reduce or avoid the adverse effects of chemotherapy and radiation treatments. More contemporary interventions include hyperthermia, high-intensity focused ultrasound, low-intensity pulsed ultrasound, and photodynamic therapies.[32] All carry their unique disadvantages but are being explored further as treatment options for many different cancers.

Genetic engineers have created advances in immunotherapy and chimeric antigen receptor (CAR)-T cells. Immunotherapy stimulates the PLWBC's innate immune system to attack cancer, and CAR-T cell therapy transfers tumor-specific cytotoxic T-cells to the PLWBC to help their immune system attack the sarcomas.[25] These advances are beginning to show promise in the fight against chondrosarcoma, osteosarcoma, Ewing sarcoma, and sarcomas with possible gene mutations.[25]

When genetic mutations are responsible for the sarcomas, such as the KIT gene mutations or tyrosine kinase protein mutations, a new adjuvant form of treatment utilizes infusions of tyrosine kinase protein inhibitors. Imatinib has shown improved results to chemotherapy or when used in adjunct with chemotherapy. These infusions can help slow the growth of the stem cells and significantly limit tumor growth.[48]

Surgical Interventions

Surgical intervention is the most recommended treatment option for PWLBCs diagnosed with a sarcoma. In the past, amputation was the only available option, but the goal is to salvage as much of the limb as possible to preserve function.[69] Considerations for surgical candidacy include overall health and wellness, comorbidities, lifestyle, age, and previous surgical/medical histories, as well as the tumor's size, location, and type.[51,70,71] Risk factors for any surgical intervention apply, including blood clots, stroke, myocardial infarctions, embolisms, infections, and poor wound healing.

Depending on the size of the tumor, the surgeons and oncologists may elect neoadjuvant radiation or chemotherapy before resection to assist with limb-sparing and the provision of clear margins.[69] The degree of surgical intervention is determined by the stage, size, and grade of the tumor. Liposarcomas, leiomyosarcomas, angiosarcomas, and rhabdomyosarcomas in the abdomen, pelvis, head, and neck can all present as large and deep tumors with poor margins. They may require very extensive and complicated surgical interventions, including removing muscle, organ, bone, nerve, blood vessel, lymph node, and fascia. Complications can arise if the tumor intersects with major nerves or blood vessels.

The surgeon may choose to leave some of the tumor behind to be managed postoperatively with radiation or chemotherapy.[4]

Reconstruction

Uncomplicated surgical interventions may only require a small incision and sarcoma resection, whereas more complex surgeries may require reconstruction with skin grafts, local/regional flaps, or free flaps.[69]

There are many different types of flaps available during the reconstructive process. Bone flaps can be used to repair and fill in bone resections to make the limb functional. Soft tissue flaps can be utilized to close the incisions or over amputations to cushion the end of the residual limb and prepare for a prosthesis and weight-bearing.[72] In some cases, surgeons can restore function to the salvaged or residual limb by moving an entire muscle or muscle group. Several soft tissue flaps can come from different parts of the body. The most common flaps used are pedicle flaps, free flaps, or combining the two.[72] Pedicle flaps, also known as turn-over or rotated flaps, are pieces of adipofascial or fasciocutaneous flaps from the original site pulled over the surgical incision.[73] Free flaps are tissue taken from one part of the body and transplanted to another part of the body. Free flaps involve surgical harvesting of the tissue along with its arteries, veins, and nerves. With all of the different types of flaps, microvascular surgeons carefully create microreanastomoses of blood and lymph vessels to ensure the flaps have proper arterial and vascular profusion and proper lymphatic drainage to improve healing and eliminate waste.[72] It is important to frequently assess the flap and its donor site for necrosis, proper wound healing, infection, hematomas, and seromas. Commonly used flaps relating to removing a sarcoma include a fibular flap, latissimus dorsi flap, anterior-lateral thigh flap, vastus lateralis flap, tensor fascia lata flap, soleus flap, and sartorius flap.

Bone involvement may precipitate the need for a tumor prosthesis, biological reconstruction with bone autografting, allografting, or a composite bone prosthesis.[74] Table 20.9 explains the differences between prosthetics choices.

Limb salvaging procedures involve resecting the cancerous lesions and sparing as much of the residual limb as possible. Reconstruction for PLWBC with bone involvement may require endoprosthetic implants, rotationplasty, or tibial turn-up procedures to improve functional outcomes and restore structural integrity to the limbs.

Endoprosthetics are a new type of prosthesis that can be surgically implanted in the body to help replace bones that have deteriorated secondary to bone cancers. The prosthetist uses clinical imaging and a 3D printer to construct a titanium alloy prosthetic that will closely match the measurements, shape, and individual characteristics of the limb.[75,76] This can make the prosthetic fit better, help restore proper joint mechanics, and help PLWBCs recover

Surgical Reconstruction Option	Definition
Tumor prosthesis	A prosthetic that can be made of metal and surgically implanted to replace the shoulder girdle, femur, knee, or pelvis; sometimes referred to as a megaprosthesis or endoprosthesis.
Bone autografting	Taking bone tissue from a different part of the PLWBC's body and using it to repair structural weaknesses by transplanting it into the affected bones after cancer has been removed.
Bone allografting	Taking a bone from a donor cadaver and using it to replace the bone damaged by the sarcoma.
Composite bone prosthesis	Donor bone is cemented together with a prosthetic and then surgically implanted into the patient's bone.

TABLE 20.9 Surgical Reconstruction Options[71,74,79,80]

faster.[69,75–78] Endoprostheses can recreate cervical vertebrae, ribs, scapulas, femurs, articulating knees, pelvic bones, etc.[79] Surgeons will often use mesh, surgical screws, plates, specific cementing procedures, and other endoprosthetic devices to help reinforce the structural integrity of the endoprosthesis, autograft, or allograft prostheses with the limb. There is promising research that coating the endoprosthesis in silver may lower the risk of infection.[79] See Table 20.9 for additional information.

The goals for an endoprosthesis are osteoinduction (stimulation of new cell growth), osteoconduction (cells starting to form new bone), and osseous integration (the bone grafts integrating through a creeping phenomenon in which the allograft, composite, and residual bone grow together and intertwine).

The risks associated with these reconstruction techniques include infection, nonunion of bone grafts, fractures, poor perfusion of the muscular flaps, rejection of the allografts, and loosening of the articulation between the bone and prosthetic implant.[69,75–78] Chemotherapy and radiation can slow down the reconstruction process and prevent the bonding of bones and implants.[71,74,79] Loosening can occur if the loading stress is more than the articular surfaces can handle, as the strain causes shearing and loosening of the implant. Signs of aseptic loosening with an endoprosthesis, allograft, or autograft bone replacement include: increased pain; feeling instability in the joint or at the bone/prosthetic articulation; and signs of fracture or bone loss on imaging.[71,74,79] It is important for oncology rehabilitation (Onc R) clinicians to listen to PLWBCs and note if they are describing any of these symptoms since this can potentially lead to an infection.

Rotationplasty is a limb salvaging procedure that involves resecting the cancerous lesion around the knee region and salvaging the tibia, ankle, and foot. The tibia is rotated 180° and surgically implanted onto the residual limb of the femur.[81–85] This type of surgery is rare and used primarily in pediatric populations due to their "skeletal immaturity."[81–85] The PLWBC then receives customized prosthetics that will fit their residual limb/foot and ankle for weight-bearing. It is an "autologous reconstruction" method that may be selected by the PLWBC and/or their families as it is cost-effective, may provide increased function, and may reduce the need for reconstructive and invasive surgeries in the future.[81]

Tibial turn-up is another option after bone sarcomas of the femur or after other limb salvage surgeries have been unsuccessful. This option involves resecting the cancerous lesions and then salvaging the tibia by flipping the distal end of the tibia up to be articulated with the distal femur. It is attached with plates and screws. The goal is to extend the residual limb/femur as much as possible while also maintaining a weight-bearing surface of the proximal tibia when it is flipped down.[86]

Amputation becomes the only option available for a PLWBC in cases where the cancer is very aggressive, a flap or prosthetic surgery is unsuccessful or when limb salvage is not an option. Imaging allows surgeons to estimate the amount of the limb to be removed to achieve clear margins and precisely plan for reconstruction. This also depends on the PLWBC's overall health, comorbidities, daily activities, and goals for function. Once the limb has been removed, the surgeon will use a flap or skin grafting to cover the wound. The goals for amputation are clear margins, pain relief, prevention of infections and necrosis, and reconstructing the residual limb to wear a prosthesis to maximize function.

Pain

Phantom Limb Pain

Following surgical amputation, the PLWBC may report phantom sensations from the surgically removed limb. These symptoms include burning, itching, stinging, aching, or sharp muscle or nerve pain.[87] The phenomenon can be aggravated by improper fitting prosthetics, scar restrictions, alignment dysfunctions, contractures, spasms, and irritated nerve roots. Phantom limb pain may diminish with healing, or lead to chronic pain. Use of non-steroidal anti-inflammatory drugs (NSAIDs), opioids, antidepressants, or other medications can help control inflammation and neuropathic pain. Rehabilitative management and treatment interventions post amputation will be discussed later in this chapter.

Neuropathic Pain

Neuropathic pain is a common adverse effect after sarcoma treatment interventions. PLWBCs may report feeling tingling, numbness, diminished proprioceptive awareness, or sharp electrical pain that radiates throughout the affected region of the body. Neuropathic pain occurs due to damage to the sensory fibers, causing a delay in or over-stimulation of nerve impulses. Rehabilitative management and treatment interventions for neuropathic pain management will be discussed later in this chapter. Chapter 22 provides more information and details on this topic.

Targeted muscle reinnervation (TMR) is a surgical intervention that may help eliminate both of these pain pathways. During amputations and limb salvage surgeries, the nerves may be directly cut or transected, or during wearing a prosthetic, the injured nerves by be compressed. As these nerves try to heal, they regenerate axons that can become trapped in the scar tissue and cause "terminal neuromas." Surgeons will prepare a nearby motor nerve by dividing it to create a space where a motor segment is deinnervated. They then cut the painful terminal neuroma off until they have fresh nerve fascicles and transfer it to the newly deinnervated motor nerve. The previously injured nerve now has a place to regenerate to and it coapts with the original nerve to provide innervation to the muscle group.[88–90]

Roles of Oncology Rehabilitation Clinicians for Patients Living With and Recovering From Sarcomas

Chapter 24 is dedicated to acute care therapy, and Chapter 29 covers palliative care—it is highly recommended to reference those chapters for details on the continuum of care for PLWBCs in this domain. This section will focus on outpatient therapy.

Outpatient Rehabilitation

In the outpatient setting, rehabilitation focuses on managing PLWBCs' musculoskeletal, neuromuscular, integumentary, and cardiopulmonary rehabilitative needs.[91] Initially therapy focuses on working through the acute secondary effects of sarcoma treatment interventions. During the acute stages of outpatient therapy, goals include managing adverse effects, promoting safety, facilitating healing, restoring and improving strength, function, and endurance, and training on how to use new adaptive equipment.

Long-term management starts approximately 8 months after the interventions. During this stage of treatment, the PLWBC may start experiencing long-term adverse effects, such as neuropathy, scar tissue adhesions, pain, and aerobic deconditioning.

For those diagnosed with a terminal cancer, palliative care options exist. In this stage of rehabilitation, manual therapy and exercises can help improve quality of life (QOL), and various modalities can help decrease pain.

Subjective Assessments

Initial evaluations should be performed following a systems review framework. Identifying strengths, weaknesses, compensation patterns, functional deficits, pain, and goals are essential components to developing a patient-centered intervention plan. An overall picture of health and wellness can be further developed by reviewing the medical history, imaging, and lab results for the hematological, digestive, and endocrine systems' status. Imaging provides Onc R clinicians with insight on the structural integrity of the muscles, bones, and joints, and in some cases assess vascular integrity as well as help to assess postoperative bone remodeling. Onc R clinicians need to review the surgical history and notes and communicate closely with the surgical team to understand and focus rehab interventions as well as follow postoperative restrictions and guidelines. Onc R clinicians must also review current medications and be familiar with pharmacological adverse effects as this can inform treatment plans.

Objective Assessments: Systems Review

The initial patient evaluation should start with a systems review. This consists of different steps, each providing specific insight to inform the treatment plan for the individual PLWBC. See Table 20.10 for a quick reference on a systems review. Not everything listed will need to be assessed. Use of clinical judgment about what is appropriate for the circumstance and the PLWBC during the treatment session is recommended.

Fascial Assessments

The fascial system connects all of the muscles, joints, and tendons throughout the body. Sarcomas and the ensuing surgical and medical interventions can cause significant impairments to this system. Restrictions in one region of the body can result in global impairment of all of the overlapping lines of fascia, causing tension above and below the affected area. Increased fascial tension may cause functional limitations, increased energy expenditures, pain, postural impairments, joint hypo/hypermobility, muscle inhibition, lymphatic blockages, and visceral and craniosacral restrictions. Table 20.11 summarizes considerations and impairments due to fascial restrictions in different areas.

Compensation Patterns

While the body is "under construction," alternative motor patterns or compensation patterns may be used temporarily to help maintain function. Compensation patterns occur when one muscle or group of muscles are recruited to compensate for the lack of participation from the weakened or inhibited group of muscles. Long term compensation patterns are not energy efficient, and may lead to muscle imbalances, weakness, pain, joint instability, and spasms. Surgery, scars, hyper- or hypotonic muscles, contractures, and joint hyper- or hypomobility can further cause muscle inhibition. It is important to assess for compensation patterns during the initial evaluation and address this with motor sequencing and coordination exercises as early as possible during rehabilitation interventions. Table 20.12 has a list of common compensation patterns to avoid.

Treatment Interventions

Postreconstructive Surgery

PLWBCs who have undergone bone reconstruction surgery via any aforementioned reconstruction methods will have a list of precautions, contraindications, and therapy protocols, similar to the orthopedic population status post joint arthroplasty. For any pelvic or lower extremity reconstruction, PLWBCs typically start with at least six weeks of nonweight bearing exercises and work strictly on range of motion (ROM), based on the surgeon's prescriptions. PLWBCs will use assistive devices for gait and progress from nonweight bearing to toe touch weight bearing, partial, and full weight-bearing statuses. Full weight-bearing is generally not permitted before 6 to 8 weeks' postsurgery, and imaging is needed to confirm that healing of the extremity will tolerate eccentric and concentric loading forces required for ambulation. Hastening this timeframe can cause aseptic loosening of the articular components, shearing, fractures, or nonunions.

Weight-bearing exercises may progress slowly once the surgeon and oncologist have permitted to proceed with therapy. It is important during this time to perform work hardening therapies over the residual limb and lymphatic drainage to facilitate scar healing.

Following amputations, PLWBCs are taught during the acute stage how to wrap their residual limb with bandages to help with healing and prevent edema. When it is appropriate, compression garments are fitted and then training with a temporary prosthetic can begin. PLWBCs work with the therapist and the prosthetist to fit the temporary prosthetic properly before casting the permanent prosthetic.

It is important to check for signs of infection, wound healing, and proper circulation to the residual limb. Therapists can teach

TABLE 20.10	**Objective Assessments for PLWBC and Sarcomas**
Assessments	**Summary**
Subjective assessments	• Subjective assessments help evaluate function, level of pain, and quality of life (QOL). • The Toronto Extremity Salvage Score (TESS) is a questionnaire given to patients for them to report on their level of activity.[92] • The Musculoskeletal Tumor Society (MSTS) has two different scoring systems. They are physician rated and specific to a joint-MSTS-87, or the entire upper or lower extremity-MSTS-93.[92]
Integumentary assessments	• Always check the surgical incision, and surrounding skin integrity and temperature to monitor for infection. • Check flaps or areas of reconstruction for signs of necrosis or infection. • If the person living with and beyond cancer (PLWBC) has a prosthetic, check for pressure points, erythema, and edema. Adjustments need to be made to their compression garments or prosthetic.
Musculoskeletal Assessments	• Check strength, muscle endurance. • Assess joint range of motion, osteokinematics, and arthrokinematics. • Assess joint/capsule mobility. • Look for alignment dysfunctions of the pelvis, spine, rib cage, shoulders, hips, knees, ankles, feet, and leg length. • Orthopedic restrictions can contribute to postural dysfunctions, compensation patterns, poor body mechanics, loss of balance, decreased energy efficiency, decreased function, and pain. Drives digestion and can alter pelvic floor tone, and poor oxygen saturation can lead to pain in the spine, increased fatigue, and circulation issues. • For surgical intervention, scar tissue restrictions and leg length discrepancies should be assessed. • Review available imaging to identify proper bone regrowth and re-mineralization.

Fascial assessments	• Fascial mobility
	  • Scar tissue restrictions
	  • Pelvic diaphragm
	  • Respiratory diaphragm
	  • Thoracic inlet/outlet
	  • Hyoid
	  • Tentorium cerebelli
	• Lymphatic drainage

Psychological assessments Chapter 14 covers psychological assessments in detail.	• Assess cognition and memory. • Psychological assessments are important as the PLWBC is learning how to cope with potentially a new body image, psychogenic pain, depression, and fatigue. • PLWBCs can have a lot of additional stress due to environmental changes. They may need a referral to social work or psychology to help them manage their current status.
Cardiopulmonary assessments	• Take baseline measurements vital signs. Deconditioning is common after surgery, chemotherapy, and radiation treatments. Baseline measurements help monitor for cardiopulmonary changes and provide early indications of chemotherapy induced cardiotoxicity symptoms.
Nervous system assessments	• Assess: dermatomes, myotomes • If indicated screen the cranial nerves. • Assess coordination, balance, and motor sequencing. • Check proprioception • Check sensation of scars and surgical incisions. • Care should be taken when checking for chemotherapy and radiation neuropathies as assessments can cause increased pain and safety issues. • If the PLWBC has a residual limb, check phantom limb sensations.
Gait assessments additional tests and measures for the neurological systems are addressed in Chapter 8.	• Gait assessments such as the 10-meter walk test, Timed Up and Go (TUG), the functional gait index, or the dynamic gait index can be used to record the baseline measurements with this population. • Assess transtibial and transfemoral gait deviations and measure leg length discrepancies with a new prosthesis.

Created by Taire M. Thie, DPT. Printed with permission.

gentle lymphatic drainage techniques to limit edema and swelling and help facilitate healing, as well as dry brushing techniques to desensitize the residual limb. PLWBCs should be encouraged to touch and massage their residual limb frequently, as doing so will improve blood flow, reduce edema, and decrease pain. Evidence of pressure ulcers must be promptly communicated to the prosthetist. See Figure 20.1 for examples of dry brushing habituation over a residual limb.

Onc R clinicians help the PLWBC prepare their residual limb for the prosthetic in several ways including work hardening,

sensory habituation, scar mobilizations, lymphedema manual drainage, myofascial release, stretching, and strengthening exercises (see Figure 20.2). Good communication between the therapist and the prosthetist will significantly benefit the PLWBC. The prosthetist measures the residual limb and discusses goals for the prosthetic, including whether for aesthetics or functionality for ambulation, sports, occupation, etc. and builds a prosthetic or a series of prosthetics aligned with the goals discussed.

Onc R clinicians work with the PLWBC more frequently than the prosthetist, affording ongoing assessment through this

TABLE 20.11   Functional Limitations Due to Fascial Restrictions Secondary to Oncological Treatment Interventions

Region	Restrictions Secondary to Treatment Interventions
Head, neck and throat	• Trismus: significant limitations to the range of motion (ROM) of the jaw • Difficulty chewing and swallowing • Difficulty producing saliva • May affect cervical and shoulder ROM • May cause headaches/migraines • May affect esophageal, trachea, and hyoid mobility • May constrict craniosacral flow • May constrict lymphatic drainage
Thorax/trunk/spine	• May diminish rib cage mobility and joint mechanics effecting respiration • May affect shoulder ROM • May constrict lymphatic drainage • May constrict visceral movements • May impair bed mobility • May affect tolerance for sitting/standing/walking
Upper extremities	• Alter scapulothoracic rhythm • Alter force-couple of the upper trapezius, serratus anterior, and lower trapezius muscles • Limit patient upper extremity ROM • May affect fine motor skills such as writing, grasping, typing, and eating • May affect gross motor skills, activities of daily living, cleaning, self-care tasks, and driving • May constrict lymphatic drainage
Lower abdomen/pelvis/peritoneum	• May affect lifting • May affect forward bending, sitting, and hip flexion • May affect backward bending, standing, and hip extension • May impair bed mobility • May impair balance • May affect sexual intimacy and function • May cause constipation or bowel/bladder incontinence • May constrict lymphatic drainage • May constrict visceral mobility
Lower extremities	• May affect mobility/standing/ambulation • May impair balance • May constrict lymphatic drainage

Created by Taire M. Thie, DPT. Printed with permission.

TABLE 20.12   Common Patient Compensation Patterns

Common Patient Compensations Include

- Holding their breath while trying to recruit their core
- Over-recruiting their hip flexors to compensate for abdominal weakness
- Using a posterior pelvic tilt while trying to engage the transverse abdominis
- Tensing up their neck and pectorals while trying to engage their rectus abdominis
- Flexing their head forward with shoulder flexion or abduction
- Hiking the shoulder up during shoulder flexion or abduction
- Anteriorly tilting the shoulder forward with shoulder extension, horizontal adduction, or internal rotation
- Over-recruiting the pectoral muscles with shoulder abduction and changing the plane of motion
- Recruiting their hamstrings instead of their glutes while lifting, walking, and performing bridges
- Recruiting their hip adductors to compensate for contralateral hip abduction weakness
- Tensing their jaw to brace their body while doing activities that involve lifting, carrying, pushing or pulling
- Gait deviations

Created by Taire M. Thie, DPT. Printed with permission.

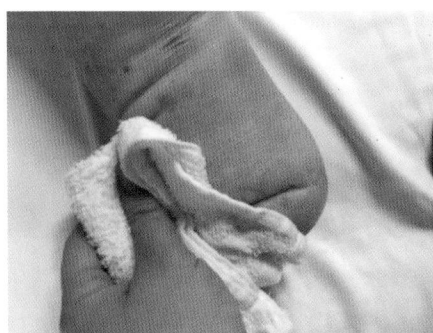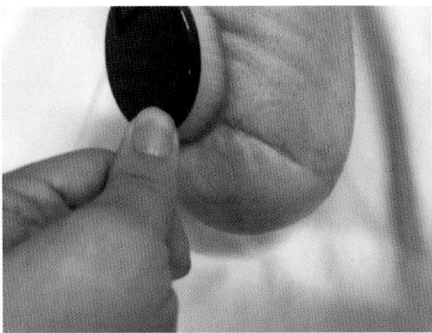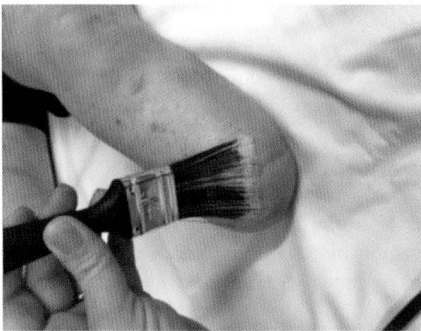

• **Fig. 20.1** An Example of Habituation Training. (Photo printed with permission by Taire M. Thie, DPT.)

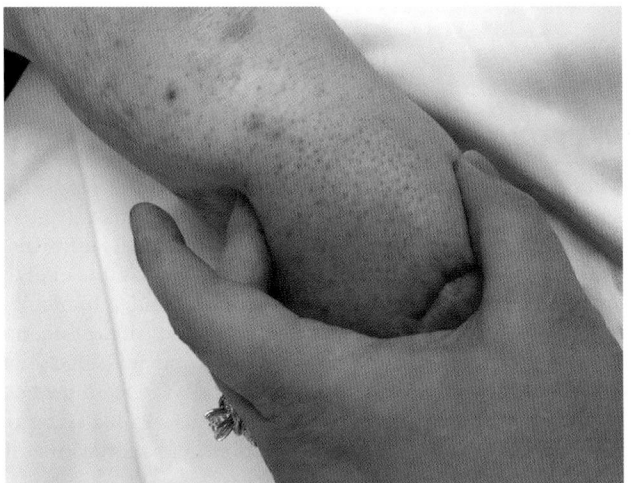

• **Fig. 20.2** Manual Therapy for a Residual Limb with Trigger Point and Myofascial Releases. (Photo printed with permission by Taire M. Thie, DPT.)

transition phase. Rehab interventions should emphasize building tolerance to wearing the prosthetic and establishing a wearing schedule that gradually helps skin, muscles, and bones acclimate to prolonged periods of contact and loading. Loading and unloading the limbs to build tolerance to functional tasks and ongoing assessment of the residual limb for erythema, bumps, rashes, and pain should be prioritized.

Onc R clinicians should tactilely evaluate the prosthetic for potential areas of elevation, ridges, lines, or bumps that could cause compression or irritation. It is equally important to observe the residual limb and prosthetic for shape compatibility. Evaluation of compression sock(s) within the prosthetic to prevent sliding down or bunching up is necessary to ensure proper fit. Identification of pain location can be made easier by using a dry erase marker to mark the inside of the prosthetic, once the PLWBC dons it and moves through loading, weight-bearing, and some functional activities, potential areas of excessive contact will leave a mark on the skin. A prosthetic with optimal fit should disperse contact universally and small areas of contact should not be present.

Pediatric PLWBCs will go through several prostheses in their lifetimes as they grow. Clinicians in this domain should educate the family on gait deviations, assessing the residual limb frequently, and identifying symptoms such as back pain as an indication that it is time to consider a new prosthetic. Properly fitted prosthetics are crucial to restoring function and decreasing their pain.

Phantom Limb and Neuropathic Pain

PLWBCs who have had amputations or reconstructive surgery after working through their sarcoma diagnosis may develop pain such as phantom limb pain, pressure sores, scar adhesions, or muscle spasms and contractures.

Rehabilitative management of phantom limb and neuropathic pain includes treating and preventing scar restrictions that can cause nerve impingements, as well as acclimating and desensitizing scar tissue. Recommended techniques include scar mobilization, positional releases with myofascial releases and soft tissue mobilization, applying Kinesiotape and modalities such as the low level laser therapy (LLLT), the 6D fascial release system, or Lymphatouch. Onc R clinicians can implement habituation retraining and skin hardening techniques to decrease noxious stimulus using everyday household tools such as washcloths, paint brushes, or make-up brushes to provide different sensations and reduce irritability when the prosthetic is donned. See Figures 20.1 and 20.2 for examples.

Other rehabilitation options for phantom limb and neuropathic pain include the use of graded motor imagery, transcutaneous electrical nerve stimulation (TENS), biofeedback retraining, and virtual reality training. Graded motor therapy has three important and sequential phases to retrain the brain.[93] Pain can alter the PLWBC's perceptions and make it difficult to discriminate between the left and right sides of their body. Phase one is a series of repetitive tests and observations that shows an image of a limb, and the PLWBC has to discriminate which side of the body the image is displaying.[93] The goal is for the PLWBC to quickly and consistently discriminate the L and the R with a minimum of 80% accuracy.[93] When the patient has met the established goals for the first phase, then they can progress to phase two which is "explicit motor imagery." The PLWBC creates a motor plan in their mind and mentally practices going through all of the steps in an organized fashion to accomplish the motor task.[93] They can choose any task they like, and can change the level of complexity, and they need to practice with both sides of the body. In the therapy setting the therapist can help the PLWBC think through different environments, distractions, perturbations, or sensory feedback and adapt their motor imagery. The PLWBC is encouraged to practice this skill often. Once the treating clinician deems it appropriate, they can initiate phase three. Phase three is called mirror therapy. Mirrors are used to reflect the body's functional side, encouraging the PLWBC to look into the mirror and imagine moving the affected side into a position of release.[93]

Virtual reality training is similar intervention, though it uses an artificial environment to deceive the brain into sensing the limb despite its absence. Virtual reality and biofeedback training use sensors on the residual limb to read its neural impulses and translate them into movement patterns on the virtual screen, giving the patient a sense of control over their limb.

Modalities

TENS can be applied to the residual or salvaged limb as long as electrode placement is not over an open wound. TENS can be used to alter the pain pathways, help ease pain, and improve circulation and proprioceptive awareness.[87]

LLLT works by emitting visible or nonvisible light, which is absorbed by the cells. The laser stimulates the mitochondria in the cells, increases cellular metabolism, clears intercellular transmission pathways, and eventually helps with RNA and DNA synthesis, which helps repair damaged tissues. Laser wavelengths vary between 600 and 1,000 nm in the visible and infrared nonvisible light spectrums. Wavelengths of 600 to 750 nm (red light) are used for treating superficial tissue, lymphedema, scars, radiation dermatitis, radiation fibrosis, and chemotherapy induced neuropathic pain while 750 to 1000 nm wavelengths in the nonvisible infrared spectrum are selected for addressing subsurface tissues, as these penetrate deeper into tissue. Laser power and energy densities are selected based on specific treatment. For oncological conditions, a power of 1 to 500 mW is typically used. For commercial lasers, energy densities can be adjusted from 1 to 40 J/cm². Wounds, oral ulcers, and blockages in the lymphatic system respond the best to 3 to 4 J/cm² in 60 second intervals, while deeper wounds typically respond better to higher energy densities in the 10 to 40 J/cm² range applied for only 30 seconds at a time to avoid damaging tissues.[87,94–96] See Figures 20.3 and 20.4 for an example of a low level laser unit.

Lasers can cause damage to the retina and should never be used over or near the eyes; both the Onc R clinician and the patient should wear protective glasses and avoid looking at the laser directly when in use. Contraindications for LLLT include using it over active infections, tumors, or metastases because of increased cellular proliferation. Precautions should be taken when treating areas with tattoos, as the ink may contain certain chemicals or metals resulting in a different rate of absorption and cause damage to the underlying tissues. LLLT can be applied along the sensory and motor pathways of the residual or salvaged limb, which helps decrease inflammatory cytokines and muscle spasms as well as improve circulation, cellular metabolism, and scar tissue pliability. When used over the temporomandibular joint (TMJ) and oral mucosa, this helps restore saliva production and reduce the effects of ulcerative mucositis (otherwise known as mouth ulcers). It can

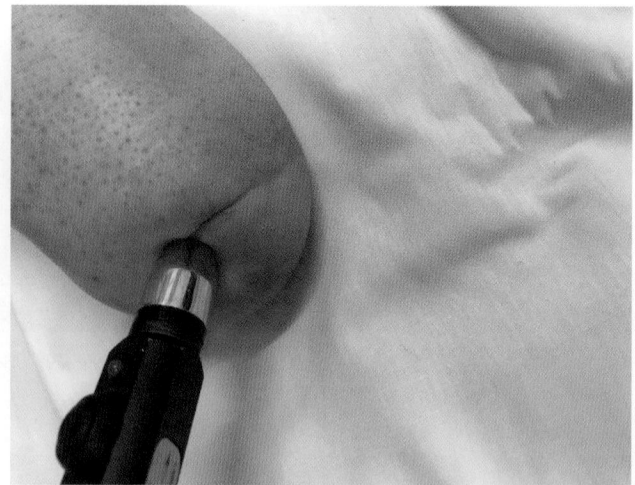

• **Fig. 20.4** An Example of Low Level Laser Therapy (LLLT) Being Used Over Scar Tissue for a Patient With a Residual Limb for Trigger Points and Phantom Limb Pain. (Photo printed with permission by Taire M. Thie, DPT.)

also be used to treat radiodermatitis after radiation therapy. LLLT also can be used for palliative care for pain and edema.

The 6D fascial release and Lymphatouch modalities utilize negative pressure to suction the skin and scar tissue off of the underlying muscles, joints, and fascia. The primary purpose is to mobilize the scar tissue, improve vascular and lymphatic circulation, and ease pain. These modalities are useful following any surgery and can be applied to areas of radiation fibrosis anywhere on the body except the carotid arteries. Contraindications include using the suction over open wounds, active infections, radiation dermatitis, or tumors.

The 6D system can apply a suction pressure of 0 to 300 mmHg and the Lymphatouch has a range of 0 to 250 mmHg, with added features of low and high vibration. Low vibrations affect deeper tissues, while higher vibrations help break up superficial scar tissue. Both systems can be adjusted to suction-release or continuous suction settings. Pictures of the 6D and Lymphatouch can be found at the end of the chapter in Figures 20.5 and 20.6.

Manual Therapy

Post radiation manual therapy in the treatment plan can be used to: (1) mobilize scars and fibrotic tissue; (2) help improve joint mechanics; (3) decrease pain; (4) improve function; (5) restore balance to the lymphatic system; and (6) improve the PLWBC's posture and help them achieve their rehabilitation goals.

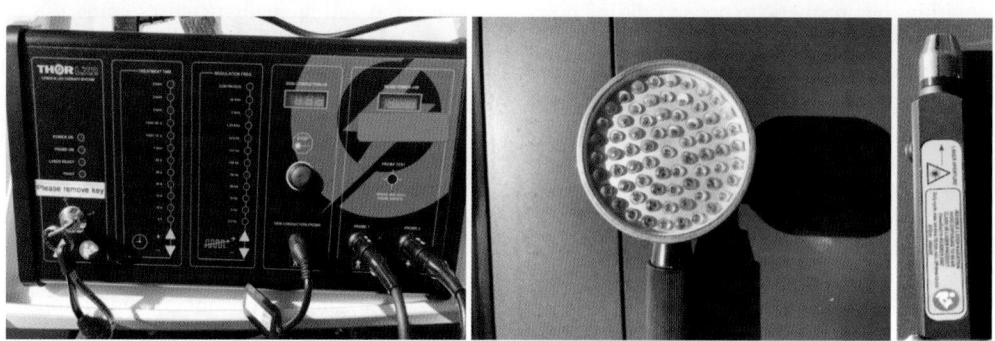

• **Fig. 20.3** An Example of an LED and Infrared Low Level Laser Machine. (Photo printed with permission by Taire M. Thie, DPT.)

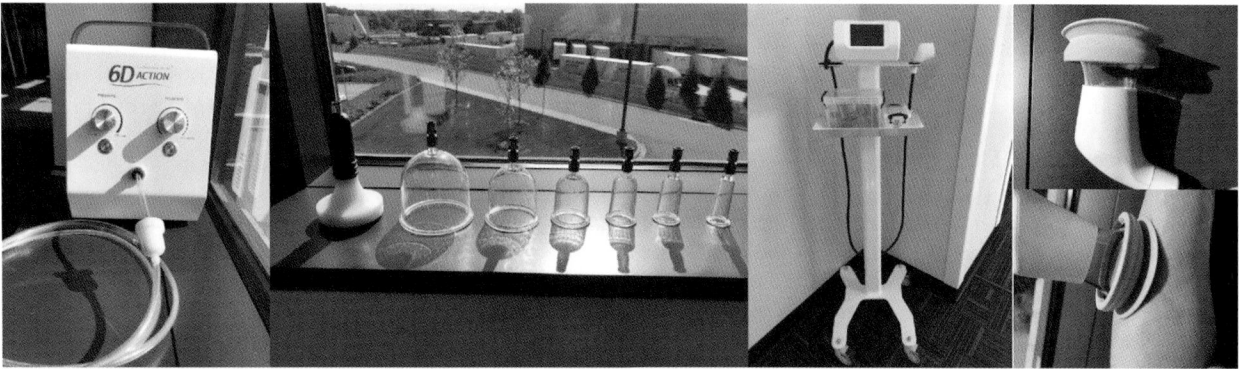

• **Fig. 20.5** An Example of the 6D Fascial Release System and the Lymphatouch. (Photo printed with permission by Taire M. Thie, DPT.)

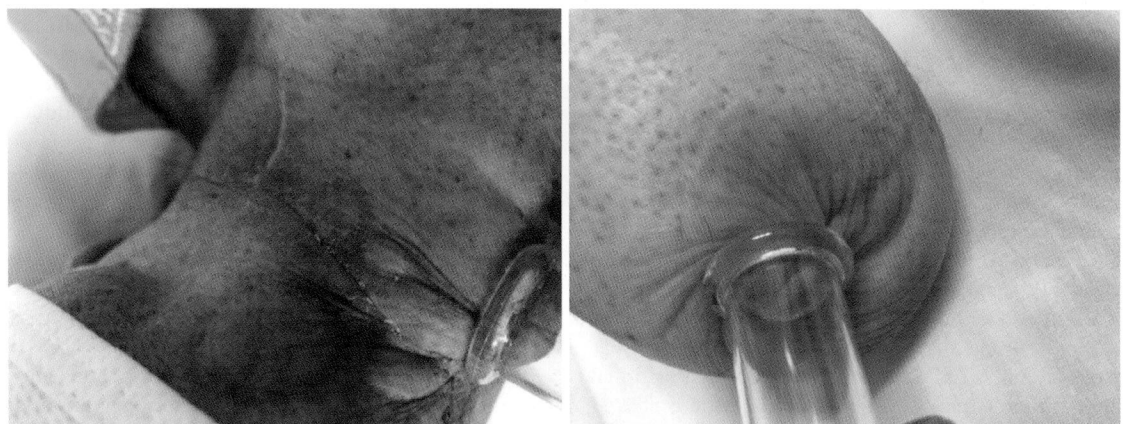

• **Fig. 20.6** An Example of the 6D Cupping Being Used for Treatment Over Scar Tissue After a Cervical Dissection and Residual Limb. (Photo printed with permission by Taire M. Thie, DPT.)

Before initiating intervention, alignment, strength, and ROM and functional movement patterns should be assessed with particular attention paid to compensation patterns, areas of inhibition, and complaints of pain or fatigue. Manipulations and high velocity-low amplitude thrusts should typically be avoided in the acute stage of recovery or with active cancer but may be used cautiously in the long-term stage depending on the patient's progress and rate of healing.

Manual therapy interventions can help improve circulation for the circulatory and lymphatic system, mobility and function of the muscles, fascia and joints, organs, craniosacral system, and decrease pain. Muscles inhibited by resection, lack of proprioception, surgical scars, or atrophy can lead other muscles to be overworked as they compensate to help the PLWBC achieve presurgical movements. Intervention begins by releasing the scars and progresses to strengthening and motor coordination exercises to decrease compensation patterns. General rules for manual therapy include communicating the intention and establishing goals for treatment, educating the patient on how the techniques and exercises should feel, and explaining clinical rationale relative to improved function. Onc R clinicians should also routinely palpate all around the affected muscles, joints, scars, etc. to assess additional fascial restrictions. Onc R clinicians should remain attentive to verbal and nonverbal communication cues to ensure comfort and safety safe throughout the entire treatment session.

Muscle Energy Techniques/Contract-Relax

Contract-relax muscle energy techniques (MET) are appropriate for use early on and throughout the entire rehabilitation

continuum to correct alignment issues. MET were developed by Fred Mitchell Sr. and Fred Mitchell Jr, and explained in by Dr. Philip Greenman in 1989. MET focuses on using three dimensions of movement to identify motion restricting barrier, and the contract-relax approach helps the body move beyond that barrier. The method works as follows: (1) the clinician moves the joint up to the soft tissue or mechanical barrier and (2) the PLWBC contracts the target muscle for 5 to 10 seconds, then relaxes on an inhale as the as the joint is passively moved past the initial barrier by the clinician.[97] Muscle tone is inhibited by initiating a hypertonic state of engagement (contract phase), or by applying ischemic pressure quickly followed by a relaxation and stretching phase. Inhibited agonist muscles are then facilitated, helping to restore balance to the system.[98] Motor sequencing and stabilization exercises to help retrain the muscles by improving motor recruitment, strength, and endurance with these techniques.

Maitland/Kaltenborn Joint Glides and Mobilization With Movement

While not encouraged during the acute stages of the patient's recovery, high velocity manipulations can be used in areas of restriction for patients with chronic conditions. These may be very helpful after radiation therapy restoring proper motion to the joints; however good clinical decision making and judgement should be exercised. If the PLWBC has any type of issue with bone or joint integrity, this type of mobilization should be avoided. Joint glides and repetitive joint compression/decompression of synovial joints helps pump synovial fluid into the joints, release the joint capsules, improve joint ROM, and warm up the muscle tissue.

Mobilization with movement techniques can help retrain movement patterns by providing assistance through the ROM and facilitating correct joint mechanics and retrain proprioceptive awareness through tactile feedback.

Positional Release Versus Stretching

It is important for the Onc R clinician to remain cognizant of goals for therapy. If trying to prevent contractures, articular or fascial adhesions, and decrease pain, stretching may be indicated. The stretching goals are to increase flexibility in stiff joints, provide proprioceptive feedback, and help the circulatory system clear deep toxins within the muscles. Benefits include increased space around joints, decompression of areas of tension on the fascia, nerves, muscles, and joints, as well as improved vascular and lymphatic circulation. Stretching should prevent scar tissue and contractures, which helps prevent scars from adhering to muscles and fascia. Stretching should be taught early in the therapy sessions, either soon after surgery or while undergoing radiation treatments, to help prevent fibrosis and puckering of scars. It is important for the Onc R clinician to manually stretch the PLWBC and help find restrictions and gently push into barriers without causing adverse effects. PLWBCs should be educated on what stretches to complete, how long to hold them, and how many repetitions to perform each day.

Stretching may be a contraindication with some limb salvage surgeries, or in areas where the scar tissue needs to be in place to create a functional or stable joint. Be sure to follow the protocols outlined by the surgeon and oncologist to prevent reconstruction failure.

If stretching is contraindicated or painful, then positional releases or strain-counterstrain techniques become the preferred approach. Easing the strain on the muscle can significantly reduce pain and is accomplished by moving the insertion of the muscle towards its origin. In some areas, such as the piriformis, the hamstrings, or the pectoral muscles, there may be several positions of ease based on the direction of the motor fibers. After positioning the entire limb in ease, the clinician can add flexion/extension, abduction/adduction, and internal/external rotation, and manually palpate the muscle fibers until less tension is noted under their fingertips. A positional release puts the hypertonic muscle fibers into a position of relaxation. After a minimum of 2 minutes, this position can be combined with either soft tissue mobilization, the Lymphatouch or 6D fascial release system, scar tissue mobilizations, or LLLT. In this state, the tissue should soften and significantly improve pliability without causing discomfort. PLWBCs should also be taught how to ease and use self-massage techniques as part of their home exercise program (HEP). An example of a positional release for the hamstrings, gluteals, and piriformis muscles would involve positioning the patient in prone with their hip extended and knee bent. An example for the pectorals is to place the patient in supine, then horizontally adduct their upper extremity across their body and bend their elbow. See Figures 20.7–20.11 for examples of positional releases.

Releasing the Diaphragms

Craniosacral therapy, visceral therapy, myofascial releases, total body balancing, lymphatic balancing, and osteopathy all focus on the importance of releasing the horizontal diaphragms of the body to restore function.

Diaphragms are areas of deep fascia or retinaculum that reinforce the structural integrity of the body regions and can tighten

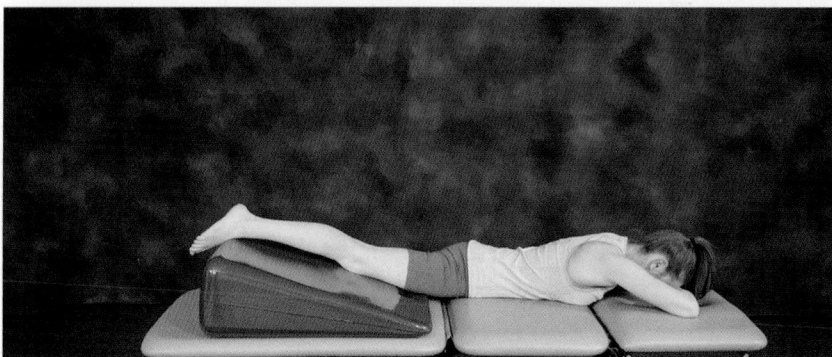

• **Fig. 20.7** Positional Release of the Posterior Hip, Hamstrings. (Photo printed with permission by John Krauss.)

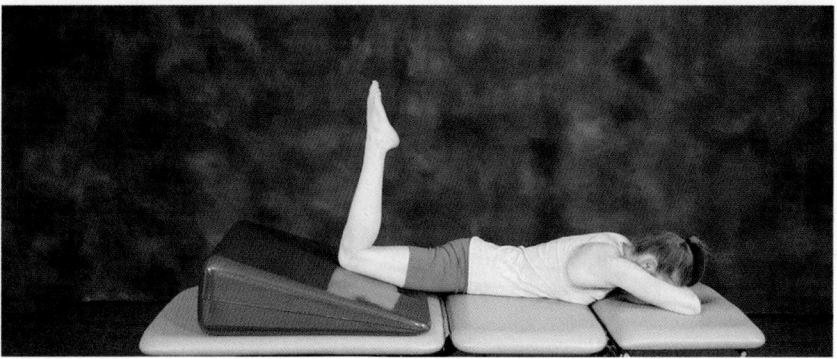

• **Fig. 20.8** Positional Release of the Posterior Leg, Gastrocnemius, and Soleus. (Photo printed with permission by John Krauss.)

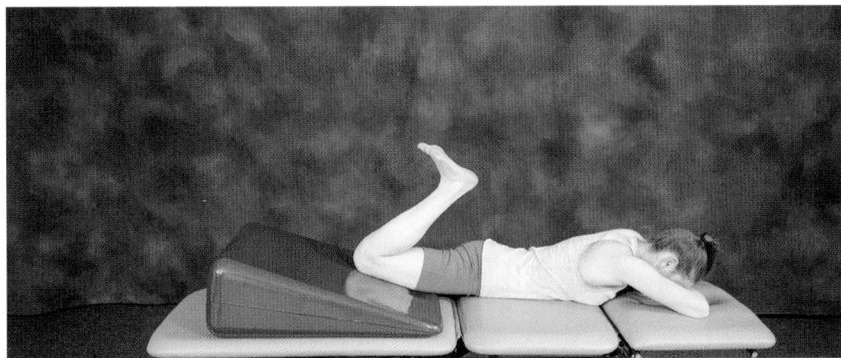

• **Fig. 20.9** Positional Release for the Posterior Hip and Anterior Tibialis. (Photo printed with permission by John Krauss.)

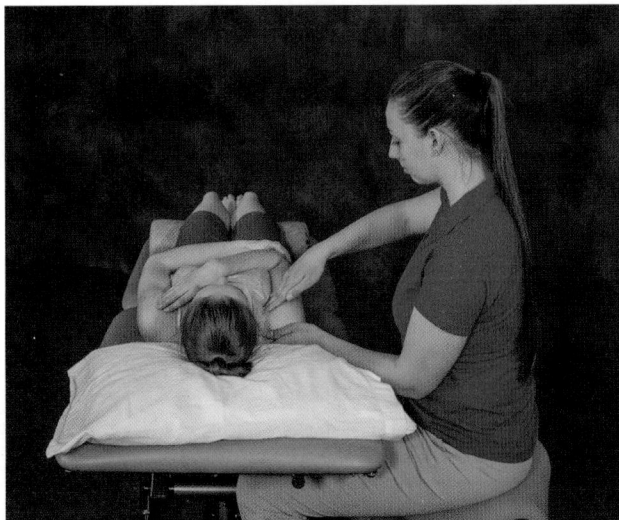

• **Fig. 20.10** Positional Release in Supine for the Pectorals. (Photo printed with permission by John Krauss.)

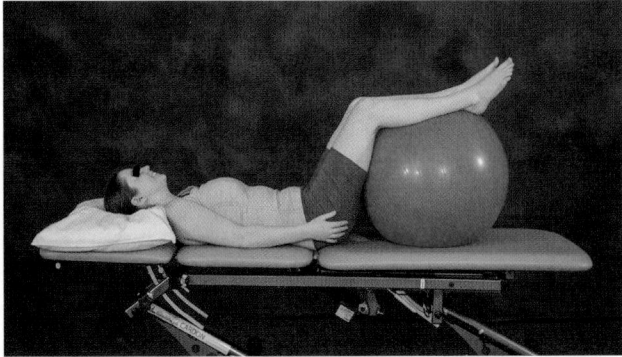

• **Fig. 20.11** Positional Release for the Hip Flexors. (Photo printed with permission by John Krauss.)

or release to change the pressure in that region.[99] The five main diaphragms are: the pelvic floor diaphragm, the respiratory diaphragm, the thoracic inlet, the hyoid, and the tentorium cerebelli. All five diaphragms can become restricted in the course of cancer treatments producing restrictions in the vertical lines of fascia.[99,100] These line up with many of the areas of watershed for lymphatic drainage; tension in the diaphragm(s) can cause back pain, impair

lymphatic drainage, and have detrimental effects on other bodily functions (e.g., digestion, circulation, respiration).[87,88] Eliminating this tension can help restore lymphatic drainage as well as function. See Figures 20.12– 20.16 for pictures of the manual diaphragm releases.

Box 20.1 highlights key details about releasing the diaphragms, and Box 20.2 describes step-by-step procedures for releasing the diaphragms. The technique is the same for the first four diaphragms and then changes for the tentorium cerebelli.

Craniosacral Therapy/Cranial Osteopathy

There is a gentle rhythm of cerebral spinal fluid pumped out of the choroid plexuses in the brain, encapsulated by the dura mater, pumped gently down into the spinal cord, and then back up into

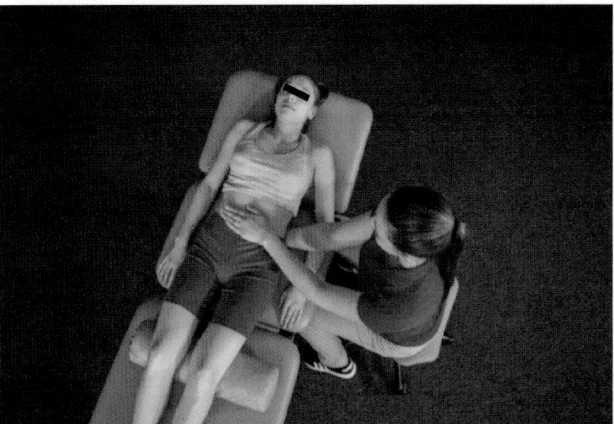

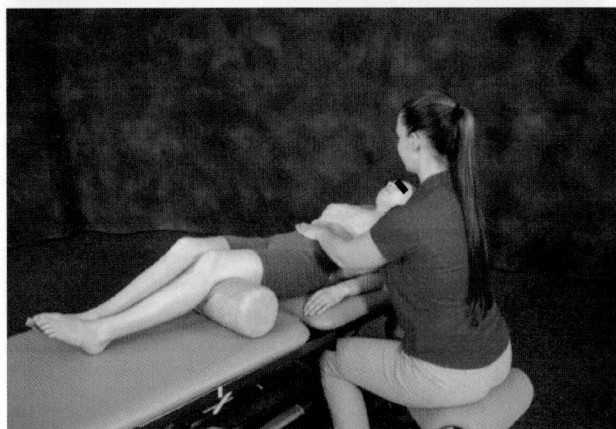

• **Fig. 20.12** Pelvic Diaphragm Release. (Photo printed with permission by John Krauss.)

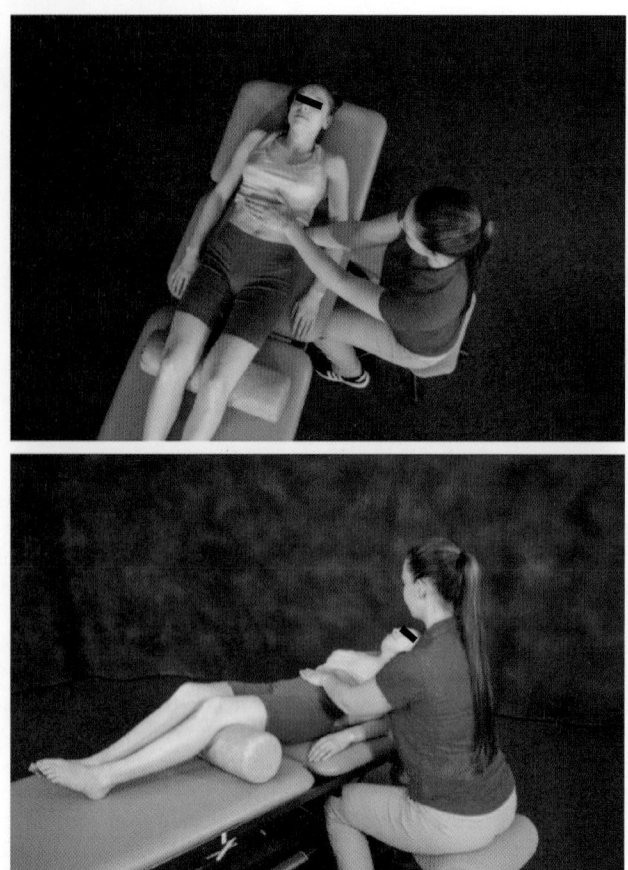

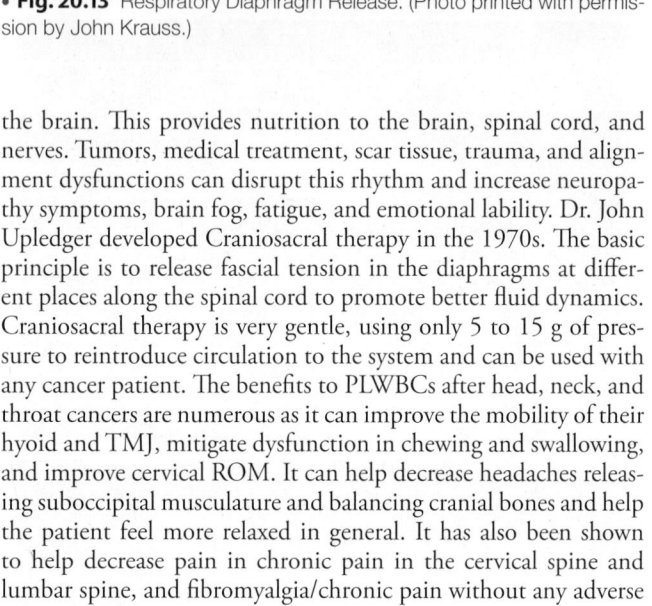

• **Fig. 20.13** Respiratory Diaphragm Release. (Photo printed with permission by John Krauss.)

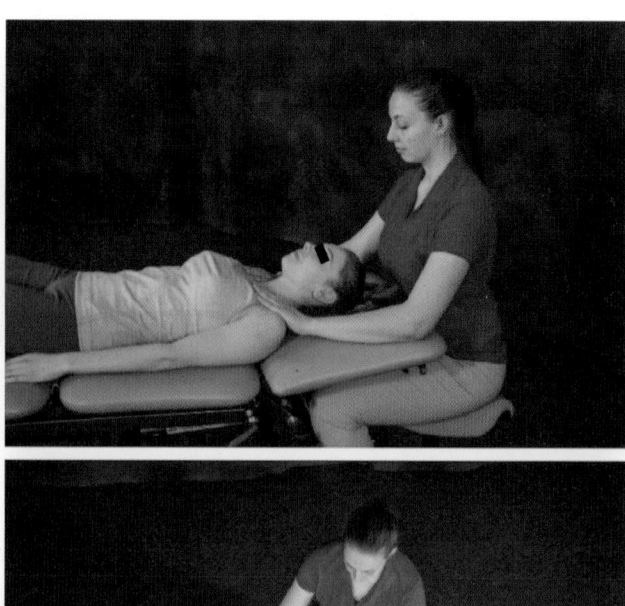

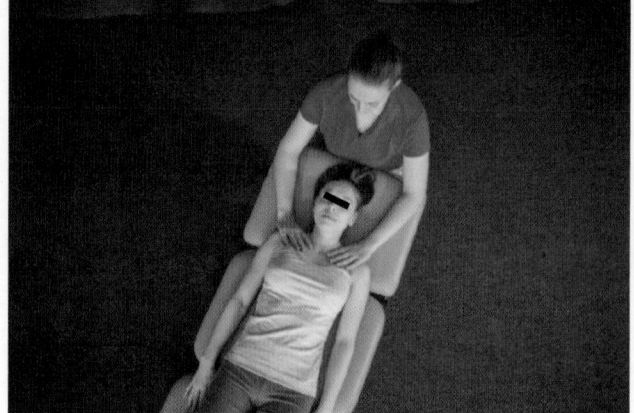

• **Fig. 20.14** Thoracic Inlet/Outlet Diaphragm Release. (Photo printed with permission by John Krauss.)

the brain. This provides nutrition to the brain, spinal cord, and nerves. Tumors, medical treatment, scar tissue, trauma, and alignment dysfunctions can disrupt this rhythm and increase neuropathy symptoms, brain fog, fatigue, and emotional lability. Dr. John Upledger developed Craniosacral therapy in the 1970s. The basic principle is to release fascial tension in the diaphragms at different places along the spinal cord to promote better fluid dynamics. Craniosacral therapy is very gentle, using only 5 to 15 g of pressure to reintroduce circulation to the system and can be used with any cancer patient. The benefits to PLWBCs after head, neck, and throat cancers are numerous as it can improve the mobility of their hyoid and TMJ, mitigate dysfunction in chewing and swallowing, and improve cervical ROM. It can help decrease headaches releasing suboccipital musculature and balancing cranial bones and help the patient feel more relaxed in general. It has also been shown to help decrease pain in chronic pain in the cervical spine and lumbar spine, and fibromyalgia/chronic pain without any adverse effects.[101–104]

Visceral Therapy

As previously mentioned in the fascial intervention section, the entire body is connected by several different layers. Organs in the body are surrounded by fascia and located close to other organs; for optimal function, organs must glide and slide relative to each other. Fascial restrictions caused by radiation, chemotherapy, or surgeries can create visceral restrictions, leading to referred pain patterns and inhibited organ function. Scar tissue can cause an increase in pressure within the thorax, abdomen, head, or pelvis,

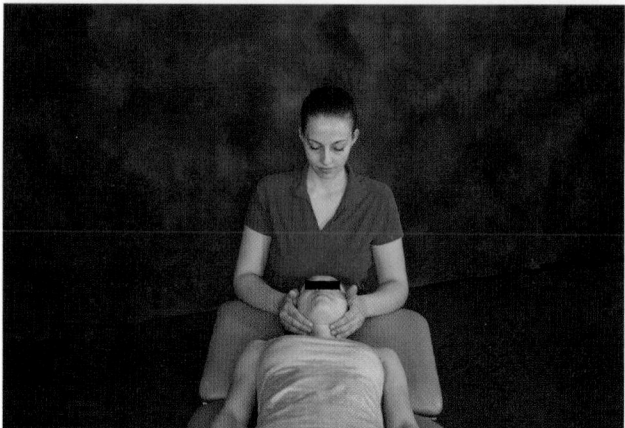

• **Fig. 20.15** Hyoid Release. (Photo printed with permission by John Krauss.)

and alter the pressure systems created by the divisions in the diaphragms. The body is then forced to compensate for these restrictions.

Visceral therapy is a type of manual release developed by Dr. Jean Pierre Barral. Each organ is innervated by specific spinal segments and fascially connected to the spine. Visceral releases are specific three-dimensional techniques used to restore fascial mobility of the organs, which results in an improved in alignment, respiration, digestion, pain, and potentially emotional tensions.[105,106] Visceral therapy is a subtle technique starting with

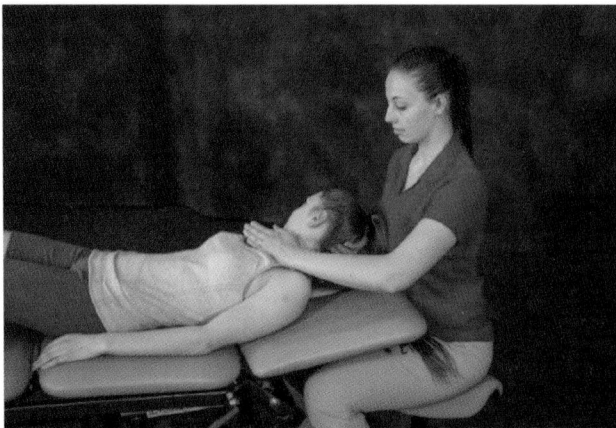

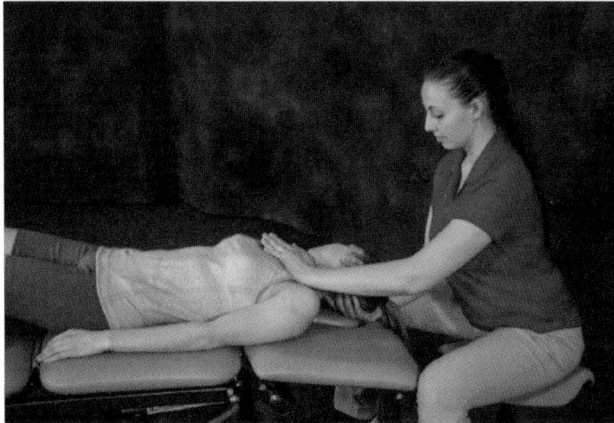

• **Fig. 20.16** Tentorium Cerebelli Release. (Photo printed with permission by John Krauss.)

• **BOX 20.1 Key Items for Successful Release of the Diaphragms**

Key items to pay attention to throughout this process include:
1. How the tissue feels: assess the tension, temperature, and movement in all planes. Temperature changes can happen as tissues are released.
2. Feedback from the patient: verbal cues, physical response, emotional response, changes in respiration, color, or eye movement. The patient should always be relaxed and not experience any pain.
3. These releases use pressures of 5–15 g and are meant to be very gentle and not painful to the patient; for reference, a nickel weighs 5 g.
4. The diaphragms should be released in order: pelvic, respiratory, thoracic inlet, hyoid, and lastly the tentorium cerebelli.
5. If there is any type of scar tissue, then it should be treated first before attempting to release the diaphragms.
6. Throughout this procedure, the therapist should think of the upper hand gently sinking into the tissue.
7. Note that movement into ease may differ with the two hands; as treatment advances and the diaphragm releases, movement becomes progressively more synchronized.

• **BOX 20.2 Details the Procedures for Releasing the Four Diaphragms**

Procedure for releasing the first four diaphragms:
1. Start with the patient in a supine position with a bolster under their knee.
2. Locate the position of the diaphragm to be released and place one hand on top of the patient and one underneath on the posterior surface of the diaphragm.
3. The clinician will gently compress their hands together and release, feeling for tension. The entire length of the diaphragm should be assessed in this way to locate specific areas.
4. Once an area has been identified, add compression and allow the hand to gently sink in.
5. The next step is to assess mobility and stack in three planes of motion, typically one direction is easier ("ease") than the other ("restricted"). The choice of whether to hold in ease or tension should be the same for 5(a)–5(c). The goal of this process is to apply constant pressure of 5–15 g in all planes identified simultaneously (5(a) + 5(b) + 5(c)).
   a. Start with gently dragging up and down and hold into either ease or tension.
   b. Then, maintaining the hold, assess side gliding with gentle left and right movements and hold based on the choice in 5(a).
   c. Finally add a clockwise and counterclockwise movement and hold based on the choice in 5(a).
6. Based on the patient's response, decide to treat into "ease" or into "tension."
   a. When treating into ease, combine the directions from step 5 where the movement is easiest. Typically treating into ease first can help the patient relax.
   b. If treating into ease does not work, attempt treating into tension; combine the directions from step 5 where movement is restricted.
7. Maintain the pressure of 5–15 grams throughout the process and follow the fascial release as it happens.
8. Repeat with the bottom hand.
9. When then the tissue softens, the clinician will release their pressure and reassess the movements. Treat any remaining barriers or move onto the next diaphragm.
10. Repeat for each diaphragm, starting from the pelvis and moving upward.
11. To release the tentorium cerebelli, flex the PLWBC's head and cervical spine, gently place a stabilizing hand over their distal anterior cervical fascia, rotate their head in the opposite direction, and slowly lower the PLWBC's head and neck back down onto the plinth. Repeat in both directions.

assessing the PLWBC's motions by gently placing their hand on their body and let the hand be pulled towards tension; the body natural tends to guard areas of restrictions and "hug the lesion." By "listening" to the body, the clinician can find the primary lesions and proceed to treat these using a combination of positional, myofascial, and energetic releases. Each organ has its own specific and precise formula for loading or unloading the fascia into ease or into tension through different planes of motion. Visceral therapy requires high precision coupled with very gentle releases. Through loading or unloading tension, the patient receives mechanical and proprioceptive input while the parasympathetic nervous system is stimulated to help the tissues relax.[107,108] This can help improve pain and ROM and restore the pressure systems for the cranium, thorax, abdomen, and pelvis.[107,108] Visceral therapy may benefit PLWBCs struggling with depression and/or anxiety by releasing somatoemotional barriers in the tissue. Finally, a combination of neurovascular and visceral lymphatic releases can mitigate neuropathic pain, lymphatic congestion, and cardiopulmonary functions.

Myofascial Release

Because fascia is a vast network of connective tissue throughout the entire body, fascial releases can and should be done over any symptomatic (pain, tension, and decreased ROM) region. There

---

• BOX 20.3   Myofascial Release Techniques

1. Find the fascial barrier/scar/trigger point.
2. Gently sink into the barrier and assess its mobility.
3. The next step is to assess mobility and stack in 3 planes of motion, typically one direction is easier ("ease") than the other ("restricted"). The choice of whether to hold in ease or tension should be the same for 3(a)–3(c). The goal of this process is to apply constant pressure of 15–30 g in all planes identified simultaneously (3(a) + 3(b) + 3(c)).
    a. Start with gently dragging up and down and hold into either ease or tension.
    b. Then, maintaining the hold, assess side gliding with gentle left and right movements and hold based on the choice in 3(a).
    c. Finally add a clockwise and counterclockwise movement and hold based on the choice in 3(a).
4. Maintaining the tension decreases your pressure and allows the soft tissues to release under your hands.
5. When the tissue softens, release the pressure and reassess.

---

are many continuing education courses to advance proficiency with this technique. Targeted myofascial release follows the same procedures as diaphragm releases but is performed in only one focused area and described step-by-step in Box 20.3. When the fascia and muscle relax, it is time to release the fascial pressure, reassess the movement restrictions/ROM, etc. The process is iterative and may need to be repeated multiple times as the barriers may change after each repetition. The PLWBC should be instructed to relax and take deep breaths throughout the process to help tap into the parasympathetic nervous system's "rest and digest" impulses. The process should be repeated into the barriers and restrictions until the tissue is soft, pliable, and can be put into a stretched or lengthened position. Once repetitions are complete and the tissue has softened, the patient should be instructed to contract the opposite muscle group; this facilitates and stimulates those motor units to retrain them, which helps the patient obtain better balance and function.

Scar Mobilizations

The four primary types of scar tissue are keloids, hypertrophic scars, contracted scars, and minor adhesions. The size, depth, and flexibility of the scars are measured, and color changes compared to the intact skin. Scar tissue can: cause muscle inhibition, ROM restrictions, and decreased motor efficiency; restrict nerve, fascia, and visceral mobility; and cause significant pain and postural impairments. Releasing scar tissue is essential for rehabilitation goal achievement.

Scars can be mobilized using the modalities of the LLLT, the 6D and Lymphatouch, and manual manipulation. Dycem can be given to patients to help with their own self-releases. Stretching the scar in several different directions should be emphasized. Stabilizing one side of the scar while move the opposite side away, up, down, diagonally, or in a twisting motion will increase pliability. Both sides of the scar can be stretched in opposite directions or towards the same direction to improve its ability to glide on the deeper tissues. Some clinicians have training and achieve good clinical outcomes using silicone taping, Kinesiotape to help lift the scar and improve mobility.[109–112] Leukotape or McConnell tape can also be used to stretch the scar in opposite directions, which allows the patient to perform self-mobilizations with functional movement as they move throughout the day.

Hydration

Scar tissue is often depleted of moisture and needs to be frequently moisturized topically with coconut oil, vitamin E oil, calendula oil, wheat germ oil, or cocoa butter. Calendula oil effectively treats radiation burns, and wheat germ oil works well over scars that pucker or scars resulting from a skin graft. Scar tissue receives hydration internally by drinking adequate amounts of water. Drinking water also helps with flushing out toxins after strengthening and stretching, and it can help patients decrease spasms and pain. Refer to Chapter 30 for additional details though general recommendations are to consume 50% of body weight (measured in pounds) in ounces of water per day (i.e., a 200 lbs [91 kg] patient should be drinking 100 oz [3 L] of water per day). If the PLWBC has a lot of scar tissue, they should add an extra 4 to 8 ounces (118 mL to 237 mL) per day depending on the depth and severity.

Therapeutic Activity

Sleep

The importance of proper sleep and sleep hygiene for persons living with sarcoma cannot be overemphasized. Fatigue and deconditioning can create a lot of emotional and physical stress. Lack of sleep also contributes to decreased pain thresholds, decreased endurance, and may impact cognition. It is important for the Onc R clinician to discuss sleep habits with the PLWBC and to help them establish good sleep techniques. Postsurgery, PLWBCs may need help identifying sleeping postures for more comfortable resting positions, and work on bed mobility for changing positions more comfortable throughout the night. For those experiencing muscle spasms at night, establishing a good stretching routine that can be performed bed can help. Others may require night splints or learn techniques such as dry brushing or wrapping their sensitive extremities in soothing fabric to avoid irritation to help with their neuropathic pain. Lymphatic balancing exercises may also be useful to help them find rest. Refer to Chapter 30 for additional ideas to promote health and wellness.

Deep Breathing/Meditation

Deep breathing is often overlooked as a therapeutic process, but it is essential to restoring function. The diaphragm is connected to most of the abdominal organs, the spine, the rib cage, the hips, and the pelvis. Inhibition of the respiratory diaphragm can cause pelvic floor dysfunctions and increase thoracic pressure which often leads to compensation patterns in the lungs and heart—the lungs work harder due to increased resistance during inhalation, and the heart in turn increases blood pressure and heart rate to oxygenate the blood. While manual therapy can be used to release all of the transverse diaphragms, PLWBCs need to be trained to avoid holding their breath while performing stretches and exercises—rather, they should be encouraged to take deep breaths while doing so. This helps avoid compensation patterns, eliminate toxins from the body via expiration, stimulate the deep lymphatics, and engage the parasympathetic nervous system, which helps the body "rest and digest." Added benefits of deep breathing include help easing into and progressing through stretches during yoga, improving flexibility and decreasing pain. It can also help restore and maintain visceral mobility, which helps with spinal alignment. Combined with meditation, it can calm the mind and decrease anxiety and depression. Therefore, deep breathing should be included with every stretch, exercise, and manual release prescribed for the PLWBC.

Exercise Therapy

Neuromuscular Re-Education

Scar tissue can cause muscle inhibition, such that patients may have had to adapt and change their movement patterns for function. Compensation patterns and new habits may have formed out of necessity; however, as recovery progresses proper body mechanics, sequencing, and movement patterns are essential to improve energy efficiency, endurance, strength, and ROM and decrease pain tension. Following scar tissue release, proprioceptive neuromuscular facilitation and yoga can be used to retrain movement patterns and motor sequencing to help coordinate retraining and strengthening. This process is called "structural integration," and it can be very useful with helping patients with balance and coordinated functional movements such as lifting, turning over in bed, transferring from sitting to standing, going up and down stairs, and walking household and community distances.

Proper motor sequencing is crucial to restoring normal movement patterns. The frontal lobe of the brain is in charge of creating motor plans, and it will alter movement patterns when dysfunctions are present. Practicing proper motor sequencing can help the body with proprioceptive retraining, stabilization, and improved balance. Progress into balance exercises to help patient safety during static and dynamic movements follows proper motor sequencing.

Gait Training

After surgery, chemotherapy, and radiation treatments, patients may have restrictions with mobility and need assistive devices such as canes, walkers, ankle-foot orthoses (AFO), heel lifts, or prostheses. For patients to achieve the safest and most energy-efficient gait pattern, extremity and core stabilization exercises and static and dynamic balance exercises must be emphasized. Appropriate fit of the assistive device is essential to ensuring proper gait mechanics and should be evaluated as needed. Compensatory patterns can indicate a poorly fitting AFO or prosthesis, such as a Trendelenburg gait pattern indicating gluteus medius weakness, hip hike or circumduction patterns indicating a leg length discrepancy or poor joint articulations. Joint alignment should be evaluated throughout the gait cycle; the patient should be stable in the stance phase and move properly during the swing phase absent of safety issues. A heel-to-toe gait pattern and a reciprocal arm swing should be encouraged, as these mechanics assist with balance and safety and promote a more energy efficient motor pattern. PLWBCs can be trained in the clinic using walking sticks to help proprioceptive retraining for the reciprocal arm swing and coordination of movements.

Therapeutic Exercise

Therapeutic exercise should include strengthening, flexibility and muscle lengthening, cardiovascular aerobic reconditioning, and endurance training. Onc R clinicians should combine therapeutic exercise with the neuromuscular re-education and prescribe stabilization exercises before initiating mobility exercises. Closed chain exercises assist with eccentric contractions on both sides of the joint to improve stability, and open chain exercises can be used for early strengthening and ROM. It is optimal to avoid compensation patterns with therapeutic exercise. When deconditioning leads to poor core and gluteal muscle recruitment, the body compensates by over-recruiting or substituting using the hip flexors, respiratory diaphragm, hamstrings, hip internal rotators, adductors, pectorals, and anterior cervical and TMJ muscles. This compensatory pattern can lead to straining, spasms, postural and gait deviations, fatigue, and decreased proprioceptive input.

PLWBCs should work on abdominal isometrics in a hook lying position with a resistance band across their thighs to help with their motor sequencing and coordination. The patient then engages their transverse abdominus towards midline, and then towards their spine, while simultaneously keeping their pelvis in neutral and avoiding a posterior pelvic tilt all while not holding their breath. Next, they should pull their ribs down towards their pelvis to recruit their rectus abdominis, and then abduct their knees to recruit their gluteus medius. The key is for their feet to be shoulder width apart, and their knees should be flexed so their heels are resting as close to the gluteals as possible to avoid recruitment and spasms of the hamstrings. Refer to Figure 20.17 for an example of an abdominal isometric. This basic abdominal isometric helps them properly recruit their core and hip stabilizers. Alternating or bilateral shoulder flexion while keeping their core engaged, or bridging progression can be introduced once the isometric sequence is mastered. They should be taught how to keep their core engaged by working on clamshells without allowing spinal rotations. The abdominal isometric with the serratus anterior can help with scapular stabilization and restoring the force couple between the upper trapezius, lower trapezius, and serratus anterior. These exercises assist with stabilization, proprioceptive retraining, and motor recruitment, and they can all be incorporated into the patient's balance, postural, and gait retraining.

Yoga is a great way to incorporate stretches with balance retraining, joint stabilization, and breathing techniques. Yoga also helps to maintain flexibility and improved ROM after manual releases.

Aerobic fitness and the PLWBC's endurance can be improved by slowly increasing their aerobic activity to their tolerance with walking, using the recumbent bike and the upper body ergometer, and incorporating circuit training. In the event of cardiopulmonary comorbidity, breathing exercises and use of an incentive spirometry will provide pulmonary excursion and endurance training. The length of time and the amount of resistance on these should be slowly increased over time to progress aerobic capacity. For additional information regarding exercise prescription, refer to Chapter 23. See Figures 20.17–20.20 for an example of

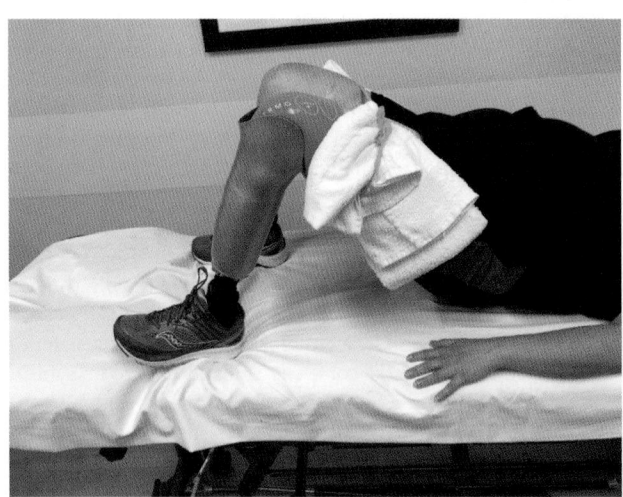

• **Fig. 20.17** A Person Living With and Beyond Cancer (PLWBC) Demonstrating the Abdominal Isometric With Hip Abduction. (Pictures printed with permission by Taire M. Thie, DPT.)

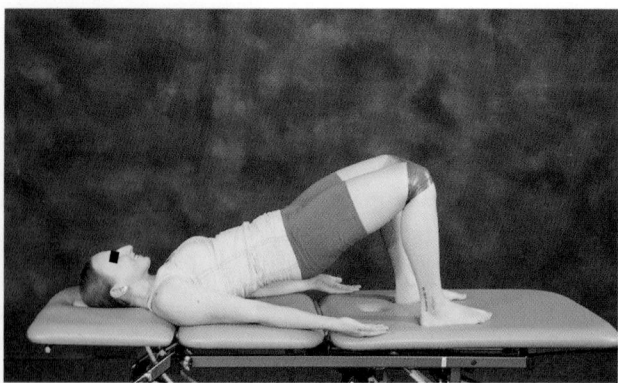

• **Fig. 20.18** Abdominal Isometric With a Bridge. (Photo printed with permission by John Krauss.)

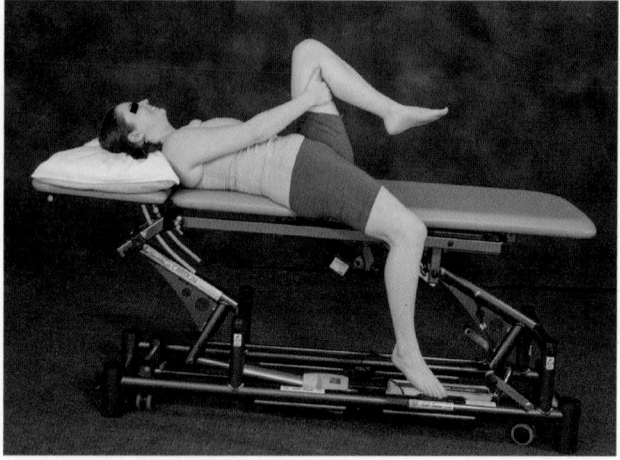

• **Fig. 20.19** Edge of Bed Hip Flexor Stretch. (Photo printed with permission by John Krauss.)

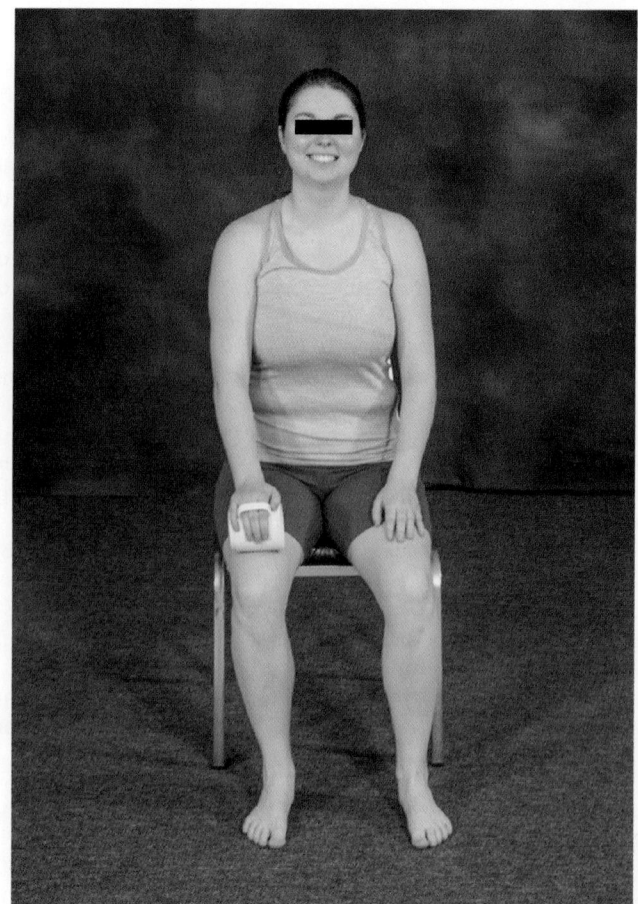

• **Fig. 20.20** Coffee Mug Self Massage. (Photo printed with permission by John Krauss.)

useful exercises that can be used to help reduce pain and improve strength, stabilization, and flexibility.

Conclusion

PLWBCs who have been diagnosed with either a bony or soft tissue sarcoma have a substantial amount of treatment and rehabilitation options. The options described above are only brief descriptions of the interventions available to help this patient population. It is highly recommended to seek out up-to-date research and continuing education courses that are complimentary towards helping each Onc R clinician develop their critical thinking skills and apply the appropriate treatment strategies.

Critical Research Needs

Areas for additional research that were identified during the writing of this chapter include:
• Long term studies children growing up with fascial restrictions causing musculoskeletal compensations after sarcoma and/or muscle resections.
• Fatigue related to scar restrictions after surgical interventions after sarcomas.
• Hyperbaric oxygen chamber therapy in conjunction with physical therapy for recovery after radiation and surgery after sarcomas.

• Using calendula oil versus vitamin E oil post radiation and after surgery for sarcoma patients.
• Discussing patient positioning during radiation to protect their alignment, reduce adhesions, and help prevent radiation fibrosis.
• Using the 6D myofascial release system to promote better tissue/fascial mobility for head, neck and throat cancers, postsurgery, with skin grafts etc. to decrease pain, improve lymphatic drainage, and improve neuromuscular retraining.
• Higher quality studies are needed regarding on how visceral restrictions after surgery, chemotherapy, and radiation cause functional deficits and back pain, and how osteopathic and visceral therapy treatment options can help restore function.

Case Study

A 47-year-old man was diagnosed with a 4.5 cm, grade II fibrosarcoma of the right (R) anterior tibialis. The patient was treated with radiation and surgical resection, followed by six rounds of chemotherapy infusions of doxorubicin, actinomycin D, and ifosfamide. A soleus muscle flap was used to cover the anterior lower 2/3 of his leg while the incision was covered with a split-thickness skin graft mesh harvested from the patient's left (L) anterior thigh. The patient received acute care physical therapy and occupational therapy before being discharged to home therapy, and eventually progressing to outpatient physical therapy for approximately 4.5 months before being discharged. At the time of discharge, he was able to ambulate with a quad cane and fixated AFO.

TABLE 20.13 **Functional Limitations**

Functional Limitation	Evaluation	Progress Note Visit #8	Progress Note Visit #13	Discharge Summary Visit #17
Walking household distances	SD with quad cane; Mild with 2WW	ND with quad cane or 2WW	ND	ND
Walking community distances	Unable with quad cane; SD with 2WW	Mod with quad cane with frequent rests; Mild with 2WW	Mild with quad cane; ND with 2WW	ND
Walking over uneven terrain	Unable with quad cane and 2WW	Unable with quad C cane; Mod with 2WW	Mod with quad cane; ND with 2WW	ND with quad cane
Standing for less than 10 min	Mod with quad cane; Mild with 2WW	Mild with quad cane; None with 2WW	ND	ND
Standing for 10–20 min	SD with quad cane; Mod with 2WW	Mod with quad cane; Mild with 2WW	ND	ND
Standing 20–30 min	Unable with quad cane; SD with 2WW	SD with quad cane; Mod with 2WW	Mild with quad cane; ND with 2WW	ND
Standing 30+ min	Unable with quad cane or 2WW	Unable with quad cane; SD with 2WW	Mild with quad cane; ND with 2WW	ND
Static balance on the R lower extremity	Unable with quad cane or 2WW	SD with quad cane; Mod with 2WW	Mod with quad cane; ND with 2WW	Mild with standard cane
Transferring from sitting to standing	Mod	ND	ND	ND
Driving	Unable	Unable	SD	Mild
Sleeping	SD due to spasms in his R LE waking him 2–3× per night.	Mild due to spasms waking him up intermittently	ND	ND
Turning over in bed	SD	ND	ND	None
Climbing a ladder	Unable	Unable	SD	Mild

Mod, Moderate difficulty; *Mild*, mild difficulty; *ND*, no difficulty; *SD*, significant difficulty; *Unable*, unable to perform the task; *2WW*, two wheeled walker.
Created by Taire M. Thie, DPT. Printed with permission.

The patient returned to outpatient physical therapy a year and 3 months (15 months) post surgery presenting regression in function and severe pain. He presented to therapy with a walker complaining of feeling "a tourniquet" around his lower leg with a constant 6 to 8/10 pain. He reported frequent muscle spasms that affected his sleep, gait, and ability to work. While he exhibited good vascular perfusion and nerve function, the scar tissue was severely restricted and adhered to the soleus and the anterior surface of the tibia. The patient worked as insurance claims adjuster, but was on disability due to his inability to traverse uneven ground, climb a ladder, or stand for prolonged periods.

His functional limitations are recorded in Table 20.13. See Tables 20.13–20.16 for baseline and ensuing objective measurements for range of motion (ROM), strength, scores for the lower extremity functional scale (LEFS), and subjective pain scores.

His goals for therapy were: (1) Return to work; (2) Ambulate with an assistive device over uneven terrain; (3) Return to driving; (4) Tolerate standing for a minimum of 60 minutes without requiring rest; and (5) Sleep through the night without muscle spasms. He was scheduled for treatment 2× per week for 60 minutes for eight sessions, then 1× per week for 60 minutes for the remaining nine sessions.

TABLE 20.14 **Range of Motion (ROM)**

Right Lower Extremity	Initial Evaluation	Progress Note Visit #8	Progress Note Visit #13	Discharge Summary Visit #17
Hip and Knee	WNL	WNL	WNL	WNL
Dorsiflexion	5° PROM/0°AROM	9° PROM/4° AROM	15° PROM & 8°AROM	20° PROM & 15°AROM
Plantar flexion	12° PROM & AROM	20° PROM & AROM	30° PROM & AROM	50° PROM & AROM
Inversion	10° PROM & AROM	18° PROM & AROM	25° PROM & AROM	35° PROM & AROM
Eversion	20° PROM & AROM	20° PROM & AROM	20° PROM & AROM	25° PROM & AROM

AROM, Active range of motion; *PROM*, passive range of motion; *WNL*, within normal limits.
Created by Taire M. Thie, DPT. Printed with permission.

TABLE 20.15   **Manual Muscle Testing for Strength**

Right Lower Extremity	Initial Evaluation	Progress Note Visit #8	Progress Note Visit #13	Discharge Summary Visit #17
Abdominals	3+/5	3+/5	4/5	5/5
Hip flexors	3+/5	3+/5	4/5	5/5
Hip extensors	3+/5	3+/5	4/5	5/5
Hip abductors	3/5	3+/5	4/5	5/5
Hip adductors	5/5	5/5	5/5	5/5
Hip external rotators	3/5	3+/5	4/5	5/5
Hip internal rotators	5/5	5/5	5/5	5/5
Knee flexion	5/5	5/5	5/5	5/5
Knee extension	5/5	5/5	5/5	5/5
Dorsiflexion	1/5	2+/5	3-/5	3+/5
Plantar flexion	2+/5	3/5	3+/5	5/5
Inversion	2+/5	3/5	3+/5	5/5
Eversion	3/5	3/5	3+/5	5/5

Created by Taire M. Thie, DPT. Printed with permission.

TABLE 20.16   **Pain Scales and Lower Extremity Functional Scale (LEFS) Scores**

	Initial Evaluation	Progress Note Visit #8	Progress Note Visit #13	Discharge Summary
LEFS	28/80	40/80	53/80	69/80
Pain intensity 1–10	6–8/10	5/10 (also reported decreased need for pain medications)	2/10, but occasional spasms would increase to 6/10	No pain

Created by Taire M. Thie, DPT. Printed with permission.

TABLE 20.17   **Positional Releases Used During the First 6 Sessions of Outpatient Therapy 15 Months' Postoperation**

Positional Releases	

Supine	• Iliopsoas and Iliacus hip releases over a physioball.
	  • Lumbar traction.
	  • Soft tissue mobilization over the distal iliopsoas, pectineus, hip adductors, and medial gastrocnemius.
	  • Scar mobilizations with manual manipulations and the Lymphatouch.
	  • LLLT.
	• L lower extremity on the ball, R lower extremity extended, hip externally rotated, knee extended, and ankle positioned into dorsiflexion to release scar tissue over the anterior tibia.

Prone	• R hip extended over a wedge, knee in flexion. • Soft tissue mobilization over the R gastrocnemius, hamstrings, piriformis, and quadratus femoris.

L, Left; LLLT, low level laser therapy; R, right.
Created by Taire M. Thie, DPT. Printed with permission.

The therapy goals were to: (1) reduce his pain by improving the mobility and flexibility of his scar tissue; (2) reduce his pain by correcting his alignment; (3) reduce his pain and improve his function by working on core stabilization and gluteus medius and maximus strengthening; (4) improve his ROM with passive ROM and active assisted strengthening; (5) improve his tolerance for standing, (6) improve his functional movement and balance; and (7) discontinue use of fixated AFO and two-wheeled walker.

Sessions 1 to 6, started by using MET called the pubic "shot gun" and R anterior innominate rotation correction, and over the R proximal and distal tibia-fibula joint to improve ROM and standing balance. To decrease fascial tension and the "tourniquet" sensation, positional releases were used in conjunction with the LLLT, the LED laser and the Lymphatouch to mobilize scar, soft tissue, and trigger points. See Table 20.17 for the positional releases used.

The infrared 810 nm low level laser set on a continuous frequency was used for 30 seconds total, one inch (2.54 cm) apart over the border of his scar, to aid in the mobility of his scar tissue, treat trigger points, and decrease his pain.

Edema was addressed by using an LED laser with 850 nm infrared LEDs and 10 mW, 660 nm red light LEDs at 2.5 Hz for 1 minute each from the proximal to distal anterior tibia, over the center portions of the scar to decrease inflammation and improve circulation.

The Lymphatouch fascial cupping system was also used starting over the border of the scar and then progressing to over the center of the scar itself to reduce adhesions and improve pliability. The suction was adjusted to his tolerance anywhere from 20 to 80 mmHg.

After using modalities, manual lymphatic drainage techniques were used starting with the inguinal node and moving distally along his R lower extremity and returning to the proximal starting position. The patient was taught how to continue these techniques at home.

Therapeutic activity focused on adding a heel lift to his L shoe to help balance his alignment in standing and account for the leg length discrepancy resulting from the AFO on his R foot. Bilateral arch support was provided using leukotape placed along the borders of the scar to add tension and stretch the scar when in weight-bearing. He was educated on getting better supporting shoes and purchased over-the-counter wide width Powerstep orthotics and a pair of the Brooks Dyad shoes.

Therapeutic exercises were taught and practiced with the goal of promoting better core recruitment as opposed to using compensation patterns. He was taught and practiced the pelvic brace and abdominal isometric exercises and was provided with a moderate resistance band to help with gluteus medius strengthening.

Sessions 7 to 13 focused on the next several goals of therapy, which included improving his strength and function, along with gentle ROM activities with weight-bearing.

Manual therapy was added in order to stretch and mobilize his scar tissue. A dry brushing technique over his scar was used to improve its tolerance to stimulus, and calendula and wheat germ oil was used for hydration. Contract-relax techniques were used to improve ankle ROM into dorsiflexion and progressed to gentle isometrics. Instrument-assisted friction massage was also used over his right gastrocnemius and peroneal muscles to help with the spasms. Modalities such as the low level laser were added as previously described. The patient was able to tolerate progressing the strength of the suction on the Lymphatouch up to 100 to 120 mmHg.

For therapeutic activity he purchased an Ossur Foot-up orthotic to assist him with dorsiflexion during the gait cycle and allow him to activate his plantar flexors. It was placed in distal portion of his laces to add the maximum amount of assistance. This led to discontinuing use of the two-wheeled walker and progression to exclusively using a quad cane.

The goals for developing his home education program (HEP) was to improve his strength, mobility, balance, stabilization, and endurance. See Table 20.18 for therapeutic exercise and neuromuscular re-education.

During sessions 14 to 16, focus was placed on strengthening, endurance, balance retraining, and improving tolerance for standing and walking. Walking outside over different terrains which included grass, gravel, and small and large inclines was added to the sessions for increased variety and to aid in improving function. He was able to use his quad cane and progressed to using a standard cane by session 16. Heel raises to tolerance were added followed immediately by standing calf stretch using a wooden wedge. The addition of a wooden wedge to carry with the patient upon his return to work was discussed to allow stretching of his calf muscles in the event of spasms. The patient was shown how to use towel rolls, the wooden handle on a shovel, and a mallet to replace the wooden wedge if needed. He was instructed to practice going up and down a ladder at home and to practice driving with his R foot on the accelerator pedal.

At discharge, 19 months' postoperation, the patient reported no functional limitations. He was able to return to driving and ambulating without an assistive device. He was taken off of disability and was able to return to working part time, with the goal of slowly returning to work full time. He no longer had ROM or strength deficits (see Table 20.12 for this summary).

TABLE 20.18	Home Exercise Program
	Pelvic Brace
Sessions 1–6	Abdominal Isometric With Hip Abduction Using a Moderate Resistance Band isometric with hip abduction using a moderate resistance band
Sessions 7–12	Continued original home exercise program Bridges Clamshells Core and hip stabilization with heel slides Bridges without upper extremity support Bridges with manual perturbations (provided by patient's wife) Side lying dorsiflexion for right lower extremity Standing balance for endurance (eyes open, closed, head moving through different motions to challenge his balance) Tandem stance Seated gastrocnemius and soleus towel stretch
Sessions 13–16	Bridges with significant resistance band for abduction Bridges with significant resistance band for abduction with significant resistance band across the hips for added hip extension resistance Clamshells with moderate resistance band Single limb balance with contralateral hip movements into flexion, abduction Dynamic balance training with upper extremity proprioceptive neuromuscular techniques (PNF) diagonals, arm swings, catching a 3 lb (1.4 kg) ball Balance star Heel raises (to tolerance) Standing gastrocnemius and soleus wedge stretch

Created by Taire M. Thie, DPT. Printed with permission.

Review Questions

Reader can find the correct answers and rationale in the back of the book.

1. Deshawn is a 14-year-old male, diagnosed with stage 3 Ewing sarcoma in his R femur. He had neo-adjuvant chemotherapy and was treated with vincristine (Oncovin, Vincasar PFS), doxorubicin (Adriamycin), and cyclophosphamide (Cytoxan) for 9 weeks before and after surgery. Limb sparing surgery was performed. He reports to therapy 1.5 years after surgery with difficulty walking, going up and down stairs, and pain 6/10 in his R groin, bilateral SI joints, and lower back. His X-rays are unremarkable. Which of the following is MOST likely to be causing his pain?

   A. He has aseptic loosening of his endoprosthesis

   B. His alignment of his pelvis is off causing increased pain in his back and hips

   C. He likely has a secondary sarcoma that wasn't found on the X-ray and he needs an MRI

   D. He is having neuropathic pain as an adverse effect from his chemotherapy
   Rationale: Signs of aseptic loosening include: feeling unstable, increased pain at the bone/prosthetic articulation and signs of fracture or bone loss on imaging. His images were clear, and he was having more global pain versus focused pain at the prosthetic articulation. Bone sarcomas can usually be seen on X-ray as they cause osteolysis of the bone. His images were clear. Neuropathic pain does not cause global pain up into the spine.

2. Violet is a 69-year-old female with a prior medical history of grade 2 chondrosarcoma of the left glenohumeral joint diagnosed and treated 3 years ago. She had surgery to remove the tumor and adjuvant radiation therapy. She is returning to therapy with a gradual onset and worsening of stiffness, edema, and decreased ROM in her left shoulder. She says that her left arm feels very heavy, and that the tension and weight increase throughout the day. She notes difficulty with dressing, doing her hair, sleeping, cleaning, and picking up her grandchildren. Imaging has ruled out a reoccurrence of cancer. Which of the following should be included in your plan of care?

   A. Plyometric exercises to increase her tolerance for weight bearing and activity

   B. Send her to an orthopedic specialist for joint injections for adhesive capsulitis

   C. Refer her to a lymphedema specialist for assessment

   D. Refer her to a cardiologist to rule out cardiomyopathy and increased risk of heart attack
   Rationale: While she had edema and swelling and symptoms in her left arm, they are not consistent with symptoms of cardiomyopathy, which has swelling of the lower extremities, and symptoms of fainting, fatigue, and changes in heart rhythm. Onset of lymphedema can take place any time after surgery and other treatment interventions.

3. Charlie is a 17-year-old male, who was diagnosed with osteosarcoma at the age of 14. He was treated with chemotherapy to reduce tumor size. Two years ago, patient underwent a transfemoral amputation with a flap. With therapy, he was able to walk with a prosthetic, and discontinued using any other assistive device. He is returning to therapy 24 months after surgery with a chief complaint of pain and irritation in his residual limb with use of his prosthetic. He describes

difficulty with standing, balance, walking, and doing stairs. He says that the pain is gone when he takes the prosthetic off, but immediately returns when he puts the prosthetic on. What is likely contributing to his pain?

   A. He has neuropathic pain causing tingling and numbness in his residual limb

   B. He has outgrown his prosthetic socket and needs to be measured for a new one

   C. He has weakness in his hip extensors and abductors and needs strengthening

   D. He has an infection in his residual limb and needs to be put on antibiotics
   Rationale: While difficulty with function can occur with neuropathic pain, those are not consistent with pain that goes away when the prosthetic is taken off. Weakness in his hips might contribute to functional limitations, but again would not relieve his pain if his prosthetic is taken off. If he had an infection in his limb, he would have other signs and symptoms such as edema, fever, and severe pain. As a growing young man, he might be experiencing growth spurts, weight gain, or leg length differences that are causing him to have pain in his residual limb when wearing his prosthetic.

4. Danielle is a 62-year-old female diagnosed with a GIST on the left anterior and inferior surface of her stomach, pyloric sphincter, and duodenum. It was surgically removed and treated with radiation. She was also put on imatinib (Gleevec). The GIST tumor returned 5 years later and was found on her distal ileum and large omentum. They repeated the surgery and radiation and underwent internal heated chemotherapy. She has a small, but restricted scar in her L upper abdomen, and a large scar in her lower abdomen from her umbilicus down to her pubic symphysis. She is reporting to therapy 3 years after her most recent surgery with significant pain in her back, hips, and ribs. She has fallen three times in the past 6 months. She notes shortness of breath, and pain with standing, ambulation, and bed mobility. Which technique should the clinician start with to help her with her pain and function?

   A. Scar releases, with manual therapy, fascial releases, and modalities such as the low level laser and 6D fascial release system

   B. Aquatic therapy for back decompression and balance retraining

   C. Manual therapy using high velocity, low amplitude mobilizations to improve her joint mobility for her ribs, spine, pelvis, and hips

   D. Balance star exercises
   Rationale: Scar releases with manual fascial releases and modalities is the best choice for starting her treatment sessions. Scars can impair muscle function, alignment, balance, and cause significant pain and restrictions. High velocity, low amplitude mobilizations are grade 5 mobilizations and should not be used. Aquatic therapy for back decompression and balance retraining is a great treatment option but should be used later on in her plan of care.

5. Gerimo is a 50-year-old man reporting to physical therapy for his initial evaluation 8 months after limb sparing surgery with bone autograft covered with a pedicle flap for a stage 3

Fibrosarcoma in his R lower extremity. He has had inpatient, home and one course of outpatient physical therapy. He said he is doing well but reports constant fatigue and lack of confidence in stability to perform prolonged activities. He denies falls but reports feeling off balance and a buckling sensation. Which of the following is MOST appropriate to be included in your initial screening?

A. Educating him on cognitive and psychological strategies to help him accept his new leg and get over the stress of surgery and learn how to trust his limb again

B. Check his strength, leg length, scar mobility, and look for compensation patterns

C. Check his cranial nerves, dermatomes, myotomes, and check for a stroke

D. Check his ROM, and vestibular system for impairments
Rationale: Compensation patterns can be exhausting as they can change motor patterns, inhibit muscles, and can cause balance issues. A leg length difference and muscle weakness can contribute to his feeling of being off balance. While educating patients is highly valued and may need to be addressed at some point, the initial evaluation is not the optimal time to start addressing this. While the nerve assessments are a part of the systems review, they are not necessary at this time, and nothing indicates that he had a stroke. He does not note dizziness with his feeling off balance, so vestibular assessments would not be a high priority to screen.

6. Signs and symptoms of phantom limb pain include:
A. Pressure ulcers, scars that will not heal, and bruises
B. Muscle spasms, difficulty breathing, and edema
C. Fever and throbbing pain
D. Tingling and numbness, sensations of itching, sharp/shooting pain, feeling like the limb is still present
Rationale: After the limb is amputated, the nerves that are trying to regenerate have no place to go. The axons can become trapped in the scar tissue and create significant pain or phantom sensations.

7. Common compensation patterns secondary due to fascial restrictions include:
A. Holding their breath while trying to recruit their core, over recruiting their hip flexors to compensate for abdominal weakness, using a posterior pelvic tilt while trying to engage the transverse abdominis
B. Using an assistive device, and orthotics
C. Hyperventilation, phantom limb pain, and loss of balance
D. Recruiting the pelvic floor to help recruit the hip flexors, engaging the serratus anterior, multifidus and rotatores for cervical rotation, and hyperextending the knees to preserve balance

Rationale: Compensation patterns are often used as substitutions for areas that exhibit weakness or loss of function. Releasing the fascial restriction and avoiding compensation patterns can restore function and reduce pain, fatigue, and spasms.

8. Target muscle reinnervation is used for:
A. Fascial restrictions
B. Radicular nerve pain
C. Phantom limb and neuropathic pain
D. Cranial nerve stimulation
Rationale: Target muscle reinnervation is a surgical procedure that finds the nerve responsible for phantom limb pain, locates another nerve close by and has it donate a motor point to give to the hypersensitive nerve. This allows the nerve to heal.

9. Graded motor imagery includes which of the following to help with sensorimotor retraining after amputations or limb salvage surgeries.
A. Coordination retraining with neuroplasticity
B. Left and Right Discrimination, Explicit Motor Imagery, Mirror Therapy to help with phantom limb pain
C. Graded strengthening with virtual reality to meet patient goals to return to functional activities
D. Using different slopes or "grades" for motor planning with ambulation and gait retraining
Rationale: Graded motor imagery is three sequential phases that help retrain the brain to recognize between the right and left sides of the body with all of its individual parts and uses repetitive training to help improve speed and accuracy. Then it assists with concentrated and explicit motor imagery where the PLWBC is taught how to think through all of the different parts of a task and mentally perform the task in their mind in an organized fashion. The final phase includes mirror therapy that helps the PLWBC perceive their lost limb as being present by presenting an image of it using mirrors and the intact extremity.

10. The goals for an endoprosthesis are
A. Osteoinduction, osteoconduction, osseous integration
B. Osteoporosis and osteopenia prevention
C. Prevent endosteal scalloping for PLWBC with chondrosarcomas
D. Using a 3D printer to create assistive devices such as walkers, canes, orthotics to help with functional movements
Rationale: The goals for an endoprosthesis are osteoinduction (stimulation of new cell growth), osteoconduction (cells starting to form new bone), and osseous integration (the bone grafts integrating through a creeping phenomenon in which the allograft, composite, and residual bone grow together and intertwine).

References

1. American Cancer Society. Cancer facts & figures 2020. https://www.cancer.org/content/dam/cancer-org/research/cancer-facts-and-statistics/annual-cancer-facts-and-figures/2020/cancer-facts-and-figures-2020.pdf. Accessed March 1, 2021.
2. Mariotto AB, Siegel RL, Lin CC, et al. Cancer treatment and survivorship statistics, 2014. *CA Cancer J Clin.* 2014;64(4):252–271.
3. PDQ® Adult Treatment Editorial Board. PDQ Soft Tissue Sarcoma Treatment. Bethesda, MD: *National Cancer Institute.* Updated 2015. Available at https://www.cancer.gov/types/soft-tissue-sarcoma/hp/adult-soft-tissue-treatment-pdq. Accessed 03/01/2021.
4. Nystrom LM, Reimer NB, Reith JD, et al. Multidisciplinary management of soft tissue sarcoma. *Sci World J.* 2013:852462. doi:10.1155/2013/852462.

5. Amankwah EK, Conley AP, Reed DR. Epidemiology and therapies for metastatic sarcoma. *Clin Epidemiol.* 2013;5(1):147–162.

6. Princic N, McMorrow D, Chan P, Hess L. Evaluation of the accuracy of algorithms to identify soft tissue sarcoma (STS) in administrative claims. *Clin Sarcoma Res.* 2020;10(1):1–9.

7. O'Neill JP, Bilsky MH, Kraus D. Head and neck sarcomas: epidemiology, pathology, and management. *Neurosurg Clin N Am.* 2013;24(1):67–78.

8. Breakey RWF, Crowley TP, Anderson IB, Milner RH, Ragbir M. The surgical management of head and neck sarcoma: the Newcastle experience. *J Plast Reconstr Aesthetic Surg.* 2017;70(1):78–84.

9. Neragi-Miandoab S, Kim J, Vlahakes GJ. Malignant tumours of the heart: a review of tumour type, diagnosis and therapy. *Clin Oncol.* 2007;19(10):748–756.

10. Waszczynskyi CHS de O, Guimarães MD, Franco LFS, Hochhegger B, Marchiori E. Primary undifferentiated sarcoma in the thorax: a rare diagnosis in young patients. *Radiol Bras.* 2016;49(6):409–410.

11. Levy AD, Manning MA, Al-Refaie WB, Miettinen MM. Soft-tissue sarcomas of the abdomen and pelvis: radiologic-pathologic features, part 1—common sarcomas: from the radiologic pathology archives. *RadioGraphics.* 2017;37(2):462–483.

12. Levy AD, Manning MA, Miettinen MM. Soft-tissue sarcomas of the abdomen and pelvis: radiologic-pathologic features, part 2—uncommon sarcomas. *RadioGraphics.* 2017;37(3):797–812.

13. American Cancer Society. About soft tissue sarcomas. https://www.cancer.org/cancer/soft-tissue-sarcoma/about/key-statistics.html. Accessed March 1, 2021.

14. Siegel RL, Miller KD, Jemal A. Cancer statistics, 2020. *CA Cancer J Clin.* 2020;70(1):7–30.

15. PDQ Adult Treatment Editorial Board. Adult soft tissue sarcoma treatment (PDQ®): patient version; 2002. https://pubmed.ncbi.nlm.nih.gov/26389216/. Accessed March 2021.

16. PDQ Pediatric Treatment Editorial Board. Childhood Soft Tissue Sarcoma Treatment (PDQ®): Health Professional Version. [June 9, 2020]. In: *PDQ Cancer Information Summaries* [Internet]. National Cancer Institute (US); 2002. https://www.ncbi.nlm.nih.gov/books/NBK65923/. Accessed March 1, 2021.

17. National Cancer Institute Surveillance, Epidemiology, and End Results Program. Bone and Joint Cancer. Cancer stat facts. https://seer.cancer.gov/statfacts/html/bones.html. Accessed November 10, 2020.

18. Nagar SP, Mytelka DS, Candrilli SD, et al. Treatment patterns and survival among adult patients with advanced soft tissue sarcoma: a retrospective medical record review in the United Kingdom, Spain, Germany, and France. *Sarcoma.* 2018:5467057.

19. Grimer R, Judson I, Peake D, Seddon B. Guidelines for the management of soft tissue sarcomas. *Sarcoma.* 2010;2010:506182.

20. Kirsanov KI, Lesovaya EA, Fetisov TI, Bokhyan BY, Belitsky GA, Yakubovskaya MG. Current approaches for personalized therapy of soft tissue sarcomas. *Sarcoma.* 2020:6716742. doi:10.1155/2020/6716742.

21. Dickie C, O'Sullivan B. Soft tissue sarcoma. *Med Radiol.* 2015;67:515–530.

22. PDQ Pediatric Treatment Editorial Board. Ewing Sarcoma Treatment (PDQ®): Health Professional Version; 2002. https://www.cancer.gov/types/bone/patient/ewing-treatment-pdq#:~:text=in%20younger%20patients.-,Signs%20and%20symptoms%20of%20Ewing%20sarcoma%20include%20swelling%20and%20pain,chest%2C%20back%2C%20or%20pelvis. Accessed March 1, 2021.

23. Choi EYK, Gardner JM, Lucas DR, McHugh JB, Patel RM. Ewing sarcoma. *Semin Diagn Pathol.* 2014;31(1):39–47.

24. Gaspar N, Hawkins DS, Dirksen U, et al. Ewing sarcoma: current management and future approaches through collaboration. *J Clin Oncol.* 2015;33(27):3036–3046.

25. Folkert IW, Devalaraja S, Linette GP, Weber K, Haldar M. Primary bone tumors: challenges and opportunities for CAR-T therapies. *J Bone Miner Res.* 2019;34(10):1780–1788.

26. Soft Tissue Sarcoma—Symptoms and Causes. Mayo clinic. https://www.mayoclinic.org/diseases-conditions/soft-tissue-sarcoma/symptoms-causes/syc-20377725. Accessed September 25, 2020.

27. Soft Tissue Sarcomas. NHS. https://www.nhs.uk/conditions/soft-tissue-sarcoma/. Accessed October 11, 2020.

28. American Academy of Orthopaedic Surgeons. Chondrosarcoma. OrthoInfo—AAOS. https://orthoinfo.aaos.org/en/diseases-conditions/chondrosarcoma/. Accessed October 14, 2020.

29. Reed DR, Hayashi M, Wagner L, et al. Treatment pathway of bone sarcoma in children, adolescents, and young adults. *Cancer.* 2017;123(12):2206–2218.

30. Widhe B, Widhe T. Initial symptoms and clinical features in osteosarcoma and Ewing sarcoma. *J Bone Jt Surg Ser A.* 2000;82(5):667–674.

31. Allison DC, Carney SC, Ahlmann ER, et al. A meta-analysis of osteosarcoma outcomes in the modern medical era. *Sarcoma.* 2012:704872. doi:10.1155/2012/704872.

32. Carina V, Costa V, Sartori M, et al. Adjuvant biophysical therapies in osteosarcoma. *Cancers (Basel).* 2019;11(3):348. doi:10.3390/cancers11030348.

33. Longhi A, Ferrari S, Tamburini A, et al. Late effects of chemotherapy and radiotherapy in osteosarcoma and Ewing sarcoma patients: The Italian Sarcoma Group Experience (1983–2006). *Cancer.* 2012;118(20):5050–5059.

34. Jackson TM, Bittman M, Granowetter L. Pediatric malignant bone tumors: a review and update on current challenges, and emerging drug targets. *Curr Probl Pediatr Adolesc Health Care.* 2016;46(7):213–228.

35. Ludwig J. Ewing sarcoma family of tumors *Bone Cancer: Primary Bone Cancers and Bone Metastases.* 2nd ed., Elsevier Inc., 2015.

36. Grünewald TGP, Cidre-Aranaz F, Surdez D, et al. Ewing sarcoma. *Nat Rev Dis Prim.* 2018;4(1):5. doi:10.1038/s41572-018-0003-x.

37. Wang Z, Chen G, Chen X, et al. Predictors of the survival of patients with chondrosarcoma of bone and metastatic disease at diagnosis. *J Cancer.* 2019;10(11):2457–2463.

38. Yuan Z, Yu M, Shen K, et al. Uterine adenosarcoma: a retrospective 12-year single-center study. *Front Oncol.* 2019;9:237. doi:10.3389/fonc.2019.00237.

39. Nathenson MJ, Ravi V, Fleming N, Wang WL, Conley A. Uterine adenosarcoma: a review. *Curr Oncol Rep.* 2016;18(11):68. doi:10.1007/s11912-016-0552-7.

40. Ricci S, Stone RL, Fader AN. Uterine leiomyosarcoma: epidemiology, contemporary treatment strategies and the impact of uterine morcellation. *Gynecol Oncol.* 2017;145(1):208–216.

41. National Cancer Institute. Treating uterine sarcomas. https://www.cancer.org/cancer/uterine-sarcoma/treating/by-stage.html. November 13, 2017. Accessed May 15, 2021.

42. Neragi-Miandoab S, Kim J, Vlahakes GJ. Malignant tumours of the heart: a review of tumour type, diagnosis and therapy. *Clin Oncol.* 2007;19(10):748–756.

43. National Cancer Institute. Angiosarcoma. https://www.cancer.gov/pediatric-adult-rare-tumor/rare-tumors/rare-vascular-tumors/angiosarcoma. Accessed March 1, 2021.

44. Augsburger D, Nelson PJ, Kalinski T, et al. Current diagnostics and treatment of fibrosarcoma: perspectives for future therapeutic targets and strategies. *Oncotarget.* 2017;8(61):104638–104653.

45. PDQ Pediatric Treatment Editorial Board. Childhood soft tissue sarcoma treatment (PDQ®): health professional version. http://www.ncbi.nlm.nih.gov/pubmed/26389361. 2002. Accessed March 1, 2021.

46. Dickey I, Floyd JG. Fibrosarcoma. Medscape emedicine. https://emedicine.medscape.com/article/1257520/2020. Accessed September 14, 2020.

47. Alghamdi H, Amr S, Shawarby M, et al. Gastrointestinal stromal tumors: a clinicopathological study. *Saudi Med J.* 2019;40(2):126–130.

48. Laurent M, Brahmi M, Dufresne A, et al. Adjuvant therapy with imatinib in gastrointestinal stromal tumors (GISTs)—review and perspectives. *Transl Gastroenterol Hepatol.* 2019;4:24–24.

49. Ozkan EE. Radiotherapy for gastrointestinal stromal tumors. *Chin Med J (Engl)*. 2018;131(2):235–240.

50. National Cancer Institute. Childhood gastrointestinal stromal tumors treatment PDQ. https://www.cancer.gov/types/soft-tissue-sarcoma/hp/child-gist-treatment-pdq. October 22, 2019. Accessed May 15, 2021.

51. Van Houdt WJ, Zaidi S, Messiou C, Thway K, Strauss DC, Jones RL. Treatment of retroperitoneal sarcoma: current standards and new developments. *Curr Opin Oncol*. 2017;29(4):260–267.

52. Greto D, Saieva C, Loi M, et al. Influence of age and subtype in outcome of operable liposarcoma. *Radiol Medica*. 2019;124(4):290–300.

53. Knebel C, Lenze U, Pohlig F, et al. Prognostic factors and outcome of liposarcoma patients: a retrospective evaluation over 15 years. *BMC Cancer*. 2017;17(1):410.

54. National Cancer Institute. Malignant peripheral nerve sheath tumor. https://www.cancer.gov/pediatric-adult-rare-tumor/rare-tumors/rare-soft-tissue-tumors/mpnst. Accessed September 14, 2020.

55. National Cancer Institute. Childhood rhabdomyosarcoma treatmen (PDQ)—patient version. https://www.cancer.gov/types/soft-tissue-sarcoma/patient/rhabdomyosarcoma-treatment-pdq. December 22, 2020. Accessed May 15, 2021.

56. Soft Tissue Cancer. Cancer stat facts. https://seer.cancer.gov/statfacts/html/soft.html. Accessed October 14, 2020.

57. Mai PL, Best AF, Peters JA, et al. Risks of first and subsequent cancers among TP53 mutation carriers in the National Cancer Institute Li-Fraumeni syndrome cohort. *Cancer*. 2016;122(23):3673–3681.

58. Bone and Joint Cancer. Cancer stat facts. https://seer.cancer.gov/statfacts/html/bones.html. Accessed October 11, 2020.

59. Schonfeld SJ, Merino DM, Curtis RE, et al. Risk of second primary bone and soft-tissue sarcomas among young adulthood cancer survivors. *JNCI Cancer Spectr*. 2019;3(3):pkz043. doi:10.1093/jncics/pkz043.

60. Wibmer C, Leithner A, Zielonke N, Sperl M, Windhager R. Increasing incidence rates of soft tissue sarcomas? A population-based epidemiologic study and literature review. *Ann Oncol*. 2009;21(5):1106–1111.

61. PDQ Adult Treatment Editorial Board. Uterine sarcoma treatment (PDQ®): patient version. PDQ cancer information summaries. http://www.ncbi.nlm.nih.gov/pubmed/26389379; June 12, 2019. Accessed October 14, 2020.

62. Cates JMM. The AJCC 8th edition staging system for soft tissue sarcoma of the extremities or trunk: a cohort study of the SEER database. *J Natl Compr Cancer Netw*. 2018;16(2):144–152.

63. Tumor Grade Fact Sheet. National Cancer Institute. https://www.cancer.gov/about-cancer/diagnosis-staging/prognosis/tumor-grade-fact-sheet. Accessed October 14, 2020.

64. Definition of Low Grade. NCI Dictionary of Cancer Terms. National Cancer Institute. https://www.cancer.gov/publications/dictionaries/cancer-terms/def/low-grade. Accessed October 14, 2020.

65. Paoluzzi L, Maki RG. Diagnosis, prognosis, and treatment of alveolar soft-part sarcoma. *JAMA Oncol*. 2019;5(2):254–260.

66. Steen S, Stephenson G. Current treatment of soft tissue sarcoma. *Baylor Univ Med Cent Proc*. 2008;21(4):392–396.

67. Smrke A, Wang Y, Simmons C. Update on systemic therapy for advanced soft-tissue sarcoma. *Curr Oncol*. 2020;27(Suppl 1):25–33.

68. Schwartz A, Rebecca A, Smith A, et al. Risk factors for significant wound complications following wide resection of extremity soft tissue sarcomas. *Clin Orthop Relat Res*. 2013;471(11):3612–3617.

69. Götzl R, Sterzinger S, Arkudas A, et al. The role of plastic reconstructive surgery in surgical therapy of soft tissue sarcomas. *Cancers (Basel)*. 2020;12(12):3534. doi:10.3390/cancers12123534.

70. Yao W, Cai Q, Wang J, et al. Biological reconstruction in the treatment of extremity sarcoma in femur, tibia, and humerus. *Medicine (Baltimore)*. 2020;99(27):e20715. doi:10.1097/MD.0000000000020715.

71. San-Julian M, Vazquez-Garcia B. biological reconstruction in bone sarcomas: lessons from three decades of experience. *Orthop Surg*. 2016;8(2):111–121.

72. López JF, Hietanen KE, Kaartinen IS, et al. Primary flap reconstruction of tissue defects after sarcoma surgery enables curative treatment with acceptable functional results: a 7-year review. *BMC Surg*. 2015;15(1):71. doi:10.1186/s12893-015-0060-y.

73. Spera LJ, Danforth RM, Pittelkow E, Hadad I. A review of local soft tissue coverage options for oncologic defects of the distal lower extremity. *Oper Tech Orthop*. 2020;30(2):100802. doi:10.1016/j.oto.2020.100802.

74. Wang C-S, Wu P-K, Chen C-F, Chen W-M, Liu C-L, Chen T-H. Bone–prosthesis composite with rotating hinged-knee prosthesis in limb salvage surgery for high-grade sarcoma around the knee. *J Arthroplasty*. 2015;30(1):90–94.

75. Lu Y, Chen G, Long Z, et al. Novel 3D-printed prosthetic composite for reconstruction of massive bone defects in lower extremities after malignant tumor resection. *J Bone Oncol*. 2019;16:100220. doi:10.1016/j.jbo.2019.100220.

76. Guo W. Using 3D printing endoprosthesis for reconstruction after resection of bone tumor. *Chinese J Orthop*. 2020;40(12):755–759.

77. Irtan S, Hervieux E, Boutroux H, et al. Preoperative 3D reconstruction images for paediatric tumours: Advantages and drawbacks. *Pediatr Blood Cancer*. 2020;68(1):e28670. doi:10.1002/pbc.28670.

78. Xu N, Wei F, Liu X, et al. Reconstruction of the upper cervical spine using a personalized 3D-printed vertebral body in an adolescent with ewing sarcoma. *Spine (Phila Pa 1976)*. 2016;41(1):E50–E54. doi:10.1097/BRS.0000000000001179.

79. Smolle MA, Andreou D, Tunn PU, Leithner A. Advances in tumour endoprostheses: a systematic review. *EFORT Open Rev*. 2019;4(7):445–459.

80. Gautam D, Malhotra R. Megaprosthesis versus allograft prosthesis composite for massive skeletal defects. *J Clin Orthop Trauma*. 2018;9(1):63–80.

81. Grimsrud C, Killen C, Murphy M, Wang H, McGarry S. Long-term outcomes of rotationplasty patients in the treatment of lower extremity sarcomas with cost analysis. *J Clin Orthop Trauma*. 2020;11:S149–S152.

82. Benedetti MG, Coli M, Campanacci L, Manfrini M. Postural control skills, proprioception, and risk of fall in long-term survivor patients treated with knee rotationplasty. *Int J Rehabil Res*. 2019;42(1):68–73.

83. Compston AM, Zak J, Alexander JH, et al. Rotationplasty rehabilitation protocol: a complex case report. *Rehabil Oncol*. 2020;38(2):E32–E40.

84. Mahmoud A, Aboujaib MF, Meda MR. Long-term follow-up of patients with rotationplasty. *Int J Surg Case Rep*. 2021;79:295–298.

85. Bernthal NM, Monument MJ, Lor Randall R, Jones KB. Rotationplasty: beauty is in the eye of the beholder. *Oper Tech Orthop*. 2014;24(2):103–110.

86. Lim CY, Katagiri H, Murata H, et al. Solution to a complex problem after failed limb salvage surgery of the distal femur: a case report describing the tibial turn-up procedure. *J Orthop Sci*. 2019;S0949-2658(19)30267-2. doi: 10.1016/j.jos.2019.08.016.

87. Kaur A, Guan Y. Phantom limb pain: a literature review. *Chinese J Traumatol English Ed*. 2018;21(6):366–368.

88. Dumanian GA, Potter BK, Mioton LM, et al. Targeted muscle reinnervation treats neuroma and phantom pain in major limb amputees. *Ann Surg*. 2019;270(2):238–246.

89. Mioton LM, Dumanian GA. Targeted muscle reinnervation and prosthetic rehabilitation after limb loss. *J Surg Oncol*. 2018;118(5):807–814.

90. Chappell AG, Jordan SW, Dumanian GA. Targeted muscle reinnervation for treatment of neuropathic pain. *Clin Plast Surg*. 2020;47(2):285–293.

91. Punzalan M, Hyden G. The role of physical therapy and occupational therapy in the rehabilitation of pediatric and adolescent patients with osteosarcoma. *Cancer Treat Res*. 2009;152:367–384.

92. Ramu EM, Houdek MT, Isaac CE, Dickie CI, Ferguson PC, Wunder JS. Management of soft-tissue sarcomas; treatment strategies, staging, and outcomes. *SICOT-J.* 2017;3:20.

93. Butler D, Moseley L, Beames T, Giles T. *The Graded Motor Imagery Handbook*: NOI Group; 2012. http://www.gradedmotorimagery.com/. Accessed February 4, 2021.

94. Robijns J, Censabella S, Bulens P, Maes A, Mebis J. The use of low-level light therapy in supportive care for patients with breast cancer: review of the literature. *Lasers Med Sci.* 2017;32(1):229–242.

95. Rezk-Allah SS, Elshafi HMA, Farid RJ, Hassan MAE, Alsirafy SA. Effect of low-level laser therapy in treatment of chemotherapy induced oral mucositis. *J Lasers Med Sci.* 2019;10(2):125–130.

96. Freitas CP, Melo C, Alexandrino AM, Noites A. Efficacy of low-level laser therapy on scar tissue. *J Cosmet Laser Ther.* 2013;15(3):171–176.

97. Thomas E, Cavallaro AR, Mani D, Bianco A, Palma A. The efficacy of muscle energy techniques in symptomatic and asymptomatic subjects: a systematic review. *Chiropr Man Therap.* 2019;27(1):35. doi:10.1186/s12998-019-0258-7.

98. Nagrale AV, Glynn P, Joshi A, Ramteke G. The efficacy of an integrated neuromuscular inhibition technique on upper trapezius trigger points in subjects with non-specific neck pain: a randomized controlled trial. *J Man Manip Ther.* 2010;18(1):37–43.

99. Bordoni B. The five diaphragms in osteopathic manipulative medicine: myofascial relationships, part 1. *Cureus.* 2020;12(4):e7794. doi:10.7759/cureus.7794.

100. Bordoni B, Marelli F, Morabito B, Sacconi B, Caiazzo P, Castagna R. Low back pain and gastroesophageal reflux in patients with COPD: the disease in the breath. *Int J COPD.* 2018;13:325–334.

101. Haller H, Lauche R, Cramer H, et al. Craniosacral therapy for the treatment of chronic neck pain. *Clin J Pain.* 2016;32(5):441–449.

102. Haller H, Lauche R, Sundberg T, Dobos G, Cramer H. Craniosacral therapy for chronic pain: a systematic review and meta-analysis of randomized controlled trials. *BMC Musculoskelet Disord.* 2020;21(1):1. doi:10.1186/s12891-019-3017-y.

103. Matarán-Peñarrocha GA, Castro-Sánchez AM, García GC, Moreno-Lorenzo C, Carreño TP, Zafra MDO. Influence of craniosacral therapy on anxiety, depression and quality of life in patients with fibromyalgia. *Evidence-Based Complement Altern Med.* 2011;2011:1–9.

104. Castro-Sánchez AM, Lara-Palomo IC, Matarán-Peñarrocha GA, Saavedra-Hernández M, Pérez-Mármol JM, Aguilar-Ferrándiz ME. Benefits of craniosacral therapy in patients with chronic low back pain: a randomized controlled trial. *J Altern Complement Med.* 2016;22(8):650–657.

105. Barral J-P, Mercier P. *Visceral Manipulation*. Revised ed. Eastland Press; 2006.

106. Barral J-P. *Visceral Manipulation II*. Revised ed. Eastland Press; 2007.

107. Lagrange A, Decoux D, Briot N, et al. Visceral osteopathic manipulative treatment reduces patient reported digestive toxicities induced by adjuvant chemotherapy in breast cancer: A randomized controlled clinical study. *Eur J Obstet Gynecol Reprod Biol.* 2019;241:49–55.

108. Silva AC de O, Biasotto-Gonzalez DA, Oliveira FHM, et al. Effect of osteopathic visceral manipulation on pain, cervical range of motion, and upper trapezius muscle activity in patients with chronic nonspecific neck pain and functional dyspepsia: a randomized, double-blind, placebo-controlled pilot study. *Evidence-Based Complement Altern Med.* 2018;2018:1–9.

109. Monstrey S, Middelkoop E, Vranckx JJ, et al. Updated scar management practical guidelines: non-invasive and invasive measures. *J Plast Reconstr Aesthetic Surg.* 2014;67(8):1017–1025.

110. Hautmann G, Mastrolorenzo A, Menchini G, Lotti TM. (2003) Keloids and hypertrophic scars. In: Katsambas A.D., Lotti T.M. (eds) *European Handbook of Dermatological Treatments.* Springer, Berlin, Heidelberg. https://link.springer.com/chapter/10.1007/978-3-662-07131-1_46.

111. Karwacińska J, Kiebzak W, Stepanek-Finda B, et al. Effectiveness of Kinesio Taping on hypertrophic scars, keloids and scar contractures. *Polish Ann Med.* 2012;19(1):50–57.

112. Zurada JM, Kriegel D, Davis IC. Topical treatments for hypertrophic scars. *J Am Acad Dermatol.* 2006;55(6):1024–1031.

21

Hematological Cancers

AMANI ALJOHI, PT, MSc, KELLY CHAPLIN, PT, DPT, CLT

CHAPTER OUTLINE

Introduction

Hematologic diseases are a varied heterogenetic group of malignancies raised up from hematopoietic tissue that affect people worldwide such as leukemia, lymphoma, and multiple myelomas. This category of cancers can be quite aggressive and vary in their clinical presentation. This chapter will review the medical and physical presentation for people living with and beyond hematological cancer to assist the oncology rehabilitation (Onc R) clinician in providing quality care.

Leukemia

Leukemia is a type of hematological malignancy that describes the production of abnormal numbers of and dysfunctional white blood cells. This disease is classified into several categories relative to how quickly it develops and what type of cell is involved. The type of leukemia is named based on which cell line the malignancy originates from.[1]

Types of Leukemia and Risk Factors

There were 474,519 new leukemia cases diagnosed globally in 2020, with a global mortality of 311,594 (3.1%).[2] Acute leukemia includes acute myeloid leukemia (AML), acute lymphoblastic leukemia (ALL), and acute promyelocytic leukemia (APL), and is characterized by the presence of blasts in the blood and tissues. AML is the most common form of acute leukemia in adults, typically presents in those over 65 years of age,[3,4] and is more common in males than females.[4] AML has the highest number of annual deaths of all leukemia diagnoses.[3] ALL is the most common form of childhood leukemia (aged 21 and younger) and is uncommon in adults.[1] ALL accounts for 35% of all pediatric cancers, and 80% are B cell precursors.[5] APL is another form of acute leukemia with a high cure rate when therapy is initiated quickly.[6] APL occurs with a genetic mutation that stops cell differentiation into neutrophil granulocytes, so they remain as promyelocytes (for details see Table 21.1).[7]

Chronic leukemia occurs more commonly in adults and includes chronic myeloid leukemia (CML) and chronic lymphoblastic leukemia (CLL). These diseases proliferate slowly, and CML is often asymptomatic and can progress to acute leukemia or a blast crisis.[7] Blast crisis occurs when myeloblasts make up 20% or more of the bone marrow, slowing the production of red blood cells and platelets.[4] CLL is the most common adult leukemia in the industrialized world[7,8] and comprises 30% of all leukemia diagnoses in the United States (US).[1]

Signs and Symptoms

The signs and symptoms of leukemia are mainly constitutional symptoms, including fever, weight loss, night sweats, fatigue, weakness, and asthenia.[9] CML can cause abdominal discomfort due to enlargement of the spleen.[7] Fever is one of the most common symptoms in patients with acute leukemia and is associated with infection most of the time.[10] Three percent of patients with ALL have central nervous system (CNS) disease at diagnosis.

Diagnosis

Blood testing may include a complete blood count (CBC) with platelets and differential of white blood cells, serum uric acid, and lactate dehydrogenase.[3] CBC is vital to determine the acuity of disease and prognosis.[9] Bone marrow aspiration or bone marrow biopsy are used to determine cytology and cytochemistry in leukemia.[4,5,11] Lumbar puncture (LP) is recommended if there are any neurological signs or symptoms. Other diagnostic modalities include positron emission tomography (PET), computed tomography (CT), and magnetic resonance imaging (MRI).[3,4,5,7,11] Echocardiogram may be performed if administration of a cardiotoxic agent is planned. Refer to Table 21.2 for a summary of common diagnostic tests for hematological malignancies.

Management

Leukemia is managed with chemotherapy. Induction chemotherapy is high-dose chemotherapy aimed at achieving complete disease remission and is followed by a consolidation regimen and/or by a hematopoietic stem cell transplant (HSCT).

Management of AML

Induction chemotherapy for AML consists of cytarabine (Cytosar-U), daunorubicin (Cerubidine),[6] and gemtuzumab ozogamicin (Mylotarg).[4,10] Response to induction chemotherapy is assessed via bone marrow aspirate between day 14 and day 21.[4,10] A person living with and beyond cancer (PLWBC) with 5% or

TABLE 21.1	Leukemia Type, Incidence, Risk Factors, and Prognosis				
Leukemia Type	Age at Diagnosis	Incidence per 100,000	5-Year Survivor Rate	Risk Factors	Prognosis
Acute myeloid leukemia (AML)[4,10]	Older adults, median age is 67	5.06	17%	Previous chemotherapy, total body irradiation,[3] exposure to radiation, or benzene and organochlorine insecticides, autoimmune conditions.[4,10] Being male, Caucasian, overweight, smoking, having Down syndrome.[10]	Older age, comorbidities, poor tolerance to chemotherapy, therapy-related AML, and previous history of myelodysplastic syndrome have a poor prognosis.[10]
Acute lymphoblastic leukemia (ALL)[10]	Children, median age 14	1.28	41.4%	Hispanic, exposure to ionizing radiation, childhood.[10]	Infants or between 10 and 21 years old, with initial white blood cell count >50,000/μL, CNS involvement, T-cell involvement.[5] 15%–20% will relapse.[5]
Chronic myeloid leukemia (CML)[9]	Adults	1–1.5	—	Ionizing radiation exposure, first-degree relatives with myeloprolifer 15%–20% will relapseative disorders.[11]	Based on age, spleen size, and blood counts/differential. Larger spleen size and higher blood basophil percentage determines a poorer prognosis.[9]
Chronic lymphoblastic leukemia (CLL)[7]	Older adults	4.2, 30 after age 80	—	European ancestry, increased age, exposure to Agent Orange.[8]	Early evaluation is associated with improved prognosis. Transformation into lymphoma is associated with a poorer prognosis.[7]

Created by Kelly Chaplin.

TABLE 21.2 Common Diagnostic Assessments for Hematological Malignancies

Physical examination	Peripheral lymph nodes, liver, spleen
Laboratory	Blood cell and differential count, serum uric acid, renal and liver function, lactate dehydrogenase
Serology	Hepatitis B (including HBsAg, anti-HBs, and anti-HBc antibodies) and C, human immunodeficiency virus.
Bone marrow	Histology, the study of cell morphology, immunophenotype, genetics/cytogenetics (fluorescence in situ hybridization), and genomics
Imaging	PET/CT/MRI, echocardiogram
Others	Lumbar puncture (LP)

CT, Computed tomography; *PET*, positron emission tomography; *MRI*, magnetic resonance imaging.
Created by Kelly Chaplin. Printed with permission.

more blasts present, will require another induction cycle. The second cycle may be given 3 weeks after the beginning of the first cycle.[10]

Once the PLWBC is in remission following induction chemotherapy, they can proceed to consolidation treatment.[4,10] Consolidation consists of either chemotherapy or HSCT, and is determined based on risk of relapse.[10] Those at low risk are consolidated with chemotherapy[7] or autologous hematopoietic stem cell transplantation (auto-HSCT). Those at moderate or high risk should undergo allogenic hematopoietic stem cell transplantation (allo-HSCT).[4] AML is the most common indication for allo-HSCT.[4] Consolidation consists of 1 to 3 cycles of chemotherapy and occurs 4 to 6 weeks after induction chemotherapy.[10] PLWBCs may receive oral midostaurin (Rydapt) or subcutaneous azacitidine (Vidaza, Onureg; a hypomethylating agent) as maintenance treatment after induction and consolidation therapy.[4]

PLWBCs not eligible for induction chemotherapy based on age greater than 75 years or overall health may receive azacitidine and decitabine (Dacogen) on a 5-day schedule.[12] PLWBCs should be treated for four cycles and be re-evaluated eligibility to receive allo-HSCT.[4]

The only cure for relapse or refractory patients with leukemia is allo-HSCT. Non-HSCT candidates will begin palliative care with some evidence of effectiveness of 5-azacitidine and decitabine (hypomethylating agents).[10]

Management of CML

Medical management of CML is with tyrosine kinase inhibitors (TKI). Imatinib (Gleevec) is the gold standard for treatment, along with nilotinib (Tasigna) and dasatinib (SPRYCEL) as second line treatments.[9,11] Allo-HSCT can be considered for patients who fail initial and secondary treatment or are in a blast crisis.[9,11]

Management of ALL

Treatment for childhood ALL includes induction chemotherapy lasting 4 to 6 weeks. 95% of patients achieve remission afterward.[5] Most regimens use vincristine (Oncovin, Vincasar PFS), corticosteroids (prednisone or methotrexate), and anthracyclines.[5,10] Allo-HSCT is attempted if remission is not achieved.[5] Consolidation is performed on an outpatient basis and includes a combination of drugs not previously utilized such as mercaptopurine (6-MP, Purinethol), thioguanine (Tabloid), methotrexate (Otrexup [PF], Xatmep, Trexall), cyclophosphamide (Cytoxan), etoposide (Toposar, VePesid), and cytarabine.[5] Maintenance chemotherapy is the longest treatment stage and can last 2 years. Maintenance chemotherapy consists of antimetabolite with methotrexate and

mercaptopurine.[5] Intrathecal chemotherapy is common in most treatment performed on an outpatient basis and protocols for ALL.[6]

Management of adult ALL is with corticosteroids, intrathecal chemotherapy, and radiation therapy as a CNS prophylaxis.[6] Intrathecal medications include methotrexate, cytarabine, prednisone, or dexamethasone.[5,10] TKIs are typically used.[5,10] Immunotherapy using rituximab (Rituxan) is used in induction/consolidation treatment for ALL for persons younger than 55.[6] For adult ALL, HSCT is recommended after a poor response to treatment.[13]

Management of CLL

Chronic lymphoblastic leukemia is managed with a "watch and wait" approach for early signs of disease.[7] Treatment is initiated with advanced disease, particularly symptomatic and active disease. The FCR combination regiment (fludarabine [Fludara], cyclophosphamide, and rituximab) is used in the first line treatment. CLL is incurable, so lifelong management is recommended, which includes blood testing and a physical exam at regular intervals (every 3–12 months).[7] Infections are a common complication of CLL[7] and transformation to lymphoma occurs in 2% to 15% of cases during the course of the disease.[7]

Lymphoma

Lymphoma is diagnosed when malignant neoplasms of lymphoid origin are present in the blood. There are two main varieties of lymphoma: Hodgkin lymphoma (HL) and non-Hodgkin lymphoma (NHL). 10% of cases are HL and 90% of cases are NHL[14] (Table 21.3).

Hodgkin Lymphoma

Hodgkin lymphoma (HL) is an uncommon type of B cell lymphoma. Globally, there were 83,087 (0.4%) new registered cases and 23,376 (0.2%) deaths in 2020.[2] HL has two histological subtypes: classical HL and nodular lymphocyte predominant HL.[15,16] Classical HL is more common while lymphocyte-predominant HL is rare.

Non-Hodgkin Lymphoma

Non-Hodgkin lymphoma (NHL) is the 13th most common cancer type amongst all cancer diagnoses globally. There were 544,000 (2.8%) new cases in 2020 and mortality was 260,000 (2.6%).[2] NHL is

TABLE 21.3	Lymphoma Histological Subtypes, Incidence, and Survival Rate[14,17,128,129]				
Lymphoma Type	Histological Classification		Prevalence	Incidence per 100,000	Survival Rate for 5 Years
Hodgkin lymphoma (HL) 10% from lymphoma	Classical HL		About 95% of all HL	2.8	85.7%
	Nodular lymphocyte-predominant HL		About 5% of all HL		
Non-Hodgkin lymphoma (NHL) 90% from lymphoma	B cell NHL	Diffuse large B-cell lymphomas Aggressive B cell NHL Adult: median age 70 years	30% of NHL	7.2	63.2%
		Follicular lymphoma Indolent B cell NHL Median age is 60 years	20% of all non-Hodgkin lymphomas	3.5	88.4%
		Marginal-zone lymphoma Indolent B cell NHL	5%–10% of all NHL	2.2	90.3%
		Burkitt lymphoma Aggressive B cell NHL	1% of NHL adult, 30% for Pediatric	0.4	64.1%
		Mantle cell lymphoma Indolent B cell NHL in the early stage and aggressive in late grade Median age is 58 years	6% of NHL	–	–
	T-NK cell NHL	Peripheral T-cell Aggressive type	10%–15% of NHL	1.2	58.4%
		Mycosis fungoides Indolent types	–	0.6	90.9%

NK, Natural killer.
Created by Amani AlJohi. Printed with permission.

diagnosed when there is a presence of large type lymphoid neoplasms. Most lymphoma cases derive from B-cells (85%), while the remaining arise from T-cell or natural killer cells (15%).[14] NHL can be classified clinically as indolent and aggressive lymphoma. Indolent cases progress slowly and are not curable. Indolent lymphomas include: follicular lymphoma, marginal-zone lymphoma, and mantle cell lymphoma at Stage I and II (mantle cell lymphoma but can transform into more aggressive forms if not treated).[17,18] Aggressive lymphoma rapidly progresses and requires urgent tumor management. Examples of aggressive NHL are diffuse large B-cell lymphomas (DLBCLs), Burkitt lymphoma, and mantle cell lymphoma in late stage.[17,18]

Risk Factors

Worldwide, HL incidence is increased for ages 20 to 39 years and age 60 or more. With NHL, the incidence increases for those 65 and older. The incidence and mortality rate is higher in males.[19–21] Incidence rate is higher in developed countries such as Australia/New Zealand, North America, and Europe.[2] The occurrence rate can increase 3.1-fold and 1.7-fold with first-degree family history of HL and NHL, respectively.[22] Moreover, infection-related lymphomas have been linked with certain viral infections such as human T-cell lymphotropic virus (adult T-cell lymphoma), Epstein-Barr virus (Hodgkin and Burkitt lymphoma), hepatitis C virus (NHL), and *Helicobacter pylori* (gastric lymphoma). Lymphoma occurs more commonly among HIV-infected individuals due to immunosuppression.[23,24] Autoimmune diseases such as rheumatoid arthritis, systemic lupus erythematosus, Sjögren disease, and celiac disease increase the risk of NHL.[25] Additionally, lifestyle factors such as cigarette smoking and increased body mass index (BMI) increase NHL risk.[25]

Diagnosis and Staging

Gold standard assessment is surgical biopsy, analysis by flow cytometry, immunohistochemistry, and molecular diagnostics.[18,26,27] Determination of the disease stage requires further imaging studies that may include: CT, MRI, PET scan, and bone marrow biopsy.[18,26,27] LP may be required for diagnosis of aggressive NHL (see Table 21.2).

Disease staging is recommended prior to the initiation of medical management. The Ann Arbor system is used for staging the diseases in lymphoma for both HL and NHL[28] (Table 21.4).

Management

Depending upon the type of lymphoma, the treatment protocol can involve active surveillance of the condition, chemotherapy, radiation therapy, auto-HSCT, and allo-HSCT.[26,27] Chemotherapy is the first line treatment for lymphoma.

Chemotherapy

Common chemotherapy regimens for HL are ABVD (doxorubicin [Adriamycin], bleomycin [Blenoxane], vinblastine [Alkaban-AQ, Velban], dacarbazine [DTIC-Dome], or Stanford V (doxorubicin, vinblastine, mechlorethamine [Mustargen], etoposide, vincristine, bleomycin, prednisone), or less frequently Escalated-BEACOPP chemotherapy (bleomycin, etoposide, doxorubicin, cyclophosphamide, vincristine, procarbazine [Matulane], prednisone).[16,26]

NHL chemotherapy regimens include CHOP and R-CHOP. CHOP consists of cyclophosphamide, doxorubicin hydrochloride (hydroxydaunorubicin), vincristine (Oncovin), prednisone.[27]

TABLE 21.4	Ann Arbor Staging Classification[28]
Stage I	Involvement of a single lymph node region or lymphoid structure.
Stage II	Involvement of ≥2 lymph node regions on one side of the diaphragm.
Stage III	Involvement of ≥2 lymph node regions on both sides of diaphragm.
Stage IV	Disseminated involvement of a deep, visceral organ.

Reprinted with permission from Steinberg A, Rao P. Hodgkin lymphoma. In: *Atlas of Diagnostic Hematology*. Elsevier; 2021:211–216.

R-CHOP includes the addition of rituximab to CHOP.[27] Intrathecal chemotherapy can be used prophylactically for aggressive lymphoma when the risk of CNS involvement is high.[27]

Radiation Therapy

Some cases of indolent lymphoma may be managed with a single treatment in early-stage presentation or include field radiotherapy for HL cases. Moreover, radiation therapy can be the only treatment for relapsed lymphoma during palliative treatment for symptom management.[17,26] Consolidation radiation therapy can be used with NHL and bone or mediastinal involvement for DLBCL and primary bone lymphoma with chemotherapy.[27] Whole brain radiotherapy may be used for young patients with CNS involvement, or for palliative management for older PLWBCs who are not candidates for chemotherapy.[27]

Surgery

Surgical management is used with specific types of lymphoma. Those with marginal-zone lymphoma may require a splenectomy and/or gastric surgery if they have bleeding.[17] Spinal surgery may be used for motor impairment with primary or secondary NHL due to mechanical instability and neurological symptoms.[29,30]

Hematopoietic Stem Cell Transplantation

Advanced disease or relapse requires high dose chemotherapy with auto-HSCT to improve survival rate.[15,16] If treatment with high dose of chemotherapy and auto-HSCT fails, allo-HSCT can be an option. Allo-HSCT may improve survivorship after risk assessment.

Multiple Myeloma

Multiple myeloma (MM) is a hematological malignancy that is characterized by uncontrolled growth of plasma cell in bone marrow. MM is not curable, but survival rates have been improving.[31,32] The prognosis of multiple myeloma has improved, with between 21.1% and 61.8% of diagnosed patients surviving 5 years.[33]

Risk Factors

Worldwide, incidence rate for MM from all cancers was 176,404 new cases (0.9%) in 2020, while the mortality rate was reported at 117,077 (1.2%).[2] MM occurs slightly more in men (1.7%) than women (1.3%), with a median age of diagnosis at 65 years.[34] The highest age-standardized incidence rate are Australia, followed by North America and Western Europe.[34]

Diagnosis and Staging

Diagnosis of MM requires bone marrow biopsy, blood tests, urinary tests, and radiological assessment for bone lesions. Baseline values need to be taken for serum and/or urine M-protein, clonal plasma cells, serum free light chain, and extramedullary involvement, as well as presence and degree of end-organ damage. According to the International Myeloma Working Group, MM is diagnosed by the presence of plasma cell infiltration plus one of Myeloma Defining Events (MDE) which includes (CRAB: calcium, renal failure, anemia, and bone lesions).[31,35] Staging is determined by the revised international staging system for MM, which uses disease biology, including levels of serum albumin, and serum beta-2-microglobuli, lactase dehydrogenase and high-risk cytogenetics from bone marrow.[36]

Symptoms

The most common symptoms for MM include pain, fatigue, constipation, and tingling sensation in hands and/or feet. In addition, decreased physical and cognitive function can occur.[37]

Medical Management

Patients with MM are commonly treated with chemotherapy, radiation, auto-HSCT, and surgical intervention for pathological fracture.[32,35]

Chemotherapy

Patients with newly diagnosed MM who are eligible for transplants are advised to receive chemotherapy, which includes an immunomodulatory medication, proteasome inhibitor (PI), and steroids.[32,35] Triplet regimen therapies for people newly diagnosed with MM who have a standard risk for HSCT can be treated with bortezomib (Velcade), lenalidomide (Revlimid), examethasone (VRd) or by bortezomib-thalidomide-dexamethasone (VTd) for presence of renal failure. If a PLWBC is determined to be at high risk for HSCT, recommendations include three to four cycles of daratumumab (Darzalex), bortezomib, thalidomide, dexamethasone (Dara-VTd) or VRd.[32,35] If the PLWBC is determined to be low risk for HSCT, this treatment is followed by maintenance therapy before and after transplant, which includes lenalidomide maintenance therapy.[35] PLWBCs who are transplant ineligible can receive the same medication of high risk HSCT which include Dara-VTd or VRd.[2]

Radiation Therapy

Low dose radiation therapy is recommended to manage compression fractures, long bone fractures, and/or pain for PLWBCs with MM, according to the bone health guidelines.[38] In addition, radiotherapy used for pain management also has been found to improve neurological symptoms and pain in cases of spinal fracture.[39,40]

Hematological Stem Cell Transplantation

This management used for eligible PLWBCs with MM is based on age and severity of comorbidity.[32,41] Auto-HSCT methods used as first line management of eligible people with MM can improve the survival rate and rate of long-term survivorship.[41]

Surgery and Procedure

Surgical intervention is performed with MM cases to manage spinal cord compression and fractures. Minimally invasive surgery such as kyphoplasty or vertebroplasty can be performed to manage symptoms with less adverse effects for PLWBCs without neurological complication after pathological spine fracture.[40,42] The International Myeloma Working Group Recommendations for the Treatment of MM considered balloon kyphoplasty better management for symptom control when compared to vertebroplasty.[40]

Hematopoietic Stem Cell Transplantation

HSCT is a medical procedure used to treat and/or cure hematological malignancies and some inherited conditions. Greater than 20,000 HSCT procedures are performed annually in the US.[43] Patients with leukemia, lymphoma, and MM can be treated with a HSCT. This procedure involves replacement of the person's malignant cells with healthy stem cells via IV infusion a few days after receiving final chemotherapy or radiation treatments to cause pancytopenia to destroy existing bone marrow.[44] The new stem cells engraft for the next 2 to 3 weeks where they will start to produce healthy blood cells.[43] This process can cause many health complications and can result in reduced physical function. There are two kinds of HSCT: autologous and allogenic.

Autologous Hematopoietic Stem Cell Transplantation

Auto-HSCT includes collecting the PLWBC's own stem cells followed by administering high doses of chemotherapy to destroy malignancy. Following chemotherapy treatment, the person becomes unable to produce additional abnormal blood cells. The PLWBC's own healthy cells are reintroduced to grow in the absence of the neoplastic cells. Blood counts typically recover in 3 weeks.[45]

Allogenic Hematopoietic Stem Cell Transplantation

Allo-HSCT is the most advantageous approach to prevent recurrence in acute leukemia. This treatment has a similar protocol to auto-HSCT, except the cells that are re-introduced to the patient are from a donor. PLWBCs with an unfavorable risk profile are candidates for allo-HSCT.[10] In addition to a healthy immune system being introduced, the PLWBCs benefit from new immune cells attacking the malignancy.[45] AML is the most frequent diagnosis to receive allo-HSCT.[4] Eligibility criteria includes intermediate or adverse risk AML and age ≤75 years.[4] A donor needs to be a Human Leukocyte Antigen match identical (9/10 or 10/10 match) for the transplant to be successful.[4]

During treatment with HSCT, patients will receive high-dose chemotherapy with the intention to reduce all blood cell counts to destroy the malignancy and then build back a healthy immune system. HSCT regimen typically includes total body irradiation, and some combination of cyclophosphamide, fludarabine, and cytarabine.[46]

Rehabilitation Considerations in the Hematological Cancers

Hematological Compromise

Bone marrow suppression during the process of HSCT increases the risk of bleeding, infection, and anemia.[47] Onc R clinicians need to pay close attention to recent blood counts to assess the safety of an exercise or physical activity intervention. Some safety recommendations concerning blood cell counts will be dictated by individual institutions. See Table 21.5 for general evidence-based guidelines for platelet counts. PLWBCs may be cytopenic for weeks following HSCT.[47] Refer to Table 21.6 for rehabilitation considerations for various lab values.

TABLE 21.5	Summary of Evidence for Exercises Versus Platelet Count				
Platelet Count	**Fu 2018[131]**	**ACSM[132]**	**Mohammed 2019[58]**	**Morishita 2020[133]**
20,000–50,000 µL	>20,000 platelets/µL No restrictions	Exercise should be limited to resistance training using elastic bands, stationary cycling, range-of-motion exercises, and walking.	31,000–50,000 µL Moderate to Intensive can include progressive resistive exercises, stretching, jumping 21,000–30,000 µL Moderate Dynamic balance, unlimited ambulation.	Resistance equipment such as weights
10,000–20,000 µL	No resistive exercise. Fall precautions.		Light to moderate transfers, limited ambulation, static balance training	Exercise gently, without resistance. Sitting or standing exercises, gentle stretching, and walking may be allowed
5,000–9,999 µL	No resistive exercises and bed/chair exercise			<10,000 µL Limit activity. Patients may require a platelet transfusion, before resuming exercise.
<5,000 µL	Discuss with oncology team or consider deferring treatment		Very light therapeutic activity in the bed, sitting at the edge of the bed or in the bed/chair, active range of motion	

ACSM, American College of Sports Medicine
Created by Kelly Chaplin. Printed with permission.

TABLE 21.6	Lab Values and Rehabilitation Considerations[47,133,134]	
	Lab Value	**Rehabilitation Considerations**
Hemoglobin	Hemoglobin <8 g/dL	– Communicate with physicians before providing intervention if 7 g/dL or lower – Onc R clinicians should monitor vital signs and signs of adverse events
Platelets	Platelets below 10,000 µL	– Communicate between physicians and rehabilitation clinician about benefit and risk of exercise/physical activity to prevent functional decline – Follow your facility's guidelines
Neutropenia	Absolute neutrophil count <500 c/mm³	– Increased risk of infection. Should take precautions to decrease risk – Observe symptoms and perform session per patient preferences – Neutropenic fever is considered an emergency
Hypercalcemia	Total albumin-corrected calcium above 10.5 mg/dL	– Assess mental status changes. – Therapy session can be continued in mild to moderate cases – Observe symptoms and perform session per patient preferences

Created by Kelly Chaplin. Printed with permission.

Adverse effects of HSCT, often severe,[48] occur due to high dose chemotherapy, isolation due to immunosuppression, bedrest, chronic use of steroids, anemia, and other factors. Adverse effects commonly experienced include: cancer related fatigue, decreased physical function, loss of muscle mass, and decreased cardiovascular function.[49]

Graft-Versus-Host Disease

One significant potential complication of allo-HSCT is the risk that the grafted cells will attack the host, causing Graft-Versus-Host Disease (GVHD). Incidence of GVHD can be as high as 40% to 60%[50] and moderate to severe disease occurs in 20% of PLWBCs regardless of human leukocyte antigen matching.[51] It reduces physical performance and functional ability and can be life threatening.[52] GVHD is commonly seen in the skin, liver, and gastrointestinal tract (Table 21.7).[50,53] See to Figure 21.1 for a summary of complications of HSCT and GVHD.

Immunosuppressants are used to reduce the chances of developing GVHD; however, they place PLWBCs at higher risk of infection. Systemic corticosteroids are a type of immunosuppressant that commonly the first line of treatment for GVHD. They are effective in managing the disease for 50% of PLWBCs.[50,53] Bortezomib and spleen tyrosine

kinase can also be effective in preventing or treating GVHD for other PLWBCs.[50,51] GVHD is classified according to clinical presentation, and is considered acute if disease presents within 100 days post allo-HSCT and is considered chronic if it presents after 100 days.[50,53] For more information about GVHD refer to Chapter 13.

Pain

Pain can be due to bone disease or due to treatment related adverse events such as chemotherapy induced polyneuropathy (CIPN), or a postsurgical procedure.[38] Prevalence of pain in this population is between 50% and 70%.[37,54] Medical management for pain can include chemotherapy, radiation therapy, pain medication, or surgical intervention for pathological fractures.[38] Nonpharmacological management includes exercises and alternative therapy such as reflexology, acupuncture, and acupressure.[38,55,56]

Cancer Related Fatigue

Increased dosage of chemotherapy is associated with higher levels of fatigue reported. Cancer related fatigue (CRF) is common, with more than half of people living with or beyond hematological

TABLE 21.7	Common Symptoms in Each Classification of Graft-Versus-Host Disease[50,53]			
Organ	**Cutaneous/Fascia**	**Gastrointestinal**	**Liver**	**Other Organs**
Acute	Erythematous, maculopapular rash involving palms and soles; may become confluent. Severe disease: Bullae	Nausea, vomiting, abdominal cramps, diarrhea, ileus, distension, bleeding	Jaundice due to hyperbilirubinemia and increased alkaline phosphatase	—
Chronic	Cutaneous: Erythematous maculopapular rash, pain, desquamation Fascia: Contracture, edema	Dysphagia, odynophagia, heartburn, anorexia, nausea, vomiting, abdominal pain, cramping, diarrhea, weight loss and malnutrition	—	Pulmonary: Bronchiolitis obliterans, airflow obstruction Ocular: Dryness, conjunctivitis Genitalia: Women vaginal scarring and clitoral/labial agglutination —men phimosis and urethral/meatus scarring

Created by Amani AlJohi. Printed with permission.

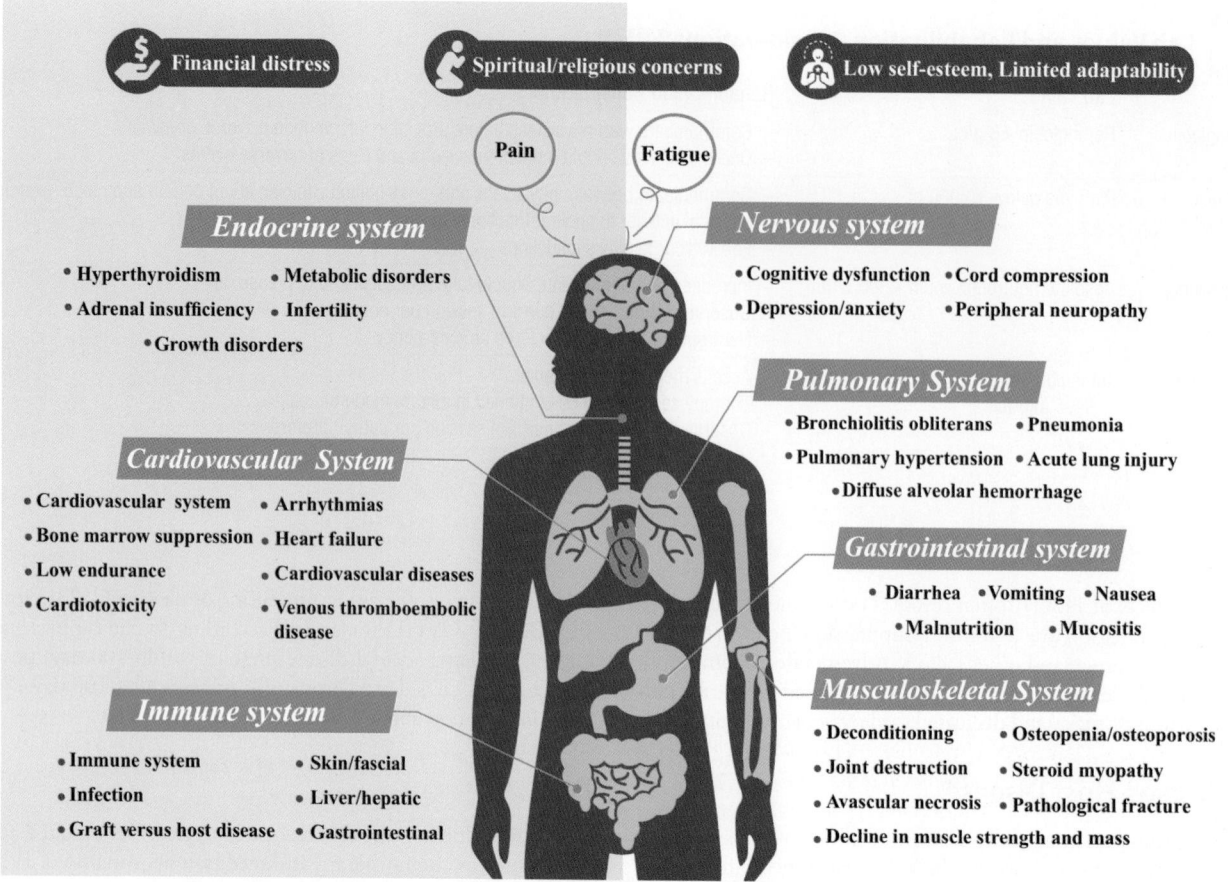

Financial distress   **Spiritual/religious concerns**   **Low self-esteem, Limited adaptability**

Pain   Fatigue

Endocrine system
- Hyperthyroidism
- Adrenal insufficiency
- Growth disorders
- Metabolic disorders
- Infertility

Nervous system
- Cognitive dysfunction
- Depression/anxiety
- Cord compression
- Peripheral neuropathy

Pulmonary System
- Bronchiolitis obliterans
- Pulmonary hypertension
- Diffuse alveolar hemorrhage
- Pneumonia
- Acute lung injury

Cardiovascular System
- Cardiovascular system
- Bone marrow suppression
- Low endurance
- Cardiotoxicity
- Arrhythmias
- Heart failure
- Cardiovascular diseases
- Venous thromboembolic disease

Gastrointestinal system
- Diarrhea
- Vomiting
- Nausea
- Malnutrition
- Mucositis

Musculoskeletal System
- Deconditioning
- Joint destruction
- Avascular necrosis
- Decline in muscle strength and mass
- Osteopenia/osteoporosis
- Steroid myopathy
- Pathological fracture

Immune system
- Immune system
- Infection
- Graft versus host disease
- Skin/fascial
- Liver/hepatic
- Gastrointestinal

• **Fig. 21.1** Complication of Blood and Marrow Transplantation and Graft-Versus-Host Disease. (Created by Amani AlJohi and Shadia Aljuaid. Printed with permission.)

cancer experiencing CRF during and post cancer management.[52] CRF is associated with biological markers such as increased cytokines, particularly interleukin 6 (IL-6) and tumor necrosis factor alpha (TNF alpha).[57] Up to 44% of PLWBCs experience moderate to severe fatigue following HSCT.[57]

Rehabilitation interventions play a principal role in managing fatigue. Physical activity is effective in reducing fatigue after HSCT, even more than pharmacological interventions.[58] Initiating exercise prior to HSCT has been shown to have a positive effect in reducing fatigue.[52,58] Exercise has also demonstrated improved biomarkers that play a role in fatigue.[52,59] According to a recent meta-analysis, PLWBCs with lymphoma had decreased fatigue when they performed mind-body exercises during physical activity.[60,61] Alternative medicine such as massage, music therapy, and foot reflexology has been found to improve fatigue.[55,62]

Musculoskeletal Complications

Bone loss commonly occurs with hematologic malignancy. Osteoporosis and osteopenia are adverse effects of systemic management, and HSCT impacts bone mineral density.[63,64]

Pharmacologic management of osteoporosis and osteopenia includes vitamin D and calcium supplementation, bisphosphonates, and hormonal therapy.[65] Nonpharmacological management includes high impact physical activity with weight bearing, resistive exercises, aerobic exercises, adequate dietary intake of calcium and vitamin D, and avoiding smoking and excessive alcohol.[65–67]

Bone lesions are common with MM and sometimes with lymphoma. Secondary bone lymphoma incidence was 16% to 20%,

while primary bone lymphoma incidence was 1% from all NHL. The highest incidence of bone fracture was in lower extremity bones (49%) and then the spine (38%).[68–70] Spine lymphoma or pathologic fracture from MM can lead to spinal cord compression.[70] Bone lesions are not always contraindications for physical activity and exercise, but do require program modifications to decrease pathologic fracture risk[70] (Figure 21.2).

Steroid myopathy is a complication of chronic corticosteroid use, and is commonly indicated following allo-HSCT and to manage GVHD.[71] Symptoms include muscle weakness and decreased functional level.[72] Adequate physical activity and exercise in mild cases may have a positive effect; however, those receiving prolonged steroid treatment may consider rehabilitation to regain muscle power.[51]

Avascular necrosis (AVN) is a late complication post allo-HSCT with incidence of 4% to 19% with 5-year survival rate. This incidence correlated with prevention and treatment of GVHD and total body irradiation. The head of the femur is the most common site for AVN.[73,74]

Chemotherapy Induced Polyneuropathy

Chemotherapy neurotoxicity is a common adverse effect of hematological malignancy management with proteasome inhibitors, immunomodulatory drugs, and vinca alkaloids. The incidence of chemotherapy induced polyneuropathy (CIPN) is high in MM, at 50%. The symptoms impact quality of life (QOL) and increase the risk for falls.[75,76] Onc R clinicians should include sensory assessments and fall risk assessments as well as education to manage comorbidities such as diabetes mellitus (DM), hypothyroidism,

Rehab Considerations for Multiple Myeloma and Bone Lesions

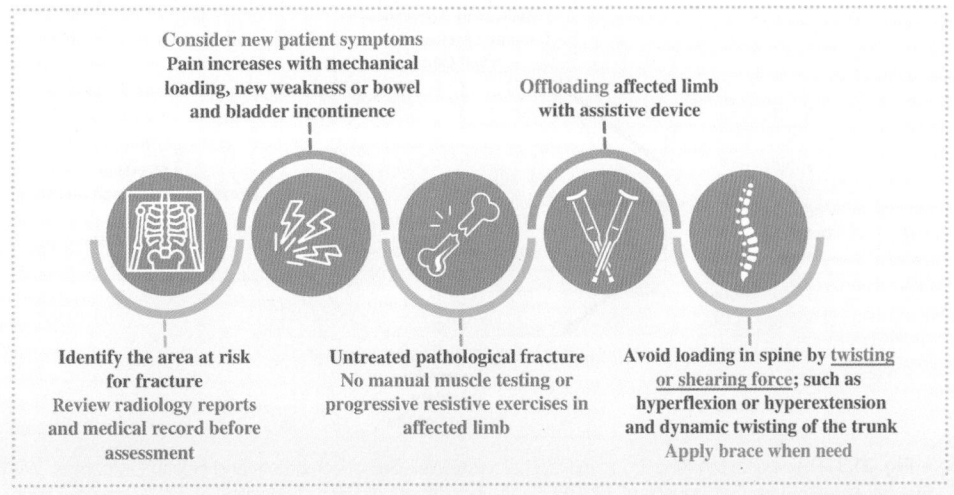

Consider new patient symptoms
Pain increases with mechanical loading, new weakness or bowel and bladder incontinence

Offloading affected limb with assistive device

Identify the area at risk for fracture
Review radiology reports and medical record before assessment

Untreated pathological fracture
No manual muscle testing or progressive resistive exercises in affected limb

Avoid loading in spine by twisting or shearing force; such as hyperflexion or hyperextension and dynamic twisting of the trunk
Apply brace when need

• **Fig. 21.2** Rehabilitation Considerations for Multiple Myeloma and Bone Lesions. (Created by Amani AlJohi and Shadia Aljuaid. Printed with permission.)

and nutritional deficiencies.[75,76] Antidepressive medications such as gabapentin, pregabalin, and tricyclic antidepressants can be prescribed to reduce sensory symptoms.[75,77] Evidence is growing for the purpose of nonpharmacological management of CIPN including transcutaneous electrical nerve stimulation, acupuncture, and exercise training.[76,78–80]

Cardiovascular and Pulmonary Complications

HSCT can be associated with increased risk for cardiovascular events due to cardiotoxic chemotherapy and radiation treatments. Anthracyclines can be associated with congestive heart failure due to their cardiotoxic adverse effects.[81] Risk of heart failure is high in patients with NHL receiving CHOP and R-CHOP regimens.[81] PLWBCs who receive radiation to the thorax can also develop restrictive cardiomyopathy, valve disease, and coronary artery disease.[81] GVHD after allo-HSCT in pediatric PLWBCs can cause cardiotoxicity.[81] Reducing the dose of chemotherapy or adding heart failure medications can help reverse cardiomyopathy,[82] but the impairments still exist. The effect of exercises in deconditioning will be discussed later in this chapter.

Pulmonary dysfunction can be a result of immunosuppression, of steroid myopathy that decreases respiratory muscle strength, or as a direct effect of chronic GVHD of the lung. Bleomycin may cause pulmonary toxicity.[83] Additionally, PLWBCs exposed to radiotherapy to the mid-sternum for lymphoma management are at risk for lung fibrosis.[83] The incidence of pulmonary complications was 37% with HSCT, which may occur from infectious or noninfectious causes. See Table 21.8 for common noninfectious pulmonary complications post HSCT. This complication increases the mortality for PLWBCs post HSCT; however, the mortality rate is decreased with advanced treatment.[84,85]

Nutritional Considerations

Nutritional intake for PLWBCs in this domain can be complicated by infections, mucositis, and poor digestive absorption.[86] Acute and chronic GVHD of the digestive tract as well as infections and digestive abnormalities can reduce nutritional absorption. There is a negative correlation between poor nutritional status and survival.[86]

A recent study reported that PLWBCs were found to lose 5% to 10% of their baseline body weight after HSCT.[86] Enteral nutrition is as effective as parenteral nutrition and should be the first choice for supplementation.[86] A neutropenic diet that includes restrictions on fresh fruits and vegetables, raw and undercooked meat as well as raw grains, smoked fish, and unpasteurized dairy products showed no benefit and had higher infection rates. Lack of support for this diet has led to fewer restrictions, although safe food handling and washing fresh produce is recommended.[86] Supplements (except for vitamin D) have no proven benefits on overall nutritional status in this population.[86] Future research including robust studies and randomized controlled trials are needed to further establish nutritional recommendations for this patient population.

TABLE 21.8 Common Noninfection Pulmonary Complication Post-HSCT[89,90]

Common Pulmonary Complications Post-HSCT	Incidence	Onset
Diffuse alveolar hemorrhage	2%–14% of HSCT	Acute/first month post HSCT
Idiopathic pneumonia syndrome	2%–17% more common after allogeneic HSCT.	Subacute/first 120 days after HSCT
Bronchiolitis obliterans syndrome	10% after allogeneic HSCT	Late/presents after the first 100 days
Cryptogenic organizing pneumonia	0.9%–10.3% post HSCT	Late/after 100 days

HSCT, Hemopoietic stem cell transplant.
Created by Amani AlJohi. Printed with permission.

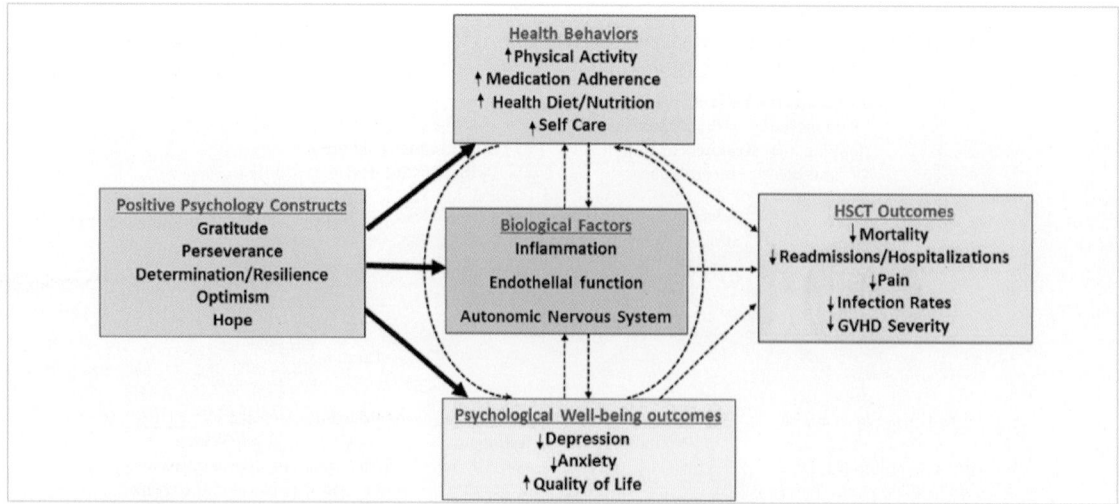

• **Fig. 21.3** Theoretical Model of Positive Psychological Well-Being Constructs and Health Outcomes. With Hematopoietic Stem Cell Transplant. *GVHD,* Graft-versus-host disease; ↑, positive effect; ↓, negative/unfavorable. (Reprinted with permission. Amonoo HL, Barclay ME, El-Jawahri A, Traeger LN, Lee SJ, Huffman JC. Positive psychological constructs and health outcomes in hematopoietic stem cell transplantation patients: a systematic review. *Biol Blood Marrow Transplant.* 2019;25(1):e5-e16. doi:10.1016/j.bbmt.2018.09.030.)

Sexual Impairment

The prevalence of sexual dysfunction generally varies between 23% and 90% in people with cancers, Women are affected greater than men, however both sexes often report symptoms of a lack of sexual desire, painful intercourse, or both.[87,88]

Sexual impairment is often due to treatment related complications, such as GVHD, chronic genital GVHD, hormonal disorders, and impaired psychological wellbeing.[87,89,90] Erectile dysfunction and ejaculatory changes are common, while women report vaginal dryness and dyspareunia.[87,91]

Sexual health issues should be screened by the Onc R clinician and referred to needed services based on the assessment, which may include: clinical nurse specialists, social workers, psychologists, sex therapists, pelvic floor physical therapists, gynecologists, and urologists.[91] A multimodal treatment approach inclusive of patient education and psychosocial interventions can improve sexual function.[91]

Psychosocial Health

Incidence of psychological disorders (depression, anxiety, posttraumatic stress) with hematologic malignancies is about 20%, though this incidence increases in adolescent and young adult populations to 39% and the severity is increased during active treatment phases.[92,93] Half of PLWBCs report anxiety and depression before stem cell transplant due to the extent of the journey and the intensive management. This statistic is impactful for the PLWBC and their support person(s)/caregiver, potentially resulting in negative psychological wellbeing consequences for both individuals.[94,95] PLWBCs have reported feeling trapped, fearful, guilty, discouraged, and powerless throughout their journeys.[94]

Different psychological approaches can be used with PLWBCs in this domain as well as their support persons/caregivers. These include mindfulness-based therapy malnutrition, and impaired lymphocyte management, positive psychology, relaxation techniques, psychological therapy, peer support groups, and cognitive reframing.[96–99]

Onc R clinicians need to enhance and educate their PLWBCs and caregivers on the positive psychological concepts which include "positive constructs such as optimism, gratitude, hope, and perseverance" in addition to working to optimize the physical symptoms and disease processes in order to facilitate overall well-being.[98,99] A recent systematic review of eighteen studies supported the impact of positive psychological well-being constructs for PLWBCs in this domain who received HSCT.[98] There was evidence of improved QOL and healthy behaviors, in addition to decreased depression and anxiety (Figure 21.3).[98]

Inclusion of psychosocial interventions for caregivers of PLWBCs including psychoeducation, and cognitive behavioral strategies to decrease burden and psychological distress as well as improve QOL has been reported to be beneficial.[100,101] Figure 21.4 summarizes the benefits of physiological interventions for the caregiver.

Cognitive Impairment

Cognitive impairment with hematologic malignancy management may result from whole brain radiation, high doses of chemotherapy, or HSCT.[102–105] In PLWBCs with hematological malignancies who had received chemotherapy, 62% demonstrated cognitive impairments.[104] Figure 21.5 summarizes factors that play a role in cognitive disorders and Onc R intervention.[105]

One method that has demonstrated improvements in cognitive function in hematologic survivors after auto-HSCT was utilizing an online computer cognitive rehabilitation program for retraining cognitive skill.[106] Participants demonstrated improvement in cognitive function and self-perceived physical well-being after this intervention.

Assessment

Assessment includes collecting information from the medical record such as malignancy type, medical management, as well as any complications postmanagement and/or relapse. Laboratory values including CBC (see Tables 21.5 and 21.6), serum creatinine, and albumin need to be reviewed before each treatment session during an inpatient hospitalization. Review of radiological investigation is also necessary for people with MM or lymphoma that have brain, bone, or spine involvement. Additionally, physical performance level, including pain, psychological well-being, QOL, and patient lifestyle should be included in assessment (for details, refer to Tables 21.9 and 21.10).

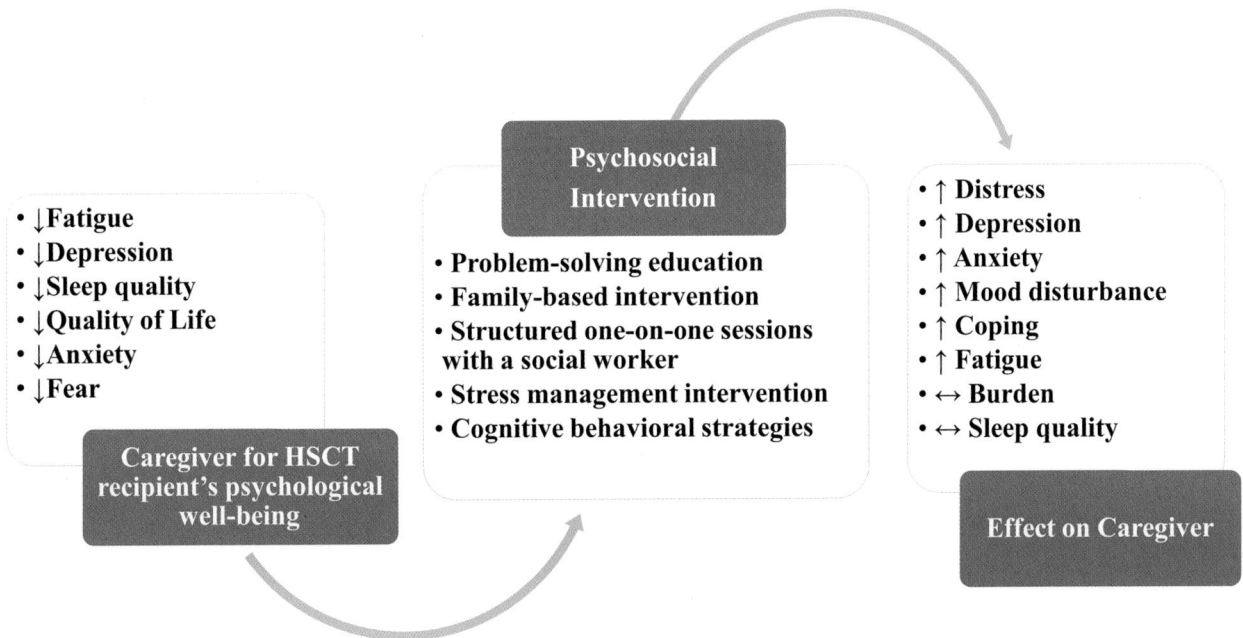

• **Fig. 21.4** Summary of Intervention Effectiveness on Caregivers' Psychological Well-Being for Hematopoietic Cell Transplantation (HCT) Patients, ↑, Positive effect; ↔, no effect; ↓, negative/unfavorable effect.[100,101] (Created by Amani AlJohi. Printed with permission.)

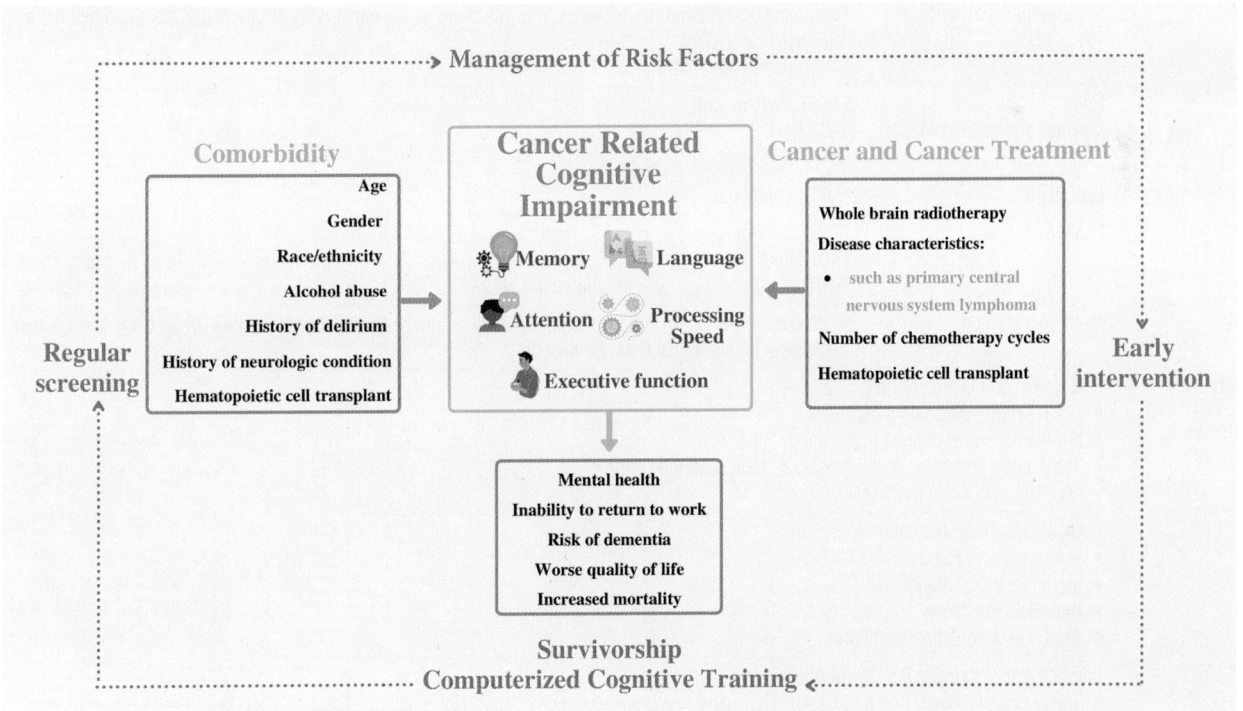

• **Fig. 21.5** Summary of Evidence Bases regarding Cognitive Impairment and the Rehabilitation Clinician's Role With the Hematology Population. (Created by Amani AlJohi and Shadia Aljuaid. Printed with permission.)

Differential Diagnoses

When evaluating people with hematologic malignancies, Onc R clinicians will be faced with diagnosing the main movement issue and establishing a therapy diagnosis. PLWBCs in this domain often present with deconditioning. The physical manifestations of these treatments will result in muscle weakness, cardiovascular dysfunction, and neurological deficits. Appropriate examination techniques provide information that the clinician will use to determine which of these movement diagnoses cause activity limitations and participation restrictions. Force production is a possible movement diagnosis where treatments will focus on specific muscle strengthening as well as functional mobility. This approach would be best for PLWBCs who have experienced long hospital stays while receiving chemotherapy or HSCT. Onc R clinicians also need to consider blood counts as resistance training is added, especially thrombocytopenia. Cardiovascular dysfunction may be resultant of chemotherapy regimens or long-term hospital stays. Onc R clinicians treating PLWBCs with cardiovascular dysfunction should carefully monitor vital signs and use short bouts of endurance activity to increase mobility and activity tolerance.

Neurological deficits may be the main movement disorder when patients have chronic CIPN related to their treatments. Additionally, balance and coordination deficits fall into this category which should prompt an Onc R clinician to include stability and balance exercises. Sensory information can be manipulated to make stability training appropriate to their functional level. For example, a PLWBC would benefit from balance training under conditions where lighting and surfaces are varied.

Rehabilitation Interventions

Acute Care Rehabilitation

Exercise training for PLWBCs in this domain during inpatient hospitalization chemotherapy or HSCT is safe and effective. Typical exercise interventions include exercises at the bedside or walking, aerobic training, balance training, and resistance training.[44,49,107–110] Exercise training during acute hospitalization has been found to enhance recovery for PLWBCs undergoing chemotherapy and decrease the potential adverse effects of their management. Many factors strongly correlate to muscle dysfunction during an inpatient hospitalization for chemotherapy and include inactivity, malnutrition, and impaired lymphocyte counts.[111] Onc R clinicians in the hospital setting need to prioritize improving a PLWBC's activity levels and minimizing bed rest and its negative multisystem implications.

Resistive exercises have been reported to positively maintain and improve the functional capacity for PLWBCs hospitalized

---

TABLE 21.9   A Summary of Evidence-based Patient Reported Assessment Tools for the Hematology Population

	Tools	
Quality of life[135]	Frequently used general tools:	• Short-Form 36-dimension (SF-36) • EuroQoL-5-dimension (EQ-5D)
	Tools applicable with hematological cancers	The Functional Assessment of Cancer Therapy-General (FACT-G) European Organization for Research and Treatment of Cancer Quality of Life Group Core questionnaire (EORTC-QLQ-C30) FACT-anemia (FACT-AN)
	Bone marrow transplant (BMT)	EORTC BMT module, FACT-BMT QoL-BMT
	Lymphoma	FACT-lymphoma
	Leukemia	EORTC leukemia FACT-leukemia EORTC-QLQ-chronic myeloid leukemia (CML24)
	Multiple myeloma	• European Organization for Research and Treatment of Cancer Quality of Life Group Core questionnaire-Multiple Myeloma (QLQ-MY24 & MY20)
Fatigue[52,136]	• Brief Fatigue Inventory (BFI) • FACT-Fatigue subscale (FACT-F) • Multidimensional Fatigue Inventory (MFI) • The fatigue subscales of the Profile of Mood States (POMS) • FACT-Anemia scale (FACT-AN)	
Pain[137,138]	• McGill Pain Questionnaire–Short Form • Numeric Rating Scale • McGill Pain Questionnaire • Brief Pain Inventory • Brief Pain Inventory–Short Form	
	Chemotherapy-Induced Peripheral Neuropathy • The Functional Assessment of Cancer Therapy/Gynecologic Oncology Group-Neurotoxicity (FACT-GOG-NTX) subjective assessment • Total Neuropathy Score (TNSr) objective scoring	

EORTC-QLQ, European Organization for Research and Treatment of Cancer Quality of Life Group Core questionnaire; *FACT,* functional assessment of cancer therapy. *QOL,* quality of life.
Created by Amani AlJohi. Printed with permission.

TABLE 21.10	A Summary of Evidence-based Physical Assessment Tools for the Hematology Population	
Rang of motion[58,121]	Photographic range of motion, goniometry, inclinometers Flexibility assessment: • Trunk lateral flexibility test
Muscle[52,57,58,108,139]	Lower limb • Dynamometer • 1-Rep max (1-RM) • Timed stair climb • 30-Second Chair Stand test /Five Times Sit to Stand Upper limb • Grip strength • Dynamometry • 1-RM
Balance[57,108,109,139,140]	• Gait speed (10-m walk test) • Fullerton Advanced Balance Scale • Timed Up and Go (TUG) • Five Times Sit to Stand
Mobility level and functional assessment/activities of daily living[43,130,141,142]	• De Morton Mobility Index (DEMMI) • Short Physical Performance Battery (SPPB) • Functional Independence Measure: • Activities of Daily Living (ADL) • Instrumental Activities of Daily Living (IADL)
Cardiorespiratory[58,120,143]	• 6-Minute walk test (6MWT)/6-minute bicycle test. • 6-Minute step test • Incremental shuttle walk test (ISWT) • VO$_2$ max and VO$_2$ peak • Lung function
Cognitive[103,105,144]	• Mini-Mental Status Exam • Montreal Cognitive Assessment • Orientation-Memory-Concentration Test
Nutritional[86,114,119,145]	• Weight loss • Body mass index • Body composition • Percentage of body fat (%) and muscle mass (kg)
Physical activity[112,113,145–147]	• Godin Leisure-Time Exercise Questionnaire • International Physical Activity Questionnaire (IPAQ) • Freiburg Questionnaire on Physical Activity • Objective: Accelerometer
Psychological[52,145,146,148,149]	• Self-rating Depression Scale (SDS) • Cancer and Treatment Distress (CTXD) • Hospital Anxiety and Depression Scale (HADS)

Created by Amani AlJohi and Shadia Aljuaid. Printed with permission.

with ALL for intensive chemotherapy.[112] Exercise intervention during and after HSCT has been widely studied. Exercise intervention can help prevent or improve functional ability,[57,108] depression,[49] and strength.[57,113] Studies which focused on exercise interventions after discharge reported improvement in physical fitness[113] as well as prevention of weight loss.[114] Typical exercise interventions included aerobic training[44,49,107,108] and resistance training.[44,57,107,113] Refer to Figure 21.6 for a summary of inpatient rehabilitative interventions for HSCT.

Aerobic exercise intensity should be monitored using the Borg Rating of Perceived Exertion Scale with a target intensity level of 10 to 13 (light to somewhat hard).[107] In general, the duration of exercise should be 30 minutes in length.[44,49,107] A walking program should be a staple of care during an inpatient stay.

Resistance training can be incorporated safely for PLWBCs undergoing HSCT two to three times per week.[44,57,113] Exercise should engage the upper body, the lower body, and abdominal muscle groups. Exercises such as the leg press and bench press can be used after HSCT[113] and exercises such as a chest fly, biceps curl, triceps extension, shoulder shrug, shoulder upright row, shoulder lateral raise, knee flexion, knee extension, wall push-ups, squats, and bed sit-ups can be used while inpatient and during HSCT.[57] Refer to Figure 21.7 for images of recommended exercises. Exercise training has been demonstrated to be safe with high levels of adherence.[44,107,113] A common limiting factor for exercise participation interventions is nausea.[44,107]

Inpatient Rehabilitation

An inpatient rehabilitation (IPR) facility offers comprehensive, high intensity, multidisciplinary treatment for a person with a hematologic malignancy. The percentage of people with hematologic malignancy who received IPR services ranges from 7% to 22%.[115–118] PLWBCs who were admitted to IPR required multiple rehabilitation disciplines. Studies reported improvement in function, symptoms, and psychological distress as a result of participation in inpatient cancer rehabilitation facilities.[115,118] See Chapter 24 for specific considerations for IPR in persons with cancer. However, proper timing for inpatient rehabilitation needs to be studied for this population.

Outpatient Rehabilitation

Treating people with hematologic malignancies in the outpatient (OP) setting allows for a series of more focused, tailored, and sustainable interventions. At the OP stage, patients are less acutely ill, but continue to have impairments and movement problems related to their treatments which warrant rehabilitation intervention. Balance deficits, chronic fatigue, cardiovascular deconditioning, proximal muscle weakness, and limitations in work and ADLs are common presenting characteristics of people after cancer treatment.[58] These individuals report limitations in their physical ability even 2 to 6 years after diagnosis and treatment.[58]

An OP Onc R clinician also must be adept at screening for possible recurrence, oncological emergencies, and early identification of GVHD[58] as they may arise. Pain that does not behave like mechanical pain should be referred to the physician. Constitutional symptoms such as fever, unexplained change in weight, night sweats, and other general health issues are critical to identify early on given the PLWBC's past medical history.

Typical outpatient treatments will address the PLWBC's presenting impairments, functional limitations, and activity limitations.[58] Chronic issues such as cancer related fatigue and falls may not be the patient's main complaint, but are important to address for a comprehensive approach. Steroid myopathy commonly occurs due to prednisone use as an immunosuppressant after HSCT and can manifest as lower extremity weakness.[58] Similarly, bone health can be improved using weight bearing exercise.[58] Aerobic and resistance exercises can be prescribed at a frequency of two to three times per

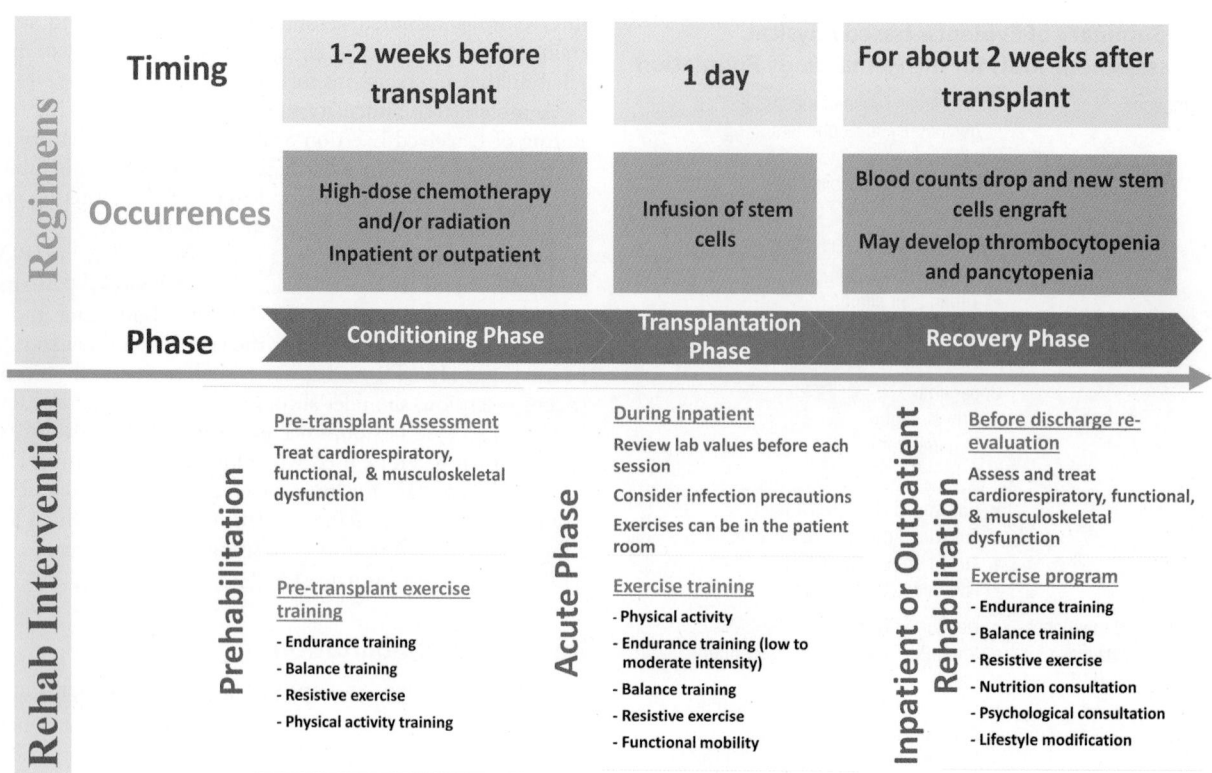

• **Fig. 21.6** Examples of Hematopoietic Stem Cell Transplantation Regimens and Exercise Training in Each Stage. Created by Amani AlJohi. Printed with permission.

week and which has demonstrated evidence of improvement in fatigue, QOL, cardiovascular fitness, strength, and body composition.[113,119] Examples of resistance exercises include rows, leg press, bench press, and flies (see Figure 21.7).[113] A systematic review evaluating the effects of exercise on QOL and fatigue among this population found significant benefits with short-term exercise training.[60] Exercise has a positive effect on fatigue for those undergoing treatment for hematological cancer.[52,110,120,121]

Bracing/Splinting

Spine bracing can be provided for spine involvement and abnormal neurological symptoms to minimize mechanical loading on vertebral bodies and reduce pain.[122] Onc R clinicians and orthotists are integral in the management of chronic GVHD for sclerodermatous or peripheral neuropathy post-HSCT to decrease joint deformity in the hands. Stretching exercises, range of motion, heat, massage, edema management, and splinting can be used to prevent joint dysfunction and regain functional ability. Review Table 21.11 for examples of splinting.[58,123,124]

Cancer Survivorship Rehabilitation Program

Survival rates for those with hematologic malignancies have increased with advancements in medical treatments, and ranges from 50% to 90% as seen in Table 21.3. A survivorship program is designed to optimize physical function, decrease symptoms, improve nutritional status with the end goal of optimizing QOL.[125] Figure 21.8 depicts a survivorship care routine for routine follow-up for a person with hematological cancer.[126] Positive effects of telephone consultations that promoted a healthy lifestyle have also been shown to improve QOL and exercise habits.[127]

Conclusion

Management of hematological malignancy depends on the type and stage of the disease. Treatments often involve chemotherapy, radiotherapy, and/or autologous or allogeneic stem cell transplantation. Adverse effects of the hematological cancer and its treatments will impact several domains of health. These include impacts to the physiological, physical, psychological, and cognitive domains, which will have a negative impact on the QOL of the PLWBC and their caregiver(s). Common adverse effects include pain, fatigue, bone lesions (especially with MM), malnutrition, sexual dysfunction, psychological distress, and cognitive impairment. In addition, acute or chronic dysfunctions can negatively impact several body systems such as the immune system with GVHD, as well as the cardiac, neurological, and pulmonary systems. Onc R clinicians need to understand these complications and the adverse effects of cancer treatment to provide tailored proactive Onc R interventions and exercise programs. For optimal outcomes, an early comprehensive survivorship rehabilitation program and exercise interventions for this population of PLWBCs are safe and effective, but more studies are still needed in the area.

Critical Research Needs

- There is limited evidence for prehabilitation prior to treatment for hematological malignancy.
- Clinical Onc R guidelines for different hematological diagnoses: lymphoma, leukemia, MM, which includes a multidisciplinary assessment, nonpharmacological management, and safety considerations for rehabilitation.
- Dietary considerations for people with hematological cancer: before, during, and after cancer treatment; randomized

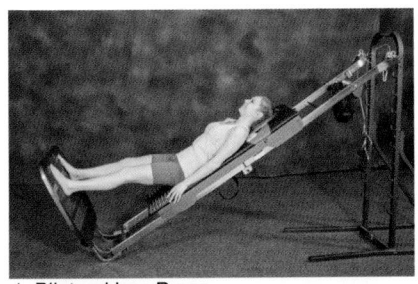
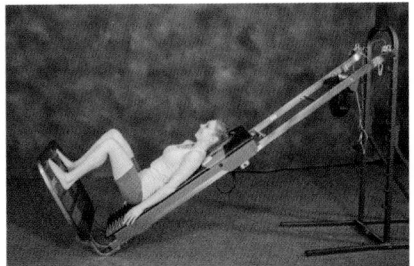

1. Bilateral Leg Press

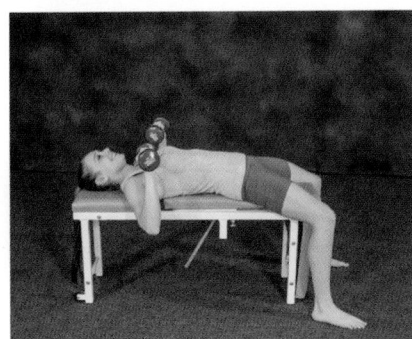
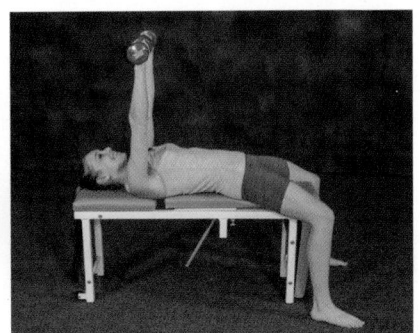

2. Bench Press

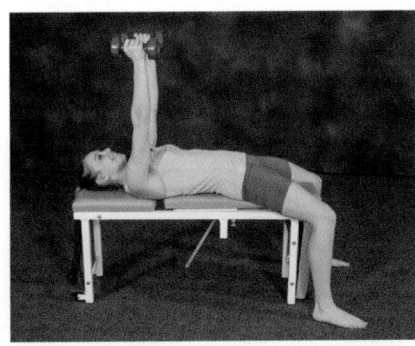
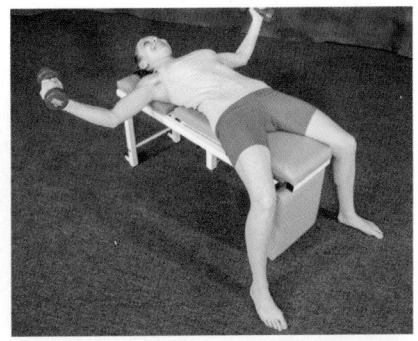

3. Shoulder Flies

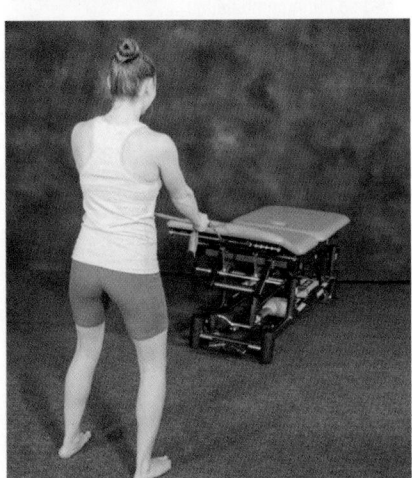
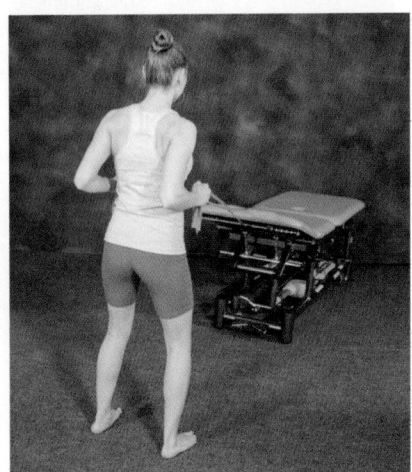

4. Shoulder Rows with Exercise Band

• **Fig. 21.7** Strengthening Exercises. (Photos printed with permission by John Krauss.)

TABLE 21.11	**Examples of Splinting Used in the Treatment of Chronic GVHD**[123]	
Name	Picture	Pros/Cons
Resting hand splint	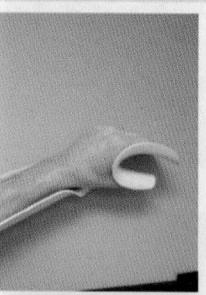	Pros: Holds fingers and hand in extension, easy to put on and take off Cons: Does not provide an active stretch, unclear if it prevents contractures
Dynamic hand splint	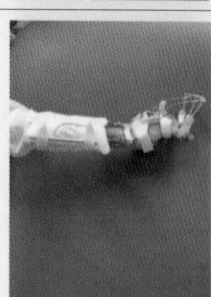	Pros: Provides a stretch in addition to limiting flexion Cons: More difficult to put on and fabricate, unclear efficacy
Ankle foot orthosis	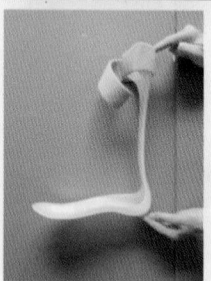	Pros: Holds ankle in dorsiflexion, prevents foot drop/drag Cons: Not effective at night, patient may need gait training in physical therapy
Multipodus (L'nard) boot	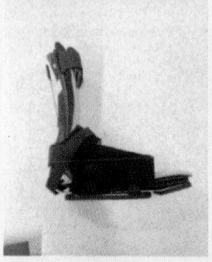	Pros: Provides dorsiflexion stretch at night, may prevent plantarflexion contracture Cons: Unclear efficacy, not for use during ambulation

GVHD, Graft-versus-host disease.
Reprinted with permission from Smith SR, Haig AJ, Couriel DR. Musculoskeletal, neurologic, and cardiopulmonary aspects of physical rehabilitation in patients with chronic graft-versus-host disease. *Biol Blood Marrow Transplant*. 2015;21(5):799–808.

controlled trials are needed to further establish nutritional recommendations.

- Examining the efficacy of multimodal intervention for bone marrow transplant populations and their caregivers.

Case Studies

Case 1

A 54-year-old white male with AML presented in the hospital for an allo-HSCT. The oncologist placed a referral reading: "Physical therapy – evaluate and treat." His allo-HSCT was planned for day 7 after his admission day. His past medical history included controlled hypertension and a knee arthroscopy for a meniscus tear. He lives at home with his wife and two high school aged children. He works in marketing and reported he plan to work while admitted to the hospital.

Examination data:

Functional mobility: Independent with all mobility

ROM (range of motion): upper extremities (UEs) and lower extremities (LEs) are within normal limits (WNL)

MMT (manual muscle test): 5/5 UEs and LEs

Berg Balance Scale: 50/56

Six-minute walk test (6MWT): >1000 feet (304 m)

He reported that he was not currently exercising and did not exercise before coming to the hospital.

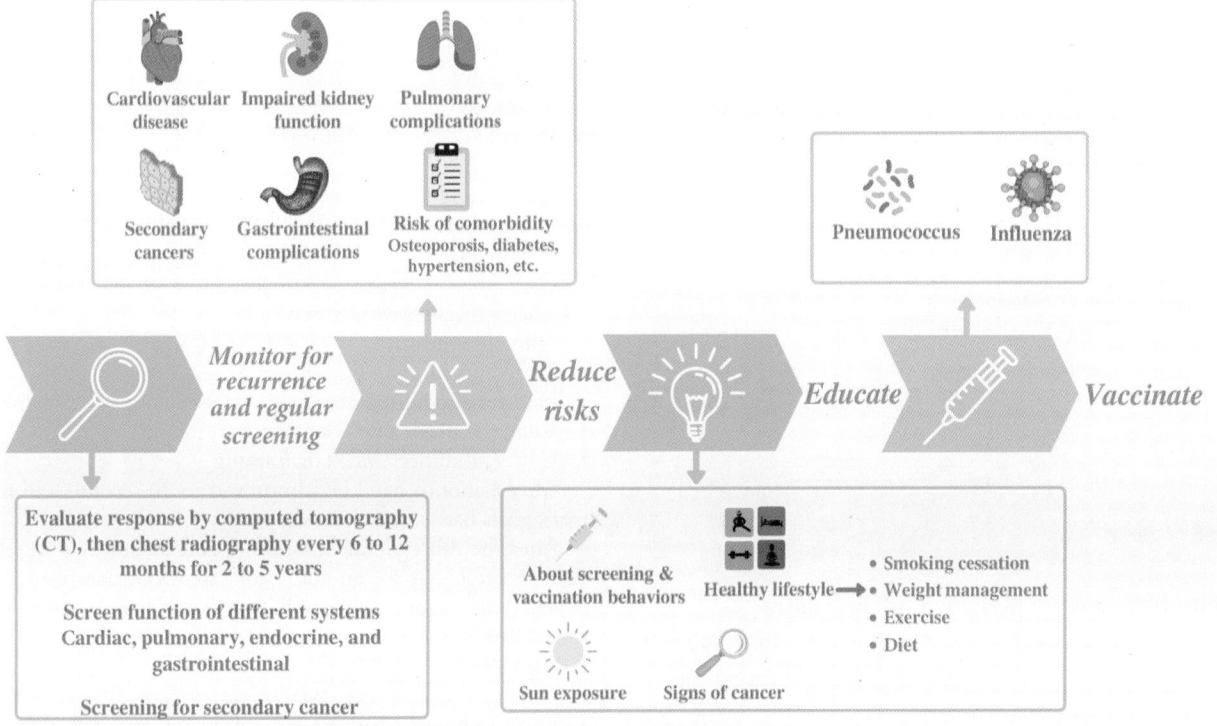

• **Fig. 21.8** Survivor Care for Routine Follow-up for Hematological Cancer. Created by Amani AlJohi and Shadia Aljuaid. Printed with permission.

Day 1 Intervention:
1. Education: Importance of exercise while admitted for his HSCT. How/where to exercise: stationary bike or treadmill versus walking the hallways. Three exercise sessions per day. How to monitor his exertion using the Borg Rate of Perceived Exertion scale.
2. Education: To modify exercise based on his blood counts, hold resistance exercises if platelets are below 20,000 µL.
3. Education: To advocate for exercise and get in contact with the physical therapist.
4. Education: Proper footwear for fall safety while exercising in the hospital.

As the patient was independent in all these tasks, he was scheduled to be seen again in 1 week.

Day 7 after his allo-HSCT:
His blood counts were as follows: hemoglobin = 9 g/dL; platelets = 40,000 µL; white blood count = 3.0 × 10⁹/L. He had a fever at 102.8°F (39.3°C) and therefore was not treated on this date due to his neutropenic fever.

Day 10 after allo-HSCT:
The physical therapist (PT) returns on day 10 after his allo-HSCT. His blood counts are as follows: hemoglobin = 10 g/dL; platelets = 80,000 µL, white blood count = 3.5 × 10⁹/L. He is afebrile. He presents in the bed and reports feeling weakened after a few days with a fever. He has not been out of bed in 3 days. The PT made the decision to treat the patient because due to his appropriate lab values via the CBC. The patient performed a 5-minute walk at a slow pace with one sitting rest break. The PT provided a series of functional strengthening exercises targeting large muscle groups: squats at the counter, single leg stance, and wall push-ups. The PT noted that he has losses of balance with turns and changing his gait speed. The patient was again provided with education and coaching to perform mobility with the nursing team when the PT was not present.

Day 20 after allo-HSCT:
The PT returned at day 20 after the patient's allo-HSCT. His blood counts have returned to his previous level without signs of disease. He has minimal GVHD in his skin. The PT worked with him to transition to a home exercise program. The patient was able to safely perform two flights of stairs without the need for assistance. He performed all his home exercises without symptoms. He was then provided with written instructions for his home exercise program that included body weight resistance exercises and cardiovascular exercise.

Discharge Assessment:
Functional mobility: Independent with all mobility
ROM: Upper Extremities (UEs) and Lower Extremities (LEs) WNL
MMT: 4/5 UEs and LEs
Berg Balance Scale: 45/56
6MWT: 800 feet (243 m)
He was referred to outpatient therapy for ongoing strengthening and balance needs that were identified when compared to his baseline evaluation.

Case 2
A 68-year-old female was diagnosed with Light Chain Multiple Myeloma Revised International Staging System (R-ISS) Stage II 2 years ago. She has had normal cytogenetics recently. She had a fall at home that resulted in low back pain and bilateral lower extremity weakness. She was admitted to the acute care hospital for investigation and suspicion of cord compression. MRI results showed multiple spinal lytic lesions and a pathological fracture at T10 with a T8 cord compression, resulting in paraplegia. Findings: fragile vertebral bodies, pathological fracture at T10, infiltration of bone and epidural space by greyish-pink fragile vascularized tissue. She underwent a T8 to L2 posterior decompression and single fraction

8 Gy spinal radiation. She was prescribed with a thoraco-lumbar-sacral orthosis (TLSO) back brace. She received adjuvant chemotherapy which consisted of 6 cycles of the CVD (cyclophosphamide, vincristine, and dacarbazine) regimen, then bortezomib and dexamethasone for eight cycles. She was transferred from acute care to IPR for 6 weeks.

Upon PT assessment:

Sensation impaired below T6, coordination intact.

ROM: UEs and LEs WNL

Muscle power:

Myotomal Strength	Initial Assessment		Discharge Assessment	
	Right	Left	Right	Left
L2	2+/5	3+/5	3/5	5/5
L3	3/5	3+/5	4/5	5/5
L4	2/5	3/5	4/5	5/5
L5	2/5	3/5	4/5	5/5
S1	2/5	3/5	4/5	5/5

Functional Independence Measure (FIM) assessment

		Initial Assessment	Discharge Assessment
Self-care	Eating	7	7
	Grooming	7	7
	Bathing	3	6
	Dressing upper	7	7
	Dressing lower	3	6
	Toileting	3	6
Sphincter control	Bladder and bowel	7	7
Transfer	Bed chair, wheelchair	4	5
	Toilet	5	5
	Tub	4	5
Locomotion	Walk/wheelchair	3	5
	Stairs	2	5
Communication	Comprehension	7	7
	Expression	7	7
Social cognition	Social interaction	7	7
	Problem solving	7	7
	Memory	7	7

7 = Complete independence; 6 = Modified independence; 5 = Supervision; 4 = Minimal assistance; 3 = Moderate assistance; 2 = Maximal assistance; 1 = Total assistance

Functional examination

Bed mobility: Independent, but required increased time

Standing balance: Static = fair, dynamic = poor

Goals:

- Patient to be independent with bed mobility
- Patient to be able to walk for more than 300 feet using a wheeled walker with supervision
- Patient to be able to ascend and descend 24 steps with supervision
  Interventions to address mobility impairment:
- Strengthening exercises for LEs
- Bed mobility training
- Endurance training (e.g., knee marches)

- Sit to stand training with deep breathing exercise and balance training
- Gait training
- Stair training
- Safety education to prevent falls
- Patient and family education

After 2 weeks of intensive training for five times per week the patient showed improvement in:

- Bed mobility, muscle power and standing balance, static and dynamic fair
- Gait: able to walk for 328 feet (100 m) without rest using wheeled walker with supervision.
  Outcome measure:
- Timed up and go (TUG) test: 32 seconds.
  Her treatment program was progressed, and exercises included:
- Isometric pelvic and core exercises, stability exercises
- Gait, endurance, and stair training

After 1 month her TUG improved to 20 seconds and her primary goals had been achieved.

After the 8th cycle of bortezomib and dexamethasone, the recommendation was for an autologous stem cell transplant, but the patient declined the procedure. She continued to receive maintenance lenalidomide and zoledronic acid (Zometa) for 2 years.

Discussion:

Her bone health was reviewed by the orthopedic and spine team and no specific precautions were provided. She had a lytic lesion in right femur and spine but was permitted to be full weight-bearing. Patient received bortezomib which increased the risk of CIPN in addition to the complication of the fractured spine and the incomplete spinal cord injury; all of which caused neurological involvement and weakness. The TUG outcome measure showed improvement but she was still at risk for falls. Safety instruction and education was given to the patient and her family to prevent falls at home. There was a delay with initiating physical therapy due to episodes of neutropenia during chemotherapy.

Case 3

A 65-year-old female presents to the outpatient clinic for a right humeral fracture status post open reduction internal fixation (ORIF) after a fall outside 5 months ago. She has a past medical history of lymphoma 3 years ago and was treated with chemotherapy. She is unsure which chemotherapy she received. She is in remission.

Examination Data:

Shoulder ROM: (in degrees)

Right (R):	**Left (L):**
Flexion: 150 degrees	Flexion: 165 degrees
Abduction: 140 degrees	Abduction: 140 degrees
ER: 70 degrees	ER: 90 degrees
IR: 45 degrees	IR: 60 degrees

Shoulder Strength: L: 4/5 all directions; R: 3+/5 all directions

Hip Strength: Bilateral (B): 3-/5 hip abductors, 3/5 hip extensors

Incision appears well healed with minimal swelling in her anterior R shoulder. No signs of infection

TUG: 22 seconds

Five times sit to stand: 20.4 seconds

Gait: shortened step length, slowed cadence, bilateral hip drop, 2 losses of balance in 150 feet

Sit to stand: two attempts to initiate, uses legs on the back of the chair to achieve standing. Lack of anterior translation of her trunk.

Assessment: Decreased functional mobility due to high levels of chemotherapy and deconditioning. Likely presents with hip weakness due to her difficulty rising from a chair. She has decreased scores on the TUG and five times sit to stand. Although she is there for her shoulder ROM and strength, she likely fell due to limitations from her cancer treatments. She would benefit from providing the exact chemotherapy regimen she was on so the therapist can anticipate any cardiovascular or neurological issues she may be Experiencing.

Interventions: Therapeutic intervention would include regular cardiovascular conditioning at a moderate level (Borg Scale of 12-13/20), for 150 minutes per week as she tolerates. To reduce her fall risk, balance training with emphasis on dynamic gait activities wound be included. Exercises for her shoulder range of motion and strength deficits would be vital for improved upper extremity function.

Discussion: PLWBCs will benefit from a multisystemic approach to deficits related to cancer treatment. Addressing the orthopedic deficits in her shoulder as well as her endurance and balance deficits will give her the best outcome with her recovery. Rehabilitation clinicians are recommended to perform a comprehensive evaluation and treatment plan to address all of her needs.

Review Questions

Reader can find the correct answers and rationale in the back of the book.

A 53-year-old male with AML is admitted to the hospital for induction chemotherapy using the 7+3 regimen (cytarabine daily for 7 days with an anthracycline [e.g., daunorubicin] on each of the first 3 days). He has a past medical history significant for hypertension, migraines, and irritable bowel syndrome. You see him immediately following his admission. He is walking independently but reports that he has increased fatigue from the high dose of chemotherapy he has received during induction chemotherapy.

1. The MOST important intervention for him is the following:
   A. Nutritional information
   B. Education about performing a walking program during admission
   C. Fatigue management strategies
   D. Stretching

2. When you return 1 week later to deliver resistance exercises, he reports increased fatigue and nausea. His current platelets are 15,000 µL. Which of the following is the MOST appropriate course of action?
   A. Do not treat, let him rest
   B. Continue with exercise intervention but monitor symptoms
   C. Continue with exercise intervention but omit resistance exercise
   D. Talk with his nurse

3. Your patient has a fever while he is neutropenic. You are safe to perform your planed therapy session:
   A. Always
   B. Never
   C. Only if they agree to participate
   D. Only if you focus on gait training

4. When he is ready for discharge, you return to evaluate his ability to go home. You find that he has proximal muscle weakness, but otherwise is independent with mobility. What would be the best intervention?
   A. Referral to outpatient physical therapy
   B. Prescribe strengthening exercises for home
   C. Educate him to about proper nutrition
   D. Fatigue management strategies

   A 29-year-old female is newly diagnosed with NHL and presents in the hospital to receive high-dose chemotherapy. She has an insignificant past medical history and is independent with all mobility.

5. She most likely is diagnosed with the most common form of NHL which is:
   A. Hodgkin lymphoma
   B. Diffuse large B-cell lymphomas
   C. Burkitt lymphoma
   D. Peripheral T-cell

6. She is most likely going to receive this treatment regimen:
   A. HSCT
   B. Dexamethasone
   C. CHOP and R-CHOP
   D. Radiation alone

   A 67-year-old male with MM presents in the emergency room with low back pain. Upon CT scan, he was found to have multiple bone lesions in his spine. He does not have any pathological fractures currently.

7. Which of the following is true?
   A. Light physical activity is prescribed, and resistive exercise is contraindicated
   B. There are contraindications for weight bearing exercises until patient receives vitamin D and bisphosphonates
   C. Onc R clinicians need to avoid movements that place excessively high loads on fragile skeletal sites such as hyperflexion, hyperextension, or trunk rotation
   D. Only supine exercises allowed, and moderate intensity exercises aerobic from sitting such as cycling for 60% VO_2 peak

8. Due to his condition, he most likely is experiencing what main symptom:
   A. Headache
   B. Constipation
   C. Nausea and vomiting
   D. Pain

9. What oncologic emergency needs to be ruled out before this patient is safe to be seen by a rehabilitation clinician?
   A. Spinal cord compression
   B. Superior vena cava syndrome
   C. Nausea
   D. Neutropenic fever

10. The diagnosis of MM is determined by the presence of plasma cell infiltration plus one of the Myeloma Defining Events (MDE) which uses the abbreviation CRAB. CRAB refers to.
   A. Cardiac, renal failure, anemia, and back pain
   B. Coronary artery disease, renal failure, anemia, and back pain
   C. Cardiac, renal failure, anemia, and bone lesions
   D. Calcium, renal failure, anemia, and bone lesions

References

1. Baima J, Khanna A. *Cancer Rehabilitation*: Baima J, Khanna A, eds Springer International Publishing; 2020.

2. Sung H, Ferlay J, Siegel RL, et al. Global cancer statistics 2020: GLOBOCAN estimates of incidence and mortality worldwide for 36 cancers in 185 countries. *CA Cancer J Clin*. 2021;71(3): 209–249.

3. O'Donnell MR, Tallman MS, Abboud CN, et al. Acute myeloid leukemia, version 3.2017: clinical practice guidelines in oncology. *JNCCN J Natl Compr Cancer Netw*. 2017;15(7):926–957.

4. Heuser M, Ofran Y, Boissel N, et al. Acute myeloid leukaemia in adult patients: ESMO Clinical Practice Guidelines for diagnosis, treatment and follow-up. *Ann Oncol*. 2020;31(6):697–712.

5. Cooper SL, Brown PA. Treatment of pediatric acute lymphoblastic leukemia. *Physiol Behav*. 2016;176(1):139–148.

6. Dicato MA. *Side Effects of Medical Cancer Therapy: Prevention and Treatment*. 2013.

7. Eichhorst B, Robak T, Montserrat E, et al. Chronic lymphocytic leukaemia: ESMO Clinical Practice Guidelines for diagnosis, treatment and follow-up. *Ann Oncol*. 2015;26(suppl 5):v78–v84.

8. Olin JL, Canupp K, Smith MB. New pharmacotherapies in chronic lymphocytic leukemia. *P T*. 2017;42(2):106–115.

9. Baccarani M, Pileri S, Steegmann JL, Muller M, Soverini S, Dreyling M. Chronic myeloid leukemia: ESMO clinical practice guidelines for diagnosis, treatment and follow-up. *Ann Oncol*. 2012;23(suppl 7):vii72–vii77.

10. W. Hiddemann. *Handbook of Acute Leukemia*; Springer International Publishing, 2016. doi: 10.1007/978-3-319-26772-2.

11. Hughes TP, Ross DM, Melo JV. Handbook of Chronic Myeloid Leukemia; Springer International Publishing. 2014.

12. Glen F, Rall MJSBMD. Treatment with a 5-day versus a 10-day schedule of decitabine in older patients with newly diagnosed acute myeloid leukaemia: a randomised phase 2 trial. *Lancet Haematol*. 2019;6(1):e29–e37.

13. Hoelzer D, Bassan R, Dombret H, et al. Acute lymphoblastic leukaemia in adult patients: ESMO clinical practice guidelines for diagnosis, treatment and follow-up. *Ann Oncol*. 2016;27(suppl 5): v69–v82.

14. S.H. Swerdlow, E. Campo, N.L. Harris, et al. *WHO Classification of Tumours of Haematopoietic and Lymphoid Tissues*. World Health Organization, Lyon, France: IARC, 2017.

15. Harris NL, Campo E, Jaffe ES. Introduction to the WHO classification of tumours of haematopoietic and lymphoid tissues. In: *WHO Classification of Tumours of Haematopoietic and Lymphoid Tissues*; World Health Organization, 2008.

16. Ansell SM. Hodgkin lymphoma: a 2020 update on diagnosis, risk-stratification, and management. *Am J Hematol*. 2020;95(8):978–989.

17. Younes A. *Handbook of Lymphoma*. Springer International Publishing. 2016:1–112.

18. EN Mugnaini, N Ghosh Lymphoma. *Prim Care*. 2016;43(4):661–675.

19. Zhang S, Gong TT, Liu FH, et al. Global, regional, and national burden of endometrial cancer, 1990–2017: results from the Global Burden of Disease Study, 2017. *Front Oncol*. 2019;9:1440.

20. Fitzmaurice C, Abate D, Abbasi N, et al. Global, regional, and national cancer incidence, mortality, years of life lost, years lived with disability, and disability-adjusted life-years for 29 cancer groups, 1990 to 2017: a systematic analysis for the global burden of disease study. *JAMA Oncol*. 2019;5(12):1749–1768.

21. Thieblemont C, Bernard S, Molina T. Management of aggressive lymphoma in very elderly patients. *Hematol Oncol*. 2017;35:49–53.

22. Cerhan JR, Slager SL. Familial predisposition and genetic risk factors for lymphoma. *Blood*. 2015;126(20):2265–2273.

23. de Martel C, Georges D, Bray F, Ferlay J, Clifford GM. Global burden of cancer attributable to infections in 2018: a worldwide incidence analysis. *Lancet Glob Heal*. 2020;8(2):e180–e190.

24. Shiels MS, Engels EA. Evolving epidemiology of HIV-associated malignancies. *Curr Opin HIV AIDS*. 2017;12(1):6–11.

25. Morton LM, Slager SL, Cerhan JR, et al. Etiologic heterogeneity among non-Hodgkin lymphoma subtypes: the interLymph non-Hodgkin lymphoma subtypes project. *J Natl Cancer Inst Monogr*. 2014;2014(48):130–144.

26. Eichenauer DA, Aleman BMP, André M, et al. Hodgkin lymphoma: ESMO Clinical Practice Guidelines for diagnosis, treatment and follow-up. *Ann Oncol*. 2018;29(suppl 4):iv19–iv29.

27. Vitolo U, Seymour JF, Martelli M, et al. Extranodal diffuse large B-cell lymphoma (DLBCL) and primary mediastinal B-cell lymphoma: ESMO clinical practice guidelines for diagnosis, treatment and follow-up. *Ann Oncol*. 2016;27(suppl 5):v91–v102.

28. Steinberg A, Rao P. Hodgkin lymphoma. In: *Atlas of Diagnostic Hematology*: Elsevier. 2021:211–216.

29. Akgül T, Bilgin Y, Karademir G. The great mimicker at thoracolumbar spine: non-Hodgkin's lymphoma. *Int J Surg Case Rep*. 2017;39:267–270.

30. Hashi S, Goodwin CR, Ahmed AK, Sciubba DM. Management of extranodal lymphoma of the spine: a study of 30 patients. *CNS Oncol*. 2018;7(2):CNS11.

31. M. Mohty, J.L. Harousseau. *Handbook of Multiple Myeloma*. Cham: Springer International Publishing, 2015.

32. Mikhael J, Ismaila N, Cheung MC, et al. Treatment of multiple myeloma: ASCO and CCO joint clinical practice guideline. *J Clin Oncol*. 2019;37(14):1228–1263.

33. Costa LJ, Brill IK, Omel J, Godby K, Kumar SK, Brown EE. Recent trends in multiple myeloma incidence and survival by age, race, and ethnicity in the United States. *Blood Adv*. 2017;1(4):282–287.

34. Cowan AJ, Allen C, Barac A, et al. Global burden of multiple myeloma: a systematic analysis for the global burden of disease study 2016. *JAMA Oncol*. 2018;4(9):1221–1227.

35. Rajkumar SV. Multiple myeloma: 2020 update on diagnosis, risk-stratification and management. *Am J Hematol*. 2020;95(5):548–567.

36. Palumbo A, Avet-Loiseau H, Oliva S, et al. Revised international staging system for multiple myeloma: a report from international myeloma working group. *J Clin Oncol*. 2015;33(26):2863–2869.

37. Ramsenthaler C, Kane P, Gao W, et al. Prevalence of symptoms in patients with multiple myeloma: a systematic review and meta-analysis. *Eur J Haematol*. 2016;97(5):416–429.

38. Coluzzi F, Rolke R, Mercadante S. Pain management in patients with multiple myeloma: an update. *Cancers (Basel)*. 2019;11(12):2037.

39. Rades D, Conde-Moreno AJ, Cacicedo J, Segedin B, Rudat V, Schild SE. Excellent outcomes after radiotherapy alone for malignant spinal cord compression from myeloma. *Radiol Oncol*. 2016;50(3):337–340.

40. Terpos E, Morgan G, Dimopoulos MA, et al. International myeloma working group recommendations for the treatment of multiple myeloma-related bone disease. *J Clin Oncol*. 2013;31(18):2347–2357.

41. Lehners N, Becker N, Benner A, et al. Analysis of long-term survival in multiple myeloma after first-line autologous stem cell transplantation: impact of clinical risk factors and sustained response. *Cancer Med*. 2018;7(2):307–316.

42. Yao X, Xu Z, Du X. PKP/PVP combine chemotherapy in the treatment of multiple myeloma patients with vertebral pathological fractures: minimum 3-year follow-up of 108 cases. *J Orthop Surg Res*. 2019;14(1):1–8.

43. Rindflesch AB, Hake MP, Spiten MA, et al. Physical performance following hematopoietic stem cell transplantation: a prospective observational study. *Rehabil Oncol*. 2020;38(3):122–126.

44. Rexer P, Kanphade G, Murphy S. Feasibility of an exercise program for patients with thrombocytopenia undergoing hematopoietic stem cell transplant. *J Acute Care Phys Ther*. 2016;7(2):55–64.

45. Steinberg A, Asher A, Bailey C, Fu JB. The role of physical rehabilitation in stem cell transplantation patients. *Support Care Cancer*. 2015;23(8):2447–2460.

46. Wakasugi T, Morishita S, Kaida K, et al. Impaired skeletal muscle oxygenation following allogeneic hematopoietic stem cell transplantation is associated with exercise capacity. *Support Care Cancer.* 2018;26(7):2149–2160.

47. Maltser S, Cristian A, Silver JK, Morris GS, Stout NL. A focused review of safety considerations in cancer rehabilitation. *PM&R.* 2017;9(1):S415–S428.

48. Abo S, Ritchie D, Denehy L, Panek-Hudson Y, Irving L, Granger CL. A hospital and home-based exercise program to address functional decline in people following allogeneic stem cell transplantation. *Support Care Cancer.* 2018;26(6):1727–1736.

49. Schumacher H, Stüwe S, Kropp P, et al. A prospective, randomized evaluation of the feasibility of exergaming on patients undergoing hematopoietic stem cell transplantation. *Bone Marrow Transplant.* 2018;53(5):584–590.

50. Ramachandran V, Kolli SS, Strowd LC. Review of graft-versus-host disease. *Dermatol Clin.* 2019;37(4):569–582.

51. Hamada R, Kondo T, Murao M, et al. Effect of the severity of acute graft-versus-host disease on physical function after allogeneic hematopoietic stem cell transplantation. *Support Care Cancer.* 2020;28(7):3189–3196.

52. Liang Y, Zhou M, Wang F, Wu Z. Exercise for physical fitness, fatigue and quality of life of patients undergoing hematopoietic stem cell transplantation: a meta-analysis of randomized controlled trials. *Jpn J Clin Oncol.* 2018;48(12):1046–1057.

53. Aladağ E, Kelkitli E, Göker H. Acute graft-versus-host disease: a brief review. *Turkish J Hematol.* 2020;37(1):1–4.

54. Shaulov A, Rodin G, Popovic G, et al. Pain in patients with newly diagnosed or relapsed acute leukemia. *Support Care Cancer.* 2019;27(8):2789–2797.

55. Rambod M, Pasyar N, Shamsadini M. The effect of foot reflexology on fatigue, pain, and sleep quality in lymphoma patients: a clinical trial. *Eur J Oncol Nurs.* 2019;43:101678.

56. He Y, Guo X, May BH, et al. Clinical evidence for association of acupuncture and acupressure with improved cancer pain: a systematic review and meta-analysis. *JAMA Oncol.* 2020;6(2):271–278.

57. Hacker ED, Collins E, Park C, Peters T, Patel P, Rondelli D. Strength training to enhance early recovery after hematopoietic stem cell transplantation. *Biol Blood Marrow Transplant.* 2017;23(4):659–669.

58. Mohammed J, Smith SR, Burns L, et al. Role of physical therapy before and after hematopoietic stem cell transplantation: white paper report. *Biol Blood Marrow Transplant.* 2019;25(6):e191–e198.

59. Sitlinger A, Brander DM, Bartlett DB. Impact of exercise on the immune system and outcomes in hematologic malignancies. *Blood Adv.* 2020;4(8):1801–1811.

60. Liu L, He X, Feng L. Exercise on quality of life and cancer-related fatigue for lymphoma survivors: a systematic review and meta-analysis. *Support Care Cancer.* 2019;27(11):4069–4082.

61. Zhou Y, Zhu J, Gu Z, Yin X. Efficacy of exercise interventions in patients with acute leukemia: a meta-analysis. *PLoS One.* 2016;11(7):1–16.

62. Bates D, Bolwell B, Majhail NS, et al. Music therapy for symptom management after autologous stem cell transplantation: results from a randomized study. *Biol Blood Marrow Transplant.* 2017;23(9):1567–1572.

63. Ruchlemer R, Amit-Kohn M, Tvito A, Sindelovsky I, Zimran A, Raveh-Brawer D. Bone loss and hematological malignancies in adults: a pilot study. *Support Care Cancer.* 2018;26(9):3013–3020.

64. Khan Z, Agarwal NB, Bhurani D, Khan MA. Risk factors for haematopoietic stem cell transplant (HSCT) associated bone loss. *Transplant Cell Ther.* 2021;27(3):212–221.

65. Kendler DL, Body JJ, Brandi ML, et al. Bone management in hematologic stem cell transplant recipients. *Osteoporos Int.* 2018;29(12):2597–2610.

66. Yu PA, Hsu WH, Bin Hsu W, et al. The effects of high impact exercise intervention on bone mineral density, physical fitness, and quality of life in postmenopausal women with osteopenia: a retrospective cohort study. *Medicine (Baltimore).* 2019;98(11):e14898.

67. Dalla Via J, Daly RM, Fraser SF. The effect of exercise on bone mineral density in adult cancer survivors: a systematic review and meta-analysis. *Osteoporos Int.* 2018;29(2):287–303.

68. Keilani M, Kainberger F, Pataraia A, et al. Typical aspects in the rehabilitation of cancer patients suffering from metastatic bone disease or multiple myeloma. *Wien Klin Wochenschr.* 2019;131(21–22):567–575.

69. Messina C, Christie D, Zucca E, Gospodarowicz M, Ferreri AJM. Primary and secondary bone lymphomas. *Cancer Treat Rev.* 2015;41(3):235–246.

70. Jeevanantham D, Rajendran V, McGillis Z, Tremblay L, Larivière C, Knight A. Mobilization and exercise intervention for patients with multiple myeloma: clinical practice guidelines endorsed by the Canadian Physiotherapy Association. *Phys Ther.* 2021;101(1):pzaa180.

71. Imahashi N, Inamoto Y, Seto A, et al. Impact on relapse of corticosteroid therapy after allogeneic hematopoietic stem cell transplantation for acute myeloid leukemia. *Clin Transplant.* 2010;24(6):772–777.

72. Lee HJ, Oran B, Saliba RM, et al. Steroid myopathy in patients with acute graft-versus-host disease treated with high-dose steroid therapy. *Bone Marrow Transplant.* 2006;38(4):299–303.

73. McClune B, Majhail NS, Flowers MED. Bone loss and avascular necrosis of bone after hematopoietic cell transplantation. *Semin Hematol.* 2012;49(1):59–65.

74. Kaya AH, Namdaroğlu S, Kayıkcı Ö, et al. Impact of guideline-driven approach in follow-up of long-term complications after allogeneic hematopoietic cell transplant: single center experience. *Exp Clin Transplant.* 2020;18(3):359–367.

75. Chakraborty R, Majhail NS. Treatment and disease-related complications in multiple myeloma: implications for survivorship. *Am J Hematol.* 2020;95(6):672–690.

76. Li T, Timmins HC, Lazarus HM, Park SB. Peripheral neuropathy in hematologic malignancies – past, present and future. *Blood Rev.* 2020;43:100653.

77. Delforge M, Ludwig H. How I manage the toxicities of myeloma drugs. *Blood.* 2017;129(17):2359–2367.

78. McCrary JM, Goldstein D, Sandler CX, et al. Exercise-based rehabilitation for cancer survivors with chemotherapy-induced peripheral neuropathy. *Support Care Cancer.* 2019;27(10):3849–3857.

79. Wong R, Major P, Sagar S. Phase 2 study of acupuncture-like transcutaneous nerve stimulation for chemotherapy-induced peripheral neuropathy. *Integr Cancer Ther.* 2016;15(2):153–164.

80. Bao T, Goloubeva O, Pelser C, et al. A pilot study of acupuncture in treating bortezomib-induced peripheral neuropathy in patients with multiple myeloma. *Integr Cancer Ther.* 2014;13(5):396–404.

81. Rotz SJ, Ryan TD, Hlavaty J, George SA, El-Bietar J, Dandoy CE. Cardiotoxicity and cardiomyopathy in children and young adult survivors of hematopoietic stem cell transplant. *Pediatr Blood Cancer.* 2017;64(11). doi:10.1002/pbc.26600.

82. Heckmann MB, Doroudgar S, Katus HA, Lehmann LH. Cardiovascular adverse events in multiple myeloma patients. *J Thorac Dis.* 2018;10(suppl 35):S4296–S4305.

83. Guner SI, Yanmaz MT, Selvi A, Usul C. Chemotherapy and radiation induced pulmonary dysfunction in Hodgkin lymphoma patients. *Indian J Hematol Blood Transfus.* 2016;32(4):431–436.

84. Diab M, ZazaDitYafawi J, Soubani AO. Major pulmonary complications after hematopoietic stem cell transplant. *Exp Clin Transplant.* 2016;14(3):259–270.

85. Pham J, Rangaswamy J, Avery S, et al. Updated prevalence, predictors and treatment outcomes for bronchiolitis obliterans syndrome after allogeneic stem cell transplantation. *Respir Med.* 2020;177:106286.

86. Baumgartner A, Bargetzi A, Zueger N, et al. Revisiting nutritional support for allogeneic hematologic stem cell transplantation: a systematic review. *Bone Marrow Transplant.* 2017;52(4):506–513.

87. Karacan Y, Yildiz H, Demircioglu B, Ali R. Evaluation of sexual dysfunction in patients with hematological malignancies. *Asia Pac J Oncol Nurs.* 2020;8(1):51–57.

88. Greaves P, Sarker SJ, Chowdhury K, et al. Fertility and sexual function in long-term survivors of haematological malignancy: using patient-reported outcome measures to assess a neglected area of need in the late effects clinic. *Br J Haematol.* 2014;164(4):526–535.

89. Thygesen KH, Schjødt I, Jarden M. The impact of hematopoietic stem cell transplantation on sexuality: a systematic review of the literature. *Bone Marrow Transplant.* 2012;47(5):716–724.

90. Booker R, Walker L. Raffin Bouchal S. Sexuality after hematopoietic stem cell transplantation: a mixed methods study. *Eur J Oncol Nurs.* 2019;39:10–20.

91. Eeltink CM, Incrocci L, Verdonck-De Leeuw IM, Zweegman S. Recommended patient information sheet on the impact of haematopoietic cell transplantation on sexual functioning and sexuality. *Ecancermedicalscience.* 2019;13:987.

92. Clinton-Mcharg T, Carey M, Sanson-Fisher R, Tzelepis F, Bryant J, Williamson A. Anxiety and depression among haematological cancer patients attending treatment centres: prevalence and predictors. *J Affect Disord.* 2014;165:176–181.

93. Muffly LS, Hlubocky FJ, Khan N, et al. Psychological morbidities in adolescent and young adult blood cancer patients during curative-intent therapy and early survivorship. *Cancer.* 2016;122(6):954–961.

94. Amonoo HL, Brown LA, Scheu CF, et al. Beyond depression, anxiety and post-traumatic stress disorder symptoms: qualitative study of negative emotional experiences in hematopoietic stem cell transplant patients. *Eur J Cancer Care (Engl).* 2020;29(5):e13263.

95. Seo HJ, Baek YG, Cho BS, Kim TS, Um YH, Chae JH. Anxiety and depression of the patients with hematological malignancies during hospitalization for hematopoietic stem cell transplantation. *Psychiatry Investig.* 2019;16(10):751–758.

96. Zhang R, Yin J, Zhou Y. Effects of mindfulness-based psychological care on mood and sleep of leukemia patients in chemotherapy. *Int J Nurs Sci.* 2017;4(4):357–361.

97. Lamers J, Hartmann M, Goldschmidt H, Brechtel A, Hillengass J, Herzog W. Psychosocial support in patients with multiple myeloma at time of diagnosis: who wants what? *Psycho-oncology.* 2013;22(10):2313–2320.

98. Amonoo HL, Barclay ME, El-Jawahri A, Traeger LN, Lee SJ, Huffman JC. Positive psychological constructs and health outcomes in hematopoietic stem cell transplantation patients: a systematic review. *Biol Blood Marrow Transplant.* 2019;25(1):e5–e16.

99. Troke R, Andrewes T. Nursing considerations for supporting cancer patients with metastatic spinal cord compression: a literature review. *Br J Nurs.* 2019;28(17):S24–S29.

100. El-Jawahri A, Jacobs JM, Nelson AM, et al. Multimodal psychosocial intervention for family caregivers of patients undergoing hematopoietic stem cell transplantation: a randomized clinical trial. *Cancer.* 2020;126(8):1758–1765.

101. Bangerter LR, Griffin JM, Langer S, et al. The effect of psychosocial interventions on outcomes for caregivers of hematopoietic cell transplant patients. *Curr Hematol Malig Rep.* 2018;13(3):155–163.

102. Ichikawa T, Kurozumi K, Michiue H, et al. Reduced neurotoxicity with combined treatment of high-dose methotrexate, cyclophosphamide, doxorubicin, vincristine and prednisolone (M-CHOP) and deferred radiotherapy for primary central nervous system lymphoma. *Clin Neurol Neurosurg.* 2014;127:106–111.

103. Koll TT, Sheese AN, Semin J, et al. Screening for cognitive impairment in older adults with hematological malignancies using the Montreal Cognitive Assessment and neuropsychological testing. *J Geriatr Oncol.* 2020;11(2):297–303.

104. Kotb MG, Soliman AER, Ibrahim RI, Said RMM, El Din MMW. Chemotherapy-induced cognitive impairment in hematological malignancies. *Egypt J Neurol Psychiatry Neurosurg.* 2019;55(1). doi:10.1186/s41983-019-0104-9.

105. Nakamura ZM, Deal AM, Rosenstein DL, et al. Cognitive function in patients prior to undergoing allogeneic hematopoietic stem cell transplantation. *Support Care Cancer.* 2021;29(4):2007–2014.

106. Gates P, Renehan S, Ku M. Examining the feasibility of an online cognitive rehabilitation program in haematology survivorship care to reduce chemotherapy-related cognitive impairment. *Aust J Cancer Nurs.* 2018;19(1):10–18.

107. Takekiyo T, Dozono K, Mitsuishi T, et al. Effect of exercise therapy on muscle mass and physical functioning in patients undergoing allogeneic hematopoietic stem cell transplantation. *Support Care Cancer.* 2015;23(4):985–992. doi:10.1007/s00520-014-2425-7.

108. Rothe D, Cox-Kennett N, Buijs DM, et al. Cardiac rehabilitation in patients with lymphoma undergoing autologous hematopoietic stem cell transplantation: a cardio-oncology pilot project. *Can J Cardiol.* 2018;34(10):S263–S269.

109. Duregon F, Gobbo S, Bullo V, et al. Exercise prescription and tailored physical activity intervention in onco-hematology inpatients, a personalized bedside approach to improve clinical best practice. *Hematol Oncol.* 2019;37(3):277–284.

110. Gheyasi F, Baraz S, Malehi AS, Ahmadzadeh A, Salehi R, Vaismoradi M. Effect of the walking exercise program on cancer-related fatigue in patients with acute myeloid leukemia undergoing chemotherapy. *Asian Pacific J Cancer Prev.* 2019;20(6):1661–1666.

111. Fukushima T, Nakano J, Ishii S, et al. Factors associated with muscle function in patients with hematologic malignancies undergoing chemotherapy. *Support Care Cancer.* 2020;28(3):1433–1439.

112. Wehrle A, Kneis S, Dickhuth HH, Gollhofer A, Bertz H. Endurance and resistance training in patients with acute leukemia undergoing induction chemotherapy: a randomized pilot study. *Support Care Cancer.* 2019;27(3):1071–1079. doi:10.1007/s00520-018-4396-6.

113. Persoon S, ChinAPaw MJM, Buffart LM, et al. Randomized controlled trial on the effects of a supervised high intensity exercise program in patients with a hematologic malignancy treated with autologous stem cell transplantation: results from the EXIST study. *PLoS ONE.* 2017;12(7):1–14.

114. Hung YC, Bauer JD, Horsely P, Coll J, Bashford J, Isenring EA. Telephone-delivered nutrition and exercise counselling after auto-SCT: a pilot, randomised controlled trial. *Bone Marrow Transplant.* 2014;49(6):786–792.

115. Riedl D, Giesinger JM, Wintner LM, et al. Improvement of quality of life and psychological distress after inpatient cancer rehabilitation: results of a longitudinal observational study. *Wien Klin Wochenschr.* 2017;129(19–20):692–701.

116. Mix JM, Granger CV, LaMonte MJ, et al. Characterization of cancer patients in inpatient rehabilitation facilities: a retrospective cohort study. *Arch Phys Med Rehabil.* 2017;98(5):971–980. doi:10.1016/j.apmr.2016.12.023.

117. AlJohi A, Javison S, Lubbada S, Beshawri Y, Hamdan AB. Impact of inpatient rehabilitation services on the functional levels of cancer patients at King Fahad Medical City, Riyadh, Saudi Arabia. *Saudi Med J.* 2020;41(9):984–989.

118. Gallegos-Kearin V, Knowlton SE, Goldstein R, et al. Outcome trends of adult cancer patients receiving inpatient rehabilitation. *Am J Phys Med Rehabil.* 2018;97(7):514–522.

119. Furzer BJ, Ackland TR, Wallman KE, et al. A randomised controlled trial comparing the effects of a 12-week supervised exercise versus usual care on outcomes in haematological cancer patients. *Support Care Cancer.* 2016;24(4):1697–1707. doi:10.1007/s00520-015-2955-7.

120. van Haren IEPM, Staal JB, Potting CM, et al. Physical exercise prior to hematopoietic stem cell transplantation: a feasibility study. *Physiother Theory Pract.* 2018;34(10):747–756.

121. Fischetti F, Greco G, Cataldi S, Minoia C, Loseto G, Guarini A. Effects of physical exercise intervention on psychological and physical fitness in lymphoma patients. *Medicina (Kaunas).* 2019;55(7):379.

122. Molloy S, Lai M, Pratt G, et al. Optimizing the management of patients with spinal myeloma disease. *Br J Haematol.* 2015;171(3):332–343.

123. Smith SR, Haig AJ, Couriel DR. Musculoskeletal, neurologic, and cardiopulmonary aspects of physical rehabilitation in patients with chronic graft-versus-host disease. *Biol Blood Marrow Transplant*. 2015;21(5):799–808.

124. Molés-Poveda P, Comis LE, Joe GO, et al. Rehabilitation interventions in the multidisciplinary management of patients with sclerotic graft-versus-host disease of the skin and fascia. *Arch Phys Med Rehabil*. 2021;102(4):776–788.

125. Ray H, Beaumont A, Loeliger J, et al. Clinical medicine implementation of a multidisciplinary allied health optimisation clinic for cancer patients with complex needs. *J Clin Med*. 2020;9(8):2431. doi:10.3390/jcm9082431.

126. Faiman B, Faiman M. Living with hematologic cancer: recommendations, solutions. *Cleve Clin J Med*. 2017;84(7):528–534.

127. Vallerand JR, Rhodes RE, Walker GJ, Courneya KS. Feasibility and preliminary efficacy of an exercise telephone counseling intervention for hematologic cancer survivors: a phase II randomized controlled trial. *J Cancer Surviv*. 2018;12(3):357–370. doi:10.1007/s11764-018-0675-y.

128. Chihara D, Nastoupil LJ, Williams JN, Lee P, Koff JL, Flowers CR. New insights into the epidemiology of non-Hodgkin lymphoma and implications for therapy. *Expert Rev Anticancer Ther*. 2015;15(5):531–544.

129. Singh R, Shaik S, Negi B, et al. Non-Hodgkin's lymphoma: a review. *J Fam Med Prim Care*. 2020;9(4):1834.

130. Fraz MA, Warraich FH, Warraich SU, et al. Special considerations for the treatment of multiple myeloma according to advanced age, comorbidities, frailty and organ dysfunction. *Crit Rev Oncol Hematol*. 2019;137:18–26. doi:10.1016/j.critrevonc.2019.02.011.

131. Fu JB, Tennison JM, Rutzen-Lopez IM, et al. Bleeding frequency and characteristics among hematologic malignancy inpatient rehabilitation patients with severe thrombocytopenia. *Support Care Cancer*. 2018;26(9):3135–3141.

132. G. Moore, J. Durstine, P. Painter, American College of Sports Medicine. *ACSM's Exercise Management for Persons With Chronic Diseases and Disabilities*. 4th ed.; American College of Sports Medicine, 2016.

133. Morishita S, Nakano J, Fu JB, Tsuji T. Physical exercise is safe and feasible in thrombocytopenic patients with hematologic malignancies: a narrative review. *Hematology (United Kingdom)*. 2020;25(1):95–100.

134. Koth J. Diagnosis and treatment of oncologic emergencies. *Radiol Technol*. 2019;91(2):161–172.

135. Goswami P, Khatib Y, Salek S. Haematological malignancy: are we measuring what is important to patients? A systematic review of quality-of-life instruments. *Eur J Haematol*. 2019;102(4):279–311.

136. Fisher MI, Davies C, Lacy H, Doherty D. Oncology section EDGE Task Force on Cancer: measures of cancer-related fatigue–a systematic review. *Rehabil Oncol*. 2018;36(2):93–105.

137. Harrington SE, Gilchrist L, Lee J, Westlake FL, Baker A. Oncology section EDGE Task Force on Cancer: a systematic review of clinical measures for pain. *Rehabil Oncol*. 2018;36(2):83–92.

138. Azoulay D, Giryes S, Nasser R, Sharon R, Horowitz NA. Prediction of chemotherapy-induced peripheral neuropathy in patients with lymphoma and myeloma: the roles of brain-derived neurotropic factor protein levels and a gene polymorphism. *J Clin Neurol*. 2019;15(4):511–516.

139. Bewarder M, Klostermann A, Ahlgrimm M, et al. Safety and feasibility of electrical muscle stimulation in patients undergoing autologous and allogeneic stem cell transplantation or intensive chemotherapy. *Support Care Cancer*. 2019;27(3):1013–1020.

140. Huang MH, Hile E, Croarkin E, et al. Academy of Oncologic Physical Therapy EDGE Task Force: a systematic review of measures of balance in adult cancer survivors. *Rehabil Oncol*. 2019;37(3):92–103.

141. Cha S, Kim I, Lee S-U, Seo KS. Effect of an inpatient rehabilitation program for recovery of deconditioning in hematologic cancer patients after chemotherapy. *Ann Rehabil Med*. 2018;42(6):838.

142. Laine J, D'Souza A, Siddiqui S, Sayko O, Brazauskas R, Eickmeyer SM. Rehabilitation referrals and outcomes in the early period after hematopoietic cell transplantation. *Bone Marrow Transplant*. 2015;50(10):1352.

143. De Almeida LB, Mira PADC, Fioritto AP, et al. Functional capacity change impacts the quality of life of hospitalized patients undergoing hematopoietic stem cell transplantation. *Am J Phys Med Rehabil*. 2019;98(6):450–455.

144. van der Meulen M, Dirven L, Habets EJJ, van den Bent MJ, Taphoorn MJB, Bromberg JEC. Cognitive functioning and health-related quality of life in patients with newly diagnosed primary CNS lymphoma: a systematic review. *Lancet Oncol*. 2018;19(8):e407–e418.

145. Koutoukidis DA, Land J, Hackshaw A, et al. Fatigue, quality of life and physical fitness following an exercise intervention in multiple myeloma survivors (MASCOT): an exploratory randomised Phase 2 trial utilising a modified Zelen design. *Br J Cancer*. 2020;123(2):187–195.

146. Cenik F, Keilani M, Hasenöhrl T, et al. Relevant parameters for recommendations of physical activity in patients suffering from multiple myeloma: a pilot study. *Wien Klin Wochenschr*. 2020;132(5–6):124–131.

147. Vermaete N, Wolter P, Verhoef G, Gosselink R. Physical activity, physical fitness and the effect of exercise training interventions in lymphoma patients: a systematic review. *Ann Hematol*. 2013;92(8):1007–1021.

148. Wingard JR, Wood WA, Martens M, et al. Pretransplantation exercise and hematopoietic cell transplantation survival: a secondary analysis of blood and marrow transplant clinical trials network (BMT CTN 0902). *Biol Blood Marrow Transplant*. 2017;23(1):161–164.

149. Fukushima T, Nakano J, Ishii S, Natsuzako A, Sakamoto J, Okita M. Low-intensity exercise therapy with high frequency improves physical function and mental and physical symptoms in patients with haematological malignancies undergoing chemotherapy. *Eur J Cancer Care (Engl)*. 2018;27(6):1–10.

UNIT **IV**

Important Considerations

22

Cancer Pain

DAVID J. SCHWARZ, PT, DPT, LMT, BBA

CHAPTER OUTLINE

Introduction

A new father is waking up in the intensive care unit (ICU) the morning following a second resection of an astrocytoma when the physical therapist (PT) walks in. His head is pounding as the PT says "Good morning! I am your physical therapist and am here to assess how you are moving following surgery." Possible thoughts from this person living with and beyond cancer (PLWBC): *Will walking hurt this more? Will I be able to do this?*

A middle-aged person with chronic back pain undergoes imaging and discovers they might have colon cancer. They are hoping that it might account for their pain. Following surgery, they still have back pain as well as the pain from the surgery. Possible thoughts from this PLWBC: *What part of the new pain is now going to stay?*

An elderly woman with a remote history of breast cancer previously treated with a double mastectomy sits in her car outside of the physical therapy clinic. She has had pain on and off over several years since her cancer treatments. The nerves down her arm are "on fire." Possible thoughts from this PLWBC: *Are they going to talk again about how she should "stick her chest out" to help with her posture?*

There are many stories of pain for the PLWBC. The pain may be acute from treatment, chronic from late effects of treatment, or other pain that is affected by treatment. These issues are important for the oncology rehabilitation (OncR) clinician to be able to address. Pain is common in the PLWBC, can lead to long-term disability, and can be a difficult aspect of the recovery process as will be demonstrated throughout this chapter.

Chapter Aims

The goal of this chapter is to present necessary knowledge of terminology, physiology, viewpoints, assessment, and interventions related to caring for the PLWBC that is experiencing pain. Refer to Table 22.1 for basic terminology regarding pain.[1] This will be an inclusive focus on pain to allow for integration within each person's journey.

Statistics

As medical management for cancer advances, the importance of diagnosing and treating cancer pain similarly advances. From the recognition of pain as the "fifth vital sign" to the opioid epidemic, pain has also become culturally relevant in healthcare. In the PLWBC, cancer-associated pain is very common with estimates of prevalence ranging from 50% to 90%.[2,3] Cancer treatment has the potential to manifest persistent pain sequelae throughout the continuum including long-term survivorship.

Cancer treatments are important but carry significant consequence to local and systemic structures. Effects can range from acute surgical pain to chronic chemotherapy-induced polyneuropathy (CIPN) pain. Additionally, the effects following cancer treatments affect the PLWBC in a variety of ways, including via postural changes or chronic pain syndromes, like phantom limb pain. Pain

is classified in different ways, though the most consistent way is presentation through the lens of the person's medical history.

Physiology of Pain

Systemic Contributions

Nervous

The nervous system has an important role to play in the presence of pain, as it is the fast communication system when a threat occurs to allow for a rapid response and resolution. The acute phase of pain occurs in order to address the need for a rapid protective response.[4] However, hypersensitivity of the peripheral nervous system (PNS) and/or central nervous system (CNS) can modify this response to something that is not consistent with the expected effect. *Peripheral sensitization* is the terminology used to describe an increase in sensory signal reception that is relatively larger than expected for that region which can increase pain.[5] This can be the result of an increase in the number of peripheral nerves, demyelination, or modulation of the associated ion channels that are represented.[4,6] *Central sensitization* is the terminology used to describe an altered processing of the signals that were received.[7] This can be related to a variety of different areas of the brain as well as past experiences related to these issues.[7]

Peripheral sensitization can occur at any time during the course of treatment. There are many very important ways in which cancer treatment affects the peripheral nerves to cause increased sensitivity. As demyelination is one factor that can increase peripheral sensitization, the response to chemotherapy and radiation needs to be assessed in both acute and chronic phases of care for a PLWBC. Clinical signs of peripheral sensitivity can include but are not limited to mechanical sensitivity to passive and active movement as well as a localized hyperalgesia response.

Central sensitization is an important factor that can be overlooked or downplayed related to physical rehabilitation. Central sensitization can happen in a variety of ways for a PLWBC. One significant effect is related to the emotional aspects of care, especially stress.[8–10] As stress elevates, a potential modulation of the pain response occurs.[9,11,12] This can have effects of either hyperalgesia or analgesia.[13,14] Both responses can increase confusion related to pain and elevate certain characteristics of the responses of other elements of the system.[14]

Endocrine

In contrast to the speed and specificity of the nervous system, the endocrine system presents with longer term and more global aspects related to pain.[15] There are numerous endocrine processes that directly relate to the adverse effect of pain because of cancer and cancer treatment.[3] Cancerous lesions themselves can be responsible for the release of hormones such as cytokines that can stimulate immune responses.[15] Additionally, each system has its own hormonal activities that can be represented in painful outcomes. This could be related to surgical procedures, such as testosterone reduction postorchiectomy from testicular cancer, or medication use, such as alterations of cortisol that occurs with corticosteroid withdrawals.[15] A firm understanding of the roles of the systems affected by cancer, cancer treatment, and comorbidity are important to properly understand endocrine processes affecting pain.

Immune

The immune system plays important roles in both the response to pain related processes and effect on pain, especially inflammatory

TABLE 22.1	Pain Terminology[1]
Term	**Definition**
Nociceptive pain	Nociception is the sensation related to noxious stimuli from tissues. Nociceptive pain is pain that is directly resulting from those noxious signals.
Neuropathic pain	Neuropathic pain is derived from an altered peripheral nervous system, often from injury or disease processes.
Nociplastic pain	Nociplastic pain is pain that occurs when there is no discernable structural reason for the pain.
Peripheral sensitization	Peripheral sensitization is increased peripheral nerve reactivity as the result of structural or physiological changes to the peripheral nerves (e.g., demyelination, nerve sprouting) that are beyond the expectations for the given stimuli.
Central sensitization	Central sensitization is related to the processing of signals received from the peripheral nervous system which recognizes increased levels of threat compared to what might be considered functionally beneficial.

Created by David J. Schwarz. Printed with permission.

effects. Inflammation is an important part of the healing response; however, it can also instigate pain responses.[16] Inflammatory chemicals can increase ion channel activation and elicit elevated peripheral signaling beyond that of the physical stimuli presented by tumor presence or by surgery.[17,18]

Systemic Integration

Interactions between the neurologic, endocrine, and immune systems are important for understanding the complexities of pain. These systemic processes will continue to compound the pain experience as they interact. The neurologic system delivers fast signals which induce a systemic endocrine response at the CNS level along with the endocrine responses locally from the presence of a tumor.[16,19] The inflammatory immune response builds based on cytokines and other factors.[20] The signals back to the brain continue to elevate as this process continues and the processing of these signals in the brain similarly continue to elevate and increase the pain experience. Another important factor requiring consideration in the pain experience is that of executive function and emotional regulation, which are both substantial elements.[20–22] This includes what pain means to each person and the goals that a person develops in response.

Tissue Damage

Surgery

The necessity of surgery for tumor resection can overshadow the negative consequences of tissue damage. The initial pain phases of tissue damage related to nerve impulses and inflammatory responses will decrease as healing occurs. However, damage does occur to the nerves which can create pain syndromes or can create maladaptive healing potentials.[18]

An appropriate example of this is that of an above-knee amputation for a lower leg malignant tumor (Figure 22.1). There are a few potential issues regarding pain following surgery. The healing

response during the initial phase will result in pain at the site of amputation. However, as the leg heals, there can be maladaptive healing such as the potential development of a sciatic neuroma,[2] which can increase locations for ion channel placements as well as increased potential for nerve compression. Additionally, this circumstance provides increased opportunities for issues such as phantom limb pain and heterotrophic ossification.[23–25] These aberrant processes may precipitate the need for additional surgery as well as complex rehabilitation interventions to improve both pain and function.

Another example of a pain syndrome resulting from surgery that is more chronic is complex regional pain syndrome (CRPS). CRPS currently is classified as type 1 and type 2. CRPS type 1 assumes no specific tissue damage while CRPS type 2 assumes injury to a specific nerve.[11,17,26,27] Tissue resection during oncologic surgery can cause damage to many nerves. Examples of this include breast, axillary, or posterior brachial CRPS following breast lumpectomies and/or mastectomies.[27] Due to signs and symptoms that can be quite traumatic for the PLWBC, these cases require extensive understanding of pain physiology for the clinician to provide beneficial education to the patient.

Chemotherapy

Chemotherapy has the potential to induce structural changes throughout the body that can lead to increased pain relative to peripheral nerve cytotoxicity (e.g., CIPN). Changes in myelin, ion channels, or other parts of the cells can increase risk for developing CIPN (Figure 22.2).[11,17,26] These issues can change the presence and expression of ion channels as well as enhance inflammatory processes, cumulatively altering sensory reception and increasing sensitivity resulting in allodynia (the perception of pain from a stimulus that does not normally cause pain).[17,26]

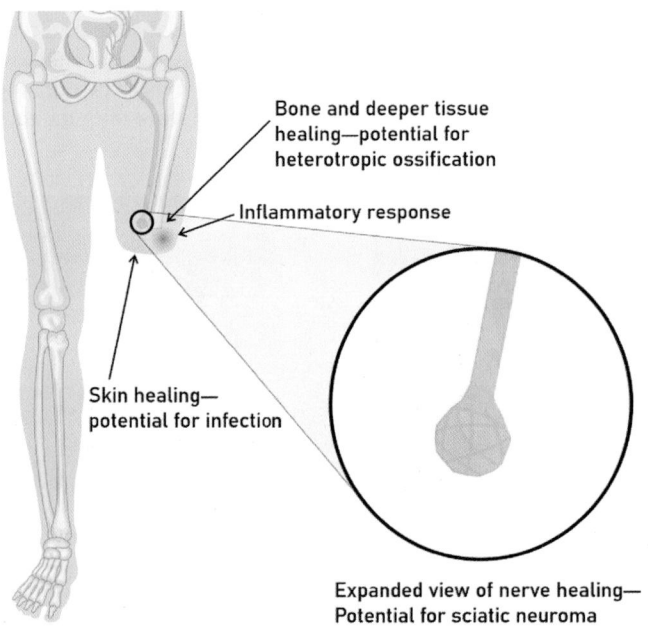

• **Fig. 22.1** Structural Contributors to Pain Post-Above Knee Amputation. (Created by David J. Schwarz and Debbie Jo Schwarz. Printed with permission.)

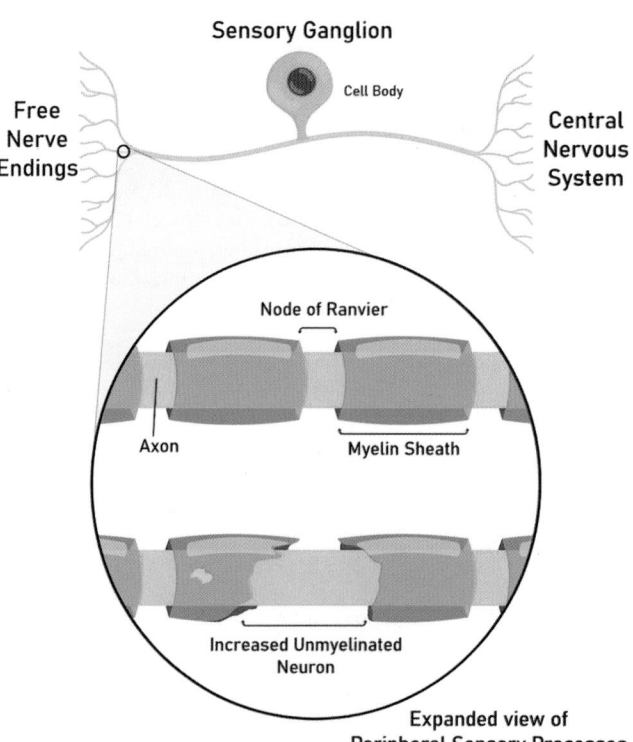

• **Fig. 22.2** Peripheral Nerve Changes From Chemotherapy-Induced Peripheral Neuropathy (CIPN).[11,17,25] (Created by David J. Schwarz and Debbie Jo Schwarz. Printed with permission.)

Central sensitization can increase due to psychosocial factors as well as cytotoxicity. Chemotherapy has the potential to affect many areas of a PLWBC's psychosocial status.[20] A PLWBC with risk factors for central sensitization therefore has increased potential for these issues to compound. Additionally, the elevated inflammatory responses resultant of astrocyte cell cytotoxicity can adversely affect CNS responses.[26] This cascade can further instigate changes to gray and white matter in areas of the brain responsible for emotional regulation, which can alter processing of the pain experience.[28–30]

Radiation

Radiation treatment can have deleterious effects on the human body. With respect to pain, the primary and secondary effects of radiation can be detrimental to the nervous system. Primary effects include tissue damage, inflammation, and demyelination.[6] These can cause acute pain as well as long-term pain if the nerve tissue is damaged. The secondary effects of radiation can be much more insidious. Radiation fibrosis, for example, prompts loss of tissue extensibility and development of contractures, and when paired with neuronal damage, can lead to changes in proprioception and postural and kinesthetic sense.[6] These sequelae have the potential to reduce mobility and postural variability which can, in turn, increase long-term structural changes, noxious shear forces, and reduce options for movement-based analgesia.

Models of Understanding Pain

Biomedical Versus Biopsychosocial

The traditional biomedical model of care focuses on anatomical and measurable physiologic factors for treating the pathological condition, which are important during rehabilitation.[31] This model is most relevant during the treatment of the initial condition; however, it lacks the insight regarding the person's behavioral responses which are important during rehabilitation. First introduced in Chapter 2 is the biopsychosocial model of cancer care. This approach is important in understanding how pain is more than a single sided problem but rather is multifaceted and requires a commensurate approach.

The biopsychosocial model (BPS) (Figure 22.3) includes the biology, anatomy and physiology, as well as psychosocial factors. Further, the BPS can be divided into the psychology or internal focus of thoughts and feelings as well as the social aspects of life such as interaction with other people and environments.[14,21,32] This holistic approach is representative of the International Classification of Functioning, Disability, and Health (ICF) model regarding environmental and personal factors,[33] however, BPS brings the psychosocial factors to the forefront of rehabilitation strategies regarding pain with relative equivalence to the anatomy and physiology as a more integrative approach.

Another important element to BPS can be the addition of spiritual aspects. A PLWBC may have a spiritual crisis that goes beyond that of standard psychosocial aspects.[34] Recognition of the pain that this can cause in a person's life is important, especially within the context of a life-threatening or terminal disease.

Cartesian Model

Cartesian dualism (Figure 22.4) as created by Rene Descartes postulates that there are two distinct systems of a person—mind and body. Modern healthcare focuses on mind versus body as factors for whether there is something that can be done about a specific health related issue.[31] Cartesian dualism in healthcare lacks the recognition that there are many additional potential effects on pain and not merely a cause-and-effect relationship. It creates unnecessary silos in integrative care that increase potential for confusion on pain etiology.

Gate Control Theory

The *gate control theory* (GCT) (Figure 22.5) contends that peripheral signals are regulated at the junction of the PNS and CNS. Central factors such as interneurons are the gatekeepers to pain and when the signals reach a certain threshold related to balance of large and small fiber responses, they allow for the signal to pass.[35] The GCT is still a relevant theory in the domain of cancer pain; however, it is not an encompassing theory as it acknowledges neither the nuances of peripheral experiences such as varied ion channels nor the responses of the CNS to higher-level threat context.[10]

Neuromatrix/Mature Organism Models

The Neuromatrix (Figure 22.6) is a pain model which recognizes that a signal reaching the brain is processed using multiple factors including sensory, cognitive, as well as current and past emotional experiences.[10] In the Neuromatrix model, these are the routine factors for processing that return with three outputs: pain

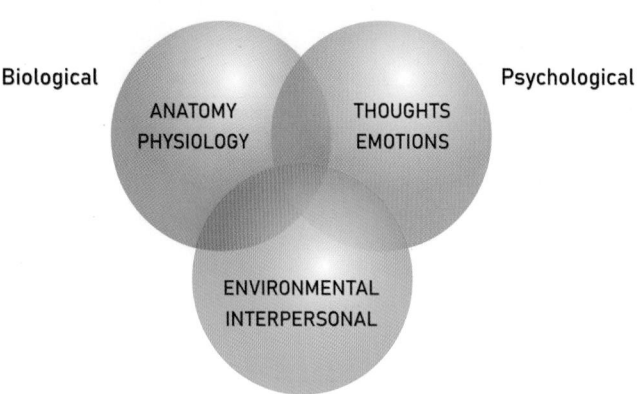

• **Fig. 22.3** BioPsychoSocial Model.[14,21,32] (Created by David J. Schwarz and Debbie Jo Schwarz. Printed with permission.)

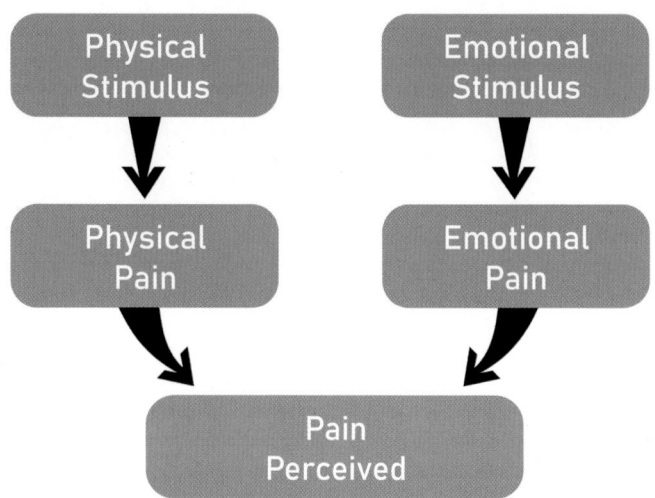

• **Fig. 22.4** Cartesian Model.[31] (Created by David J. Schwarz and Debbie Jo Schwarz. Printed with permission.)

GATE CONTROL THEORY

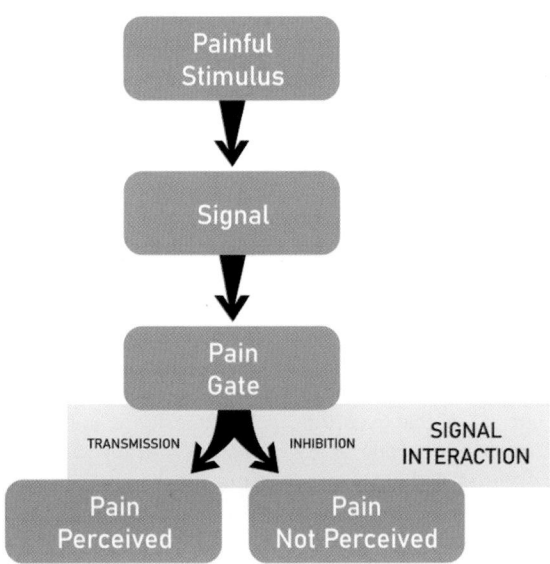

• **Fig. 22.5** Gate Control Theory.[35] (Created by David J. Schwarz and Debbie Jo Schwarz. Printed with permission.)

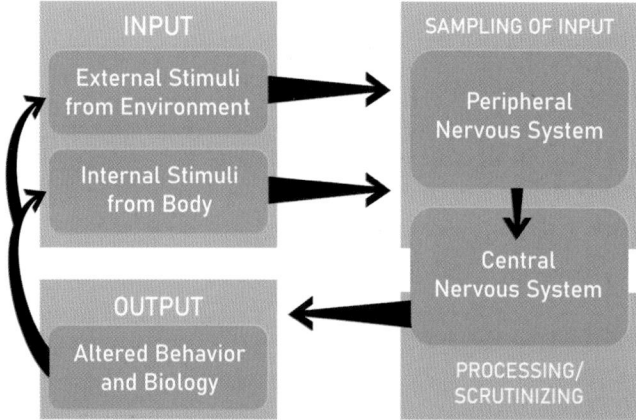

• **Fig. 22.7** Mature Organism Model.[9] (Created by David J. Schwarz and Debbie Jo Schwarz. Printed with permission.)

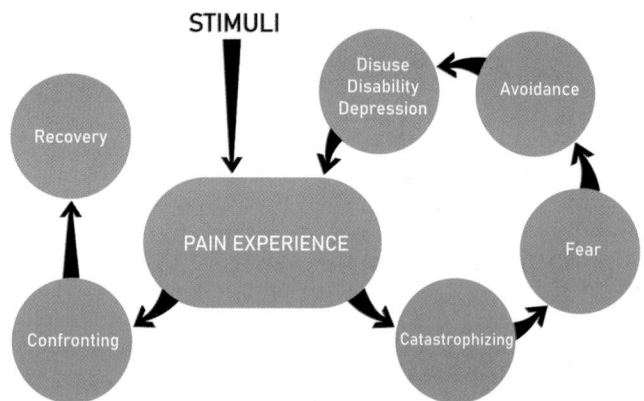

• **Fig. 22.8** Fear-Avoidance Model.[14,22,36,37] (Created by David J. Schwarz and Debbie Jo Schwarz. Printed with permission.)

perception, a response to the stimuli, and the internal regulation that the human system needs to perform for optimal function.[10]

The Mature Organism Model (Figure 22.7) from Louis Gifford takes the Neuromatrix and recognizes it as a feedback loop. Information from the external and internal environments are received at the spinal cord and "sampled" to pass along the relevant information.[9] This information is then processed or "scrutinized" in the higher levels of brain creating cognitive and emotional outputs related to pain which change our behavior and response to the situation.[9] This is a much more comprehensive model for understanding pain. For example, if a PLWBC has postsurgical pain from a tumor resection, this may draw most of their attention toward one area of the body versus another that was previously painful. This did not change the prior structural issues, but it does change the attention given to certain danger signals that are more immediately relevant.

Fear-Avoidance Model

Fear affects our planning of movement. This is seen in all normally developing humans from a young age. The fear-avoidance model (Figure 22.8) demonstrates the aversion to danger and the limiting

problems that can occur.[36] There are numerous psychological and behavioral principles represented in this model, but the simplicity of the pathway toward aberrant pain behavior is helpful in education and behavior change. The goal of this model is to demonstrate the importance of active engagement during the pain experience toward rehabilitation rather than creating an avoidant reaction.[36,37]

Emerging Models

Emerging rehabilitation models for understanding and treating pain are evolving in the direction of improved behavioral understandings. These include uses of cognitive behavioral therapy (CBT) and acceptance and commitment therapy (ACT). CBT is

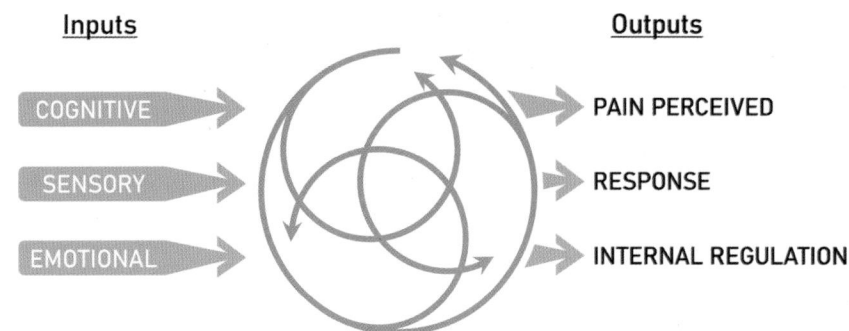

• **Fig. 22.6** Neuromatrix Pain Model.[10] (Created by David J. Schwarz and Debbie Jo Schwarz. Prined with permission.)

a broad term for the understanding of the changing brain and influence on behavior.[38–40] ACT uses Relational Frame Theory to identify and recognize individual context and the relationship to behavior which occasionally changes in ways beyond human control. Increased understanding of the human experience through scientific discovery promotes development of more models for understanding pain, which is especially relevant in the domain of oncology care. However, the landscape of pain management will be determined based on the psychological flexibility of the clinicians providing care and their ability to help patients shift their perspective as more accurate and sophisticated models of pain understanding are developed.[38]

Assessment

Subjective Assessment

Subjective assessments related to pain are important components of a holistic evaluation. A PLWBC may have had pain prior to their initial diagnosis of cancer. If this is not revealed or recognized, misunderstandings can result for the patient as well as the clinician. For example, if an individual had low back pain prior to a cancer diagnosis and it continued, the person may link the back pain to their cancer. This can create overall confusion because they may be missing out on important educational factors related to their pain physiology. In this case, identifying the presence or absence of red flags are important. For example, monitoring for new back pain in a PLWBC can indicate the development of metastatic bone disease and needs to be monitored closely, especially in cancers of the breast, lungs, and prostate due to the likelihood of metastases from these cancers.[41]

Descriptors of pain are important in that they help guide clinical decision making, however they are not always beneficial beyond initial recognition.[42] Overemphasis on pain descriptors can increase cortical sensitivity resulting in further risk for heightened central sensitization. Additionally, with alteration of the global system of the PLWBC, there is increased potential for diminished reliability regarding the sensation relating directly to the tissue or structure involved.

Pain mapping can be a useful tool for recognition and tracking of symptoms, especially related to affected areas requiring rehabilitative care.[42] Specifically, pain mapping can provide for a relevant discussion and create opportunities to discover new aspects related to the individual's pain. For example, allowing a person to develop a visual narrative may allow for greater opportunities for them to convey all the information they are concerned about, including comorbid pain problems or locations that may be spatially significant, such as along the path of a nerve. A written, graphic format of the pain map is recommended to allow the person time to consider the affected areas, though this should always be followed up by the PLWBC pointing to the correlating areas on their person because a PLWBC may have a distorted sense of their body position including potential issues pertaining to laterality.

Temporal characteristics are important for determination of when supportive measures may be needed, such as biophysical agents, as well as identification of functional modifications that can be made.[42] Symptom journaling is an excellent example of this because it allows for a reduction in subjective analysis on the part of the PLWBC and focuses on the immediate response to life activities. Journaling can be done in several different ways. One option is journaling by subjective, reflective recording of how activities went through the day related to pain presence, relative intensity, and interference with activities. A second option is using a log to identify when pain was most burdensome relative to time of day and activity, which might include various pieces of information at regular intervals (e.g., every hour) including activity type, numerical pain rating scale, other clinically relevant ordinal scales. The Onc R clinician can use this as a guide to help determine rehabilitative options such as pacing or use of biophysical agents.

Pain Measurement Scales

Single construct scales for measuring pain intensity are not an effective stand-alone tool. They can also increase the potential for a PLWBC to become overly worried about or become defensive of their pain. When a PLWBC is continually asked for their pain intensity score, they can become conflicted on what they are to say in a conscious or subconscious manner. This can lead to inaccurate responses as well as misunderstandings by the clinician. This does not mean that recording pain intensity is not important, but it needs to be done in a way that is clinically meaningful to guide decision-making rather than just for the sake of scoring the PLWBC's current condition. For example, knowing that someone has a certain level of intensity may not have any meaning, but knowing that they are struggling with their pain during a particular activity does. Pain intensity as an ordinal measure has little meaning other than to measure change over time.

There are three main scales that are used for measuring pain: Numerical Pain Rating Scale (NPRS), Visual Analog Scale (VAS), and Faces Pain Scale-Revised (FPS-R).[42–44] The NPRS uses numbers from 0 to 10 to quantify the pain experience. This is an easy way to quantify a person's pain numerically but does not comprehensively measure all aspects of pain. The NPRS is appropriate for use with most adults and is widely known. The utilization of the NPRS may be limited for PLWBCs who are demonstrating symptoms consistent with central sensitization. The VAS is a widely accepted scale that uses a single line measuring 100 mm that may or may not have demarcated intensities. After the person marks their pain on the line, it should be measured using a ruler by the clinician. This provides a higher level of accuracy and may be easier for a person to mark a line as opposed to deciding on a specific numerical pain value. The VAS is limited in its utility for those with a visual impairment. The FPS-R is a tool designed to assist a PLWBC in rating the intensity of pain who may also have communication or cognitive issues. It uses six different faces with progressive expressions of distress that are measured at 0, 2, 4, 6, 8, and 10.

Movement Assessment

Observation of Movement and Posture

It is important for the Onc R clinician to recognize the movement signs of pain related to rigidity, muscle guarding and inhibition, cogwheel-like movement (in absence of a medical condition that would cause this to happen), lack of coordination, nonfunctional asymmetries, and subjective reporting of feeling weak while observing the PLWBC sit, stand, lay down, and ambulate. While these movement disorders can be representative of other issues, the recognition of these pain triggers can indicate substantial and functionally disruptive pain. This is especially important in the absence of a structural issue that is obligating specific motions (e.g., multilevel vertebral reconstruction that is limiting spinal extension following excision of a vertebral body sarcoma) or other disease process. This is especially relevant if the movement disorder is beyond the area of main impairment, but the muscle might be bracing or protecting that area and can potentially indicate areas of spreading pain due to neural mechanical irritation or altered blood flow to an area.

Patient-Initiated Movement (Active Provoking)

Actively provoking symptoms is an important aspect of pain assessment. This can be done with simple measures such as active range of motion (AROM) and myotome testing, but to improve the understanding of the quality of the movement is more important than the range of the motion itself relative to pain assessment. Beyond identifying red flags, the goal of the pain assessment is to recognize and identify protective reactions in local areas that may be limiting to function. Additionally, assessing through targeted palpation can provide more information about how the human movement system is responding to external stimuli. For example, to assess for pain with cervical spine motion following healing from the resection of a neck tumor, it can be helpful to palpate the superficial and deep cervical muscles during the painful movements to evaluate how the muscles are reacting to the motion.

Therapist-Initiated Movement (Passive/Assisted Provoking/Evoking)

Patient-initiated pain provocation can be important toward identification of local sensitivity, but evoking pain via external means can be more functionally relevant. The difference between these two evaluative strategies is that provoking helps to find the pain response, while evoking aims to elicit pain through more expansive efforts. Pain provocation can provide useful information, but that information might not always be functional or what the PLWBC generally experiences. Evoking pain takes function into consideration and aims for anticipated response of the PLWBC. An example of this might be performing passive range of motion (PROM) following the typical active motion. For example, in a PLWBC who had radiation therapy for breast cancer targeted toward the upper quadrant combined with pain, provocation of their symptoms is accomplished by passively moving their shoulder through a plane of motion. However, evoking their symptoms is accomplished by passively moving their shoulder while passively promoting normalized scapulothoracic motion. Both assessments will elicit pain but evoking their symptoms might allow for understanding what pieces of the movement system are limiting their active, functional motion.

Deep tendon reflexes (DTRs) are an additional important assessment related to cancer pain; they provide a deeper understanding of potential nerve damage from the result of tumor infiltration, surgery, and/or other treatment.[45] Similarly, assessment of tone and upper motor neuron signs like the Babinski reflex and Hoffman's reflex provide additional clinical context.[45] Cumulatively, these neurologic tests will also provide prognostic information as well as information for potential need of referrals to other healthcare providers.

Functional Assessments Related to Pain

Observation of functional mobility provides added context to the holistic pain assessment and can allow for rehabilitative treatment interventions that modifies internal and external factors. For example, if a PLWBC reports pain during full shoulder flexion that limits their ability to reach into their cupboard, the clinician should observe this motion to determine if the angle of their reach is optimal for the situation. If not, the clinician needs to determine if this is modifiable by using a different strategy to obtain the required

shoulder motion. Furthermore, the clinician is advised to carefully assess for any potential strength or coordination limitations. In the absence of modifiable internal factors, functional assessments allow for temporary or permanent changes to the external factors to achieve the task. For example, can the commonly used items be moved to a lower, more comfortably achievable height? Modifications such as these can be helpful to reduce the ongoing exacerbations of the PLWBC's pain, instead of allowing them to successfully achieve a functional movement at the edge of tolerance. Additionally, function-based interventions have the potential to naturally require repetition, improving the likelihood for exercise-induced analgesia as well as increased task confidence.[46]

Central Sensitization

Central Sensitization Inventory

A standard measure for establishing the likelihood of developing central sensitization is the central sensitization inventory (CSI). The CSI Part A measures the prevalence of 25 biopsychosocial factors that can influence or be indicative of sensitivity of the CNS. Some of these factors include childhood trauma, bruxism (clenching or grinding teeth), achiness, headaches, and the anatomic extent of the PLWBC's pain. These items are rated on a 0-to-4-point ordinal scale (0 = never having, 4 = always having). Part B of the CSI asks for the presence of 10 health conditions, such as anxiety, depression, and irritable bowel syndrome (IBS). A score on Part A of greater than 40 indicates high likelihood for developing or having central sensitization.[47,48]

Yellow Flags

Yellow flags can include items representative of psychosocial factors that may lead to disability.[49] These are factors such as anxiety, depression, childhood trauma, financial concerns, and family problems. This assessment is primarily recommended for individuals with chronic pain. The identification of these concerns for a PLWBC can be helpful to decrease the likelihood of pain becoming a larger more profound influence on their life.[50,51]

Peripheral Sensitization

Neurodynamic Testing

Testing for neurodynamic tension indicates peripheral sensitivity and guides the Onc R clinician to the sensitive pathway.[52] It is also commonly known as nerve tension testing. Neurodynamic testing guides gross movement assessment through differences in nerve excursion.[53] Palpating for guarding responses and assessing for subjective changes in symptoms can help the clinician to evoke symptoms based on the motion and provide clinically relevant information for treatment planning.

Hyperalgesia

Due to increased sensitization, moderately noxious stimuli can become substantially more painful, which is appropriately termed hyperalgesia. Appropriately increasing shear forces to specific tissues during the pain assessment can assist the clinician's understanding of symptoms. To this end, the techniques of palpation and pressure provide evidence of potential hyperalgesia and are helpful for guiding and recognizing the mechanical sensitivity in the assessed area. The PLWBC may report excessive pain with the administration of these techniques and/or reflexively guard against

TABLE 22.2	Sensory Assessment Stimuli With Selection Rationale	
Sensory Stimulus	**Reason for Testing**
Localization	Determines peripheral sensory changes and cortical mapping problems related to the sensory homunculus
Two-point discrimination	Objective measure of aspects of cortical mapping, local dissociation, and sensory processing attention
Light touch	Quick and easy screen for sensory changes
Deep pressure	Helps determine presence of deeper stimuli or if there is significant sensory loss
Vibration	Assists with screening for stress fractures and small fiber changes
Sharp/dull	Useful for checking small fiber changes along dermatomes
Proprioception	Provides deeper understanding of kinesthetic sense and pain with movement and positioning

Created by David J. Schwarz. Printed with permission.

them. For example, if assessing joint motion in midrange is painful, this would be considered hyperalgesia and might occur with an excessive guarding response.

Allodynia

Light touch or a gliding touch of smooth or slightly coarse material across the skin (e.g., facial tissue) can help identify the presence of allodynia in a PLWBC. Just as with hyperalgesia, the subjective response is clinically important, though another important response with allodynia is the individual's physical withdrawal from the stimulus. The subjective response may also be that of disgust accompanied by a facial expression of disgust.

Sensory Assessment

Appropriate and comprehensive assessment of the sensory system provides improved understanding of the PNS and CNS changes that have affected the physiology of the PLWBC system as well as how their pain experience might have developed. Refer to Table 22.2 for a list of various sensory assessments and rationale for clinical selection.[45]

Interventions

Education

Pain Neuroscience Education

Pain neuroscience education (PNE) is the generally accepted term for the educational intervention for the PLWBC relative to the neuroscience of pain. PNE generally consists of condensed narratives and descriptors of complex neurologic processes related to pain. This includes an emphasis on somatosensory processing, but also addresses motor and autonomic effects.[16] This education utilizes a biopsychosocial approach to pain, rather than a pathoanatomical approach and can help guide the PLWBC away from a fear-avoidance pathway and toward goal-oriented pain management.[16] Refer to Box 22.1 for a clinical example of pain neuroscience patient education.

• BOX 22.1 Pain Neuroscience Education Example

An example of a conversation to shift a PLWBC's focus from a pathoanatomical understanding of pain to a biopsychosocial understanding:

Onc R clinician: "Is it okay if we talk about pain? Let's talk about something as simple as stubbing your toe. It hurts right? However, the signal that occurs is related to a large compressive force, it is not yet pain. That signal travels up your nerves to your low back where at the spinal cord it recognizes that large force and sends a reflex back to your leg that causes you to pull back. It still is not the full experience of pain at this point."

"The signal continues to travel up to the brain where it travels in many different areas and it asks questions of what is going on such as 'where was that signal from?,' 'How strong was the signal?,' 'What type of signal?,' 'Have I felt that before?,' 'What happened last time?,' 'What am I worried about right now?,' 'What is going on around me?,' etc. Then the signal can finally decide if stubbing your toe was a threat or not. If it is, then the experience will be one of pain. However, there are other effects of movement such as muscle guarding and inhibition that occur as well, which is why you limp after you stub your toe. Now, consider that you are out on a nature walk and a bear surprises you on the trail. If you stub your toe at this point, the threat is different than if you were walking around at home. The focus is going to be on the bear."

"Recognizing that you have something that is much more threatening than stubbing your toe; you have cancer, and it is affecting every part of your life. It makes sense that you would feel stiff and uncomfortable and that other areas may hurt even if there is not always a clearly recognizable reason. Not all of this pain is a direct cause of the cancer tissue. Pain is a much bigger issue than just the tissue."

Motivational Interviewing

Motivational interviewing is helpful when a PLWBC is experiencing ambivalence related to their pain experience (see Chapter 30: Wellness, Health Promotion, and Prevention for expanded content on motivational interviewing). This is a common tool for Onc R clinicians to use to help evoke a response when a PLWBC struggles to make a change on something they have determined that they want to change.[54,55] This approach may be applied when a PLWBC decides that they want to walk in a charity 5k, but they are unsure if this is possible due to pain. The PLWBC wishes to avoid increasing their pain, but they also want to walk the 5k. So far, they have only tried intermittently to do the things that are necessary to move forward but have been limited by discomfort and patterns of behavior. Motivational interviewing is an evidence-based method for assisting with behavior change such as this example. This approach allows a PLWBC to choose where they want to put their energy/efforts and identify where pain is in their hierarchy of needs and wants, increasing the likelihood of their success in goal achievement.

Goals and Function Despite Pain

Collaboratively developing goals is an important intervention for pain; although simply choosing to reduce pain is a goal that should be avoided and should be shared openly with the PLWBC. The overarching goals of rehabilitation for cancer-related pain should be that of improving quality of life (QOL) and the finding of the meaning behind the pain. Pain cannot always be changed or modulated, therefore setting goals based on improvement of functional tasks that are painful and objective sensitivity measurements can be more beneficial as it does not require constant reminders of pain intensity.[36,37]

Medication and Medical Treatments

An Onc R clinician caring for a PLWBC with cancer pain should always be ready to answer questions regarding the pain modulating effects of medication and medical treatments. This education is important for decreasing concerns and improving communication and compliance related to the treatment plan as well as presenting opportunities for the PLWBC to make informed choices in their care. Additionally, this education allows the PLWBC to focus on their goals related to pain rather than focus on what the pain means related to their condition.

Manual Therapies

Manual therapies for the management of pain have limitations for PLWBCs for two main reasons. First, there is limited potential to directly change a structure that has an underlying systemic pathology. Second, there are precautions and/or contraindications to providing some manual interventions while a PLWBC is receiving certain medical treatments to manage their cancer, especially radiation. These are two important rationales that additionally clarify rehabilitation objectives for a PLWBC that is experiencing cancer pain.

Using the Neuromatrix or the Mature Organism Model for understanding, no change of tissue needs to occur for change in the pain experience. A clinician can apply numerous hands-on sensory and interpersonal inputs away from the area of pain and still have an effect.[56,57] Gentle, skilled touch for a PLWBC with allodynia and/or hyperalgesia or who is lacking social contact can have substantial influences on the autonomic nervous system (ANS) as well as within the CNS.[58–61] During later stages of healing, more aggressive manual therapies can be performed, though the intent should not be for direct tissue change to improve pain intensity but rather for improved kinesthetic sense and cortical mapping.

Movement

Graded Motor Imagery

Graded motor imagery (GMI) is an important tool for pain management for a PLWBC who has dissociated from an area of their body and/or cannot functionally use the associated extremity/body part.[62] The three most relevant phases of GMI exposure categories in this domain are laterality preference recognition, watching and imagining activities, and mirror therapy. These techniques can be conducted in different sequences, but generally the aforementioned order is most effective unless the PLWBC reports difficulty or disgust with a particular activity. Refer to Box 22.2 for a clinical example of these techniques.

Progressive Loading

The human body is built to tolerate load and it responds to increasing load as demonstrated in Wolff's Law.[63] However, reduced loads combined with changes to the neuro-endocrine-immune response similarly changes perception of pain tolerance as well as the subconscious and unconscious protective brain work through inhibition of movement. This is especially relevant in PLWBCs during and after treatment. Increased time lying in bed can increase load sensation in nonfunctional positions, such as the shear forces when laying supine. Once the PLWBC attempts to increase activity, fatigue will increase but so will pain due to a change in tolerance to loads. Creating gradual, safe loading programs can assist with improving confidence despite pain, but over time pain should improve as systemic tolerance to load improves.

Aerobic Activity

Aerobic activity increases systemic circulation which improves nerve healing and sensitivity. The repetitive movements that are synonymous with aerobic activities also are found to have an

---

• BOX 22.2 Graded Motor Imagery (GMI) Progression Related to Development of Post Mastectomy Pain Syndrome Example

Jill underwent a mastectomy due to breast cancer and is already struggling with moving her arm due to pain. There was potential nerve damage during surgery due to complications and there is concern for development of complex regional pain syndrome. Jill's rehabilitation is not progressing quickly, and she is struggling to perform any arm movement at home even though she wants to move her arm. While more active movement is encouraged in the therapy clinic with support, she is taught how to perform GMI activities.

Laterality: Jill is given a stack of flashcards to separate into piles of left and right necks, shoulders, and hands. She gets some correct and some incorrect, but she is struggling with identifying her affected side more than her less affected side. She is also encouraged to flip through magazines at home and circle the affected shoulders in order to encourage her to draw attention to that area and how people are performing with that part of their body.

Observing and Imagining Activities: Jill loves to play tennis, but the affected arm is her dominant arm for playing tennis and she really wants to get back to that activity. She is assigned the activity of watching a tennis game of someone using the same arm to play with. Every round of volleys she is to pause the video and imagine herself performing that motion.

Mirror Therapy: Shoulder abduction and flexion is a hard motion for Jill, but she knows she needs those motions for playing tennis. In front of a mirror, she is instructed to stand so that her opposite arm looks like her affected arm and perform flexion and abduction movements without and with her racket.

As Jill progresses with the GMI, it is anticipated that she will be progress in the clinic and should be able to start tolerating more motions and decreasing fear related to motions.

---

analgesic effect.[64] Nerve healing and repair resultant of increased blood flow takes longer to occur, though the analgesic effects from repeated movement occur more quickly.

Mind–Body Care

Mindfulness Integration

Improved awareness and meaning through movement have important effects on the pain experience of the PLWBC.[65] The first benefit is that of improving descriptors and recognition of what they feel, which may better guide the clinician caring for them, improving their overall care. Mindfulness can also assist with recognition of the choices made related to pain. A principal example of this is pacing. A PLWBC who is experiencing pain and fatigue with ambulation sees a chair 10 feet away. They may rush to the chair, limping harder and faster with degrading functional posture during the movement which increases their exertion and pain. Mindfulness and openness to the situation prompts them to pace themself with a standing rest break, shifting off the painful side to relieve pressure before continuing with less pain toward the same chair. There is evidence that mindfulness-based stress reduction programs may have measurable CNS changes that can assist with processing related to cancer pain.[66,67]

Breathing Techniques

Teaching breathing techniques is an important source of regulation of the ANS. There are many breathing techniques that are beneficial for the PLWBC in the domain of cancer pain management. Generally, for pain management, a down-regulation of the sympathetic nervous system is beneficial, but sometimes elevating it can improve tolerance to a modulating system. Breathing techniques have been found to accomplish this needed down-regulation.[68] Conversely, the fight, flight, or freeze response is important regarding pain especially as a PLWBC on current treatment may not have the capacity for fight or flight and instead they freeze with increased tension and decreased motion which can further exacerbate a pain state.

Biophysical Agents

There are many concerns related to the use of biophysical agents with a PLWBC. However, an important biophysical agent to recognize is electrical stimulation. Both transcutaneous electrical nerve stimulation (TENS) and spinal cord stimulators have a benefit in very specific and controlled circumstances with a PLWBC.[69,70] Currently, evidence for the benefit of electrical stimulation in cancer pain is lacking.[70] Electrical stimulation is an especially relevant intervention for a PLWBC with metastatic bone disease and intractable pain as the pain reduction outweighs the risks.

Coordination of Care and Patient Education

Medicine

Numerous options for managing pain exist, though it is appropriate to recognize the scope of care that rehabilitation clinicians can provide. Recognition of opportunities for pain relief for a PLWBC is informed by comprehensive review of medication lists and medical histories, as well as conversations about the expectations for pain management and balancing other aspects of their lives. Collaboration with physicians and other providers as well as providing functional education and referrals are an important part of rehabilitation.

Opioids have a substantial effect on a PLWBC though are an important part of acute pain management (see Chapter 6: Pharmacology Principles in Cancer Care). Opioid use does carry the potential for increasing opioid induced hyperalgesia as well as opioid induced mood disorders which can have a secondary effect on condition perception and pain.[71] The Onc R clinician should discuss opioid use with the PLWBC in a manner conducive to improving functional outcomes. As a point of more routine engagement on this potential issue, the clinician should also recognize risk factors for development of a substance use disorder.

Initially, there was some hope that medical marijuana would be an alternative medicine for modulating pain. However, evidence has not met those expectations thus far. Marijuana may have some beneficial effects for some PLWBCs secondarily affecting their pain experience though there is limited direct effect, and unfortunately for some, there is worsening of symptoms.[72] Additionally, mood alteration can also affect the PLWBC and how they experience their life in a harmful way.

Referrals and Recommendations

Referrals or recommendations for other services are an important component of comprehensive care for a PLWBC. Crying and other signs of depression evident during a rehabilitation session are opportunities to not only listen (guiding improved treatment options), but also to consider and attempt referral to an appropriate counseling or mental health therapist or recommend they discuss the situation with their counseling or mental health therapist if they already have one. Another option is to join a support group so as to improve active engagement (see Chapter 3 for more information).

Other important roles of the Onc R clinician include interprofessional communication and professional recommendations. Onc R clinicians suspecting central sensitization or peripheral neuropathy should discuss findings and recommendations with the referring physician and advocate for consideration of modalities and medications that could assist with and improve pain and function objectives.

Complementary and Alternative Medicine

Complementary and alternative medicine (CAM) services are a growing area of cancer care; many PLWBCs may inquire about efficacy and utility of various CAM modalities. Motivational interviewing is a useful strategy for discussion of these services, after ensuring that the PLWBC understands that they should consult with their medical oncologist prior to receiving any CAM treatments. Guiding the PLWBC to make informed decisions about implementing CAM interventions to supplement care without imparting bias is important so as not to foster false or lost hope. With respect to the cancer pain domain, there are a few instances where the Onc R clinician can and should make recommendations. Massage and aromatherapy constitute medically cleared relaxation services found helpful in improving cancer pain.[57] Reiki and other energy therapies are CAM therapies can provide a calming effect for a PLWBC which can also improve the pain experience.[73] Some CAM treatments can increase pain, such as acupuncture which has been used for many people with good benefit but also may increase sensitivity for some PLWBCs.[74] Overall, listening to the PLWBC and providing guidance relative to areas of importance can allow for whatever benefit a CAM therapy might afford for them.

Conclusion

Pain is a much more complex issue than a simple physiologic cause and effect response. It requires recognition of the whole person and the factors that affect them. Considering the substantial effects that cancer has on the biologic, psychological, social, and spiritual elements of the PLWBC, rehabilitation requires recognition of these factors as well as addressing of them to be effective.

Critical Research Needs

- Effectiveness of a functional contextual physical therapy treatment for cancer related pain conditions that have traditionally utilized a pathoanatomic approach, such as chemotherapy induced poly neuropathy.
- Measuring comparative fear avoidance beliefs and characteristics with cancer associated pain with acute and chronic symptomatology.
- Quantifying effects of comorbid chronic pain syndromes on acute cancer care and cancer associated pain management.

Case Study

History

A 70-year-old male presented to a physical therapy clinic with low back pain 5 years after a vertebroplasty due to loss of bone mass from a diagnosis of multiple myeloma. He had an initial treatment with stem cells and had continued to receive thalidomide (Thalomid). His initial diagnosis occurred after follow-up imaging by a spinal surgeon related to a long history of low back pain and concern for lumbar foraminal stenosis. He did not have a surgical need related to his stenosis though some stenosis was identified. He was initially receiving physical therapy for his low back pain, but he was told by his oncologist that physical therapy needed to be discontinued due to concern for structural integrity of the spine and recommended lifting restrictions of no more than 10 lb. After his cancer treatment stabilized, the patient was referred to physical therapy by a physiatrist at a pain management clinic. Upon initial examination, he reported a history of stress at home that had increased during this period and he reported not having a strong support system. He reported that he no longer worked in manufacturing but that he misses working.

Past Medical History: Multiple myeloma, depression, lumbar spinal stenosis

Examination

Central Sensitization Inventory Score: 55 [0 = lowest risk of central sensitization, 100 = highest risk of central sensitization, Cutoff Score = 40) *Item marked indicating frequent childhood trauma.

Observation: Static standing posture demonstrated age-appropriate thoracic kyphosis with a rigid upper lumbar spine with a flattened lordosis and substantial loss of lower lumbar extension movement. The patient was able to reach his toes without a significant effort. His gait revealed shortened strides with substantially limited transverse or frontal plane motion of spine.

Range of Motion: The patient demonstrated difficulty with mobility coordination and guarding behavior. These factors resulted in variable range of motion (ROM) across standing, sitting, and passive palpation of his lumbar spine. During seated trunk flexion, he demonstrated erector spinae guarding. He demonstrated decreased lumbar segmental muscular activity via palpation when the trunk was supported by the clinician; conversely during unsupported active segmental movement, there was increased erector spinae muscular activity. The quality of this muscular behavior was guarding/splinting in nature and was clinically relevant as it prevented accurate measurement of ROM.

Palpation: Superficial and deep tissue and joint guarding of lumbopelvic region with hyperalgesia present. Gentle posterior/anterior pressure at the upper lumbar region was firmly rigid with substantial hypomobility upon joint play testing at the lower lumbar or thoracic regions.

Neurodynamic Testing: Slump test was positive bilaterally. Femoral nerve neurodynamic testing was negative.

DTRs at his knees and ankles were normal.

Myotomes were normal though increased pain was reported with proximal loading.

Dermatomes were normal though upon light touch; the patient indicated that the left side felt different than the right, though no defined quality could be made. There was mild diminished sharp/dull sense distally.

2-Point Discrimination at Lumbar Spine: Left = 90 mm, Right = 75 mm

Balance testing was normal and there was no recent history of falls reported. However, his 30-second Chair Rise Test score was 9 repetitions with slightly increasing dyspnea as he was observed holding his breath. He also reported low back pain with subsequent repetitions. At the last 5 seconds of the test, he discontinued his effort and rested.

Assessment: This patient's chronic low back pain appeared to have several contributing factors including his cancer treatment and the history of progressive lumbar stenosis. This resulted in mobility and motor coordination deficits and central sensitization. He demonstrated decreased pressure pain thresholds, a central sensitization inventory score of >40, sensory and lateralization discrimination deficits, neurodynamic sensitivity, and a history associated with central sensitization neuroplastic changes. Yellow flags existed including depression, fear of loading demonstrated through a modified lifting technique as well as avoidance of completing a repeated task due to pain. He also worked in a job where there was a standard perception of low back pain being caused by the work tasks (i.e., nocebo effect). Finally, he had a history of childhood trauma which is associated with central sensitization.

Treatment options for this person included:
- Pain neuroscience education to decrease his fear of pain and improve engagement in activity.
- Breathing activities to modulate his ANS and improve his somatic response to loading activities.
- Functional loading activities integrated with mindfulness to assist with his kinesiophobia.
- Manual treatments including massage and other gentle treatments to encourage movement and decrease aberrant muscle guarding behavior.
- Referral to counseling services with a therapist that is skilled in working with pain within the context of trauma.
- Establishing a progressive home exercise program to improve his functional capacity and decrease neurodynamic tension.

Review Questions

Reader can find the correct answers and rationale in the back of the book.
Scenario #1:

A 24-year-old male presents to outpatient physical therapy with low back pain and intermittent pelvic pain that occurred one year prior as a result of treatment for recurrent testicular cancer. An orchiectomy with resection of retroperitoneal lymph nodes was performed along with radiation. Repeated imaging and testing have demonstrated no return of cancer, but the patient still reports worries. He sees no other healthcare providers other than the oncologist, his primary care physician, a pain specialist, and now a physical therapist. He is relatively healthy with no prior injuries and the only health

conditions are depression and anxiety. He currently takes no medications. He notes that his diet is poor and has been for a while. He would like to get back to activities, but his pain is limiting him. He used to like to play baseball but has not been able to in a while due to pain.

1. This patient demonstrates potential need for referral to assist with his pain. Which of the following providers/services would be the MOST indicated first referral in this situation:
   A. Dietitian/nutritionist
   B. Massage therapist
   C. Counselor
   D. Group fitness class

2. Sitting has been difficult for this patient especially at work. He has a nice office chair and tries to follow the workplace ergonomic specialist suggestions, but he continues to have issues with sitting for a functional length of time. Which of the following is LEAST likely to be a contributor for his pain problem?
   A. Increasing the lumbar support on his chair and sitting as upright as he can
   B. Occasional "slouching" in chair causing decreased lumbar lordosis
   C. Shearing forces along the distribution of the inferior cluneal nerve
   D. The current stressful work environment

3. Given this case, which of the following rehabilitation paths would be the BEST course for long-term recovery of this patient?
   A. Work on skills toward playing baseball again
   B. Strengthen the back and core
   C. Stretching hamstrings and lumbar spine
   D. Utilize soft tissue mobilization of the adductors and hamstrings and joint mobilization of the lumbar spine along with other appropriate manual techniques

Scenario #2

A 45-year-old female presents in a subacute rehablition unit following an above knee amputation due to a large, spreading osteosarcoma from the lower leg. Chemotherapy was done for 3 months prior to surgery and the chemotherapy is planned to continue for 3 to 6 months after surgery.

4. The patient reports that she has phantom limb pain. What would be the BEST first rehabilitative treatment for phantom limb pain.
   A. Mirror therapy
   B. Aerobic activity
   C. Breathwork
   D. Pain neuroscience education

5. This patient was cleared by the surgeon for use of a prosthetic. Which of the following is NOT a structural contributor to pain to consider/assess for?
   A. Inflammatory response
   B. Sciatic neuroma
   C. Skin integrity
   D. Heterotropic ossification

Scenario #3

A 77-year-old female presents to outpatient physical therapy with chronic low back pain with pain down each leg and in both feet. She has a history of recurrent breast cancer with bilateral mastectomy, chemotherapy, and radiation. She has numerous health issues including lumbar stenosis, depression, anxiety, hypertension, and diabetes mellitus type 2. She does not like to go out very much but does like to play with her dogs outside. She has not been able to do that as much in the last couple of years due to increases in falls.

6. CIPN is a likely issue in this case and is compounded with age and a history of diabetes. When tested, she has relatively intact sensory integrity to light touch on her feet but she demonstrates sensitivity and withdrawal when gently touching along portions of her foot. What is the peripheral factor that might be the MOST relevant consideration first in this case regarding pain related to her feet?
   A. Poor vasculature
   B. Peripheral nerve demyelination
   C. Axonal degeneration
   D. Lumbar stenosis

7. What is indicated in the prior question when there was sensitivity and withdrawal?
   A. Allodynia
   B. Hyperalgesia
   C. Laterality
   D. Cortical mapping

8. There are likely multiple central nervous system effects on her pain. Which of the following is the LEAST likely effect related to central sensitization?
   A. Age-related demyelination
   B. Reactive microglia
   C. Mitochondrial changes in astrocytes
   D. Chronic stress

9. What is the MOST likely behavioral contributor to this patient's back pain due to sequalae from treatment?
   A. Limited stride length and gait speed
   B. Post-radiation fibrosis limiting upright posture
   C. Forward rounding posture to disguise the lack of breast tissue
   D. Radiation-related demyelination

10. If you needed to provide a referral to another provider to assist in treating for the behavioral contributor above, who would be the BEST fit?
    A. Massage therapist
    B. Acupuncturist
    C. Counselor
    D. Pain management physician

References

1. International Association for the Study of Pain. IASP terminology; 2017. https://www.iasp-pain.org/Education/Content.aspx? Accessed May 24, 2021.
2. Russo MM, Sundaramurthi T. An overview of cancer pain: epidemiology and pathophysiology. *Semin Oncol Nurs*. 2019;35(3):223–228.
3. Leysen L, Adriaenssens N, Nijs J, et al. Chronic pain in breast cancer survivors: nociceptive, neuropathic, or central sensitization pain? *Pain Pract*. 2019;19(2):183–195.
4. Danchalski K. Treating pain. *Rehab Manag*. 2020;33(5):10.
5. Rodriguez L. Pathophysiology of pain: implications for perioperative nursing. *AORN J*. 2015;101(3):338–344.
6. Magee D, Bachtold S, Brown M, Farquhar-Smith P. Cancer pain: where are we now? *Pain Manag*. 2019;9(1):63–79.
7. Nijs J, Leysen L, Adriaenssens N, et al. Pain following cancer treatment: guidelines for the clinical classification of predominant neuropathic, nociceptive and central sensitization pain. *Acta Oncol*. 2016;55(6):659–663.
8. Smith EML, Bridges CM, Kanzawa G, et al. Cancer treatment-related neuropathic pain syndromes—epidemiology and treatment: an update. *Curr Pain Headache Rep*. 2014;18(11):1–10.
9. Gifford L. Pain, the tissues and the nervous system: a conceptual model. *Physiotherapy*. 1998;84(1):27–36.
10. Melzack R. From the gate to the neuromatrix. *Pain*. 1999;82(1):S121–S126.

11. Shim HS, Bae C, Wang J, et al. Peripheral and central oxidative stress in chemotherapy-induced neuropathic pain. *Mol Pain*. 2019;15:1744806919840098.

12. Melzack R. Pain and the neuromatrix in the brain. *J Dent Educ*. 2001;65(12):1378–1382.

13. Lai H, Lin Y, Hsieh C. Acupuncture-analgesia-mediated alleviation of central sensitization. *Evid Based Complement Altern Med*. 2019:1–13.

14. Carlino E, Frisaldi E, Benedetti F. Pain and the context. *Nat Rev Rheumatol*. 2014;10(6):348–355.

15. Tennant F. The physiologic effects of pain on the endocrine system. *Pain Ther*. 2013;2(2):75–86. doi:10.1007/s40122-013-0015-x.

16. Nijs J, Leysen L, Pas R, et al. Treatment of pain following cancer: applying neuro-immunology in rehabilitation practice. *Disabil Rehabil*. 2018;40(6):714–721.

17. Aromolaran KA, Goldstein PA. Ion channels and neuronal hyperexcitability in chemotherapy-induced peripheral neuropathy; cause and effect? *Mol Pain*. 2017;13:1744806917714693. doi:10.1177/1744806917714693.

18. Rawson R, Miller M. Chronic pain in breast cancer survivors. *Cancer Nurs Pract*. 2012;11(4):14–18. doi:10.7748/cnp2012.05.11.4.14.c9093.

19. Yoon SY, Oh J. Neuropathic cancer pain: prevalence, pathophysiology, and management. *Korean J Intern Med*. 2018;33(6):1058–1069. doi:10.3904/kjim.2018.162.

20. Sforzini L, Nettis MA, Mondelli V, Pariante CM. Inflammation in cancer and depression: a starring role for the kynurenine pathway. *Psychopharmacology*. 2019;236(10):2997–3011. doi:10.1007/s00213-019-05200-8.

21. De Laurentis M, De Laurentis M, Rossana B, et al. The impact of social-emotional context in chronic cancer pain: patient-caregiver reverberations: social-emotional context in chronic cancer pain. *Support Care Cancer*. 2019;27(2):705–713.

22. Linton SJ, Flink IK, Schrooten MGS, Wiksell R. Understanding co-occurring emotion and pain: the role of context sensitivity from a transdiagnostic perspective. *J Contemp Psychother*. 2016;46(3):129–137.

23. Minarelli J, Davis EL, Dickerson A, et al. Characterization of neuromas in peripheral nerves and their effects on heterotopic bone formation. *Mol Pain*. 2019;15:1744806919838191 doi:10.177/744806919838191.

24. Cruz E, MD, Dangaria HT, MD. Phantom limb pain from spinal sarcoma: a case report. *PM R*. 2013;5(7):629–632.

25. Chapman S. Chronic pain syndromes in cancer survivors. *Nurs Stand*. 2011;25(21):35–41.

26. Gordon-Williams R, Farquhar-Smith P. Recent advances in understanding chemotherapy-induced peripheral neuropathy. *F1000Res*. 2020;9.

27. Mewa Kinoo S, Singh B. Complex regional pain syndrome of the breast and chest wall. *Breast J*. 2016;22(3):366–368.

28. Pomykala KL, de Ruiter MB, Deprez S, McDonald BC, Silverman DHS. Integrating imaging findings in evaluating the post-chemotherapy brain. *Brain Imaging Behav*. 2013;7(4):436–452.

29. McDonald BC, Saykin AJ. Alterations in brain structure related to breast cancer and its treatment: chemotherapy and other considerations. *Brain Imaging Behav*. 2013;7(4):374–387.

30. Menning S, de Ruiter MB, Veltman DJ, et al. Changes in brain white matter integrity after systemic treatment for breast cancer: a prospective longitudinal study. *Brain Imaging Behav*. 2018;12(2):324–334.

31. Quintner JL, Cohen ML, Buchanan D, Katz JD, Williamson OD. Pain medicine and its models: helping or hindering? *Pain Med*. 2008;9(7):824–834.

32. Jorn A. Elements of the biopsychosocial interview of the chronic pain patient: a new expanded model using rational emotive behavior therapy. *J Ration Emot Cogn Behav Ther*. 2015;33(3):284.

33. ICF, World Health Organization. Towards a common language for functioning, disability and health; 2002.

34. Hanmod SS, Gera R. Oncologic pain in pediatrics. *J Pain Manage*. 2016;9(2):165–175.

35. Melzack R, Wall PD. Pain mechanisms: a new theory. *Science*. 1965;150:971–979.

36. Claes N, Karos K, Meulders A, Crombez G, Vlaeyen JWS. Competing goals attenuate avoidance behavior in the context of pain. *J Pain*. 2014;15(11):1120–1129.

37. Volders S, Meulders A, De Peuter S, Vlaeyen JWS. The reduction of fear of movement-related pain does motivational context matter? *Clin J Pain*. 2015;31(11):933–945.

38. Yu L, Norton S, McCracken LM. Change in "Self-as-context" ("Perspective-taking") occurs in acceptance and commitment therapy for people with chronic pain and is associated with improved functioning. *J Pain*. 2017;18(6):664–672.

39. Hadlandsmyth K, Dindo LN, Wajid R, Sugg SL, Zimmerman MB, Rakel BA. A single-session acceptance and commitment therapy intervention among women undergoing surgery for breast cancer: a randomized pilot trial to reduce persistent postsurgical pain. *Psycho-oncology*. 2019;28(11):2210–2217.

40. Law E. Psychological interventions for parents of children and adolescents with chronic illness. *Cochrane Database of Syst Rev*. 2019;3:CD009660.

41. Finucane L, Greenhalgh S, Selfe J. Which red flags aid the early detection of metastatic bone disease in back pain? *Physiother Pract Res*. 2017;38(2):73–77.

42. Gallagher E, Rogers BB, Brant JM. Cancer-related pain assessment: monitoring the effectiveness of interventions. *Clin J Oncol Nurs*. 2017;21(3):8–12.

43. Caraceni A, Shkodra M. Cancer pain assessment and classification. *Cancers*. 2019;11(4):510.

44. Nadella S, Patel DR. Neuropathic pain pediatrics: an introductory overview. *J Pain Manage*. 2016;9(2):87–90.

45. Young AC, Wainger BJ. Neurological exam and neurophysiologic evaluation for the pain patient. In: *Spine Pain Care*. Springer International Publishing; 2019:115–131.

46. Roberts KE, Rickett K, Feng S, Vagenas D, Woodward NE, Roberts KE. Exercise therapies for preventing or treating aromatase inhibitor-induced musculoskeletal symptoms in early breast cancer. *Cochrane Database Syst Rev*. 2020;1(1):CD012988.

47. Scerbo T, Colasurdo J, Dunn S, Unger J, Nijs J, Cook C. Measurement properties of the central sensitization inventory: a systematic review. *Pain Pract*. 2018;18(4):544–554.

48. Mayer TG, Neblett R, Cohen H, et al. The development and psychometric validation of the central sensitization inventory. *Pain Pract*. 2012;12(4):276–285.

49. Nicholas MK, Linton SJ, Watson PJ, et al. Early identification and management of psychological risk factors ("Yellow flags") in patients with low back pain: a reappraisal. *Phys Ther*. 2011;91(5):737–753.

50. Poleshuck EL, Katz J, Andrus CH, et al. Risk factors for chronic pain following breast cancer surgery: a prospective study. *J Pain*. 2006;7(9):626–634.

51. Leysen L, Beckwée D, Nijs J, et al. Risk factors of pain in breast cancer survivors: a systematic review and meta-analysis. *Support Care Cancer*. 2017;25(12):3607–3643.

52. Smoot B, Boyd BS, Byl N, Dodd M. Mechanosensitivity in the upper extremity following breast cancer treatment. *J Hand Ther*. 2014;27(1):4–11.

53. Shacklock M. Neurodynamics. *Physiotherapy*. 1995;81(1):9–16.

54. Brodie DA, Inoue A. Motivational interviewing to promote physical activity for people with chronic heart failure. *J Adv Nurs*. 2005;50(5):518–527.

55. Vong SK, Cheing G, Gladys L, Chan F, So EM, Chan CC. Motivational enhancement therapy in addition to physical therapy improves motivational factors and treatment outcomes in people with low back pain: a randomized controlled trial. *Arch Phys Med Rehabil*. 2011;92(2):176–183.

56. Rossettini G, Carlino E, Testa M. Clinical relevance of contextual factors as triggers of placebo and nocebo effects in musculoskeletal pain. *BMC Musculoskel Dis.* 2018;19(1):27.

57. Sundaramurthi T, Gallagher N, Sterling B. Cancer-related acute pain: a systematic review of evidence-based interventions for putting evidence into practice. *Clin J Oncol Nurs.* 2017;21(3):13–30.

58. Diego MA, Field T, Sanders C, Hernandez-Reif M. Massage therapy of moderate and light pressure and vibrator effects on EEG and heart rate. *Int J Neurosci.* 2004;114(1):31–44.

59. Field T, Diego M, Hernandez-Reif M. Moderate pressure is essential for massage therapy effects. *Int J Neurosci.* 2010;120(5):381–385.

60. Diego MA, Field T. Moderate pressure massage elicits a parasympathetic nervous system response. *Int J Neurosci.* 2009;119(5):630–638.

61. Shin E, Seo K, Lee S, et al. Massage with or without aromatherapy for symptom relief in people with cancer. *Cochrane Database Syst Rev.* 2016(6):CD009873. doi:10.1002/14651858.CD009873.pub3.

62. Kaur J, Ghosh S, Sahani AK, Sinha JK. Mental imagery training for treatment of central neuropathic pain: a narrative review. *Acta Neurol Belg.* 2019;119(2):175–186.

63. Teichtahl AJ, Wluka AE, Wijethilake P, Wang Y, Ghasem-Zadeh A, Cicuttini FM. Wolff's law in action: a mechanism for early knee osteoarthritis. *Arthritis Res Ther.* 2015;17(1):207.

64. Segal R, Zwaal C, Green E, Tomasone JR, Loblaw A, Petrella T. Exercise for people with cancer: a clinical practice guideline. *Curr Oncol.* 2017;24(1):40–46.

65. Mikolasek M, Berg J, Witt CM, Barth J. Effectiveness of mindfulness- and relaxation-based eHealth interventions for patients with medical conditions: a systematic review and synthesis. *Int J Behav Med.* 2018;25(1):1–16.

66. Mioduszewski O, Hatchard T, Fang Z, et al. Breast cancer survivors living with chronic neuropathic pain show improved brain health following mindfulness-based stress reduction: a preliminary diffusion tensor imaging study. *J Cancer Surviv.* 2020;14(6):915–922.

67. Hatchard T, Mioduszewski O, Khoo E, et al. Reduced emotional reactivity in breast cancer survivors with chronic neuropathic pain following mindfulness-based stress reduction (MBSR): an fMRI pilot investigation. *Mindfulness.* 2021;12(3):751–762.

68. Busch V, Magerl W, Kern U, Haas J, Hajak G, Eichhammer P. The effect of deep and slow breathing on pain perception, autonomic activity, and mood processing—an experimental study. *Pain Med.* 2012;13(2):215–228.

69. Hurlow A, Bennett MI, Robb KA, Johnson MI, Simpson KH, Oxberry SG. Transcutaneous electric nerve stimulation (TENS) for cancer pain in adults. *Cochrane Database Syst Rev.* 2012;3:CD006276. doi:10.1002/14651858.CD006276.pub3.

70. Flagg A II, McGreevy K, Williams K. Spinal cord stimulation in the treatment of cancer-related pain: "Back to the origins." *Curr Pain Headache Rep.* 2012;16(4):343–349.

71. Wiffen PJ, Wee B, Derry S, Bell RF, Moore RA. Opioids for cancer pain: an overview of Cochrane Reviews. *Cochrane Database Syst Rev.* 2017;7(7):CD012592. doi:10.1002/14651858.CD12592.pub2.

72. Häuser W, Welsch P, Klose P, Radbruch L, Fitzcharles M. Efficacy, tolerability and safety of cannabis-based medicines for cancer pain: a systematic review with meta-analysis of randomised controlled trials. *Schmerz.* 2019;33(5):424–436.

73. Behzadmehr R, Dastyar N, Moghadam MP, Abavisani M, Moradi M. Effect of complementary and alternative medicine interventions on cancer related pain among breast cancer patients: a systematic review. *Complement Ther Med.* 2020;49:102318.

74. Deng G, Bao T, Mao JJ. Understanding the benefits of acupuncture treatment for cancer pain management. *Oncology.* 2018;32(6):310–316.

23

Exercise Testing, Prescription, and Intervention

ANDREW CHONGAWAY, PT, DPT, DEBORAH J. DOHERTY, PT, PhD

CHAPTER OUTLINE

Introduction

The Role of Exercise/Physical Activity

Exercise has numerous benefits in promoting an enhanced quality of life (QOL) by improving the multiple systems (musculoskeletal, neurological, cardiovascular, pulmonary, endocrine, and integumentary) that work together within the human body. Unfortunately, there is a significant percentage of the adult population across the lifespan that does not meet the minimum physical activity guidelines set by the American College of Sports Medicine (ACSM) of at least 150 minutes of moderate intensity, 75 minutes of vigorous intensity, or a combination moderate and

vigorous intensity activities per week.[1-3] This is especially true for a person living with and beyond cancer (PLWBC) as only roughly 35% to 40% of PLWBCs are meeting minimum physical activity guidelines.[4-6] Although differing definitions exist, in research the two terms—exercise and physical activity (E/PA)—are often used interchangeably. In this chapter the terms will be combined—E/PA. Fortunately, research has shown numerous benefits of frequent engagement in E/PA across the health and wellness spectrum. There is strong evidence that E/PA has been shown to reduce the risk of certain cancers (colorectal, breast, bladder, kidney, endometrial, and gastric cancers).[7] In addition to reducing the risk for certain cancers, E/PA has the potential to improve treatment (surgery, chemotherapy, radiotherapy, and immuno therapy) outcomes and reduce the chance or severity of adverse effects of treatment.[8] Altogether, the benefits of consistent E/PA from prevention through the spectrum to end-of-life has the ability to promote an optimal QOL.[9–11] Many PLWBCs have comorbidities which can affect numerous body systems that have the potential to negatively affect treatment tolerance, physical function, and disease-free and overall survival.[12] By engaging in E/PA, not only can a person move beyond their diagnosis of cancer but can also move beyond other comorbidities affecting their QOL. This chapter will provide a brief background on molecular physiology, examine the evidence on the benefits of E/PA for PLWBCs, and provide a framework/background on evaluating and developing individualized exercise prescriptions for PLWBCs across various settings.

Molecular Physiology of Mitochondrial Biogenesis, Muscle Hypertrophy, and Muscle Atrophy

Mitochondria play significant roles in energy production and cellular homeostasis within skeletal muscles via oxidative phosphorylation.[12] Mitochondrial biogenesis is mediated by the expression of peroxisome proliferator-activated receptor-gamma coactivator 1 alpha (PGC-1α).[12,13] PGC-1α also potentially plays important roles in muscle fiber specificity, angiogenesis, and GLUT4 receptor expression which is responsible for insulin flux into skeletal muscle cells.[12,14] Expression of PGC-1α is mediated through various primary signaling pathways which are dependent on nutrient and energy status, as well as cellular damage.[13,15] These primary pathways activate various downstream secondary signaling pathways to promote mitochondrial biogenesis.[13]

Movement of calcium from the sarcoplasm to the cytoplasm to promote muscle contraction, production of free radicals resulting in generation of antioxidants, and the activation of 5′ AMP-activated protein kinase (AMPK) due to reduced muscle energy levels from an increased ratio of AMP/ATP result in secondary signaling.[13,15] The shift of calcium activates calmodulin-dependent kinase (CaMK) which upregulates PGC-1α and calcineurin which promotes a shift of skeletal fiber type from fast twitch to slow twitch, as well as skeletal fiber growth and regeneration via downstream activation of NFAT (nuclear factor of activated T cells) and MEF2 (myocyte enhancer factor 2).[12,13,15]

The production of oxidative stress from exercise results in the activation of p38 mitogen activated protein kinase (MAPK) which promotes antioxidant production to protect against cellular damage. MAPK is also implicated in the upregulation of PGC-1α.[12,13]

An increased ratio of NAD+/NADH (nicotinamide adenine dinucleotide) during endurance exercise also increases expression of PGC-1α via activation of downstream signaling of SIRT1 (a nicotinamide adenosine dinucleotide [NAD]-dependent deacetylase) which promotes activation of PGC-1α via peroxisome proliferators-activated receptor α (PPARα).[12,13,15,16] SIRT1 also has been indicated in numerous other roles involved with insulin sensitivity, cancer proliferation, oxidative stress, cell aging, and environmental stress.[16] These pathways are the major contributors to the development of mitochondrial biogenesis as well as other beneficial pathways for homeostasis.[12,13,16]

Muscle hypertrophy occurs through appropriate stimulus resulting in increased sarcomeres in parallel.[17] For these sarcomeres

to form and muscle mass to be added, muscle protein synthesis must occur.[12] The main pathway for muscle protein synthesis is the IGF1-PI3K-Akt-mTOR pathway.[18] This pathway is activated when appropriate stimulus is provided and is mainly seen with resistance training due to the mechanical stretch across the skeletal muscle membrane.[13] This mechanical stretch results in insulin-like growth factor 1 (IGF-1) binding to its respective receptor on the cell membrane which initiates a cascade within the cytoplasm.[12,13] This cascade activates phosphoinositide 3-kinase (PI3K) which induces phosphoinositide dependent kinase 1 (PDK).[18] PDK then activates Akt inhibiting tuberous sclerosis complex 1 and 2 (TSC 1/2). TSC1/2 is also inhibited by extracellular regulated kinase (Erk).[12,13] This inhibition of TSC1/2 and activation of Akt initiates mTOR (mammalian target of rapamycin) promoting Rheb (Ras homolog enriched in the brain) which acts on mTOR at the lysosome.[12,13] Phosphatidic acid (PA) which is at low levels at rest or with usual activity is increased during resistance exercise due to mechanical stimuli and is able to activate mTOR.[12,13] mTOR then phosphorylates eukaryotic translation initiation factor 4E binding protein 1 or activates p70S6K kinase resulting in protein synthesis and muscle hypertrophy.[12,13] Akt has been implicated in the downstream activation of myogenic regulatory factors (MRFs) which are responsible for muscle maintenance. Akt is responsible for the downstream regulation of other multiple pathways that have inhibitory effects such as the ubiquitin-proteasome pathway (UPP) which will be explained in a later section.[12,13,19] There are other inhibitory or facilitatory effects downstream of the Akt that do not directly relate to muscle protein synthesis and will not be discussed here. Figure 23.1 depicts these pathways and their relation to mitochondrial biogenesis and muscle hypertrophy.

Pathways That Affect Skeletal Muscle/Protein Synthesis and Increased Oxidative Stress Mitochondrial Biogenesis

The human body is constantly in a state of breaking down and then rebuilding structures. However, at times the pathways breaking down structures are upregulated causing a shift to an increased catabolic state that is not held in check by anabolic pathways.[20] This shift can be due to age, increased sedentary time, disuse of skeletal muscle, disease, reduced anabolic hormone concentrations, increased oxidative stress and/or systemic inflammation, medications, and malnutrition to name a few.[17,20–26] These factors do not singularly act alone in the development of a catabolic state but are intertwined to upregulate specific catabolic pathways.[23–25] For the purpose of this book we will not delve into the intricacies of these factors though the pathways that result in mitochondrial and skeletal muscle dysfunction and breakdown will be briefly discussed.

Aging diseases including cancer, reduced E/PA, medications, and pro-inflammatory cytokines (Interleukin-1, Tumor Necrosis Factor alpha, C-Reactive Protein) are all factors that affect the function and quality of mitochondria and skeletal muscle.[13,24–27] This dysfunction leads to reduced quality of mitochondria which produces less energy and more reactive oxidative species (ROS).[12,13,25,27] An increase in ROS acts in a cyclical manner that causes further damage and dysfunction in the mitochondria leading to disruption in the mitochondrial membrane potential, signaling the mitochondria to release apoptotic factors.[12,13,25–27] This results in depletion of subsarcolemmal (SS) and intermyofibrillar (IFM) mitochondria content along with poorer quality in the remaining mitochondria.[28] This is caused by damage to mitochondrial DNA (mtDNA) and altered fusion and fission of established mitochondrial matrixes.[28] These altered pathways and quality control mechanisms lead to further mitochondrial dysfunction and increased amounts of ROS.[26,28] The continued increase in ROS affects skeletal muscle tissue content and quality as muscle atrophy pathways such as the UPP are upregulated which is usually inhibited via the IGF-1-Akt-mTOR pathway.[25-28] Akt normally inhibits Forkhead box O (FOXO) from remaining in the nucleus by phosphorylation which moves FOXO into the cytoplasm.[12,13] However, with reduced activity and increased ROS there is upregulation of NF-kB and proteins of the transforming growth factor beta (TGF-b) family which inhibit the IGF-1-Akt-mTOR pathway via FOXO.[25-29] This inhibition of Akt allows FOXO to remain in the nucleus and upregulates MAFbx/atrogin-1 and muscle RING finger-1 (MuRF1) resulting in skeletal muscle cell atrophy.[25,27,28] Myostatin also plays a potential role in inhibiting Akt resulting in upregulation of Smad 2/3 which also is implicated in muscle atrophy.[25] Figure 23.1

portrays the relation of these pathways and muscle atrophy. These altered pathways in mitochondrial function and quality control lead to reduced energy production, impaired antioxidant production, increases in systemic inflammation and ROS, diminished immune responses, and muscle atrophy due to the increase in systemic inflammation and ROS inhibiting the IGF-1-Akt-mTOR pathway.[12,13,25,27-29]

Skeletal muscle atrophy is often classified as either sarcopenia or cachexia.[22,29] Primary sarcopenia is the age-related loss of muscle mass while secondary sarcopenia is the disease-associated loss of muscle mass.[22] Along with the sarcopenic loss of muscle mass, there are associated reductions in quality of skeletal muscle, lipid infiltration of skeletal muscle, denervation of motor units, and anabolic resistance and can be seen with individuals with cancer.[22,29] A term that is a bit more synonymous with cancer is cachexia which is also the loss of skeletal muscle mass along with loss of adipose tissue due to an elevated resting metabolic rate.[29] This hypermetabolic state leads to "wasting" with reduction in body weight and cannot be corrected with nutritional support

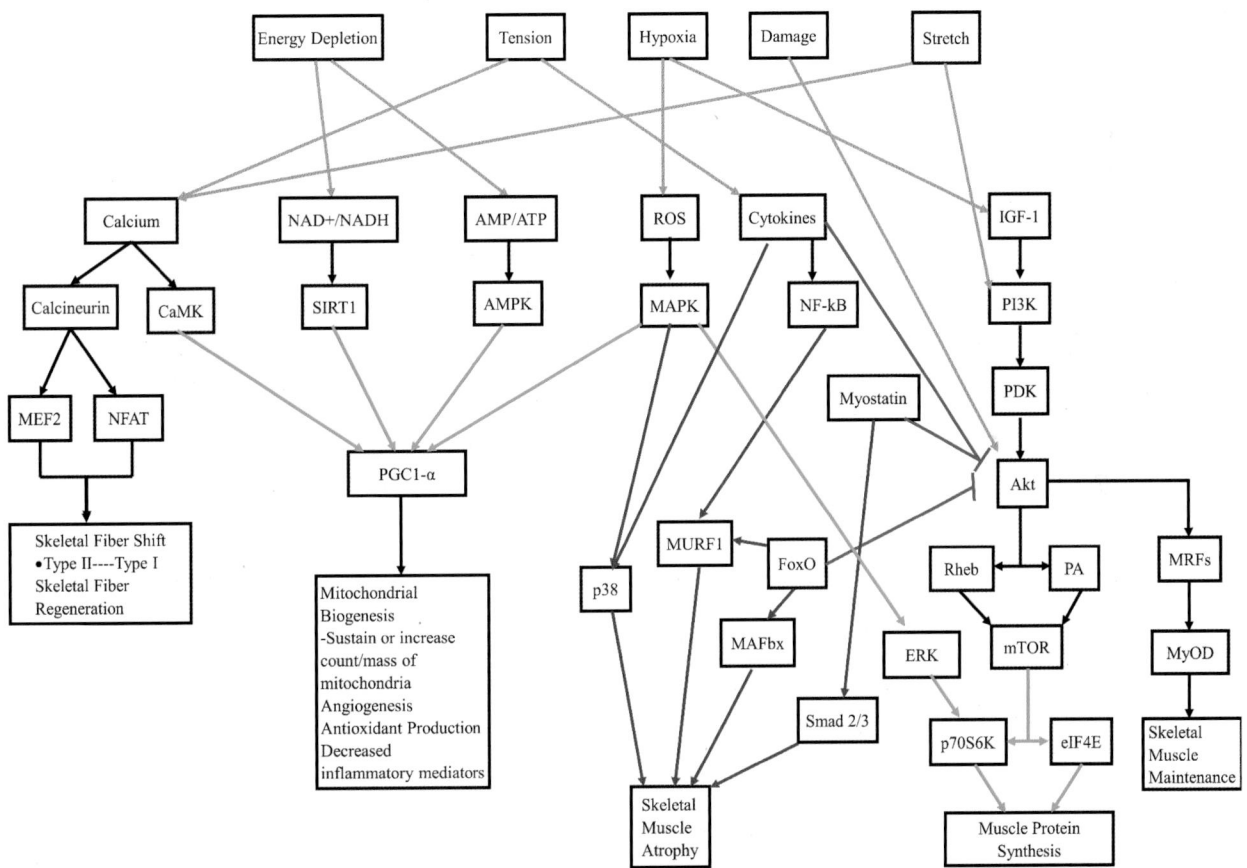

• **Fig. 23.1** Molecular Pathways of Mitochondrial Biogenesis, Muscle Protein Synthesis, and Muscle Atrophy. *Akt*, Protein kinase B; *AMP*, adenosine monophosphate; *AMPK*, AMP-activated protein kinase; *ATP*, adenosine triphosphate; *CaMK*, Ca²⁺/calmodulin-dependent protein kinase; *eIF4E*, eukaryotic Translation Initiation Factor 4E; *ERK*, extracellular signal regulated kinases; *FoxO*, Forkhead box proteins; *IGF-1*, insulin-like growth factor 1; *MAFbx*, muscle atrophy F-box/atrogin-1; *MAPK*, mitogen-activated protein kinase; *MEF2*, myocyte enhancer factor 2; *MRFs*, myogenic regulatory factors; *mTOR*, mammalian target of rapamycin; *MURF1*, muscle RING finger 1; *MyOD*, myoblast determination protein 1; *NAD+*, nicotinamide adenine dinucleotide; *NFAT*, nuclear factor of activated T-cells; *NF-κB*, nuclear factor kappa B; *PA*, phosphatidic acid; *PDK*, pyruvate dehydrogenase kinase; *PGC1-α*, peroxisome proliferator-activated receptor-gamma coactivator alpha; *PI3K*, phosphoinositide 3-kinases; *p70S6K*, ribosomal protein S6 kinase beta-1; *Rheb*, Ras homolog enriched in brain; *ROS*, reactive oxidative species; *SIRT1*, sirtuin 1. (Created by Andrew Chongaway, PT, DPT. Printed with permission.)

alone.[29] While there is the delineation between sarcopenia and cachexia there are varying stages of each and the possibility of sarcopenia to precede cachexia.[22,29]

As shown in Figure 23.1, there are numerous pathways involved in maintaining, building, and breaking down vital organelles (mitochondria) and structures (sarcomeres) that are essential in being able to carry out everyday tasks and engage in hobbies, activities, and the ability to work. Aging, disease (cancer, chronic obstructive pulmonary disease, diabetes, hypertension, etc.), and reduced physical activity intertwine in a vicious cycle that leads to a disruption in the maintenance and building of mitochondria and skeletal muscle resulting in atrophy and reduced quantity and quality of both mitochondria and skeletal muscle.[12–14,20,25,27–29] Appropriate E/PA in regard to amount and intensity, which will be described later in the chapter, can potentially reduce the effects of catabolic pathways and stimulate anabolic pathways resulting in the maintenance and increased quantity and quality of mitochondria, sarcomeres, and motor units.[12–14]

National and International Recognition for the Benefits of E/PA

E/PA is recommended and strongly encouraged by numerous United States (US) and international organizations to be implemented for not only primary prevention of cancer but to mitigate and attenuate the adverse effects from the treatments for cancer. E/PA has shown to be a valuable intervention throughout the cancer journey.

Although there is a wealth of evidence confirming the benefits of E/PA in cancer care, it is still not a standard of practice in the US. However, Australia has demonstrated a commitment to exercise for every person diagnosed with cancer. The Clinical Oncology Society of Australia (COSA)[30] released a position statement in 2018 stating that "exercise should be prescribed to all cancer patients as a standard part of their cancer care to help counteract the effects of cancer and its treatment;" Professor Prue Cormie, Chair of the COSA Exercise and Cancer Care Group stated that "the evidence to support the recommendation that every person diagnosed with cancer should be prescribed exercise medicine in addition to their other cancer treatments is overwhelming," and that "…evidence suggests that withholding exercise from people with cancer is harmful."[30]

The National Cancer Institute (NCI) confirms that evidence is strong linking higher levels of E/PA to lower risks of cancers including bladder (13%–15%), breast (12%–21%), colon (19%), endometrial (20%), esophageal adenocarcinoma (21%), kidney/renal cell (12%), and stomach/gastric (19%); there is some evidence for reduced risk of lung cancer. They also report that exercise lowers levels of sex hormones (estrogen, growth factors) that may contribute to cancer in the breast and colon; prevents high blood levels of insulin, reduces inflammation, improves immune system function, alters metabolism of bile acids, reduces time for food to travel through gastrointestinal tract, and helps prevent obesity.[31]

The ACSM International Multidisciplinary Roundtable on exercise and cancer concluded that there is strong evidence to warrant an exercise prescription to reduce anxiety, depressive symptoms, and fatigue and improve health-related QOL, lymphedema and physical function; and moderate evidence to warrant a prescription for improving bone health and sleep.[32]

There is now strong evidence that E/PA lowers the risk of seven types of cancer (colon, breast, kidney, endometrium, bladder, and stomach, and esophageal adenocarcinoma) from 10% to 24%, and moderate evidence that E/PA lowers the risk for lung cancer. The Roundtable concluded that "Being physically active is one of the most important steps people of all ages and abilities can take for cancer prevention, treatment, and control."[33] The evidence is even more promising in prostate cancer (PC). When physically active, all-cause death in PC is lowered by 33% from PC and lowers risk of any cause of death by 45%.[9,34] The American Cancer Society (ACS) affirms the evidence that moderate intensity (walking 3 mph/20 minutes per mile at least 150 minutes each week) exercise lowers the risk of 13 specific types of cancers including: colon, breast, endometrial, esophageal, liver, stomach, kidney, myeloid leukemia, multiple myeloma, cancers of the head and neck, rectum, bladder, and lung (in current and former smokers).[35]

The American Institute for Cancer Research (AICR) recognizes that E/PA has a positive effect on the endocrine, immunologic, and metabolic processes which affects the risk for cancer. Being physically active helps to maintain a healthy weight, decreases the risk of colon, endometrial, and pre- and post-menopausal breast cancer.[36] Furthermore, AICR concluded that E/PA lowers the risk of cancer-specific mortality for a variety of cancer types from 21% to 35%. E/PA decreases cancer-related fatigue, decreases distress, anxiety, depression, stress, improves emotional well-being and mental health issues, sleep, body image, and physical health.[37] Exercise directly lowers insulin-like growth factor (IGF-1), and influences epigenetic (gene expression) changes that leads to DNA repair, especially BRCA1 and BRCA2 genes, which are particularly sensitive to exercise. E/PA improves immunity in all age groups, reduces chronic inflammation, helps maintain a healthy weight, and lowers cholesterol, which is associated with increased risk of cancer. E/PA is correlated with a higher sunlight exposure leading to higher levels of Vitamin D which is known to modify cell proliferation.[38]

With these examples of endorsements, it is unclear why E/PA is not part of every cancer plan of care and a standard of practice in the US and globally. Onc R clinicians are perfectly positioned to offer education and interventions at all five levels of prevention throughout the cancer continuum. E/PA improves both physical and mental health during every phase of cancer treatment and even if a person was sedentary prior to treatment for cancer, it is safe to exercise during and after treatment with a program individually designed to meet each person's unique needs. Exercise should be initiated at the time of diagnosis and prescribed as "exercise medicine." One author eloquently described a successful exercise program utilizing Social Cognitive Theory (SCT) to ensure sustainability and efficacious results. This program is based on "structured, individualized, well-defined exercise regimens; convenient and accessible locations, easily mastered exercise components to build self-efficacy, monitored exercise sessions with positive feedback and achievable goal setting, and an established exercise community to provide accountability and inspiration to succeed."[39] See Box 23.1 for overall benefits of exercise.[40]

Five Levels of Prevention

Prevention can be categorized in five levels: Primordial, Primary, Secondary, Tertiary, and Quaternary. Please see Chapter 2 for full

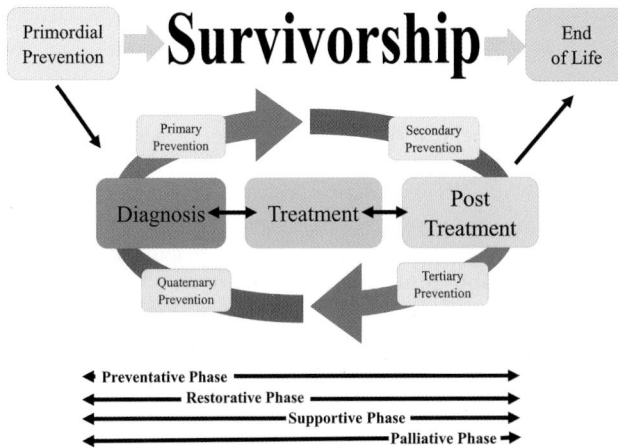

● **Fig. 23.2** The Oncology Rehabilitation and Wellness Nexus Model. (Created by Deborah J. Doherty, PT, PhD, Amy Litterini, PT, DPT, and Andrew Chongaway, PT, DPT. Printed with permission.)

political, environmental, and institutional factors influencing human health and well-being.[41] Societal issues include but are not limited to environmental contamination, conditions that are unsafe for E/PA as well as food deserts.[41]

The Office of the Surgeon General in the US Department of Health and Human Services released their "Step It Up"—Call to Action to promote walking and walkability for all Americans in 2015.[42] The strategic goals are to: "make walking a national priority, design communities that make it safe and easy to walk for people of all ages and abilities, promote programs and policies to support walking where people live, learn, work and play, provide information to encourage walking and improve walkability and to fill surveillance, research and evaluation gaps related to walking and walkability."[42] The World Health Organization (WHO) stated that globally 23% of adults and 81% of adolescents (aged 11–17 years) do not meet the WHO global recommendations on E/PA for health. Significant inequities in the opportunities for E/PA are prevalent by gender and social position, within and between various nations. WHO specifically identifies the social injustices: "Girls, women, older adults, people of low socioeconomic position, people with disabilities and chronic diseases, marginalized populations, indigenous people, and the inhabitants of rural communities often have less access to safe, accessible, affordable and appropriate spaces and places in which to be physically active."[43] Thus, a global action plan on E/PA was created to be implemented from 2018 to 2030. Four strategic objectives were identified including the creation of: (1) active societies; (2) active environments; (3) active people; and (4) active systems. Twenty policy actions coincide with the objectives providing specific measurable goals where E/PA is a necessary component for success. Actions included: ending malnutrition; reducing premature mortality; ensuring quality education from preprimary to secondary (which includes safe, inclusive, effective learning environments); ending discrimination against females within E/PA; promoting development of E/PA related jobs; developing infrastructure that provides easy cycling and walking opportunities for pleasure or work; empowering and promoting total inclusion into PA programs and sports which promotes fairness; promoting increased walking, including walking and cycling in communities and in nature; and improving overall health and nurturing positive social values.[43]

Primary Prevention

Primary prevention interventions aim to provide risk reduction to prevent cancer from ever occurring by altering the person's current habits or lifestyle behaviors that are known to increase the risk for and potentially lead to cancer. It is also important to address the broader, social determinants of health, including lifestyle behaviors, actions and decisions that inhibit the establishment of good habits. These may include nutrition, sleep hygiene, stress reduction, social relationships, and spirituality. However, the focus here will be on the E/PA evidence that lowers the risk for cancer. The Center for Disease Control (CDC) refers to sedentary behavior as a low level for energy expenditure (less than or equal to 1.5 METs) while sitting, reclining, or lying. This behavior increases risk of colon, endometrial, and lung cancer. However, they also promote that moderate intensity E/PA lowers the risk of bladder, breast, colon, endometrial, esophageal, kidney, lung, and stomach (cardia and noncardia adenocarcinoma). Moderate intensity E/PA also decreases the risk of death from colon, prostate, and breast cancer while improving health related and fitness.[44]

explanation of the Nexus Model Figure 23.2. This model aims to demonstrate how E/PA can and should be incorporated into every level of prevention. Currently Onc R clinicians primarily practice at the tertiary prevention level. True patient and family-centered care requires that increased time and energy is also spent in primordial, primary, secondary, and quaternary prevention to decrease the occurrence of cancer and prevent adverse effects thus improving QOL.

Primordial Prevention

Primordial prevention consists of risk reduction in population and community health domains targeting social and environmental conditions that improve access to increased E/PA with the goal of decreasing the risk factors for cancer but also decreasing the risk factors for obesity and type 2 diabetes (also risk factors for cancer). A transdisciplinary and multifaceted approach is needed to prevent cancer including changes to the social, economic,

There is an abundance of evidence that examines and confirms how sedentary behavior increases our risk for cancer and moderate to vigorous exercise will prevent cancer from ever developing as well as recurring. A meta-analysis of 43 studies (68,936 cancer cases) concluded that each 2 hour per day increase in sitting time increased the risk for colon cancer by 8%, endometrial cancer by 10%, and lung cancer by 6%.[45] Another study of 1.44 million participants from 12 prospective US and European cohorts found that that high versus low levels of leisure time PA were associated with a lower risk for 13 out of 26 types of cancer including: bladder, breast, colon, endometrium, esophageal adenocarcinoma, gastric cardia, head and neck, liver, lung, kidney, myeloid leukemia, myeloma, and rectal. The higher levels of leisure time PA were described by these authors as 3 to 6 metabolic equivalent for task (MET) hours per week for moderate intensity and over 6 MET hours per week for vigorous intensity. This is equivalent to 150 minutes/week of moderate intensity activity, such as walking. These associations were able to be correlated regardless of smoking history or body size. This level of PA could lower the risk for these cancers by 10% to 30%.[46]

Secondary Prevention

Secondary prevention refers to the participation in exercise for persons already diagnosed with cancer that either have not started cancer treatment or have just started treatment but have not experienced any adverse effects yet. There is evidence that demonstrates that exercise can prevent or decrease the severity of the adverse events that occur from the medical treatments for cancer.

These interventions can be classified in two categories: (1) prehabilitation (see Chapter 27) provided prior to treatment, as well as (2) rehabilitation provided from the moment of diagnosis throughout cancer treatment aimed at preventing the adverse effects of cancer treatment.

Eighteen studies with a combined 966 participants diagnosed with cancers of the lung, prostate, and abdomen (e.g., colorectal and liver cancers), were provided with aerobic and strength training that varied by mode, intensity, frequency, and duration. Significant improvement in rate of return to continence, functional walking capacity, cardiorespiratory fitness, and decreased hospital stay were evidenced.[47] Another study analyzed persons diagnosed with prostate, lung, breast, and bladder cancers and compared those who participated in prehabilitation versus those who did not. The prehabilitation groups found that pelvic floor muscle training for persons diagnosed with PC demonstrated a 60% reduction the incidence of incontinence at 1 and 3 months compared to a control group. Presurgical pulmonary exercises for persons with lung cancer reduced the number of days spent in the hospital postsurgically (4.4 vs. 6.9) and lowered the odds of postsurgery complications; a preoperative exercise group that participated in high-intensity interval training (HIIT) had fewer number of days with a chest tube (4.3 vs. 8.8) and reduced hours spent in recovery from anesthesia (17 vs. 25) compared to a nonexercise control group.[48]

In a study of 230 persons diagnosed with breast or colon cancer, a low-intensity, home-based, individualized E/PA program (30 minutes for 5×/wk) called Onco-Move was compared to a moderate- to high-intensity aerobic and resistance training program called OnTrack where participation was 2 times per week. These were contrasted with usual care or no exercise program. This program started with the first cycle of chemotherapy and lasted until 3 weeks post chemotherapy. Both exercise interventions

demonstrated less decline in cardiorespiratory fitness and better physical functioning with less nausea and vomiting compared to usual care. However, the group that completed On-Track also was found to have less pain and better outcomes for muscle strength and decreased physical fatigue.[49]

When persons diagnosed with breast cancer cycled 5 times per week for 6 weeks, 1 hour before radiotherapy, the intervention group had a statistically significant decrease in diastolic blood pressure (DBP) and heart rate as well as an increase in the 6-minute walk distance (6MWD), while the control group demonstrated an increase in heart rate and dyspnea.[50]

Tertiary Prevention

Tertiary prevention focuses on exercise that helps to manage the adverse events and effects of cancer treatment that impact function and QOL. The goal of this level of treatment is to reduce disability and restore function to the highest level possible. Common adverse effects that can result from the treatment for cancer include: axillary web syndrome (cording), balance impairment, cancer related cognitive impairment (CRCI), cancer related fatigue (CRF), cardiotoxicity, chemotherapy induced polyneuropathy (CIPN), lymphedema, muscle weakness, postural changes, muscular imbalances, decreased joint mobility, pain/tenderness, scar tissue adhesions, psychosocial issues (i.e., fear of movement, fear of recurrence, depression, anxiety, negative body image, etc.) pelvic floor dysfunction, and radiation induced fibrosis (RIF)/radiation fibrosis syndrome (RFS). Evidence is clear that exercise can eliminate or decrease the intensity of these symptoms and can assist in managing these adverse effects. Most importantly, there are little or no adverse effects to the performance of exercise. The authors of this chapter highly recommend that each person diagnosed with cancer receive a screening, consultation, or Onc R intervention as needed to provide the education and exercise prescription that is safe for each individual. This personalized care is essential as each person's cancer diagnosis, treatments, physical, mental, and emotional abilities as well as the cancer treatment's adverse effects and events they experience are uniquely individual. Unfortunately, there is not a definitive method to determine what adverse effects someone will experience from treatment for cancer. Thus, education on possible effects is imperative. Three objectives are necessary for every PLWBC to preserve their QOL throughout the cancer journey: (1) understanding of the potential adverse effects; (2) having knowledge regarding the interventions for those adverse effects; and (3) being able to access exercise interventions through physician referral and financial support. To further explore the benefits of exercise for some of the common adverse effects from the treatment for cancer, see Table 23.1 which summarizes the benefits of E/PA for these adverse effects.

1. Balance/Chemotherapy-induced polyneuropathy—Balance impairments are resultant of polyneuropathy in the feet, damage to the vestibulocochlear nerve (cranial nerve VIII), as well as generalized deconditioning. Several systematic and integrative reviews demonstrate that the proper interventions can result in increases in both static and dynamic balance, decreases in numbness, tingling and pain, decrease risk of falls and improvements in physical functioning and QOL for persons experiencing CIPN. Exercise programs differed among studies but were focused on balance and sensorimotor training, postural and stabilization exercises, core strengthening exercises and lower limb closed kinetic chain exercises, as well as endurance.[51-53]

TABLE 23.1	Benefits of E/PA on Cancer Treatment Adverse Effects								
Adverse Effects	Increase Joint Motion	Increase Strength	Decrease Pain	Improve Function	Decrease Fatigue	Improve Balance	Improve Cognition	Decrease Numbness/ Tingling	Improve Cardio Respiratory Fitness
Balance	X	X	X	X	X	X		X	
Cardiotoxicity				X	X	X		X	X
CIPN		X	X	X		X		X	
CRCI				X			X		
CRF		X		X	X				X
Lymphedema	X	X	X	X					
Muscle weakness	X	X	X	X	X	X		X	
Pain	X	X	X	X					X
RFI/RFS	X	X	X	X					

AWS, Axillary web syndrome (cording); *CRCI*, cancer related cognitive impairment; *CIPN*, chemotherapy induced peripheral neuropathy; *CRF*, cancer related fatigue; *RIF/RFS*, radiation-induced fibrosis/radiation fibrosis syndrome.
Created by Deborah J. Doherty, PT, PhD. Printed with permission.

It is clear that there is not one exercise that is best for CIPN but multimodal and closed-chain exercises appear to be more beneficial than singular and open-chain exercises. The authors of this text advocate for individualized, patient-centered treatment regimens as each person's symptomology and adverse effects combined with their preexisting co-morbidities are not conducive to a one-size-fits-all exercise program.[53]

2. Cardiotoxicity—Cancer treatment-induced damage to the heart is a serious adverse effect of several chemotherapeutic agents, including but not limited to anthracyclines, fluorouracil, taxanes, monoclonal antibodies, and tyrosine kinase inhibitors as well as radiotherapy to the thorax.[54] The damage can be classified as reversible, irreversible, acute, chronic, and late onset (see Chapters 5 for more information). Studies are showing very positive results in preventing and treating cardiotoxicity. Numerous studies confirm the benefits of a variety of E/PA in counteracting the negative effects that cancer treatment induces on the cardiovascular system. Thirty minutes of vigorous intensity treadmill walking 24 hours prior to four doxorubicin-containing chemotherapy treatments appeared to prevent changes in hemodynamics (increased cardiac output, resting heart rate, decreased systemic vascular resistance) and reduced body weight gain, prevalence of depressed mood, sore muscles, and low back pain compared to usual care which did not include exercise.[55] Survey results of 4015 breast cancer survivors found that greater than 9 MET-hours/week of exercise was associated with decreased risk of cardiovascular events and coronary artery disease in the year after breast cancer diagnosis and treatment.[56] Investigators completed a very comprehensive review of the effects of exercise to mitigate cardiotoxicity and mortality. They describe how without exercise, a 4-month period of anthracycline-based chemotherapy can decrease the peak VO_2 so significantly that it nears what is expected after 15 years of aging; however, with a 16-week exercise program of 30 minutes of exercise three times per week at a minimum intensity of 50% heart rate reserve, VO_{2peak} was improved.[23]

Furthermore, in a study of 55 breast cancer survivors with no cardiovascular risk factors, only 19.45% of participants in the physical exercise group demonstrated symptoms of heart failure as compared to 68.42% of the control or inactive group.[23]

3. Chemotherapy-related cognitive impairment—CRCI is a common adverse effect of non-CNS-related cancers. Numerous murine studies and studies with healthy elderly subjects show significant 4015 reduction in cognitive decline as well as increased cognition with aerobic exercise. Now there is evidence to demonstrate the great potential in exercise to prevent and treat cognitive impairment caused from the treatment of some chemotherapeutic interventions. Two systematic reviews[57,58] found improved cognitive function resultant of aerobic and/or resistance exercises, mind-body interventions, and/or mindfulness-based exercises following cancer treatment. The challenge is heterogeneity of the interventions reported in terms of types of exercise, duration, frequency, intensity, supervision, control group, self-reported cognitive function, and neurophysiological assessments.[58] A 2016 systematic review (19 studies) examined the prefrontal cortex-dependent cognitive abilities (e.g., executive functions) which are frequently impaired in patients experiencing CRCI. Combinations of aerobic, resistance exercises, and/or cognitive training as well as yoga and YOCAs (combination of breathing exercise, Hatha Yoga, and meditation) demonstrated improved cognitive function. Benefits of these interventions included improved hippocampus-dependent cognitive functions, improved cognitive functions of the prefrontal cortex, elevation of levels of neurotransmitters like dopamine (associated with prefrontal cortex function), and increased lactate. Lactate is used as an energy substrate by neurons as it crosses the blood-brain barrier. It has been known to ameliorate neuronal function, inducing an increase in synaptic plasticity and reducing chronic inflammation, which is associated with cognitive impairment. It should be noted that yoga or YOCA exercises also improves mood, motivation, and mindfulness and should be considered as an intervention to

improve cognition. Other confounding variables that could affect cognition and ought to be considered are anxiety, post-traumatic stress, increasing age, intelligence quotient, symptoms of depression, sleep behaviors, and fatigue.[59]

4. Cancer-related fatigue—CRF is the most reported adverse effect of cancer treatment with a prevalence of 25% to 99% of persons diagnosed with cancer.[60] The evidence is overwhelming for the efficacy of exercise in reducing CRF. A meta-analysis analyzed the evidence of mixed interventions (supervised high and low intensity, resistance and aerobic exercise) provided during and following both chemotherapy and/or radiation. These programs lasted an average of 21 weeks (45 minutes; 2–3 times per week) and worked patients to 50% to 80% of their maximum heart rate. Outcomes included a statistically significant reduction in moderate and severe fatigue.[61] In another meta-analysis, treatments including exercise, psychological intervention, a combination of both, or pharmaceutical intervention were analyzed. CRF was improved significantly with exercise, psychological intervention, or both during and after treatment for cancer. However, pharmaceutical intervention did not demonstrate any decrease in fatigue.[62] Regardless of the type of exercise, the general concept of physical movement can decrease fatigue. Twelve different interventions were utilized throughout 245 studies including aerobic, resistance, combined aerobic and resistance exercises, cognitive behavior therapy (CBT), relaxation, yoga, massage, combined exercise and CBT, healing touch, dance, music therapy, and tai chi. There was a statistically significant decrease in fatigue both during and after cancer treatment.[60] Lastly, a meta-analysis of 31 randomized control trials found aerobic and/or resistance exercise all demonstrated statistically significant improvements in CRF as compared to normal care (no exercise prescribed). Interestingly, supervised exercise was found to be more effective than unsupervised.[63]

5. Lymphedema—A systematic review and meta-analyses of 29 studies investigating resistance exercise with breast cancer-related lymphedema (BCRL) concluded that prior to earlier beliefs, resistance exercise not only does not negatively affect BCRL, in fact, it decreases BCRL. Exercise protocols included both upper and lower extremity and core resistance exercises of various types, duration, and frequency. Protocols varied from 2 to 3 sets, 5 to 20 reps, 2 to 52 weeks, supervised and unsupervised sessions, and with exercise equipment as well as body weight. Examples of exercises included chest press, latissimus pulldown, bicep curls with free weights, leg press, abdominal crunches, and resistance band exercises for shoulder motions. All exercise programs are easily reproducible in any clinic, gym, or hospital setting.[64] A systematic review evaluating different types of physical exercise (aqua lymph training, swimming, resistance exercise, yoga, aerobic, and gravity-resisted exercise) on women who had BCRL demonstrated that a variety of E/PA types improves BCRL.[65] It is important to note that the training programs need to be supervised, individually designed, and always with safety in mind. The exercise interventions varied significantly from progressive resistance, gravity-resistive upper extremity flexibility or isotonic exercises, diaphragmatic breathing, progressive muscle relaxation, qigong, tai chi, and may or may not include manual lymphatic drainage and compression. It is noteworthy that regardless of the heterogeneity of exercise programs, positive results were yielded. This provides a wonderful opportunity to advocate for PLWBCs to participate in a variety of exercise programs to improve their physical functioning. Lastly, the effects of Pilates exercises delivered in a clinical setting with women developing lymphedema after treatment for breast cancer was studied.[66] A group of women who participated in an 8-week (1 hour, 3 days per week) program of clinical Pilates exercises was compared to a control group. The theory behind clinical Pilates is that through spinal stabilization and abdominal and upper extremity exercises, lymphatic flow will be stimulated to the ductus thoracicus. This study resulted in a greater reduction in lymphedema, as well as improvements in anxiety, QOL, and upper extremity function in the intervention group as compared to the control group. These are just a few studies highlighting evidence available to assist Onc R clinicians in advocating for exercise programs for women diagnosed with BCRL.[66]

6. Muscle weakness—Evidence has demonstrated that exercise increases muscle strength in PLWBCs. More recently, evidence exists defining the molecular changes to muscle with exercise during treatment for cancer. This is groundbreaking news for clinicians and will help in advocating for all patients diagnosed with cancer to also receive exercise training as standard of care. Muscle biopsies were obtained from 10 females before and after 4 to 7 weeks of chemotherapy and again after 10 weeks of continued chemotherapy in combination with exercise training. These results were compared to those of 10 healthy subjects.[67] The exercise intervention (90-minutes sessions, 3 times per week) included both aerobic and resistance training with progressive increases in intensity of both resistance and aerobic exercise continued throughout the research. In normal muscles, skeletal muscle mass is regulated by the balance between protein synthesis and degradation. Chemotherapy disrupts this balance. However, exercise was able to bring the system back into balance. The investigators also demonstrated that although chemotherapy alone disrupted molecular signaling pathways involved in adaptation to exercise training, exercising during chemotherapy prevented further disruption.[67]

Another study demonstrated that a 1-year resistance training program improved muscle strength in androgen-deprived PC survivors. The Prevents Osteoporosis With Impact + Resistance (POWIR) program consisted of supervised classes twice per week and a home program once per week for 12 months. Free weights, multi-joint movements (e.g., sits, squats, bent knee raises, pushups) and resistance band exercises for the home program were included with the control group completing flexibility exercises.[68] Achievements were encouraging with a noted decrease in androgen deprivation therapy-related bone loss which likely reduced fracture risk. In addition, significant gains were noted in strength, self-reported physical function, walking speed and decreased disability. In another randomized control trial, the control group demonstrated significant positive changes in lean body mass, muscle strength, maximal muscle power, self-reported fatigue, and physical performance as compared to the control group. The 12-week (3 times per week) resistance training protocol included: three sets (8–12 repetitions per set) of each exercise (leg extension, leg curl, calf raise, 45-degree leg press) with an estimated load of 80% of one-repetition maximum.[69] These studies are just a small sample of the evidence for strength training in PLWBCs.

7. Pain—Pain is one of the most common adverse effects of cancer treatment (please see Chapter 22 for more information on cancer pain). Not only is pain identified as moderate to intense in 30% to 60% of persons treated for breast cancer but half of them receive inadequate treatment to address their pain. Exercise is one intervention that shows excellent promise in

mitigating the intensity of pain.[70] A 12-week (3 times per week) supervised aerobic and resistance training program complemented by unsupervised flexibility exercises were completed by females diagnosed with breast cancer undergoing chemotherapy and radiation therapy. Aerobic training (30 minutes on a cycle ergometer) was followed by resistance training (30 minutes) including hip flexion, extension, shoulder exercises, squatting with a Swiss ball, French presses, and lifting exercises. This resulted in reduced total pain points, pain intensity, and interference of pain in patients' daily lives, as well as increased maximum oxygen uptake, flexibility, and strength.[70] Exercise has also been proven to reduce pain and other musculoskeletal symptoms (stiffness, weak grip strength, and reduced QOL) in persons diagnosed with breast cancer taking aromatase inhibitors (AIs).[71] This study evaluated pain and found a statistically significant difference in exercise versus usual care in reducing pain caused from AIs. The authors theorized that AIs decrease estrogen which is known to attenuate pain via opioid neurons in the spinal cord, therefore the quick depletion of estrogen from AIs could make the patient more sensitive to pain. Exercise increases anti-inflammatory cytokines which theoretically also reduces pain. Exercise also increases circulation and skeletal muscle volume, which makes activities of daily living (ADLs) and easier, range of motion easier, and increases muscle strength—all of which would likely decrease pain. A 10-year longitudinal study[72] followed women diagnosed with breast cancer to determine if E/PA would reduce pain. Not only did PA reduce pain but it also highlighted how weight gain and lack of PA increased risk for pain long after the treatment ended. After 10 years, 24% of participants reported improved pain, 9% maintained above-average pain, 33.1% reported worsened pain. The participants who met the criteria for being overweight/obese and those who did not meet the PA guidelines were the participants who reported worsened pain. These studies highlight the efficacy, feasibility, convenience, and potentially long-term sustainability of nonpharmacologic interventions for pain.

Quaternary Prevention

Quaternary prevention is defined as "an action taken to protect individuals (persons/patients) from medical interventions that are likely to cause more harm than good."[73] The concept of quaternary prevention helps to identify risk of over-medicalization. This requires a dynamic balance between assessment and the health activities that achieve more benefit than harm. The concept of quaternary prevention is inter-related with the nonmaleficence principle of medical ethics known as *primum non nocere* (first, do no harm) by protecting PLWBCs from an excess of medicine. Movement is essential throughout life in one form or another and is one of the few interventions that improves QOL and does no harm. However, it is important to have reassessment and modification of an E/PA prescription to meet the needs of each person at each stage of their lifespan.

Goals and Benefits of Exercise/Physical Activity

E/PA can play a vital role in ameliorating adverse effects from cancer and related treatments while improving overall survival and QOL.[8–10] The goals and direction of an exercise program may change as the person moves within survivorship to address their current concerns and limitations, and to optimize the person's QOL throughout the stages of prehabilitation, treatment, post-treatment, survivorship, and palliation.[4,34] Regardless of the direction of the disease and treatment, the E/PA program should promote whole person care. This program should always encompass what is meaningful to the person and address potential or current deficits in physical function in order to optimize treatment adherence, overall survival, and QOL while attempting to meet the recommended guidelines for E/PA.

Caring for the Whole Person; Not Just the Diagnosis

When designing an E/PA program or plan of care for a PLWBC, simply treating the diagnosis, like a joint limitation or tissue restriction brings a siloed approach resulting in suboptimal care. The aspect of patient-centered care is a staple and promoting optimal health and wellness for a PLWBC is essential to facilitate an optimal QOL. There are numerous factors that are important to consider when designing, prescribing, and providing education for E/PA. Not only the diagnosis but the person's entire biopsychosocial emotional medical history (diagnosis, past, current, and future treatment history, comorbid conditions, current medications, and prognosis) must be considered when developing an E/PA program.[74,75] A PLWBC can have significant multisystem (cardiovascular, pulmonary, endocrine, musculoskeletal, integumentary, neurological, psychoemotional) impairments that may limit their activity participation which would require special considerations with E/PA modality and intensity.[74,75] Furthermore, the person's anticipated or planned cancer treatment regimen must also be considered when developing an E/PA program. If the person is actively going through chemotherapy and/or radiation therapy, they may experience fatigue, myelosuppression, decreased appetite, myalgias, or arthralgias; these factors can affect the person's E/PA participation and their ability to tolerate a higher intensity or volume of E/PA.[76,77] In contrast, a person who has not yet commenced their cancer treatment may be able to engage in more E/PA at higher intensity.[76,78]

Each individual's previous and current level of physical function, as well as their goals of care is a key consideration. Adverse effects of cancer and treatment (weakness, fatigue, CIPN, cardiotoxicity, etc.) can hinder the person's physical function resulting in a lower QOL and potentially poorer treatment and health outcomes.[74,76,79] An E/PA program can be developed for a multitude of reasons whether to improve the functional status of a person (optimize movement such as range of motion of the shoulder or gait mechanics), to improve overall strength and muscle mass, to amplify cardiorespiratory fitness, and more. Optimization of these factors can result in an enhanced recovery from surgery, improved tolerance to treatment (systemic/radiation therapy), and improved overall survival leading to a better QOL.[76,79] By listening and engaging a PLWBC with the whole-person care approach and addressing their goals related to E/PA, a plan of care and exercise program can be developed to empower them and allow them to reach their goals.

There are numerous factors that need to be considered when educating about E/PA along with developing an individualized plan for each PLWBC. This plan should include the entire cancer journey, from the point of diagnosis through the remainder of life and between the acute care, home care, and outpatient settings. Figure 23.3 demonstrates numerous factors that could motivate

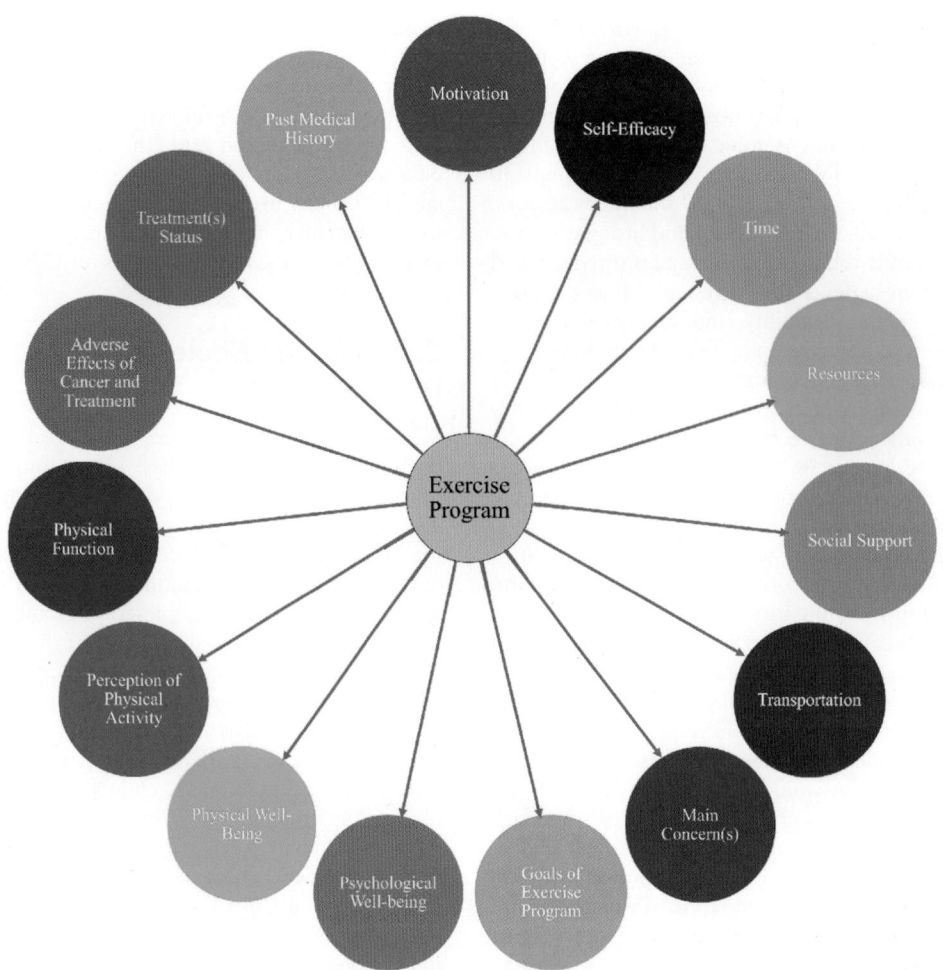

• **Fig. 23.3** Factors to Consider When Developing an Individualized Exercise Program. (Created by Andrew Chongaway, PT, DPT. Printed with permission.)

and facilitate adherence to an E/PA program or inhibit and deter in engaging in E/PA.[80–86]

Often, time and resources can be barriers to care and E/PA.[80–86] Time may be limited due to ongoing treatments, numerous doctors' visits, work, caregiver roles, etc. In these situations where a PLWBC attends formal rehabilitation weekly, providing education about how to incorporate E/PA into their day can provide meaningful change to a person's health and wellbeing.[87] However, the ability to provide in-person education may be limited due to a scarcity of Onc R clinicians who are fully integrated within the cancer care teams and various settings limiting the skilled provision and education regarding safe E/PA.[35] Further, if qualified Onc R clinicians are available, they may only be practicing in one setting or location (e.g., within a local cancer center) which may limit patient access due to transportation and time issues.[80,81] Even with the ability to provide education, resources within the community, such as safe outdoor exercise areas (tracks, parks, sidewalks) or public wellness centers/gyms, may not be available further limiting the ability for this population to safely engage in E/PA.[80–83] Other barriers for PLWBCs include limited financial resources, transportation, and equipment available in the home.[85,86]

Motivation and self-efficacy play an important role in accepting and adhering to an E/PA program. PLWBCs may experience feelings of depression, anxiety, hopelessness, frustration, and may feel as though they will not be able to return to their previous lifestyle or activities.[35,82,83] This can be a barrier to E/PA and should

be routinely screened and addressed prior to and throughout an E/PA program with appropriate referrals as needed to other qualified professionals.[82–84] Additionally, social and caregiver support needs must be considered, as having strong social support has been shown to promote adherence to engaging in E/PA.[88] There may be periods of time when a person is not interested in engaging in E/PA or is unmotivated to participate. Discussion, education, and shared decision making is important to understand the person's current QOL, how it may have been affected since their cancer diagnosis, what their perception of E/PA is, and how E/PA could potentially play a role in improving their QOL.[82–84]

Screening and Assessing Functional Performance Status

The person's medical status, adverse effect burden, and impairments in physical function all need to be considered during the prescription and delivery of exercise. For example, a person with stable disease and low symptom burden with no functional impairments may be suitable to participate in supervised exercise at a wellness center/gym with a cancer exercise trainer. A person who has significant functional impairments (gait abnormalities, limited range of motion, CIPN, pain, etc.) or advanced disease (bone metastasis) should be receiving supervision from an Onc R clinician with specialty training.[4,35,89,90] Figure 23.4 shows a

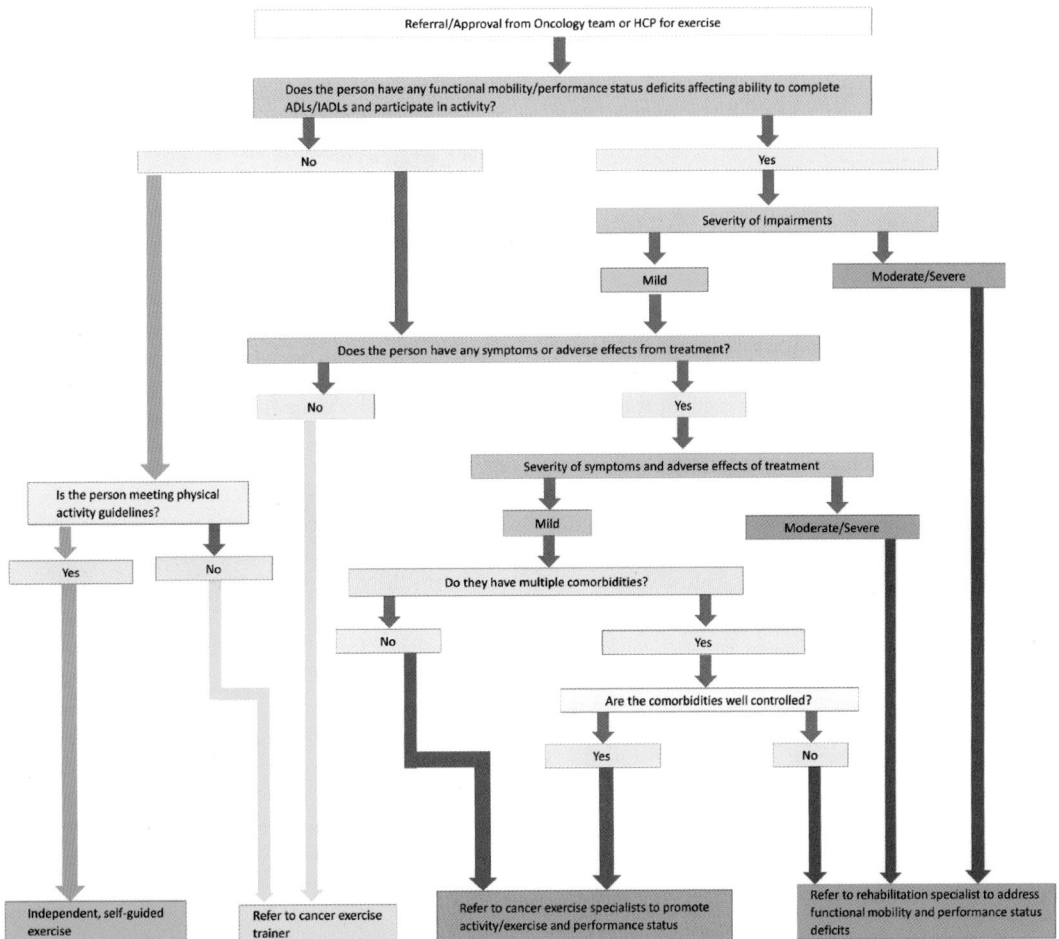

• **Fig. 23.4** Screening and Referral Algorithm. (Adapted from Stout NL, Brown JC, Schwartz AL, et al. An exercise oncology clinical pathway: Screening and referral for personalized interventions: Screening and referral for exercise. *Cancer*. 2020;126(12):2750–2758; Schmitz KH, Campbell AM, Stuiver MM, et al. Exercise is medicine in oncology: Engaging clinicians to help patients move through cancer. *CA Cancer J Clin*. 2019 Nov;69(6):468–484; Suderman K, McIntyre C, Sellar C, McNeely ML. Implementing cancer exercise rehabilitation: An update on recommendations for clinical practice. *Curr Cancer Ther Rev*. 2019;15(2):100–109. Created by Andrew Chongaway, PT, DPT. Printed with permission.)

referral decision-making algorithm for PLWBCs based on complexity (disease state, functional impairments, adverse effects of treatment, comorbid conditions) to ensure appropriate screening and referral. In most situations, a referral from the person's medical team (oncologist, primary care provider, cardiologist, pulmonologist) is also recommended prior to initiation of an E/PA program. By considering the whole-person care approach, proper direction and referral can be completed to develop and provide a safe, individualized E/PA program to optimize physical function. Due to the potential for a sudden and unexpected reduction in physical function, objective physical function screening should be completed periodically throughout the person's cancer journey.[90–92]

Physical Function, Functional Mobility, or Physical Status?

An individual with better overall physical function will often exhibit improved treatment adherence, postsurgical recovery, QOL, and overall survival rates, as well as reduction of symptoms and late-effects from cancer treatments.[34] Unfortunately, physical function is often inconsistently defined, assessed, and classified across settings, demographics, and diagnoses.[90] Physical function is defined as "the ability to perform the basic actions (get out of bed, walk, climb stairs) that are essential for maintaining independence and carrying out more complex activities."[93] With this definition, there are two different subgroups of function: performing basic tasks and carrying out more complex activities.[93] The ability to complete basic functions such as being able to stand up, walk safely, and complete the necessary day-to-day tasks could be classified as functional mobility. Although a person may be "independent" with functional mobility, they may still exhibit a slow gait speed, lower extremity weakness, limited cardiorespiratory fitness, or impaired balance—all of which may limit their ability to participate in hobbies or return to work. Any of these factors may also affect overall treatment adherence, outcomes, and QOL.[94]

The terminology "performance status" has been used in the oncology field since the development of the Karnofsky Performance Status (KPS) to quantify the person's ability to complete ADLs.[95] The Eastern Cooperative Oncology Group (ECOG) Performance Status quantifies the person's ability to care for themselves (ADLs/instrumental activities of daily living [IADLs]) as well as their ability to work, walk, and participate in E/PA.[96] As the KPS and ECOG are used to quantify the person's ability to complete ADLs/IADLs, neither truly assesses an individual's physical function. To address this shortcoming, the KPS or ECOG can be used to identify persons that are exhibiting or reporting adverse effects from cancer and treatment; it is recommended to establish and utilize a predetermined cut-point to initiate a referral to an Onc R clinician.[97] This will allow the Onc R clinician to conduct a formal assessment of adverse effects and how they affect mobility, cardiorespiratory status, strength, and balance[97] (see Chapter 2 for a KPS/ECOG comparison).

Within this chapter the use of the term functional performance status is globally described as the amount of upper and lower extremity strength/endurance, cardiorespiratory fitness, and balance measured via established and accepted assessment tools. The need for a consistent definition of physical function along with sub-definitions to capture the whole person is needed in the Onc R setting. This is due to the fact that a person's functional mobility does not always correlate to their functional performance status and vice versa, though it is less common for a high functional performance to result in lower functional mobility. Figure 23.5 demonstrates what encompasses functional mobility and functional

performance status and how both combine to ensure physical function.

Assessing Functional Performance Status Across the Settings

Onc R refers to restoring motion, reducing pain, exercise prescription, and optimizing movement to improve QOL. This coincides with the American Physical Therapy Association's (APTA)[98] vision statement "Transforming society by optimizing movement to improve the human experience." Oftentimes the focus of restoring functional mobility (getting out of or into a bed, being able to stand up from a chair, ambulating safely and efficiently, navigating stairs/curbs) or reducing pain requires skilled interventions. These may include manual therapy, blocked practice of movements, passive/active-assisted/active range of motion exercises, or relearning motor pathways. An appropriate E/PA program to strengthen weakened muscles, promote cardiorespiratory fitness, and improve balance in PLWBCs should not be overlooked.

Across the various Onc R settings, the initial focus may be evaluating the person's ability to get out of bed, assess gait mechanics,

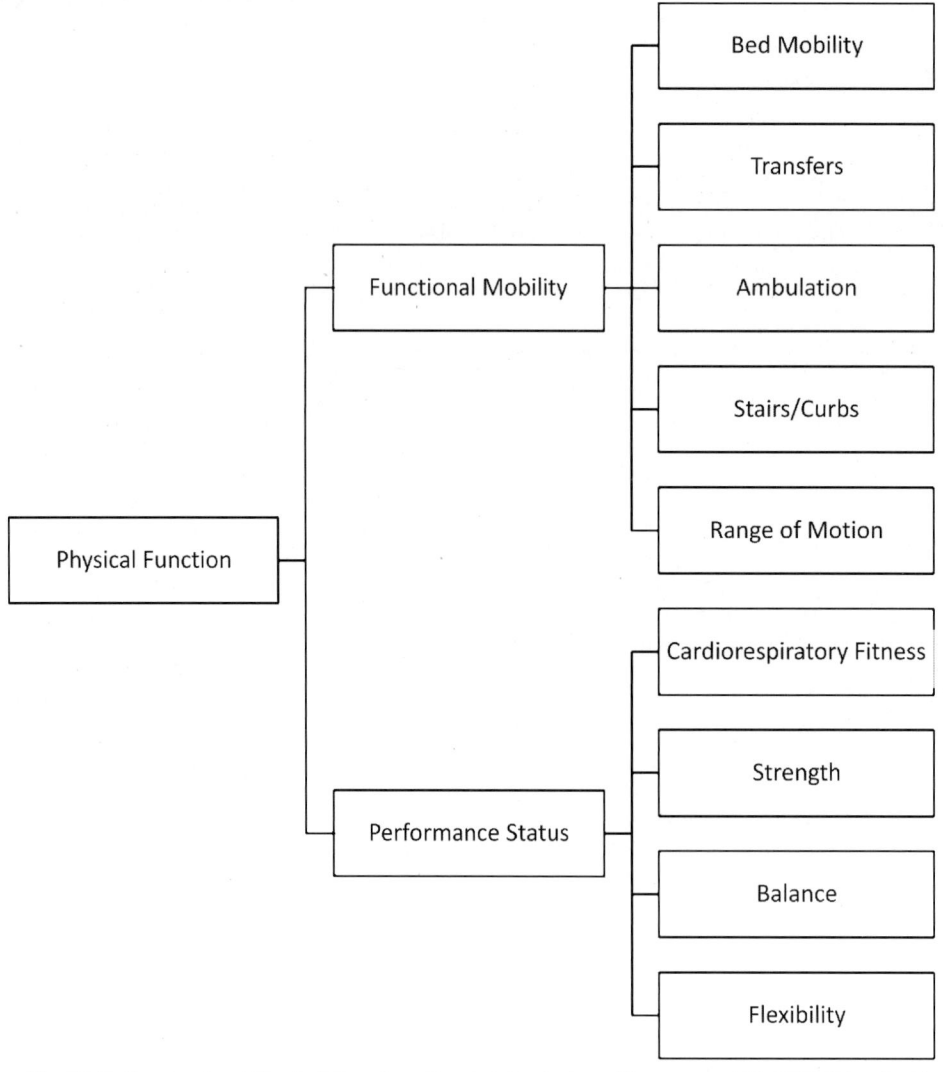

• **Fig. 23.5** Constructs of Physical Function. (Created by Andrew Chongaway, PT, DPT. Printed with permission.)

ability to complete tasks within the home, range of motion, girth, and/or sensation. This is important as limitations in functional mobility can limit functional performance status which in turn hinders E/PA participation. If deficits in functional mobility are present then the focus of sessions should be to promote improvements in functional mobility, though this does not mean an E/PA program cannot be established to promote overall strength, improve CRF, and increase balance. For example, if a person is unable to ambulate safely over significant distances, supine, seated, or standing exercises using resistance bands or bodyweight could be utilized to promote lower extremity strength and endurance; this would logically translate to improving a person's ability to ambulate.

Prior to starting the initial session, the Onc R clinician should have a sound understanding of the person's medical history (cancer diagnosis, previous/current/future treatments, comorbid conditions, and medications).[74–76,79] Once the initial session has started, evaluating cognition, assessing pain at rest and with movement, and measuring vitals should be completed (vitals should be assessed at the start and end of every session).[79,99] In order to understand each person's response to activity, vitals (blood pressure [BP], heart rate [HR], oxygen saturation [SpO2]) should also be assessed following positional changes, functional mobility tasks, assessment measures (e.g., 5× sit to stand, 2- or 6-minute walk test [2MWT/6MWT]), and throughout exercise performance.[99] See Box 23.2 for reference on when to assess vitals.

In the following section there are three algorithms, acute care (Figure 23.6), home care (Figure 23.7), and outpatient/wellness (Figure 23.8), to help guide the Onc R clinician in assessing functional performance status of a PLWBC in these different settings. Each algorithm utilizes a variety of different assessment tools to be able to assess the person's functional performance status in the situation of significant weakness, fatigue, balance, etc. It should be noted that these algorithms do not include assessment tools for persons who may have a higher functional performance status at

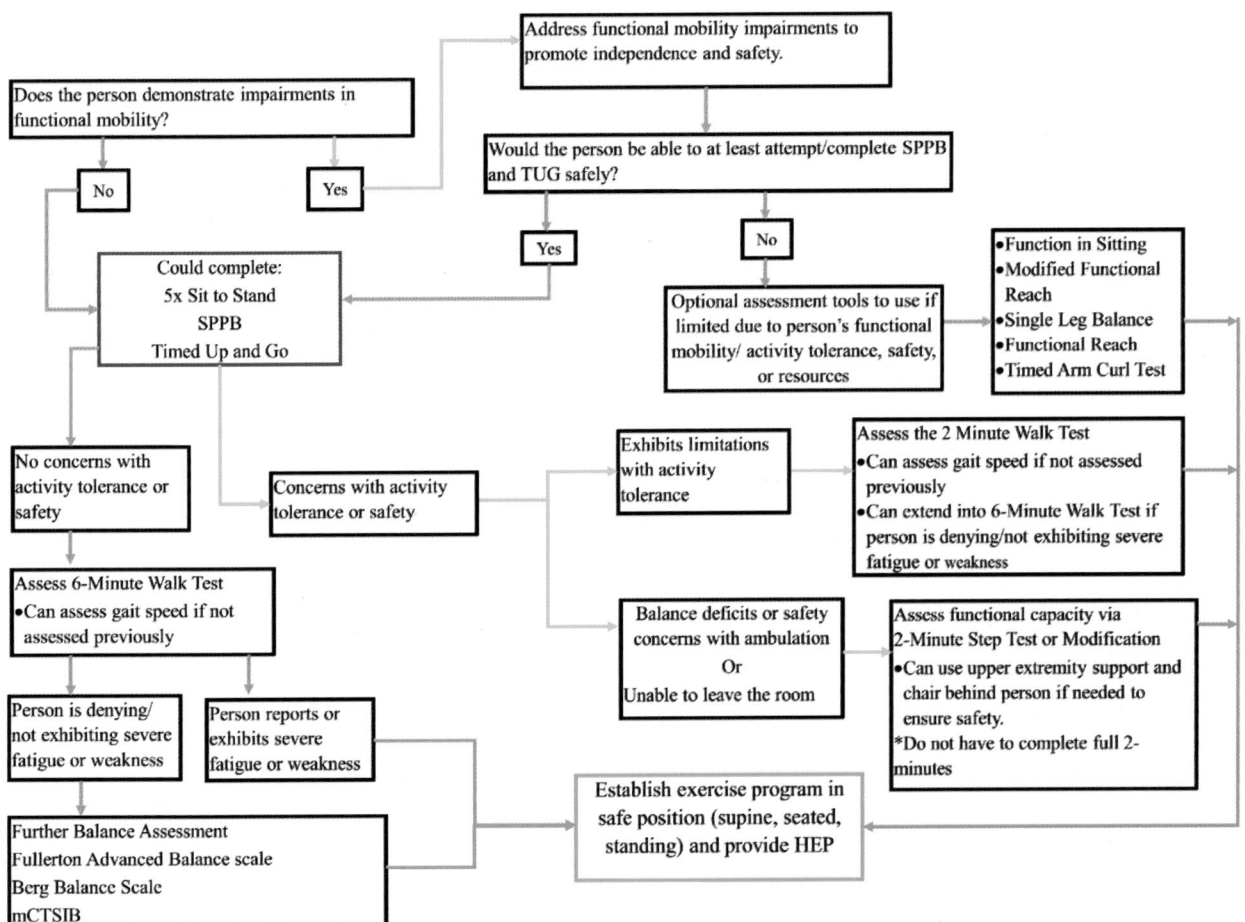

● **Fig. 23.6** Acute care functional performance status evaluation algorithm. *mCTSIB*, modified Clinical Test of Sensory Interaction in Balance; *SPPB*, Short Physical Performance Battery; *TUG*, Timed Up and Go. (Created by Andrew Chongaway, PT, DPT. Printed with permission.)

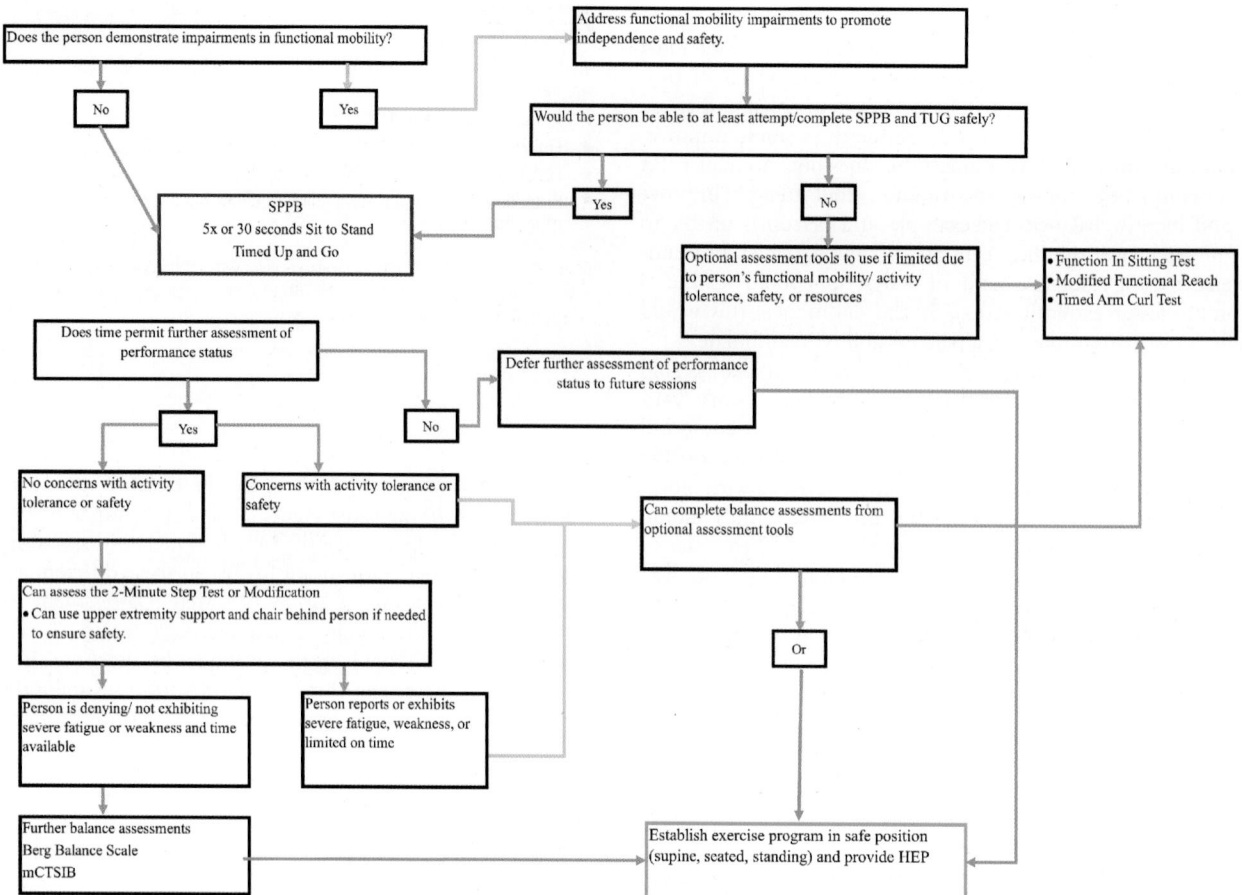

- **Fig. 23.7** Home care functional performance status evaluation algorithm. *mCTSIB*, modified Clinical Test of Sensory Interaction in Balance; *SPPB*, Short Physical Performance Battery; *TUG*, Timed Up and Go. (Created by Andrew Chongaway, PT, DPT. Printed with permission.)

baseline and would be able to tolerate a greater intensity of E/PA. The majority of the assessment tools included in these algorithms were recommended for clinical use by APTA Oncology EDGE Task force.[100–102] By assessing the person's balance, strength, and cardiorespiratory fitness/functional capacity, the Onc R clinician is able to develop an appropriate E/PA program to meet the person's needs and address deficits in functional mobility and functional performance status. As demonstrated in each algorithm, functional mobility is assessed first prior to moving into the person's functional performance status. Further, each one of these algorithms does not need to be completed in their entirety during the initial evaluation or in future sessions. The Timed Up and Go (TUG) and Short Physical Performance Battery (SPPB) are utilized as the first two assessment tools for all three algorithms as these assessment tools require minimal equipment, space, and time to administer (SPPB: 10 minutes/TUG: Up to 5 minutes). In addition they both assess aspects of lower extremity strength, balance, and functional mobility and are applicable in all clinical settings.[103,104]

With respect to the Outpatient/Wellness algorithm there are a few assessment tools that are not commonly used or well-known such as the Steep Ramp Test and University of North Colorado Cancer Rehabilitation Institute (UNCCRI) Treadmill Test to assess VO_{2peak} and 1/5/8/10 repetition maximum for strength assessment.[105–107]

Measuring CRF is important as research has demonstrated that persons with a higher VO_{2max} or functional endurance/capacity

have lower cancer-mortality and all-cause mortality rates.[35,87] Also, comorbidities that affect the cardiopulmonary system (congestive heart failure, coronary artery disease, chronic obstructive pulmonary disease) are common and can greatly affect CRF leading to a reduced functional performance status and an impaired QOL. The 2MWT, 6MWT, and 2-minute step test (2MST) have been included in this algorithm as space is usually available, they require little equipment, and can be safely completed with most PLWBCs in an outpatient setting.[108–111] However, these tests do not measure VO_{2peak} but rather assess functional endurance/capacity. It should be noted that prior to assessing functional endurance/VO_{2peak}, the person should be screened for cardiovascular risk and whether medical clearance is recommended prior to assessing cardiorespiratory fitness and engaging in aerobic exercise.[113] Please refer to Chapter 10 for details.

Aside from the Steep Ramp Test and the UNCCRI Protocol requiring equipment, both have specific parameters to complete the measures.[105,107] The Steep Ramp Test is performed with a cycle ergometer and the UNCCRI protocol is a treadmill-based test. Both of these tests have the ability to predict VO_{2peak} through formulas.[106,107] As the UNCCRI uses a treadmill, it might not be suitable for persons with neuropathy or gait instabilities, in which case the Steep Ramp Test may be more appropriate. Before utilizing either the Steep Ramp or UNCCRI in clinical practice, the Onc R clinician should be able to proficiently execute all aspects of the test in a simulated environment.

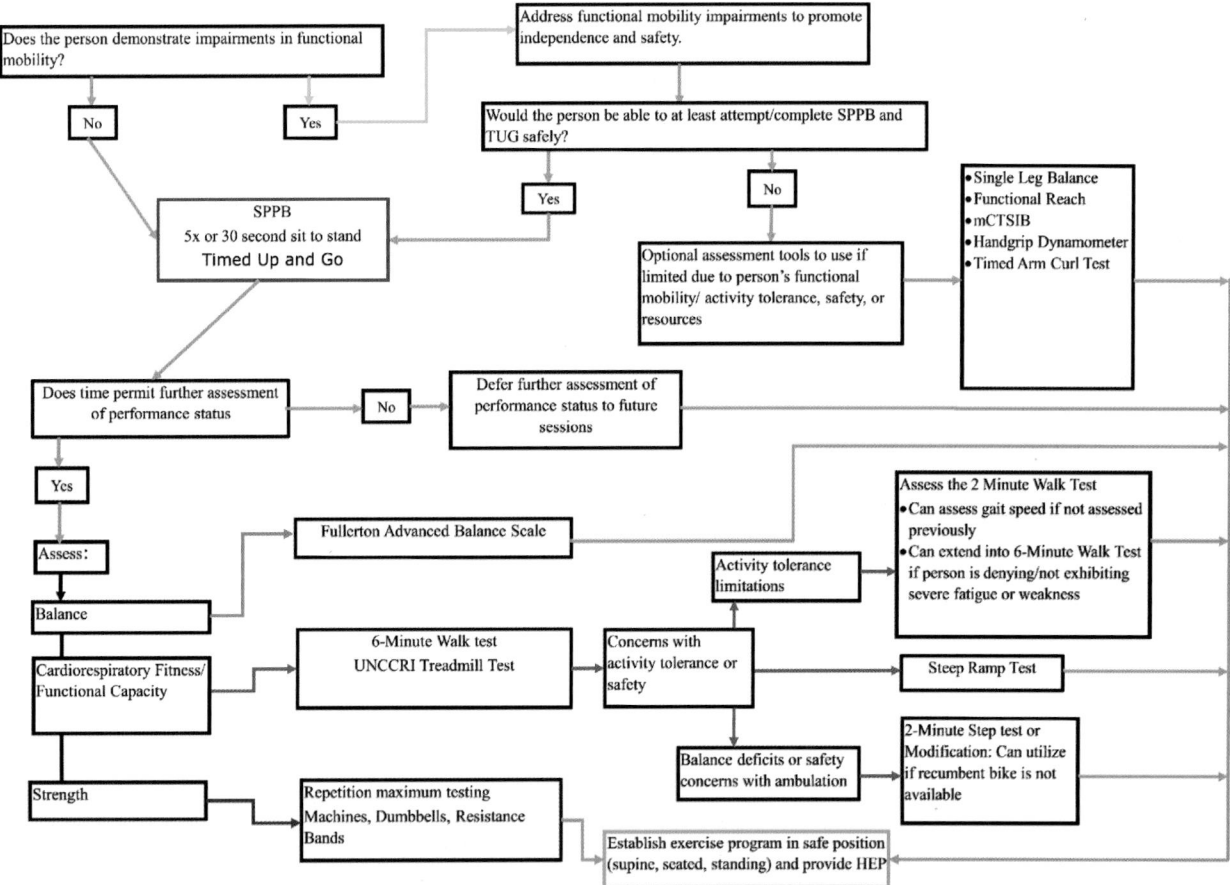

• Fig. 23.8 Outpatient/Community-based functional performance atatus evaluation algorithm. *mCTSIB*, modified Clinical Test of Sensory Interaction in Balance; *SPPB*, Short Physical Performance Battery; *TUG*, Timed Up and Go. (Created by Andrew Chongaway, PT, DPT. Printed with permission.)

BP, HR, SpO_2, and RPE should be taken at the beginning and end of the measures and should be attempted during as able (HR and SpO_2).[99]

Steep Ramp Test[105,106]

This is a cycle ergometer-based maximal exercise capacity test. This quick test allows for predicted VO_{2peak} and maximum workload (measured in watts [W_{peak}]) to be measured from maximal short exercise capacity (MSEC).

A short 2 to 3 minute warm-up needs to begin the process. The person is then instructed to pedal the ergometer between 70 and 80 revolutions per minute (rpms). After the warm-up, pedaling continues for 30 seconds at 25 watts. The load is increased by 25 watts every 10 seconds until the individual reports that they can no longer maintain pedaling at minimum of 60 rpms. MSEC is calculated by taking the last stage completed plus 2.5 watts for every second completed in the last stage.[105,106] This test is a fairly new measure used in persons diagnosed with cancer and further research is warranted on the Steep Ramp Test. Results are individually based on the formulas listed below:

- VO_{2peak}: 676.8+3.92*MSEC+5.02*weight (kg)–327.6*female (using 1 for "female" and 0 for "male")
- W_{peak}: 0.33*MSEC+124*height(m)–22.4*female–0.47*age–107

University of Northern Colorado Cancer Rehabilitation Institute VO_{2peak} Protocol[107]

For this protocol the resting BP, HR, SpO_2, and body weight are all measured before all tests are administered. During the test, SpO_2 and HR are taken every minute, while RPE and BP are taken every 3 minutes. The person's maximal heart rate needs to be determined prior to initiation. Before the test begins, instructions should be provided, including: (1) educating the person on the Modified Borg Scale (0–10); (2) recruit a clinician to assist in recording all test data, as well as changing the speed and grade of the treadmill; and (3) make sure someone is available to stand behind the treadmill for safety purposes. See Table 23.2 for the testing protocol. During the test, the person should be encouraged to attempt to push to their maximum exertion, however, they can ask to stop at any time. The clinician should also recommend that handrails are not used unless necessary. If the person chose not to use handrails, they are not allowed to use them later in the test, and vice versa if they chose to use handrails. After perceived maximal exertion is attained, a cool-down phase is completed until vitals are returned to near resting values.

If any participant was able to complete stage 20, the speed is increased by 0.1 mile per hour (mph) and the grade is increased by 1% every minute until fatigue is elicited. The test is terminated when the person has reached their maximum threshold of exertion and cannot continue or when: the HR did not increase with

TABLE 23.2	**UNCCRI Treadmill Protocol**							
Stage	**Speed (mph)**	**Grade (%)**	**Time (min)**	**Stage**	**Speed (mph)**	**Grade (%)**	**Time (min)**
0	1.0	0	1	11	3.8	8	1
1	1.5	0	1	12	3.9	9	1
2	2.0	0	1	13	4.0	10	1
3	2.5	0	1	14	4.1	11	1
4	2.5	2	1	15	4.2	12	1
5	3.0	2	1	16	4.3	13	1
6	3.3	3	1	17	4.4	14	1
7	3.4	4	1	18	4.5	15	1
8	3.5	5	1	19	4.6	16	1
9	3.6	6	1	20	4.7	17	1
10	3.7	7%	1	Cooldown	–	0	–

Created by Andrew Chongaway, PT, DPT. Printed with permission.

TABLE 23.3	**UNCCRI Treadmill Protocol VO$_{2peak}$ Formulas**	
Walking **without** handrail usage during the last competed stage	$VO_{2peak} = (0.1 \times S) + (1.8 \times S \times G) + 3.5$
Running **without** handrail usage during the last competed stage	$VO_{2peak} = (0.2 \times S) + (0.9 \times S \times G) + 3.5$
Walking **and holding onto** the handrails during the last competed stage	$VO_{2peak} = 0.694\,[(0.1 \times S) + (1.8 \times S \times G) + 3.5]$
Running **and holding onto** the handrails during the last competed stage	$VO_{2peak} = 0.694\,[(0.2 \times S) + (0.9 \times S \times G) + 3.5]$

G, Grade; *S*, speed.
Created by Andrew Chongaway, PT, DPT. Printed with permission.

increased intensity, systolic blood pressure (SBP) did not increase with increased intensity, DBP oscillated more than 10 mmHg from resting measure, or SpO$_2$ dropped below 80%, and/or the participant requested the test to end.[107] At the point of the test being terminated, final HR, BP, SpO$_2$, and treadmill time should be taken. A test is deemed a VO$_{2peak}$ test if at least two of the following criteria are met: A person terminated the test due to perceived maximal effort and fatigue, the HR was elevated to within 10 beats per minute of the individual's estimated maximal heart rate, or a person verbalized an RPE value on the modified Borg scale of at least eight out of 10.[107] Formulas to calculate VO$_{2peak}$ based on the person's performance are shown in Table 23.3.[107]

The last step of the outpatient algorithm would be to assess strength of the upper and/or lower extremity. There are a number of ways to assess the strength of a PLWBC. Traditionally to assess strength, a 1-repetition maximum (1-RM) will be assessed for various muscles where the person will move the heaviest load possible through a full ROM.[3,112,113] However, this may be daunting for individuals that are significantly debilitated or do not have a background in exercising. In this scenario, a higher number of repetitions could be used (e.g., 5, 8, or 10 repetitions) as an estimation of 1-RM and plugged into an equation such as the Bryzcki Equation (1-RM = W/[102.78– 2.78(R)]/100, where W is the weight used and R is the maximal number of repetitions performed) to estimate the individual's 1-RM.[114] This will still give a suitable measurement of the person's strength and allow for targeted prescription of exercises.[3,4,114] The main caveat to this method is having the appropriate equipment available (machines, barbells, dumbbells, or kettlebells) to be able to assess the person's true or calculated 1-RM.

Use of a barbell or dumbbell requires the individual to stabilize the weight which can affect form, the amount of load able to be lifted through the ROM, and ultimately the safety of the individual.[3] This is where the use of machines, when available may be more advantageous as the weight is stabilized which can allow novice lifters to move a greater load through the appropriate range or motion.[3] Other supplemental exercises can be included into the exercise prescription to allow for focus of stabilization of targeted musculature if deemed necessary. The focus initially should be on optimizing form then appropriately adding load to the movement. See Box 23.3 for the ACSM protocol for assessing the 1-RM along with examples of movements/exercises that can be tested to establish baseline data.[3] Other optional tests for determining strength include the timed arm curl test or use of a handgrip dynamometer.

While most facilities will not have some or all of the machines listed above, it is likely that elastic resistance bands are generally universally available for resistance training. When using resistance bands, the choice in band resistance should be tailored to the person's strength capacity.[115] The person should first be instructed in the exercise to ensure the movement is completed correctly. Then

- Ten-minute warm-up consisting of low intensity aerobic exercise, dynamic stretching, and the specific movements to be tested at a light load.
- Initial load should be around 50%–70% of individual's anticipated max.
- If lift is successful a rest period of 3–5 minutes should be given.
  - Resistance should be progressed in increments of 5–40 lbs until the individual cannot complete the lift.
    Should not exceed four sets to prevent neural and muscular fatigue. With the use of estimated 1-repetition max using the Bryzcki Equation, at most two working sets should be completed.
  - For each set no more than 10 repetitions should be completed to prevent overexertion.
- Movements may be single joint or multi-joint although multi-joint is preferred, from a functional standpoint.
  - Can use machines, barbells, free weights, or medicine balls based on equipment available or person's functional performance status.
  - With a barbell, dumbbells, kettlebells, or medicine balls: Squat, Deadlift, Step Up, Press, Row, Sit to Stand, Squat to Press.
  - With machines: Leg Press, Leg Extension, Leg Flexion, Chest Press, Machine Row, Lat Pulldown.

Created by Andrew Chongaway, PT, DPT. Printed with permission.

determine the number of repetitions that the person can complete before fatigue or significant form breakdown with resistance. For example: The person can complete 10 repetitions of a standing row with no form breakdown or fatigue with a "light" resistance band and an RPE of 2/10. Rest is given then the movement is repeated for 10 reps with a "light-moderate" resistance band with minimal form breakdown on the last two reps and an RPE of 5/10.[115] Rest is given, and the person completes the movement with a "moderate" resistance band where the person completes 10 repetitions and demonstrates significant form breakdown on the final two reps and reports an RPE of 8/10.[115] In this situation the use of the "moderate" resistance band would be the most appropriate due to the person completing the required repetitions, with appropriate form and fatigue.[115] Not every section of the algorithm (balance, strength, functional capacity) must be completed during the initial assessment and instead can be completed as warranted during follow up sessions if the clinician chooses to do so.

Assessing Functional Performance Status in the Acute Care Setting

Assessing functional mobility (bed mobility, transfers, gait, stairs) is the first step. During assessment of functional mobility and functional performance status, evaluation of mechanics, sequencing, strength, balance, or capacity for activity should occur with each task. Safety is paramount and in a situation when high risk therapeutic activities are provided, the Onc R clinician should focus on educating, assessing, and providing the appropriate assistive device and safety measures (e.g., gait belt) as necessary.

In the situation where an individual exhibits poor sitting postural control, difficulty with transfers, or significant impairments with standing postural control, the Function in Sitting Test (FIST) may be applicable.[116] The FIST is an assessment tool that can be used to assess static and dynamic sitting balance tasks providing information about deficits allowing for targeted interventions.[116]

The FIST is relatively quick, requiring about 10 minutes to complete. However, if there is difficulty with command following, the Modified Functional Reach Test could also be used.[117]

If impairments with functional mobility are observed during assessment, a clinical decision should be made on whether assessing functional performance status is safe and feasible. If deemed appropriate, then completing the SPPB and TUG would be the first steps. If the person is able to complete these tests safely then further assessing CRF/functional capacity and balance can be completed.

Further, assessing functional performance status can be interwoven into evaluating functional mobility safely to maximize time, as the person may be experiencing pain, fatigue, or debility limiting their capacity to participate. A possible examination sequence would be to first evaluate the person's ability to stand; if person is able to stand safely, next the 5× sit to stand could be assessed. During a rest period after the 5× sit to stand, the person's RPE and vitals could be assessed. After this rest, the TUG can then be assessed while evaluating gait over the short distance. After the TUG, another rest period can occur while assessing RPE and vitals. If deemed safe, more advanced testing of functional capacity and balance can occur.

Short Physical Performance Battery[103]

Balance

The three balance tests used are close (feet together), semi-tandem, and tandem stance in progressive sequence. Each stance is held for a maximum of 10 seconds, though if a person is unable to maintain one of the stances then the balance assessment is over. For each balance test only one trial is administered, and the person can place either foot in front of the other during semi-tandem and tandem stance.

Gait Speed[103,118]

Gait speed is measured over 3 or 4 m (~10 feet and ~13 feet). Two trials are measured and both trials are at the person's usual gait speed. The fastest trial recorded is the time used for scoring this domain. To determine the person's gait speed (meters/second), the distance used divided by the person's score will provide gait speed (meters/second) which is not included in the SPPB. Usual and fast gait speed can also be captured individually if not utilizing SPPB.

5x Sit to Stand[119]

The 5× sit to stand can be performed independently or as a component of the SPPB. Preferably the 5× sit to stand is completed from a chair but can be completed from the edge of the bed. The first trial with the sit to stand should be attempted without the use of upper extremities. If the person is unable to complete without use of their arms, use of upper extremities is allowable but this modification must be noted (If the 5× sit to stand is scored as a component of the SPPB, the use of hands results in a 0 score). If the person's knees are above their hips, the Onc R clinician can adjust bed or chair to have the knees and hips at the same level. If the person is unable to complete the 5× sit to stand, use of the 30 seconds sit to stand is appropriate but is not applicable within the SPPB.[120]

Timed Up and Go (TUG)[104]

The TUG is valuable in assessing functional mobility quickly over a short distance as it incorporates a sit-to-stand transfer, gait speed, and the ability to complete multiple turns. A Dual Task

TUG can also be completed to assess cognition with mobility via cognitive or other psychomotor tasks (e.g., counting backwards by 3s from 100 or carrying a cup of water). If a person requires more than two minutes to complete the TUG trials, additional formal assessment of functional capacity may not be clinically impactful as their 2MST results may not differ significantly. Following the completion of the SPPB and TUG, if time is still available, assessing functional capacity would be the next assessment.

2- or 6-Minute Walk Test or 2-Minute Step Test[108–111]

For all of the following tests, vital signs should be taken before and after testing. When assessing functional capacity, the attempt to assess 6MWT is preferred, though if limited on time, the 2MWT is appropriate. During the 6MWT, it is advised to mark the 2MWT distance in the event that the patient is unable to ambulate for 6 minutes.

In the situation where neither the 2MWT nor 6MWT are able to be completed safely either due to impaired balance, poor gait mechanics, or safety (no wheelchair or help available to follow behind with a chair for seated rests) then completing the 2MST may be an appropriate clinical modification. In this test, the person will march standing in place for 2 minutes and the clinician will count the number of times the right knee reaches the goal height (midway between the patella and iliac crest). In this test, the person is able to use upper extremity support and a chair or bed can be behind the person. Many PLWBCs may not be able continuously march for 2 minutes therefore the time when the person requested to rest along with repetitions completed should be recorded similar to the 2MWT or 6MWT. Following the completion of either the 2MWT, 6MWT, or 2MST, more advanced balance assessments may be administered such as assessment on unstable surfaces, external perturbations, or with eyes closed.

Formal Balance Assessments

The Fullerton Advanced Balance scale (FAB scale), Berg Balance Scale (BBS), or Modified Clinical Test of Sensory Interaction in Balance (mCTSIB) can be used to assesses varying domains of balance (base of support, sensory, vestibular, visual, and static/dynamic).[102] These assessment tools require some equipment (foam pad, step, object to pick up, etc.) which may limit the ability to utilize them in the acute care setting. The FAB scale may also require higher level balance capacity due to the nature of some of the tasks (hopping, tandem walk, reactive postural control); this may result in reluctance to administer this assessment. However, the Onc R clinician may choose to adapt or exclude certain portions (e.g., hopping) to assure safety. The BBS is appropriate to utilize and assesses a variety of balance domains including static, dynamic, anticipatory, and with varying base of supports. The mCTSIB is a static balance assessment that utilizes a foam pad where impairments in sensory, vestibular, or visual integration can be assessed.

Other optional assessment tools that could be utilized depending on factors such as functional mobility level, resources, space, or fatigue are the single leg balance test, functional reach, and timed arm curl test.[117,121,122]

Assessing Functional Performance Status in the Home Care Setting

In the home care setting, there are often numerous confounding variables and constraints to time, space, and equipment. Due to these variables, assessing the person's functional performance status may not be as extensive, though it is still crucial in developing

an exercise program that improves the person's ability to be safe within the home, complete ADLs/IADLs and hopefully, return to community ambulation. Vitals should be recorded prior to the initiation of assessing functional mobility and functional performance status.[99]

If there are impairments with functional mobility, addressing these impairments first is important to promote independence and safety with ADLs/IADLs and activity participation. The FIST can be utilized to assess sitting postural control static and dynamically if the person demonstrates difficulty in unsupported sitting.[116] If the person does have impairments with functional mobility but the clinician deems it safe to assess functional performance status, the next step would be to assess the person via the SPPB and TUG. If the person can complete these assessment tools, then progressing to assess CRF, functional capacity, and balance would be warranted.

If there are no significant or limiting functional mobility impairments, then the SPPB and TUG are recommended to be completed first as these tools require little time and space to complete. Following the completion of both assessment tools, the next step would be to complete the 2MST. The 2MWT and 6MWT were not selected for the home care algorithm due to potential space limitations, however they should be completed if space permits. Finally, if time and resources are available, the FAB, BBS, or mCTSIB can be used to assess balance.

Points to Remember About the Various Setting Algorithms

These algorithms are created to help guide the Onc R clinician in assessing a person's functional performance status in a variety of settings, however a clinical situation may require elimination, supplementation, or replacement of some assessments based on clinical judgment. Not every section of the algorithm (balance, strength, functional capacity) must be completed during the initial assessment and instead can be completed as warranted during follow up sessions. The majority of assessment tools throughout these algorithms were chosen as they are at least "recommended for clinical use" by APTA Oncology Section EDGE Taskforce.[100–102] There are some exceptions which includes the FIST, 2MST, Mini-BESTest (though the BESTest is recommended), timed arm curl test, 12-Minute Walk Test, UNCCRI Treadmill Test, Steep Ramp Test, and 1-Rep Max Testing. By completing these assessment tools, baseline data is gathered allowing for appropriate exercise can be prescribed and improvement can be tracked through an exercise program.

Exercise Prescription

E/PA can play a vital role in the prevention of cancer or adverse events, improving QOL through addressing impairments in physical function, and maintaining QOL even at the end-of-life. The ACSM recommends that adults engage in aerobic exercise for at least 150 minutes of moderate intensity, 75 minutes of vigorous intensity, or a mix of the two intensities each week.[3] This should be supplemented by resistance training at least twice a week.[9,112] Flexibility/mobility and balance exercises should also be included within the exercise program as able.[3,123]

It is estimated that only approximately 33% of PLWBCs are meeting the recommended exercise guidelines.[4] As with other clinical tasks, developing individualized exercise programs that meet the recommended parameters is a skill that can be learned.

In some cases, barriers to providing exercise prescriptions may lie within the Onc R provider themselves.[124] In one survey, 60% of Onc R clinicians correctly identified the E/PA guidelines for adults while 37% correctly identified the E/PA guidelines for older adults.[124] Further, the majority of clinicians acknowledged their job included prescribing aerobic (75%) and resistance training (89%).[124] However, only 38% to 50% were confident in prescribing aerobic exercises and 49% to 70% were confident in prescribing resistance training.[124] This lack of confidence may be due to a lack of education or training in designing an E/PA program which at times can seem daunting. The following section aims to provide a useful and clinically applicable approach to utilizing the data collected and designing an E/PA program for PLWBCs in any setting. As described above, evaluating functional performance status is a necessary first step in order to establish baseline measures to facilitate the development of a precise individualized E/PA program.[100,125,126] Additionally, as depicted in Figure 23.3, the PLWBC's goals, treatment status, physical function, comorbidities, and adverse effects of treatment must be considered when developing the E/PA program.

First, the pillars that hold structure to an exercise program involve frequency, intensity, type, time (FITT).[3] Figure 23.9 provides an overview of FITT for aerobic, resistance, flexibility, and balance training. An individualized exercise prescription for a PLWBC should meet the minimum requirements of: (1) engaging in aerobic exercise 3 to 5 times per week for a total of 150 minutes of moderate-intensity or 75 minutes of vigorous-intensity; (2) resistance training for 2 to 3 times per week on nonconsecutive

Aerobic Training[9,80,115]

- Frequency: 3–5x per week
- Intensity:
  - 40%–90% of VO2max or HRR
  - METs: Moderate – 3 to 6 METs (walking 3.0 mph, stationary bicycling at 100 watts with light effort, light effort calisthenics)
  - Vigorous - >6 METs (jogging, jumping rope, heavy effort calisthenics)
  - RPE 11–16/20 or 5–8/10.
- Type: Continuous, rhythmic movement involving large muscle groups, though can involve rounds of moderate to vigorous intensity with recovery–rest periods of light intensity (walking, jogging, stationary bike, recumbent bike, NuStep, Rower, etc.)
- Volume: A minimum of 30 minutes 3 times per week but should try to complete 150 minutes of moderate intensity, 75 minutes or vigorous, or a mix of both.
- Time/Duration: Can be as little as 10 minutes up to 60 minutes depending on the person's physical function, fatigue, etc.

Resistance Training[3,9,115,118,142]

- Frequency: 2–3x per week on non-consecutive days
- Volume: 1–2 sets of 8–15 repetitions have been demonstrated in literature with the oncology and geriatric populations to promote positive physiological adaptations while.
  - Power: 3–5 sets of 1–5 repetitions
  - Strength: 2–6 sets of ≤ 6 repetitions
  - Hypertrophy: 3–6 sets of 6–12 repetitions
  - Endurance: 2–3 sets of ≥ 12 repetitions
- Intensity: Dependent upon the set and repetition scheme being utilized. The minimal load to induce positive physiologic adaptations is roughly 60% of the 1RM, though with severely unconditioned persons starting at 40% is appropriate. RPE can also be used where a 3/10 would equate to 55%–60% of maximal effort where the person may be able to complete 12–15 repetitions prior to fatigue.
- Rest: May vary between 30 seconds up to 4 minutes between sets
- Type: Large, multi-joint movements should be complete prior to single joint movements. Can utilize free weights, machines, bodyweight, isometrics, or resistance bands.
- Volume: The combination of sets and repetitions. Volume will vary based on the intensity of the exercises being performed.

Flexibility Training[3]

- Frequency: 2–3x per week
- With stretching should avoid ballistic or bouncing movement
- 2–3 repetitions with holds of 30–45 seconds with a total time spent of 10 minutes.

Balance Training[143]

- Frequency: 2–3x per week has been shown to be beneficial in literature
- Intensity: Using the RPS for intensity; moderate 4–6/10, high 7–9/10, and all-out effort 10/10.
- Time: 20–45 minutes has shown to be beneficial, but evidence is still limited.

• **Fig. 23.9** FITT principles of exercise programming. (Created by Andrew Chongaway, PT, DPT. Printed with permission.)

days for major muscle groups for 1 to 2 sets of 8 to 15 reps; and (3) flexibility and balance exercise should be included at least 2 to 3 times per week (increased frequency may be warranted depending on the focus of the exercise program).[3,9] Some PLWBCs may find it difficult to meet these guidelines, especially for frequency and time. In 2019, a roundtable by the ACSM specifically evaluating exercise for PLWBCs established a minimum dose of aerobic training 3 times per week for 30 minutes and resistance training at least 2× per week.[9] In the event that the recommended frequency and time cannot be met, the PLWBC is encouraged to remain as active as possible. Furthermore, ACSM recommends that adults with chronic conditions should engage in regular PA to their abilities and should avoid inactivity even if that means walking for 5 to 10 minutes a day.[3,112]

There are numerous ways to measure intensity of an E/PA program whether it be aerobic or resistance. More of the common methods to measure intensity with aerobic exercises is with using a percentage of VO_{2max} or VO_{2peak}, heart rate reserve (HRR), RPE, or MET.[3,112,113] For resistance exercises, a percentage of 1-RM or RPE can be used to prescribe intensity.[127,128] With balance exercises the use of rate of perceived stability (RPS) can be utilized to ensure appropriate intensity.[129]

There is a wide range of E/PA intensities that have been shown to yield positive physiologic benefits in the literature for both aerobic and resistance training. For aerobic training, the intensity may be as low as 40% of VO_{2max} or HRR.[3,112] However, VO_{2max} or even VO_{2peak} in most situations are not easily assessable and HRR may not be suitable to use depending on factors such as medications and altered physiologic variables like hemoglobin and hematocrit.[130] With resistance training, at least 60% of a 1-RM has resulted in positive physiologic adaptations to skeletal muscle (increased strength, quality, hypertrophy),[3,128] though as low as 30% to 40% of a repetition maximum has shown positive benefits in strength gains in severely deconditioned persons.[131,132]

The use of VO_{2max}, VO_{2peak}, HRR, and percentage of a 1-RM may not be applicable across the various settings depending on resources such as space and equipment. For these reasons, RPE may be more useful in monitoring the intensity of aerobic training and is also quite useful in monitoring resistance training.[3,9,133] Often RPE for aerobic training is prescribed between 11 to 16/20 and 5 to 8/10 depending on the scale used. With resistance training a range of 11 to 17/20 or 3 to 7/10 can be used.[3,112]

Appropriate intensity depends on several other variables such as: the goal of the specific E/PA and E/PA program, number of sets and repetitions per set, rest given between each set, and how the program for the session is set up (e.g., whether it focuses only on the lower extremities, encompasses the whole body, or is designed to be completed as a circuit or as intervals).[3,113,134] Additionally, the person's physiologic and psychologic status needs to be considered to meet the PLWBC's abilities on a daily basis.[135]

The FITT principle can be extended to include volume and progression (FITT-VP).[3,113,128] Volume for aerobic exercise should attempt to meet a minimum of 30 minutes of moderate-intensity E/PA for 3 times per week with the aim to build to 150 minutes of moderate-intensity, 75 vigorous-intensity, or a mix of both. Resistance training should aim to complete 1 to 2 sets of 8 to 15 repetitions for major muscles of the body.[3,9] It should be noted that it has been demonstrated in literature that more E/PA generally yields greater physiologic benefits.[136,137] In addition to appropriate volume, the exercises within the program should progress to continue to promote positive physiologic adaptations and challenge the person.[3,113] This allows the person to become comfortable with

the movement patterns, improve neuromuscular control, and progress with volume and/or intensity[3,13] (see Figure 23.10).

In many cases, these FITT-VP variables are under-prescribed and undervalued in E/PA programs.[115,138] Often, the intensity of aerobic and resistance training is prescribed arbitrarily, and the person is provided generic exercises for minimal repetitions or provided no guidance.[138] In some cases, the resistance or volume is not adjusted to the patient's new physical capacity. Finally, in some cases, resistance training is not prescribed at all.[115,138] Due to these factors, there may not be an appropriate stimulus (tension, cellular damage, energy shift) to promote signaling to induce positive adaptations.[13,115,130,136,139] Therefore, when developing an E/PA program, the intensity and volume must be prescribed appropriately to promote positive physiological adaptations while allowing the person to engage in E/PA frequently and consistently.[13,130,132,139]

Along with the E/PA program meeting the appropriate FITT-VP, the exercises need to address the PLWBC's main concern and address the deficits noted from assessing strength, balance, cardiorespiratory fitness, and/or functional capacity.

Throughout their cancer journey, each PLWBC may not participate in Onc R for the majority of the week (≥4x/week) which results in barriers to implementing a multimodal training program that incorporates everything needed to optimize the person's physical function. For this reason, prioritizing E/PAs within an Onc R session and developing a home exercise program (HEP) is important. If the person is able to walk daily but does not have access to resistance/strength equipment, then focusing on resistance training during Onc R sessions would be ideal to promote a well-rounded multimodal training plan.[140] When developing an E/PA program, there are numerous ways to integrate aerobic, resistance, and balance activities while embracing a whole-body training program. Some styles that can be used across all settings include complete body workouts or upper body, lower body splits, or focusing solely on specific muscles (e.g., back/parascapular muscles), lower extremities (e.g., glutes, quadriceps, hamstrings), while incorporating aerobic and balance exercises on varying days. Within these routines various set structures can be used like traditional sets, super sets, cluster sets, and even high-speed resistance training (HSRT).[3,133,141–144] Further, depending on the person's functional performance status, goals, and preferences, HIIT can be utilized.[145]

It is important to remember that when performing resistance/loading exercises, proper form should be established first to prevent compensatory movements/recruitment which may result in an injury. Once the person is able to perform the exercise with proper form, resistance/loading can be increased based off a percentage of 1-RM or RPE and the person should be monitored for compensatory movements/recruitment and breakdown in form to reduce the chance of injury.

Complete Body Workout

A complete body workout lends itself well into a multimodal approach as there are numerous ways to incorporate aerobic, resistance, and balance exercises into each session or week. Within each session, a circuit style of aerobic, resistance, and balance exercises can be used.[3] If a more directed focus is warranted, each session could focus on either resistance, aerobic, or balance exercises. A focused session approach can reduce the chance of overtraining, allow for proper recovery, and maximize supervised sessions for safety, monitoring of vitals, and appropriate progression

Borg RPE Scale	Modified Borg RPE Scale	Perceived Effort	Relative Percentage of Effort (%)
6		No Exertion	20
7			30
8		Extremely Light Effort	40
9	1		45
10	2		50
11		Light Effort	55
12	3		60
13			65
14	4		70
15	5	Moderate Effort	75
16	6		80
17	7		85
18	8	Vigorous Effort	90
19	9		95
20	10	Maximum Effort	100

• **Fig. 23.10** 6–20 and 1–10 Rate of perceived exertion scale with perceived effort. (Created by Andrew Chongaway. PT, DPT. Printed with permission.)

of exercises.[136,138] In the scenario where a person may only participate in Onc R for 2–3x per week, a HEP could focus on aerobic training or resistance training depending on the person's confidence and resources while each supervised session could focus on a complete body resistance program with incorporation of balance exercises.[140]

Upper/Lower Body Splits

This style allows for a more precise focus on specific muscles and can allow for the incorporation of multi-joint and single-joint exercises. This style can blend itself well into the traditional rehabilitation plan of care where there may be specific weakness(es) or dysfunctions within the upper and/or lower body musculature/joints.[141,146] Using a targeted split, time can be spent restoring neuromuscular control, strength, and endurance to restore appropriate function.[141,146] Within the Upper/Lower Body Split, exercises can be paired into a push/pull style to maximize time and reduce the chance of early onset fatigue within the session. The movements are completed back-to-back with minimal rest between movements with a longer rest period following the completion of the second movement. Just as with circuit training, the use of bodyweight exercises, resistance bands, free weights, weight machines, or even isometrics can be utilized to provide the appropriate intensity and volume.[113]

Set and Repetition Structure

Exercises are traditionally completed in a manner where the repetitions within each set are completed in their entirety prior to resting for a predetermined interval.[143] Once this rest interval is over another set of the same movement is completed and so on until the desired number of sets is completed. An example would be complete 3 sets of 10 repetitions of sit to stands with 1 minute of rest between sets then moving to the next exercise in the session. In this style, as the number of sets and repetitions are greater (high-volume), the resistance is often lower (low-load) and vice versa as the volume is less the resistance is greater (low-volume/high-load).[143,147] These exercises are also usually completed with an equal tempo (ex. 3 seconds for concentric and eccentric phases) for the concentric and eccentric phase to promote control and ensure form.[143] While this method has demonstrated how to promote strength and hypertrophy gains, it may not always be the most efficacious depending on the presentation of the person.[143,148]

Other options that could be beneficial depending on the clinical scenario include the superset style, cluster sets, and/or high-speed resistance training (HSRT). With "supersetting," exercises are paired together.[113] The exercises will be paired together and of opposite movements (push/pull) or will be a primary movement followed by an accessory movement with rest following the completion of the second exercise. This may be beneficial as it could reduce the onset of muscular fatigue within the session as there is the extended rest period between each set. However, due to the short transitional rest between the two exercises this may increase perceived effort resulting in a greater psychological or mental fatigue. A possible solution to this is to allow a longer transitional rest between movements to focus on recovery. If able, balance exercises can be incorporated into the transitional rest period. An example of this could be completing upper extremity rows, then 60 seconds of tandem stance, followed by chest press with a 60 to 180 second rest after.

Cluster sets are a bit different as rest is given within the set. The rest interval can be between 2 to 4 repetitions (intra-set rest), between each repetition (inter-rep rest), or after the person reaches a failure point within the set (rest pause).[142,143] In the scenario where intra-set rest is used, the person may complete 4 repetitions, rest 30 seconds, complete 4 repetitions, rest 30 seconds, and then complete 4 more repetitions before resting for 90 to 180 seconds (inter-set rest).[143] With inter-rep rest style, a rest interval is given between each repetition and can range from 3 seconds to upwards of 45 seconds if necessary.[143] The person would then complete the required repetitions within the set before taking the inter-set rest interval. Rest pause is utilized as an intra-set rest interval when the person reaches a point of failure.[143] The person would then rest a predetermined amount of time whether it be 15 seconds or 60 seconds then continue with the set till another failure point is met or the set is completed. The use of cluster sets can employ the principles of HSRT in which the concentric phase is completed as fast as possible with a controlled eccentric phase.[144] This style has the capacity to maximize motor unit recruitment of Type II (fast twitch) fibers leading to an increase in force development and muscular power.[134] Further, cluster sets can maximize volume as the additional rest given within each set possibly reduces the development of muscular fatigue.[143,144] Additionally, the increased rest given can reduce cardiopulmonary demands leading to diminished perceived effort and anxiety further increasing adherence, comfort, and self-efficacy with exercise.[148] As demonstrated, the utilization of cluster sets may be beneficially employed in exercise programming for PLWBC. This is due to the fact that a substantial portion of PLWBCs have poor muscular strength and power, experience adverse effects of cancer and treatments, or have other comorbidities affecting the cardiopulmonary or nervous systems which can result in a lower tolerance to the traditional exercise sets.[9,125,126,136]

High Intensity Interval Training

This style uses work intervals of high intensity broken up with either active or passive recovery periods at a lower intensity. The benefit of HIIT is that it maximizes the time with the person and has demonstrated similar or greater improvements in physical function compared to other various exercise routines.[145,149] Interval style training is extremely adaptable to the person and the setting. Exercises may be prescribed in supine, sitting, or standing and may employ the use of resistance bands, weights, or machines or may simply use the person's own bodyweight. Depending on the person's perceived effort of the E/PA (which may change daily or weekly depending on physiologic and psychologic variables), alterations to the duration of work and recovery intervals may be instituted.[145] Functional training such as bed mobility, transfers, and stairs may also be completed utilizing a HIIT approach. Work-to-recovery interval ratios can range from 1:10 to as little as 1:1.[145] Commonly, the intervals will be shorter with passive recovery as compared to an active recovery period, however this is

variable depending on the person's functional status, intensity, and volume of the prescribed exercises.[3,137] Again, even within HIIT, HSRT training can be employed to promote the development of muscular power.

Eccentric/Isometric Exercise Training

Cancer cachexia can severely affect a PLWBC's well-being and QOL.[22,29] PLWBCs that have been diagnosed with cachexia are already at a point where there is a significant imbalance in metabolic function in that muscle wasting and energy depletion are rapidly occurring resulting in reduced physical function.[25,150] These persons can still benefit from individualized exercise programs to maintain or optimize physical function, thereby allowing the person to optimize QOL and participate in their desired hobbies/tasks.[22] In the setting of reduced metabolic reserve, eccentric/isometric-focused exercise(s) may be efficacious to promote strength and hypertrophy gains as both are less metabolically demanding as compared to traditional concentric movements.[151–154] Further, it has been demonstrated that eccentric exercises/movements produce greater gains compared to concentric exercises/movements.[153] In the presence of cachexia, close coordination with the patient's physician or oncology nutritionist is imperative to avoid exacerbating a potential nutritional deficiency further by expending more calories than are taken in.

Even if the person is not cachectic, incorporating eccentric/isometric-focused exercises may be beneficial to the person in the presence of fatigue or pain.[151] More research is needed in this area of exercise oncology to continue to assess the efficacy and overall benefits of eccentric and isometric exercises. Care should be taken though with the use of strenuous eccentric/isometric exercises in the setting of low platelet counts due to a chance for increased muscle cell damage due to strain and potential for increased intra-abdominal pressure.

Home Exercise Program (HEP)

Aside from developing an individualized exercise program, a HEP should be developed to promote exercise outside of formal Onc R sessions. This will facilitate empowerment, self-efficacy, and independence with exercise.[155–157] The HEP exercises can reinforce key aspects completed during an Onc R session or focus on other aspects (aerobic, balance, flexibility) based on the person's resources, time, and confidence.[155] One example of HEP complimenting an Onc R session is the HEP including a regular walking program and previously-taught stretches, which allows for more time for clinician-provided manual therapy and/or strengthening during the Onc R session. Although most research studies evaluated E/PA programs that are completed in the standing position, the development of HEP for sitting and supine positions may be a valuable adaptation. This is especially relevant in the acute care setting as the majority of the day is spent in these positions and the person may spend only a fraction of the day standing or ambulating.[138] This situation may also occur within the home setting in the presence of fatigue, pain, and poor sleep. By providing a HEP for all situations, adherence to daily physical activity may be maintained which will provide positive impact to the person's physical function and QOL.

Exercise and the Person With Advanced Cancer

A person living with advanced cancer may be suffering from significant functional mobility impairments secondary to pain, fatigue, weakness, or other debilitating symptoms which negatively impacts their QOL.[158,159] There may be concern for these persons to be engaging in E/PA in fear of an injury or an adverse event during exercise.[159] However, these people can benefit from an individualized exercise prescription to optimize physical function and QOL.[159] It has been established that E/PA can be safe for persons with advanced cancer and can be beneficial in reducing symptom burden such as fatigue, anxiety, depression, and dyspnea.[159] Care does need to be taken with a person with advanced stage disease; thus it is recommended to review A Focused Review of Safety Considerations in Cancer Rehabilitation,[160] Exercise Preserves Physical Function in Prostate Cancer Patients with Bone Metastases,[161] and Spinal Stabilization Exercises for Cancer Patients with Spinal Metastases of High Fracture Risk: Feasibility of the DISPO-II Training Program.[162] These articles provide a solid foundation to apply safe exercise especially in relation to bone metastases. In these situations, care needs to be taken to closely monitor for tolerance to the exercise prescription and frequent assessments or refinements are recommended to ensure safety. Further, the aim of the exercise prescription may not be to improve strength or VO_2 but to enable the person to be able to maintain independence with ADLs/IADLs or partake in hobbies/family roles as they choose. A HEP should still be prescribed and encouraged to optimize/maintain physical performance as able, though this may be limited due to contextual factors such as nutrition. Caregiver training can be easily incorporated into an Onc R session so the caregiver can assist with the HEP as well as being able to assist the person in completing mobility safely through body mechanics and education on safe movement patterns.

Conclusion

Exercise can improve physical function for PLWBCs by promoting the maintenance/increase of VO_2, strength, and balance while reducing the impact of comorbidities (e.g., metabolic syndrome, heart failure, chronic obstructive pulmonary disorder, muscle atrophy) and adverse effects of cancer treatment (e.g., weakness, muscle atrophy, CIPN, lymphedema).[4–6,9–11] As PLWBCs continue through the care continuum, the goals of exercise and level of supervision necessary may change depending on the cancer diagnosis, adverse effects, physical function, competing comorbidities, motivation, and barriers/facilitators.[80–83,85,86,163] This is why routine screenings of physical function and performance status via standardized assessment tools in any setting is vital in order to assess the person's ability to complete ADLs/IADLs and participate in hobbies and activity.[74,97,126] Based on the person's functional status and outcomes of these assessment tools, a referral to an appropriate Onc R clinician can be made. Factors impacting E/PA performance include impairments, severity of adverse effects, and progression of disease and comorbidities. These factors need to be addressed to optimize the person's physical function and QOL.[89,90] Each person's E/PA program should be individualized and address their individual goals and main concerns while being enjoyable and providing the appropriate stimulus.[4,9,130] At a minimum, each person should be participating in E/PA 5 times per week and should attempt to engage in aerobic exercise 3×/week for 30 minutes and resistance training 2x/week focusing on major muscles of the body.[9]

Education on the importance of E/PA is critical and development of a HEP and resources for each person is important to encourage independence and promote self-efficacy in continuing to meet the minimum dosage and push to achieve the goal of 150 minutes of moderate or 75 minutes of vigorous exercise per week.[3,9] As the number of PLWBC continue to increase, so will the specialty fields of Onc R and exercise oncology evolve and grow. For this reason, Onc R clinicians educated in exercise prescription and implementation are critical to help prevent cancer, improve cancer treatment outcomes, and optimize QOL. This will help to further establish the benefits of exercise prior to, during, and after cancer treatments to build evidence for exercise and rehabilitation to support these persons along their journey.

Critical Research Needs

- Utilization of the exercise prescription algorithm including piloting and assessing feasibility, validity/reliability
- Effectiveness and safety of exercise with bone metastases (QOL, performance status, cardiorespiratory fitness, pain)
- Short-course exercise effectiveness of prehabilitation as well as sustained changes during treatment and 1-year post. This would include assessing variables such as inflammatory markers, length of stay, QOL, pain, adverse events, failure to thrive, and readmissions.
- Early initiation (immediately post-op) of endurance exercises for head and neck and breast cancer to improve pain, fatigue, and physical activity (steps per day). Possibly including a wearable activity monitor, in-person, or via group classes. Outcomes might include impact on healing, QOL, increased circulation, without adversely affecting surgical intervention.
- Telerehabilitation for exercise. Examples include a variety of populations for outcomes including functional capacity, strength, and balance, safely with no adverse events. Variables may include a single face-to-face session and then telerehab, or weekly phone calls, in-person monthly recheck as compared to a control group.
- Utility of HIIT in acute care setting. Outcomes include performance status, functional status, length of stay, adverse events, and safety

Case Studies

Case Study 1: Acute Care

Patient A is a 72-year-old male who was admitted to the hospital due to fever, dyspnea, generalized weakness, and fatigue that he reports started about 2 weeks prior. He was previously diagnosed with Stage IIB non-small cell lung cancer 4 years ago and underwent lobectomy with adjuvant chemotherapy (cisplatin [Platinol] and pemetrexed [Alimta] for 4 cycles). His past medical history also includes: hypertension, coronary artery disease, and stage III chronic kidney disease. His vitals at rest are BP = 124/60 mmHg, HR = 79 beats per minute, SpO_2 = 96% on room air, and respiratory rate = 14 breaths per minute. With functional mobility, he can get out of bed with modified independence using the bed rail. He can stand with minimal assist, which is mainly impacted due to balance impairment; when he stands he loses his balance posteriorly requiring assistance to maintain balance. When transferring from the bed to the bedside commode, he demonstrates poor eccentric control when sitting. When walking he is impulsive, often forgetting he still is attached to an IV. He refuses to use an assistive device and prefers to push the IV pole. He has difficulty with managing the IV pole and turning and often hits his foot on the base of the IV pole when navigating around objects in the halls. His gait does improve when he does not have to manage the IV pole with no significant deviations observed. His functional performance assessment demonstrated a SPPB score of 6/12 with 12 being the best possible score (close stance [feet together]: 10 seconds, semi-tandem stance: 10 seconds, tandem stance: 3 seconds, gait speed: 0.56 m/s, 5× Sit to Stand: 32 seconds). His vitals after the 5× sit to stand were HR = 94 bpm; SpO_2 = 97%; RPE = 7/10. He then completes two trials of the TUG with scores of 25 and 23 seconds. Lastly, he scores 36/56 on the BBS. Based on his performance status assessment, he is appropriate for an exercise program utilizing an interval-style routine focusing on lower extremity strength and balance. When he reports worse fatigue at the start of the session, passive recovery can be used instead of active recovery. An example of a session is shown below where static and dynamic balance activities were used as the rest period followed by passive recovery of 2 to 3 minutes following the completion of each interval superset.

- 5 rounds of 5 sit-to-stands with a 5-second eccentric phase into 1 minute of close stance (feet together) with eyes closed.
- 4 rounds of 10 mini lunges without support into 2 laps of marching (20 feet).
- 3 rounds of 10 single leg heel raises with support into 4 laps of tandem walking (20 feet).
- 2 rounds of 15 bridges into 2 minutes of close stance with moderate/maximum external perturbations.

Case 2: Outpatient

Patient B is a 56-year-old male diagnosed with metastatic colon cancer 1 year prior. He underwent a right hemicolectomy and received adjuvant FOLFOXIRI (folinic acid, 5-fluorouracil, oxaliplatin, and irinotecan) plus bevacizumab. He was referred to outpatient rehabilitation due to chemotherapy-induced polpheral neuropathy (CIPN) affecting his balance and gait. His main objective is to be able to return safely back to work as a sales associate at a local hardware store. His other past medical history is significant for hypertension, Type 2 diabetes, and he recently sprained his left ankle while working in his yard two weeks ago. His vitals taken at rest are BP = 136/82 mmHg, HR = 71 beats per minute, SpO_2 = 99%, and respiratory rate of 14 breaths per minute. His assessment for functional performance demonstrated a usual gait speed of 1.02 m/s (fast gait speed was not assessed.) He completed the 5× Sit to Stand in 21 seconds with use of his hands on knees with limited hip-hinge, early knee extension, and delayed hip extension. His weight was shifted posteriorly toward his heels during four of the sit-to-stands repetitions with a slight loss of postural

control though he was able to maintain balance independently. He also demonstrated poor eccentric control (e.g., uncontrolled descent into chair) which worsened by the fifth repetition. He rated his effort during the 5× sit to stand a 4/10. Next, he completed the FAB scale and scored a 23/40. He scored poorly on items 1, 6, 7, and 10. He chose not to attempt item 8. The 6MWT was the last assessment tool completed. He ambulated 248 meters during the 6 minutes and took two standing rest breaks for ~20 seconds each time due to shortness of breath. Discussion during the initial evaluation revealed that he was motivated to increase his E/PA and started walking daily for at least 30 minutes (multiple intervals or in one interval) and was open to moving the focus of his Onc R sessions to improving his balance and strength. The initial HEP consisted of toe yoga, foot towel scrunches, close stance with eyes closed, tandem stance with eyes open, and single leg balance. For both the toe yoga and towel scrunches, a time frame of spending 2 to 3 minutes on each daily was given. For the other three exercises he was asked to accumulate up to 2 minutes of each in as many repetitions as needed. Each session followed a more traditional split session where the beginning focused on balance and transitioned into resistance training. Through the sessions his 8-rep max on the leg press was assessed with a max weight of 160 lbs. Prior to exercises, he performed a 5- to 7-minute aerobic warm-up with the NuStep recumbent exercise stepper focusing on maintaining a low MET level range for the entirety of the time. The following depicts a sample session with flexibility, balance, and strengthening exercises following several sessions.

Flexibility:
- Static stretching of the calves, quadriceps, hamstrings, and hips

Balance:
- Tandem stance while throwing/catching a 5 lbs. medicine ball from varying angles: 4 sets for 1 minute.
- Static stagger stance on foam resisting against moderate external perturbations: 3 sets for 2 minutes.
- On command tapping appropriate colored disc w/ single leg while standing on foam pad: 4 sets for 2 minutes.
- Standing in tandem stance on foam plank with eyes closed: 3 sets for 1 minute.

Resistance Training:
- Leg Press: 4 sets of 6 repetitions at 205 lbs. with a focus on a powerful concentric phase and 3-second tempo eccentric phase
- Reverse Lunges with weight in opposite hand: 4 sets of 10 repetitions for each leg with 20 lb dumbbell
- Standing hip abduction with 3-second tempo eccentric phase: 3 sets of 12 each leg repetitions with moderate resistance band
- Full squat with 45 lbs. weighted crate: 5 sets of 5 repetitions

Review Questions

Reader can find the correct answers and rationale in the back of the book

1. Muscle hypertrophy and increased muscle mass occurs when:
   A. Stimulus increases sarcomeres in a perpendicular fashion
   B. There is muscle protein synthesis activated by resistance training
   C. A mechanical stretch across the skeletal muscle inhibits insulin-like growth factor 1
   D. Through the inhibition of phosphatidic acid during resistance exercise

2. The loss of skeletal muscle mass along with loss of adipose tissue due to an elevated resting metabolic rate is classified as:
   A. Primary sarcopenia
   B. Secondary sarcopenia
   C. Cachexia
   D. Frailty

3. A patient is diagnosed with breast cancer. Surgery consisting of a right mastectomy is completed and radiation will begin in 2 weeks. She has limited motion to the right glenohumeral joint. Exercises that are prescribed to increase shoulder flexion and abduction before radiation to the breast area is a form of:

A. Primordial prevention
B. Primary prevention
C. Secondary prevention
D. Tertiary prevention

4. The outpatient clinic decided to run a fundraiser to raise money to help extend the paving of an old railroad track for walkers, runners, and bikers in the community. Community healthy lifestyle behaviors are a form of:
A. Primordial prevention
B. Primary prevention
C. Secondary prevention
D. Tertiary prevention

5. A prostate cancer survivor is 2 months post robotic prostatectomy and has just completed pelvic radiation. He has some radiation induced fibrosis. The most appropriate initial functional capacity test in the outpatient clinic setting would be:
A. 2MWT
B. 2MST
C. 6MWT
D. TUG

6. The best measure of intensity for balance is:
A. Repetition maximum
B. Repetitions in reserve
C. Rate of perceived exertion
D. Rate of perceived stability

7. Which patient diagnosed and treated for breast cancer and who is receiving Onc R for the first time would be the most appropriate to prescribe an HIIT program to?
A. 75-year-old female Stage 4 with metastases to the bone in palliative care
B. 60-year-old female Stage IIB post mastectomy with reports of cardiotoxicity
C. 52-year-old female with Stage IIIA, post mastectomy and radiation with CRF
D. 35-year-old female with Stage 2 B post chemotherapy reporting severe CIPN

8. Every person diagnosed with cancer needs to make sure that each aspect of their functional performance status is assessed and treated as needed. This includes all of the following EXCEPT?
A. Cardiovascular fitness
B. Strength
C. Ambulation
D. Balance

9. 50-year-old female diagnosed with melanoma on her upper back. She has completed surgical removal of the cancer including axillary lymph node removal (8 on left and 10 on right). She presents 2 years post surgery with bilateral lymphedema. She has had MLD, wears compression sleeves bilaterally 24 hours/day. She complains of fatigue, insomnia. Her body mass index (BMI) is 30. She has no other comorbidities. She has had rehab in two different places with upper extremity exercise and manual lymphatic drainage with no change in status. Her goals are to decrease weight and which workout program would be the most appropriate.
A. HIIT
B. Upper/lower body split
C. Complete Body Program
D. Yoga

10. A 60-year-old woman with ovarian cancer is 1 year post surgery and chemotherapy. She reports that she hasn't been able to ride her horses since her surgery and her goal is to return to that lifestyle. She still has some minor abdominal discomfort with palpation but is able to walk around the yard and feed her dogs and horses. She feels too weak to ride the horses as yet, has difficulty sleeping, but is happy her hair has grown back. Which workout program would be the most appropriate?
A. HIIT
B. Upper/lower body split
C. Complete Body Workout
D. Yoga

References

1. Centers for Disease Control and Prevention. Trends in meeting physical activity guidelines, 2008–2018. https://www.cdc.gov/physicalactivity/downloads/trends-in-the-prevalence-of-physical-activity-508.pdf. Accessed May 22, 2021.
2. Centers for Disease Control and Prevention. CDC behavioral risk factor surveillance survey. http://www.cdc.gov/brfss/. Accessed May 22, 2021.
3. American College of Sports Medicine. *ACSM's Resources for the Exercise Physiologist.* 2nd ed.: Lippincott Williams and Wilkins; 2017.
4. Suderman K, McIntyre C, Sellar C, McNeely ML. Implementing cancer exercise rehabilitation: an update on recommendations for clinical practice. *Curr Cancer Ther Rev.* 2019;15(2):100–109.
5. Blanchard CM, Courneya KS, Stein K. American Cancer Society's SCS-II. Cancer survivors' adherence to lifestyle behavior recommendations and associations with health-related quality of life: results from the American Cancer Society's SCS-II. *J Clin Oncol.* 2008;26(13):2198–2204.
6. Webb J, Foster J, Poulter E. Increasing the frequency of physical activity very brief advice for cancer patients: development of an intervention using the behaviour change wheel. *Public Health.* 2016;133:45–56.
7. Patel AV, Friedenreich CM, Moore SC, et al. American College of Sports Medicine Roundtable report on physical activity, sedentary behavior, and cancer prevention and control. *Med Sci Sports Exerc.* 2019;51(11):2391–2402.
8. Bland KA, Zadravec K, Landry T, Weller S, Meyers L, Campbell KL. Impact of exercise on chemotherapy completion rate: a systematic review of the evidence and recommendations for future exercise oncology research. *Crit Rev Oncol Hematol.* 2019;136:79–85.
9. Campbell KL, Winters-Stone KM, Wiskemann J, et al. Exercise guidelines for cancer survivors: consensus statement from International Multidisciplinary Roundtable. *Med Sci Sports Exerc.* 2019;51(11):2375–2390.
10. Gerritsen JKW, Vincent AJPE. Exercise improves quality of life in patients with cancer: a systematic review and meta-analysis of randomised controlled trials. *Br J Sports Med.* 2016;50(13):796–803.

11. Edwards BK, Noone A-M, Mariotto AB, et al. Annual Report to the Nation on the status of cancer, 1975–2010, featuring prevalence of comorbidity and impact on survival among persons with lung, colorectal, breast, or prostate cancer. *Cancer.* 2014;120(9):1290–1314.

12. Wackerhage H. *Molecular Exercise Physiology: An Introduction*: Routledge; 2014.

13. Powers SK, Howley ET. *Exercise Physiology: Theory and Application to Fitness and Performance*. 10th ed.: McGraw-Hill Education; 2017.

14. Assi M, Dufresne S, Rébillard A. Exercise shapes redox signaling in cancer. *Redox Biol.* 2020;35(101439):101439.

15. Drake JC, Wilson RJ, Yan Z. Molecular mechanisms for mitochondrial adaptation to exercise training in skeletal muscle. *FASEB J.* 2016;30(1):13–22.

16. Cantó C, Auwerx J. PGC-1alpha, SIRT1 and AMPK, an energy sensing network that controls energy expenditure. *Curr Opin Lipidol.* 2009;20(2):98–105.

17. Hojman P, Gehl J, Christensen JF, Pedersen BK. Molecular mechanisms linking exercise to cancer prevention and treatment. *Cell Metab.* 2018;27(1):10–21.

18. Fruman DA, Chiu H, Hopkins BD, Bagrodia S, Cantley LC, Abraham RT. The PI3K pathway in human disease. *Cell.* 2017;170(4):605–635.

19. Stitt TN, Drujan D, Clarke BA, et al. The IGF-1/PI3K/Akt pathway prevents expression of muscle atrophy-induced ubiquitin ligases by inhibiting FOXO transcription factors. *Mol Cell.* 2004;14(3):395–403.

20. Wilkinson DJ, Piasecki M, Atherton PJ. The age-related loss of skeletal muscle mass and function: measurement and physiology of muscle fibre atrophy and muscle fibre loss in humans. *Ageing Res Rev.* 2018;47:123–132.

21. Wall BT, Dirks ML, van Loon LJC. Skeletal muscle atrophy during short-term disuse: implications for age-related sarcopenia. *Ageing Res Rev.* 2013;12(4):898–906.

22. Bauer J, Morley JE, Schols AMWJ, et al. Sarcopenia: a time for action. An SCWD position paper. *J Cachexia Sarcopenia Muscle.* 2019;10(5):956–961.

23. D'Ascenzi F, Anselmi F, Fiorentini C, Mannucci R, Bonifazi M, Mondillo S. The benefits of exercise in cancer patients and the criteria for exercise prescription in cardio-oncology. *Eur J Prev Cardiol.* 2019:2047487319874900.

24. Thomas RJ, Kenfield SA, Jimenez A. Exercise-induced biochemical changes and their potential influence on cancer: a scientific review. *Br J Sports Med.* 2017;51(8):640–644.

25. Cole CL, Kleckner IR, Jatoi A, Schwarz EM, Dunne RF. The role of systemic inflammation in cancer-associated muscle wasting and rationale for exercise as a therapeutic intervention. *JCSM Clin Rep.* 2018;3(2):1–19. doi:10.17987/jcsm-cr.v3i2.65.

26. Koelwyn GJ, Quail DF, Zhang X, White RM, Jones LW. Exercise-dependent regulation of the tumour microenvironment. *Nat Rev Cancer.* 2017;17(10):620–632.

27. Malavaki CJ, Sakkas GK, Mitrou GI, et al. Skeletal muscle atrophy: disease-induced mechanisms may mask disuse atrophy. *J Muscle Res Cell Motil.* 2015;36(6):405–421.

28. Calvani R, Joseph A-M, Adhihetty PJ, et al. Mitochondrial pathways in sarcopenia of aging and disuse muscle atrophy. *Biol Chem.* 2013;394(3):393–414.

29. Ali S, Garcia JM. Sarcopenia, cachexia and aging: diagnosis, mechanisms and therapeutic options—a mini-review. *Gerontology.* 2014;60(4):294–305.

30. COSA. Exercise prescription for all cancer patients. https://www.cosa.org.au/media/332487/media-release-exercise-prescription-for-all-cancer-patients-final.pdf. Accessed May 22, 2021.

31. Physical Activity and Cancer. National Cancer Institute. National institute of health. https://www.cancer.gov/about-cancer/causes-prevention/risk/obesity/physical-activity-fact-sheet. February 10, 2020. Accessed December 20, 2020.

32. Campbell KL, Winters-Stone KM, Patel AV, et al. An executive summary of reports from an International Multidisciplinary Roundtable on Exercise and Cancer: evidence, guidelines, and implementation. *Rehabil Oncol.* 2019;37(4):144–152.

33. Patel AV, Friedenreich CM, Moore SC, et al. American College of Sports Medicine Roundtable Report on physical activity, sedentary behavior, and cancer prevention and control. *Med Sci Sports Exerc.* 2019;51(11):2391–2402.

34. Schmitz KH, Campbell AM, Stuiver MM, et al. Exercise is medicine in oncology: engaging clinicians to help patients move through cancer. *CA Cancer J Clin.* 2019;69(6):468–484.

35. American Cancer Society. Physical activity and cancer. https://www.cancer.gov/about-cancer/causes-prevention/risk/obesity/physical-activity-fact-sheet.NCI. Accessed April 1, 2021.

36. Physical Activity and the Risk of Cancer. American institute for cancer research. https://www.aicr.org/wp-content/uploads/2020/01/Physical-activity.pdf. Accessed May 25, 2021.

37. Exercise Helps Cancer Patients and Survivors, New research reviews. American institute for cancer research. https://www.aicr.org/news/exercise-helps-cancer-patients-and-survivors-new-research-reviews/. Accessed May 25, 2021.

38. Review: Howe Exercise Leads to Anti-Cancer Effects. American institute for cancer research. https://www.aicr.org/news/review-how-exercise-leads-to-anti-cancer-effects/. Accessed May 25, 2021.

39. Kimmel GT, Haas BK, Hermanns M. The role of exercise in cancer treatment bridging the gap. *Current Sports Med Rep.* 2014;13(4):246–252.

40. Exercise During Cancer Treatment. Cancer.net. https://www.cancer.net/survivorship/healthy-living/exercise-during-cancer-treatment#:~:text=Benefits%20of%20exercise&text=Lower%20the%20chance%20of%20having,balance%20to%20reduce%20fall%20injuries. April 2019. Accessed May 25, 2021.

41. White MC, Peipins LA, Watson M, Trivers KF, Holman DM, Rodriguez JL. Cancer prevention for the next generation. *J Adolesc Health.* 2013;52(50):S1–S7.

42. Centers for Disease Control and Prevention. *Status Report for Step It Up! The Surgeon General's Call to Action to Promote Walking and Walkable Communities*: Centers for disease control and prevention, US dept of health and human services; 2017. https://www.cdc.gov/physicalactivity/walking/call-to-action/pdf/status-report.pdf. Accessed April 1, 2021.

43. Global Action Plan on Physical Activity 2018–2030. World Health Organization. https://www.who.int/ncds/prevention/physical-activity/global-action-plan-2018-2030/. Accessed December 20, 2020.

44. Physical Activity and Cancer. Centers for disease control. https://www.cdc.gov/physicalactivity/basics/pa-health/physical-activity-and-cancer.html. Updated December 15, 2020. Accessed December 20, 2020.

45. Schmid D, Leitzman MF. Television viewing and time spent sedentary in relation to cancer risk: a meta-analysis. *J Natl Cancer Inst.* 2014;106(7):dju098. doi:10.1093/jnci/dju098.

46. Moore SC, Lee IM, Weiderpass E, et al. Association of leisure-time physical activity with risk of 26 types of cancer in 1.44 million adults. *JAMA.* 2016;176(6):816–825.

47. Singh F, Newton RU, Galvão DA, Spry N, Baker MK. A systematic review of pre-surgical exercise intervention studies with cancer patients. *Surg Oncol.* 2013;22(2):92–104.

48. Treanor C, Kyaw T, Donnelly M. An international review & meta-analysis of pre-habilitation compared to usual care for cancer patients. *Cancer Surviv.* 2018;12:64–73.

49. van Waart H, Stuiver MM, van Harten WH, et al. Effect of low-intensity physical activity and moderate- to high-intensity physical exercise during adjuvant chemotherapy on physical fitness, fatigue, and chemotherapy completion rates: results of the PACES randomized clinical trial. *J Clin Oncol.* 2015;33(17):1918–1927.

50. Milecki P, Hojan K, Ozga-Majchrzak O, Molińska-Glura M. Exercise tolerance in breast cancer patients during radiotherapy after aerobic training. *Contemp Oncol (Pozn).* 2013;17(2):205–209.

51. Brayall P, Donlon E, Doyle L, Leiby R, Violette K. Physical therapy-based interventions improve balance, function, symptoms, and quality of life in patients with chemotherapy-induced peripheral neuropathy: a systematic review. *Rehabil Oncol.* 2018;36(3):161–166.

52. Duregon F, Vendramin B, Bullo V, et al. Effects of exercise on cancer patients suffering chemotherapy-induced peripheral neuropathy undergoing treatment: a systematic review. *Crit Rev Oncl Hematol.* 2018;21:90–100.

53. Kanzawa-Lee GA, Larson JL, Resnicow K, Smithe EML. Exercise effects on chemotherapy-induced peripheral neuropathy. *Cancer Nurs.* 2020;43(3):E172–E185.

54. Thomas SA. Chemotherapy agents that cause cardiotoxicity. *US Pharm.* 2017;42(9):HS24–HS33.

55. Kirkham AA, Eves ND, Shave RE, et al. The effect of an aerobic exercise bout 24 h prior to each doxorubicin treatment for breast cancer on markers of cardiotoxicity and treatment symptoms: a RCT. *Breast Cancer Res Treat.* 2018;167:719–729.

56. Palomo A, Ray RM, Johnson L, et al. Associations between exercise prior to and around the time of cancer diagnosis and subsequent cardiovascular events in women with breast cancer: a Women's Health Initiative (WHI) analysis. *J Am Coll Cardiol.* 2017;69(suppl):1774. doi:10.1016/S0735-1097(17)35163-X.

57. Campbell KL, Zadravec K, Bland KA, Chesley E, Wold F, Janelsins MC. The effect of exercise on cancer-related cognitive impairment and applications for physical therapy: systematic review of randomized controlled trials. *Phys Ther.* 2020;100(3):524–542.

58. Myers JS, Erickson KI, Sereika SM, Bender CM. Exercise as an intervention to mitigate decreased cognitive function from cancer and cancer treatment. *Cancer Nurs.* 2018;41(4):327–343.

59. Zimmer P, Baumann FT, Oberste M, et al. Effects of exercise interventions and physical activity behavior on cancer related cognitive impairments: a systematic review. *Biomed Res Int.* 2016;2016:1820954. doi:10.1155/2016/1820954.

60. Hilfiker R, Meictry A, Balfe LN, Knowls RH, Verra ML, Taeymans J. Exercise and other non-pharmaceutical interventions for cancer-related fatigue in patients during or after cancer treatment: a systematic review incorporating an indirect-comparisons meta-analysis. *Br J Sports Med.* 2018;52(10):651–658.

61. Meneses-Echávez JF, González-Jiménez E, Ramírez-Vélez R. Effects of supervised exercise on cancer-related fatigue in breast cancer survivors: a systematic review and meta-analysis. *BMC Cancer.* 2015;15:77. doi:10.1186/s12885-015-1069-4.

62. Mustian KM, Alfano CM, Heckler C, et al. Comparison of pharmaceutical, psychological, and exercise treatments for cancer-related fatigue: a meta-analysis. *JAMA Oncol.* 2017;3(7):961–968.

63. Van Vulpen JK, Peeters PHM, Velthuis MJ, van der Wall E, May AM. Effects of physical exercise during adjuvant breast cancer treatment on physical and psychosocial dimensions of cancer-related fatigue: a meta-analysis. *Maturitas.* 2016;85:104–111.

64. Hasenoehrl T, Palma S, Ramazanova D, et al. Resistance exercise and breast cancer-related lymphedema: a systematic review update and meta-analysis. *Support Care Cancer.* 2020;28(8):3593–3603.

65. Bauman FT, Reike A, Reimer V, et al. Effects of physical exercise on breast cancer-related secondary lymphedema: a systematic review. *Breast Cancer Res Treat.* 2018;170(1):1–13.

66. Sener HO, Malkoc M, Ergin G, Karadibak D, Yavuzsen T. Effects of clinical Pilates exercises on patients developing lymphedema after breast cancer treatment: a randomized clinical trial. *J Breast Health.* 2017;13:16–22.

67. Moller AB, Lanbro S, Farup J, et al. Molecular and cellular adaptations to exercise training in skeletal muscle from cancer patients treat with chemotherapy. *J Cancer Res Clin Oncol.* 2019;145:1449–1460.

68. Winters-Stone KM, Dobek JC, Bennett JA, et al. Resistance training reduces disability in prostate cancer survivors on androgen deprivation therapy: evidence from a randomized controlled trial. *Arch Phys Med Rehabil.* 2015;96(1):7–14.

69. Sangagnello SB, Martins FM, de Oliveira Junior GN, et al. Improvements in muscle strength, power, and size and self-reported fatigue as mediators of the effect of resistance exercise on physical performance breast cancer survivor women; a randomized controlled trial. *Support Care Cancer.* 2020;28:6075–6084.

70. Reis AD, Pererira PTVT, Diniz RR, et al. Effect of exercise on pain and functional capacity in breast cancer patients. *Health Qual Life Outcomes.* 2018;16:58. https://doi.org/10.1186/s12955-018-0882-2.

71. Lu G, Zheng J, Zhang L. The effect of exercise on aromatase inhibitor-induced musculoskeletal symptoms in breast cancer survivors: a systematic review and meta-analysis. *Support Care Cancer.* 2020;28:1587–1596.

72. Forsythe LP, Alfano CM, George SM, et al. Pain in long-term breast cancer survivors: the role of body mass index, physical activity, and sedentary behavior. *Breast Cancer Res Treat.* 2013;137(2):617–630.

73. Martins C, Godycki-Cwirko M, Heleno B, Brodersen J. Quaternary prevention: reviewing the concept. *Eur J Gen Pract.* 2018;24(1):106–111.

74. McNeely M, Dolgoy N. Principles of physical and occupation therapy in cancer. In: Stubblefield MD, ed. *Cancer Rehabilitation: Principles and Practice.* 2nd ed. Springer Publishing; 2018.

75. Fowler H, Belot A, Ellis L, et al. Comorbidity prevalence among cancer patients: a population-based cohort study of four cancers. *BMC Cancer.* 2020;20(1):2.

76. Campbell K, Kirkham A. During infusion therapy. In: Schmitz KH, ed. *Exercise Oncology: Prescribing Physical Activity before and after a Cancer Diagnosis.* Springer International Publishing; 2020.

77. Brown JM, Shackelford DYK, Hipp ML, Hayward R. Evaluation of an exercise-based phase program as part of a standard care model in cancer survivors. *Trans J Am Coll Sports Med.* 2019;4:45–54.

78. Wiskemann J. During radiation therapy. In: Schmitz KH, ed. *Exercise Oncology: Prescribing Physical Activity before and after a Cancer Diagnosis.* Springer International Publishing; 2020.

79. Gilchrist LS, Galantino ML, Wampler M, Marchese VG, Morris GS, Ness KK. A framework for assessment in oncology rehabilitation. *Phys Ther.* 2009;89(3):286–306. doi:10.2522/ptj.20070309.

80. Weller S, Oliffe JL, Campbell KL. Factors associated with exercise preferences, barriers and facilitators of prostate cancer survivors. *Eur J Cancer Care (Engl).* 2019;28(5):e13135.

81. Courneya KS, McKenzie DC, Reid RD, et al. Barriers to supervised exercise training in arandomized controlled trial of breast cancer patients receiving chemotherapy. *Ann Behav Med.* 2008;35:116–122.

82. Eng L, Pringle D, Su J, et al. Patterns, perceptions, and perceived barriers to physical activity in adult cancer survivors. *Support Care Cancer.* 2018;26(11):3755–3763.

83. Blaney J, Lowe-Strong A, Rankin J, Campbell A, Allen J, Gracey J. The cancer rehabilitation journey: barriers to and facilitators of exercise among patients with cancer-related fatigue. *Phys Ther.* 2010;90(8):1135–1147.

84. Pudkasam S, Polman R, Pitcher M, et al. Physical activity and breast cancer survivors: importance of adherence, motivational interviewing and psychological health. *Maturitas.* 2018;116:66–72. doi:10.1016/j.maturitas.2018.07.010.

85. Ashton LM, Hutchesson MJ, Rollo ME, et al. Motivators and barriers to engaging in healthy eating and physical activity. *Am J Mens Health.* 2017;11(2):330–343.

86. Joseph RP, Ainsworth BE, Keller C, et al. Barriers to physical activity among African American women: an integrative review of the literature. *Women Health.* 2015;55(6):679–699.

87. Rock CL, Doyle C, Demark-Wahnefried W, et al. Nutrition and physical activity guidelines for cancer survivors. *CA Cancer J Clin.* 2012;62(4):243–274.

88. Barber FD. Effects of social support on physical activity, self-efficacy, and quality of life in adult cancer survivors and their caregivers. *Oncol Nurs Forum.* 2013;40(5):481–489.

89. Brown JC, Winters-Stone K, Lee A, Schmitz KH. Cancer, physical activity, and exercise. *Compr Physiol*. 2012;2(4):2775–2809.

90. Stout NL, Brown JC, Schwartz AL, et al. An exercise oncology clinical pathway: screening and referral for personalized interventions: screening and referral for exercise. *Cancer*. 2020;126(12):2750–2758.

91. Stout NL, Binkley JM, Schmitz KH, et al. A prospective surveillance model for rehabilitation for women with breast cancer. *Cancer*. 2012;118(suppl 8):2191–2200. doi:10.1002/cncr.27476.

92. Harrington SE, Stout NL, Hile E, et al. Cancer rehabilitation publications (2008–2018) with a focus on physical function: a scoping review. *Phys Ther*. 2020;100(3):363–415.

93. Painter P, Stewart AL, Carey S. Physical functioning: definitions, measurement, and expectations. *Adv Ren Replace Ther*. 1999;6:110–123.

94. L'Hotta AJ, Varughese TE, Lyons KD, Simon L, King AA. Assessments used to measure participation in life activities in individuals with cancer: a scoping review. *Support Care Cancer*. 2020;28(8):3581–3592.

95. O'Toole DM, Golden AM. Evaluating cancer patients for rehabilitation potential. *West J Med*. 1991;155:384–387.

96. Azam F, Latif MF, Farooq A, et al. Performance status assessment by using ECOG (Eastern Cooperative Oncology Group) score for cancer patients by oncology healthcare professionals. *Case Rep Oncol*. 2019;12(3):728–736. doi:10.1159/000503095.

97. Scott JM, Stene G, Edvardsen E, Jones LW. Performance status in cancer: not broken, but time for an upgrade? *J Clin Oncol*. 2020;38(25):2824–2829.

98. Vision Statement for the Physical Therapy Profession. Apta.org. https://www.apta.org/apta-and-you/leadership-and-governance/policies/vision-statement-for-the-physical-therapy-profession; September 25, 2019. Accessed September 27, 2020.

99. O'Sullivan SB, Schmitz TJ, Fulk GD. *Physical Rehabilitation*. 6th ed. F.A. Davis Company; 2013.

100. Fisher M, Lee J, Davies C, Geyer H, Colon G, Pfalzer L. Oncology section EDGE task force on breast cancer outcomes: a systematic review of outcome measures for functional mobility. *Rehabil Oncol*. 2015;33(3):19–31.

101. Davies C, Colon G, Geyer H, Pfalzer L, Fisher M. Oncology EDGE task force on prostate cancer outcomes: a systematic review of outcome measures for functional mobility. *Rehabil Oncol*. 2016;34(3):82–96.

102. Huang MH, Hile E, Croarkin E, et al. Academy of oncologic physical therapy EDGE task force: a systematic review of measures of balance in adult cancer survivors. *Rehabil Oncol*. 2019;37(3):92–103.

103. Short Physical Performance Battery. Sralab.org. https://www.sralab.org/rehabilitation-measures/short-physical-perfromance-battery. Accessed September 27, 2020.

104. Timed Up and Go. Sralab.org. https://www.sralab.org/rehabilitation-measures/timed-and-go. Accessed September 27, 2020.

105. De Backer IC, Schep G, Hoogeveen A, Vreugdenhil G, Kester AD, van Breda E. Exercise testing and training in a cancer rehabilitation program: the advantage of the steep ramp test. *Arch Phys Med Rehabil*. 2007;88(5):610–616.

106. Stuiver MM, Kampshoff CS, Persoon S, et al. Validation and refinement of prediction models to estimate exercise capacity in cancer survivors using the steep ramp test. *Arch Phys Med Rehabil*. 2017;98(11):2167–2173.

107. Kee Shackelford DY, Brown JM, Peterson BM, Schaffer J, Hayward R. The University of Northern Colorado Cancer Rehabilitation Institute Treadmill Protocol accurately measures VO$_2$peak in cancer survivors. *Int J Phys Med Rehabil*. 2017;5:437. doi:10.4172/2329-9096.1000437.

108. 2 Minute Walk Test. Sralab.org. https://www.sralab.org/rehabilitation-measures/2-minute-walk-test. Accessed September 27, 2020.

109. 6 Minute Walk Test. Sralab.org. https://www.sralab.org/rehabilitation-measures/6-minute-walk-test. Accessed September 27, 2020.

110. Bohannon RW. Normative reference values for the two-minute walk test derived by meta-analysis. *J Phys Ther Sci*. 2017;29(12):2224–2227. doi:10.1589/jpts.29.2224.

111. Bohannon RW, Crouch RH. Two-minute step test of exercise capacity: systematic review of procedures, performance, and clinimetric properties. *J Geriatr Phys Ther*. 2019;42(2):105–112.

112. Irwin ML. *ACSM's Guide to Exercise and Cancer Survivorship*: Human Kinetics; 2012.

113. Haff G, Travis Triplett N. National Strength & Conditioning Association. *Essentials of Strength Training and Conditioning*. 4th ed. Human Kinetics; 2016.

114. Abdul-Hameed U, Rangra P, Shareef MY, Hussain ME. Reliability of 1-repetition maximum estimation for upper and lower body muscular strength measurement in untrained middle aged type 2 diabetic patients. *Asian J Sports Med*. 2012;3(4):267–273. doi:10.5812/asjsm.34549.

115. Avers D, Brown M. White paper: strength training for the older adult. *J Geriatr Phys Ther*. 2009;32(4):148–152, 158.

116. Gorman S. *Function in Sitting Test (FIST)*: Samuel Merritt University; 2017. https://www.samuelmerritt.edu/fist. Accessed 20 September 2020.

117. Functional Reach Test/Modified Functional Reach Test. Sralab.org. https://www.sralab.org/rehabilitation-measures/functional-reach-test-modified-functional-reach-test. Accessed September 27, 2020.

118. Middleton A, Fritz SL, Lusardi M. Walking speed: the functional vital sign. *J Aging Phys Act*. 2015;23(2):314–322. doi:10.1123/japa.2013-0236.

119. Five Times Sit to Stand Test. Sralab.org. https://www.sralab.org/rehabilitation-measures/five-times-sit-stand-test. Accessed September 27, 2020.

120. 30 Second Sit to Stand Test. Sralab.org. https://www.sralab.org/rehabilitation-measures/30-second-sit-stand-test. Accessed September 27, 2020.

121. Single Leg Stance or "One-Legged Stance Test". Sralab.org. https://www.sralab.org/rehabilitation-measures/single-leg-stance-or-one-legged-stance-test. Accessed September 27, 2020.

122. Jones CJ, Rikli RE. Measuring functional fitness of older adults. *J Active Aging*. 2002;2:24–30.

123. ACSMIrwin ML. *ACSM's Guide to Exercise and Cancer Survivorship*: Human Kinetics; 2012.

124. Barton CJ, King MG, Dascombe B, et al. Many physiotherapists lack preparedness to prescribe physical activity and exercise to people with musculoskeletal pain: a multi-national survey. *Phys Ther Sport*. 2021;49:98–105.

125. Crandell CE, Quinn SE, Wingard CJ, et al. A physical assessment tool to evaluate functional status compared to ECOG scores in cancer outpatients. *J Clin Oncol*. 2018;36(30_suppl):135–135.

126. Pergolotti M, Sattar S. Measuring functional status of older adults with cancer with patient and performance-based measures, a how-to guide: a young society of geriatric oncology and nursing and allied health initiative. *J Geriatr Oncol*. 2021;12(3):473–478. doi:10.1016/j.jgo.2020.09.025.

127. Helms ER, Cronin J, Storey A, Zourdos MC. Application of the repetitions in reserve-based rating of perceived exertion scale for resistance training. *Strength Cond J*. 2016;38(4):42–49. doi:10.1519/SSC.0000000000000218.

128. Schoenfeld BJ, Ratamess NA, Peterson MD, Contreras B, Sonmez GT, Alvar BA. Effects of different volume-equated resistance training loading strategies on muscular adaptations in well-trained men. *J Strength Cond Res*. 2014;28(10):2909–2918.

129. Espy D, Reinthal A, Meisel S. Intensity of balance task intensity, as measured by the rate of perceived stability, is independent of

physical exertion as measured by heart rate. *J Nov Physiother.* 2017;7(S4). doi:10.4172/2165-7025.1000343.

130. Kirkham AA, Bland KA, Zucker DS, et al. Chemotherapy-periodized" exercise to accommodate for cyclical variation in fatigue. *Med Sci Sports Exerc.* 2020;52(2):278–286.

131. Mayer F, Scharhag-Rosenberger F, Carlsohn A, Cassel M, Müller S, Scharhag J. The intensity and effects of strength training in the elderly. *Dtsch Arztebl Int.* 2011;108(21):359–364.

132. Silva NL, Oliveira RB, Fleck SJ, Leon ACMP, Farinatti P. Influence of strength training variables on strength gains in adults over 55 years-old: a meta-analysis of dose-response relationships. *J Sci Med Sport.* 2014;17(3):337–344.

133. Helms ER, Byrnes RK, Cooke DM, et al. RPE vs. Percentage 1RM loading in periodized programs matched for sets and repetitions. *Front Physiol.* 2018;9:247.

134. Galloza J, Castillo B, Micheo W. Benefits of exercise in the older population. *Phys Med Rehabil Clin N Am.* 2017;28(4):659–669.

135. Lopez P, Pinto RS, Radaelli R, et al. Benefits of resistance training in physically frail elderly: a systematic review. *Aging Clin Exp Res.* 2018;30(8):889–899.

136. Losa-Reyna J, Baltasar-Fernandez I, Alcazar J, et al. Effect of a short multicomponent exercise intervention focused on muscle power in frail and pre frail elderly: a pilot trial. *Exp Gerontol.* 2019;115: 114–121.

137. Falvey JR, Mangione KK, Stevens-Lapsley JE. Rethinking hospital-associated deconditioning: proposed paradigm shift. *Phys Ther.* 2015;95(9):1307–1315. doi:10.2522/ptj.20140511.

138. Tufano JJ, Brown LE, Haff GG. Theoretical and practical aspects of different cluster set structures: a systematic review. *J Strength Cond Res.* 2017;31(3):848–867.

139. Kirkham AA, Bonsignore A, Bland KA, et al. Exercise prescription and adherence for breast cancer: one size does not FITT all. *Med Sci Sports Exerc.* 2018;50:177–186.

140. De Backer IC, Schep G, Backx FJ, Vreugdenhil G, Juipers H. Resistance training in cancer survivors: a systematic review. *Int J Sports Med.* 2009;30(10):703–712.

141. Lesinski M, Hortobágyi T, Muehlbauer T, Gollhofer A, Granacher U. Effects of balance training on balance performance in healthy older adults: a systematic review and meta-analysis. *Sports Med.* 2015;45(12):1721–1738.

142. Thomas MH, Burns SP. Increasing lean mass and strength: a comparison of high frequency strength training to lower frequency strength training. *Int J Exerc Sci.* 2016;9(2):159–167.

143. Latella C, Peddle-McIntyre C, Marcotte L, Steele J, Kendall K, Fairman CM. Strengthening the case for cluster set resistance training in aged and clinical settings: emerging evidence, proposed benefits and suggestions. *Sports Med.* 2021. doi:10.1007/s40279-021-01455-4.

144. Sayers SP, Gibson K. High-speed power training in older adults: a shift of the external resistance at which peak power is produced. *J Strength Cond Res.* 2014;28(3):616–621.

145. Mugele H, Freitag N, Wilhelmi J, et al. High-intensity interval training in the therapy and aftercare of cancer patients: a systematic review with meta-analysis. *J Cancer Surviv.* 2019;13(2):205–223.

146. Hurst C, Weston KL, Weston M. The effect of 12 weeks of combined upper- and lower-body high-intensity interval training on muscular and cardiorespiratory fitness in older adults. *Aging Clin Exp Res.* 2019;31(5):661–671. doi:10.1007/s40520-018-1015-9.

147. Fairman CM, Hyde PN, Focht BC. Resistance training interventions across the cancer continuum: a systematic review of the implementation of resistance training principles. *Br J Sports Med.* 2017;51(8):677–685.

148. Fairman CM, Nilsen TS, Newton RU, et al. Reporting of resistance training dose, adherence, and tolerance in exercise oncology. *Med Sci Sports Exerc.* 2019;52(2):315–322.

149. Gomes-Neto M, Durães AR, Reis HFCD, Neves VR, Martinez BP, Carvalho VO. High-intensity interval training versus moderate-intensity continuous training on exercise capacity and quality of life in patients with coronary artery disease: a systematic review and meta-analysis. *Eur J Prev Cardiol.* 2017;24(16):1696–1707.

150. Belloum Y, Rannou-Bekono F, Favier FB. Cancer-induced cardiac cachexia: pathogenesis and impact of physical activity (Review). *Oncol Rep.* 2017;37(5):2543–2552.

151. Lastayo PC, Larsen S, Smith S, Dibble L, Marcus R. The feasibility and efficacy of eccentric exercise with older cancer survivors: a preliminary study. *J Geriatr Phys Ther.* 2010;33(3):135–140.

152. LaStayo P, Marcus R, Dibble L, Frajacomo F, Lindstedt S. Eccentric exercise in rehabilitation: safety, feasibility, and application. *J Appl Physiol.* 2014;116(11):1426–1434.

153. Lum D, Barbosa TM. Brief review: effects of isometric strength training on strength and dynamic performance. *Int J Sports Med.* 2019;40(6):363–375.

154. Hedayatpour N, Falla D. Physiological and neural adaptations to eccentric exercise: mechanisms and considerations for training. *Biomed Res Int.* 2015;2015:193741.

155. Yang M, Liu L, Gan CE, et al. Effects of home-based exercise on exercise capacity, symptoms, and quality of life in patients with lung cancer: a meta-analysis. *Eur J Oncol Nurs.* 2020;49:101836. doi:10.1016/j.ejon.2020.101836.

156. Pinto BM, Rabin C, Dunsiger S. Home-based exercise among cancer survivors: adherence and its predictors: home-based exercise adherence. *Psychooncology.* 2009;18(4):369–376.

157. Lee DH, Kim JY, Lee MK, et al. Effects of a 12-week home-based exercise program on the level of physical activity, insulin, and cytokines in colorectal cancer survivors: a pilot study. *Support Care Cancer.* 2013;21(9):2537–2545.

158. Dittus KL, Gramling RE, Ades PA. Exercise interventions for individuals with advanced cancer: a systematic review. *Prev Med.* 2017;104:124–132.

159. Heywood R, McCarthy AL, Skinner TL. Safety and feasibility of exercise interventions in patients with advanced cancer: a systematic review. *Support Care Cancer.* 2017;25(10):3031–3050.

160. Maltser S, Cristian A, Silver JK, Morris GS, Stout NL. A focused review of safety considerations in cancer rehabilitation. *PM R.* 2017;9(9S2):S415–S428.

161. Galvão DA, Taaffe DR, Spry N, et al. Exercise preserves physical function in prostate cancer patients with bone metastases. *Med Sci Sports Exerc.* 2018;50(3):393–399.

162. Rosenberger F, Sprave T, Clauss D, et al. Spinal stabilization exercises for cancer patients with spinal metastases of high fracture risk: feasibility of the DISPO-II training program. *Cancers (Basel).* 2021;13(2):201.

163. Edgington A, Morgan MA. Looking beyond recurrence: comorbidities in cancer survivors. *Clin J Oncol Nurs.* 2011;15(1):E3–E12.

24

Acute Care and Inpatient Management

COURTNEY WITCZAK, PT, DPT, GCS, GRACE BURNS, PT, DPT, AND
CYNTHIA BARBE, PT, DPT, MS

CHAPTER OUTLINE

Introduction

Oncology rehabilitation (Onc R) in the inpatient setting requires the professional to possess a unique skillset in order to navigate the diverse and complex issues inherent to the setting. Although not every Onc R clinician will practice in inpatient or acute settings, it is imperative to understand the challenges and experiences that patients and clients encounter during an inpatient stay in order to support them physically and emotionally. While some persons with cancer (PWCs) may experience a planned admission for chemotherapy, others present with an emergency because of various treatments- or disease-related sequalae. Still others receive a new cancer diagnosis after presenting to the hospital with unexplained symptoms. If the hospitalization is prolonged and significant functional impairments result, the client may be discharged to a postacute rehabilitation setting (e.g., subacute rehab facility [SAR], inpatient rehabilitation [IPR], long term acute care hospital [LTACH]) prior to returning home. All Onc R clinicians will benefit from understanding the patient's unique journey through hospitalization as new complications require modifications to established treatment plans as well as holistic, patient-centered approaches to multisystem involvement.

The Varied Inpatient Journey

Approximately 4.2% of emergency visits were made by persons with a cancer diagnosis, with the most common cancers including breast, prostate, and lung cancer.[1] While many strategies are in place to reduce emergency department (ED) utilization by oncology teams, there are still several reasons that a PWC would find themselves there.[1] Symptoms commonly reported include nausea, vomiting, dehydration, pain, fever, cough, and shortness of breath. The most common diagnoses included pneumonia, nonspecific chest pain, and urinary tract infections.[2] Over half of these cases resulted in admissions, where noncancer-related ED presentations held around a 16% admission rate.[2]

A hospital admission from the ED frequently results in transfer to a general oncology medical floor if a person has a known cancer diagnosis. With or without a known cancer diagnosis, patients may find themselves transferred to a general medical floor, intensive care unit (ICU), or surgical floor depending on the admitting diagnosis, its severity, and the urgency of medical interventions required.

During a planned hospitalization, specific cancer treatments will be delivered to a PWC after being directly admitted to the oncology medical floor. Most commonly, planned admissions center around high-dose chemotherapy, invasive chemotherapy, or surgery. As it relates to chemotherapy, an expected decline in blood levels or infection risk may necessitate an acute care stay to closely monitor and manage the pancytopenia.

Patients who experience life-threatening complications related to cancer or its treatments are most likely to be transferred to the ICU. These complications include severe infections, decompensation of comorbidities, or postoperative care after major surgery.[3] A study found 17.9% of ICU admissions were PWCs.[3]

A well-planned cancer treatment regimen may be disrupted due to the hospitalization, which may result in delays to chemotherapy, surgery, or radiation. In addition, many individuals are at risk for a decline in functional status from a hospitalization, often from prolonged immobilization, as a result of the admitting medical condition, or via an acquired comorbidity. If a patient's functional status does not allow the patient to safely return home, he or she may be discharged to an IPR unit, SAR, or extended care facility (ECF). Less often, a stable but acutely ill PWC may be transferred to a long term acute care hospitals LTACHs. These settings are discussed more thoroughly in the discharge disposition section of this chapter.

Patients can also be admitted to the oncology acute care setting for other reasons. Those coming in from the ED may present with symptoms requiring a workup of lab tests and diagnostics in order to move towards treatment. For instance, a patient may present with a seizure, and workup may suggest a brain tumor etiology. This would lead to a neurology and oncology consult to determine a cancer treatment plan. Another patient may present with bruising, fatigue, and shortness of breath. Their workup may suggest hematologic involvement, thus requiring an oncology consult to determine the type and extent of hematologic involvement and to establish a requisite plan of care.

Depending on the type of cancer and plan of care, patients can be categorized as medical oncology or surgical oncology patients. Patients with hematologic cancers are those diagnosed with leukemias, lymphomas, and multiple myeloma, and most often, they are categorized as medical oncology patients requiring systemic therapies. These patients primarily receive treatments such as chemotherapy, bone marrow transplants, stem cell transplants, and/or immunotherapy. In this population, there exists a sequelae of adverse effects that are synergistic with the disease process of cancer such as fatigue, nausea, anemia, low platelet count, bruising, decreased appetite, changes in white blood cell counts (WBC), decreased activity tolerance, pain, decreased sleep, changes in mental health (anxiety, depression), changes in cognition, declines in functional mobility and activity, changes in balance, and decreased overall quality of life (QOL). Whether patients are admitted for a planned chemotherapy cycle or urgently for chemotherapy, there is often a resulting drop in blood count levels (pancytopenia) from the treatment itself; thus, knowing the PWC's lab values and activity tolerance plays an integral part of developing and updating the plan of care throughout one's admission as well as facilitating timely communication with the interdisciplinary care team.

As described in Chapter 5, surgical oncology includes those PWCs whose solid tumor(s) may be resected, debulked, or otherwise surgically treated. If hospitalization is required for surgery, it can be expected that these PWCs may require major surgical intervention, and thus, are at an increased risk for a prolonged length of stay (LOS), complications, or functional debility after the procedure. In addition to surgical intervention to remove the tumor and attempt to get clean or negative margins, patients may also receive chemotherapy, radiation, or immunotherapy. These treatments may be administered neoadjuvantly to attempt to shrink the tumor(s) so that the surgical procedure need not be as extensive. The adverse effects of these neoadjuvant or adjuvant treatments remain impactful and may further complicate recovery through pancytopenia or malnutrition, which may result in delayed surgical healing times.

As a hospital admission may be unanticipated or radiation may be newly required during hospitalization, the acute care clinician will need to consider the adverse effects of radiation during their acute care treatment planning. Those patients receiving radiation treatment may also exhibit signs and symptoms of myelosuppression as well as burns and/or skin fragility at the irradiated location. As integumentary effects of external beam radiation do not occur immediately after the initiation of treatment, the acute care Onc R clinician may note changes to the skin approximately 10 days after delivery of the radiation therapy, which may occur during the hospitalization. In some cases, there are efforts to continue with radiation during a hospitalization, but this can vary greatly based on the reason for admission. As mentioned, knowing the patient's lab values and activity tolerance plays an integral part of the plan of care and communication with the interdisciplinary care team.

Patients who are candidates for bone marrow transplants frequently require a longer hospital stay, mainly due to initial efforts of myeloablation, the suppression of bone marrow activity in preparation for stem cell transplantation. This generally involves high-dose chemotherapy and/or total body irradiation prior to the transplant of the bone marrow cells. This myeloablation greatly reduces a person's ability to synthesize new blood cells resulting in pancytopenia, increasing the risk of infection, hemorrhage, and critical illness, hence the need for hospitalization and monitoring.

After myeloablation, new noncancerous bone marrow cells are implanted in the patient to proliferate; if the cells are from the patient, it is autologous. Transplantation of cells from a donor is termed allogenic, which further increases the risk of complications, notably graft-versus-host disease (GVHD). Refer to Chapter 21 on this topic for further details. GVHD can affect the skin, gut, and/or lungs. This can be difficult to manage because these hospitalized patients are already at risk of skin involvement, edema, and/or contractures; this may require proactive positioning and/or splinting. Research has shown that GVHD is often associated with malnutrition, protein-losing enteropathy, as well as deficiencies of zinc, vitamin B12, and vitamin D. If there is gut involvement, nutrition can be an issue with absorption, frequency of defecation, nausea, and appetite, all of which may require an alternative source of nutrition (e.g., total parenteral nutrition).[4] These individuals may require more frequent, shorter bouts of exercise due to changes in activity tolerance. With lung involvement, shortness of breath, oxygen requirements, and activity tolerance may be affected. In these cases, shorter bouts of more frequent activity may be better tolerated with this patient population.

Lastly, there are people who come to the hospital with a known history of cancer. There may be a consult placed for rehabilitation while in the ED or when the patient is admitted to the acute care setting. In either case, the Onc R clinician should perform a comprehensive chart review and examination to identify the admitting condition, the primary cancer and any metastatic sites, relevant medications, prior treatments, and their adverse effects. This knowledge will guide the examination and is critical to developing a safe, patient-centered plan of care. For example, a person with a history of prostate cancer who is presenting to the ED with a new onset of low back pain should be examined for possible metastatic involvement or pain as an adverse effect of previously administered treatment. Being able to recognize the metastatic patterns of common cancers can assist a clinician in differentiating between symptoms of cancer and its treatment or other biomechanical causes of the patient's symptoms.

When evaluating, assessing, and treating any of the aforementioned patients, considerations will include the patient's goals while focusing on functional mobility, addressing cancer-related fatigue, reducing risk of falls, communicating as part of an interdisciplinary team (IDT), educating family members or caregivers, and recognizing physiologic changes in patients during exercise due to the cancer itself and/or its treatments. As patients may be newly diagnosed or returning for follow-up treatment, current or new medications or medical issues may result in a dynamic and unpredictable symptom presentation, which may fluctuate on a daily (or even hourly) basis. In addition, the concepts of prehabilitation remain important in the inpatient setting as well. Key skills of an inpatient Onc R clinician are flexibility, adaptability, and having a safety-focused clinical approach to address the patient's medical, functional, and psychosocial needs.

The Role of the Oncology Rehabilitation Clinician in the Acute Care Setting

Four key themes have been identified that influence acute care clinical practice: (1) the environment; (2) communication and relationships; (3) the clinician as a person; and (4) the professional role of the clinician.[5] The environment and circumstances of a patient's hospitalization make efficiency and efficacy challenging at times. This is certainly true when working with PWCs as there are often competing priorities for the patient's time, attention, and emotions, impacting the prioritization of physical activity and Onc R.

The role of an Onc R clinician in the acute care setting is unique in that it requires adaptation to a challenging and dynamic environment in a relatively abbreviated time period. Simultaneously, many PWCs in the hospital are experiencing a pivotal moment in their cancer journey with a variety of emotional responses and fluctuating personal goals. Biopsies, chemotherapy infusions, radiation therapy, imaging studies, and other procedures and tests all compete for a patient's focus and energy. An acute care clinician who exhibits emotional intelligence and flexibility will be better able to adapt their plan of care to accommodate the needs of the medical team and the patient simultaneously.

Patients who feel heard and understood are more likely to hear and understand the purpose of rehabilitation while hospitalized. It is important for an Onc R clinician to not only be knowledgeable in Onc R, but also cognizant of the patient's goals, social barriers, and emotional issues. Empathy and acknowledgement of a patient's frustrations will help to build trust and a therapeutic relationship, which is especially important during this pivotal moment in their cancer journey.

While the patient may be his or her own advocate and decision maker, families, and caregivers are often involved during a hospitalization and should be considered an equal partner in care. In some cases, a PWC may make a medical decision based on what their partner or child is advising, even if the goal may be different from theirs. Skilled Onc R clinicians should navigate these conversations carefully to ensure all parties are supportive of the collective goals while advocating for the patient. See Chapter 29 for considerations in communication. Onc R clinicians should include both the patient and their partners in care to assist with setting goals and ensuring a safe discharge. Family meetings, virtual conferences, and collaborative multidisciplinary team meetings have been successful in navigating the care for the patient.

One of the advantages to the Onc R clinician in the inpatient or acute setting is the accessibility of key members of the IDT. Frequent communication with the medical team is essential to optimize timing of a rehabilitation session. For example, if a patient was just notified that their cancer diagnosis was terminal, receipt of this critical piece of information from the IDT members can help the Onc R clinician to adapt their approach or intervention. This situation would certainly be approached differently than that of a patient who is well acquainted with their diagnosis undergoing their third round of inpatient chemotherapy. In both cases, the clinician would introduce themselves as part of the care team in the hospital who assists in optimizing treatment plans and the patient's response to those plans. In the former situation, an Onc R clinician would need to approach the patient with more sensitivity and consideration of the patient's psychological response, which can be variable. Ongoing consultation with the patient's nurse is critical to establishing medical stability, determining levels of anxiety, and any other contextual considerations that may impact a rehabilitation session. Four different coping styles have been described for patients who were given a new cancer diagnosis.[6] These coping styles included: (1) positive/confronting; (2) fatalistic; (3) hopeless-helpless; and (4) denial/avoidance. Additionally, the patient's health locus of control will influence the starting point of any clinician-patient conversation. Regardless of coping style or locus of control, a skilled Onc R clinician should strive to navigate these initial conversations by helping the PWC to understand how Onc R can allow for an optimal QOL and improved clinical outcomes throughout the cancer continuum. In the author's experience, when explained with skill and honesty, most patients will "buy into" the benefits of strengthening the body in order to optimize its response to what is to come.

The professional role of an acute care or inpatient Onc R clinician includes a variety of responsibilities which will vary based upon the needs or wishes of the patient as well as the dynamics of the evolving medical situation. Their role includes not only providing direct interventions, education, and information to the patient, but also acting as an essential IDT member in guiding the medical plan of care. For example, a physical therapist (PT) or occupational therapist (OT) may identify a scenario where the medical team is focused on medical management but increasing a physical activity level may require clarification of a weight bearing status in the presence of metastatic bone disease. The inpatient Onc R clinician will also utilize the patient's current mobility status and trajectory to advise on discharge disposition and options to transition patients to their home environment. In addition, the OT and/or speech language pathologist (SLP) may work with the IDT to assist with tasks or techniques to maximize the patient's ability to eat, swallow, and perform basic activities of daily living (ADLs) while hospitalized.[7] All of these Onc R clinicians should strive to anticipate the needs of a patient and prepare for them, in order to reduce the care burden of the patient and family. This often includes patient and family training for tasks that will be done frequently throughout the day such as bathing, dressing, toileting, and eating. In addition, the OT can identify and recommend useful adaptive equipment needed to facilitate independence with ADLs. Furthermore, the SLP will also evaluate and develop an intervention plan for cognitive impairments, communication, as well as effective swallowing and nutritional intake. Finally, as with almost any hospitalized patient, promoting and facilitating mobility and participation in ADL performance is key. There are well-known, negative effects of bedrest such as muscle atrophy, delirium, pneumonia, and significant functional decline—all of which can be detrimental to function and may increase healthcare costs through delaying discharge and increasing LOS. Onc R clinicians in the acute setting should emphasize and promote mobility and patient independence to reduce the risk and impact of these negative effects.

As it relates to communication within the inpatient IDT, the SBAR method is commonly utilized. This technique includes conveying the situation, background, assessment, and recommendations from one provider to another. It is intended to facilitate patient handoff by conveying concise and clear information among healthcare team members. For example, this may be especially useful when communicating with a physician colleague to clarify restrictions related to weight bearing or specialized mobility procedures (e.g., mechanical lifts) in the presence of bone metastases. Additionally, open communication with the palliative or hospice IDT can assist the Onc R clinician in the development of therapy goals that align with the PWC's current situation, disease trajectory, and wishes.[8] In addition, it is essential to communicate with other critical team members, including, but not limited to, social workers, pastoral care professionals, physical medicine, and rehabilitation physicians (or physiatrists), and, of course, the attending physician, who often serves as the conduit for communication with other consulting physicians such as, orthopedic surgeons, neurosurgeons, or oncology specialists.

Establishing Medical Stability in the Acutely Ill Person With Cancer

Upon initiating a rehabilitation examination in an acute care setting, a thorough understanding of the patient's current status needs to be established. This is initially conducted via a chart review and then via interviews with the patient, family, and/or aforementioned healthcare team members. Identification of the presence and extent of conditions impacting the Onc R clinician's examination is crucial in the acute care setting, where medical instability is the norm.

Common Conditions Impacting Oncology Rehabilitation

Orthostatic Hypotension

One condition that should be recognized for its impact on Onc R is orthostatic hypotension. Normal blood pressure is defined as less than 120 mmHg/80 mmHg.[9] In orthostatic hypotension, a patient's blood pressure falls significantly with a change of position due to the effects of gravity and the body's inability to quickly compensate for the distal shift in blood volume. According to the Centers for Disease Control and Prevention, orthostatic hypotension is identified as a drop in systolic blood pressure by 20 mmHg or a drop in diastolic blood pressure by 10 mmHg, which often is accompanied by dizziness or lightheadedness.[10] Most patients with orthostatic hypotension experience this when performing a sit to stand activity. Common causes for orthostatic hypotension in a PWC are older age, hypovolemia, dehydration, immobility, anemia, and medications such as diuretics, beta blockers, calcium channel blockers, ACE inhibitors, nitrates, and angiotensin II blockers.[11]

The main symptom of orthostatic hypotension is feeling dizzy or lightheaded upon sitting up or standing. In some cases, patients may also experience nausea, confusion, or blurred vision. If this condition is not addressed, orthostatic hypotension may result in syncope and the possibility of fall related injury. Monitoring hemodynamics throughout the entire physical activity session is important during an acute care evaluation and treatment. Nonpharmacological approaches to the management of orthostatic hypotension include ongoing mobilization and early lifestyle changes as well as using elastic abdominal binders or lower extremity compression garments.[12,13] In attempts to abort an impending syncopal event, physical counterpressure maneuvers (mass isometric contractions of the arms or legs) can help to force the return of blood to the brain in an emergent situation (Figure 24.1).[14] Quickly returning the patient to a seated position then transitioning to supine (ideally in a trendelenburg position) is also a staple of care in presyncopal situations. In addition, educating the patient on self-monitoring their exercise tolerance, recommending slow progression of transitional movements, and performing isometric exercises prior to mobility can help stabilize blood pressure and prevent the significant drop in blood pressure, seen with orthostatic episodes. Most symptoms resolve after a few minutes of sitting or lying down and elevating the legs may also assist in symptom resolution. Individuals with persistent symptoms require pharmaceutical therapy to increase blood volume and peripheral vascular resistance.[15,16]

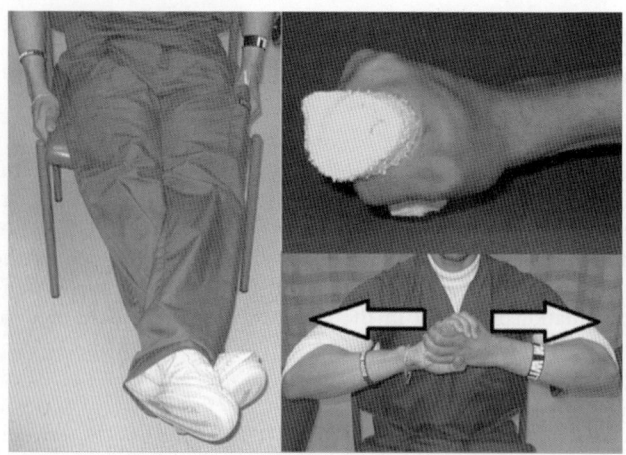

• **Fig. 24.1** Physical Counterpressure Maneuvers. (Reprinted with permission from Wilson CM, Kline JJ, Cook ME, et al. Therapist perceptions of physical counterpressure maneuvers for the management of pre-syncope. *J Acute Care Phys Ther.* 2015;6(3):102–115.)

Tumor Lysis Syndrome (TLS)

TLS is the most common disease-related emergency encountered by physicians caring for patients diagnosed with hematologic cancers. This occurs when tumor cells release their contents into the bloodstream leading to characteristic findings of excessive potassium phosphate, increased uric acid, and hypocalcemia (Figure 24.2).[17] These abnormalities most likely occur between three days prior to and 7 days after starting chemotherapy. TLS develops most often in patients with non-Hodgkin lymphoma or acute leukemia. The clinical presentation of this syndrome is cardiac arrhythmias, seizures, renal insufficiency, and multi-system organ failure.[18] Other

possible symptoms of TLS include lethargy, nausea, edema, syncope, fluid overload, and heart failure. Common treatment of TLS focuses on maintaining a normal balance of electrolytes in the blood to maximize kidney function, prevent uric acid formation, and facilitate breakdown or excretion of existing uric acid. Hydration via IV is the cornerstone of TLS prophylaxis.[17,18] While treating a PWC in an acute setting, paying close attention to the uric acid, calcium, and potassium lab values, in conjunction with symptom monitoring, can alert a therapist to the presence of TLS. This information would then be provided to the multidisciplinary team for further work up.

Acute Confusional States

An acute confusional state can present in multiple forms while a patient is hospitalized, such as delirium, encephalopathy, reversible dementia, organic brain syndrome, and terminal restlessness (referring to the agitated delirium often seen in the last days of life). In PWCs, many things can cause confusion including metastatic brain disease, brain anoxia, anemia, hypoglycemia, infection, fever, electrolyte imbalances, pain, or certain cancer treatments and medications.[19]

Confusion is the most common neurologic symptom in cancer and may be directly related to the cancer itself or to cancer treatment.[19] Confusion is common in persons diagnosed with advanced cancer during a hospitalization, especially older adults or those with underlying cognitive issues, metabolic abnormalities, or brain metastases. Cognitive status is imperative to functional learning, patient and family education, and end-of-life planning. Confusion can be associated with significant morbidity, mortality, and prolonged hospitalization, resulting in increased LOS in an acute setting and increased health care costs. Confusion can be very unsettling for the patient as well as the family or caregiver.

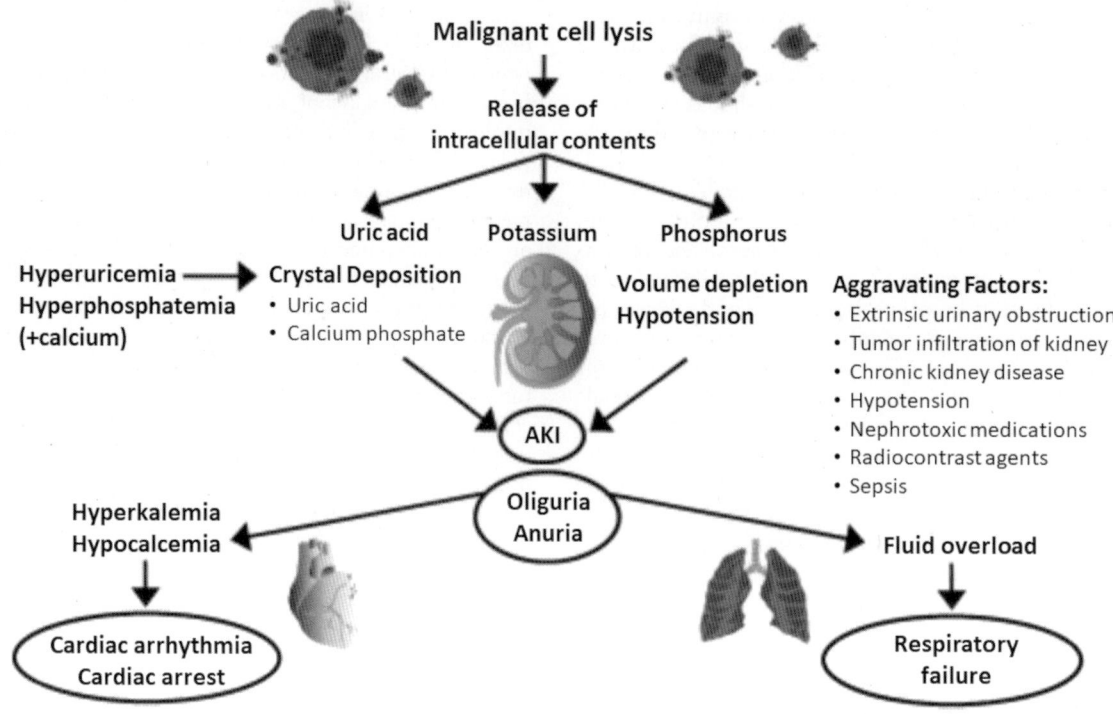

• **Fig. 24.2** Tumor Lysis Syndrome. (Reprinted with permission from Abu-Alfa AK, Younes A. Tumor lysis syndrome and acute kidney injury: evaluation, prevention, and management. *Am J Kidney Dis.* 2010;55(5 suppl 3):S1–13; quiz S14-9. doi:10.1053/j.ajkd.2009.10.056.)

Delirium is common in the ICU and one of the most common causes of acute confusion seen during hospitalizations. Early recognition and treatment of delirium is essential to improve clinical outcomes and determine accurate discharge dispositions. In an acute care setting, this requires Onc R clinicians to screen for cognitive impairments upon evaluation and treatment. Onc R clinicians often utilize orientation questions to screen for confusion; however, utilization of a standardized, evidence-based outcome measure is preferred due to validity in the patient population, as well as sensitivity and specificity. Common assessments utilized in the acute care setting are the Confusion Assessment Measure (CAM)-ICU, Short Blessed Test, Mini-Cog, Saint Louis University Mental Status (SLUMS), and Mini Mental State Exam. Once identified, SLPs and OTs can provide interventions to assist with delirium reduction and optimizing cognitive status. Interventions may include simple memory tasks or problem-solving skills. Interventions may be focused on increasing attention span or alertness using meaningful activities to facilitate cognitive return. Activities may include introducing family photographs, familiar television shows, or integration of established routines specific to the PWC.

The Importance of Lab Values

PWCs frequently have alterations in lab values which impact their participation in rehabilitation. These alterations may be related to the cancer diagnosis, its treatments (e.g., chemotherapy, a concurrent medical diagnosis, infection). Laboratory tests are helpful in determining the patient's medical stability, tolerance to treatment, and even overall prognosis. Although these lab values are readily accessible, referenced, and examined in the acute care setting, their impact often extends to non-inpatient settings, impacting the clinical approach to care outside the hospital. Onc R clinicians, understanding the pertinence of these values, should seek out and request these values, especially if warranted by symptom presentation. The American Physical Therapy Association's Academy of Acute Care Physical Therapy (APTA-AACPT) maintains an extremely useful series of resource guides on the interpretation of lab values (https://www.aptaacutecare.org/page/ResourceGuides).[20]

The most common lab value test is a complete blood count (CBC). Although there are nearly a dozen tests reported in a CBC, each with its own utility, this chapter will highlight the importance of those most relevant to the Onc R professional. In addition to their utility to the medical team and to prognostication, lab values also guide the intensity and volume of rehabilitation intervention and should be reviewed prior to initiating an evaluation or treatment session. It is important to note, however, that some PWCs possess chronically low lab values and may be able to physiologically compensate for such abnormal counts. Ongoing conversations with the physician may allow for activities outside traditional guidelines; however, the patient should always be monitored for symptoms caused by abnormal lab values, especially with exertion or physical activity. It is not unusual to observe a person diagnosed with leukemia with a chronically low hemoglobin of less than 8.0 g/dL walking the hallways of the hospital, but it is highly advisable to clarify activity parameters with the attending physician or consult department guidelines prior to initiation of this activity. An important term when considering lab values is *nadir*, where blood count(s) reach the lowest point. RBCs take longer to reach their *nadir* than WBCs.[21] This timeframe generally poses the highest risk for infections or adverse events and, depending on the drug administered and the specific blood count/lab value, often occurs during the 7 to 14 days following the administration of chemotherapy.[21]

Hemoglobin (Hgb)

Hgb is a protein that transports oxygen within the blood. The APTA-AACPT 2017 Laboratory Values Interpretation Resource defines the normal range of Hgb for a female as 12 to 16 g/dL and for males as 14 to 17 g/dL.[20] An increase in Hgb may indicate dehydration and polycythemia. Symptoms of this may include blurred vision, dizziness, seizure, headache, or symptoms similar to a transient ischemic attack (TIA). More commonly, PWCs present with low Hgb. Common causes of low Hgb in PWCs include hemorrhage, lymphoma, stress to the bone marrow, heart failure, and systemic therapy such as chemotherapy.[22] If a patient's Hgb is low, their endurance and tolerance to physical activity may be limited. Therefore, a clinician may need to recommend modifications to activity levels, such as limiting the patient's activity to only performing essential ADLs, to prevent any safety issues. These patients also may require assistance with ADLs to ensure safety and mitigation of fall risks. Low Hgb has also been associated with increased fatigue and tachycardia.[22] Due to the decreased oxygen carrying capacity within the body, the person's heart rate and cardiac output needs to increase to supply tissues with oxygen, thereby causing an increased workload on the heart. Clinical presentation of patients with low Hgb may include decreased endurance, decreased activity tolerance, and pallor.[20] It is important to consider that some physical activity remains warranted even in the case of low Hgb; however, activity restrictions to in-bed or open-chain exercises may be warranted in cases of symptomatically low Hgb. See Table 24.1 for considerations.

Hematocrit

Hematocrit represents the total percentage of whole blood volume that is composed of erythrocytes (red blood cells or RBCs). Hematocrit can be used to assess for overall blood loss and fluid balance.[20] Normal range for females is 37% to 47% and for males is 42% to 52%. Decreased levels of hematocrit can be associated with anemia, which commonly occurs in patients with cancers that involve the bone marrow. A hematocrit value of less than 15% to 20% is indicative of an increased risk of cardiac failure or imminent death.[20] If this occurs, the medical team will need to monitor tissue perfusion. A hematocrit between 25% and 37%

TABLE 24.1	Physical Activity in the Presence of Low Hemoglobin
Hgb Level	**Physical Activity Considerations**
Less than 7 g/dL	Bed exercises only
7–8 g/dL (severe anemia)	Close monitoring of symptoms and vital signs Short period of intervention, symptom limited Education on energy conservation
8–10 g/dL	Symptom monitoring of vital signs
Greater than 11 g/dL	Establish baseline vitals and utilize symptom-based intervention while measuring rating of perceived exertion

Reprinted with permission from Myszenski A. The role of lab values in clinical decision making and patient safety for the acutely ill patient lecture. http://www.PhysicalTherapy.com. Accessed October 4, 2020.

should prompt a symptom-based approach when determining appropriateness for physical activity or physical rehabilitation.[20] This should occur in collaboration with the IDT as a transfusion may be required prior to engaging in certain activities. A hematocrit level of greater than 60% may result in spontaneous blood clotting which can increase the risk of stroke or pulmonary embolism.[20]

White Blood Cells (WBCs)

WBCs are part of the immune system, and as with RBC, the term WBCs can mean either white blood count or white blood cells. These cells are responsible for fighting infections. Some common types of WBCs are neutrophils, lymphocytes, monocytes, and macrophages. A reduced WBCs count can result in an increased vulnerability to infection and may occur due to immunosuppression. Normal values for WBC are 5.0 to 10.0 10^9/L.[20] The term leukopenia refers to a decrease in WBCs, most commonly neutrophils, which are phagocytic cells that ingest or kill microorganisms that cause infection.[23,24] Leukopenia is a reduction in WBCs of less than 4.0×10^9/L.[20,23] A deficiency in neutrophils to less than 1.5×10^9/L indicates a patient is neutropenic.[20,23] Having a low neutrophil count substantially increases the risk of developing a serious infection. Common causes of having a lower WBC include chemotherapy, radiation, or a stem cell transplant. Symptoms that may present include weakness, fatigue, fever, and headache. The APTA-AACPT recommends Onc R clinicians use a symptom-based approach and monitor for a patient's fever when performing clinician evaluation and treatments in the setting of leukocytosis, neutropenia, and leukopenia.[20]

Leukocytosis is when a patient has an elevated WBC level of greater than 11.0×10^9/L.[20] Common causes of leukocytosis include infection, leukemia, and surgery. Clinical presentation includes fever, lethargy, and malaise.[20] Leukocytosis is frequently a sign of an inflammatory response, commonly the result of infection, but may also occur in the setting of certain bone tumors and leukemia.[23]

Neutrophils

Neutrophils are the first cell types to travel to the site of an infection.[24] Neutrophils help fight infection by ingesting microorganisms and releasing enzymes that kill the microorganisms.[25] Health care providers utilize the absolute neutrophil count (ANC) as a proxy measure of a patient's immune system function. The ANC is found by multiplying the WBC count by the percent of neutrophils in the blood. For example, if the WBC count is 7000 and 40% of the WBCs are neutrophils, the patient's ANC would be 2800 (7000 × 0.40 = 2800).[20]

Neutropenia is marked by an ANC of less than 1500 per microliter (1500/μL). Severe neutropenia is defined as less than 500 per microliter (500/μL).[26] As ANC decreases, the risk of infection increases. Neutropenia generally occurs a week after administration of myelosuppressive chemotherapy and may last up to 6 weeks following chemotherapy.[27] Patients who are at a higher risk for neutropenia are those who are receiving certain chemotherapy and radiation treatments or steroids, and those following bone marrow transplant.[20] Symptoms of neutropenia include fever, chills, mouth sores, difficulty breathing, coughing, abdominal pain, and rectal pain.[20,27] In some cases, a fever may be the only symptom of neutropenia, as other commonly encountered symptoms may not occur when the immune system is unable to generate a substantive immune response. Patients hospitalized with neutropenia are often placed on neutropenic precautions, with specific parameters varying by health system. Common precautious include excellent hand hygiene and environment sanitation, avoiding exposure to other patients and potentially ill people, and wearing a mask and gloves to decrease the risk of transmission of infection to the patient while participating in rehabilitation interventions. Some patients with neutropenia may develop a neutropenic fever, which can be identified by a single oral temperature greater than 101°F (38.3°C) or an oral temperature of 100.4°F (38.0°C) lasting longer than an hour.[28] A neutropenic fever requires prompt attention with initiation of antibiotics within 1 hour of presenting symptoms. If antibiotics are delayed, there is a substantially increased risk of sepsis and death.[29]

Treatment of neutropenia varies. Myeloid growth factors are proteins that stimulate the bone marrow to produce more WBCs available to fight infections. There are some medications known to increase growth factors such as filgrastim (Neupogen), tbo-filgrastim (Granix), and pegfilgrastim (Neulasta).[29] See Chapter 6 for more information on colony stimulating factors.

Platelets

Platelets or thrombocytes are critical in blood clotting. Platelets help form blood clots to slow or stop bleeding and to help wounds heal. Patients with leukemias and lymphomas are at a higher risk of experiencing thrombocytopenia. Thrombocytopenia may also be caused by myelosuppression from chemotherapy and radiation. A platelet count of less than 150,000/μL is generally considered as the cutoff range for thrombocytopenia.[20] The main concern with thrombocytopenia is the risk for excessive bleeding and inability to stop bleeding during a traumatic event. Signs and symptoms of low platelets are frequent bruising, bloody or dark urine, stool, or sputum, weakness, blurred vision, and pain in the joints. Patients who exhibit thrombocytopenia are at increased risk for bleeding, therefore during mobility and exercise intervention, Onc R clinicians should ensure proper guarding and fall risk mitigation to prevent injurious falls and trauma, including intracerebral hemorrhage.[30]

Thrombocytopenia is common following chemotherapy, with the nadir expected 7 to 10 days after chemotherapy and recovery is generally expected within 2 to 3 weeks.[30] A variety of safety precautions may be employed in the presence of thrombocytopenia, from activity restrictions to complete bedrest. Although bedrest can temporarily reduce the risk of falls and hemorrhage, it must be weighed with the risk of functional decline from immobilization.[30] Evidence is somewhat variable with rehabilitation guidelines related to thrombocytopenia.[30–32] Patients with low platelets under 50,000/μL should not perform strenuous resistive exercises to decrease risk of bleeding within the muscle belly.[30,31] Between 30,000/μL and 50,000/μL, progressive resistive exercises should be avoided but active range of motion or aquatic therapy may be beneficial if the PWC's immune status allows.[31] For platelet levels between 20,000/μL and 50,000/μL, light exercises without strenuous effort using elastic bands are appropriate if no signs of bleeding are present.[32] When platelet levels are between 10,000/μL and 20,000/μL, there is a risk of bleeding from high exertional blood pressure with aggressive exercise; in this case, gentle range of motion, ADLs, ambulation, and exercise without resistance is recommended.[30,31] It is also recommended that exercises be performed without strain to avoid bleeding due to possible spikes in blood pressure.[30] The APTA-AACPT 2017 Laboratory Values Interpretation Resource recommends a symptoms-based approach is necessary as well as partnership with the medical multidisciplinary team.[20]

When considering prescribing exercises, Onc R clinicians should screen for signs of bleeding. In addition, these patients should be educated about these signs and to self-monitor during performance of home exercises. Discretion and clinical judgment should be used in collaboration with the medical team as appropriate.[30–32]

Electrolyte Disorders

Electrolyte disorders are common in PWCs. These conditions can be associated with a worsening outcome, from an unrelated medical issue, or as an adverse effect of cancer treatment and can negatively impact QOL or survival. Common conditions affecting electrolytes include paraneoplastic syndrome, TLS or anticancer therapies.[33] Electrolyte disorders in patients diagnosed with cancer depend on several causes: cancer pathophysiology, anti-tumor treatments, concomitant clinical conditions, or therapies. Some cancer treatments or drugs such as chemotherapy, immunotherapies, osmotic diuretics, corticosteroids, and enteral or parenteral nutrition can also cause electrolyte imbalance.[33] However, electrolyte imbalances often have a multifactorial etiology and may be both secondary to and responsible for multiple organ system's dysfunction. A prompt correction of electrolyte disorders is associated with a better prognosis.[27]

Sodium

Sodium (Na+) is an essential electrolyte that helps muscles to function and controls fluid balances. Normal values for Na+ are 134 to 142 mEq/L.[34] Hypernatremia is categorized as >145 mEq/L.[20] Causes for hypernatremia include increased sodium intake, dehydration, renal insufficiency, and diabetes.[20] Hypernatremia can be seen in PWCs who exhibit cancer cachexia, kidney damage, brain metastasis, and gastrointestinal disorders due to cancer infiltration. Clinical presentation includes irritability, agitation, increased fluid retention, edema, impaired cognition, seizure, and coma. Onc R clinician considerations for treatment include seizure precautions.[20,35]

Hyponatremia is categorized as low Na+ with a value of <130 mEq/L.[20] Common causes are gastrointestinal impairments and cirrhosis. Among PWCs, hyponatremia occurs most frequently with small cell lung cancer (SCLC). Most cases of hyponatremia are caused by the syndrome of inappropriate antidiuretic hormone (SIADH), with higher rates of SIADH found with SCLC than with other malignancies.[33] Clinical presentation includes headache, lethargy, impaired cognitive status, diarrhea, impaired reflexes, seizure, and coma. Onc R clinician considerations for treatment include seizure precautions and monitoring for orthostatic hypotension.[20]

Potassium

Elevated or decreased potassium can interfere with muscle contractility and cardiac conductivity causing an arrhythmia. The normally accepted range for potassium is 3.7 to 5.1 mEq/L.[35] Increased potassium is known as hyperkalemia and is marked by potassium levels greater than 5.5 mEq/L.[20] Hyperkalemia can lead to serious cardiac issues. The APTA-AACPT recommends a symptom-based approach is warranted when determining the appropriateness for activity.[20] TLS represents an important cause of acute hyperkalemia in cancer patients. Falk et al. found a strong association between elevated serum potassium levels and long-term cancer risk in healthy individuals.[36] Muscle weakness is a common symptom of hyperkalemia.

Hypokalemia, defined as less than 3.5 mEq/L, can also be a medical emergency.[20] If potassium is trending down, a symptoms-based approach is also recommended as best practice.[20] Electrocardiograms or EKGs should be monitored in patients with hypokalemia. Common causes of hypokalemia in PWCs are prolonged vomiting or diarrhea, trauma, alkalosis, hyperglycemia, or subarachnoid hemorrhage. Medications such as diuretics can also cause hypokalemia.

Calcium

Calcium is a cation with a normal range of 8.6 to 10.3 mg/dL.[35] It plays a role in the formation of bone, cell division, blood coagulation, muscular function, and cell growth.[20] Hypocalcemia is defined as less than 8.5 mg/dL and is common in cancer from the cancer treatment itself or as an adverse effect. It is found in anorexia, cachexia, bowel obstruction, and hepatic dysfunction.[32] Some cancer treatments may cause hypocalcemia including bisphosphonates, denosumab (Prolia), and some chemotherapeutic agents.[27] Symptoms may include hyper-excitability of the neuromuscular system, spasms, cramps, parkinsonism, and in severe cases, arrhythmias may occur.[33]

Hypercalcemia is characterized by a value over 10.5 mg/dL. Hypercalcemia (as with hyponatremia) is found in breast, renal, and prostate cancers and is associated with a poor prognosis. A key cause of hypercalcemia is hormonal factors, including hyperparathyroidism, though it may also arise from osteolysis, kidney failure, fracture, immobilization, and some drugs.[33] Symptoms found with hypercalcemia include lethargy, weakness, excessive thirst (polydipsia), and confusion.[33] In severe cases, delirium, psychosis, and cardiac arrhythmias may be noted.[33]

Glucose

Glucose is an essential component of cellular operations, including cancer cells. There is increasing evidence suggesting a link between cancer and diabetes.[37] High glucose and high insulin levels can induce cancer cell proliferation through different mechanisms. Pancreatic cancer is more likely to occur in patients who have long standing diabetes.[37] Controlling blood glucose and insulin levels is extremely important in patients with cancer.[38] Normal values for blood glucose are 70 to 100 mg/dL.[39] Hyperglycemia, or high blood glucose, is a condition in which an excessive amount of glucose circulates in the blood, a condition which develops when the body has too little insulin or when the body cannot use insulin properly. Some brain tumors such as brain metastases and astrocytomas, can precipitate hyperglycemia with a clinical presentation of extreme fatigue.[40] Evidence shows that having an elevated blood sugar increases the risk of cancer at several sites including the colon, breast, and bladder.[38]

Hyperglycemia is defined as >200 mg/dL, and when considering therapy indications for exercise, a symptoms-based approach to appropriateness of activity is warranted.[20] In patients with hyperglycemia, clinician should be aware of a decreased activity tolerance and fatigue. Steroid medications can raise blood glucose levels by reducing the action of insulin.[41] Even in those without a history of diabetes, Onc R clinicians should be vigilant to identify signs of hyperglycemia in those receiving steroids.[41] Hypoglycemia is generally considered to be less than 70 mg/dL.[20] Patients diagnosed with hypoglycemia may not tolerate therapy until their glucose level increases. A glucose target between 140 mg/dL and 180 mg/dL is recommended for most patients in noncritical care units while hospitalized.[39] Patients diagnosed with malignancy may exhibit hypoglycemia with a clinical presentation of lethargy, irritability, shaking, extremity weakness, and loss of consciousness.

Other Pertinent Lab Values

Other values may be pertinent to the Onc R clinician and the care they provide across the broad array of patient presentations seen in the acute setting. Albumin and prealbumin, seen in complete metabolic panels, are composites of a patient's nutritional status and reflect levels of protein in the blood.[20] Normative values are noted below, with deficiencies identifying the extent of protein depletion. Elevated levels may be seen in severe infections or dehydration and kidney disease.[20] Down-trending values, correlated with nutritional compromise and malnutrition may be accompanied by peripheral edema and hypotension.[20] Serum bilirubin correlates with liver function, with aberrancies inducing metabolic sequalae that may impact therapy participation and approach. While elevated bilirubin may result from a number of medical conditions, in oncology, hepatotoxicity, or liver dysfunction, may result from damage caused by chemotherapy agents.[20] Clinical presentations include jaundice, activity-limiting fatigue, nausea, and generalized weakness. Ammonia also evaluates liver function and metabolism, and in cases of hepatitis, hepatotoxicity or kidney failure, may present in patient confusion, encephalopathy, lethargy, and peripheral nerve impairments. Blood urea nitrogen, or BUN, and serum creatinine represent kidney function, and when elevated, may present clinically in peripheral or generalized edema, fatigue, and possible cognitive changes.[20] It is imperative that the Onc R clinician examines the breadth of the patient's laboratory workup in order to best tailor, modify, and prescribe exercise intervention for the medically complex patient. For additional insight into the interpretation of these and other lab values, see the referenced interpretation resource guide of the APTA-AAACPT (Table 24.2).

Anticoagulation

Patients who require anticoagulation for various reasons during a hospitalization will require close monitoring of lab values the partial thromboplastin time (PTT), activated partial thromboplastin time (aPTT), and International Normalized Ratio (INR). INR assesses blood clotting time in patients who are on medications for anticoagulation like warfarin (Coumadin).[20] A normal range for INR is 0.8 to 1.2.[20] Although patients may participate with therapy without substantive restriction when achieving a therapeutic range between 2.0 and 3.0, if INR is >5.0, the person is at a higher risk of bleeding and a risk-benefit discussion for proceeding with or holding mobility should occur

TABLE 24.2	Normative Lab Values for Kidney Function[20]
Normative Lab Values for Kidney Function	**Normative Range**
Serum Albumin	3.5–5.2 g/dL
Serum Prealbumin	19–39 mg/dL • 0–5 mg/dL = severe protein depletion • 5–10 mg/dL = moderate protein depletion • 10–15 mg/dL = mild protein depletion
Bilirubin	0.3–1.0 mg/dL; Critical value: > 12mg/dL
Ammonia	15–60 µg/dL
Blood Urea Nitrogen (BUN)	6–25 mg/dL
Serum Creatinine	Male: 0.7–1.3 mg/dL; Female: 0.4–1.1 mg/dL

Created by Courtney Witczak, Grace Burns, and Cynthia Barbe. Printed with permission.

with the medical team.[42] If the INR is >6.0 bedrest is be indicated until the INR is back within an acceptable range.[42] This is imperative to protect those patients with a high fall risk. It is imperative to review all anticoagulation medications prior to mobilizing/treating the patient, particularly if the patient is not therapeutic. Timing of medications and nature of the specific anticoagulants may be used as a guide for safe mobility (Figure 24.3). PTT also measures clotting time for persons on warfarin, with a normal range of 21 to 35 seconds.[35] Similar to INR, there is a therapeutic range for PTT, which is generally 2 to 2.5 times the reference range, specifically between 60 and 109 seconds.[35] If the PTT is greater than 70 seconds, there is an increased risk of spontaneous bleeding.[20] The aPTT measures clotting time for patients on heparin with a normal range between 11 seconds and 13 seconds. If the aPTT is >70 seconds, there is an increased risk of spontaneous bleeding.[20]

A Venous Thromboembolism (VTE) Clinical Practice Guideline (CPG) that assists with decisions regarding physical activity and mobility with an individual receiving anticoagulation has been developed (see Figure 24.3).[42]

Medication Review

Prior to treating a PWC in the acute care setting, the Onc R clinician must perform an extensive review of the patient's medications in order to best inform the evaluation and subsequent treatment sessions. This action alone is invaluable in piecing together a past medical history in a patient who may not be able to communicate their medical history. Although a PWC can be on a wide variety of medications during an acute or inpatient stay, below are some of the most commonly encountered medications in PWCs that may affect rehabilitation. See Chapter 6 for additional information on medications and their adverse effects.

Antiemetics

Many disease- or treatment-related sequalae can cause nausea and vomiting, which impair the patient's ability to participate in rehabilitation evaluations and treatments while in the hospital. These symptoms also impair the patient's ability to perform basic ADLs. Nausea and vomiting (N/V) can contribute to weakness, malnourishment, electrolyte imbalances, vitamin deficiencies, and weight loss. Ondansetron hydrochloride (Zofran) is a common medication provided to patients to decrease the symptom of N/V caused by radiation therapy, chemotherapy, and surgery. Zofran is a serotonin receptor antagonist.[43] It blocks the action of serotonin, a natural substance that may cause N/V.[43] The key to preventing vomiting is to be proactive by taking steps before the N/V becomes uncontrollable. It is a key role of the acute care clinician to proactively anticipate and collaborate with the care team in order to curtail the N/V that may be elicited by rehabilitation or may be a barrier to starting a therapy intervention. Collaboration with the medical team and bedside nurses is needed as this medication can be provided to the patient intravenously for a prompt decrease in the symptoms of N/V, allowing the patient to participate fully in the rehab treatment. Zofran is also available in a tablet, an oral solution, or a dissolvable film taken orally.[43]

Agents for Neutropenia

As noted previously, colony-stimulating factors are often used to treat neutropenia. Patients receiving chemotherapy or those undergoing treatment with a bone marrow or stem cell transplant

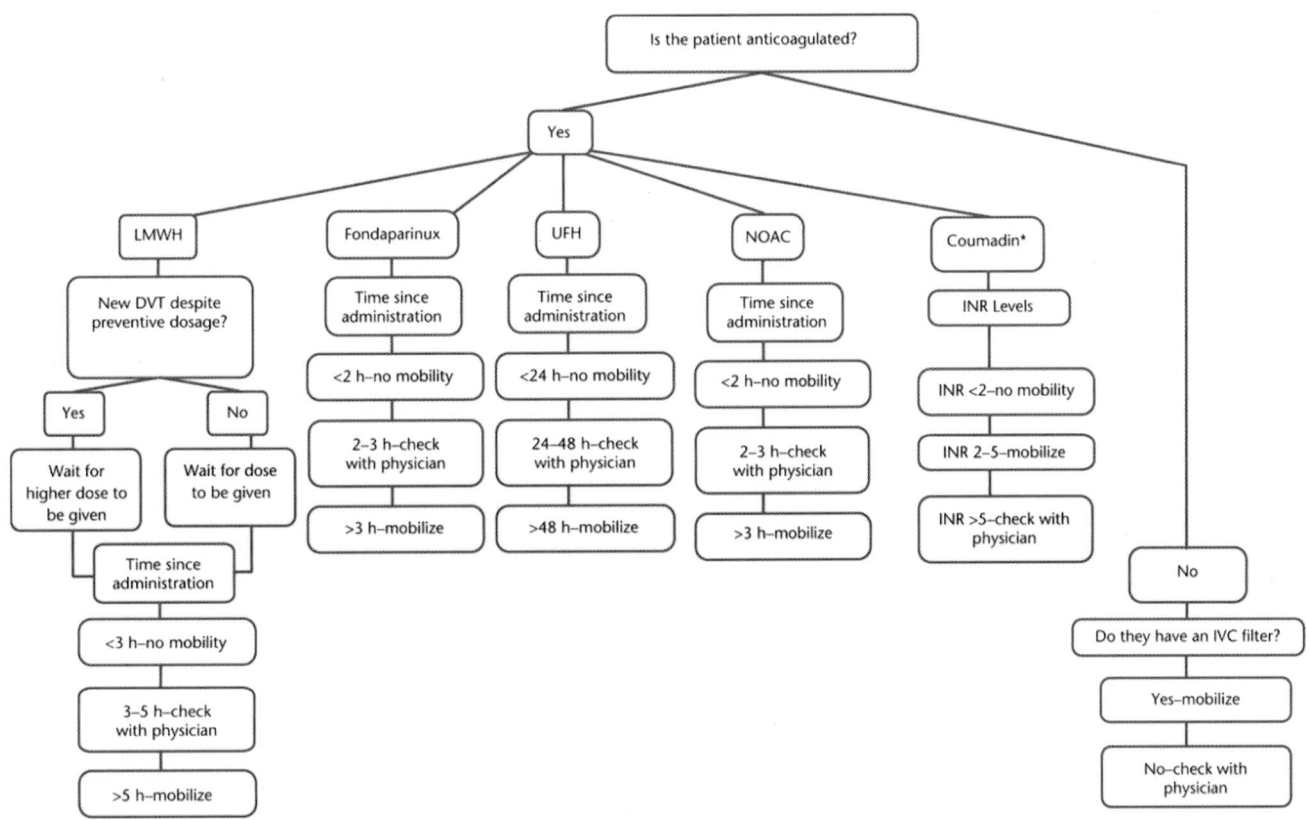

• **Fig. 24.3** Algorithm for Mobilizing Patients With Known Lower Extremity Deep Vein Thrombosis. *If started on Coumadin, LMWH usually also started. Use LMWH guidelines for mobilization decision in these situations. DVT, deep vein thrombosis; INR, international normalized ratio; IVC, inferior vena cava; LMWH, low-molecular-weight heparin; NOAC, novel oral anticoagulants; UFH, unfractionated heparin.* (Reprinted with permission from Hillegass E, Puthoff M, Frese EM, Thigpen M, Sobush DC, Auten B. Guideline Development Group. Role of physical therapists in the management of individuals at risk for or diagnosed with venous thromboembolism: evidence-based clinical practice guideline. *Phys Ther.* 2016;96(2):143–166. doi:10.2522/ptj.20150264.)

commonly receive filgrastim injection products (Granix, Neupogen, Nivestym, Zarxio).[44] A typical administration of this drug is a daily injection over a short period of time or IV infusion. In most cases, neutrophils are restored within 14 days but may take longer depending on the severity of the disease.[44] During this time, the aforementioned neutropenic precautions will likely be warranted.

Corticosteroids

Corticosteroids are medications commonly used to reduce inflammation and lower the body's immune response.[45] Common corticosteroids used in the hospital setting are prednisone, dexamethasone, and methylprednisolone. Steroids can be used to treat anemia, nausea, headaches, hypercalcemia, thrombocytopenia, and adverse drug reactions. Many PWCs are prescribed corticosteroids for a variety of reasons. For example, a person receiving palliative and hospice care may benefit from corticosteroids to attempt to reduce the symptoms produced by brain or bone metastases.[46] These medications cause an anti-inflammatory response in the body and are widely used in diagnoses such as including acute lymphoblastic leukemia (ALL), chronic lymphocytic leukemia (CLL), acute myeloid leukemia (AML), chronic myelogenous leukemia (CML), and Hodgkin and non-Hodgkin lymphoma.[47] These medications may be administered orally by liquid or tablet, intravenously, or topically. Common adverse effects that may

affect an acute rehabilitation evaluation or treatment may include increased blood pressure, weight gain, osteoporosis, and increased circulating blood glucose.[46]

Reviewing Diagnostic Imaging

While patients are admitted to the hospital, a variety of imaging tests may be performed with material relevance to Onc R. It is critical to review these imaging studies when performed to have a clear understanding of any new findings warranting modification to rehabilitation (e.g., metastatic disease of the brain, bones, or lungs, or tumors obstructing the gastrointestinal system). In some cases, it may be necessary to postpone a rehabilitation session if a test is ordered but incomplete or unread, especially those related to the musculoskeletal, nervous, and cardiopulmonary systems. In addition, repeated images may be able to assist the medical team in determining the effectiveness of cancer treatments and to determine if a cancer regimen is effective by reducing tumor size or slowing its growth. Common imaging tests used to evaluate the presence and extent of cancer include computerized tomography (CT) scan, bone scan, magnetic resonance imaging (MRI), positron emission tomography (PET) scan, ultrasound, and X-rays.[48]

CT scans examine the tumor's shape and size as well as the extent to which proximate structures are impacted by the tumor. CT scans can be performed with or without contrast. The scan causes no direct pain to the patient and takes about 10 to 30 minutes to complete. Patients with musculoskeletal or neuromuscular dysfunctions (e.g., low back pain, axial bone metastasis) may report difficulty achieving or sustaining the requisite supine positioning for examination. In those scans with contrast, contrast media must be injected, giving the potential for injection site or allergic reactions in some (a small percentage) patients. CT scans with contrast can also identify blood vessels that may be feeding the cancer or tumor.[48] In some cases, a biopsy may be completed via CT guidance to assist in collecting a sample of cells without inadvertently damaging other surrounding vital organs or tissues. In addition, CT scans may be done in conjunction with PET scans to assess for extent of tumor metabolic activity and spread.[48]

Nuclear medicine exams such as PET scans, bone scans, thyroid scans, multigated acquisition (MUGA) scans, and gallium scans assist the medical team in finding tumors and assessing their spread in the body. Nuclear scans assist with body imaging through the use of liquid substances called radionuclides in which low levels of radiation are released. Radioactivity is picked up where the tracer, or radionuclide, travels throughout the body. If cancer is present, pending the sensitivity or specificity of the imaging modality as well as the behavior of the specific tumor type, the tumor may show up on the scan as an area of increased cell activity. Bone scans, for instance, are more sensitive in identifying osteoblastic lesions whereas PET-CT scans are more readily able to identify osteolytic lesions.

A PET scan is an imaging scan that is useful in detecting cancer, determining cancer spread, and evaluating for cancer recurrence or treatment efficacy.[48] In this procedure, a small amount of a radioactive glucose analogue, ^{18}F-FDG, is injected into a vein. Because cancer cells are more metabolically active thus utilizing more glucose, they are contrasted with noncancerous tissues. Cancer cells that show higher chemical activity on a PET scan exhibit a higher metabolic rate than normal cells. However, it is imperative to consider that some areas are normally quite metabolically active, and therefore, are also more highly contrasted on a PET. These sites include the cerebrum, liver, and spleen. In addition, the urinary system also looks brighter because of the excretion of the ^{18}F-FDG.

Bone scans identify if cancer has spread and metastasized from other places to the bones.[49] Bone scans may provide an improved ability to identify metastatic change as opposed to regular X-rays as bone lesions are often not visible on radiographs until after cortical bone disruption or involvement has occurred. Onc R clinicians must be aware of bone scan results prior to initiating physical activity in weight bearing bones to avoid pathologic fracture or unnecessary pain. Thyroid scans are performed as the radioactive iodine (iodine-123 or iodine-131) is swallowed and goes into the bloodstream of the patient. This scan can be utilized to assess for thyroid cancer.

MRIs can also be used to evaluate the extent and spread of cancer. They can also assist the medical team to plan treatments such as surgery or radiation. MRIs use strong magnets to create images as opposed to a CT scan which utilizes radiation.[48] In addition, MRIs are more advantageous in assessing the intricacies of soft tissues than CTs or X-rays. MRIs with contrast dye may be utilized to locate brain and spinal cord tumors. MRIs can also be used to look for signs that the cancer may have metastasized from where it started to another part of the body. Patients with

metal components in their bodies, not limited to implanted infusion ports, metal pins or screws, pacemakers, clips used for brain aneurysms, cochlear implants, or arterial or vascular stents, are not candidates for an MRI.

Additional Procedures to Review

Angiography can be utilized to identify arteries throughout the body including those in the brain, kidneys, and lungs. In order to complete an angiogram, a catheter with dye is inserted into the blood vessel. After the dye is injected, X-rays are then performed. After the catheter is removed, Onc R clinicians may have to delay treatment as firm pressure is required to ensure bleeding does not occur. Patients are instructed to maintain strict bedrest and elevate their legs for a few hours following the procedure. Angiography usually takes 1 to 2 hours to complete.

A lumbar puncture (LP) is also known as a spinal tap. This diagnostic test collects cerebrospinal fluid (CSF) which may be analyzed to assist in the diagnostic workup for brain and spinal canal cancers. Blood cancers can also be identified in CSF. Typical bedrest times after a LP is 4 hours. Patients will receive their test results approximately 1 to 2 weeks after their LP. Onc R clinicians must be vigilant for spinal headaches after a LP procedure and monitor cognition.

Vital Sign Assessment

Close monitoring of vital signs is essential in an acute care or inpatient setting. In order to promptly recognize abnormal responses to activity and exercise in PWCs, baseline vital signs should be taken, especially in individuals with concurrent abnormal lab values. Abnormal vital signs alone might be a reason to modify the therapeutic intervention, but Onc R clinicians must consider the compound effects of the vital signs and lab values. A patient with anemia may be more likely to have an adverse event in the presence of low oxygen saturation or low blood pressure as compared to a patient with normal hemoglobin and hematocrit. See Table 24.3 for normal resting values that have been determined based on evidence.[50,51]

Termination of exercise is a key component in the clinical decision making for a physical rehabilitation intervention. In general, Onc R clinicians should not initiate mobility or physical activity with persons whose vital signs are outside of normal parameters without consultation with the patient's physician. This is important as a deviation from expected values may reflect the patient's inability to tolerate undue physical stressors, mobility, or intervention.[52] Other signs and symptoms to terminate a therapy session based on abnormal vital signs include an increase in heart rate greater than 30 beats/minute over baseline, an increase in SBP

TABLE 24.3	Normative Values for Vital Signs[50,51]
Vital Sign	**Normative Range**
Heart rate (HR)	60–100 beats/min
Blood pressure (BP)	Systolic blood pressure (SBP): <120 mmHg Diastolic blood pressure (DBP): <80 mmHg Mean arterial pressure (MAP): 70–110 mmHg
Oxygen saturation (SaO$_2$)	>95%
Respiratory rate (RR)	12–18 breaths per minute

Created by Courtney Witczak, Grace Burns and Cynthia Barbe. Printed with permission.

by 30 mmHg or a decrease in SBP by 20 mmHg.[52] Additional reasons for ceasing a therapy session include a change in DBP of 10 mmHg from resting value with mobility, new onset dizziness or lightheadedness that can be indicative of orthostatic hypotension, shortness of breath, blurred vision, anginal pain, or dilated pupils.[52] These signs and symptoms could be reflective of activity-limiting orthostasis, neurological aberrations or cardiac abnormalities, warranting additional examination and workup. Mean arterial pressure (MAP) is significant because it measures the pressure necessary for adequate perfusion of the organs of the body and a value of less than 60 mmHg may indicate decreased perfusion.[50]

Line and Lead Management

Within the acute care setting, tubes and lines are common and the Onc R professional must demonstrate proficiency at maintaining the safety and patency of these external devices as a key member of the healthcare team and to ensure patient safety during mobility efforts. Onc R clinicians in other settings must also be versed in the roles and management of these devices as it is not uncommon for these to be present in PWCs who present to other care settings. Common tubes, lines, ports, and catheters might be needed to give cancer treatments, supportive drugs, fluids, blood products, oxygen, and liquid nourishment. Some tubes, lines, ports, and catheters may be used to administer cancer medications, fluids, and blood products. In addition, supplemental oxygen and nutrition are administered by external lines. These lines and tubes may be temporary or permanent depending on the patient's medical status, stage on the treatment continuum, and level of medical fragility. With lines and leads, Onc R clinicians must be vigilant in reviewing what is present and identifying requisite modifications or contraindications to movement-based interventions. Specific to mobility in the acute care setting, gait belts are widely utilized to maintain patient safety and clinician support during the patient encounter and must be implemented with informed consideration of the patient's lines and leads to avoid interfering with medication or supplement administration or vital readings (e.g., positioned inferior to or superior to a patient's access points, with lines and leads unhindered by belt placement). Gait belt placement is a key consideration to avoid entangling or dislodging lines, tubes, and ports. Gait belts should never be placed on or around lines, tubes, or ports and when able, the belt can be positioned superiorly or inferiorly to the line in question.

As medical interventions, lines, leads, and tubes differ with respect to medical acuity and clinical environment, this section is not intended to be a comprehensive list but an overview of relevant and commonly encountered medical devices.

Supplemental Oxygen (O₂)

Several types of O_2 delivery systems are available to administer supplemental O_2 in a healthcare setting. Invasive ventilation modalities include endotracheal/oral or tracheal ventilation. The following O_2 delivery systems are listed in the order from least intensive to most intensive: nasal cannula, high-flow nasal cannula (NC), high-flow high humidity nasal cannula (also known as Vapotherm), face tent, Venturi mask (aka venti mask), nonrebreather (NRB), and noninvasive ventilation that includes BiPAP (bilevel positive airway pressure). Onc R clinicians are instrumental in identifying, modifying, and educating patients and providers alike on situational O_2 needs through the skilled monitoring of vitals and patient response during activity.[50] This information

is often utilized by the care team to prescribe supplemental O_2 and to ensure the patient has adequate resources available upon discharge to their home environment or another care setting. Supplemental O_2 is initiated by physician order and may require titration, an increase or decrease in provided O_2 in liters per minute to maintain adequate oxygenation, during activity. Titration occurs within the parameters of the prescribing physician's order and the patient response at rest and with activity, with examination not limited to the patient's vital signs, subjective symptoms or signs of breathlessness, or dyspnea on exertion. The ability to titrate supplemental oxygen varies by profession, organization, and jurisdiction. Onc R clinicians are advised to review their respective situation, the prescription or order, and the patient's needs before titrating O_2. Generally, supplemental O_2 should be titrated to keep SpO_2 levels above 90% with activity and should be returned to baseline dosages once the activity is completed and the patient's vitals have returned to baseline levels. Variations in this protocol exist and are specific to the patient's medical status. CO_2 retainers, or patients with hypercapnia, represent one such instance whereby special consideration and consultation with the medical team is needed, as increased oxygen supplementation may result in worsened oxygenation, vitals, and patient response to treatment.[53]

Nonspecific signs and symptoms of hypoxemia include dyspnea, breathlessness, palpitations, angina, restlessness, headaches, and tremors. Severe hypoxemia may be marked by confusion, cognitive and motor changes, and lightheadedness, culminating in eventual loss of consciousness. Periodic assessment of the signs and symptoms of hypoxemia are important during physical activity as the ability to continuously monitor oxygen saturation via pulse oximetry regularly may not be feasible.

Dyspnea, difficult breathing, or labored breathing is one of the most common and distressing symptoms of advanced lung cancer and other cancers of the thoracic cavity. In addition to generalized deconditioning and poor cardiorespiratory endurance, postural dysfunction, myopathy, sarcopenia and muscle weakness, and poor positioning in the acute care environment contribute to dyspneic presentations. Underlying lung disease, chronic obstructive pulmonary disorder (COPD) or other pulmonary complications or adverse effects related to oncologic or medical treatments may also contribute to labored breathing in the PWC. To safely optimize the functional ability of the patient, the Onc R clinician must: (1) assure adequate O_2 saturation and appropriate titration of supplemental O_2; (2) discuss safety considerations for mobilization, exercise, and activity interventions; (3) administer appropriate exercise regimens focusing on functional performance; and (4) provide thorough instruction on breathing exercises, energy conservation, and pacing strategies to optimize functional activity tolerance and supplemental O_2 usage and decrease breathlessness.

At times O_2 delivery can be palliative rather than utilized as a treatment. Supplemental O_2, much like rehabilitation intervention, is administered in accordance with the needs of the patient and may be initiated for restorative or supportive means, as noted above, or for palliative means, as needed for patient comfort. As O_2 needs readily change in conjunction with the patient's medical status, O_2 flow, and oxygen delivery systems may fluctuate between treatment sessions. Therefore, a clinician must readily adapt their rehabilitation approach and goals, assess the patient's readiness and appropriateness for therapy, and continuously monitor vital signs, specifically O_2 saturation, in order to maintain patient safety and prescribe the most pertinent interventions specific to the patient's presentation. Secondary to pulmonary compromise and O_2 desaturation, a patient with lung cancer may regress from needing 2 L/minute via nasal cannula one session to subsequently requiring 60% Venturi mask FiO_2; a condition representing a deterioration in patient status and a significant increase in O_2 need. This worsening respiratory status will warrant a re-examination of the patient's functional activity tolerance before a rehabilitation intervention is initiated. Clinical intervention, in this situation, may shift from progressive cardiorespiratory and muscle endurance intervention to tailored education on activity pacing, breathing strategies including pursed lip breathing, and airway clearance techniques as well as utilization and self-monitoring of rating of perceived exertion (RPE).

Implanted Ports

There are a variety of locations and types of central lines (Figure 24.4). Central venous catheters (CVCs) or central lines, narrow, soft tubes generally terminating in a large vein in the thorax, are used widely in oncologic settings for the administration of medications and chemotherapeutic agents in patients with prolonged need for systemic versus venous access. These catheters are more robust than peripheral IVs and are frequently utilized in patients with fragile or hard to find veins. These may be utilized in upper extremity access restrictions as in patients at risk for breast cancer-related lymphedema, and those receiving hyperalimentation therapy (total parenteral nutrition or TPN), which is nourishment delivered via IV that bypasses the digestive system. Many medications and antineoplastic agents damage thin, peripheral veins. Thus, central lines provide a consistent, proximal access point for medical treatment over an extended period of time.

Some kinds of CVCs are implanted ports and peripherally inserted central catheters (PICC). An implanted port is inserted into the large vein near the heart with an access port underneath

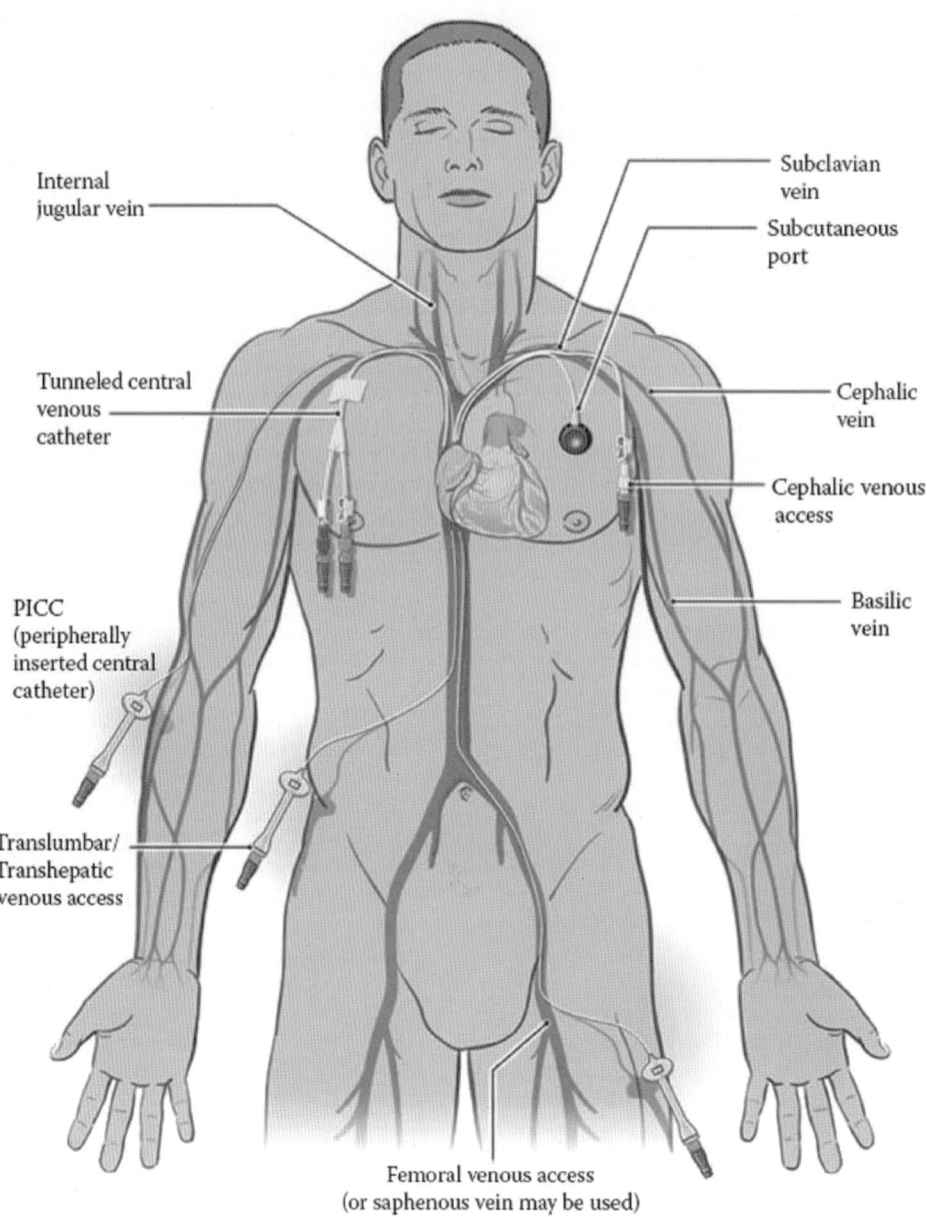

Internal jugular vein

Tunneled central venous catheter

PICC (peripherally inserted central catheter)

Translumbar/ Transhepatic venous access

Subclavian vein

Subcutaneous port

Cephalic vein

Cephalic venous access

Basilic vein

Femoral venous access (or saphenous vein may be used)

• **Fig. 24.4** Examples of Central Venous Access Ports. (Reprinted with permission from Kirby DF, Corrigan ML, Speerhas RA, Emery DM. Home parenteral nutrition tutorial. *J Parenter Enteral Nutr.* 2012;36:632–644. doi:10.1177/0148607112460397.)

the skin. A small bulge is often visible under the skin where the port is located, frequently in the upper chest. Dressings usually cover this port when accessed and care should be taken to avoid pressure or excessive contact over the port. PICC lines are inserted into the arm, often by interventional radiologists, and are threaded through the venous system to terminate in the thorax. The distal aspect of the PICC line remains outside the skin as an access point for delivering medications and fluids. Patients may be on mobility restrictions, including lifting limited to 5 to 10 pounds and limits to repetitive or excessive upper extremity movements. Blood pressure measurement should be performed on the contralateral extremity as indicated.

Urinary Drainage

Closed catheter drainage systems reduce the incidence of bacteriuria and have become a standard of care. Urinary catheters are common in the acute hospital setting but may also be utilized in patients with genitourinary or gynecological cancers as a more long-term solution for physiologic urinary drainage in the setting of anatomical genitourinary compromise. Foley catheters are the most widely used indwelling urinary drainage systems and are inserted through the urethra into the bladder. After insertion, a small balloon is filled with fluid within the bladder to maintain the placement of the device.

A suprapubic catheter is a thin, long sterile tube that is surgically placed in the lower abdomen, superior to the pubic rami, to drain urine from the bladder when patients cannot urinate independently or are not appropriate for indwelling (Foley) catheters. Nephrostomy tubes are utilized in patients with urinary tract obstructions or following cystectomies and are surgically placed to drain urine before it would typically reach the bladder. These may be indicated as a result of disease- or treatment-related sequalae in gastrointestinal or genitourinary cancers. In each instance, urine drains into an exterior bag usually fastened to the patient's upper thigh. Onc R clinicians should note the placement of the catheter bag(s) prior to mobilization to ensure positioning below the level of the bladder, ensuring proper drainage. Condom catheters, those surrounding the penis, or female external catheters (e.g., PrimaFit) may also be utilized in the setting of urinary incontinence, though are not appropriate in the setting of urinary retention given their distal positioning. The PrimaFit is a relatively new device that adheres to the vaginal area with an adhesive and is attached to a suction canister to collect excreted urine. With all peripherally inserted or positioned urinary drainage systems, patients are at increased risk for urinary tract infections. Avoiding excessive tension on the system, as well as promoting regional hygiene is paramount for patient comfort and safety. A major challenge for Onc R professionals during patient mobilization is maintaining the location of these devices. Pending patient status and medical clearance, it may be best to remove external devices prior to mobilization. Strategies to maintain patient safety and a clean environment include having a patient wear an incontinence brief or allowing them to void completely prior to out of bed activity.

Fluid Drainage Tubes

Several drainage tubes may be utilized in PWCs to drain excess fluid that builds up after surgery or as a result of tumor obstruction. A nasogastric (NG) tube can be used if there is a blockage or obstruction in the upper gastrointestinal tract. The NG tube is inserted through the nasal passages and is placed in the stomach or the small intestine to drain excess fluid with suction or to deliver some medications directly to an area. In some cases, the NG tube may be disconnected from wall suction allowing for progressive mobility during rehabilitation efforts; however, the Onc R clinician should consult with the bedside nurse and physician for medical clearance as indicated.

Ostomies, or content diversion procedures, may be utilized in patients with gastrointestinal disease and those with dysfunctional urinary or digestive systems to assist with collecting intestinal fecal material. Onc R clinicians need to be aware of the location of ostomies, stomas, and other abdominal drainage systems to ensure that gait belts, clinician hands, and other supportive devices do not hinder, alter, or compromise system patency with mobility. Onc R clinicians can also work on cleaning and emptying collection containers and set goals for patient and family education while in the acute care setting. Partnership with bedside nurses and wound care specialists is essential in obtaining the requisite resources and ensuring the educational needs for the patient are met. In addition to the cardiorespiratory, musculoskeletal, and neuromuscular benefits of mobility and physical rehabilitation, physical activity, mobility, and skilled exercise intervention serves a key role in encouraging gut peristalsis and gastrointestinal motility.

Jackson-Pratt (JP) drains are frequently encountered soft plastic drainage bulbs that are attached to surgical drainage tubes during a surgical procedure. This drain operates by a self-suction vacuum that is initiated when the bulb is compressed and sealed, thereby creating negative pressure. The associated drainage tubes are secured externally by a surgical stitch, with duration of use often dependent on the type of surgery performed and the amount of drainage present. Patients diagnosed with breast cancer commonly have JP drains following mastectomy. Typically, JP drains are removed once drainage is less than 30 mL of fluid in a 24-hour period. During acute care rehabilitation, common practice is to pin or fasten the JP drain to the patient's gown or clothes to ensure it does not hang or become dislodged with mobilization. In addition to mindfulness regarding drain location and tensioning, clot management is an important component of patient education postoperatively and involves teaching the patient to "milk" the tube, working proximal to distal, to help mobilize clots forming within the tubes. Pending functional cognition and fine motor abilities, patients may require assistance with emptying their drains, though many patients are able to independently manage these devices. Frequent cleaning, skin checks, and emptying of the JP drain are required to prevent infection and promote postoperative recovery. Patients must be educated on signs and symptoms of site infection. These include the following: warmth, pus or discharge, redness, swelling, and tenderness around the incision(s).

Chest tubes are utilized to remove air and fluid from the thoracic cavity in the pleural space, often in the setting of pneumothorax, pleural effusion, hemothorax, empyema, chylothorax, or following cardiothoracic surgery. These collection containers must stay below the site of insertion and should be secured and monitored regularly to prevent spilling or tipping. While the patient is at rest, drains are commonly placed on the floor for gravity-assist with site drainage. In some cases, wall suction will be applied to further assist with drainage. As with a NG tube, it may be permissible to disconnect the device from wall suction temporarily for optimal rehabilitation performance; however, consultation with the nurse or physician is necessary beforehand. If a chest tube reservoir tips over, it should be immediately placed upright, and the levels of the fluid should be checked. The bedside nurse should be informed in order to perform necessary assessments to assure continued proper functioning of the chest tube. Clamping or kinking of the chest tube should be avoided and promptly rectified if noted. Poor patency of a chest tube can lead to insufficient drainage, resulting in tension pneumothorax, excessive cardiac pressure, and ultimately, a mediastinal shift which may be fatal.

Other fluid accumulations may occur prompting the use of more emergent drainage solutions. Malignant pleural effusions (MPE) are abnormal, excessive collections of pleural fluid in pleural space, leading to reduced functional lung volumes, and eventually, impaired air exchange. MPEs represent an untoward complication of cancer and its treatment and are most likely to develop in individuals with advanced lung cancer, breast cancer, and lymphoma. MPEs are associated with a shortened life expectancy.[54] A thoracentesis involves needle aspiration of the pleural cavity and is a common procedure implemented to relieve pressure in the pleural cavity. With symptomatic fluid accumulations, thoracenteses may result in immediate improvement in dyspnea and resting and exercise aerobic capacity. Treatment of MPEs is typically palliative and most MPEs do not respond to systemic therapy. In order to control pleural effusions and avoid excessive thoracentesis, a PleurX drainage catheter can be placed. This drainage catheter is inserted surgically in the chest to address pleural effusions or in the abdomen to address malignant ascites. Patient and family training of PleurX use is warranted in the acute setting as patients may be discharged with a PleurX due to its small size and ease of use. As with a chest tube, PleurX position must be considered prior to gait belt placement. Pending body habitus and insertion site, the gait belt frequently is placed superior to the insertion point of the PleurX catheter. As an essential component of rehabilitation, thorough education on proper breathing techniques is important to optimize airway exchange and promote safe exercise progression. Incentive spirometers and postural awareness strategies are often employed as interventions by Onc R clinicians to assist in chest wall expansion and lung aeration within patient tolerance.

Similarly, malignant ascites are collections of abnormal, excessive fluid within the abdominal cavity. Malignant ascites are a sign of advanced cancer and represent an overall poor prognosis. Abdominal distension in the setting of ascites is often accompanied by decline in QOL. Supportive treatments are often employed to reduce the burden of fluid accumulation. Ascites may be drained by paracentesis, percutaneously implanted catheters (CVC), peritoneal ports, or peritoneovenous shunts.[55] To reduce the impact of symptoms associated with abdominal ascites, the rehabilitation team can offer education to facilitate optimal bowel and bladder function and breathing strategies to promote relaxation and pain management. Educational topics may include positioning for bowel movements, colonic massage, benefits of mobility, and hydration/nutrition guidelines. Diaphragm position and function may be adversely impacted by abdominal distension. Diaphragmatic breathing and other breathing strategies are beneficial in maximizing lung volumes and reducing thoracic cage and abdominal discomfort associated with distension, constipation, and immobility. Pending the patient's presentation, pain management status and symptoms, it may be necessary to delay or modify rehabilitation interventions until the ascites are reduced or pain is managed.

Nutritional Support

Nutritional status and maintenance of adequate intake are instrumental in prognosis, treatment, and activity tolerance, and often, QOL in PWCs. Medications, treatment options, tumor bulk and location, and dysgeusia or loss of taste can impair a person's ability and willingness to eat and maintain the nutrition that is needed to optimize healing and recovery along the cancer continuum. In patients with difficulty maintaining adequate intake or those with dysphagia, conversion to liquid medicines or parenteral feedings may be beneficial or necessary. Liquid nutrition may be administered through NG tubes or other aforementioned access devices and are often termed tube feedings, a usually temporary form of nutritional support. If supplemental nutrition is needed for a longer period of time, a tube or access site will be surgically placed through the abdominal wall directly into the stomach called a gastrostomy tube or G tube. It may also be placed in the small intestine and thus termed a jejunostomy tube, or J tube. Percutaneous endoscopic gastrostomy (PEG) tubes and percutaneous endoscopic jejunostomy (PEJ) tubes may erroneously be referenced interchangeably as "PEG tubes" as, exteriorly, they appear the same. However, each access method possesses unique roles and uses for the benefit of the patient. Skin checks around the PEG/PEJ tube, ensuring proper flushing, and site cleaning need to be performed routinely. Gait belt placement must be superior to the site to ensure surgically inserted feeding tubes are not dislodged or compromised. With nursing guidance and medical clearance, common practice is to pause feeding tube delivery machines if the patient must lay supine to reduce the risk of aspiration.

The use of TPN in persons with advanced disease or terminal illness is controversial in many settings.[56] Malnutrition, a common manifestation in patients with cancer, often presents with loss of appetite and ineffective utilization of nutrients. Many PWCs develop cachexia, a syndrome of bodily wasting, as a result of poor caloric and nutritional intake and increased metabolic requirements due to the disease process. Presently, the guidelines for the use of TPN include: (1) patients who cannot eat or cannot use their gastrointestinal tract and who have reasonable life expectancy; (2) malnourished patients who cannot eat or cannot use their gastrointestinal tract who are undergoing surgery, chemotherapy, or radiation therapy; and (3) malnourished patients in whom severe gastrointestinal or treatment toxicity preclude adequate enteral intake.[57]

Central Nervous System (CNS) Access

Many chemotherapeutic agents and medications do not cross the blood–brain barrier (BBB) with conventional administration devices. As such, access to the CNS is pivotal for the successful management of a variety of oncologic processes. An Ommaya reservoir is a synthetic dome surgically placed beneath the scalp that is attached to a catheter inserted into an intracranial ventricle. The purpose of the Ommaya reservoir is to deliver medication, including antibiotics or chemotherapy drugs, directly into the CSF. This method is effective in the management of certain types of brain cancer as well as for CNS prophylaxis in subtypes of leukemia and lymphoma. With an Ommaya reservoir, chemotherapy is delivered directly to the CSF to attack malignant cells in the area, thereby bypassing the BBB. In addition, an Ommaya reservoir may be used for diagnostic workup to collect samples of CSF to further examine for the presence of infection or cancerous cells. Beyond noting its presence and purpose, an Ommaya reservoir generally has very little impact on a therapy session. See Chapter 5 for more information and an image of the Ommaya reservoir.

An external ventriculostomy device (ventric) is a drain or shunt in the CNS that drains CSF and is also used to measure intracranial pressure (ICP). A ventric is common in those with hydrocephalus caused by malignant brain lesions, subarachnoid hemorrhage, and infection. Metastatic disease in the periventricular brain tissue can obstruct the flow of CSF throughout the CNS, including the subarachnoid space, resulting in obstructive or noncommunicating hydrocephalus, which may induce neurological changes not limited to altered mental status, severe headaches, nausea, vomiting, and possibly, impaired functional mobility. Shah et al. demonstrated that therapy intervention in patients with a ventriculostomy was safe and feasible.[58] Partnership with bedside nursing is key in ventric management as clamping the device and navigating positioning restrictions is necessary prior to initiating physical mobility. Once the treatment session is completed, additional coordination and follow-up with the bedside nurse will be necessary to restore function to the ventric.[58]

Pain Management

Pain management is vital in PWCs as pain represents one of the most common symptoms patients encounter along the cancer continuum. This section will explore the medical interventions utilized in the treatment of cancer-related pain that are unique to the acute setting. A thorough understanding of these devices and their implications is paramount for the Onc R clinician to best optimize their unique skills in conservative, nonpharmacologic pain management strategies. Common pain management systems implemented in PWCs include patient-controlled analgesia (PCA) device, peripheral nerve blocks, and epidural steroid injection (ESI). A PCA is a method of pain control that gives alert and oriented patients the ability to control their pain within established parameters. With a PCA, the medical team sets an amount of medication that can be released with each dose. Utilizing an IV or other venous access point, the patient, and only the patient, may administer the dose through pushing a button located at the bedside. These pumps are used for patients with significant cancer-related, postsurgical, or other pain.

A peripheral nerve block can be delivered by a catheter to a painful peripheral nerve to anaesthetize and reduce the painful sensation. This can be delivered by a medication delivery device and can also be provided for short-term relief by a direct anesthetic injection. Care must be taken with nerve blocks to ensure patient safety and promote rehabilitation tolerance, as the sensory threshold used to target or control pain may inadvertently affect the motor nerves, thereby increasing weakness and resulting in a fall.

In the event that subacute or chronic pain is not well controlled, an intrathecal (IT) drug delivery system may be recommended. Oral or intravenous administration of medications does not pass the BBB. IT drug delivery delivers medication directly into the IT space of the spinal column for immediate bioavailability to target tissues. These may be delivered via programmable pumps, either implanted or external.[59] A pain management team is able to monitor the device and can adjust dosages through program alterations, independent of the location of the device. During mobility and positioning or repositioning, care should be taken to minimize pressure around the device and the affected area and potentially noxious stimuli should be removed from the affected area as a blunted pain response is inherent in IT pain management. IT therapy can improve pain management and function in patients whose pain is not well controlled with conventional pain medications including opioids.[60]

Key implications for Onc R clinicians working with PWCs and navigating these pain management devices include gait belt placement, skilled line and lead management during mobility, and maintenance of pain management regimen prior to and during mobilization to ensure treatment efficacy and promote patient

tolerance for intervention. Of note, many patients may request assistance with utilizing and pressing the button for PCAs; however, Onc R clinicians must ensure patients are the only ones administering the medication when pain is present to ensure patient safety and adequate medication dosing.

An ESI is the delivery of anti-inflammatory medicine directly into the epidural space surrounding the spinal cord. Some PWCs may find benefit from an ESI for chronic pain. These injections can be used for cancers that press on the spine such as liver, breast, colon, kidney, and pancreas.

Physical Assessments and Selected Interventions in the Inpatient Setting

Physical Assessments

Physical assessments are performance-based outcome measurements used to determine the patient's functional limitations/deficits and guide treatment interventions. These objective tests provide a baseline level of function, track changes throughout the course of care as a result of therapeutic interventions, assist with discharge planning, and provide a standardized approach to quantifying clinically important changes in a patient's status. These outcome measures also inform treatment and prognostic decisions as well as goals of care.

LOS, baseline functional performance, and medical treatment in the acute care setting can vary depending on the level of impairment and medical status of the patient, requiring the Onc R clinician to carefully choose the appropriate test(s) to capture and track the PWC's performance status with respect to oncologic treatment and rehabilitation intervention. The Academy of Oncologic Physical Therapy publishes and updates guidelines for utilization of outcomes for PWCs.[61] See Table 24.4 for a summary of valid and reliable tests and measures that can be used in the acute care setting—taking into consideration patient's status, abilities, time to perform, and equipment needed to perform.

Patient-reported outcome measures are utilized to capture the subjective patient experience and help define the extent of patient-specific experiences regarding fatigue during an activity, and QOL. The EDGE Task Force highly recommended the following for Fatigue: Modified Brief Fatigue Inventory (mBFI), Cancer-Related Fatigue Distress Scale, 10-point Rating Scale for Fatigue, and the Multidimensional Fatigue Symptom Inventory.[61]

Assistive Devices and Durable Medical Equipment Assessment and Interventions

A frequently necessary intervention for a PWC is the prescription and utilization of durable medical equipment (DME) to assist with mobility, performing ADLs, or patient safety or comfort. Often, it is in the acute care setting where a patient is first introduced to an assistive device for safe transfers or ambulation. The PT may be the first to provide a recommendation for an assistive device to enhance mobility and mitigate fall risk. This may necessitate close coordination with the OT, as the OT will assist in skill transference and device utilization to facilitate patient performance of ADLs and self-care tasks. Common ambulatory aids utilized for gait training in an acute care setting include walkers (standard, hemiwalkers, pyramid canes, walkers with platform attachments, rolling including two-wheeled and 4-wheeled seated), canes (standard, quad canes including large-base and small base), crutches (axillary, Lofstrand/

			Functional Ability**		
Outcome Measure	**Clinical Relevance**	**EDGE Recommendation*[61]**	**Low**	**Moderate**	**High**
Short Physical Performance Battery (includes 3 or 4 meter walk test, 10 second standing in 3 different positions and 5 times sit to stand)	Proxy measure of overall health and function	Highly Recommend		X	X
10 Meter Walk Test	Proxy measure of overall health and function	Highly Recommend		X	X
6 Minute Walk Test	Walking distance and cardiopulmonary endurance	Highly Recommend		X	X
5 Times Sit to Stand	Fall risk	Highly Recommend		X	X
30 Second Sit to Stand	Lower extremity strength and endurance	Recommended as Reasonable to Use		X	X
AMPAC 6-Clicks	Prediction of destination of discharge	Recommended	X	X	X
Balance Evaluation Systems Test	Static and dynamic balance	Recommended		X	X
Berg Balance Scale	Static and dynamic balance	Recommended as Reasonable to Use		X	X
Fullerton Advanced Balance Scale	Static and dynamic balance	Highly Recommended		X	X
Function in Sitting Test	Sitting balance	Not assessed	X		
Functional Status Score-ICU	Improvements in ICU setting	Not assessed	X	X	
Tinetti Balance and Gait Assessment	Fall risk	Recommended as Reasonable to Use		X	X
Timed Up & Go	Fall risk	Highly Recommended		X	X

TABLE 24.4   Performance-Based Outcome Measures Applicable in the Acute Care Setting

AMPAC, activity measure for post-acute care; *ICU*, intensive care unit.

*Some EDGE recommendations are for specific cancer types or symptoms and may not be specifically validated in the acute care setting.

**Author's experiential recommendations.

Created by Courtney Witczak, Grace Burns, and Cynthia Barbe. Printed with permission.

forearm), pneumatic support walkers (PSW), thoracic walkers, and wheelchairs (manual and power). While assistive devices may increase energy expenditure and the functional cognitive burden for the PWC, risks and benefits must be considered in order to optimize patient independence and reduce caregiver burden both in the acute care setting and with subsequent discharge. Regular assessment of a patient's functional status and supportive need is recommended to ensure the appropriate device is prescribed as a patient progresses or declines along the disease trajectory and during the hospital stay.

In addition, orthoses and prostheses are important to consider in assuring functional mobility, safety, and comfort. In the inpatient setting, administrative and medical challenges may hinder coordination, access, acquisition and fit of a prosthesis or orthosis, including wound and skin integrity. Prostheses may be utilized to improve or support functional mobility, QOL, and aesthetics and positive body images.[62] Limb prostheses include leg, arm, hand, and foot with the nature of use dependent on the location, level of impairment, prior level of function, potential to return to a more advanced level of function, patient's acuity, and the type of cancer. A range of devices, prosthetics, and orthotics must be considered from posterior leaf spring ankle-foot orthoses to lower limb prothesis with dynamic, microprocessor joint components. In addition, laryngeal prostheses can be utilized when the larynx, or voice box, is removed with a laryngectomy. These electronic devices help restore speech. Ocular prostheses can be utilized in the loss of an eye for PWCs with ocular melanoma, ocular lymphoma, and retinoblastoma.[62]

Helmets are employed in the acute neurologic setting to provide enhanced protection to the cranium in patients following a surgical intervention on the brain. Tumor resections requiring a craniectomy may necessitate wearing a helmet to prevent cerebral injury, as structural and anatomic integrity is disrupted when a bone flap is removed to manage cerebral edema or promote improve access. If external protection is prescribed, the rigid or semi-rigid helmet should be donned when performing functional mobility, self-care, ADLs, and rehabilitation activities.

Safety is key in ensuring that PWCs remain as functionally independent as possible as they near discharge from the acute setting. As such, assistive device management is a chief priority for the rehabilitation team. Acute care Onc R clinicians are responsible for training and educating patients on all mobility devices with the aim of preparing the patient for their anticipated discharge disposition. Each DME should be precisely chosen to enhance the long-term functional independence of the patient. Typically, insurance covers one new ambulatory or mobility device every 5 years, therefore it is imperative the clinician appropriately selects the device based on the current needs of the patient as well as the anticipated needs of the patient and family upon returning home. For example, if a patient diagnosed with advanced cancer, and a projected lifespan of approximately 1 to 2 months, is expected to experience further functional decline, procuring a rolling walker, or other least restrictive mobility device, based on their current mobility status may not be prudent, considering they may necessitate greater levels of assistance with mobility in the coming days to weeks. In this instance, the DME focus may need to shift toward more supportive DME (e.g., bedside commode, hospital bed, or manual wheelchair) to allow for decreased caregiver burden and optimization of patient and caregiver safety. Encompassing the present and future needs of the patient and family is paramount, but feasibility of clinician recommendations must be weighed. Home access and navigation is another important consideration and may include a recommendation for a wheelchair ramp if a wheelchair is prescribed. Engaging with a discharge planner, case manager, or social worker will help ensure needs are met, recommendations are carried through, and needed equipment or home modifications are completed. In end-of-life situations, home modifications requiring a substantial amount of time or financial investment may not be feasible or practical. Assessing the impact of DME recommendations, the feasibility and investment required, as well as the timeframe and patient prognosis are key components to informed care.

Assessment for Assistive Devices (AD) and DME

Prior to determining the appropriate AD and DME to be used for ambulation, a comprehensive mobility and balance assessment needs to be performed to ensure that the patient utilizes the device properly after discharge. Static and dynamic balance in sitting and standing should be screened to establish risk of falls and to provide a foundation for intervention. A history of cancer and its treatments can increase fall risk at any age. Many factors of cancer affect a patient's balance such as fatigue, weakness, neuropathy, and vision or vestibular impairments.[63] Older adults diagnosed with cancer have a higher risk of falls and may be predisposed to other serious injuries as a result of a fall. Many patients report having difficulty walking during treatments such as chemotherapy. Maintaining balance is a complex process that involves multiple body systems which can be affected by cancer treatments. Various domains of postural control, including base of support configuration, postural alignment, lower extremity muscle strength, stability limits, anticipatory and reactive responses, sensory integration, stability during walking, and dual-task walking, are important factors in the maintenance of balance. Motor learning and motor control also are key components necessary in the maintenance of independence with transitional movements. Evidence-based outcome measures such as the Timed Up and Go (TUG) and the short physical performance battery are quick, easy, and valid assessments to utilize with PWCs in the acute care setting to assess balance and fall risk.[61] These risk factors, when known, provide a foundation for patient education regarding home and community safety, as well as inform possible interventions ranging from cardiorespiratory endurance to gait on even and uneven terrains, and possibly vestibular rehabilitation.[64,65]

In addition to static and standing balance assessments, comprehensive physical assessments of PWCs in the acute care setting call for a neurological assessment of sensation as neurotoxic chemotherapeutic agents, like plant alkaloids (taxanes and vinca alkaloids) and platinum-based compounds, used to treat cancer damage peripheral nerves causing chemotherapy-induced polyneuropathy (CIPN).[66] CIPN can present as numbness and tingling, pain, weakness, changes in temperature, or cramping in the hands or feet. CIPN can cause severe pain with movement and ADL performance. The duration of CIPN varies between patients with some cases resolving in a few months to others with long term or permanent impairments. If neuropathic pain is too high, systemic issues may arise including an increased heart rate, increased blood pressure, falls, and difficulty breathing. Onc R clinicians should perform a brief screen of sensory integrity and if impairments are noted, standard evaluation by the use of monofilaments is recommended, with the inability to detect a 5.07 monofilament at 1 or more sites indicative of a loss of protective sensation.[67]

Pain Assessment and Interventions

Pain assessments are important for all patients while hospitalized, and especially important in PWCs. According to a recent meta-analysis, pain is reported in 59% of patients undergoing cancer treatment, in 64% of patients with advanced disease, and in 33% of patients after curative treatment.[68] While hospitalized, patients may experience pain in various scenarios. It is important to consider pain in terms of etiology (e.g., disease-related, treatment-related, or noncancerous source of pain) in order to determine the most effective interventions to treat the pain. Most commonly, patients experience postsurgical pain, chemotherapy-related pain, or pain associated with end of life.

Interventions for postsurgical pain include education for patients regarding postsurgical restrictions, bed mobility, positioning, and breathing. PTs and OTs are skilled in the treatment and management of acute and postoperative pain. Education specific to the analgesic effects of tailored and gradual aerobic activity, as well as evidenced-based education on the use of biophysical agents (modalities) and other topical pain-relievers may be beneficial. Advocating for mobility early in the postoperative period, with surgeon guidance and clearance is foundational in establishing a positive relationship with mobility and exercise, as fear of movement and fear of falls are inadvertently associated with increased risks of falls and injurious falls.

Chronic pain is more challenging to address with many factors contributing to a patient's pain presentation. In some cases, a person may have unresolved pain from a preexisting condition that may become exacerbated from cancer treatment or stress. A skilled differential diagnosis using imaging, history, and evaluation techniques, such as provocation-alleviation testing, may inform the clinician's approach to intervention. Chronic pain requires a well-informed biopsychosocial approach to care, considering the psychological, diagnosis-specific, biomechanical, and neuromusculoskeletal components of the patient's pain. While flexibility tasks, soft tissue mobilization, or positioning strategies may alleviate or reduce pain in the acute setting, cognitive behavioral approaches, including cognitive reframing and strategies to promote self-management and patient autonomy, are often cornerstones in the management of chronic and persistent pain presentations. See Chapter 22 for additional considerations related to pain management.

Pain Assessment

In order to establish an effective plan of care to address complex pain, it is imperative to have a thorough understanding of the patient's source and extent of pain.[69] If pain is nociceptive, the treatment plan is targeted at the symptomatic tissue. Neuropathic pain may require inhibition techniques or neuromuscular reeducation targeted at the pain pathway. If upon examination, it is determined that the patient's pain has a psychogenic or nociplastic component, cognitive reframing and pain neuroscience education and resources may prove beneficial. Often pain is a result of mixed pathophysiology and generally diaphragmatic breathing is a beneficial first step. Upon initiation of rehabilitation, a comprehensive pain assessment is necessary, specifically as it relates to function. The APTA Oncology EDGE Task Force highly recommends the McGill Pain Questionnaire–short form, numeric rating scale, visual analog scale and recommends the brief pain inventory, brief pain inventory–short form, McGill Pain Questionnaire, and the pain disability index.[61] If pain is a barrier to the most basic of functions, the patient will be unable to be successful at the next level of care. Education provided to the patient on the benefits of activity or exercise in terms of tissue mobility or endorphin release may be enough to allow a patient to participate in therapy when pain may have otherwise been a prohibiting factor.

It is important to recognize atypical pain presentations that may be indicative of referred pain or signs of progressing disease. Examples include back pain with neurological signs indicating possible spinal cord involvement or new onset of pain with weightbearing that could indicate bone metastases. In cases where new metastases are discovered, further discussion should occur with the medical team regarding possible radiographic studies or protective weight bearing strategies.

Postural assessment often provides information on the patient's pain as well. If primarily confined to bed, a PWC may have posture and positioning needs that may benefit from the use of pillows, wedges, or ankle-foot orthotic devices to reduce pain, as well as prevent pressure ulcers or contractures. Seating postural assessments may result in lumbar or head support in addition to initiation of an exercise program. Manual facilitation to optimize seated posture may dramatically improve respiratory or cognitive status as well. Finally, standing posture may be impacted by lack of mobility including tight pectoral muscles, hip flexors, hamstrings, or gastrocnemius soleus muscles. A postsurgical patient may benefit from manual facilitation and neuromuscular reeducation to progress toward their presurgical posture.

If pain, posture, or any other impairment is likely to prevent a hospitalized PWC from completing their ADLs, an OT can utilize their knowledge and skillset to facilitate performance of these tasks. While many disciplines can positively impact a patient's emotional well-being, occupational therapy may be the link to providing the patient the fastest route to independence in the safest manner. Coordination between rehabilitation services will assist in prioritizing short-term goals for safety and social-emotional well-being by facilitating progression to the next level of care.

Integumentary and Wound Assessment and Intervention

Depending on each individual's functional mobility and activity capabilities, in conjunction with any cancer treatment history and consideration of medical status, skin and wound inspections should be performed with each treatment session. The most common scale used for pressure ulcer risk is the Braden Scale.[70] The following should be noted: discoloration of the skin, integrity of the skin (e.g., supple, firm, fibrotic, the presence or absence of hair, shine, flakiness), presence and quality of any swelling (e.g., fluctuating, firm, pitting, bogginess), wrinkles, bruising, scarring, surgical incisions, and/or reddened pressure points (occiput, scapulae, spinal processes, elbows, sacrum, heels, ears, greater trochanters, iliac crests, condyles, and malleoli). Based on any findings, interventions can be implemented to prevent decubiti and infections such as positioning and/or pressure redistribution. Education should also be provided to the client, family members, and care team such as performing self-assessments, moisturizing for skin care, using electric razors, and avoiding needle sticks (blood draws or administration of medications) on affected limbs, as able.

For some individuals who have limited ability to self-position or perform physical mobility, a turning schedule may be necessary with the assistance of the healthcare team. This involves turning the patient at designated intervals, typically every 2 hours, onto each side and supine, as well as elevating extremities to assist with pressure relief and edema. Care should be taken to avoid friction and shear forces when re-positioning individuals, as these forces can lead to skin breakdown and perhaps infection. Several external positioning devices are available, and can be classified as soft, firm, or rigid. Soft devices include hospital pillows, towel rolls, and elbow/heel protectors. Firm devices include gel pillows, foam wedges, elbow/knee immobilizers (medial and lateral support), certain ankle-foot orthoses (medial and lateral support to achieve dorsiflexion), and seizure pads. Finally, rigid positioning devices include ankle-foot orthoses with a metal posterior upright which offloads the heel (commonly called multi-podus boots) as well as custom thermoplastic splints. For those individuals requiring pressure redistribution, specialty beds may be provided to simulate their body being immersed in a fluid medium, as well as turn assist mattresses for re-positioning of the clients. Individuals are at risk for delayed wound healing due to low blood counts, fevers, decreased nutrition, changes in functional status and cognition, and overall medical status.

Edema and Lymphedema Management

There are instances where the IDT will consult a PT or OT for lymphedema evaluation and treatment in the acute care setting. Treating lymphedema is a specialized skill, requiring advanced training and certification. However, this does not preclude acute care Onc R clinicians from proactively screening their patients for lymphedema and other edematous pathologies or presentations. While the principles of protection, rest, elevation, ice, compression, and exercise (PRICE) are utilized in the management of postoperative and edematous conditions, lymphedema represents a distinct pathology of the lymphatic system, resulting in a protein-rich fluid accumulation, often leading to reactive fibrosis and inflammation and necessitating a distinct approach to treatment. Typically, lymphedema is unilateral and demonstrated varying degrees of pitting, associated with a cancer diagnosis and treatment effects (radiation, lymph node removal, surgery), has a positive Stemmer's sign (Figure 24.5), and presents with feelings of heaviness or fullness, poor fitting clothing or jewelry, and skin changes, including hypomobility and thickness. While some edema may be reduced, lymphedema is often not responsive to diuretic medication. In contrast, systemic or generalized edema may be bilateral, fluctuating, and often decreases with elevation and/or diuretics. Management of lymphedema involves a comprehensive approach termed complete decongestive therapy or CDT. The components of CDT include skin care and hygiene, manual lymphatic drainage, compression garments or bandaging as indicated, and exercise prescriptions. Manual lymphatic drainage is the skilled, gentle manipulation of the patient's skin in a specific sequence to facilitate the natural drainage of lymph fluid out of the edematous area. A variety of compression garments and stockings may be employed and are specific to the patient's presentation, skin integrity and tolerance to wear. Skilled exercise intervention in patients with edematous conditions may be specific to promoting peripheral circulation in an edematous limb, strengthening proximal muscle groups to assist in extremity function and posturing, and/or enhancing aerobic capacity through repetitive, cyclical motions. Addressing barriers to mobility and optimizing the patient's tolerance for and engagement

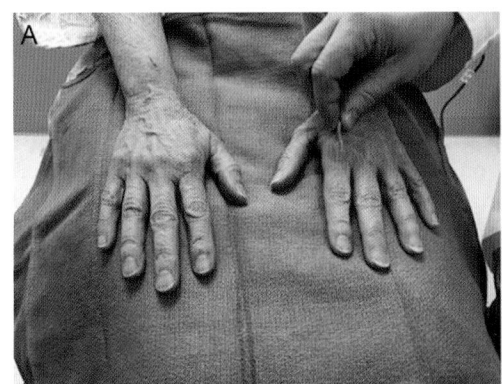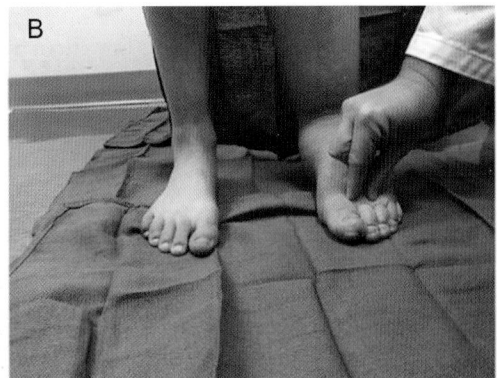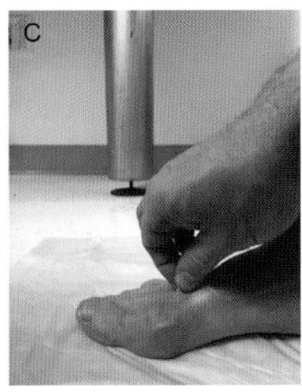

• **Fig. 24.5** Stemmer Sign Result Examples. **A.** True-negative Stemmer sign (examiner is able to pinch the skin in a patient without lymphedema). **B.** True-positive Stemmer sign (skin is unable to be pinched in an individual with lymphedema). **C.** False-negative Stemmer sign (the skin is able to be pinched in a subject with lymphedema). (Reprinted with permission from Goss JA, Greene AK. Sensitivity and specificity of the stemmer sign for lymphedema: a clinical lymphoscintigraphic study. *Plast Reconstr Surg Glob Open*. 2019;7(6):e2295.)

with exercise should be prioritized. Reducing a patient's risk for infection and edema exacerbation is fundamental in the long-term successful management of lymphedema.

Compression and supportive garments are common amongst those with cancer, especially as it relates to lymphedema, and may include variations in bandages and garments or stockings. The pressure provided by external support or compression softens indurated tissue and assists the innate muscle pump of the patient's extremities, thus facilitating the proximal return of fluid out of the edematous limb. Screening is performed and treatment may be initiated in the acute setting; however, challenges to initiating a comprehensive lymphatic treatment in the acute or inpatient setting exist, including cost and definitive diagnosis of lymphedema. Efficiency can be improved by coordinating with nursing to have supplies at the bedside or by asking family to bring lymphedema wraps to the bedside if the patient has been wrapped in the past.

In acute care, patients exhibit a wide variety of medical conditions that may mimic lymphedema to the untrained eye. Establishing an accurate diagnosis is key in successful edema management as treatment will differ pending the cause of the edematous condition. Some of these conditions, including congestive heart failure, renal insufficiency, and cellulitis or other active infection can be exacerbated by compression and decongestive therapy if not properly implemented. Where precautions or relative contraindications stand, not limited to the presence of acute infection, respiratory distress, or congestive heart failure, a clear discussion with a referring provider, including a risk-benefit analysis, should be initiated before beginning therapy. Successful management of lymphedema is predicated on the establishment of self-management strategies and patient diligence in their home program. Given the chronic, persistent nature of lymphedema and the need for lifelong management, education must reflect the importance of patient independence in CDT treatment. Partnership between the acute clinician and the receiving outpatient clinician should be priority to assist in a seamless transition and continuation of skilled management of edema in the outpatient setting. See Chapter 9 for additional insight into lymphedema management.

Scrotal and genital edema can often be a painful barrier to mobility in genitourinary cancers, including renal cell carcinoma. This problem is often treated medically with diuretics depending on the initial cause of the edema. A supportive garment or

simply a support sling with pillowcases may help with positioning in bed. Body-assist scrotal supporters can be ordered or a stockinette converted to a sling may be utilized as a softer, more convenient option. Patient comfort and consent may dictate the level of assessment and intervention, however, with consent, supportive treatment is often well tolerated and successful in mitigating symptoms associated with scrotal and genital edema.

Safe Patient Handling and Mobility (SPHM)

Patient handling and mobilization activities in acute care hospitals are fundamental aspects of patient care and rehabilitation. The concepts and equipment utilized to assure safe mobility in acutely ill individuals are termed SPHM. Generally, SPHM is considered to be the liberal application of mechanical lifts and standing frames in the acute setting but ultimately it represents the comprehensive approach to patient safety and mobility by all healthcare team members with associated training, policies, and procedures. Hands-on instruction to the patient and family is critical in preventing injury and decreasing risk to the patient while mobilizing in a hospital setting. Safe patient handling equipment can aid Onc R clinicians to assist a patient with their personal mobility as well as to optimize safety and trust with necessary rehabilitation techniques.

Early and frequent patient mobilization can assist in maintaining patient hygiene, preventing physical deconditioning, and reducing serious complications of immobility in the PWC. The Onc R clinician should consider physical characteristics such as the patient's weight, level of functioning, weight-bearing status, and the patient's physical status, not limited to fatigue, balance, tone, joint issues, posture, and strength in their decision-making. The presence of wounds, surgeries, lines, and leads also needs to be considered when selecting the piece of SPHM equipment that is best for the patient.[71] Cachexic or deconditioned PWCs may require increased levels of assistance initially for safe out of bed mobility. Family training on various types of equipment can be performed to assist the patient and family in returning home by facilitating supported functional independence.

Needham described the importance of "early mobilization" as a critical component of patient care in ICUs that emphasize early physical medicine and rehabilitation.[71] Early mobilization is quickly becoming standard of practice and is usually started as soon as a patient is physiologically stable enough to tolerate mobility. This may include progressive transfers, bed mobility, standing, in bed exercises, getting into a chair, and walking.[72] Pending institutional protocols and patient-specific considerations, these activities may be performed while the patient is on a ventilator or other external devices. In these and other situations of high patient acuity, close collaboration and monitoring by the interdisciplinary ICU team is paramount. Neuromuscular complications after critical illness are common and can be severe and persistent.[72] Items such as an upper and lower body cycle exerciser (MOTOmed), tilt table (Figure 24.6), and stretcher chairs (Moveo XP, Barton chair [Figure 24.7]) are common pieces of equipment utilized in the ICU for mobility and are applicable to PWCs who do not exhibit contraindications to these devices. In addition, simply positioning the ICU

bed in a chair position is an excellent way to start encouraging upright activity after critical illness after cancer. Cycle ergometers were designed to be applied within the ICU setting and can be used sitting in a wheelchair or chair or lying supine in bed. Neuromuscular electrical stimulation therapy creates passive contraction of muscles through low-voltage electrical impulses delivered through skin electrodes placed over target muscles (Figure 24.8).

The partnership between SPHM techniques with proper ergonomics and the proper equipment can maximize mobility by reducing risk. Patients requiring two-person assistance or dependent care, including at end of life or in the ICU, can benefit from devices such as mechanical patient lifts and inflatable lateral transfer pads (e.g., Hovermatt, Air Pal) (Figure 24.9). For example, a patient with a new spinal cord compression as a result of metastatic prostate cancer may have difficulties transferring out of bed if the patient is unable to transfer on a slide board due to poor trunk control.[73] In order to increase out of bed sitting time in a wheelchair or stretcher chair (e.g., Moveo XP, Barton chair) be facilitated by the PWC being transferred from bed to chair with an electronic mechanical lift (Figure 24.10) or an inflatable lateral transfer pad.

Patients with cancer experiencing low muscular endurance and/or rapid onset of fatigue may also benefit from standing devices to perform assisted transfers and gradually increase standing duration and tolerance. As both devices require weight bearing through the tibias and femurs, patients with weight bearing restrictions, lower extremity fractures, or extensive lower extremity metastases may not be candidates for these devices. A nonmechanical standing aid (Arjo Stedy) facilitates upright semi-standing and has a seat

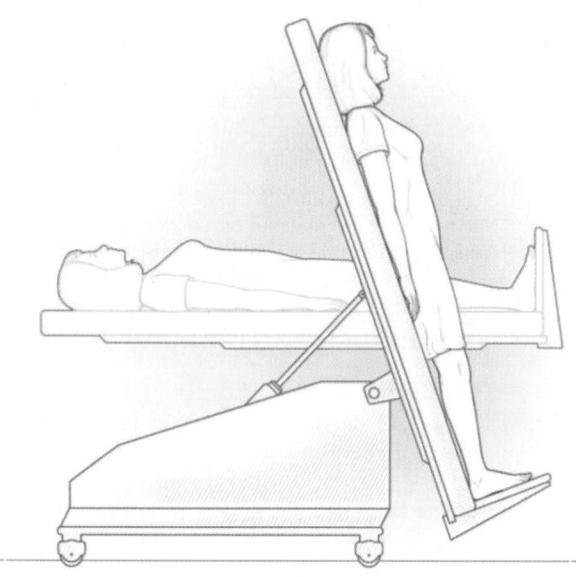

• **Fig. 24.6** Tilt Table. (Reprinted with permission from Cronin H, Anne Kenny R. Cardiac causes for falls and their treatment. *Clin Geriat Med.* 2010;26(4):539–567.)

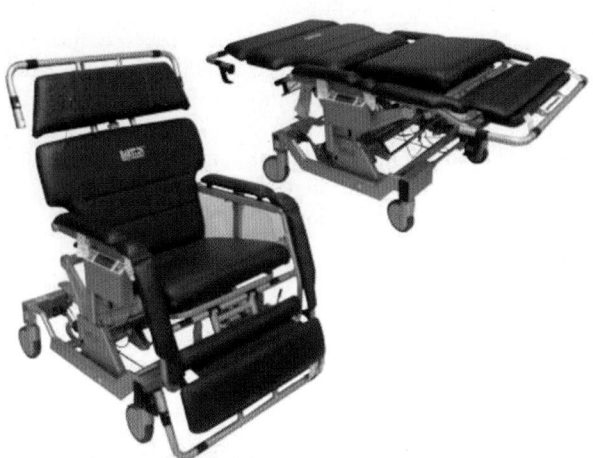

• **Fig. 24.7** Stretcher Chair. (Courtesy of Arjo Inc.)

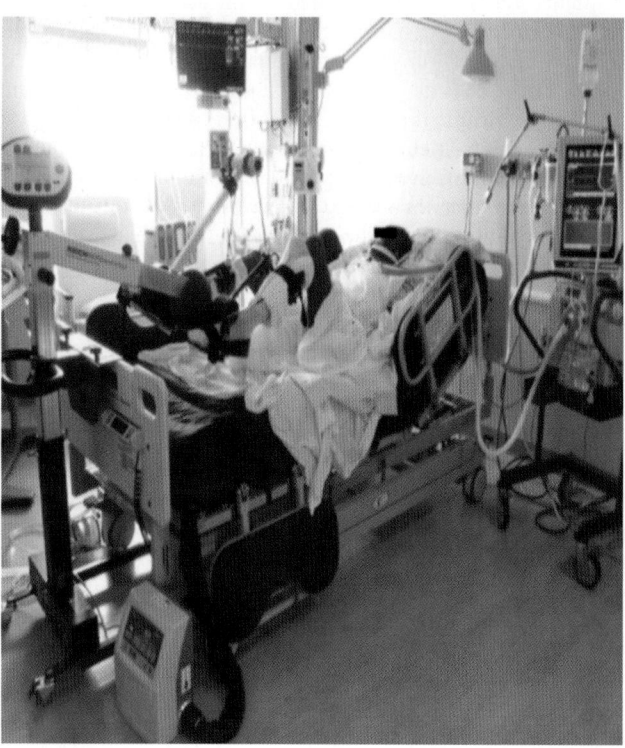

• **Fig. 24.8** Example of Patient Receiving Mechanical Ventilation and In-Bed Cycling in the ICU. (Reprinted with permission from Kho ME, Martin RA, Toonstra AL, et al. Feasibility and safety of in-bed cycling for physical rehabilitation in the intensive care unit. *J Crit Care.* 2015;30(6):1419.e1–e5.)

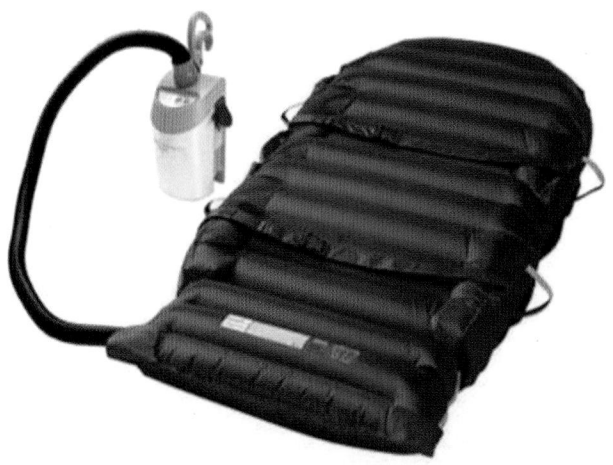

• **Fig. 24.9** Inflatable Lateral Transfer Mat. (Courtesy of Arjo, Inc.)

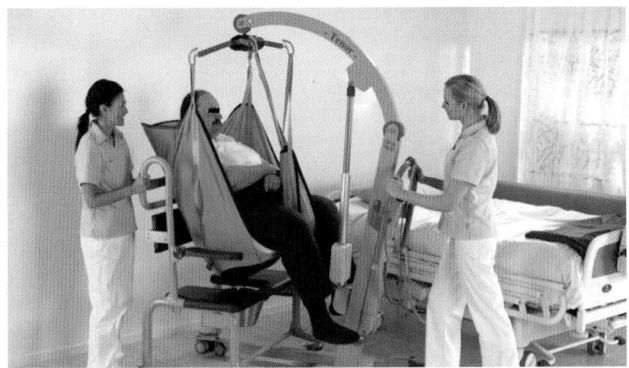

• **Fig. 24.10** Mechanical Bariatric Dependent Lift System. (Courtesy of Arjo, Inc.)

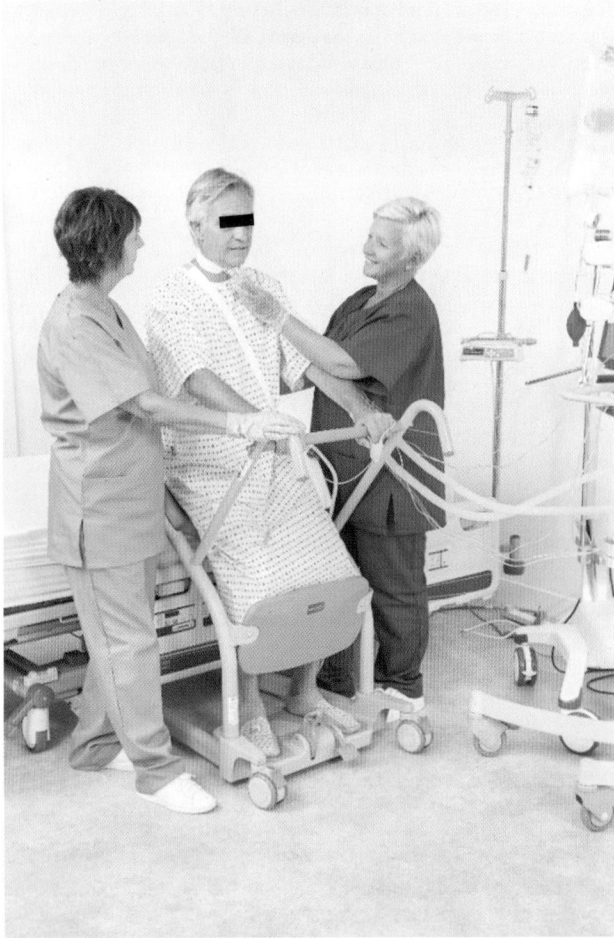

• **Fig. 24.11** Nonmechanical Standing Frame. (Courtesy of Arjo, Inc.)

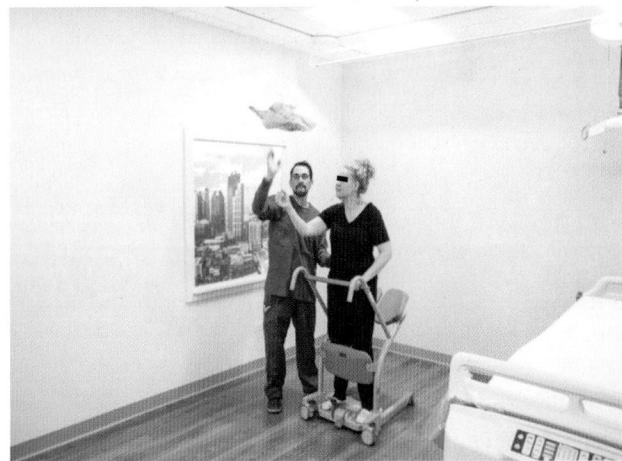

• **Fig. 24.12** Therapeutic Use of Nonmechanical Standing Aid. (Courtesy of Arjo, Inc.)

feature to allow the patient to rest (Figure 24.11). Nonmechanical standing aids offer another option to transfer to and from the commode or wheelchair. This device allows the patient to utilize their upper extremities for external support on the device while continuing to weight bear through both legs, a therapeutic benefit for the musculoskeletal and neuromuscular systems (Figure 24.12). A mechanical standing platform (Arjo Sara Plus) can assist with transfers, balance education, and gait (Figure 24.13). The detachable footplate allows for gait training while supported in a walking sling (Figure 24.14).

Rehabilitation Interventions in the Acute Setting

As each hospitalized PWC is unique, specific rehabilitation interventions will vary; however, in the acute environment, interventions frequently focus on optimizing the functional mobility and independence of patients as required to safely discharge home or to the next level of care. Bed mobility, transfers, gait/locomotion, stairs, and associated ADLs are essential to address for optimization of patient QOL and a safe discharge plan. Creativity and the prioritization of impairments and associated interventions are fundamental in a setting where limitations in time, space, and resources often affect the therapy plan of care.

A primary goal of acute or inpatient rehabilitation is to optimize and increase safe mobility for medically complex patients in order to improve health and equip patients and families for the next step of their journeys. Patients hospitalized with cancer benefit from increased time out of bed thus reducing risk for blood clots, pressure injuries, and cognitive decline. Upright positioning for those with respiratory compromise is especially important. This facilitation may

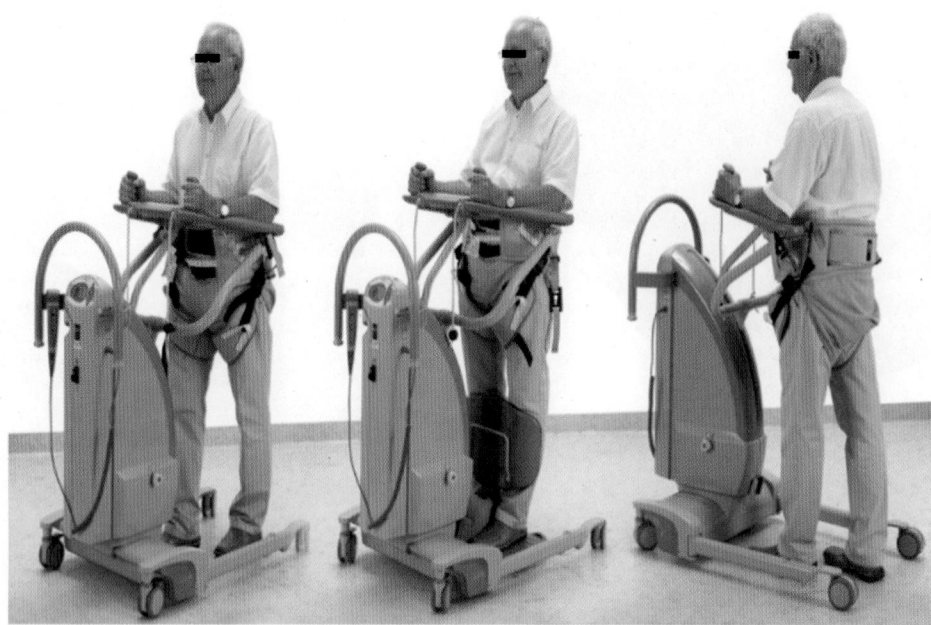

• **Fig. 24.13** Mechanical Standing Frame Used for Gait Training. (Courtesy of Arjo, Inc.)

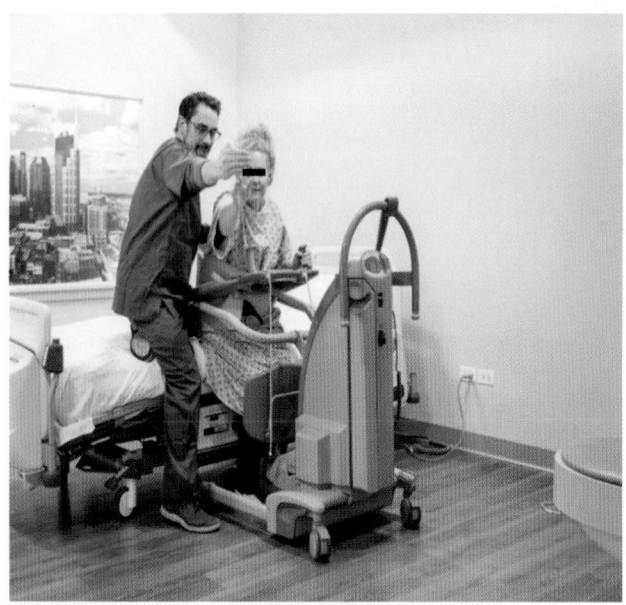

• **Fig. 24.14** Mechanical Standing Frame Used for Rehabilitation for Reaching. (Courtesy of Arjo, Inc.)

include education focused on breathing techniques, strengthening of core and postural musculature, and optimizing balance. Manual therapy including percussion or vibration to assist with airway clearance is useful in patients with significant bronchial secretions; however, modifications may be warranted in the case of metastatic spread to bone, osteopenia or osteoporosis, or in cases of thrombocytopenia.

In patients with neurological impairments from cancer or its treatments, facilitation of midline positioning and normal movement patterns may be prioritized over strengthening. Once the patient is able to tolerate out of bed activity for meals and use of the bathroom, progression of aerobic exercise, and strengthening can be introduced with

introduction of the RPE scale and exercise guidelines as described in Chapter 23. Communication with and recommendations for nursing and support staff to facilitate safe advancement of mobility should be clearly documented in the medical record and should be visible in the patient's room for any healthcare provider to access quickly to safely assist with mobility. This may be accomplished through reader-friendly handouts, institutional protocols and resources, or, simply, as written notes on a dry-erase board in the patient's room. Communication of mobility protocols and recommendations should be relayed with the patient and the patient's caregiver(s) given their partnership in the care plan and functional outcomes of the patient. Surgical patients often benefit from instruction in safe mobility and ADLs related to their specific surgery. For example, patients after spinal or abdominal surgery should be educated on how to log roll to get out of bed, various techniques to ease transitions and mitigate painful postures, including log rolling for supine to sit transfers and splinting during mobility, to mitigate pain exacerbation and complications during the postoperative period. In addition, some individuals after colorectal cancer may experience pain and nausea after postostomy placement. While coordination with nursing around nausea and pain control is important, the patient may need significant encouragement and education on abdominal bracing, breathing techniques, and activity recommendations to initiate and progress mobility. Clinical practice guidelines have been developed for enhanced recovery as a standardized order set of procedures before, during, and after surgery. These enhanced recovery protocols are geared toward improving patient outcomes, minimizing complications, reducing hospital lengths of stay, and decreasing risk of readmissions to positively impact health care costs, and more importantly, patient outcomes. Ahn and colleagues described a supervised inpatient exercise program for persons with colorectal cancer after ostomy which reduced hospital LOS and time to flatus.[74] The patients participating in this postoperative exercise regimen performed a series of stretching, core, balance, and light resistance exercises twice per day (Table 24.5).

After neurosurgery, a significant amount of neuromuscular reeducation may be needed with facilitation of normal movement patterns

TABLE 24.5   Inpatient Exercise Program for Colorectal Cancer

	Exercise Program	Conventional Care
The first phase	Supervised exercise (twice/day)	Unsupervised sitting or walking in the ward
Lying on the bed (POD 1)	Stretching (neck, shoulder, wrist, ankle, and pelvis)	
	Core exercise (pelvic tilt: isometric contraction)	
	Resistance exercise (ankle dorsi- and plantar flexion against the hand of the clinician)	
	Unsupervised sitting or walking in the ward	
The second phase	Supervised exercise (twice/day)	Unsupervised walking in the hallway
Limited ambulation (POD 1~3)	Stretching (whole body, leg, and shoulder)	
	Core exercise (pelvic tilt and thrust, one leg raise, crunch)	
	Resistance exercise (chest, shoulder, arm, thigh, and calf)	
	Unsupervised walking on the hallway	
The third phase	One supervised and one unsupervised exercise	Unsupervised walking in the hallway
Ambulation without discomfort (POD 2~discharge)	Stretching (whole body, leg, and shoulder)	
	Core exercise (pelvic tilt, bridge, one leg raise, and crunch)	
	Resistance exercise (chest, shoulder, arm, thigh, and calf) (12 repetitions × 3 sets)	
	Supervised balance exercise (once/day)	
	One leg standing	
	One leg calf raise	
	Hip adduction	
	Hip abduction	
	Hip flexion with knee bent	
	Hip extension	
	Unsupervised walking on the hallway	

POD, post op day.
Reprinted with permission from Ahn KY, Hur H, Kim DH, et al. The effects of inpatient exercise therapy on the length of hospital stay in stages I-III colon cancer patients: randomized controlled trial. *Int J Colorectal Dis.* 2013;28(5):643–651. doi:10.1007/s00384-013-1665-1.

to achieve independence in bed mobility, transfers, and gait. Finally, as many PWCs will often experience ongoing physical deficits beyond the hospitalization, a clinician may find it efficacious to initiate caregiver training at the start of care. This shift in focus and early recruitment of caregivers is essential for successful discharge dispositions and ensuring the comprehensive management of the patient's medical and functional situation. Clarity of roles and responsibilities is vital, as increasing caregiver involvement and family training are complementary and essential to long-term safety and functional outcomes and do not necessarily negate goals for patient independence.

Exercise for the "Well" PWC in Acute Care

A PWC who is admitted for monitoring during cancer treatments may well end up hospitalized for a prolonged period of time. These "well" PWCs are often referred to rehabilitation services to optimize their physical activity and exercise programs during their stay. These patients are from various backgrounds in terms of physical activity, and a PT or OT can help guide them to an appropriate exercise program and ADL performance during the stay. See Chapter 23 for specific recommendations, precautions, and contraindications to exercise. An individualized program can be tailored to meet the goals and comfort level of the PWC, whether it includes a simple cardiorespiratory endurance program using a recumbent bike or walking, body weight exercise, or even, resistance exercises using

weights or elastic exercise bands where not contraindicated. Given the inherent complexities of scheduling associated with inpatient acute care, a program that is given and taught to a patient to perform on their own with periodic advancements is ideal. The foundations of the program should include education on RPE and energy conservation and activity modification strategies, heart rate guidelines, and symptom monitoring to help the PWC monitor and progress their mobility efforts.

Discharge Considerations for PWCs

Determining discharge disposition and ensuring a seamless hand-off of care is a primary role of Onc R clinicians in the acute care setting, especially in caring for a PWC where care coordination and the minimization of treatment interruptions has prognostic ramifications. Foundational considerations include: What is the optimal destination for the patient to continue recovery and receive the treatment they were prescribed? What equipment and services will they need upon getting there? Determining the appropriate adaptive equipment recommendations is imperative to maintaining physical independence and safety (Figure 24.15). These items also will make the transition from life-altering treatment or surgery more manageable for the patient as they re-integrate with society.

While a patient may require extended rehabilitation after a hospitalization, the goal should always be focused on returning the

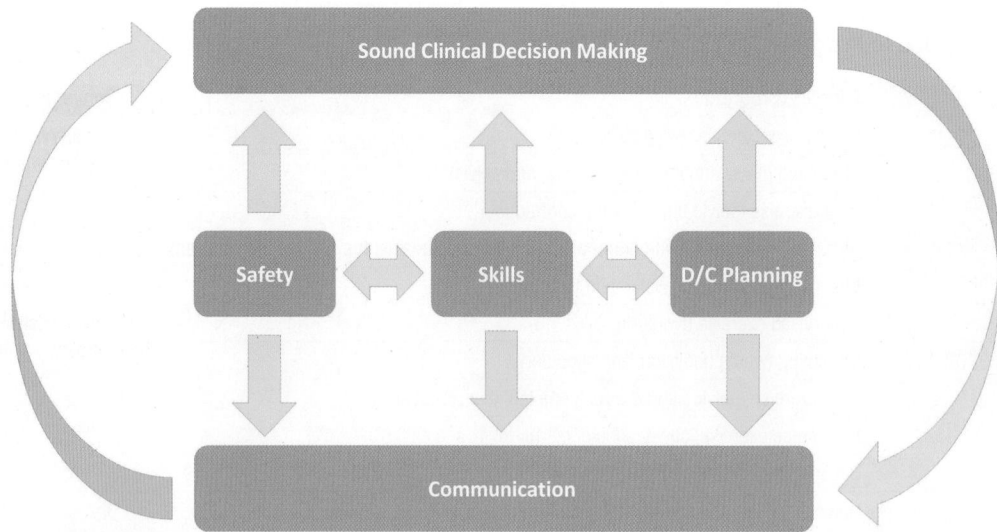

• **Fig. 24.15** Considerations When Making Discharge Recommendations. (Reprinted with permission from Greenwood K, Stewart E, Hake M, Milton E, Mitchell L, Sanders B. Defining entry-level practice in acute care physical therapist practice. *J Acute Care Phys Ther*. 2017;8(1):3–10. doi:10.1097/JAT.0000000000000048.)

patient home with adequate support while receiving rehabilitation services. Many PWCs will require frequent follow-up appointments and outpatient treatments including radiation, chemotherapy, or transfusions. Whether home care or outpatient rehabilitation is recommended, close collaboration with the social worker or discharge planner will assist in coordination of support services.

Considerations for Discharge Home

If a patient is able to safely manage their impairments and self-care and mobility needs at home, and the recommended equipment and services are available, a discharge home is generally the location of choice. Whereby a patient may be unable to leave their home without undue burden, homecare services, including nursing and rehabilitation, may be initiated.

Other patients who are physically able to leave their home and have adequate transportation are good candidates for outpatient services, including rehabilitation. Education on the benefits of ongoing rehabilitation services is often needed as patients may not fully grasp the benefits and role of rehabilitation in the post-acute transition and the need to prioritize such services in addition to other high priority appointments related to oncologic treatment may not be fully realized. The acute care Onc R clinician should assure appropriate referrals are initiated prior to discharge. In some institutions the clinician can initiate an electronic referral via the electronic medical record (EMR) or a traditional paper referral to outpatient therapy services can be signed in preparation for discharge. If the goal of a patient is to remain physically active and they are appropriate for community-based exercise, a clinician can also provide resources to community-based resources, exercise classes, and support groups in their area.

A patient diagnosed with advanced cancer may consider palliative or hospice care to help transition to the home environment. An IDT approach to goal setting and decision-making is critical. While a PT or OT consult may seem counterintuitive when a hospice decision is pending, a clinician should realize the valued role they provide in assisting with medical decision making, optimizing patients' function, decreasing caregiver burdens, and enhancing patient QOL, regardless of prognosis or level of ability. Often, these goals of care discussions are centered around individualized

goals and fears and are navigated by the patient's care team. As an expert of the movement system, safety devices, and strategies for promoting mobility and managing functional impairments, the Onc R clinician is well positioned to inform and contribute to these discussions. Onc R professionals can outline practical expectations and the functional implications or requirements for a patient and their caregivers, as well as provide supportive strategies to address some of the patient's and caregiver's fears, including concerns regarding caregiver burden. A patient with mobility concerns may benefit from education regarding home modifications, DME, adapted ADL performance, and wheelchair or assistive device use at home to reduce caregiver burden and optimize patient independence. Conversely, a person with delirium may demonstrate improved alertness and orientation with increased upright positioning, time out of bed and increased physical activity, thereby improving their QOL and reducing caregiver burden. In some cases, if a patient requires inpatient hospice within the hospital, some therapy services may not be warranted as the expected life expectancy is a matter of days or the symptoms may require close control; however other patients may still appreciate substantial benefit from Onc R in hospice. Further discussion with the medical team is recommended prior to speaking to the patient or family for an evaluation in the case of rehabilitation within inpatient hospice. See Chapter 29 for additional information on palliative care and end-of-life.

Communication During Care Coordination

A key consideration in assuring safe transition to the next level of care is effectively communicating the myriad barriers and challenges to assure a patient-centered discharge. Ensuring consistency with and clarity among the medical team can be achieved through regular team updates, as well as through direct communication and reflection with the patient and their family. Careful questioning regarding the discharge plan is an effective strategy in promoting patient understanding and ensuring the treatment plan and recommendations are communicated accurately. When a debilitated patient is focused on returning home, a treatment plan designed around caregiver training will be needed. This

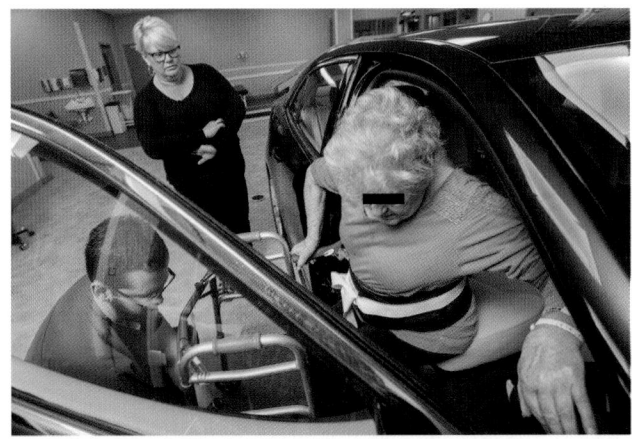

• **Fig. 24.16** Practicing Car Transfers Prior to Discharge Home. (Photo printed with permission by Courtney Witczak PT, DPT, GCS.)

may include education on positioning, equipment recommendations, use of lifts, wheelchair safety, safe transfer techniques, and activity recommendations. The role of the OT is essential to focus on environmental modifications and energy conservation in these cases as caregivers can easily become overwhelmed or injured when a patient requires significant assistance. Additionally, hands on practice should occur as soon and as frequently as possible during the hospitalization to ensure full understanding of the patient's physical assistance requirements and allow for alternative rehabilitation or care options to be arranged if needed (Figure 24.16).

Options for Discharge

Some patients and family may not understand why discharge discussions are occurring despite significant illness persisting. This is especially true in patients diagnosed with advanced cancer nearing the end of life. See Chapter 29 for approaches and decision making toward end-of-life care.

If the patient is unable to safely return home with services at discharge or requires a higher level of rehabilitation or skilled nursing, alternative discharge dispositions include IPR, subacute rehab, or a LTACH with 24-hour medical support. An assisted living facility (ALF) or ECF are alternative discharge options for longer-term residence.

IPR provides the highest intensity of skilled services including PT, OT, and SLP services as well as recreational therapy, with average LOS of 12.7 days per U.S. Centers for Medicare & Medicaid Services (CMS).[75] Patients need to be able to tolerate at least 15 hours of intensive rehabilitation therapy within a 7-consecutive day period, beginning with the date of admission, which may be achievable and beneficial for many PWCs. Home safety needs and caregiver support may preclude a patient's safe transition to the home environment. These barriers have been addressed in some institutions through a short stay program in the IPR setting. The primary focus of these stays is caregiver training, including the use of SPHM equipment, guarding techniques, and direct patient care activities. A program entitled Short Stay Family Training was described by Smith and colleagues in 2020.[76] In this program, a shorter LOS in IPR can be arranged with the caveat that caregivers are present throughout every therapy session to receive education, hands-on training, and discharge support to prepare the patient for return home with the caregiver's

assistance. A key consideration is that the person who is available for training must be the person who will be providing care after the return home.

A patient who would benefit from a slower paced, longer rehabilitation may require SAR (often used interchangeably with ECF) which provides some of the same therapies as IPR, though at a reduced intensity and duration. Both settings require active participation from the patient and rehabilitation potential; however, in SAR, the patients typically undergo 1 hour, versus the aforementioned 3 hours in IPR, of rehabilitation, allowing patients with more limited activity tolerance to still participate in rehabilitation services. A patient who is continuing with ongoing cancer treatment such as chemotherapy or radiation may be faced with transportation issues from an SAR or ECF that is not affiliated with their healthcare system. Discussion of car transfers and feasibility of attending these appointments should always be considered when guiding the patient and family these locations.

In certain situations, a PWC may need to transition to an ALF where various levels of support are available. Options for this vary widely in level of assistance available and cost. Whether it is simply medication management or more frequent assistance for toilet transfers or ADLs, the financial burden can escalate quickly and be a barrier for many. In addition, it often takes a substantial amount of time to arrange an ALF stay and this may not be feasible during some shorter hospital stays.

A long-term care facility may be best suited for select critically ill PWCs with advanced disease and a limited expected lifespan who required specialized skills and care. LTACHs are often separate facilities from the acute care hospital that provide extensive support for critically ill but medically stable individuals. Candidates for LTACHs include those who are chronically ventilator dependent or are weaning off of the ventilator, those who need ongoing dialysis, frequent and intensive respiratory care, complex or intensive medication regimens, or those with extensive burns.[77] PWCs who are appropriate for LTACH include those whose care requires a higher intensity of medical management than a SAR can provide but less than that required in the acute or emergent setting as per Medicare guidelines, the patient must need more than 25 days of hospitalization.[77] The average LOS of a person in an LTACH is approximately 30 days.[78]

Given the complexity of discharge planning, the Onc R clinician should always work closely with the discharge planner and social worker to best institute the safest and most beneficial discharge recommendation, skillfully integrating the patient's goals, values, and desires. In each of these settings, rehabilitation services may be indicated, especially in settings of hospice or palliative care, and should be advocated for to reduce likelihood of readmission to the hospital to maximize patient function and mobility, and to facilitate access to and participation in those tasks important to the patient and their family.

Conclusion

A hospitalization often represents a divergence in the trajectory of one's medical journey and represents a unique juncture in the life of PWCs. Whether a short stay for medical supplementation or a prolonged admission managing emergent treatments or unfortunate complications, the Onc R clinician must be well prepared to assist in navigating the complex acute care environment and facilitating the transition of patients beyond their service. An integral part of the interdisciplinary medical team, the Onc R clinician is invaluable in screening, assessing and stratifying risk, as well as intervening upon present and anticipated deficits stemming from oncologic processes or treatment-related sequalae. This promotes function, patient independence, and QOL for persons living with and beyond cancer. The Onc R clinician is a key stakeholder in managing a patient's a safe and satisfactory discharge, as well as establishing and preparing the patient for their next steps. Through skilled navigation of the acute care environment, the patient's cancer journey and medical trajectory, and the complexities of care continuity and discharge dispositions, the Onc R clinician stands as a vital member of the patient's care team and is essential at the juncture of acute care and the cancer care continuum.

Critical Research Needs

- Guidelines to advise therapists on when to proceed with evaluation and/or treatment if the patient has abnormal lab values, bone metastases, brain metastases, and pending scans.
- Defining a therapist's role in the continued rehabilitation process when the patient is transitioning to palliative care and hospice.
- Defining the role of the clinician in early mobility in terms of exercise prescription, interventions, and plan of care for patients with an oncology diagnosis in the ICUs and inpatient units.

Case Study

A 57-year-old female was admitted to the hospital with bilateral thigh pain. Her medical history was significant for recurrent breast cancer. A review of her oncologic history included a bilateral mastectomy at age 50 after being diagnosed with left breast cancer. Surgery was followed by adjuvant chemotherapy including doxorubicin (Adriamycin) and cyclophosphamide (Cytoxan). This recent recurrence of breast cancer was also found in a lymph node, and doxorubicin was recommended, however the patient adamantly refused due to her concern for cardiotoxicity. Instead, she was started on docetaxel (Taxotere) and Cytoxan every 21 days. She received pegfilgrastim (Neulasta) with the second cycle of chemotherapy.

After the second cycle of chemotherapy, she required a visit to the emergency center due to thigh pain that started 3 days after this cycle began. She could find no relief with pain medications. Pain was located primarily in bilateral quadriceps muscles with strength graded at 3+/5 for right knee extension, 3–/5 for the left leg. Her creatinine phosphokinase (CPK) was noted to be over 3000 at the time of her admission and the patient was diagnosed with rhabdomyolysis.

The PT evaluated the patient 2 days after admission, however the patient requested to be discharged from therapy services on the follow-up treatment session, as she did not feel she needed physical therapy. The patient was discharged after 2 weeks in the hospital. Upon entering her home, she fell trying to ascend the steps. She was readmitted for a total of 2 weeks which consisted of 11 sessions of therapy in the acute and IPR settings.

Rehabilitation included multiple disciplines and various interventions focused on strengthening, education, neuromuscular reeducation, safety, and pain management. All outcome measures improved including 5 times sit to stand, timed up and go, and activity measure for post-acute care (AMPAC) 6-clicks, which supported a plan to discharge home safely.

In this case, the patient was experiencing significant physical and emotional stress which must be addressed within the traditional course of rehabilitation. Helping a patient understand the barriers he or she may face before, during, or after this setback is a skill in itself to help empower the patient to meet this new challenge with the support of the entire IDT.

Review Questions

Reader can find the correct answers and rationale in the back of the book.

1. A hospitalized patient with acute leukemia initiated chemotherapy 3 days prior to your scheduled therapy evaluation. Upon chart review, the PWC presents with hyperkalemia and reports new flank pain with dysuria. How would a therapist address the order for eval and treat?
   A. Proceed with eval and treat if potassium values fall within an acceptable range
   B. Ask the PWC to hydrate well and follow up in the afternoon
   C. Defer eval and treat given PWC isn't feeling well
   D. Discuss symptoms and lab value changes with the physician prior to initiating evaluation

2. An order to evaluate and treat a 57-year-old female is placed postostomy surgery. You find the patient up in the bathroom with the nursing assistant who states the patient is doing well. The PWC states she does not need therapy and "does everything on her own."
   How do you proceed?
   A. Return later to provide education on specific goals of therapy postostomy as it has been shown to reduce the length of stay
   B. Ensure the patient is up and walking several times a day, and with respect to the request of the PWC sign off of therapy services
   C. After seeing the patient is moving independently in the bathroom, collect objective information, leave a handout, and sign off

   D. Put the patient on the schedule for the next day for a second attempt

3. A person with end stage renal cancer has been on therapy services for over 3 weeks without progress. The PWC consistently states the goal to be able to walk, however most scheduled sessions are declined secondary to uncontrolled pain and the treatment sessions are limited to bed mobility and sitting tolerance at the edge of the bed. The intrathecal pain pump the PWC has is being managed by the surgical team and therapy is timing sessions around pain management. How would you proceed when a re-evaluation is completed?
   A. Continue with the current goals and plan of care as it is the wish of the PWC to walk
   B. Discuss the lack of progress and pain barrier with the interdisciplinary team with recommendation to support palliative goals
   C. Sign off secondary to lack of progress
   D. Suggest family comes to help motivate the PWC to work through the pain

4. A person admitted to the oncology unit for her third round of chemotherapy treatment for lymphoma has platelet levels at 17,000/µL over the last 4 days but wants to come down to the therapy gym. How do you respond?
   A. Defer exercise in the gym and encourage patient to sit up in chair as much as possible until lab values improve

B. Bring PWC down to use the NuStep and light weights as long as she feels okay

C. Suggest interval training ambulation with symptom-limited intensity and vital monitoring throughout

D. Page the physician to get clearance to work with PWC

5. You receive a therapy consult on a PWC in the ICU who currently has a ventriculostomy. Immediately you realize you will need to do the following:

A. Limit your evaluation and treatment to bed/edge of bed given the invasive line

B. Hold therapy

C. Proceed with evaluation and treatment, carefully clamping the ventriculostomy then unclamping at the end of the session

D. Arrange your session around nursing availability in order to clamp the ventriculostomy for mobility

6. A hospitalized PWC is nearing discharge, but lives alone and has a flight of stairs to an upstairs apartment. He currently needs moderate physical assist to stand from a chair. What outcome measure would best indicate his most appropriate discharge disposition?

A. AMPAC 6-clicks

B. 5 Times sit to stand test

C. 6-minute walk test

D. TUG

7. A 71-year-old PWC has been hospitalized for over a week with acute myeloid leukemia. When vitals are taken at the onset of your treatment session, she becomes upset at her elevated blood pressure. This, combined with weight gain and increased insulin needs for blood glucose regulation is upsetting for her. What is the best way to respond when she expresses her frustration?

A. Reassure her that the fluctuations in these factors are likely related to decreased mobility then progresses her exercise program

B. Acknowledge her frustration and proceed with the session

C. Encourage her to speak with her physician about the side effects of corticosteroids

D. Use this opportunity to open dialogue regarding healthy nutrition

8. A 68-year-old female is hospitalized with pneumonia and a therapy consult is placed as she has been having difficulty making it up a flight of stairs to her bedroom at home. She is a breast cancer survivor and received cisplatin (Platinol) as part of her chemotherapy treatment. Which impairment would most likely be related to long-term adverse effects of her cancer treatment?

A. Dyspnea with exertion

B. Decreased bilateral lower extremity sensation

C. Lower extremity weakness

D. Decreased endurance

9. A therapy consult is placed for a 72-year-old man, newly diagnosed with metastatic prostate cancer. He presents with lesions in the thoracic and lumbar spine resulting in spinal cord compression and max physical assistance is required to maintain sitting at the edge of bed, despite being independent with ambulation 1 month prior to admission. His family is very supportive and he is planning on following up with palliative radiation for the spine. What is the most appropriate discharge recommendation?

A. Subacute rehab to maximize the independence for the PWC

B. Inpatient rehabilitation to train the PWC and family on transfer techniques

C. Home with hospice

D. Defer the decision to the medical team

10. A therapy consult is placed for a patient with back pain in the emergency center. The patient indicates the back pain started about a month ago after moving furniture, but this morning he woke up with extreme pain preventing him from walking. His surgical history includes resection of the lung 6 years prior, but he states he has not followed up with his oncologist in the last 2 years. Which of the following would most likely lead you to ask the medical team for further imaging?

A. Sustained clonus with rapid manual stretch of the ankle

B. Bilateral lower extremity weakness

C. History of lung cancer

D. Pain unable to be relieved with position changes

References

1. Philip T, Gleason K, Nekola C, et al. Reducing emergency department utilization by improving patient access to their oncology care team. *J Clin Oncol.* 2019;37(27_suppl) 77.
2. Rivera DR, Gallicchio L, Brown J, Liu B, Kyriacou DN, Shelburne N. Trends in adult cancer-related emergency department utilization: an analysis of data from the nationwide emergency department sample. *JAMA Ondol.* 2017;3(10):e172450.
3. Soares M, Bozza FA, Azevedo LC, et al. Effects of organizational characteristics on outcomes and resource use in patients with cancer admitted to intensive care units. *J Clin Oncol.* 2016;34(27):3315–3324.
4. Van der Mejj BS, DeGraff P, Wierdsma NJ, et al. Nutritional support in patients with GVHD of the digestive tract: state of the art. *Bone Marrow Transplant.* 2012;48(4):474–482.
5. Lau B, Skinner EH, Lo K, Bearman M. Experiences of physical therapists working in the acute hospital setting: systematic review. *Phys Ther.* 2016;96(9):1317–1332.
6. Burgess C, Morris T, Pettingale KW. Psychological response to cancer diagnosis—II. Evidence for coping styles (coping styles and cancer diagnosis). *J Psychosomatic Res.* 1988;32(3):263–272.
7. Adler J, Malone D. Early mobilization in the intensive care unit: a systematic review. *Cardiopulm Phys Ther J.* 2012;23(1):5–13.
8. Wilson CM, Mueller K, Briggs R. Physical therapists' contribution to the hospice and palliative care interdisciplinary team: a clinical summary. *J Hospice Palliat Nurs.* 2017;19(6):588–596.
9. Whelton PK, Carey L, Aronow WS, et al. 2017 ACC/AHA/AAPA/ABC/ACPM/AGS/APhA/ASH/ASPC/NMA/PCNA Guideline for the prevention, detection, evaluation, and management of high blood pressure in adults: executive summary: a report of the American College of Cardiology/American Heart Association Task Force on Clinical Practice Guidelines. *Hypertension.* 2018;71(6):1269–1324.
10. Center for Disease Control and Prevention. Measuring orthostatic blood pressure; 2017. https://www.cdc.gov/steadi/materials.html. Accessed April 8, 2021.
11. Pepersace T, Gilles C, Petrovic M, et al. Prevalence of orthostatic hypotension and relationship with drug use amongst older patients. *Acta Clinica Belgica.* 2013;68(2):107–112.
12. Fanciulli A, Goebel G, Metzler B, et al. Elastic abdominal binders attenuate orthostatic hypotension in Parkinson's disease. *Mov Disord Clin Pract.* 2015;3(2):156–160. doi:10.1002/mdc3.12270.
13. Mills PB, Fung CK, Travlos A, Krassioukov A. Nonpharmacologic management of orthostatic hypotension: a systematic review. *Arch Phy Med Rehabil.* 2015;96(2):366–375.

14. Wilson CM, Kline JJ, Cook ME, et al. Therapists perceptions of physical counterpressure maneuvers for the management of pre-syncope. *J Acute Care Phys Ther*. 2015;6(3):102–115.

15. Ali A, Ali N, Waqas N, et al. Management of orthostatic hypotension: a literature review. *Cureus*. 2018;10(8):e3166. doi:10.7759/cureus.3166.

16. Frith J, Parry SW. New horizons in orthostatic hypotension. *Age Ageing*. 2017;46(2):168–174. doi:10.1093/ageing/afw211.

17. Mullen EA. Chapter 122: Oncologic emergencies. In: Zaoutis LB, Chiang VW, eds. *Comprehensive Pediatric Hospital Medicine*. Mosby; 2007:767–773.

18. Howard SC, Jones DP, Pui CH. The tumor lysis syndrome. *N Engl J Med*. 2011;364(19):1844–1854.

19. Nolan C, DeAngelis LM. The confused oncologic patient: a rational clinical approach. *Curr Opin Neurol*. 2016;29(6):789–796.

20. Tompkins J, Norris T, Levenhagen K, et al. Laboratory Values Interpretation Resource. Academy of acute care physical therapy-APTA task force on lab values; 2017. https://cdn.ymaws.com/www.apta-acutecare.org/resource/resmgr/docs/2017-Lab-Values-Resource.pdf. Accessed August 27, 2020.

21. Canadian Cancer Society. Low blood cell counts. https://www.cancer.ca/en/cancer-information/diagnosis-and-treatment/managing-side-effects/low-blood-cell-counts/. Accessed May 8, 2021.

22. American Cancer Society. https://www.cancer.org/treatment/treatments-and-side-effects/physical-side-effects/low-blood-counts/anemia.html. February 1, 2020. Accessed April 21, 2021.

23. Territo M. Overview of Leukopenias. Merck manual professional version. https://www.merckmanuals.com/professional/hematology-and-oncology/leukopenias/overview-of-leukopenias. January 2020. Accessed April 21, 2021.

24. National Cancer Institute. Neutrophil. National Cancer Institute website. https://www.cancer.gov/publications/dictionaries/cancer-terms/def/neutrophil. Accessed April 21, 2021.

25. Mayadas TN, Cullere X, Lowell CA. The multifaceted functions of neutrophils. *Ann Rev Pathol Mech Dis*. 2014;9(1):181–218.

26. American Academy of Allergy Asthma and Immunology. Neutropenia definition. https://www.aaaai.org/conditions-and-treatments/conditions-dictionary/Neutropenia. Accessed April 21, 2021.

27. Vioral AN, Wentley D. Managing oncology neutropenia and sepsis in the intensive care unit. *Crit Care Nurs Quart*. 2015;38(2):165–174.

28. National Comprehensive Cancer Network. NCCN clinical practice guidelines in oncology: prevention and treatment of cancer-related infections. Version 2-2020. https://www.nccn.org/professionals/physician_gls/pdf/infections.pdf. Accessed April 21, 2021.

29. Gabriel J. Acute oncological emergencies. *Nurs Stand*. 2012;27(4):35–41.

30. Jeevanantham D, Rajendran V, McGillis Z, Tremblay L, Larivière C, Knight A. Mobilization and exercise intervention for patients with multiple myeloma: clinical practice guidelines endorsed by the Canadian Physiotherapy Association. *Phys Ther*. 2021;101(1):pzaa180. doi:10.1093/ptj/pzaa180.

31. Maltser S, Cristian A, Silver JK, Morris GS, Stout NL. A focused review of safety considerations in cancer rehabilitation. *Phys Med Rehabil*. 2017;9(9S2):S415–S428. doi:10.1016/j.pmrj.2017.08.403.

32. Lucelia LM. Thrombocytopenia and physical activity among older adults: the tenuous line between bleeding prevention physical functional decline. *OAJ Gerontol Geriatric Med*. 2017;1:555571.

33. Berardi R, Torniai M, Lenci E, Pecci F, Morgese F, Rinaldi S. Electrolyte disorders in cancer patients: a systematic review. *J Cancer Metastasis Treat*. 2019;5:79. doi:10.20517/2394-4722.2019.008.

34. Fischbach FT, Dunning MB. *A Manual of Laboratory and Diagnostic Tests*. 9th ed.: Wolters Kluwer Health; 2015.

35. Castillo JJ, Vincent M, Justice E. Diagnosis and management of hyponatremia in cancer patients. *Oncologist*. 2012;17(6):756–765.

36. RS Falk, T Heir, TE Robsahm, et al. Fasting serum levels of potassium and sodium in relation to long-term risk of cancer in healthy men, Clin Epidemiol 2020;12:1–8.

37. Suh S, Kim K-W. Diabetes and cancer: is diabetes causally related to cancer? *Diabetes Metab J*. 2011;35:193–198.

38. Bernardo BM, Orellana RC, Lowneberg Weisband Y, et al. Association between prediagnostic glucose, triglycerides, cholesterol and meningioma, and reverse causality. *Brit J Cancer*. 2016;115(1):108.

39. American Diabetes Association. Position statement: standards of medical care in diabetes—2016. *Diabetes Care*. 2016;39(suppl. 1):S1–S112.

40. Alexandru O, Ene L, Purcaru OS, et al. Plasma levels of glucose and insulin in patients with brain tumors. *Curr Health Sci J*. 2014;40(1):27–36.

41. Brady VJ, Grimes D, Armstrong T, LoBiondo-Wood G. Management of steroid-induced hyperglycemia in hospitalized patients with cancer: a review. *Oncol Nurs Forum*. 2014;41(6):E355–E365. doi:10.1188/14.ONF.E355-E365.

42. Hillegass E, Puthoff M, Frese EM, Thigpen M, Sobush DC, Auten B. Guideline Development Group. Role of physical therapists in the management of individuals at risk for or diagnosed with venous thromboembolism: evidence-based clinical practice guideline. *Phys Ther*. 2016;96(2):143–166. doi:10.2522/ptj.20150264.

43. MedlinePlus. Ondansetron. MedlinePlus website. https://medlineplus.gov/druginfo/meds/a601209.html. November 15, 2019. Accessed April 21, 2021.

44. Thom KA, Kleinberg M, Roghmann MC. Infection prevention in the cancer center. *Clin Infect Dis*. 2013;57(4):579–585. doi:10.1093/cid/cit290.

45. Matsuo N, Morita T, Matsuda Y, et al. Predictors of responses to corticosteroids for cancer-related fatigue in advanced cancer patients: a multicenter, prospective, observational study. *J Pain Symptom Manage*. 2016;52(1):64–72. doi:10.1016/j.jpainsymman.2016.01.015.

46. Denton A, Shaw J. Corticosteroid prescribing in palliative care settings: a retrospective analysis in New Zealand. *BMC Palliat Care*. 2014;13:7. doi:10.1186/1472-684X-13-7.

47. McKay LI, Cidlowski JA, et al. Corticosteroids in the treatment of neoplasms. In: Kufe DW, Pollock RE, Weichselbaum RR, et al. eds. *Holland-Frei Cancer Medicine*. 6th ed.: BC Decker; 2003. https://www.ncbi.nlm.nih.gov/books/NBK13383/.

48. National Cancer Institute. *Cancer Imaging Basics*. National Cancer Institute; 2020. https://imaging.cancer.gov/imaging_basics/cancer_imaging.htm. November 6, Accessed April 21, 2021.

49. Suh CH, Shinagare AB, Westenfield AM, Ramaiya NH, Van den Abbeele AD, Kim KW. Yield of bone scintigraphy for the detection of metastatic disease in treatment-naive prostate cancer: a systematic review and meta-analysis. *Clin Radiol*. 2018;73(2):158–167.

50. Joint Task Force of APTA Acute Care and the Academy of Cardiovascular & Pulmonary Physical Therapy of the American Physical Therapy Association. Adult Vital Sign Interpretation in Acute Care Guide 2021. APTA Acute Care and APTA Cardiovascular and Pulmonary Physical Therapy; April 2021.

51. Sapra A, Malik A, Bhandari P. Vital sign assessment. [Updated May 23, 2020] In: *StatPearls [Internet]*: StatPearls Publishing; 2021. https://www.ncbi.nlm.nih.gov/books/NBK553213/.

52. Myszenski A. The role of lab values in clinical decision making and patient safety for the acutely ill patient. https://www.physicaltherapy.com/articles/essential-role-lab-values-and-3637. September 7, 2017. Accessed April 21, 2021.

53. Abdo WF, Heunks LM. Oxygen-induced hypercapnia in COPD: myths and facts. *Crit Care*. 2012;16:323. doi:10.1186/cc11475.

54. Zamboni MM, da Silva Jr CT, Baretta R, Cunha ET, Cardoso GP. Important prognostic factors for survival in patients with malignant pleural effusion. *BMC Pulm Med*. 2015;15:29. doi:10.1186/s12890-015-0025-z.

55. Stukan M. Drainage of malignant ascites: patient selection and perspectives. *Cancer Manag Res*. 2017;9:115–130.

56. Dincer M, Kahveci K, Doger C. An examination of factors affecting the length of stay in a palliative care center. *J Palliat Med*. 2018;21(1):11–15.

57. Mitchell J, Jatoi A. Parenteral nutrition in patients with advanced cancer: merging perspectives from the patient and healthcare provider. *Semin Oncol*. 2011;38(3):439–442.

58. Shah SO, Kraft J, Ankam N, et al. Early ambulation in patients with external ventricular drains: results of a quality improvement project. *J Intensive Care Med.* 2018;33(6):370–374.

59. Bruel BM, Burton AW. Intrathecal therapy for cancer-related pain. *Pain Med.* 2016;17(12):2404–2421.

60. Pope JE, Deer TR. Guide to implantable devices for intrathecal therapy. *Pract Pain Manag.* 2013;3(8):1–11.

61. Inscore E, Litterini, A. Academy of oncologic physical therapy EDGE task force report summaries. https://oncologypt.org/wp-content/uploads/2019/10/EDGE-Annotated-Bibliography-8.19-update.pdf. Accessed May 9, 2021.

62. American Cancer Society. Prostheses. American Cancer Society website. https://www.cancer.org/treatment/treatments-and-side-effects/physical-side-effects/prostheses.html. Accessed April 21, 2021.

63. Winters-Stone KM, Torgrimson B, Horak F, et al. Identifying factors associated with falls in postmenopausal breast cancer survivors: a multidisciplinary approach. *Arch Phys Med Rehabil.* 2011;92(4):646–652.

64. Huang MH, Shilling T, Miller KA, et al. History of falls, gait, balance, and fall risks in older cancer survivors living in the community. *Clin Interv Aging.* 2015;10:1497–1503.

65. Wechsler S, Wood L. The effect of chemotherapy on balance, gait, and falls among cancer survivors: a scoping review. *Rehabil Oncol.* 2021;39(1):6–22.

66. Tofthagen C, Overcash J, Kip K. Falls in persons with chemotherapy-induced peripheral neuropathy. *Support Care Cancer.* 2012;20:583–589.

67. Dros J, Wewerinke A, Bindels PJ, van Weert HC. Accuracy of monofilament testing to diagnose peripheral neuropathy: a systematic review. *Ann Fam Med.* 2009;7(6):555–558.

68. van den Beuken-van Everdingen MH, Hochstenbach LM, Joosten EA, Tjan-Heijnen VC, Janssen DJ. Update on prevalence of pain in patients with cancer: systematic review and meta-analysis. *J Pain Symptom Manage.* 2016;51(6):1070–1090.e9.

69. Portenoy RK, Dhingra LK. Assessment of cancer pain. https://www.uptodate.com/contents/assessment-of-cancer-pain. February 28, 2019. Accessed April 21, 2021.

70. Wake WT. Pressure ulcers: what clinicians need to know. *Perm J.* 2010;14(2):56–60.

71. Dennerlein JT, O'Day ET, Mulloy DF, et al. Lifting and exertion injuries decrease after implementation of an integrated hospital-wide safe patient handling and mobilisation programme. *Occup Environ Med.* 2017;74:336–343.

72. Needham DM, Truong AD, Fan E. Technology to enhance physical rehabilitation of critically ill patients. *Crit Care Med.* 2009;37(10):S436–S441.

73. Nelson A, Owen B, Lloyd JD, et al. Safe patient handling and movement: preventing back injury among nurses requires careful selection of the safest equipment and techniques. The second of two articles. *AJN Am J Nurs.* 2003;103(3):32–43.

74. Ahn KY, Hur H, Kim DH, et al. The effects of inpatient exercise therapy on the length of hospital stay in stages I–III colon cancer patients: randomized controlled trial. *Int J Colorectal Dis.* 2013;28(5):643–651.

75. The Medicare Payment Advisory Commission. Chapter 10. Inpatient rehabilitation facility services. Report to the congress: medicare payment policy. http://www.medpac.gov/docs/default-source/reports/mar20_medpac_ch10_sec.pdf. March 2020.

76. Smith S, Wilson CM, Lipple C, et al. Managing palliative patients in inpatient rehabilitation through a short stay family training program. *Am J Hospice Palliat Med.* 2020;37(3):172–178.

77. Center for Medicare and Medicaid Services. Long term care hospital services. https://www.medicare.gov/coverage/long-term-care-hospital-services. Accessed April 21, 2021.

78. American Speech Language and Hearing Association. Long-term acute care hospitals. https://www.asha.org/slp/healthcare/ltac/. Accessed October 5, 2020.

25
Pediatric Cancer Management

SHARA CREARY-YAN, PT, BSc, GCOR, CLWT, HALLIE LENKER, PT, DPT

CHAPTER OUTLINE

Introduction

Given the incidence of pediatric cancer and the improvement in overall survival rates, oncology rehabilitation (Onc R) is essential in the treatment of the whole child beginning at time of diagnosis. Onc R intervention is essential across the continuum of care in children diagnosed with cancer. Rehabilitative focus should include improving activity tolerance, providing patient-specific interventions, as well as educating the children, family, and medical team. Treatment for pediatric cancer impacts participation, quality of life (QOL), and the entire family unit, The Onc R clinician is integral in the evaluation and treatment of these impairments. This chapter will review common pediatric diagnoses including childhood leukemias, central nervous system (CNS) tumors, nephroblastoma, and neuroblastoma including the rehabilitative implications of cancer treatment for children living with and beyond cancer.

Childhood Leukemias

The three most common pediatric leukemias include acute lymphoblastic leukemia (ALL), acute myeloid leukemia (AML), and chronic myeloid leukemia (CML).

Acute Lymphoblastic Leukemia (ALL)

ALL is the most common childhood cancer at 25% to 35% of overall diagnoses and accounts for 80% of childhood leukemia diagnoses.[1,2] AML, which is less common as a primary cancer, has a higher incidence as a secondary cancer for children previously treated for cancer.[1,3,4] The 5-year survival rate for ALL is 90% with low risk ALL as high as 92%.[5] AML demonstrates a slightly decreased survival rate at 60% to 70%[2,5] though patients with acute promyelocytic leukemia (APL), a subset of AML, typically have 5-year survivals at 82%.[6,7] Higher incidences of leukemia have been demonstrated in children with chromosomal abnormalities, identical twins, and individuals with Down syndrome have a 10 to 20 times higher risk.[5,8] Given the higher rate of incidence of leukemia in the pediatric population, it is imperative that all Onc R clinicians are versed in the signs and symptoms as first-line providers.

Leukemia starts in the bone marrow where new blood cells are created; as the leukemia cells, increase they crowd out the other, normal blood cells as depicted in Figure 25.1. As the bone marrow begins to produce less normal, healthy blood cells, there is a decrease in red blood cells (RBCs), also referred to as anemia, white blood cells WBCs) or (neutropenia, and/or platelets

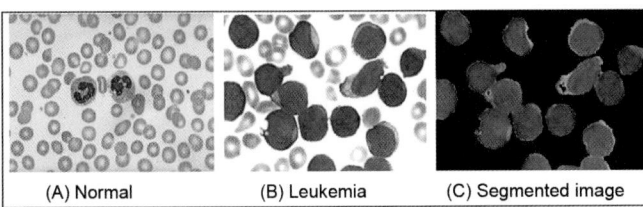

• **Fig. 25.1** Image Segmentation of Blood and Bone Marrow Smear With Emphasis to Automated Detection of Leukemia. (Reprinted with permission from Anilkumar KK, Manoj VJ, Sagi TM. A survey on image segmentation of blood and bone marrow smear images with emphasis to automated detection of leukemia. *Biocybern Biomed Eng.* 2020;40(4):1406–1420.)

TABLE 25.1	Leukemia Phases
Leukemia Phase	**Definition**
Untreated leukemia	Not yet received treatment
Leukemia in remission	No detectable leukemia
Recurrent leukemia	Relapse after a period of remission
Refractory leukemia	Remission not achieved during induction

Created by Hallie Lenker. Printed with Permission.

(thrombocytopenia). Pancytopenia, a deficiency in RBCs, WBCs, and platelets, typically accounts for initial leukemia symptoms. eFigure 25.1 displays some symptoms that children often complain of namely weakness, fatigue, shortness of breath, pallor (associated with anemia), and infections or fevers of unknown origin (associated with neutropenia); easy bruising or nosebleeds (thrombocytopenia) are also common.[8,9] Bone and joint pain are often caused by overcrowding of the cells within the bone.[5] If there is any concern of new onset of symptoms the child should always be referred to the referring provider to determine the need for further workup.

Differential diagnoses for the primary care provider may include non-Hodgkin lymphoma, juvenile rheumatoid arthritis (JRA), mononucleosis, or idiopathic thrombocytopenic purpura.[5] Typically, the first test for leukemia involves a blood test to check a child's complete blood count (CBC), which demonstrates increased WBCs called lymphocytes. To determine the cause of the increase in peripheral WBCs, called blasts in the blood, a bone marrow biopsy and aspirate is completed to examine the bone and liquid bone marrow. The bone marrow biopsy determines hyper- and hypocellularity of the blood-forming cells. The aim for these tests is to determine whether the child has leukemia and to diagnose the type and subtype which dictates the type of treatment the child will receive.[10] Flow cytometry is completed to differentiate between the type of leukemia to determine if the child has ALL, AML, or CML as well as a subset such as T-cell or B-cell ALL.[2] For leukemia, children are also classified as standard versus high risk. This classification drives treatment regimens and is determined by age at diagnosis, with ages 1 to 9 years old categorized as standard risk while children less than 1 year or greater than 10 years old are placed in a high-risk category. Initial WBC count at diagnosis with children that have very high WBCs (greater than 50,000 cells per cubic meter) are also placed in the high-risk group.[11,12] See Table 25.1 for the phases of leukemia during diagnosis and treatment.

Once a child has been diagnosed with leukemia, the child begins treatment. Outside of the type/subset of treatment, the treatment plan depends on the child's leukemia treatment status, risk group, age, immunophenotype, and presence of CNS involvement.[5] During leukemia treatment, children undergo five treatment phases: induction, consolidation, interim maintenance, delayed intensification, and maintenance. After the initial diagnosis, the child undergoes induction therapy which is approximately 4 weeks of intensive chemotherapy after which the child will undergo a bone marrow biopsy. Currently, 98% of children achieve remission after induction.[13,14] If remission is achieved, most standard-risk children undergo consolidation for 12 to 16 weeks which destroys any remaining leukemia and prophylactically prevents CNS growth with a drug regime that

includes intrathecal (IT) methotrexate.[13,15] Interim maintenance follows consolidation and is 8 weeks to maintain remission and allow the bone marrow to recover. After interim maintenance, children undergo delayed intensification with 8 weeks of chemotherapy to prevent recurrence of their leukemia. The longest, and final, phase of treatment is maintenance which is typically 2 to 3 years in length with less frequent, mostly oral chemotherapies.[13,15,16]

In children, most leukemia is treated primarily with chemotherapy; however, children with CNS involvement can receive radiation to the brain as chemotherapy does not cross the blood–brain barrier. Males who demonstrate testicular involvement after induction may receive testicular radiation. Radiation is often received five times per week for 2 weeks.[13] Surgical interventions are usually only for central line placement and biopsies. The chemotherapy a child receives often drives its initial and long-term physical and functional impairments. For most standard-risk children the chemotherapies used during induction includes L-asparaginase (Elspar, Kidrolase), vincristine (Oncovin, Vincasar PFS), and a corticosteroid with most treatment regimens adding an anthracycline.[12,13] High-risk leukemia also receives an anthracycline class of chemotherapy, often daunorubicin (Cerubidine).[15,17,18] During consolidation, children receive cyclophosphamide (Cytoxan), cytarabine (Cytosar-U), and mercaptopurine (6-MP, Purinethol) and transition to high dose methotrexate toward interim maintenance. During the maintenance phase, children receive oral chemotherapies such as 6-MP and low dose methotrexate as well as intermittent vincristine and steroid pulses.[12,19]

Due to the prolonged and multidrug treatment plan for the child undergoing leukemia treatment, the Onc R clinician needs to be mindful of the anticipated adverse effects of chemotherapy both medically and physically. The child's current treatment status and full treatment plan must be considered when initiating an Onc R plan of care (POC). For a child early in the treatment course, intervention should be around education and prevention of known physical adverse effects of the chemotherapy regimen. Due to the prevalence of vincristine-related neuropathy, the Onc R POC should include fine motor, balance, and range of motion (ROM), with special attention to ankle dorsiflexion due to ankle ROM deficits and gait deviations associated with vincristine.[20,21] Formal gait assessments and home exercise programs (HEPs) should be provided to maintain or improve these areas.[20] There is a risk of osteonecrosis, with higher rates in the adolescent population especially females, due to prolonged and frequent steroid administration, therefore, safe weight-bearing (WB) activities should be included especially early on in treatment courses. While chemotherapy regimens are advancing to decrease the dosing and use of anthracyclines, such as daunorubicin/doxorubicin (Adriamycin), they are still used in the pediatric population. Due

TABLE 25.2	World Health Organization Classification of Central Nervous System Tumors			
Tumor Type		**Grading**	**Tumor Type**	**Grading**
Diffuse astrocytic and oligodendroglia tumors			**Embryonal tumors**	
Diffuse astrocytoma		II	Medulloblastoma	IV
Oligodendroglioma		II	Embryonal tumor with multiple layers	IV
Anaplastic astrocytoma		III	Medulloepithelioma	IV
Anaplastic oligodendroglioma		III	CNS embryonal tumor	IV
Glioblastoma		IV	Atypical teratoid/rhabdoid tumor	IV
Other astrocytic tumors			**Meningiomas**	
Pilocytic astrocytoma		I	Meningiomas	I
Ependymal tumors			Atypical mengioma	II
Subependymoma		I	Anaplastic mengiomas	III
Myxopapillary ependymoma		I		
Ependymoma		II or III		
Anaplastic ependymoma		III		

Adapted from 2016 CNS WHO Grading Scale. Created by Hallie Lenker. Printed with permission.

to the predisposition of cardiotoxicity with use of anthracyclines, the child's cardiac status is evaluated during and post-treatment. Results of echocardiograms should be known, and the cardiopulmonary system should be monitored during exercise.[22]

Acute Myeloid Leukemia (AML)

The incidence of AML is 13% of childhood leukemia diagnoses between the ages of 0 and 10 years old and increases substantially as a child ages, accounting for 36% of leukemia diagnoses in adolescents and young adults aged 15 to 19.[2] While ALL is diagnosed with increased lymphocytes in the bone marrow, AML demonstrates myeloid blasts. Treatment differences include a decreased overall treatment time for children undergoing AML treatment as there is no prolonged maintenance phase, this therefore decreases the treatment duration to 6 to 8 months in total. Chemotherapies in AML treatment include cytarabine, etoposide (Toposar, VePesid), and anthracyclines. While the treatment is typically shorter in duration, the overall intensity of the chemotherapy regimen is higher, requiring more frequent inpatient admissions during cycles for hydration and for monitoring acute medical adverse effects. CML has an even lower incidence in children and is treated with an oral tyrosine kinase inhibitor.[2,23]

Central Nervous System (CNS) Tumors

This section reviews the more common childhood CNS tumors and treatment strategies. Brain tumors discussed include astrocytomas and medulloblastomas, while spinal cord tumors include both intramedullary spinal cord tumors and astrocytomas of the spine.

Pediatric Brain Tumors

Pediatric brain tumors are the second most common pediatric cancer (5%–17%),[5,24,25] the most common pediatric solid tumor and the cause of 25% of pediatric cancer-related deaths.[6,26,27] Brain tumors are graded using the World Health Organization (WHO) grading scale (Table 25.2). The most common pediatric brain tumors are astrocytomas (Grade I and II—low grade gliomas) with pilocytic astrocytoma accounting for 50% of astrocytomas diagnosed, either benign or malignant.[25,27] Most pilocytic astrocytomas are in the cerebellum and supratentorial structures.[27,28] Ependymal astrocytomas are often diagnosed in children under three years old and can block the fourth ventricle resulting in hydrocephalus, similar to congenital teratoma which occurs in the first year of life.[29] The 5-year survival rate for low-grade gliomas and medulloblastoma is 75%.[30] High-grade gliomas (WHO Grade III/IV) are rarer at 20% of brain tumors and they account for 44% of brain tumor-related death in children under 14 years old.[26,27] Medulloblastomas are the most common, aggressive, malignant brain tumors in children, located in the posterior fossa and can also result in hydrocephalus if obstructive. Males are at a higher risk for malignant tumors, with high-grade gliomas more commonly diagnosed in males by 60%; females are at a higher risk for nonmalignant tumors as they are twice as likely to develop nonmalignant meningiomas.[31]

Precipitating factors for medical workup for pediatric brain tumors include macrocephaly, irritability, failure to thrive, regression of developmental milestones, nausea, vomiting, headaches, and/or altered mental status (AMS).[27,29] Onc R clinicians can be initial providers for children who have a slow onset of symptoms. Symptom progression or loss of milestones should result in referral to a pediatrician. If a child is demonstrating neurologic symptoms, initial testing is typically via a computed tomography (CT) scan which can demonstrate intracranial hemorrhage, mass effect, midline shift of the anatomic structures, or edema. If a mass is noted or suspected a magnetic resonance imaging (MRI) is performed for the anatomical extent of the tumor and to aid differential diagnosis (Figure 25.2).[27] While total resection is the goal, surgical options are dependent on the location of the tumor and the neurologic risk.[32] A tumor biopsy is needed as the pathology, histology, and molecular makeup drive both diagnosis and therapeutic management.

Treatment for pediatric brain tumors is multimodal. Children who have not previously been followed by a Onc R clinician should have an evaluation completed prior to biopsy or resection during

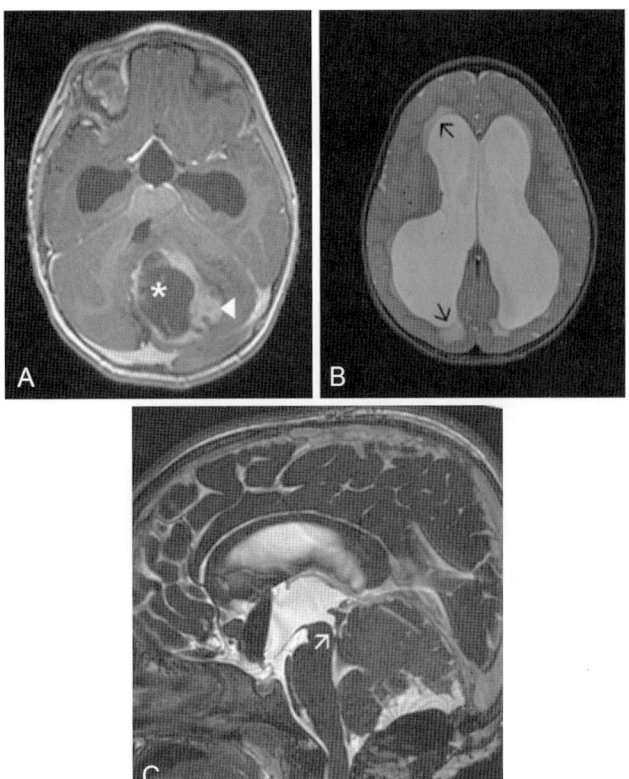

• **Fig. 25.2** Post-Gadolinium Image of a Cerebellar Pilocytic Astrocytoma, in a 3-Year-Old Boy. (Reprinted with permission from Pediatric Surgery, licensed content authors Eamon J. McLaughlin, Michael J. Fisher, Leslie N. Sutton, and Phillip B. Storm. Coran AG, Caldamone AN, Scott A, et al. Post-gadolinium image of a cerebellar pilocytic astrocytoma, in a 3-year-old boy. In: *Pediatric Surgery*. 2012:595.) (A) Axial T1WI post-gadolinium image of a cerebellar pilocytic astrocytoma, in a 3-year-old boy, showing a large cyst *(white asterisk)* and enhancing mural nodule *(white arrowhead)*. (B) Axial T2WI image showing markedly dilated lateral ventricles and transependymal flow of cerebral spinal fluid (CSF) out of the ventricles into the surrounding brain parenchyma *(black arrows)*. The obstructive hydrocephalus is a result of the cerebellar astrocytoma. (C) Sagittal T2WI postoperative image showing resection of tumor and flow through the floor of the third ventricle *(white arrow)* after the endoscopic third ventriculostomy done at the time of tumor resection. Reprinted with permission.

the acute hospitalization; however, due to timing and urgency the evaluation may be more appropriate postoperatively. Children undergoing resection of medulloblastomas in the posterior fossa may experience a sequela of symptoms from a disruption of the cerebellum referred to as posterior fossa syndrome. Posterior fossa syndrome has symptoms of mutism, ataxia, hypotonia, behavioral changes, and emotional lability that occurs in 25% of children postoperatively. Most recover their speech abilities although ongoing dysarthria may occur.[33] Cranial radiation and/or proton radiation is standard and comes with high risk for short- and long-term adverse effects.[32] There are clinical trials attempting to maximize the efficacy of chemotherapy regimens and targeted cell therapies to limit the initiation and/or duration of radiation though most have mixed response and there is difficulty crossing the blood-brain barrier.[32]

Intramedullary Spinal Cord Tumors

Intramedullary spinal cord tumors in pediatrics are rare, accounting for 1% to 10% of pediatric CNS tumors.[34] As with brain tumors, astrocytoma tumors of the spine are the most common (1 child in 100,000) followed by ependymomas (0.06 children in 100,000).[34,35] Due to the overall low incidence, prognosis is

difficult to report but spinal cord astrocytomas reported from 1973 to 2013 were noted to have survival rates of 85.3% at one year, 79.5% at two years, and 75.8% at five years (74.8%).[34,36] Older age (15–21 years), non-White races, high tumor grade, nonfocal tumors, and need for radiation all resulted in decreased survival. Gradual onset is likely, typically presenting with pain, sensory/motor deficits, and gastrointestinal symptoms.[34,37] For astrocytoma spinal cord tumors, retrospective patient analysis has shown the incidence is higher in the thoracic region and in males. Males have a higher incidence of ependymoma spinal cord tumors while females have higher recurrence rates.[35] The first line of treatment is resection with gross total resection being standard. Radiation and chemotherapy are prescribed for inoperable or high-grade tumors. See Table 25.3 for characteristics of CNS cancers.

Nephroblastoma

Renal tumors are the third most common pediatric solid malignancy with a global age-standardized incidence rate of 8.2 per million persons per year.[41] Nephroblastoma or Wilms tumor is the most common primary renal neoplasm while the other three diagnoses are relatively rare. These include: rhabdoid renal tumor (RRT), renal carcinoma, and renal sarcoma/peripheral primitive

TABLE 25.3   Characteristics of CNS Cancers[38,39,39]

Location	Tumor Type	Clinical Presentation	Pathologic Subtype	Grading Scale	Treatment	Prognosis
Posterior fossa Spinal cord Supratentorial	Cerebellar astrocytoma	Headaches, macrocephaly, visual impairment, location of tumor key	Pilocytic astrocytoma Diffuse astrocytoma	I—low grade II—low grade	Observation/resection Partial resection may receive chemotherapy (carboplatin, vincristine, vinblastine, temozolomide) and/or RTx[146]	I/II: favorable prognosis if easily resected, metastases are uncommon
		Headaches, macrocephaly, visual impairment, location of tumor key	Anaplastic astrocytoma Glioblastoma	III—high grade IV—high grade	Resection if operable, radiation, chemotherapy (temozolomide); may receive high dose chemotherapy and stem cell transplant	Worse prognosis than low grade, improved with gross total resection
Posterior fossa	Medulloblastoma	80% of tumors in fourth ventricle – hydrocephalus – headaches – nausea/vomiting – lethargy – ataxia – nystagmus – papilledema		Malignant	≤3 years old: surgery and chemotherapy >3 years old: surgery, chemotherapy and RTx (4–6 weeks postoperative) Chemotherapy can include cyclophosphamide, etoposide, cisplatin, vincristine, methotrexate	40%–90% depending on subtype, degree of resection, dissemination throughout CNS
Posterior fossa Supratentorial Spinal cord	Ependymomas	Posterior fossa: hydrocephalus symptoms, ataxia, neck pain, cranial nerve palsies Supratentorial: headache, seizures, focal neurologic deficits Spinal cord: back pain, LE weakness, bowel/bladder dysfunction	Grades I–III	Malignant	Dependent on grading, location and age Resection Radiation Chemotherapy-recurrent or noncomplete resections	Genetic makeup changes prognosis Posterior fossa: 35%–90% Supratentorial 80%–100% Poorer prognosis: younger age, anaplastic histology, partial resection, lower dose/no radiation
	Brainstem glioma	Cranial nerve deficits, hypertonia, ataxia, hydrocephalus, change in behavior	Diffuse intrinsic pontine glioma (DIPG)	Malignant	Radiation	Aggressive, typically <1 year, 2-year survival rate 10% Progression typically occurs by 1-year post-RTx
		Cranial nerve deficits, hypertonia, ataxia, hydrocephalus, change in behavior	Low grade brain stem glioma		Resection, observation Nonoperable: radiation/chemotherapy	5-year survival rate 90%
Posterior fossa Supratentorial	Atypical teratoid rhabdoid tumors (ATRT)	Quick progression of symptoms – headaches – vomiting – lethargy – regression of motor skills – macrocephaly		Malignant	Resection, radiation (age dependent), chemotherapy (high dose and intrathecal)	Rare and aggressive, poor outcomes when germline mutation, <2 years old, metastases at diagnosis, partial resection
spinal cord	Vertebral hemangiomas			Benign		Asymptomatic: incidental finding on imaging Aggressive: typically, in thoracic spine, can cause spinal cord compression

CNS, Central nervous system; LE, lower extremity; RTx, radiation therapy.
Created by Hallie Lenker. Printed with permission.

neuroectodermal tumors. The highest incidence occurs in African and the lowest in East Asian territories and racial groups. Europe, Australia, and North America display similar trends with recent studies highlighting a lower incidence of nephroblastomas and excellent survival rates in countries with a high and middle human development index (HDI) compared to those with a lower HDI (http://hdr.undp.org/en/content/human-development-index-hdi).[42,43] Nephroblastomas are also the most common pediatric abdominal malignancies and possess a better prognosis in children less than 5 years old with a median age at diagnosis being 3.5 years.[44]

These tumors are thought to develop from persistent metanephric tissue or nephrogenic rests with abnormal metanephric cells found in up to 100% of cases of bilateral nephroblastomas but only in 35% of unilateral tumors.[45] Genetic alterations occurring in the normal embryological development of the genitourinary tract are regarded as strong predisposing factors for nephroblastomas. Some of the genetic markers that have been associated with Wilms tumor include *WT1*, *CTNNB1*, and *WTX*, and gene alterations that have been found in about one-third of all Wilms tumors. Other associated genes include *MYNC* and *TP53*, the latter which is linked to poorer prognosis along with the loss of heterozygosity at chromosomes 1p, 1q, 11p15, and 16q. Renal tumors are also found in sequela of congenital anomalies, including Beckwith-Wiedemann syndrome, isolated hemihypertrophy, neurofibromatosis, Denys-Drash syndrome, Perlman syndrome, and an increased familial gene loci (familial WT1 and WT2).

The most common first signs of nephroblastomas are swollen, distended, hard abdomens with some parents able to palpate a hard mass within the child's abdomen (Figure 25.3 displays characteristics and clinical features). This mass is often not painful, and most children will continue to play with no apparent discomfort. Other features include fever, abdominal pain, constipation, loss of appetite, hematuria, urinary tract infections, varicocele, anemia (especially in advanced cases), or metastasis to the lungs. The child may also present with dyspnea, tachypnea, and hypotension or more commonly hypertension in children with renin-producing tumor cells. In most cases, a return to normal blood pressure

occurs following nephrectomy. Initial laboratory tests include a CBC investigating anemia, renal function, urinalysis, chemistry profile, coagulation studies, and cytogenetic studies. Imaging studies are integral in surgical planning to aid in tumor size and extension and the displacement of large vessels. A renal ultrasound may be among the first scans performed, though abdominal and chest CTs or MRIs may replace the ultrasound in some settings. Metastasis patterns for nephroblastomas include the lungs, liver, lymph nodes, bone, and brain. Often a chest X-ray is ordered to examine the mediastinum. Biopsy of the tumor retrieved during surgical removal is instrumental in staging, identifying histology, and treatment.

The National Wilms Tumor Staging Group and the Children's Oncology Group (COG) staging system divides nephroblastomas into five stages (Table 25.4).

There are vast differences in international treatment practices, though a multidisciplinary approach is integral in ensuring rehabilitation of these children. Primarily, surgical resection or neoadjuvant (for tumor regression and reduction of intraoperative tumor rupture) is considered based on tumor appearance and preliminary staging. Radical nephrectomy, regional lymph node sampling, and thorough examination of the organs in the abdominal cavity with biopsy of suspicious areas are instrumental for accurate staging and treatment of the disease. The thoracic cavity may be explored if imaging showed signs of metastasis with tumor excisions carried out under more minimally invasive techniques such as video assisted thoracoscopic surgery (VATS). Careful selection of chemotherapy drugs are ordered based on staging, histology, and likelihood of relapse (Table 25.5).

External beam radiation therapy is used with surgery in more advanced cases of nephroblastoma (Stages III, IV, and V) that have spread beyond the kidney or are not fully resectable. This form of treatment is also used in unfavorable histology profiles for tumors of Stages I and II disease. Common adverse effects from treatment that are targeted in rehabilitation include many of the initial symptoms such as fatigue, nausea, and pain in addition to those typical of postmedical and surgical management. Comprehensive Onc R across the survivorship continuum must include identification

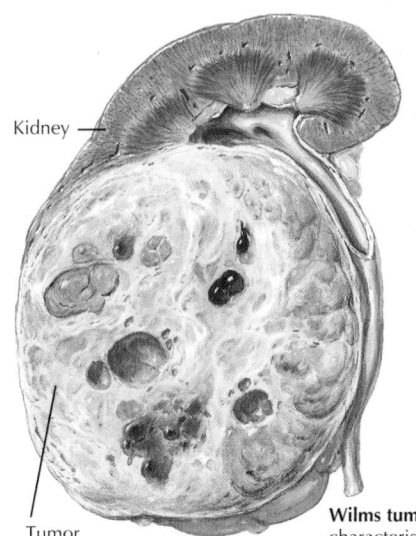

Clinical features of Wilms tumor

Occurs in infants and young children

Mass in loin or abdomen often first manifestation (differentiate from solitary cyst or multicystic kidney, large hydronephrosis, neuroblastoma)

Pressure phenomena may occur; gastrointestinal, venous (edema), respiratory

Metastasizes chiefly to local nodes, lungs, and liver; rarely to bone, in contrast to neuroblastoma where bone is principal site

Fever in many cases

Loss of weight, anemia, cachexia may appear late; hematuria absent; hypertension may appear

Kidney

Tumor

Wilms tumor. With pseudocapsule and characteristic variegated structure

Stroma of sarcoma-like spindle cells. With islands of malignant columnar cells in irregular tubular arrangements typical of Wilms tumor

• **Fig. 25.3** Characteristics and Clinical Features of Wilms Tumors. (Reprinted with permission from Florin TA, Ludwig S. Renal neoplasms. In: *Netter's Pediatrics*. 1st ed. Elsevier; 2011: 361.)

TABLE 25.4	Wilms Tumor Staging[43,45]
Stage I	Tumor completely resected and confined to the kidney. No involvement of the renal sinus vessels or capsule. 40% of all Wilms tumors are found at this stage.
Stage II	Tumor is completely resected but extended beyond the kidney. Penetration of the renal capsule, invasion of the renal sinus vessels, biopsy of tumor before removal or spillage of tumor locally during removal may have occurred. 20% of Wilms tumors.
Stage III	Tumor remains postoperatively, including at surgical margins, an inoperable tumor, abdominal and or pelvic lymph node metastasis and tumor spillage involving peritoneal surfaces. 20% of Wilms tumors.
Stage IV	Metastases; hematogenous or lymph nodes outside of the abdomen including lung, liver, bone, or brain. 10% of Wilms tumors.
Stage V	Bilateral Wilms tumors, often from primitive abnormal tissue on both kidneys and not spread from one to the other. 5% of Wilms tumors.

Adapted from the National Wilms Tumor Staging Group and the Children's Oncology Group Staging System.
Created by Shara Creary-Yan. Printed with permission.

TABLE 25.5	Nephroblastoma Stages and Common Chemotherapy Agents Used[47–49]
Stage I and II	Treated intravenously vincristine and dactinomycin. initially on a weekly schedule and then every 2–3 weeks. Some settings may allow for this to be done as an outpatient as the adverse effects are usually mild and not requiring hospitalization. In the presence of chromosomal changes doxorubicin may also be given as well. Stage II with diffuse anaplastic histology more aggressive combinations following radiation therapy include the use of vincristine, doxorubicin, etoposide, cyclophosphamide, and carboplatin, along with mesna (helps protect the bladder from the effects of cyclophosphamide), which is given for about 6 months.
Stage III–V	In cases of very large tumors, biopsy followed by radiation and or chemotherapy before and or after surgery may be utilized. Chemotherapy may be given as an outpatient, however, treatment for these stages of disease often requires hospitalization and is often associated with more serious adverse effects. Various treatment protocols utilizing vincristine, dactinomycin, doxorubicin, cyclophosphamide, carboplatin, etoposide or ifosfamide (rarely). Mesna is also given as indicated.
Recurrent	Treatment at this point depends on histology, location of return and prior treatment. Treatment for these children may include surgery if possible to remove the recurrent cancer, radiation therapy (if not already given to the area), and chemotherapy, often with drugs different from those used during first treatment. For more aggressive tumors protocols such as the ICE regimen (ifosfamide, carboplatin, and etoposide) or others being studied in clinical trials may be utilized. These protocols of management followed by a stem cell transplant might also be an option, although this is still being studied.

Created by Shara Creary-Yan. Printed with permission.

of adverse effects and the treatment of late and long-term adverse along with continuous patient and family education (Table 25.6).

Neuroblastoma

Neuroblastoma is commonly used to reference an umbrella of neuroblastic tumors that arise from primitive sympathetic ganglion cells (including neuroblastomas, ganglioneuroblastomas, and ganglioneuromas). Across decades, neuroblastomas hold a global reputation for being the most common extracranial tumor, ranging from 7% to 9% of childhood cancers in regions such as France, United States (US), Japan, sections of the Caribbean, and Africa.[44–49] In the developing embryo, these primitive sympathetic ganglion cells invaginate, migrate along the neuraxis, and populate the sympathetic ganglia, adrenal medulla, and other sites.[47] Though not all autonomic nervous system tumors are malignant, they may exhibit malignant and nonmalignant cells within the same tumor. Ganglioneuroma is a benign tumor made up of mature ganglion and nerve sheath cells. A ganglioneuroblastoma is a tumor that has both malignant and benign parts, with neuroblasts that can grow and spread abnormally, similar to neuroblastoma, as well as areas of more mature tissue that are similar to ganglioneuroma.[48]

TABLE 25.6	Summary of Late and Long-Term Adverse Effects of Nephroblastoma Treatment[49,50,51]
Late and Long-Term Effects	
Reduced kidney function and premature failure	
Damage to the musculoskeletal and nervous system	
Cardiac toxicity and pulmonary complications	
Developmental delay, regression, and cognitive disabilities	
Reproductive changes, challenges, and infertility	
Increased risk of secondary cancers	

Created by Shara Creary-Yan. Printed with Permission.

The neuroectodermal cells that comprise neuroblastic tumors originate from the neural crest during fetal development. Most neuroblastomas begin in abdominal sympathetic nerve ganglia with about half originating in the adrenal gland, followed by sympathetic ganglia near the spine, in the chest, neck, or pelvis (see Figure 25.4). Transformation of undifferentiated sympathoadrenal progenitor cells results in tumor formation in the adrenal medulla in the abdomen and sympathetic ganglia along the sympathetic chains. Notable characteristics of these tumors implicate their heterogeneous and complex biology. These include a high incidence of spontaneous regression and differentiation to a benign tumor in infants less than 12 months of age with a stage 4S on the International Neuroblastoma Staging System (INSS), whereas in children older than 18 months of age and in the advanced stages, neuroblastoma proves extremely malignant often requiring systemic therapy.[52–54] In the advanced stages, neuroblastoma cells metastasize widely to the bone marrow, bone, lymph nodes, liver, intracranial and orbital sites, lung, CNS, and skin resulting in long-term survival rates less than 40%, even with intensive treatment.[55,51]

Many sources regard neuroblastomas as a disease of unknown etiology, with continued research highlighting variable risk factors. Neuroblastomas have been shown to be associated with other pathologies derived from the neural crest called neurocristopathies. These diseases display an abnormally high frequency of neuroblastic tumors compared to the general population.

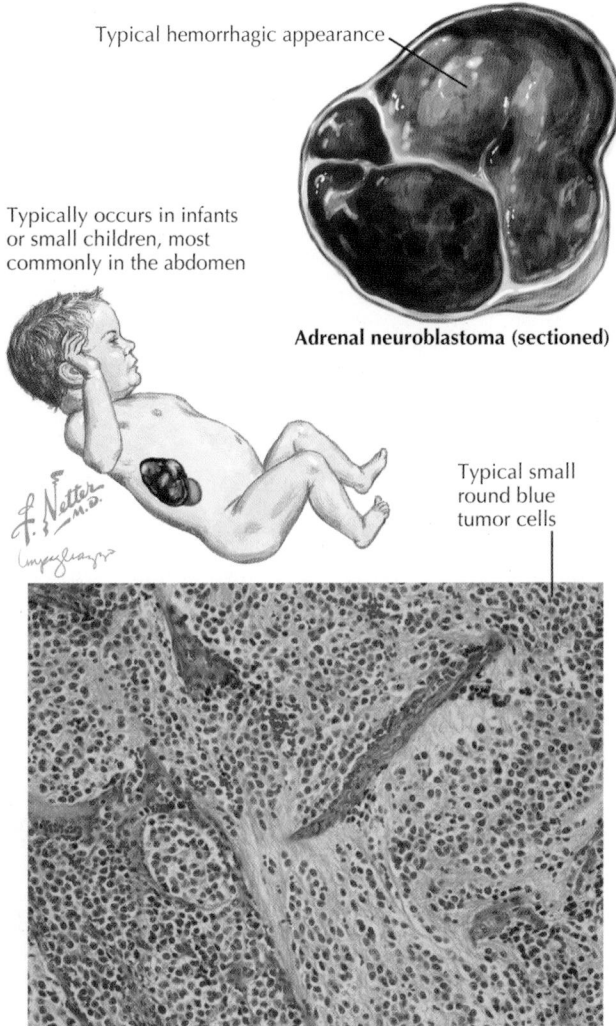

Typical hemorrhagic appearance

Typically occurs in infants or small children, most commonly in the abdomen

Adrenal neuroblastoma (sectioned)

Typical small round blue tumor cells

Histopathology, poorly differentiated adrenal neuroblastoma
(Courtesy of Bruce Pawel, MD, Children's Hospital of Philadephia)

• **Fig. 25.4** Overview of Neuroblastomas. (Reprinted with permission from Florin TA, Ludwig S. Neuroblastoma. In: *Netter's Pediatrics*. 1st ed. Elsevier; 2011: 356)

These include Hirschsprung disease, Type 1 neurofibromatosis, heterochromia iridis, and congenital central hypoventilation syndrome (CCHS), also called Ondine's curse.[58,59] Other characteristic features of neuroblastomas include a slightly higher male preponderance, higher incidence in non-African/Black racial groups and global trends of higher incidence in countries with a HDI.[60] These diverse clinical phenotypes and characteristics of neuroblastomas demonstrate an urgent need for comprehensive management and relentless medical and scientific research.

Neuroblastomas may be identified as early as in-utero ultrasounds and during urine testing at three weeks and six months old. Though a large portion of these tumors may self-resolve or are favorable to treatment, urinary catecholamine metabolite analyses are useful tumor markers. Other laboratory tests may include CBC, liver and kidney function tests including electrolyte analysis with serum ferritin levels often elevated. Imaging procedures include an X-ray or an ultrasound if a tumor in a specific area is highly suspected. Further steps include the use of MRIs (with or without contrast) and CT scans with a guided biopsy (see Figure 25.2).

A meta-iodobenzylguanidine (MIBG) scan may be ideal as it locates the tumor and extent of metastatic spread, and if absorbed by the mass, this radioactive molecule can be used at higher doses to treat the neuroblastoma. Bone and positron emission tomography (PET) scans are widely used in many settings, with some machines capable of producing PET and CT scans at the same time. Biopsies, though more invasive, are integral in confirming a diagnosis. The clinical manifestation of neuroblastomas may be grouped into categories based on classical signs, symptoms linked to the primary tumor, symptoms associated with catecholamine production, and metastasis (Table 25.7).

Once diagnosed, staging and risk groups are instrumental in identifying medical management. The International Neuroblastoma Risk Group Staging System (INRGSS; Stages L1, L2, M, and MS) uses results from imaging and a stage can be determined before treatment has started, whereas the International Neuroblastoma Staging System (INSS; Stages 1, 2A, 2B, 3, 4, 4S, *recurrent*) uses biopsy or resection to determine staging. The COG uses prognostic factors combined with the INRGSS stage of the disease, to place children into three different risk groups: low, intermediate, and high. Table 25.8 shows a comparison of risk group, staging, possible treatment, and adverse effects that these patients may experience. It is important that Onc R clinicians understand staging and to anticipate likely treatment adverse effects to effectively rehabilitate these children and their families across the continuum of care.

Hematopoietic Stem Cell Transplant (HSCT)

HSCT is a treatment for both malignant and nonmalignant diseases in pediatric patients. Twenty percent of allogenic HSCTs occur in children.[62] In pediatrics, HSCT can be used as a curative treatment for hematological diseases such as ALL, AML, severe combined immunodeficiency (SCID), chronic granulomatous disease (CGD), Wiskott-Aldrich syndrome (WAS), hemophagocytic lymphohistiocytosis (HLH), Fanconi anemia, black diamond anemia, congenital amegakaryocytic thrombocytopenia, sickle cell disease (SCD), aplastic anemia, and thalassemia.[63,64] HSCT is used as a rescue for solid tumors to treat the cellular hypoplasia

TABLE 25.7 **Neuroblastoma Spectrum of Symptoms**[50–52,54,58]

Local Classic Signs	Primary Tumor Symptoms	Catecholamine Associated Symptoms (Paraneoplastic Syndromes)	Metastasis Signs
Weight loss (supressed appetite, complaints of feeling full, anorexia) Irritability Fever Abdominal pain bloating Gastrointestinal disturbances (vomiting and diarrhea) Pallor Fatigue Palpable mass, may be irregular and painless Bone pain and limping	Chest/neck: Problems with breathing and coughing, difficulty swallowing, lumps or visible mass, edema and skin changes (blue-red color) to upper extremities and face, changes in consciousness and motor skills, drooping eyelids, small pupil. Abdomen/pelvis: Marked hepatomegaly, enlarged abdomen with palpable mass, painful and/ or full feeling abdomen, edema to lower extremities, neurological dysfunction, bladder and bowel disturbances. Eyes: Periorbital edema, swelling, and yellow-brown ecchymoses (aka raccoon eyes) Skin: Subcutaneous nodules of blue color which become reddish and then white commonly observed in neonates or infants with disseminated neuroblastoma. Bones: Common in long bones and skull. On X-rays, seen as lytic defects with irregular margins and periosteal reactions	Constant watery diarrhea Fever High blood pressure (causing irritability) Rapid heartbeat Reddening (flushing) of the skin Sweating Anemia, thrombocytopenia and leukocytopenia may occur with bone marrow infiltration or massive intratumoral haemorrhage Opsoclonus-myoclonus-ataxia syndrome or "dancing eyes, dancing feet"	Enlarged lymph nodes, liver or tumor size Blue or purple bumps that look like small blueberries may be a sign of spread to the skin Consumption coagulopathy Complaints of bone pain with associated neurologic changes

Created by Shara Creary-Yan. Printed with permission.

from the high dose of chemotherapy. This treatment involves taking the stem cells from either the peripheral blood (PBSCT) or bone marrow (BMT) from the child (autogenic) or donor (allogenic). HSCT requires prolonged hospitalizations for pretransplant conditioning with high dose chemotherapy, potential total body irradiation (TBI), and medications for immunosuppression and eradication of the bone marrow tissue.[63,64] Children remain hospitalized during the neutropenic phase of the transplant while they await neutrophil recovery—typically 7 to 14 days for autogenic and 20 to 30 days of allogeneic transplants.

While HSCTs can be curative for a variety of conditions there are transplant-related morbidity and mortality risks. After HSCT, children are at risk for acute complications within the first 90 days such as infection from myelosuppression, veno-occlusive disease (VOD), mucositis, and acute graft-versus-host disease (aGvHD). Chronic complications are measured at ≥90 days and can include chronic GvHD (cGvHD) and opportunistic infections.[64] Rehabilitation evaluations prior to HSCT in children improve delivery of care during and post-transplant as patients can be screened and pre-existing cognitive or activity limitations can be identified.[65]

Musculoskeletal pain, muscle weakness, reduced cardiovascular capacity and metabolic syndromes can arise from the transplant or disease relapse.[64] GvHD should be monitored as it can cause both acute and long-term functional complications. One retrospective

study of 476 patients with ALL found that children 2 to 12 years old demonstrated lower rates of GvHD (3% acute, 8% chronic).[67] This may be detrimental as GvHD has an anti-leukemic effect. GvHD was found to be higher in children younger than 2 years. One study demonstrated late effects of HSCT that occurred years after transplant and most notably endocrine dysfunction was exhibited such as hypothyroidism and gonadal failure.[68]

Rehabilitation Management of Pediatric Oncology

Developing a Comprehensive Multidisciplinary Rehabilitation Program

Implementing a comprehensive Onc R program is essential to optimizing the QOL of the pediatric population. Pediatric cancer occurs during a crucial phase of human development. This, coupled with the adverse effects of both cancer and its treatment, undoubtedly predisposes these children to immediate and long-term negative effects in overall health, physical functioning, as well as social and cognitive abilities.[67] This section will focus on creating a comprehensive multidisciplinary rehabilitation program including: prehabilitation and screening, acute, chronic, home, school-based intervention, palliative, and end of life management.

TABLE 25.8   Neuroblastoma Staging, Treatment, and Adverse Effects[52,60,61]

COG	INRGSS	Treatment	Adverse Effects of Treatment Targeted in Rehabilitation
Low Stage 1 Stage 2A or 2B <1 year old Stage 2A or 2B, >1 year old, no extra copies of the MYCN gene Stage 2A or 2B, >1 year, extra copies of the MYCN gene and favorable histology Stage 4S <1 year old, favorable histology, hyperdiploid, no extra copies of the MYCN gene	Stage 1—Small localized tumor, no MYCN amplification or chromothripsis Stage 2—Localized tumor, some lymph node involvement, no MYCN amplification or chromothripsis Stage 4S—Localized primary tumor, metastasis to liver, skin, bone marrow; diagnosed <12 months of age, no MYCN amplification	Mainstay: *Stage 1 and 2* Surgery and Chemotherapy *(common and combination drugs include cyclophosphamide, cisplatin, doxorubicin, epipodophyllotoxin, topotecan with G-CSF support according to international protocols)* Stage 4S—Observation Multidisciplinary rehabilitation inclusive of as indicated: Physical therapy, occupational therapy, respiratory therapy, speech and language therapy, nutrition, alternative medicine, psychologist, social worker, teacher or child lifestyle/ developmental specialist.	Loss of appetite, Nausea and vomiting, diarrhea and constipation, fatigue, pain, immunocompromised state, cardiac toxicity, cardiopulmonary deficits and disease, peripheral neuropathy, musculoskeletal deficits and decreased mobility, wounds, delayed milestones, hearing impairment, cognitive regression and disability, secondary cancers, psychological issues, caregiver burden.
Intermediate Stage 3, <1 year old, no extra copies of the MYCN gene or Stage 3, >1 year old, no extra copies of the MYCN gene, favorable histology Stage 4, <1 year old, no extra copies of the MYCN gene Stage 4S <1 year old, no extra copies of the MYCN gene, normal DNA ploidy, unfavorable histology	Stage 3—Tumor infiltrating across midline, regional or contralateral lymph node involvement, no MYCN amplification. Stage 4—Primary tumor, metastasis to lymph nodes, bone marrow, skin, liver; diagnosed <12 months of age, no MYCN amplification	Mainstay: *Stage 3 and 4* Surgery and Chemotherapy. Multidisciplinary rehabilitation inclusive of as indicated: Physical therapy, occupational therapy, respiratory therapy, speech and language therapy, nutrition, alternative medicine, psychologist, social worker, teacher or child lifestyle/ developmental specialist.	Loss of appetite, nausea and vomiting, diarrhea and constipation, fatigue, pain, immunocompromised state, cardiac toxicity, cardiopulmonary deficits and disease, peripheral neuropathy, musculoskeletal deficits and decreased mobility, wounds, delayed milestones, hearing impairment, cognitive regression and disability, secondary cancers, psychological issues, caregiver burden.
High Stage 2A or 2B, >1 year old, extra copies of the MYCN gene, unfavorable histology Stage 3, <1 year old, extra copies of the MYCN gene or >1 year, has extra copies of the MYCN gene or >18 months, unfavorable histology Stage 4, extra copies of the MYCN gene regardless of age or Stage 4 and older than 18 months or Stage 4 and between 12 and 18 months old, extra copies of the MYCN gene, unfavorable histology, and/or normal DNA ploidy Stage 4S >1 year old, extra copies of the MYCN gene	Stage 3—as above with MYCN amplified Stage 4—as above but with diagnosis >12 months of age, MYCN amplified	Mainstay: *Stage 3 and 4* Surgery, chemotherapy and high dose chemotherapy with autologous stem cell rescue, radiotherapy, biologic and immunotherapeutic maintenance therapy, retinoids. Multidisciplinary rehabilitation inclusive of as indicated: Physical therapy, occupational therapy, respiratory therapy, speech and language therapy, nutrition, alternative medicine, psychologist, social worker, teacher or child lifestyle/ developmental specialist. Palliative management	Loss of appetite, nausea and vomiting, diarrhea and constipation, fatigue, pain, immunocompromised state, cardiac toxicity, cardiopulmonary deficits and disease, peripheral neuropathy, musculoskeletal deficits and decreased mobility, wounds and lymphedema, delayed milestones, hearing impairment, cognitive regression and disability, secondary cancers, psychological issues, caregiver burden. Skin and nail changes inclusive of burn/wounds and lymphedema, growth retardation or slowing increased risk for scoliosis.

COG, Children's Oncology Group; BHLH, transcription factor; DNA, deoxyribonucleic acid; G-CSF, granulocyte colony-stimulating factor; INRGSS, International Neuroblastoma Risk Group Staging System; MYCN, MYCN Proto-Oncogene.
Created by Shara Creary-Yan. Printed with permission.

The measure of an optimal pediatric Onc R program lies in its ability to prevent negative impacts where possible, educate, monitor, treat and optimize outcomes across the continuum of care, while focusing on the universal development of children and their families. At the core of creating such a program is the aim of increasing the knowledge and confidence for referral and treatment as well as integrating Onc R in the cancer continuum. Importantly, the goal is to improve and increase the QOL and lifespan of these children and their families.

Globally, varying programs have been developed in order to provide pediatric Onc R. Best practice as it relates to interdisciplinary team membership includes a nurse navigator (a healthcare professional who coordinates multidisciplinary services for the patient), oncologist (medical, surgical, and radiation), physical therapist, occupational therapist, speech and language pathologist, integrative medicine, prosthetist, nutritionist, a learning specialist or teacher, music and/or play/recreational therapist, child life specialist, psychologist, social worker, financial advisor, and a spiritual advisor. Though not every setting may be able to fully integrate all of the professionals listed above, especially in the early phases of development, it is encouraged to pursue integration of as many of these team members as possible at the inception of the team to aid in program efficacy and longevity. Where this is not possible, it is imperative to understand each professional's role in rehabilitation and to be aware of and utilize referral sources. Key factors to consider in developing or enhancing a comprehensive multidisciplinary Onc R program include[68]:

1. Onc R clinicians. These personnel can improve program visibility and boost referrals to rehabilitation through attendance and active participation in medical/ward rounds and clinics. These Onc R clinicians will also increase their level of skill with the pediatric oncology population as well as maximize their schedules in treating both inpatients and outpatients which will significantly improve efficiency and the transition of these children across the continuum.

2. Diverse work/treatment schedules. The US-based Children's Hospital Colorado- Center for Cancer and Blood Disorders' rehabilitation programs have seen positive gains through implementing staggered work schedules. They noted that this allowed for flexibility of treatment times and is beneficial in promoting attendance, compliance, as well as improving the total number of patients that are treated over time. Coordinating therapy appointments with clinic visits will also aid in attendance compliance and in decreasing some burden on caregivers.

3. Dedicated treatment areas. In settings with outpatient treatment where a dedicated area is not available for the sole treatment of persons diagnosed with cancer, consider creating a treatment block dedicated to only these persons or provide treatment in low traffic times (such as the early morning or late evening). Utilizing the oncology clinic where patients are being evaluated by other members of the team is also a strategy where possible and maximizes infection control measures.

4. Prospective surveillance model. This proactive model of therapy facilitates early detection of impairments and timely intervention through ongoing assessment at specific intervals during and after treatment, even when impairments are not present. This model is cost-effective, improves continuity of care, and when incorporated early in rehabilitation can help improve the acceptance of rehabilitation services among patients and families.[71] Improved motor function outcomes were observed in children with ALL via the implementation of a prospective model in the Stoplight Program.[68,71,72] This proactive physical therapy intervention directed at improving physical impairment and activity limitation found that those who completed the program tested within healthy norms.

5. Survivorship program. Based on the setting, the creation of a system that will allow patients to be monitored, screened, and treated periodically is essential to sustaining an optimal QOL. Re-educating children and their families on the late-term effects of cancer and its treatment, while screening for deficits and relapse over time aids in promoting exercise, healthy lifestyle practices, and cancer prevention. Important components may include familial genetic counseling, adolescent therapy (emphasis on self-image and coping with the social and nutritional adverse effects), life skills training groups, reproductive health guidance and therapy post-cancer treatment as well as support groups.

6. Specialized programs or components based on setting and patient population. These may include collaborating with a learning therapist or social worker for the transition to home or school, intensified therapy for specific diagnoses or phases, group caregiver training sessions, and support group facilitation. A financial advisor or social worker is instrumental in securing funding, transportation, and even housing opportunities for children and their families providing much-needed respite and improved compliance to treatment and its outcomes. These professionals may work toward securing resources such as donations, grants, and even equipment that may aid in the growth and sustainability of the rehabilitation program.

7. Strategies to monitor outcomes and evaluate program efficacy. This will provide the basis not only for research and the dissemination of standard of care but also for the universal implementation of comprehensive pediatric Onc R programs.

Prehabilitation and Screening in Pediatric Oncology

Prehabilitation and screening children for Onc R is an integral facet in achieving optimal rehabilitation outcomes as well as decreasing overall healthcare costs. Prehabilitation occurs during the time of cancer diagnosis and the beginning of acute treatment. Evidence indicates that those who receive intervention of prehabilitation prior to surgery have superior outcomes (see Chapter 27). This emerging field of practice relies on multidisciplinary baseline assessments to establish the current level of function, identify impairments, and highlight anticipatory concerns and other comorbidities that may negatively influence recovery. It also serves to introduce and prepare the family to the rehabilitation and survivorship continuum and to provide interventions aimed at promoting physical and psychological health in order to reduce the incidence or severity of future and long-term impairments as a result of cancer treatment. Gains from prehabilitation are notably not limited to use before cancer treatment begins but positively influences the entire survivorship continuum.[73]

Research in pediatric oncology prehabilitation is quite limited. However, reflecting on the growing body of evidence from adult oncology prehabilitation, promising results have been established. As Onc R clinicians, it is our duty to advocate, innovate, implement, and research prehabilitation protocols for children in order to establish a standard of practice. Prehabilitation programs for children diagnosed with cancer should include multi-system baseline assessments (Table 25.9) and patient and family education on the adverse effects of cancer and its treatment.

A 2018 prospective clinical trial examined the feasibility and functional outcome of adding prehabilitation during the 10-to 12-week period prior to surgery for tumor removal in children and adolescents with a lower extremity sarcoma. Set at a 50% feasibility rate, significant improvement was noted in physical function (via the Functional Mobility Assessment [FMA]) for the intervention group who received strengthening exercise interventions three times per week for 30 to 60 minutes.[75] In creating individualized or general prehabilitation programs, consider Table 25.10 as a potential template.

Screening children with cancer is an effective tool to be utilized in advocating for Onc R referrals and in raising prehabilitation program awareness. The St. Jude Children's Research Hospital developed an Early Childhood Clinic in hopes of ensuring that children specifically younger than 3 years old, who are at great risk for developmental delays, could be screened by a psychologist and referred to the relevant multidisciplinary team (MDT) members during active cancer treatment.[75] Depending on the available scope of each practice setting, an Onc R clinician should consider administering screenings using standardized assessment tools or a novel tool/form at oncology clinics, wards, offices or other available instances or locations. In addition, novel/self-created screening tools in the form of a quick questionnaire ascertaining the presence of specific symptoms may also be administered by other members of the MDT or given to parents to complete. This will also educate and guide MDT members as to the symptoms that can be addressed in prehabilitation. Clear instructions need to be provided to the Onc R clinician administering the screening on what results necessitate referral for specialist screening or a direct referral to commence prehabilitation or acute rehabilitation treatment. Refer to Table 25.11 for a summary of standardized and population-specific screening and assessment tools.

Acute Management

Hospitalizations are often inevitable in the diagnosis and treatment of pediatric cancers for most children. Many children require hospitalization at initial diagnosis with the child's length of stay and medical POC being highly individualized and cancer specific. In the US, between 2007 and 2014 there were 104,315 admissions for neutropenic fever, with mean length of stay 5 days.[91] As pediatric cancer treatments advance, the focus has shifted toward supportive care throughout the treatment continuum. Children diagnosed with leukemia typically require hospitalization during

TABLE 25.9	Key Components in Prehabilitation Programs for Children Diagnosed With Cancer	
Baseline Assessment of Global Development	Balance and Coordination Assessment
Cardiopulmonary status and aerobic capacity	Sensory testing
Functional mobility testing	Cognition assessment
Strength and ROM assessment	Patient and family education

ROM, Range of motion.
Created by Shara Creary-Yan. Printed with permission.

TABLE 25.10	Template Guide to Developing a Comprehensive Individualized Prehabilitation Program
Patient Diagnosis: Schedule and Plan for Medical and Surgical Cancer Treatment	
Patient's Individualized Factors	Onc R Clinician's Response/ Plan of Care
1. System(s) affected by cancer	
2. System(s) to be affected per cancer treatment	
3. Expected impairments	
4. Required prehabilitation interventions	
5. Level of supportive care, frequency, and mode of intervention as well as assistive devices needed post-acute cancer treatment	
6. Referrals required to other multidisciplinary members (social worker, nutritionist, psychologist, prosthetist, occupational therapist, speech and language pathologist, play therapist, developmental specialist, etc.)	
Individualized Prehabilitation Program	

Created by Shara Creary-Yan. Printed with permission.

chemotherapy induction while children with solid tumors may be hospitalized for chemotherapy or surgical interventions. A study compared physical activity in 80 healthy, age-matched controls to children with cancer; the study demonstrated a significant decline in the children with cancer's level of activity in both the home and inpatient setting. Children with cancer reached 23% of the controls' gait cycles per day during inpatient stays and 40% during home stays. During hospitalizations, the patients reached 58% of their activity levels at home.[92] Another study found that 50% of pediatric inpatients left their bed less than 1 hour/day and only 2% of children were out of bed more than 10 hours/day.[93] These findings suggest the necessity of increased opportunities and education for physical activity in the acute setting.

The need for increased Onc R services has been established in critically ill patients and has demonstrated decreased rehabilitation-based consultation in children with higher baseline functions.[94] A meta-analysis of children with cancer in the pediatric ICU (PICU) found that 40% of children with cancer required at least one PICU admission often for acute respiratory distress (ARDs) and sepsis.[95] Mortality was found to be 28%, which is five times higher than typical PICU rates; mortality was further increased in children requiring continuous renal replacement therapy (CRRT), mechanical ventilation, or inotropic support.[95] A retrospective analysis of sarcopenia in children diagnosed with ALL after induction examined the cross-sectional area of bilateral psoas muscles on CT in 47 patients. Thirty percent of these patients were classified as sarcopenic. A 35% incidence of invasive fungal infections was found in children diagnosed with sarcopenia, while the nonsarcopenic children demonstrated these infections of only 6%.[98]

TABLE 25.11	Summary of Pediatric Standardized Assessment Tools and Screening Resources
Target Assessment or Area of Concern	**Assessment/ Screening Tool**
Quality of life	Pediatric Quality of Life Inventory (PedsQL)[78] Pediatric Quality of Life (PedsQL Core)[77] Child Health Questionnaire (CHQ)[78] DISABKIDS[78]
Fatigue	PedsQL Multidimensional Fatigue Scale, Childhood Cancer Fatigue Scale (CCFS)[77] Fatigue Scale for a child (FS-C)[79–83] Fatigue Scale for adolescents (FS-A)[83] Fatigue Scale for parents (FS-P)[83]
Pain	Visual Analog Scale (VAS)[86]
Peripheral neuropathy	Pediatric Modified Total Peripheral Neuropathy Score (ped-mTNS)[87] Total Neuropathy Score-Pediatric Vincristine (TNS-PV)[84,86] Total Neuropathy Score (TNS)
Balance	Bruininks Osteretsky Test of Motor Proficiency (BOTMP)[87] Balance Subtest[125] Bruininks Osteretsky Test of Motor Proficiency Second Edition (BOT-2) Balance Subtest Berg Balance Scale (BBS) Alberta Infant Motor Scale (AIMS)[88] Romberg Test Pediatric Balance Scale (PBS)
Gait	Assessed descriptively or by use of a computerized electronic gait analysis
Range of motion	Goniometry
Strength	Hand-held dynamometer[89] Lateral step up test Sit-to-stand test
Endurance/ participation	Timed Up and Go (TUG)[76] 6-minute walk test (6MWT)[89,91] 30-second walk test[92]

Created by Hallie Lenker and Shara Creary-Yan. Printed with permission.

Often Onc R clinicians can be unsure of safety parameters in relation to exercise for children with cancer, especially in the acute setting. A randomized controlled trial (RCT) examined 49 children with solid tumors (mean age of 10 ± 4) years old during hospitalization for chemotherapy. The experimental intervention consisted of three weekly sessions of aerobic and strength training. The study demonstrated no adverse events with exercise training in the intervention group and improvement in strength testing, especially in those children that had lower baseline scores and no changes in fatigue scores.[99] Another study measured mobility, cognition, and activities of daily living (ADL) independence in children during chemotherapy admissions and the effect of exercise interventions. There were significant changes in the total, motor, and locomotion scores with no adverse events; however, this was a retrospective study with no control and the type and intensity of intervention was unclear.[100] Furthermore, a systematic review of literature of exercise interventions for children with pediatric cancer during inpatient admissions, including children undergoing HSCT which also confirmed positive outcomes. Ten

studies were reviewed which included 204 patients. In all studies no adverse events were observed within the intervention groups.[100] The children undergoing HSCT did not demonstrate a decrease in immune recovery with exercise intervention.

Another study demonstrated the benefit of flexibility in treatment intervention during inpatient admissions. They offered sessions twice daily to allow for deferrals or refusal. In the 16 children that completed the intervention, 50% achieved 60 minutes of low to moderate exercises (with rating of perceived exertion [RPE] of 3–4/10) for 5 out of 7 days/week. The study demonstrated no adverse events. They found a stabilization or no change in strength in the intervention group while the control group demonstrated a decline in strength with repeated testing. After the interventions, repeated testing demonstrated a decline in the 6-minute walk test (6MWT) and balance scores in both groups.[102]

Onc R clinicians should aim to provide the same quality of care when children are in the PICU as well. Children who require PICU admission may have increased medical acuity given their cancer diagnosis and treatment. Anthracycline chemotherapies are cardiotoxic and can lead to heart failure. There is increased risk of electrolyte imbalances with multiple oncology treatment regimens that can lead to tumor lysis syndrome (TLS), VOD, and pancytopenia (see leukemia section for definition) from chemotherapy, therefore lab monitoring is crucial with PICU admissions. Tumor lysis syndrome occurs when many cancer cells breakdown and release their contents into the blood in a very short period of time.[103] VOD occurs when the small blood vessels leading to and within the liver become blocked after HSCT.[104] Due to the potential for multiple inpatient admissions, family education and buy-in to Onc R services is important especially when children are critically ill. Outcome measures can be challenging to implement in the inpatient pediatric population due to the wide range of ages and medical acuity. The Functional Independence Measure (FIM) and weeFIM have been used to measure mobility, cognition, and ADL independence.[100] Inpatient pediatric interventions can adapted to the individual using the RPE scale.[101] A 6MWT is often used in the acute setting for submaximal exercise testing and was feasible with children undergoing HSCT without an adverse response.[105]

Home-Based Management

Throughout the continuum of care, Onc R within the home is critical. This form of treatment serves to empower the family unit, create a bridge between the medical world and home, and most importantly promote healing, adaptation, and a healthy lifestyle. As Onc R clinicians, the goal of treatment is to respect the family dynamic, while guiding caregivers, family members, and patients on effective methods of symptom control and management, improving and safeguarding function, as well as optimizing ADLs to increase the QOL of these children. Unnecessary modifications and high-demand HEPs must be critically assessed and with the aim to alleviate stress within the home and boost compliance to therapy principles. Home care also provides a very valuable opportunity for family education and training, which when properly adopted will significantly improve quality of care of children and parents.[106]

The most prevalent symptoms that Onc R clinicians will encounter within home care are pain, decreased mobility, fatigue, decreased strength, difficulties performing ADLs, impaired cognitive function, and depression. Childhood cancers lead to significant levels of pain which are often managed at home. This can increase the burden on caregivers who become tasked with pain management.[107] Onc R clinicians must acknowledge and attempt to address pain with both physical and psychological approaches through conventional, integrative, and newer approaches in chronic pain management. Among the most researched home-based interventions are HEPs in patients with leukemia. A 2020 randomized control trial in Spain revealed that a HEP resulted in changes in measures of VO_2 peak (peak oxygen uptake), V_E(minute ventilation),VCO_2 (output of carbon dioxide), and functional capacity during a Timed Up and Down Stairs (TUDS) test and a Timed Up and Go (TUG) test over the 16-week intervention period in childhood survivors of ALL.[108] Similar trends were observed in children with ALL, ages 5 to 10 years, receiving maintenance therapy. A 6-month home-based intervention, with written and video instruction, was supervised with weekly calls from an exercise coach and demonstrated improvement in knee and grip strength, hamstring/low-back pain, and ankle flexibility, as well as improvement on the 6MWT and the Bruininks-Oseretsky Test of Motor Proficiency Version 2 (BOT-2).[73,109] Current comprehensive home rehabilitation trends include proper nutrition and detoxification, complete decongestive therapy (CDT), diverse exercise and movement-based activities, yoga, music, and play therapy.

Play and socialization are very instrumental in the global development of children. These two components are even more critical for children with cancer in supporting age-appropriate developmental progression and in combating developmental regression. Opportunities for continued play and socialization with same-aged peers must be safely encouraged and facilitated. An optimal way of doing this may be through incorporating siblings in treatment sessions and activities. Research on siblings of children with cancer emphasizes their ability to adapt to the cancer experience through recognition and active management (social support and therapeutic interventions) of their response to this disruption in their family life as well as inclusion rather than exclusion in the cancer process. This inclusion has been proven to be mutually beneficial with the sharing of experiences such as healing gardens, animal-facilitated therapy (AFT), and play therapy.[110–112] For the child diagnosed with cancer, these experiences have led to the improvement in pain reported, adjustment difficulties, mood changes, and overall symptom management thereby improving QOL. Technological advancements such as supervised social media, video calls, and digital games can be mechanisms to promote age-based relationships and interactions with family and friends when immunocompromised or hospitalized.

Outpatient and School-Based Interventions

In the outpatient and school settings, children living with and beyond cancer can demonstrate overall deconditioning, myopathy, balance, and ROM deficits that result in gait disturbances and gross and fine motor deficits that impact their participation. Given the multisystem impact of the medical components of cancer treatment as well as the functional impacts, it is expected that children undergoing cancer treatment will have a lower level of physical fitness. The medical treatment can negatively impact the neurologic, cardiovascular, pulmonary, and musculoskeletal systems. A systematic review of 22 studies was completed with children undergoing treatment for non-CNS cancers. Gait impairments were demonstrated in multiple studies including sequelae from CIPN, which can cause gait changes impacting velocity, step-length, foot slap, and base of support (BOS).[113,114] There was

a decline in endurance in three studies as demonstrated by a reduction in 6MWT distance. Balance deficits are common given that treatment regimens often impact the neurologic, neuromuscular, and musculoskeletal systems. These children demonstrate a decline in balance scores on the BOT-2 especially those with neuropathy.

Muscle weakness in children undergoing cancer treatment is often related to immobility and disuse, as well as impact from chemotherapy causing neurotoxicity and steroid-induced myopathy. A reduction in muscle strength leads to a decline in physical function as it impacts the cardiovascular reserve, gross and fine motor strength, gait, and mobility. High dose steroids during induction, and throughout treatment, lead to myopathy causing weakness in the proximal muscle groups in the lower and upper extremities. Anterior tibialis strength was impacted in 92% of patients undergoing chemotherapy that included vincristine in one study.[20] Children undergoing cancer treatment reported activity challenges affected by a change in perspective of independence with ADLs and a loss of physical strength.[113] ROM is impacted with cancer treatment. ROM can be limited due to surgical interventions such as sarcoma lesions or due decreased muscle strength. Many children with ALL demonstrate a reduction in ankle and hip ROM whereas children with lower extremity sarcoma lesions often demonstrate ROM impairments in the affected extremity.[114]

Fatigue is the most reported adverse effect of cancer treatment. The cause of fatigue in a person with cancer can be either central or peripheral. Five studies in a systematic review investigated the effect of improving functional activity and whether this impacted reports of fatigue.[114] Overall, the studies were small, and the research studies had limitations but there were positive trends in fatigue in the studies that had longer exercise times and with the use of ankle-foot-orthoses (AFOs) in children with ankle weakness.[114] Measuring physical fitness can be challenging in children undergoing cancer treatment with submaximal outcome measures often required given the complex medical status of the child. Improvements were noted in two studies relating to improving the number of gait cycles and minutes of physical activity per day in long term exercise programs.[114] Onc R intervention in the outpatient setting for children diagnosed and living with cancer often involves increasing activity tolerance and should include initiation of exercise interventions and education at appropriate levels. Physical activity during cancer treatment has demonstrated an improvement in QOL and decreased the decline of physical function.[115]

There are few studies that are intervention-specific within pediatric Onc R. Regarding interventions aimed at improving gait mechanics, results have been mixed with 2 of 3 studies in a systematic review demonstrating an improvement in walk distance in the 6- and 9-minute walk tests.[114] Strength improvements are feasible using specifically prescribed interventions (see Chapter 23). Interventions to improve ROM have demonstrated positive results with the initiation of a HEP. Improvements were impacted by whether the patient was monitored by a nurse versus a physical therapist when comparing two separate studies.[114] Yoga has demonstrated some efficacy with adolescents undergoing cancer treatment to improve anxiety, mood, and fatigue, however studies have been limited in the younger population.[116] Measuring physical fitness can be challenging with children undergoing cancer treatment with submaximal exercise testing measures being generally preferred (vs. exercising to exhaustion) given the complex medical factors.

As previously discussed, a team approach is recommended for children undergoing cancer treatment including the Onc R clinician and neuropsychological testing. In a survey study, nearly half of parents reported receiving little to no information on the impact of cancer treatment on school performance.[119] In a separate study, oncology providers were surveyed and 77% reported a need for increased training around the cognitive effects and school reentry.[116] While the role of the Onc R clinician in school reentry may be understood, the role of the Onc R clinician in providing education to families undergoing school transition is less appreciated. Improvement in education allows parents to take on the new parental role of advocate and should be included within all disciplines who provide care to these children.[118] Onc R clinicians should provide education in their roles related to school reentry and the functional effects of pediatric cancer treatment to their provider colleagues. See Table 25.12 for treatment intervention suggestions based on clinical presentation.

Cognitive deficits, along with physical impairments, impact a child's success in the school environment by impacting performance, learning, and social functioning. Attendance at school for a child with cancer can be impacted due to physical, emotional, and behavioral adverse effects of treatment including the child's perception of the treatment itself. Children may have difficulty completing work in the classroom and may spend substantially more time completing homework assignments. There may be difficulties with handwriting, fine motor activities, organizing content and lining up columns, or diagrams for arithmetic problems. Interestingly, adults living beyond childhood leukemia who did not receive radiation were found to also display alterations in functional connectivity in the brain, as well as difficulties on a set-shifting task compared to controls, but no changes in white or gray matter volume were found; a relationship was identified between earlier treatment and a worse outcome in cognitive performance.[119] Peer-to-peer relationships can be difficult to maintain given the cognitive impairments, frequent school absences, and impaired concentration which leads to decreased social QOL.[120] Children who were receiving inpatient care report concerns related to disconnection from the school environment and isolation from peers. Onc R clinicians are crucial in limiting the impact of the physical and cognitive adverse effects of treatment such as assisting physical negotiation of the school environment through recovery or adaptation. Prior to or during the school reentry phase, treatment interventions should include activities that mimic the school day in an opening environment such as carrying a backpack, attending to cognitive tasks, or opening/closing lunch boxes or bags (Video 25.1).

Developmental Progression and Cognition

International collaborative studies have found that infants and toddlers living with and beyond cancer displayed delayed developmental milestones when compared to their same aged healthy peers. Children treated before age four were found to progress more slowly in areas including vocabulary, cognitive functions such as attention and memory, as well as motor skills; social and emotional development delays were also noted, but to a lesser extent. These findings suggest that children may benefit greatly from early intervention of physical therapy, occupational therapy, and speech/language pathology.[121] Declines in intellectual functioning, including impairments in working memory and inhibition, are common for children who receive CNS-directed cancer therapies.[122] The following specific factors can also cause CNS-related cognitive impairments: CNS tumors, CNS prophylaxis via chemotherapy or radiation for children with leukemia or non-Hodgkin lymphoma, brain tumors requiring localized external beam radiation therapy, whole body radiation, and myeloablative chemotherapy in preparation

for allogenic bone marrow transplant and, lastly, solid tumors or leukemia treated during critical developmental periods and with prolonged or repeated hospitalizations.[123]

Children who undergo radiation and chemotherapy treatment for cancer demonstrate cognitive impairments including decreased IQ, processing speed, working memory, executive functioning, and attention deficits.[123] Persons living with and beyond pediatric malignant brain tumors or ALL have demonstrated increased risk for cognitive difficulties with nonverbal abilities being most impaired such as short-term memory, processing speed, visual-motor integration, sequencing ability, attention, and concentration.[103,122,123] Younger children who received high doses of cranial radiation demonstrated decreased IQ, working memory, and processing speeds 3 years postradiation as compared to older children and children of all ages that receive focal, proton radiation.[122] Persons living with and beyond ALL may demonstrate cognitive deficits but not to the extent of children after treatment for CNS tumors.[120] More research into these findings is warranted given the complexities of cancer treatment and their vast potential to impact brain volume and cognitive functioning especially in the developing brain.

Research has evolved which utilize cognitive training programs to increase attention, memory, and cognitive flexibility in pediatric cancer survivors. These children are often unable to use stimulant medications due to medical contraindications, adverse effects, or poor tolerance. Thus, either therapist-delivered or computer-delivered cognitive training provides a viable alternative capable of yielding positive results.[125] A study of an 8-week online cognitive rehabilitation program yielded increased activation in the inferior frontal gyrus, medial frontal gyrus, and superior frontal gyrus post intervention and had higher scores on standardized cognitive testing.[126]

Not all children with CNS exposure to radiation and chemotherapy will experience neurocognitive effects, and currently there is no certain way to predict which children will be affected. Preoperative cognitive assessments can help to identify pre-existing cognitive deficits as long-term impairments are often associated as treatment effects, especially in children with brain tumors. Specific factors that have been found to be associated with higher risk for cognitive impairment include younger age at the time of diagnosis, treatment intensity, and duration of time between treatment and evaluation.[123] Prolonged hospitalization, absences from school, and lack of other age-appropriate developmental opportunities can also contribute to impaired academic performance and developmental delays.

Palliative and End of Life Care

The American Academy of Pediatrics (AAP) professional guidelines endorse concurrent pediatric palliative care and disease-directed care as best practice.[125] Studies have compared the symptom distress and QOL experience for children who received concurrent end-of-life care from a pediatric palliative care home care program with that of those who died without exposure to these programs.[73] The results revealed that children who received pediatric palliative care were significantly more likely to have fun (70% vs. 45%), to experience events that added meaning to life (89% vs. 63%), and to die comfortably at home (93% vs. 20%). Parents and healthcare professionals have reported on the effectiveness of pediatric palliative care rehabilitation and its beneficial effect on improving the basic life functions, comfort, and QOL.[73]

The main needs of a home-based palliative rehabilitation program are to decrease pain and suffering, while improving family education and training.[104] Onc R clinicians should also educate

TABLE 25.12 Clinical Presentations and Onc R Treatment Interventions

Clinical Presentation	Cancer Related Adverse Effect Cause	Treatment Interventions
Steppage gait or toe walking gait	Peripheral neuropathy Anterior tibialis weakness	– Normalize gait pattern for heel toe pattern – Trial AFOs – Ankle strengthening – Gastroc and hamstring ROM assessment – EMG Biofeedback
Foot slap	Decreased anterior tibialis eccentric strength	– Ankle strengthening – AFOs – Functional electrical stimulation
Difficulty transitioning floor to stand	Impaired core strength with steroids Deconditioning	– Core and gluteal strengthening – Postural training and biomechanical education
Difficulty opening bottles or buttoning buttons	Peripheral neuropathy Intrinsic hand weakness	– Grip strengthening – Gross and fine motor hand exercises – Sensory exposure with various textures and desensitization as necessary
Difficulty with coloring or handwriting	Intrinsic hand weakness or acquisition of skills	– Exposure to fine motor activities – Kneading and gripping exercises – Hand and finger manipulation activities
Decreased or resistance to oral intake	Oral aversion	– Oral desensitization – Sensory diet – Facial exercises
Frequent tripping	Neuropathy Deconditioning Decreased coordination	– Exposure to different terrain and surfaces – Fall prevention and safety training – Modified strength and aerobic exercise – Balance and coordination activities *Aquatic training may be an optimal treatment modality – Anterior tibialis strengthening – Gastroc stretches
Difficulty with single leg stance or kicking	Decreased coordination Weakness	– Dynamic balance and coordination training – Aerobic, LE, and core strengthening
Fatigue	Global and cardiopulmonary deconditioning	– Cardiopulmonary endurance training – Treadmill, aquatic and Wii therapy-based exercises
Hand and/or foot burning, tingling pain	Peripheral neuropathy	– Desensitization training – Gentle stretching – Progressing weight bearing – Coordination with pain management medications
Decreased sensation in feet or hands	Peripheral neuropathy – Team should rule out CNS involvement if acute and abrupt onset	– Monofilament testing – Fall prevention techniques – Education on skin checks – Sensory retraining

AFO, Ankle foot orthoses; *CNS,* central nervous system; *EMG,* electromyography; *LE,* lower extremity; *ROM,* range of motion; Wii, Nintendo video game.
Created by Hallie Lenker and Shara Creary-Yan. Printed with permission.

and train the family on energy conservation strategies, the use of assistive devices, proper positioning, preserving muscle and joint integrity, importance of breathing techniques, and chest physical therapy interventions when appropriate. Comprehensive Onc R should also facilitate appropriate psychological/emotional processing for the impact of palliative and end-of-life care among immediate family members. For siblings of all ages, this period may be met with a unique bereavement trajectory. Parents and siblings of children with cancer were found to greatly benefit from inclusion and participation in the care of their loved one during the terminal process of illness.[127] Honest and open communication between healthcare providers and family members is essential in the bereavement process. Consideration must also be made to

familial, spiritual, and cultural preferences to ensure the provider is respecting and practicing family-centered care.

Studies within the US and Australia have revealed significant gains in the use of music therapy as an integrated component in palliative care as measured by the PedsQL Family Impact Module.[128] Parents described observing physical improvements in their child during music therapy, by providing comfort and stimulation; additional positive feedback shared by the family was that sessions were strength and family centered. Aromatherapy is another intervention studied with some studies showing lasting effects of lower symptom burden up to 60 minutes postintervention for pain, nausea, and depressed mood.[129] Caution must be utilized in using aromatherapy as some patients sustained pulmonary and allergic adverse effects.

Engagement in various local or international outreach opportunities designed for children with critical illnesses, such as Make-A-Wish America, will also support the goal of empowering these children and their families with a sense of fulfillment, joy and in leaving a legacy of their lives.

Pediatric and Treatment Specific Considerations

Bone Health

Acquisition of bone mass and bone strength is crucial in development as bone mass peaks between 20 and 30 years of age. During treatment there is concern for both bone loss due to treatment, especially with corticosteroid use, as well as decreased formation due to impaired mobility and decreased muscle mass. Factors that decrease bone health in children with cancer include use of corticosteroids, IT methotrexate, ifosfamides, HSCT, cranial radiation, malnutrition, vitamin D deficiencies, decreased physical activity, and limited weight bearing.[130] Long bones and spinal vertebrae are often where the largest decrease in bone mineral density (BMD) is observed, resulting in osteoporosis. BMD measures the amount of mineral in a bone. There are some reports of increased incidence of vertebral fractures in the first year of treatment.[131] Female adolescents may be at highest risk due to lower levels of vitamin D.[132,133] Children in impoverished areas demonstrate suboptimal vitamin D levels at diagnosis, with 64% having deficient or insufficient values.[133] In a study comparing pediatric patients with mixed cancers to healthy controls, the children with cancer demonstrated decreased blood calcium and phosphorus levels at time of diagnosis. Fifteen of their nineteen patients received corticosteroids and at one month of treatment all showed a decrease in BMD z-scores.[130] Children with hematological cancers demonstrated the greatest decline in BMD during the first 6 months of treatment with the greatest loss in the first month, whereas children with solid tumors did not show a BMD decline until 6 to 12 months of treatment.[130] A prospective RCT with 36 children with ALL examined the effects a home-based physical activity program on BMD.[134] Unsurprisingly, both the intervention and control groups demonstrated decreases in activity intensity during treatment, and the intervention group had no improvement in BMD with unsupervised exercise, likely due to decreased compliance. This reinforces the need for intensive follow up by Onc R providers throughout cancer treatment for assessment and to modify interventions as appropriate. Children with cancer are at high risk for loss or decreased formation of BMD therefore swift consultation is imperative to minimize controllable effects such as decreased physical activity and minimized weightbearing unless medically indicated.

Corticosteroids are prescribed as both pediatric cancer treatment and for the management of treatment complications. Children with cancer are, therefore, at higher risk of osteonecrosis (ON) or avascular necrosis (AVN). ON is due to infarction or bone ischemia due to the loss of blood supply to the bone.[135] AVN occurs when there is bone death in a segment. ON and AVN impacts function when weight bearing joints are affected and especially if symptomatic. High dose glucocorticoids increase the risk of ON due to a hypercoagulable state, microthrombi, and suppression of osteoblasts that compromise bone blood circulation.[135] Overall prevalence has mixed results with 0.5% to 17% reported in children 10 to 20 years old, and there may be increased risk due to the

rapid acquisition of skeletal growth during puberty.[132,135] Asymptomatic presentations may lead to potentially higher incidence at 53% of children. Symptomatic children often report pain, demonstrate decreased participation and QOL, and require surgical intervention with unsuccessful conservative management or for decreased structural integrity.[132,136] There is minimal conservative treatment to offer children with symptomatic ON. Bisphosphonate treatment can decrease reports of pain as it decreases bone resorption.[132] Analgesia, decreasing WB physical and/or occupational therapy are typically recommended.[131] Children who demonstrate AVN should be referred to orthopedics to determine potential WB or activity restrictions prior to Onc R intervention. Orthopedic surgical interventions include core decompressions or total joint replacements.

Chemotherapy-Induced Polyneuropathy (CIPN)

CIPN is an adverse event due to neurotoxic properties of chemotherapy. Vincristine is used within the treatment regimens for leukemia, lymphomas, Wilms tumors, Ewing sarcoma, rhabdomyosarcoma, and gliomas.[137] Vincristine restricts tumor growth and has less myelosuppression than other chemotherapies therefore it is used more frequently in children.[137] Other neurotoxic chemotherapies include cisplatin, carboplatin, and etoposide.[138,139] The English and Dutch versions of the pediatric-modified total neuropathy score (peds-mTNS) has been validated for use to measure CIPN in children.[140]

CIPN can result in pain, sensory, and motor loss, and autonomic symptoms such as autonomic polyneuropathy, orthostatic hypotension, and constipation.[141] Thirty-six percent of children with ALL report musculoskeletal pain at diagnosis while 78% of children who receive vincristine get some symptoms of vincristine-induced peripheral neuropathy (VIPN), according to one study.[119] Within three days of vincristine administration, children may demonstrate neuropathic symptoms such as areflexia, weakness, atrophy, and muscle pain/cramps.[134] Within 4 to 5 months of vincristine administration children may demonstrate decreased dorsiflexion and quadricep weakness.[134] Longer neurons are most affected resulting in more distal than proximal involvement with lower extremities most impacted. High rates of CIPN can lead to a dose reduction or cessation of use which can lessen treatment effect and/or lead to questionable treatment efficacy.[137,142,143] Most children with sensory and motor symptoms from VIPN resolve a few months after completion of chemotherapy. There has been indication of increased incidence in older and Caucasian children though there is risk of underreporting in younger children given the difficulty reporting symptoms.[141]

Low grade gliomas (LGG) often require chemotherapy when total resection is not possible due to the location of the tumor. The standard first round of chemotherapy includes carboplatin and vincristine. While vincristine is neurotoxic due to its effects on the mitotic spindles, carboplatin inhibits DNA synthesis and can lead to CIPN by damaging the DNA in the sensory neurons.[139] One study investigated the incidence of neuropathy in 15 children with pilocytic astrocytomas who received chemotherapy.[139] The children demonstrated most neuropathy symptoms during the first cycle of chemotherapy with nearly all demonstrating distal weakness and some reporting pain. Forty-seven percent of children had sensory and motor symptoms and 9% had residual weakness 12 months post treatment.[139] Electrophysical studies were used to further investigate incidence of motor neuropathy by conducting electrophysical testing on 27 patients prior to initiation of chemotherapy and after at least four induction doses. After induction only 19% of children were neuropathy-free with highest neuropathy complaints of paresthesia and constipation and the most common neuropathic sign of loss of deep tendon reflexes (DTR).[143] Children undergoing treatment with carboplatin and cisplatin are at higher risk for hearing loss.[139] Children with hearing loss should be additionally screened for vestibular involvement.

With multiple systems involved, activity participation can be limited due to decreased coordination, fine motor, and gross motor activities.[137] Forty-six percent of children with ALL demonstrated below average motor proficiency measures after cancer treatment.[137] CIPN impacts balance due to the impact on the somatosensory system and distal strength.[138] When considering long-term effects, 11.5% of children with ALL, 57% of children with lymphoma, and 60% with solid tumors demonstrated abnormal CIPN scores 6 months post treatment. Of these children, 53% of children demonstrate scores 1 standard deviation (SD) below age-based normative values on the BOT-2 despite near normal neuropathy scores and regular physical therapy intervention while 6% scored 2 SDs below the norm.[138] Fine motor deficits occur due to the distal muscle weakness or atrophy. This weakness can result in difficulty in self-care and dressing activities.[144] One study used the Canadian Occupational Performance Measure (COPM) and BOT-2 to determine whether task specific training on ADLs resulted in improved ability compared to the control group of only HEP.[145] The intervention group demonstrated significant improvement in all areas indicating improvement of both physical ability as well as patient perception.

Pediatric Braces/Prosthetics Considerations

Children undergoing cancer treatment may benefit from bracing for a variety of cancer-related adverse effects. One study revealed children receiving vincristine demonstrated dorsiflexor weakness, loss of DTRs, and reduced light touch and vibration scores on peds-mTNS. Gait changes included decreased velocity and decreased step length.[40] A smaller study demonstrated improvement in step length and ankle dorsiflexion ROM in children wearing solid ankle foot orthoses (AFOs) for approximately 1 month during one full cycle of chemotherapy.[20,146] Given the incidence of foot drop and decreased ROM in children with CIPN, orthotics should be considered to promote age-appropriate biomechanics and participation. Orthoses are used to improve or maximize alignment such as improvement of hindfoot collapse or increased pronation or supination.[145] Children that are undergoing surgical procedures may require postoperative bracing to guard the surgical site such as knee immobilizers or hip braces after resection. Nighttime or positioning splints may also be used to maintain or improve ROM in a less mobile child, such as during a hospitalization. While limb sparing procedures have become more common in sarcoma management, some children continue to require amputation and prosthetics. Bracing should be considered throughout the continuum of care including during a transition to palliative treatment if it maximizes comfort and soft tissue integrity. The Onc R clinician should work with the child, family, and treatment team to provide appropriate options while allowing for adaptation for both the family and medical team goals. review

Secondary Lymphedema

The progression of lymphedema in children, regardless of origin, follows a similar trajectory to that of adults with lymphedema. Children with secondary lymphedema are found to receive a diagnosis and treatment sooner than those with primary lymphedema[145] (Figure 25.5).

Though secondary lymphedema is relatively rare, late diagnosis and treatment can carry a significant burden for lifelong management and risk of secondary complications.[147] In children, lymphedema may emerge due to malignant tumors which physically interfere with lymphatic function, in response to cancer treatment (often with lymph node dissections, radiation, and chemotherapy), and during palliative and end of life care.[148]

Stemmer's sign is a useful screening tool that may be used by all Onc R clinicians to definitively identify lymphedema and has a very low false positive rate. The test consists of trying to pinch and lift a skin fold at the base of the second toe or middle finger. The inability to lift the skin results in a positive sign confirming the presence of lymphedema. A negative test does not rule out the presence of lymphedema. Recently developed, the Bjork Bow Tie Test[149] has expanded on Stemmer's Sign to include testing on any area of the body as well as in identifying soft tissue changes that may signal interventions needed to help remodel soft tissue back to its normalized state. The test is done in one maneuver of gently pinching, rolling, and twisting the skin between the thumb and pointer finger assessing the presence of a bow tie and wrinkles when twisted. The absence of the bow tie appearance indicates a positive test for the presence of lymphedema. If lymphedema is suspected and/or confirmed, the Onc R clinician should refer the child for further assessment and staging by a certified lymphedema professional. The standard of practice treatment is CDT which consists of family education, meticulous skin care, manual lymphatic drainage, exercises, and use of compression garments and bandages. The lymphedema therapist will be able to guide family members and children in ongoing measurement and monitoring as well as self- or co-management in order to control the lymphedema and flare-ups.

Common complications of secondary lymphedema (particularly if untreated) include cellulitis and, in rare cases, lymphangitis. In a 2018 study, the incidence rate for cellulitis in children was similar to rates in adults with a median age of 11.5 years at first incidence. Of the children who experienced cellulitis, 29% had a second episode and 26% a third.[150] Other complications include upslanting toenails, skin changes and ulcerations, lymphorrea, psychological distress due to self-consciousness of the swelling, and local system disturbances such as genitourinary or oral motor symptoms if lymphedema is present in the area.

Nutrition

Overall, the amount of research around specific nutritional interventions with children during cancer treatment is limited. With the increase of childhood obesity, persons diagnosed with cancer are at higher risk of obesity at time of diagnosis. Diet and nutrition are often suboptimal in these children and can be exacerbated by steroid treatment regimes.[113] A meta-analysis demonstrated an overall increase in body mass index (BMI) in ALL patients during induction and maintenance.[151] Poor nutrition resulting in low calcium and vitamin D can exacerbate already low BMD from corticosteroid and methotrexate regimes. While BMI acknowledgment is important, some diet strategies can result in loss of muscle bulk.

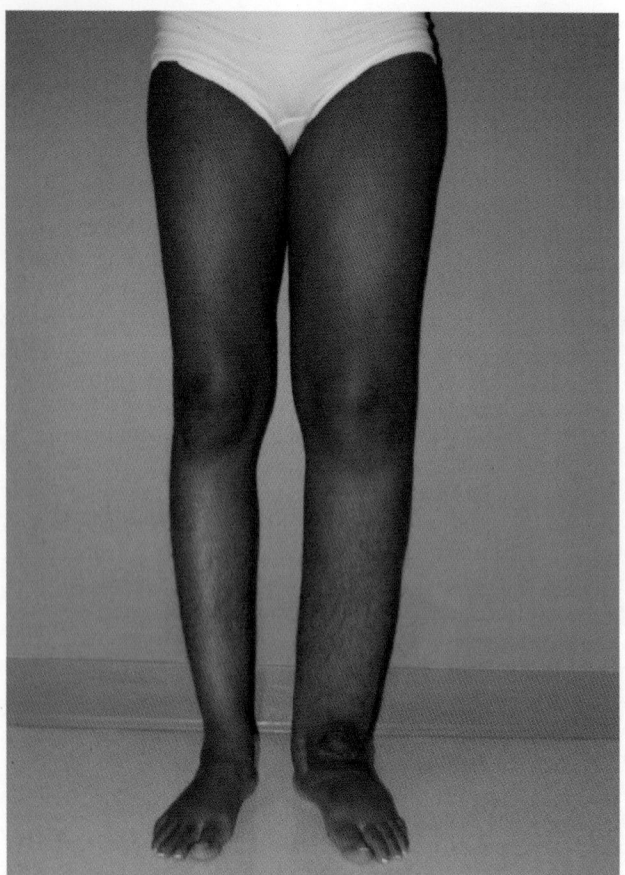

• **Fig. 25.5** Left Lower Extremity Secondary Lymphedema in a Pediatric Patient. (Reprinted with permission from Chang. Cheng MH, Chang D, Patel K. Left lower extremity secondary lymphedema in a pediatric patient. In: *Principles and Practice of Lymphedema Surgery*. Elsevier; 2015. ISBN: 9780323322638.)

Physical activity, exercise, and close monitoring of nutrition status work together toward a more equal energy balance.

Cancer Prevention

This rapidly emerging field of study attempts to uncover the factors that may prevent, delay, or reverse the development of carcinogenesis. Global experts have shared their perspective that cancer prevention may be required in as early as the preconception stage. This lends greatly to the role of epigenetics in cancer. A physical or chemical exposure can interact with an organism leading to a series of signaling events culminating in an epigenetic change.[108,109]

Prenatal supplementation has been shown to decrease the risk of several congenital malformations with more recent studies highlighting a potential protective effect of folic acid on certain pediatric cancers. A 2006 meta-analysis revealed an apparent protective effect for leukemia, pediatric brain tumors, and neuroblastoma.[152] However, at that time, it was not known which constituent(s) of the multivitamin were responsible for this protective effect. A more recent review published in 2019, revealed a protective association between maternal folic acid supplementation and childhood ALL. There was, however, no significant association between maternal folic acid supplementation and AML or childhood brain tumors.[153] Maternal folate metabolic genotype may be associated

with DNA methylation patterns for ALL in their offspring. Therefore, the effect of maternal genotypes on ALL susceptibility may act through aberrant promoter methylation, which may contribute to the in-utero origins of ALL.[154] According to Dr. Mukesh Verma of the US National Cancer Institute's Division of Cancer Control and Population Sciences, "Cancer epigenetics is important for prevention because we may be able to use methylation markers to identify people at higher risk of cancer and perhaps detect cancer earlier."[155] Though gene mutation reversal may not be possible at this time, it is hoped that drugs may be able to reverse changes in methylation which holds significant promise in cancer prevention.

Diet also influences epigenetics and specifically methylation. Though studies reviewed for this chapter have not been conclusive in human subjects, pregnant mice provided with diets rich in methyl donors, including folic acid, choline, methionine, and genistein (an ingredient in soy) can modify the methylation patterns of a certain gene in offspring.[155] Dr. Paul Rogers, a pediatric oncologist at British Columbia Children's Hospital and Professor at the University of British Columbia in Vancouver, Canada noted that "A fundamental mistake when considering the impact of nutrition on cancer prevention is ignoring that prevention should start before conception, continue during pregnancy, infancy, childhood and adolescence, to have maximum optimal benefits at all ages."[156]

Prenatal and early life exposure to chemical and environmental carcinogenic factors has been a consistent base in the pyramid of cancer prevention. These include exposure to varying infections, heavy metals, industrial solvents, and other known teratogens such as alcohol, cigarette smoking, and assorted narcotics. Maternal exposure to industrial solvents is also linked to development of ALL in their offspring.[157] More recent trends aimed at exploring these factors consider global climate change, such as an increased run off of toxins in the water to which bottle-fed babies are more susceptible, increasing their risk of cancer. Increased air pollution, a depleted planetary stratosphere, and increase in ultraviolet radiation predisposes this population to higher susceptibility of cancers. Children are at greater risk of sun exposure and sun burns through play and outdoor activities, increasing the risk of melanoma and other skin cancers before the age of 20 years.

Measures to decrease these risks calls for Onc R clinicians to further integrate and align with community-based medicine in order to create an active cancer prevention strategy. While this may not prevent all pediatric cancers, it will significantly strengthen the efforts of eliminating preventable cancers. This includes the provision of regular education and health promotion aimed at:

- Promoting balanced meals and active healthy lifestyles
- Educating on the role of genetic testing and counseling
- Promotion of prenatal supplementation and the benefits of folic acid
- Advocating for increased testing of environmentally used chemicals in reproductive toxicity or hormonal activity as well as in enforcing strict protocols for reduced workplace exposures to carcinogens
- Emphasis on breast feeding and breast milk supplementation
- Sunscreen use and/or clothing and shielding
- Educating on their choice to seek cancer preventative vaccines

Conclusion

Pediatric cancers and their treatment affect multiple systems within the body at various points in time across the lifespan.

This field of medicine necessitates collaboration across a MDT to ensure treatment of the whole child, with significant consideration of managing immediate as well as later term adverse effects. Empowering and partnering with family members and caregivers is crucial for effective lifestyle modifications and treatment carryover across and between sessions, geared at maximizing rehabilitation goals. Prioritizing rehabilitation during a pediatric cancer diagnosis facilitates the child's ability to achieve and maintain their optimal development and QOL.

Critical Research Needs

- Prehabilitation in pediatric oncology
- The effects of consistent and long-term structured exercise programs in multimodal settings
- The role of therapeutic modalities in pediatric oncology; safety, efficacy and determining protocols for use
- Aquatic therapy in improving cancer treatment adverse effects in the pediatric population
- The role of CDT in treating secondary lymphedema in pediatric oncology patients
- Cognitive baseline assessments and further research on "chemo brain" and its response to exercise prescription

Case Studies

Case Study #1

Presentation: A 7-year-old presents to outpatient rehabilitation during consolidation treatment for ALL with concern for vincristine-induced peripheral neuropathy. The child continues to undergo chemotherapy including intrathecal methotrexate and vincristine with steroid pulses.

ASSESSMENT

Physical Therapy:
- Gait analysis demonstrates steppage gait pattern with flat foot contact and decreased terminal hip extension during stance phase.
- Manual muscle testing demonstrates weakness in the abdominals, hip extensors, hip abductors, gastrocnemius, and anterior tibialis.
- Range of motion:
  - Dorsiflexion: passive ROM: right (R) 3 degree, left (L) 4 degree, active ROM: -3 strength bilaterally.
  - Hamstring popliteal angle 50 degree bilaterally.
- BOT-2 balance subtext: 22/47 (4.5 age equivalent) indicating well below age matched normals.
- Single leg stance time: <5 second bilaterally.
- 6MWT: 1130 feet (344 m) with one standing rest break, SaO_2 100% throughout test, HR increased from 83 to 130 beats per minute indicating good effort, Borg fatigue at rest: 3/10, posttest: 5/10, Borg shortness of breath at rest: 2/10, posttest: 7/10, decreases to 3/10 within 2 minutes of rest; steppage gait, decreased step length and speed.
- Stairs: Step-to pattern left foot leading on stairs with bilateral handrails, lateral step downs to descend with two hands on handrail. Caregiver reports the child often bumps down the stairs at home.
- Peds-mTNS: 8/40 indicating peripheral neuropathy with >5 score.

Occupational Therapy (OT):
- BOT-2 manual dexterity score: 16/45 (5 year old equivalent).

- Grip strength: R = 8 lbs (3.6 kg), L = 6 lbs (2.7 kg). R hand dominant.
- Dressing: total assist for shoe tying with caregiver reporting prior independence.
- Unable to open water bottles, difficulty with buttons, independent with zippers.
- Holds crayon and markers with immature grasp with atrophy noted within hand intrinsic muscles.

INTERVENTION

Physical Therapy
- Obstacle course focusing on dynamic balance, strengthening, and stretching with balance beam, ramps, and various height steps.
- Core strength with animal walks, prone and sitting on scooter.
- Balance training with single leg stance training, standing on foam dynamic and static.
- Ankle strengthening with heel raises and using toes to pick up cotton balls and place in cone; sitting and standing with support.

Physical Therapy HEP: Hamstring and gastroc stretches, core strengthening with bridges, side lying clam shells, straight leg raise, modified plank on knees and elbows.

Occupational Therapy:
- Fine motor activities with coloring on vertical surface with easel and wall.
- Shoulder and hand strengthening using trapeze swing.
- Upper extremity WB with animal crawls and crawling up ramp.
- Fine motor training with large button buttoning and stringing activities.

Occupational Therapy HEP: Putty hand strengthening with grip, finger extension, and pinch; wall pushups, and climbing on playground equipment.

OUTCOME

The patient participated in physical therapy 2 times per week and OT 1 time per week for 10 weeks with improvement in fine motor coordination (BOT-2 manual dexterity 24/45), ambulation (heel toe gait pattern), 6MWT 1870 ft (570 m), balance (BOT-2 balance subtext 32/47), and ROM. The patient and their family were provided with an HEP at discharge. The physical therapist checked in on a bimonthly basis during oncology clinic appointments to determine progress or regression.

Case Study #2

Presentation: 3-year-old admitted to inpatient pediatric ICU for new onset of lethargy, vomiting, and gait difficulties. Found to have posterior fossa tumor, now 2 days out after resection. Physical Therapy, OT, and speech language pathology (SLP) was consulted for evaluation and treatment. The team is concerned for posterior fossa syndrome.

ASSESSMENT

Speech Language Pathology:
- Coughs with drinking water on bedside swallow evaluation.
- Word finding difficulty with the patient tearful with eyes closed throughout evaluation with slowed speech pattern.

Occupational Therapy:
- Limited vision assessment as patient prefers eyes closed with report of double vision.
- Positive dysmetria with reaching for stuffed animal.
- Decreased grasp bilaterally.

Physical Therapy:
- Decreased cervical rotation and side bending: preferred cervical posture right rotation (toward family sitting beside) unable to maintain midline without reports of pain.
- Minimal assistance for sitting at the edge of bed, moderate assist with standing and a standing pivot transfer to the bedside chair to sit on caregiver's lap. Ataxia with ambulation.
- Vestibular assessment limited due to patient's tolerance to maintain eyes open.

INTERVENTION following initial evaluation:

Speech Language Pathology:
- Schedule video fluoroscopy study to evaluate for dysphagia.
- Picture communication board for ease of communication.

Occupational Therapy:
- Recommend team consult ophthalmology due to reports of double vision, consider sunglasses or eye patching after evaluation.
- Putty and building blocks (e.g., Lego) exercises for fine motor strengthening.

Physical Therapy:
- Encourage active cervical rotation towards midline; recommend family sitting on other side of bed if able to encourage rotation to left.
- Out of bed to chair twice daily to improve tolerance for upright activities.
- Standing with assist to play with toys on bed.
  Discharge recommendations: Inpatient rehabilitation.

OUTCOME

Patient was discharged to acute inpatient rehabilitation two weeks postoperatively. Six weeks after discharge from rehab the patient was walking with handhold assistance of one hand from a parent, ascending stairs with a step to pattern, visual acuity and oral intake returned to baseline, mild fine motor deficits, and continued dysarthria. The patient was referred to outpatient physical therapy, OT, and SLP to continue their rehabilitation.

Review Questions

Reader can find the correct answers and rationale in the back of the book.

1. In children, leukemia is treated primarily with chemotherapy though children with CNS involvement may receive radiation therapy to the brain. With the prevalence of vincristine-induced polyneuropathy, an Onc R POC should prioritize sensory assessment and treatment. Which of the following would be MOST appropriate to be prioritized as well?
   - **A.** Ankle range of motion
   - **B.** Muscular pain
   - **C.** Pulmonary decompensation
   - **D.** Vertigo

2. Late and long-term adverse effects of the treatment of nephroblastomas include reduced kidney function and premature failure, cardiac toxicity and pulmonary complications. They also include a higher incidence of all the following EXCEPT:
   - **A.** Secondary leukemias
   - **B.** Secondary solid tumors
   - **C.** Breast cancer
   - **D.** Squamous cell carcinoma

3. Hematopoietic stem cell transplant (HSCT) is a treatment for both malignant and nonmalignant diseases in pediatric patients. In pediatrics, HSCT can be used as a curative treatment for hematological diseases such as ALL. After HSCT, children are at risk for acute complications within the first 90 days with symptoms . Which of the following is LEAST likely to be an acute complication after HSCT?
   - **A.** Infections
   - **B.** Acute Graft Versus Host Disease
   - **C.** Seizures
   - **D.** Myelosuppression

4. Which of the following is the MOST important key factor to consider in developing or enhancing a comprehensive multidisciplinary Onc R program?
   - **A.** Diverse treatment schedules
   - **B.** Open, busy treatment areas
   - **C.** Patient only/restricted access to support groups

   - **D.** Rigid work schedules for therapists

5. Pediatric standardized assessment tools are valuable screening resources. A 7-year-old boy diagnosed with ALL displays symptoms of fatigue with walking to clinic appointments post chemotherapy treatment cycle 1. Which of the following is the MOST appropriate tool for assessing his fatigue?
   - **A.** Romberg test
   - **B.** 6 Minute walk test
   - **C.** Child health questionnaire
   - **D.** Pediatric modified total peripheral neuropathy

6. The need for increased Onc R services has been established in critically ill patients. Research shows that 40% of children with cancer will require at least one PICU admission. Which of the following is MOST likely to be the condition that will require a PICU admission?
   - **A.** ARD and sepsis
   - **B.** Exercise-induced asthma
   - **C.** Emphysema
   - **D.** Chronic obstructive pulmonary disease

7. Childhood cancers lead to significant levels of pain which are often managed at home. This can increase the burden on caregivers who become tasked with pain management. Which of the following statements is MOST accurate related to pain relief measures?
   - **A.** Only be administered by a member of the Onc R MDT
   - **B.** Be addressed by both physical and psychological approaches
   - **C.** Be prescribed instead of a HEP
   - **D.** Utilize pharmaceutical agents only.

8. Muscle weakness in children undergoing cancer treatment is related to immobility and disuse, as well as impact from chemotherapy causing neurotoxicity and steroid-induced myopathy. High dose steroids during induction, and throughout treatment, is MOST likely to lead to which of the following?
   - **A.** Seizure disorders
   - **B.** Peripheral neuropathy of the lower extremities
   - **C.** Myopathy in the proximal muscle groups
   - **D.** Gross increase in muscle tone

9. Children who undergo radiation and chemotherapy treatment for cancer demonstrate cognitive impairments. Younger children who received high doses of cranial radiation demonstrate decreased IQ, working memory, and processing speeds _____ postradiation than older children and children of all ages that receive focal, proton radiation.
   A. 1 month
   B. 3 years
   C. 5 years
   D. 8 years

10. Factors that decrease bone health in children with cancer include use of corticosteroids, IT methotrexate, ifosfamides, HSCT, cranial radiation, malnutrition, vitamin D deficiencies, decreased physical activity and limited weight bearing. _____ are often where the largest decrease in bone mineral density (BMD) is observed, resulting in osteoporosis.
   A. Upper extremity bones
   B. Pelvic bones
   C. Bones of the feet
   D. Long bones and spinal vertebrae

References

1. Santiago R, Vairy S, Sinnett D, et al. Novel therapy for childhood acute lymphoblastic leukemia. *Expert Opin Pharmacother.* 2017;18:1081–1099.
2. Madhusoodhan PP, Carroll WL, Bhatla T. Progress and prospects in pediatric leukemia. *Curr Probl Pediatr Adolesc Health Care.* 2016;46:229–241.
3. Hunger SP, Mullighan CG. Acute lymphoblastic leukemia in children. *N Engl J Med.* 2015;373(16):1541–1552.
4. Ishida Y, Maeda M, Adachi S, et al. Secondary cancer after a childhood cancer diagnosis: viewpoints considering primary cancer. *Int J Clin Oncol.* 2018;23(6):1178–1188.
5. SR Ambati, F Boulad, Evaluation and management of pediatric cancers, in: MD Stubblefield (Ed.), Cancer Rehabilitation: Principles and Practice, 2nd ed., Springer Publishing Company, 2018.
6. Rubnitz JE. Current management of childhood acute myeloid leukemia. *Paediatr Drugs.* 2017;19(1):1–10.
7. Kutny MA, Geyer S, Laumann KM, et al. Outcome for pediatric acute promyelocytic leukemia patients at Children's Oncology Group sites on the Leukemia Intergroup Study CALGB 9710 (Alliance). *Pediatr Blood Cancer.* 2019;66(3):e27542.
8. Imbach P. General aspects of childhood leukemia. In: Imbach P, Kuhne T, Arceci R, eds. *Pediatric Oncology: A Comprehensive Guide.* 3rd ed.: Springer International Publishing; 2014:12–16.
9. Imbach P. Acute lymphoblastic leukemia. In: Imbach P, Kuhne T, Arceci R, eds. *Pediatric Oncology: A Comprehensive Guide.* 3rd ed.: Springer International Publishing; 2014:16–30.
10. Mohseni M, Uludag H, Brandwein JM. Advances in biology of acute lymphoblastic leukemia (ALL) and therapeutic implications. *Am J Blood Res.* 2018;8(4):29–56.
11. American Cancer Society. Survival rates for childhood leukemias https://www.cancer.org/cancer/leukemia-in-children/detection-diagnosis-staging/survival-rates.html; Updated February 12, 2019. Accessed August 7, 2020.
12. Cooper SL, Brown PA. Treatment of pediatric acute lymphoblastic leukemia. *Pediatr Clin North Am.* 2015;62(1):61–73. doi:10.1016/j.pcl.2014.09.006.
13. COG-AALL0331. *Phase III Randomized Study of Different Combination Chemotherapy Regimens in Pediatric Patients with Newly Diagnosed Standard Risk B-Precursor Acute Lymphoblastic Leukemia*: Ped-Onc Resource Center; 2006. http://www.ped-onc.org/diseases/ALLtrials/COG0331.html: Accessed August 10, 2020.
14. O'Connor D, Bate J, Wade R, et al. Infection-related mortality in children with acute lymphoblastic leukemia: a retrospective analysis of infectious deaths on UKALL 2003. *Blood.* 2014;124:1056–1061.
15. Kato M, Manabe A. Treatment and biology of pediatric acute lymphoblastic leukemia. *Pediatr Int.* 2018;60(1):4–12.
16. Gaynon PS, Angiolillo AL, Carroll WL, et al. Long-term results of the children's cancer group studies for childhood acute lymphoblastic leukemia 1983–2002: a Children's Oncology Group Report. *Leukemia.* 2010;24(2):285–297.
17. American Cancer Society. Test for childhood leukemia. https://www.cancer.org/cancer/leukemia-in-children/detection-diagnosis-staging/how-diagnosed.html; Updated February 12, 2019. Accessed August 7, 2020.
18. Pui CH, Pei D, Sandlund JT, et al. Long-term results of St Jude Total Therapy Studies 11, 12, 13A, 13B, and 14 for childhood acute lymphoblastic leukemia. *Leukemia.* 2010;24(2):371–382.
19. Pui CH, Campana D, Pei D, et al. Treating childhood acute lymphoblastic leukemia without cranial irradiation. *N Engl J Med.* 2009;360(26):2730–2741.
20. Gilchrist L, Tanner L. Gait patterns in children with cancer and vincristine neuropathy. *Pediatr Phys Ther.* 2016;28(1):16–22.
21. Tanner LR, Hooke MC, Hinshon S, et al. Effect of an ankle foot orthosis intervention for children with non-central nervous system cancers: a pilot study. *Pediatr Phys Ther.* 2015;27(4):425–431.
22. Bansal N, Amdani S, Lipshultz ER, Lipshultz SE. Chemotherapy-induced cardiotoxicity in children. *Expert Opin Drug Metab Toxicol.* 2017;13(8):817–832.
23. Imbach P. Acute myeloid leukemia. In: Imbach P, Kuhne T, Arceci R, eds. *Pediatric Oncology: A Comprehensive Guide.* 3rd ed.: Springer International Publishing; 2014:21–34.
24. Imbach P. Brain tumor. In: Imbach P, Kuhne T, Arceci R, eds. *Pediatric Oncology: A Comprehensive Guide.* 3rd ed.: Springer International Publishing; 2014:95–117.
25. Bhatia A, Pruthi S. Pediatric brain tumors: a different ball game. *Semin Roentgenol.* 2018;53(53):77–100.
26. Grob ST, Mulcahy Levy JM. Improving diagnostic and therapeutic outcomes in pediatric brain tumors. *Mol Diagn Ther.* 2018;22:25–29.
27. Jaimes C, Poussaint TY. Primary neoplasms of pediatric brain. *Radiol Clin N Am.* 2019;57:1163–1175.
28. Curtin SC, Minino AM, Anderson RN. Declines in cancer death rates among children and adolescents in the United States, 1999–2014. *NCHS Data Brief.* 2016(257):1–8.
29. Koeller KK, Sandberg GD. From the archives of the AFIP. Cerebral intraventricular neoplasms: radiologic-pathologic correlation. *Radiographics.* 2015;64(2):1203–1213.
30. Pollack IF, Agnihotri S, Broniscer A. Childhood brain tumors: current management, biological insights, and future direction. *J Neurosurg Pediatr.* 2019;23:261–273.
31. Ostrom QT, Fahmideh MA, Cote DJ, et al. Risk factors for childhood and adult primary brain tumors. *Neuro-Oncology.* 2019;21(11):1357–1375.
32. Udaka YT, Packer RJ. Pediatric brain tumors. *Neurol Clin.* 2018;36:533–556.
33. Guerreiro AS, Ramaswamy V, Daniels C, et al. Review of molecular classification and treatment implications of pediatric brain tumors. *Curr Opin Pediatr.* 2018;30:3–9.
34. Lanier JC, Annah AN. Posterior fossa syndrome: review of the behavioral and emotional aspects in the pediatric cancer patients. *Cancer.* 2017;123:551–559.
35. Luksik AS, Garzon-Muvdi T, Yang W, et al. Pediatric spinal cord astrocytomas: a retrospective study of 348 patients from the SEER database. *J Neurosurg Pediatr.* 2017;19:711–719.
36. Szathmari A, Zerah M, Vinchon M, et al. Ependymoma of the spinal cord in children: a retrospective French study. *World Neurosurg.* 2019;126:e1035–e1041.

37. Azad TD, Pendharkar AV, Pan J, et al. *J Neurosurg Pediatr.* 2018;22:404–410.

38. PDQ Pediatric Treatment Editorial Board. Childhood Astrocytomas Treatment (PDQ®): Health Professional Version. [Updated November 25, 2020]. In: *Cancer Information Summaries* [Internet]. US: National Cancer Institute; 2002. https://www-ncbi-nlm-nih-gov.proxy1.library.jhu.edu/books/NBK65944/s.

39. Joaquim AF, Ghizoni E, Valadares MGC, Appenzeller S, Aguiar SDS, Tedeschi H. Spinal tumors in children. *Rev Assoc Med Bras.* 2017;63(5):459–465. doi:10.1590/1806-9282.63.05.459.

40. Jones BC, Youlden DR, Cundy TP, et al. Renal tumours in Australian children: 30 years of incidence, outcome and second primary malignancy data from the Australian Childhood Cancer Registry. *J Pediatr Child Health.* 2020;56(6):908–916.

41. Cunningham ME, Klug TD, Nuchtern JG, et al. Global disparities in Wilms tumor. *J Surg Res.* 2020;247:34–51.

42. Kamihara J, Ma C, Fuentes Alabi SL, et al. Socioeconomic status and global variations in the incidence of neuroblastoma: call for support of population-based cancer registries in low-middle-income countries. *Pediatr Blood Cancer.* 2017;64(2):321–323.

43. Steliarova-Foucher E, Colombet M, Ries LAG, et al. International incidence of childhood cancer, 2001–10: a population-based registry study. *Lancet Oncol.* 2017;18:719–731.

44. Xie W, Wei L, Guo J, Guo H, Song X, Sheng X. Physiological functions of Wilms' tumor 1-associating protein and its role in tumourigenesis. *J Cell Biochem.* 2019. doi:10.1002/jcb.28402.

45. Children's Oncology Group. Wilms tumor staging. https://childrensoncologygroup.org/index.php/newly-diagnosed-with-kidneywilms-tumor-#:~:text=The%20staging%20system%20used%20to,V%20(1%20to%205); Updated July, 2011. Accessed June 24, 2020.

46. Nakagawara A, Li Y, Izumi H, Muramori K, Inada H, Nishi M. Neuroblastoma. *Jpn J Clin Oncol.* 2018;48(3):214–241.

47. Traoré F, Eshun F, Togo B, Yao JJA, Lukamba MR. Neuroblastoma in Africa: a survey by the Franco-African Pediatric Oncology Group. *J Glob Oncol.* 2016;2(4):169–173.

48. Desandes E, Clavel J, Berger C, et al. Cancer incidence among children in France, 1990–1999. *Pediatr Blood Cancer.* 2004;43(7):749–757.

49. Bishop KL, Hanchard B, Gibson TN, et al. Incidence of childhood cancer in Kingston and St. Andrew, Jamaica, 1983–2002. *West Indian Med J.* 2012;62(7):575–581.

50. Shohet JM, Nuchtern JG. Epidemiology, pathogenesis, and pathology of neuroblastoma. In: Shah S, Park JR, eds. *UpToDate*; 2021. https://www.uptodate.com/contents/epidemiology-pathogenesis-and-pathology-of-neuroblastoma#H16. Accessed May 23, 2021.

51. American Cancer Society. What is Neuroblastoma? https://www.cancer.org/cancer/neuroblastoma/about/what-is-neuroblastoma.html; Updated March 19, 2018. Accessed June 20, 2020.

52. Imbach P, Neuroblastoma, Imbach P, Kuhne T, Arceci R. *Pediatric Oncology: A Comprehensive Guide.* 3rd ed.: Springer International Publishing; 2014:1119–1132.

53. Brodeur GM, Bagatell R. Mechanisms of neuroblastoma regression. *Nat Rev Clin Oncol.* 2014;11(12):704–713. doi:10.1038/nrclinonc.2014.168.

54. Cohn SL, Pearson AD, London WB, et al. The International Neuroblastoma Risk Group (INRG) classification system: an INRG Task Force report. *J Clin Oncol.* 2009;27(2):289–297.

55. Adamson PC, Houghton PJ, Perilongo G, Pritchard-Jones K. Drug discovery in paediatric oncology: roadblocks to progress. *Nat Rev Clin Oncol.* 2014;11(12):732–739.

56. Maris JM, Hogarty MD, Bagatell R, Cohn SL. Neuroblastoma. *Lancet.* 2007;369(9579):2106–2120.

57. Qualman SJ, Green WR, Brovall C, Leventhal BG. Neurofibromatosis and associated neuroectodermal tumors: a congenital neurocristopathy. *Pediatr Pathol.* 1986;5(1):65–78.

58. Roshkow JE, Haller JO, Berdon WE, Sane SM. Hirschsprung's disease, Ondine's curse, and neuroblastoma—manifestations of neurocristopathy. *Pediatr Radiol.* 1988;19:45–49.

59. Kamihara J, Ma C, Fuentes Alabi SL, et al. Socioeconomic status and global variations in the incidence of neuroblastoma: call for support of population-based cancer registries in low-middle-income countries. *Pediatr Blood Cancer.* 2017;64(2):321–323.

60. American Cancer Society. Neuroblastoma: detection, diagnosis, and staging. https://www.cancer.org/cancer/neuroblastoma/detection-diagnosis-staging/risk-groups.html; Updated March 19, 2018. Accessed June 22, 2020.

61. Salazar BM, Balczewski EA, Ung CY, Zhu S. Neuroblastoma, a paradigm for big data science in pediatric oncology. *Int J Mol Sci.* 2016;18(1):37. doi:10.3390/ijms18010037.

62. Galgano L, Hutt D. HSCT: how does it work? In: Kenyon M, Babic A, eds. *The European Blood and Marrow Transplantation Textbook for Nurses.* Springer; 2018:23–36.

63. Khaddour K, Hana CK, Mewawalla P. Hematopoietic stem cell transplantation. In: *StatPearls*: StatPearls Publishing; 2022.

64. Lenker H, Foley M. Pre-bone marrow transplant physical therapy evaluations in pediatric oncology. *Rehabil Oncol.* 2019;37(4):e9–e11.

65. Dirou S, Chambellan A, Chevallier P, et al. Deconditioning, fatigue, and impaired quality of life in long-term survivors after allogenic hematopoietic stem cell transplantation. *Bone Marrow Transplant.* 2018;53(3):281–290.

66. Qayed M, Wang T, Hemmer MT, et al. Influence of age on acute and chronic GVHD in children undergoing HLA-identical sibling bone marrow transplantation for acute leukemia: implications for prophylaxis. *Biol Blood Marrow Transplant.* 2018;24:521–528.

67. Marinho D, Ribeiro L, Nichele S, et al. The challenge of long-term follow-up of survivors of childhood acute leukemia after hematopoietic stem cell transplantation in resource-limited countries: a single-center report from Brazil. *Pediatr Transplant.* 2020;24:e13691.

68. Oeffinger KC, Mertens AC, Sklar CA, et al. Chronic health conditions in adult survivors of childhood cancer. *N Engl J Med.* 2006;355(15):1572–1582. doi:10.1056/NEJMsa060185.

69. L'Hotta AJ, Beam IA, Thomas KM. Development of a comprehensive pediatric oncology rehabilitation program. *Pediatr Blood Cancer.* 2020;67(2):e28083. doi:10.1002/pbc.28083.

70. Stout NL, Binkley JM, Schmitz KH, et al. A prospective surveillance model for rehabilitation for women with breast cancer. *Cancer.* 2012;118(8 suppl):2191–2200.

71. Tanner L, Sencer S, Hooke MC. The Stoplight Program: a proactive physical therapy intervention for children with acute lymphoblastic leukemia. *J Pediatr Oncol Nurs.* 2017;34(5):347–357.

72. Macartney G, Harrison MB, VanDenKerkhof E, Stacey D, McCarthy P. Quality of life and symptoms in pediatric brain tumor survivors: a systematic review. *J Pediatr Oncol Nurs.* 2014;31(2):65–77.

73. Shun SC. Cancer prehabilitation for patients starting from active treatment to surveillance. *Asia Pac J Oncol Nurs.* 2016;3(1):37–40.

74. Corr AM, Liu W, Bishop M, et al. Feasibility and functional outcomes of children and adolescents undergoing preoperative chemotherapy prior to a limb-sparing procedure or amputation. *Rehabil Oncol.* 2017;35(1):38–45.

75. Meyer AC, Thomas K. Screening for early childhood intervention in oncology. *Rehabil Oncol.* 2019;37:83–85.

76. Varni JW, Burwinkle TM, Katz ER, Meeske K, Dickinson P. The PedsQL in pediatric cancer: reliability and validity of the Pediatric Quality of Life Inventory Generic Core Scales, Multidimensional Fatigue Scale, and Cancer Module. *Cancer.* 2002;94(7):2090–2106. doi:10.1002/cncr.10428.

77. Raat H, Bonsel GJ, Essink-Bot ML, Landgraf JM, Gemke RJ. Reliability and validity of comprehensive health status measures in children: The Child Health Questionnaire in relation to the Health Utilities Index. *J Clin Epidemiol.* 2002;55(1):67–76. doi:10.1016/s0895-4356(01)00411-5.

78. Sandeberg M, Johansson EM, Hagell P, Wettergren L. Psychometric properties of the DISABKIDS Chronic Generic Module (DCGM-37) when used in children undergoing treatment for cancer. *Health Qual Life Outcomes*. 2010;8:109. doi:10.1186/1477-7525-8-109.

79. Mandrell BN, Yang J, Hooke MC, et al. Psychometric and clinical assessment of the 13-item reduced version of the Fatigue Scale Adolescent instrument. *J Pediatr Oncol Nurs*. 2011;28:287–294.

80. Hinds PS, Yang J, Gattuso JS, et al. Psychometric and clinical assessment of the 10-item reduced version of the Fatigue Scale-Child instrument. *J Pain Symptom Manage*. 2010;39:572–578.

81. Mahdizadeh F, Mehraban AH, Faranoush M, Amini M, Mehdizadeh M. Fatigue in children with cancer: reliability and validity of the Persian Version of Child, Parent, and Staff Fatigue Scale. *Asia Pac J Oncol Nurs*. 2020;7(2):174–179. doi:10.4103/apjon.apjon_44_19.

82. Perdikaris P, Merkouris A, Patiraki E, Tsoumakas K, Vasilatou-Kosmidis E, Matziou V. Evaluating cancer related fatigue during treatment according to children's, adolescent's and parents's; perspectives in a sample of Greek young patients. *Eur J Oncol Nurs*. 2009;13(5):399–408.

83. Collins JJ, Byrnes ME, Dunkel IJ, et al. The measurement of symptoms in children with cancer. *J Pain Symptom Manage*. 2000;19(5):363–377.

84. Lavoie Smith EM, Li L, Hutchinson RJ, et al. Measuring vincristine-induced peripheral neuropathy in children with acute lymphoblastic leukemia. *Cancer Nurs*. 2013;36(5):E49–E60.

85. Habib Z, Westcott S. Assessment of anthropometric factors on balance tests in children. *Pediatr Phys Ther*. 1998;10(3):101–109.

86. Dumas HM, Fragala-Pinkham MA, Rosen EL, Lombard KA, Farrell C. Pediatric Evaluation of Disability Inventory Computer Adaptive Test (PEDI-CAT) and Alberta Infant Motor Scale (AIMS): validity and responsiveness. *Phys Ther*. 2015;95(11):1559–1568.

87. Beenakker E, Van der Hoeven J, Fock J, Maurits N. Reference values of maximum isometric muscle force obtained in 270 children aged 4–16 years by hand-held dynamometry. *Neuromuscul Disord*. 2001;11:441–446.

88. Okuro RT, Schivinski CI. Six-minute walk test in pediatrics: the relationship between performance and anthropometric parameters. *Fisioter Mov*. 2013;26:219–228.

89. Bartels B, de Groot JF, Terwee CB. The six-minute walk test in chronic pediatric conditions: a systematic review of measurement properties. *Phys Ther*. 2013;93(4):529–541.

90. Van Brussel M, Helders PJ. The 30-second walk test (30sWT) norms for children. *Pediatr Phys Ther*. 2009;21:244.

91. Lekshminarayanan A, Bhatt P, Gandhi Linga V, et al. National trends in hospitalization for fever and neutropenia in children with cancer, 2007–2014. *J Pediatr*. 2018;202:231–237.

92. Winter C, Müller C, Brandes M, et al. Level of activity in children undergoing cancer treatment. *Pediatr Blood Cancer*. 2009;53(3):438–443.

93. Götte M, Kesting S, Winter C, et al. Comparison of self-reported physical activity in children and adolescents before and during cancer treatment. *Pediatr Blood Cancer*. 2014;61:1023–1028.

94. Kudchadkar SR, Nelliot A, Awojoodu R, et al. Physical Rehabilitation in Critically Ill Children: A Multicenter Point Prevalence Study in the United States. *Crit Care Med*. 2020;48(5):634–644.

95. Wösten-van Asperen RM, van Gestel JPJ, van Grotel M, et al. PICU mortality of children with cancer admitted to pediatric intensive care unit a systematic review and meta-analysis. *Crit Rev Oncol Hematol*. 2019;142:153–163.

96. Suzuki D, Kobayashi R, Sano H, et al. Sarcopenia after induction therapy in childhood acute lymphoblastic leukemia: its clinical significance. *Int J Hematol*. 2018;107(4):486–489.

97. Morales JS, Padilla JR, Valenzuela PL, et al. Inhospital exercise training in children with cancer: does it work for all? *Front Pediatr*. 2018;6:404.

98. Taguchi K, Ueno T, Shimizu Y, Ishimoto R, Hada Y. Effect of inpatient rehabilitation on activities of daily living in pediatric cancer patients in Japan. *Int J Rehabil Res*. 2018;41(2):146–151.

99. Rustler V, Hagerty M, Daeggelmann J, Marjerrison S, Bloch W, Baumann FT. Exercise interventions for patients with pediatric cancer during inpatient acute care: a systematic review of literature. *Pediatr Blood Cancer*. 2017;64:e26567.

100. Bogg TF, Broderick C, Shaw P, Cohn R, Naumann FL. Feasibility of an inpatient exercise intervention for children undergoing hematopoietic stem cell transplant. *Pediatr Transplant*. 2015;19(8):925–931.

101. Gupta A, Moore JA. Tumor lysis syndrome. *JAMA Oncol*. 2018;4(6):895.

102. Veno-Occlusive Disease (VOD). *Survival Rates for Childhood Leukemias*: American Cancer Society. Veno-occlusive disease (VOD). Canadian Cancer Society; 2021. www.cancer.ca Accessed February 21, 2021.

103. Wallek S, Senn-Malashonak A, Vogt L, et al. Impact of the initial fitness level on the effects of a structured exercise therapy during pediatric stem cell transplantation. *Pediatr Blood Cancer*. 2018;65(2). doi:10.1002/pbc.26851.

104. Rico-Mena P, Palacios-Ceña D, Martino-Alba R, et al. The impact of home-based physical rehabilitation program on parents' experience with children in palliative care: a qualitative study. *Eur J Phys Rehabil Med*. 2019;55(4):494–504.

105. Money S, Smith S, Clark M, et al. Cancer pain management. In: Mitra R, ed. *Principles of Rehabilitation Medicine*: McGraw-Hill; 2019.

106. Manchola-González JD, Bagur-Calafat C, Girabent-Farrés M, et al. Effects of a home-exercise programme in childhood survivors of acute lymphoblastic leukaemia on physical fitness and physical functioning: results of a randomised clinical trial. *Support Care Cancer*. 2020;28(7):3171–3178.

107. Gillis C, Li C, Lee L, et al. Prehabilitation versus rehabilitation: a randomized control trial in patients undergoing colorectal resection for cancer. *Anesthesiology*. 2014;121(5):937–947.

108. Lima KY, Santos VE. Play as a care strategy for children with cancer. *Rev Gaucha Enferm*. 2015;36(2):76–81.

109. Urbanski BL, Lazenby M. Distress among hospitalized pediatric cancer patients modified by pet-therapy intervention to improve quality of life. *J Pediatr Oncol Nurs*. 2012;29(5):272–282.

110. Sherman S, James WV, Ulrich R, et al. Post-occupancy evaluation of healing gardens in a pediatric cancer center. *Landscape Urban Plan*. 2005;73(2–3):167–183.

111. Kuntz N, Anazodo A, Bowden V, et al. Pediatric cancer patients' treatment journey: child, adolescent, and young adult cancer narratives. *J Pediatr Nurs*. 2019;48:42–48.

112. Wacker K, Tanner L, Ovans J, Mason J, et al. Improving functional mobility in children and adolescents undergoing treatment for non-central nervous system cancers: a systematic review. *PM R*. 2017;9(9S2):S385–S397.

113. Schadler KL, Kleinerman ES, Chandra J. Diet and exercise interventions for pediatric cancer patients during therapy: tipping the scales for better outcomes. *Pediatr Res*. 2018;83(1–1):50–56.

114. Stein E, Rayar M, Krishnadev U, et al. A feasibility study examining the impact of yoga on psychosocial health and symptoms in pediatric outpatients receiving chemotherapy. *Support Care Cancer*. 2019;27(10):3769–3776.

115. Ruble K, Paré-Blagoev J, Cooper S, et al. Parent perspectives on oncology team communication regarding neurocognitive impacts of cancer therapy and school reentry. *Pediatr Blood Cancer*. 2019;66(1):e27427.

116. Ruble K, Paré-Blagoev J, Cooper S, et al. Pediatric oncology provider perspectives and practices: supporting patients and families in schooling after cancer diagnosis. *Pediatr Blood Cancer*. 2020;67:e28166.

117. Billiet T, Elens I, Sleurs C, et al. Brain connectivity and cognitive flexibility in nonirradiated adult survivors of childhood leukemia. *J Natl Cancer Inst*. 2018;110(8):905–913.

118. Wengenroth L, Rueegg CS, Michel G, et al. Concentration, working speed and memory: cognitive problems in young childhood cancer survivors and their siblings. *Pediatr Blood Cancer*. 2015;62(5):875–882.

119. Eunice Kennedy Shriver National Institute of Child Health and Human Development (NICHD). NIH study links childhood cancer to delays in developmental milestones. https://www.nih.gov/news-events/news-releases/nih-study-links-childhood-cancer-delays-developmental-milestones; Published March 9, 2012. Accessed October 1, 2020.

120. Mulhern RK, Merchant TE, Gajjar A, Reddick WE, Kun LE. Late neurocognitive sequelae in survivors of brain tumours in childhood. *Lancet Oncol.* 2004;5(7):399–408.

121. Institute of Medicine (US) and National Research Council (US). National Cancer Policy Board. In: Hewitt M, Weiner SL, Simone JV, eds. *Childhood Cancer Survivorship: Improving Care and Quality of Life.* US: National Academies Press; 2003.

122. Hutchinson AD, Pfeiffer SM, Wilson C. Cancer-related cognitive impairment in children. *Curr Opin Support Palliat Care.* 2017;11(1):70–75.

123. Esbenshade AJ, Friedman DL, Smith WA, et al. Feasibility and initial effectiveness of home exercise during maintenance therapy for childhood acute lymphoblastic leukemia. *Pediatr Phys Ther.* 2014;26(3):301–307.

124. Kesler SR, Lacayo NJ, Jo B. A pilot study of an online cognitive rehabilitation program for executive function skills in children with cancer-related brain injury. *Brain Inj.* 2011;25(1):101–112.

125. Section on Hospice and Palliative Medicine and Committee on Hospital Care. Pediatric palliative care and hospice care commitments, guidelines, and recommendations. *Pediatr.* 2013;132(5):966–972.

126. Corr A, Thomas K. Screening for early childhood intervention in oncology. *Rehabil Oncol.* 2019;37(2):83–85.

127. Varni JW, Sherman SA, Burwinkle TM, Dickinson PE, Dixon P. The PedsQL Family Impact Module: preliminary reliability and validity. *Health Qual Life Outcomes.* 2004;2:55. doi:10.1186/1477-7525-2-55.

128. Weaver MS, Robinson J, Wichman C. Aromatherapy improves nausea, pain, and mood for patients receiving pediatric palliative care symptom-based consults: a pilot design trial. *Palliat Support Care.* 2020;18(2):158–163.

129. Choi HS, Chang EJ, Lee EH, et al. Changes in bone health during the first year of cancer treatment in children. *J Clin Densitom.* 2017;20(1):25–31.

130. Mostoufi-Moab S, Ward LM. Skeletal morbidity in children and adolescents during and following cancer therapy. *Horm Res Paediatr.* 2019;91(2):137–151.

131. Mogensen SS, Harila-Saari A, Mäkitie O, et al. Comparing osteonecrosis clinical phenotype, timing, and risk factors in children and young adults treated for acute lymphoblastic leukemia. *Pediatr Blood Cancer.* 2018;65(10):e27300.

132. Aristizabal P, Sherer M, Perdomo BP, et al. Sociodemographic and clinical characteristics associated with vitamin D status in newly diagnosed pediatric cancer patients. *Pediatr Hematol Oncol.* 2020;37(4):314–325.

133. Cox CL, Zhu L, Kaste SC, et al. Modifying bone mineral density, physical function, and quality of life in children with acute lymphoblastic leukemia. *Pediatr Blood Cancer.* 2018;65(4). doi:10.1002/pbc.2692910.1002/pbc.26929.

134. Amin N, Kinsey S, Feltbower R, et al. British OsteoNEcrosis Study (BONES) protocol: a prospective cohort study to examine the natural history of osteonecrosis in older children, teenagers and young adults with acute lymphoblastic leukaemia and lymphoblastic lymphoma. *BMJ Open.* 2019;9(5):e027204.

135. Ali N, Gohar S, Zaky I, et al. Osteonecrosis in children with acute lymphoblastic leukemia: a report from Children's Cancer Hospital Egypt (CCHE). *Pediatr Blood Cancer.* 2019;66(1):e27440.

136. Nama N, Barker MK, Kwan C, et al. Vincristine-induced peripheral neurotoxicity: a prospective cohort. *Pediatr Hematol Oncol.* 2020;37(1):15–28.

137. Gilchrist LS, Tanner LR. Short-term recovery of balance control: association with chemotherapy-induced peripheral neuropathy in pediatric oncology. *Pediatr Phys Ther.* 2018;30(2):119–124.

138. Rosca L, Robert-Boire V, Delisle JF, et al. Carboplatin and vincristine neurotoxicity in the treatment of pediatric low-grade gliomas. *Pediatr Blood Cancer.* 2018;65(11):e27351.

139. Gilchrist LS, Tanner L. The pediatric-modified total neuropathy score: a reliable and valid measure of chemotherapy-induced peripheral neuropathy in children with non-CNS cancers. *Support Care Cancer.* 2013;21(5):847–856.

140. van de Velde ME, Kaspers GL, Abbink FCH, et al. Vincristine-induced peripheral neuropathy in children with cancer: a systematic review. *Crit Rev Oncol Hematol.* 2017;114:114–130.

141. Lopez-Lopez E, Gutierrez-Camino A, Astigarraga I, et al. Vincristine pharmacokinetics pathway and neurotoxicity during early phases of treatment in pediatric acute lymphoblastic leukemia. *Pharmacogenomics.* 2016;17(7):731–741.

142. Kavcic M, Koritnik B, Krzan M, et al. Electrophysiological studies to detect peripheral neuropathy in children treated with vincristine. *J Pediatr Hematol Oncol.* 2017;39(4):266–271.

143. Tanner L, Keppner K, Lesmeister D, et al. Cancer rehabilitation in the pediatric and adolescent/young adult population. *Semin Oncol Nurs.* 2020;36(1):150984.

144. Sahin S, Semin Akel B, Huri M, et al. Investigation of the effect on task-orientated rehabilitation program on motor skills of children with childhood cancer: a randomized-controlled trial. *Int J Rehabil Res.* 2020;43:167–174.

145. Ibanez K, Andrews CC, Daunter A, et al. Chapter 63: Pediatric oncology rehabilitation. In: Mitra R, ed. *Principles of Rehabilitation.* McGraw-Hill Education; 2019.

146. Tanner LR, Hooke MC, Hinshon S, et al. Effect of an ankle foot orthosis intervention for children with non-central nervous system cancers: a pilot study. *Pediatr Phys Ther.* 2015;27(4):425–431.

147. Phillips JJ, Gordon SJ. Conservative management of lymphoedema in children: a systematic review. *J Pediatr Rehabil Med.* 2014;7(4):361–372.

148. Davey L. Comprehensive guide to lymphedema in children. Toronto Physiotherapy. https://torontophysiotherapy.ca/comprehensive-guide-lymphedema-in-children/#I_How_does_pediatric_secondary_lymphedema_occur; Updated May 24, 2018. Accessed October 1, 2020.

149. Bjork R, Ehman S, S.T.R.I.D.E Professional guide to compression garment selection for the lower extremity. *J Wound Care.* ;28(6a)(2019)1–44.

150. Quere I, Nagot N, Vikkula M. Incidence of cellulitis among children with primary lymphedema. *N Engl J Med.* 2018;378(21):2047–2048.

151. Zhang FF, Liu S, Chung M, Kelly MJ. Growth patterns during and after treatment in patients with pediatric ALL: a meta-analysis. *Pediatr Blood Cancer.* 2015;62(8):.

152. Guerrero-Preston R, Herbstman J, Goldman LR. Epigenomic biomonitors: global DNA hypomethylation as a biodosimeter of lifelong environmental exposures. *Epigenomics.* 2011;3(1):1–5.

153. Goh YI, Bollano E, Einarson T, et al. Prenatal multivitamin supplementation and rates of pediatric cancers: a meta-analysis. *Clin Pharmacol Ther.* 2007;81(5):685–691.

154. Schraw JM, Yiu TT, Lupo PJ, et al. Maternal folate genes and aberrant DNA hypermethylation in pediatric acute lymphoblastic leukemia. *PLoS ONE.* 2018;13(5):e0197408. doi:10.1371/journal.pone.0197408.

155. National Cancer Institute. Epigenetics and cancer. https://prevention.cancer.gov/news-and-events/news/epigenetics-and-cancer; March 13, 2007. Accessed October 1, 2020.

156. Rogers P. *Cancer prevention must begin in pregnancy and childhood*: World Cancer Research Fund International; 2019. https://www.wcrf.org/int/blog/articles/2019/02/cancer-prevention-must-begin-pregnancy-and-childhood; Accessed October 1, 2020.

157. Abadi-Korek I, Stark B, Zaizov R, Shaham J. Parental occupational exposure and the risk of acute lymphoblastic leukemia in offspring in Israel. *J Occup Environ Med.* 2006;48(2):165–174.

26

Young Cancer Survivors

SCOTT J. CAPOZZA, PT, MSPT, ALLISON J. L'HOTTA, PhD, OTD, OTR/L, AND
URSULA SANSOM-DALY, PhD

CHAPTER OUTLINE

Introduction

Definition of the Young Adult

To understand the needs of adolescent and young adults (AYAs), we must first define who is an AYA. The AYA is too old to be considered a pediatric person living with and beyond cancer (PLWBC), but they also do not fall within the typical age demographic of the majority of PLWBCs later in life. Within the United States (US), an AYA is defined in the literature and clinical practice as someone between the ages of 15 and 39 years old.[1]

When delivering care to AYAs, oncology rehabilitation (Onc R) clinicians need to be aware of the cognitive function and developmental stage of the AYA. Young people develop cognitively, emotionally, and socially during this period from being dependent children to capable, independent adults. AYAs' emerging capabilities during this life stage, combined with the transitions they undergo in every domain of their lives, have important implications for the focus of treatment with Onc R clinicians. As AYAs transition from childhood to adulthood, developmentally-normative concerns about establishing identity and independence, peer and romantic relationships, and longer-term decision-making about education, vocation, and family intersect with ongoing physical, cognitive, and psychosocial development.[2-4] The diagnosis and treatment of cancer at this life-stage complicate these maturational processes.[5] These developmental disruptions are a core reason why AYAs diagnosed and living with cancer are a uniquely vulnerable cohort. See Table 26.1 for more extensive details of the social issues and concerns by age grouping within the AYA timespan.

Cancer in the Young Adult

In 2020, there will be approximately 89,500 new cases of young adults diagnosed with cancer in the US,[6] accounting for approximately 5% of all cancer diagnoses in the US. Compared to pediatric cancers, the prevalence of cancer in the young adult is six times higher than in children 0 to 14 years old.[1,7] AYAs are often diagnosed at a later stage compared to non-AYA patients; less than half

TABLE 26.1	Social Issues for Adolescents and Young Adults With Cancer	
Age	**Social and Developmental Concerns**
<18 y/o: Mid-adolescent	• Interrupted social skills development • High school achievement/graduation delays • Delays in living independently • Difficulty establishing or maintaining employment
18–25 y/o: Emerging Adulthood	• Delays in higher education • Interruptions in employment • Barriers to achieving financial independence • Difficulties obtaining health insurance • Difficulty establishing and maintaining relationships with significant others/spouses
26–39 y/o: Young adulthood	• Difficulty establishing and maintaining relationships with significant others/spouses • Difficulties with intimate relationships and sexual function • Fertility issues impacting parenthood • Challenges managing a multitude of life roles (parent, spouse, co-worker, etc.) • Barriers to achieving or maintaining financial independence • Difficulties obtaining or maintaining health insurance

Adapted from Close AG, Dreyzin A, Miller KD, Seynnaeve BKN, Rapkin LB. Adolescent and young adult oncology—past, present, and future. *CA Cancer J Clin.* 2019;69(6):485–496; Warner EL, Kent EE, Trevino KM, Parsons HM, Zebrack BJ, Kirchhoff AC. Social well-being among adolescents and young adults with *cancer.* A systematic review. Cancer. 2016;122(7):1029–1037. Created by Scott Cappoza, Allison L'Hotta, and Ursula Sansom-Daly. Printed with permission.

of AYA women diagnosed with breast cancer (47%) are diagnosed at a local stage compared to 60% in women 45 to 54 years old and 65% in women 55 to 64 years old.[8] Factors contributing to this disparity include that routine mammographic screening is not recommended to AYAs who are not in a high-risk category for breast cancer and that there is a higher proportion of more aggressive tumor type (e.g., triple-negative breast cancer) at younger ages.[9] Because of these factors, the 5-year survival rate for female breast cancer in the AYA patient is lower than in older populations (86% compared to 91% in women ages 45–64).[8] See Table 26.2 for the most commonly diagnosed cancers in AYAs.

While the long-term outcomes of people with a history of childhood cancer are well documented,[10] there is limited data on the late and long-term adverse effects in AYAs. Concerns such as fertility preservation, financial toxicity, and developing a secondary cancer are more unique to AYAs, yet these areas of concern have not been as extensively studied as their pediatric[11] or older population counterparts. Overall, the 5-year survival rate for AYAs with cancer has shown a slow increase since the mid-1970s.

Building a Therapeutic Working Relationship

Getting to Know the AYA With Cancer

Age-appropriate care tailored to AYAs' unique needs requires that healthcare providers ground their practice in the development of a strong therapeutic relationship.[12,13] The first step in building a strong therapeutic relationship is developing a good understanding of who the AYA sitting in front of you is. Using the biopsychosocial approach,[14] which highlights that AYAs with cancer are young people first and foremost, develops a good understanding of the uniqueness and individuality of the AYA presenting for care.

Clinical Assessment

The AYA years are the peak time of onset for most mental health disorders[14]; therefore, a cancer diagnosis during this period can mean that AYAs experience a *'double whammy'* in terms of their psychological distress and challenges with coping and adaptation.[2] Best-practice clinical work with AYAs involves healthcare clinicians understanding that while AYAs face numerous psychosocial risks, the AYA years can also be a unique window of opportunity for young people to learn about, and become engaged in, their own healthcare.[13,15–18] Taking a competency-focused approach can help Onc R clinicians support and work with AYAs. Starting with the working assumption that AYAs bring strengths, skills, and potential with them, and working with AYAs to help them identify and harness these skills to the benefit of their physical and mental health and rehabilitation post-cancer.

As reviewed in *Chapter 14:*, patient reported outcome measures such as the National Comprehensive Cancer Network (NCCN) Distress Thermometer[19] can be used to assess overall distress as well as specific physical, emotional, and financial concerns of the AYA living with or beyond cancer. Other assessments that are more specific to the unique psychosocial, daily life and other practical needs of AYAs include the Cancer Needs Questionnaire-Young People (CNQ-YP).[20] The CNQ-YP was recently updated to link assessment findings to health services through the Needs Assessment &

TABLE 26.2	Leading Sites of New Cancer Cases in AYAs, Both Sexes Combined – 2020 Estimates					
Ages 15–19		**Ages 20–29**		**Ages 30–39**	
Thyroid	800	Thyroid	4,600	Breast (female)	11,100
Hodgkin lymphoma	800	Testicular germ cell tumor	3,000	Thyroid	9,000
Brain and other nervous system	500	Melanoma (skin)	2,200	Melanoma (skin)	5,500
Non-Hodgkin lymphoma	500	Hodgkin lymphoma	2,000	Colon and rectum	4,100
Testicular germ cell tumor	400	Breast (female)	1,500	Testicular germ cell tumor	3,100

Adapted from American Cancer Society. Cancer facts and figures 2020. https://www.cancer.org/content/dam/cancer-org/research/cancer-facts-and-statistics/annual-cancer-facts-and-figures/2020/cancer-facts-and-figures-2020.pdf. Published 2020. Accessed August 10, 2020. Printed with permission.

Service Bridge.[21] In a hospital-based medical setting with shared electronic medical records, a thorough review of the AYA's medical record should include the review of any cardiac and pulmonary function assessments, current lab work, and any reporting of physical adverse effects in the past; in a community-based rehabilitation facility, initiating a dialogue with the referring oncology team member will be imperative to obtain this information.

The "How": Setting Up the Right Dynamic

To motivate and mobilize AYAs in taking responsibility for managing their care and rehabilitation post-treatment, Onc R clinicians must approach them as active, autonomous partners in decision-making and care planning rather than passive recipients of treatment.[22] One powerful strategy to establishing a strong therapeutic rapport with an AYA is to level the unspoken power imbalance that can often exist in clinician-patient interactions. This can be achieved by explicitly acknowledging that while the caring Onc R clinician may be an 'expert on physical rehabilitation after cancer treatment,' the young person is also an 'expert' in their own right—on their own life, on their body, and what works for them in terms of their healthcare, mental health, and wellbeing. Thus, the clinician invites the young person to feel comfortable enough to actively bring the expertise of their lived experience to the working relationship and their therapy sessions and to continue to provide feedback to the clinician about their ways of working together. This simple acknowledgment can go far in engaging AYAs and can help lay the foundation for them to take ownership over their rehabilitation.

Depending on where in the AYA spectrum an individual is, their cognitive and/or emotional capacity to understand, digest, and retain complex health-related information may still be in development. An individual's ability to process information will also be impacted by their fatigue, pain, levels of distress, and any ongoing treatment/medication-related adverse effects.[16,17] Psychological distress, including symptoms of depression, anxiety, and stress, can significantly impact AYAs' working-memory capacity, attention, and concentration.[2] Assessment of psychological distress within a broader evaluation is critical at the start of the working relationship. Speaking directly to AYAs using clear, easy-to-understand language such as *"What questions do you have?"* (rather than the more common, *"Do you have any questions?"*) is more direct and concise.[23,24] Where more complex information (or behavioral/rehabilitation-related instructions) also needs to be discussed, clinicians can summarize what they understood from the consultation using techniques such as the "teach-back" method, which has been shown to enhance information comprehension and retention.[13,16,24–27] See Box 26.1 for more practical tips on communication strategies when working with AYAs.

The "Who": Who to Involve in the Assessment?

Depending on an AYA's age, cultural and community-related background, and other personal circumstances, it may be appropriate and recommended to involve others in an AYA's rehabilitation care. Best practice care for younger AYAs (including AYAs still living in the family home) requires a "family systems" approach, where parents and/or other immediate family members are involved in the provision of information, therapeutic recommendations, and are generally provided the opportunity to contribute to the process in support of the AYA with cancer.[4,28] Older and/or more independent AYAs may wish for a partner, spouse, or other support people to be involved in consultations. AYAs should still be consulted as the leader of their care and afforded

---

> ### • BOX 26.1 Practical Tips for Communicating With AYAs
>
> **Building Your Working Relationship**
> - Acknowledge the young person as an expert on their life, body, and experiences.
> - How would you like us to share information about your physical therapy home program? With whom should we share this information?
> - Ask: What questions do you have? (vs. Do you have any questions?)
> - Use the teach-back method
>
> **To Understand Hopes and Motivation**
> - What are you hoping that physical therapy will change for you?
> - What have you heard about physical therapy?
> - What are you hoping we can achieve together?
> - What matters most to you to be able to do in your life?
>
> **Blue Sky Questions**
> - If our work together was successful beyond your wildest dreams, where would you hope to be in 3 months' time? What would that look like? What would be different for you?
>
> **When There Are Challenges in Therapy**
> - Normalize feelings of distress as an acceptable/expected response to their circumstances.
> - How do you feel things are going in physical therapy? What is working/ what isn't working?
> - What can I do to better support you?
>
> Created by Sansom-Daly U. Printed with permission.

the opportunity to make the final decision about who may be involved in their healthcare consultations.[4,29] Involving AYAs in their rehabilitation care helps promote autonomy and can support their independence.[15]

The "What": Questions to Ask/Domains to Assess

Given the complex psychosocial factors that can contribute to AYAs' engagement with care, Onc R clinicians should complete a psychosocial screening. A general psychosocial screening can help gauge how the individual's physical and rehabilitation concerns fit into their broader needs, experiences, and ongoing challenges following treatment. Brief tools exist that may enable this. In Australia, the Youth Cancer Services[2] has developed a simple 1-page screening assessment for AYAs post-treatment, adapted from the validated Distress Thermometer.[30] This tool has a "problem checklist" with concerns tailored to the unique spectrum of concerns for AYAs living beyond cancer, including emotional, social, lifestyle, educational, and vocational concerns.

The "Why": Getting to the Heart of an AYA's Goals and Motivations

AYAs can be wonderfully honest, frank, and forthright, and so many will come with a good idea of what they hope to achieve from their clinical interactions with the Onc R clinician. Asking AYAs to express their hopes and motivations in their own words can be informative. For other AYAs, motivation may be more challenging; some AYAs may experience a disconnect between intellectually understanding why they need the intervention and feeling emotionally invested in doing the work this entails. For these individuals, asking more directed open-ended questions, such as *"How can I help you achieve your goals"* or *"What would like to get out of rehab?,"* can be useful to elicit AYAs' goals.

Rehabilitation Considerations for the AYA Living With or Beyond Cancer

Breast Cancer

Chemotherapy treatment of breast cancer can commonly include doxorubicin (Adriamycin). which can have long-term cardio toxic adverse effects. Additionally, if the breast tumor is HER2 positive, treatment will include trastuzumab (Herceptin) monthly for 12 months. As a HER2/neu receptor inhibitor, it can also cause cardio toxic adverse effects, which will require early and frequent cardiac screenings. There is a two-fold cardiovascular disease (CVD) risk increase for survivors of AYA cancer when compared with demographically matched patients without cancer.[31] Furthermore, survivors of AYA cancer who developed CVD had a 10-fold increased risk of dying compared with survivors without CVD.[31]

Often in the case of the young female with breast cancer, a medical oncologist will recommend dose-dense administration of chemotherapy. This entails that the patient receives their chemotherapy infusion every 2 weeks instead of the more traditional 3 weeks.[32] The thinking among some medical oncologists is a dose-dense administration that allows for faster completion of chemotherapy, thus a faster "return to normalcy" for the patient. The feeling is also that because these patients are younger, and presumably in better health, than older adults with breast cancer, they can sustain the adverse effects more easily than someone in their 60s or 70s. However, this dose-dense administration of chemotherapy does not properly allow for the bone marrow to recover from each chemotherapy cycle, and thus young people with breast cancer often experience a more sudden and severe onset of physical adverse effects.[32]

While the onset of menopause does not typically occur until the late 40s or early 50s, some young adults with breast cancer may be placed on hormone suppression if their breast cancer is estrogen and/or progesterone positive. Additionally, younger patients with breast cancer may undergo a hysterectomy with bilateral salpingo-oophorectomy to remove their ovaries and thus further decrease their levels of estrogen and progesterone. Either or both of these scenarios will biologically thrust the young female with breast cancer into menopause. In this case, women will be placed on an aromatase inhibitor (AI); the three common AIs are letrozole (Femara), anastrazole (Arimidex), and exemestane (Aromasin). The adverse effects of these AIs include joint pains (primarily at the hips, knees, and first metacarpophalangeal joint) and accelerated bone loss. Due to these adverse effects, AYAs with breast cancer are less likely to adhere to endocrine therapy, which can adversely impact overall survival.[33] For these reasons, weight-bearing cardiovascular exercises (e.g., walking, hiking, jogging, running) plus strength training incorporating the use of resistance bands, free weights, or cable column machines for core and upper extremity strengthening are optimal to address these concerns (see Table 26.3).

Rehabilitation considerations involve assessment of strength including the use of the handgrip dynamometer for the upper extremities and a 5-time sit-to-stand test for the lower extremities.[32] Special consideration for balance screening and functional mobility should be incorporated in a physical therapy evaluation if the young person with breast cancer has received paclitaxel (Taxol). or similar taxane-based chemotherapy. Assessments such as the more traditional Timed Up and Go can provide a quick assessment of balance, whereas the Fullerton Advanced Balance (FAB) scale can provide a more detailed assessment of balance including standing on non-compliant surfaces.[32] Due to the increased incidence of advanced stage breast cancer in the AYA population,

an axillary lymph node dissection may be indicated or required to surgically remove involved lymph nodes. In this case, careful screening for the development of axillary web syndrome (AWS), and lymphedema will be required by the treating Onc R clinician.

Young people living with or beyond breast cancer also need to be screened for cardio-pulmonary endurance. Coordinating with the oncology team, including cardio-oncology if available, will be important for consistent surveillance of cardiovascular function. Young people with breast cancer should be educated on establishing or reestablishing cardiovascular exercise to mitigate potential myocardial damage from both Adriamycin and Herceptin, following current exercise guidelines for PLWBCs.[34]

Testicular Cancer

The typical treatment for testicular germ cell tumors (GCT) is orchiectomy, which will require lifting restrictions for the AYA patient for 4 to 6 weeks post-operatively to avoid increased intra-abdominal pressure. Metastases to the retroperitoneal lymph nodes may require a retroperitoneal lymph node dissection (RPLND), which also requires restricted lifting for 4 to 6 weeks post-operatively. As most people living beyond GCTS will prefer to resume or initiate strength training,[35] careful education following surgery is imperative and will require the development of a gradual return to a prior level of function guided by an Onc R clinician. Many previously active and physically fit people with a history of GCTs may be anxious to return to their prior level of exercise such as strength training at a gym or competitive sports at the high school or collegiate level. Establishing realistic expectations, defining clear benchmarks for achieving cardiovascular exercise and resistance training, and close monitoring during this post-operative phase are vital for acceptance and implementation of the rehabilitation plan. Following clearance from the surgical team, the Onc R clinician can safely re-introduce strength training sessions and progress cardiovascular exercise to assist the AYA in returning to their prior level of function and fitness.

If the GCT is caught early enough requiring only orchiectomy, survival rates are >95%[7] and the person may not require chemotherapeutic intervention. However, if the tumor has metastasized to the retroperitoneal lymph nodes or other parts of the body, the medical oncologist may recommend several cycles of etoposide (Etopophos, Toposar) and cisplatin (Platinol). Acoustic nerve damage may occur due to cisplatin exposure. Both cisplatin and etoposide exposure increase the risk of developing secondary leukemia; additionally, cisplatin exposure also increases the risk for developing a second solid cancer including bladder, kidney, thyroid, and soft tissue including rhabdomyosarcomas.[31]

People with a history of testicular cancer who have received cisplatin are also at increased risk of developing CVD. The prevailing theory is that cisplatin causes direct damage to the vascular endothelium.[36] Incorporating high intensity interval training (HIIT) into a structured rehabilitation program can help strengthen the cardiovascular system and has demonstrated a longer lasting benefit.[37]

Less contemporary chemotherapy regimens would have also included bleomycin (Blenoxane), which can lead to pulmonary fibrosis in some patients. AYAs previously treated with bleomycin should be regularly assessed for declining pulmonary function.[37] Both bleomycin and cisplatin can also cause cold sensitivity in the fingers and toes due to vascular changes, thus mimicking a Raynaud's phenomenon sequelae.[38] This chemotherapy-induced Raynaud's phenomenon can last for over 20 years in up to 25% of AYAs with GCTs.[38] In this case, ice and other traditional cold modalities should be avoided for musculoskeletal injuries of the distal extremities.

TABLE 26.3 Common Cancers in the AYA Population With Incidence, Adverse Effects, and Rehabilitation Considerations

Cancer Type	Incidence in AYAs	Oncologic Treatment	Potential Adverse Effects	Rehabilitation Considerations/ Interventions
Breast (See Chapter 15 for more details)	1,500 cases annually in ages 20–29, up to 11,100 in ages 30–39[7]	- Taxane-based chemotherapy, often given in dose-dense administration (infusions every 2 weeks vs. every 3) - Herceptin for HER2+ breast tumors; ovarian suppression/BSO - Surgical interventions (e.g., mastectomy with or without reconstruction) - Axillary lymph node dissection	- CIPN in hands and feet - Early-onset of menopause (accelerated bone loss) - Joint pain - Cardiotoxicity - Fatigue - Upper extremity range of motion restrictions, strength limitations, and pain due to surgery and/or development of AWS - Adverse effects accumulate faster with dose-dense administration	- Static/dynamic balance retraining - Weight-bearing cardiovascular exercise (walking, jogging) and strength training (resistance bands, free weights) - Emphasize the importance of cardiovascular training - Scar massage - Range of motion - Screen for AWS + manual therapy to address
Testicular (See Chapter 16 for more details)	Highest incidence in males 20–39 (est. 6,100 in 2020); highly curable (>95%) if caught early[6]	- Orchiectomy - Retroperitoneal lymph node dissection when metastasis has occurred - Platinum-based chemotherapy with possibility of bleomycin	- Lifting restrictions 4–6 weeks post-surgery - CIPN with the possibility of Raynaud's phenomenon - Hearing loss - Pulmonary fibrosis	- Static/dynamic balance retraining - Progressive CV exercise program including HIIT - Gradual return to prior level of function post-operatively - Support in return to baseline exercise - Avoid ice and other cold modalities to the distal extremities for individuals with Raynaud's phenomenon
Melanoma	3rd most common form of cancer in AYAs; est. 7,900 cases in 2020[7]	Surgical resection with the potential removal of involved lymph nodes	- Lymphedema - AWS	- Complete decongestive therapy - Manual therapy to release AWS
Colorectal (See Chapter 17 for more details)	4,100 cases in 30–39-year olds; incidence increasing by 3%–6% per year[6]	- Platinum-based chemotherapy - Surgery	- CIPN - Fatigue	- Static/dynamic balance retraining - Progressive CV exercise program

AWS, Axillary web syndrome; *AYA,* adolescent and young adult; *BSO,* bilateral salpingo-oophorectomy; *CIPN,* chemotherapy-induced polyneuropathy; *CV,* cardiovascular; *HER2,* human epidermal growth factor receptor 2; *HIIT,* high intenisty interval training. Adapted from: American Cancer Society. Cancer facts and figures 2020. https://www.cancer.org/content/dam/cancer-org/research/cancer-facts-and-statistics/annual-cancer-facts-and-figures/2020/cancer-facts-and-figures-2020.pdf. Published 2020. Accessed August 10, 2020.
Miller KD, Fidler-Benaoudia M, Keegan TH, Hipp HS, Jemal A, Siegel RL. Cancer statistics for adolescents and young adults, 2020. *CA Cancer J Clin.* 2020. Printed with permission.

Melanoma of the Skin

In the AYA population, melanoma is more commonly diagnosed in women compared to men[7]; this trend reverses in the older population. The incidence of melanoma in the AYA population continues to steadily decline in the 15 to 19- and 20- to 29-year age groups.[7] Incidence rates have remained relatively stable for female AYAs aged 30 to 39, but have shown some decrease in similarly aged males.

The treatment for melanoma can include surgical resection of the suspected lesion, chemotherapy, radiation therapy, and lymphadenectomy. Depending on the size and extent of surgical resection and the total volume of lymphadenectomy involved, AYAs are at an increased risk of developing AWS. Similar to breast cancer, AWS and lymphedema can develop soon after surgery or may not develop for years following surgery.

Colorectal Cancer

While the incidence of colorectal cancer (CRC) is declining in the older (>65-year-old) population, the opposite is true for the AYA population.[6] Prevailing theories about this rise in CRC in the AYA population could be attributed to the finding that CRC tumors in AYAs generally are more poorly differentiated compared to older adults.[39] AYAs are more likely to have mucinous CRC, signet ring cell carcinoma, and/or poorly differentiated tumors.[39]

AYAs fall below age-based screening guidelines for CRC, which begins at age 50 in the US. Even with lowering the threshold for screening to 45 years of age based on revised guidelines,[40] this still does not lend itself to routine screening of AYAs in their 20s and 30s.

Due to the often-advanced stage of CRC in the AYA population, aggressive adjuvant chemotherapy typically follows surgical resection of the tumor. CRF is also commonly experienced by the AYA with a history of CRC, which has been reported to affect 17% to 29%[41] to as high as 80%[42] of all people with CRC. Following clearance from the surgical team, a gradual introduction (or return to activity) will be required to attain American College of Sports Medicine (ACSM) exercise recommendations.[34] For the AYA with a history of CRC who requires the placement of an ostomy, special attention to progressive core stabilization exercises will be required to assist with return to typical activities, such as work or school.[43]

Supporting Participation in Life Activities and Roles

AYAs experience cancer during a time in life when they are typically working towards or achieving critical developmental milestones[44] and have a variety of life roles. For many AYAs, active cancer treatment may lead to de-prioritization of, and even inability to, engage in many life roles (e.g., student, athlete, relationship development). This absence from the normal spheres of their lives is compounded by the dominance of their new "patient" role; as a person with an illness who is dependent on others for care and survival. This "sick role" can be very disempowering, can contribute to low mood and self-esteem, and for some AYAs can make it difficult to re-imagine their new future realities once cancer treatment is finished.[3,5]

Managing a cancer diagnosis associated treatment and potential adverse effects presents a unique challenge for AYAs to fully engage in life. The 2018 NCCN guideline for AYA oncology identifies the need to evaluate AYAs' (1) relationships with parents, spouse/partner, siblings, children, and peers; (2) sexual orientation; (3) participation in community and social activities;

and 4) communication with health care clinicians.[45] These guidelines for a comprehensive evaluation of AYAs highlight the unique needs of this population and the multitude of life roles they are balancing. The NCCN guidelines also identify the importance of evaluating exercise needs, hobbies, and recreational activities,[45] which are prime areas for intervention by rehabilitation clinicians.

Understanding what life roles and activities are most meaningful to an AYA is essential when designing their treatment plan. Life roles can be relational (e.g., brother, mother), functional (e.g., related to a job or student role), cultural or community-based (e.g., member of a religious or faith-based group), and activity or interest-focused (e.g., sport, activity, hobby-related). Table 26.4 highlights ways in which a cancer diagnosis and treatment may impact these different role types along with implications for clinical practice.

TABLE 26.4	Sources of Identity for AYAs Living With or Beyond Cancer and Their Implications for Assessment and Intervention			
Role Type	**Examples**	**Potential Impact of Cancer**	**Assessment Questions**	**Potential Interventions**
Relational	• Brother/sister • Son/daughter • Friend, best friend, acquaintance, part of a particular group at school • Boyfriend, girlfriend, partner, spouse • Mother, father • Other perceived "roles" (e.g., the "class clown" at school; the person who always organizes get-togethers)	Relationships may be strained or put under pressure as some people are perceived not to "get" the cancer experience or appear to "disappear". Other relationships may become stronger, and people may choose to spend more time with family. There may be missed opportunities that may take on a lot of meaning in the context of a relationship (e.g., missed milestones, events, holidays, or missed windows for things such as purchasing a house or starting a family	• Who are the key people in your life I should know about? • Who is in your family? • Who are your closest friends? • "go-to" people when you're having a rough time? • Have you noticed any changes in the people you are close to since your diagnosis?	• Consider engaging support people as part of goal setting and rehabilitation planning • Consider what social outcomes may be important for the AYA as part of their rehabilitation—particular relationships or groups may need attention • Identify what skills or adaptations are needed to support engagement in important relational roles (e.g., energy to attend a child's soccer game)
Educational/ Vocational	High school student, college senior; work roles (e.g., retail assistant, computer technician, teacher)	Stalled progress; missed opportunities; altered future potential (e.g., cognitive impact of cancer/treatment) Refer to the chapter text on work/school challenges	• Tell me about your work-life/experiences. • What work roles have you felt fulfilled in? • Describe the layout of your high school/ college campus?	• Consider what skills or supports are needed to help AYAs transition back into work/school • Consider whether the AYA will be able to return to their previous job/ career trajectory or whether they will need assistance in pivoting to a new vocation/career • Identify academic/workplace accommodations
Recreational	• Guitar player • Football player • Gardener • Baker, cook • Painter, sketcher, cartoonist, artist • Craft, sewing • Surfer, beach-goer • Traveler	Physical, cognitive, and emotional adverse effects of treatment can make it challenging to engage in a variety of preferred activities. These challenges may result in disconnection with previously meaningful and/or enjoying activities. Cancer may result in individuals identifying new areas of interest and a strengthened source of meaning from activities.	• Tell me about what you like doing? • If you have a weekend day to yourself, what would you be doing? • What activities/hobbies feel like they most reflect who 'you' are? • What skill or hobby would your family/ friends say you are famous for?	• Encourage continued engagement in enjoyable hobbies and activities, as these aspects of their lives are critical for mental health, wellbeing, and self-esteem. • Consider whether any new hobbies could be further cultivated, potentially also achieving new social goals (e.g., making new friends, reconnecting with existing relationships) or learning new skills (e.g., learning to cook or do grocery shopping for healthy foods as a stepping-stone to independence) • Strategize how to modify activities to meet their current functional skills.

TABLE 26.4 **Sources of identity for AYA survivors and their implications for assessment and intervention—Cont'd**

Role Type	Examples	Potential Impact of Cancer	Assessment Questions	Potential Interventions
Cultural	• Religion • Ethnic or cultural community • Sororities and fraternities • Clubs and societies, interest groups • Language communities (e.g., Brazilian Portuguese-speaking community; Spanish-speaking community).	These community groups may have become a source of strength, meaning, and support during treatment. They could also be a source of distress (e.g., if they are not understanding of the person's needs, or if there is perceived shame/stigma around cancer, or if the AYA's belief systems differ from their community). Some AYAs may rely heavily on their faith as a source of support when dealing with a life-threatening illness, while others may question their faith through these challenges.	• How did you make meaning of your whole cancer diagnosis and experiences so far? • What groups of people around you have played a big role in how you've dealt with your cancer experiences, either for better or worse? • What different groups or communities would I need to know about to truly 'get' who you are? • What does that community represent for you?	• Consider whether and how AYAs can be supported to reconnect with those communities via meaningful shared activities/experiences. • Consider whether any key supports can be engaged from different communities around the person to help them in pursuing rehabilitation goals. • Consider whether any community-based systems or behaviors may be less helpful in the AYA's rehabilitation goals (e.g. is the person perceived as a fragile patient who needs to simply rest and avoid exerting themselves?) or whether they understand ways in which the person may need to make lifestyle changes to achieve their rehabilitation goals. • Consider whether AYAs need support in communicating their needs and new goals/aspirations with different communities/groups in their lives.
Past, experience-based	• Cancer survivor • Graduate/alumni of specific school(s), colleges • Survivor of other types of life stressors, traumas	AYAs may feel disconnected from some of their past identities (e.g., on the same trajectory as the rest of their graduating class); they may also have developed new identities that may be a source of strength, purpose, or resilience (e.g., some AYAs identify strongly as 'survivors' or 'fighters'). It is important to note that not all AYAs like or identify with the term 'survivor' so this should not be assumed. An AYA's cancer experiences may also seem to them to continue a running 'theme' for them in their lives in terms of roles/identities (i.e., if they have experienced other life stressors or traumas, they may connect these events into a bigger picture/meaning).	• What have been some of the other key roles you have had in your life? • Before cancer, what events or experiences would you have said defined who you are? • How does your cancer diagnosis fit in with the story of your life?	• Understanding the AYA's history to some degree, including the impact on how the cancer experience has led to meaning and/or distress, is helpful for clinicians to inform their interventions in sensitive ways. (e.g., if a person tends to see themselves as a 'victim', as someone who always has bad luck, or who has no control), a rehabilitation care clinician can gently help the AYA to notice any times when they do something well, take initiative, and exert control over a situation. However, for the most part, it will be more appropriate for psychosocial care clinician colleagues to address concerns around these past experiences if they appear to be a source of ongoing distress.
Aspirational/future-oriented	• Future study and/or career aspirations • Future family-oriented aspirations (e.g., meet a partner, get married, have a child/children)	Stalled progress or missed opportunities (e.g., may have missed critical exams); altered future potential (e.g., if the cognitive impact of cancer/treatment, or if the cancer experiences have diminished their financial savings). Some AYAs can find thinking and planning for the future anxiety-provoking after cancer due to the level of uncertainty the cancer has introduced.	• Where do you see yourself in 1 year's time? In 5 years? • Before cancer, what was your biggest dream/hope for yourself? • What does 'success' mean to you? • Are there particular things you are hoping to achieve by the time you are 20/25/30 years old? • Has cancer gotten in the way of particular goals/plans you had made for your future?	• Normalize and provide support when AYAs have no plans/goals for the future or when they prefer to avoid thinking about the future • Clinicians can gently explore and normalize experiences with survivor guilt and explore how actions and behaviors can be meaningful, positive, and inspirational in the world (e.g., helping an elderly neighbor can be as meaningful and inspirational as starting a charity or becoming a surgeon). Depending on an AYA's degree of distress about these things, consider exploring if they may benefit from seeing a psychologist also to address this further.

(Continued)

TABLE
26.4**Sources of identity for AYA survivors and their implications for assessment and intervention—Cont'd**

Role Type	Examples	Potential Impact of Cancer	Assessment Questions	Potential Interventions
Aspirational/ future-oriented continued.	• Future status/ social mobility related aspirations (e.g., salary/ earning aspirations, financial savings aspirations; asset attainment goals such as car or homeownership, or moving to a different neighborhood/city)	• Some AYAs can experience 'survivor guilt' (i.e., distress around the fact that they survived their cancer while peers they may know did not) and this can lead to some AYAs putting a great deal of pressure on themselves to achieve great and inspirational things with their 'second chance' at life. (Society can also contribute to this pressure through traditional and social media channels).		• Consider encouraging the AYA to engage in self-compassion (kindness) around changes to their future plans and encourage them to permit themselves to 'scale back' their future plans (e.g., thinking about their plans for next week or next month, rather than trying to plan big over the next year or 5 years) • Support AYAs in identifying realistic future goals.

Created by Sansom-Daly U. Printed with permission.

School and Work Pursuits

While the life roles of AYAs are highly variable and frequently evolving, the majority of AYAs are involved in academic and/or career pursuits. Returning to a previous academic/career setting or transitioning into a new vocational environment presents numerous challenges for AYAs. More than 50% of AYAs experience challenges with work or school after their cancer diagnosis.[46] Fostering success in educational and occupational pursuits is essential to enhancing self-efficacy and motivating AYAs to participate in educational and employment activities.[7] Engaging in work-related pursuits can have a broader impact on an AYA's participation in the home, community, and social and leisure pursuits.[7]

Some groups of AYAs are at higher risk for employment and academic challenges. These groups include individuals with acute lymphoblastic leukemia and non-Hodgkin lymphoma,[46] non-Hispanic Black people, and AYAs who receive more intensive treatment,[46] such as hematopoietic stem cell transplant.[47] To ensure these groups succeed in employment and school, rehabilitation services must be prioritized.

Treatment Adverse Effects and Work/School

Returning to work/school can highlight or exacerbate treatment adverse effects. While physical limitations present a clear challenge in a variety of vocational environments, many AYAs may experience hidden deficits such as fatigue and cognitive changes.[48] When returning to a work/school environment, AYAs will have to contend with the potential long-term cognitive impact of treatment as they realize their impairments may be worsening over time rather than improving.[4]

How to Support Participation in Work/School

Onc R clinicians have a critical role in supporting AYAs in their return to work and school. AYAs typically receive clearance from their medical team to return to pre-cancer activities, yet they receive minimal guidance or support on how to participate in previous activities given any new cancer-related impairments.[47] University personnel[49] and employers may not have the training necessary to capably support individuals with cancer.[4,5] Onc R clinicians have a unique combination of medical training, experience with patient-centered care, and focus on functional goals, which

can help bridge this gap and support the academic and vocational development of AYAs.

Each discipline within the rehabilitation team, including physical therapy, occupational therapy, speech-language pathology, and neuropsychology, can support AYAs in their academic and career pursuits. Onc R clinicians must be aware of how important return to school and work are for many AYAs. Individuals with cancer may hold onto the return to school or work as an opportunity to return to a sense of normalcy or their lives pre-cancer.[48] Consequently, many may return to school or work before they are ready for the increased demands of engaging in an academic or work environment.[47] When AYAs rush back into these settings they may be unprepared emotionally and physically; some AYAs acknowledge that they needed a longer period of physical and psychological rehabilitation before returning to work or school.[47] See Box 26.2 for ways Onc R clinicians can support AYAs in return to work or school. The return to school/work transition needs to start long before the AYA makes this transition[47] and ongoing support is needed to support academic/career maintenance.[50]

AYAs are in the prime of their work lives and the inability to return to work or school poses a challenge to gaining financial independence[51] and risk of financial losses at the individual, family, and societal levels.[52] Collaboration and open communication between AYAs, healthcare clinicians, and employers/schools improves support for AYA in all of these domains.[52,53] Consistent communication can support the implementation of accommodations that match the AYA's current skill level and improve the overall return to work/school experience.[52,54] Work and school environments must accommodate changes in medical and functional status and implement supports and modifications to optimize strengths and adapt to areas of impairment.[55] To support AYAs in a survivorship clinic, an occupational therapist can serve as a communication and coordination liaison between key stakeholders in the return to work/school transition.[52]

Many AYAs with cancer experience impairments that limit essential vocational skills and can present barriers to participation. AYAs need to manage associated stresses, enact appropriate functional and social skills, and adapt to personal and environmental demands in academic/work settings.[50] As AYAs better understand the long-term impact of their treatment, they may need support with identifying a new academic or career focus.

• BOX 26.2 **Ways Rehabilitation Clinicians Can Facilitate Return to Work/School/Vocational Activities for AYAs**

- Assist in planning the transition back to school or work
- Provide direct interventions and home exercise programs to increase endurance, strength, and other job-related skills
- Educate on potential accommodations or recommend changes in job tasks
- Assess cognitive skills and educate clients on adaptive strategies, such as scheduling and note taking skills[43]
- Prepare clients for the high likelihood of fatigue when they return to work/school[4] and discussing fatigue management strategies
- Educate on available resources and their legal rights
- Assist in problem solving through challenges that arise after returning to work/school
- Conduct vocational assessments to help identify a good job/skill match

Adapted from Wiskemann J, Schommer K, Jaeger D, Scharhag-Rosenberger F. Exercise and cancer: return to work as a firefighter with ostomy after rectal carcinoma—a case report. *Medicine (Baltimore)*. 2016;95(29):e4309.
Zebrack B, Santacroce SJ, Patterson P, Gubin A. Adolescents and young adults with cancer: a biopsychosocial approach. In: *Pediatric Psychosocial Oncology: Textbook for Multidisciplinary Care*. Springer; 2016:199–217. Printed with permission.

Individual awareness is a key factor in career development for AYAs.[50] Awareness encompasses an individual's understanding of their own skills, abilities, and interests.[50] Onc R clinicians can implement the Cognitive Orientation to daily Occupational Performance (CO-OP) approach[56] to facilitate the guided discovery of an individual's strengths and limitations to help support them in academic and work pursuits. CO-OP supports clients in identifying strategies that will promote successful performance of client-identified goals.[56] Clinicians guide clients in the problem-solving process of applying the Goal-Plan-Do-Check strategy.[56] In this process, clients identify a goal, develop a plan, do/carry out the plan, and check to see if the plan worked.[56] Through a collaborative discussion, clinicians guide the problem-solving process of understanding why/how a plan did or didn't work.[56] The process of guided discovery helps clients independently identify challenges and solutions.[56] Ultimately, identifying strategies on their own will promote the generalizability of skills to other tasks.[56]

Mental Health, Motivation, and Engagement: Issues for Clinical Practice

Mental Health, Self-Esteem, and Adjustment in Survivorship

While cancer is devastating at any age, AYAs' pre-existing mental health vulnerabilities contribute to the unique challenges that they experience.[2,57] Additionally, AYAs remain at lifelong risk for mental health disorders even after the completion of successful cancer treatment and remission has been achieved. In fact, despite the considerable joy and relief associated with this celebrated milestone, AYAs living beyond cancer and their families also often experience peak distress during this period.[2,58,59] Clinical-level psychological distress is seen in about a quarter of AYAs in the first 12 months post-diagnosis,[60,61] which does not decrease meaningfully over the following year.[57] AYAs are significantly more at risk for suicidal behavior in the year post-diagnosis and up to 5 years later, relative to control cancer-free peers.[62] Even beyond 5 years, 25% to 40% of AYAs experience ongoing unmet needs related to their

identity, social isolation, difficult emotions, survivorship, and life direction.[63] The rehabilitation approach needs to be informed by AYAs' psychosocial history and mental health functioning in two ways: (1) by understanding how their mental health may impact clinical interactions; and (2) by recognizing how the focus of the rehabilitation work may be integrally connected to the source of any current distress and levels of self-esteem.

Trouble Shooting Roadblocks

Low Mood, Apparent Lack of Engagement/Motivation

Depending on the unique physical sequelae, some AYAs may lose significant aspects to their previous identity—who they were, according to themselves or the world. AYAs' perceived and actual social and emotional isolation can compound this, contributing to low mood and poor self-esteem. This may make engaging in rehabilitation more challenging for some as feelings of hopelessness for the potential of rehabilitation to lead to improved physical function and participation in life can impede their progress in rehabilitation.

Connecting with peers also living beyond cancer has been highlighted as a core developmental need by AYAs,[64] and is an important focus of distress-reducing interventions in this group.[12] A strategy to address hopelessness around future change is to situate an AYA's experiences into the broader group experience of AYAs living with and beyond cancer. Clinicians can talk with AYAs about common physical, emotional and social challenges, and about the experiences of other AYAs they may have worked with. Connecting AYAs with a history of cancer or those attending a survivorship clinic/Onc R service can also be a powerful source of motivation and comfort for AYAs. Many AYAs may not have opportunities to meet other AYAs living with or beyond cancer due to their dispersion across hospital sites (and their relative rarity as a group), as such, AYAs may lack contact with peers who have been through a similar experience.[65-67] AYAs, particularly those with a history of GCTs, are more likely to engage in socially-focused physical activity if the activity is outside of the hospital setting, involves group settings such as an organized sport, and is age-specific.[35] Other community resources that combine both physical activity and socialization for AYAs, including First Descents, should be recommended to AYAs when it is not possible to connect AYAs in clinical settings; for more resources for AYAs, please see Table 26.5. Concerns about mental health always warrant discussions relative to clinical psychologist referral for further assessment and treatment.

Rehabilitation Considerations: Resistance, Poor Attendance, and 'Non-Compliance'

Engaging AYAs in clinical settings can be difficult, particularly if they are experiencing feelings of anger, fear, or intimidation.[68] AYAs may disengage when discussing sensitive or personal areas of their life (e.g., emotional problems, family issues, peer and romantic relationships, sexual behavior, drug use) and/or when exploring topics that evoke feelings of personal shame, embarrassment, guilt, or anxiety.[22] AYAs may fear being misunderstood, ridiculed, or judged in some way,[69] while clinicians' feelings of embarrassment, awkwardness, and uncertainty may likewise prevent them from initiating these conversations or persisting with them.[22] Many AYAs also report feeling angry or disappointed with one's body due to perceiving that their body "betrayed them" by getting cancer at such a young age in the first place.[70,71] For some AYAs, this can become a barrier to engaging with rehabilitation if the very act of focusing on their body triggers distress. In these instances, it is important to normalize these feelings as natural responses to an unexpected and relatively uncommon event. Onc R Clinicians can also gently support AYAs in noticing what they can do (rather than cannot), what is in their control (rather than what is not) and how far they may have come already in rehabilitation to assist them in productively refocusing their attention. For Onc R clinicians, this can be achieved through assisting AYAs to reflect on concrete gains towards activities and functioning that have been made, and realistic steps towards future short- and medium-term rehabilitation goals. For some AYAs, concurrent support from a psychologist may also be useful to assist in working through these feelings of anger, disappointment, and changed self-image.

For some AYAs, the disruptions caused by cancer may lead them to resist and react against this sudden lack of control in their lives; this can include resisting clinical interventions. After experiencing an unexpected cancer diagnosis, and a cancer treatment period likely largely out of their control, AYAs may choose to exert control in apparently self-defeating or counter-productive ways. For example, an AYA may choose not to take some of their medications (perhaps less 'vital' ones) or may miss/avoid healthcare appointments that clash with social events.[13] Whilst this behavior is quite developmentally normal, it can create challenges for care clinicians by complicating the delivery and efficacy of care outcomes.[4]

AYAs tend to value honesty and being provided real choices in their healthcare interactions. Consequently, it is important to address perceived 'non-compliance' with rehabilitation recommendations in such a way that these elements of the therapeutic relationship are preserved. Firstly, care clinicians can consider using a moment of progress stalling (or regressing/reversing) by taking stock of the therapeutic working relationship: what is working well for the AYA, and what is not? It is also critical to get a sense of how the AYA feels they are doing—they may not perceive that progress has stalled, and/or they may not necessarily perceive this as a negative thing in the same way as the clinician. Naming what the clinician has observed objectively and taking the opportunity to 'reality test' this with the AYA's own experiences and feelings about progress is crucial.

Several interventions may be useful in addressing poor adherence to therapeutic recommendations depending on the 'root cause' that a clinician discovers in collaboration with the AYA. These would include:

- Provide further information, clarification, and discussion to develop simple, practical, and logistical solutions[13]
- Assess for developmentally normative health risk behaviors (e.g., alcohol and drug use) which could interfere with rehabilitation interventions[13]
- Assess for signs of distress including depression, anxiety, and low self-esteem
- Collaborate with and/or provide a referral to appropriate mental health and psychosocial support services to further address these concerns

Other Needs of AYAs

Financial Challenges and Insurance

Cancer treatment is incredibly costly, and some individuals have to limit interventions because of the high cost of treatment.[72] Cancer results in lost time from school and work, in turn compounding financial hardships during a time when economic independence is

a primary goal.[73] Missing out on early career opportunities impacts long-term career opportunities, financial status, and lifetime earnings of AYAs.[74] More than 75% of AYAs diagnosed with cancer at older ages (26–39) reported cancer had a negative impact on their financial situation.[75] AYAs with a history of cancer without a chronic condition have an average of $5468.00 in annual medical expenditures; having at least one chronic condition increases the annual average medical expenditure by $2777.00[76] Insufficiency of financial resources can be incredibly stressful for AYAs.[77] Financial challenges tend to distract from other life priorities, make it challenging for AYAs to move beyond their cancer, and can prevent AYAs from living a fulfilling life after cancer.[77] Onc R clinicians can improve client outcomes by providing appropriate supports/recommendations to facilitate success in their academic/career pursuits, including organizations such as the SamFund.[77] Helping AYAs achieve success in work/school is an optimal strategy in supporting their financial growth and independence. Onc R clinicians should work with the care team to connect AYAs to financial resources when financial concerns warrant. The rehabilitation team can also help AYAs identify low-cost medical equipment and develop fiscally mindful strategies to fully engage in life. For a more detailed list of financial resources for AYAs, please see Table 26.5.

When AYAs are dependent on employment for health insurance, this can present several challenges. Due to high rates of unemployment in AYAs,[46] they may have difficulty accessing more affordable health insurance, further restricting their access to essential medical services. In the US, if a parent has health insurance, AYAs are eligible to stay on their parent's insurance policy until the age of 26.[78] After aging out of parental insurance coverage, some AYAs may still be in school and have limited access to employer-sponsored health insurance benefits.[75] Health insurance coverage is important for Onc R clinicians to be aware of in determining an appropriate rehabilitation care delivery model. For AYAs with limited insurance coverage for rehabilitation services, a clinician may need to develop a comprehensive home program following a one-time evaluation. Physical inactivity was associated with additional medical expenditures ($3558) and health care use,[76] which further demonstrates that Onc R clinicians may need to address physical activity in a concise and thorough manner to help reduce financial burden on the AYA. Alternatively, when an individual has ongoing coverage there is an opportunity for ongoing education/training and continued adaptation of the therapy approach to meet an individual's evolving needs.

Loss of Independence

AYAs are at a time in their life when they are establishing independence and their sense of self. However, when faced with cancer, many AYAs regress developmentally and put plans for their future on hold. They may have to move back in with their parents or rely more on their parents or spouse than they are used to.[74] These dramatic shifts in how AYAs live their lives can lead to a multitude of inter- and intrapersonal challenges. Rehabilitation clinicians have a key role in supporting the independence of AYAs. Clinicians can support AYAs in developing goals for the future and creating action plans to progress towards those goals. Therapists can also help AYAs identify goals that are realistic based on their individual skill levels. Onc R clinicians can identify impairments that limit independence[79] and help empower AYAs to gain independence by supporting their function, activity performance, and participation in life by planning and implementing activities that engage the AYA in meaningful person-centered care.

TABLE 26.5   Helpful Resources/Reference Sites/Supportive Services for AYA

Resources for AYAs	Resources Offered	Website/Contact Information
Adolescent and Young Adult (AYA) Cancer Societal Movement	Monthly online chats for both AYAs and providers	#AYACSM (Twitter)
Cancer and Careers	Financial support, assistance with job placement, employee rights	www.cancerandcareers.org
Elephants and Tea	Online and in-print magazine, including survivor stories and resources	www.elephantsandtea.com
First Descents	Outdoor experiences ranging from hiking to surfing in a small group setting	www.firstdescents.org
Imerman Angels	Online one-on-one, cancer-specific support network	www.imermanangels.org
Lacuna Loft	Online group support	www.lacunaloft.org
LIVESTRONG Fertility	Fertility support, assistance with financial burden of fertility preservation	https://www.livestrong.org/we-can-help/livestrong-fertility
National Comprehensive Cancer Network (NCCN) Guidelines	Patient-friendly guidelines for surveillance and recommendations	https://www.nccn.org/patients/guidelines/content/PDF/aya-patient.pdf
Stupid Cancer	Online support groups/live chats, plus AYA-specific conferences and symposiums	www.stupidcancer.org
The SamFund	Financial support, treatment-related scholarships, employee rights	www.thesamfund.org

Created and curated by Capozza S, L'Hotta A, Sansom-Daly U. Printed with permission.

When AYAs become more dependent on their family or partner they may lose their voice both in medical care settings and in daily life. AYAs may struggle with communication with peers[48] and employers[49] and face ongoing challenges in advocating for their own needs and desires.[74,75] Therefore, AYAs would benefit from education on self-advocacy skills to support their participation in daily life. Onc R clinicians can incorporate education on self-advocacy strategies into therapy sessions and can develop interventions focused on self-advocacy in daily life.

Oncology Care Setting and Care Transitions

AYAs typically fall in the gap between care provided at pediatric centers and adult facilities.[53] Whether treated in a pediatric or adult facility, neither care setting is designed to meet the unique needs of AYAs. Some hospitals have developed specialty centers for AYAs[45] to better meet their needs. While there is advocacy for pediatric Onc R specialization,[80] similar recommendations have not yet been made for AYAs, but they too have a distinct set of rehabilitation needs, which have been highlighted throughout this chapter.

Transitioning care between facilities and clinicians poses another potential challenge for AYAs. To help AYAs advocate for their unique needs during a care transition or following treatment completion, the AYA and new medical team need to be provided with a detailed treatment summary and care plan.[81,82] Currently the rehabilitation needs of AYAs are not a standard component of transition summaries. Care summaries need to outline the AYA's current rehabilitation needs, as well as potential future needs due to late effects. To help AYAs identify future rehabilitation and supportive care needs they need, to understand what potential late effects can be experienced after active cancer treatment[53] and how late effects can impact their function.

Ongoing surveillance by rehabilitation clinicians, either in a traditional rehabilitation setting or in collaboration with a multidisciplinary survivorship program, is critical to identifying new impairments in function resulting from late effects.[79] Multidisciplinary team monitoring of AYAs throughout the entire trajectory of their cancer journey provides opportunities to effectively support transitions in care.[79] Onc R clinicians need to work with the medical team to develop a comprehensive transition plan to support the long-term function, well-being, and quality of life of AYAs.

Awareness of Rehabilitation Services

Rehabilitation services are underutilized in oncology.[83,84] Most AYAs with cancer are unaware of rehabilitation services or do not believe these services support PLWBCs.[85] Advocating for and educating medical clinicians as well as AYAs about the potential need for and benefit of Onc R services is of paramount importance. Many AYAs continue to live with deficits that are amenable to rehabilitation interventions. AYAs and even clinicians may accept these adverse effects as an inevitable component of fighting cancer and do not recognize that working with Onc R clinicians can help improve QOL.

Conclusion

The developmental needs of AYAs are dynamic. A cancer diagnosis during the AYA timespan can delay the achievement of important developmental and societal milestones. Many AYAs may subjectively appear healthy, but they often experience premature aging and can more commonly experience physical impairments observed in older adults. The implications of long-term adverse effects can persist for decades. Furthermore, AYAs may have increased challenges in engaging in rehabilitation due to a multitude of factors including financial, psychosocial, and a clear understanding of the importance of rehabilitation services. AYAs with a history of cancer should be thoroughly assessed based on their oncology treatment history in addition to their unique needs during this timeframe in their lives.

Critical Research Needs

- Identify and validate functional assessments relevant to AYAs with cancer.
- Determine how physical sequelae in AYAs with cancer are similar and different from other age groups affected by cancer, including assessing the role of the vestibulocochlear, phrenic, or pudendal nerves in CIPN.
- Develop and test strategies to integrate rehabilitation assessments into routine clinical care through the electronic medical record.
- Establish guidelines for consistent rehabilitation and psychosocial evaluations and interventions for potential late and long-term adverse effects of treatment through long-term survivorship for AYAs.
- Foster support for AYAs with cancer as they transition care from specialized oncology clinicians to primary care physicians.
- Determine the impact of psychosocial factors on utilization of and engagement in rehabilitation services.
- Develop and evaluate programs to support AYAs with cancer in gaining, maintaining, and returning to work during and after treatment.

Case Study

Emily is a 31-year-old female who was diagnosed with left-sided breast cancer 2 years ago. She has undergone a bilateral mastectomy with tissue expander placement, followed by placement of an implant. Her breast cancer was diagnosed as ER(+)/PR(+), as well as HER2(+). She received 6 cycles of docetaxel (Taxotere), carboplatin (Paraplatin), trastuzumab (Herceptin) and pertuzumab (Perjeta) (TCH+P) followed by monthly Herceptin for an additional 6 months. Cycle 4 of chemotherapy was delayed due to detection of atrial thrombus on echocardiogram, which required a short course of enoxaparin sodium (Lovenox). Following the completion of chemotherapy, she began ovarian suppression together with letrozole. She soon developed osteopenia and began taking denosumab (Prolia) every 6 months. Six months ago, she experienced a non-traumatic left 6th rib fracture due to worsening osteopenia. She also reported decreased tolerance of letrozole and was switched to exemestane 4 months ago.

She presents to an outpatient physical therapy clinic reporting continued joint pains from exemestane. She also reports dissatisfaction with her body image, as she has gained 35 pounds since being put on ovarian suppression. Her most recent dual-energy X-ray absorptiometry (DEXA) scan revealed osteopenia in her left iliac crest and thoracic spine. While she elected not to pursue fertility preservation at the time of beginning chemotherapy, she admits to the rehabilitation clinician that she is experiencing sadness in watching her friends have children. She also reveals during the subjective history that she recently had a break-up with her long-time boyfriend, who had been with her during her treatments but told her that 'I expected you to be back to normal now, and I can't wait around anymore for you to feel better.'

She scores a 6 on the NCCN Distress Thermometer, checking off 'Ability to Have Children,' 'Sadness,' 'Fatigue,' 'Body Image,' and 'Pain.' Physical assessment includes the following:

Assessment	Value	Comments
L shoulder flexion	135°	'Pulling' in the lateral chest wall
L shoulder abduction	123°	'Pulling' in the lateral chest wall
Grip strength	R hand: 57 psi; L hand: 48 psi	Right hand dominant
Timed Up and Go	9.7 seconds	
5 time sit to stand	10.9 seconds	'Achy' feeling in B knees
Pain Visual Analog Scale	4/10	L lateral chest wall

L, left; R, right; psi, pounds per square inch; B, bilateral. Created by Scott Cappoza, Allison L'Hotta, and Ursula Sansom-Daly. Printed with permission.

Based on this patient's subjective and objective findings, the physical therapist initiated soft tissue mobilization and myofascial techniques to the left lateral chest wall, axilla, and upper left chest. Given the history of the non-traumatic rib fracture, joint mobilizations to the rib cage were not used. Muscle energy techniques into shoulder extension and horizontal abduction were used which helped to increase active range of motion. Following manual work, the patient was progressed to active assisted range of motion activities including pulleys. She was able to quickly advance to active range of motion stretching including side-lying on her right side (with a pillow supporting her right thoracic area) and horizontally abducting her left arm.

Due to her history of atrial thrombus, communication was initiated with cardio-oncology. Cardio-oncology cleared her for progressive exercise, so a progressive cardiovascular exercise program was initiated beginning with walking for 15 minutes three times a week. As the patient increased her walking duration to 30 minutes, interval training in the clinic was initiated. Additionally, communication was initiated with the referring oncologist to suggest a referral to a registered dietitian who could address weight loss strategies to compliment the patient's increase in exercise. The patient expressed interest in meeting with the dietitian.

Additionally, the physical therapist reached out to the referring oncologist to suggest a referral to social work to help the patient's distress about fertility, social life/dating, and body image. A referral was placed, although the patient was initially hesitant to meet with the social worker. The physical therapist supported the patient by stating that the social worker would have resources and suggestions for psycho-social support.

At this patient's 2-month follow-up, physical assessment was the following:

Assessment	Value	Comments
L shoulder flexion	155°	'Doesn't feel as bad as it was'
L shoulder abduction	142°	'Doesn't feel that bad'
Grip strength	R hand: 61 psi; L hand: 54 psi	Right hand dominant
Timed Up and Go	9.2 seconds	
5 time sit to stand	10.3 seconds	
Pain Visual Analog Scale	2/10	L lateral chest wall

L, left; R, right; psi, pounds per square inch. Created by Scott Cappoza, Allison L'Hotta, and Ursula Sansom-Daly. Printed with permission.

The patient reports a 13-pound intentional weight loss. She credits this to walking 6 days a week for 30 to 45 minutes per session, as well as increased awareness of portion control and eliminating late night snacking per recommendations from the dietitian.

NCCN Distress score has decreased to a 3. She reports that she initially was resistant to the social worker's suggestions to join a larger support group for other AYAs living with or beyond cancer, but was ultimately put in touch with another AYA with a history of breast cancer through the social worker's recommendation of connecting with Imerman Angels. The patient also reports that, with the support of the social worker, that she has recently returned to online dating. She reports that she did not put in her profile that she had cancer, but thinks that 'at some point, I will add that in.'

Review Questions

Reader can find the correct answers and rationale in the back of the book.

Scenario #1:

A 34-year-old female presents to an outpatient physical therapy clinic. She was diagnosed with stage II colon cancer 9 months ago. She has undergone surgery to remove one-third of her distal colon followed by six cycles of FOLFOX chemotherapy in combination with gemcitabine. She reports that her feet feel like 'lead bricks' and is also having difficulty with fine motor tasks such as picking up paper clips. She reports that she has not experienced any falls in the last 6 months but has had several episodes when she experienced a momentary loss of balance. She expressed challenges with engaging in work activities and exercise due to her need to frequently use the bathroom urgently. Her score on the NCCN Distress Thermometer is a 6. While she elected not to pursue fertility preservation at the time of beginning chemotherapy, she admits to the rehabilitation clinician that she is experiencing sadness in watching her friends have children.

1. Which chemotherapy agent is most likely responsible for the decreased sensation in this patient's hands and feet?
   A. Gemcitabine
   B. Fluorouracil (5-FU)
   C. Leucovorin
   D. Oxaliplatin

2. What would the most appropriate balance screening tool to use for this patient?
   A. Berg Balance Score
   B. FAB Scale
   C. Romberg Balance Test
   D. Tinetti Performance-Oriented Mobility Assessment (POMA)

3. What is the first step you should take as a clinician to support this client in their daily participation in activities such as work and exercise?
   A. Discuss workplace accommodations with their manager
   B. Develop a home strengthening program to address potential fall concerns
   C. Interview the client to better understand their daily routine as well as barriers and supports to participation
   D. Recommend they avoid all exercise at this time because they are a fall risk

4. This woman has scored above the clinical threshold for distress on the NCCN Distress Thermometer. How would you assess if this woman might benefit from seeing a clinical psychologist?
   A. If her distress has persisted for at least 2 weeks or more
   B. If her distress is interfering with her ability to participate in productive activities (e.g., work, study, socializing)
   C. If she feels she would find it helpful to learn adaptive coping strategies to process and manage her emotional responses in survivorship
   D. If she endorses any of the above

Scenario #2:

A 28-year-old male is seen in an outpatient physical therapy clinic for a fracture of his first metatarsal bone on his right foot. He has been in a walking boot for the past 6 weeks and has now been cleared to participate in physical therapy. He presents with restricted range of motion of the great toe as well as ankle dorsiflexion. The chart review reveals that the patient was diagnosed with stage II testicular cancer 2 years ago and received three cycles of bleomycin, etoposide, and cisplatin (Platinol) (BEP) chemotherapy. On the NCCN Distress Thermometer, he scores a 3 and checks off 'Insurance/Financial' as a concern. When asked about employment status, he states that he is between jobs at this time and had to stop his previous job because he couldn't keep up with job tasks.

5. In developing a comprehensive plan of care for this patient, which of the following treatment strategies is most likely to be contraindicated?
   A. Cardiovascular exercise incorporating high-intensity interval training one to two times a week
   B. Ice pack to the great toe following activity
   C. Open chain ankle strengthening exercises
   D. Passive range of motion to the great toe

6. How can you support this client with their insurance/financial challenges?
   A. Connect them with relevant resources, such as First Descents
   B. Connect them with relevant resources, such as the Sam Fund
   C. Encourage them to work on gaining new skills to be eligible for more job opportunities
   D. Suggest they apply for more job opportunities

7. Young men often minimize their distress and can be reluctant to seek help for it. How might you approach assessing further psychosocial needs with this young man?
   A. Start by exploring the 'Insurance/Financial' concerns he has indicated, explore further what factors led to him stopping his previous job, and provide education around how low mood and anxiety can impact attention, concentration, and the ability to switch quickly between tasks in the workplace
   B. Tell him that because he scored a 3 (under the clinical threshold) he is doing great and doesn't need to speak to a psychologist
   C. Ask him if he would find it beneficial to learn some strategies to manage his cognitive impacts and the stress this is causing, and discuss possible psychologist options with him
   D. Option A followed by C

Scenario #3:

A 23-year-old female with a history of melanoma is seen in an outpatient physical therapy clinic. She was diagnosed with a basal cell carcinoma on her left scapular region which metastasized to the left axillary lymph nodes. She underwent an axillary lymph node dissection (3/16 LNI) 5 months ago, followed by 6 weeks of radiation therapy to the left axilla completed 3 months ago. She is left hand dominant and presents with limited range of motion of her left shoulder: flexion to 110 degrees, abduction to 80 degrees. Circumferential measurement of the left upper extremity is within 5% of her right upper extremity. She lives alone in a one-bedroom apartment and enjoys cooking her meals but is having difficulty with meal preparation due to her restricted range of motion. She reveals to the physical therapist that she feels that she is all alone and cannot relate to her friends.

8. What would be the most important part of the musculoskeletal assessment for this patient?
   A. Assessing for the presence of AWS
   B. Assessing tissue pliability of axially incision
   C. Manual muscle testing of shoulder flexors and abduction
   D. Supraspinatus test (empty can test)

9. To best support, this patient's independence in cooking and meal preparation, what is the most likely recommendation the clinician can discuss with her?
   A. Stop cooking until her range of motion improves
   B. Have somebody else help her cook meals
   C. Recommend that all cooking tasks are completed with her right upper extremity only because her left upper extremity needs to heal from the surgery
   D. Rearrange the location of essential cooking items in her kitchen so she can easily reach them

10. In terms of ensuring her wellbeing, what would be the three most appropriate psychosocial issues to explore as a priority with this young woman?
    A. Current mood and coping strategies, social supports and networks, and occupational/financial status
    B. Dietary intake, exercise routine, and leisure preferences
    C. Coping strategies, exercise/sport history, and capability of undertaking activities of daily living
    D. Social supports and networks, income, and sun-safe behaviors

References

1. National Cancer Institute. Adolescents and young adults with cancer. https://www.cancer.gov/types/aya. Published 2020. Accessed August 9, 2020.
2. Sansom-Daly UM, Wakefield CE. Distress and adjustment among adolescents and young adults with cancer: an empirical and conceptual review. *Transl Pediatr.* 2013;2(4):167–197.
3. Sansom-Daly UM, Wakefield CE, Robertson EG, McGill BC, Wilson HL, Bryant RA. Adolescent and young adult cancer survivors' memory and future thinking processes place them at risk for poor mental health. *Psycho-Oncol.* 2018;27(12):2709–2716.
4. Zebrack B, Santacroce SJ, Patterson P, Gubin A. Adolescents and Young Adults with Cancer: A Biopsychosocial Approach. In: *Pediatric Psychosocial Oncology: Textbook for Multidisciplinary Care*: Springer; 2016:199–217.
5. Lindsay T. *Cancer, Sex, Drugs and Death: A Guide for the Psychological Management of Young People with Cancer.* Samford, QLD, Australia: Australian Academic Press; 2017.
6. American Cancer Society. Cancer facts and figures 2020. https://www.cancer.org/content/dam/cancer-org/research/cancer-facts-and-statistics/annual-cancer-facts-and-figures/2020/cancer-facts-and-figures-2020.pdf. Published 2020. Accessed August 10, 2020.
7. Miller KD, Fidler-Benaoudia M, Keegan TH, Hipp HS, Jemal A, Siegel RL. Cancer statistics for adolescents and young adults, 2020. *CA Cancer J Clin.* 2020;70(6):443–459. doi:10.3322/caac.21637.
8. Siegel RL, Miller KD, Jemal A. Cancer statistics, 2019. *CA Cancer J Clin.* 2019;69(1):7–34.
9. Ruddy KJ, Gelber S, Tamimi RM, et al. Breast cancer presentation and diagnostic delays in young women. *Cancer.* 2014;120(1):20–25.
10. Armstrong GT, Chen Y, Yasui Y, et al. Reduction in late mortality among 5-year survivors of childhood cancer. *New Engl J Med.* 2016;374(9):833–842.
11. Berkman AM, Livingston JA, Merriman K, et al. Long-term survival among 5-year survivors of adolescent and young adult cancer. *Cancer.* 2020;126(16):3708–3718.
12. McGill BC, Sansom-Daly UM, Wakefield CE, Ellis SJ, Robertson EG, Cohn RJ. Therapeutic Alliance and Group Cohesion in an Online Support Program for Adolescent and Young Adult Cancer Survivors: Lessons from "Recapture Life". *J Adolesc Young Adult Oncol.* 2017;6(4):568–572.
13. Robertson E, Wakefield CE, Marshall K, Sansom-Daly U. Strategies to improve adherence to treatment in adolescents and young adults with cancer: a systematic review. *Clin Oncol Adolesc Young Adult.* 2015;2015:35–49.
14. Auerbach RP, Mortier P, Bruffaerts R, et al. WHO World Mental Health Surveys International College Student Project: Prevalence and distribution of mental disorders. *J Abnorm Psychol.* 2018;127(7):623–638.
15. Fardell JE, Patterson P, Wakefield CE, et al. A narrative review of models of care for adolescents and young adults with cancer: barriers and recommendations. *J Adolesc Young Adult Oncol.* 2018;7(2):148–152.
16. Lin M, Sansom-Daly UM, Wakefield CE, McGill BC, Cohn RJ. Health literacy in adolescents and young adults: perspectives from Australian cancer survivors. *J Adolesc Young Adult Oncol.* 2017;6(1)150–158. doi:10.1089/jayao.2016.0024.
17. Sansom-Daly UM, Lin M, Robertson EG, et al. Health literacy in adolescents and young adults: An updated review. *J Adolesc Young Adult Oncol.* 2016 Jun;5(2)106–18. doi:10.1089/jayao.2015.0059.
18. McDonald FEJ, Patterson P, Costa DSJ, Shepherd HL. Validation of a health literacy measure for adolescents and young adults diagnosed with cancer. *J Adolesc Young Adult Oncol.* 2016;5(1):69–75.
19. National Comprehensive Cancer Network. NCCN distress thermometer. https://www.nccn.org/patients/resources/life_with_cancer/pdf/nccn_distress_thermometer.pdf. Published 2020. Accessed September 15, 2020.
20. Clinton-McHarg T, Carey M, Sanson-Fisher R, D'Este C, Shakeshaft A. Preliminary development and psychometric evaluation of an unmet needs measure for adolescents and young adults with cancer: the Cancer Needs Questionnaire—Young People (CNQ-YP). *Health Qual Life Outcomes.* 2012;10(1):13.
21. Haines ER, Lux L, Smitherman AB, et al. An actionable needs assessment for adolescents and young adults with cancer: the AYA Needs Assessment & Service Bridge (NA-SB). *Support Care Cancer.* 2021 Aug;29(8): 4693–4704. doi:10.1007/s00520-021-06024-z.
22. Kim B, White K. How can health professionals enhance interpersonal communication with adolescents and young adults to improve health care outcomes?: systematic literature review. *Int J Adolesc Youth.* 2018;23(2)198–218. doi:10.1080/02673843.2017.1330696
23. Palmer S, Mitchell A, Thompson K, Sexton M. Unmet needs among adolescent cancer patients: A pilot study. *Palliat Support Care.* 2007;5(2):127–134.

24. Gessler D, Juraskova I, Sansom-Daly U, Shepherd HL, Patterson P, Muscat DM. Clinician-patient-family decision-making and health literacy in adolescents and young adults with cancer and their families: A systematic review of qualitative studies. *Psycho-Oncol.* 2019;28(7):1408–1419.

25. May EA, McGill BC, Robertson EG, Anazodo A, Wakefield CE, Sansom-Daly UM. Adolescent and young adult cancer survivors' experiences of the healthcare system: a qualitative study. *J Adolesc Young Adult Oncol.* 2018;7(1):88–96.

26. Kane HL, Halpern MT, Squiers LB, Treiman KA, McCormack LA. Implementing and evaluating shared decision making in oncology practice. *CA Cancer J Clin.* 2014;64(6):377–388.

27. Dinh HTT, Clark HR, Bonner HA, Hines HS. The effectiveness of health education using the teach-back method on adherence and self-management in chronic disease: a systematic review protocol. *JBI Database Syst Rev Implement.* 2013;11(10):30–41.

28. Patterson P, Hardman F, Cheshire J, Sansom-Daly UM. Balancing risk with resilience: using holistic screening and assessment tools effectively with adolescents and young adults with cancer. In: Olsen PR, Smith S, eds. *Nursing Adolescents and Young Adults with Cancer: Developing knowledge, competence and best practice.* London: Springer; 2018.

29. CanTeen. *Adolescent and Young Adult Oncology Psychosocial Care Manual (Rev. Ed.).* Australia: CanTeen; 2015.

30. Patterson P, McDonald F, Anazodo A, et al. Validation of the distress thermometer for use among adolescents and young adults with cancer in Australia: a multicenter study protocol. *Clin Oncol Adolesc Young Adult.* 2015;5:51–62.

31. Chao C, Xu L, Bhatia S, et al. Cardiovascular disease risk profiles in survivors of adolescent and young adult (AYA) cancer: the Kaiser Permanente AYA cancer survivors study. *J Clin Oncol.* 2016;34(14):1626–1633.

32. Litterinin A. EDGE Task Force Report Summaires. https://oncologypt.org/wp-content/uploads/2019/10/EDGE-Annotated-Bibliography-8.19-update.pdf. Published 2019. Accessed September 15, 2020.

33. Cathcart-Rake EJ, Ruddy KJ, Bleyer A, Johnson RH. Breast cancer in adolescent and young adult women under the age of 40 years. *JCO Oncol Pract.* 2021:Op2000793.

34. Campbell KL, Winters-Stone KM, Wiskemann J, et al. Exercise Guidelines for Cancer Survivors: Consensus Statement from International Multidisciplinary Roundtable. *Med Sci Sports Exerc.* 2019;51(11):2375–2390.

35. Petrella AR, Sabiston CM, O'Rourke RH, Santa Mina D, Matthew AG. Exploring the survivorship experiences and preferences for survivorship care following testicular cancer: a mixed methods study. *J Psychosoc Oncol Res Pract.* 2020;2(4):e038.

36. Fung C, Dinh PC, Fossa SD, Travis LB. Testicular Cancer Survivorship. *J Natl Compr Canc Netw.* 2019;17(12):1557–1568.

37. Adams SC, DeLorey DS, Davenport MH, Fairey AS, North S, Courneya KS. Effects of high-intensity interval training on fatigue and quality of life in testicular cancer survivors. *Br J Cancer.* 2018;118(10):1313–1321.

38. Feldman DR, Schaffer WL, Steingart RM. Late cardiovascular toxicity following chemotherapy for germ cell tumors. *J Natl Compr Canc Netw.* 2012;10(4):537–544.

39. Khan SA, Morris M, Idrees K, et al. Colorectal cancer in the very young: a comparative study of tumor markers, pathology and survival in early onset and adult onset patients. *J Pediatr Surg.* 2016;51(11):1812–1817.

40. American Cancer Society. Colorectal Cancer Early Detection, Diagnoisis, and Staging. Published 2020. Updated June 29, 2020. Accessed February 7, 2021.

41. Ahmad SS, Reinius MA, Hatcher HM, Ajithkumar TV. Anticancer chemotherapy in teenagers and young adults: managing long term side effects. *BMJ (Clinical research ed).* 2016;354:i4567.

42. Berger AM, Mooney K, Alvarez-Perez A, et al. Cancer-related fatigue, version 2.2015. *J Natl Compr Canc Netw.* 2015;13(8):1012–1039.

43. Wiskemann J, Schommer K, Jaeger D, Scharhag-Rosenberger F. Exercise and cancer: return to work as a firefighter with ostomy after rectal carcinoma—a case report. *Medicine (Baltimore).* 2016;95(29):e4309.

44. Abrams AN, Hazen EP, Penson RT. Psychosocial issues in adolescents with cancer. *Cancer Treat Rev.* 2007;33(7):622–630.

45. Coccia PF, Pappo AS, Beaupin L, et al. Adolescent and young adult oncology, version 2.2018, NCCN clinical practice guidelines in oncology. *J Natl Compr Canc Netw.* 2018;16(1):66–97.

46. Parsons HM, Harlan LC, Lynch CF, et al. Impact of cancer onwork and education among adolescent and young adult cancersurvivors. *J Clin Oncol.* 2012;30(19):2393–2400.

47. Brauer ER, Pieters HC, Ganz PA, Landier W, Pavlish C, Heilemann MV. From snail mode to rocket ship mode: adolescents and young adults' experiences of returning to work and school after hematopoietic cell transplantation. *J Adolesc Young Adult Oncol.* 2017;6(4):551–559.

48. Elsbernd A, Pedersen KJ, Boisen KA, Midtgaard J, Larsen HB. On your own: adolescent and young adult cancer survivors' experience of managing return to secondary or higher education in Denmark. *J Adolesc Young Adult Oncol.* 2018;7(5):618–625.

49. Blanch-Hartigan D, Kinel J. Addressing career-related needs in adolescent and young adult cancer survivors: university careerservice professionals' experience and resources. *J Adolesc Young Adult Oncol.* 2018;7(2):245–248.

50. Strauser DR, Jones A, Chiu C-Y, Tansey T, Chan F. Career development of young adult cancer survivors: A conceptual framework. *J Vocat Rehabil.* 2015;42:167–176.

51. Fardell JE, Wakefield CE, Patterson P, et al. Narrative review of the educational, vocational, and financial needs of adolescents and young adults with cancer: recommendations for support and research. *J Adolesc Young Adult Oncol.* 2018;7(2):143–147.

52. Gupta AA, Papadakos JK, Jones JM, et al. Reimagining care for adolescent and young adult cancer programs: Moving with the times. *Cancer.* 2016;122(7):1038–1046.

53. Fernandez C, Fraser GAM, Freeman C, et al. Principles and recommendations for the provision of healthcare in Canada to adolescent and young adult-aged cancer patients and survivors. *J Adolesc Young Adult Oncol.* 2011;1(1):53–59.

54. Lindbohm ML, Viikari-Juntura E. Cancer survivors' return to work: importance of work accommodations and collaboration between stakeholders. *Occup Environ Med.* 2010;67(9):578–579.

55. Doidge O, Edwards N, Thompson K, Lewin J. Conceptual framework to identify and address the education and vocational barriers experienced by adolescents and young adults with cancer. *J Adolesc Young Adult Oncol.* 2019;8(4):398–401.

56. Dawson D, McEwen S, Polatajko H. *Cognitive Orientation to daily Occupational Performance in Occupational Therapy: Using the CO-OP Approach to Enable Participation Across the Lifespan,* AOTA Press. 2017.

57. Kwak M, Zebrack BJ, Meeske KA, et al. Prevalence and predictors of post-traumatic stress symptoms in adolescent and young adult cancer survivors: a 1-year follow-up study. *Psycho-Oncol.* 2013;22(8):1798–1806.

58. Wakefield C, McLoone J, Butow P, Lenthen K, Cohn R. Support after the completion of cancer treatment: Perspectives of Australian adolescents and their families. *Eur J Cancer Care.* 2013;22(4):530–539.

59. Wakefield CE, McLoone JK, Butow P, Lenthen K, Cohn RJ. Parental adjustment to the completion of their child's cancer treatment. *Pediatr Blood Cancer.* 2011;56(4):524–531.

60. Kwak M, Zebrack BJ, Meeske KA, et al. Trajectories of psychological distress in adolescent and young adult patients with cancer: a 1-year longitudinal study. *J Clin Oncol.* 2013;31(17):2160–2166.

61. Zebrack BJ, Corbett V, Embry L, et al. Psychological distress and unsatisfied need for psychosocial support in adolescent and young adult cancer patients during the first year following diagnosis. *Psycho-Oncol.* 2014;23(11):1267–1275.

62. Lu D, Fall K, Sparen P, et al. Suicide and suicide attempt after a cancer diagnosis among young individuals. *Ann Oncol.* 2013;24:3112–3117.

63. Millar B, Patterson P, Desille N. Emerging adulthood and cancer: how unmet needs vary with time-since-treatment. *Palliat Support Care.* 2010;8(2):151–158.

64. Olsson CA, Boyce MF, Toumbourou JW, Sawyer SM. The role of peer support in facilitating psychosocial adjustment to chronic illness in adolescence. *Clin Child Psychol Psychiatry.* 2005;10(1):78–87.

65. Roberts CS, Piper L, Denny J, Cuddeback G. A support group intervention to facilitate young adults' adjustment to cancer. *Health Soc Work.* 1997;22(2):133–141.

66. Anazodo A, Chard J. Medical and psychosocial challenges in caring for adolescent and young adult patients with cancer. Paper presented at: Cancer Forum; 2013.

67. White V, Skaczkowski G, Thompson K, et al. Experiences of care of adolescents and young adults with cancer in Australia. *J Adolesc Young Adult Oncol.* 2018.

68. Korsvold L, Mellblom AV, Lie HC, Ruud E, Loge JH, Finset A. Patient-provider communication about the emotional cues and concerns of adolescent and young adults patients and their family members when receiving a diagnosis of cancer. *Patient Educ Couns.* 2016;99(10):1576–1583.

69. Binder PE, Moltu C, Hummelsund D, Sagen SH, Holgersen H. Meeting an adult ally on the way out into the world: adolescent patients' experiences of useful psychotherapeutic ways of working at an age when independence really matters. *Psychother Res.* 2011;21:554–566.

70. Lathren C, Bluth K, Campo R, Tan W, Futch W. Young adult cancer survivors' experiences with a mindful self-compassion (MSC) video-chat intervention: A qualitative analysis. *Self Identity.* 2018;17(6):646–665.

71. Tindle D, Denver K, Lilley F. Identity, Image, and sexuality in young adults with cancer. *Semin Oncol.* 2009;36(3):281–288.

72. Zafar SY, Abernethy AP. Financial toxicity, Part I: a new name for a growing problem. *Oncology (Williston Park, NY).* 2013;27(2):80–149.

73. Bleyer A. Young adult oncology: the patients and their survival challenges. *CA Cancer J Clin.* 2007;57(4):242–255.

74. Zebrack B, Isaacson S. Psychosocial care of adolescent and young adult patients with cancer and survivors. *J Clin Oncol.* 2012;30(11):1221–1226.

75. Kaddas HK, Pannier ST, Mann K, et al. Age-related differences in financial toxicity and unmet resource needs among adolescentand young adult cancer patients. *J Adolesc Young Adult Oncol.* 2020;9(1):105–110.

76. Abdelhadi OA, Joseph J, Pollock BH, Keegan THM. Additional medical costs of chronic conditions among adolescent and young adult cancer survivors. *J Cancer Surviv.* 2021.

77. Johnson RH, Landwehr MS, Watson SE, Stegenga K. "Aftermath": financial resource requirements of young adults moving forward after cancer treatment. *J Adolesc Young Adult Oncol.* 2020;9(3):354–358.

78. U.S. Department of Health and Human Services. Young adult coverage. https://www.hhs.gov/healthcare/about-the-aca/young-adult-coverage/index.html. Published 2021. Accessed May 30, 2022.

79. Tanner L, Keppner K, Lesmeister D, Lyons K, Rock K, Sparrow J. Cancer Rehabilitation in the pediatric and adolescent/young adult population. *Semin Oncol Nurs.* 2020;36(1):150984.

80. L'Hotta AJ, Beam IA, Thomas KM. Development of a comprehensive pediatric oncology rehabilitation program. *Pediatr Blood Cancer.* 2020;67(2):e28083.

81. Nathan PC, Hayes-Lattin B, Sisler JJ, Hudson MM. Critical issues in transition and survivorship for adolescents and young adults with cancers. *Cancer.* 2011;117(S10):2335–2341.

82. Freyer DR, Brugieres L. Adolescent and young adult oncology: transition of care. *Pediatr Blood Cancer.* 2008;50(S5):1116–1119.

83. Cheville AL, Beck LA, Petersen TL, Marks RS, Gamble GL. The detection and treatment of cancer-related functional problems in an outpatient setting. *Support Care Cancer.* 2009;17(1):61–67.

84. MD Stubblefield, Hubbard G, Cheville A, Koch U, Schmitz KH, Dalton SO. Current perspectives and emerging issues on cancer rehabilitation. *Cancer.* 2013; 119(S11):2170–2178.

85. Scardaville MC, Murphy KM, Liu F, et al. Knowledge of legal protections and employment-related resources among young adults with cancer. *J Adolesc Young Adult Oncol.* 2019;8(3):312–319.

27

Prehabilitation

LORI E. BORIGHT, PT, DPT, DScPT

CHAPTER OUTLINE

Introduction

Prehabilitation, also referred to as pretreatment optimization, can encompass physiological as well as psychological measures to fortify the reserve status of persons living with cancer (PLWCs). Prehabilitation has been described as "a process on the cancer continuum of care that occurs between the time of cancer diagnosis and the beginning of acute treatment and includes physical and psychological assessments that establish a baseline functional level, identify impairments, and provide interventions that promote physical and psychological health to reduce the incidence and/or severity of future impairments."[1] More contemporary definitions of prehabilitation additionally include the domain of nutritional status assessment and intervention.

Prehabilitation has been commonly and routinely employed in the orthopedic domain for decades though is gaining traction for efficacy with various cancer populations over the last decade.[2–4] The noted benefits of prehabilitation are many and include reduced postsurgical complications as well as overall disablement, though benefits also extend beyond improved clinical outcomes to encompass administrative benefits by way of reduced length of hospital stays, reduced hospital readmissions, reduced days requiring intensive care, and reduced overall healthcare costs.[5,6] Evidence for the efficacy of oncology prehabilitation is most robust with gastrointestinal/colorectal, breast, and prostate cancer populations.[7–9]

Components

Unimodal Versus Multimodal

Prehabilitation programs that employ one intervention modality (physical, psychological, or nutrition) are termed unimodal; whereas programs that employ multiple modalities are termed multimodal. Evidence suggests that multimodal programs correlate more positive clinical and administrative outcomes for some cancer diagnoses.[7,10,11]

Patient Education

Patient education is an essential component of prehabilitation and is the responsibility of every member of the multidisciplinary care management team to prepare the PLWC for their respective cancer journey. Presentation of a timeline, even in very general terms, of who and what the PLWC will likely encounter and when, provides a roadmap and sense of clarity for this journey. It is recognized that a significant amount of information is provided at a time when the stress of a potentially life-threatening cancer diagnosis might preclude full attention to volume and specifics of detail; it is therefore recommended that a support person accompany the PLWC to all initial appointments to assist with retention of information.

Additional, helpful resource information for PLWCs before initiation of treatment includes: red flags (e.g., when and who to call for a variety of potential adverse effects); contact information for all providers in the respective care team (including rehabilitation services); cancer center resources and programs, if applicable; survivorship information pertaining to general exercise recommendations for wellness and prevention; and any contact information for local cancer support groups. Above all, oncology rehabilitation (Onc R) clinicians should impart the importance and necessity of self-advocacy with PLWCs and ideally their support person(s).

Exercise Intervention

Modes of exercise interventions relative to prehabilitative programming encompasses prescribed cardiovascular, resistance, and flexibility training in keeping with American College of Sports Medicine (ACSM) guidelines of either 75 minutes of vigorous or 150 minutes of moderate intensity exercise per week.[12] It is important to note that specific recommendations for frequency, duration, mode, and intensity of prehabilitation protocols do not presently exist in the literature. Onc R clinicians are well positioned to help define these parameters.

Many studies support the benefits of conducting at least some exercise sessions in-person to support compliance. Following up via telehealth-type check-ins and use of exercise logs to promote at-home compliance with home exercise programs (HEPs) can also help improve safety and performance accuracy.[13]

Nutritional Intervention

Nutritional interventions provided by qualified members of the multidisciplinary team including registered dietician nutritionists (RDN) comprise a multimodal approach to prehabilitative efforts and have potential to positively impact outcomes of quality of life (QOL) and reduced post-treatment complications. It is now within the scope of professional practice for the physical therapist (PT) to screen for nutritional deficits as well as provide basic nutritional information to patients within the clinical setting. The American Physical Therapy Association (APTA) supports interdisciplinary collaboration among physical therapy professionals and RDNs to promote prevention efforts at all levels, including in the prehabilitation domain.[14] A randomized controlled trial reported that PLWCs of the colon who received nutrition counseling and whey supplementation in the preoperative period demonstrated improved functional walking capacity.[15]

Psychosocial Intervention

The addition of psychosocial interventions additionally qualifies prehabilitative efforts as multimodal and is provided by qualified members of the multidisciplinary team including medical social workers and by psychologists and psychiatrists upon appropriate referral. There is no question that embarking on an unwanted and unanticipated cancer journey evokes a multitude of emotions and stress for the PLWC and interventions aimed at ameliorating the negative consequences stand to benefit the person throughout their treatment trajectory. A systematic review reported benefits of prehabilitative psychosocial interventions for multiple cancer diagnoses (breast, gynecologic, colorectal, and prostate) that included bolstered immunologic function as well as a variety of patient reported outcomes that included improved psychological, QOL, and somatic symptoms.[16] Specific interventions suggested to comprise an effective psychological prehabilitative protocol

include relaxation techniques, guided imagery, stress management, as well as psychotherapeutic interventions. An additional randomized controlled trial reported significant reductions in anxiety and depression on the Hospital Anxiety and Depression Scale (HADS) for participants who received a 90-minute consultation with a trained psychologist who included anxiety reduction and relaxation (visualization) techniques as well as breathing exercises as part of a multimodal presurgical prehabilitation protocol for PLWC of the colon or rectum.[17]

Outcome Measures

The outcome measures employed during the prehabilitative phase will largely be dictated by the cancer diagnoses and are utilized to establish baseline demographic, anthropometric, physiologic, and functional performance data, among others, that becomes the basis for individualized prescriptive interventions that will be discussed in the next section. Assessments typically take the form of screens or brief assessments that perhaps evaluate several domains at once to minimize impact on busy multidisciplinary or similar clinical settings.

Demographic and anthropometric measurements provide helpful information for longitudinal observation. Measurement of vital statistics such as blood pressure, heart rate, and oxygen saturation yields information that will assist the One R clinician in prescribing exercise interventions that are appropriate and safe for the PLWC. This also allows for identification of abnormal exercise response and detection of the development of medical treatment toxicity when longitudinally assessed and compared to baseline values. Recording and referencing of laboratory values initially and across the continuum provides similar utility and value. Range of motion (ROM) assessments are useful to predict potential functional deficits and/or to identify areas that may require intervention attention, through either formal prescriptive rehabilitation or HEP intervention to mitigate the development of anticipated adverse effects. For example, shoulder ROM measurement is relevant in a PLWC of the breast who will undergo radiation and therefore has the potential to develop radiation induced fibrosis of the soft tissues of the upper quarter. ROM may be screened grossly through function or assessed more empirically with goniometry when specificity is required and as deficits are identified.

Muscular strength can be screened grossly through functional mobility and assessed with greater specificity with manual muscle testing or dynamometry. Handgrip dynamometry has been shown is recent evidence to be a valid and reliable method in determining weakness in the upper extremity which may also be generalized to overall strength as well as used as a measure of frailty in older PLWCs.[18] The five times sit to stand test or 30-second chair rise test may also be used as screening measures for lower extremity strength and endurance. These tests are especially useful for older PLWCs.[19]

Standing balance screening is an important component of prehabilitation to elucidate baseline deficits, especially for those PLWCs who will undergo chemotherapeutic intervention and are therefore at risk for developing cancer-related polyneuropathy. The Timed Up and Go test (TUG) and the 30-second chair rise test are effective and brief screens for balance deficits as is the four stage balance test.[20] Gait speed is most often assessed via the 10-meter walk test, and cardiorespiratory fitness is frequently assessed in the clinic setting via the six minute walk test (6MWT).[21] Emerging evidence supports the use of the two minute walk test as a quicker and more efficient alternative, thereby minimizing impact on the clinical setting.[22] Additional screening and assessment alternatives are presented in Chapter 23.

Pretreatment assessment of QOL is an additional important component of prehabilitation. Valid and reliable tools for this purpose include the Functional Assessment of Cancer Therapy-General (FACT-G),[23] the HADS, and the European Organization for Research and Treatment of Cancer Quality of Life Questionnaire-c30 (EORTC-QLQ-c30).[24]

Additional outcome assessments that yield meaningful data when tracked longitudinally include: prehabilitation program compliance, rate of postoperative complications, hospital length of stay (LOS), 30-day hospital readmission, length of time to return to work, discharge disposition, and financial metrics inclusive of health care cost savings. A systematic review and meta-analysis reported decreased postoperative complications for patients requiring intra-abdominal surgery following prehabilitation that consisted of inspiratory muscle training, aerobic exercise, and/or resistance training.[25] Another systematic review reported that higher preoperative levels of physical activity were positively associated with significantly decreased hospital LOS.[26] An additional study reported decreases in both postoperative complications and LOS for PLWCs of the lung following preoperative moderate to high intensity exercise training using a stationary bike or treadmill.[27]

Interventions

Recommended prehabilitation interventions, similar to outcome assessments, may vary relative to cancer diagnosis. Prehabilitation programs should be designed to achieve (or progress toward achievement) of ACSM guidelines including resistance and flexibility training.[12]

Mode

Intervention mode defines the way in which exercise is delivered. The intended setting of the exercise can be a major factor in the type of exercise that is prescribed and will be discussed later in this section. Cardiovascular exercise can be accomplished in a variety of ways, including: walking programs, use of treadmill, stationary or free bike, stationary recumbent stepper (e.g., Nustep™), or circuit training. Chapter 23 discusses prescription, including dosing, in greater detail.

Resistance exercises should supplement the cardiovascular components of a prehabilitation intervention program and can be accomplished with free weights, cable systems, resistance bands, and bodyweight exercises. Evidence supports incorporating

resistance exercises 2 to 3 days per week.[12] Additionally, flexibility exercises in targeted areas (e.g., gluteal, quadriceps, hamstring, and gastrocnemius stretching following a lower extremity resistance and/or cardiovascular session) are an important component of a well-rounded prehabilitation exercise program. Flexibility exercises should be encouraged during each exercise session.

Diagnosis Specific Considerations

Exercise prescription will vary depending on the specific cancer diagnosis owing to anticipated treatment adverse effects and the potential consequence to mobility and function. For example, PLWC of the head and neck will require prehabilitative exercises prescribed to address anticipated reduced cervical and shoulder ROM, decreased trunk strength and posture, and reduced functional walking capacity. Specific exercises that meet these criteria include multiplanar cervical and shoulder ROM exercises, shoulder and trunk strengthening with resistance bands, and a graduated walking program (e.g., The Otago Walking Program).[28] See Figures 27.1 and 27.2 for examples of prehabilitation exercises for PLWCs of the head and neck.

Additionally, PLWCs of the gastrointestinal (GI) and genitourinary (GU) systems should receive prehabilitative exercises tailored to meet the potential consequences of bladder and bowel incontinence. A systematic review has reported improved post-treatment continence in these populations following prehabilitation participation,[11] and a randomized controlled study of males undergoing radical prostatectomy concurs that pretreatment pelvic floor exercises improve post-treatment continence.[29] See Chapter 16 for additional information on appropriate interventions for PLWC of the GI and GU systems.

One further example of targeted prescriptive prehabilitative exercise is for the PLWC of the breast whose treatment plan includes radiation. It is important to educate the person on the potential of reduced shoulder ROM as a consequence of radiation-induced fibrosis affecting joint mobility and to prescribe multiplanar exercises (e.g., shoulder flexion, extension, abduction, internal rotation, external rotation) that will mitigate the development of this function–limiting adverse effect. Addressing the potential of reduced shoulder ROM can facilitate medical management without delay, ideally ensuring that the PLWC can attain the required overhead positioning of the arm for radiation therapy.

Frequency

As previously mentioned, ACSM guidelines are the benchmark for the metric of exercise frequency in the oncology rehabilitation

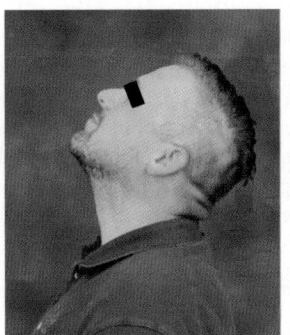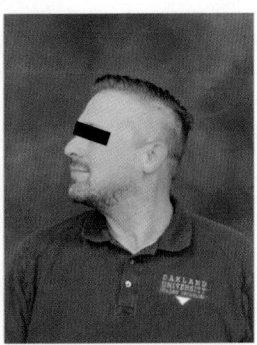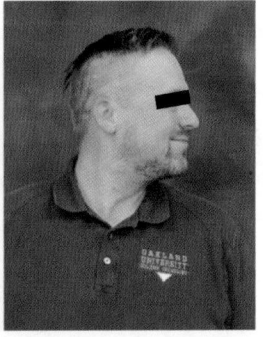

• **Fig. 27.1** Multiplanar Cervical Range of Motion Exercises. (From Boright L, Doherty DJ, Wilson CM, Arena SK, Ramirez C. Development and feasibility of a prehabilitation protocol for patients diagnosed with head and neck cancer. *Cureus*. 2020;12(8):e9898. doi:10.7759/cureus.9898. Reprinted with permission.)

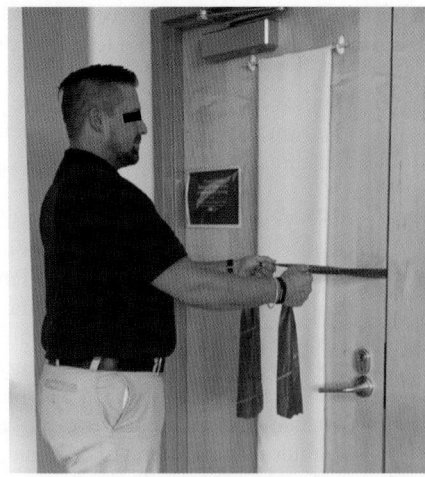 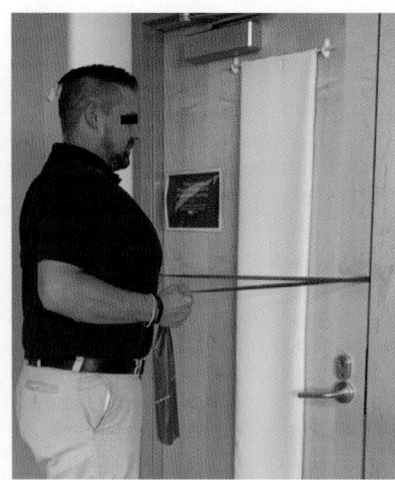

• **Fig. 27.2** Resisted Scapular Retraction Exercise. (From Boright L, Doherty DJ, Wilson CM, Arena SK, Ramirez C. Development and feasibility of a prehabilitation protocol for patients diagnosed with head and neck cancer. *Cureus*. 2020;12(8):e9898. doi:10.7759/cureus.9898. Reprinted with permission.)

domain inclusive of prehabilitation. It is important to note that many PLWCs begin their cancer journey in a deconditioned state and therefore are unable to achieve that benchmark. The emphasis for prehabilitation is to obtain a baseline status and to prescribe an appropriately dosed exercise prescription that will enhance cardiorespiratory endurance and therefore aim to optimize physiological condition over the course of the prehabilitation program. Beginning a walking program, for example, to the current level of tolerance and encouraging the PLWC to increase the duration of each bout of walking by up to five minutes per session until the desired time per bout of walking is achieved. A well-rounded prehabilitation program will also include strengthening/resistance exercises and flexibility exercises that are appropriate for identified or anticipated areas of deficit relative to the treatment trajectory.

Duration

Duration is the metric of widest variability relative to prehabilitation programs and varies largely by cancer diagnoses. Many cancers require urgent medical intervention and therefore the window for prehabilitation intervention is much shorter than ideal (e.g., lung, breast). Other cancers grow more slowly and/or require more extensive presurgical work-up, and therefore afford increased time for the prehabilitation window to occur (e.g., gastrointestinal, head and neck). Additionally, the time between cancer diagnosis and the onset of medical treatment is often a very unsettling time for PLWCs and their support systems. Accommodating many appointments inclusive of additional opinions on diagnosis presents additional challenges to prehabilitation adherence. In any case, however, it is generally expected that prehabilitation programs span between 2 to 4 weeks and encompass multidisciplinary interventions to maximize results as mentioned previously.

Compliance

Strategies to enhance compliance include supervised training, effective patient education, journaling or use of an exercise log, and telehealth or telecoaching. Evidence suggests that supervised exercise programs in the prehabilitation domain correlate improved compliance and outcomes.[13] Providing early and recurrent education as well as encouragement to empower the PLWC to optimize the prehabilitation timeframe and have control over an element of a potentially seemingly out of control life circumstance. Equipped with rationale that supports reducing risk of morbidity and mortality as well as improved clinical outcomes, PLWCs can make informed decisions related to program compliance. Corresponding HEPs produce varied compliance success, though use of tracking mechanisms such as exercise journaling or use of an exercise log are suggested strategies to empower PLWCs to track progress, gain control, and ultimately achieve frequency metrics. Emerging evidence suggests that telehealth and telecoaching are useful strategies to enhance prehabilitation program compliance, weekly phone call check-ins is one very low impact way to accomplish this objective.[30] A novel approach in one study that demonstrated success with compliance, and is worthy of continued employment and investigation, included a digital companion to alert patients when it was time to exercise.[31]

Conclusion

The time between cancer diagnosis and the onset of medical treatment can be wrought with challenges as the PLWC navigates many appointments to coordinate care and also works to manage feelings of uncertainty and distress. However, this time can also be effectively used to gather baseline health data, identify areas requiring immediate and/or potential future rehabilitation, fortify physiologic reserves via targeted rehabilitative interventions, provide information that will inform next phases of the person's journey, and afford a sense of greater control over some aspects of a seemingly out-of-control life circumstance. Onc R clinicians are key advocates for the development of rehabilitative programming in their respective institutions and for informing key research in this domain.

Critical Research Needs

- Unify theory relative to frequency, duration, mode, and intensity of prehabilitation interventions in the oncology domain
- Clarify optimal timing of prehabilitative assessments and reassessments

- Investigate the role and impact of prehabilitation on lesser-studied cancer diagnoses, including liver, lung, gastric, and head and neck

Case Study

A 72-year-old male received a diagnosis of invasive adenocarcinoma of the pancreas. He underwent multiple diagnostic procedures including surgical biopsy. The PLWC was screened for prehabilitation in the multidisciplinary clinic, where the gastrointestinal oncologic surgeon consulted along with other members of the care team. A Whipple procedure was planned for 30 days later, affording an approximate 4-week window for prehabilitative interventions to occur. Screening revealed deficits in overall function, most notably reduced core strength as well as endurance via the 6MWT. The PLWC and his spouse were receptive to a course of prehabilitation to address these deficits. Nutritional prehabilitation was provided through nutrition services by a RDN which included dietary assessment and prescription which included a nutrition shake supplement.

The PLWC participated in six Onc R treatment sessions over the course of 3 weeks. These sessions consisted of a variety of targeted cardiovascular, extremity, and core strengthening exercises, flexibility exercises, and appropriate education. Vital signs were monitored throughout each clinic session to ensure safety. The PLWC was compliant with a progressive HEP inclusive of

walking for 30+ minutes, five times per week, cycling to tolerance, and exercises that corresponded to the prescribed clinic-based program.

Refer to Table 27.1 for initial and discharge assessment data. The participant's body mass index (BMI) was reduced from a 39 to a 36, and his albumin was improved from 3.1 to 4.4. Later the PLWC underwent the Whipple procedure and was discharged home on postoperative day 12 without complications.

TABLE 27.1 Case Study Initial and Discharge Assessments		
	Initial Assessment	Discharge Assessment
Anthropometrics		
Body mass index (BMI)	39	36
Labs		
Albumin	3.1	4.4
Outcome Measures		
Six-minute walk test	1244 feet	1489 feet
Functional Assessment of Cancer Therapy-General (FACT-G)	66	86

Review Questions

Reader can find the correct answers and rationale in the back of the book.

Use this vignette for Questions 1-3: A 45-year-old female was just diagnosed with ductal carcinoma in situ of the left breast. She was screened by a colleague at the multidisciplinary clinic earlier this week and is presenting to a PTs clinic today due to identified shoulder strength and range of motion impairment as well as a below normative result on her two-minute walk test.

1. What is the most appropriate mode of exercise to initiate and prescribe for her home exercise program to address her reduced functional walking capacity?
   A. NuStep for 10 minutes in clinic and ergometer for 10 minutes at home
   B. Assess treadmill tolerance for walking in clinic and progressive walking program, increasing by 5 minutes in duration each day
   C. Arm bike for 5 minutes in clinic and wall push ups for 5 minutes at home
   D. Shoulder flexion for 10 repetitions with cane in clinic and at home
2. What targeted exercise will most optimally benefit her reduced shoulder function?
   A. Arm bike
   B. Wall washing (shoulder flexion, scaption, and horizontal/abduction with a towel on the wall and against gravity)
   C. Pulleys
   D. Supine cane flexion bilaterally
3. What is the MOST appropriate assessment to obtain baseline information for this patient?
   A. Cranial nerve testing

B. Circumferential bilateral upper extremity lymphedema measurement
C. Balance assessment
D. Bilateral hand grip testing

Use this vignette for Questions 4-6: A 63-year-old male is being evaluated by the oral maxillofacial surgeon in the office today, the Onc R clinician will have 15 minutes to perform a pretreatment screen of function to identify any potential issues and prescribe a targeted home exercise program for him to work on prior to his surgical procedure which will be scheduled in 14 days.

4. What is the most appropriate way to assess functional walking capacity?
   A. Six minute walk test
   B. Bruce treadmill protocol
   C. Timed Up and Go test
   D. Two Minute walk test

Use this vignette for Question 5: The Onc R clinician's screening assessments reveal poor seated and standing posture as well as upper posterior trunk weakness.

5. What targeted exercise would you prescribe as a component of his home exercise program?
   A. Body mechanics handout
   B. Resistance band exercises for the upper back musculature
   C. Cervical range of motion exercises
   D. Progressive walking program

Use this vignette for Question 6: Your QOL screen with the Functional Assessment of Cancer Therapy-Head and Neck (FACT H&N) reveals that the PLWC is not coping well initially with his diagnosis and that he lacks social support.

6. Which clinician is the most appropriate referral source for him?
   A. The oral maxillofacial surgeon
   B. The head and neck nurse navigator
   C. The licensed medical social worker
   D. The registered dietician nutritionist

Use this vignette for Questions 7 and 8: A 67 year old male presents to outpatient PT via direct referral from a gastrointestinal oncologic surgeon following a diagnosis of esophageal cancer. The patient is set to begin radiation therapy for the purpose of reducing tumor size prior to surgical intervention. The referral indicates that the PLWC is referred for pretreatment optimization.

7. What is the MOST appropriate assessment to obtain baseline information for this PLWC?
   A. Six minute walk test
   B. Monofilament testing of bilateral feet
   C. Circumferential measurements of bilateral lower extremities
   D. Abdominal muscle strength

8. The PLWC reveals that he has been increasingly more tired and irritable, frequently feels cold, and additionally has been experiencing loss in appetite. Physical exam correlates some of these subjective reports with a loss of upper trunk and extremity muscle mass. Malnutrition is suspected. Which is the MOST appropriate multidisciplinary team member to refer this PLWC to for this problem?
   A. Oncology nurse navigator
   B. Radiation oncologist
   C. Registered dietician nutritionist
   D. Gastrointestinal oncologic surgeon

9. Which component has been found in the literature to yield MOST positive clinical and administrative outcomes with respect to prehabilitation programming?
   A. Unsupervised exercise
   B. Telehealth services
   C. Unimodal
   D. Multimodal

10. Which cancer diagnosis is LEAST likely to have robust prehabilitation evidence in the current literature?
   A. Head and neck
   B. Prostate
   C. Colorectal
   D. Breast

References

1. Silver JK, Baima J, Mayer RS. Impairment-driven cancer rehabilitation: an essential component of quality care and survivorship. *CA Cancer J Clin*. 2013;63(5):295–317.

2. Nielsen PR, Jorgensen LD, Dahl B, et al. Prehabilitation and early rehabilitation after spinal surgery: randomized clinical trial. *Clin Rehabil*. 2010;24(2):137–148.

3. Topp R, Swank AM, Quesada PM, et al. The effect of prehabilitation exercise on strength and functioning after total knee arthroplasty. *PM&R*. 2009;1(8):729–735.

4. Carli F, Silver JK, Feldman LS, et al. Surgical prehabilitation in patients with cancer: state-of-the-science and recommendations for future research from a panel of subject matter experts. *Phys Med Rehabil Clin N Am*. 2017;28(1):49–64.

5. Silver JK. Cancer rehabilitation and prehabilitation may reduce disability and early retirement. *Cancer*. 2014;120(14):2072–2076.

6. Silver JK. Cancer prehabilitation and its role in improving health outcomes and reducing health care costs. *Seminars Oncol Nurs*. 2015;31(1):13–30.

7. Minnella EM, Carli F. Prehabilitation and functional recovery for colorectal cancer patients. *Eur J Surg Oncol*. 2018;44(7):919–926.

8. Yang A, Sokolof J, Gulati A. The effect of preoperative exercise on upper extremity recovery following breast cancer surgery: a systematic review. *Int J Rehabil Res*. 2018;41(3):189–196.

9. Santa Mina D, Matthew AG, Hilton WJ, et al. Prehabilitation for men undergoing radical prostatectomy: a multi-centre, pilot randomized controlled trial. *BMC Surg*. 2014;14(1):89. doi:10.1186/1471-2482-14-89.

10. Bousquet-Dion G, Awasthi R, Loiselle S, et al. Evaluation of supervised multimodal prehabilitation programme in cancer patients undergoing colorectal resection: a randomized control trial. *Acta Oncologica*. 2018;57(6):849. doi:10.1080/0284186x.2017.1423180.

11. Faithfull S, Turner L, Poole K, et al. Prehabilitation for adults diagnosed with cancer: a systematic review of long-term physical function, nutrition and patient-reported outcomes. *Eur J Cancer Care*. 2019;28(4):e13023. doi:10.1111/ecc.13023.

12. Campbell KL, Winters-Stone KM, Wiskemann J, et al. Exercise guidelines for cancer survivors: consensus statement from international multidisciplinary roundtable. *Med Sci Sports Exerc*. 2019;51(11):2375–2390.

13. Awasthi R, Minnella EM, Ferreira V, Ramanakumar AV, Scheede-Bergdahl C, Carli F. Supervised exercise training with multimodal pre-habilitation leads to earlier functional recovery following colorectal cancer resection. *Acta Anaesthesiol Scand*. 2019;63(4):461–467.

14. American Physical Therapy Association. The role of the physical therapist and the American Physical Therapy Association in diet and nutrition [HOD P06-19-08-44]. https://www.apta.org/siteassets/pdfs/policies/role-of-pt-diet-nutrition.pdf. September 20, 2019. Accessed October 31, 2020.

15. Gillis C, Loiselle SE, Fiore JF Jr., et al. Prehabilitation with whey protein supplementation on perioperative functional exercise capacity in patients undergoing colorectal resection for cancer: a pilot double-blinded randomized placebo-controlled trial. *J Acad Nutr Diet*. 2016;116(5):802–812.

16. Tsimopoulou I, Pasquali S, Howard R, et al. Psychological prehabilitation before cancer surgery: a systematic review. *Ann Surg Oncol*. 2015;22(13):4117–4123.

17. Santa Mina D, Scheede-Bergdahl C, Gillis C, Carli F. Optimization of surgical outcomes with prehabilitation. *Appl Physiol Nutr Metab*. 2015;40(9):966–969.

18. Bohannon RW. Muscle strength: clinical and prognostic value of hand-grip dynamometry. *Current Opinion Clin Nutr Metabolic Care*. 2015;18(5):465–470.

19. Goldberg A, Chavis M, Watkins J, et al. The five-times-sit-to-stand test: validity, reliability and detectable change in older females. *Aging Clin Exp Res*. 2012;24:339–344.

20. Panel on Prevention of Falls in Older Persons, American Geriatrics Society and British Geriatrics Society. Summary of the Updated American Geriatrics Society/British Geriatrics Society clinical practice guideline for prevention of falls in older persons. *J Am Geriatr Soc*. 2011;59(1):148–157.

21. Schmidt K, Vogt L, Thiel C, Jäger E, Banzer W. Validity of the six-minute walk test in cancer patients. *Int J Sports Med*. 2013;34(7):631–636.

22. Bohannon RW. Normative reference values for the two-minute walk test derived by meta-analysis. *J Phys. Ther Sci*. 2017;29:2224–2227.

23. List MA, D'Antonio LL, Cella DF, et al. The performance status scale for head and neck cancer patients and the Functional Assessment of Cancer Therapy-Head and Neck FACT-H&N scale: a study of utility and validity. *Cancer*. 1996;77:2294–2301.

24. Yun-Jen Chou, Kuo H, Shun S. Cancer prehabilitation programs and their effects on quality of life. *Oncology Nursing Forum*. 2018;45(6):726–736.

25. Jonathon Moran, Guinan E, McCormick P, et al. The ability of prehabilitation to influence postoperative outcome after intra-abdominal operation: a systematic review and meta-analysis. *Surgery*. 2016;160(5):1189–1201.

26. Daniel Steffens, Beckenkamp P, Young J, et al. Is preoperative physical activity level of patients undergoing cancer surgery associated with postoperative outcomes? A systematic review and meta-analysis. *Eur J Surg Oncol*. 2019;45(4):510–518.

27. Cavalheri V, Granger C. Preoperative exercise training for patients with non-small cell lung cancer. *Cochrane Database Syst Rev*. 2017;6(6):CD012020. doi:10.1002/14651858.CD012020.pub2.

28. Boright L, Doherty DJ, Wilson CM, Arena SK, Ramirez C. Development and feasibility of a prehabilitation protocol for patients diagnosed with head and neck cancer. *Cureus*. 2020;12(8):e9898. doi:10.7759/cureus.9898.

29. Centemero A, Rigatti L, Giraudo D, et al. Preoperative pelvic floor muscle exercise for early continence after radical prostatectomy: a randomised controlled study. *Eur Urol*. 2010;57(6):1039–1043. doi:10.1016/j.eururo.2010.02.028.

30. Moug SJ, Mutrie N, Barry SJE, et al. Prehabilitation is feasible in patients with rectal cancer undergoing neoadjuvant chemoradiotherapy and may minimize physical deterioration: results from the Rex trial. *Colorectal Dis*. 2019;21(5):548–562.

31. Bruns ERJ, Argillander TE, Schuijt HJ, et al. Fit4SurgeryTV at-home prehabilitation for frail older patients planned for colorectal cancer surgery: a pilot study. *Am J Phys Med Rehabil*. 2019;98(5):399–406.

28

Long-Term Survivorship and Late Effect Management

MARY ALICE HEWELT, PT, MPT, CLT[a], MEGHAN HUBER, PT, DPT, CLT[a], AND
CYNTHIA MARSILI, PT, CLT[a]

CHAPTER OUTLINE

Long-Term Survivorship

Cancer has become a chronic illness as opposed to a terminal disease for many people due to advances in diagnosis and treatment. Cancer survivorship entails much more than simply surviving the diagnosis. For many persons living with and beyond cancer (PLWBCs), it means living with the chronic conditions that can result from the actual cancer as well as its various treatments. This can include the physical adverse effects that arise during and after treatments, resultant financial toxicity, underemployment, loss of employment, social/emotional challenges that can lead to changes in relationships, psychological impairments including depression and anxiety, as well as fear of recurrence. All of these factors contribute to surviving cancer under new normal pretenses.

The National Coalition for Cancer Survivorship (NCCS) is credited with establishing the most widely accepted definition of cancer survivorship in 1986 as the period from diagnosis until death.[1] Since then the definition of survivor has been expanded to include family, friends, and caregivers and is endorsed by such organizations as the American Society of Clinical Oncology (ASCO) in its Survivorship Compendium and the National Comprehensive Cancer Network (NCCN) in the General Survivorship Principles in the NCCN Guidelines that serve as resources for health professionals.[2,3] This chapter will focus on the portion of time defined by the National Academies of Sciences, Engineering and Medicine (NASEM) perspective (formerly the Institute of Medicine [IOM]), as that which begins following completion of active treatment and continues until the end of life.[4,5] It is

---

[a]Board Certified Clinical Specialist in Oncologic Physical Therapy

recognized that the terms survivor and survivorship are not consistently utilized outside of the United States (US), though they will be used throughout this chapter and in the context of a PLWBC as well as the process on the continuum of cancer care by which one with cancer experiences life.

History of Survivorship

Since the first National Cancer Policy Forum (NCPF) of the NASEM in 1999 that brought awareness to the long-term functioning and well-being of those with cancer, to the 2011 American Cancer Society interdisciplinary team of stakeholders developing the Prospective Surveillance Model (PSM) as a best practice framework for rehabilitation, access to Onc R from the time of diagnosis through treatment and beyond has been identified as the standard of care.[4,6] The National Institutes of Health (NIH) updated recommendations from 2018 to indicate that prehabilitation and Onc R services are necessary to optimize tolerance to adjuvant treatment, minimize toxicity, and improve outcomes. This publication also emphasizes the need for all cancer care team members, including Onc R clinicians, to have the necessary education and training.[5]

In Box 28.1, the timeline of when Onc R services are integrated into the multidisciplinary care team emphasizes the importance of the role Onc R clinicians play in cancer survivorship. Of all of the care team members, Onc R clinicians have the privilege of devoting a significant amount of time to the clients in their care. As a result, these clinicians are not only able to identify dysfunctions and impairments in a timely fashion, they are also often the first to identify changes in signs and symptoms, sequelae of treatment effects, and potentially unaddressed psychosocial deficits that necessitate referral to other care team members.

Initiation of the Rehabilitation Role in Survivorship

Onc R clinicians have the opportunity to impact the health and well-being of PLWBCs at various times throughout the spectrum of oncology care. The historical significance of the decades of work by pioneering professionals in this domain allows clinical specialists to appreciate the tremendous impact their value-added services can have on PLWBC. Dietz's seminal work established the taxonomy known as the Classification of Cancer Rehabilitation.[13–15] Briggs outlined the various physical therapy practice patterns for persons with advanced cancers in 2000 that can be utilized when establishing plans of care that may change and be modified throughout the continuum of care as the patient's needs change.[16] Colombo and Wilson identified the PRISM Rehab Model of Survivorship in 2015 (see Chapter 31).[11] In 2019, Stout et al. established a call to action that emphasizes the importance of a Prospective Functional Screening and Assessment Model (Prospective Surveillance Model is the proposed framework outlined by ASCO) and the necessity to have specialized education and training that provides professionals with the tools to safely and effectively administer the model in the cancer population.[6]

The four categories of Onc R services identified by Dietz and described in the Description of Specialty Practice (DSP) published by the American Physical Therapy Association (APTA) that occur throughout the continuum of cancer survivorship include preventative, restorative, supportive, and palliative services.[13,14,17] Preventative services have a primary function to screen and

---

| • BOX 28.1 | Timeline of Integration of Rehab Services Into Cancer Survivorship |

1922 American College of Surgeons (ACoS) established the Commission on Cancer (CoC) to "establish standards to ensure quality, multidisciplinary, and comprehensive cancer care delivery in health care settings; conduct surveys in health care settings to assess compliance with those standards; collect standardized data from CoC-accredited health care settings to measure cancer care quality; use data to monitor treatment patterns and outcomes and enhance cancer control and clinical surveillance activities; and develop effective educational interventions to improve cancer prevention, early detection, cancer care delivery, and outcomes in health care settings."[7]

1999 First National Cancer Policy Forum (NCPF) of the Institute of Medicine (IOM) brought forth awareness of long-term functioning and well-being of individuals with cancer.[4]

2004 American Society of Clinical Oncology (ASCO) developed a Survivorship Task Force.

2006 IOM was the first to identify rehabilitation as part of survivorship care.[8]

2007 IOM's report that established a treatment model for distress based on National Comprehensive Cancer Network's (NCCN) guidelines.[9]

2011 ASCO established a formal Cancer Survivorship Committee that created the Cancer Survivorship Compendium which defined, developed guidelines around, and outlined models of survivorship care; it developed templates for survivorship care plans (SCPs) and provides resources and tools for building and implementing a survivorship program.[2]

2011 American Cancer Society (ACS) facilitated the development of the Prospective Surveillance Model as the best practice framework for cancer rehabilitation.[6]

2013 NCPF report emphasized the integral role rehabilitation providers play in the coordinated oncology care team.[10]

2015 Colombo and Wilson introduced the PRevention Intervention Sustainable Wellness Model of care (PRISM model) as a roadmap for how rehabilitation professionals can carry out their role in facilitating the health and functional well-being of persons living with and beyond cancer.[11]

2016 CoC Standard 3.3 established the requirement that SCPs and follow-up plans be provided to patients.[2,12]

2018 NCPF report highlights the critical role of the rehabilitation provider in prehabilitation as well as "to maintain and restore function, reduce symptom burden, maximize independence, and improve quality of life."[5]

2019 CoC Standard 4.8 acknowledges the barriers in executing Standard 3.3 including the lack of reimbursement for the time-consuming completion and distribution of the SCP and who is responsible. While it encourages SCPs, the emphasis is on documenting a minimum of three services that are offered each year to better support patients. These services may include but are not limited to summaries or SCPs, seminars for survivors, Onc R services, or nutritional and psychological services.[2]

Created by Mary Alice Hewlett, Meghan Huber, and Cynthia Marsili. Printed with permission.

---

provide activity recommendations and a secondary function to facilitate prospective surveillance for subacute and late effects of cancer treatment. Restorative services aim to address the physical impairment and functional limitations of the patient and restore them to a prior level of function. Supportive Onc R promotes accommodation of disabilities, teaches compensatory strategies, and provides ongoing therapy during disease recurrence or temporization efforts; these efforts may include short or medium-term provisional restorative options that are needed in preparation for a more permanent treatment plan. While the primary goal of palliative rehabilitation is to "mitigate the impact of symptoms of advanced cancer and its adverse effects," the National Cancer Institute (NCI) indicates that the palliative approach aims to provide more holistic care which should occur throughout the entire continuum of care.[18]

Briggs has further expanded on the physical therapy model in palliative care which is applicable to those with advanced cancers, noting six different practice patterns that can be utilized independently or concurrently throughout the duration of advanced disease.[16] They include traditional Onc R services, rehabilitation light, rehabilitation in reverse, case management, skilled maintenance, and supportive care. See Chapter 29 for more on these models. Traditional care focuses on improvement in function in a shorter time with increased frequency of interventions. Rehabilitation light can follow a more gradual trajectory when gains are anticipated but require an extended length of time to achieve with less frequent visits. Rehabilitation in reverse allows clinicians to provide education and skilled care that anticipates progressive decline; this may include the use of assistive devices, caregiver training, and modifications to an exercise program that may focus on mobility and comfort more than progress. Skilled maintenance is necessary when PLWBCs who require complex assistance and/or have comorbidities requiring skilled monitoring need the expertise of movement experts, such as physical therapists, to optimize functional movement. A PLWBC may require skilled care to achieve goals focusing on quality of life (QOL) even though an increase in function is not anticipated. Case management allows rehabilitation clinicians to supervise a care plan being followed by unskilled caregivers; while this is no longer reimbursable under home health care, it is valid under the Medicare Hospice Benefit (the program available for patients with a life expectancy of 6 months or less and who are no longer seeking curative treatment). Supportive care is the primary model provided during hospice care but can be secondary at any of the other levels of care. These services occur when family or other medical professionals are unable to safely and confidently mobilize the PLWBC or when gentle range of motion (ROM), massage, and positioning education can meet comfort goals during end-of-life care. Having a keen understanding of the skills and interventions available and knowledge of reimbursement options and requirements allows Onc R clinicians to provide care from early diagnosis until the end of life. A plan of care that thoroughly documents deficits, goals, and recommended interventions is key to communicate to peers, managers, and intermediaries the medical necessity of the care being provided within each practice pattern.

Colombo and Wilson were instrumental in introducing the PRISM Rehab Model of Survivorship that encompasses the Onc R clinician's ability and necessity of participating in the continuum of care from the time of diagnosis through survivorship to end of life. PRISM stands for (PR)evention (I)ntervention (S)ustainable wellness (M)odel of care.[11] It emphasizes the importance of Onc R clinicians having an active role in influencing the health and functional well-being of a PLWBC. In short, that means establishing a baseline level of function at the time of diagnosis, providing recommendations to improve that level of function and facilitate optimal outcomes of the anticipated medical interventions, intervening with traditional rehabilitation services when the adverse effects of treatment lead to impairment and functional decline, and finally, facilitating lasting lifestyle adjustments and opportunities to promote ongoing health and wellness following completion of cancer and/or rehabilitation treatment.

In 2012, the direct costs of cancer care provided over 1 year of a PSM were compared to the traditional model of care.[19] It demonstrated a significant reduction in direct costs for the single breast cancer-related impairment of lymphedema. While the authors acknowledged the need for further investigation of the cost effectiveness from a societal perspective and a cost benefit analysis, they proposed a shift in the medical paradigm in which rehabilitation reimbursement is dictated by impairment-based procedural interventions instead of secondary prevention. A focus on secondary prevention may very well mitigate the likely impairments before they occur, thereby improving QOL and potentially avoiding the secondary deficits of decline in function with activities of daily living (ADLs) and the tertiary consequences of limitations in fulfilling familial and work-related roles.[19]

There has been a direct call to action emphasizing the need to implement prospective functional screening and assessment in Onc R care, to increase educational opportunities for clinicians, and to facilitate additional research opportunities that investigate the value of health promotion activities.[20] When Onc R clinicians can demonstrate skills in screening, risk assessment, and triage, health care administrators can advocate for the shift in the payment structure that is reflective of a proactive model of oncology care.[20]

Both of these models parallel the Medical Model of Survivorship identified as the Survivorship Care Plan (SCP).[21] An SCP includes prevention, surveillance for recurrence or new primary cancers, interventions for psychosocial factors, and coordination of care. Its purpose is to provide a bridge of communication between the multidisciplinary team and the primary care provider outlining the details of the cancer treatment, outcomes, and effects. It may be administered by physicians, nurses, or advanced practice registered nurses. While the completion of the SCP is time consuming and in many locations is not fully integrated into the electronic medical record, it has been documented to improve patient satisfaction and QOL.[22]

Quality of Life

Through the course of providing patient/family centered care that focuses on the multi-faceted well-being of PLWBCs, it is incumbent upon the Onc R clinician to screen for all factors that affect QOL. Many tools are available to assess distress and QOL and are well documented in the literature for their reliability, specificity, validity, and ease of use. Two such tools include the NCCN Distress Thermometer and Problem List and the Functional Assessment of Cancer Therapy (FACT).[23,24] When such tools are incorporated into the survivorship care model, the psychological, social, emotional, and spiritual problems that can accompany the physiological challenges are effectively monitored. They can also facilitate referrals to the multidisciplinary team members that are best equipped to address these deficits. Failure to address high levels of distress can affect decision-making and adherence to treatment as well as the ability to maintain healthy lifestyle choices such as exercising and smoking cessation. This may lead to poor management of pain and increased utilization of the medical system as noted by more frequent physician and emergency room visits.[25]

The NCCN is a not-for-profit alliance of 30 leading cancer centers established in 1993 that is focused on improving the quality and accessibility of cancer care. For this chapter, the focus will be the NCCN Distress Thermometer and Problem List for Patients that are typically utilized by the advanced practice registered nurse to identify the level and reasons for the distress (see Chapter 14). The Problem List allows the PLWBC to identify the practical, family, emotional, and spiritual problems as well as physical problems that may not be mentioned to the provider during a particular encounter. An algorithm allows the practitioner to determine if an individual will benefit from a referral for a more thorough psychological assessment.

The FACIT Group (FACIT.org) is the licensing entity that was formed based on the work of David Cella, whose research developed the FACT questionnaire.[26] His work was the foundation for what has become over 100 self-reported measures that have been translated and linguistically validated in over 80 languages as well as each item being part of a national statistical database that allows Onc R clinicians to create patient-specific tools. The transition from the FACT, which was specific to cancer diagnoses, to the Functional Assessment Chronic Illness Therapy (FACIT) reflected innovative advancements that identified that QOL is vitally important to well-being not only of a PLWBC, but also those experiencing impairments caused by numerous other chronic health conditions. The FACIT questionnaires can be general as well as specific for disease, symptoms, or treatment. For example, the FACIT-F is a general tool that includes a domain assessing the impact of fatigue, a common adverse effect of numerous cancer treatments, upon daily activities and function. Additional resources can be found at www.facit.org.[24] The scoring resources allow Onc R clinicians to identify areas of concern that allow them to establish goals within their area of expertise as well as when to refer to other members of the multidisciplinary team. This can include referrals to the physician for management of physical signs and symptoms, other Onc R clinicians to address functional limitations outside the scope of the referring Onc R clinician. In addition, referrals may be indicated for integrative medicine for complementary and alternative treatments, nutrition services, social work, spiritual support, and referral to cancer centers that can provide community-based resource information. See facit.org or the enhanced eBook for eFigure 28.1 and eFigure 28.2, the FACIT F tool and scoring.

Long-Term Survivorship Summary

The unique opportunity to spend a significant amount of time with the PLWBC is a privilege that can be likened to a long-term caregiver role akin to that of the primary care physician. The Onc R clinician has the ability to "leave the door open" for future opportunities to intervene. When inevitable setbacks occur due to a new diagnosis, recurrence, injury, late effect, gradual decline, or any combination of these, the survivor should feel as though they have a resource to facilitate the re-entry into the active rehabilitative process. This demonstrates the cyclical intervention that the PRISM model advocates for when identifying the role of the Onc R clinician to meet the PLWBC wherever they are in the survivorship continuum of care.

Late Effects

While the primary focus of medical intervention for cancer diagnoses is survival, PLWBCs often experience physical impairments including but not limited to ROM, weakness, discomfort, pain, and fatigue during and following treatment. Acute adverse effects occur as a direct consequence of medical treatment and can limit tolerance to the medical interventions (chemotherapy, radiation therapy, or surgery).[27] Long-term adverse effects begin during cancer treatment and extend beyond the treatment window; whereas, late effects occur months to years following completion of cancer related medical treatment.[27,28] Late and long-term adverse effects of cancer treatment are becoming more prevalent because of the

increased long-term survival rates.[29] Late effects not only occur in the tissue diagnosed with cancer, but they also involve other organs/systems in the body that were not directly affected by the primary cancer diagnosis.[29] Late effects often negatively impact an individual's employment, education, finances, and social relationships.[27] A general overview of late effects specific to surgery, chemotherapy, and radiation therapy can be found below in Table 28.1.

Childhood Cancers

Cancer is the leading cause of death in children worldwide.[30] Up to 80% of children diagnosed in high-income countries will survive the cancer diagnosis, but only 20% in low to middle-income countries will experience long-term survival.[30] The survival discrepancy between countries is attributed to the accuracy of diagnosis, access to appropriate medical care, affordable treatment options, and appropriate surveillance for adverse effects as well as relapse. Many childhood cancers cannot be prevented or adequately screened for. As most are not the result of lifestyle or environmental factors, they develop idiopathically. Genetic etiology in childhood cancers remains unclear and remains a topic for investigation. Children in low- to middle-income countries may be exposed to chronic infections such as human immunodeficiency virus (HIV), Epstein-Barr virus, and malaria which increase the risk of childhood cancer.[30] Children in high-income countries have greater access to receive medical treatment for these infections, which may decrease the risk of cancer development resulting from each infection.

In the US there are approximately 17 million cancer survivors, with many experiencing diagnoses as a child.[31] Childhood cancer survivors include individuals diagnosed from birth to age 14, while teenage and young adult cancer survivors include individuals diagnosed at the age of 15 to 24 years old.[32,33] There are inconsistencies in the literature as not all definitions of teenage and young adult are consistent. Some sources define adolescent and young adult cancer survivors as the age 15 to 39.[32]

The most commonly diagnosed childhood cancer is leukemia including acute lymphocytic leukemia (ALL) and acute myelogenous leukemia (AML). Other types of prevalent childhood cancer diagnoses include brain tumors (26%), lymphoma (Hodgkin 3% and non-Hodgkin 5%), neuroblastoma (6%), Wilms tumor (5%), rhabdomyosarcoma (3%), bone cancers (osteosarcoma and Ewing sarcoma 3%), and retinoblastoma (2%).[34] Due to improved medical treatment and availability, it is expected that 80% of individuals diagnosed with childhood or young adult cancer will survive longer than 5 years in the US.[33] Currently, it is estimated that there are 270,000 survivors of childhood cancer between age 20 and 39 in the US.[35] Despite increasing survival rates for childhood and young adult cancers, the risk of morbidity is significantly increased in these individuals, both immediately following diagnosis and treatment as well as years into survival. Approximately 40% of childhood and young adult survivors experience comorbidities 10 years following diagnosis, compared to 20% of peers with no history of cancer.[32]

Many factors influence the development and severity of long-term and late effects of childhood cancer with the most prominent factors being the type and location of cancer diagnosis, treatment plan, dosage of medical treatment, age, genetics, and other underlying health conditions/comorbidities.[31] Generally, the severity of comorbid conditions increases in those surviving a primary diagnosis of Hodgkin lymphoma or brain tumors, which will be discussed in more detail below.[36,37]

TABLE 28.1	Adverse Effects of Cancer-Related Medical Interventions	
Interventions/Effects	Short- and Long-Term Adverse Effects During and Immediately Following Cancer Treatment	Late Effects Up To 5 Years or Beyond
Surgery	Delayed healing Swelling (surgical) Pain Muscle guarding Cording after breast cancer treatment Decreased ROM	Myofascial restrictions Decreased scar mobility and/or presence of keloid scars Postmastectomy pain (3 months) Shoulder dysfunction Postmastectomy syndrome Continued ROM limitations
Radiation Therapy	Erythema Burned radiated tissue Blistering Muscle tightness Fatigue	Sexual dysfunction RTx fibrosis Vaginal stenosis Chronic radiation enteritis Micro-vessel disease Cardiomyopathy
Hormonal	Joint pain Hot flashes Vaginal dryness Fatigue Erectile dysfunction	Weight gain Increased risk of thromboembolic events Osteoporotic fractures
Chemotherapy	Peripheral neuropathy Fatigue Hair loss Weakness	Continuation of neuropathy Fatigue Cardiomyopathy Hypogonadism Premature aging Sarcopenia Cachexia

ROM, Range of motion.

Created by Mary Alice Hewelt, Meghan Huber, and Cynthia Marsili. Printed with permission.

Most Common Childhood Cancer Diagnoses

Leukemia

Long-term and late effects following childhood leukemia can range from mild to severe. Childhood leukemia survivors may experience an array of long-term adverse effects that may include but are not limited to: fatigue, cardiovascular disease, growth and developmental delays, infertility, and a secondary cancer diagnosis. They are at an increased risk for heart failure, myocardial infarction, and valvular disease.[38] Due to the cardiotoxic effects of treatment regimens utilized in this population, heart transplantation demands have similarly increased.

Sarcopenic obesity is a phenomenon experienced in many long-term survivors of childhood ALL.[39] Sarcopenic obesity is identified by an increase in body fat with a decrease in fat-free mass. This combination increases body fat and subsequently the adverse effects resultant of obesity, as well as frailty and the associated adverse effects from decreased skeletal muscle mass. Sarcopenic obesity seen in ALL survivors may be a factor of premature aging.[40]

Survivors of leukemia treated with total body radiation therapy followed by hematopoietic stem cell transplant are at an increased risk of obesity, though this is physiologically different when compared to obese individuals with no history of cancer or cancer treatment. The survivors of hematopoietic stem cell transplant with total body irradiation experience a significant decrease in fat-free mass with abnormal fat distribution (increased central fat deposition, decreased subcutaneous fat, increased visceral fat,

and increased intramuscular fat mass proportions).[40] Visceral fat is more detrimental to cardiovascular health when compared to subcutaneous fat and may be one of many factors contributing to long-term cardiovascular effects.[41]

Brain Tumors

A malignant brain tumor is the most commonly seen solid tumor in childhood.[42] Table 28.2 describes the most common brain tumors experienced during each age. The most common brain tumors in children are pilocytic astrocytoma and embryonal tumors. Pituitary tumors are more common in the age range of 15 to 34 while meningiomas and glioblastomas are the most commonly seen in the adult population.[42,43] Medical management for brain tumors can consist of surgery, radiation therapy, and/or chemotherapy.

Radiation therapy to brain tumors can lead to hypothalamic-pituitary dysfunction which results in early or late puberty in children.[44] Cognitive impairment is common following medical treatment of childhood brain tumors, especially following cranial radiation therapy. Cognitive impairments typically become most evident 1 to 2 years after radiation therapy.[37] Cognitive impairments are considered progressive because PLWBCs are typically not able to acquire new abilities at a rate comparable to healthy, age-matched peers.[37] Other long-term and late effects inclusive to survivors of childhood brain tumors involve impairments related to psychological, vocational, community integration, physical performance, and fitness.[42]

TABLE 28.2	Most Common Brain Tumors by Age
Age (Years)	**Most Common Brain Tumors**
0–4	Embryonal tumors (medulloblastoma), pilocytic astrocytoma
5–9	Pilocytic astrocytoma, embryonal tumors
10–14	Malignant glioma
15–19	Pituitary tumors (craniopharyngioma and germ cell)
20–34	Pituitary, meningioma
34–74	Meningioma, glioblastoma multiforme

Created by Mary Alice Hewelt, Meghan Huber, and Cynthia Marsili. Printed with permission.

Hodgkin Lymphoma

Those surviving Hodgkin lymphoma are at higher risk for the development of second malignancy as well as cardiovascular disease, each of which substantially reduces lifespan.[45] Alkylating chemotherapy regimens used to treat Hodgkin lymphoma are attributed to an increased risk of developing AML later in life.[45] AML is most likely to occur within the first 10 years following Hodgkin lymphoma diagnosis.[46,47] The overall risk of AML as a secondary cancer is declining due to advances and changes in chemotherapy medications. Radiation therapy has been attributed to an increase in secondary solid tumors of the lung, breast, stomach, and pancreas with a higher radiation therapy dose increasing the risk of developing the solid tumor later in life.[45]

Long-Term and Late Effects by System

Cardiovascular

Damage to the cardiovascular system is emerging as one of many causes of morbidity and mortality in survivors of childhood and young adult cancer diagnoses. Childhood cancer survivors at the highest risk for cardiotoxic long-term and late effects include individuals who are female, children who were diagnosed and treated before the age of seven, received chest radiotherapy, completed high doses of anthracyclines, and had higher body fat.[48] The increase in cardiovascular risk is four to six times higher in childhood and young adult cancer survivors when compared to non-cancer peers. This risk is increased in survivors of lymphoma, those receiving mediastinal radiation therapy, or those receiving anthracycline chemotherapy.[33] Anthracycline chemotherapy can result in acute cardiac complications during infusion as well as long-term cardiac damage resulting in heart failure. Coupled with cardiovascular risk, this population is at a ninefold risk for cerebrovascular accidents in adulthood.[37] Given the increased cardiovascular risk in childhood cancer survivors, screening for comorbidities including hypertension, diabetes, dyslipidemia, and obesity become of high importance with goals of decreasing morbidity and mortality.

Pulmonary

Radiation therapy and chemotherapy can result in permanent damage to the pulmonary system. Radiation exposure to the lungs, especially in young children, can result in respiratory damage. Most often, this lung damage results in decreased total lung capacity and forced vital capacity as well as poorer diffusion capability due to damage of the lung parenchyma.[37]

High doses of bleomycin (Blenoxane), which may be used in combination therapies to treat Hodgkin lymphoma or germinative cancers, result in pulmonary dysfunction and damage later in life.[37] Approximately 10% to 20% of individuals treated with bleomycin will experience pulmonary toxicity, which can be fatal.[49] The most common symptoms present in bleomycin-induced pulmonary damage include nonproductive cough and exertional dyspnea.[49] As pulmonary damage progresses, the person living beyond cancer may experience dyspnea at rest, tachypnea, and cyanosis.[49] Bleomycin can lead to long-term pulmonary fibrosis. Pulmonary fibrosis occurs when lipid peroxidation causes interstitial swelling and an inflow of inflammatory cells which can lead to fibrosis of the tissue.[25]

Pulmonary comorbidities remain a significant impairment for individuals after allograft hematopoietic stem cell transplant due to the intensive treatment course before and during the transplant.[37] An estimated 25% of PLWBC of childhood allograft hematopoietic stem cell transplant endure pulmonary complications.[50]

Endocrine and Reproductive

The most common endocrine-related long-term effect following a cancer diagnosis is hypothalamic-pituitary dysfunction and metabolic syndrome.[44] The dysfunction of the metabolic endocrine system develops over time. Individuals who receive radiation for brain tumors may experience endocrine dysfunction most frequently due to deficiencies in growth hormone followed by follicle stimulating hormone, luteinizing hormone, thyroid stimulating hormone, and adrenocorticotropic hormone.[44] Shifts in these hormones affect puberty development in children, increase the risk of cardiovascular disease, and result in comorbidities. Obesity and diabetes following the treatment of Hodgkin lymphoma and central nervous system (CNS) cancers also increase the risk of further endocrine dysfunction in these survivors.[33] High doses of chemotherapy and radiation to the pelvis including the gonads may result in primary hypogonadism which can lead to infertility and sexual dysfunction. Reproductive and sexual dysfunction is prevalent in childhood and young adult cancer survivors. Male PLWBCs are four times more likely to experience erectile dysfunction when compared to peers without a history of cancer.[33]

The severity of endocrine deficiencies depends on the total radiotherapy dosage, fraction size, and the schedule of radiation therapy. Growth hormone deficiencies typically appear first, with an average of 2.8 years following treatment.[44] The effects from radiotherapy are anticipated to decrease with the improvements in technology for the treatment and more prevalent use of proton beam therapies for brain tumors.

Auditory and Vestibular

Ototoxicity is a significant long-term effect of childhood cancer treatment. Sensorineural hearing loss can be experienced by those treated with high doses of platinum-based chemotherapy (cisplatin [Platinol] dose >360 mg/m^2), a combination of platinum-based chemotherapy with concurrent cranial radiation therapy, a combination of platinum-based chemotherapy, or if the person's treatment was delivered before 5 years of age.[37]

Cognitive Function

Children living with and beyond cancer and treatment experience disruptions in educational pursuits, vocational endeavors, and relationships leading to distress, depression, anxiety, and potentially harmful behavior. PLWBCs of the CNS are at risk for impairments in intelligence, processing speed, and executive function followed by deficits in memory and attention.[51] These deficits impact daily activities and interactions in the family, school, and community. Cranial radiation therapy can result in cognitive impairments, and usually presents 1 to 2 years after the final dose of radiation.[37] Cranial radiation has led to a decline in white matter integrity (as evidenced by brain imaging) with increasing age which suggests accelerated aging and may increase the risk of early onset dementia.[51] No clear indicators of accelerated aging following chemotherapy have been discovered or reported.[51]

Larger cranial radiation fields, specifically whole brain radiation, result in greater neurocognitive impairments. Corticosteroids and antimetabolite chemotherapy exacerbates cognitive impairments.[37] People living beyond childhood brain tumors and ALL are at the highest risk for neurocognitive impairments including processing speed, executive function, memory, inattention, and complex fine-motor functioning.[37]

Many interventions are utilized to assist compensation or recovery of cognitive deficits in childhood cancer survivors. Among these are behavioral and cognitive strategies and exercise have proven as beneficial. Following a 12-week group exercise program, white matter and hippocampal volume increased resulting in improved reaction times of children following cranial radiation for brain tumors.[52]

Childhood Cancers Summary

The Children's Oncology Group has developed screening guidelines and recommendations entitled *Long-Term Follow-Up Guidelines for Survivors of Childhood, Adolescent, and Young Adult Cancers.*[36,37] These guidelines provide an appropriate screen for asymptomatic individuals in remission from childhood malignancy. Should an individual exhibit symptoms, further medical evaluation is warranted via a specialized pediatric oncologist. Since 2010, all major pediatric survival cancer guideline groups worldwide have been collaborating to unify surveillance recommendations for the most prevalent late effects of childhood cancers.[53] The goal of providing standardized surveillance and survivorship cancer screenings is to improve early detection resulting in timely treatment initiation, should this be warranted.[53]

Adult Cancers

Late and long-term effects also occur in diagnoses of adult cancers. The 10-year survival rate for the 20 most common types of cancers is approximately 50% but increases to 80% with selective cancers inclusive of breast, lymphoma, melanoma, and uterine.[48] The 5-year survival rate has improved in the various forms of breast cancer due to the advances made in early detection and treatment protocols.[54]

Long-Term and Late Effects by System

Cardiovascular

Cardiovascular toxicity is a late adverse effect notably observed following the use of chemotherapy drugs, hormone suppression drugs, and radiation therapy. Anthracycline-based agents (e.g., doxorubicin [Adriamycin], epirubicin [Ellence], daunorubicin [Cerubidine], idarubicin [Idamycin]) are commonly used in the treatment of breast, lymphoma, ovarian, sarcoma, and myeloma. Brown et al. reported a higher risk of cardiotoxicity in those receiving anthracycline as compared to a control group.[55] Anthracycline-induced cardiomyopathy causes heart failure by free radicals damaging cardiac muscle and is most commonly observed more than 1 year after completion of treatment which occurs in up to 65% of childhood cancer survivors. It is a dose-dependent phenomenon that has a greater effect on right ventricle function with a chronic progression.[25] Trastuzumab (Herceptin) is a monoclonal

antibody linked to cardiac adverse effects, causing heart failure 20 years following administration.[56] Combining trastuzumab with anthracyclines interferes with the growth, repair, and survival of cardiomyocytes and immune-mediated destruction. This medication is commonly used to treat stomach and HER2+ breast cancer. Hormonal suppression and iatrogenic menopause and andropause can contribute to the progression of atherosclerosis.[25] Radiation therapy contributes to the development and progression of coronary artery disease by causing microcirculatory damage that advances atherosclerosis and induces clotting leading to myocardial fibrosis and reduced cardiac efficiency.[25] Despite new techniques to reduce dosage to cardiac tissue, those treated for left side breast cancer and with mantle radiation therapy for Hodgkin lymphoma sustain the greatest risk for long-term and late effects. Hypertension is a significant consideration in managing cardiac toxicity due to the increased stress, the increased fluid volumes incurred during chemotherapy infusions, and the renovascular dysregulation that can occur when trying to manage changes in fluid volume.

It has become standard of care for patients to receive a cardiac evaluation to determine baseline cardiac function. While many use 2D echocardiograms for monitoring cardiac functioning, the maximal exercise stress test with electrocardiogram is a useful tool to identify heart abnormalities with physical exertion. A resting echocardiography of the left ventricular ejection fraction is not sensitive to detect early cardiomyopathy that is a result of chemotherapy. The baseline evaluation allows for the medical team to identify any pre-existing conditions that may affect optimal outcomes as well as monitor for changes/deviations from the baseline cardiac function that indicate cardiotoxicity. However, VO_2 max is a criterion standard of cardiopulmonary reserve. A decline in VO_2 max is a normal physiological aging process observed in the noncancer population, yet the decline is more rapid in cancer survivors.[25] See Chapter 23 for further explanation regarding rehabilitation and exercise implications.

Pulmonary

A variety of pulmonary adverse effects are the possible result of cancer and cancer treatment. Following radiation therapy, the lungs may become inflamed and result in radiation pneumonitis. Radiation pneumonitis generally appears 1 to 3 months following radiation, although may appear up to 6 months after radiation therapy. Individuals may experience dyspnea, low-grade fever, cough, or chest pain/congestion; more severe cases demonstrate permanent scarring resulting in pulmonary fibrosis.[57] Mild symptoms are often treated with supportive treatments inclusive of inhaled corticosteroids, while severe cases may lead to long-term disability. An estimated 5% to 15% of individuals diagnosed with lung cancer receiving high dose external beam radiation will experience radiation pneumonitis.[25]

Chemotherapy regimens also result in pulmonary toxicity. The pulmonary adverse effects of chemotherapy are drug and dose dependent and increase with concurrent radiation treatment. Interstitial lung injury is often categorized in the early onset of pulmonary toxicity whereas late effect pulmonary toxicity includes pulmonary fibrosis. Bleomycin and small molecule tyrosine kinase inhibitors (TKIs) are considered the main causative agents inducing pulmonary disease. Adverse effects can be early onset (prior to 2 months following therapy) or late onset (longer than 2 months following treatment).[58,59]

Musculoskeletal

PLWBCs may present to Onc R services with complaints of non-specific pain that are difficult to associate with causative sources.

Physicians may provide a generic diagnosis or diagnoses that are often used broadly aligned to their very specific patterns of criteria or behavior (e.g., fibromyalgia, adhesive capsulitis). The Onc R clinician should identify the historical cancer-specific information that will lead to a more precise rehab diagnosis. In the absence of degenerative or event-based circumstances, identifying the history of cancer and the subsequent treatment interventions can allow the clinician to conclude that the late effects of those treatments could be the causative agent leading to dysfunction. Joint arthrosis, tissue fibrosis, and nonspecific pain are common presentations following radiation therapy and chemotherapy in addition to the myofascial changes that can happen over time following surgical interventions. Once these latent changes present themselves and the clinician has established a correlation with the late effects of cancer and its treatment, then the clinician can proceed with a sense of awareness of the most appropriate interventions to utilize and caution for the relative or absolute contraindications.

Living with cancer increases the likelihood of diagnosed or undiagnosed bone metastases. The presence of bone metastases may indicate the spread of disease or recurrence. When a patient has a history of cancer and is experiencing unpredictable pain (e.g., no mechanical explanation, no identifiable relieving, or aggravating factors) and the pain is solely present with weight-bearing activities, the Onc R clinician should be prompted to inquire about recent oncologic follow-up if ongoing surveillance is occurring.

Hormonal suppression not only has cardiotoxic effects as noted previously but negatively influences the integrity of the bone. Postmenopausal women on aromatase inhibitors (AI) for breast cancer are at an increased risk of osteoporosis given the disruption of hormonal levels resulting in bone loss that carries an associated increased risk of fracture.[54,60] Generalized joint pain is also commonly seen with treatment using AIs.[54] Men that are receiving androgen deprivation therapy for the treatment of prostate cancer are at an increased risk for bone loss. Relative to anti-hormonal therapy such as tamoxifen (Nolvadex) used for premenopausal women with estrogen receptor positive cancer, there is a dose-dependent increased risk of endometrial cancer, pulmonary embolism, and deep vein thrombosis.[25]

Sexual dysfunction is a long-term adverse effect of gynecological cancers.[61] Radiation therapy may result in vaginal stenosis and damage of the mucosal lining and vaginal tissue resulting in fibrotic changes with decreased elasticity. Fibrotic changes may occur years after radiation treatment. Surgical interventions for vulvar, vaginal, and cervical cancer often result in loss of anatomy and clitoral tissue leading to vaginal stenosis and sexual dysfunction. Chemotherapy can induce premature menopause which will affect vaginal tissue and therefore sexual function.

Patients with head and neck cancer (HNC) can experience late pharyngeal-laryngeal toxicity as well as oral toxicity.[62] When chemotherapy is utilized with the HNC population the risk for late effects increases, furthering the importance of follow up assessments even 5 years after cessation of treatment.[62]

Neurological
Many chemical agents affect neurological functioning including memory, cognition, concentration, balance, sensory, and gross/fine motor control. During treatment, individuals experience sensory impairments such as numbness and tingling, cold sensitivity, and extremity weakness. Although many of these symptoms dissipate following completion of treatment, the individual may experience long-term adverse effects from the chemotherapy that persist for an extended time. Cancer-induced peripheral neuropathy (CIPN) is a commonly experienced long-term effect following interventions with vinca alkaloids, platinum-based compounds, and taxanes. It directly affects proprioception and sensation thereby increasing fall risk, especially in those populations that have comorbidities such as but not limited to: diabetes, vertigo, visual impairments, peripheral vascular disease, and age-related decline.

Endocrine
Endocrine and metabolic disorders can be seen commonly after cancer treatments. Hypopituitarism is a common endocrine disorder that can lead to conditions such as adrenal insufficiency, hypogonadism, hypothyroidism, and growth hormone deficiency.[44] Metabolic disorders can contribute to a high risk for cardiovascular issues.[44] The survival rate has improved significantly over the years for brain tumors, including malignant tumors. Cranial radiation therapy can cause hypothalamic-pituitary dysfunction which can impact QOL.[44]

Cognitive Function
The most common dysfunctions in cognition that PLWBCs report are forgetfulness, distractibility, attention deficits, and difficulty multitasking. Not only is it common to have cognitive deficits as an adverse effect during treatment, but PLWBCs of the breast and lymphoma have also demonstrated long-term deficits with concentration and attention up to 10 years following chemotherapy treatment.[63]

Cognitive rehabilitation involves specific training and/or education of PLWBCs on how to compensate for deficits in cognition. Cognitive training includes many techniques such as practicing certain skills in an attempt to work on building up their attention and improving their memory as well as psychomotor development.[63] The Onc R clinician needs to remain aware of cognition during all phases of the person's rehabilitation treatment. There is no specific pharmacological treatment presently known to target cancer associated cognitive decline (CACD). The NCCN recommends that nonpharmacological interventions are preferred over pharmacologic treatments for CACD.[63]

Rehabilitation Implications for Long-Term Survivorship and Late Effects

Subjective History

It is common for PLWBCs to be referred to Onc R services with a generic diagnosis (e.g., shoulder stiffness, generalized weakness, gait dysfunction, spinal pain), or specific diagnoses such as impingement, adhesive capsulitis, and bursitis that may be consequential to the underlying source of the impairment. The cancer diagnosis is often not mentioned in a referral and is only exposed via a thorough evaluation completed by the Onc R clinician. The importance of taking a thorough history during an initial evaluation should not be understated and should include a cancer history, current medications, symptoms, and functional limitations.

A comprehensive cancer history and a thorough systems review are crucial and necessary steps when identifying the source of the impairment. A thorough cancer history includes the cancer type and stage, timeline of medical treatments utilized (chemotherapy regimen, radiation dose, surgical interventions), complications experienced during medical treatment, and scheduled follow-up. Ongoing medical management of cancer and other comorbidities can be gleaned from a review of current medications. Some individuals receive long-term administration of chemotherapy or hormonal suppression therapy for many years after diagnosis. Comorbidity awareness and knowledge of the potential late effects of these treatments are essential when providing rehabilitation interventions. The late effects of both cancer and the type of medical treatment utilized will heavily influence the plan of care the evaluating Onc R clinician develops. Barriers to obtaining a thorough history include accessibility to medical records, the time allotted for an Onc R evaluation, and decreased cognitive recall of cancer treatments.

As with any population, patient specific goals provide a foundation for Onc R interventions. Onc R clinicians must also be alert to signs and symptoms that may indicate a recurrence, secondary cancer, or metastasis. Secondary cancer can be in the same area as the original cancer but have a completely different cellular makeup.

Critical Decision Making

Critical decision making to determine the efficacy and appropriateness of Onc R intervention is paramount when specialized care is required and when the PLWBC requires assistance from other multidisciplinary team members. These referrals can include physical therapy specialists (oncology, pediatric, pelvic health, or lymphedema), occupational therapy, speech language pathology, nutrition, social work, psychiatry, physiatry, or return to their referring physician for further assistance with medical management. PLWBCs may benefit from referral to local, community-based services for support and resources including but not limited to: transportation, household assistance, meal preparation, support groups, educational retreats, and acquisition of self-care items (e.g., hats, wigs, prosthetics, compression garments, clothing).

Goals of Interventions

The direction of the plan of care will be dictated by the timing and circumstances that the PLWBC is currently experiencing. As noted earlier, this chapter intends to emphasize the time following completion of cancer treatment. However, reviewing the goals of rehabilitation intervention throughout the continuum of care provides continuity of care from initial diagnosis, through treatment, into disease free/managed survivorship.

When Onc R clinicians perform screening and functional assessments at the time of diagnosis, baseline measurements are obtained and goals are established to achieve optimal health prior to medical interventions, improve tolerance to treatment regimens and promote healthy lifestyle modifications (e.g., smoking cessation, low fat diet, regular physical activity, optimal water intake). The frequency of visits is typically limited with an emphasis on education and home exercise program instruction. Onc R clinicians need to be mindful of insurance benefits and be fiscally responsible to reserve resources for when more formal intervention may be required during and/or after cancer treatment.

PLWBCs may be referred to rehabilitation during cancer treatments for symptom management, mitigating mobility deficits, and preventing functional decline. Previous chapters have discussed the immediate adverse effects that can occur consequential to active medical treatment. Onc R clinicians should play an active role in providing physical interventions that can help reduce

the need for pharmacological treatment of pain and empower the PLWBC to take an active role in their symptom management. The Onc R clinician may utilize treatment modalities such as exercise, sleep hygiene, stress management, postural corrections, activity modifications, energy conservation, and improvement in body awareness and mechanics.

Onc R management of the person living with the long-term and/or late effects of cancer may incorporate any or all of the above activities in addition to facilitating the PLWBC's ability to maintain ongoing exercise and wellness goals. The interventions that are needed may be based on whether or not the PLWBC had access to these services previously during their survivorship. Even in optimal settings where Onc R clinicians are active participants in the multi-disciplinary teams from the time of diagnosis, each PLWBC's experience is unique and requires skilled and specialized care that is tailored to their needs at that moment in time.

Exercise Prescription

During exercise testing, an Onc R clinician should monitor vital signs of blood pressure, heart rate, pulse oximetry, and rate of perceived exertion in conjunction with obtaining a baseline exercise stress test to safely design and administer an appropriate exercise program that incorporates all FITT-VP (flexibility, intensity, time, type, volume, progression) principles. Chapter 23 provides further details regarding specific exercise principles, prescription, and precautions.

Physical activity during and following cancer diagnosis provides numerous benefits to the PLWBC. These benefits include increasing strength, mobility, and aerobic capacity; improving survival and QOL, and decreasing the risk of recurrence or new occurrence.[55] Each individual should be encouraged to participate in physical activity, whether structured or unstructured, according to the American College of Sports Medicine guidelines and is discussed in further detail in Chapter 23.[64]

Weight-bearing exercises play an important role in bone health and fracture prevention for PLWBCs. Prior to weight bearing and resistive exercises, the presence of bone metastasis should be ruled out or cleared by oncologic/orthopedic physicians. Refer to Chapter 7 for more information regarding the management of bone metastases and activity guidelines.

Considerations During Treatment Interventions

Skin integrity can be compromised during radiation therapy and modifications will be necessary for some manual therapy interventions to allow for the necessary tissue healing and remodeling to occur. It is important that the PLWBC performs active mobility but avoids overstretching radiated tissue. The onset of tissue tension following radiation therapy can be immediate or present months later. The initiation or resumption of therapy can be patient specific based on skin reactions, tissue healing, and tolerance to recommended treatment activities. Muscle imbalances and scarring following surgical intervention and/or radiation therapy can lead to kinematic dysfunction caused by inflammation, weakness, tightness, and loss of excursion. These may lead to joint dysfunction or joint impingement from altered movement patterns. Refer to Chapter 9 for more information regarding tissue healing.

Nitric oxide, which acts as a signaling molecule and a free radical scavenger, is released in response to stretching the striated muscle. Therefore, stretching prior to and following radiation therapy of up to 70 Gy is beneficial for patients with cancer of the head and neck.[25] This same principle can be applied to cardiac tissue in the presence of aerobic exercise in addition to the modulation of oxidative stress.[25] This supports the importance of establishing routine exercise programs to mitigate the effects of these treatment modalities.

Impaired venous return and lymphedema may also occur as acute, long-term, or late effects from cancer treatments. Causative factors can include the number of lymph nodes resected, field extent and dosage of radiation delivered, and the effects of increased fluid volume during chemotherapy infusion. An impaired venous return may be addressed with compression and more complicated situations may benefit from referral to a certified lymphedema therapist (CLT) to provide complete decongestive therapy (CDT).

Outcome Measures

Please refer to previous chapters included in this text as well as the APTA Oncology Edge Task Force for direction on specific subjective and functional tools that are most appropriate for common cancer diagnoses.[65]

Conclusion

It is paramount for Onc R clinicians to have an active role in empowering each PLWBC's ability to achieve the healthiest version of themselves possible throughout their cancer survivorship journey, especially considering the increased population of cancer survivors and improved life expectancy. Onc R clinicians in this domain need to advocate for participation in the multidisciplinary team with emphasis on early intervention at the time of diagnosis followed by ongoing surveillance and potential intervention throughout a patient's life.

Critical Research Needs

- Identify the benefits and determine the cost-effectiveness of multidisciplinary rehabilitation programs and if there are any differences based on which health professional provides delivery of the interventions.[66,67]
- Determine if the completion of the time-consuming survivorship care plan actually yields the intended results of improving patient-reported outcomes and facilitating communication between health care professionals regarding the long-term management of PLWBCs.[68]
- Investigate the benefits and/or risks of complementary and alternative therapies for management of long-term effects.

- Examine the efficacy of acupuncture and/or the use of nonsteroidal anti-inflammatories for the management of AI-induced musculoskeletal symptoms.
- Identify optimal treatments for the management of cancer induced cognitive decline.

Case Study

A 39-year-old female was diagnosed with invasive ductal carcinoma of the right breast. Approximately 3 months after initial diagnosis, she had a right nipple sparing mastectomy and immediate reconstruction with an expander. The procedure included a sentinel lymph node biopsy of a singular lymph node that was negative for metastases.

The patient was screened by the physical therapist in the multidisciplinary clinic setting 1 month following surgical intervention; subsequently, physical therapy was recommended to address the deficits of pain, decreased ROM and strength, and functional limitations. She was seen intermittently for five visits during the first episode of care. Progress toward her rehabilitation goals was limited due to concurrent management of other comorbidities including pain with positioning, gastroesophageal reflux disorder (GERD), bronchospasm, and scheduling of her final reconstruction. Surgical exchange of the expander for a breast implant occurred 1 month after discharge from this initial physical therapy episode.

As part of the patient's prospective surveillance, she was screened 6 months after her final reconstructive surgery by the same physical therapist in the cancer survivorship clinic. Once again, therapy was recommended to address the exacerbated deficits of pain, decreased ROM and strength, and functional limitations. The second episode of care included 14 consistently scheduled visits, and the patient achieved decreased pain, increased ROM and strength throughout the upper quadrant and improved functional abilities as noted with the Patient Specific Functional Scale and Upper Extremity Functional Index.

This case reflects the necessity of prospective surveillance for PLWBCs. QOL and functional abilities can be significantly diminished in the time following medical interventions. Without rehabilitation interventions scheduled at regular intervals, this person may not have otherwise received physical therapy and its associated benefits. Even though she did not receive chemotherapy or radiation, she would also benefit from inclusion in a rehabilitation-based long-term surveillance program as part of her SCP to monitor the potential for the deleterious effects that scar tissue and neuromuscular dysfunction can have on her functional abilities in the future.

Review Questions

Reader can find the correct answers and rationale in the back of the book. A 64-year-old male is referred for outpatient physical therapy by his oncologist with a diagnosis of stage 4A nonsmall cell lung cancer with metastasis to the lymph nodes and liver that was diagnosed 10 months ago. His treatments have consisted of palliative radiation and chemotherapy consisting of gemcitabine (Gemzar) and paclitaxel (Taxol). The rehabilitation diagnosis on the referral form is generalized weakness. The patient reports he enjoys walking his dog and gardening. He is becoming discouraged that he can only walk his dog or garden for a short time due

to fatiguing quickly and also reports he is tripping over his feet more frequently. He lives alone in a ranch-style home with no basement.

1. All of the following should be the primary physical therapy goals EXCEPT:
   A. Reducing fall risk within the home
   B. Instructing the patient in the use of an appropriate assistive device
   C. QOL activities
   D. High intensity strengthening

2. What questionnaire would be the most efficient tool to assess how his fatigue has affected his QOL?
   A. Patient pain questionnaire (PPQ)
   B. FACT-G
   C. FACIT-F
   D. NCCN Distress Thermometer and Problem List

An 18-year-old female is referred to physical therapy for evaluation and treatment of generalized fatigue, deconditioning, and limited cardiovascular endurance. She has a history of intermediate-risk Hodgkin lymphoma which was diagnosed at 15 years old. She completed 4 cycles of doxorubicin (Adriamycin), bleomycin (Blenoxane), vincristine (Oncovin), etoposide (VePesid), prednisone (Deltasone), and cyclophosphamide (Cytoxan). Mantle radiation was also completed. She is currently in remission. Before her diagnosis, she was very active and competed in volleyball. Following treatment, she was able to remain active recreationally, though she did not participate competitively. At her medical follow-up, she informed her oncologist of her fatigue and inability to keep up with her friends. She was medically cleared for therapy.

3. Which secondary cancer is the patient at the highest risk for?
   A. Acute lymphocytic leukemia (ALL)
   B. Acute myelogenous leukemia (AML)
   C. Non-Hodgkin lymphoma
   D. Chronic lymphocytic leukemia (CLL)

4. What medical interventions would most likely be contributing to her cardiovascular dysfunction?
   A. Vincristine, prednisone, etoposide, and radiation
   B. Doxorubicin and radiation
   C. Radiation, doxorubicin, and bleomycin
   D. Bleomycin and radiation

5. When do the late and long-term effects of cancer treatment begin?
   A. Long-term and late effects begin during treatment and extend beyond treatment completion
   B. Long-term effects begin immediately after cancer treatment, but late effects start years following completion of cancer treatment
   C. Long-term effects begin during cancer treatment and late effects arise months to years following completion of cancer treatment
   D. Long-term effects begin weeks to months following treatment whereas late effects begin months to years following treatment

A 54-year-old female is referred to physical therapy for right shoulder pain and right upper extremity lymphedema with a past medical history of stage III right breast cancer (ER+, PR+, HER2-) 2 years ago. She received neoadjuvant chemotherapy consisting of doxorubicin (Adriamycin), cyclophosphamide (Cytoxan), and paclitaxel (Taxol). She underwent a lumpectomy with 7 lymph nodes removed followed by radiation therapy. She reports that 3 weeks ago she sustained a burn to the lateral aspect of her right hand. She is currently taking the aromatase inhibitor letrozole (Femara). She presents to therapy with achiness in multiple joints, right shoulder pain, chest tightness with reaching, and weakness of the right upper extremity. Last week she noticed mild swelling of the right hand which is progressively worsening with no signs of erythema or pain.

6. What treatment regimen for her breast cancer is most likely the primary cause of her ongoing generalized joint achiness?
   A. Chemotherapy drugs
   B. Letrozole
   C. Radiation to the right upper quadrant
   D. Surgical intervention

7. Which of the following factors in combination present the highest risk of her development of lymphedema?
   A. Removal of 7 lymph nodes, radiation therapy, local burn
   B. Removal of 7 lymph nodes, radiation therapy, letrozole
   C. Doxorubicin, radiation therapy, local burn
   D. Doxorubicin, removal of 7 lymph nodes, local burn

8. What treatment technique is the top priority for this patient?
   A. Arm strengthening
   B. Modalities such as ultrasound and moist heat pack
   C. CDT
   D. Joint manipulation

9. When considering the differential diagnosis, the cause of chest pain could include all of the following EXCEPT:
   A. Doxorubicin
   B. Radiation therapy
   C. Cyclophosphamide
   D. Surgical intervention

10. According to Briggs, which palliative care practice pattern would be the most appropriate for this patient?
    A. Restorative
    B. Rehabilitation light
    C. Rehabilitation in reverse
    D. Supportive care

References

1. National Coalition for Cancer Survivorship. Our history. https://canceradvocacy.org/about/our-history/. Accessed February 7, 2021.
2. American Society of Clinical Oncology. Survivorship compendium. https://www.asco.org/practice-policy/cancer-care-initiatives/prevention-survivorship/survivorship/survivorship-compendium. Accessed February 7, 2021.
3. National Comprehensive Cancer Network. NCCN® guidelines version 2.2020. General survivorship principles. https://www.nccn.org/professionals/physician_gls/default.aspx#site; July 14, 2020. Accessed February 7, 2021.
4. Institute of Medicine and National Research Council. *Ensuring Quality Cancer Care*: National Academies Press; 1999.
5. National Academies of Sciences, Engineering, and Medicine. *Long-Term Survivorship Care After Cancer Treatment: Proceedings of a Workshop*: National Academies Press; 2018.
6. Stout NL, Binkley JM, Schmitz KH, et al. A prospective surveillance model for rehabilitation for women with breast cancer. *Cancer*. 2012;118:2191–2200.
7. American College of Surgeons. https://www.facs.org/quality-programs/cancer/coc. Accessed February 7, 2021.
8. Hewitt M, Greenfield S, Stovall S. *From Cancer Patient to Cancer Survivor: Lost in Transition*: National Academies Press; 2006.
9. Institute of Medicine. In: Adler N, Page A, Eds. Cancer Care for the Whole Patient: Meeting Psychosocial Health Needs. The National Academies Press; 2008.

10. Institute of Medicine. *Delivering High-Quality Cancer Care: Charting a New Course for a System in Crisis*: National Academies Press; 2013.

11. Colombo R, Wilson C. PRevention, Intervention, and Sustained Wellness Model (PRISM) care philosophy in cancer survivorship, palliative care, and chronic disease management in the era of healthcare reform: a perspective paper. *Rehabil Oncol.* 2015;33(2):45–51.

12. Blaes AH, Adamson PC, Foxhall L, Bhatia S. Survivorship care plans and the commission on cancer standards: the increasing need for better strategies to improve the outcome for survivors of cancer. *JCO Oncol Pract.* 2020;16(8):447–450.

13. Dietz JH Jr. Rehabilitation of the cancer patient. *Med Clin North Am.* 1969;53:607–624.

14. Dietz J. *Rehabilitation Oncology*: John Wiley & Sons; 1981.

15. Chowdhury RA, Brennan FP, Gardiner MD. Cancer rehabilitation and palliative care—exploring the synergies. *J Pain Symptom Manage.* 2020;60(6):1239–1252.

16. Briggs RW. Models for physical therapy practice in palliative medicine. *Rehabil Oncol.* 2000;18(2):18–19, 21.

17. American Physical Therapy Association. *Oncologic Description of Specialty Practice*: American Physical Therapy Association; 2017.

18. National Cancer Institute. Palliative care in cancer. https://www.cancer.gov/about-cancer/advanced-cancer/care-choices/palliative-care-fact-sheet; October 20, 2017. Accessed February 21, 2021.

19. Stout NL, Pfalzer LA, Springer B, et al. Breast cancer-related lymphedema: comparing direct costs of a prospective surveillance model and a traditional model of care. *Phys Ther.* 2012;92:152–163.

20. Stout NL, Silver JK, Alfano CM, Ness KK, Gilchrist LS. Long-term survivorship care after cancer treatment: a new emphasis on the role of rehabilitation services. *Phys Ther.* 2019;99:10–13.

21. Mayer DK. Using survivorship care plans to enhance communication and cancer care coordination: results of a pilot study. *Oncol Nurs Forum.* 2016;43(5):636–645.

22. Spears JA, Craft M, White S. Outcomes of cancer survivorship care provided by advanced practice RNs compared to other models of care: a systematic review. *Oncol Nurs Forum.* 2017;44(1):E34–E41.

23. National Comprehensive Cancer Network. Distress thermometer and problem list. https://www.nccn.org/about/permissions/thermometer.aspx. Accessed on February 21, 2021.

24. FACIT Group; 2020. https://www.facit.org/. Accessed on February 21, 2021.

25. Stubblefield MD. *Cancer Rehabilitation Principles and Practice* 2nd ed. Springer Publishing Company; 2019.

26. Cella DF, Tulsky DS, Gray G, et al. The functional assessment of cancer therapy (FACT) scale: development and validation of the general measure. *J Clin Oncol.* 1993;11(3):570–579.

27. Treanor C, Donnelly M. Late effects of cancer and cancer treatment: the perspective of a patient. *Support Care Cancer.* 2016;24:337–346.

28. Shapiro CL. Cancer survivorship. *N Engl J Med.* 2018;379:2438–2450.

29. Marchese VG, Morris S, Gilchrist L, et al. Screening for chemotherapy adverse late effects. *Top Geriatr Rehabil.* 2011;27(3):234–243.

30. World Health Organization. Childhood cancer. https://www.who.int/news-room/fact-sheets/detail/cancer-in-children; January 2021. Accessed May 10, 2021.

31. American Society of Clinical Oncology. Late effects of childhood cancer. https://www.cancer.net/navigating-cancer-care/children/late-effects-childhood-cancer; June 2019. Accessed February 2021.

32. Newton H, Friend A, et al. Survival from cancer in young people; an overview of late effects focusing on reproductive health. *Acta Obstet Gynecol Scand.* 2019;98:573–582.

33. Chao C, Bhatia S, Xu L, et al. Chronic comorbidities in survivors of AYA cancer. *J Clin Oncol.* 2020;38(27):3161–3174.

34. American Childhood Cancer Organization. About the most common types of childhood cancer. https://www.acco.org/blog/about-the-most-common-types-of-childhood-cancers/; January 2021. Accessed May 10, 2021.

35. American Childhood Cancer Organization. US childhood cancer statistics. https://www.acco.org/us-childhood-cancer-statistics/; January 2021. Accessed May 10, 2021.

36. Children's Oncology Group. Long-term follow-up guidelines for survivors of childhood, adolescent, and young adult cancers. https://www.childrensoncologygroup.org/index.php/research-257/survivorship-guidelines. Accessed May 10, 2021.

37. Landier W, Armenian S, Bhatia S, et al. Late effects of childhood cancer and its treatment. *Pediatr Clin N Am.* 2015;62:275–300.

38. Ness KK, Armenian SH, Kadan-Lottick N, Gurney JG. Adverse effects of treatment in childhood acute lymphoblastic leukemia: general overview and implications for long-term cardiac health. *Expert Rev Hematol.* 2011;4(2):185–197.

39. Marriott CJC, Beaumont LF, Farncombe TH, et al. Body composition in long-term survivors of acute lymphoblastic leukemia diagnosed in childhood and adolescence: a focus on sarcopenic obesity. *Cancer.* 2018;124(6):1225–1231.

40. Wei C, Thyagarajan MS, Hunt LP, Shield JP, Stevens MC, Crowne EC. Reduced insulin sensitivity in childhood survivors of hematopoietic stem cell transplantation is associated with lipodystropic and sarcopenic phenotypes. *Pediatr Blood Cancer.* 2015;62(11):1992–1999.

41. Gruzdeva O, Borodkina D, Uchasova E, Deyleva Y, Barbarash O. Localization of fat depots and cardiovascular risk. *Lipids Health Dis.* 2018;17:218. doi:10.1186/s12944-018-0856-8.

42. Vargo MM. Brain tumors and metastasis. *Phys Med Rehabil Clin N Am.* 2017;28:115–141.

43. Merchant TE, Pollack IF, Loeffler JS. Brain tumors across the age spectrum: biology, therapy and late effects. *Semin Radiat Oncol.* 2010;20(1):58–66.

44. Han T, Gleeson H. Long-term and late treatment consequences: endocrine and metabolic effects. *Curr Opin Support Palliat Care.* 2017;11:205–213.

45. Ng A, Leeuwen FE. Hodgkin lymphoma; late effects of treatment and guidelines for surveillance. *Semin Hematol.* 2016;53(3):209–215.

46. Cancer Connect. Declining risk of AML after Hodgkin's lymphoma. https://news.cancerconnect.com/hodgkins-lymphoma/declining-risk-of-aml-after-hodgkin-s-lymphoma-ZQ3I7CP-h0etDW-geX3hPmA. March 8, 2009. Accessed February 2021.

47. Schonfeld SJ, Gilbert ES, Dores GM, et al. Acute myeloid leukemia following Hodgkin lymphoma: a population-based study of 35,511 patients. *J Nat Cancer Inst.* 2006;98:215–218.

48. McGowan JV, Chung R, Maulik A, Piotrowska I, Walker M, Yellon D. Anthracycline chemotherapy and cardiotoxicity. *Cardiovasc Drugs Ther.* 2017;31:63–75.

49. Reinert T, Baldotto C, Nunes F, Scheliga A. Bleomycin induced lung injury. *J Cancer Res Clin Oncol.* 2013;480608:1–9. doi:10.1155/2013/480608.

50. Quigg TC, Kim YJ, Goebel WS, Haut PR. Lung function before and after pediatric allogeneic hematopoietic stem cell transplantation: a predictive role for DLCOa/VA. *J Pediatr Hematol Oncol.* 2012;34(4):304–309.

51. Krull KR, Hardy KK, Kahalley LS, Schuitema I, Kesler SR. Neurocognitive outcomes and interventions in long-term survivors of childhood cancer. *J Clin Oncol.* 2018;36(21):2181–2189.

52. Riggs L, Piscione J, Laughlin S, et al. Exercise training for neural recovery in a restricted sample of pediatric brain tumor survivors: a controlled clinical trial with crossover of training versus no training. *Neuro Oncol.* 2017;19(3):440–450.

53. Landier W, Skinner R, Wallace WH, et al. Surveillance for late effects in childhood cancer survivors. *J Clin Oncol.* 2018;36(21):2216–2222.

54. Kenyon M, Mayer DK, Owens AK. Late and long-term effects of breast cancer treatment and surveillance management for the general practitioner. *J Obstet Gynecol Neonatal Nurs.* 2014;43:382–398.

55. Brown JC, Winters-Stone K, Lee A, Schmitz KH. Cancer, physical activity and exercise. *Compr Physiol.* 2012;2(4):2775–2809.

56. Okwousa TM, Anzevino S, Rao R. Cardiovascular disease in cancer survivors. *Postgrad Med J.* 2017;93:82–90.

57. Canadian Cancer Society. Managing adverse effects: radiation pneumonitis. https://www.cancer.ca/en/cancer-information/diagnosis-and-treatment/managing-side-effects/radiation-pneumonitis/?region=on. Accessed on March 7, 2021.

58. Abid SH, Malhotra V, Perry MC. Radiation-induced and chemotherapy-induced pulmonary injury. *Curr Opin Oncol.* 2001;13:242–248.

59. Shah RR. Tyrosine kinase inhibitor-induced interstitial lung disease: clinical features, diagnostic challenges and therapeutic dilemmas. *Drug Saf.* 2016;39:1073–1091.

60. American Cancer Society. Hormone therapy for breast cancer. https://www.cancer.org/cancer/breast-cancer/treatment/hormone-therapy-for-breast-cancer.html. Accessed on March 7, 2021.

61. Andrews S, von Gruenigen VE. Management of the late effects of treatments for gynecological. *Cancer Curr Opin Oncol.* 2013;25:566–570.

62. Dong Y, Ridge JA, Li T, Lango MN, Churilla TM, Bauman JR. Long term toxicities in 10-year survivors of radiation treatments for head and neck cancer. *Oral Oncol.* 2017;71:122–128.

63. Ahles TA, James C, Root JC. Cognitive effects of cancer and cancer treatments. *Annu Rev Clin Psychol.* 2018;14:425–451.

64. American College of Sports Medicine. *Trending Topic: Physical Activity Guidelines*: American College of Sports Medicine; 2021. https://www.acsm.org/read-research/trending-topics-resource-pages/physical-activity-guidelines. Accessed May 9, 2022.

65. Inscore E, Litterini A. *Academy of Oncologic Physical Therapy EDGE Task Force Report Summaries*: APTA Oncology; 2021. https://oncologypt.org/wp-content/uploads/2019/10/EDGE-Annotated-Bibliography-8.19-update.pdf. Accessed May 9.

66. Khan F, Amatya B, Ng L, Demetrios M, Zhang NY, Turner-Stokes L. Multidisciplinary rehabilitation for follow-up of women treated for breast cancer. *Cochrane Database Syst Rev.* 2012;12:CD009553. doi:10.1002/14651858.CD009553.pub2.

67. Scott DA, Mills M, Black A, et al. Multidimensional rehabilitation programmes for adult cancer survivors. *Cochrane Database Syst Rev.* 2013;3:CD007730. doi:10.1002/14651858.CD007730.pub2.

68. Hill RE, Wakefield CE, Cohn RJ, et al. Survivorship care plans in cancer: a meta-analysis and systematic review of care plan outcomes. *Oncologist.* 2020;25:e351–e372.

29

Palliative and End of Life Care

CHRISTOPHER M. WILSON, PT, DPT, DScPT, BOARD CERTIFIED GERIATRIC PHYSICAL THERAPIST

CHAPTER OUTLINE

Cancer Remains a Terminal Illness for Some

Despite the best efforts and advances in cancer care and treatment, some cancers will remain undetected until an advanced stage or will be unresponsive to conventional treatments. In these circumstances, individuals will experience increasing challenges to staying healthy and functional, particularly as their disease process advances. This may also occur if their cancer treatments are progressively taxing on their physiologic systems.

While very few oncology rehabilitation (Onc R) clinicians chose their profession with the initial intention to provide care for individuals with a life-limiting illness, it can be a very rewarding and essential component of Onc R practice.[1] Although palliative care (PC) and hospice care philosophies evolved out of necessity based on the care needs of people with a terminal illness, it also behooves the Onc R clinician who integrates into PC or hospice interdisciplinary team PC or hospice interdisciplinary team (IDT)

to understand how that team collectively manages the care of persons with other advanced life-limiting or chronic diseases besides cancer. These individuals will invariably experience exacerbations and remissions in their disease process and subsequent functional decline—all conditions that are often amenable to improvement or mitigation by the Onc R clinician. Finally, essential components of caring for those with a terminal illness are the concepts of a good death and death with dignity. Again, Onc R professionals can utilize their skillsets to reduce pain, improve remaining function, and optimize quality of life (QOL) to assist individuals to live until the end of life (EOL) on their terms.[2] This can only occur if the clinician has the unique skills and knowledge that this chapter will impart.

The Palliative Care Philosophy and Approach

Since human beings have developed civilizations, they have dedicated substantial resources, knowledge, and skills toward caring for

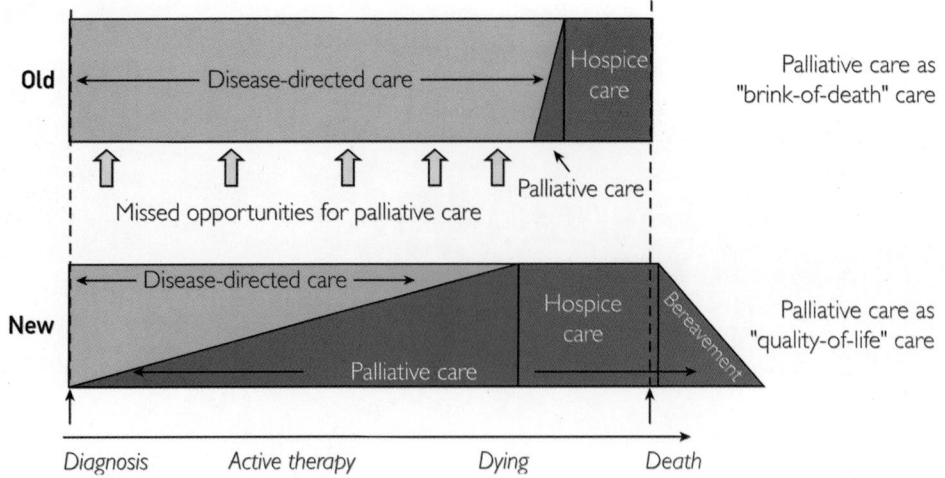

• **Fig. 29.1** Benefits of Early Implementation of Palliative Care.[6] (Reprinted with permission from Buss MK, Rock LK, McCarthy EP. Understanding palliative care and hospice: a review for primary care providers. *Mayo Clin Proc.* 2017;92(2):280–286.)

those at or near death. This may be, in part, due to the inevitability of death for every person. PC is a medical specialty aimed at meeting the unique holistic needs of persons with advanced or life-threatening diseases. PC focuses on improving the QOL of persons with cancer (PWCs) and their families by providing relief from severe disease symptoms and easing the psychosocial burden at any stage of the disease continuum. In general, PC is ideally aimed at the early stages of disease alongside curative treatment but should be under consideration once symptoms begin to affect functional performance.

The World Health Organization defines PC as an "approach that improves QOL for patients and families facing life-threatening illness."[3] The definition emphasizes its applicability early in the course of a disease and that it can be provided concurrently with other curative (e.g., radiation, surgery, chemotherapy) or rehabilitative treatments. A key focus of PC is preventing or facilitating relief from suffering from sources such as physical, psychosocial, or spiritual pain.[3] PC is often perceived as a spectrum of care starting with a minimal role during curative treatment attempts through its primary aim during hospice services occurs at the EOL. Due to the patient-centered approach of PC, it is also applicable for individuals with incurable chronic diseases (e.g., history of stroke, chronic kidney disease) who are not considered to have a terminal illness but would benefit from the aforementioned holistic, patient-centered approach.[4] Since 2000, there has been a rapid proliferation of PC programs, in part due to the improvements in QOL afforded by this clinical approach, as well as the potential cost savings to the healthcare system.[5] Unfortunately, because of misconceptions related to PC's role and services, PC is often not initiated early enough to improve QOL significantly but is instead used as "brink-of-death" or prehospice care. In contrast, if started earlier, it would likely have a more substantive impact on a person's wellbeing and symptom burden (Figure 29.1).[7,8]

To facilitate these improvements to symptoms and QOL, Onc R clinicians should strive to consider the entire disease trajectory and what interventions can assist the PWC's immediate issues and prepare them for future needs. See Figure 29.2 for a staging system to assist in considering the disease trajectory and some clinical implications.

The Differences Between Palliative Care and Hospice Services

One of the critical challenges to understanding and working with persons with advanced or terminal cancer toward the EOL is

understanding the key differences between PC and hospice care (Table 29.1). A common misconception among laypersons and some healthcare professionals is that the terms are equivalent, and while they have similar philosophies, there are several differences in administration and treatment approaches. In the United States (US), a crucial difference between PC and hospice is that in hospice a person must have a life expectancy of less than 6 months, but with PC, there is no specific limitation on life expectancy. In many other areas of the world, the term hospice frequently refers to a building or location where PC or EOL care is provided (i.e., the person receives PC in a hospice facility). An Onc R clinician providing care and support to an individual with a terminal illness needs to understand the similarities and differences between PC and hospice as it relates to payment and regulatory structures. As this payment methodology varies by nation, this description will highlight the US payment system.

Within the US Medicare system, the payment methodology remains the same for PC with the traditional Medicare Part A or B conventions (including payment for rehabilitation services). However, Medicare's payment methodology for hospice services is via a *per diem* rate (a set amount of money provided to the agency per day). In 2016 the US Centers for Medicare and Medicaid Services (CMS) modernized the hospice service payment methodologies. This established a two-tiered payment model where hospice agencies will be paid a higher rate for the first 60 days of hospice care and a lower rate for subsequent days in hospice care. As of 2021, the per diem rate for routine hospice care is $199 for the first 60 days of care and then adjusts to $157 for any remaining days.[8] In addition, CMS established a service intensity add-on payment to account for patients receiving visits conducted by a nurse or social worker during the week of life before death when more intensive services are needed.[9]

A key consideration in this *per diem* is that it is used to cover all services (such as rehabilitation) that are necessarily administered during hospice care. The hospice agency does not receive more funds to pay for Onc R services but would come out of the per diem. This factor makes the administration of ongoing intensive rehabilitation more challenging (but not impossible) in the hospice setting. It is up to the IDT to determine the needs of the person, including Onc R needs. Although Onc R clinicians are not defined as a "core" team member, their participation in the IDT remains essential to assure appropriate utilization of these services.

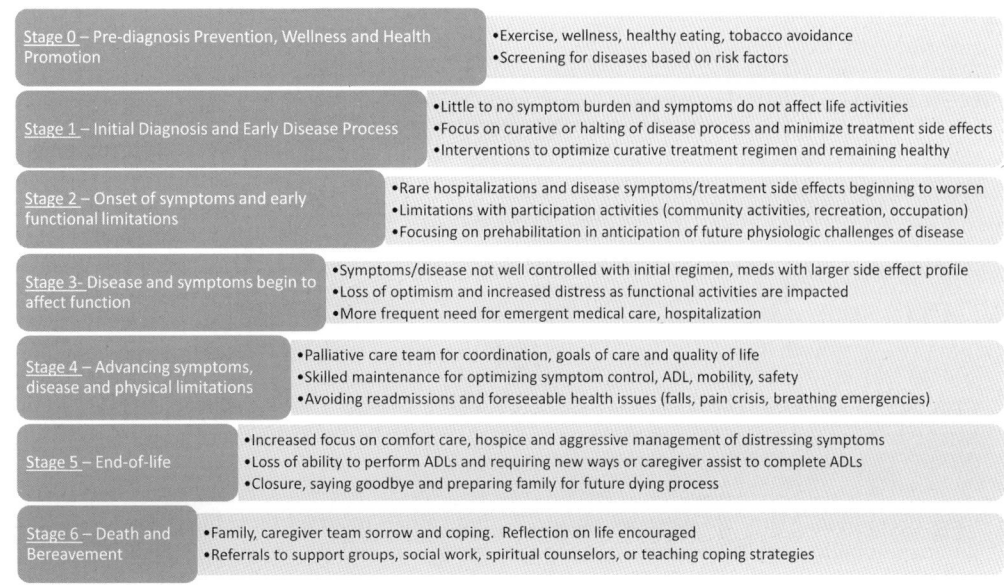

Stage 0 – Pre-diagnosis Prevention, Wellness and Health Promotion
- Exercise, wellness, healthy eating, tobacco avoidance
- Screening for diseases based on risk factors

Stage 1 – Initial Diagnosis and Early Disease Process
- Little to no symptom burden and symptoms do not affect life activities
- Focus on curative or halting of disease process and minimize treatment side effects
- Interventions to optimize curative treatment regimen and remaining healthy

Stage 2 – Onset of symptoms and early functional limitations
- Rare hospitalizations and disease symptoms/treatment side effects beginning to worsen
- Limitations with participation activities (community activities, recreation, occupation)
- Focusing on prehabilitation in anticipation of future physiologic challenges of disease

Stage 3- Disease and symptoms begin to affect function
- Symptoms/disease not well controlled with initial regimen, meds with larger side effect profile
- Loss of optimism and increased distress as functional activities are impacted
- More frequent need for emergent medical care, hospitalization

Stage 4 – Advancing symptoms, disease and physical limitations
- Palliative care team for coordination, goals of care and quality of life
- Skilled maintenance for optimizing symptom control, ADL, mobility, safety
- Avoiding readmissions and foreseeable health issues (falls, pain crisis, breathing emergencies)

Stage 5 – End-of-life
- Increased focus on comfort care, hospice and aggressive management of distressing symptoms
- Loss of ability to perform ADLs and requiring new ways or caregiver assist to complete ADLs
- Closure, saying goodbye and preparing family for future dying process

Stage 6 – Death and Bereavement
- Family, caregiver team sorrow and coping. Reflection on life encouraged
- Referrals to support groups, social work, spiritual counselors, or teaching coping strategies

• **Fig. 29.2** Stages of Disease Progression. *ADLs*, Activities of daily living. (Reprinted with permission from Litterini A, Wilson CM. *Physical Activity and Rehabilitation in Life Threatening Illness*. Routledge; 2021.)

TABLE 29.1 Differences Between Hospice and Palliative Care Payment Systems in the United States

Hospice	Palliative Care
• Covered under a separate hospice benefit • Hospice receives ~$199 per day flat rate (called a per diem rate) • Pay nurses, drugs, therapy, and equipment out of the same $199 • Care for unrelated conditions will still come out of the PWC's traditional medical insurance	• Covered under traditional Medicare inpatient or outpatient insurance regulations • Same OASIS, IPR Care Item Set, or conventional insurance (e.g., Medicare part A or B) therapy rules apply • Skilled maintenance codes may be utilized • PT must be homebound to receive homecare services

IPR, Inpatient rehabilitation; *OASIS*, Outcome and Assessment Information Set.
Created by Chris Wilson, PT, DPT, DScPT. Printed with permission.

An example depicting this is shown in eFigure 29.1. One exception to this is that if the Onc R service is needed for a condition outside of the expected scope of the terminal diagnosis, it may be covered under the PWC's "non-hospice" health insurance.[10] An example is a person enrolled in hospice with a diagnosis of Stage IV lung cancer who sustains an ankle sprain and requires outpatient rehabilitation; these services would likely be covered by the PWC's conventional rehabilitation benefit as opposed to the hospice benefit. A proactive consultation with the person's insurance company is highly recommended when exploring the provision of these services to avoid delays or denials in insurance payment.

To optimize the quality of remaining life while concurrently containing healthcare costs, PC should focus on avoiding unwarranted or avoidable medical care or hospitalizations. For example, near the EOL, 74% of individuals with a life-threatening disease preferred not to spend their remaining time in a hospital.[11] Yet 50% of people will visit an emergency room 30 days before death and 75% will visit in the 6 months preceding death.[12] In addition, a substantial amount of healthcare costs over a lifetime are spent at the EOL. In 2010, Medicare beneficiaries incurred 25% of their costs in the year preceding death.[13] See Figure 29.3 for a visual depiction of healthcare cost expenditures over a lifespan.

Studies have shown that PC improves outcomes for families, as well as the PWC themselves. Caregivers of persons receiving PC were shown to have a better QOL, experienced less regret, and demonstrated improvements in physical and mental health.[14] When compared to dying at home with hospice, dying in a hospital is associated with a nine fold increased risk of prolonged grief disorder in caregivers. In addition, dying in an intensive care unit was associated with a five fold increased risk of post-traumatic stress disorder (PTSD) in caregivers.[15]

A key benefit to a PC approach is that it concurrently improves outcomes and contains costs. In a study of 151 persons with lung cancer, patients were randomized to usual care (without PC) versus those who received a PC consultation. Compared to usual care, persons receiving PC had less depression, fewer unwarranted tests, fewer invasive treatments, had better QOL, and lived an average of 11 weeks longer.[16] One of the voiced concerns of patients, families, and caregivers is that PC will speed an unhindered dying process; however, there is evidence that palliative symptom management does not shorten life.[17]

As an Onc R clinician integrating into a PC team, one of the challenges is determining a lifespan prognosis and a functional prognosis within that lifespan prediction. This is especially important as Onc R clinicians are often requested to provide input on

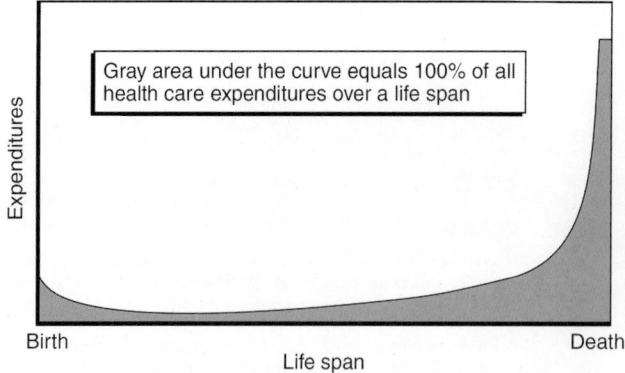

Gray area under the curve equals 100% of all health care expenditures over a life span

Expenditures

Birth

Life span

Death

• **Fig. 29.3** Americans' current Health care Expenditures are Concentrated in the Final Part of the Life Span. (Lynn J, Adamson DM. *Living Well at the End of Life*. RAND Corporation; 2003. Reprinted with permission.)

home safety and discharge disposition. Many late-stage diseases are characterized by significant morbidity and fluctuations in symptoms from a disease or its treatments, making the prognostication of functional decline more challenging. Also, these individuals experience an increasing rate of hospitalization with an advancing disease process. This results in a cycle of hospitalization, discharge to a rehabilitation facility, and then hopefully back home before another exacerbation with a resultant readmission starts the cycle again. Breaking this cycle is a key goal of PC (and Onc R within PC) as this cycle is detrimental to the person's QOL and also results in a significant increase in care and associated treatment costs.[18]

As the goal of PC is to have a "big picture," holistic approach toward patient management, a PC specialist will evaluate and address the patient/family's emotional and psychosocial status while also focusing on the overall disease trajectory. A primary focus of the PC IDT is symptom management in coordination with other specialists' curative management. Additional concerns include evaluating and addressing the goals of care, advance care planning (ACP), and discussing *do not resuscitate* (DNR) preferences. During the specialist training in PC, practitioners receive education on how to proactively address suffering and symptoms. PC specialists also address the distress of chronic illness including physical, emotional, spiritual, and practical sources of this distress. A key goal is to partner with PWCs and families to achieve *their* hopes within the context of the medical reality. An essential skill of a PC provider is to provide communication that illuminates the "big picture." This will empower PWCs and families to clarify their goals, values, and wishes, and recognize how they may be enhanced or diminished by any future treatments. Finally, an important role of the PC team member is to coordinate care with the aim of assisting these individuals and their families with transitions—especially to hospice, as treatment options become recognized as futile and the benefits of more comfort-focused care are apparent.

Burden of Chronic Diseases

As of 2014, about 60% of all adults in the US were living with at least one chronic health condition and 42% of adults had two or more chronic health conditions.[19] Seven of the top ten causes of death in 2014 were chronic diseases.[20] Two of these chronic diseases—heart disease and cancer—together accounted for nearly half of all deaths.[20] Five percent of the sickest Medicare beneficiaries account for approximately half of all healthcare spending in the US. Also, most people with serious illnesses have high healthcare costs over an extended period[21]; only 11% of terminally ill

individuals incurred these high costs in the last year of life.[22] For the 5% of individuals with the highest costs, approximately 40% of them incur high costs for several years and are affected by multiple comorbidities, hospitalizations, functional impairments, or cognitive impairments, all of which increase the cost and reduce QOL.[21–23] As much of the healthcare costs are focused on a small percentage of the population, even minor systematic improvements in the management of those with advanced disease can be reflected in large improvements in cost savings as well as QOL. To accomplish this goal, a well-trained and organized IDT is needed to clarify realistic, patient-centered goals of care, and work together cohesively toward those care goals.

Integrating With the PC Team

PC is a consultative service similar to many other medical specialties within the hospital setting. In home care or ambulatory/outpatient settings, an agency may be providing community PC services, often branded with a program name to differentiate it from conventional home care or outpatient services. There are several similarities between the composition and roles of the cancer IDT members described in Chapter 2 to the PC IDT; however, the PC team's focus is often more holistic and symptom-driven. In these advanced cases, the focus will shift away from curative care toward optimization of QOL and expert symptom management. IDT members often include attending physicians, PC specialists (physicians and mid-level providers such as physician assistants or nurse practitioners), social workers, nurse case managers, occupational therapists (OTs), physical therapists (PTs), pastoral care professionals/clergy, and most importantly, the PWC and their family/caregivers. In some larger institutions, it may be beneficial to designate a "lead" therapist to coordinate care with other therapists and represent the Onc R disciplines among the PC team.

Home Palliative Care Services

Many home care agencies have established a PC service in partnership with local hospitals to provide proactive symptom management and prevent unwarranted readmissions. These PC homecare programs are specialty programs within a home healthcare agency (like wound care or pediatrics programs). In general, these programs are designed for people that are not yet ready or perhaps not yet eligible for hospice care. As with any other home care services, payment and regulatory issues still apply including the requirement that a person

The Medicare Coverage Criteria for home care patients indicates that:
- The patient must be homebound.
- Leaving the home requires a considerable and taxing effort.
- Absences from home for medical reasons are allowed and nonmedical reasons are allowed if infrequent for short periods of time.
- There is a normal inability to leave home without assistance.
- The person does not need to be confined to bed.

be homebound. As with PC in general, curative treatments can continue in the home setting but must be able to be administered in the home or via transportation services. See Box 29.1 for Medicare criteria for homebound status to be eligible to receive home healthcare services.[24]

The Process of Advance Care Planning

As PC services are aimed at clarifying and directing care toward the person's goals and wishes, a foundational concept is that of ACP. ACP "enables individuals to define goals and preferences for future medical treatment and care, to discuss these goals and preferences with family and health care providers, and to record and review these preferences if appropriate."[25,p546] See Box 29.2 for the extended definition of ACP.

The ACP conversation is often initiated by a specialist and will often revolve around the person's and family's wishes and further clarify the medical realities of the situation. As can be imagined, these conversations are often difficult and wrought with emotion. If these conversations and decisions do not occur, it may result in unclear care goals, unnecessary or painful tests or procedures, or attempts at lifesaving interventions that have little to no chance of success. After these discussions occur, decisions are documented as an advance care directive. This is usually a standardized form that will have clear documentation of the wishes of the PWC, their family members, and an ACP specialist or physician. The advance directive documentation often includes whether cardiopulmonary resuscitation should be initiated in the event of a life-threatening emergency or whether the person wishes for nature to take its course —often termed a DNR status. Additional components include whether the individual wishes to have various medical interventions such as mechanical ventilation and if they become unable to voice their own medical decisions, who would be the designated person to carry out their wishes. The best practice is for the PWC to have a series of thorough discussions with the decision-maker (often a

close family member or friend) as to what they wish in the event of various scenarios. This will assist in reducing uncertainty and guilt if the designated person must try to guess what their loved one might have wished in a specific scenario.

One key challenge to ACP is that historically the documentation of the person's wishes was often only confined to one health system, or in some cases, only applicable for one hospitalization or stay. The administrative barriers to transferability of the ACP documentation are currently being addressed by a variety of means with the goal that if a person has a documented ACP, it will be legally binding and upheld at any time or in any location. In some locales, this is being completed via jurisdictional, statewide, or national legislation for a universal advance care directive document that is applicable in any healthcare setting. Within the US, a national movement called Physician Orders for Life-Sustaining Treatment (POLST): Portable Medical Orders aims to translate an individual's choices into a group of actionable medical orders and is incorporated in some capacity throughout all 50 states within the US.[26] A second initiative called Respecting Choices is a collaborative effort between healthcare institutions in La Crosse, Wisconsin, and is also gaining momentum in additional regions of the nation. As with POLST, the Respecting Choices initiative is aimed at advance directives being recognized by all healthcare practitioners in the community and region.[27]

Although Onc R clinicians are not often the individuals who have these formal key discussions on ACP, as a trusted healthcare professional this topic may come up during patient care procedures.[28] Onc R clinicians should have knowledge of their institutions' processes for establishing an advance directive and should be able to speak to the ACP process if this topic arises. A PWC may also ask the Onc R clinician's opinion regarding various aspects of the ACP process, including what effect this may have on rehabilitation efforts. Realistic information should be consistently provided about the person's rehabilitation potential within the context of the disease trajectory and situation.[28] If the Onc R clinician determines that the rehabilitation process may be extensive, painful, or unlikely to be effective, this should be gently but clearly stated o allow the person make informed choices regarding any future care. It should also be clarified that the PWC may continue to participate in rehabilitation or receive other treatments (e.g., chemotherapy, radiation) even if they change their code status to DNR (with the exception of enrolling in hospice services as described previously). Finally, as medical emergencies such as cardiac arrest may occur during rehabilitation interventions, the Onc R clinician must understand the person's wishes to know whether to call emergency services or not, depending on the person's DNR status. Even if the person has a DNR in place, prompt notification of the individual's nurse or physician remains important to assure that procedures are being followed per the person's wishes.

"Advance care planning enables individuals who have decisional capacity to identify their values, to reflect upon the meanings and consequences of serious illness scenarios, to define goals and preferences for future medical treatment and care, and to discuss these with family and health care providers. ACP addresses individuals' concerns across the physical, psychological, social, and spiritual domains. It encourages individuals to identify a personal representative and to record and regularly review any preferences, so that their preferences can be taken into account should they, at some point, be unable to make their own decisions."

Rehabilitation in Palliative and End of Life Care

Rehabilitation services within PC have gained substantial momentum and growth concurrently with the institutional growth of PC programs. This was not the case in the past, as historically a person might not have received extensive rehabilitation services in the presence of significantly advanced cancer. Onc R clinicians should strive to modify their clinical practice to achieve these key goals of improved care continuity and communication.

The Role of the Onc R Clinician in Palliative Care and End of Life

Many foundational rehabilitation concepts are applicable in PC, but there are some differences as well. In two studies published in 2017[1] and expanded upon in 2020,[2] PTs were interviewed who provided care for those with life-threatening or terminal illnesses from 10 different nations that had PC services highly integrated into their national medical system. From these studies, a conceptual framework was developed to assist in the operationalization and role clarification of PC clinicians. Although the research study focused on PT practice, Figure 29.4 has applicability for a variety of rehabilitation professions within PC.

Within the large oval at the top are the roles of the Onc R clinician in patient/family management, as an IDT member, and their professional responsibilities. In the bi-directional arrow are the considerations for Onc R clinician services along the disease continuum from initial diagnosis through the end of life, with the aim of optimizing QOL and facilitating a *good death*. The concept of a good death is highly individualized but generally involves the person finding satisfaction in the remaining part of life with dignity, comfort being surrounded by loved ones, engaging in enjoyable activities, and living in a preferred location such as their home. Within the box below are numerous influences on rehabilitation participation in PC, including internal factors such as the clinician's perceptions of their role in PC and EOL care and external factors such as payment, administrative, and governmental factors.

Physical Therapist (PT) Quote Related to the PT's role in PC[1]

"Patient and family quality of life, I have always defined my interventions—safety first; second, comfort; and third, mobility. Safety for the patient and caregiver, then comfort issues—pain, edema, dyspnea, and third is mobility. How are they with driving, doing transfers, mobility? I have often felt safety has to be what drives what I do. The worst thing is having a patient fall and fracture a hip or be hospitalized and in more pain or family members injure themselves when caring for a loved one. It creates so much unneeded stress and discord at end of life."

As there are often multiple interacting clinical factors for a PWC, Onc R clinicians must carefully weigh which of those should be prioritized during their care delivery. Box 29.3 illustrates considerations for prioritization of rehabilitation in PC, with safety being a high priority, followed closely by optimizing QOL. Often in traditional (non-PC) rehabilitation, there is a consideration for temporarily inducing discomfort or fatigue to rebuild the body stronger, however, this *no pain, no gain* philosophy should be carefully considered and used very judiciously in PC rehabilitation as the primary emphasis should always be focusing on QOL. If the intervention risks outweigh the person's immediate or long-term QOL outcomes, then alternatives to that intervention would be warranted. Such a model to consider is the *no pain —> gain* approach (e.g., devising a treatment approach where pain is not induced, yet through some effort, gains can be achieved).

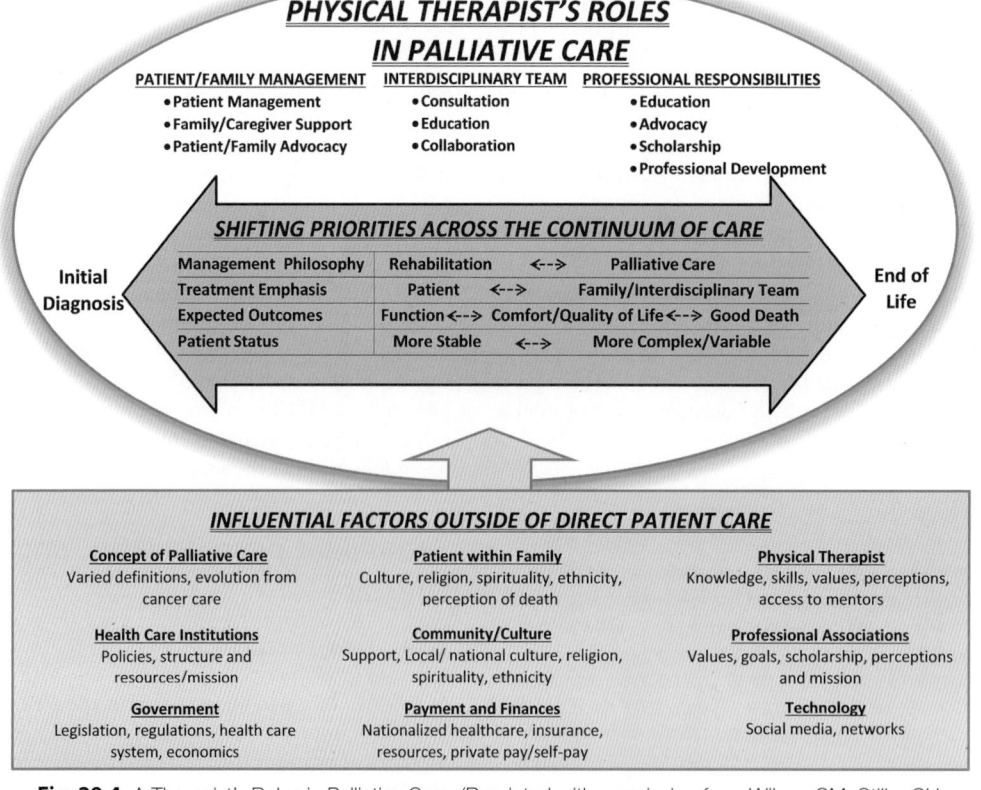

● **Fig. 29.4** A Therapist's Roles in Palliative Care. (Reprinted with permission from Wilson CM, Stiller CH, Doherty DJ, et al. Physical therapists in integrated palliative care: a qualitative study. *BMJ Support Palliat Care.* 2022;12(e1):e59–e67. doi:10.1136/bmjspcare-2019-002161.)

Professional Roles Within Palliative Care and End of Life Care

Despite the value of potential rehabilitation interventions, several barriers may prevent or limit the integration of Onc R clinicians into the interdisciplinary HPC team. At the policy level, the most significant challenge may lie in section 481.64 of Medicare's *Conditions of Participation* (COP*) In Hospice.*[29] Within the "core services" section of this document, essential disciplines that every person in hospice must receive are identified. Onc R clinicians, such as PTs, OTs, or speech-language pathologists (SLPs) are not identified as members of the core IDT. This omission may be due in part to the perception that rehabilitation services are not frequently employed in palliative situations, rather are consistently employed to facilitate the improvement of function. Despite these professionals not being defined as mandatory, their services remain circumstantially essential, and their level of involvement is left to the autonomy of the IDT. In 2008, the Medicare hospice COP was updated to include section 418.72: *Condition of Participation: Physical Therapy, Occupational Therapy and Speech-Language Pathology.*[30] This section states that PT, OT and SLP "services must be available, and when provided, offered in a manner consistent with accepted standards of practice." Unfortunately, the term "made available" is not clearly defined and therefore open for interpretation, often resulting in very limited utilization of these services within hospice. This update does identify the comprehensive assessment skills of Onc R clinicians which enhance the IDT and should be included for a complete and accurate picture of a person's needs. Referrals for Onc R services are left to the IDT or their referring physicians, neither of whom may be aware of the scope of services that can be provided by these professionals, thus the importance of rehabilitation representation at IDT meetings for care planning and decision making. Furthermore, advocacy efforts should include reducing administrative barriers to therapy evaluations, such as establishing automatic or standing orders when indicated by the person's condition.

One of the key challenges for Onc R clinicians working with individuals at the EOL is the common perception that persons could not receive Onc R services if they did not demonstrate improvement or demonstrate the capacity for improvement. If the Onc R clinician were to administer rehabilitation services and the PWC did not demonstrate improvement, then there was a perceived risk of being denied payment for these services by the PWC's insurance company. One landmark settlement helped to dissuade this common dilemma. In 2014, *Jimmo vs. Sebelius* was a US Federal Court settlement that clarified the prevalent misperception that patients are not eligible for skilled care such as rehabilitation or nursing unless their condition was amenable to improvement.[31] As most insurance companies, inclusive of Medicare, utilize clinical documentation to establish medical necessity, to assure the provision of skilled services, and to assess for reasonable and customary services, the provider's clinical documentation is critical in these cases. In the past, Onc R clinicians were often discouraged by mentors and colleagues to avoid using "red flag" words such as *stable, maintenance,* or *declining* as these terms might indicate that the clinician's services might be futile or not medically necessary, therefore risking an insurance denial. The clinical documentation must justify why the Onc R clinician's skill was required to slow physical decline or maintain safe functional performance. Under the Medicare Hospice Benefit, the expectation of functional improvement is not required so skilled rehabilitation services to achieve care-appropriate goals can more easily be provided. See Box 29.4 for some useful key phrases to include in the clinical documentation for these circumstances.

As an individual with an advancing disease such as cancer faces more frequent hospital readmissions, multiple co morbidities, and declining function, they would benefit from the expert, proactive care coordination offered by the PC team. Also, these individuals would benefit from conversations related to EOL planning in anticipation of the expected and unexpected events that may occur. For the individual with a life-limiting illness such as advanced cancer, each Onc R discipline has an opportunity to apply their unique skills to improve QOL, including recreation therapy, exercise specialists, nurses, and rehabilitation physicians. The three most common rehabilitation disciplines—PTs, OTs, and SLPs all have unique contributions to the rehabilitation continuum of a person with advanced cancer and will be described below in more detail.

Physical Therapy

In 2011, the American Physical Therapy Association (APTA) established a position statement regarding the role of PTs within PC and EOL via unanimous endorsement through the APTA House of Delegates.[32] The position emphasized the importance of continuity of care and the active, compassionate role of PTs and physical therapist assistants (PTAs), as well as emphasizing "the rights of all individuals to have appropriate and adequate access to PT services regardless of medical prognosis or setting."[32] In addition, a key aspect was also related to the therapists' being integrated into the IDT to avoid delays in involvement by the PT/PTA, especially during transitions of care or during a physical or medical change in status. Advancement in this area would be achieved by educating PTs, PTAs, and students in the concepts related to treating an individual while in hospice and PC. Finally, the APTA advocated for fair and adequate payment structures for PT services.

To further enshrine this concept within PT care, in 2015, the APTA House of Delegates amended its principle on the Delivery of Value-Based Physical Therapist Services to clarify the definition of medical necessity to include that PT services may be necessary to "maintain the current level of function or to prevent, minimize, maintain, slow the decline of, or eliminate impairments, activity limitations, or participation restrictions."[33]

Occupational Therapy

The American Occupational Therapy Association (AOTA) emphasizes the role of OTs within PC and has established a Fact Sheet to discuss key contributions of OTs.[34] These include the OTs' role in optimization of activities of daily living (ADLs) such as dressing, bathing/showering, functional mobility, and safety, as well as addressing instrumental ADLs such as meal preparation, home

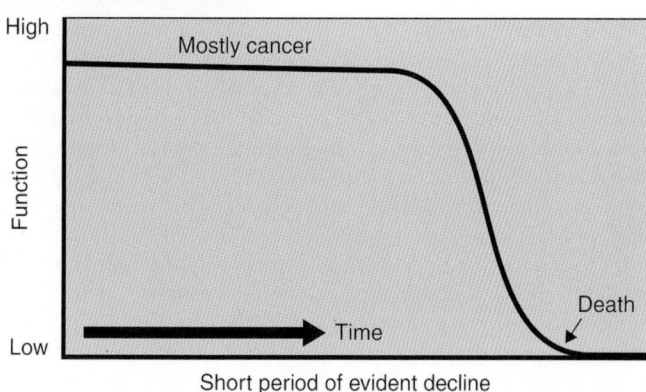

Short period of evident decline

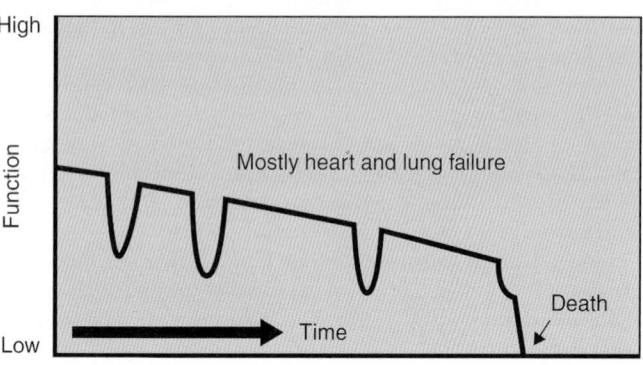

Long-term limitations with intermittent serious episodes

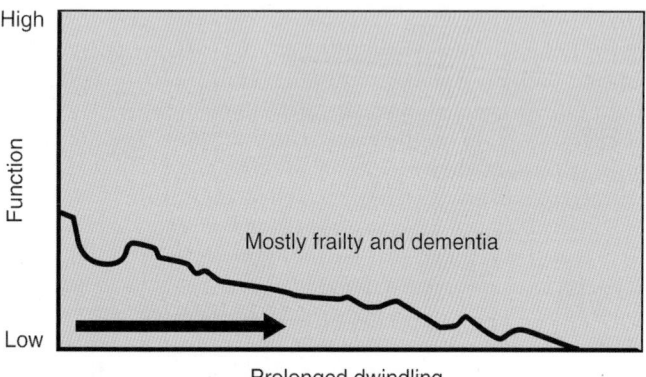

Prolonged dwindling

• **Fig. 29.5** Functional Trajectories of Terminal Illnesses. (Reprinted with permission from RAND Corporation.)[5]

management, health management, and religious/spiritual activities.[35] Furthermore, OTs should also address rest, sleep, and relaxation habits in addition to participation in leisure and recreational activities. Finally, the AOTA states that OTs can be facilitators of communication and supporting the PWC's caregivers by avoiding musculoskeletal injury or burnout.

Speech-Language Pathology

Communication, eating, and drinking are fundamental skills for every person at all stages of life. Especially in times when a person becomes more dependent in functional mobility or self-performance of ADLs, they continue to require engagement in these activities. The American Speech-Language-Hearing Association (ASHA) has established a website to discuss key considerations

for SLPs working with individuals at EOL.[36] If a person has a swallowing difficulty, the SLP should facilitate the development of compensatory strategies which may allow the person to maintain safe oral intake. Additionally, a role of the SLP is to participate in the decision-making discussions as to when and if alternative nutrition (e.g., tube feeding) may be appropriate. Finally, if the person is having difficulty with communication due to shortness of breath or cognition, the SLP can use their expertise to help develop alternative communication strategies to allow for the expression of wishes and desires. All of these strategies by the SLP would be focused on optimizing the abilities they still possess to facilitate interaction and communication or enjoy foods and drinks with the ultimate goal of assuring QOL and dignity.

Courses of Disease Processes

Rehabilitation professionals are experts in establishing predictive care plans for individuals to improve their impairments, functional limitations, and participation restrictions, but this process becomes more challenging when the person is facing an imminent and unpredictable physical decline. Some notable patterns of physical decline for some common conditions have been characterized to assist healthcare providers to anticipate functional changes.[6] See Figure 29.5 for visual depictions of the most frequently occurring functional changes.

The most applicable to cancer is the *Short period of evident decline*, which is characterized by a relatively high level of functioning until the disease process or treatment effects overwhelm the system and a precipitous decline in function is experienced. This precipitous decline in function may result in or occur concurrently with a hospitalization. Onc R clinicians can utilize this information to anticipate this precipitous physical decline and assist in facilitating a safe location for discharge. In the author's clinical experience in the acute PC setting, some PWCs who wished to spend their remaining days at home were not able to obtain an efficient discharge from the hospital, and when the "window of opportunity" closed and the PWC's medical status worsened, they were not able to achieve their goal of being at home with their family for their remaining life. As acute care PTs and OTs are actively involved with discharge planning from the hospital, their input and advocacy are essential to assist these persons in achieving one of their final life goals.

The next pattern of functional decline is *Longer term limitations with intermittent exacerbations and sudden dying*, which is common with organ system failure pathologies such as chronic obstructive pulmonary disorder and congestive heart failure.[5] The last pattern of functional decline to be discussed is *Prolonged dwindling* which is typical of central nervous system failure with a generally slow decline in physical or mental capacity that may require long-term institutional care.[5] Such conditions may include frailty, dementia, or Parkinson's disease. As many PWCs also have a variety of co morbidities, these additional practice patterns are valuable to consider when establishing a treatment plan.

Palliative Rehabilitation Care Models

Five patient management models beyond "traditional rehabilitation" for treating the person with a life-threatening or terminal illness have been proposed.[37] A person can go back and forth between the models or be receiving more than one at the same time. These models can be used to establish care plans, justify appropriate therapy intervention, and educate PWCs, referral sources, and payers about these therapy services. These models are *Rehabilitation Light, Rehabilitation in Reverse, Case Management, Skilled Maintenance,* and *Supportive Care.*[37] In the author's experience, most Onc R clinicians have employed some of these treatment paradigms during their clinical practice. A key value of these PC rehabilitation models is their usefulness in communication among Onc R colleagues and IDT members the variety of approaches that Onc R clinicians can employ in different palliative scenarios.

Rehabilitation Light

In some cases, a PWC has the physical capacity and motivation to participate in rehabilitation and demonstrate some potential for improvement, but their advancing disease process may limit their ability to tolerate intensive rehabilitation. In fact, an excessive amount of physical rehabilitation may even overtax the body systems and cause a delay in recovery or a functional regression. In the *Rehab Light* treatment paradigm, a slower, more gentle rehabilitation regimen with a reduced intensity of visits is beneficial. This may include reducing the number of visits, reducing the total treatment time in a session, or refocusing treatment sessions toward education as opposed to only physical exercise activities. For example, a normal treatment regimen may be three to four times per week but in *Rehab Light*, the frequency may be reduced to once or twice a week. This rehabilitation program may be supplemented by a highly individualized home exercise program (HEP), with careful avoidance of prescribing an excessive amount of exercise. During rehabilitation, as improvements or an increased capacity or tolerance of rehabilitation are noted, clinical adjustments can be made to the therapy plan of care.

Case Management

The next treatment paradigm, entitled *Case Management*, may be a relatively novel approach for Onc R clinicians who might be accustomed to a brief but regular episode of care, but it is a common approach employed in medicine and dentistry. It involves regular, periodic re-evaluations with targeted interventions if impairments are identified. Within Onc R, the *Case Management* paradigm is similar to the concept of *Prospective Surveillance* as described in Chapter 2. This is often applied early in a disease process when a PWC is stable or functionally doing well, but there is a likelihood of functional decline or development of impairments. Clinically, this involves visits on a monthly, bi-monthly, or on an as-needed basis. In some cases, it may involve updating a HEP and re-assessing some baseline measurements. In other cases, if functional changes are noted or regular rehabilitation is indicated, treatment can be initiated via establishing a traditional rehabilitation plan of care. In the earlier stages of a disease process, this may involve an exercise or activity prescription that the person could execute in a community exercise or wellness setting. Within this exercise prescription, clear details of any limitations or things to avoid should be conveyed, including any immunosuppressive precautions or activities that may be unsafe (e.g., advanced balance activities in a person with high fall risk).

This paradigm may also be applied in the later stages of a disease where the person's disease process is advancing but the benefit of ongoing skilled rehabilitation may be limited. For example, a person with progressive weakness who was ambulatory for several months will have periodic assessments by an Onc R clinician but if the person's ambulatory status declined, a reassessment may indicate a new need for training in adaptive equipment or family training (perhaps moving to *Rehab in Reverse*, which follows below). Furthermore, some individuals who may be receiving hospice care may be able to progress enough or have their medical condition stabilized enough to be discharged while living from hospice service. In 2018, the National Hospice and Palliative Care Organization (NHPCO) estimated that 1.55 million people enrolled in hospice and that 17% were discharged from hospice care alive for reasons including an extended prognosis or a desire for curative or rehabilitative treatment.[38]

Rehabilitation in Reverse

In traditional rehabilitation, patients are progressed from a lower functional status to a higher functional status. However, with *Rehab in Reverse*, there is the anticipation of functional decline and as such, the Onc R clinician should anticipate this and prepare the PWC for the next steps in the disease progression and subsequent functional regression as they occur (Box 29.5). For example, in traditional rehabilitation, a patient may start in a wheelchair, progress to a walker or a cane, and then possibly eliminate the need for an assistive device as they recover from their condition. For the person with declining function, assistive technology needs may change often in the reverse direction and more intensive skilled training with compensatory strategies will be necessary (Box 29.6). Onc R clinicians are the experts on assessing for need and appropriateness of the devices and predicting the physical, functional, cognitive, and oral motor dysfunctions that will result from an advancing disease process. It is imperative that this is communicated to the IDT and concurrently adapting the rehabilitation plan of care, especially if there are increasing risk factors for hospitalization, falls, uncontrolled pain, or other manageable issues that may arise. A key consideration is preventing unwarranted hospital admissions, especially if the PWC's goal is to remain safe at home; therefore, proactive education on the potential issues that may arise should be clear, though sensitively addressed. This may be more feasible for an Onc R clinician who has established a long-term longitudinal relationship with a person as they will have a more thorough grasp of the PWC's baseline functional status, life goals, personal situation, and medical trajectory.

• BOX 29.5   Importance of Considering the Functional and Disease Trajectory[1]

"The therapist needs to be ready for the patient's condition to change and fluctuate over days and therapists may be ordering things that are inappropriate. A therapist got the family to put in a stair glide for a dying patient and the therapist didn't realize the disease progression. The family used the glide once, but the patient couldn't get off it. The rehab therapist didn't do the wrong thing. He had good intentions, but the family was in a jumble. Education and communication are critical."

• BOX 29.6   Physical Therapist (PT) Quote Related to the PT's role in Palliative Care[1]

"[Educating the family/caregiver] further helps the family be prepared for the decline in the patient…it starts when they were doing sliding board transfers and then went to a Hoyer Lift then we went to bed positioning at all times, so through the whole decline, I think it is so helpful. Having that relationship with the family where they trust you at a time when their emotional resources are limited, I think is important."

PC outcome measures often include a focus on pain reduction, reducing re-hospitalizations, and preparing the PWC in the event of dyspnea. For example, an Onc R clinician may be able to reduce future pain by educating the individual in joint protection techniques as opposed to needing more pain medications. Successful outcomes within the *Rehab in Reverse* model are highly individualized but may include the PWC's ability to stay safely stay at home, that caregivers have a good understanding on the use of the equipment, and minimizing the risk of falls.

Skilled Maintenance

Recently clarified via the aforementioned Jimmo settlement, *Skilled Maintenance* is required when a person with an advancing illness would functionally decline at a more rapid rate without the clinician's unique skills and services (Figure 29.6). "*In the case of maintenance therapy, the skills of a therapist are necessary to maintain, prevent, or slow further deterioration of the patient's functional status, and the services cannot be safely and effectively carried out by the beneficiary personally, or with the assistance of non-therapists, including unskilled caregivers.*"[39]

For skilled maintenance services to be applicable, the key tasks required to manage the PWC's condition would be too complex or unsafe for unskilled caregivers to perform. Medicare clarified that payment for these services are not available "in a situation where the beneficiary's maintenance care needs can be addressed safely and effectively through the use of nonskilled personnel."[39] Some examples of this might include when muscle facilitation or inhibitions, limb assist, or weight shifting for balance will make the difference in functional performance for the PWC but are too technical for the family member.

Consider the case of a 74-year-old male diagnosed with Stage IV lung cancer with a metastatic bone lesion to the left femur that is 3 cm in diameter. Due to the high risk of pathologic fracture, the orthopedic surgeon recommended that the PWC only be 5% partial weight bearing of his left leg during ambulation. The PWC was not a candidate for prophylactic surgical fixation due to the expectation of a limited lifespan. Due to brain metastases and the related cognitive impairment, the PWC is not able to maintain this restricted weight-bearing. In this case, the PWC's condition may decline more quickly if the person is sedentary, however, the PWC requires the ongoing coaching and patient handling skills of a licensed PT or OT to preserve ADL and ambulatory performance and enhance QOL—a primary goal at the EOL.

To justify skilled maintenance, the clinical documentation must reflect that the Onc R services required the skills of a qualified healthcare professional and that they were medically necessary. Within the skilled maintenance model, clinician visits can be delivered intermittently and coordinated among the IDT care team. Topics such as ongoing support and preparation for the impending natural dying process must be considered and addressed. Key considerations include emphasizing rehabilitation interventions to slow the person's debility and optimizing ADLs and QOL. Skilled maintenance may also facilitate spreading out visits over time and among Onc R disciplines so clinicians can be another set of eyes on the case.

For different insurance companies, skilled maintenance may not be a viable option as it may not be in their coverage criteria. The Onc R clinician should consult with the patient's insurance provider guidelines to clarify the coverage for these services. In the outpatient Medicare Part B settings, the conventional common procedural terminology (CPT) codes that are traditionally used for billing remain viable and applicable in skilled maintenance scenarios. Within the homecare setting in Medicare Home Health Part A, the Medicare Claim should show that the services were established and are being carried out for skilled maintenance. See Box 29.7 for applicable skilled maintenance codes for rehabilitation professionals within home health.[40] Finally, skilled maintenance fits well within the hospice setting.

Supportive Care

As the person nears the EOL, they may benefit from a variety of interventions provided and facilitated by Onc R clinicians. *Supportive care* primarily focuses on symptom management/relief and the focus often shifts to the caregivers when the PWC is severely debilitated or impaired cognitively. Clinical aims are to attempt to ease terminal discomfort, mitigate some of the negative effects of immobility, and assist in allowing a death with dignity to occur. A key intervention may include teaching caregivers about injury

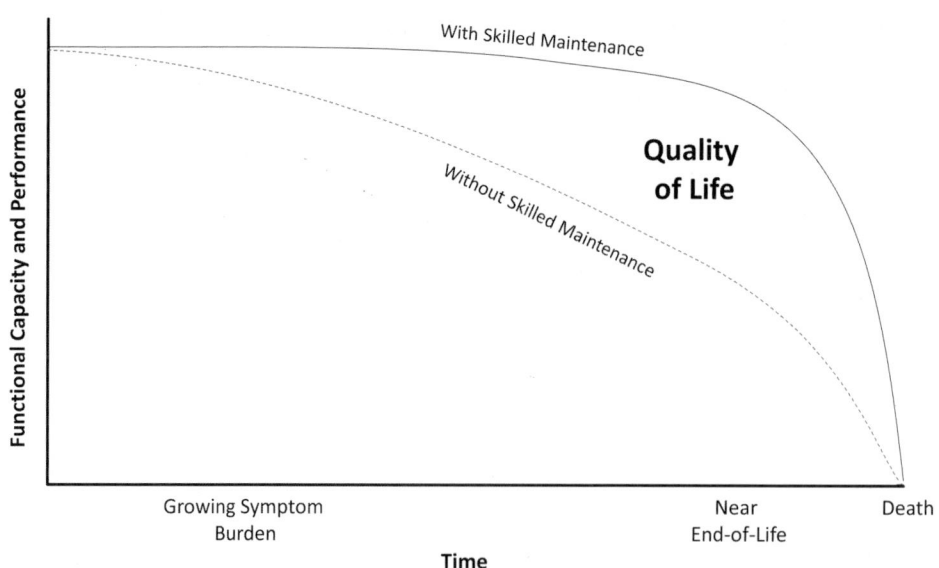

• **Fig. 29.6** With and Without Skilled Maintenance. (Reprinted with permission from Litterini A, Wilson CM. *Physical Activity and Rehabilitation in Life Threatening Illness*. Routledge; 2021.)

prevention, education on body mechanics, and how to reposition their loved ones safely and effectively. These may not be ongoing interventions delivered by Onc R clinicians directly to a PWC, but to educate caregivers in the performance of these care activities. This may include educating caregivers in performing gentle passive range of motion to reduce the symptoms of stiffness or pain and prevent contractures. It also may include teaching proper positioning to reduce the risk of skin breakdown or pressure ulcers. If the person develops edema or lymphedema, the Onc R clinician can teach skills in edema management such as manual lymphatic drainage and applying compression wrapping. As oral intake may be one of the last functional activities to be lost, a person may benefit from the skills of a SLP to educate in alternative strategies to eat or drink, or also educating the family when the risk of aspiration may be too high and oral intake may need to be minimized. Finally, supportive care should also include education to family members to provide meaningful ways to comfort their loved one in hospice. This may include means to ease the discomfort of inactivity or restlessness with gentle rocking for vestibular stimulation.

Palliative Prehabilitation

A relatively novel concept is the consideration of implementation of prehabilitation within the context of a terminal disease. Although prehabilitation is often described within the context of physically preparing the body for the physiologic insults to be incurred by cancer treatments, this same concept can be applied to prepare the body in anticipation of functioning during the end stages of a terminal illness. Refer to Chapter 27 for information on prehabilitation. A key time for this *palliative prehabilitation* is early within the disease process while there is little to no symptom burden (Figure 29.7). This will improve the PWC's physiologic reserve capacity, strength, and reduce the risk of falls during an advancing disease which will assist in preserving the remaining QOL.

Operationalizing Palliative Rehabilitation and Chronic Disease Management

In order to provide high-quality, longitudinal services to individuals with advanced cancer, Onc R services may require some administrative modifications and adaptations to clinical practice to manage common palliative scenarios. Within a hospital or an inpatient setting, it is advised that there is a core group of clinicians who are dedicated to PC as their primary practice area and to be the liaison between the Onc R team and the PC IDT. In addition to diagnosis-specific rehabilitation specialists (e.g., cancer, cardiopulmonary, neurologic), the PC rehabilitation specialists can coordinate the care of persons in PC and provide some direct treatments. Also, the PC rehabilitation specialist can communicate situational details to and from the rehab team as to any material updates to the PWC's plan of care, situational changes, and overall goals of care for individuals with a terminal illness.

For the PC rehabilitation specialist, a strong personal relationship and trust with physicians, nurses, PWCs, and all members of the IDT is a valued and critical skill. Challenges to overcome when working in PC is that the coordination of care, facilitating optimum transitions in care, and communicating with the IDT are not often considered to be "billable" time in routine therapy, and may be restricted due to administrative or productivity concerns. This may include an Onc R clinician attending regularly scheduled rounds and huddles with IDT members and coordinating discharge planning. In some cases, these may be walking rounds where key IDT members can go from room to room and

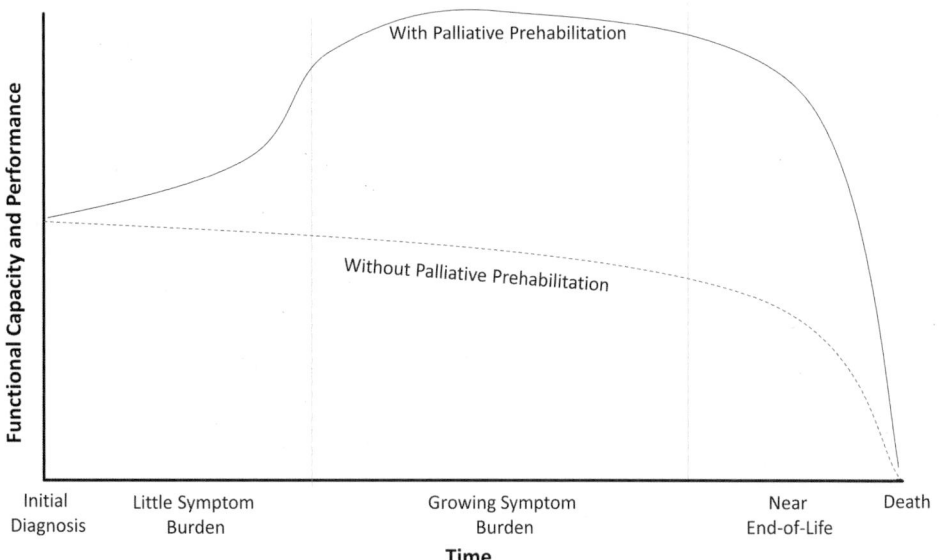

• **Fig. 29.7** Palliative Prehabilitation. (Reprinted with permission from Litterini A, Wilson CM. *Physical Activity and Rehabilitation in Life Threatening Illness*. Routledge; 2021.)

at times, may even incorporate the family into the conversation. Other institutions with a more decentralized PC population may choose to collaborate in a central location like a conference room.

As the increasingly complex care and the likelihood of costly readmissions are major considerations, nondirect care time should be just as valued as direct treatment time to avoid unwarranted admissions. In addition, the Onc R clinician should consider additional reasons for possible readmissions (e.g., inability to complete home ADLs, aspiration, confusion, pain crisis, dehydration, nausea, diarrhea, vomiting, weakness, falls) and proactively providing interventions to minimize the occurrence or impact of these events. It is in the prevention of these events that PC rehabilitation services hold their true value within the healthcare system and to the quality of remaining life of the PWC. The challenge is to capture the value and return-on-investment of these nonbillable procedures as it is not often easy to establish a direct correlation between these essential care activities with a reduction in hospital length of stay or a reduced readmission rate.

Care Differences Between Rehabilitation and Palliative Therapy[41]

To provide quality PC and EOL rehabilitation services, all parties should have a clear understanding of the adaptations in approach and interventions that Onc R clinicians can employ and how services are aimed at optimizing QOL, improving safety and function, preventing falls and readmissions, and ultimately facilitating a good death. Misperceptions remain regarding rehabilitation interventions for those in PC, including that Onc R clinicians' interventions are always difficult, exhausting, or painful. Accordingly, a 2012 survey of 395 oncologists and physiatrists found 8% of oncologists would refer patients with advanced terminal cancer for rehabilitation services while 35% of physiatrists recommended rehabilitation services, further highlighting the inconsistent referral patterns in this patient population.[42]

Some providers and patients may consider that "aggressive therapy" and "no therapy" are the only options for rehabilitation. The author has found that communication of the role of a discipline like PT could be illustrated in the following way: "PT in PC is not a light switch, but more like a dimmer switch. Instead of intensive therapy or no therapy, we are able to adjust our services based on how the person is feeling each day. If the person is having a good spell, we can turn the dimmer up or if the person is

having a rough patch, the dimmer can be turned to low and more education on topics such as pacing or energy conservation would be applied." This strategy will help to avoid interruption in rehabilitation care and carefully modulate the frequency and intensity and transition from each of the PC rehab models as the patient situation requires until the EOL.

Even though a cornerstone of rehabilitation services is the individualization of care and sensitivity to a person's life situation, this is especially important in patient-and family-centered palliative rehabilitation, and the Onc R clinician should be even more sensitive to the person's wishes and comfort. This will include a shift in focus to QOL, anticipating future disability and equipment needs, and even assistance with "bucket list" assistance—generally life goals that a person might wish to complete during their remaining time. Bucket list items may include going on a trip, visiting a favorite location or loved ones, holding a grandchild, walking a child down the aisle at their wedding, or simply sitting up for one last holiday meal. As one can imagine, opportunities for an Onc R clinician to assist with the achievement of these activities can be extremely satisfying and enriching for all involved. Finally, PC rehabilitation services should emphasize the prevention of pressure ulcers, contractures, immobility pain as well as providing family/caregiver education, support, and consultation in unique or specialized circumstances. See Table 29.2 for clinical differences between Onc R services for PC and traditional, restorative rehabilitation.

An overarching theme of PC rehabilitation is the expectation that physical variability will occur including functional capacity, strength, pain, and ADL performance. Even if physical status temporarily remains stable, therapy services may be negatively affected by the person's emotional states or ability to participate. This may even be affected by the person getting good or bad news, which may require the clinician to modify or delay their intended therapeutic interventions to address the PWC's current state of being.

Facilitating Transitions in Care

Before enrolling in PC or hospice services, a PWC may be undergoing rehabilitation. Especially in hospice situations, the person may be arbitrarily discharged from rehabilitation services or other administrative barriers may arise that limit the person's ability to access skilled rehabilitation services. In these cases, a key role of the care team is proactive advocacy to assist with the transition of rehab services. In some cases, the person may choose to remain comfortable and no longer wish to participate in active therapy. Of course, this person's decision should be respected, however, it

TABLE 29.2	Differences Between Traditional Restorative Rehabilitation and Palliative Therapy
Traditional Restorative Rehabilitation	**Palliative Care Therapy**
• Push patients closer to their physical tolerance or pain threshold	• Balance function and participation with comfort and preserving some strength
• More aggressive with treatment compliance	• More willing to accept a "refusal" or physical variability
• Focus on ADL function over temporary pain management	• Focus on pain control with modified ADLs
• Generally, have clarity with care goals	• Anticipate unclear care goals
• Little to no existential anxiety	• Patient and family distress
• More fact-based interactions	• Emotion-based interactions
• Procure durable medical equipment with the intent of improvement or long-term stability	• Procure durable medical equipment in anticipation of functional decline or "bad days"

ADLs, Activities of daily living.
Created by Christopher Wilson, PT, DPT, DScPT. Printed with permission.

should be clearly stated that therapy services are available if circumstances arise where they are needed and the PWC should be provided with clear means to contact the Onc R clinician to resume these services.

Additional administrative barriers that may be encountered are the aforementioned payment barriers (e.g., limited therapy payment in hospice scenarios) as well as clinical barriers. These individuals may now have a new, unfamiliar care team which may also not have a clear understanding of the rehabilitation goals and aims to optimize QOL. Finally, there may be misunderstandings by the PWC's family, the PWC themself, or other care team members. Despite all of these factors, the PWC may still have the same physical needs and potential for actively participating in life events as when they were undergoing active treatment, and therefore they should, by principle, have the same access to Onc R clinicians who can assist with these goals.

Palliative Care Within Inpatient Rehabilitation (IPR)

In general, a traditional IPR unit often requires 3 hours of skilled therapy per day between PT, OT, and SLP, if appropriate, for approximately 15 hours/week. This presents some increased challenges to persons with advanced cancer within PC. Some useful considerations include adjusting the frequency of visits from 5 to 7 days/week to decrease the amount of therapy required per weekday by spreading the 15 hours across the entire week. In this care setting, the physical decline is a large confounding variable. Common deficits/barriers to therapy in IPR may include depression, anxiety, low endurance, low insight, or even a poor understanding of their underlying medical condition. Even with the decreased duration of treatment sessions, it may be important to slowly implement physical interventions and providing frequent rest breaks. One additional approach that may be considered in IPR is the concept of a short stay family training program developed in 2019.[43] Although described in more detail in Chapter 24, this care model focuses on training key caregivers of people with advanced disease in the IPR setting. Topics to be taught to the PWC and caregiver may include safe patient handling, adapted ADL techniques (dressing, bathing, feeding, grooming), modified communication and oral intake techniques, and safe use of durable medical equipment (DME). As both the PWC and caregiver are involved with the physical tasks and educational process, this is a financially viable model as long as the clinical documentation reflects the skilled care of instruction. By providing this training, it will increase the caregiver's and PWC's confidence and skills to achieve a successful, longer-term transition to home.

Care Transitions Within PC

The care coordination and stability of persons with advanced cancer is more challenging during care transitions and this may be a vulnerable and stressful time for the PWC, family, and caregiving team. Especially as PTs and OTs are integrally involved in pursuing a safe and appropriate discharge, these disciplines must be involved in care well before an imminent discharge to facilitate the logistics and training required, such as procuring and educating on needed DME. Patient handoff, especially from setting to setting, has emerged as a key step in successful medical care. In general, Onc R clinicians do not often engage in a clear purposeful handoff from setting to setting. Ideally, this might be a phone call between the PWC's acute care clinician and homecare clinician after hospital discharge or between the homecare clinician and the outpatient clinician after the PWC can safely get to outpatient rehabilitation. See Table 29.3 for examples of topics to be discussed during a rehabilitation professional handoff of care.

To improve access and timeliness of Onc R services for persons in PC, it is highly recommended that a proactive screening and referral process occur. Unfortunately, in some settings where a variety of diagnostic service lines are served, persons in PC or at EOL may not be prioritized as highly as other diagnostic categories such as orthopedics or neurology. While providing rehabilitation to a person after a joint replacement or a stroke is important to clinical outcomes, persons in PC should also be highly prioritized to meet their need as the window of opportunity may be limited, to minimize costly readmissions, and assure that a comprehensive, successful discharge plan is achieved. In some situations, a formal referral to Onc R from an IDT member may arrive too late and may cause a rushed, incomplete, or stressful discharge planning process. To mitigate this, in an inpatient setting like a hospital or a subacute rehabilitation setting, a three-step process is recommended to be undertaken by the rehabilitation department to proactively identify needs for all Onc R disciplines; (1) screening

TABLE 29.3	Topics for Discussion During a Care Transition Handoff Between Therapists
Current Mobility, Functional, Communication, or Oral Motor Status	
Overall tolerance to treatment and treatment focus during the previous rehabilitation setting (including vital sign responses)	
How much physical activity should the PWC get besides PT/OT?	
Are there any equipment needs identified?	
What symptoms might be an early warning sign of medical instability or risk of the condition worsening? What would be the plan if these were identified?	
ADL performance status as compared to baseline	
What are the risk factors for this patient to hospital readmission?	
Social barriers to activity or safety?	
Any other needs that the person requires to be successful in this new therapy setting?	
Barriers remaining or additional services needed (e.g., PT, OT, SLP, pulmonary rehab, pastoral care, social work)	

ADLs, Activities of daily living; *OT*, occupational therapy; *PT*, physical therapy; *PWI*, person with cancer; *SLP*, speech language pathology.
Created by Christopher Wilson, PT, DPT, DScPT. Printed with permission.

through chart review of all patients that have current PC consultations (with appropriate permissions to access the health records); (2) If the chart review indicates possible needs, communicate with either the attending physician or another IDT member who can provide context as to the appropriateness of the identified service need; and (3) If needs exist and the patient is appropriate, initiate referral through a pre-established protocol (e.g., medical executive protocol) or direct consultation through referral.

Considering When to Initiate a PC Consult

As Onc R clinicians develop close relationships with PWCs and are highly attuned to physical, cognitive, or oral motor functioning, they may have the ability to identify if a person might benefit from a PC consult. Symptoms may include unrelieved or unmanaged pain, worsening symptoms of the underlying condition, repeated hospitalizations, difficult family relations or coping, or identification of suffering or spiritual distress. Additional areas that the Onc R clinician may notice include if the clinician's treatments/curative measures are losing effectiveness or causing distressing symptom burden, or if the person has multiple comorbidities that need expert management. Finally, a key question that the Onc R clinicians should ask themself is, "Would you be surprised if you learned this patient passed away within the next 12 to18 months?" If the answer is that you would not be surprised, a consultation with PC should be strongly considered.

Individuals who may also be appropriate for PC include those with unplanned weight loss or loss of appetite, declining cognitive abilities, a request for "Comfort Care Only," or declining functional ability. Finally, PC may be beneficial if there is family disagreement or lack of knowledge about care goals, where family meetings could help, and before invasive or life-prolonging procedures (e.g., before feeding tube placement in a person with advanced dementia). In general, if the PWC is having challenging pain or symptoms, if there is a feeling that curative treatment options could do more harm than good, or if the PWC would benefit from goals-of-care discussions, the Onc R clinician should reach out to the person's attending/primary physician or the PC team to discuss a consultation. This may be accomplished by written or verbal communication. A useful phrasing might include "Dr. [attending], based on the rehab evaluation, problems identified indicate this patient might benefit from an additional discussion of long-term care goals for their life-threatening condition, which might be accomplished by a PC consult. Please order if you agree. Thank you."

Communication Keys With Palliative Care

One of the concerns of many healthcare providers is that they do not get substantial training in core PC concepts and an often-voiced area of concern for Onc R clinicians is regarding communication with individuals with a life-threatening disease.[44] Within this section, some useful strategies will be shared to assist the Onc R clinician in the initiation of these difficult conversations. A very useful resource is the Vital Talk website (www.vitaltalk.org) which provides a variety of communication guides and strategies to employ during difficult conversations. Many of the strategies are represented by acronyms which are designed to be easy to remember and employed in a clinical context.

The Ask-Tell-Ask method is a useful tool to convey information by first gathering information, then conveying the critical information, and then finally asking for understanding and input on the next steps.[45]

- Ask—The first *Ask* is to ascertain the PWC's understanding of the situation and assist in determining what additional information the person will require. An Onc R clinician may ask, "Please tell me what your medical oncologist has told you about the extent of your cancer." An additional question should include asking permission to share the upcoming information with them; sometimes even the request to provide this information helps to reduce the anxiety and defensiveness that may arise from a difficult conversation and returns some locus of control to the person.
- Tell—Provide clear, straightforward information in small doses. Only one or two pieces of information should be delivered at a time while avoiding medical jargon. This information should be delivered succinctly without lecturing. After telling the information, you should pause to allow the PWC to comprehend the information and its implications.
- Ask—The second *ask* is to ascertain if the person understood what was said and also allows the person to ask questions. Finally, another useful question is "How can I help you with the steps that are to come next?"

Additional useful communication strategies include using *I wish...* statements and *tell me more*.[45] *I wish* statements can be useful when starting a conversation to provide empathy and provide a prelude to the next steps. For example, "I wish that the rehabilitation you have been performing was making you stronger, but it appears that your strength is not progressing as we had hoped. Let's discuss how to approach this new information." The *tell me more* approach can assist in asking the PWC to elaborate on statements or questions that have come up in the conversation. For example, "You said that you are worried about your family after you are gone. Please tell me more about that."

Communication With Patients: CLASS

The CLASS (Content, Listen, Acknowledge, STrategy, Summary) acronym provides a solid foundation for any discussion or communication strategy during patient care, especially within the context of PC.[46]

- Context: This includes your body language and the environment that is chosen to have this discussion. A private, quiet setting should be chosen and if there are others (e.g., family members, friends) in the room, ask if it is okay if they remain or would the PWC prefer to have the conversation alone. The clinician should also be seated and allow adequate time for the conversation. Additionally, attempts to minimize distractions are important and may require silencing electronic devices that may cause disruptions so that the PWC feels he or she has the clinician's full attention. After conveying the critical information, stop and allow the person to process it.
- Listen: Some Onc R clinicians think that listening takes a long time and delays the conveying of critical medical information but if allowed to finish, most patients will complete talking in less than 2 minutes. Be patient, be comfortable with pauses or silence, and seek to clarify information that may be unclear.
- Acknowledge: It is important to state what might be obvious, including emotions and fears. The Onc R clinician should acknowledge the reactions that the person displays or voices.
- Strategy: After explaining the situation, encourage the person to provide their input into the treatment plan or to assist them in understanding the implications of the various choices. Incorporating the individual's input will assist in the adherence and understanding of the plan.

- Summary: Provide a summative conclusion as to what was discussed and what the next steps are. This may also include what input or further steps are needed or expected from the person. Also, provide information as to how to contact the provider if needs or concerns arise between the next steps.

In addition to the CLASS approach, VitalTalk offers the GUIDE steps which may be more applicable in PC or EOL situations. GUIDE is short for *Get ready, Understand, Inform, Dignify,* and *Equip.*

- Get ready: The clinician should assure that they have all the necessary information needed and obtain any information that may not be available.
- Understand: Establish what the patient already knows about the situation to not contradict or inadvertently deliver unintended information.
- Inform: Provide the needed information to the person, starting with the most important information first; do not bury the headline. After sharing this information, pause to allow the individual to consider this information.
- Dignify: Acknowledge and recognize the validity of emotional response; "I can imagine that this must be very upsetting information for you, please talk to me about that."
- Equip: Provide the person with the tools, knowledge, and support to undertake the next steps and to establish a plan.

Confusion and Delirium

At the EOL, many people experience confusional states from a variety of causes, including brain metastases, metabolic changes, delirium, or dementia. The Alzheimer's Association estimates that 33% of people will have some form of dementia at or near death.[47] Common clinical presentations include problems finding the right words, lack of coherence or logic in speech, emotional lability, repetition of ideas, a decreased attention span, or regularly forgetting recent events, names, and faces. These issues may be compounded by other factors including sensory deficits (hearing or vision loss) or external factors including unfamiliar surroundings or caregivers.

A major challenge for Onc R clinicians in providing care for these individuals is related to communication and conveying information. This is in a large part due to some clinicians attempting to apply communication strategies that work well for cognitively unimpaired patients, which will not be successful for those with confusion or disorientation.[45] A series of communication strategies that are effective when communicating with those with memory loss or confusion have been identified.[48] These include eliminating outside distractions, approaching the person from the front with a friendly face, and with good eye contact. Additionally, communications should be conveyed via short and clear sentences. The caregiver is recommended to avoid open-ended questions, asking multiple questions at a time, or avoid giving multiple instructions at a time. In some cases, repeating messages with the same wording or paraphrasing instructions may be helpful. Finally, the provider should attempt to not interrupt or rush the person but if there are word-finding difficulties, the person should be encouraged to try to find alternate words or "talk around or describe" the words.

To facilitate therapeutic success for those with confusional states, there are several options available to Onc R clinicians. A key goal of providing therapeutic interventions to those with confusion is having the environment facilitate the practice of the task without an excessive cognitive demand. For example, instead of complex balance tasks, the clinician could have the person retrieve a cup

of water but be required to navigate a series of obstacles to do so. Alternatively, colleagues could be stationed around a therapy gym and the patient could be encouraged to go greet each person or give them an item to facilitate endurance, ambulation, and balance.

One additional useful communication tool for individuals with cognitive impairment is the concept of vanishing cues.[49] This is useful when teaching a task or a new process. This involves a full instruction the first time teaching the task using a clear demonstration, but with subsequent instructions, components of the instruction or the demonstration are eliminated, with prompts for the person to fill in the blanks from memory. See Box 29.8 for an example of vanishing cues. Refer to Chapter 8 for additional discussion on communication and interventions in those with confusion.

Saying Goodbye as a Healthcare Provider

An important but often intimidating consideration for those practicing with individuals at EOL is the concept of having to say goodbye for the last time to one of your patients. Within the context of communication in the PC and EOL care, this is often cited by clinicians to be an uncomfortable possibility, with very few conventions or best practices.[50,51] Yet this is important for Onc R clinicians because they often develop a strong personal relationship with their patients and not saying goodbye may be confusing or upsetting to the patient or family. Given the uncertain timing of death, it is helpful to always appreciate and acknowledge the time of each interaction or visit, and verbalize looking forward to the next encounter, without the certainty that either the patient or clinician will be there. This can allow a conversation to arise of the true nature of living and dying and provide closure regardless of what subsequently occurs. Some of the best practices recommended include showing your gratitude to the patient for what they have taught you or what you will miss about them.[51] A useful conversation starter is, "I'm not sure when we will see each other again as our rehab sessions are going to be put on the back burner for now but I wanted to thank you for your [humor, kindness, sharing your family story]." Simple phrases such as this can assist the Onc R clinician and the patient in obtaining closure and begin the process of letting go and bereavement.

In some cases, the Onc R clinician may be invited to funeral services or invited into the person's home for a personal visit before death. These opportunities should be met with gratitude and should reflect the strong personal relationship that you have built with them and acknowledge the impact that they have made on your life. One other uncomfortable scenario that may

---

• BOX 29.8 Vanishing Cues for Teaching a Person How to Safely Stand Up

1. When standing up, push up from the armrests with both hands. (With therapist demonstration)
2. What should you do with your hands when you stand up? (With therapist demonstration)
3. What should you do with your hands when you stand up? (Without demonstration)
4. What should you do with the armrests when you stand up? (With therapist demonstration)
5. What should you do with the armrests when you stand up? (Without demonstration)
6. When standing up, you should… (With therapist demonstration)
7. When standing up, you should… (Without demonstration)

Created by Christopher Wilson PT, DPT, DScPT. Printed with permission.

be encountered is seeing family members at funeral services or in the community after the PWC has passed away. Useful words that might assist in this scenario are, "It is wonderful to see you again. How are you holding up these days? I still think about your [family member] from time to time and I remember what a great and fun person they were."

Functional Outcome Measures

Within rehabilitation, patient-reported and functional outcomes are a necessary component of care to document response to treatment. It is common practice (and an expectation of insurance payers) that the Onc R clinician employs established, evidence-based, researched *functional outcome measures* to establish the need for service and any improvements made.

Quantifying Physical Performance Status

One of the challenges in PC or EOL care is that most outcome measures are designed to demonstrate improvement in function. Additionally, in some cases, if a patient's functional status worsens, even if it worsens at a slower rate with skilled maintenance via rehabilitation services, this may be misperceived by insurance companies or payers that the services were ineffective, and therefore not eligible for payment. In PC cases, clinicians may need to be more deliberate and careful when choosing outcome measures, including those related to physical performance, the patient-reported outcome measures (i.e., questionnaires), and PC-specific measures. In hospice, declining performance scores can be used to affirm qualification for care and re-certification when other subjective measures or patient self-report do not indicate changing or declining status. An example would be during *case management,* the PWC is without complaint, but monthly re-assessment shows steadily worsening Timed-Up-and-Go scores indicating physical deficits and fall risk.

One clinically applicable measure is the Palliative Performance Scale (PPS) developed in 1996.[52] It uses five observer-rated domains from the Karnofsky Performance Scale (100-0). Its reliability and validity have been established and it has been used for correlations with the duration of remaining life.[53] The PPS may be used to monitor for potential care needs of persons with advanced

---

TABLE 29.4　**Palliative Performance Scale Version 2**[54]

Palliative Performance Scale Level	Ambulation	Activity and Evidence of Disease	Self-Care	Intake	Conscious Level
100%	Full	Normal activity and work No evidence of disease	Full	Normal	Full
90%	Full	Normal activity and work Some evidence of disease	Full	Normal	Full
80%	Full	Normal activity with effort Some evidence of disease	Full	Normal or reduced	Full
70%	Reduced	Unable to perform normal job/work Significant disease	Occasional assistance necessary	Normal or reduced	Full
60%	Mostly sit/lie	Unable to perform hobby/housework Significant disease	Considerable assistance required	Normal or reduced	Full or confusion
50%	Mainly in bed	Unable to do any work Extensive disease	Mainly assistance	Normal or reduced	Full or confusion
40%	Totally bed bound	Unable to do most activity Extensive disease	Total care	Normal or reduced	Full or drowsy ± confusion
30%	Totally bed bound	Unable to do most activity Extensive disease	Total care	Normal or reduced	Full or drowsy ± confusion
20%	Totally bed bound	Unable to do most activity Extensive disease	Total care	Minimal to sips	Full or drowsy ± confusion
10%	Totally bed bound	Unable to do most activity Extensive disease	Total care	Mouth care only	Drowsy or coma ± confusion
0%	Death				

disease, particularly as additional needs emerge during the progression of cancer (Table 29.4).[54]

An additional PC specific tool is the Edmonton Functional Assessment Tool (EFAT-2) which is specially designed to measure physical impairment and functional performance of patients with advanced cancer or in PC.[55] As this measure can be administered by Onc R clinicians such as PTs and OTs, it has utility in quantifying outcomes for rehabilitation. An additional advantage is its simplicity and brevity, and it does not require substantial training to apply. It also displays sensitivity to identify changes in symptoms such as pain, fatigue, and motivation, all of which may impact a PWC's functional performance. Categories that are quantified include communication, mental status, pain, dyspnea, sitting/standing balance, bed mobility and transfers, locomotion via ambulation/wheelchair, fatigue, motivation, ADL status, and performance status. Each category is quantified from 0 = functional, 1 = minimal dysfunction, 2 = moderate dysfunction, and 3 = severe dysfunction. In addition to its utility in quantifying functional performance, the EFAT-2 has demonstrated discriminatory ability for discharge location for persons in PC.[55]

Quantifying Quality of Life

A key focus of Onc R services in PC and EOL is the optimization of QOL. Due to this focus, it is prudent to quantify a person's QOL objectively using valid, reliable patient-reported outcome measures. Several QOL measures will be introduced here. Especially in cases where the PWC is not expected to demonstrate physical or functional gains, if a valid, reliable outcome measure can demonstrate maintenance of or improvement in QOL, it provides additional evidence of the efficacy of palliative rehabilitation services. The European Organization for Research and Treatment of Cancer Quality of Life Questionnaire encompasses 30 items for PWC (EORTC QLQ-C30) and can be found at https://qol.eortc.org/. It has external validity for a variety of cancer diagnoses and has been translated into over 100 languages and is used in thousands of peer-reviewed publications annually.

Another widely researched QOL measure is the group of measures entitled the Functional Assessment of Cancer Therapy (FACT)/Functional Assessment of Chronic Illness Therapy (FACIT) which can be found at www.facit.org. These measures are appropriate for all cancer diagnoses and chronic diseases. There are a wide variety of diagnosis-specific measures for a large number of cancer and noncancer diagnoses. See Chapter 28 for information on the FACT/FACIT scales and their applicability.

Family and Caregiver Issues

At times, near the end stage of life, Onc R services are often fixated on as "the last hope" or when rehab is not tolerated, as the final catalyst to transition to hospice/PC. This often puts the Onc R clinicians in a difficult situation where rehab services may demonstrate some clinical gains, but it should be emphasized these are only temporary. Despite their temporary status, the PWC's hard work and efforts should be recognized and provide opportunities for the person to get home (if able and desired) or to perform new functional tasks with more independence. Despite these gains, it is imperative that the Onc R clinician be forthright and reminds the person that these gains are only temporary and the patient's disease process will continue to advance despite these gains.

An additional challenge for the Onc R clinician working with a person in PC or at the EOL is that there may not be an agreement between PWCs and their families regarding rehabilitation goals. This may be compounded by the circumstances that some family members may have underlying or unresolved issues or conflicts that may arise in times of stress. In an advanced disease process, some family members who have not seen each other for years will come together to support their loved ones during this difficult time. In some scenarios, this can result in a touching, emotional, positive experience—in other cases, it may result in frequent conflict and disarray. The Onc R clinician is encouraged to leverage their interdisciplinary resources such as social workers, pastoral care chaplains, or PC providers to help mitigate conflict and assist in aligning goals for all parties.

Terminal Cancer Pain

Pain at EOL is common and complex. It is not always a nociceptive condition that is easily treated with pain medications or anti-inflammatory medications. Pain at the EOL does not only occur because of the underlying diagnosis or as a consequence of underlying pathology. Before the EOL, many PWCs report moderate to severe pain, and 30% report pain as severe and approximately 25% of PWCs will die in pain.[56] The prevalence of pain ranges from 50% to 90%; 40% to 50% rated it as severe while 25% to 30% reported very severe pain.[57]

The *biopsychosocial model* has been detailed in Chapters 2 and 22 and should be applied as a multidimensional framework that incorporates not just the biomedical issues that a PWC is encountering but also the psychological and social factors that influence health.[58] Onc R clinicians should consider all of the possible pain sources or influences when preparing to address terminal cancer pain. In the biological domain, pain causes may include inflammation, tissue damage, or the advancing disease process. In the psychological domain, influences include pain beliefs, coping abilities, the PWC's loss of locus of control, lack of self-efficacy, and the emotions encountered during the disease journey and the circumstances therein. Finally, social aspects include cultural influences on pain, learning mechanisms, or social relationships. It is the role of the Onc R clinician to consider all domains of pain and either provide direct treatment, education, or referral after identification of the various sources and causes of the pain. Psychological pain may be a result of biological pain from nociceptive sources; psychological pain can also exacerbate or amplify biological pain. In addition, underlying psychosocial diagnoses (anxiety, depression, etc.) can increase the risk for more frequent or intense pain can further influence the PWC's perception of pain.[57,59]

One useful model to consider is Saunders' Model of Total Pain.[60] It is similar to the concept of the biopsychosocial model. By addressing the many contributions to distress, the PWC's emotional resources can then be reserved for meaningful and comforting activities, thus enhancing their QOL.

In the palliative management of pain, pharmacologic and non-pharmacologic measures should be encouraged proactively rather than reactively. Furthermore, referrals should be made to address any sources of pain. For example, a hospice chaplain could address spiritual pain, a social worker might mitigate issues of bureaucratic pain (e.g., frustration of filling out endless and tedious forms required for insurance claims), and rehabilitation can assist in the treatment of physical pain and the emotional/psychosocial pain of the loss of independence.

Other sources of Total Pain may include distress from financial toxicity (see Chapter 33) as well as pain from the loss of hope. A key goal for Onc R clinicians is to anticipate issues and prepare the

PWC, family, and care team to address these issues. For example, a person lung cancer will likely have dyspnea issues, a person with a large metastatic bone lesion will have a pain crisis, and a person with a lesion near the spinal cord may progressively lose strength, and chemotherapy may cause weakness, cognitive impairments, deconditioning, and may fall. Instead of waiting for these events to transpire in a palliative or EOL situation, the Onc R clinician can proactively educate the PWC and caregivers. This may reduce the distress and increase self-efficacy, which may avoid unwarranted readmissions or hospitalizations at the EOL. Additionally, as a PWC progressively becomes weaker, caregivers may try to help with physical mobility tasks and may sustain a musculoskeletal injury. Proactive education and training in safe patient handling and safe transfer techniques can reduce the risk of caregiver injuries.

Caregiver Burden and Burnout

Especially in scenarios where the PWC's disease is advancing, the family caregivers often take on more of the care tasks for these individuals. This may result in a stressful situation and set up the family or caregivers for burnout. Symptoms of burnout may include ignoring their health problems or symptoms (including putting off seeing their doctor), eating poorly, feeling tired all the time, or poor sleep hygiene habits. Burnout behaviors may also include overusing tobacco, alcohol, or other substances, or giving up exercise and hobbies. Due to the amount of time caring for their family member or loved one, they may lose contact with friends. These individuals may be bottling up feelings of sadness and frustration, demonstrating angry outbursts, feeling resentful toward others or unreasonably annoyed by them, as well as feeling anxious, depressed, or hopeless. This may also result in blaming the PWC or healthcare providers for the situation. These symptoms must be recognized, and the caregiver is encouraged to take time for themselves. A social worker or another community resource may be useful to procure respite services allowing the caregiver to have some restorative time or complete needed errands and doctors' appointments. Regardless, if the family caregiver suffers burnout, both the caregiver and the PWC themselves will likely have negative health outcomes. In addition to burnout being possible in family caregivers, healthcare team members are susceptible to burnout. A key role of the Onc R clinician is to monitor oncology staff and clinician colleagues for emotional overload, including themself. We should watch for burnout, as it likely will negatively affect patient care. During times of loss and death, a mourning process is important for everyone, and sharing with colleagues, friends, or even speaking with the team's social worker or chaplain should be encouraged. See Chapter 33 for additional considerations in caregiver burnout.

Conclusion

Onc R clinicians have been working with persons with incurable or terminal conditions since the start of our respective professions; the difference is a shift in philosophy. These PWCs can present in any care setting including outpatient, skilled nursing, IPR, acute care, and homecare. Services provided by Onc R clinicians in PC or EOL are specific, safe, and can improve the QOL, dignity, and comfort of the person with terminal disease. The frequency and intensity of services should be reasonable and skilled rehabilitation

services should require the complexity of each disciplines' domain to warrant payment. During this time in a person's life, they need a home and a reason to go on. Onc R can provide such, assisting the person to have an enriching and meaningful time of remaining life.

Critical Research Needs

- Effect of Onc R clinician involvement in palliative multidisciplinary team
- Randomized controlled trials of quality of life for terminally ill individuals with and without therapist services based on cancer type
- Do Onc R services in acute care for individuals with advanced cancer shorten hospital length of stay or reduce preventable readmissions?
- What knowledge, skills, and interventions are necessary for an Onc R clinician to care for an individual in palliative care or at the end of life?

Case Study

TS was a 63-year-old male who was diagnosed 9 months ago with metastatic lung cancer. He was recently in the hospital for three weeks with an exacerbation of his breathlessness and weakness for advanced lung cancer compounded by bacterial pneumonia. Prior to this hospitalization, TS was ambulating with a two-wheeled walker at home and was on 2 L of O_2 via nasal cannula. The PWC elected to go home on hospice with supplemental oxygen at 3 to 6 L based on his oxygen saturations and an antibiotic. During this time, he was not able to get out of bed for 2 weeks. At 2 weeks, TS became more alert and began to request to get out of bed. The hospice physician and nurse placed a consult for a PT to evaluate him.

Upon examination, TS was able to tolerate supine to sit to stand with minimal assistance but was only able to stand for 40 seconds. He was able to do this twice before he reported a need to rest. After a rest, the PWC was able to tolerate transfer training with his wife from bed to a wheelchair and he was able to tolerate sitting in wheelchair for 5 minutes. His vitals were monitored closely through all transitions. He did demonstrate some fluctuation in oxygen saturation where it reached 90% but never went below 90% as he was able to improve his oxygen levels after 1 minute of rest and deep breathing.

In evaluating the PWC's status and rehabilitation potential, the PT considered that some patients experience ups and downs while in disease progression and that a patient may experience a set-back, followed by an improvement with the desire to regain a small amount of strength, even with the knowledge that their illness may not be cured. This clinician chose to apply the palliative rehabilitation concept of *Rehab Light* with the aim to prescribe limited and targeted exercise with the aim to improve his strength without overwhelming his system or negatively affecting his QOL. The PT would return weekly for a short bout of physical therapy and to update or modify TS's HEP. In addition, the PT closely coordinated with the nurse case manager to discuss the plan of care, the amount of assistance needed and the level of safe mobility that TS could perform with assistance.

During the 1-week follow up, TS was now able to ambulate with a rolling walker for the first time in over a month. His first bout was 10 feet and he was able to walk 20 feet on his second bout. After this physical therapy session, the PWC started expressing the desire to sit at his dining table to eat at least one meal per day. In addition, he started expressing a desire to leave his home via wheelchair. The PT incorporated these patient-centered goals into the plan of care as they were important to

TS' remaining QOL and engagement in life activities. Although the rehabilitation services did not appreciably lengthen TS's life, he was now able to engage in some remaining meaningful life events that may have otherwise not been possible.

Review Questions

Reader can find the correct answers and rationale in the back of the book.

1. Which of the following statements is not matched with its appropriate definition?
   A. Rehabilitation light—Anticipate functional decline, procures needed equipment beforehand, teaches family positioning and safe patient handling before physical decline
   B. Case management—Providing training, follow up care, instruction for individuals with long term chronic conditions—update home programs, preventing complications
   C. Skilled maintenance—Where ehabilitation service is required to maintain or slow decline of a condition
   D. Supportive care—Psychosocial support, range of motion, massage, pain management techniques

2. A 78-year-old male diagnosed with Stage 4 lung cancer was referred to the health system's outpatient PC service. He demonstrates severe difficulty with performing his ADLs and demonstrates dyspnea during ambulation of household distances. His doctor referred him to outpatient physical therapy and occupational therapy to improve his performance status. Which of the following is MOST ACCURATE regarding this person's eligibility for skilled PT/OT?
   A. The person's PC consultation excludes his ability to receive skilled PT/OT
   B. He is eligible for skilled PT/OT which would be covered by Medicare Part B for therapy services
   C. This person is eligible for skilled PT/OT but it is not appropriate due to his imminent death
   D. This person is eligible for limited skilled PT/OT but the amount will be limited by Medicare's "per diem" payment structure

3. An Onc R clinician is working with a 67-year-old female with Stage IV colorectal cancer for lower extremity lymphedema management. Over the first month, her leg volume decreased significantly but this is beginning to plateau. The person does not have a strong social support network, lives alone, and has rheumatoid arthritis of the hands and cannot apply a custom lymphedema garment herself. Due to her medical issues, the clinician deems that if she does not receive her manual lymph drainage and application of wrapping bandages, her condition will get worse. This clinician is considering keeping the PWC on schedule for skilled maintenance. Which of the following is the MOST accurate as it relates to skilled maintenance in this case?
   A. Medicare will pay for maintenance services when they require the skill of a licensed therapist/assistant
   B. Medicare will only pay for maintenance services when it does not require the skill of a licensed therapist
   C. As this person has Stage IV cancer, her limb swelling is not a primary focus of care

D. This person should be advised to go on hospice as she is too ill for outpatient therapy

4. A 81-year-old male with a primary brain tumor is being seen by a PT for an unrelated low back pain issue. During the course of PT treatment, he states he is really upset because his doctor mentioned that he should talk to a PC specialist. The patient states "palliative care is only for dying people and I didn't think I was dying." He asks the therapist about what PC is and why it might be helpful. Which of the following statements is LEAST accurate for PC.
   A. This person is right, hospice and PC are the same things
   B. PC uses a holistic team approach to proactively address symptoms
   C. PC emphasizes optimizing remaining QOL
   D. PC is not only for those who terminally ill and is appropriate for those with chronic or incurable illnesses

5. A hospital system is considering implementing regular rehabilitation professional representation on the PC team. The managers are considering designating one key person as the lead therapist. Which of the following is a benefit to designating a "lead" therapist to PC services?
   A. The lead therapist can see every patient on palliative service themselves to not bother the other therapists
   B. Makes sure that PC patients are not evaluated by the rehabilitation team until they are ready for discharge
   C. Serves as a resource person for other therapists who also care for patients with palliative diagnoses during challenging situations
   D. Prevents the need to have the therapists treat patients with major issues to maximize efficiency

6. An OT is providing care for a 76-year-old male with Stage IV metastatic prostate cancer. The OT is going to be off for a week and is handing off care to a colleague and notes that the current care plan is using a "Rehab Light" approach. What statement does NOT accurately describe the "Rehab Light" component of the Palliative Care Model?
   A. PWCs experience ups and downs while in chronic disease progression
   B. A PWC may experience a set-back, followed by an improvement with the desire to regain small amount of strength, even with the knowledge that their illness may not be cured
   C. In order to optimize insurance reimbursement, a PWC should always have a minimum of 5 visits per week
   D. Communication with the IDT is essential

7. Which statement most accurately describes "skilled maintenance" rehab philosophy?
   A. It can be easily performed by family members and general caregivers
   B. Skilled maintenance is needed when tasks are to complex or unsafe for caregivers to perform

C. Formal documentation is not required for this type of care

D. Visits should be coordinated with other disciplines so that you meet with the patient at the same time

8. A therapist is treating a 45-year-old female who has just completed surgery and radiation and is currently undergoing chemotherapy for her Stage IV pancreatic cancer. She is a single mother of with three children, she works full time and has no family in the area. She confides to you that she is worried about losing her job and her associated health benefits. She also admits she is running out of money and her credit cards are overextended. She is thinking of stopping her cancer treatment because she cannot afford it. Clinically, she has a minimal balance impairment, cancer related fatigue rated as a 4/10 (10 being the worst), and decreased strength to both arms and legs to 4+/5. As a therapist, which of the following would be the HIGHEST priority intervention?

A. Contact the person's doctor or cancer center to begin to address her financial toxicity

B. Begin basic balance exercises for fall prevention

C. Discuss energy conservation techniques for her fatigue

D. Initiate an aerobic exercise program to start working on her cardiopulmonary fitness

9. An Onc R clinician is beginning outpatient treatment of a 78-year-old female for general strengthening when undergoing palliative chemotherapy for her Stage IV colon cancer. The clinician is very interested in quantifying the person's report of QOL to justify to the insurance company that rehab services were needed. Which of the following would be the MOST APPROPRIATE outcome measure for quantifying QOL?

A. FACT-G

B. Timed up and go

C. Lower extremity functional scale

D. Handgrip dynamometry

10. A 63-year-old male is being treated for Stage III bladder cancer. He complains of pain 10/10 "all over" but upon the Onc R clinician's evaluation there is very little palpatory tenderness, and his pain is not provocable or alleviated with special testing or ROM or MMT. He rates his distress as a 9/10 on the distress thermometer. He also rated a low overall QOL on the FACT-G especially mainly in the domains of psychosocial and emotional. He is also reporting that he is having issues with being intimate with his wife since the cancer started. Based on the information presented in the case, which of the following is MOST LIKELY to be a key component of his pain?

A. Hip flexor muscle spasm

B. Emotional and psychosocial distress

C. Metastatic bone pain

D. Sacroiliac pain

References

1. Wilson CM, Stiller CH, Doherty DJ, Thompson KA. The role of physical therapists within hospice and palliative care in the United States and Canada. *Am J Hospice Palliat Med.* 2017;34(1):34–41.

2. Wilson CM, Stiller CH, Doherty DJ, Thompson KA, Smith AB, Turczynski KL. Physical therapists in integrated palliative care: a qualitative study. *BMJ Support Palliat Care.* 2020. doi:10.1136/bmjspcare-2019-002161.

3. World Health Organization. WHO definition of palliative care. https://www.who.int/cancer/palliative/definition/en/. Accessed October 25, 2019.

4. Lynn J, Adamson DM. *Living well at the end of life: adapting health care to serious chronic illness in old age.* RAND Corp; 2003.

5. Center to Advance Palliative Care. Palliative care continues its annual growth trend, according to latest center to advance palliative care analysis; 2018. https://www.capc.org/about/press-media/press-releases/2018-2-28/palliative-care-continues-its-annual-growth-trend-according-latest-center-advance-palliative-care-analysis/; Accessed October 26, 2019.

6. Buss MK, Rock LK, McCarthy EP. Understanding palliative care and hospice: a review for primary care providers. *Mayo Clin Proc.* 2017;92(2):280–286.

7. Scibetta C, Kerr K, Mcguire J, Rabow MW. The costs of waiting: implications of the timing of palliative care consultation among a cohort of decedents at a comprehensive cancer center. *J Palliat Med.* 2016;19(1):69–75.

8. Healthcare Financial Management Association. Medicare program; FY 2021 hospice wage index and payment rate update [CMS-1733-F]: summary of final rule. https://www.hfma.org/content/dam/hfma/Documents/industry-initiatives/fact-sheets/fy2021-hospice-wage-index-payment-rate-update-final-rule-summary.pdf. Accessed January 23, 2021.

9. Center for Medicare and Medicaid Services. Medicare program; FY 2016 hospice wage index and payment rate update and hospice quality reporting requirements. Federal Register. 2015(80 FR 47141):47141–47207. https://www.federalregister.gov/articles/2015/08/06/2015-19033/medicare-program-fy-2016-hospice-wage-index-and-payment-rate-update-and-hospice-quality-reporting.

10. Center for Medicare and Medicaid Services. How hospice works. https://www.medicare.gov/what-medicare-covers/what-part-a-covers/how-hospice-works. Accessed January 23, 2021.

11. Burge F, Lawson B, Johnston G, Asada Y, McIntyre PF, Flowerdew G. Preferred and actual location of death: what factors enable a preferred home death? *J Palliat Med.* 2015;18(12):1054–1059.

12. Smith AK, McCarthy E, Weber E, et al. Half of older Americans seen in emergency department in last month of life; most admitted to hospital, and many die there. *Health Aff.* 2012;31(6):1277–1285.

13. Riley GF, Lubitz JD. Long-term trends in Medicare payments in the last year of life. *Health Serv Res.* 2010;45(2):565–576.

14. Wright AA, Zhang B, Ray A, et al. Associations between end-of-life discussions, patient mental health, medical care near death, and caregiver bereavement adjustment. *JAMA.* 2008;300(14):1665–1673.

15. Wright AA, Keating NL, Balboni TA, Matulonis UA, Block SD, Prigerson HG. Place of death: correlations with quality of life of patients with cancer and predictors of bereaved caregivers' mental health. *J Clin Oncol.* 2010;28(29):4457.

16. Temel JS, Greer JA, Muzikansky A, et al. Early palliative care for patients with metastatic non-small-cell lung cancer. *N Engl J Med.* 2010;363(8):733–742. doi:10.1056/NEJMoa1000678.

17. Connor SR, Pyenson B, Fitch K, Spence C, Iwasaki K. Comparing hospice and nonhospice patient survival among patients who die within a three-year window. *J Pain Symptom Manage.* 2007;33(3):238–246.

18. Miranda DG, Peces EMS, Babarro AA, Sánchez MCP, Cerdeira MV. HOLD study (home care obstructive lung disease): natural history of patients with advanced COPD. *BMC Palliat Care.* 2016;15(1):1–9.

19. Buttorff C, Ruder T, Bauman M. *Multiple Chronic Conditions in the United Sates:* RAND Corporation; 2017. doi:10.7249/TL221. https://www.rand.org/pubs/tools/TL221.html.

20. Xu J, Murphy SL, Kochanek KD, Arias E. *Mortality in the United States,* 2018. NCHS Data Brief, No. 355. National Center for Health Statistics; 2020.

21. Aldridge MD, Kelley AS. The myth regarding the high cost of end-of-life care. *Am J Public Health.* 2015;105(12):2411–2415.

22. Schoenman JA, Chockley N. *The concentration of health care Spending:* National Institute for Health Care Management Research Educational Foundation (NIHCM) Foundation; 2012 Data Brief.

23. Meier DE, Back AL, Berman A, Block SD, Corrigan JM. Sean Morrison R. A national strategy for palliative care. *Health Aff.* 2017;36(7):1265–1273.

24. Center for Medicare and Medicaid Services. Certifying patients for the medicare home health benefit; 2015. https://www.cms.gov/Outreach-and-Education/Outreach/NPC/Downloads/2014-12-16-HHBenefit-HL.pdf; 2015. Accessed January 24, 2021.

25. Rietjens JA, Sudore RL, Connolly M, et al. Definition and recommendations for advance care planning: an international consensus supported by the European Association for Palliative Care. *Lancet Oncol.* 2017;18(9):e543–e551.

26. Meier DE, Beresford L. POLST offers next stage in honoring patient preferences. *J Palliat Med.* 2009;12(4):291–295.

27. Hammes BJ, Rooney BL, Gundrum JD. A comparative, retrospective, observational study of the prevalence, availability, and specificity of advance care plans in a county that implemented an advance care planning microsystem. *J Am Geriatr Soc.* 2010;58(7):1249–1255.

28. Wilson CM. Advance directives, advance care planning, and the physical therapists' role in these challenging conversations. *Rehabil Oncol.* 2016;34(2):72–74.

29. Mueller K, Wilson CM, Briggs R. Chapter 27: Hospice and end of life. In: Avers D, Wong R, eds. *Guccione's Geriatric Physical Therapy.* 4th ed. Mosby; 2019.

30. Center for Medicare and Medicaid Services. Condition of participation: physical therapy, occupational therapy, and speech-language pathology. https://www.govinfo.gov/app/details/CFR-2016-title42-vol3/CFR-2016-title42-vol3-sec418-72/summary. Accessed March 26, 2021.

31. Gladieux JE, Basile M. Jimmo and the improvement standard: implementing Medicare coverage through regulations, policy manuals and other guidance. *Am J Law Med.* 2014;40(1):7–25.

32. American Physical Therapy Association. The role of physical therapy in palliative care and hospice; 2019. https://www.apta.org/apta-and-you/leadership-and-governance/policies/role-of-physical-therapy-in-palliative-care-and-hospice. Accessed March 26, 2021.

33. American Physical Therapy Association. Amend: delivery of value-based physical therapy services; 2019. https://www.apta.org/apta-and-you/leadership-and-governance/policies/delivery-value-based-pt-services. Accessed March 26, 2021.

34. American Occupational Therapy Association. The role of occupational therapy in palliative and hospice care; 2015. https://www.aota.org/-/media/Corporate/Files/AboutOT/Professionals/WhatIsOT/PA/Facts/FactSheet_PalliativeCare.pdf. Accessed March 26, 2021.

35. Pizzi MA, Briggs R. Occupational and physical therapy in hospice: the facilitation of meaning, quality of life, and well-being. *Top Geriatr Rehabil.* 2004;20(2):120–130.

36. American Speech-Language-Hearing Association. *End-of-life issues in speech-language pathology*; 2021. https://www.asha.org/slp/clinical/endoflife/. Accessed March 26.

37. Briggs RW. Clinical decision making for physical therapists in patient-centered end-of-life care. *Top Geriatr Rehabil.* 2011;27(1):10–17.

38. National Hospice and Palliative Care Organization. *NHPCO facts and figures 2020 Edition.* https://www.nhpco.org/wp-content/uploads/NHPCO-Facts-Figures-2020-edition.pdf. Accessed March 26, 2021.

39. Center for Medicare and Medicaid Services. *Jimmo v. Sibelius settlement agreement program manual clarifications fact sheet*; 2014. https://www.cms.gov/Medicare/Medicare-Fee-for-Service-Payment/SNFPPS/Downloads/jimmo_fact_sheet2_022014_final.pdf. Accessed March 26, 2021.

40. Medicare Learning Network. *MM7182—New home health claims reporting requirements for G Codes related to therapy and skilled nursing services.* Center for Medicare and Medicaid Services; Center for Medicare and Medicaid Services; 2011. https://www.cms.gov/Outreach-and-Education/Medicare-Learning-Network-MLN/MLNMattersArticles/Downloads/MM7182.pdf Accessed March 26, 2021.

41. Wilson CM, Mueller K, Briggs R. Physical therapists' contribution to the hospice and palliative care interdisciplinary team: a clinical summary. *J Hospice Palliat Nurs.* 2017;19(6):588–596.

42. Spill GR, Hlubocky FJ, Daugherty CK. Oncologists' and physiatrists' attitudes regarding rehabilitation for patients with advanced cancer. *PMR.* 2012;4(2):96–108.

43. Smith S, Wilson CM, Lipple C, et al. Managing palliative patients in inpatient rehabilitation through a short stay family training program. *Am J Hospice Palliat Med.* 2020;37(3):172–178.

44. Back AL, Fromme EK, Meier DE. Training clinicians with communication skills needed to match medical treatments to patient values. *J Am Geriatr Soc.* 2019;67:S435–S441.

45. Back AL, Arnold RM, Baile WF, Tulsky JA, Fryer-Edwards K. Approaching difficult communication tasks in oncology. *CA: Cancer J Clin.* 2005;55(3):164–177.

46. Buckman R. Communication skills in palliative care: a practical guide. *Neurol Clin.* 2001;19(4):989–1004.

47. Alzheimer's Association. 2019 Alzheimer's disease facts and figures; 2019. https://www.alz.org/media/documents/alzheimers-facts-and-figures-2019-r.pdf. Accessed March 26, 2021.

48. Small JA, Gloria G, Saskia M, Beth H. Effectiveness of communication strategies used by caregivers of persons with Alzheimer's disease during activities of daily living. *J Speech Lang Hear Res.* 2003;46(2):353–367.

49. Glisky EL. Method of vanishing cues. In: Kreutzer JS, DeLuca J, Caplan B, eds. *Encyclopedia of Clinical Neuropsychology.* New York: Springer; 2011:1586–1587.

50. Mott FE, Marcus JD. The final goodbye. *Palliat Support Care.* 2013;11(3):277–279.

51. Back AL, Arnold RM, Tulsky JA, Baile WF, Fryer-Edwards KA. On saying goodbye: acknowledging the end of the patient–physician relationship with patients who are near death. *Ann Intern Med.* 2005;142(8):682–685.

52. Anderson F, Downing GM, Hill J, Casorso L, Lerch N. Palliative Performance Scale (PPS): a new tool. *J Palliat Care.* 1996;12(1):5–11.

53. Wilner LS, Arnold R. The Palliative Performance Scale: fast facts and concepts #125: Palliative Care Network of Wisconsin; 2015. https://www.mypcnow.org/wp-content/uploads/2019/02/FF-125-PPS.-3rd-Ed.pdf Accessed March 26, 2021.

54. Reville B, Axelrod D, Maury R. Palliative care for the cancer patient. *Prim Care.* 2009;36(4):781–810.

55. Kaasa T, Wessel J, Darrah J, Bruera E. Inter-rater reliability of formally trained and self-trained raters using the Edmonton Functional Assessment Tool. *Palliat Med.* 2000;14(6):509–517.

56. Leleszi JP, Lewandowski JG. Pain management in end-of-life care. *J Am Osteopath Assoc.* 2005;105(3 suppl):6S–11S.

57. Fink RM, Brant JM. Complex cancer pain assessment. *Hematol Oncol Clin.* 2018;32(3):353–369.

58. Smith RC, Fortin AH, Dwamena F, Frankel RM. An evidence-based patient-centered method makes the biopsychosocial model scientific. *Patient Educ Couns.* 2013;91(3):265–270.

59. Bennett MI, Eisenberg E, Ahmedzai SH, et al. Standards for the management of cancer-related pain across Europe—a position paper from the EFIC task force on cancer pain. *Eur J Pain.* 2019;23(4):660–668.

60. Clark D. Total pain: the work of Cicely Saunders and the hospice movement. *Am Pain Society Bulletin.* 2000;10(4):13–15.

30

Wellness, Health Promotion, and Prevention

SUZETTE SMITH, PT, DPT, CLT, RYT200 (BOARD CERTIFIED ONCOLOGIC PHYSICAL THERAPY CLINICAL SPECIALIST), ERIN DAIEK, RDN

CHAPTER OUTLINE

Wellness Scope of Practice

Oncology rehabilitation (Onc R) clinicians have the expertise to be at the forefront of the wellness, health promotion, and prevention movement. In the past, the role of rehabilitation clinicians focused on treatment of an existing condition; however, increasingly, Onc R clinicians are using patient care time to educate on prevention and mitigation of disease. Currently, the Centers for Disease Control and Prevention (CDC) lists heart disease and cancer as the top two causes of death in the United States (US). Onc R clinicians are positioned to educate patients to engage in activities known to reduce disease risk, such as exercise; disengage in activities known to increase risk, such as smoking; provide prehabilitation interventions to improve outcomes during cancer treatment; and provide care through a prospective surveillance model to identify early onset of functional impairments, resolving issues before they become chronic and mitigating adverse treatment effects. The American Physical Therapy Association (APTA) scope of practice statement supports physical therapists' (PTs') involvement in wellness and prevention and indicates that they are vital and essential providers of rehabilitation and habilitation, performance

enhancement, prevention, and risk-reduction services.[1] The APTA supports the PTs' role in the promotion of health and wellness and states that "identifying contributing lifestyle factors such as weight, exercise, and stress reduction are integral components of the PT practice."[1] Onc R clinicians have the ability to significantly impact public health in this regard. Onc R clinicians have more time with patients than most other healthcare providers and can provide services both in person and remotely via telehealth.

A survey study identified that PTs believe that they have a role in promotion of prevention and wellness in the cancer population. This study demonstrated a disconnect between how PTs who treat patients diagnosed with cancer see their role in health promotion and wellness and the education provided to patients. It was found that PTs provide information to persons living with and beyond cancer (PLWBCs) regarding exercise, nutrition, and stress management. Although in this study, PTs rated it important to educate patients regarding smoking and alcohol cessation, substance abuse, and sleep, this education is often not provided during therapy sessions. Some of the reasons cited for this disconnect were time constraints, perceived lack of patient interest, and inadequate practitioner education.[2] This chapter discusses components of cancer prevention, wellness and health promotion that can be addressed by Onc R clinicians to improve community health and patient care.

Prevention

Onc R clinicians have a role in disease prevention across the continuum of care throughout the lifespan. The nexus model of cancer prevention (see Chapter 2) includes five levels of prevention and their relationship to survival: primordial, primary, secondary, tertiary, and quaternary. Primordial prevention involves community level intervention to prevent cancer and other diseases and negative health effects, primary prevention involves individual intervention in prevention of cancer and other diseases before a health effect occurs, secondary prevention involves screening for early onset of disease to allow for early intervention with emphasis on prehabilitation to prevent and mitigate the adverse effects caused from the treatments for cancer, tertiary prevention involves an intervention to slow or manage the adverse effects caused from the treatment for cancer, and quaternary prevention involves avoiding over medicalization when more harm than good may come from treatment.[3,4] The CDC includes rehabilitation as a component of tertiary prevention. However, the scope of practice of Onc R clinicians has the potential to have an impactful role in all levels of cancer prevention. At the primordial level of cancer prevention, Onc R clinicians may participate in community outreach to promote healthy lifestyles and allow the community to engage in safe physical activity such as fall prevention clinics, helmet and bike fittings, and community walking programs. In terms of primary prevention for Onc R, clinicians can educate and provide personalized plans of care to alter lifestyles or behaviors, promote adequate physical activity (PA), encourage smoking cessation, and provide nutrition counseling to reduce disease risk. Onc R clinicians are involved in secondary prevention by completing rehabilitation tests and measures, neurological screenings, assessing medical history, asking red flag questions, and implementing cancer screening protocols and prehabilitation programs to improve physical function prior to treatment for cancer. See Chapter 27 for more information on prehabilitation. Onc R clinicians contribute to tertiary prevention by providing services to mitigate adverse effects of cancer treatment and encourage behavior development that will assist with improved outcomes and quality of life (QOL), as well as decreased propensity for recurrence of disease. In quaternary prevention clinicians can assist with pain modulation, durable medical equipment recommendations, as well as caregiver training and movement modifications to maximize QOL. These interventions may also contribute to decreased hospitalization near the end of life or improved function when a medical intervention is contraindicated, for example, in the case of nonsurgical bone metastasis.

An estimated 42% of cancer cases are attributable to modifiable lifestyle changes; two of the top modifiable behaviors pertaining to mortality are smoking and body weight. Other contributing modifiable behaviors include consumption of red and processed meat, inadequate fruit and vegetable consumption, alcohol intake, and physical inactivity.[5] Five key health behaviors have been associated with chronic disease prevention: negative smoking history, achieving the recommended amount of PA (defined as at least 150 minutes/week of moderate-intensity PA or 75 minutes/week of vigorous-intensity PA), consuming little to no alcohol (defined as maximum one drink per day for women and two a day for men), maintaining body weight in normal body mass index (BMI range

of 18.5–24.9, and getting sufficient daily sleep (at least 7 hours). Only 6.35% of Americans practice all five key health behaviors regularly.[6] There is ample opportunity for Onc R clinicians to educate and engage patients in these lifestyle modifications to prevent cancer and other chronic diseases. These factors are important education topics for PLWBCs that can be easily integrated into clinical practice.

Prevention Screening

Cancer screening protocols are available for multiple cancer types to detect cancer before symptoms appear. Early detection allows for early intervention which equates to improved clinical outcomes and less invasive treatment options. Screening parameters for average-risk persons are an important piece of cancer prevention and include breast, cervical, colorectal, and prostate cancers (Table 30.1). There are heightened screening measures for these cancers for people at higher risk. For certain cancers, such as lung cancer, screening protocols are only recommended for individuals with high risk and not the general population. Specific screening and surveillance recommendations exist for PLWBCs relative to early detection of recurrent disease. There is often a lack of consensus on screening recommendations among cancer experts, therefore PLWBCs are encouraged to speak with their respective medical team for individualized screening recommendations. The risk to benefit ratio requires consideration when determining screening recommendations for any cancer.

TABLE 30.1	Screening Recommendation by Cancer Type
Cancer Type	**Screening Recommendations**
Breast[7,8]	American Cancer Society: annual mammogram from age 45 to 55 years and then every 2 years from age 55 to 75 years. Women should continue to receive screening throughout life as long they have a 10-year life expectancy. National Comprehensive Cancer Network: annually starting at age 40 years. U.S. Preventative Service Task Force: from age 50 to 74 years mammograms every 2 years with an option to discuss earlier screenings with healthcare providers.
Prostate[9,10]	American Cancer Society: prostate-specific antigen blood test and rectal exam in men over age 50 years with at least 10 years life expectancy.
Cervical[11]	HPV and PAP every 3 years beginning at age 21 years.
Colorectal[12,13,14]	Starting at age 45 to 50 years Stool based tests: Fecal occult blood test annually Fecal immunochemical test annually Multitarget stool DNA test every 1–3 years Structural tests: Colonoscopy every 10 years Flexible sigmoidoscopy every 5 years CT colonography every 5 years

CT, Computed tomography; *DNA,* deoxynucleic acid; *HPV,* human papillomavirus; *PAP,* Papanicolaou.
Created by Suzette Smith. Printed with permission.

Breast

There is lack of consensus between the American Cancer Society (ACS), National Comprehensive Cancer Network (NCCN), and the United States Preventive Task Force (USPTF) relative to breast cancer screening parameters.[15,16] Mammogram imaging is the recommended screening assessment for women of average risk and offers the advantage of cancer detection up to 3 years before it can be palpated manually.[16]

The NCCN recommends annual mammograms for *women starting* at age 40 years. Testing is recommended to continue as long as the woman has a 10-year life expectancy. Whereas the USPTF recommends starting testing at age 50 years as the risk may outweigh the benefit in average-risk women aged 40 to 49 years.[7] Women with higher risk stratification (those with genetic *BRCA1* or *BRCA2* mutations, who received chest or mantle radiation before the age of 30 years, or who have a family history that places them in a higher risk bracket) will have more stringent screening recommendations.[17]

Prostate

The ACS and American Urological Association (AUA) recommend prostate-specific antigen blood test (PSA) and digital rectal examination beginning at age 50 years for the average-risk male with a life expectancy of at least 10 years. The USPTF recommends that for men aged 55 to 75 years, the decision to have PSA screening should be individualized between the patient and physician, and it is not believed that benefits outweigh the potential harm of the test for men aged over 75 years.[24]

Colorectal

Ninety percent of colon cancer cases occur in persons over the age of 50 years, and one-third of adults in this age bracket do not get tested as recommended. The indications for screening persons under the age of 50 years include the following: inflammatory bowel disease, a close relative with colorectal polyps or colorectal cancer, or a genetic syndrome such as Lynch syndrome or familial adenomatous polyposis.[18] The CDC and USPTF recommend structural testing, tests that show the inside of the colon, begin at age 50 years and is repeated every 10 years until the age of 75 years. CDC, USPTF, and ACS recommend the decision for continued screening from age 75 to 85 years be based on general health and past testing results.[19–20]

ACS recommends screening begin at age 45 years with an occult blood test or structural test and continue through the age of 75 years if life expectancy is greater than 10 years. ACS recommends any positive non-colonoscopy testing, such as stool-based tests, be followed up with a colonoscopy. ACS discourages testing in people over age 85 years. See Table 30.2 for a list of structural and stool-based tests.[22]

Cervical

Cervical cancer screening recommendations differ between the American College of Obstetricians and Gynecologists (ACOG) and the ACS. The ACOG recommends Papanicolaou (PAP) testing begin at age 21 years and continue every 3 years until the age of 29 years. For persons aged 30 to 65 years a primary human papillomavirus (HPV) test or co-testing with PAP and HPV test is recommended every 3 years. Testing may continue past the age of 65 years if certain risk criteria are present.[23,24] ACS recommends starting at age 25 years with primary HPV testing every 5 years until the age of 65 years. Testing may continue past the age of 65 years if certain risk criteria are present.[25]

TABLE 30.2	BMI Weight Categories[31]
Weight Category	**BMI**
Underweight	Below 18.5
Normal	18.5–24.9
Overweight	25.0–29.9
Obesity	30.0 and above

BMI, Body mass index.
Created by Suzette Smith and Erin Daiek. Printed with permission.

Lung Cancer

Currently, lung cancer screening is not recommended for the average-risk person. Candidates for yearly lung cancer screening are between age 55 and 74 years, in relatively good health and have a 30-pack year history of tobacco use, currently smoking tobacco, or have quit within the last 15 years.[26,27] Screening with low-dose computed tomography (LDCT) has been shown to reduce lung cancer mortality by identifying early stage asymptomatic disease. Commonly, incidental findings of lung nodules, defined as a rounded opacity measuring up to 3 cm in diameter, are discovered during these screenings, as well as during unrelated chest X-ray and CT scans.[28] The majority of these nodules are benign, however Fleischner Society, NCCN, and others have released specific guidelines for management of these cases. Guidelines consider lung cancer risk factors such as smoking history, age, cancer history, history of lung disease, family history, and occupational history, or carcinogenic exposure. These factors along with imaging studies and possible biopsies guide management.[21] Many hospital systems provide specialty lung nodule clinics for proper management of these cases.

Endometrial Cancer

The ACS does not recommend screenings for endometrial cancer unless the woman has Lynch syndrome, thereby placing her in a higher risk category. Recommendations for women at menopause include comprehensive education relative to signs and symptoms of endometrial cancer inclusive of risk factors (women who have taken hormone replacement therapy, late menopause, tamoxifen [Nolvadex] therapy, nulliparity, infertility, and obesity), and the importance of reporting any unexpected bleeding or spotting to a physician.[20]

Weight Control

Maintaining a normal body weight is a component of wellness that contributes to the prevention of major chronic diseases, including cancer, diabetes, heart disease, and cerebral vascular accident. This not only contributes to cancer risk reduction, but also improves survival and prognosis for certain cancer types and decreases the risk of disease recurrence.[29] There are many mechanisms at play in the causal relationship between obesity and increased risk for cancer, and the following is not an all-inclusive list. Obesity is linked to insulin resistance, which indicates the body has elevated insulin and insulin-like growth factor in the bloodstream which may promote cancer cell growth and inhibit apoptosis. Obesity is associated with chronic low-grade levels of local and systemic inflammation which can cause DNA damage. Adipose tissue produces an excess amount of estrogen which is associated with increased risk of certain cancers. Increased leptin levels is associated with obesity and may promote cell growth while inhibiting apoptosis.[30]

Being overweight or obese, as defined by BMI categories, is an established overall risk factor for cancer, and is calculated by dividing weight in kilograms by height in meters squared. The range of normal BMI for adults is 18.5 to 24.9. A BMI of 25 or higher is directly related to increased cancer risk.[31] Table 30.2 indicates BMI ranges for individuals who are underweight, normal, overweight, and obese.[21]

Clinical use of BMI is a screen with limitations for determining amount of body fat, as it does not account for amount of muscle mass or body fat distribution. For example, a fit person with increased muscle mass can assess as overweight on the BMI scale and not assess into an at-risk weight category due to fitness level. Clinically it may be used in conjunction with waist circumference and waist to hip ratio for a more complete clinical picture of risk. This addresses the distribution of excess weight, as it is possible to have a normal BMI, but have increased risk secondary to higher waist circumference and hip to waist ratio. Evidence demonstrates that obesity-associated disease risk, including cancer, increases with a waist circumference measurement that is greater than 35 inches for women or greater than 40 inches for men.[31] If a person is above or below normal BMI, it would be beneficial to discuss weight loss and or gain, provide an exercise program, and possibly provide a referral to a dietitian or medical doctor for professional weight management services.

There is growing evidence linking youth obesity to adult cancer risk.[32] Almost 32% of children and adolescents are overweight or obese.[32] Adults who are in overweight or obese BMI categories have increased risk compared to adults with normal BMI for the following cancers: endometrial, esophageal adenocarcinoma, gastric, breast cancer in postmenopausal women, liver, kidney, multiple myeloma, meningioma, pancreatic, colorectal, gallbladder, ovarian, and thyroid cancers. The degree of correlation between above normal BMI and cancer risk varies by cancer type and the extent of excess body weight.[33] Overweight and obesity BMI categories are associated with 55% of all cancer types diagnosed in women and 24% of those diagnosed in men.[34] According to research from the ACS, excess body weight is thought to be responsible for approximately 11% of cancers in women and about 5% of cancers in men in the US, as well as about 7% of all cancer deaths.[35]

Weight loss is most strongly associated with decreased risk of endometrial, colon, and breast cancers in postmenopausal women.[36] Additionally, weight loss needs to be maintained to maintain health benefits. "Among individuals who are overweight or obese, losing weight—even if reductions are small and regardless of age or the degree of excess weight—is beneficial for reducing cancer risk."[37] Recommendations for weight loss include consumption of a balanced and nutrient-rich diet and increased PA.[38]

Physical Activity (PA)

PA is a principal modifiable lifestyle factor in cancer prevention. Regular PA impacts risk reduction and improved cancer outcomes by lowering estrogen levels, preventing high blood insulin levels, strengthening the immune system, decreasing inflammation, improving efficiency of food transit time in the gastrointestinal (GI) tract leading to less carcinogen exposure, decreasing cell proliferation and increasing apoptosis.[39,40] PA activity does reduce

risk by decreasing obesity, it lowers the risk of cancer in people of all weight categories.[39,41]

Onc R clinicians have the expertise to guide patients with safe and effective exercise. Regular exercise is linked to improved cancer outcomes, decreased treatment adverse effects, improved treatment tolerance, reduced risk of recurrence and improved overall prognosis.[42] Regular PA before, during, and after cancer treatment decreases anxiety, fatigue, and depression, and improves physical function, QOL, and improves cardiovascular function.[42,43] Multiple studies support the finding that exercise helps in the prevention of cancer. The American College of Sports Medicine (ACSM) reports that regular exercise reduces the risk of the following seven cancers: colon, stomach, breast, esophageal, bladder, endometrial, and kidney cancers.[44] The 2019 Roundtable on Exercise and Cancer included researchers from ACSM, ACS, National Cancer Institute (NCI) among other experts in the field and established a link between PA and decreased risk of 13 different cancers, among them: esophageal, liver, stomach, myeloid leukemia, kidney, head and neck, rectal, bladder and lung cancers.[39] A systematic review reports that getting the recommended amount of PA can reduce overall cancer risk by 10% to 20%.[44] Exercise following a cancer diagnosis was associated with a 28% to 44% reduced risk of cancer-specific mortality, a 21% to 35% lower risk of cancer recurrence, and a 25% to 48% decreased risk of all-cause mortality.[41] Exercise has an even greater impact on the mortality rate for breast, colorectal, and prostate cancer, reducing the relative mortality risk from all causes and cancer-related mortality by 40% to 50%.[44]

Regular moderate PA is shown to reduce fatigue, anxiety, improve self-esteem, strength, and cardiovascular fitness.[45,46] It also reduces cancer-related fatigue (CRF) and psychosocial distress in PLWBCs. Fatigue is the number one reported adverse effect in persons with cancer (PWCs) ranging from 59% to 100%.[48] The NCCN guidelines for managing fatigue recommend exercise as the number one approach for reducing CRF. Exercise has also been shown to improve sleep and body image during cancer treatment.[41] Regular PA improves physical function, immune system functioning, muscle strength, and range of motion.[41] In the absence of adequate PA, reducing time spent sedentary may also reduce the risk of endometrial, colon, and lung cancers. The exact dose of PA needed to reduce cancer-specific or all-cause mortality is not known, but generally more activity appears to lead to improved risk reduction.[39]

Currently ACSM guidelines for exercise in PLWBCs are: 150 minutes/week of moderate-intensity exercise or 75 minutes/week of vigorous-intensity aerobic exercise, as well as twice per week strength training.[48] Exercise parameters do not change when a person has a cancer diagnosis in terms of recommended time and type of exercise. What is considered moderate and vigorous exercise will fluctuate depending on the person's endurance, strength, overall health, and adverse effects from cancer treatment. Moderate and vigorous intensities are recommended and are gauged by percent of an individual's heart rate reserve; ACSM defines moderate intensity as 40% to 59% heart rate reserve and vigorous-intensity as 60% to 89% heart rate reserve.[49] The percentage of heart rate reserve is measured by the Karvonen formula; refer to Box 30.1.

Exercise is generally considered safe during treatment for cancer and improves QOL both during and post treatment. There are circumstances when PA is contraindicated or needs to modified and/or carefully monitored for treatment response. This includes, but is not limited to, anemia, thrombocytopenia, high fracture

Max HR = 220–age
Heart rate reserve = max HR – resting HR
Percent of heart rate reserve: (percentage) (max heart rate–resting heart rate) + resting heart rate

HR, Heart rate.

risk, postsurgical restrictions, unstable vitals in response to exercise, tumor lysis syndrome, and neutropenic fever.[51] Exercise is contraindicated in cases of oncologic emergencies such as spinal cord compression, superior vena cava syndrome, venothrombolic event, and severe hypercalcemia.[51] The parameters for starting and maintaining PA during and after cancer treatment should be individualized for safety and optimal clinical outcomes. However, cancer treatments can increase the risk for exercise-related injuries. An individualized plan with an Onc R clinician with specialty training can ensure that necessary precautions are followed as it relates to cancer and cancer treatments, such as surgical precautions, radiation precautions, bone health, polyneuropathy, and cardiopulmonary health.

Prudent exercise prescription requires that the Onc R clinician understand the type and stage of cancer, surgical history, additional treatment approaches, presenting adverse effects and symptoms from medical management, and the impact of these factors on exercise tolerance to guide clinical decision making. Exercise should be modified to fit the PLWBC's current goals, health needs, and exercise preference. Exercise prescription should be feasible to implement within a PLWBC's life without adding increased stress/burden and should also account for prognosis and current symptom burden.[42]

Several other specific considerations should be taken into account when prescribing exercise for PLWBCs. One is the PLWBC's bone health, especially if the patient is currently taking or has taken medications that negatively impact osseous integrity or have known metastatic bone disease. Additionally, cardiac health should be noted, as many medical treatments cause cardiotoxicity and negatively impact exercise tolerance. Chemotherapy-induced polyneuropathy (CIPN) is another important consideration for exercise prescription. Moreover, PLWBCs may have diagnostic echocardiograms, DEXA (dual energy X-ray absorptiometry) scan scores, various imaging, and/or nerve conduction studies to provide Onc R clinicians with valuable information to guide treatment planning efforts that aim to mitigate issues as well as prescribe safe and effective exercise parameters. Onc R clinicians, especially PTs, are highly regarded as movement experts and ensure that PLWBCs have access to individualized and safe exercise plans to improve QOL that additionally decreases cancer incidence through exercise promotion and education.

The publication entitled *Exercise is Medicine in Oncology* indicates that despite the research that supports the benefits of exercise before, during, and after cancer treatment for improved health, most PLWBCs do not engage in regular PA. It is reported that only 30% to 47% of PLWBCs get the recommended amount of PA.[52] Research additionally shows 80% of PLWBCs would like advice from their oncology care team on how to safely exercise. This gap in care is partially resultant of unclear expectations "on the part of those who work in oncology clinical settings of their role in assessing, advising, and referring patients to exercise."[52] Healthcare providers should assess a PLWBC's PA at regular intervals, advise on how to meet their current and desired levels of PA, and refer to appropriate exercise programs or the appropriate healthcare professionals for exercise evaluation.[52]

Nutrition and Diet

The APTA supports collaboration between PTs and registered dietitian nutritionists (RDNs) to promote education, research, and practice that elevates the health and well-being of society. Diet and nutrition are components of prevention that affect Onc R practice and patient care. APTA states that within specific state guidelines, it is within the professional scope of PT practice to screen for and to provide basic information on diet and nutritional issues including appropriate consultation or referral to an RDN.[53]

Proper nutrition is essential to remaining strong and healthy before, during, and after cancer treatment. Many PLWBCs experience unintentional weight loss preceding diagnosis and during treatment due to changes in metabolism, decreased appetite/anorexia, nausea/vomiting, constipation, mouth sores, chewing/swallowing difficulty, changes in taste/smell, pain, and depression. Malnutrition occurs in up to 80% of PLWBCs and greater than 50% have a nutritional deficiency at the time of diagnosis.[54] Protein-calorie malnutrition (PCM) is the most common secondary diagnosis in PLWBCs, due to inadequate caloric intake to meet metabolic requirements and/or the reduced absorption of macronutrients.[55] Malnutrition increases the risk for disease complications, leads to longer hospital length of stay and hospital readmissions, and has been associated with increased risk of mortality and decreased QOL.[56,57] The multiple causes and serious consequences of malnutrition in cancer include anorexia, cachexia, and sarcopenia.[58] It is also important to recognize that obesity and malnutrition can coincide. Obesity can affect clinical outcomes during treatment by masking malnutrition.[59] Early nutrition screening is essential to identify PLWBCs who are at risk for malnutrition. Identifying at-risk patients leads to early nutrition intervention by a RDN and has the potential to improve clinical outcomes. Based on current evidence, the Malnutrition Screening Tool (MST) is a simple screening tool validated by the Academy of Nutrition and Dietetics to determine adults at risk for malnutrition.[60] Refer to Figure 30.1. All PLWBCs should be screened for malnutrition on their initial visit and routinely throughout treatment. The Academy of Nutrition and Dietetics/American Society of Parenteral and Enteral Nutrition (ASPEN) guidelines indicate that the presence of two or more of the following criteria supports a diagnosis of malnutrition in adult PLWBCs: unintended weight loss (>2% over 1 week, 5% over 1 month, 7.5% over 3 months), inadequate energy intake, loss of subcutaneous fat, loss of muscle mass, localized or generalized fluid accumulation, and reduced grip strength.[62] All at-risk PLWBCs should be referred to an RDN for nutrition support. An RDN will review current height/weight and weight history, dietary habits/diet history, medical history, food allergies, and nutrition-related symptoms to assist in the identification of nutritional deficiencies and nutrition risk. The RDN will provide nutrition recommendations and design a diet plan tailored to specific needs, including strategies to meet elevated calorie and protein requirements and dietary tips to curb the adverse effects of treatment. Proper nutrition will support tolerance to cancer treatments, assist in controlling adverse effects of treatment, and may prevent further illness. In light of the considerable evidence of exercise in PLWBCs, exercise professionals should be

MALNUTRITION SCREENING TOOL (MST)	
Have you lost weight recently without trying?	
No	0
Unsure	2
If yes, how much weight (kilograms) have you lost?	
1–5	1
6–10	2
11–15	3
>15	4
Unsure	2
Have you been eating poorly because of a decreased appetite?	
No	0
Yes	1
Total	

Score of 2 or more = patient at risk of malnutrition.

• **Fig. 30.1** Malnutrition Screening Tool (MST).[61] (Reprinted with permission from Ferguson M, Capra S, Bauer J, Banks M. Development of a valid and reliable malnutrition screening tool for adult acute hospital patients. *Nutrition.* 1999;15(6):458–464.)

working closely with the RDN. This is imperative in those at risk of malnutrition who are increasing their exercise or activity levels in order for appropriate dosing and modulation of activity and nutritional intake. If exercise is initiated in a person who is malnourished or at risk of malnourishment, a caloric deficit may result and further complicate the cancer treatment process.

Diet, as defined as a habitual eating pattern, plays a major role in the prevention of cancer. There is no specific food that will prevent cancer, overall risk is reduced by adhering to a healthy eating pattern. Many specific diets claim to prevent cancer, some with minimal or limited research (Table 30.3). Major cancer organizations promote dietary guidelines based on foods to consume, limit, and avoid rather than strict adherence to a specific diet. The American Institute for Cancer Research (AICR) and World Cancer Research Fund International (WCRF) have developed recommendations based on evidence-based, peer-reviewed literature on diet, exercise, and cancer. Their recommendations include maintaining a healthy weight, being physically active, eating a diet rich in whole grains, vegetables, fruits and beans while limiting consumption of red meat, processed foods, sugar-sweetened drinks, and alcohol (Box 30.2).[69] Many studies strongly suggest that consuming a primarily plant-based diet significantly protects against breast, prostate, colorectal, and GI cancers.[65] There are some differences in the public health guidelines from major organizations for cancer prevention but they all share the recommendation of consuming mostly plant-based foods (including nonstarchy vegetables, whole fruits, whole grains, legumes, and nuts/seeds) and limiting red meat consumption, intake of added sugar, and excess calories.[66]

Alcohol Cessation

Excess alcohol consumption is linked to 6% of cancers including cancers of the mouth, larynx, pharynx, esophagus, liver, colorectal, and breast. Alcohol consumption increases risk by DNA

TABLE 30.3 Diets That Claim to Support Cancer Prevention

Mediterranean diet	• Primary plant-based, high in vegetables, fruits, whole grains, beans, nut and seeds, and olive oil • Moderate in poultry, eggs, and dairy • Limits red meat consumption	• Mediterranean diet follows many of the AICR/WCRF guidelines for cancer prevention. • Several studies have demonstrated a strong and inverse relationship between consuming a Mediterranean diet and cancer.[63] • Studies have shown that consuming a primarily plant-based diet significantly protects against breast, prostate, colorectal, and gastrointestinal cancers.[64]
Ketogenic diet	• High fat, moderate protein, low carbohydrate	• Limited research regarding cancer treatment and weight loss when body uses ketones instead of glucose for energy. • Diet should only be followed with medical doctor recommendation and with RDN guidance and monitoring.[65] • Short-term and long-term health risks, very restrictive, high in saturated fats, deficient in several nutrients, often requires supplementation.[66]
Fasting	• Limits all nutrient intake for 24 hours to several daily	• Limited research studies demonstrate that short-term fasting may protect healthy cells from chemotherapy.[67]
Vegetarian (lacto, ovo, or lacto-ovo)/Vegan diet	• Vegetarian (avoids all animal products except may include eggs and/or dairy) or • Vegan (excludes all animal products)	• Academy of Nutrition and Dietetics' official position on vegetarian diets "appropriately planned vegetarian, including vegan, diets are healthful, nutritionally adequate, and may provide health benefits for the prevention and treatment of certain diseases including ischemic heart disease, type 2 diabetes, hypertension, certain types of cancer, and obesity."[68]

AICR, The American Institute for Cancer Research; *RDN,* registered dietitian nutritionist; *WCRF,* World Cancer Research Fund.
Created by Erin Daiek. Printed with permission.

• BOX **30.2** **General Diet Guidelines for Disease Prevention**[64,72–76]

- Achieve calorie balance to maintain a healthy body weight throughout lifetime.[64,71]
- Consume a predominantly plant-based diet—whole grains, consume a variety of vegetables (dark green, red, and orange), whole fruits, and beans.[64]
- Limit red meat consumption >350–500 g/week.[71]
- Minimizing or avoiding consumption of processed foods, sugary drinks (usually calorie-dense, deficient in essential nutrients).[70–72]
- Limit sodium intake to <2300 mg/day.[70]
- Limit intake of solid fats (<10% calories per day) and added sugars (<10% calories per day).[70]
- Eliminate/minimize alcohol consumption (daily maximum, 1 drink daily for women/2 drinks for men).[71,73]
- Aim to meet all nutrients from food before using nutrition supplements.[64] However, in patients with chronic illnesses, oral nutritional supplementation has been shown to be beneficial in terms of physical function and weight gain.[74]

• BOX **30.3** **American Cancer Society Lung Screening Guidelines**[84]

LDCT is recommended for people that meet the following criteria:
1. Age 55–74 years
2. Current smoker or have smoked in last 15 years
3. Have at least a 30-pack-year smoking history

LDCT, Low-dose computed tomography.

damage via the production of acetaldehyde.[75] Research indicates the amount of alcohol consumed over time, not the type of alcohol is linked to an increased risk of cancer. The more alcohol consumed, the higher the risk. It is postulated that alcohol combined with smoking has a synergistic effect and overall risk is greatly increased.[76] One theory for this synergistic effect is that alcohol has the ability to increase the permeability of oral mucosa and therefore may "act as a solvent to tobacco products potentially increasing its carcinogenic effects."[71,75] Referral back to the primary care provider for appropriate care is warranted if a PLWBC consumes tobacco products and excess alcohol during cancer treatment, as intervention beyond the education of the health risks of these combined behaviors will likely require a multimodal intervention approach beyond the scope of the Onc R clinician alone.

Tobacco Cessation

Tobacco contains carcinogens that cause damage to DNA and therefore tobacco consumption, via smoking, smokeless tobacco, or secondhand smoke, is a risk factor for multiple cancers. Smoking tobacco products is the underlying cause of 30% of all cancer deaths in the US and 80% of all lung cancer deaths.[79] Smokeless tobacco also elevates the risk for certain head and neck cancers and pancreatic cancer. Tobacco causes a variety of other health consequences that can affect health and ability to heal from cancer diagnosis and treatment including decreased immune system function, bone density, wound healing, and increased risk of developing type 2 diabetes, cardiovascular disease, and chronic obstructive pulmonary disease (COPD). Smoking increases the risk of the following cancers: lung, mouth, larynx, pharynx, esophagus, kidney, cervix, liver, bladder, pancreas, stomach, colorectal, and myeloid leukemia. Smoking at the time of prostate cancer diagnosis is associated with an increased mortality rate and an increased risk of overall cancer recurrence.[80] Lung cancer risk dramatically drops in heavy smokers (≥15 cigarettes a day) 5 years after quitting but remains threefold higher than people who never smoked for up to 25 years later.[81] Onc R clinicians need to know that former heavy smokers still have an elevated risk. Current USPSTF guidelines include data to support that former smokers are eligible to receive lung cancer screenings up to 15 years after quitting.[82] See Box 30.3

for ACS lung screening guidelines. Furthermore, people diagnosed with head and neck cancer were more likely to recognize smoking as a risk to their survival if they had quit smoking before diagnosis than those currently smoking, and this perception of smoking not being problematic was cited as a barrier in smoking cessation programs.[85] Education on the adverse effects of smoking upon one's health risk reduction and healing should be provided. If a patient is ready to quit, a referral to a primary care doctor is warranted.

Sleep

Sleep is a critical component of health and wellness, and sleep disturbance negatively affects QOL in PLWBCs. The CDC recognizes sleep deprivation as a public health problem. Adults require 7 to 8 hours of sleep each night, children require more; see Table 30.4 for recommendations. Only 63.9% of Americans reported getting regular adequate sleep (at least 7 hours per 24-hour period).[88] The American Academy of Sleep Medicine (AASM) reports that sleep is essential and as important as nutrition and PA for health. Sleep disturbance affects up to 75% of PLWBCs, with the US National Institute of Health (NIH) reporting it as 50%.[89,90] Adequate sleep is necessary for proper immune function, hormone balance, blood sugar regulation, pain modulation, and brain health. Deficient sleep is linked to accidents, poor problem-solving skills, and chronic health issues. PLWBCs have rated sleep disturbance as the second-most bothersome symptom of cancer or its treatment.[89] For example, impaired sleep is one of the most common complaints of persons diagnosed with breast cancer and affects 20% to 40% of them versus only 10% of their peers.[91] Cancer-related sleep issues can be confounded by premorbid untreated or undiagnosed sleep disorders. Sleep issues are also more prevalent in the cancer population compared to the general population, which is of particular concern because inadequate sleep has been found to negatively affect cancer outcomes and increase the risk of cancer recurrence.[90]

TABLE **30.4** **Amount of Sleep Recommended by Age**[86,87]

Age	Recommended Hours of Sleep Per 24-hour Period for Optimal Health
4–12 months	12–16 hours
1–2 years	11–14 hours
3–5 years	10–13 hours
6–12 years	9–12 hours
13–18 years	8–10 hours
Adults	7 or more hours

Created by Suzette Smith. Printed with permission.

Sleep involves two cycles: rapid eye movement (REM) and non-REM sleep. In the event of frequent wakening, the body is unable to complete the cycles and hinders the body's ability to adequately heal and recover from the activities of the previous day. PLWBCs are prone to experiencing sleep issues for a variety of reasons, including pain, anxiety regarding diagnosis, tumor effects, medication or treatment adverse effects, nausea, shortness of breath, physical changes from cancer or surgery, GI issues, bladder issues, and more. Another barrier to sleep that many PLWBCs experience is related to hospital admissions. Sleep disturbances that occur in the hospital should be discussed with the care team to determine if lighting, noise, comfort, decreased disruptions for medications, and roommate/visitors can be addressed. Types of sleep issues include insomnia, (which is most common in PLWBCs), narcolepsy, restless leg syndrome, parasomnia, hypersomnia, and circadian rhythm disorders, as well as sleep apnea. The collective consequences of sleep issues are decreased sleep duration, increased sleep latency increased sleep disruption, and daytime dysfunction. Sleep hygiene education is widely recommended to decrease sleep issues (Box 30.4).

Additionally, adults of childhood cancer are more at risk for sleep disturbance. PLWBCs with premorbid sleep disorders (e.g., sleep apnea, restless leg syndrome) may be at particular risk as these disorders may be confounded by the stress of a cancer diagnosis, or the effects of cancer and/or cancer treatment. Referral to the primary care provider is warranted in these circumstances.

Although sleep deprivation is a common issue for PLWBCs, referrals for sleep evaluations are often overlooked when the healthcare team is planning and implementing holistic cancer care. Onc R clinicians can be of value to these patients by providing screenings to determine if referrals are necessary as well as addressing

---

• BOX 30.5   Relaxation Exercise for Sleep

Begin by supporting body in a comfortable position and try one of the following exercises:

- Take slow deep breaths while intentionally relaxing areas of tension in the body.
- Incrementally relax body parts from head to toe (body scan) can be guided or patient can perform independently.
- Count backward from 100, decreasing one number with each exhale and intentionally relaxing body with each number, count down toward zero.

---

underlying issues related to pain and positioning to allow for reduced discomfort and improved breathing (Table 30.5). Onc R clinicians can provide interventions to address strengthening and bed mobility techniques to allow for more independent repositioning. Training in the use of wedges and pillows may be employed to support improved sleeping posture. Bladder training or bladder/bowel programs can be implemented to decrease awakening for toileting overnight. Onc R clinicians are also able to provide sleep hygiene protocols, educate on lifestyle behaviors that support sleep, educate on avoidance of behaviors that impair sleep, or refer to the additional members of the medical team if the problem is beyond the scope of their practice. Ensuring adequate sleep will help reduce symptoms of CRF, pain, and brain fog. Although CRF may persist despite adequate sleep, sleep deprivation is often one component of CRF. Pain is also closely related to sleep disturbances and the treatment of pain should be prioritized to assist in addressing sleep issues. Evaluation of sleeping positions and modifying accordingly is a beneficial component of an Onc R treatment session by optimizing comfort, preventing pressure sores, and facilitating adequate breathing and pain reduction. Refer to Table 30.5 for common symptoms impacting sleep and solutions.

Motivational Interviewing

"How you talk with patients about their health can substantially influence their motivation for behavior change."[95] Motivational interviewing (MI), a clinical intervention used to promote behavior change, has evidence for its efficacy as an intervention method with growing evidence for its use by Onc R clinicians in promoting positive health behavior change.[96,97] The Self-Determination Theory[96] is one of the foundational principles from which MI emerged as a clinical practice model, and asserts that change comes about from an individual's intrinsic motivation and willingness to self-regulate their own lifestyle choices. Additionally, the Transtheoretical Model provides a framework for appreciating an individual's readiness to change a behavior.[98] The five stages of readiness for change described by detailed in Table 30.6.[98]

Key features of the MI style of health coaching are: (1) a nonjudgmental approach; (2) use of open-ended, nonthreatening questions; (3) intention toward reflective listening; and (4) exploration of an individual's ambivalence. This is referred to as the RULE principle: **R**esist the righting reflex, **U**nderstand patients' motivations, **L**isten with empathy, **E**mpower with optimism and hope.[94] Onc R clinicians should avoid taking the "expert role" when using this approach. The aim is to have ideas for change come from the individual being coached, as this approach asserts that they would be the "expert" for the context in which a change would occur. Miller and Rollinick provide a comprehensive book

---

• BOX 30.4   Sleep Hygiene Techniques[92–94]

1. Go to sleep and wake up at the same time every day. This allows the body to find the sleep-wake rhythm. This may involve setting an alarm to awaken at the same time every day, even on the weekends.
2. Decrease caffeine intake and avoid caffeine for at least 6 hours before bed.
3. Keep room dark.
4. Keep room temperature cool.
5. Get adequate exercise during the day, but avoid moderate to vigorous exercise 3 hours before sleep (American Cancer Society recommends aerobic exercise 3–4x/week for 30–40 minutes per session of moderate-intensity to improve sleep in cancer patients)
6. Eliminate tobacco and alcohol use, or at least avoid it for 3–4 hours before bed.
7. Avoid naps.
8. Avoid large meals and spicy food before bed, instead opt for light high protein, or a high fiber snack.
9. Avoid loud noise or screens before bed. Screens should be turned off 30 minutes before bed as blue light disrupts sleep quality.
10. Avoid liquids and empty your bladder before bed.
11. Only lay down when sleepy.
12. Only use the bedroom for sleep and sex.
13. Set bed up for comfort.
14. Establish a relaxing bedtime routine.
15. Get out of bed if you do not fall asleep within 20 minutes and do not return until feeling sleepy. If unable to leave bed for mobility reasons, try meditation or deep breathing exercises in the bed (see Box 30.5 for relaxation exercise suggestions).

TABLE 30.5	Common Symptoms Impacting Sleep and Modifications

Symptom	Possible Solutions
Feelings of breathlessness	Positioning for breath support during sleep • Use of wedge or pillows to support in either elevated supine or side-lying position • Semi-electric hospital bed to assist with positioning
Back pain	Positions for back support. • Side-lying with a pillow between knees • Supine with a pillow under knees
Difficulty with bed mobility	Props to allow for more independent mobility and positioning • Semi-automatic hospital bed • Bed assist rails
Pressure sores and edema	If a patient is unable to reposition independently the following techniques can help prevent pressure sores: • Assist to reposition every 2 hours • Float heels off the bed with a pillow or PRAFO boots • Position with pillows or wedge in one-fourth turned position to unweight sacrum • When positioning, attention must be paid to bony prominences like sacrum, heels, elbows Ensure that edematous limbs are elevated on pillows
Anxiety	The following techniques may reduce anxiety and help promote sleep • Guided imagery • Body scan • Breathing techniques • Restorative yoga before bed
Bowel/bladder issues	• Empty bladder before bed and get on bowel/bladder program during the day with the goal of voiding every 2–3 hours • Do not drink 3 hours before bed • Avoid bladder irritants such as coffee, tea, cigarette smoking, and citrus fruits • Refer to a physical therapist specialized in pelvic floor therapy

PRAFO, Pressure relief ankle foot orthosis.
Created by Suzette Smith: Prined with permission.

TABLE 30.6	Stages of Readiness for Behavior Change

Stage of Change	Description
Precontemplation	Individual is not intending to take action in the foreseeable future, usually measured as the next 6 months.
Contemplation	Individual is intending to change in the next 6 months.
Preparation	Individual is intending to take action to change in the immediate future, usually measured as the next month.
Action	Individual has made specific overt modifications in their life styles within the past 6 months.
Maintenance	Individual is working to prevent relapse but they do not apply change processes as frequently as do people in action. They are less tempted to relapse and increasingly more confident that they can continue their changes.

Modified from Prochaska JO, Velicer WF. The transtheoretical model of health behavior change. *Am J Heal Promot.* 1997;12(1):38–48.

TABLE 30.7	A's to Successful Motivational Interviewing

5 "A's" of Motivational Interviewing	Expanded Description of Each "A"
ASK	Screen patients for health risk behaviors such as smoking, sedentary lifestyle and poor nutritional balances resulting in underweight, overweight, and obesity.
ADVICE	Provide specific information regarding health risks and the benefits of recommended changes in behavior.
ASSESS	Ask questions to obtain further insight into the patient's personal beliefs, intentions, outcomes, expectations, and readiness for change.
ASSIST	Help the patient to identify barriers and potential impediments to the new behavior in order to uncover problem-solving techniques, strategies, and source of social and environmental support.
ARRANGE	Establish a specific plan for patient follow up, including opportunities to renew performance feedback and revise goals and strategies.

Modified from Pignataro RM, Huddleston J. The use of motivational interviewing in physical therapy education and practice: empowering patients through effective self-management. *J Phys Ther Educ.* 2015;29(2):62–71.

outlining each aspect of the MI approach from its foundational mindset through clinical examples.[95] A rehabilitation provider focused manuscript outlining the "5 A's to successful MI"[99] is very helpful and detailed in Table 30.7. Furthermore, it is notable that MI techniques are now commonly incorporated into entry level occupational therapist and PT curriculum.[100,101] Furthermore, health coaching certifications (which includes competency in the use of the MI technique) are now widely available to clinicians seeking continuing education on this topic.

MI can be a useful tool for Onc R clinicians to incorporate in most patient populations including PLWBCs. However, a clinician must be mindful of the individual's stage of change readiness as a new cancer diagnosis may present both facilitators and barriers to a person's willingness to change current behaviors. For example, a new lung cancer diagnosis may facilitate a person's desire to stop smoking while another individual may be unwilling to consider smoking cessation as they identify it as an essential coping strategy. In the later scenario, an Onc R clinician may need to engage the patient in reflective conversation to uncover another positive health change (e.g., engaging in PA, improving hydration, etc.) the individual would be potentially more willing and confident to commence.

The potential barriers to the use of MI among the PLWBC population are highlighted in a randomized controlled trial which identified low recruitment and compliance among the PLWBCs assigned to the 12-week intervention group time frame. The study found a 3-month protocol was not feasible to bring about change as attrition was high; therefore, the potential efficacy of a MI intervention to increase PA behavior among individuals with a gynecologic cancer diagnosis could not be confirmed.[102] Exercise barriers have been reported which hindered adoption and adherence among individuals with breast cancer. These barriers included include low confidence, lack of exercise prior to diagnosis, less education, being postmenopausal, as well as the presence of physical and psychological problems.[103] However, another study examining the use of MI on individuals with breast cancer found the technique to have positive outcomes toward improving sexual satisfaction among women who had undergone mastectomy.[104] Finally, a systematic review of the use of MI interventions among PLWBCs concluded MI to be a promising technique, but that Onc R clinicians should be mindful of intervention design to assure sensitivity to cancer type, phase of care, and complexity of desired behavior.[105]

Wellness (Supportive Care) and Symptom Reduction

Complementary and alternative medicine (CAM) techniques are techniques that are not considered part of standard medical care. These techniques are used by approximately 50% of PLWBCs during their cancer journey, and often they do not feel it is important to discuss these therapies with their medical providers.[106] However, this can be detrimental as certain herbs or therapies may have drug interactions or cause medical treatment to be less effective. Many academic centers are offering integrative medical care for PWCs. CAM therapies are not designed as lifesaving therapies, but rather serve as additional treatment options to decrease symptom burden and improve QOL.[107] CAM therapies include but are not limited to herbal remedies, mind/bodywork such as meditation, yoga, tai chi, acupressure/acupuncture, and massage. Although it is beyond the scope of this chapter to discuss all CAM therapies, select studies will be presented which have preliminary results pointing to CAM's safety and effectiveness in decreasing the symptom burden of cancer or the medical management of cancer. There is a paucity of evidence on the efficacy of CAM for PLWBCs as high-quality research efforts are rare and have focused primarily on breast cancer which limits generalizability to other cancer populations. The Society of Integrative Oncology (SIO) recommends specific CAM therapies as it relates to breast cancer (Table 30.8).[107]

Emotional Freedom Technique

"Emotional freedom techniques (EFT) comprise a novel intervention that combines elements of exposure, cognitive and other

TABLE 30.8	American Society of Integrative Oncology Complementary and Alternative Therapy Recommendations for Breast Cancer
Stress and anxiety	Music therapy, meditation, yoga
Depression/mood disorders	Meditation, relaxation, yoga, massage, and music therapy
Improve the quality of life	Meditation and yoga
Cancer-induced nausea and vomiting	Acupressure and acupuncture

Created by Suzette Smith. Printed with permission.

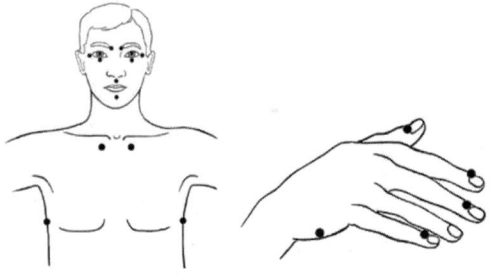

EFT on a Page

1. **Where in your body** do you feel the emotional issue most strongly?

2. **Determine the distress level** in that place in your body on a scale of 0 to 10, where 10 is maximum intensity and 0 is no intensity:

    10, 9, 8, 7, 6, 5, 4, 3, 2, 1, 0

3. **The Setup:** Repeat this statement three times, while continuously tapping the Karate Chop point on the side of the hand (large dot on hand diagram below):

    "Even though I have _____ (name the problem), I deeply and completely accept myself."

4. **The Tapping Sequence:** Tap about 7 times on each of the energy points in these 2 diagrams, while repeating a brief phrase that reminds you of the problem.

5. **Determine your distress level** again on a scale of 0 to 10 again. If it's still high, say:

    "Even though I have some remaining _____ (problem), I deeply and completely accept myself."

6. **Repeat from Step 1** till your distress level is as close to 0 as possible.

Find dozens of tap-along videos at EFTuniverse.com

• **Fig. 30.2** Emotional Freedom Technique on a Page.[108] (Reprinted with permission from Church D. *EFT MINI-MANUAL*. 2nd ed. Energy Psychology Press. evidencebasedeft.com/wp-content/uploads/2017/02/EFTMiniManual.pdf. Accessed October 31, 2020.)

conventional therapeutic techniques with the somatic stimulation of acupressure points."[108] EFT involves tapping acupressure points on the face, collar bone, axilla, and hand while repeating a specific affirmation statement regarding the symptom being experienced. EFT can be done independently by the PLWBC, quickly and with little to no adverse effects (Figure 30.2). Please see ebook Ch30 for a video example of EFT. EFT has been shown to decrease symptoms of post traumatic stress disorder (PTSD), anxiety, pain, and depression in the general population.[109] Few preliminary studies looking at the effects of EFT specifically for PLWBCs exist, though data is warranted as PLWBCs often experience PTSD, anxiety, and pain.

Additionally, EFT has been shown to improve mood and QOL in older adults when provided by nursing staff.[110] An internal service evaluation of 41 women with breast cancer taking tamoxifen or aromatase inhibitors reporting symptoms of hot flashes, myalgias, or mood disturbances reported a significant reduction in all symptoms when measured at 6 and 12 weeks of treatment (Video 30.1).[111]

Emotional Freedom Technique and Yoga

Massage is a form of bodywork involving pressing, rubbing and manipulating skin and muscles. Oncology massage is similar in technique to general massage techniques; however, trained Onc R clinicians account for the complete clinical picture of the PLWBC when determining how the techniques are applied. Contraindications for oncology massage include avoiding techniques directly over: tumor sites, areas with a known thrombosis, sensitive areas after radiation exposure, areas of bruising, and open wounds.[112] Additionally, surgical precautions and pressure may need to be modified pending platelet counts and in the circumstance of anticoagulant use.[113]

Massage is generally considered to be safe for PLWBCs and numerous studies have shown beneficial trends not only in decreased anxiety but also in nausea, pain, fatigue, and depression.[113,114]

Although evidence is limited, two RCTs demonstrated that oncology massage reduced reported CIPN symptoms and improved QOL for patients receiving taxanes. CIPN is one of the most common and dose-limiting toxicities related to paclitaxel (Taxol); approximately 32% to 98% of the breast cancer patients receiving paclitaxel suffer from CIPN.[115] Participants with breast cancer receiving paclitaxel study were provided a 30-minute massage session (20 minutes for their feet and 10 minutes for their hands) before infusions and were measured with European Organization for Research and Treatment of Cancer's Quality of Life Quotient Chemotherapy-Induced Peripheral Neuropathy-20 (EORTC QLQ CIPN20) questionnaire at 0, 4, 8, and 12 weeks of infusion treatment and pre-treatment and post treatment nerve conduction studies. The study showed that massage, when given concurrently with paclitaxel, seemed to reduce CIPN and improved QOL.115 In addition, persons with colorectal cancer being treated with oxaliplatin also demonstrated a reduction in CIPN symptoms and improved QOL.[116]

Yoga

Yoga involves a combination of breath work, mindfulness work, and postures. This combination offers a unique form of exercise that has the added benefits of relaxation, strengthening, and stretching in one session. Yoga is an integrative therapy that offers a nonpharmacological option for treating certain cancer-related adverse effects and cancer treatment-related toxicities.[117] There is a growing body of evidence supporting the use of yoga as a supportive treatment throughout the cancer continuum. The majority of these studies have been conducted specifically in the breast cancer population. Yoga practice has been linked to overall improved QOL, decreased sleep disturbance, improved mood, and decreased anxiety.[118] The benefits of yoga for the breast cancer population includes the improved psychological health outcomes of reduced anxiety, depression, and distress.[48] A review of RCTs on the impact of yoga on symptom management in oncology populations indicated efficacy in improving overall QOL with signifi-

cant improvements reported for fatigue and cognition, as well as decreased sleep issues and stress. Some studies also reported improvements in biomarkers that indicate improved immune function as well as decreased cortisol levels.[119] Yoga has also been found to diminish some musculoskeletal pain and discomfort related to cancer.[117]

Acupuncture

Acupuncture is a traditional Chinese medicine technique that works by stimulating certain energy lines within the body. It involves placing thin needles into the skin at specific points in the body. Research has shown this technique is effective in decreasing nausea and vomiting in PLWBCs.[120] Evidence is limited relative to other cancer-related adverse effects such as pain, insomnia, and hot flashes. Currently, research is being conducted in these areas to determine efficacy. Acupuncture is generally considered safe for oncology populations if proper sterilization techniques are employed.[121]

Mindfulness-Based Stress Reduction

Mindfulness-based stress reduction (MBSR) is a technique developed by Jon Kabat-Zin and is used as a nonpharmacological treatment for chronic stress, pain, and other symptoms of chronic disease. The technique focuses on "nonjudgmental awareness" of the body. It has been found to alleviate stress, anxiety, and sleep issues as well as improving general mood.[122] MBSR has been mostly studied with early stage breast cancer.[123] Several meta-analyses of RCTs employing MBSR have been conducted with the oncology population to determine efficacy. MBSR was reported to have a significant positive effect on stress, QOL, depression, anxiety, and CRF as compared to control groups.[123,124]

Social Wellness

A growing body of literature is demonstrating the value of social supports in oncology outcomes. The NCI defines social supports as a "network of family, friends, neighbors, and community members that is available in times of need to give psychological, physical, and financial help."[125] Social wellness is a component of overall wellness and social support has been found to be essential for the wellbeing of PLWBCs. The size and extent of social networks can be predictive factors in health and wellness.[126] The needs from a social support system will likely change when PLWBCs experience different issues across the continuum of a cancer diagnosis.

Coping with cancer may be particularly difficult for PLWBCs that lack strong social support prior to diagnosis. It is important for PLWBCs that lack an adequate support system from family and friends to procure this resource elsewhere. It should also be noted that often those who need more psychosocial support do not always know how to find this type of support.[127] Oncology nurse navigators and oncology social workers are positioned to guide PLWBCs to quality care including access to psychosocial support.[128]

Studies have shown correlations between social support and depression, QOL, stage of cancer at diagnosis, and even mortality rate. Women with colorectal cancer with more intimate social ties and who were more socially integrated experienced lower all-cause mortality and colorectal cancer mortality when compared to those that were more isolated.[129,130]

Inadequate social networks and support have also been shown to be a risk factor for anxiety and depression in women with breast cancer.[131] Conversely, adequate social support was correlated to improved resilience to cancer adversity.[132] For example, men with prostate cancer with adequate social support had improved QOL and decreased stress levels in multiple studies.[133,134] Inadequate social support can cause distress. The NCCN defines distress as "an unpleasant experience of mental, social, spiritual or physical nature." The NCCN distress thermometer can be used as a screening tool to determine if a PLWBC needs more support or possibly a referral to social work, nurse navigator, or mental health professional.

Furthermore, social support has a protective effect on older adults with cancer.[136] Inadequate social support has been linked to higher rates of depression, possibly poorer tolerance to cancer treatment, and poorer survival in older PLWBCs. Some interventions to help improve social support include in-person support, telephone-based support, tech-based video conferencing, as well as animal-assisted therapy. Patient navigation programs and peer support networks have also been found to adequately meet support needs.

It is also important to consider the caregiver burden and caregiver support when providing interventions. Caregivers may also need support or may not be able to provide adequate support to their PLWBC without additional assistance.[136]

Conclusion

Onc R clinicians have the opportunity to provide education on cancer prevention and health promotion to the PLWBCs they serve. By integrating this education into clinical practice, clinicians can positively impact cancer outcomes. Lifestyle behaviors such as proper nutrition, maintaining a healthy weight, adequate PA, adequate sleep, smoking cessation, and limited intake of alcoholic beverages can reduce cancer risk, all of which can be addressed by Onc R clinicians. Prevention screening tools are able to detect cancer prior to symptom development and therefore improve outcomes. CAM therapies may be a useful and valuable adjunct to conventional cancer care and knowledge of the major therapies may be helpful in reducing symptom burden from cancer or cancer treatment adverse effects.

Critical Research Needs

- Effect of providing modified yoga practice in the acute care setting for persons diagnosed with cancer on distress levels and/or length of stay.
- Effect of group relaxation or MBSR for persons diagnosed with cancer in the acute care setting on social wellness/distress level/QOL.
- Impact of Onc R clinician referrals to RDNs for nutrition counseling on tolerance to therapy for inpatient and outpatient PLWBCs.

Review Questions

Reader can find the correct answers and rationale in the back of the book.

Scenario 1: A 63-year-old male diagnosed with Stage III small cell lung cancer, currently being treated with etoposide (Etopophos, Toposar) and cisplatin (Platinol), is receiving outpatient physical rehabilitation for strengthening and balance training. He reports he has been taking echinacea for his immune system and an herbal blend to increase energy with little improvement.

Case Study

A 40-year-old female was in the acute care setting 2 days after a lumbar laminectomy to the L3–L5 levels. She was seen by a PT in the acute care setting for her second treatment. Her past medical history included HPV, a loop electrosurgical excision procedure (LEEP) to her cervix, back pain, anxiety, and a BMI of 28.2. Patient presented with anxiety 6/10 and low back pain rated at 8/10 upon the Onc R clinician's arrival. She initially reported that she was unable to participate in rehabilitation due to pain. The Onc R clinician offered to try an EFT, a CAM therapy, to help her relax and possibly reduce her pain. The patient was agreeable. The therapist talked the patient through three rounds of tapping with the method shown in Figure 30.2, with the key statement "even though I have this 8/10 pain, I love and accept myself" repeated three times while tapping on the side of her hand at the initiation of each round. Then the patient repeated "8/10 pain" while tapping the remainder of tapping points. At the completion of each round, the patient was instructed to take a deep breath through her nose and slowly exhale out her mouth. She rated her pain after each round. After the third round was completed, she rated her anxiety 3/10 and pain 4/10.

After the EFT session, the patient was agreeable to the spine mobility and education treatment. During therapy, the patient discussed her anxiety regarding her health with the therapist; she reported that in the last year she had a LEEP procedure to remove abnormal cervical cells related to her HPV diagnosis and now this back surgery. She reported feeling that she had no control over her health. She said she was afraid of getting cancer from her HPV. She stated she lives a relatively sedentary life and she mentioned that she wants to lose weight but does not know where to start. In addition to postoperative spine education and mobility training per the surgical protocol, the therapist provided general preventative health information. This included education that lifestyle choices such as nutrition and regular PA can impact her cancer risk. The therapist encouraged the patient to be diligent with her doctor-recommended screening protocols, as early detection is related to improved outcomes. The therapist provided information for an RDN referral as the patient was interested in nutrition education and a personalized eating plan to improve her health. She was also advised to increase her PA safely with the guidance of a PT as she heals from surgery. After the session, the patient reported feeling hopeful and more at ease with regard to her health and excited to try EFT on her own to help manage her pain. In an acute care setting, within one short treatment session, it is still possible to provide prevention and wellness education that may impact a patient's cancer risk and health choices going forward. Although this setting does not often lend itself to follow up visits, the patient is given the opportunity to make better informed choices about their health and have resources to help guide them in improving their health.

He also reports he has not been eating well because foods he usually enjoys taste like metal. The patient reports that he has had difficulty sleeping since his diagnosis and often falls asleep in his recliner chair because he finds it easier to breathe. He said he has anxiety regarding his diagnosis, and he is hesitant to talk to his doctor about this as he does not want to take more medications.

1. Are there any concerns that would warrant referral to different medical providers?

A. No referrals are necessary. The patient is taking measures to manage his health and cancer/treatment adverse effects

B. A referral to a dietitian is warranted to address decreased food intake. A referral back to the primary care physician is warranted to address anxiety and concerns for decreased energy

C. A referral back to the primary care physician to address anxiety and concerns for decreased energy. A referral to dietician is not warranted as the PT will be able to adequately address general nutrition concerns

D. No referrals are warranted at this point in care, it is within the PTs scope of practice to fully manage these issues

2. How can the therapist address this patient's complaints of difficulty sleeping and why is this important?

A. Unfortunately, sleep disturbance is a common experience for PLWBC and they should be referred back to the doctor for a prescription for sleep medication

B. Work on positioning techniques and use of wedges to improve ease of breathing in his bed

C. Provide a list of sleep hygiene techniques for him to try for improved sleep

D. Provide him with a list of herbal supplements that may improve sleep, as he reported he is not interested in taking more medication

3. How can the therapist address the patient's concern regarding supporting his immunity and possible concerns for how the patient is currently addressing this issue in his life?

A. Educate on the importance of informing oncologists of all supplements he is consuming as there is a potential for interaction with chemotherapeutic agents. Discuss the importance of a patient-specific exercise program, nutritious diet, and adequate sleep for improved immunity

B. Provide a list of herbal supplements that don't have known drug interactions with current chemotherapeutic regimen. Discuss the importance of a patient-specific exercise program, nutritious diet, and adequate sleep for improved immunity

C. Educate that immunity will be reduced while receiving chemotherapeutic agents, and there is little that can be done to improve upon this

D. Refer back to primary care doctor as this discussion is out of the PT's scope of practice

4. How can the therapist address the patient's concern about boosting his energy level?

A. Educate on the importance of informing oncologists of all supplements he is consuming as there is a potential for interaction with chemotherapeutic agents. Educate on CRF and the evidence for a patient-specific exercise prescription to improve energy levels

B. Educate the patient that fatigue is to be expected during cancer treatment, and is usually managed successfully with sleep hygiene protocols

C. Create a patient-specific exercise program and provide a list of the best natural supplements to improve energy naturally

D. Commend the patient for finding natural sources of energy, and provide resources for sleep hygiene protocols

5. How can the therapist address the patient's concern regarding anxiety?

A. Encourage him to talk to his doctor. Provide resources for meditation and support groups

B. Reinforce that speaking with doctor will likely result in taking more medications

C. Instruct the patient in mindfulness based stress reduction and use of herbal supplements for anxiety management

D. Provide therapeutic listening for the patient but make no suggestion because this is out of the rehabilitation clinician's scope of practice

6. During the initial evaluation the patient reports that he smokes 1 pack of cigarettes daily. He does not see the point of quitting because he already has a cancer diagnosis. Should the therapist provide any education regarding smoking cessation?

A. No. Smoking cession will not change the patient's prognosis or outcomes

B. Yes. The therapist should encourage smoking cessation and provide the patient with resources

C. Educate patient that stress reduction is important for healing and if smoking reduces stress, that now is not the right time to quit

D. Provide therapeutic listening for the patient but make no suggestion because this isout of the rehabilitation clinician's scope of practice

Scenario 2: A 55-year-old female with a new diagnosis of Stage II breast cancer was admitted to outpatient PT due to weakness and decreased range of motion. Prior to cancer diagnosis, the patient had no notable medical history, lived a moderately active lifestyle and BMI is currently 28. During the initial evaluation, the patient mentions that her appetite has significantly decreased over the past month. She is unsure of her usual body weight but believes she has lost weight because her clothes are loose-fitting. She states that she is happy to finally be losing weight.

1. Would a referral to an RDN be warranted?

A. No, the patient's BMI is 28, indicating the patient is overweight. Weight loss is beneficial

B. Complete Malnutrition Screening Tool. If the score is over 2, refer to RDN. Provide patients with information on healthy diet guidelines and exercise

C. Provide this patient with information on healthy diet guidelines and exercise instead of refeering to the RDN

D. No, the patient is not concerned about this weight loss and there is no reason for the PT to be concerned

2. How can the therapist address her sleep issues?

A. Explain that watching the screen 30 minutes before bed reduces sleep quality. Educate on sleep hygiene techniques and specific relaxation techniques to assist with falling asleep. Refer to the physician to address anxiety and to ensure there are no premorbid or underlying sleep issues.

B. Suggest the patient take melatonin to help her fall asleep and improve sleep quality.

C. Suggest a calming television channel to watch before bed to help deactivate the sympathetic nervous system and activate the parasympathetic nervous system.

D. The patient reports that sleep issues are not new for her, and she has struggled with sleep most of her life. This does not need to be addressed because it is a chronic issue.

Scenario 3: A 65-year-old woman presents to physical therapy status post knee replacement. When asked about her general health, the patient reports that she is hoping she can improve her health now that she has had her knee surgery. She reports a 10-pound weight gain over the past year that she attributes to decreased activity from her knee pain. She is interested in starting an exercise program once she heals from her surgery. She reports that her body "gets confused sometimes" because although she has been in menopause for many years, she has had intermittent vaginal bleeding over the last several months.

1. Which of the following would be the MOST appropriate course of action for the PT?

    A. No action is needed, she has a good plan to improve her health after healing from her knee surgery

    B. A referral to an RDN is warranted as she experienced a 10-pound weight gain over the last year

    C. A referral to the medical doctor as postmenopausal bleeding is a concern for uterine cancer

    D. Recommend a reduced calorie diet plan

2. During a treatment session, the patient reports that she normally drinks 2 bottles of beer with dinner daily, but she switched to red wine daily because "it's healthier". Should the therapist provide any education regarding alcohol consumption?

    A. The therapist should agree with the patient. Red wine is a better choice

    B. Yes. The therapist should encourage the patient to reduce alcohol consumption to 0-1 drinks per day and provide the patient with resources

    C. Educate patient that light beer would be a better choice because it is lower in calories

    D. Provide therapeutic listening for the patient but make no suggestion because this isout of the rehabilitation clinician's scope of practice

References

1. American Physical Therapy Association. Introduction to the guide to physical therapist practice. https://guide.apta.org/introduction. Accessed September 29, 2021.

2. Wilson CM, Lucado AM, Wendland DM, Taylor DW, Black B. Health promotion, wellness, and prevention practice in oncologic physical therapy. *Rehabil Oncol.* 2021;39(3):E51–E57. doi:10.1097/01.reo.0000000000000244.

3. Centers for Disease Control and Prevention. Primary prevention. https://www.cdc.gov/pictureofamerica/pdfs/picture_of_america_prevention.pdf. Accessed October 30, 2021.

4. Pandve HT. Quaternary prevention: need of the hour. *J Family Med Prim Care.* 2014;3(4):309–310.

5. Islami F, Goding Sauer A, Miller KD, et al. Proportion and number of cancer cases and deaths attributable to potentially modifiable risk factors in the United States. *CA Cancer J Clin.* 2017;68(1):31–54.

6. Liu Y, Croft JB, Wheaton AG, et al. Clustering of five health-related behaviors for chronic disease prevention among adults, United States. *Prev Chronic Dis.* 2013;2016(13):E70. doi:10.5888/pcd13.160054.

7. Muhsen S Pilewoskie M. Principles of breast surgery in cancer. In: Stubblefield MD, ed. *Cancer Rehabilitation: Principles and Practice.* 2nd ed.: Springer Publishing Company; 2018:61.

8. Centers for Disease Control and Prevention. What is a mammogram? https://www.cdc.gov/cancer/breast/basic_info/mammograms.htm. Accessed October 30, 2020.

9. Centers for Disease Control and Prevention. Breast Cancer Screening Guidelines for Women. https://www.cdc.gov/cancer/breast/pdf/breast-cancer-screening-guidelines-508.pdf Accessed October 30, 2020.

10. Centers for Disease Control and Prevention. What Should I Know About Screening for Colorectal Cancer? https://www.cdc.gov/cancer/colorectal/basic_info/screening/index.htm. Accessed September 28, 2020.

11. US Preventative Services Task Force. Recommendation: Colorectal cancer: screening | United States. https://www.uspreventiveservicestaskforce.org/uspstf/recommendation/colorectal-cancer-screening, Published June 15, 2016. Accessed October 31, 2020.

12. Nikolian VC, Hardiman KM. Evaluation and management of gastrointestinal cancer. In: Stubblefield MD, ed. *Cancer Rehabilitation: Principles and Practice.* 2nd ed.: Springer; 2018:271.

13. Wolf AMD, Fontham ETH, Church TR, et al. Colorectal cancer screening for average-risk adults: 2018 guideline update from the American Cancer Society. *CA Cancer J Clin.* 2018;68(4):250–281.

14. American Cancer Society. Guideline for colorectal cancer screening. https://www.cancer.org/cancer/colon-rectal-cancer/detection-diagnosis-staging/acs-recommendations.html. Accessed February 25, 2021.

15. American College of Obsetricians and Gynecologists. ACOG: Home. https://www.acog.org/. Accessed September 28, 2020.

16. Aviki EM, Mueller JJ. Evaluation and management of gynecologic cancers. In: Stubblefield MD, ed. *Cancer Rehabilitation: Principles and Practice.* 2nd ed.: Springer; 2018:298.

17. Fontham ET, Wolf AM, Church TR, et al. Cervical cancer screening for individuals at average risk: 2020 guideline update from the American Cancer Society. *CA Cancer J Clin.* 2020; 70(5):321–346.

18. Wender R, Fontham ET, Barrera E Jr. American Cancer Society lung cancer screening guidelines. *CA Cancer J Clin.* 2013;63(2):107–117.

19. Smith RA, Andrews KS, Brooks D, et al. Cancer screening in the United States, 2018: a review of current American Cancer Society guidelines and current issues in cancer screening. *CA Cancer J Clin.* 2018;68(4):297–316.

20. Antoniou KM, Tomassetti S, Tsitoura E, Vancheri C. Idiopathic pulmonary fibrosis and lung cancer: a clinical and pathogenesis update. *Curr Opin Pulm Med.* 2015;21(6):626–633.

21. Koehne G. Principles of Immunotherapy. In: Stubblefield MD. *Cancer Rehabilitation: Principles and Practice.* 2nd ed.: Springer; 2018:61.

22. Centers for Disease Control and Prevention. Breast cancer screening guidelines for women. cdc.gov.

23. Slovin SF. Evaluation and management of prostate and genitourinary cancer. In: Stubblefield MD, ed. *Cancer Rehabilitation: Principles and Practice.* 2nd ed.: Springer; 2018:278.

24. American Cancer Society. Screening tests for prostate cancer. https://www.cancer.org/cancer/prostate-cancer/detection-diagnosis-staging/tests.html. Revised January 4, 2021. Accessed May 17, 2021

25. Locati L, Lim SH, Patel S, Pfister DG. Evaluation and Treatment of Head and Neck Cancer. In: Stubblefield MD. *Cancer Rehabilitation: Principles and Practice.* 2nd ed.: Springer Publishing Company; 2018:298.

26. Grimm, SA, DeAngelis LM. Evaluation and Treatment of Primary Central Nervous System Tumors. In: Stubblefield MD. *Cancer Rehabilitation: Principles and Practice.* 2nd ed.: Springer Publishing Company; 2018:271.

27. United States Preventive Services Taskforce. Home Page. https://uspreventiveservicestaskforce.org/uspstf/home. Accessed October 31, 2020.

28. National Cancer Institute. Obesity and cancer. https://www.cancer.gov/about-cancer/causes-prevention/risk/obesity/obesity-fact-sheet; January 17, 2017. Accessed November 1, 2020.

29. Stone TW, McPherson M, Gail Darlington L. Obesity and cancer: existing and new hypotheses for a causal connection. *eBioMedicine.* 2018;30:14–28.

30. Hales CM, Carroll MD, Fryar CD, Ogden CL. Prevalence of obesity and severe obesity among adults: United States, 2017–2018. *NCHS Data Brief.* 2020;(360):1–8.

31. Centers for Disease Control and Prevention. Assessing your weight. https://www.cdc.gov/healthyweight/assessing/index.html, Reviewed September 17, 2020. Accessed October 18, 2020.

32. United States Preventive Services Taskforce. Recommendation: obesity in children and adolescents: screening www.uspreventiveservicestaskforce.org. https://www.uspreventiveservicestaskforce.org/uspstf/recommendation/obesity-in-children-and-adolescents-screening. Accessed October 30, 2020.

33. National Cancer Institute. Obesity and cancer; 2017. https://www.cancer.gov/about-cancer/causes-prevention/risk/obesity/obesity-fact-sheet, Accessed October 30, 2020.

34. Centers for Disease Control and Prevention. More than 630,000 in the U.S. affected. https://www.cdc.gov/media/releases/2017/p1003-vs-cancer-obesity.html; Published June 3, 2017. Accessed October 31, 2020.

35. American Cancer Society. Does body weight affect cancer risk? https://www.cancer.org/cancer/cancer-causes/diet-physical-activity/body-weight-and-cancer-risk/effects.html. Accessed October 31, 2020.

36. Luo J, Hendryx M, Manson JE, et al. Intentional weight loss and obesity-related cancer risk. *JNCI Cancer Spectr*. 2019;3(4):pkz054. doi:10.1093/jncics/pkz054.

37. Arnold M, Freisling H, Gunter MJ. Intentional weight loss and cancer risk: never too late to lose weight. *JNCI Cancer Spectr*. 2019;3(4):pkz059. doi:10.1093/jncics/pkz059.

38. American Cancer Society. What does the American Cancer Society recommend about body weight? https://www.cancer.org/cancer/cancer-causes/diet-physical-activity/body-weight-and-cancer-risk/acs-recommendations.html, Reviewed January 22, 2021. Accessed October 31, 2020.

39. Patel AV, Friedenreich CM, Moore SC, et al. American College of Sports Medicine roundtable report on physical activity, sedentary behavior, and cancer prevention and control. *Med Sci Sports Exerc*. 2019;51(11):2391–2402.

40. McTiernan A, Friedenreich CM, Katzmarzyk PT, et al. Physical Activity in Cancer Prevention and Survival: A Systematic Review. Med Sci Sports Exerc. 2019;51(6):1252-1261. doi:10.1249/MSS.0000000000001937

41. Cormie P, Zopf EM, Zhang X, Schmitz KH. The impact of exercise on cancer mortality, recurrence, and treatment-related adverse effects. *Epidemiol Rev*. 2017;39(1):71–92.

42. National Cancer Institute. Physical activity and cancer fact sheet; 2015. https://www.cancer.gov/about-cancer/causes-prevention/risk/obesity/physical-activity-fact-sheet, Accessed October 30, 2020.

43. Campbell KL, Winters-Stone KM, Patel AV, et al. An executive summary of reports from an international multidisciplinary roundtable on exercise and cancer: evidence, guidelines, and implementation. *Rehabil Oncol*. 2019;37(4):144–152.

44. American College for Sports Medicine. Exercise for cancer prevention and treatment. https://www.acsm.org/read-research/resource-library/resource_detail?id=d081604d-aff3-4961-bbe8-4e4220193c54. Accessed October 24, 2020.

45. McTiernan A, Friedenreich CM, Katzmarzyk PT, et al. Physical activity in cancer prevention and survival: a systematic review. *Med Sci Sports Exerc*. 2019;51(6):1252–1261.

46. Lugo D, Pulido AL, Mihos CG, et al. The effects of physical activity on cancer prevention, treatment and prognosis: a review of the literature. *Complement Ther Med*. 2019;44:9–13.

47. Kokila G, Smitha T. Cancer and physical activity. *J Oral Maxillofac Surg Med*. 2017;21(1):4–7.

48. Weis J. Cancer-related fatigue: prevalence, assessment and treatment strategies. *Expert Rev Pharmacoecon Outcomes Res*. 2011;11(4):441–446.

49. American College of Sports Medicine. Effects of exercise on health-related outcomes in those with cancer. https://www.acsm.org/docs/default-source/files-for-resource-library/exercise-guidelines-cancer-infographic.pdf?sfvrsn=c48d8d86_4. Accessed October 11, 2020.

50. Ignaszewski M, Lau B, Wong S, Isserow S. The science of exercise prescription: Martti Karvonen and his contributions. *B C Med J*. 2017;59(1):38–41. https://bcmj.org/articles/science-exercise-prescription-martti-karvonen-and-his-contributions.

51. Maltser S, Cristian A, Silver JK, Morris GS, Stout NL. A focused review of safety considerations in cancer rehabilitation. *PM R*. 2017;9(9S2):S415–S428.

52. Schmitz KH, Campbell AM, Stuiver MM, et al. Exercise is medicine in oncology: engaging clinicians to help patients move through cancer. *CA Cancer J Clin*. 2019;69(6):468–484.

53. American Physical Therapy Association. The role of the physical therapist and the American Physical Therapy Association in Diet and Nutrition [HOD P06-19-08-44]. https://www.apta.org/site-assets/pdfs/policies/role-of-pt-diet-nutrition.pdf, Updated September 20, 2019. Accessed October 31, 2020.

54. Trujillo EB, Dixon SW, Claghorn K, Levin RM, Mills JB, Spees CK. Closing the gap in nutrition care at outpatient cancer centers: ongoing initiatives of the oncology nutrition dietetic practice group. *J Acad Nutr Diet*. 2018;118(4):749–760.

55. PDQ Supportive and Palliative Care Editorial Board. Nutrition in cancer care (PDQ®): health professional version. In: *PDQ Cancer Information Summaries*. National Cancer Institute (US); 2020.

56. McCauley SM, Barrocas A, Malone A. Hospital nutrition care betters patient clinical outcomes and reduces costs: the malnutrition quality improvement initiative story. *J Acad Nutr Diet*. 2019;119(9):S11–S14.

57. Zhang X, Edwards BJ. Malnutrition in older adults with cancer. *Curr Oncol Rep*. 2019;21(9):80. doi:10.1007/s11912-019-0829-8.

58. Muscaritoli M, Lucia S, Farcomeni A, et al. Prevalence of malnutrition in patients at first medical oncology visit: the PreMiO study. *Oncotarget*. 2017;8(45):79884–79896. doi:10.18632/oncotarget.20168.

59. Greenlee H, Santiago-Torres M, McMillen KK, Ueland K, Haase AM. Helping patients eat better during and beyond cancer treatment. *Cancer J*. 2019;25(5):320–328.

60. Skipper A, Coltman A, Tomesko J, et al. Position of the Academy of Nutrition and Dietetics: malnutrition (undernutrition) screening tools for all adults. *J Acad Nutr Diet*. 2020;120(4):709–713.

61. Ferguson M, Capra S, Bauer J, Banks M. Development of a valid and reliable malnutrition screening tool for adult acute hospital patients. *Nutrition*. 1999;15(6):458–464.

62. Thompson KL, Elliott L, Fuchs-Tarlovsky V, Levin RM, Voss AC, Piemonte T. Oncology evidence-based nutrition practice guideline for adults. *J Acad Nutr Diet*. 2017;117(2):297–310. e47.

63. World Cancer Research Fund/American Institute for Cancer Research. Diet, nutrition, physical activity and cancer: a global perspective. Continuous update project expert report 2018. http://www.dietandcancerreport.org. Accessed October 20, 2020.

64. Madigan M, Karhu E. The role of plant-based nutrition in cancer prevention. *J Unexplored Med Data*. 2018;3(11):9. doi:10.20517/2572-8180.2018.05.

65. Rock CL, Thomson C, Gansler T, et al. American Cancer Society guideline for diet and physical activity for cancer prevention. *CA Cancer J Clin*. 2020;70(4):245–271.

66. Mentella MC, Scaldaferri F, Ricci C, Gasbarrini A, Miggiano GAD. Cancer and Mediterranean diet: a review. *Nutrients*. 2019;11(9):2059. doi:10.3390/nu11092059.

67. Oliveira CLP, Mattingly S, Schirrmacher R, Sawyer MB, Fine EJ, Prado CM. A nutritional perspective of ketogenic diet in cancer: a narrative review. *J Acad Nutr Diet*. 2018;118(4):668–688.

68. Li Z, Heber D. Ketogenic diets. *JAMA*. 2020;323(4):386. doi:10.1001/jama.2019.18408.

69. de Groot S, Pijl H, van der Hoeven JJM, Kroep JR. Effects of short-term fasting on cancer treatment. *J Exp Clin Cancer Res*. 2019;38(1):209. doi:10.1186/s13046-019-1189-9.

70. Melina V, Craig W, Levin S. Position of the academy of nutrition and dietetics: vegetarian diets. *J Acad Nutr Diet*. 2016;116(12):1970–1980.

71. Office of Disease Prevention and Health Promotion, U.S. Department of Health and Human Services. 2020–2025 Dietary Guidelines for Americans, 9th Edition; 2020. https://www.dietaryguidelines.gov/resources/2020-2025-dietary-guidelines-online-materials Published December 2020. Accessed May 25, 2022.

72. Shams-White MM, Brockton NT, Mitrou P, et al. Operationalizing the 2018 World Cancer Research Fund/American Institute for Cancer Research (WCRF/AICR) cancer prevention recommendations: a standardized scoring system. *Nutrients.* 2019;11(7):1572. doi:10.3390/nu11071572.

73. Fiolet T, Srour B, Sellem L, et al. Consumption of ultra-processed foods and cancer risk: results from NutriNet-Santé prospective cohort. *BMJ.* 2018;360:k322. doi:10.1136/bmj.k322.

74. World Cancer Research Fund. Alcoholic drinks and risk of cancer. https://www.wcrf.org/dietandcancer/exposures/alcoholic-drinks; Accessed September 25, 2020.

75. Nicolini A, Ferrari P, Masoni MC, et al. Malnutrition, anorexia and cachexia in cancer patients: a mini-review on pathogenesis and treatment. *Biomed Pharmacother.* 2013;67(8):807–817.

76. Mello FW, Melo G, Pasetto JJ, Silva CAB, Warnakulasuriya S, Rivero ERC. The synergistic effect of tobacco and alcohol consumption on oral squamous cell carcinoma: a systematic review and meta-analysis. *Clin Oral Investig.* 2019;23(7):2849–2859.

77. Viner B, Barberio AM, Haig TR, Friedenreich CM, Brenner DR. The individual and combined effects of alcohol consumption and cigarette smoking on site-specific cancer risk in a prospective cohort of 26,607 adults: results from Alberta's Tomorrow Project. *Cancer Causes Control.* 2019;30(12):1313–1326.

78. U.S. Department of Health and Human Services. *A Report of the Surgeon General: How Tobacco Smoke Causes Disease: What It Means to You.* U.S. Department of Health and Human Services, Centers for Disease Control and Prevention, National Center for Chronic Disease Prevention and Health Promotion, Office on Smoking and Health; 2010.

79. Darcey E, Boyle T. Tobacco smoking and survival after a prostate cancer diagnosis: a systematic review and meta-analysis. *Cancer Treat Rev.* 2018;70:30–40.

80. Tindle HA, Shiffman S. Smoking cessation behavior among intermittent smokers versus daily smokers. *Am J Public Health.* 2011;101(7):e1–e3. doi:10.2105/ajph.2011.300186.

81. United States Preventive Services Taskforce. Lung cancer: screening. https://www.uspreventiveservicestaskforce.org/uspstf/recommendation/lung-cancer-screening, Published March 9, 2021. Accessed May 17, 2021.

82. Hamant C, Deneuve S, Albaret M-A, et al. Accompagnement des dépendances à l'alcool et au tabac des patients atteints d'un cancer des voies aérodigestives supérieures. [Smoking and alcohol cessation programs in patients with head and neck cancer]. *Bull Cancer.* 2018;105(11):1012–1019. doi:10.1016/j.bulcan.2018.07.006.

83. American Cancer Society. Health risks of smoking tobacco; 2000. https://www.cancer.org/cancer/cancer-causes/tobacco-and-cancer/health-risks-of-smoking-tobacco.html, Accessed October 14, 2020.

84. Liu Y, Croft JB, Wheaton AG, et al. Clustering of five health-related behaviors for chronic disease prevention among adults, United States. *Prev Chronic Dis.* 2013;2016(13):160054. doi:10.5888/pcd13.160054.

85. Otte JL, Carpenter JS, Manchanda S, et al. Systematic review of sleep disorders in cancer patients: can the prevalence of sleep disorders be ascertained? *Cancer Med.* 2014;4(2):183–200.

86. O'Donnell JF. Insomnia in cancer patients. *Clin Cornerstone.* 2004;6(1):S6–S14.

87. Zeichner SB, Zeichner RL, Gogineni K, Shatil S, Ioachimescu O. Cognitive behavioral therapy for insomnia, mindfulness, and yoga in patients with breast cancer with sleep disturbance: a literature review. *Breast Cancer (Auckl).* 2017;11:1178223417745564. doi:10.1177/1178223417745564.

88. Siengsukon CF, Al-Dughmi M, Stevens S. Sleep health promotion: practical information for physical therapists. *Phys Ther.* 2017;97(8):826–836.

89. Maness DL, Khan M. Nonpharmacologic management of chronic insomnia. *Am Fam Physician.* 2015;92(12):1058–1064.

90. Center for Disease Control and Prevention. Tips for better sleep. https://www.cdc.gov/sleep/about_sleep/sleep_hygiene.html, Reviewed July 15, 2016. Accessed October 10, 2020.

91. Paruthi S, Brooks LJ, D'Ambrosio C, et al. Recommended amount of sleep for pediatric populations: a consensus statement of the American Academy of Sleep Medicine. *J Clin Sleep Med.* 2016;12(6):785–786.

92. Watson NF, Badr MS, Belenky G, et al. Recommended amount of sleep for a healthy adult: a joint consensus statement of the American Academy of Sleep Medicine and Sleep Research Society. *J Clin Sleep Medicine.* 2015;11(6):591–592. doi:10.5664/jcsm.4758.

93. Miller WR, Rollinick S. *Motivational Interviewing: Helping People Change.* 3rd ed.: Guilford Press; 2012.

94. Teixeira PJ, Palmeira AL, Vansteenkiste M. The role of self-determination theory and motivational interviewing in behavioral nutrition, physical activity, and health: an introduction to the IJBNPA special series. *Int J Behav Nutr Phys Act.* 2012;9(1):17. doi:10.1186/1479-5868-9-17.

95. Dunn C, Deroo L, Rivara FP. The use of brief interventions adapted from motivational interviewing across behavioral domains: a systematic review. *Addiction.* 2001;96(12):1725–1742.

96. Prochaska JO, Velicer WF. The transtheoretical model of health behavior change. *Am J Heal Promot.* 1997;12(1):38–48.

97. Pignataro RM, Huddleston J. The use of motivational interviewing in physical therapy education and practice: empowering patients through effective self-management. *J Phys Ther Educ.* 2015;29(2):62–71.

98. Fortune J, Breckon J, Norris M, Eva G, Frater T. Motivational interviewing training for physiotherapy and occupational therapy students: effect on confidence, knowledge and skills. *Patient Educ Couns.* 2019;102(4):694–700.

99. Schoo AM, Lawn S, Rudnik E, Litt JC. Teaching health science students foundation motivational interviewing skills: use of motivational interviewing treatment integrity and self-reflection to approach transformative learning. *BMC Med Educ.* 2015;15(1):228. doi:10.1186/s12909-015-0512-1.

100. Lion A, Backes A, Duhem C, et al. Motivational interviewing to increase physical activity behavior in cancer patients: a pilot randomized controlled trials. *Integr Cancer Ther.* 2020;19:153473542091497. doi:10.1177/1534735420914973.

101. Pudkasam S, Polman R, Pitcher M, et al. Physical activity and breast cancer survivors: importance of adherence, motivational interviewing and psychological health. *Maturitas.* 2018;116:66–72. doi:10.1016/j.maturitas.2018.07.010.

102. Zangeneh F, Masoumi SZ, Shayan A, Matinnia N, Mohagheghi H, Mohammadi Y. The effect of motivational interviewing-based counseling on women's sexual satisfaction and body image. *Evid Based Care J.* 2019;9(3):58–62.

103. Spencer JC, Wheeler SB. A systematic review of motivational Interviewing interventions in cancer patients and survivors. *Patient Educ Couns.* 2016;99(7):1099–1105.

104. Buckner CA, Lafrenie RM, Dénommée JA, Caswell JM, Want DA. Complementary and alternative medicine use in patients before and after a cancer diagnosis. *Curr Oncol.* 2018;25(4):e275–e281.

105. Lopez G, Guttierez C. Complimentary therapies in cancer rehabilitation and symptom management. In: Stubblefield MD, ed. *Cancer Rehabilitation: Principles and Practice.* 2nd ed.: Springer; 2018:938.

106. Greenlee H, DuPont-Reyes MJ, Balneaves LG, et al. Clinical practice guidelines on the evidence-based use of integrative therapies during and after breast cancer treatment. *CA Cancer J Clin.* 2017;67(3):194–232.

107. Feinstein D. Energy psychology: efficacy, speed, mechanisms. *Explore (NY).* 2019;15(5):340–351.

108. Bach D, Groesbeck G, Stapleton P, Sims R, Blickheuser K, Church D. Clinical EFT (Emotional Freedom Techniques) improves multiple physiological markers of health. *J Evid Based Integr Med.* 2019;24. doi:10.1177/2515690X18823691110 2515690X18823691.

109. Harbottle L. Potential of emotional freedom techniques to improve mood and quality of life in older adults. *Brit J Community Nurs.* 2019;24(9):432–435.

110. Baker BS, Hoffman CJ. Emotional Freedom Techniques (EFT) to reduce the side effects associated with tamoxifen and aromatase inhibitor use in women with breast cancer: a service evaluation. *Eur J Integr Med.* 2015;7(2):136–142. doi:10.1016/j.eujim.2014.10.004.

111. Church D. EFT Mini Manual. 2nd ed. Energy Psychology Press. evidencebasedeft.com/wp-content/uploads/2017/02/EFTMini-Manual.pdf. Accessed October 31, 2020.

112. Collinge W, MacDonald G, Walton T. Massage in supportive cancer care. *Semin Oncol Nurs.* 2012;28(1):45–54. doi:10.1016/j.soncn.2011.11.005.

113. Qin S, Xiao Y, Chi Z, et al. Effectiveness and safety of massage in the treatment of anxiety and depression in patients with cancer. *Medicine.* 2020;99(39):e22262. doi:10.1097/md.0000000000022262.

114. Lopez G, Liu W, Milbury K, et al. The effects of oncology massage on symptom self-report for cancer patients and their caregivers. Support Care Cancer. 2017;25(12):3645-3650. doi:10.1007/s00520-017-3784-7.

115. Izgu N, Metin ZG, Karadas C, Ozdemir L, Çetin N, Demirci U. Prevention of chemotherapy-induced peripheral neuropathy with classical massage in breast cancer patients receiving paclitaxel: an assessor-blinded randomized controlled trial. *Eur J Oncol Nurs.* 2019;40:36–43.

116. Coşkun HŞ, Arikan F, Gökdoğan F. Effect of massage therapy on peripheral neuropathy and life quality of colorectal cancer with patient receiving chemotherapy. *Ann Oncol.* 2014;25:iv533. doi:10.1093/annonc/mdu356.49.

117. Lin PJ, Peppone LJ, Janelsins MC, et al. Yoga for the management of cancer treatment-related toxicities. *Curr Oncol Rep.* 2018;20(1):5. doi:10.1007/s11912-018-0657-2.

118. NIH. Yoga: what you need to know. https://www.nccih.nih.gov/health/yoga-what-you-need-to-know. April 2021. Accessed May 25, 2022.

119. Danhauer SC, Addington EL, Cohen L, et al. Yoga for symptom management in oncology: a review of the evidence base and future directions for research. *Cancer.* 2019;125(12):1979–1989.

120. Rithirangsriroj K, Manchana T, Akkayagorn L. Efficacy of acupuncture in prevention of delayed chemotherapy induced nausea and vomiting in gynecologic cancer patients. *Gynecol Oncol.* 2015;136(1):82–86. doi:10.1016/j.ygyno.2014.10.025.

121. National Center for Complementary and Integrative Health. *Cancer: In Depth National Institutes of Health*; 2014. https://www.nccih.nih.gov/health/cancer-in-depth Accessed October 23, 2020.

122. Norouzi E, Gerber M, Masrour F, Vaezmosavi M, Pühse U, Brand S. Implementation of a mindfulness-based stress reduction (MBSR) program to reduce stress, anxiety, and depression and to improve psychological well-being among retired Iranian football players. *Psychol Sport Exerc.* 2000;47:101636.

123. Xunlin NG, Lau Y, Klainin-Yobas P. The effectiveness of mindfulness-based interventions among cancer patients and survivors: a systematic review and meta-analysis. *Support Care Cancer.* 2020;28(4):1563–1578.

124. Compen F, Bisseling E, Schellekens M, et al. Face-to-face and internet-based mindfulness-based cognitive therapy compared with treatment as usual in reducing psychological distress in patients with cancer: a multicenter randomized controlled trial. *J Clin Oncol.* 2018;36(23):2413–2421.

125. National Cancer Institute. Social support. https://www.cancer.gov/publications/dictionaries/cancer-terms/def/social-support. February 2, 2011. Accessed February 25, 2021.

126. Lin S, Faust L, Robles-Granda P, Kajdanowicz T, Chawla NV. Social network structure is predictive of health and wellness. *PLoS ONE.* 2019;14(6):e0217264. doi:10.1371/journal.pone.0217264.

127. Raphael D, Frey R, Gott M. Maintaining psychosocial wellbeing for post-treatment haematological cancer survivors: strategies and potential barriers. *Eur J Oncol Nurs.* 2019;38:36–41.

128. Reed LM, Rua K. Defining the role of the oncology nurse navigator. *J Oncol Navigation Surviv.* 2020;11(3). jons-online.com/issues/2020/march-2020-vol-11-no-3/2842-defining-the-role-of-the-oncology-nurse-navigator.

129. Sarma EA, Kawachi I, Poole EM, et al. Social integration and survival after diagnosis of colorectal cancer. *Cancer.* 2018;124(4):833–840.

130. Kroenke CH, Paskett ED, Cené CW, et al. Prediagnosis social support, social integration, living status, and colorectal cancer mortality in postmenopausal women from the women's health initiative. *Cancer.* 2020;126(8):1766–1775.

131. Puigpinós-Riera R, Graells-Sans A, Serral G, et al. Anxiety and depression in women with breast cancer: social and clinical determinants and influence of the social network and social support (DAMA cohort). *Cancer Epidemiol.* 2018;55:123–129.

132. Aizpurua-Perez I, Perez-Tejada J. Resilience in women with breast cancer: a systematic review. *Eur J Oncol Nurs.* 2020;49:101854. doi:10.1016/j.ejon.2020.101854.

133. Jan M, Bonn SE, Sjölander A, et al. The roles of stress and social support in prostate cancer mortality. *Scand J Urol.* 2015;50(1):47–55.

134. Capistrant BD, Lesher L, Kohli N, et al. Social support and health-related quality of life among gay and bisexual men with prostate cancer. *Oncol Nurs Forum.* 2018;45(4):439–455.

135. Kadambi S, Soto-Perez-de-Celis E, Garg T, et al. Social support for older adults with cancer: young International Society of Geriatric Oncology review paper. *J Geriatr Oncol.* 2020;11(2):217–224.

Administrative Aspects of Oncology Rehabilitation

31

Building and Sustaining an Oncology Rehabilitation Program

HOLLY LOOKABAUGH-DEUR, PT, DSc, GCS, CEEAA BOARD CERTIFIED GERIATRIC CLINICAL SPECIALIST, REYNA COLOMBO, PT, MA, AND CHRISTOPHER M. WILSON, PT, DPT, DScPT, BOARD CERTIFIED GERIATRIC CLINICAL SPECIALIST

CHAPTER OUTLINE

Introduction

There is a vast body of evidence described in previous chapters reaffirming the benefits of oncology rehabilitation (Onc R) for persons with cancer (PWCs) as well as those living with lingering sequelae, as a person living with and beyond cancer (PLWBC). Through the years, foundations and organizations have been promoting the importance of addressing the comprehensive care that PWCs need. Yet today, comprehensive Onc R services are not available to many PLWBC due to the limited offerings of their local institutions. Thus, the objective of this chapter is to guide oncology leaders and administrators in designing sustainable Onc R services for individuals across the cancer journey. In addition, it is hoped that Onc R clinicians who read this chapter will have a better understanding of the depth and breadth of the influences on their clinical practice, and they will work in synergy with their managers to provide high-quality, inclusive Onc R. By providing these necessary services across the continuum of care, Onc R clinicians will become an important force in the future of community health.

Health services evolve in response to ever-changing community and population needs. As public health priorities shift, so does the rehabilitation market respond, focusing on prevention, intervention, and lifestyle-related services. In the 1970s and 80s, rehabilitation efforts focused on orthopedics and neurological programs, which resulted in these service lines being fine tuned into well-oiled machines for these patient populations. The 90s brought in-depth programming at abating heart disease, the nation's leading killer, followed by the immersion and growth of specialty skills in the 2000s, such as women's health (now pelvic health), vestibular care, sports medicine, and more. While oncologic care has been a major health challenge for decades, Onc R has experienced rapid growth over the past 15 years. Recognized as a specialty of the physical therapy profession since 2016, with its first board certified oncology specialists in 2019; Onc R is an essential component of the cancer care process, with growing evidence supporting its value and role on the oncology team.[1]

Establishing a Philosophy of Care

When establishing, supporting, or growing an Onc R program, it all starts with a clear, concise mission and vision. This is especially important as leadership of an Onc R specialty service requires more than a perfunctory knowledge of all aspects of this complex medical condition and its course of care. Cancer affects people of any age, sex, economic status, social status, ethnicity, lifestyle, and educational level. Therefore, it requires a broad, proactive, holistic vision and understanding of consumer needs in a complicated healthcare system. Due to the breadth of service possibilities, it is imperative that each program has a clearly articulated mission, vision, and set of values that will serve to guide the program and its clinicians. This mission serves as the guiding force in all administrative infrastructure decisions.

Establishing a program's mission will hinge greatly on the scope and resources of the team, geographical and competitive considerations, and the local and regional healthcare needs. This essential step of creating a framework for the program can also be an important "team-unifying" exercise, which requires a consensus-driven focus developed by exploring the following[2]:

- A **mission statement** describes why the organization exists. As a team, ask "what is our purpose?" "Why will this program benefit our community?"
- An organization's **vision statement** describes the ideal future state of the organization, articulating what the organization is trying to accomplish. More details of who, how, and other parameters are defined in this step.
- A **values statement** describes and lists the fundamental values and principles that guide the organization in the pursuit of its vision and mission. Examples include teamwork, interdisciplinary communication, integrity, growth, and service to others.

As it is a relatively new or nonexistent service for many institutions, there may not be consensus on what an Onc R program should entail. As more programs evolve, a gold standard is likely to emerge in the literature that will guide us to more standardized programming. Additionally, the spectrum of opportunities to touch the PWC at multiple points throughout the journey adds another level of complexity to the planning process. Onc R planning considerations may include the wide variety of program components based on the key factor that Onc R during active treatment is different from survivorship/surveillance programs.

- Therapy during active treatment may include inpatient/acute care management, outpatient management of adverse effects of treatment, or even prevention of potential issues. Necessary skills and program development include knowledge and care for the unique aspects of bone marrow transplants, cancer related fatigue (CRF), skin care, lymphedema prevention and early management, balance, and prevention of falls while adapting to chemotherapy induced polyneuropathy (CIPN). Other team interventions include nutrition and other essential wellness habits vital for optimal recovery such as sleep and stress management.
- Onc R posttreatment, referred to as the "survivorship" period (in some countries) incorporates all of the skill sets mentioned previously, but also adds important adjuncts to prevention and early recognition of lingering adverse effects. Sequelae of cancer treatment may include: CRF, CIPN and related risks, lymphedema, tissue restriction and fibrosis, and mild to profound functional losses, to name a few. Self-awareness is a key focus in survivorship programs, with attention to cancer

recurrence signs and symptoms as well as maximizing full potential with appropriate manual techniques, patient education, strengthening, and aerobic and endurance progression. Program goals are different during this phase of programming; avid cancer prevention and thorough education, and restoration of physical and cognitive abilities as well as leisure skills and instrumental activities of daily living (iADLs) should be emphasized.

Clarity in the intent and purpose of the mission and vision of the program is a critical step prior to creation of a business plan.

The Impetus for Developing an Oncology Rehabilitation Program

A key consideration in developing the mission and subsequent program development is understanding the needs of the local community it will serve. A United States (US) poll in 2004 gave voice to more than 2300 cancer survivors, which revealed that about half (49%) of these individuals felt that their nonmedical needs were not being met.[3] In addition, 70% of respondents indicated that they did not feel that their oncologists offered support in dealing with their nonmedical needs. The remaining 30% responded that their physicians were willing to talk about their needs but felt that the resources were not available to address them.[3] Furthermore, another study found that treatment for cancer-related disability was only provided to 1% to 2% of individuals.[4] Why then, after nearly two decades of a growing body of literature related to the rehabilitative needs of individuals with cancer, do we still have barriers to access rehabilitation services? Factors may include a shortage of Onc R clinicians, poor knowledge and recognition among the cancer community to refer for Onc R, and the limited capacity of PLWBCs to seek Onc R as an additional healthcare venue due to internal or external factors.

In 2006, The US Institute of Medicine (IOM—now named the National Academy of Medicine) released a report, *From Cancer Patient to Cancer Survivor: Lost in Transition*, which focused on survivors of adult cancer during the phase of care that follows primary treatment.[5] The IOM reported that, "Too many survivors are lost in transition once they finish treatment. They move from an orderly system of care to a 'nonsystem' in which there are few guidelines to assist them through the next stage of their life or help them overcome the medical and psychosocial problems that may arise."[5] This challenge can provide an opportunity for rehabilitation professionals to assist in provision of these cancer survivorship services. Therapy professionals can affect change by building their own skill sets, offering effective care, measuring outcomes, and increasing awareness of available services to all members of the medical community.

Value-Based Oncology Rehabilitation

The availability and accessibility of oncology care for PLWBCs is heavily influenced by a nation's public policy as will be described further in Chapter 32. For example, within the US, the implementation of the Affordable Care Act brought with it the concept of healthcare reform and a new system of delivery and payment reform known as *value-based purchasing*. Under this model, payment from Medicare was defined by quality, accountability, and outcomes. This model of care promoted sharing of risk between payers and providers with the intention of providing better outcomes for defined populations (especially patients with chronic diseases, such as cancer). Furthermore, the concept of value-based competition is critical to drive improvements in quality, safety, and efficiency. These principles have been highlighted in the book *Redefining Health Care: Creating Value-Based Competition on Results*.[6] The authors' argument is that the failure of competition is evidenced by large and inexplicable differences in cost and quality for the same type of care across providers and across geographic areas. They proposed to shift the conversation from competition to fundamental value of the healthcare service for the patient. They postulated that value in healthcare can be best achieved by addressing the individuals' medical condition over the full cycle of care, from monitoring and prevention to treatment to ongoing disease management.[6] According to the authors, the accountability of the physician is expanding to also include the responsibility for the integration of the total care of the medical condition. Accountability for value is then shared among the providers involved. Value is measured by tracking a person's outcomes longitudinally across their disease journey. When considering value, two terms are important to consider: *process outcomes* and *actual outcomes*. Process outcomes may or may not be related to delivery of quality of care and may be exemplified by a metric such as number of persons on a waiting list. There may be many means to improve this process metric (e.g., discharging patients prematurely to schedule more patients) but this may not be tied to value-based outcomes. Instead, actual outcomes tend to focus on what a PLWBC values, such as accessible care that is convenient, patient-centered, and relevant to improving their life situation. In addition, actual outcomes often introduce innovations in the care of PLWBC while process outcomes are less likely to do so. Institutions and healthcare personnel often improve and adapt innovative clinical processes to improve care delivery to PWC, but a key component of this improvement is the emphasis on *patient experience* rather than process-driven procedures. Persons diagnosed with cancer perceive value in their cancer care in a stepwise manner: (1) years of survivorship; (2) relative freedom from disease and return to functional status. (e.g., How long to recovery? How much recovery?); and (3) the sustainability of their health, functional recovery, and independence. Among common predictors of the overall quality perception by PLWBC, four should be of particular interest because individuals perceived them as relatively problematic aspects of care. These were identified related to communication and information exchange: (1) perception of if the PWC was well informed about follow-up care after treatment; (2) the PWC understood the next steps for care; (3) the PWC knew who the right resource for questions was; and (4) providers were aware of test results and were up to date on the PWC's case.[7] Each of these concepts needs to be integrated into an Onc R program during its development. Unfortunately, most institutions struggle in the measurement of these metrics and have failed to prioritize value-based, outcome-driven improvement and innovation.[8]

Due to recent attempts to reform healthcare payment, alternate payment models have heavily influenced cancer care and Onc R. For example, the concept of bundled payments has grown widely in the US; bundled payment programs generally provide a single, comprehensive payment to an institution that covers all the services involved in a patient's episode of care. Traditionally, Medicare has made separate payments to providers for each of the individual services that are furnished to beneficiaries for a certain illness or course of treatment. However, policymakers and providers have become increasingly concerned that this approach may result in fragmented care coordination across providers and healthcare settings. Bundled payments can align incentives for providers—hospitals, postacute care providers, physicians, and other practitioners—and encourage them to work together to improve the quality and coordination of care. This model of payment is viewed as somewhat of a "middle ground" between traditional fee-for-service payments, which entails very little financial risk for providers, and full capitation, in which a provider assumes almost full financial risk.[9] A key consideration of bundled payments is that if predetermined "bundles" are established without key services (for example, Onc R), these services will be harder to administer (and be paid for) after the proverbial "ship has sailed." In addition, a concern with bundled payments is that it may favor early providers and more intensive services. For example, if an institution is required to provide more early care (e.g., intensive care unit or acute care services) or is relatively inefficient with early hospital-based services, there may be insufficient funds available to provide downstream services such as outpatient rehabilitation.

In the midst of a very complex healthcare environment, national organizations such as the American Physical Therapy Association (APTA) have shifted their visions to consider their positive, proactive impact on society at large. This vision, "*Transforming society by optimizing movement to improve the human experience*" was adopted in 2013 and aligns well with the needed approach to building and sustaining an Onc R program. As this transformative vision focuses on the role of clinicians within society (as opposed to focusing solely on individual patients), rehab leaders and administrators are tasked with finding a way to put this vision into practice, including the need to impact and transform the experiences of individuals, communities, and populations.[10] Through this vision, clinicians can add value to PLWBCs by not only treating impairments and disabilities but also preventing physical limitations and promoting safe activity and mobility, all of which will result in improving a PLWBC's ability to participate in life activities and integration into society.

In order to achieve these goals, clinicians must advocate to achieve clear understanding of the role and value of Onc R to key stakeholders such as state and local agencies, payers, healthcare leaders, and professional organizations. This is especially important to Onc R as these clinicians are not often considered to be integral team members in the management of individuals with a chronic disease such as cancer, therefore current payment models may not provide for preventative or case management services of rehabilitation professionals. Financial considerations are essential components of any new service line planning process. Gathering information such as case mix of payer types and any policy limitations for an individual with a diagnosis of cancer are examples of fact-finding to supplement critical conversations regarding funding. New partnerships may emerge with nonprofit organizations and foundations to supplement and support services for those with limited financial means. Additionally, research is clear and emerging about needing to address health disparities, particularly with the LBGTQIA+ communities—both in treatment and rehabilitation access.[11]

The Science of Program Implementation

Through the years, healthcare delivery has become more complex and Onc R clinicians must ask themselves, "*What business are we in?*" This question helps by guiding us in defining who our customer is, what their needs are, and how we should organize our operations to deliver services to meet their needs. Defining these questions will further assist Onc R clinicians in creating value for PLWBC by building Onc R programs around value-driven outcomes and working backward from there to establish processes to best achieve these outcomes. This is especially important as it has been cited to take nearly two decades for research findings to be integrated into clinical practice and improve the value provided to PWCs.[12]

To develop these value-based services, it is important understand the relatively new concept of *implementation science*. This is an empirical, scientific approach to development and implementation, including examining and validating theories and models for creating the framework for implementation and sustainability of programs and policies. Similar to the concept of evidence-based clinical practice, it is equally important for administrators and leaders in the field of oncology to utilize scientific evidence to design Onc R programs. Armed with a rapidly growing body of knowledge, administrators and oncology leaders must use evidence and research to implement programs. They must translate research into practice and knowledge into action.

The Role of Implementation Science

Implementation science is defined as the scientific study of methods to promote the systematic uptake of research findings and evidence-based practice (EBP) into routine practice to improve the quality and effectiveness of the health services and care.[13] Implementation science has been informed by disciplines, such as sociology, psychology, and organizational theories, all with the end goal to create a framework in which the program's implementation is most likely to succeed. Administrators and/or oncology leaders may benefit from applying the following principles: (1) describing and/or guiding the process of translating research into practice; (2) understanding and/or explaining what influences implementation outcomes; and (3) evaluating the implementation.[14] These steps are important during development and implementation because it gives leaders the opportunity to describe the purpose of their program/project, thereby influencing implementation outcomes and the adoption of evidence-based interventions.

Oncology leaders and administrators need to be aware of the difference between knowledge transfer (KT) and knowledge exchange (KE). Both need to occur as they move forward toward implementation of an oncology program. Internally, within their department there is a need to transfer knowledge to staff, preparing them and empowering them to deliver evidence-based care. In a system, the concept of KE is also important as leaders need to exchange knowledge with other administrators and oncology partners to understand the interconnectivity of their goals, to increase the utility of their research, and ultimately the implementation of goals.

Knowledge Exchange

A key consideration for oncology leaders is the concept of partnership in research to affect policy and practice. Today, healthcare researchers are developing partnerships with decision makers to effectively exchange and transfer empirical knowledge into practice. There is a growing exchange between knowledge producers and knowledge users.[15] This KE is evident by the partnership created in the landmark publication "Toward a National Initiative in Cancer Rehabilitation: Recommendations from a Subject Matter Expert Group."[16] In this article, a group of subject matter experts in cancer came together to inform government, healthcare providers, and the general public about the need to integrate Onc R models into oncology care from the point of diagnosis through survivorship. They advocated for incorporating

evidence-based rehabilitation clinical assessment tools into routine practice as well as including rehabilitation professionals in shared decision-making.[16]

A useful example of this interconnectivity is the conceptual framework depicting the numerous moving parts and pieces that make up Beaumont Health's (Troy, MI, USA) Cancer Survivorship Program Model (Figure 31.1). During the development of this model and the corresponding survivorship program, leaders needed to learn from each other during the development process. Some critical components during the development of the model were relationship building, reciprocity, collaboration, and trust. After establishing these components, they were leveraged during the implementation of the actual processes. Using the concepts of KE, the project planning leaders carefully selected taskforce members to help develop the program model. As this diagram depicts all of the components and services offered to patients and families, it is especially helpful when orienting new team members and sharing with accrediting agencies (e.g., Commission on Cancer [CoC]). As an example, this institutions' program includes six major components as well as program coordination with other services offered within the health system. One of the earliest components of this overall survivorship program initiative was the inclusion of oncology rehabilitation Onc R. Due to the fluctuating nature of healthcare, this model underwent 37 revisions over nearly a decade; many revisions resulting from the evolution and expansion of the oncology rehabilitation program under the name of *Exercise and Wellness Program*. A key skill of the Survivorship Program team members was adaptability, as any program will likely undergo many changes and setbacks during the creative process. As each institution's cancer services may vary, leaders will need to strategically assess what services and resources are available within their healthcare system and what might need to be supplemented, supported, or offered through strategic partnerships outside the organization.

Oncology leaders can collaborate within their institution but may need to establish partnerships with other institutions or among the private sector to provide the comprehensive services required by PWCs. Oncology leaders should also pursue partnerships with state and local governments, agencies, physicians, and universities to facilitate KE and services that will be effective in adding value to the practice of Onc R.

Knowledge Transfer

Another helpful concept for oncology leaders is KT. The Canadian Institutes of Health Research defined the term in 2000 as "the process to address the gap between what is known from research (knowledge synthesis) and implementation of this knowledge by key stakeholders with the intention of improving health outcomes."[17] One author stated that the scientific research which is produced does not add inherent value to the patient or the healthcare system until that knowledge is applied clinically to direct patient care.[17] Thus, various terms applied to Knowledge Transfer Applications (KTA) include: (1) knowledge translation; (2) knowledge transfer; (3) knowledge exchange; (4) research utilization; (5) implementation; (6) dissemination; (7) diffusion; (8) continuing education; and (9) continuing professional development. Transferring abstract knowledge into action is a required skill of administrators and rehab leaders who aim to develop Onc R programs that support evidence-based, cost-effective, and accountable healthcare. Responsible leaders who make decisions on the direction of rehabilitation programs must seek opportunities to use research in an actionable form.

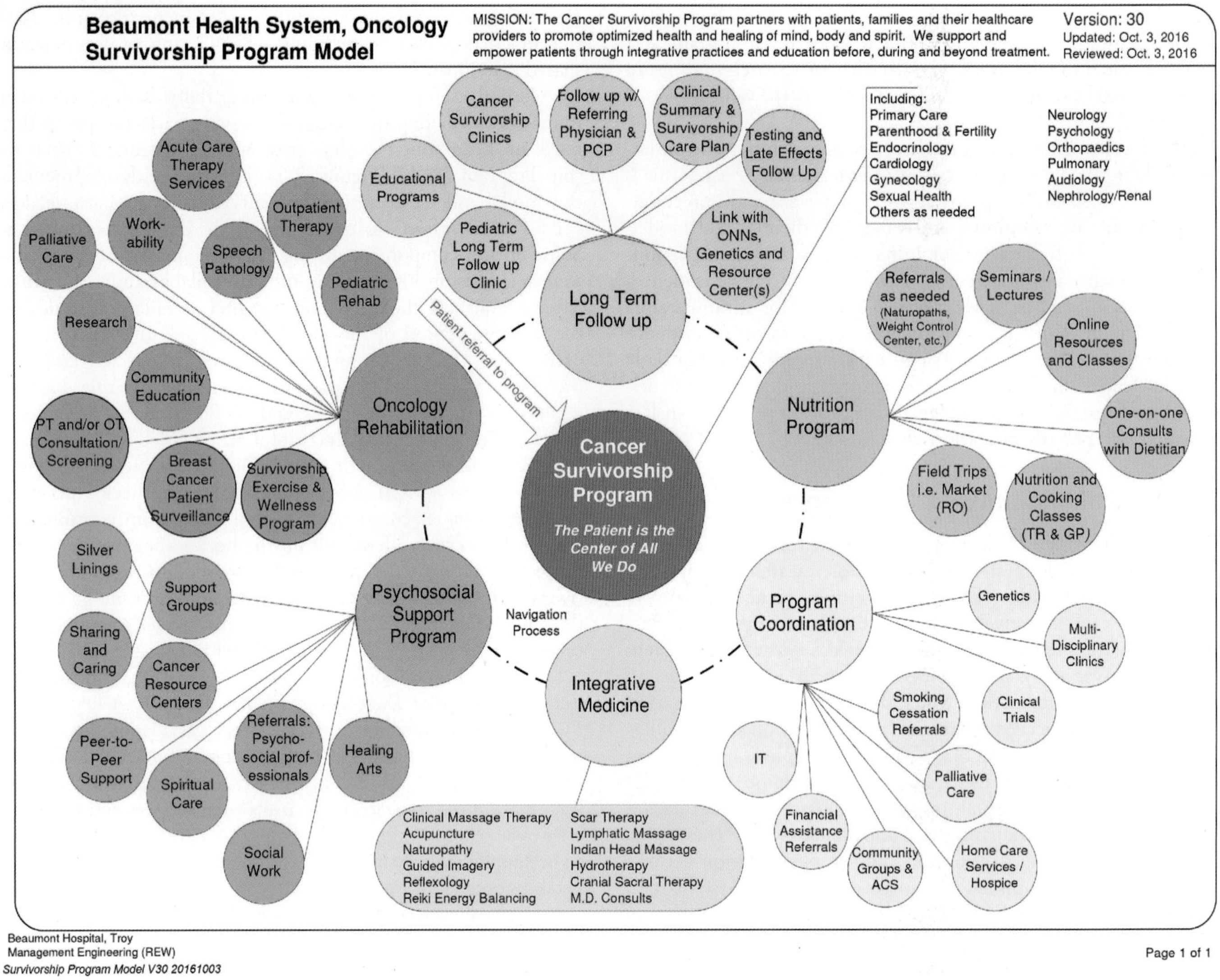

Beaumont Health System, Oncology Survivorship Program Model

MISSION: The Cancer Survivorship Program partners with patients, families and their healthcare providers to promote optimized health and healing of mind, body and spirit. We support and empower patients through integrative practices and education before, during and beyond treatment.

Version: 30
Updated: Oct. 3, 2016
Reviewed: Oct. 3, 2016

Cancer Survivorship Clinics

Follow up w/ Referring Physician & PCP

Clinical Summary & Survivorship Care Plan

Testing and Late Effects Follow Up

Including:
Primary Care
Parenthood & Fertility
Endocrinology
Cardiology
Gynecology
Sexual Health
Others as needed

Neurology
Psychology
Orthopaedics
Pulmonary
Audiology
Nephrology/Renal

Acute Care Therapy Services

Educational Programs

Outpatient Therapy

Pediatric Long Term Follow up Clinic

Long Term Follow up

Link with ONNs, Genetics and Resource Center(s)

Referrals as needed (Naturopaths, Weight Control Center, etc.)

Seminars / Lectures

Palliative Care

Work-ability

Speech Pathology

Pediatric Rehab

Patient referral to program

Nutrition Program

Online Resources and Classes

Research

Community Education

Oncology Rehabilitation

Cancer Survivorship Program

The Patient is the Center of All We Do

Field Trips i.e. Market (RO)

Nutrition and Cooking Classes (TR & GP)

One-on-one Consults with Dietitian

PT and/or OT Consultation/ Screening

Breast Cancer Patient Surveillance

Survivorship Exercise & Wellness Program

Silver Linings

Support Groups

Psychosocial Support Program

Navigation Process

Program Coordination

Genetics

Multi-Disciplinary Clinics

Sharing and Caring

Cancer Resource Centers

Integrative Medicine

Smoking Cessation Referrals

Clinical Trials

Peer-to-Peer Support

Spiritual Care

Referrals: Psycho-social professionals

Healing Arts

IT

Financial Assistance Referrals

Palliative Care

Social Work

Community Groups & ACS

Home Care Services / Hospice

Clinical Massage Therapy
Acupuncture
Naturopathy
Guided Imagery
Reflexology
Reiki Energy Balancing

Scar Therapy
Lymphatic Massage
Indian Head Massage
Hydrotherapy
Cranial Sacral Therapy
M.D. Consults

Beaumont Hospital, Troy
Management Engineering (REW)
Survivorship Program Model V30 20161003

Page 1 of 1

• **Fig. 31.1** Example of Conceptual Framework for a Cancer Survivorship Program. Beaumont Health. (Reprinted with permission).

An example of KTA was the development of PRevention, Intervention, and Sustained wellness Model (PRISM), a visual depiction and acronym which attempts to rapidly convey the growing role of rehabilitation professionals not just as interventionists but also key stakeholders in prevention and sustainable wellness.[18,19] During initial implementations of a an Onc R program, the rehabilitation department's administrator shared this framework to highlight the therapists' role in the PRISM in the care of PLWBCs and chronic diseases. Although simplistic by design, behind the visual depiction is the large body of research clearly establishing the key role and benefits of rehabilitation professionals across the entire disease journey. The developers of the PRISM concept used this model when orienting staff members and hospital administrators to the novel care philosophy of cancer rehabilitation (and chronic disease management) as compared to other diagnoses that rehabilitation professionals have traditionally cared for (e.g., orthopedics, neurology). PRISM was designed to be a simple, concise, and user-friendly conceptual model, but it conveyed explicit recommendations to influence stakeholders based on synthesis of the literature (Figure 31.2).

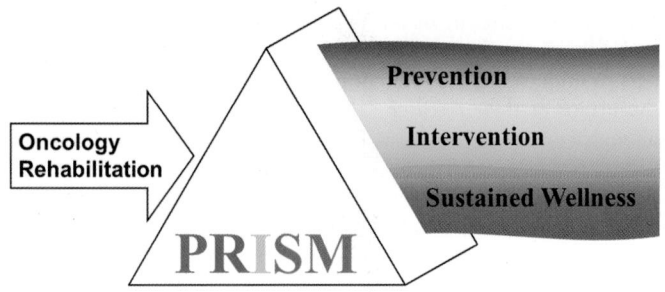

• **Fig. 31.2** PRevention, Intervention, and Sustained wellness Model (PRISM) Visual Depiction to Facilitate Knowledge Translation into Practice. Reprinted with permission from Colombo R, Wilson C. PRevention, Intervention, and Sustained wellness Model (PRISM) care philosophy in cancer survivorship, palliative care, and chronic disease management in the era of healthcare reform: a perspective paper. *Rehabil Oncol.* 2015;33(2):45–51.

For each of the three categories, the administrator outlined the key steps and institutional support structure to facilitate the delivery of care to patients with chronic conditions, and in particular for PWCs. PRISM represented a new treatment paradigm.

Prevention: The administrator set the expectation for the provision of prospective surveillance, early prevention of functional limitations, and preventive care in PWCs. This required a modification in the rehabilitation department's care approach, visit appointment structure, and therapist training.

Intervention: As Onc R clinicians are already experts in the provision of interventions to treat movement and functional disorders, this area required very little modification beyond additional education in foundational cancer concepts. Areas of emphasis included the need to intervene proactively and in collaboration with the interdisciplinary team to avoid underutilization of Onc R services for PLWBCs.

Sustainable wellness: The administrator emphasized the need to support individuals whose cancer treatment had been completed or had stabilized (often termed *cancer survivorship*). These services would allow them to maintain an optimal level of activity and health behaviors. This would facilitate the highest quality of life (QOL) for as long of a duration as possible. This might require periodic reassessments, updating of exercise prescriptions, and early resumption of skilled interventions to mitigate any health issues that arise. A key concept of this phase was conveying the need for a clinician to maintain a lifelong relationship with their patient—a *Therapist for Life*, if you will.

Strategies for Integration of Rehabilitation Into the Cancer Team

Parallel to the purposeful, deliberate actions to implement a new program and its associated practices and services, it is important to recognize that first the Onc R administrator and/or Onc R clinical leader must be "at the table" where decisions are made in order to avoid inequities in implementation outcomes (e.g., assuring appropriate access to Onc R services for all PWCs). Without rehabilitation representation at the table during key meetings, there is a risk of decisions being made by those who have not considered or do not have a thorough understanding of the role of Onc R in the cancer continuum. This is especially important given the fact that Onc R clinicians have not always been included in the foundational development of cancer programs. This often results in an underutilization of services and inequity in representation as compared to other healthcare providers. As there is an ethical imperative to provide these rehabilitative services to PWCs, the Onc R leader should not wait for an invitation to "sit at the table" but must exhibit professional courage to *invite themselves to the table* to be integrally involved with the decision-making process. Onc R clinicians can show their value through service to organizations that have embraced their value, such as the CoC, cancer roundtable for the American College of Sports Medicine (ACSM) and more local opportunities, such as the Komen Foundation, Gilda's Club, and other visible, sustainable organizations serving PLWBCs.

Once administrators and leaders are established as a part of the multidisciplinary cancer team, a similar framework can be utilized to address inequities in healthcare delivery. Previously established frameworks have been refined for implementation science to specifically address inequities in healthcare.[16] The principles included: "(1) focus on reach from the beginning; (2) design and select interventions for vulnerable populations and low-resource communities with implementation in mind; (3) implement what works and develop implementation strategies that can help reduce inequities in care; (4) develop the science of adaptations;

and (5) use an equity lens for implementation outcomes." See Chapter 32 for additional considerations for addressing care inequities.

Logistical Considerations

Essential to any program development, beyond the establishment of the mission, vision, and values, the program administrator is responsible for creating and implementing a work plan for Onc R, a road map to initiation of services as well as an ongoing assessment and reflection process. Periodic assessments to measure success are suggested at quarterly intervals.[20]

A simple timeline with the following considerations (at a minimum) are recommended for planning and collaborative development as seen in eTable 31.1.

Although this table serves as a foundational guideline for program development, it does not imply that all of these components must exclusively exist within the rehabilitation domain. Depending on size and structure of the program and its institution, social workers, oncology nursing staff, and others may be the right fit for leadership and execution. With clear communication of expectations as well as anticipating and navigating forthcoming roadblocks, the Onc R program developers are better equipped to adapt and maintain progress toward the goal of opening the program.

Programmatic Needs Assessment

The *needs assessment* phase is essential to gathering objective data that will ultimately drive the development of philosophy and scope of services.[21] Oncology leaders should use these principles early in the design of Onc R programs, especially in the needs assessment phase, to design programs that are valuable to multiple communities and service sectors. Key metrics include:

- Customer demographics
- Referral source perceptions and opportunities to build relationships
- Prevalence of cancer-related conditions
- Challenges of PLWBCs that could benefit from Onc R services
- Geographic considerations
- Barriers to accessing care
- Financial/payer profile, including special payment programs (e.g., bundling)

Conducting focus groups with key stakeholders such as referral sources, community members, strategic partners, and PWCs provides an opportunity for early brainstorming. This will subsequently lead to improved clarity in purpose and focus. This should include all members of the oncology team most certainly, but also business leaders from the community such as local chambers of commerce, health insurance representatives, local law firm leadership, emergency medical service providers, and alternative living environments such as assisted living facilities and retirement communities.

Once again, with information from multiple levels such as patients, organizations, policy makers, regulators, and state and local agencies, Onc R leaders can incorporate the important elements and tailor the program to meet the needs of the PLWBCs that they serve.

One way to initiate the needs assessment is through a support group that serves persons living beyond cancer (i.e., cancer survivors), and/or via physician and nurse navigator meetings. In addition, helpful information can be found within regulations

TABLE 31.1	Characteristics of an Effective Multi-Disciplinary Team for Cancer Care[23]

I. The team
   Level of expertise and specialization
   - Attendance of multidisciplinary meetings (MDMs)
   - Leadership (e.g., chair or leader of the MDMs)
   - Teamwork and culture (e.g., mutual respect and trust, equality, resolution of conflict, constructive discussion, absence of personal agendas, ability to request and provide clarification)
   - Personal development and training
II. Infrastructure for MDM
   - Appropriate meeting room
   - Availability of technology and equipment
III. MDM organization
   - Regular meetings
IV. Logistics
   - Preparation for meetings
   - Organization during meetings
   - Postmeeting coordination of services for the patient
V. Patient-centered clinical decision-making
   - Who to discuss (e.g., having local mechanisms in place to identify all patients where discussion at MDM is needed)
   - Patient-centered care (e.g., patient's views and preferences are presented by someone who has met the patient, and the patient is given sufficient information to make a well-informed decision on their treatment and care)
   - Clinical decision-making process
   - The information the team needs to make informed decisions/recommendations at team meetings are as follows: pathological, radiological, comorbidities, psychosocial, palliative care needs, patient history, and patient views
   - The decisions/recommendations at team meetings need to be evidence-based (in line with NICE [the United Kingdom's National Institute for Health and Care Excellence] and/or cancer network guidelines), patient-centered, and in line with standard treatment protocols (unless there is a good reason against this)
VI. Team governance
   - Organizational support (e.g., funding and resources)
   - Data collection during team meetings, analysis, and audit of outcomes (e.g., patient experience surveys); the results of these investigations are fed back to multidisciplinary teams (MDTs) to support learning and development
   - Clinical governance (e.g., there are agreed policies, guidelines, and protocols for MDTs; performance assessment and peer review against similar MDTs using cancer peer review processes and other tools)

Created by Holly Lookabaugh-Deur, PT, DSc, GCS, CEEAA. Printed with permission.

such as the accreditation standards from the CoC.[22] Further, useful information includes system-level data including the goals and vision of the health system's oncology program (via health system leaders) and reviewing demographic data from state and local agencies on the incidence of cancer in their respective communities.

Staff Selection and Development

One of the most important roles of the administrator is creating the most cohesive and collaborative team possible.[23] Perhaps there is no other rehabilitation setting that staff selection and development are more important than Onc R. Demonstration of professional maturity, interpersonal skills, and excellence in communication match well with the expected demands of the Onc R clinician. The ability to balance empathy, compassion, and coping strategies are as important as the scientific knowledge necessary for treatment. Entry-level professional education does not prepare the therapist for the depth of knowledge necessary for independent, comprehensive care delivery in the oncology environment. Investment in highly motivated individuals is needed, and self-directed learning as well as advanced professional education are necessary to meet essential competencies (e.g., the American Board of Physical Therapy Specialties' Description of Specialty Practice for Oncology as well as available Oncology Residency programs).[1–24] As the

multi-disciplinary team often makes decisions about care of the PWC together, the dynamics of this team has been subject to study. Components of an effective team are described in Table 31.1.[23]

Clinician longevity and experience in the oncology setting is incredibly valuable to the entire team. Research directs managers to identify and foster internal motivators for retaining high performing, engaged employees.[25] The five ways that *intrinsic motivation* can be used to increase employee engagement in the workplace are (1) creating a safe environment; (2) creating a sense of purpose; (3) trust; (4) belonging; and (5) achievement. Creating opportunities to recognize professional growth and progressive autonomous practice needs to be a priority of an institution's human resource department.[26] To that end, consideration of establishing a Clinical Career Ladder as an administrative priority fits nicely with efforts to build both a sense of belonging and achievement with the oncology clinician.[27] An example of a Career Ladder is outlined in Table 31.2.

In addition to offering education and performance incentives, another management strategy related to staffing might be addressing the psychological support needs of the team. Coping with continued loss and the emotional demands that the oncology environment provides can take a silent toll on the clinician.[20] Arranging for frequent individual "check ins" and periodic psychological services for the team may contribute to a spirit of support that builds trust and a sense of personal safety.

TABLE 31.2 Clinical Career Ladder Model

Clinician Level	Steps or Tasks to Achieve	Recognition or Compensation
Entry level clinician	• Assigned to a mentor • Continuing education allowance • Achieved a level one certification	• Consideration to advance toward advanced clinician
Advanced clinician	• Clinical education: Served as mentor or clinical instructor • Achievement of a specific level of clinical outcomes • Achievement of specific level of net promoter score or customer satisfaction • Successful completion of level 1 and level 2 certifications	• Reward: 1.5 times education allowance • Additional education days • Professional membership reimbursement
Expert clinician	• Clinical education: Served as mentor or clinical instructor • Achievement of specific level of promotion or customer satisfaction scores • Successful completion of advanced certification or specialist board certification	• Reward: 2 times education allowance • Additional education days • Professional membership reimbursement

Created by Holly Lookabaugh-Deur, PT, DSc, GCS, CEEAA. Printed with permission.

• BOX 31.1 Examples of Training Modules

1. Clinical: Lymphedema management
2. Clinical: Exercise and activity guidelines; management of cancer related fatigue
3. Clinical: Laboratory values and implications to activity
4. Clinical: Pelvic floor therapy
5. Clinical: Balance and chemotherapy-induced peripheral neuropathy
6. Clinical: Nutrition and hydration during chemotherapy
7. Clinical: Pain science and management of central sensitization
8. Interpersonal: Ethics refresher
9. Interpersonal: Patient communication
10. Interpersonal: End of life; grief management
11. Operations: Documentation of medical necessity
12. Operations: Infection control

An administrator is expected to assess the team's ability to execute and operate at the highest level of efficiency and effectiveness. Assessing gaps in talent is an important role of the manager and then is followed by creating a plan for recruitment, education, and training to address identified gaps. Using a multi-dimensional approach to talent development is suggested. Examples of training modules and certifications to include in building a competency checklist can be found in Box 31.1.

Finally, as there are a variety of advanced certifications in oncology, lymphedema, and cancer exercise, Onc R clinicians should be actively encouraged and supported to pursue these skills, not only for garnering employee loyalty but also to increase the credibility of the program to referral sources, patients, the community, and the profession. If resources are available and the oncology patient caseload is adequate, some institutions may consider establishing a clinical residency in oncologic physical therapy.

Building the Program Processes and Procedures

In order to provide focus toward a workplan and program development, the oncology leader should do a gap analysis and use a work plan to ensure success in implementation. This serves as a checkpoint in facilitating the process of completion. To orient the team members to the various updated processes and procedures,

the use of flowcharts or diagrams is recommended to visualize the flow of activities resulting in utilization of rehabilitation services (Figure 31.3). In addition, these are helpful to transfer and disseminate information. As an example, the diagram below shows a general flow of Onc R clinician involvement across a patient's disease journey, which is useful to educate key stakeholders in implementation of a new process.

The diagram also defines the screening and consultation phase; the screening leads to the follow-up care based on the PWC's need. At this point, the Onc R clinician would select the type of intervention ranging from conventional therapy, a supervised exercise and wellness program, or a home exercise program via an independent, individualized wellness program.

Of significant importance is to define the role of the oncology nurse navigators (ONNs) within the Onc R care continuum as these professionals can be key allies in establishing new services or navigating PLWBCs to Onc R clinicians. According to the Oncology Nursing Society (ONS), the "role of navigation is to reduce cancer morbidity and mortality by eliminating barriers to timely access to cancer care, which may be financial, psychological, logistical, or related to communications or the healthcare delivery system."[28] Navigation services should begin with prevention and screening activities and facilitate care transitions through diagnosis, treatment, survivorship, and end-of-life care. Once the barriers are identified, the ONN follows with an intervention and documents the time needed to resolve the issues. Typically, the ONN is a professional registered nurse with oncology-specific clinical knowledge who offers individualized assistance to patients, families, and caregivers to help overcome health system barriers. In 2015, the ONS defined the role and qualifications of ONNs by stating that they shall possess a national certification, contribute to (or conduct) nurse-sensitive, patient-specific outcome research, uphold a core competency of care, provide care across the continuum, and monitor navigation in conjunction with the interprofessional team.[29]

Accreditation Guidelines and Supporting Organizations

Administrators and oncology leaders need to become familiar with many national, state, and local organizations and associations that

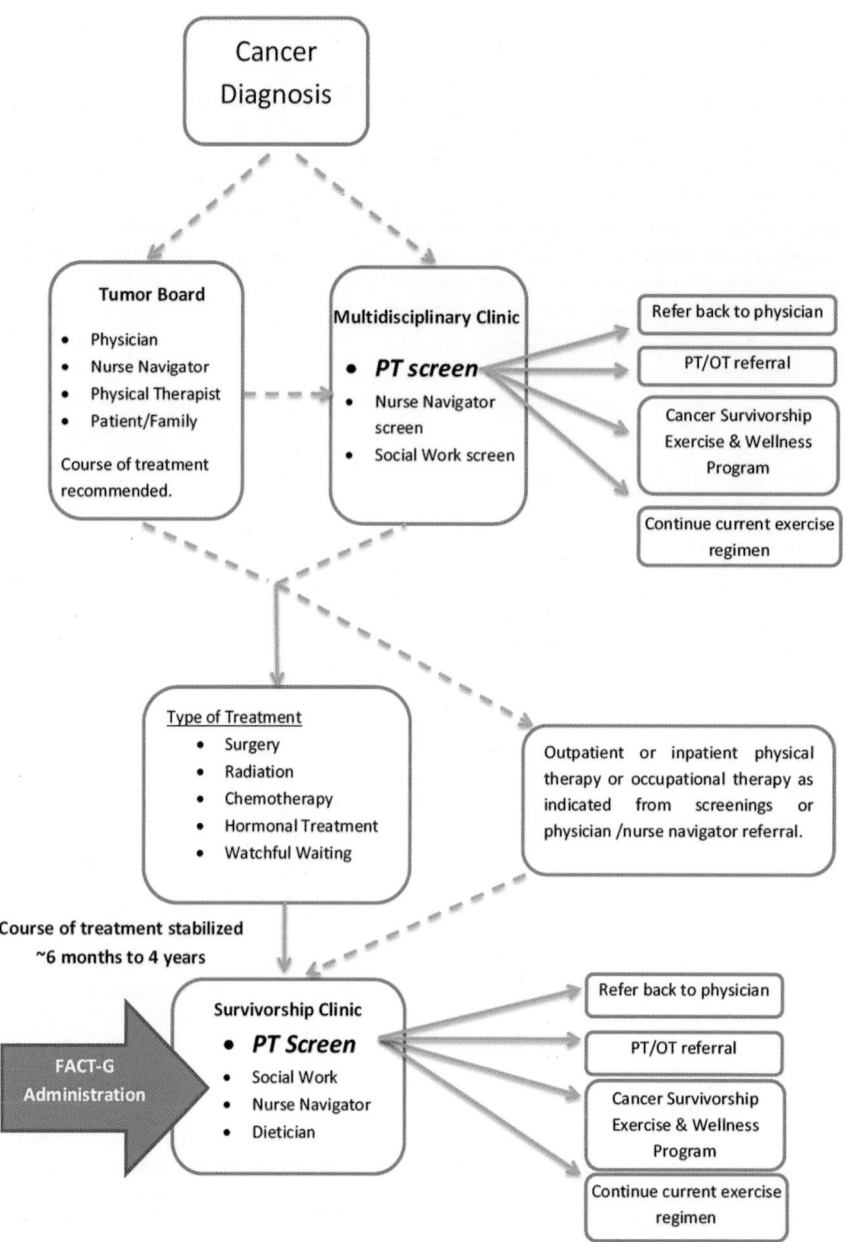

• **Fig. 31.3** Workflow of Cancer Screening by Physical Therapist. Reprinted with permission from Colombo R, Doherty DJ, Wilson CM, et al. Implementation and preliminary analysis of FACT-G quality of life questionnaire within an oncology survivorship clinic. *Cureus.* 2018;10(3):e2272. doi:10.7759/cureus.2272.

serve PLWBCs. Naming all of the relevant organizations would be a daunting task; however, there are a few which are key in the development and implementation of an Onc R program. For example, the CoC is a consortium of professional organizations dedicated to improving survival and QOL for PWC by improving healthcare, prevention, research, and education by the monitoring of comprehensive quality care. It was established by the American College of Surgeons (ACoS) in 1922. The CoC establishes standards to ensure quality, multidisciplinary, and comprehensive cancer care delivery in healthcare settings; conducts surveys in healthcare settings to assess compliance with those standards; collects standardized data from CoC-accredited healthcare settings to measure cancer care quality; uses data to monitor treatment patterns and outcomes and enhance cancer control and clinical surveillance activities; and develops effective educational interventions to improve cancer prevention, early detection, cancer care delivery, and outcomes in healthcare settings.[30]

In 2020, the CoC updated its quality standards by including Standard 4.6 which defined and established the rehabilitation requirements. Standard 4.6 stated that policies and procedures must be in place to guide referrals to appropriate rehabilitation care services, either on-site or by referral. This standard stressed that the availability of rehabilitation care services is an essential component of comprehensive cancer care, beginning at the time of diagnosis and that it should be continuously available throughout treatment, surveillance, and, when applicable, through the end of life. CoC Standard 4.6 further required that institutions specify in a policy which rehabilitation services are provided onsite and which are available by referral. Rehabilitation services that are not available at the facility must be provided through a referral relationship to other facilities and/or agencies. In addition, there must be written criteria for performing functional assessments and criteria for referral to a rehabilitation care specialist. Each calendar year, the cancer committee should provide evidence that it has monitored, evaluated, and made recommendations for improvements, as needed, to rehabilitation care services and/or referrals. The content of the review and any recommendations for improvement must be documented in the cancer committee minutes. Lastly, the CoC makes a strong recommendation that a rehabilitation leader attends each meeting and report on Onc R services. This may be one of the most important roles for the Onc R representative and ensures a *seat at the table*. In order to provide evidence of this participation, as a measure of compliance, these tasks are monitored and reviewed by the cancer committee and documented in meeting minutes.[22]

The ACoS also accredits two other specific cancer programs. The National Accreditation Program for Breast Centers (NAPBC) is "focused on breast health and dedicated to the improvement of quality care and outcomes of patients with diseases of the breast through evidence-based standards and patient and professional education." Programs accredited with the NAPBC voluntarily agree to meet the standards outlined in the *NAPBC Standards Manual*.[31] Similarly, the National Accreditation Program for Rectal Cancer's (NAPRC) goal is to ensure that patients with rectal cancer receive appropriate care using a multidisciplinary approach. The NAPRC is based on programs that have demonstrated successful outcomes which provides best practices for clinical pathways and process improvement, to optimize future outcome. Programs accredited by the NAPRC voluntarily agree to meet the standards outlined in the *NAPRC Standards Manual*.[32]

The Commission on Accreditation of Rehabilitation Facilities (CARF) is an international agency that offers voluntary accreditation to a variety of medical rehabilitation facilities (www.carf.org). In 2014, CARF published Cancer Rehabilitation Specialty Program standards in their *Medical Rehabilitation Standards Manual*. Key principles of these Onc R standards include a person-centered approach to care, collaboration across the continuum of care to improve functional independence, establishing a framework for continuous process improvement, and providing a holistic interdisciplinary team approach.[33]

Understanding the requirements needed for accreditation, leaders in Onc R are better able to support their institutions to achieve national recognition for their cancer programs. Furthermore, it provides them with information specific to certain types of cancers. For example, many institutions around the country aspire to be NAPBC certified and, most recently, there is also a move to acquire NAPRC certification. The important implication here is that Onc R clinicians can play a pivotal role in the rehabilitation of these two types of cancer. Therefore, surgeons, medical oncologists, and radiation oncologists are generally interested in providing comprehensive services, including integrating rehabilitation in their plan of care since it provides concrete evidence of program enhancement.

It is also important to consider other organizations that provide excellent information and support to cancer survivors and administrators designing oncology programs. As cancer is a

global issue, each nation likely has key governmental or regulatory agencies that often provide guidance and resources, many that are freely available, For example, within the US, the National Academy of Medicine (formerly the IOM) is a nonprofit organization established in 1970 as a component of the US National Academy of Sciences that works outside the framework of government to provide evidence-based research and recommendations for public health and science policy. (www.nam.edu) A notable publication by this organization was proceedings of an expert panel workshop entitled *Long-term Survivorship Care and Cancer Treatment*, which highlighted potential opportunities to improve the planning, management, and delivery of cancer survivorship care.[34] See Box 31.2 for additional organizational resources for cancer clinicians.

It is also important to identify regional or local cancer organizations that support PLWBCs. For example, the Michigan Cancer Consortium is tasked with "Unifying public and private organizations to reduce the burden of cancer for all people by addressing health disparities through a commitment to collaboration, evidence-based practices, and improved quality of care." The Michigan Department of Health and Human Services, through a federal grant, provides administrative support to the Michigan Cancer Consortium (www.michigan.gov/michigancancer). Readers are encouraged to find, and then actively pursue involvement in their state, provincial, or regional cancer advocacy group.

Oncology leaders, now armed with clear information related to organizational infrastructure, the concepts of implementation science, the identified needs of their local community, their health system's mission, and an understanding of the capacity and resources of their own department are now ready to enact the guiding policies to establish or enhance their Onc R program.

Building the Program for the Entire Disease Journey

In order to build a program that meets the needs of the PLWBC across their entire journey, a visual depiction such as Figure 31.4 may be useful to share with staff members to assist them in grasping the patient's entire journey. In this depiction, the patient is at the center of the program and the phases include prediagnosis, diagnosis, treatment including multimodal treatment protocols (inclusive of Onc R), completion of treatment, follow up, and lastly palliative care and/or end of life care.

Individuals with cancer (or those at risk of cancer) experience a journey that requires a longitudinal approach with

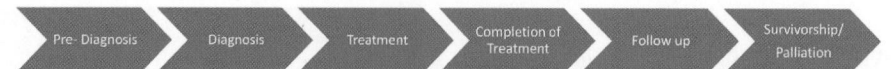

• **Fig. 31.4** Building the Program for the Entire Disease Journey. Created by Reyna Colombo, PT, MA. Printed with permission.

close collaboration with the interdisciplinary team. During the *Prediagnosis* phase, persons may undergo genetic testing and other cancer-specific screens or preventive measures to minimize the risk of a cancer diagnosis. Individuals may receive education, counseling, and instructions in nutrition, fitness, and wellness, of which rehabilitation professionals can and should be integrally involved.

At the *Diagnosis* stage, rehabilitation professionals need to understand what is important to the patient at this point. It is important to respect and honor the PWCs' wishes and stresses by planning treatment around their individual goals. At this point, cancer treatment begins, including multimodal treatment protocols and rehabilitation. At this phase, PWCs need emotional and psychological support as well as education on the disease and treatments. During the *Treatment* stage, patients may be connected to their local cancer center where patients will have access to tumor boards and/or multidisciplinary clinics. At some facilities, therapists are part of the multidisciplinary clinics which are generally cancer diagnosis specific. Screening patients at this stage can result in early identification to determine if the patient requires conventional rehabilitation or other interventions such as exercise prescription.

Prior to initiation of cancer treatment (e.g., chemotherapy, radiation, and/or surgery), a structured prehabilitation program may be indicated and the providers should be ready to initiate these services. Prehabilitation should include rehabilitation involvement in performing includes physical and psychological assessments to establish a baseline functional level, identify impairments, and provide targeted interventions that improve patient outcomes (see Chapter 27 for more on Prehabilitation). Specific interventions such as guided motor imagery, practicing movement patterns, postsurgical airway clearance techniques, and pain management strategies have been proven to enhance patient outcomes.[35] Equally important to the physical preparation is the psychological impact of learning and clarifying expectations.[36]

During cancer treatment, patients are in active recovery and usually supported by the oncology team, including ONNs, physicians, social workers, registered oncology dieticians, spiritual care professionals, integrative medicine, and rehabilitation professionals. *Completion of Treatment* (often termed *survivorship*) is often considered to be one of the most anxiety producing times in the cancer journey as the person will not be supported regularly by the entire cancer team by in-person appointments and diagnostic tests; now their treatment is completed or stabilized and for the most part they must manage their own recovery. This is an optimal time for the Onc R clinicians to provide an ongoing connection and support to facilitate return to function. This may be administered with in-person therapy as well as telehealth.[37] Connection via telehealth therapy sessions can make the difference between a rapid decline due to inactivity as compared to a structured, supported recovery from commonly encountered adverse effects such as cancer-related fatigue, balance, and strength deficits. This connection is also useful in combatting the stress and anxiety of isolation.

Many cancer centers facilitate and perform *Follow Up* visits often established by a *survivorship care plan*. Although this care plan includes a clinical summary of the person's treatment and future diagnostic testing for recurrence, it should also include additional rehabilitation interventions or periodic screenings. It is at this stage that Onc R clinicians should be providing screenings to monitor changes via functional outcome measures as well as elevating awareness and educating patients on potential future health risks.

As some PWCs may be diagnosed at advanced stages or their conditions may not be amenable to treatments, the *Palliative Care/End of Life* phase includes providing necessary ongoing support and advance care planning. The emphasis of care during this stage is to optimize remaining QOL for patients and families facing life-threatening illness. See Chapter 29 for Palliative and End of Life Care and the Onc R professionals' role within this practice area.

Key Components for a Cancer Rehabilitation Policy Oncology

In order to convey the key concepts of an Onc R program, a well written, comprehensive policy should be crafted. This document will be used to support and develop clinical operations as well as to share with external agencies and regulatory bodies to convey the scope and services of the program. This policy should include key concepts of a department's clinical operations and will certainly be unique to each department or health system. If the department has any special relationships or unique offerings, they should be included. See Box 31.3 for specific components of an Onc R policy. In general, transient or temporary initiatives are not appropriate to include in policies. A contingency plan or emergency plan to sustain services during healthcare disruptions may be advisable (e.g., COVID-19). See Appendix 1 in the enhanced eBook for a downloadable, customizable policy template.

Financial Sustainability

Looking back at some of the principles of implementation science, it is important to create a framework in which the Onc R program's implementation is most likely to succeed. At this phase, the oncology leader aims to ensure the adaptability and sustainability of the program to facilitate and serve as many PWCs as possible with the highest quality of care. To accomplish this, a program developer should employ well established financial tools and budget strategies to sustain the program. These tools vary among settings; however, it is important to use a few financial tools such as establishing the *break-even point* and developing a long-term budget to predict sustainability beyond the implementation phase. In order to establish the break-even point for an Onc R program, the first goal would be to determine the total expenses from providing oncology services and computing how many visits are required by the therapist providers to break even financially. This scenario considers the revenue generated by patients' visit and the hourly cost of the clinician (salary and benefits). In general, the break-even

1. The purpose/mission of the program
2. The vision/mission of the healthcare system/institution
3. The vision of the rehabilitation department
4. Scientific and community/population needs justifying the program
5. Relationship with any key internal or external departments or agencies and what they entail
6. Scope and offerings of the cancer rehab program (e.g., prehab, prospective surveillance)
7. Interventions available and disciplines (physical therapy, occupational therapy, speech language pathology, etc.)
8. Points of entry into the program
9. Unique programs (support groups, aftercare programs, wellness services)
10. Representation on the health system's cancer oversight committee
11. Staff qualifications, preparation, continuing education, residencies, specialist certification support
12. Which rehabilitation services are offered internally versus which require offsite referral (and to whom, if applicable)

point is the point where the revenue generated by the clinician's treatments is equal to the variable costs and fixed costs (e.g., rent, utilities, insurance). See Figure 31.5, and eTables 31.2 and 31.3 are examples of a financial pro-forma or budget to project the future implementation of the program.

Of equal importance, leaders should collect data and maintain metrics on the services provided to the PWC. This should include billable and unbillable time (e.g., time spent at tumor boards or doing screenings). Metrics regarding number of screens, consultations, number of conventional (billable) visits, and after care services should be closely tracked. Other considerations such as insurance payer mix and reimbursement are important to monitor on an ongoing basis. Senior healthcare system administrators and physicians are interested in reviewing the financial performance of the rehab program; therefore, it is important to demonstrate that the oncology rehab program adds financial value to the institution

or clinic in addition to its inherent value to the PWC and the clinician.

Oncology Program Settings

Let us now explore the unique clinical applications and associated financial viability of oncology programs across the continuum of care. In general, at the institutional health system level, services are broadly organized as acute and postacute care (PAC), which also includes ambulatory (also known as outpatient) services. Cancer survivor treatment can be provided in the acute or postacute care setting as well as ambulatory centers offering services such as rehabilitation services, chemotherapy and infusion therapy, integrative medicine, psychosocial support services, and radiation therapies. PWCs enter each of these settings based on their individual medical and support needs.

The coordination of care, hand off instructions, and documentation amongst these clinicians is paramount in facilitating the journey of the PWC. Figure 31.6 shows the connectivity between acute and PAC. At each of these settings, administrators and rehab leaders need to translate the evidence-based research and the clinical science to develop clinical pathways and treatment regimens with consideration of the needs and capacity of the individual clinical facility. As many clinicians only practice in one clinical area, it is important to have an understanding of the various payment influences that the cancer care team may have to navigate across the continuum of care. As the US Medicare system is one of the more complex and universal systems for care provision and a majority of US PWCs have some form of Medicare, it will be used as an example for describing the various payment methodologies for these settings. Payment means vary greatly for private insurances and the reader is encouraged to consult directly with a specific payer for guidelines on how and what is covered by each individual insurance company.

Acute Care

Hospitalization services are compensated by Medicare and some private health insurance companies by using the payment system

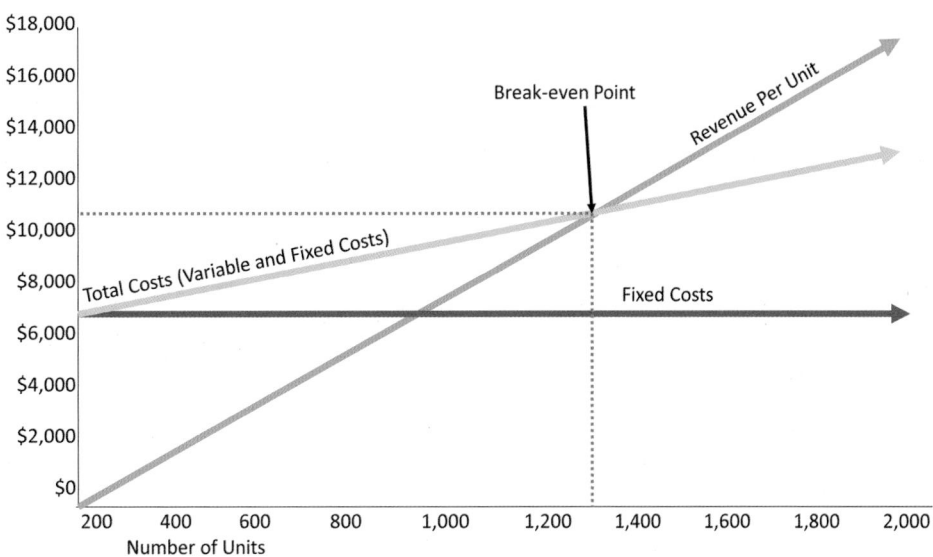

• **Fig. 31.5** Establishing the Break-even Point for Establishing a Budget. Created by Chris Wilson, PT, DPT, DScPT. Printed with permission.

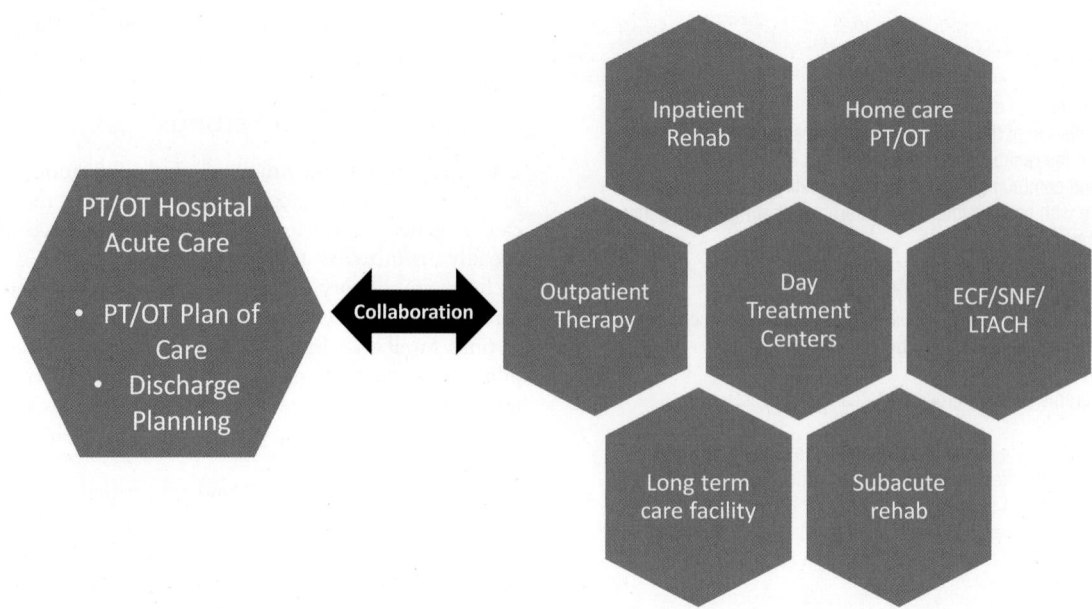

• **Fig. 31.6** Acute and Postacute Care Settings. Created by Reyna Colombo, PT, MA. Printed with permission. *ECF*, extended care facility; *LTACH*, long-term acute care hospital; *OT*, occupational therapy; *PT*, Physical therapy; *SNF*, skilled nursing facility.

known as Diagnosis Related Groups (DRG). Under the DRG payment methodology, the patient's expected hospital length of stay (LOS) is a deciding factor on the total revenue that the hospital appreciates during the stay; regardless how much money a hospital spends providing care to the patient, the hospital gets paid a fixed amount for that DRG (this is similar to the bundling concept described earlier but the DRG only considers services incurred during the hospitalization). Hospitalized PWCs who receive rehabilitation have the potential to spend less time at the hospital, thus decreasing LOS, incurring less costs, and maximizing function and revenue. A key consideration in acute care is navigating the complex discharge needs and facilitating discharge to reduce hospital LOS. For example, provision of additional physical therapy can shorten LOS by 0.6 days in acute care and by 3 days in a subacute setting.[38] Furthermore, increased spending on occupational therapy (OT) in the acute care setting was significantly correlated with reduced hospital readmission rates.[39] Utilization of a standardized outcome measure such as the AM-PAC "6-clicks" outcome tool has been established as a useful tool to help clinicians predict and choose a safe and appropriate discharge setting.[40]

Postacute Care

After hospitalization, PAC includes services in inpatient rehabilitation (IPR) facilities, long-term acute care hospitals (LTACHs), skilled nursing facilities (SNFs), home health agencies, and outpatient providers.

Inpatient Rehab Facilities

IPR facilities are compensated based on rates under the prospective payment system (PPS). Medicare adjusts the Federal rates to reflect a series of factors, the first being *patient case mix* which is "the relative resource intensity typical for each patient's clinical condition identified by the patient assessment process."

Based on the primary IPR diagnosis, Medicare groups cases into *rehabilitation impairment categories*. These categories are further grouped into *case-mix groups* (CMGs), according to their functional, motor, and cognitive scores as well as age. Within each CMG, four tiers are established according to patient comorbidities beyond the primary IPR diagnosis (with higher payment for higher tiers). Finally, additional adjustments are made for interrupted stays, short stays (<3 days), short-stay transfers to another facility, and high-cost outlier cases.[41]

Within the US Medicare System, one confounding factor for providing IPR with PWC is the 60/40 rule (also known as the 60% rule) where 60% of patients in an IPR must have the following conditions: amputation, burns, hip fracture, spinal cord injury, arthritis or arthropathies, neurologic disorders, brain injury, congenital deformity, major trauma, stroke, or joint replacement. As cancer is not a listed condition of the 60%, it often is considered to fall under the remaining 40%; however, many of these conditions may occur in PWCs as well (e.g., brain tumors may be considered brain injuries, amputations may result from sarcomas).[42] Evidence shows that PWCs who were deconditioned were more likely to require a readmission to acute care from IPR as compared to a person without cancer.[42] Acute care readmission rates from IPR were found to be between 11% and 14%. Infection was one of the primary reasons for needing a readmission to the hospital.[42] As it relates to persons with advanced cancer, a novel concept of a short stay family training program in IPR with an average length of IPR stay of 6 days is being implemented in some healthcare organizations.[43] Instead of focusing on Onc R of a medically fragile patient who may not tolerate it, this program focused the resources of the IPR team to train family caregivers with the aim to achieve a safe and stable discharge home for the remainder of a person's life.[43] Despite the increased medical complexity of this patient population, there are substantial benefits to clinical outcomes and administrative outcomes in this patient population. Finally, key considerations for administration of PWC in IPR include controlling the length of stay and minimizing the need for readmission to the acute care setting, when possible.

Long-Term Acute Care Hospitals

There may be a limited need for LTACH with PWCs, especially those with advanced disease, due to most of these individuals having a terminal illness and most individuals reporting that they prefer home to an institution to receive their care. One study noted that 74% of individuals with terminal illness preferred to die at home, 16% preferred to die in the hospital, and only 10% preferred to have their remaining care provided in a long-term care facility.[44] Furthermore, only 40% of people who preferred to die at home achieved this goal.[44] Despite the patient preference, the care needs of some PWCs may be too complex or symptom control may be too multifaceted to manage at home, therefore there is a need for provision of care in LTACHs and SARs. Under the PPS, discharges are assigned to case-mix groups containing patients with similar clinical problems who are expected to require similar amounts of resources. Each case-mix group has a national relative weight reflecting the expected costliness of treatment for a patient in that category compared with that for the average LTACH patient.[45]

Skilled Nursing Facilities

One might first expect that a skilled nursing facility may be a challenging setting to implement a successful oncology program. Tens of thousands of PWCs, representing 10% to 15% of nursing home residents, are admitted to nursing facilities every year.[45] However, with the density of cancer survivors with lingering symptoms contributing to their disability, the SNF might be an ideal location for some aspects of Onc R, especially for individuals who may not be strong enough to return home or do not have the functional reserve capacity to tolerate three hours of IPR.[46] Research indicates that individuals in SNF were less likely to receive high quality cancer care which may lead to limited outcomes.[47] As there is a substantial and growing population of PWCs who require SNF services, there is substantial opportunity to provide specialty services for Onc R to optimize care for these individuals. Specific screenings and interventions that are appropriate for implementation might include:

- Chronic lymphedema management, collaborating with nursing care
- Group activity design for strengthening and treatment of CRF
- Balance and fall prevention intervention for residents with CIPN
- Postmastectomy rehabilitation such as posture training, breathing, and upper extremity exercise instruction, and self-care manual lymph drainage

In 2020, the SNF payment methodology was revised to utilize the *patient-driven payment model* (PDPM). The model is based on a resident's classification among five components (including rehabilitation) that are adjusted based on the case mix of residents. In addition, it employs a *per diem* system that adjusts payment rates over the course of the stay.[48] Payments under the SNF PPS are case mix adjusted to reflect the relative resource intensity that would typically be associated with a given patient's clinical condition, as identified through the resident assessment process.

Home Health

Home health is also a key environment for provision of Onc R. For example, early intervention for persons after mastectomy through recommendations for sleeping positions, early self-mobilization

strategies, and early mobility and activity are useful to be introduced in the home setting. Postprostatectomy management of urinary incontinence and management of home safety and efficiency are examples of other specialty interventions. Caregiver education and functional carryover is optimized in the patient's environment.[49]

Under prospective payment, Medicare pays home health agencies (HHAs) a predetermined base payment. The payment is adjusted based on a classification system called the *patient-driven groupings model* (PDGM).[50] These categories are based on the source of HHA admission (ambulatory or institutional/hospital), timing of the admissions, 12 clinical group categories, and the patient's functional impairments. Finally, adjustments are made for the extent and severity of clinical comorbidities. The home health PDGM model provides HHAs with payments for each 30-day periods of care for each beneficiary.

Outpatient or Ambulatory Setting

A common setting for the Onc R treatment of PWCs is in the outpatient ambulatory setting. Unless an organization exclusively works with PWCs, these services will require a balance between the noncancer population and the cancer population. Especially in busy clinics, this may require an algorithm or decision-making process for prioritizing PWCs so they do not have to wait an inordinate amount of time to access Onc R clinician services.

Payment for this setting for those who are over 65 in the US is under Medicare Part B, which is the segment of Medicare benefits that includes outpatient Onc R services. Medicare Part B covers the evaluation and treatment of injuries and diseases affecting function. One key consideration in outpatient Medicare Part B rehabilitation was the repeal of "hard" therapy caps for annual services in 2018.[51] Previously these therapy caps would not allow for payment and provision of additional services beyond an arbitrary dollar amount. Now the hard therapy cap is an annual threshold that therapists can exceed if accompanied by the KX modifier to confirm the services are medically necessary. In 2021, this threshold is $2110 for PT/SLP and an additional $2110 for OT. Finally, a perpetual concern for outpatient services is payers' continual attempts to adjust their payment fee schedules, which tends to reduce payments for medical services, often in contrast to economic inflation. These issues require the continual advocacy of Onc R clinicians to assure appropriate payment to assure financial stability to continue to offer services to PWCs as described further in Chapter 32.

Marketing Oncology Rehabilitation Services

As Onc R is not yet a mainstream healthcare service, deliberate and strategic marketing is required. This plan should be multi-dimensional, focusing first on general awareness and understanding and then narrowing the focus on specific diagnoses and physician referrers. To some extent, Onc R is still in its infancy stage with respect to consumer and health professional awareness.[25] There is limited understanding by most health providers and consumers about why lingering symptoms following cancer treatment persist and what resources and treatment interventions can effectively improve function and QOL. Increasing this level of awareness needs to occur simultaneously with the deliberate, targeted promotion of the intuition's Onc R program. As awareness about Onc R increases, so will opportunities to attract direct access clients for Onc R services such as PT or OT. Similarly, physicians are often eager to offer solutions to problematic symptoms to PLWBCs so they should be provided with an easy means to address these issues

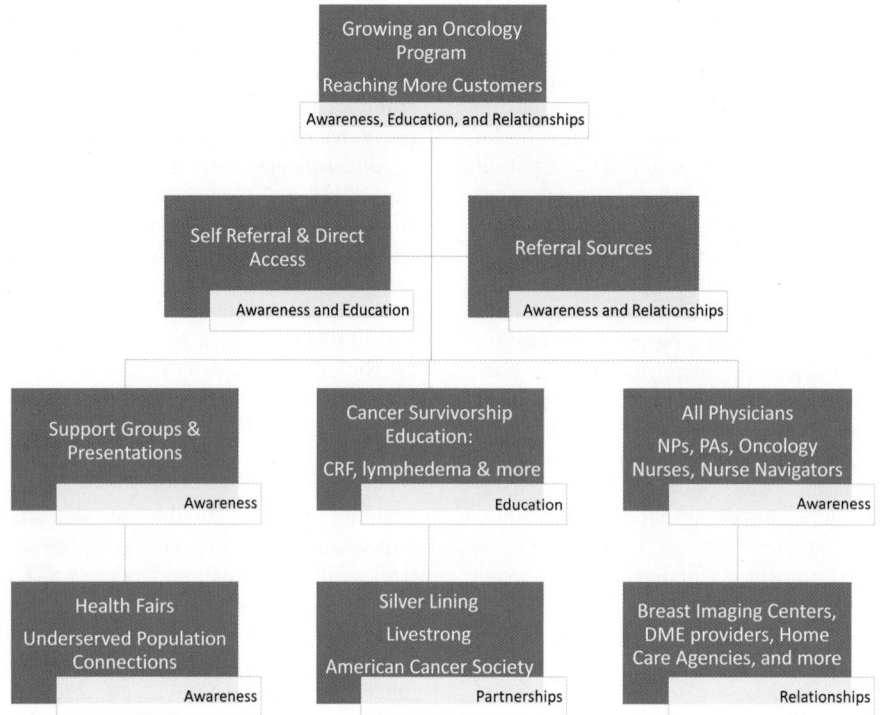

• **Fig. 31.7** Aspects of a Comprehensive Marketing Plan. Created by Holly Lookabaugh-Deur, PT, DSc, GCS, CEEAA. Printed with permission. CRF, cancer-related fatigue; NPs, nurse practicioners; PAs, physician assistants; DME, durable medical equipment.

as they arise. Approaching healthcare professionals who may refer to Onc R will require succinct summaries of the evidence, as well as barrier-free systems for streamlined referrals. Opportunities to reach both consumers and referrals sources are limitless in the hands of a creative, resourceful Onc R manager. See Figure 31.7 for key aspects of a marketing plan for an Onc R program.

As with any comprehensive marketing plan, a multi-media plan is most effective, including print, visual ads (billboards), social media, and sponsorships. Patient and family testimonials and stories are particularly poignant and meaningful in healthcare marketing. Due to the power of word-of-mouth marketing, the most impactful customer reach is generated from an exceptional patient experience; without this, any public relations initiative may not be an effective investment.

Conclusion

The need for quality, sustainable Onc R programs is clearly evident. With the increasing prevalence of cancer in our communities, advances in treatment impacting survivorship, and growing expertise of therapy professionals, and limited availability of Onc R programs across the continuum of care, there is a vast opportunity for passionate and talented leaders and clinicians to make a lasting impact on the QOL of countless PWC and the surrounding communities.[52] By assessing all potential barriers—regulatory, talent, organizational structure, team communication and others—as a part of a systematically planned program, a critical new service for PWCs may be created with successful individual and institutional outcomes. Inspired and resourceful leaders can make a lasting impact on the QOL in their community by gathering critical information through research and needs assessments, establishing a mission, vision, and values to guide the program, assembling and developing talent, constructing and executing a realistic work plan, and increasing awareness of the benefit of Onc

R services to consumers and referring professionals. Each of these steps is essential for the creation of a comprehensive Onc R program. Successful leaders should strive to be committed to a shared mission, passionate about providing care to PWC, and fearless of hard work and the occasional failure. Coaching an inspired Onc R team and being a part of changing lives can be deeply fulfilling for the right leader.

Critical Research Needs

- The science of program implementation in oncology rehabilitation disciplines.
- Financial implications of developing an oncology rehab program.
- Which setting (acute, inpatient rehabilitation, outpatient, etc.) has been most successful in implementing an oncology rehab program—consistency, compliance, cost management, etc.—and possible reasons/rationale.

Case Study

A rehabilitation manager at a medium-sized community health system is called into a meeting with the physician system lead for oncologic services. The physician began by voicing concerns as to why his cancer patients are not prioritized as highly as orthopedic or neurologic patients in the hospital and in the outpatient setting. He provided a directive that this should be improved, and the rehabilitation department's therapists need to be trained in Onc R to have a fully-fledged program.

This was a difficult conversation for the rehabilitation manager. Initially she was offended and frustrated that her hard work and prioritization was not being appreciated but upon further reflection, she determined that this physician was right. Shortly after that, she gathered a team of her team leaders and staff therapists to discuss this idea and how to best offer these services to this patient population. The team decided that they needed to establish a workplan that included operational modifications to the department's prioritization system, providing and supporting therapists in employing core concepts of oncology rehabilitation, and increasing the awareness of these services to the interdisciplinary team. This was agreed upon by all of the team members and the rehabilitation manager shared this with her administrator who was in support of this recommendation and was also interested in expanding to a new untapped market for rehabilitation services.

In line with knowledge translation concepts, the team members began to explore the literature to provide guidance as to where to start with a rehabilitation oncology program, especially as it related to the services already offered by this institution. In this case, they had a solid core group of experienced lymphedema therapists in the outpatient setting as well as several therapists with some oncology experience and interest in the acute hospital setting. The manager brought in a nationally known expert in Onc R to provide a continuing education seminar in order to build a foundation for all providers. The manager deliberately invited key therapists to the team with a variety of specialty training, including neurology, geriatrics, palliative care, ICU, orthopedics, and pelvic health in order to prepare for the wide variety of diagnoses and conditions that would come from accepting referrals. After this training, some therapists were provided additional funds to take more oncology continuing education courses. Therapists were recognized and rewarded by the department's career ladder based upon the number of courses they have completed and their roles in furthering the program development.

Concurrently, a strategic awareness plan was developed to increase the visibility of the newly offered Onc R program.

Therapists were encouraged and supported to present at interdisciplinary cancer conferences within and external to the organization. Therapists were also allotted time to attend tumor boards and multidisciplinary clinics. At first this was mainly as a passive participant but as the therapists' confidence and knowledge grew, they began to be more active participants. Not long after, these professionals were an invaluable member of the team. As the oncology rehabilitation program organically grew and became fully integrated within the oncology operations, the administrators and rehabilitation managers hardwired these Onc R operations into the institution's core policies and procedures to be shared with accrediting agencies. This helped to ensure sustainability and long-term viability of the program. Finally, as this program continued to grow, the managers began to focus on a retention plan to ensure that these now highly trained clinicians remained with the institution. In addition, a legacy plan was also established so that when inevitable staff turnover occurred despite the retention plan, the program would be self-sustaining and not person-dependent. This involved recording processes and procedures as well as having the current content experts mentor their colleagues and identify a backup person in the event that the primary therapist took time off or went on a leave. This ensured long term sustainability and continuity of care. Finally, to increase the institution's leadership in this area and to continue to train future healthcare providers, an annual Onc R symposium was established. All of these deliberate steps helped to grow the oncology rehabilitation program from its infancy into a nationally known provider of Onc R services which earned the institution several awards and recognitions.

Review Questions

Reader can find the correct answers and rationale in the back of the book.

1. A rehabilitation manager is in the early stages of developing a cancer rehabilitation program. The manager recalls a course attended on value-based case. Which of the following best defines value-based healthcare services?
   A. Integrating concepts of quality and accountability within the context of cost and patient-centered outcomes
   B. Dedicating a physical therapist to provide free screenings for a population with low risk of cancer or adverse effects
   C. Ensuring each patient receives the maximal amount of rehabilitation visits that their insurance allows so they get the most face-to-face time with the therapists
   D. Limiting rehabilitation services to only those with severe impairments to utilize the therapists' skills to the highest level within their scope of practice

2. A rehabilitation manager is working with the hospital administration to develop a clinical career ladder. Which of the following is the LEAST likely to be a key aim of the implementation of the career ladder?
   A. Demonstrating the organization's commitment to quality care
   B. Providing team members with recognition for pursuing additional clinical skills
   C. Improving recruitment and retention
   D. Ensuring that a clinician does not take any leaves of absence

3. Which is the best example of knowledge translation?

A. Conducting a well-structured, randomized controlled trial using a new piece of technology in a research laboratory setting
B. Facilitating a journal club with team members to review new literature and identifying ways to implement these new findings into routine clinical practice
C. Mandating that each clinician provide a modality/biophysical agent treatment on the patient to help strengthen the evidence for the use of these treatments
D. Referring every cancer patient for a 12-visit episode of physical therapy care for prehabilitation as there is evidence that prehabilitation helps with cancer outcomes

4. A 75-year-old male is admitted into the hospital for a colon resection and ostomy for colorectal surgery. He is not sure if he wants to participate in rehabilitation during his acute care stay. He is concerned as to how much extra it will cost him as he is on Medicare. Which of the following best describes the payment mechanism when a patient is admitted to the hospital?
   A. Fee for service where each rehabilitation visit will cost more for the patient
   B. This hospitalization will not be covered by his Medicare insurance as it was not medically necessary
   C. Acute care hospitalizations are covered under a DRG where the hospital gets a lump sum based on the patient's diagnosis and length of stay
   D. His rehabilitation during the acute care stay will be covered under Medicare Part B

5. A rehabilitation manager is considering starting a new clinic specifically related to oncology rehabilitation. After establishing startup costs and beginning to calculate ongoing costs to establish the break-even point, the manager first considers the stable ongoing costs to the daily operations before any revenue is generated. What is the best term for these stable ongoing costs?
   A. Taxes
   B. Gross revenue
   C. Fixed costs
   D. Salary cost per procedure

6. A 67-year-old female is in the acute care hospital setting after a diagnosis of advanced Stage IV lung cancer. She had been receiving radiation and chemotherapy, which has now concluded. Her condition is considered terminal and her goal is to get home safely to spend her remaining time with her supportive family and visiting friends and sitting outside on her porch. She is very weak and is unable to move out of the bed without maximum assistance of two but is otherwise currently medically stable and her symptoms are controlled. Based on the patient's clinical situation, potential discharge options, and goals of care, which would be the MOST appropriate discharge plan?
   A. Admit to inpatient hospice for ongoing symptom control
   B. Discharge home immediately after hospitalization
   C. Admit to IPR for a short stay of family training before home
   D. Admit to a long-term acute care facility in case her symptoms worsen

7. Defining a clear mission for a new oncology rehabilitation program is:
   A. Best suited as a final step prior to opening, once funding and referral opportunities have been identified
   B. An early step in the development process, driving all aspects of the organization, such as the funding process and direction for marketing
   C. Constantly changing and evolving as operations of the oncology rehab program are refined
   D. Dependent on the administrator, and should change as people are recruited and exit the organization

8. The phrase "use an equity lens" in the development of an oncology rehab program refers to the need for program pioneers to consider the importance of:
   A. Having close controls of who is able to access the oncology rehabilitation program to highly target care to specific needed populations
   B. Recognizing the existing inequities within the current healthcare system and consciously creating opportunities to proactively address these inequities
   C. Focusing on the populations that have good insurance in order to stay financially viable
   D. Making sure that there are enough therapists to see a volume of patients to achieve the break-even point

9. Creating and sustaining a dynamic team is a critical step in the development and ongoing operation of an oncology rehab program. What administrative methods may be helpful in this process?
   A. Requiring all personnel to hold the highest level of credential prior to employment
   B. Offering career mentorship, clinical career ladders, and ongoing financial support for lifelong learning in the field
   C. Building a sturdy program structure so that it is essentially the same years later as when it was built
   D. Knowing that the privilege of working in oncology rehabilitation is sufficient to assure good recruitment and retention to sustain a program

10. A health system is exploring developing a new oncology rehabilitation program. Which of the following statements will be LEAST likely to assist the program development team?
    A. Due to the wide variety of rehabilitation needs for the PWC across the oncology journey, oncology rehab programs may vary greatly with size of scope of service
    B. Rehabilitation during active cancer treatment may be vastly different than outpatient survivorship programs focusing on full restoration of function and optimum QOL, identification of red flags for reoccurrence and prevention strategies
    C. With enough searching and investigation, the team members will be able to find another program that is an exact fit for their program to emulate it to grow their program
    D. Translating foundational oncology knowledge into practice will be a fundamental step in developing a cancer rehab program

References

1. American Board of Physical Therapy Specialties. *Oncologic Physical Therapy Description of Specialty Practice.* American Physical Therapy Association. http://www.abpts.org/Specialist_Certification/Oncology/Specialist_Certification_Examination_Outline__Oncology/. Accessed May 5, 2021.

2. Cady SH, Wheeler, JV, DeWolf J, Brodke M. Mission, vision, and values: what do they say? *Organ Dev J.* 2011;29:63–78.

3. Wolff SN, Nichols C, Ulman D, et al. Survivorship: an unmet need of the patient with cancer-implications of a survey of the Lance Armstrong Foundation (LAF). *J Clin Oncol.* 2005;23(16_suppl):6032–6032.

4. Cheville AL, Mustian K, Winters-Stone K, Zucker DS, Gamble GL, Alfano CM. Cancer rehabilitation: an overview of current need, delivery models, and levels of care. *Phys Med Rehabil Clin.* 2017;28(1):1–7.

5. Institute of Medicine and National Research Council. *From Cancer Patient to Cancer Survivor: Lost in Transition.* The National Academies Press; 2006. https://doi.org/10.17226/11468.

6. Porter ME, Teisberg EO. *Redefining Health Care: Creating Value-based Competition on Results.* Harvard Business Press; 2006.

7. Porter ME. What is value in health care. *N Engl J Med.* 2010;363(26):2477–2481.

8. Sandoval GA, Brown AD, Sullivan T, Green E. Factors that influence cancer patients' overall perceptions of the quality of care. *Int J Quality Health Care.* 2006;18(4):266–274.

9. American Hospital Association. Bundled payment: results from 2018 member survey; 2018. https://www.aha.org/bundled-payment. Accessed October 27, 2020.

10. American Physical Therapy Association. Vision, Mission and Strategic Plan. https://www.apta.org/apta-and-you/leadership-and-governance/vision-mission-and-strategic-plan. June 2013. Accessed October 27, 2020

11. Boehmer U. LGBT populations' barriers to cancer care. *Semin Oncol Nurs.* 2018;34(1):21–29.

12. Campione E, Wampler-Kuhn M, Fisher MI. Translating evidence into practice through knowledge implementation. *Rehab Onc.* 2021;39(2):103–110.

13. Eccles MP, Miittman S. Welcome to implementation science. *Implement Sci.* 2006;1:1. doi:10.1186/1748-5908-1-1.

14. Nilsen P. Making sense of implementation theories, models and frameworks. *Implement Sci.* 2015;10:53. doi:10.1186/s13012-015-0242-0.

15. Mitchell P, Pirkis J, Hall J, Haas M. Partnerships for knowledge exchange in health services research, policy and practice. *J Health Service Res Policy.* 2009;14(2):104–111.

16. Stout NL, Silver JK, Raj VS, et al. Toward a national initiative in cancer rehabilitation: recommendations from a subject matter expert group. *Arch Phys Med Rehabil.* 2016;97(11):2006–2015.

17. Graham ID, Logan J, Harrison MB, et al. Lost in knowledge translation: time for a map? *J Contin Educ Health Prof.* 2006;26(1):13–24.

18. Colombo R, Wilson CM. PRevention, Intervention, and Sustained wellness Model (PRISM) care philosophy in cancer survivorship, palliative care, and chronic disease management in the era of healthcare reform: a perspective paper. *Rehabil Oncol.* 2015;33(2):45–51.

19. Baumann AA, Cabassa LJ. Reframing implementation science to address inequities in healthcare delivery. *BMC Health Serv Res.* 2020;20(1):1–9.

20. Bauer P. Building a comprehensive oncology rehabilitation program. *Oncology Issues.* 2014;29(6):24–31.

21. Carlton R, Singh, S. Erik L. Joint community health needs assessments as a path for coordinating community-wide health improvement efforts between hospitals and local health departments. *Am J Publ Health.* 2018;108:676–682.

22. Commission on Cancer. 2020 Program Standards. American College of Surgeons website. https://www.facs.org/quality-programs/cancer/coc/standards/2020; 2020. Accessed October 28, 2020.

23. Soukup T, Lamb BW, Arora S, Darzi A, Sevdalis N, Green JS. Successful strategies in implementing a multidisciplinary team working in the care of patients with cancer: an overview and synthesis of the available literature. *J Multidiscip Healthc.* 2018;11:49–61.

24. American Board of Physical Therapy Residency and Fellowship Education. Oncologic description of residency practice. https://abptrfe.apta.org/for-programs/clinical-programs/oncology. Accessed March 3, 2022.

25. Tremblay MA, Blanchard CM, Taylor S, Pelletier LG, Villeneuve M. Work Extrinsic and Intrinsic Motivation Scale. *Can J Behav Sci.* 2009;41(4):213–226.

26. Drenkard K, Swartwout E. Effectiveness of a clinical ladder program. *J Nurs Admin.* 2005;35(11):502–506.

27. Wilson CM, Schwartz KK, Malushi V, et al. Development and implementation of a professional advancement program for physical therapists and occupational therapists: an administrative case report. *Phys Ther J Policy, Administration, Leadership (PTJ-PAL).* 2018;18(1):5–15.

28. Oncology Nursing Society. Oncology nurse navigation role and qualifications. *Oncol Nurs Forum.* 2015;42(5):447–448.

29. Baileys K, McMullen L, Lubejko B, et al. Nurse navigator core competencies: an update to reflect the evolution of the role. *Clin J Oncol Nurs.* 2018;22(3):272–281.

30. Commission on Cancer. About the commission on cancer. American College of Surgeons. https://www.facs.org/quality%20programs/cancer/coc/about. Accessed October 27, 2020.

31. National Accreditation Program for Breast Cancers. National Accreditation Program for Breast Centers Standards Manual 2018 Edition. American College of Surgeons; 2018. https://www.facs.org/quality-programs/napbc/standards. Accessed October 30, 2020.

32. National Accreditation Program for Rectal Cancers. Optimal resources for rectal cancer care 2020 standards. American College of Surgeons; 2018. https://www.facs.org/quality-programs/napbc/standards. Accessed October 30, 2020

33. Commission on Accreditation of Rehabilitation Facilities. Integrating rehabilitation into cancer care. http://www.carf.org/cancercare. July 23, 2014. Accessed February 19, 2021.

34. National Academies of Science Engineering Medicine. Long-Term Survivorship Care and Cancer Treatment. In: Proceedings of a Workshop. National Academies Press; 2017. http://www.nationalacademies.org/hmd/Activities/Disease/NCPF/2017-July-24.aspx. Accessed August 15, 2019.

35. Silver J. Cancer prehabilitation and its role in improving health outcomes and reducing healthcare costs. *Semin Oncol Nurs.* 2015;31(1):13–30.

36. Silver J, Baima J. Cancer prehabilitation: an opportunity to decrease treatment-related morbidity, increase cancer treatment options, and improve physical and psychological health outcomes. *Am J Phys Med Rehabil.* 2013;92(8):715–727.

37. Sirintrapun SJ, Lopez AM. Telemedicine in cancer care. *Am Soc Clin Oncol Educ Book.* 2018;38:540–545.

38. Peiris CL, Shields N, Brusco NK, Watts JJ, Taylor NF. Additional physical therapy services reduce length of stay and improve health outcomes in people with acute and subacute conditions: an updated systematic review and meta-analysis. *Arch Phys Med Rehabil.* 2018;99(11):2299–2312.

39. Rogers AT, Bai G, Lavin RA, Anderson GF. Higher hospital spending on occupational therapy is associated with lower readmission rates. *Med Care Res Rev.* 2017;74(6):668–686.

40. Jette DU, Stilphen M, Ranganathan VK, Passek SD, Frost FS, Jette AM. AM-PAC "6-Clicks" functional assessment scores predict acute care hospital discharge destination. *Phys Ther.* 2014;94(9):1252–1261.

41. Center for Medicare and Medicaid Services. Inpatient rehabilitation facility prospective payment system. https://www.cms.gov/outreach-and-education/medicare-learning-network-MLN/MLNProducts/downloads/inpatrehabpaymentfctsht09-508.pdf. March 2020. Accessed February 19, 2021.

42. Fu JB, Raj VS, Guo Y. A guide to inpatient cancer rehabilitation: focusing on patient selection and evidence-based outcomes. *PM&R.* 2017;9(9):S324–334.

43. Smith S, Wilson CM, Lipple C, et al. Managing palliative patients in inpatient rehabilitation through a short stay family training program. *Am J Hospice Palliat Med.* 2020;37(3):172–178.

44. Burge F, Lawson B, Johnston G, Asada Y, McIntyre PF, Flowerdew G. Preferred and actual location of death: what factors enable a preferred home death? *J Palliat Med.* 2015;18(12):1054–1059.

45. Center for Medicare and Medicaid Services. Long term care hospital prospective payment system. https://www.cms.gov/outreach-and-education/medicare-learning-network-MLN/MLNProducts/downloads/long-term-care-hospital-pps-fact-sheet-ICN006956.pdf. March 2020. Accessed February 19, 2021.

46. Rodin MB. Cancer patients admitted to nursing homes: what do we know? *J Am Med Dir Assoc.* 2008;9(3):149–156.

47. Fennell ML. Nursing homes and cancer care. *Health Serv Res.* 2009;44(6):1927–1932.

48. American Physical Therapy Association. Patient driven payment model. APTA. https://www.apta.org/your-practice/payment/medicare-payment/coding-billing/skilled-nursing-facilities/patient-driven-payment-model. Accessed December 25, 2020.

49. Tralongo P, Ferraù F, Borsellino N, et al. Cancer patient-centered home care: a new model for health care in oncology. *Ther Clin Risk Manage.* 2011;7:387–392.

50. Center for Medicare and Medicaid Services. Home health patient-driven groupings model. https://www.cms.gove/Medicare/Medicare-Fee-for-Service-Payment/HomeHelahtPPS/HH-PDGM; March 2020. Accessed February 19, 2021.

51. American Physical Therapy Association. Medicare payment thresholds for outpatient therapy services; 2018. https://www.apta.org/your-practice/payment/medicare-payment/coding-billing/therapy-cap. Accessed February 19, 2021.

52. Silver JK, Stout NL, Fu JB, Pratt-Chapman M, Haylock PJ, Sharma R. The state of cancer rehabilitation in the United States. *J Cancer Rehabil.* 2018;1:1–8.

32

Advocacy and Public Policy

JENA COLON, PT, DPT, MBA, APRIL GAMBLE, PT, DPT, CLT

CHAPTER OUTLINE

Describing Advocacy

Many oncology rehabilitation (Onc R) clinicians have the professional role of advocacy embedded within their scope of practice. The American Physical Therapy Association's Code of Ethics states that physical therapists (PTs) "shall advocate to reduce health disparities and healthcare inequities, improve access to healthcare services, and address the health, wellness, and preventive healthcare needs of people."[1] Advocacy is described in the literature in a variety of ways: (1) fighting with and/or on behalf of an individual, family, or community to ensure access to healthcare, support, and important life opportunities; (2) navigating a system to obtain needed resources and to serve the individual's best interests; (3) using knowledge, skills, and position to secure the best services consistent with the constraints of the service; (4) a combination of individual and social actions to gain policy support and social acceptance for a specific goal.[2–5]

In this chapter, advocacy will be operationally defined as "activities carried out at various levels of the healthcare system, by a variety of people—persons living with and beyond cancer (PLWBCs), clinicians, advocacy groups, legislators, national and international associations – and through the use of a variety of skills alongside and/or on behalf of others to support an idea or a cause."[6] The role of advocacy for promoting the health and function of persons impacted by cancer is increasingly vital with the ongoing changes in healthcare, including medical advances, increased health inequities, increased survivorship, and significant changes in healthcare,

delivery strategies and methods of reimbursement. Onc R clinicians are uniquely positioned to work alongside persons impacted by cancer to perform effective advocacy efforts. Advocacy efforts by these professionals are grounded in the fact that they have witnessed the importance of not just surviving cancer, but surviving well. Therefore, this chapter aims to catalyze the Onc R clinician to engage in advocacy by presenting practical strategies, key principles, relevant examples, and conceptual frameworks that the Onc R clinician can utilize in a variety of contexts, cultures, and professional settings to promote equitable and just opportunities for health and functioning for persons and communities impacted by cancer.

The Current State of the Field of Oncology Rehabilitation

Specific to the state of Onc R services, there is lack of accessible and equitable Onc R services globally.[7–9] Advances in early detection and treatment have resulted in a growing number of persons living beyond cancer (PLBCs) (i.e., cancer survivors) and persons living with cancer-related disability throughout the world.[10,11] Cancer-related disability has significant consequences on the person living with cancer, their family, community, and the greater society (Figure 32.1). These impacts of cancer survivorship have catalyzed the growth of the field of Onc R globally over the past 10 years.

As an example of the recent evolution of the Onc R field in the United States (US), numerous US national organizations

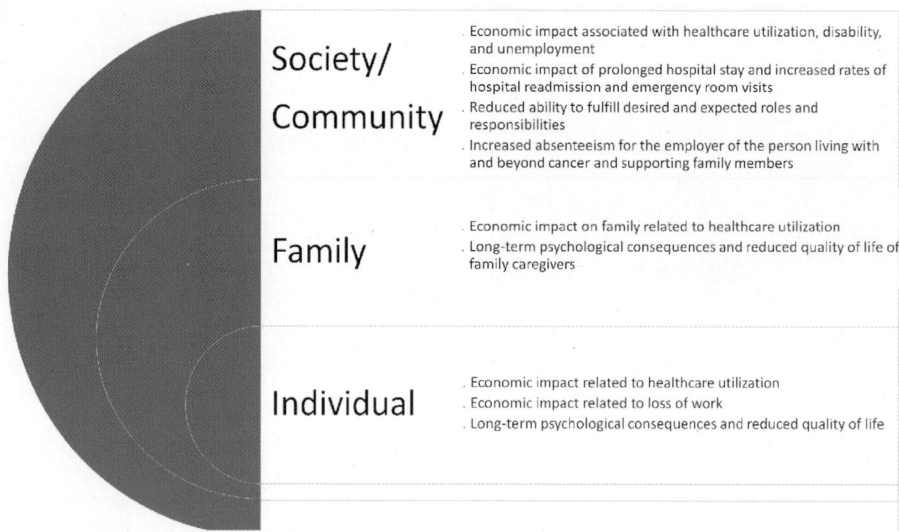

Society/
Community
- Economic impact associated with healthcare utilization, disability, and unemployment
- Economic impact of prolonged hospital stay and increased rates of hospital readmission and emergency room visits
- Reduced ability to fulfill desired and expected roles and responsibilities
- Increased absenteeism for the employer of the person living with and beyond cancer and supporting family members

Family
- Economic impact on family related to healthcare utilization
- Long-term psychological consequences and reduced quality of life of family caregivers

Individual
- Economic impact related to healthcare utilization
- Economic impact related to loss of work
- Long-term psychological consequences and reduced quality of life

• **Fig. 32.1** Impact of Cancer-Related Disability[13–19] (Created by Jena Colon and April Gamble.)

have begun issuing guidelines for Onc R research and post cancer treatment healthcare.[12] Many academic hospital departments in physical medicine and rehabilitation recognize Onc R as a standard of care and are actively recruiting researchers and clinical faculty.[12] Concurrently, entry-level and postgraduate education for Onc R clinicians are striving to catch up with anticipated clinical demand by increasing the number of cancer rehabilitation training programs as well as introducing Onc R/prehabilitation concepts earlier in entry-level educational programs.[12] Efforts such as these have been made to standardize Onc R and its integration into the course of oncology care. These collaborative approaches to delivery of optimal cancer care aim to enhance treatment of not only the cancer disease, but also any short-term or long-term adverse effects of the cancer and its treatments that may be experienced.

Throughout the world there is a growing number of organizations that are advocating for increased delivery of just and equitable Onc R services. The National Comprehensive Cancer Network (NCCN) Clinical Practice Guidelines, the American College of Surgeons Commission on Cancer Program Standards, the American Cancer Society (ACS), and the Association of Community Cancer Centers (ACCC) Cancer Program Guidelines now identify rehabilitation as a crucial, if not mandatory, component of cancer care. The ACCC's Cancer Program Guidelines call for comprehensive rehabilitation services and provides 14 exemplars of elements of comprehensive services.[12] The Commission on Accreditation of Rehabilitation Facilities (CARF), the main accrediting organization for inpatient rehabilitation facilities, initiated accreditation for inpatient and outpatient Onc R units. Professional organizations such as the World Health Organization (WHO), Oncology Nursing Society, and the American Society of Clinical Oncologists (ASCO) that traditionally focus on the medical treatment of cancer are also now promoting the efficacy of Onc R.[12] Importantly, the US National Institutes of Health (NIH) held the first ever Cancer Rehabilitation Summit in June 2015.[12] In that same year, the Rehabilitation Medicine Department of the Clinical Center at the NIH established a panel of interdisciplinary experts to review current research and typical practice patterns, identify opportunities to address gaps in Onc R, and make recommendations for future efforts that promote better quality Onc R overall.

Onc R is severely underutilized in all phases of the disease process despite these professional evidence-based guidelines and the large amount of evidence demonstrating the benefits of Onc R for reducing cancer-related disability.[12] There are insufficient services in communities around the world to meet the overall patient need for therapeutic interventions related to the type of cancer itself and/or the effects of the treatment for their cancer[13] (Table 32.1). Based on this lack of Onc R services globally, all clinicians and stakeholders are called to be advocates for Onc R. Access to beneficial healthcare at the appropriate time is a human right required to support the quality of life (QOL) for individuals and our greater society.[25]

Unjust Oncology Rehabilitation Services

When considering advocacy, it is not enough to define it, but rather the reason behind why advocacy is needed must be explored; this centers on concepts of health equity and justice (Figure 32.2). Healthy People 2020, the US national health objectives, define health equity as the "attainment of the highest level of health for all people."[26] It goes on to further describe that this pursuit requires "focused and ongoing societal efforts to address avoidable inequality, historical, and contemporary injustices, and the elimination of health and healthcare disparities."[26] It is well established that eliminating health disparities at a clinician, hospital, subnational (e.g., state, local, regional, provincial, etc.), national, and global level cannot be achieved without addressing social determinants of health (SDH). SDH are nonmedical factors that influence health outcomes and contribute to unjust health disparities.[27] Research has shown that SDHs, like education, food insecurity, and secure housing, can account for 30% to 55% of health outcomes.[27] It is important to name that the existence and perpetuation of SDH and the associated health disparities are the result of economic, social, and political policies and systems that reflect racism, colonialization, discrimination, and oppression.[28]

Various international associations have goals and long-term strategic plans to address disparities and the underlying social determinants of health including the WHO "Rehabilitation 2030" and "Global Action Plan for Healthy Lives and Well-Being for All."[29,30] Some nations, including the United Kingdom (UK),

TABLE 32.1 Summary Research by Pergolotti et al. in Evaluating the Needs of Rehabilitation[8]

Authors	Patient Population	Needs Identified	Results
Cheville et al.[14]	Community-dwelling adults in the US with metastatic breast cancer	Of 163 patients, 92% had at least 1 impairment, 88% required OT/PT, only 21% received treatment	Impairments are poorly addressed, even in centers with access to therapy
Cheville et al.[15]	Community-dwelling adults in the US with cancer, over the age of 18	Of 202 patients, 67% with functional problems, 1 in 5 reported a cognitive issue	No functional problems were addressed by therapy and only 1 patient received OT/PT
Cheville et al.[16]	Adults with Stage IV breast cancer still receiving chemotherapy in the US	The majority of 163 patients had 3 or more physical impairments	Disability occurs with a number of physical impairments and adverse symptoms accumulate slowly, making them more difficult to find and treat
Holm et al.[17]	Community-dwelling adults from Southern and Central Denmark with cancer	Of 3439 patients, one-half reported sexual problems and one-third reported a need for physical rehabilitation at 14 months after cancer diagnosis	Compared with women with breast cancer, those with colorectal, gynecological, and head and neck cancers reported more needs
Hansen et al.[18]	Danish population-based adults with cancer	Of 3439 patients, 60% had an unmet rehabilitation need, 40% had an unmet physical need	Perceived unmet need is related to decreased quality of life
Lehman et al.[19]	Community-dwelling adults with cancer in the US	Of 805 patients, 35% had weakness, 30% had an ADL impairment, 25% had difficulty walking	Mental health issues were common and related to those with physical health issues
Movsas et al.[20]	Community-dwelling adults in the US with cancer in acute care setting	Of 55 patients evaluated, 87% had rehabilitation needs, 76% had deconditioning, 58% had mobility impairment, 22% had ADL deficits	Of the 87% who had rehabilitation needs on admission, 9% received therapy
Pergolotti et al.[21]	Community dwelling older adults in the US, 63% married with postsecondary education with cancer in outpatient setting	Of 529 patients, 65% had an identified functional deficit (physical health, IADL, falls, cognition)	Only 9% received OT/PT in 1 year of identified deficit
Ross et al.[22]	Danish adults with cancer	Of 1490 patients, 39% reported they were not offered needed physical rehabilitation	Younger patients and those who are divorced or single were more likely to have difficulty returning to everyday life
Söderback et al.[23]	Swedish community-dwelling adults with cancer	Of 102 patients, 56% reported a perceived need for OT; only 7 were referred	59% of the patients would need a referral
Veloso et al.[24]	Community-dwelling male and female adults with cancer	Of 4346 patients, 19% needed physical rehabilitation, 17% needed practical help, 14% needed information on how to return to work	Young age, male sex, low educational level, and living alone increased risk for unmet needs

ADL, Activity of daily living; *IADL*, Instrumental activity of daily living; *OT*, Occupational therapy; *PT*, Physical therapy; *US*, United States.
Reprinted with permission from Pergolotti M, Williams GR, Campbell C, Munoz LA, Muss HB. Occupational therapy for adults with cancer: why it matters. *Oncologist*. 2016;21(3):314–319. doi:10.1634/theoncologist.2015-0335.

have developed standards to work toward achieving health equity related to Onc R.[31]

When implementing strategic plans and standards such as these to strive for health equity within Onc R, it is essential to understand the barriers related to accessing or benefiting from Onc R (Table 32.2). Before expounding on these barriers, it is vital to name that most of this research has been conducted in the US or other high-income countries and with predominantly white heterosexual populations. Consequently, these barriers to Onc R may or may not apply in other contexts. Further research and reporting that focus on the needs and experiences of communities that are not historically dominant are necessary to facilitate the advancement of Onc R globally.

Barriers to Onc R contribute to the prevalence of cancer-related disability within many communities and populations globally.

The impact of these barriers is greater for populations that are historically marginalized, like **B**lack, **I**ndigenous, and **P**eople **of** **C**olor (BIPOC), resulting in cancer-related health disparities.[40–46] It is well established that systemic racism, defined as an organized political and economic system that categorizes, ranks, and differentially allocates societal resources to population groups, results in these racial and ethnic health disparities.[46] An example of a cancer-related health disparity is the effective assessment and treatment of cancer-related pain, as persons from BIPOC communities consistently receive less effective pain management treatments compared to white counterparts.[40,41] It is has also been described that due to the impact of systemic racism, there is a greater prevalence of and more severe physical functioning limitations in people with breast cancer who were African American and other BIPOC in comparison to white counterparts.[41–44] Similarly, the relationship between

Status Quo

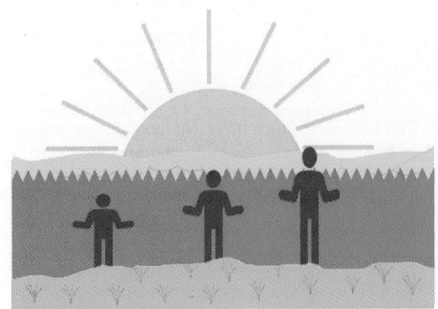

Equality

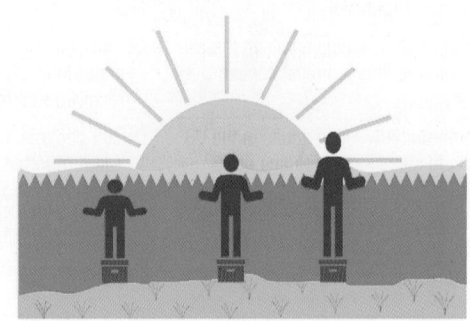

Equity

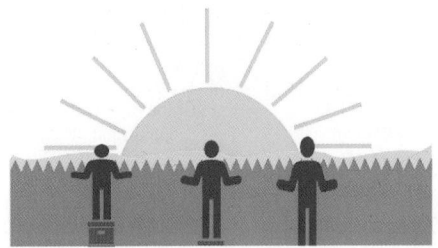

Justice

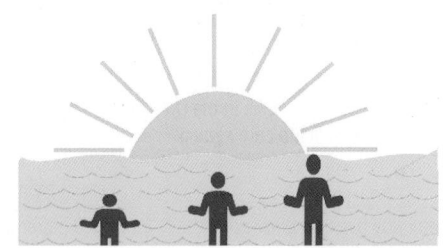

• **Fig. 32.2** Equality, Equity Versus Justice. Equality: The assumption that everyone benefits from the same supports. This is equal treatment. Equity: Everyone gets the supports they need, thus producing equity. Justice: All three people can see the sunrise without accommodations because the cause of the inequality was addressed. The systematic barrier was removed. (Created by Christopher Wilson. Adapted with permission from avarna.com)

socioeconomic status and health disparities has been demonstrated as evidenced by persons with low-income levels having a greater prevalence of breast cancer-related physical impairments, coupled with lower utilization of rehabilitation services due to environmental barriers restricting access.[46]

The root cause of these Onc R health disparities are not related to the individual choices or biology of PLWBCs but rather are caused by unjust systems of healthcare and research that thrive throughout the world.[47] These unjust systems, by design, marginalize and restrict access to maximal health and functioning for populations based on race, socioeconomic status, gender identity, immigration status, location (e.g., rural living), and other unearned determinants.[48] For example, unjust processes and policies within health systems contribute to greater under-utilization of cancer treatments and Onc R within marginalized populations.[13,28–31,34–36,48] Advocacy efforts should aim to address the various root causes of health disparities so that all persons have the opportunity to achieve maximal physical and social functioning during and after cancer and cancer treatment.

Advocating for Just Oncology Rehabilitation Services

To work toward equitable and just Onc R services (see Figure 32.2), the Onc R clinician can engage in a variety of advocacy activities across all levels of healthcare delivery from the individual patient to the healthcare institution, within their community, nation, and globally (Table 32.3). Skills required to practice critical advocacy

effectively across all levels of the health system include the following: (1) exceptional communication skills; (2) ability to collaborate and form strategic partnerships; (3) ability to understand and clearly communicate current research evidence; (4) commitment to improving equity of healthcare through a justice-centered approach; (5) an understanding of inequity, health disparities, and social determinants of health; (6) a recognition of personal positions of privilege and power; (7) skills to work in solidarity and collective action on systems of inequity; (8) perseverance; (9) passion; (10) humility; and (11) resourcefulness.[49,50]

All advocacy efforts should embody a justice-centered approach. Justice-centered advocacy can be described as "working towards eliminating root causes of inequity in solidarity with persons and communities that experience the impact of health injustices." Only through justice-centered advocacy, will *all* persons impacted by cancer, regardless of unearned disadvantages like race and location, obtain benefit from Onc R services. Only when unjust systems are comprehensively rebuilt can Onc R services be consistently person-centered, culturally responsive, and human rights oriented so as to effectively respond to a person's personal goals, values, preferences, and desires.

Applied specifically to Onc R, justice-centered advocacy can be described as working under the leadership and stewardship of persons impacted by cancer to address the root causes of unjust access to equitably beneficial Onc R services. See Table 32.4 for key principles of justice-centered advocacy. It is important to acknowledge that to effectively practice justice-centered advocacy, requires significant life-long personal development that aims to contribute to significant systemic changes.[53] It is outside the

TABLE 32.2 Documented Barriers to Oncology Rehabilitation[32]

Persons are not referred to oncology rehabilitation (Onc R) services due to the following factors:

Cancer-related disability and cancer-related physical impairments are a gradual process, rarely with acute and readily detected declines, so the decline goes unnoticed by referring providers[32]	• Oncology clinicians wrongly believe that treating cancer is the most effective way to minimize functional decline.[32] • Oncology training programs and the scope of oncology practice do not include topics of Onc R and functional issues.[32–34] • Oncology clinicians lack training and understanding about Onc R and functional assessments.[19,32–34] • Oncology clinicians lack knowledge, time, resources, and training to assess for physical rehabilitation needs and to coordinate rehabilitation services.[32,34–36] • Limited clear guidelines and care pathways to identify who is responsible to make a referral to Onc R.[32] • Limited use of screening guidelines and tools for identifying persons that would benefit from Onc R are lacking.[32] • Rehabilitation professionals lack adequate training, knowledge, and evidence specific to Onc R.[32,36,37] • Persons during and after cancer treatment may underreport functional impairments due to their perception that it will limit their future treatment options.[32] • There is a lack of public and private funding and resources dedicated to the development, maintenance, and promotion of Onc R services.[32,33,37] • Within healthcare systems that rely on insurance coverage, there is limited payment for Onc R services.[32,37]
There is a lack of knowledge available to persons during and after cancer treatment due to the following factors[32]:	• Oncologists and other clinicians rarely provide educational information about Onc R to persons during and after cancer treatment.[38] • Websites dedicated to cancer lack educational information related to Onc R.[39] • Education resources for persons during and after cancer treatment often have inaccurate and incomplete information about Onc R.[39]
Many social, environmental, and systemic factors make accessing, adhering, and benefiting from Onc R difficult for persons impacted by cancer include the following[32]:	• Lack of available time due to family, social, and employment roles and responsibilities. • Inadequate financial resources. • Transportation challenges including a financial burden and long distances to commute to an Onc R provider. • Inadequate insurance coverage of Onc R (when applicable within the health system). • Illness. • Fear of injury, illness, and/or fatigue. • Lack of social and emotional support. • Fear of experiencing discrimination related to race, gender expression, or other unearned disadvantages. • Lack of Onc R providers available from their community, especially for historically marginalized groups.

Created by Jena Colon and April Gamble.

TABLE 32.3 Roles and Responsibilities of the Oncology Clinician as Described in the *Oncologic Physical Therapy Description of Specialty Practice*[51] and the *Description of Residency Practice Oncology*[52]

- Assists oncologic population in obtaining access to healthcare needs across the continuum of care.
- Aids persons living with and beyond cancer (PLWBCs) in developing the skills to advocate for themselves by identifying supportive services through programs such as Five Wishes.
- Assists oncologic patients in gaining access to resources that help them understand their health condition and manage it with consideration for late effects of cancer treatment.
- Provides health promotion information to patients and clients regarding cancer screening, cancer prevention, cancer impairment secondary prevention, and wellness throughout the cancer care continuum.
- Assists oncologic patients in gaining access to resources that help them understand their health condition and manage it with consideration for late effects of cancer treatment.
- Provides health promotion information to the general public regarding cancer screening, cancer prevention, cancer impairment, secondary prevention, and wellness throughout the cancer care continuum.
- Seeks opportunities to advocate for cancer-related issues with policy and law-making bodies (e.g., Women's Health and Cancer Rights Act, Agency for Health Care Research and Quality guidelines, Centers for Medicare and Medicaid Services).
- Utilization of global events like World Cancer Day, Cancer awareness months, etc.
- Culturally responsive public service announcements, patient testimonial videos, etc.
- Free cancer screenings and education within community and wellness events.

Created by Jena Colon and April Gamble.

scope of this chapter to provide comprehensive skill development in this area; however, Table 32.5 presents additional educational resources. This is not a comprehensive list but rather a starting point to learn about health justice and its applications within rehabilitation. If you are working alongside specific communities that are historically marginalized, it is essential to learn from them and clinicians should seek out the resources that they produce.

As Onc R clinicians strive to engage in justice-centered advocacy efforts to promote just and equitable rehabilitation services, it is important to consider two common advocacy approaches:

TABLE 32.4	Educational Resources Related to Justice-Centered Advocacy[45,46,50,53–55]

- Blake T. In the fight for racial justice, the sidelines are no longer an option. *Brit J Sports Med.* 2020;54(21):1245–1246. doi:10.1136/bjsports-2020-102894.
- Colombo DG. Closing the gap in a generation: health equity through action on the social determinants of health. Final report of the Commission on Social Determinants of Health. *Revista De Direito Sanitário.* 2010;10(3):253. doi:10.11606/issn.2316-9044.v10i3p253-266.
- Jaffe KM, Jimenez N. Disparity in rehabilitation: another inconvenient truth. *Arch Phys Med Rehabil.* 2015;96(8):1371–1374. doi:10.1016/j.apmr.2015.04.017.
- Nixon SA. The coin model of privilege and critical allyship: implications for health. *BMC Public Health.* 2019;19(1):1637. doi:10.1186/s12889-019-7884-9.
- Roush SE, Sharby N. Disability reconsidered: the paradox of physical therapy. *Phys Ther.* 2011;91(12):1715–1727. doi:10.2522/ptj.20100389.

TABLE 32.5	Key Principles to Embody When Striving to Practice Justice-Centered Advocacy

- The root causes of why some do not access or get equal benefits from rehabilitation services are social, cultural, political, environmental, economic, and systemic as opposed to an individual's behavior or biology.
- The goal of advocacy efforts is to dismantle systems that cause inequities rather than to help or save those that experience the unearned disadvantages of these systems.
- Health justice can only occur when persons with power actively and purposefully step back and practice humility to make room for the actions of those that experience the impact of health disparities.
- We build our capacity to effectively work alongside communities to disrupt unjust structures that produce health inequities.
- We each recognize and take responsibility for our own positions of privilege, power, and race and our role in upholding systems of oppression that create health inequities.
- We continuously evaluate, acknowledge, and take responsibility for the inevitable impact of our biases, attitudes, and beliefs in our work and within the communities we work alongside.
- It is the impact of our actions, rather than our intention, that matter the most when working to eliminate disparities.
- We celebrate differences and recognize that they contribute to enriched discussion, creativity, and innovative solutions, policies, and operational processes.
- We recognize that feelings of discomfort are different than feelings of being unsafe/physically threatened—feelings of discomfort commonly arise when: (1) engaging in self-reflection and personal growth; (2) when discussing the impact of race, privilege, and oppression; (3) when your ideas or beliefs are challenged; and (4) during honest and brave discussions related to justice
- We recognize the negative consequences of elevating the position of power and the "expert" role of oncology clinicians—it directly minimizes, weakens, or even replaces a person's and community's strengths, resources, and unique traditional strategies that positively contribute to heath and function.

Created for the APTA Michigan Fall Conference 2020 by Binkley J, Cleaver, S, Collins P, et al. Working towards health equity and justice within the world of rehabilitation. October 10, 2020. Reprinted with permission.

(1) professional-oriented advocacy; and (2) community-oriented advocacy. In the scope of Onc R, professional-oriented advocacy can be defined as "activities that seek to elevate the position of power and influence of Onc R clinicians so as to improve their ability to provide clinical services." This would include professional bodies, like physical therapy associations, lobbying for increased insurance coverage of Onc R services, or working to recognize a defined scope of practice within licensing authorities. Another example of professional-oriented advocacy is clinicians working with physicians to facilitate more Onc R referrals of persons during and after cancer treatment.

Community-oriented advocacy, within the scope of Onc R, can be defined as working under the leadership of and in collaboration with persons impacted by cancer so as to work toward the goals and needs that they articulate. Onc R clinicians can engage in community-oriented advocacy in a countless number of ways as each community directs their advocacy efforts specific to their needs, context, and culture. To prevent contributing to greater health disparities, harm, and oppression, an effective community-oriented advocacy can only occur when the community directly invites the clinician to support their efforts and the clinician mobilizes under their leadership. An example of community-oriented advocacy is an Onc R clinician delivering lymphedema prospective surveillance programs and educational sessions upon the request of a local breast cancer support group. Community-oriented advocacy would also be working with PLWBC within the LGBTQIA+ community to change national policy to increase safe access to community-based survivorship services.

When advocacy efforts consistently embody justice-centered practices, then both professional-oriented and community-oriented activities can effectively work toward eliminating disparities related to Onc R. It is essential to recognize that if advocacy is not rooted in practices of justice, including a personal awareness of privilege and the clinician's role in contributing to disparities, then efforts performed even with the best intentions will only contribute to further disparity. The risk of contributing to disparities is higher when engaging in professional-oriented advocacy, as the efforts are led by clinicians with the emphasis on providing opportunities for the clinicians rather than on the direction and needs of those who experience the impact of health disparities.

In the book *Pink Ribbon Blues*, Sulek postulated that early advocacy efforts by the ACS were professional-oriented with the primary aim being to elevate the expert role of the oncology healthcare team.[55] This orientation was rooted in the intention to contribute to increased survival from cancer. However, the author described that the actual impact of the activities was further marginalization of and harm to persons impacted by cancer.[55] Their professional-oriented advocacy efforts involved volunteer survivors of breast cancer being primarily paraded in front of the media to serve as direct evidence of the power of the medical field to cure cancer.[55] The survivors were even forbidden to discuss medical information. Furthermore, healthcare professionals strongly fought against the establishment of peer-to-peer support groups as they feared relinquishing these positions of power would result in a loss of privileges and opportunities awarded to them by being in this expert role.[56] These historical examples reveal that some advocacy efforts do not embody justice—and inadvertently marginalize and minimize the contribution of groups—which ultimately produces poorer health outcomes and greater health disparities.

Opportunities for Advocacy

We will now discuss how Onc R clinicians can effectively engage in advocacy efforts at different levels of health systems—including alongside the individual PLWBC, the healthcare institution, communities, subnational, and national entities, and globally.

Advocating Alongside the Person Living With and Beyond Cancer

The Onc R clinician has an important role in performing advocacy related to individual PLWBCs. This can be described as a clinician responsibly using their knowledge and positions of power to promote the health and well-being of individual PLWBCs. This often involves supporting a person by actively acquiring resources for them or on their behalf, assuring quality of care, guaranteeing their rights as a patient, and serving as a liaison between the person and the healthcare system.[57,58]

Cancer and cancer treatment can result in long-term impairments that benefit from lifelong access to rehabilitation and healthcare services, as well as to services that support the performance of self-care and self-management activities that reduce the impact of cancer treatment effects. The Onc R clinician is not only uniquely poised to equip an individual with knowledge and skills to bolster their self-management, but also to support their access to resources, services, and support. For example, specific to lymphedema self-management, persons with cancer-related lymphedema have expressed that they would like clinicians to advocate for them to access: (1) tangible physical assistance in the home; (2) support groups; (3) resources like insurance coverage for supportive services; (4) educational resources; (5) self-care supplies like bandages and compression sleeves; and (6) fast and affordable antibiotics to reduce the impact of infections.[59]

Another important advocacy opportunity for the Onc R clinician is assessing, advising, and referring people to programming to support their participation in physical activity and exercise at every stage of cancer care. Considering the strong evidence for the impact of exercise and physical activity presented throughout this text, it is vital that Onc R clinicians support PLWBC to access the benefits of safe, effective, and culturally relevant exercise programming. To advocate for patients in this realm, clinicians must have: (1) knowledge of the benefits of exercise and physical activity within this population; (2) the skills to assess and advise regarding physical activity's impact, safety, and suitability, (3) awareness of available programming; and (4) skills for making referrals and connecting the person to beneficial and culturally relevant services.[60]

The Onc R clinician is responsible for performing justice-centered advocacy so that all PLWBCs receive the same benefits from healthcare, rehabilitation, and supportive services. The specific actions taken by an Onc R clinician in regard to PLWBC advocacy should always be in response to the expressed needs of the person. Considering that each person will have different needs, conditions, preferences, and past experiences, effective advocacy requires patient-centered communication and the time and skills to foster a trusting therapeutic relationship. It requires the ability to conduct a comprehensive assessment specific to advocacy needs with subsequent shared decision making.[61,62]

The Onc R clinician should act from the understanding that persons belonging to historically marginalized and oppressed groups will commonly present with greater advocacy needs. This is not due to individual choices, behaviors, or biology, but rather this is caused by the impact of unjust healthcare systems that create significant systemic barriers for certain populations in accessing quality services, information, and support. Research has established that people from marginalized groups frequently encounter discrimination in healthcare experiences.[63] This has a deleterious impact on the care provided and the level of patient-centered communication, shared decision-making, patient self-advocacy, and advocacy efforts.[63] Therefore, the Onc R clinician should be equipped with the skills to effectively advocate on behalf of persons from historically marginalized communities. The aim of advocacy efforts is to support people to navigate unjust barriers to care. The aim is not to treat everyone equally but rather to treat everyone *equitably*—so everyone has the effective support required to achieve their desired health, functioning, and QOL.

Empowering Self-Advocacy

Onc R clinicians also have a unique opportunity to promote self-advocacy by PLWBCs. Self-advocacy is a commonly used term, but literature reveals that it has varying understandings and definitions amongst clinicians and PLWBCs.[64,65] In a 2013 analysis that aimed to clarify the concept, self-advocacy was described as "a process (by the PLWBC) of internalizing and activating resources into actions to overcome cancer and treatment-related obstacles."[66] Possible outcomes of self-advocacy include decreased healthcare utilization, more patient-centered care, improved symptom management, enhanced satisfaction with care and QOL, as well as improved adherence to treatment, exercise, rehabilitation, and self-management activities.[67,68]

In an article published in 2010, Judith Wagner shared her personal experiences that illustrated how self-advocacy efforts can sometimes move beyond advocating for their own personal healthcare and needs: *"My personal journey into breast cancer advocacy resulted from a diagnosis of low-grade DCIS (ductal carcinoma in situ). I joined with others throughout the world in turning adversity into advocacy to support endeavors which further public and professional education, political change, and scientific research. This path took me from a mere one-woman networking effort to addressing national panels of experts in Washington, D.C. charged with improving quality of breast care. It often became more than a full-time job, but the rewards were worth it. My family also supported my mission and the potential impact that advocacy could make on both a personal and community level. So, I follow in the footsteps of other tenacious advocates and always keep in mind the singular focus of improving standards for quality breast care now and in the future."*[68]

Self-advocacy is a very personal and highly individualized practice that is greatly influenced by a person's personality, social and physical environment, culture, and context.[69] PLWBC in high income countries, where the majority of cancer self-advocacy research has been conducted, have expressed that their primary goals in performing self-advocacy include: (1) maintaining a positive outlook on life; (2) connecting and communicating effectively with their healthcare team; (3) making informed decisions; (4) joining support groups; (5) educating themselves; (6) working with their employers; (7) managing their health information; and (8) managing symptoms and adverse effects.[64–66] For a person to engage in self-advocacy, it requires internal resources including personal awareness and an openness to try new experiences, as well as learned skills in self-reflection, communication, problem solving, and information seeking.[64–66] It is hypothesized that oncology clinicians can work with PLWBC to develop skills that enhance the effectiveness of self-advocacy, but the evidence-based recommendations for this are almost nonexistent at this time.[64,66]

Impactful self-advocacy relies on the availability of resources in the community that provide options for relevant emotional, tangible, and informational support.[65,66] Furthermore, a person's self-advocacy efforts will not result in improved access to or benefit from services and resources if the system which they are engaging in has practices and policies that reflect racism, sexism, ableism (discrimination against people with physical disabilities), and other forms of discrimination and biases. One author reported that when women demonstrated the same clinical findings, reported self-advocating more and used a greater diversity of self-advocacy strategies during physician interactions than men, women still received less medical treatment for pain control than men and had poorer clinical outcomes.[69] Beside the impact of gender biases, a well-documented barrier to self-advocacy for non-English speakers in the US is a lack of professional language interpretation services made available during healthcare experiences.[70] As these examples highlight, a lack of self-advocacy behaviors are unlikely to be the only reason why there are poorer clinical outcomes for persons who belong to marginalized groups. Consequently, coaching persons to be better self-advocates will not always mitigate health inequities or result in increased access to and benefits from services.

In addition to systemic factors, the impact of self-advocacy relies on the response of the clinician. When persons during and after cancer treatment attempt to perform self-advocacy with members of their healthcare team, they reported that the clinician

can unintentionally silence them or not respond effectively to these efforts by their use of the following actions described in Box 32.1.[50,62,63,71]

PLBCs report that Onc R clinicians can better support their self-advocacy efforts by doing the following: (1) increasing available culturally congruent resources in the community; (2) responding to the PLBC's specific requests for information and providing information that is clear and culturally relevant; (3) being knowledgeable and compassionate; (4) discussing and engaging in collaborative problem solving in regards to symptom management; (5) supporting access to external resources; and (6) respecting that the individual expression of self-advocacy is diverse and based on environmental, cultural, societal factors and a person's internal resources, needs, and preferences.[64–66] Working alongside PLWBCs to enhance self-advocacy skills and efforts will only be effective if clinicians and organizations systematically remove the barriers that prevent clinicians from justly responding to the needs expressed by individuals.

Advocacy Within the Healthcare Institution

The Onc R clinician can contribute to changes within their healthcare institution to retain and/or develop just and equitable beneficial rehabilitation services. This is an integral part of the continuum of cancer care and can increase access to Onc R services for PLWBC.[48] When engaging in advocacy efforts within an institution, the emphasis is shifting beyond the "fight" against cancer to a dual message of surviving and thriving at a macro level that includes not only the individual person but all persons with cancer. A three-pronged approach has been proposed in which a QOL-focused pathway within an institution can be implemented.[72] To drive an effective QOL initiative, it is recommended to focus on three key areas: clinical practice, messaging, and research.

Regarding clinical practice, a focus is on creating greater system efficiencies that increase the likelihood of patient referrals to Onc R services. These impairment screening tools should be embedded in the electronic health records of health systems and independent clinical practice sites (oncology and primary care sites).[32] This makes rehabilitation referrals more feasible and easier for providers, as well as can reduce the impact of provider bias. Another way to promote enhanced QOL-oriented services is by rehabilitation healthcare professionals contributing to the institution's multidisciplinary tumor board. The tumor board is an integrative care delivery approach toward the evaluation, management, and treatment of all types of cancers and is an important part of best practices for the treatment of cancer and improved survival rates.[34] Becoming an integral part of the tumor board, that is, having a "seat at the table," is just the first step in advocating in your institution. To effectively advocate within a tumor board, the Onc R clinician must develop effective communication skills and confidence related to their unique expertise in the care and treatment of PLWBC. Simply attending tumor board meetings without the confidence and/or communication skills to deliver a meaningful message in both context and strategy will often lead to little or no change in the multidisciplinary process or outcomes for the patient. Examples of advocating within the multidisciplinary team and on the tumor board include educating other healthcare providers on the functional limitations that can occur with radiation, chemotherapy, and surgical interventions, and how these impairments can be addressed with rehabilitation and community-based services.

Related to messaging, it is vital that advocacy efforts within an institution include discussions of the various benefits for the

---

• BOX 32.1 **Actions by a Healthcare Provider That May Negatively Affect a Person's Self-Advocacy**

1. Discouraging information seeking behavior and shared decision making by ignoring a person's question, giving an ambiguous answer, or even changing the topic.
2. Providing health information that is not culturally designed to attract or be relevant to racial, ethnic, or other populations.
3. Not prioritizing time for listening to and not encouraging the person to share their needs and to engage equally in decision making.
4. Not responding to different communication styles, perceptions, and preferences related to health decision making.
5. Lacking skills in cross-cultural communication.
6. Lacking a culturally congruent approach to patient-centered care.
7. Not providing professional interpretation services and carelessly proceeding with the provision of services despite a significant language barrier being present.
8. Not taking actions on behalf of the patient's stated needs because of falsely attributing adherence challenges to the individual traits of the person rather than to environmental and societal factors.

Created by April Gamble and Jena Colon.

institution and the specific communities that it serves. For example, it can be helpful to discuss how Onc R is primarily completed on an outpatient basis, which saves costs when compared to the cost of treatment received during inpatient rehabilitation and can potentially reduce readmission rates. Within institutions, oncologists and other healthcare specialists may focus on treating the disease without considering the PLWBC's perception of their QOL and daily struggles with functional limitations that may result from the treatments for their cancer.[38] Therefore, when crafting advocacy messages within an institution, the Onc R clinician is uniquely poised to increase awareness on this topic, which may contribute to changing the institution's processes related to services that promote rehabilitation and QOL.

Lastly, advocating for institutions to contribute to research is especially important as advances in research have led to earlier detection of cancer and improved treatments. According to the American Society of Clinical Oncology, the 5-year survival rate has increased from less than 63% in the 1960s to 99% today with breast involvement alone.[73] The success of research and advocacy efforts in prolonging survival has paved the path for high-quality care that reflects the PLWBC's priority for survival and QOL. This has inspired researchers, PLWBCs, and healthcare providers to advocate for enhanced interventions related to mitigating treatment-related adverse effects alongside disease-directed treatments as a core part of care. When advocating for institutions to contribute to research, it is vital to embody a justice-centered approach. Justice-centered research involves working alongside communities that are historically marginalized to ensure that they direct research agendas and that their needs, experiences, and preferences are reflected in the research that will ultimately be utilized to direct changes in care within an institution and beyond.

Patient Navigators

An important model of care that can be implemented within healthcare institutions is the use of patient navigators (PNs). Onc R clinicians can utilize their positions within institutions to advocate for integrating PNs into the cancer care continuum to improve patient outcomes and reduce health disparities for persons impacted by cancer. Patient navigation is a barrier-focused intervention where PNs work alongside individual patients to eliminate any barrier they encounter when attempting to access or benefit from health services. The goal of PN services is to ensure that everyone has equitable opportunities to benefit from timely, quality, coordinated, multidisciplinary, and patient-centered care. Barriers that PNs respond to can be related to a variety of systemic factors including financial, communication, medical system, informational, and emotional/fear.[74]

The literature reveals that PN models of care are very diverse as each model is designed based on the: (1) specific needs, cultures, and preferences of the particular community it is serving; (2) the infrastructure and services of the healthcare system; (3) the barriers that persons face; (4) the resources available within the community and healthcare system; and (5) the specific outcome of interest.[75] Although each PN's role is dependent on the aforementioned variables, the literature reveals that PNs often perform the following: (1) bridging language and cultural differences between patients and providers; (2) providing emotional and social support; (3) providing culturally relevant education; (4) trouble-shooting with the patient and their family as problems arise; (5) arranging transportation, (6) performing appointment reminders and follow-ups via telephone calls; (7) hosting educational events within community spaces; (8) arranging and/or performing interpreting services; (9) facilitating referrals to support services in the healthcare system and the community; (10) mobilizing financial assistance; (11) offering psychosocial support and advocacy; and (12) coordinating multidisciplinary services and appointments.[75–77]

Persons that serve as PNs can be lay persons or a range of healthcare professionals including nurses and rehabilitation professionals. Lay PNs are persons without professional training and are ideally from the specific communities that experience health disparities within the healthcare system.[75] The lay PNs are often survivors of cancer, and in some contexts may be traditional healers within the community. They often receive on-the-job training to perform their responsibilities and work closely with case managers, patient advocates, or other support personnel. Lay PN programs should strive to match PLWBCs with PNs that align with their racial, ethnic, or cultural background.[76] Lay PNs from the community, rather than trained professional PNs, have greater potential to impact health disparities specific to systemic barriers that impact persons based on unearned disadvantages such as race, ethnicity, sexual preferences, culture, and religion.[76]

The literature is lacking in regard to the use of PNs to support people to access and benefit from Onc R.[59] In 2018, the first article was published describing the use of a professional "rehabilitation navigator" to support proactive functional assessment as well as working individually with patients to overcome barriers to rehabilitation services throughout the continuum of cancer care.[78] This article described that the rehabilitation navigator program serves to address: (1) the ongoing gap that traditional care pathways continue to have regarding identifying functional decline; (2) the making of referrals to Onc R services; and (3) patients' ability to access and benefit from those services to address their functional needs.

The literature is still emerging regarding best practice guidelines related to PN models of care, as well as the evidence for its cost-effectiveness and impact in various healthcare contexts, communities, and Onc R. However, various cancer care policies and best practice guidelines do recommend optimizing patient navigation models of care along the cancer care continuum, from diagnosis to survivorship, to improve patient and system outcomes and reduce health disparities.[74–76,78] The Onc R clinician can advocate for integrating models of patient navigation within a healthcare to promote all persons having access to and benefitting from Onc R services.

Advocacy Alongside Communities

The Onc R clinician is uniquely equipped to work alongside communities to advocate for equal access to and benefit from Onc R services, as well as community services and resources that promote physical health and functioning. Communities in this context can be defined in a variety of ways from geographical locations, such as a city, or as a group of persons self-united with a shared trait, history, or experience such as the LGBTQIA+ community. Due to the high prevalence of cancer, all communities inherently include persons that are impacted by cancer.

As described above, applying a justice-centered and community-oriented approach is essential to effectively conducting advocacy activities that result in just, meaningful, and sustainable changes. One approach for effectively mobilizing under the leadership of community members is to collaborate with community health workers (CHWs). The umbrella term *community health worker* denotes a variety of individuals, usually without formal education, that are selected, trained, and are working in the communities from which they self-identify as belonging to. Through a variety of activities and roles, CHWs serve to promote health and reduce health inequities within their communities.[78] There is robust evidence that CHWs can undertake actions that lead to improved health outcomes including cancer screening rates and levels of physical activity and exercise amongst cancer survivors.[79–81] If CHWs are not available, Onc R clinicians can also look to mobilize alongside community leaders, traditional healers, community groups, advocacy groups, or groups led by PLWBC.

Opportunities for Advocacy Within the Community

There are innumerable advocacy activities that an Onc R clinician can perform to support the health and physical functioning of members of a community. A few opportunities will be highlighted here.

Community-Based Exercise and Physical Activity Programs

The Onc R clinician is uniquely equipped to work alongside communities to advocate for, establish, and support sustainable community-based exercise and physical activity services for PLWBC. There is extensive evidence regarding the feasibility and impact of these community-based programs during and after cancer treatment (see Chapters 23 and 28). Many, if not most, communities lack exercise programs that can support the unique needs of PLWBCs. Extant research reveals some of the important considerations for ensuring the effectiveness, feasibility, and safety of community-based exercise, and physical activity programs include: (1) ensuring that persons from the community lead the design, implementation, and maintenance of the programs; (2) ensuring that programs are unique and based on the cultural and contextual needs of the participants; (3) ensuring capacity of providers to meet the distinct needs of persons impacted by cancer; (4) facilitating family members and other support persons to also participate; (5) proactively addressing social barriers like the embarrassment associated with cancer adverse effects such as urinary incontinence; (6) considering the use of technology to increase access to programs; and (7) purposefully addressing root causes that impact participant attendance like location, distance to travel, financial resources, available time, beliefs about exercise and readiness for exercise, and referral pathways.[82–84]

Education and Awareness Raising for Community Members

There is a general lack of knowledge available to PLWBCs regarding the adverse effects of cancer treatment, the benefit of physical activity, self-management strategies, available resources, and the role of Onc R.[16] Therefore, the Onc R clinician has a responsibility to provide educational information and to contribute to "awareness raising" campaigns regarding the topics about which they are uniquely informed. For example, it is a common misconception that following breast cancer, movement of the affected arm should be avoided as it causes or exacerbates lymphedema. Even though the evidence negates this, many people, including healthcare providers, continue to follow this harmful belief which contributes to reduced QOL and increased physical impairments. Additionally, after cancer treatment, people often feel that they should "just live with" debilitating long-term adverse effects of cancer treatment and not seek options for support, treatment, and management.[85] These are examples of individual health beliefs and practices that Onc R clinicians can work toward changing through community-wide educational efforts to contribute to improved health and functioning for all.

When delivering educational interventions at the community level, there must be established accountability mechanisms to ensure that all information that is delivered is accurate and unbiased. These mechanisms also ensure that the information provided does not omit negative research findings or unanticipated adverse effects so the interests of stakeholders like professional associations, advocacy groups, pharmaceutical companies, and medical technology manufacturers are protected.[56] All educational materials and activities should be developed and implemented alongside members of the community. This collaborative strategy will ensure that the preferences, values, and needs of the community members are prioritized and the resultant education and materials will effectively align to address these interests and meet their needs. Efforts should purposefully integrate traditional and cultural practices that strengthen physical, emotional, and social functioning and resiliency, but that may be not explored within research literature or be within the clinician's awareness.

Education and Increasing Awareness for Practicing Healthcare Professionals

PLWBCs have expressed frustration that the long-term adverse effects of cancer are not uniformly well understood by healthcare providers or framed as a chronic condition that requires an investment of resources. Furthermore, PLWBCs have reported that they frequently encounter the need to teach various healthcare providers about the adverse effects of cancer treatment(s), like lymphedema.[59] PLWBCs also report frustration with a lack of support and clear recommendations related to managing symptoms and adverse effects of cancer treatment.[65] These reports and the barriers to Onc R illustrate a great need for healthcare providers, including those not specifically working within the field of oncology, to increase their knowledge and skills related to the needs of PLWBC. Therefore, Onc R clinicians can educate healthcare professionals within their community, especially healthcare providers in communities that lack access to cancer specialists and cancer centers. Further, clinicians can align with educational institutions within their communities to increase content related to Onc R within various healthcare degree programs. Onc R clinicians can also use their positions of power and influence within healthcare systems to increase resources in communities to support relevant and community-centered practices of self-management and wellness.

Advocating at Subnational and National Levels via Legislation and Policy

The purpose of regulatory policymaking is to provide protection to healthcare consumers receiving services in their national or subnational (e.g., state, region, territory, province) jurisdiction. As Shoemaker[86] illustrated in the figure below for policy development, Walt and Gilson's Policy Analysis Triangle framework highlights additional factors such as social and political contexts, political processes, and primary stakeholders beyond just the policy content that can impact policy development, adoption, and implementation (Figure 32.3). The Policy Triangle framework helps explain how policy adoption and implementation attempts can fail and it also helps guide the development of new policymaking strategies.[86] Examples of policymaking strategies at subnational and national levels include: (1) patients, health care providers, and representatives from subnational-level organizations testifying in legislative hearings; (2) providing written testimony for legislative hearings; and (3) individual meetings with key legislators before

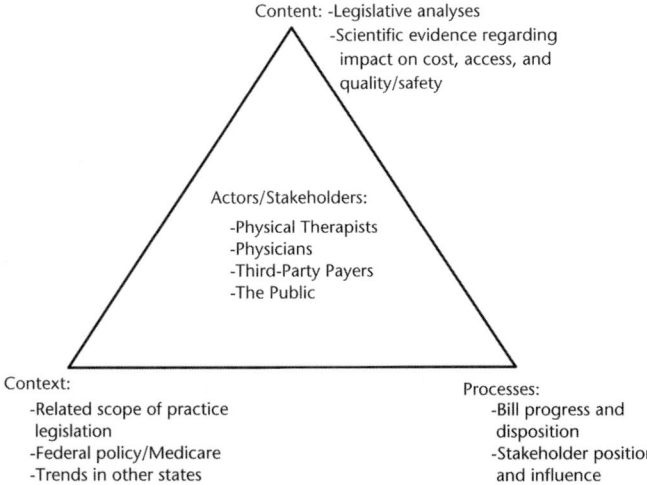

Content: -Legislative analyses
-Scientific evidence regarding
impact on cost, access, and
quality/safety

Actors/Stakeholders:

-Physical Therapists
-Physicians
-Third-Party Payers
-The Public

Context:
-Related scope of practice
legislation
-Federal policy/Medicare
-Trends in other states

Processes:
-Bill progress and
disposition
-Stakeholder position
and influence

• **Fig. 32.3** The Public Policy Triangle (Reprinted with permission from Shoemaker MJ. Direct consumer access to physical therapy in Michigan: challenges to policy adoption. *Phys Ther.* 2012;92(2):236–250.)

policies are formally presented to the legislators for consideration, debate, further legislative actions, and ultimately submitted for vote or tabled.

Limited evidence exists for the overall impact on a national level for legislation, policy, and advocacy in Onc R. There are, however, several historical examples of how legislation and advocacy played a role in recognizing the need to care for cancer patients with disabilities. The National Cancer Act of 1971 "declared cancer rehabilitation as an objective and directed funds to the development of training programs and research projects." Additionally, the National Cancer Institute sponsored its first National Cancer Rehabilitation Planning Conference in 1972 and identified key objectives for treatments of patients with cancer, including the optimization of physical functioning. There are also specific case examples from the field of physical therapy within the US that can be used to illustrate the power of advocating for legislation and policy change at the subnational and national level.

Case One: Utilizing Legislation and Policy to Increase Access

Direct access is the term describing the ability of a patient to go directly to a rehabilitation provider, including a PT, without a prescription or referral from a physician. Direct access plays a major role in Onc R, as PLWBCs learn to advocate for their own wellbeing and recognize they may benefit from Onc R as illustrated earlier in this chapter, even without a physician referral. PTs are trained to act as front-line providers for neuromusculoskeletal problems or movement disorders. They have the potential to help mitigate barriers to healthcare and decrease overall costs of expensive visits to emergency departments, unnecessary imaging, and delays in access to medical care after an acute injury. In 1973 the House of Delegates (HOD), as the decision-making body of the American Physical Therapy Association (APTA), resolved to establish the necessary "guidelines which stipulate the professional and ethical implications and responsibilities of a PT evaluation of patients without practitioner referral."[87] The HOD revised this resolution in 1978 to "devise a plan for the development of physical therapy practice (evaluation and treatment) independent of practitioner referral."[88] At that time, there were only two states

that did not require practitioner/physician referral. Therefore, the APTA began a direct access initiative to eliminate the physician referral requirement in all jurisdictions in the US.[86] Similar to the advancements in physical therapy practice and education in Onc R specialization, during that time there also were progressive changes in professional education standards to better prepare entry-level PTs to screen for the presence of medical disease and function as the patient's first point of contact with a healthcare provider in the healthcare system.[86] These advocacy efforts in advocacy have now resulted in all 50 states having some level of direct access to a PT without requiring a referral.

After achieving direct access to evaluate and treat patients without the need for gatekeepers, subsequent national advocacy efforts have focused on promoting appropriate payment for direct access services on state and local levels which have enabled better access to care both economically and without additional costs associated with a physician visit solely to obtain a referral to a PT. For this change to become permanent and legally recognized, advocacy was required to change the law at the state level as public health code. The scope of practice of any licensed health professional must follow the state's public health code. These regulatory policies are developed to protect persons receiving healthcare services in their state. Lawmakers work to develop and change policies within the public health code; therefore, they influence and determine the legal parameters within which healthcare providers can practice their professions.

This example illustrates how advocacy efforts often need to be directed at both national and subnational levels to allow for increased access to rehabilitation professionals for PLWBC. The example highlights the fact that direct access as a model of care can reduce systemic barriers to accessing and benefiting from rehabilitation services. For direct access for rehabilitation providers in the US, advocacy efforts were aimed at overcoming the long-standing misconception that only a physician can diagnose and develop a treatment plan for patients in need of rehabilitation care. This demonstrates how a major achievement was made possible by the process of clinicians being directly involved in advocacy and policymaking efforts.

Policymaking and legislative policies seek to achieve the ideal balance between diverse values, needs, and wants of its constituents and the potential consequences that may arise from whatever decision is made. The balance can often have conflicting potential outcomes and best practices can be difficult to discern. Regulatory policymaking is not free of special interest influence, but regardless of the strength of scientific evidence, nothing is enough to guide policymaking without political influence.[86] The following case example illustrates the challenges encountered with regulatory policy making across all of patient populations receiving rehabilitative services.

Case Two: How Policy Influences Patient-Centered Care

In the US, PTs in the state of Michigan have been licensed healthcare providers since 1965 because of Michigan Public Act (PA) 164. The initial scope of practice of physical therapy was restricted and not truly autonomous as it was specifically indicated to be performed under the prescription and direction of a physician. This is an example of how the specific language in every law makes a substantial difference in how a clinician may practice and what treatments they are permitted to provide to each patient. The word "direction" in this case can be defined as the PT following the instructions as written in the patient's referral—an example would be a referral for physical therapy stating the PT is to only use "ultrasound, hot pack, and massage" interventions. This does not allow for clinical decision-making or patient-centered care as the treating clinician does not have the autonomy to develop and deliver a service based on the expressed and ever-evolving needs and preferences of the patient. Nor does it reflect the advanced entry-level education that PTs in the US receive which equips them with the skills to effectively determine a plan of care. To address this challenge, the requirement for practice under the "direction" of a physician was removed because of Michigan PA 368 of 1978. Furthermore, advocacy efforts by clinicians were undertaken to change how physician referrals were to be interpreted by the PT and to what level the referral directed the care the patient was to receive during their individualized therapy sessions. Currently in the US, the most common standard referral for physical therapy now typically states "PT Eval and Treat." This example illustrates how policy and scope of practice can impact the care provided, which ultimately can reduce the effectiveness of care for persons receiving the service.

Education Regarding Public Advocacy

When considering the role of Onc R clinicians in policymaking and legislative advocacy efforts, it is essential to consider the influence of healthcare educational degree programs. The clinician has an important role in regard to advocating for legislation and policy change. However, the importance of public policy and legislation is not often emphasized in the curriculum of entry-level educational degree programs for healthcare professionals; but it is of great importance to students, practicing clinicians, and the persons that clinicians serve. Limited evidence exists illustrating the importance of and advocacy as a major part of didactic education for various healthcare professionals. But many students of rehabilitation degree programs have reported learning the importance of advocacy with and for persons with disabilities as part of their core curriculum working in both national as well as international arenas.[89] Involvement in advocacy efforts may contribute to not only professional growth, but also professional identity as rehabilitation clinicians. Benefits of involvement in advocacy include the development of leadership skills and a broader perspective of the factors that impact patient care, thereby allowing for a more comprehensive team-oriented approach to improve patient outcomes. Research shows that clinical internships/rotations increase clinical competence, promote socialization within the profession, foster the development of a positive self-image, and promote professional confidence.[89] The development of the ability to communicate confidently and with cultural competence is of paramount importance when striving for equitable and justice-centered rehabilitation services. Advocacy and the ability to influence change is a necessary skill and successfully advocating for a patient's access to care can truly make the difference between survival and surviving well.

For Onc R clinicians that seek to advocate for policy change, developing lasting relationships with their legislators and decision makers is vitally important. In many political systems, this is an ongoing endeavor as specific decision makers do not remain in their elected office or appointed positions indefinitely. As new terms of office begin, new persons are often introduced for each district or jurisdiction. The key to understanding how one individual can make a difference lies within the common thread all decision makers share regardless of how long they have been in office or whether they function at a national, subnational, or local level—the desire to make a positive impact in the lives of their constituents.

For Onc R clinicians that may not desire to be intimately involved in advocacy at the policy making level, it is still essential to recognize their role as a constituent within their subnational and national governmental systems. A constituent is described as a person who is represented by a member of government or government official. As an example, a citizen of the US has the right to vote for and ultimately elect a member of government who best represents their interests when voting on public policy and changes in law. An individual clinician advocating for their patients is also a constituent—a voter who may have voted to get this politician elected and may vote for them again. The constituents are truly the reason why elected officials are in office. The protection of the wellbeing of their constituents is one of the main drivers behind every hearing they attend and policy they vote for, against, or abstain from voting. An individual Onc R clinician *can* take responsibility for engaging with their political system in a manner that promotes health justice.

Individual clinicians advocate in so many ways that they may not even consider their actions as advocacy; writing letters of medical necessity, appealing insurance denials to both public and private insurers, and even contacting insurers by phone to complete necessary authorization requests for the appropriate number of treatment sessions. While clinicians often regard this as a "necessary evil" and simply a part of a patient's episode of care, many do not immediately consider this to be advocacy when, in effect, it is. To take this example one step further, a clinician who feels passionate about fighting the undue administrative burdens that often lead to delays in vital healthcare services may choose to engage their professional associations at both the subnational and national levels. This can be done both before and after submitting an official complaint directly to the insurer. Within the context of the US and other healthcare systems that rely on insurance mechanisms, professional organizations can help facilitate meetings with private insurance companies on the behalf of clinicians and will take the concerns and requests directly to insurance policy decision-makers. Providing this type of vital information to both local and national associations only helps to strengthen advocacy efforts for all patients. Effective changes in an insurer's policies as a result of these combined efforts help promote improved patient outcomes and drive down overall healthcare costs.

Advocacy on a Global Scale

To advocate at a global level, it is essential for the Onc R clinician to contribute to social mobilization efforts to achieve large scale change.[90] Social mobilization aims to increase visibility of an issue on a global level while simultaneously creating real change in subnational and national policies and within the structures of governments and healthcare systems.[91,92] Social mobilization can be described as an inclusive and collective societal action where all of society is mobilized to educate, raise awareness, engage, and advocate for improvements.[91] Social mobilization has been centered in many health equity initiatives around the world ranging from vaccination programs, infectious disease responses, and prevention and control initiatives of noncommunicable disease and cancers.[91–93] Global events like World Cancer Day and Cancer Awareness months are examples of global social mobilization efforts related to cancer.

Little has been reported regarding social mobilization efforts specific to rehabilitation or Onc R. However, exploration of the social mobilization literature related to disability and cancer prevention and control reveals key principles and practical strategies that can be applied (Table 32.6). Specific to the physical health and functioning needs of PLWBC, it is advantageous to integrate this topic into a current global advocacy platform like general cancer survivorship and/or the breast cancer movement.[91]

Analysis of the breast cancer movement reveals that the culture of action embodied within social mobilization efforts can inadvertently use narratives and take actions that actually replicate and maintain systems that create health inequity and barriers to cancer care and survivorship.[93] To avoid this, social mobilization efforts should be mindfully centered on inclusive and just cultures of actions. This centering serves to: (1) elevate the voices, experiences, and needs of all affected communities and especially those that are marginalized; (2) affect change in the root causes of health inequities; and (3) recognize that health and function are basic human rights.[91–93]

The literature also highlights the importance of allocating time and resources as well as building the capacity of PLWBC and "patient organizations" and elevating their contributions."[91] PLWBCs must be intimately involved in policy-making and high-level decision-making and should also be positioned to lead social mobilization efforts. Examples of unique ways that PLWBCs can lead social mobilization efforts include: (1) working with the media to mobilize public opinion and demand change; (2) serving as the "watchdog" of the political and healthcare system; (3) sharing experiences to reduce stigmas and inspire others to seek and demand services; and (4) advocating for improvements in attitudes, knowledge, practice, policy, systems, and services.[91]

The Onc R clinician has knowledge and experiences that can contribute to global social mobilization efforts. As discussed above, however, one must apply principles of justice-centered and community-oriented advocacy. History reveals additional lessons learned regarding global advocacy efforts—including that it is essential to not center the agenda, practices, and values of one homogenous group. For example, breast cancer advocacy efforts in the US in the 1970s were primarily rooted in the values and experiences of white high-income women. The efforts

TABLE 32.6	Elements of Successful Social Mobilization[91–94]
Establish sustainable multisectoral partnerships that integrate the following:	• Collaboration between all actors including governments, private sector, academia, patient groups, patient organizations, community-based organizations, professional societies, media, and others. • Emphasize working alongside established networks and community groups • Establish a nonhierarchical structure. • Clearly define mutually beneficial goals, a consensus on solutions, and convincing reasons to act. • Maintain diverse participation and leadership with opportunities for all to contribute different skills and resources to achieve the shared goals. • Establish a platform for multiple, but interrelated topics to be promoted (e.g., the historical integration of the promotion of breast cancer and cervical cancer screening into HIV/AIDS programs).[72] • Maintain organized processes, policies, and plans with reliable accountability mechanisms.[71]
Inform and engage a large number of people across many regions and sectors with a community-based and culturally relevant approach	• Recognize, embrace, and empower the diverse range of social mobilization strategies used by communities. • Recognize that not all communities will communicate, act, and mobilize in the same way so a range of different methods should be employed. • Center efforts on appropriate and community-oriented evidence, experience, traditional and community approaches to health and functioning, outcomes, and monitoring and evaluation tools. • Engage with each community, its leaders, and its champions to identify the issues the community perceives are important and their views on specific issues. • Engage with each community to ensure the use of culturally and contextually appropriate, effective, and inclusive approaches. • Utilize relevant technology and social media to share advocacy messages and mobilize grassroots support.
Ensure sustainability	• Mobilize sustainable financial resources. • Include advocacy within the mission of healthcare organizations so that resources and technical expertise will be meaningfully allocated to sustain social mobilization efforts.

Apply key theories of social mobilization including the following:	• The biopsychosocial understanding of how a community interacts with its social, economic, and political environment and the acknowledgment that social mobilization efforts will vary across cultures, countries, and contexts.
	• The understanding that participation in collective action is a physical, emotional, cognitive, mental, and social experience.
	• The application of the logics of oppression and health disparities in relation to social mobilization.[50]
	• De-center the experiences of the normative majority or one homogeneous group (e.g., Western practices, white and/or high-income communities, etc.)—rather actively center a range of diverse experiences, voices, needs, and solutions so that all can be compelled to engage in social mobilization activities.
	• The "Nothing Without Us" model which acknowledges the lived experience of oppression for people with disabilities and health conditions and demands the following:
	  • self-representation and control over the resources needed to live a decent life
	  • recognition that the experiential knowledge of the community is essential for making decisions that affect their lives
	  • all policies should be decided with full and direct participation of members of the group(s) affected by that policy
	  • disability and health conditions are a political and social condition that requires political and social solutions[94]

Created by Jena Colon and April Gamble.

TABLE 32.7	**Additional Resources for Advocacy**
Diagnosis-specific cancer advocacy and support groups	• National Comprehensive Cancer Network • https://www.nccn.org/patientresources/patient-resources/support-for-patients-caregivers/advocacy-and-support-groups

Selected professional networks to explore for advocacy opportunities	• International Physical Therapists for HIV/AIDS, Oncology, Hospice and Palliative Care (IPT-HOPE)
	  • https://world.physio/subgroups/hiv-aids-oncology-hospice-palliative
	• Critical Physiotherapy Network
	  • https://criticalphysio.net

Selected physical therapy advocacy networks specific to the United States	• American Physical Therapy Association
	  • https://www.apta.org/advocacy
	• Student Advocacy
	  • https://www.apta.org/for-students/student-involvement#advocacy
	• State Level Chapters within the United States https://aptaapps.apta.org//componentconnection/chaptersandsections.aspx
	• APTA's Global Health Special Interest Group
	  • https://www.aptahpa.org/page/GlobalHealthSIGAbout

Occupational therapy advocacy	• World Federation of Occupational Therapists
	  • https://wfot.org/programmes/leadership-advocacy
	• American Occupational Therapy Association
	  • https://www.aota.org/AboutAOTA/Membership/Advocacy.aspx

Speech therapy and speech language pathology	• Curated international resources by the American Speech and Hearing Association • https://www.asha.org/members/international/international-professional-associations/
US legislative process	• United States Government Resource Page • https://www.usa.gov/how-laws-are-made

Created by Jena Colon and April Gamble.

emphasized increasing the availability of breast prostheses, wigs, and breast reconstruction surgery to enable women to conform to the majority culture's norms related to feminine appearance and beauty.[56] This emphasis was included in global social mobilization activities and therefore had a wide-reaching impact. However, not only were these values and approaches not always culturally or contextually relevant outside of the US, but they also did not consistently capture the diverse values and experiences of women impacted by breast cancer within the US.

Furthermore, various stakeholders, including healthcare professionals and companies that profit from healthcare services, pharmaceuticals, and cosmetics, continue to collude together for their mutual advantage rather than aiming to achieve just opportunities for health and function for all PLWBC.[54] This has significant negative consequences on PLWBC and further intensifies health inequities. For example, cancer survivorship advocacy efforts often promote the belief that expert professionals and pharmaceutical and beauty products, especially from high-income Western countries, are the superior method for maintaining physical functioning and optimal QOL following cancer. This narrative undermines the ability of lay people and communities to deal with challenges in day-to-day life and to self-manage side effects of treatment. Critics of social mobilization efforts have described that cancer-related global advocacy should center on informed decision making, social justice, root causes of health inequity, public policy change, and primary prevention.[56]

Conclusion

The Onc R clinician is uniquely positioned to advocate at multiple levels of the healthcare system with the aim of all persons impacted by cancer benefiting from Onc R and community wellness services that support optimal health and functioning. Justice-centered and community-led advocacy efforts have the potential to drive sustainable changes to reduce health disparities and improve the health and wellness of all communities. Advocacy truly begins with education; education of ourselves, our patients, our providers, and our legislators (Table 32.7). As you begin to realize what advocacy means to you as an individual, you can reflect on ways in which you are already advocating for persons impacted by cancer and ways you can further make a difference in the lives of PLWBCs. It is recognized that each clinician has their own unique strengths, skills, and interest. Onc R clinicians are urged to explore what advocacy activities align with their own unique attributes and join the movement to work toward a world where all people thrive beyond cancer treatment.

Critical Research Needs

- Evidence for the gaps, needs, and effective strategies related to advocacy, legislative policy, and reimbursement specific to Onc R.
- Evidence-based national standards and advocacy action plans for working toward justice-centered Onc R.
- Current state of oncologic rehabilitation services in the US and around the world, including evidence of inequitable distribution of services and the factors contributing to this inequity specific to Onc R.
- Evidence-based best practice guidelines for implementing interdisciplinary teams for Onc R, for describing the need for cancer rehabilitation, and for establishing the role of the PT in patient advocacy.

Case Study

This case study is based on the experiences of one of the authors in working alongside communities impacted by cancer in the Kurdistan Region of Iraq.

The context:

Within this public healthcare system, the emphasis for persons impacted by cancer is on survival and the provision of physician-directed cancer treatment. Disparities in access to and benefit from cancer treatment exist and are magnified in persons that live in rural areas, people that are refugees or displaced, older persons, persons with low income, and women. Currently, in outpatient rehabilitation clinics, there are some people accessing rehabilitation services postcancer treatment. The majority are women living beyond breast cancer that present with upper extremity issues, lymphedema, and persistent infections. Across the healthcare system, access to skilled Onc R is almost nonexistent with the documented barriers including lack of trained healthcare staff, lack of supportive infrastructure, and lack of awareness of the role of rehabilitation within the medical and lay community.

Currently, there are regional standards for cancer treatment practices, but these standards do not integrate rehabilitation. Within the last few years, regionally there has been a social mobilization effort led by the health authority and healthcare professionals to increase public awareness of cancer, improve rates of cancer screenings, and decrease the stigma related to cancer. However, rehabilitation and QOL initiatives have not yet been integrated into these efforts. In the community, there is a group of women impacted by breast cancer that self-organize to engage in physical activity outings and provide peer support to those affected by breast cancer. Recently, a physiotherapist has been selected to sit on the health authority's cancer board which directs the cancer care within the public healthcare system.

When considering the advocacy efforts that could contribute to just and equitable access to Onc R services, here are some vital questions to reflect on. The aim is to engage in advocacy efforts that center justice and that mobilize under the leadership of persons impacted by cancer.

- How can I contribute to advocacy within my context? Consider your positions of power and privilege, available time, resources, knowledge, strengths, personal style, and interests.
- How can I learn more about the relevant public policy efforts, pathways to support public policy, who is involved in this, how persons impacted by cancer are informing policy, and opportunities for me to contribute?
- How can we as healthcare professionals mobilize under the leadership of the community of persons impacted by cancer?
- How can we as healthcare professionals make sure that the needs and desires of people impacted by cancer are the focus of our advocacy efforts rather than centering our needs and preferences as Onc R clinicians?
- How could rehabilitation, QOL, and the diverse needs and experiences of persons impacted by cancer be integrated and elevated within the ongoing social mobilization efforts?
- What are the barriers that may contribute to equitable access to and benefit from Onc R services within our specific context and health system? What are the root causes of these barriers in terms of social, cultural, political, environmental, and economic contributors and how can they be eliminated?
- What are culturally and contextually effective approaches for advocacy?

- Considering the presence of health disparities related to cancer treatment that are already present within the healthcare system, how may these disparities be replicated in our efforts to establish Onc R services? How can we approach the clinical service delivery to minimize this?
- Could PN or Community Health Workers be integrated into the cancer care and Onc R service delivery model?
- How can the advocacy efforts be measured to evaluate the impact and inform ongoing efforts?
- What accountability mechanisms can be put in place to ensure the key principles of justice-centered advocacy are followed and to identify and address health disparities and injustices?

Here are some examples of advocacy efforts that would be relevant within this context and that strive to center justice and the community.

Advocating Alongside the Person Living With and Beyond Cancer:

As most PLWBCs that you see in your clinical setting are women impacted by breast cancer, you decide to focus your initial advocacy efforts in this area. You recognize that your knowledge, skills, and abilities should be enhanced so that you can provide high quality rehabilitation services for this group. Therefore, you create a personal development plan that includes participating in an online course, reading resources, and establishing a mentor that has significant clinical experience in this area.

Based on the needs and experiences expressed by the women impacted by breast cancer, you also work to create some specific services in your clinic. These include: (1) establishing a feasible referral pathway for infection response and management; (2) establishing a system to follow-up with each patient on a regular basis to ensure she is able to access and benefit from the resources for persistent infections and subsequently offering support to navigate any barriers faced in health system; (3) working with a group of women impacted by breast cancer to develop an educational handout related to infection, lymphedema, and upper extremity issues; and (4) integrating this handout alongside education during individual treatment sessions that you deliver.

Advocacy Within the Healthcare Institution:

Based on what persons impacted by cancer have shared with you, you recognize that one barrier to people accessing rehabilitation during and after cancer treatment is a lack of referral pathways. Therefore, you want to engage with your healthcare institution to establish screening tools and referral pathways for rehabilitation from cancer treatment services. You start with working with a few interested colleagues to host a series of healthcare forums where healthcare professionals and persons living with and beyond cancer share experiences centered on QOL and function. From this, a coalition organically forms that includes healthcare professionals and persons impacted by cancer that want to work together to implement contextually and culturally effective screening tools and referral pathways from cancer treatment services to rehabilitation services. Over time this coalition is also able to: (1) work with the health authority and institution to allocate resources to support sustainable referrals pathways and rehabilitation services; (2) establish lay PNs within the cancer care service and train them to support referrals to rehabilitation; and (3) provide regional continuing education opportunities for rehabilitation professionals to equip them with knowledge and skills specific to Onc R.

Advocacy Alongside Communities:

You are aware of the group of women impacted by breast cancer that have self-organized their own peer support group and activities. But you do not have a relationship with them, or any others impacted by cancer except within the context of providing rehabilitation treatment to some. You know that it could cause harm to insert yourself into this community with the assumption that you know what is best. Therefore rather than focusing on delivering advocacy activities in this community, you approach this group of women and explore ways to create regular opportunities to engage with this community, build relationships, and listen and understand their experiences, needs, and their ways of approaching advocacy. As you engage with them for many months, you often find yourself feeling like you are not doing enough. But you try to stay focused on your aim to mobilize under the leadership of the community rather than directing the activities from your position of power as a healthcare professional. After 9 months of regular connection with this group of women, they ask you to contribute to a peer support event that they are organizing. They ask you to work with one of the organizers to help her better understand the role of physical activity during and after cancer treatment so that she can present the information to the attendees. You work alongside this woman to offer your knowledge while ensuring that she decides the most culturally effective way to deliver the information during the event. You do not get publicly recognized for your effort. But you feel energized as you witness this group of persons impacted by cancer leading their own advocacy and community awareness activities. You recognize that your role is to stay connected to them and contribute to their efforts as they invite you to do so.

Advocating at Subnational and National Levels via Legislation and Policy:

You do not have any experience working within public policy, so you feel nervous and unsure about how to approach this. You decide that a good first step is to meet with the PT that has been selected to sit on the health authority's cancer board which directs the cancer care within the public healthcare system. In this meeting,

you start to understand the processes of legislation and policy within your context and different ways as a constituent you can contribute to policy making. During this meeting, the PT expresses that she is trying to figure out how to best use her position to push for policies that reflect the needs of persons impacted by cancer, including QOL and rehabilitation. One idea that you both think may be helpful is to establish a community advisory board to inform her and the cancer care board of the needs of the community. You do not have experience with this type of activity, but you know colleagues that do. Therefore, you offer to support this initiative by connecting the PT to your experienced colleagues, encouraging people impacted by cancer to join the coalition, and participating as an active member of the coalition.

Advocacy on a Global Scale:

Through online research, attending events, and meeting with organizers, you learn more about the ongoing social mobilization efforts in your region related to cancer care. You observe that these efforts are effectively aligned with global events like World Cancer Day. You also observe that everything is directed by the health authority and healthcare professionals. This results in the voices and experiences of healthcare providers being elevated rather than people affected by cancer. You also observe that the focus is on survival, with no consideration for thriving and functioning during and after cancer. You recognize that this way of approaching social mobilization is causing harm and further health injustices. You are not in a position of power to influence this initiative within the health authority. So, you consider raising your observations with the newly formed cancer board coalition that you are participating on and with the group of women self-organizing peer support and advocacy activities. You hope that through raising this with these groups, changes can be catalyzed so that people impacted by cancer take a leadership role in the region's social mobilization efforts.

Review Questions

Reader can find the correct answers and rationale in the back of the book.

1. Which of the following does not accurately describe health equity and justice?
   A. Attainment of the highest level of health for all people
   B. Societal efforts to address historical and contemporary injustices
   C. Developing services based on equality as everyone benefits from the same support
   D. Providing different supports and resources so everyone has the same opportunities for health and function

2. Which of the following is not an evidence-based example of how barriers contributing to the prevalence of cancer-related disability are magnified within populations that are historically marginalized, like BIPOC?
   A. Greater prevalence of and more severe physical functioning limitations in African American and other BIPOC breast cancer survivors in comparison to white counterparts
   B. Less effective pain management treatments in persons from BIPOC communities when compared to white counterparts
   C. Lack of Onc R providers within a community that have similar racial/ethnic identities and experiences as the community that is accessing the service

   D. Women receive more and better medical treatment for pain control than men and have better clinical outcomes because they engage in greater self-advocacy

3. Which of the following is not a key principle that should inform the practice of justice-centered advocacy?
   A. We each recognize and take responsibility for our own positions of privilege, power, and race and our role in upholding systems of oppression that create health inequities
   B. We work toward eliminating root causes of inequity in solidarity with persons and communities that experience the impact of health injustices
   C. We work to primarily elevate the "expert" role of oncology clinicians so that we can have the positions of power to aide persons impacted cancer
   D. The root causes of why some do not access or get equal benefits from rehabilitation services are social, cultural, political, environmental, economic, and systemic as opposed to an individual's behavior or biology

4. Which of the following is not true regarding professional-oriented advocacy and community-oriented advocacy?
   A. Community-oriented advocacy, within the scope of Onc R, can be defined as working under the leadership of and in collaboration with persons impacted by cancer to work toward the goals and needs that they articulate
   B. The risk of contributing to health disparities is lower when engaging in professional-oriented advocacy

C. If professional-oriented advocacy or community-oriented advocacy is **not** rooted in a personal awareness of privilege and the clinician's role in contributing to disparities, then efforts performed even with the best intentions will only contribute to further disparity

D. Effective and nonharmful community-oriented advocacy can only occur when the community directly invites the clinician to support their efforts and the clinician mobilizes under their leadership

5. Which of the following is not accurate or evidence-based regarding self-advocacy?

A. Impactful self-advocacy relies on an availability of resources in the community that provide options for relevant emotional, tangible, and informational support

B. A lack of self-advocacy behaviors is likely to be the only reason why there are poorer clinical outcomes for persons, so coaching persons to be better self-advocates will always mitigate health inequities and result in increased access to and benefits from services

C. It is hypothesized that oncology clinicians can work with people impacted by cancer to develop skills that enhance the effectiveness of self-advocacy, but the evidence-based recommendations for this are almost nonexistent at this time

D. For a person to engage in self-advocacy, it requires internal resources including personal awareness and an openness to try new experiences, as well as learned skills in self-reflection, communication, problem solving, and information seeking

6. Which of the following is not one of the three key areas that Parikh et al. proposed can drive effective QOL initiatives within healthcare institutions?

A. Clinical practice
B. Financial planning
C. Messaging
D. Research

7. Which of the following is not accurate or evidence-based regarding the role and impact of PNs?

A. The goal of PN services is that everyone has equitable opportunities to benefit from timely, quality, coordinated, multidisciplinary, and patient-centered care

B. Barriers that PNs respond to can be related to a variety of systemic factors including financial, communication, medical system, informational, and emotional/fear

C. Lay PNs from the community, rather than trained professional PNs, have greater potential to impact health dis-

parities specific to systemic barriers that impact persons based on unearned disadvantages such as race, ethnicity, sexual preferences, culture, and religion

D. Specific to Onc R services, it is not the role of the PN to support timely referrals to Onc R services to prevent or minimize functional decline

8. Which of the following is a potential impact on student outcomes when integrating knowledge and skills related to policymaking and legislative advocacy within curriculums of healthcare educational degree programs?

A. Development of leadership skills
B. Development of a broader perspective of the factors that impact patient care, thereby allowing for a more comprehensive team-oriented approach
C. Decreased competence related to clinical skills and patient care
D. Improved skills to successfully advocate alongside a patient with the aim of increasing opportunities for persons to access and benefit from rehabilitation and community services

9. Which of the following is not a key element for successful social mobilization efforts related to advocacy on a global scale?

A. Maintain diverse participation and leadership with opportunities for all to contribute different skills and resources to achieve the shared goals
B. Emphasize that all communities should communicate, act, and mobilize in the same way
C. Recognize that disability and health conditions are a political and social condition that requires political and social solutions
D. Include advocacy within the mission of healthcare organizations so that resources and technical expertise will be meaningfully allocated to sustain social mobilization efforts

10. In the US and beyond, clinicians may advocate for their patients in a variety of ways discussed throughout this chapter. Professional organizations such as the American Physical Therapy Association can help facilitate patient advocacy by:

A. Providing financial resources to patients in need of assistance with healthcare costs
B. Providing financial resources to clinicians to subsidize the cost of providing rehabilitative services to patients
C. Offer legal advice to patients who are suing for medical malpractice
D. Facilitate meetings with private insurance on behalf of clinicians and voice concerns/requests directly to the insurer

References

1. Code of Ethics for the Physical Therapist. www.apta.org/ethics. Accessed July 21, 2020.
2. World Health Organization. Health promotion strategies. https://www.who.int/health-topics/health-promotion. Accessed April 14, 2021.
3. Okumura JM, Saunders M, Rehm RS. The role of health advocacy in transitions from pediatric to adult care for children with special health care needs: bridging families, provider and community services. *J Pediatr Nurs*. 2015;30(5):714–723.
4. Segesten K, Fagring A. Patient advocacy: an essential part of quality nursing care. *Int Nurs Rev*. 1996;43(5):142–144.
5. Michael L. Street-level bureaucracy: dilemmas of the individual in public services New York: Russell Sage Foundation, 1980. *Polit Soc*. 1980;10(1):116. doi:10.1177/003232928001000113.
6. Babu AS, Lopez-Jimenez F, Thomas RJ, et al. Advocacy for outpatient cardiac rehabilitation globally. *BMC Health Serv Res*. 2016;16(1):1–9. doi:10.1186/s12913-016-1658-1661.
7. Stout NL, Santa Mina D, Lyons KD, Robb K, Silver JK. A systematic review of rehabilitation and exercise recommendations in oncology guidelines. *CA Cancer J Clin*. 2021;71(2):149–175. doi:10.3322/caac.21639.
8. Albreht T, Borrás Andrés JM, Dalmas M, et al. Chapter 7: Survivorship and rehabilitation: policy recommendations for quality improvement in cancer survivorship and rehabilitation in EU member

states. In: Albreht T, Kiasuwa R, Marc Van den Bulcke M, eds. *European Guide on Quality Improvement in Comprehensive Cancer Control*. National Institute of Public Health; 2017. https://cancercontrol.eu/archived/guide-landing-page/index.html.

9. Silver JK, Stout NL, Fu JB, Pratt-Chapman M, Haylock PJ, Sharma R. The state of cancer rehabilitation in the United States. *J Cancer Rehabil*. 2018;1:1–8.

10. Sung H, Ferlay J, Siegel RL, et al. Global Cancer Statistics 2020: GLOBOCAN estimates of incidence and mortality worldwide for 36 cancers in 185 countries. *CA Cancer J Clin*. 2021 May;71(3):209–249.

11. American Cancer Society. Cancer Treatment & Survivorship Facts & Figures 2019–2021. https://www.cancer.org/content/dam/cancer-org/research/cancer-facts-and-statistics/cancer-treatment-and-survivorship-facts-and-figures/cancer-treatment-and-survivorship-facts-and-figures-2019-2021.pdf. Accessed May 21, 2021.

12. Stout NL, Silver JK, Raj VS, et al. Toward a national initiative in cancer rehabilitation: recommendations from a subject matter expert group. *Arch Phys Med Rehabil*. 2016;97(11):2006–2015.

13. Pergolotti M, Williams GR, Campbell C, Munoz LA, Muss HB. Occupational therapy for adults with cancer: why it matters. *Oncologist*. 2016;21(3):314–319.

14. Cheville AL, Troxel AB, Basford JR. Prevalence and treatment patterns of physical impairments in patients with metastatic breast cancer. *J Clin Oncol*. 2008;26:2621–2629.

15. Cheville AL, Beck LA, Petersen TL. The detection and treatment of cancer-related functional problems in an outpatient setting. *Support Care Cancer*. 2009;17:61–67.

16. Cheville AL, Kornblith AB, Basford JR. An examination of the causes for the underutilization of rehabilitation services among people with advanced cancer. *Am J Phys Med Rehabil*. 2011;90(Suppl. 1):S27–S37.

17. Holm V, Hansen DG, Johansen C. Participation in cancer rehabilitation and unmet needs: a population-based cohort study. *Support Care Cancer*. 2012;20:2913–2924.

18. Hansen DG, Larsen PV, Holm LV. Association between unmet needs and quality of life of cancer patients: a population-based study. *Acta Oncol*. 2013;52:391–399.

19. Lehmann JF, DeLisa JA, Warren CG. Cancer rehabilitation: assessment of need, development, and evaluation of a model of care. *Arch Phys Med Rehabil*. 1978;59:410–419.

20. Movsas SB, Chang VT, Tunkel RS. Rehabilitation needs of an inpatient medical oncology unit. *Arch Phys Med Rehabil*. 2003;84:1642–1646.

21. Pergolotti M, Deal AM, Lavery J. The prevalence of potentially modifiable functional deficits and the subsequent use of occupational and physical therapy by older adults with cancer. *J Geriatr Oncol*. 2015;6:194–201.

22. Ross L, Petersen MA, Johnsen AT. Are different groups of cancer patients offered rehabilitation to the same extent? A report from the population-based study "The Cancer Patient's World". *Support Care Cancer*. 2012;20:1089–1100.

23. Söderback I, Paulsson EH. A needs assessment for referral to occupational therapy. Nurses' judgment in acute cancer care. *Cancer Nurs*. 1997;20:267–273.

24. Veloso AG, Sperling C, Holm LV. Unmet needs in cancer rehabilitation during the early cancer trajectory: a nationwide patient survey. *Acta Oncol*. 2013;52:372–381.

25. World Health Organization. Human Rights and Health; 2017. https://www.who.int/news-room/fact-sheets/detail/human-rights-and-health Accessed May 21.

26. Office of Disease Prevention and Health Promotion, Healthy People 2020. Disparities. https://www.healthypeople.gov/2020/about/foundation-health-measures/Disparities. Accessed April 14, 2021.

27. World Health Organization. Social determinants of health. https://www.who.int/health-topics/social-determinants-of-health. Accessed May 21, 2021.

28. American Public Health Association. Better health through equity. https://www.apha.org/~/media/files/pdf/topics/equity/equity_stories.ashx. Accessed April 14, 2021.

29. World Health Organization. Global action plan. https://www.who.int/sdg/global-action-plan. Accessed April 14, 2021.

30. World Health Organization. Rehabilitation 2030—a call for action. Meeting Report; 2017. https://www.who.int/disabilities/care/Rehab2030MeetingReport2.pdf. Accessed April 14, 2021.

31. Welsh Assembly Government. National Standards for Rehabilitation of Adult Cancer Patients. United Kingdom National Health Service. http://www.wales.nhs.uk/sites3/Documents/322/National_Standards_for_Rehabilitation_of_Adult_Cancer_Patients_2010.pdf. Published 2010. Accessed April 14, 2021.

32. Cheville AL, Kornblith AB, Basford JR. An examination of the causes for the underutilization of rehabilitation services among people with advanced cancer. *Am J Phys Med Rehabil*. 2011;90(suppl 5). doi:10.1097/PHM.0b013e31820be3be.

33. Alfano CM, Leach CR, Smith TG, et al. Equitably improving outcomes for cancer survivors and supporting caregivers: a blueprint for care delivery, research, education, and policy. *CA Cancer J Clin*. 2019;69(1):35–49.

34. Raj VS, Balouch J, Norton JH. Cancer rehabilitation education during physical medicine and rehabilitation residency: preliminary data regarding the quality and quantity of experiences. *Am J Phys Med Rehabil*. 2014;93(5):445–452.

35. McCartney A, Butler C, Acreman S. Exploring access to rehabilitation services from allied health professionals for patients with primary high-grade brain tumours. *Palliat Med*. 2011;25(8):788–796.

36. Kristiansen M, Adamsen L, Piil K, Halvorsen I, Nyholm N, Hendriksen C. A three-year national follow-up study on the development of community-level cancer rehabilitation in Denmark. *Scand J Public Health*. 2019;47(5):511–518.

37. Sayyari S, Kin B. *Access to Oncology Physical Rehabilitation Services in British Columbia*. University of British Columbia; 2017. doi:10.14288/1.0362580.

38. McEwen S, Rodriguez AM, Martino R, et al. "I didn't actually know there was such a thing as rehab": survivor, family, and clinician perceptions of rehabilitation following treatment for head and neck cancer. *Support Care Cancer*. 2016;24(4):1449–1453.

39. Silver JK, Raj VS, Fu JB, et al. Most national cancer institute-designated cancer center websites do not provide survivors with information about cancer rehabilitation services. *J Cancer Educ*. 2018;33(5):947–953.

40. Stephenson N, Dalton JA, Carlson J, Youngblood R, Bailey D. Racial and ethnic disparities in cancer pain management. *J Natl Black Nurses Assoc*. 2009;20(1):11–18. http://www.ncbi.nlm.nih.gov/pubmed/19691179. Accessed July 22, 2020.

41. Green CR, KO Anderson, Baker TA, et al. The unequal burden of pain: confronting racial and ethnic disparities in pain. *Pain Med*. 2003;4(3):277–294.

42. Gallicchio L, Calhoun C, Helzlsouer KJ. Association between race and physical functioning limitations among breast cancer survivors. *Support Care Cancer*. 2014;22(4):1081–1088.

43. Eversley R, Estrin D, Dibble S, Wardlaw L, Pedrosa M, Favila-Penney W. Post-treatment symptoms among ethnic minority breast cancer survivors. *Oncol Nurs Forum*. 2005;32(2):250–254.

44. Paskett ED, Alfano CM, Davidson MA, et al. Breast cancer survivors' health-related quality of life. *Cancer*. 2008;113(11):3222–3230.

45. Morehead-Gee AJ, Pfalzer L, Levy E, et al. Racial disparities in physical and functional domains in women with breast cancer. *Support Care Cancer*. 2012;20(8):1839–1847.

46. Flores AM, Nelson J, Sowles L, Bienenstock K, Blot WJ. Physical impairments and physical therapy services for minority and low-income breast cancer survivors. *Springerplus*. 2016;5(1). doi:10.1186/s40064-016-2455-3.

47. Williams DR, Rucker TD. Understanding and addressing racial disparities in health care. *Health Care Financ Rev*. 2000;21(4):75–90.

48. Institute of Medicine. *The Unequal Burden of Cancer: An Assessment of NIH Research and Programs for Ethnic Minorities and the Medically Underserved.* The National Academies Press; 1999. https://doi.org/10.17226/6377.

49. Kelland K, Hoe E, McGuire MJ, Yu J, Andreoli A, Nixon SA. Excelling in the role of advocate: a qualitative study exploring advocacy as an essential physiotherapy competency. *Physiother Canada.* 2014;66(1):74–80.

50. Nixon SA. The coin model of privilege and critical allyship: implications for health. *BMC Public Health.* 2019;19(1):1637. doi:10.1186/s12889-019-7884-9.

51. American Board of Physical Therapy Specialties. Oncologic Physical Therapy Description of Specialty Practice; 2017. http://www.abpts.org/uploadedFiles/ABPTSorg/Specialist_Certification/Resources/Outlines/ABPTSOncologyDSP.pdf. Accessed April 14, 2021.

52. American Board of Physical Therapy Residency and Fellowship Education. Description of Residency Practice Oncology; 2017. https://abptrfe.apta.org/for-programs/clinical-programs/oncology. Accessed April 14, 2021.

53. Roush SE, Sharby N. Disability reconsidered: the paradox of physical therapy. *Phys Ther.* 2011;91(12):1715–1727.

54. Whitley R. Postmodernity and mental health. *Harv Rev Psychiatry.* 2008;16(6):352–364.

55. Sulik G. *Pink Ribbon Blues: How Breast Cancer Culture Undermines Women's Health.* Oxford University Press; 2010.

56. Sulik G, Zierkiewicz E. Gender, power, and feminisms in breast cancer advocacy: lessons from the United States and Poland. *J Gender Power.* 2014;1:111–145.

57. Canadian Physiotherapy Association. Essential competency profile; 2017. https://physiotherapy.ca/essential-competency-profile. Accessed August 17, 2020.

58. Negarandeh R, Oskouie F, Ahmadi F, Nikravesh M, Hallberg IR. Patient advocacy: barriers and facilitators. *BMC Nurs.* 2006;5(1):1–8. doi:10.1186/1472-6955-5-3.

59. Ridner SH, Rhoten BA, Radina ME, Adair M, Bush-Foster S, Sinclair V. Breast cancer survivors' perspectives of critical lymphedema self-care support needs. *Support Care Cancer.* 2016;24(6):2743–2750.

60. Schmitz KH, Campbell AM, Stuiver MM, et al. Exercise is medicine in oncology: engaging clinicians to help patients move through cancer. *CA Cancer J Clin.* 2019;69(6):468–484.

61. Negarandeh R, Oskouie F, Ahmadi F, Nikravesh M, Hallberg IR. Patient advocacy: barriers and facilitators. *BMC Nurs.* 2006;5(1):1–8. doi:10.1186/1472-6955-5-3.

62. Mead EL, Doorenbos AZ, Javid SH, et al. Shared decision-making for cancer care among racial and ethnic minorities: a systematic review. *Am J Public Health.* 2013;103(12):e15. doi:10.2105/AJPH.2013.301631.

63. Wiltshire J, Cronin K, Sarto GE, Brown R. Self-advocacy during the medical encounter: use of health information and racial/ethnic differences. *Med Care.* 2006;44(2):100–109.

64. Hagan TL, Medberry E. Patient education vs. patient experiences of self-advocacy: changing the discourse to support cancer survivors. *J Cancer Educ.* 2016;31(2):375–381.

65. Hagan TL, Donovan HS. Ovarian cancer survivors' experiences of self-advocacy: a focus group study. *Oncol Nurs Forum.* 2013;40(2):140–147.

66. Hagan TL, Donovan HS. Self-advocacy and cancer: a concept analysis. *J Adv Nurs.* 2013;69(10):2348–2359.

67. Hagan TL, Rosenzweig MQ, Zorn KK, Van Londen GJ, Donovan HS. Perspectives on self-advocacy: comparing perceived uses, benefits, and drawbacks among survivors and providers. *Oncol Nurs Forum.* 2017;44(1):52–59.

68. Wagner JA. The ever-changing face of breast advocacy. *Breast.* 2010;19(4):280–283. doi:10.1016/j.breast.2010.03.016.

69. Kolmes SK, Boerstler KR. Is there a gender self-advocacy gap? An empiric investigation into the gender pain gap. *J Bioeth Inq.* 2020;17(3):383–393. doi:10.1007/s11673-020-09993-8.

70. Flynn Weitzman P. Middle-aged and older Latino American women in the patient-doctor interaction. *J Cross-Cultural Gerontol.* 2004;19(3):221–239. doi:10.1023/B:JCCG.0000034220.35324.95.

71. Fazil Q, Aujla N, Hale RN C, Joe Kai P. Unequal treatment: health care experiences and needs of patients with cancer from minority ethnic communities. *Divers Equal Heal Care.* 2015;12(3):95–103. doi:10.21767/2049-5471.100036.

72. Parikh RB, Kirch RA, Brawley OW. Advancing a quality-of-life agenda in cancer advocacy: beyond the war metaphor. *JAMA Oncol.* 2015;1(4):423–424.

73. American Society of Clinical Orthopedics. Breast cancer: statistics. https://www.cancer.net/cancer-types/breast-cancer/statistics. January 2021. Accessed April 14, 2021.

74. Freeman HP. Patient navigation: a community based strategy to reduce cancer disparities. *J Urban Heal.* 2006;83(2):139–141.

75. Paskett ED, Harrop JP, Wells KJ. Patient navigation: an update on the state of the science. *CA Cancer J Clin.* 2011;61(4):237–249.

76. Dohan D, Schrag D. Using navigators to improve care of underserved patients: current practices and approaches. *Cancer.* 2005;104(4):848–855.

77. Basu M, Linebarger J, Gabram SGA, Patterson SG, Amin M, Ward KC. The effect of nurse navigation on timeliness of breast cancer care at an academic comprehensive cancer center. *Cancer.* 2013;119:2524–2531.

78. Stout NL, Sleight A, Pfeiffer D, Galantino ML, deSouza B. Promoting assessment and management of function through navigation: opportunities to bridge oncology and rehabilitation systems of care. *Support Care Cancer.* 2019;27(12):4497–4505.

79. Lehmann U, Sanders, D. Community Health Workers: What Do We Know About Them? World Health Organization; 2017. https://www.who.int/hrh/documents/community_health_workers.pdf.

80. Bollmer Dahlke D, Cho J, Gines V, St. John J, Ory M. Barriers to physical activity education for cancer survivors: a survey of English and Spanish speaking promotores/community health workers in Texas. *Texas Public Health J.* 2014;66(1):15–19.

81. Haughton J, Ayala GX, Burke KH, Elder JP, Montañez J, Arredondo EM. Community health workers promoting physical activity. *J Ambul Care Manage.* 2015;38(4):309–320.

82. Takken T, van der Torre P, Zwerink M, et al. Development, feasibility and efficacy of a community-based exercise training program in pediatric cancer survivors. *Psychooncology.* 2009;18(4):440–448.

83. Rajotte EJ, Yi JC, Baker KS, Gregerson L, Leiserowitz A, Syrjala KL. Community-based exercise program effectiveness and safety for cancer survivors. *J Cancer Surviv.* 2012;6(2):219–228.

84. Catt S, Sheward J, Sheward E, Harder H. Cancer survivors' experiences of a community-based cancer-specific exercise programme: results of an exploratory survey. *Support Care Cancer.* 2018;26(9):3209–3216.

85. Binkley JM, Harris SR, Levangie PK, et al. Patient perspectives on breast cancer treatment side effects and the prospective surveillance model for physical rehabilitation for women with breast cancer. *Cancer.* 2012;118(S8):2207–2216.

86. Shoemaker MJ. Direct consumer access to physical therapy in Michigan: challenges to policy adoption. *Phys Ther.* 2012;92(2):236–250.

87. House of Delegates Stenotypist Notes. American Physical Therapy Association; June 1973.

88. House of Delegates Stenotypist Notes. American Physical Therapy Association; June 1978.

89. Dhillon SK, Wilkins S, Law MC, Stewart DA, Tremblay M. Advocacy in occupational therapy: exploring clinicians' reasons and experiences of advocacy. *Can J Occup Ther.* 2010;77(4):241–248.

90. Cancer Control: *Knowledge Into Action: WHO Guide for Effective Programmes: Module 6: Policy and Advocacy.* ADVOCACY STEP 4: MOBILIZING SUPPORT. World Health Organization; 2008. https://www.ncbi.nlm.nih.gov/books/NBK195419/. Accessed April 14, 2021.

91. Perez CP, de Castilla Yabar EMR, Huerta E, et al. Session 2: Mobilizing "all of society" for effective cancer control. In: Conference Proceedings of the Fifth International Cancer Control Congress; 2014.

http://www.cancercontrol.info/wp-content/uploads/2014/09/Session-2.pdf. Accessed April 14, 2021.

92. Wittet S, Aylward J, Cowal S, et al. Advocacy, communication, and partnerships: mobilizing for effective, widespread cervical cancer prevention. *Int J Gynecol Obstet.* 2017;138:57–62.

93. Klawiter M. Racing for the cure, walking women, and toxic touring: mapping cultures of action within the Bay Area terrain of breast cancer. *Soc Probl.* 1999;46(1):104–126.

33

Ethical, Legal, and Financial Aspects

EMIL BERENGUT, PT, DPT, MSW, MHA, BOARD CERTIFIED ORTHOPEDIC CLINICAL SPECIALIST MANAGER, PHYSICAL THERAPY DEPARTMENT, GRAYSON STEPHEN CHAO, PT, DPT, BOARD CERTIFIED ORTHOPEDIC CLINICAL SPECIALIST ASSOCIATED FACULTY

CHAPTER OUTLINE

Introduction

Cancer begins and ends with people. In the midst of scientific abstraction, it is sometimes possible to forget this one basic fact....
— **SIDDHARTHA MUKHERJEE, THE EMPEROR OF ALL MALADIES**

In the pursuit of enhancing cancer care, our successes are often measured in increasing survival rates, new therapies, and procedures. However, it is wise to bear in mind that the human element is equally inextricable from the care of patients with cancer.

Consider the case of a patient; let us call her Kay (Box 33.1). Kay comes to the clinic with a history of childhood myosarcoma treated with a unilateral long above-knee amputation. This has resulted in decreased ambulation capacity, and she currently uses a wheelchair. The mobility limitation is exacerbated by the lack of

financial and supportive resources. This in turn limits her access to rehabilitative services, regular medical follow-ups, and home modifications to assist her with transfers, wheelchair management, and a functional prosthesis. The resultant decreased mobility and healthcare access caused health issues including obesity, heart disease, and the need for bilateral shoulder replacements and multiple spinal surgeries. These medical costs, progressive disability, and unemployment further compounded the demands on her financial resources. Unable to afford new equipment, Kay's home environment was unsafe, resulting in multiple falls and related injuries. Kay's case illustrates the complex interaction of medical, financial, and legal factors entrenched in cancer care.

Many clinicians who work with a person living with cancer (PLWC) have encountered similar complex situations. This chapter will illustrate ethical, financial, and legal concepts that will

"I just want to dance at my wedding." The person in front of the physical therapist (PT) was describing her goals. Kay's previous medical history was long and arduous. She survived childhood cancer, an above knee amputation, and multiple spine surgeries. She has been a patient at the PT clinic intermittently for many years, treated by almost the whole staff. As the PT spoke to Kay, more details about her living conditions emerged. She lived in an unpermitted, basement apartment with her fiancé and two children. The apartment was constructed illegally and was completely inaccessible to her. Kay had to be carried down the steps by her family and got around the apartment in a rolling office chair. She has suffered multiple falls and fractures while scooting around the apartment and bathing. Kay was looking forward to her wedding and simply wanted to walk out to the altar and dance with her partner. Her previous treatment at the rehabilitation clinic was an impairment-based approach which aimed to stretch, strengthen, and mobilize. Yet, as is common in survivors of cancer, she was experiencing issues in multiple systems. A direct treatment approach focused mainly on her impairments, while effective in the short-term, failed to address all the other problems affecting Kay's quality of life for the long term. She was struggling financially because she was unable to work and was on disability. This affected her ability to afford better, accessible housing and a lighter, smaller, more comfortable wheelchair. She was experiencing housing discrimination and was affected by her landlord's noncompliance with housing and employment laws.

enable the Oncology rehabilitation (Onc R) clinicians to better understand the challenges this population experience.

Ethical Considerations

> It is curious – curious that physical courage should be so common in the world, and moral courage so rare.
>
> — MARK TWAIN

The adherence to a code of ethics and governance of behavior by an established organization codifies a unique healthcare discipline into a profession. To borrow the definition from the Australian Council of Professions, a profession is defined as "…a disciplined group of individuals who adhere to ethical standards and who hold themselves out as, and are accepted by the public as possessing special knowledge and skills in a widely recognized body of learning derived from research, education, and training at a high level, and who are prepared to apply this knowledge and exercise these skills in the interest of others."[1]

Nevertheless, one can pose the question, "Why do Onc R clinicians have to practice ethically?" Some have proposed that ethical practice is the essential element that makes a specific discipline into a profession.[1] Without ethical practice, we simply learn a collection of techniques and their application. However, practicing within an ethical framework defines our collective work. As an example, physical therapist (PT) professional ethics have evolved through three overlapping periods. While initially focused on self-identity as a profession, the profession later progressed to the patient's identity. More recently, the emphasis has been on self-identity and focus on the patient within the society. As such, our code of ethics outlines our professional responsibilities in reducing the inequities in health and social justice.[2]

Onc R specialty practice occupies one of the most complex intersections of our profession. As evident in Kay's case, PLWCs present with significant multisystemic impairments and limitations. Onc R clinicians are tasked with addressing these challenges

to empower and enable our patients. An ethical framework set forth by professional associations and governing bodies equips rehabilitation clinicians that work in oncology with a professional structure to help our patients.

Ethical Practice Framework

The following framework has been proposed for ethical practice.[3]

Autonomy

The patients and their caregivers have the right to make decisions that affect their care. Onc R Clinicians are often faced with this principle when consenting their patients for treatment. This is even more critical as Onc R clinicians are becoming the first point of contact for any patients (e.g., PTs in the direct access environment). One of our professional obligations is to explain the potential harms and benefits of any rehabilitative procedure and obtain the patient's consent. This extends beyond the signed informed consent. For example, in an Onc R setting, educating the patient about potential soreness after exercise or soft tissue mobilization. This explanation enables the patient and their caregivers to participate in the decision-making process.

Case Example: A patient in your care underwent a total joint replacement following an osteosarcoma resection. You recommend inpatient rehabilitation following an extended stay at the hospital. However, the patient would like to be discharged home with services despite your recommendation. Although based on your assessment, inpatient rehabilitation would be clinically indicated, you proceed working with the patient to help them to transition to home care. (Alan Ho, PT, DPT, phone communication, January 25, 2021)

Justice

Onc R clinicians must advocate for their patients to have care regardless of their socioeconomic status, racial and ethnic background, sexual orientation, and geographic location. It is often said that cancer knows no color or income. However, access to cancer treatment and Onc R services is affected by the patient's racial, ethnic, and economic background. Evidence shows that both the incidence of cancer and survival rates are affected by the person's access to preventative care and treatment.[4] Similarly, not getting appropriate Onc R affects the patient's function and quality of life (QOL). Onc R clinicians can advocate for their patients on three different levels—individual, organizational, and societal. On an individual level, this may mean providing your patients with the resources to obtain Onc R and support services, liaising with the insurance company for additional visits, and contacting their healthcare providers to secure referrals. On an organizational level, rehabilitation clinicians can propose to their employers to start Onc R services, secure grants to begin programs, initiate research projects, and educate their colleagues and other providers about the rehabilitation needs of PLWCs. At the societal level, clinicians can participate in the local, state, and national professional and patient advocacy organizations and lobby their legislators for laws that protect the rights of PLWCs to get appropriate prevention and healthcare services.

Case Example: While working at a tertiary cancer hospital, you recognize that many patients from underserved communities have difficulties accessing the Onc R clinic. They experience long commute times and as a result many forego treatment. The local community clinics do not provide adequate services. You collect cancer treatment outcome data, interview the patients, and identify disparities in access to Onc R services. This allows you to demonstrate to the hospital leadership that there is a need for an additional Onc R clinic in the underserved community.

Beneficence

Onc R clinicians are obligated to do good for their patients. Beneficence is defined as an act of charity, mercy, and kindness with a strong connotation of doing good to others, including moral obligation. One way to think about this is striving to deliver the absolute best care for our patients. Another might be the moral imperative to exhibit kindness and patience toward all patients at all times regardless of instances of personality clashes. Patients seek our care when they are in physical and emotional pain, which influences their interactions. The clinician is obligated to exhibit constant positive regard for the patient even if the professional interaction is difficult to maintain. Another example of beneficence may be going the extra step for a patient or their family, such as taking additional time to listen to their concerns or extending the treatment session to progress their mobility goals.

Case Example: *A patient with terminal cancer in your care has quickly decompensated. You have adjusted the treatment intensity to reflect the change in status. The patient's family is very upset and feels like they are not getting the best care. In order to help the family, understand the patient's status you help to facilitate a meeting with the treatment team.*

Nonmaleficence

Onc R clinicians must do no harm. While some proposed that this duty stems from beneficence, others have argued that it is a separate obligation. Healthcare professions have widely accepted this principle since its inception. Nevertheless, an ethical challenge may emerge when the patient's autonomous decision may cause them harm. Which principle should the clinician support? It is not easy to provide a prescription for these scenarios, as the circumstances will differ for each case. The Onc R clinician is encouraged to examine all the information pertinent to the case before making a decision. One of the benefits of oncologic practice is there is often a diverse team of colleagues that may assist a clinician in navigating these ethical dilemmas.

Case Example: *A patient with spinal metastasis is determined to improve their balance so that they can go open-water fly fishing. The patient advises the Onc R that they have booked their travel regardless of whether they work with them. Should the PT attempt to minimize harm by creating dynamic balance drills that may cause a fall? Or should the PT decline to work with the patient on this functional goal to avoid a potential fall during treatment?*

Ethical Challenges

Cancer care, especially in the context of advanced cancer, is often fraught with a variety of ethical challenges. It is essential to consider key concepts pertinent to the discussion of ethics in Onc R clinical practice to better navigate them.

Informed Consent

Informed consent is the permission that the patient gives to the clinician in order to provide care with the understanding of the benefits and risks.[5] Although it is sometimes perceived as a formality, clinicians are urged to consider the consent's ethical grounding, specifically, *beneficence* and *autonomy*. As healthcare professionals, we aim to promote the well-being of our patients. Similarly, we respect the right of the patient to decide what is best for them after receiving the appropriate information. Thus, we ensure that

the patients know any potential risks and reasonable alternatives to the treatment. In Onc R, we are not only legally obligated to provide our patients with informed consent but morally as well. One example may include discussing the potential risks associated with administering manual stretching in proximity to an irradiated axilla and alternative ways of improving the range of motion. Another example may be educating the patient about the potential for delayed onset muscle soreness following their therapeutic exercise and the clinical indications to improve strength and endurance.

Privacy

Privacy is the right of every patient to keep their information from being disclosed. In 1996, The Health Insurance Portability and Accountability Act (HIPAA) was enacted in the United States (US). For the first time, the US had an established set of national standards to protect health information.[6] As Onc R clinicians, we often encounter issues related to privacy and must be ever vigilant for possible privacy breaches. For example, a PLWC who walks into a specialized Onc R facility or receives confirmation calls for their appointments can inadvertently have their cancer diagnosis revealed. Other common examples include requests to release patient health information from family members and others potentially involved in their care. It is not uncommon for patients and family members to attempt to take photographs of their rehabilitation process to share on social media, potentially exposing patients to privacy breaches. Healthcare organizations must implement strict rules and protocols to help protect patient privacy. Employees must be empowered to enforce these, as violations are illegal and undermine patient trust.[7]

Confidentiality

Onc R clinicians protect the patients' information and only share it within the patient's explicit permission and within the confines of the law. It is vital to Onc R practice because patients must be able to entrust their most private information to us during their care. Patients share their most personal details within the context of receiving Onc R. If they cannot trust us to protect the information, they will be hesitant to share it, affecting their care. Engendering a trusting relationship facilitates an effective therapeutic alliance—a key to therapeutic outcomes.[8]

Overutilization of Services and Fraud

Overutilization of service has been defined as "provision of a service that is unlikely to increase quality or quantity of life, that poses more harm than benefit, or that patients who were fully informed of its potential benefits and harms would not have wanted."[9] Onc R clinicians are frequently faced with ethical dilemmas concerning overutilization of service—for example, recommending a more intensive level of care than clinically indicated under pressure from the patient, their family, or even their facility's administrators. Patients may enter treatment with predetermined expectations for their treatment intensity. Dissonance may occur when the therapist's recommendations are different based on their evaluation. The patient may reach a therapeutic plateau, yet want to continue their rehabilitation because of perceived benefit. Similarly, the patient's caregivers or family members can attempt to exert pressure on the therapist to provide services that are not clinically appropriate. Some facilities may set productivity expectations that include prescribed treatment duration and intensity. These are all complex circumstances. However, our professional ethics dictate that we must avoid overutilization of services and base our recommendations on what is clinically appropriate and necessary.

Professional Competence

Many healthcare consumers assume that their rehabilitation and medical providers maintain some degree of professional competence. Some of it is codified through local and state regulations, others through various organizations' professional requirements. However, in the ethical discourse, we urge a different take on competence. While most Onc R clinicians share some foundational skills in diagnosis and treatment, few have had the requisite training in managing the multiple, complex, and severe impairments that often come with a cancer diagnosis. Fewer still have had advanced education and training in specialized rehabilitative treatments for these conditions. This gap in competence may emerge when a PLWC seeks treatment for an impairment related to cancer or cancer treatment at a facility without extensive professional competence in Onc R. The facility or the individual provider undoubtedly will want to help the patient. How much of their experience (or inexperience) should they disclose to the patient? Will the patient perceive them as incompetent and seek care elsewhere? What if there are no providers nearby with the necessary experience? Perhaps, the provider can explain their professional expertise to the patient and describe how they will seek guidance and education to enhance their knowledge. These challenges manifest themselves often in rehabilitative practice and are not limited to Onc R. Furthermore, unlike some other medical professions, referral to other qualified providers within a rehabilitation discipline is not considered common practice. However according to ethical principles, if a provider is not qualified to manage a patient's complex issues or knows that a colleague has adequate credentials to provide better care, it is likely that this referral would be an appropriate course of action.

Therapist Self-Care

Practicing in Onc R holds a unique weight and gravity. That weight is one that those in the world of oncology take on readily. For the initiated, the necessary scope of knowledge, breadth of skills, and proficiency level feel unparalleled to any of the other disciplines. Perhaps even more unique amongst the specialties is the individual psychological and emotional cost to the Onc R clinician. We form unique bonds with our patients, as they spend countless hours in rehabilitation to recover function during and after cancer treatment. These bonds are rewarding and help to motivate us. However, this also exposes the clinician to a unique degree of burnout and compassion fatigue.

Burnout

Burnout is a broad term to describe a psychosocial syndrome that results from exposure to chronic and interpersonal stressors in patient care. Burnout usually has three components: emotional exhaustion and reduced energy, a sense of cynicism and lack of empathy, and a sense that their accomplishments and contributions are insignificant.[10]

Compassion Fatigue

Compassion fatigue is defined as "the physical and mental exhaustion and emotional withdrawal experienced by those who care for sick or traumatized people over an extended period of time."[11] Those suffering from compassion fatigue often exhibit similar signs of burnout, such as a decreased sense of self-esteem, reduced energy, and irritability. They also may grow increasingly difficult to motivate to action with emotional or passionate appeals.

When it comes to the question of "Who helps the helpers?," the Onc R clinician must ensure that they know signs of burnout and compassion fatigue in themselves and their colleagues. Recognition of these signs is the most critical step in mitigating the impact of their work. Therapists who note they are suffering from burnout or compassion fatigue are encouraged to engage in their preferred self-care activities or seek out help from their support networks or services. For example, many employers offer no-cost, confidential employee assistance program. Engaging in self-care is critical to ensuring that Onc R clinicians remain at optimum effectiveness in their duties, which is undoubtedly part of their ethical obligation.

Conflicts of Interest

Conflicts of interest (COI) are situations in which clinicians may have ulterior motives that may impact the patient's routine care. A COI does not have to be an outward or intended act; sometimes merely the potential for a situation to possibly result in a COI or even being perceived as a COI by others may be enough to warrant proactive action to mitigate a COI.

In cases of a real or potential COI, it is important to delineate the clinician's typical role and responsibilities and how this COI may affect it. For example, an equipment vendor presents a product to your clinic, which claims to help patients manage their lymphedema at home. They offer your clinic a financial compensation each time the product is prescribed to a patient with lymphedema. If this treatment is not superior to other traditional means of lymphedema management, it would be a clear COI. Even in the event that this product is superior in managing lymphedema, the providers and the clinic stand to gain financially for recommending a device, particularly when it is not part of their typical treatment plan for lymphedema. Regardless of the treatment effectiveness, this is a clear example of a conflict of interest as the treatment decisions are not made purely for the patient's benefit.

Why is it important for clinicians to avoid conflicts of interest? The short answer is—COIs affect our professional integrity. People seek our assistance, particularly Onc R, at the most vulnerable time in their lives. They trust us to make the best possible decision in their care, unaffected by ulterior motives. This trust is essential to a therapeutic relationship. COIs and potential COIs affect the patient's confidence in us and our valued therapeutic relationship. The clinician must take at least one of the following steps in situations where there is a potential COI[12]:

1. Surrender the conflicting relationship.
2. Avoid the COI.
3. Reveal the relationship to their patient and the employer.

Underserved Populations

Healthcare in many nations, including the US, is fragmented, costly, and inequitable. The COVID-19 pandemic laid bare the ingrained inequities in our healthcare system. Despite years of warnings by various stakeholders, there was a clear failure to create a comprehensive, equitable, and affordable system. Instead, a disjointed marketplace exists that preferentially serves the interests of well-to-do in centralized, large population centers. In part, this failure contributed to thousands of deaths from preventable illnesses, including the COVID-19 health crisis. The inequity in health care access has always affected the traditionally marginalized and disadvantaged groups most.[13] PLWCs have frequently experienced difficulties with access to highly specialized Onc R services.[13] This section will review how some of these communities are affected by the lack of access to key services. We also invite the reader to consider using the novel Brief Needs Assessment Tool

TABLE 33.1	Brief Needs Assessment Tool		
Social Determinant of Health	Strengths	Deficit Areas	Description
Economic stability			
Transportation			
Community resources			
Home environment			
Health literacy			
Diet and food sources			
Social network and support			
Healthcare coverage			

(Table 33.1). Although it has not been validated, it is provided here to help evaluate the patients' psychosocial needs.

Economically Disadvantaged Groups

It has been said that one cannot live in a society but be free of it. As an example, while the PT professional ethics were initially focused on self-identity, an evolution toward an "emerging" period of societal identity was described by one author.[3] As such, PTs are tasked with improving health equity, including access to specialized care such as Onc R and reducing health disparities.[14] A significant body of research pointedly outlines the contribution of social determinants of health, social injustice to morbidity, and mortality of our patients[13] Socioeconomic status has been identified as a factor in cancer care access, affecting the QOL and survival rates. Individually, PTs may become aware of these barriers when their patients must end care prematurely for financial reasons. Some may never follow up with referrals for PT because they cannot afford it, while others may live in areas underserved by transportation or healthcare facilities.

Racial and Ethnic Minorities

Similarly, data points to the race and ethnicity of the patients as a barrier to obtaining healthcare. Individuals in historically marginalized communities struggle to get timely, quality, affordable cancer care. For example, Black women are less likely to receive recommendations for breast cancer screening.[15] White people had significantly higher odds of receiving rehabilitation in any setting compared to Black people.[16] Black patients also experienced worse functional outcomes following hip fracture.[17]

Furthermore, culturally competent care has only recently been emphasized despite years of evidence demonstrating its importance.[18] For example individuals who are not fluent in English may have a tough time receiving equitable care in some facilities.[19] Consider the difficulties that one encounters when having to coordinate appointments with a qualified interpreter. Research has suggested that some clinicians choose to forego using interpreters and try to "get by" due to resource constraints.[20] Others may misinterpret the patient's low participation with the treatment program as noncompliance when cultural barriers exist.[21]

However, cultural competence alone may be insufficient to address the dynamic and complex needs of our patients. For example, it assumes that White culture is the norm.[22] Thus, cultural incompetence is described as a lack of knowledge of the "other culture." This implies that finite attainment of this

knowledge is possible without a concordant examination and reflection of one's own biases. In their landmark 1998 paper, Tervalon and Murray-García propose an approach called *cultural humility* described as "a lifelong process of self-reflection and self-critique whereby the individual not only learns about another's culture, but one starts with an examination of her/his own beliefs and cultural identities."[23] This explorative process has been well described within palliative rehabilitation practice.[24] They suggest not only obtaining information about diversity and inclusion, but also analyzing how our "attitudes and behaviors" affect others. By engaging in this practice, we can begin to understand the historical and social context of their patient's life by reflecting on our background. This process can allow us to be better aware of how systemic racism, institutionalized violence, and oppression against certain groups have helped create current healthcare barriers. Moreover, by committing to a lifelong process, we can continue to grow as clinicians.

LGBTQIA+ Groups

Lesbian, gay, bisexual, transgender, queer, intersex, and asexual individuals (LGBTQIA+) have traditionally been marginalized in healthcare.[25] This population is at a higher risk of certain types of cancers, HIV, hepatitis B, mental illness, and substance abuse. The transgender population in particular experiences more risk of osteoporosis due to some undergoing hormone replacement therapy (HRT). Onc R clinicians must understand these high-risk factors and barriers to healthcare access in the LGBTQIA+ community to serve it better. For example, LGBTQIA+ people may be more likely to be uninsured due to systemic discrimination in the workplace and the health insurance sector. As with other marginalized groups, the LGBTQIA+ patients report greater reluctance to use healthcare when it is not culturally sensitive and higher satisfaction with care when it is.[26] This reluctance to use healthcare services may result in delays in health screenings and subsequent delays in a cancer diagnosis, which may result in diagnosis at an advanced, less curable stage.

Some examples of culturally insensitive healthcare include misgendering patients, using their "dead" names, assuming their significant other's gender, and asking for gender on the intake forms. In addition to these everyday concerns, we encourage our colleagues to learn more about the elevated health risks and access barriers for LGBTQIA+ patients, understand their own biases, and engage in a continuous self-reflective process of their practice.

Geographically Marginalized

Access to cancer care and Onc R remains limited to some populations in the US. Many PLWCs experience difficulties accessing care despite significant evidence that this negatively affects treatment outcomes. Rural residents and those in underserved communities appear to be disproportionately impacted. For example, PTs play an essential role in improving the QOL and mobility for PLWCs.[27] Yet in one study, over half of respondents with chronic, disabling illnesses could not obtain rehabilitation services.[28] This is further exacerbated by a relatively low supply of therapists trained in Onc R services. Thus, PLWCs experience increased difficulties accessing specialized care. While increasing the supply of trained Onc R providers requires a significant investment of time and resources, telehealth may be a useful stopgap measure to mitigate geographical disparities.[29] As many of us have experienced during the COVID-19 pandemic, telemedicine is a safe and effective method of delivering specialty services to geographically underserved populations.

Legal Aspects

Many nations or jurisdictions have established legal protections for those with health issues or individuals from traditionally underserved or discriminated populations. Although it is beyond the scope of this text to enumerate each legal statute from the variety of nations from which readers may originate, we will describe a few key examples from the US healthcare system. We encourage the reader to reach out to advocacy organizations for relevant statutes that may impact our patients and clients in their individual jurisdiction.

The Americans With Disabilities Act

The US Congress passed the first version of the Americans With Disabilities Act (ADA) in 1990. On July 26, 1991, it was expanded to include additional regulations for states and accommodations for public and commercial facilities. The final version of this federal law was passed in 1992, prohibiting the exclusion of people with disabilities from taking part in working, shopping, and receiving governmental or public services.[30] The ADA also requires employers with more than 15 employees to make reasonable accommodations to allow individuals to work. PLWC may have pre-existing disabilities or may experience disability because of cancer and cancer treatment. Onc R clinicians must be aware of the ADA as providers of care and as employers. They might be required to make reasonable accommodations to comply with the ADA for their employees and patients. Detailed information is available from the US federal government to guide the accommodation process.[31]

Role of Physical Therapy/Occupational Therapy in Reasonable Accommodations

Up to 70% of PLWC are of working age.[32] They may require different accommodations based on their stage in treatment and recovery. For example, some may need additional time to complete tasks due to cancer treatment-induced fatigue. Others may be unable to reach and lift after breast reconstruction surgery. In addition to helping individuals rehabilitate from these impairments, employers may ask Onc R clinicians to provide documentation about disability and functional limitations. For instance, a patient with a limited range of motion following breast cancer treatment may have trouble reaching for work tools. Their employer may request documentation "describing the impairment; the nature, severity, and duration of the impairment; the activity or activities that the impairment limits; and the extent to which the impairment limits the employee's ability to perform the activity or activities (i.e., the employer is seeking the information as to whether the employee has an ADA disability)."[31] The PT must follow their facility's guidelines on the release of information pertaining to the ADA documentation, including a written consent for information release from the patient. Moreover, the documentation must be strictly limited to the minimum required to establish the disability and the specific impairments that affect their ability to perform duties.

It is notable that despite statutes such as the ADA, PLWCs still experience high levels of workplace discrimination.[32] Up to 53% of PLWCs lost their jobs or quit working following their cancer diagnosis. Survivors were less likely to be re-employed and more likely to retire early in the first six years following diagnosis.[33] Moreover, PLWCs experience stigma related to their diagnosis. Certain cancers are associated with behavior choices, such

as lung cancer and smoking. Some individuals are stigmatized because of the lasting effects of cancer, such as colostomies and sexual functioning. In the workplace, survivors may be perceived as a burden for employers due to insurance costs. Others are seen as a drain on staff resources when their peers have to cover their work responsibilities in the event of more frequent absenteeism due to health appointments or other health-related issues.[34] It is essential for clinicians to understand the issues their patients may experience upon return to the workplace and actively screen for and address any employment issues. A high priority should be educating the patient on their rights as an employee, including leaves of absence or other entitlements assured by law or policy. On an individual level, clinicians can understand the potential negative consequences of stigma and workplace discrimination their patients may experience, particularly since some avoid seeking care due to these challenges. On a community level, Onc R clinicians can advocate for PLWCs by participating in community organizations and engaging lawmakers. See Chapter 32 for more information on advocacy within Onc R.

Women's Health and Cancer Rights Act

The Women's Health and Cancer Rights Act (WHCRA) of 1998 is a US federal law that protects patients who undergo breast reconstruction following a mastectomy.[35] The law requires insurance companies to include coverage of all reconstruction stages, including surgery, prosthesis, and rehabilitation. It is important to note that the name of the law is misleading, as cancer does not have to be the cause of mastectomy. The law also covers treatment for the contralateral breast to achieve a symmetrical appearance and is not limited to any gender.

The WHCRA covers treatment for the resultant impairments of breast reconstruction, such as physical therapy and occupational therapy to restore strength, range of motion, and lymphedema. Landmark legislation such as this assist in assuring that persons diagnosed with breast cancer have fair and adequate access to the specialized services of Onc R clinicians to return to function following breast reconstruction.

Department of Labor's Job Accommodation Network

The Job Accommodation Network (JAN) is a free service sponsored by the US Department of Labor's Office of Disability Employment Policy that provides information on specific job accommodations, including leave. The JAN can be contacted by calling 1-800-526-7234 or 1-800-ADA-WORK (1-800-232-9675) (voice/TTY).

State-Level Disability Law

A few states have laws that require employers to provide disability insurance. For those states where it is not required, employers may provide such insurance. State law may require specific provisions in a group disability policy sold by insurers. Finally, some state regulations prohibit insurers from including discretionary clauses in insurance contracts or policies.

Family and Medical Leave Act

The Family and Medical Leave Act (FMLA) is a federal law designed to help workers balance job and family responsibilities by giving employees up to 12 weeks of unpaid leave per year for specific reasons, including a serious health condition or to care for an immediate family member who has a serious health condition. During FMLA leave, employers must continue employee health insurance benefits and, upon completion of the leave, restore employees to the same or equivalent positions.

Covered Employers

The FMLA applies to private employers with 50 or more employees working within 75 miles of the employee's worksite. Employers with fewer than 50 employees can also choose to provide benefits similar to those required by the FMLA, and many find it beneficial to do so. The FMLA also applies to all public agencies and private and public elementary and secondary schools, regardless of the number of employees.

Covered Individuals

Employees are eligible to take FMLA leave if they have worked for their employer for at least 12 months and have worked for at least 1250 hours over the 12 months immediately prior to the leave, if there are at least 50 employees working within 75 miles of the employee's worksite.

Medical and Disability-Related Leave Rules

Eligible employees can take up to 12 weeks of leave for treatment of or recovery from serious health conditions. The FMLA's definition of a serious health condition is broader than the definition of a disability, encompassing pregnancy and many illnesses, injuries, impairments, or physical or mental conditions that require multiple treatments and intermittent absences. Generally, things like cosmetic surgery, colds, headaches, and routine medical and dental care are not included. FMLA leave is unpaid, but employers may require employees to concurrently take paid leave, such as accrued vacation or sick leave, or employees may elect to do so.

Financial Aspects and Considerations

The financial burden of healthcare on American society is acknowledged as one of the most prominent public health threats. In 2018 alone, healthcare expenditures increased by 4.8%, reaching $3.6 trillion or $11,172 per person. As a share of the nation's Gross Domestic Product, health spending accounted for 17.7%.[3] It is estimated that the US spends more than $200 billion on cancer care alone.[4] The cost of cancer care takes a tremendous toll on PLWCs, their loved ones, and employers and can exceed $200,000 per year.[4]

First a commonly used term vocabulary will be introduced to discuss the financial aspects of cancer care (Box 33.2).

Financial Toxicity

In healthcare, financial toxicity is the resultant problems that a patient experiences related to their medical care costs. Being uninsured or underinsured can cause financial problems and may lead to debt and bankruptcy. Financial toxicity can affect a patient's QOL and access to medical care. Many factors have been shown to influence survival, such as cancer type, age and stage at diagnosis, treatment selection and related physician biases, insurance status, competing health conditions, and financial resources.[36] However, it has also been shown that access to high-quality cancer care increases the likelihood of survival and better patient QOL.[36] Structural barriers such as being underinsured or uninsured

---

• **BOX 33.2**   **Financial Terminology**

Terminology

- Insured—party covered by an insurance policy
- Underinsured—(of a person) having inadequate insurance coverage
- Uninsured—one not covered by insurance
- Insurer—an insurer or reinsurer authorized to write property and casualty insurance under the laws of any state
- Disparity—a great distance or gap as may be in economic status, wages, or access to public services
- Health disparity—when one population group experiences a higher burden of disability or illness relative to another group
- Healthcare disparity—differences in access to healthcare services or health insurance, or the quality of care received
- Underserved—provided or accessing insufficient/inadequate services.
- Under resourced—provided or accessing insufficient/inadequate resources.
- Medically underserved areas—geographic region or segment which lacks access to skilled quality medical services
- Medically underserved populations—a segment of the population that lacks access to skilled, quality medical services
- Financial toxicity—negative impacts on a patient's health and care as a result of increasing financial burden of their care
- Financial downward spiral—a process that leads to rapid premium increases and eventual loss of coverage. Individuals most at risk to experience illness purchase coverage, while those at lower risk do not. The insurance company raises premiums to decrease risk. The cycle continues until very few people can afford to pay for their coverage.

---

frequently limit access to quality cancer care. Inadequate health insurance is a significant barrier to the receipt of timely and appropriate care. For example, uninsured patients diagnosed with Stage I colorectal cancer have lower survival than Stage II colorectal cancer patients with private insurance.[36] In addition, a patient may not take prescription medicine or avoid going to the doctor to save money. PLWCs tend to be more likely to experience financial toxicity than others who receive medical care.[37]

Let us revisit the case of Kay.

While her functional deficits were initially a result of her cancer treatment, it caused rippling effects throughout her life. Her functional capacity was reduced and, as a result, limited her ability to access educational and job resources, exacerbating her already strained economic resources. With her continued barriers to improving her socioeconomic status, she continued to face difficulties managing her health; limited access to higher quality food sources, inability to obtain supportive equipment, and unsafe home environments all served to increase health comorbidities. For example, Kay fell at home and fractured her shoulder because she could not afford home safety modifications.

There is mounting evidence that interventions targeting social, economic, and environmental factors can account for sizable reductions in morbidity and mortality.[6] In order to appreciate these gains, financial issues must be proactively identified and addressed, either through direct intervention or referral by Onc R clinicians.

The Downward Financial Spiral of Cancer and Management

Within the cancer treatment continuum, a spiraling interaction exists between exacerbating financial toxicity and the resultant impact on the patient's disease course (Figure 33.1).[36] It begins

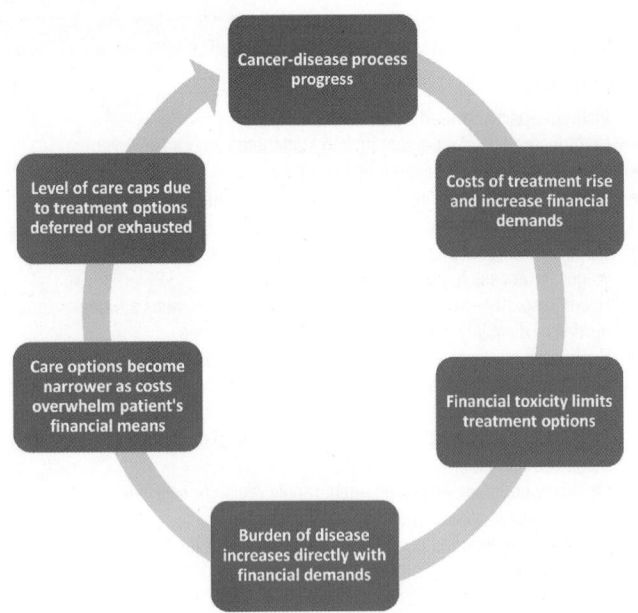

Cancer-disease process progress

Costs of treatment rise and increase financial demands

Financial toxicity limits treatment options

Burden of disease increases directly with financial demands

Care options become narrower as costs overwhelm patient's financial means

Level of care caps due to treatment options deferred or exhausted

• **Fig. 33.1** Financial Downward Spiral of Cancer. (Reprinted with permission from Lentz R; Benson AB, 3rd; Kircher S. Financial toxicity in cancer care: prevalence, causes, consequences, and reduction strategies. *J Surg Oncol.* 2019;120(1):85–92.)

with the patient's cancer diagnosis. At this stage, they must address the costs associated with treating their disease. Constraints in the ability to pay for treatments will impact care options, and health or survival outcomes may be inferior as a result. In turn, this increases the financial burden because the advanced symptoms or complex medical situation is more costly; this further limits their ability to access care, and additional treatment options further diminish. Ultimately a stalemate is reached: either the care stops because they need to prioritize other financial aspects (food, mortgage, childcare, tuition) or simply cannot afford needed medical care anymore, and the care also stops.

It is essential for Onc R clinicians to know where the patient is in this spiral to identify additional needs or areas where support can be provided. As with the concept of prehabilitation for physical health prior to initiation of cancer treatment, clinicians should strongly consider proactive or preventative educational measures to anticipate and facilitate protective financial measures—*financial prehabilitation.*

Table 33.2 describes the types of costs that can be incurred along the cancer treatment continuum. Notably, a PLWC may only incur some of these costs, and the magnitude of these can vary. Although a person's medical treatment may be relatively inexpensive, traveling to a distant specialty cancer center, co-payment, co-insurance, and lost wages can drastically increase the costs associated with

TABLE 33.2	Financial Demands Along the Cancer Treatment Continuum	
Category	**Description**	**Examples**
Travel	Dedicated cancer care is not always directly accessible and travel to specialty centers for treatment or diagnosis is often incurred by patients and their caregivers	• Taxis to appointments • Travel costs incurred to reach out of state treatment • Gas and tolls • Public transportation
Lodging	There are those that may require specialty, oncology-related services which extend beyond a day of travel and lodging may be required to stay overnight. Furthermore, additional caregiver support from out of state may be necessary and also has lodging costs associated.	• Hotel stays for out of state treatment • Lodging for caregiver • Costs for home health aide • Apartment rental
Loss of income(s)	A PLWC and their caregivers are often limited or prohibited from participating in income-generating activities as a result of their treatment or side effects.	• Loss of wages • Job loss for significant other or other family caregivers • Housing instability
Dependent care	A PLWC may require hiring private caregiver services for an adult-dependent or children during their cancer treatment	• Home health aide fees • Childcare • Adult dependent care
Medication	Costs of related medications directly related to their cancer treatment	• Direct medical costs • Supportive medication such as OTC
Resources in survivorship	Costs incurred in the period where primary cancer treatment has concluded	• Medical treatment copays/ deductibles related to secondary diagnoses (e.g., adverse effects of chemotherapy and rehabilitation) • Costs for dietary modifications • Costs from additional disease surveillance
Fees	Out of pocket financial costs. These may or may not be associated with their cancer treatment or any additional services that result from their	• Out of pocket medical fees • Copays • Legal document preparation fees (e.g., living will preparation, financial services estate planning) • Home accommodation fees

OTC, Over the counter; *PLWC,* person living with cancer.

TABLE 33.3 Select Financial Assistance Resources for PLWC

Name	Type	Resources Provided
Ronald McDonald House Coalition https://www.rmhc.org/	Lodging	• Overnight lodging for families of children undergoing treatment
American Cancer Society Hope Lodge www.cancer.org	Lodging	• Overnight lodging for individuals traveling from out of state for treatment
AvonCare CancerCare https://www.cancercare.org	Financial	• Co-payment, co-insurance, and deductible assistance for breast cancer treatment • Transportation assistance for treatment appointments
SamFund http://www.thesamfund.org/get-help/grants/	Financial	• Financial assistance for PLWCs between the ages of 21–39
Livestrong https://www.livestrong.org/	After-care	• No cost exercise and wellness programs for PLWCs with specially trained fitness trainers
CancerCare (800-813-4673)	Financial	• Co-pays, transportation, home care, and childcare
Family Reach (973-394-1411)	Financial	• National organization dedicated to eradicating the financial barriers that accompany a cancer diagnosis
HealthWell Foundation (800-675-8416)	Financial	• General assistance for patients with chronic illness
Cancer Financial Assistance Coalition http://www.cancerfac.org/	Financial	• Group of national organizations that provide financial help to patients

PLWC, Person living with cancer.

treating the disease. At present, many public and private organizations offer financial assistance according to the categories laid out in Table 33.3.

These potential resources for financial support break down into a few broad categories:
- National level resources
  - These are private or public organizations that provide services on a national level. Many nonprofit organizations like the Leukemia & Lymphoma Society which provide financial support or advisement services.
- State and local resources
  - As previously mentioned, many nonprofit organizations exist nationally but break out into local and state-level groups.
- Institutional resources
  - Some cancer care centers or hospitals have support services associated with their institution that provide financial support and counseling for PLWCs.
- Private and religious funds
  - Religious organizations and social clubs may have charitable commitments or divisions that provide financial support services to people undergoing treatment.
- Additional resources
  - Some have also turned to individual fundraising, such as their home churches, schools, or online crowdsourcing websites.

Financial Educational Interventions

Wherever possible, the patient should be educated about maximizing their existing financial resources such as health insurance, public assistance, and disability coverage. Some larger institutions may have dedicated departments to counsel patients on their insurance and financial options. Onc R clinicians at larger institutions, are advised to be familiar with such a dedicated department

or another department on this task, such as case managers, social workers, or patient services.

Clinicians are also encouraged to familiarize themselves with the patient's benefits and the options available to them:
- Do they have a health savings account (HSA) or any other pre-tax healthcare payment plan?
- Does the practice maintain a fund for them to help pay for sessions?
- Does your practice or institution allow payment plans or flexible payment arrangements?
- Are you personally aware of the local support services available in your area or network?

Strategies for Clinicians

Many Onc R clinicians may feel challenged to minimize the financial impacts on our patients. Below are some strategies we can employ to facilitate their ability to participate in rehabilitation.

Financially Conscious Scheduling

Scheduling and being financially conscious may seem unrelated, but certain financial benefits operate on temporal factors. In the US, insurances with deductibles or out of pocket maximums often reset on an annual basis. Most start on the calendar year but can also begin on the anniversary of the insurance policy's start. In either case, being conscious of how much the patient has paid toward the caps on their responsibilities can help the clinician educate the PLWC about a schedule that maximizes their insurance coverage. For example, if the patient can defer rehabilitation services until after their insurance deductible has been satisfied, they can maximize their services.

Arranging appointments in blocks can minimize the need for days off from work or travel costs. If the PLWC is to have multiple services, such as PT, occupational therapy (OT), speech language pathology (SLP), and a physician visit, it is prudent to attempt to arrange them on days where all, or most, of the visits can occur together to minimize the costs associated with the time and the travel associated with the appointments.

Lastly, understanding where the patient is in their treatment process may help to prevent last-minute cancellations and decrease exposure to cancellation fees. Many patients are not ready to participate in vigorous PT in the one to two days following their infusion.

Financially Conscious Treatment Planning

Onc R clinicians are encouraged to consider cost when planning interventions, when appropriate. For example, PTs, occupational therapists (OTs), and speech-language pathologists (SLPs) can coordinate their appointments in conjunction with each other to minimize travel. In some instances, PT or OT sessions can be spaced out farther apart with the understanding that the PLWC will participate in exercises at home to maintain progress between larger gaps in therapy.

Conclusion

Cancer remains a pervasively insidious condition. It presents PLWCs and their loved ones not only with ethical, physical, and emotional challenges, but often legal and financial ones as well. Onc R clinicians help PLWCs recover their function and

QOL, which presents challenges unique to this population. Four important ethical concepts impacting cancer and Onc R care are autonomy, justice, beneficence, and nonmaleficence. Key ethical challenges experienced by Onc R clinicians and PLWCs include such as informed consent, privacy, and confidentiality.

In order to provide just and equitable Onc R services, care must be adequately and proactively available to underserved populations. Key legal concepts include the Americans with Disabilities Act, employment law, and other legal statutes impacting healthcare access including Onc R. Cancer and cancer treatment can inflict tremendous financial damage on a PLWC. Onc R clinicians should proactively screen for financial toxicity and a downward financial spiral. Working with the cancer interdisciplinary team, Onc R clinicians can assist in addressing these various issues and assist with coping to facilitate optimal outcomes across the entire spectrum of cancer care.

Critical Research Needs

- How does race and ethnicity of the patient impact outcomes in Onc R?
- Does geographic location affect access to Onc R and how?
- Does the patients' sexual orientation/gender identity impact their experience in Onc R?

Review Questions

Reader can find the correct answers and rationale in the back of the book.

Base your response to questions 1 to 3 regarding conflict of interest in the following scenario.

You are a clinician working in a hospital-run satellite facility that offers outpatient lymphedema management services such as bandaging, decongestive therapy, and fabricating and measuring of compressive garments. You are approached by a biotechnology firm to serve on their advisory board regarding the physical design of their garment.

1. What kind of potential conflict of interest does this scenario illustrate?
   A. A dual relationship that has an implied quid pro quo
   B. A business relationship that constitutes a financial reward for preferential treatment
   C. A financial reward for access to your clientele on the part of the company
   D. No conflict exists if it is disclosed
2. They now ask you to assist their marketing team. Which of the following behaviors would represent a potential conflict of interest if committed?
   A. Serving as an advisor to the vendor representative on proper usage of the device during patient fittings. You are paid for this time and your role is described to the patient
   B. Developing descriptive content regarding the way the garment works for materials given ONLY to third party sellers of the garment and not patients
   C. Serving as an independent agent to answer patient questions on a phone hotline where only your time is compensated for monetarily
   D. Arranging a meeting with your Director of Procurement at your hospital so that they can start to have you sell these garments to your patients as a certified vendor of their company, where you will also receive a commission

3. Now imagine the scenario where it comes to your attention that a conflict of interest does, in fact, exist by participating in the development of this garment. What is the appropriate course of action?
   A. Work with your employer to modify your job description to then remove the conflict of interest
   B. You can continue to operate with the biotechnology company as long as you start disclosing your relationship moving forward
   C. Disclose all pertinent information regarding the relationship to your patients using this device as well as your employer and surrender the relationship
   D. Continue the relationship established between you and the biotechnology company but surrender your payment
4. Which of the following behaviors is most consistent with the ethical principle of *nonmaleficence*?
   A. You stay late at work to counsel your patient's family on safe transfer techniques for your patient who recently underwent a right hemipelvectomy
   B. You decline an offer from your patient to document higher functional deficits in order for the patient to qualify for higher disability benefits
   C. You perform a chart review prior to seeing a patient to ascertain any precautions that must be observed
   D. You verbally describe the procedure of soft tissue mobilization to your patient prior to initiating the treatment as permission
5. You are creating a care plan for the rehabilitation of a patient recently diagnosed with ductal carcinoma in situ (DCIS) of the right breast. They underwent a right modified radical mastectomy; no adjuvant treatment was needed. The patient has no evidence of lymphedema or difficulties using the right upper extremity. The patient reports significant anxiety related to the potential development of new functional deficits in the

future; however, is vague about specific concerns. Despite this, the patient requests that they receive a custom right upper extremity compression garment, a full round of decongestive therapy for the right upper quarter, lymph node transplantation surgery, and repeat corticosteroid injections to increase shoulder range of motion. What ethical challenge does this pose?

A. Informed consent

B. Overutilization of services

C. Privacy

D. Confidentiality

E. Fraud

6. A 22-year-old male patient who is status-post amputation of the left leg just proximal to the knee joint with a temporary prosthesis plans to progress to a permanent prosthetic. The patient, however, has been unable to receive the new prosthetic device. You find out that the patient works as a factory foreman in a rural area and must drive for over an hour each way. Therefore, he has been unable to return to the clinic for repeat fittings. In what way is this patient not having his healthcare needs met?

A. He is disadvantaged geographically

B. He is being discriminated against based on his age

C. He is being discriminated against based on his gender

D. He is refused treatment on the basis that he cannot pay

7. You are treating a person living with cancer and have a friendly relationship. One day the patient tells you that they want you to read their last computerized tomography scan and tell them if their tumor has increased in size. They insist that they do not believe what their oncologist tells them and you are the clinician that they most trust.

On what basis must you decline?

A. It would be a conflict of interest between you and the patient by reinforcing a quid pro quo

B. It would be unethical on the grounds of maintaining professional competence

C. It would be committing fraud

D. You would be overutilizing services

8. What statement best describes "Financial Toxicity"?

A. A family needing to take out a loan to pay for their cancer treatment

B. The state of being uninsured while living with cancer

C. Being discriminated against on the basis of the patient's ability to pay for their treatment

D. A physician's bias to use a less effective treatment because the patient has run out of money

9. Which factor WOULD NOT lead to healthcare disparity in the US?

A. Being uninsured or underinsured

B. Being part of a underrepresented group (e.g., LGBTQIA+, African-American, physically disabled)

C. Being geographically isolated

D. Having medical coverage through a federal program such as Medicare

10. Which of the following would be a strategy that can be employed to proactively facilitate financially protective measures thus serving as a "financial prehabilitation" intervention?

A. Checking that the patient has insurance at their first visit

B. Providing a pamphlet on financial resources supporting cancer treatments and how to qualify

C. Setting the patient up on a payment plan for services rendered

D. Choosing less expensive services to provide to the patient in an effort to reduce costs

References

1. Gabard DL, Martin MW. *Physical Therapy Ethics*. 2nd ed. F.A. Davis Company; 2011.

2. Purtilo RB. Thirty-first Mary McMillan lecture. A time to harvest, a time to sow: ethics for a shifting landscape. *Phys Ther*. 2000;80(11):1112–1119.

3. Purtilo RB. Applying the principles of informed consent to patient care. Legal and ethical considerations for physical therapy. *Phys Ther*. 1984;64(6):934–937.

4. Zhao J, Mao Z, Fedewa SA, et al. The Affordable Care Act and access to care across the cancer control continuum: a review at 10 years. *CA Cancer J Clin*. 2020;70(3):165–181.

5. Copnell G. Informed consent in physiotherapy practice: it is not what is said but how it is said. *Physiotherapy*. 2018;104(1):67–71.

6. Gostin LO, Jacobson PD, Record KL, Hardcastle LE. Restoring health to health reform: integrating medicine and public health to advance the population's well-being. *Univ Pa Law Rev*. 2011;6(159):1777–1823.

7. Shen N, Bernier T, Sequeira L, et al. Understanding the patient privacy perspective on health information exchange: a systematic review. *Int J Med Inform*. 2019;125:1–12.

8. Ferreira PH, Ferreira ML, Maher CG, Refshauge KM, Latimer J, Adams RD. The therapeutic alliance between clinicians and patients predicts outcome in chronic low back pain. *Phys Ther*. 2013;93(4):470–478.

9. Zadro JR, Décary S, O'Keeffe M, Michaleff ZA, Traeger AC. Overcoming overuse: improving musculoskeletal health care. *J Orthop Sports Phys Ther*. 2020;50(3):113–115.

10. McCormack HM, MacIntyre TE, O'Shea D, Herring MP, Campbell MJ. The prevalence and cause(s) of burnout among applied psychologists: a systematic review. *Front Psychol*. 2018;9:1897. doi:10.3389/fpsyg.2018.01897.

11. Merriam-Webster Inc. *The Merriam-Webster Thesaurus*. New ed. Merriam-Webster; 2005:668.

12. Davis M. Conflict of Interest. *Encyclopedia of Applied Ethics*: Academic Press; 1998.

13. Holm LV, Hansen DG, Larsen PV, et al. Social inequality in cancer rehabilitation: a population-based cohort study. *Acta Oncol*. 2013;52(2):410–422.

14. Edwards I, Delany CM, Townsend AF, Swisher LL. New perspectives on the theory of justice: implications for physical therapy ethics and clinical practice. *Phys Ther*. 2011;91(11):1642–1652.

15. Trivedi AN, Grebla RC, Wright SM, Washington DL. Despite improved quality of care in the Veterans Affairs health system, racial disparity persists for important clinical outcomes. *Health Aff (Millwood)*. 2011;30(4):707–715.

16. Keeney T, Jette AM, Freedman VA, Cabral H. Racial differences in patterns of use of rehabilitation services for adults aged 65 and older. *J Am Geriatr Soc*. 2017;65(12):2707–2712.

17. Graham JE, Chang PF, Bergés IM, Granger CV, Ottenbacher KJ. Race/ethnicity and outcomes following inpatient rehabilitation for hip fracture. *J Gerontol A Biol Sci Med Sci*. 2008;63(8):860–866.

18. Gwyer J, Hack L. In search of cultural competence. *J Phys Ther Educ*. 2014;28(1):3.

19. Mirza M, Luna R, Mathews B, et al. Barriers to healthcare access among refugees with disabilities and chronic health conditions resettled in the US Midwest. *J Immigr Minor Health*. 2014;16(4):733–742.

20. Mirza M, Harrison EA, Roman M, Miller KA, Jacobs EA. Walking the talk: understanding how language barriers affect the delivery of

rehabilitation services. *Disabil Rehabil.* 2020;44(2):301–314. doi:10 .1080/09638288.2020.1767219.

21. Black J, Purnell L. Cultural competence for the physical therapy professional. *J Phys Ther Educ.* 2002;16(1):3–10.

22. Kumaş-Tan Z, Beagan B, Loppie C, MacLeod A, Frank B. Measures of cultural competence: examining hidden assumptions. *Acad Med.* 2007;82(6):548–557.

23. Tervalon M, Murray-García J. Cultural humility versus cultural competence: a critical distinction in defining physician training outcomes in multicultural education. *J Health Care Poor Underserved.* 1998;9(2):117–125.

24. Barnes C, Mueller K, Fawcett L, Wagner B. Living and dying in a disparate health care system: rationale and strategies for cultural humility in palliative and hospice care physical therapy. *Rehabil Oncol.* 2020;38(1):30–38.

25. Copti N, Shahriari R, Wanek L, Fitzsimmons A. Lesbian, Gay, Bisexual, and transgender inclusion in physical therapy: advocating for cultural competency in physical therapist education across the United States. *J Phys Ther Educ.* 2016;30(4):11–16.

26. Polek CA, Hardie TL, Crowley EM. Lesbians' disclosure of sexual orientation and satisfaction with care. *J Transcult Nurs.* 2008; 19(3):243–249.

27. Onega T, Duell EJ, Shi X, Wang D, Demidenko E, Goodman D. Geographic access to cancer care in the U.S. *Cancer.* 2008; 112(4):909–918.

28. Beatty PW, Hagglund KJ, Neri MT, Dhont KR, Clark MJ, Hilton SA. Access to health care services among people with chronic or dis-abling conditions: patterns and predictors. *Arch Phys Med Rehabil.* 2003;84(10):1417–1425.

29. Lee AC, Harada N. Telehealth as a means of health care delivery for physical therapist practice. *Phys Ther.* 2012;92(3):463–468.

30. Americans with Disabilities Act. *ADA Guide for Small Businesses.* Office of Entrepreneurial Development; 1999.

31. Enforcement Guidance on Reasonable Accommodation and Undue Hardship under the ADA. U.S. Equal Opportunity Commission; 2002.

32. Stergiou-Kita M, Pritlove CBK. The "Big C"-stigma, cancer, and workplace discrimination. *J Cancer Surviv.* 2016;10(6):1035–1050.

33. Mehnert A. Employment and work-related issues in cancer survivors. *Crit Rev Oncol Hematol.* 2011;77(2):109–130.

34. Mak AK, Chaidaroon S, Fan G, Thalib F. Unintended consequences: the social context of cancer survivors and work. *J Cancer Surviv.* 2014;8(2):269–281.

35. Xie Y, Tang Y, Wehby GL. Federal health coverage mandates and health care utilization: the case of the Women's Health and Cancer Rights Act and use of breast reconstruction surgery. *J Womens Health (Larchmt).* 2015;24(8):655–662.

36. Lentz R, Benson AB 3rd, Kircher S. Financial toxicity in cancer care: prevalence, causes, consequences, and reduction strategies. *J Surg Oncol.* 2019;120(1):85–92.

37. Yu JB. The death spiral of cancer and financial hardship. *JNCI Cancer Spectr.* 2018;2(2):pky013.

34

Billing, Coding, and Documentation

RACHEL T. TRAN, PT, DPT, BOARD CERTIFIED NEUROLOGIC CLINICAL SPECIALIST, KIRK RANDALL, PT, AND CHRIS WILSON, PT, DPT, DScPT, BOARD CERTIFIED GERIATRIC CLINICAL SPECIALIST

CHAPTER OUTLINE

Introduction

Successful documentation, billing, and coding are vital components in the care of persons diagnosed with and treated for cancer. Documentation occurs in many forms throughout the continuum of patient care. It serves as a means of communication between providers and as a record to justify that all oncology rehabilitation (Onc R) services that were provided was skilled and medically necessary. To ensure full payment for services provided, it is important to understand the requirements and regulations of documentation, billing, and coding. What is documented and what is billed must align and support each other based on payable diagnostic codes. When they do not, facilities or departments are at risk of audits and/or denials, which can result in serious fines and lost revenue.

Documentation must demonstrate skill and best practice while complying with requirements dictated by regulatory bodies and third-party payers. Within the United States (US), documentation and billing are moving quickly from fee for service to value-based care. Value-based care is based on two primary components; the outcomes that have been achieved during treatment and the cost it took to achieve those outcomes. The Centers for Medicare/Medicaid Services (CMS) currently defines value-based care as paying for healthcare services in a manner that links performance to cost, quality, and the patient's experience of care.[1] This change to value-based care will hold Onc R clinicians more accountable for patient outcomes and require them to become more innovative and look at new approaches for delivering their care.[2]

A clinician's specialty knowledge of the Onc R needs of persons with cancer (PWCs) must be represented in the clinical documentation to justify the complexity of a patient's presentation, set realistic goals, and explain fluctuations that can occur from cancer and its treatments. PWCs have individualized Onc R needs dependent on their level of impairment, adverse effects of cancer treatment, and disease prognosis. According to Dietz's Model[3] for Onc R, there are four phases of care: preventative, restorative, supportive, and palliative. Each phase has its unique characteristics that need to be documented and addressed throughout a patient's rehabilitative care. A patient referred for a prospective surveillance evaluation will have different needs than a patient with terminal cancer who is receiving palliative care. As such, the plan of care (POC), goals, and treatment notes must adequately represent the different needs and disease trajectories of patients.

This chapter will explore the components of documentation throughout different phases of care with attention paid to the unique Onc R needs of PWCs. Finally, this chapter will also touch on the regulations that oversee documentation and billing and provide insights into how to avoid an audit. As you read through this chapter, it is important to understand that variances exist based on jurisdiction, setting, and payor type. These regulations also change frequently; therefore strategies will be provided to stay in alignment with current regulations and requirements.

Documentation

The documentation of patient management is a professional responsibility and a legal requirement. It is more than just a record of services provided and outcomes supporting payment for services; documentation is critical to ensure that individuals receive appropriate, comprehensive, efficient, client-centered, and high-quality healthcare services throughout the POC.[4] Documentation that lacks specificity and accuracy could be at risk for denial of reimbursement and increase a facility's risk of an insurance audit. In addition, the Onc R clinician must be able to defend the documentation if it were ever called into question.

Due to active disease or the adverse effects of treatment, PWCs often experience fluctuations in symptom severity and function. Documenting prior baseline function, chemotherapy regimens, or disease progression can help justify the need for continued treatment, even as fluctuations in a patient's presentation arise.

The requirements of the different documentation types required throughout an episode of care are described in this chapter. It is important to keep in mind that documentation requirements vary slightly by jurisdiction, setting, and insurance type. To ensure that a clinician's documentation is reimbursable and defensible, it is important to stay up to date with changes in documentation requirements set forth by local regulatory agencies and various payment sources. As it is not feasible to cover the myriad regulations and payment methods of all of its international readership in this chapter, scenarios will utilize the example of the US Medicare requirements as these tend to be the most strict and are consistent across state lines. There are over 400,000 pages of CMS regulations so this chapter will discuss regulations that are most relevant to Onc R clinicians in practice.

Examination and Evaluation

The examination and evaluation documentation sets the stage for a patient's entire treatment course. The information included in an evaluation primarily serves to defend a patient's initial need for skilled intervention. Describing the severity of impairment and

functional disability, the complexity of PWCs medical history, and personal and environmental factors that may influence a patient's recovery provides the rationale for skilled treatment. It is critical to consider that the initial examination and evaluation documentation often only justifies *initial* medical necessity; as an episode of care continues, it will be more important and more challenging to justify *ongoing* medical necessity as the patient's condition improves, stabilizes, or regresses. Thus, concrete steps should be taken to always justify ongoing medical necessity in treatment notes and interim/progress reports. In this section, we will discuss the basic components required of an evaluation and highlight the unique needs to be considered when evaluating a PWC.

Subjective History

Due to the complexity of certain cancer diagnoses, PWCs often require additional questioning to obtain all necessary information needed to inform the choice of testing, goals, and POC. It takes practice and skill to ask the right questions. A complete subjective intake should include aspects of medical history that relate to the patient's prior and current status, or aspects that can influence a patient's Onc R prognosis.[5] As such, not every component of a patient's past medical history must be reported; this will be illustrated by describing a patient referred to Onc R for shoulder pain. While this patient's history of breast cancer and surgical history of unilateral mastectomy and reconstruction using a latissimus dorsi flap are all relevant to the Onc R episode of care, the patient's co-morbidity of hyperlipidemia is less relevant. Always include a detailed report of the patient's symptoms and limitations. This should be written in the patient's voice, not converted into medical terminology.[5] As falls are a major issue in PWCs, it is important to record fall history (including near falls, fear of falling, or risk of falls) during evaluations. Third-party payers, such as Medicare, prioritize functional limitations and safety gaps. Be sure to inquire about and document how the patient's symptoms are impacting their current function such as their ability to mobilize and complete their basic activities of daily living (ADLs) and instrumental ADLs (IADLs) at home and in the community. Returning to prior function may not always be achievable but understanding one's prior functional status and life roles will drive the decision-making process behind what tests and measures need to be included in evaluation documentation. A description of the patient's previous level of function (including occupational and recreational profile) before the onset of injury or illness will further describe the current extent of dysfunction. As always, include a complete profile of a patient's home environment and social support, as these contextual factors can further justify the need for skilled Onc R.

While conducting a subjective history for a PWC, a thorough discussion should be documented to establish individualized patient and caregiver goals for rehabilitation. This history can be documented anecdotally or via patient-reported outcome (PRO) measures that the patient completes (usually before a rehabilitation session). There are five general types of PROs, including health-related quality of life (HR-QOL), functional status, symptoms/symptom burden, health behaviors, and patient experience of care.[6] The Academy of Oncologic Physical Therapy has published and regularly updates a summary of the evidence supporting a variety of these outcome measures.[7] A few notable measures of HR-QOL include the Patient-Reported Outcomes Measurement Information System (PROMIS), which is a multi-institution initiative coordinated by the National Institute of Health. The PROMIS-Cancer (PROMIS-Ca) measures were specifically selected by content experts to choose relevant cancer-specific question items, including anxiety, depression, fatigue, pain interference, and physical function. Another series of useful measures of HR-QOL is the Functional Assessment of Chronic Illness Therapy (FACIT), also known as the Functional Assessment of Cancer Therapy (FACT). These measures are free to use and apply, highly reliable and valid, and have been translated into several languages. These measures can be found on www.facit.org. See Chapter 29 for more information on quantifying quality of life.

Some diagnosis/region-specific outcome measures may include the Disability of Arm, Shoulder, and Hand (DASH) for breast cancer; the Neck Disability Index (NDI) for head and neck cancer; and the Pelvic Floor Distress Inventory-Short Form or Pelvic Floor Impact Questionnaire-Short Form for urogenital cancers. Onc R clinicians are encouraged to always apply at least a HR-QOL measure and one to two other PROs to adequately capture the breadth and depth of the PWC's limitations and restrictions. These measures can be complemented by clinician-administered functional outcome measurements such as the Activity Measure for Post-Acute Care (AM-PAC),[8] the Karnofsky Performance Scale,[8,9] or the components of a comprehensive geriatric assessment.[10] Such outcome measurements will establish a baseline for disease severity and functional deficits. Due to the late effects of cancer treatment, it is important to collect information about a patient's current and past treatment regimens, including radiation, chemotherapy, or surgical history. This information will reveal restrictions or precautions and can explain fluctuations in fatigue severity, function, and overall presentation throughout the course of care. With the availability of an integrated medical record, it may seem redundant to find information in the medical record and document it within a rehabilitation note, yet this task remains important due to the fact that when insurance companies perform medical necessity reviews of rehabilitation services, only the therapists' notes are often supplied. If a critical piece of contextual information is not within the rehabilitation notes, it may result in more thorough reviews and/or denial of payment.

Within the subjective history documentation, it is important to document screenings that were performed beyond the patient's primary impairment or concern. These might include screenings in individuals with pelvic or abdominal cancers for any issues with urination or bowel movements or experiencing pain with sex. With the prevalence of depression in PWCs reported at 8% to 24%,[11] completing a depression and/or suicide screen in the initial intake is recommended. The outcomes of these screens and the actions taken because of these screens (such as referrals to appropriate professionals) should be included in all evaluation documentation. Finally, it is important to identify the patient's

managing oncologist to establish a point of contact as medical or rehabilitation questions and concerns arise.

Systems Review

Because individuals in many jurisdictions now can seek some outpatient rehabilitation services without a physician referral, it is important to include and document a systems review in an evaluation of a PWC or someone with a history of cancer. This will rule out potential conditions that would require consultation with, or referral to, another provider. An experienced Onc R clinician can complete a systems review in a relatively short time, but failure to do so can put patients and the clinician at risk of not identifying or addressing health concerns that may be more critical than the primary impairment that prompted the pursuit of Onc R.

Impairment Testing

During the subjective history, pay attention to signs that a patient may have cancer-related cognitive impairment (CRCI) requiring attention for safety and adaptations to general interactions. Such signs may include delayed response time, word finding difficulties, or poor attention. CRCI deficits are often seen in survivors who have received neurotoxic chemotherapies, head/neck radiation therapy (RTx), RTx with a total dose over 24 Gy,[12] and patients with severe fatigue. A clinician may notice a patient exhibits tangential speech or thought processes or that their historical report was vague or inconsistent. Onc R clinicians who suspect CRCI should document the results of a basic cognitive screen. Simple orientation questions are often used to assess cognition, though this does not screen for problems with executive function or impulsive behavior. Other tools, such as the Saint Louis University Mental Status (SLUMS) Exam or the MiniCog, provide a quick and comprehensive screen of executive function. The results of a cognitive screen can help to justify a referral to an occupational therapist (OT) or speech-language pathologist. Identifying CRCI at the evaluation can also help to defend a lack of carryover seen between treatments and the need for repeated teaching and additional skilled therapy.

As impairment testing should be included in the evaluation documentation, results should only be included if they are relevant to the patient's complaints and goals. The clinician should select and document testing that will describe the severity of the patient's dysfunction and identify the cause of the patient's complaints. The results of any testing should have a clear relationship to the patient's functional limitations and participation restrictions. In caring for PWCs, Onc R clinicians should select measures based upon anticipated or likely adverse effects of each patient's past cancer treatment, objectively quantify the severity of these impairments, and document the role of these impairments within the context of the patient's current problem. Table 34.1

TABLE 34.1 Assessing Late Effects of Cancer Treatment

Late Effect of Cancer Treatment	Relevant Impairment Assessment
Chemotherapy-induced polyneuropathy	Sensory testing of distal extremities; balance assessment, vestibular function assessment
Decreased bone density	Postural assessment; height
Radiation fibrosis	Skin integrity, range of motion (ROM)
Fatigue	6-Minute Walk Test
Lymphadenectomy	Circumferential measurements

Created by Rachel Tabak Tran, PT, DPT, Kirk Randall, PT, and Christopher Wilson, PT, DPT, DScPT.

has key examples of possible late effects of cancer and means to quantify them.

Objective Tests and Measures

Standardized objective measurements are key in describing the results of the examination and the success of subsequent interventions in a language that is common across providers.[13] These measures often draw the most attention to functional deficits and can be used to inform the payer of the necessity of skilled intervention. Objective measurements can also be used to determine equipment needs (see section on Documenting Equipment Needs). When evaluating a PWC, it is recommended to document outcomes that are deficient as well as those that are normal (especially normal findings that were anticipated to be abnormal). Due to the effects of cancer treatment, "normal" measures may regress into areas of deficit during the episode of care. While the objective measures performed during an evaluation will be used to establish baseline ability, the same measures must be repeated throughout the episode of care to describe progress made as a result of care and justify the need to extend or discontinue services. Therefore, Onc R clinicians should select measures that highlight current deficits, will be responsive to change, and are easily repeatable.

Documenting the Evaluation

Complexity

From the medical history of a PWC and adverse effects of treatment, to the social strain of cancer, each PWC carries a complex presentation. In the US, therapists are asked to use different billing codes for a "low," "moderate," or "high" complexity evaluation. Justification to support the selection of each code must be embedded throughout the evaluation documentation. Below are the four main evaluation complexity factors. These factors guide the decision-making behind selecting the most appropriate evaluation complexity.

Patient History

Personal Factors

These include age, sex, social background, professional, behavior pattern, education level, coping style, social background, lifestyle, behavior patterns, and other factors that influence how a disability is experienced by the PWC. Personal factors that are prevalent in PWCs include financial strain, lack of social support, educational level, and coping style.

Comorbidities

This includes any past medical history that may impact a POC. Comorbidities potentially encountered in PWCs include the cancer diagnosis, obesity, diabetes, cognitive deficits, neuropathy, fatigue, osteopenia, cardiovascular debility, and graft-versus-host disease (GVHD). Comorbidities that may complicate rehabilitation should be emphasized or prioritized as opposed to remote past medical issues or surgeries that will not substantively impact the therapy POC.

Examination of Body Systems

This is a running total how many assessments were performed during the evaluation, including assessments of body structures and functions, activity limitations, and participation restrictions. See Box 34.1 for criteria for body system examination.

Clinical Presentation

When categorizing the clinical presentation, it is important to describe the stability of the clinical presentation, not the stability

---

• BOX 34.1	Body System Assessments When Determining Complexity[14]
Body regions	Refers to areas of the body, such as head, neck, back, lower extremities, upper extremities, and trunk
Body systems	Includes the circulatory, skeletal, muscular, nervous, respiratory, immune, excretory, integumentary, lymphatic, cardiovascular, reproductive, and digestive systems
Body structures	Refers to the body's structural or anatomical parts (e.g., organs or limbs), which are classified according to body systems
Body functions	Refers to physiological functions of body systems
Activity limitations	Difficulties an individual may have in performing a task or activity
Participation restrictions	Problems an individual may experience in involvement in life situations or life roles
Clinical presentation	Status of current condition (stable to unstable) and mechanism of current condition, described as stable/uncomplicated, evolving/changing, or unstable/unpredictable.[15]

---

of the cancer disease process. While it may be reasonable to claim that any patient with stage IV cancer has an unpredictable disease course, the clinical presentation is only considered unstable when a patient has sudden and unpredictable fluctuations in vital signs or symptoms that are progressing without clear cause. Fluctuations in presentation related to the cancer diagnosis or cancer treatment fit best into the category of *evolving clinical presentation*.

Decision Making

A skilled summary of the three prior factors, including the use of a standardized patient assessment instrument and/or measurable assessment of functional outcome. Table 34.2 describes how to calculate the overall complexity of a patient's evaluation based on the personal factors, examination of body systems, and clinical presentation.

Here are three case examples that illustrate a low, moderate, and high complexity evaluation:

Case Example 1

A 36-year-old female initially diagnosed with stage 1 breast cancer in full remission has recently experienced mild generalized weakness, causing her difficulty with managing stairs at the end of her day. She has been unable to go on her daily 10-mile bike rides, now riding only twice weekly for up to five miles. She does not report pain or any range of motion (ROM) loss. After performing several tests, you conclude that she has mild strength loss in both of her legs and core, and her 6-Minute Walk Test is diminished, yet her cardiac function is normal. See Box 34.2 for the rationale for the appropriate code.

Case Example 2

A 65-year-old right hand dominant female presents to physical therapist (PT) for lymphedema evaluation of the right upper extremity following a mastectomy with lymphadenectomy 4 months ago. She is currently on her fifth cycle of a bi-monthly chemotherapy regimen for her breast cancer. Prior to surgery and development of lymphedema, she was completely independent and working part time as a secretary. She volunteered 2 days/week,

TABLE 34.2	Evaluation Code Reference[14–16]		
	Low	Moderate	High
Physical Therapy Evaluation Codes	97161	97162	97163
Occupational Therapy Evaluation Codes	97165	97166	97167
Patient History			
No personal factors and/or comorbidities	X		
1–2 personal factors and/or comorbidities		X	
3+ personal factors and/or comorbidities			X
Examination of Body Systems			
1–2 assessments performed	X		
3+ assessments performed		X	
4+ assessment performed			X
Clinical Presentation			
Stable/uncomplicated	X		
Evolving/changing		X	
Unstable/unpredictable			X
Decision Making Complexity	Low	Moderate	High

• BOX 34.2   Rationale for Low Complexity Evaluation Code

PT Evaluation: Low Complexity CPT 97161

History	**Examination**	**Clinical Presentation**
Comorbidities/ Personal Factors:	Assessments Performed:	Stable as patient has no personal factors or current comorbidities and her strength and endurance are expected to return to prior levels of function.
1. History of breast cancer, no active disease	1. ROM 2. Strength 3. Endurance	

---

attended monthly gardening class, and enjoyed going out for coffee with her friends. Currently she is unable to lift reams of paper at work, is having difficulty with typing for data entry, reports poor balance, and has pain 6/10 at the incision site. Examination findings include edema, upper extremity weakness, and ROM loss at her shoulder, elbow, wrist, and fingers. She also indicates that she had a fall 3 weeks ago. The treatment plan is for manual lymph drainage and bandaging with home exercise program (HEP) instruction, balance training, and strengthening. See Box 34.3 for the rationale for the appropriate code.

Case Example 3

A 78-year-old male admitted to an acute rehabilitation facility with a history of head and neck cancer status-post resection with pectoral flap repair. He also has a past medical history significant for emphysema and liver dysfunction due to alcoholism. Due to fluctuating levels of ascites, this patient inconsistently requires the use of supplemental oxygen and his vitals fluctuate significantly with exertion, requiring constant monitoring with activity. This patient is widowed and lives with his family though he is usually left home alone while his daughter and son-in-law are at work. His behavior is unpredictable and at times he can become agitated and use inappropriate language. Upon examination, the Onc R clinician finds his bilateral lower extremity ROM and strength are significantly limited as is his neck mobility. He has low endurance and a shuffling gait pattern with frequent loss of balance. He is uncooperative and is not adhering to his precautions or exercise recommendations. As such, the Onc R clinician determines that he will need extensive family training for safe return home as well as functional training to improve safety and reduce his fall risk. See Box 34.4 for the rationale for the appropriate code.

• BOX 34.3   Rationale for Moderate Complexity Evaluation Code

PT Evaluation: Moderate Complexity 97162

History	**Examination**	**Clinical Presentation**
Comorbidities/Personal Factors:	Assessments Performed:	Evolving as the patient is in early stage of recovery and experiences fluctuations in symptoms related to chemotherapy treatments.
1. History of breast cancer 2. Surgical history of mastectomy and lymphadenectomy 3. Lymphedema 4. Currently receiving chemotherapy	1. ROM 2. Strength 3. Edema 4. Balance	

• BOX 34.4   Rationale for High Complexity Evaluation Code

PT Evaluation: High Complexity 97163

History	Examination	Clinical Presentation
Comorbidities/Personal Factors: 1. History of head and neck cancer 2. Emphysema 3. Liver dysfunction 4. Falls 5. Unpredictable and nonadherent behavior	Assessments Performed: 1. ROM 2. Strength 3. Balance 4. Gait analysis 5. Cardiovascular endurance	Complex due to unpredictable fluctuations in patient's vitals that require constant monitoring, unstable disease, and agitation/inappropriate behavior.

Evaluation Summary

The section is also known as the *assessment* and provides a summary of the evaluation findings, a description of these findings, and how they impact the patient's function and life roles, as well as justification of the necessity of skilled Onc R services. In addition, an astute clinician can also portray possible negative consequences to the patient if Onc R services are not administered, further justifying medical necessity for interventions. An evaluation summary or assessment should not merely list findings or repeat the subjective report. Instead, it should indicate the prior level of function before the onset of diagnosis and how this has changed. An assessment may include what support the patient will need at home, physical assistance or otherwise, to ensure safety. Other information to be included in the assessment includes potential barriers to progress, the patient's involvement in goal setting, the patient's agreement to the POC, and rationale for referrals to other disciplines. To prevent duplication of services and goals, the clinician should note if interdisciplinary discussion has occurred. Finally, an assessment should indicate the patient's rehabilitation prognosis, or what level of function the clinician expects the patient to achieve by the end of the episode of care. Not all PWCs will make progress, though this should not make a patient ineligible for Onc R services. In these situations, skilled intervention may be justified around the need for caregiver education or training, equipment allocation, or maintenance therapy to reduce functional and safety issues related to decline. Such needs must be clearly indicated in the assessment.

Goals

Goals provide an opportunity for the patient and caregivers to describe the functional changes they hope to accomplish through Onc R. Writing functional goals is important to demonstrate the medical necessity of Onc R services and the need for the skilled intervention of the Onc R clinician or support personnel (e.g., PT assistant, certified occupational therapist assistant). Goals

demonstrate a patient's prognosis and provide the foundation on which the POC is directed. To effectively use goals to direct the progression of treatment, goals should meet all of the criteria for SMART goals: Specific, Measurable by re-evaluation, Achievable, Relevant to the patient's functional deficits, and Time sensitive (Table 34.3). To comply with Medicare expectations, goals must be tied to function. This means that goals must be written around a functional task or a participation activity.

Goal writing for PWCs is challenging due to various factors, including an unclear disease course and adverse effects of treatment. When considering rehabilitation potential for PWCs, consider the following: if the PWC has active disease, their treatment course including upcoming chemotherapy regimen (including chemo holidays/vacations), previous response to treatment, and the chronicity of the late effects of cancer treatment. Many cancer treatments are associated with prolonged hospitalizations, including certain chemotherapies, hematopoietic stem cell transfers, and chimeric antigen receptor T cell (CAR-T) therapy. Aside from the numerous and severe adverse effects associated with each treatment, immobility associated with a prolonged hospitalization may challenge a patient's rehabilitation potential. Common distresses of a person living beyond cancer (PLBC), such as pain, anxiety, social isolation, lack of support, and financial strain, may also interfere with their rehabilitation prognosis.

Certification of the Plan of Care

A POC is composed upon completion of the initial evaluation. Specific requirements may vary by jurisdiction or insurance payer; for example, Medicare requires that a POC includes a medical diagnosis and a rehabilitation diagnosis; long-term goals; description of the type, amount, duration, and frequency of services to be provided; and a dated signature with the professional designations of the developer of the POC.[17-18] When selecting the most appropriate frequency of treatment for PWC, consider how many other appointments the patient has to attend. For example, if a patient has daily radiation, adding two more visits per week may

TABLE 34.3   Goal Writing

Example of Incomplete Goals	Example of Function-Based SMART Goals
PT will be able to walk with a walker.	PT will ambulate modified independently with a front wheeled walker greater than 500 feet for community activities such as going to her doctor's office in 4 weeks.
PT will have no pain with reaching.	PT will be able to reach into her cupboards at home to get plates down for meals with no pain within 3 weeks.
PT will be able to put on her socks.	PT will be able to don her socks with the use of a sock aid modified independent in 1 week.

SMART, Specific, measurable, achievable, relevant, and time-based.
Created by Rachel Tabak Tran, PT, DPT, Kirk Randall, PT, and Christopher Wilson, PT, DPT, DScPT.

be too burdensome and lead to nonadherence to the POC. In patients with active disease, it is recommended to extend the duration of care in case the patient misses treatment due to illness or hospitalization.

Diagnostic Coding for Payment

An essential component to receiving payment for Onc R services is selecting an appropriate diagnostic code for the episode of care. Many rehabilitation departments have a clerical person who assist with coding or contracts with a coding specialist. This is due to the complexities of coding and the changing regulations. Certain insurance companies may not allow for the billing of specific codes for an episode of care; therefore, an Onc R clinician must be prepared to evaluate the patient comprehensively to establish the use of another diagnostic code. A common coding system is the International Classification of Diseases (ICD), which is used nearly universally in the US and by many healthcare providers internationally. ICD-10 is the most current version of this coding system. eTable 34.1 in the enhanced eBook provides some applicable codes to be utilized in Onc R for a variety of conditions and physical impairments; however, as the reader will note, these codes are highly specific and hinge on the medical diagnosis and clinical presentation. It should also be noted that providers should not list the medical diagnosis as their primary ICD-10 code unless treating that specific condition. For example, with a person with right shoulder pain as a result of breast cancer treatment, the *shoulder pain* ICD-10 code would be applied (M25.511), not *malignant neoplasm of unspecified site of right female breast* (C50.911). Some billing systems and insurance companies may allow secondary ICD-10 codes to be supplied, in this case, it is recommended that several codes be provided to clarify that the patient's shoulder pain is a direct result of the breast cancer, providing further justification for the rehabilitation services. For direct applicability of these procedures, therapists should refer to the insurance company's individual provider guidelines.

Treatment Note

A treatment note (commonly referred to as a "daily note") must be completed for every rehabilitation interaction following the initial evaluation. The purpose of this note is to create a record of all encounters and interventions provided by the Onc R clinician and to justify the use of each billing code on the claim.[17] The contents of a complete daily note are further described below:

Subjective Report

The subjective report of a daily note should include any updates from the patient such as changes in function, symptom report, HEP compliance, incidence of a fall, or new information related to their diagnosis. For example, the patient may report that their shoulder pain has improved so that they can now sleep without interruption or that they have a follow up appointment with their oncologist next week. It is of great importance to document changes in chemotherapy regimens, new therapies such as RTx, new adverse effects of treatment, and disease progression, as these can all cause symptom exacerbation or even functional regression.

Interventions

The most important part of a treatment note is the description of interventions provided. Each note must include the specifics of all interventions performed and should describe the skill required by the therapist or therapy assistant to complete recorded interventions. Documenting the intervention performed, as well as the purpose of said intervention, justifies the billing code selected. Do not simply state what was done by the patient (e.g., "Ambulated with a wheeled walker for 100 ft.") as this does not demonstrate skill. Skilled intervention is displayed through providing evidence-based practice/clinical reasoning for engaging the patient in a specific activity in the objective and analysis sections of a note.[5] For example, "Patient participated in functional mobility using 4-wheeled walker to bathroom. Patient required mod verbal cues to stand close to walker during ambulation. Patient education provided regarding safe use and ambulation with walker to prevent falls."

The Onc R clinician should avoid using words that describe solely what the patient did such as *completed*, *practiced*, *performed*, *ambulated*, and *demonstrated*. Instead, words should be incorporated that establish the necessary therapist skills such as *modified*, *revised*, *upgraded*, *initiation*, *progressed*, and *regressed*. For example, "patient participated in standing dynamic balance and upper extremity (UE) ROM, strength, and endurance activity of placing cups in an overhead cupboard. PT required min physical assist to place cups in cupboard and min verbal cues to engage abdominals and gluteal muscles to maintain balance. Patient required tactile cues for trunk extensors and gluteal activation for improved posture. Patient also required verbal cues for proper weight shifting and stride to improve balance and speed over 100 ft." The intervention description should not be repetitive from note to note. Instead should demonstrate progress made through advancement of activity and function. When progress is not made, barriers to progress should be documented, such as CRCI, disease progression, or patient's non-compliance to treatment recommendations.

Education

Patient and caregiver education should begin at the time of evaluation and be ongoing until the patient has been discharged. The opportunities for a therapist to educate or provide resources are vast. All education, from updates to the HEP, equipment training, patient handling, fall reduction strategies, handouts on symptom management, and more should be thoroughly documented in the daily notes with extensive detail.

Assessment

The assessment included in a treatment note need not be as robust as the initial evaluation summary assessment. Rather, this is a short summary indicating how the patient performed during the treatment session and may include areas of improvement, areas that remain limited, or the need to modify planned interventions. Adverse events, safety concerns, or new findings that are affecting the desired outcome should also be included. Barriers to progress must be mentioned in this assessment to justify lack of progression or the need for repetitive treatment. For example, a PWC may be experiencing significant fatigue due to chemotherapy causing a regression in their ability to independently ascend stairs as compared to her function 2 weeks ago. To justify the need for continued Onc R in this situation, it is important to document the reason for the regression (e.g., adverse effects of chemotherapy) and a plan to ensure the patient's safety and regain function or adjust the POC, if necessary.

Plan

Many clinicians are guilty of the common errors of writing "Continue as planned" or "Plan as tol[erated]," but this is a serious error as it does not provide sufficient evidence of skill. These common phrases may prompt an insurance company to consider that if nothing will need specific advancement, monitoring, or updating, then the patient could self-administer these treatments as a part of the home program without the need of a skilled and licensed clinician. Instead, the Onc R clinician should provide key details of what treatments would be advanced, modified, regressed, or held based on the patient's current presentation or how they responded to today's treatment. This may also include any follow up, referrals, or symptoms to monitor. It may be helpful to document your plan in the event that you would not be at work the next day and a colleague had to care for your patient. The plan would be sufficiently detailed such that they would be able to advance the treatment safely, efficiently, and cohesively.

Progress Reports

Best practice in rehabilitation is to provide a periodic reassessment to re-examine the patient's status and update goals or treatment focus; however, some jurisdictions or insurance companies may require a specific timeframe for documenting a progress report (sometimes known as an interim evaluation or a "re-eval"). For example, within the US, Medicare requires a progress report to be completed after every 10th outpatient treatment, or sooner, if there is a change to the patient's POC.[17] The purpose of a progress report is to provide *ongoing* justification of medical necessity of skilled intervention.[17] Progress reports do not always require a thorough physical examination to be performed. All goals should be restated and include a description of progress made toward each goal as compared to the previous report.[17] In the oncologic population, lack of progress may be related to several factors, including disease progression, adverse effects of treatment, or cognitive deficits. Providing a rationale for the lack of progress toward a goal will help to justify the necessity of continued care. Likewise, a rationale for not addressing one of the goals in the previous treatments should also be included. An assessment will describe the patient's status, progress made to date, and plan for continuation of treatment. Specific descriptions of how the Onc R interventions have led to specific functional gains will further justify the medical necessity of an intervention. For example, "The patient has progressed from requiring moderate assistance with bilateral rail support to ascend 10 stairs to standby assist with one rail as a result of extensive bilateral lower extremity strengthening and stabilization exercises and the balance training provided during treatment." The assessment should also indicate any adverse outcomes, the need for continued skilled intervention with the frequency and duration of rehabilitation, and any changes to the POC.

Discharge Note

Upon the discontinuation of rehabilitation, whatever the reason, a discharge note must be completed. Per Medicare guidelines, the discharge includes the same requirements of the progress report and should include a summary of the entire episode of care.[17] Information to be noted in this summary can include a description of the patient's initial and current level of function, an update on relevant outcome measures, changes in participation or activity, pain, equipment allocation, and education provided. Patients with active disease or who are receiving cancer treatment often require services extended beyond what was initially expected. An Onc R clinician is advised to thoroughly justify the need for this extension in the discharge note. In patients with chronic conditions

or those who were unable to resolve all their complaints during the episode of care, the plan should also be described for ongoing progress with a home program and indicate how the patient was transitioned to the next level of care (e.g., outpatient services or homecare services). Discharge notes may also indicate the need for future Onc R intervention based on a patient's condition.

Documentation for Telehealth

While still in its infancy, telehealth is gaining traction as a necessary mode of Onc R and healthcare. Most notably, during the COVID-19 pandemic of 2020, virtual tele-rehabilitation appointments provided an opportunity for patients to access care when being face-to-face with an Onc R clinician was not deemed safe. All previously mentioned documentation requirements apply to any telehealth visit. In addition, a statement confirming that the patient requested and consented to the tele-rehabilitation appointment is required on each note. Further research is necessary to fully understand the benefits and risks of telehealth Onc R.

Billing

An Onc R clinician's skills are engaged from the moment they say hello to the PWC. As the Onc R clinician escorts the patient from the waiting room to the treatment room, assessments on the patient's movement patterns and the gathering of subjective information has begun. The clinician can observe for symmetrical weight bearing with rise to stand from the waiting room chair, gait deviations as the patient walks through the clinic, and facial grimaces with activity to clue one into pain provoking movements. When documented correctly, all this time can be billed. Understanding the most appropriate use of each Common Procedural Technology (CPT code is the first step to ensuring full reimbursement. In Table 34.4, commonly billed CPT) codes in Onc R practice are defined with examples of interventions that align with these codes.

To justify billing, daily treatment notes should elaborate on both the skill provided and the purpose of the intervention performed. Writing "sit to stands ×10 with min A[ssist]" is an incomplete justification of Therapeutic Activity. An example of a complete justification that captures the skill provided and purpose of intervention is "sit to stands from various surface heights (16–24″) performed with min A to improve independence with transfers; provided verbal cues to decrease valgus force at knees and visual demonstration of correct form to improve ease of transfer." Some CPT codes sound similar making it difficult to select the most appropriate code for each intervention. Understanding the difference between seemingly similar codes is key in ensuring full payment for services rendered. Following is additional discussion on commonly confused codes:

Therapeutic Exercise Versus Therapeutic Activity Versus Neuromuscular Re-Education

Onc R clinicians often have difficulty discerning the difference between when to use the codes for Therapeutic Exercise, Neuromuscular Re-education, and Therapeutic Activity. As defined above, Therapeutic Exercise is performed for the purpose of improving strength, ROM, or endurance, while Neuromuscular Re-education is used for specific cueing of muscle groups or kinesthetic awareness, balance, and postural awareness. These interventions are focused on a patient's impairment. Conversely,

TABLE 34.4 Commonly Billed Common Procedural Technology (CPT) Codes for Physical Therapy[19]

CPT Code Defined	Example of Intervention	Documentation Example
97110 Therapeutic Exercise: To develop strength, endurance, range of motion and flexibility, one or more areas.	Targeted strength training; endurance training; active/active assisted range of motion; self-stretching	Performed 10 reps of quad sets to improve strength, educated patient in technique, and added to home carryover program.
97140 Manual Therapy Techniques: Mobilization or manipulation, manual traction, manual lymphatic drainage, applied to one or more regions.	Joint mobilization; soft-tissue mobilization; passive range of motion; manual lymphatic drainage	Performed manual lymphatic drainage techniques to the right foot and ankle and calf region to decrease swelling.
97112 Neuromuscular Re-Education of movement, balance, coordination, kinesthetic sense, posture, and proprioception for sitting and/or standing activities, one or more areas.	Balance training; gait training with assistance or cueing; kinesiology taping; coordination training; postural training	Facilitated trunk extensor musculature through manual tapping and verbal cues to improve upright posture during standing balance activity.
97530 Therapeutic Activities: Direct (one on one), patient contact by the Onc R clinician (use dynamic activities to improve functional performance).	Bed mobility training; transfer training; functional strengthening; wheelchair skills	Patient performed transfer training from their wheelchair to the mat table with verbal cues to push from the wheelchair and to reach for the mat for controlled descent.
97014 Electrical Stimulation (Unattended): Supervised electrical stimulation provided without constant direct contact required.	Interferential current (IFC); transcutaneous electrical nerve stimulation (TENS); cyclical muscle stimulation (Russian stimulation)	Set up TENS for pain reduction to right hand program #2. Placed glove electrode on and applied negative pad over forearm. Increased intensity to sensory level only.
97032 Electrical Stimulation (Manual): Electrical stimulation provided that requires constant direct contact.	Functional electrical stimulation; neuromuscular electrical stimulation with exercise or functional activity; instructing patient on independent use of TENS device	Set up NMES to left ankle dorsiflexors in series pattern. Increased intensity until motor activity noted. Cued patient to perform ankle motion through verbal cues and tactile cues for 10 min with interval rest periods.
97116 Gait Training: For training patients whose walking abilities have been impaired by neurological, muscular, or skeletal abnormalities or trauma.	Fitting a patient for the correct assistive device; instructing ambulation for weight bearing restrictions, turns, chair transfer, or ascending/descending stairs with assistive device or prosthesis	Patient ambulated outside over a grassy surface and on the sidewalk with a single point cane, cued the patient for proper gait pattern with the use of the cane.
97535 Self-Care/Home Management Training (e.g., activities of daily living [ADL] and compensatory training, meal preparation, safety procedures, and instructions in use of assistive technology devices/adaptive equipment), direct one-on-one contact.	Retraining of ADL; instruction of energy conservation/pacing techniques; training of assistive technology to be used with ADL completion	Educated patient and spouse in lower body hemiparetic dressing techniques demonstrating increased performance with sock aid w/ minimal verbal cues. Patient performed overhead dynamic reaching tasks by retrieving items outside BOS in kitchen setting.

Therapeutic Activities are focused on function. A patient may have difficulty standing from a chair due to lower extremity weakness. For this patient, supine mat exercise performed to strengthen key muscles of the legs are best billed as Therapeutic Exercise unless the therapist performed tactile cues to facilitate/activate specific muscle groups then it would be billed as Neuromuscular Re-education. Therapeutic Activities generally involve functional tasks; repeated sit to stand performed at various height chairs and education about proper form with the transfer should be billed as Therapeutic Activity. For a PWC with urinary incontinence, the performance of pelvic floor strengthening exercise (without biofeedback) should be billed as Therapeutic Exercise while training the pelvic floor to contract during dynamic movements to decrease leakage with movement should be billed as Therapeutic Activity.

Gait Training Versus Neuromuscular Re-Education

The correct use of the Gait Training or Neuromuscular Re-education codes can also pose a challenge when ambulation activity is performed. Gait Training is to be used when the PT is

instructing a patient on how to use a new assistive device or on the proper sequencing with stairs with respect to a new injury. For example, training a patient to use crutches with partial weight bearing after a recent tibial bone biopsy. In the inpatient setting, this code can be used when the PT is progressing the total distance a patient ambulates. Neuromuscular Re-education should be used with ambulation training when the focus is on training neuromuscular activation, balance response, coordination, or postural control.

Billing for Education

Patient and/or caregiver education is billable time if the provision of said education requires the unique skills of a therapist or a licensed therapist assistant. Once the patient and/or caregiver has been educated on and demonstrates full understanding of the items presented, further education is no longer skilled or billable. While billing for education is allowable, there is no separate CPT code for education. When billing for education, the therapist should select the code that most closely aligns with the purpose of the education. For example, if an OT is providing education on safety with transfers for a patient with a brain tumor, it would be most appropriate to use the Therapeutic Activity CPT code. Similarly, if the therapist is educating on a home carryover program for the purpose of improving strength, then the Therapeutic Exercise CPT code should be used.[20] When billing for education for a specific CPT code, it is imperative that the specific topics, duration of education, strategies used during education, patient response, and carryover of education be documented. Avoid vague terms such as "Educated on exercise" as these brief, nonspecific phrases do not sufficiently substantiate billing for a 15-minute code.

Physical Therapy/Occupational Therapy Re-Evaluation (97164/97168)

In certain circumstances, a Physical Therapy/Occupational Therapy Re-Evaluation (97164/97168) is needed. The re-evaluation code should never be used as a routine, recurring service. The purpose of a re-evaluation is to gather more objective clinical information that was not included in an initial evaluation. Such information would illustrate the need for further testing and typically results in a substantive change in the POC.[17] Circumstances that may occur in the oncologic population and require a re-evaluation include relapsed disease, pathologic fracture, a fall, or treatment toxicities resulting in new symptoms causing a decline in function or rehabilitation prognosis. For example, a patient with a brain tumor had progressed to walking without an assistive device when she sustained a seizure at home resulting in a short hospitalization. Upon return to the clinic, she demonstrated significant right leg weakness and now requires a walker for ambulation, which is a clear change in status as compared to the intial examination. The findings of a re-evaluation and appropriate modifications to treatment goals will be communicated to the referring provider in the form of a recertification.

Choosing the Right Billing Codes

Some CPT codes cannot be billed in combination during the same patient encounter.[21] This changes quarterly, so it is important to reference the current National Correct Coding Initiative to be accurate. For example, the CPT code 97140-Manual Therapy, and 97124-Massage cannot be billed together, even if documentation indicates that these were performed as distinct services, independent from each other.[21] The same goes for 97014-Electrical Stimulation (Unattended) and 97032-Electrical Stimulation (Manual). Similarly, it is not allowable to combine an evaluation code (for example: 97161-PT Evaluation: Low Complexity with a Muscle Testing, ROM Testing, or Re-evaluation code [for example: 95831-Muscle Testing, Extremity [excluding Hand] or Trunk or 97164-Physical Therapy Re-evaluation]).[21] Other billing caveats exist as well. For example, Biofeedback Training for urinary incontinence is only reimbursable after a failed, 4-week trial of pelvic muscle exercise training is documented.[22]

Like documentation requirements, billing codes may change over time. One example of a recent code modification is billing Biofeedback Training as an intervention for urinary incontinence, which is a common occurrence in genitourinary and gynecological cancers.[22] Prior to 2020, CPT code 90911, "Biofeedback Training, perineal muscle, anorectal or urethral sphincter, including EMG and/or manometry," was billed as an untimed code. On January 1, 2020, this code was deleted and replaced with 90912,

"Biofeedback Training, perineal muscle, anorectal or urethral sphincter, including EMG and/or manometry, when performed; initial 15 minutes" and 90913, "Biofeedback Training, perineal muscle, anorectal or urethral sphincter, including EMG and/or manometry, when performed; each additional 15 minutes."[23] To avoid being denied reimbursement for the services provided, it is important to stay current with the policy guidelines of various revenue sources. Failure to stay current on code changes can result in using outdated codes and ultimately a denial of payment.

Maintenance Therapy

Maintenance therapy may be indicated when a patient's prognosis to restore function is poor and the individual requires skilled intervention to maintain his/her current level of function and prevent further functional decline. Maintenance therapy is not limited to patients with chronic or progressive diseases. Due to the debilitating adverse effects of cancer treatment and the progressive nature of the disease, some PWCs may be eligible for maintenance therapy. As described by CMS,[24] maintenance programs can take two forms:

1. Individual Activities Concurrent with Rehabilitative Treatment: An individualized plan of exercise and activity for persons living with and beyond cancer (PLWBCs) and their caregiver(s) may be developed to maintain and enhance an individual's progress during skilled therapy and after discharge from Onc R services. Prior to discharge, the maintenance program may be revised based on the person's attained functional status so that they do not regress or lose important functional skills, or to gain further improvement.

2. Maintenance Program without Onc R: Onc R may be covered by the patient's insurance for the establishment of a safe and effective maintenance program to maintain or prevent decline in function. Through prospective surveillance, maintenance programs with periodic monitoring may be indicated for determining the need of special equipment or establishing/revising a program. These programs are covered only when the clinical judgment of an Onc R clinician is required to design or establish the plan, assure patient safety, train the PLWBC or caregivers, and make infrequent but periodic re-evaluations of the plan. This form of maintenance therapy should be managed within two to four visits. Any further visits would require supporting documentation to justify continued visits. Another scenario where maintenance therapy is justifiable is when a patient is admitted for an allogeneic hematopoietic stem cell transplantation. Though the patient may enter the hospital walking independently, they are at high risk of functional decline related to a prolonged hospitalization, myeloablative conditioning, and the adverse effects of transplant. Maintenance therapy also plays a significant role in providing palliative care for PWCs. See Chapter 29 for more details about the role of maintenance therapy in palliative care.

There are important differences to understand when writing goals for a patient receiving a maintenance program without Onc R. Unlike typical goals which are restorative in nature, these goals are based around maintaining current levels of function. There are circumstances when you may have a combination of restorative and maintenance goals. For example, while it may not be realistic to improve a patient's ability to walk due to severe hemiparesis caused by a progressing brain tumor, it may be realistic for the patient to improve his/her ability to transfer in and out of a wheelchair. It is allowable to include both restorative and maintenance goals if such goals are associated with different tasks.[5] In the previous example, it would be permissible to add a maintenance goal for walking and a restorative goal for transfers. Once a goal is written as restorative, it cannot be modified into a maintenance goal. Likewise, if a patient's progress exceeds the initial prognosis, a maintenance goal cannot be modified to a restorative goal.[5]

Prehabilitation

Prehabilitation (prehab) plays an important role in the reduction of long-term therapy needs related to cancer treatments. Emerging evidence suggests that prehab results in improved patient outcomes when utilized prior to certain chemotherapies, RTx, and surgeries. Similarly, the prospective surveillance model is an approach that involves routine monitoring and early intervention aimed to lessen or eliminate common physical impairments that are caused by cancer treatments.[25] Prospective surveillance includes physical and psychological assessments for the purpose of establishing a baseline functional level and early identification of impairments.[26] Prehab may also provide targeted interventions to optimize a patient's health prior to cancer treatments such as chemotherapy, surgery, or hematopoietic stem cell transplantation. Prehab always involves patient education about the adverse effects of their cancer treatments, impairment mitigation, and health optimization.[27]

Currently, most insurance providers are not covering prehab without clear documentation of an impairment, functional limitation, or participation restriction. An Onc R clinician should not attempt to bill a third-party payer for prehab (without an impairment) unless they specifically have seen the patient's policy that indicates coverage of this therapy service. It is important to consider that many PWCs have underlying impairments that warrant some level of rehabilitation, and in some cases, it may require a thorough examination to identify and document these therapeutic needs. Furthermore, some patients may pay out of pocket for individual prehab while others may obtain a form of prehab by attending classes sponsored by healthcare facilities or outpatient community-based programs. While these classes offer good information, they are not specific to the individual needs of everyone attending. More research and advocacy to state lawmakers is needed to raise awareness for payment reform to facilitate the benefits of prehab in reducing long-term dysfunction related to cancer treatments.

Prehab may also have cost-saving benefits through decreasing hospital length of stays and the amount of rehabilitation needed after treatment. For example, prior to receiving head and neck RTx, a patient would benefit from prehab for education of specific neck stretches and postural exercises to lessen the onset of cervical contractures that could lead to difficulties with speech or swallowing. Likewise, a patient who is going to have a mastectomy with lymphadenectomy would benefit from prehab for instruction in shoulder ROM exercise and education on lymphedema symptom management. In this case example, early education on symptom management through prehab may decrease the severity of adverse effects following surgery, ultimately decreasing the associated costs of treatment. Some therapists have had success in completing and billing an evaluation visit and initiating an exercise prescription during that same visit. However, if the patient has no major impairments that would establish medical necessity, an ongoing prehab exercise program would not likely be paid for as a skilled therapy service.

Audits and Denials

Audits are amongst the most dreaded events by those in rehabilitation administration and should be taken seriously by all Onc R clinicians. Especially as Onc R is an emerging area of practice, relevant agencies and insurance companies may not have a clear understanding of the need and practice patterns employed for PWCs. The purpose of an audit is to ensure that there is no fraud, waste, and abuse, and to verify that all services provided have been billed appropriately. Avoiding an audit saves lost revenue and lost time. The best way to avoid an audit is to proactively and aggressively practice in compliance with the legal regulations set forth by local and national jurisdictions and insurance companies. For example, within the US, it is important to stay current with updates to Medicare's Local and National Coverage Policies to prevent arbitrary technical errors that may trigger an audit (e.g., not documenting a start and end time on each treatment). Larger rehabilitation departments may employ a compliance officer to stay informed and disseminate these rules. Some audits, such as probe audits, are truly unavoidable as these are randomly issued. Many audits for rehabilitation services are related to excessive use of the KX modifier (which signals exception of the Medicare therapy payment threshold [formerly the therapy cap] due to medical necessity, which may be necessary in PWCs), multiple therapists billing under the same provider number, and billing more than the average number of codes per date of service.[28]

In 2017, the most common cause of a claim denial was insufficient documentation, accounting for 64% of denials. This was followed by denials due to documentation lacking demonstration of medical necessary at 17% and incorrect coding at 10%.[29] Common mistakes that would fall under the category of insufficient documentation include the use of a medical diagnosis that was either not current or did not suggest a need for rehabilitation. Failing to explain the impact of the condition on function, independence, and participation in life roles is also considered insufficient documentation. (To note, Medicare and several other insurances do not consider recreational activities as medically necessary.) Other common mistakes that can lead to a denial is failing to describe a patient's prior level of function or not including impairment testing that is related to reported functional deficits. Poor goal writing can also result in a claim denial for various reasons including goals that are created from information that was not tested, goals that are unrealistic, previously met goals that have not been discontinued or revised to reflect patient's progress, and goals that are not based on function. Similarly, a therapist will be at risk of claim denials if treatment is not directed toward feasible, achievable, or realistic goals. As discussed earlier in this chapter, documentation must justify the CPT code selection. Failing to do so can result in a claim denial. Likewise, selecting different codes for similar interventions provided on different treatment encounters can result in payment denial.

Submitting fraudulent documentation or billing can not only lead to denial of claims but also can result in criminal prosecution and hefty criminal fines. Examples of fraudulent billing include billing for services not provided, using false information about credentials such as a college degree or license, duplicate payments, billing noncovered services as a covered code, and providing services that are not medically necessary.[30] Other examples of fraud are less obvious and may be unintentional. For example, most electronic medical records feature the ability to copy the contents of a previous note forward into subsequent encounters. While often praised as a time saving feature, submitting identical (or nearly identical) notes is considered a form of fraudulent documentation. Similarly, use of identical goals for patients with the same diagnosis (coined "copy-cat goals") is fraudulent.[5] See the enhanced eBook for an audit awareness checklist.

Documenting Equipment Needs

Individuals with cancer often have a need for specialty equipment such as a wheelchair, ambulatory devices (orthoses, prosthetics, etc.), special seating or positioning devices, and lymphedema supplies. A Letter of Medical Necessity (LOMN) is the document used to justify the medical necessity of equipment so that an insurance company will cover the cost of the equipment. LOMNs are comprehensive and require detailed subjective information and objective measurements. A LOMN should include the functional limitations that a PWC is experiencing without the equipment and the improved functional independence and positive physiological changes that will result from the use of such equipment. The equipment requested should always be the least expensive option that meets the patient's needs. It will not be assumed, however, that less expensive options were trialed and so, if this is not included in the LOMN, an insurance company may replace the equipment requested with a cheaper option. For this reason, always include what equipment has been tried and has failed to meet the patient's needs. Justifying the reimbursement of specialty equipment has grown more difficult over the years. Composing a LOMN that will be successful in obtaining requested equipment is time intensive. The more detailed, objective, and comprehensive that Onc R evaluations and daily notes are, the less difficult it will be to compose a LOMN. See the enhanced eBook for templates for LOMN for lymphedema garments, walkers, and wheelchairs or accessories.

Conclusion

Onc R clinicians are experts in mitigating and treating a myriad of issues that arise across the cancer journey but to provide these services, it must be done sustainably. To ensure financial stability and provide additional services for future PWCs, great care must be taken when documenting, billing, and coding for Onc R services. Onc R clinicians should always administer a strategic, comprehensive assortment of patient-reported and functional outcome measures and objective measurements. This will further justify the development of an achievable set of goals and a POC. In addition, accurate billing and coding will ensure adequate and fair payment for services rendered. As Onc R is a relatively new care model, this will further entrench this care philosophy as standard of practice and customary payment, including novel concepts such as prehabilitation and prospective surveillance.

Critical Research Needs

- Examining the difference in the length of stay following oncologic surgery for patients who receive prehabilitation
- Exploring the rate of utilization of Onc R referrals among medical oncology providers
- Assessing for the long-term difference in cost of care for patients who receive interval rehabilitation treatment throughout the course of chemo/radiation.
- What are the most common reasons for denial of Onc R claims for people seeking treatment due to cancer or treatment effects?

Case Study

An outpatient rehabilitation clinic which has been well established in orthopedics and neurology recently developed a new relationship with an oncologist who began referring patients for Onc R (physical therapy, occupational therapy, and speech language pathology). Due to time constraints, the clinic managers did not have time to coach the Onc R clinicians in the nuances of documentation. This resulted in a series of denials for payment from one insurance company. Now the clinic is on a 25% audit where a quarter of all claims will be closely audited by the insurance company before payment. This is a very distressing situation for the entire clinic team and has resulted in more denials and lost revenue.

The clinic managers requested a courtesy meeting with the reviewers from the insurance company to find out where the issues are, and several areas of deficiency were identified. The reviewers noted that there were four main areas to be addressed: (1) there was not consistent evidence of need for skilled services that appeared to be aerobic conditioning (prehab); (2) the notes were not clear as to why the patients always needed therapy; (3) sometimes it appeared the patients were getting worse with rehabilitation, thereby providing evidence that the therapy was not medically necessary; and (4) patients being seen for an "excessively long time." Based upon this meeting and a careful self-reflection and review of the notes in question, the managers developed an action plan to address these deficiencies.

The managers convened an all-staff meeting to summarize the findings and garner "buy in" from the team on an action plan. A priority was to provide or facilitate education of all team members in the nuances of Onc R by taking a continuing education course or pursuing an Onc R certification. Some Onc R clinicians with more cancer experience offered to mentor more novice clinicians in this area of practice. A check and balance process would be put in place, which included two levels of review before insurance submission: (1) peer review of medical records for all PWCs; and (2) manager review of care episodes that go beyond a set number of visits to assess if services were still medically necessary at the same intensity level.

To address these issues, the clinic managers establish the following action plan:

1) Skill of prehab care: Develop a decision-making algorithm to determine which PWCs required one-on-one skilled care during prehab and which PWCs could be prescribed and taught a HEP for doing prehab at home. Those that could do the prehab independently would have 1 to 2 visits to teach safe performance and then periodic phone calls to monitor how the HEP is going.

2) Lack of clarity of therapy needs: A root cause was identified in this case that the therapists were not providing enough detail as to the specific cancer stages or cancer treatments. The peer reviewers would look for sufficient detail of the stage of cancer, treatment course (including specific chemotherapy and RTx regimens and dosages), and medical issues affecting therapy (e.g., pancytopenia, falls, hospitalizations). Peer reviewers would also assess for a close, clear relationship between the cancer diagnosis/treatments and the persons' impairments and restrictions that required Onc R.

3) Patients getting worse during therapy: Some patients were indeed demonstrating fluctuations or regressions as expected during a course of cancer care. Upon retrospective chart review, these variations were not clearly linked to the cancer treatments or the underlying disease. The Onc R clinicians were educated

on using the Assessment/Evaluation portion of the note to make these connections clearly and thoroughly, especially in the cases of advanced cancer or palliative care.

4) Excessively long episodes of care: This was a noted issue as the clinic's noncancer episode of care was 9 visits and the episode of care for PWCs was 20+ visits. The team decided that any episodes of care beyond 12 visits would prompt a manager review to justify if skilled services continued to be needed or whether reducing the frequency or intensity of services would be warranted. In many cases, keeping the PWC on was appropriate due to the complexity of the diagnosis; however in some cases, stability was observed with the PWC's case and the frequency of visits was able to be reduced to once a week or twice a month to provide ongoing coaching and longitudinal care without overutilization of services.

After continuing to work collaboratively with the insurance company over the next 6 months, the clinic did not have any denials and the insurance company noted that overall costs of care for the PWCs that the clinic treated were slightly lower than other PWCs regarding hospital readmissions and emergency room visits. The reputation of this facility improved, and more oncologists began to refer to the clinic for their PWCs.

Review Questions

Reader can find the correct answers and rationale in the back of the book.

1. A patient's presentation is unpredictable due to fluctuations in vitals that require constant monitoring. This patient's complexity is best categorized as:
   A. Low
   B. Moderate
   C. Complex
   D. Prehabilitation

2. Which of the following is an example of a function-based goal?
   A. Patient will improve left quadriceps strength to 4/5
   B. Patient will decrease ankle pain to 0/5 at rest
   C. Patient will improve hamstring length to 60 degrees
   D. PT will be able to don her socks with the use of a sock aid modified independent in 1 week

3. A PT spent 30 minutes for teaching a patient with a left femur metastasis how to correctly sequence their ambulation while walking with crutches and weight bearing restrictions on the left lower extremity in the hallway and up/down stairs. It is most appropriate to bill this intervention as:
   A. Therapeutic activity
   B. Gait training
   C. Neuromuscular re-education
   D. Therapeutic exercise

4. Which of the followig is the LEAST likely to be a benefit of using objective tests during your evaluation?
   A. Repeating objective tests can be used to show progress
   B. Objective tests can be standardized between Onc R clinicians
   C. Objective tests can help illustrate the severity of a patient's functional deficit
   D. Objective tests will assure that an audit or denial will never occur

5. Which of the following documentation descriptors is LEAST likely to demonstrate skill?
   A. Modified
   B. Progressed
   C. Performed
   D. Revised

6. Proper documentation is important to prevent a denial of a claim. Which choice would be LEAST likely to be a flag that could trigger a denial?
   A. Providing skilled therapy outside the initial POC
   B. Copy and pasting prior assessment to indicate no change had occurred from the last visit
   C. Writing a goal to progress a sedentary PWC to get back to golfing
   D. Describing the PWC prior level of function and current limitations

7. Which of the following would be the LEAST likely situation where it would be appropriate to bill for a re-evaluation code?
   A. If the patient has a significant event such as a fall or new injury
   B. When the patient advances past their initial POC and you assess to set new goals
   C. Following a hospital stay with a noticeable change in function
   D. On visit two when the patient's status has not appreciably changed

8. When determining the appropriate evaluation complexity code, what four factors must be assessed to accurately guide you to the correct billing code?
   A. Personal factors, comorbidities, examination of body systems, participation restrictions
   B. Patient history, assessment of body regions, assessment clinical presentation, patient reported limitations
   C. Patient's history, examination, clinical presentation, clinical decision making
   D. Time to perform the examination, review of body regions, comorbidities, participation limitations.

9. A 56-year-old female was evaluated for range of motion limitations after mastectomy breast cancer surgery. Which of the following ICD codes would be the most appropriate primary code for this Onc R episode of care?
   A. 97162 Moderate complexity physical therapy evaluation
   B. Z48.3 Aftercare following surgery for neoplasm
   C. C50.919 Malignant neoplasm of unspecified site of unspecified female breast
   D. 97140 Manual therapy techniques

10. Which of the following examples is LEAST likely to result in a denial or audit from Medicare?
    A. Not documenting a start and end time for a Onc R treatment
    B. Providing skilled maintenance care to maintain or slow the decline of a condition
    C. Not using valid, reliable outcome measures to quantify the patient's issues
    D. Providing ongoing prehabilitation services by a licensed therapist when the activities can safely be performed by the patient at home

References

1. American Physical Therapy Association. Value based payment models. http://www.apta.org/Payment/ValueBasedCare/. Accessed June 12, 2020.
2. Moody-Williams JD. Center for Medicare & Medicaid Services: value based care. Health Resources and Services Administration. https://www.hrsa.gov/sites/default/files/hrsa/advisory-committees/nursing/meetings/2018/nacnep-sept2018-CMS-Value-Based-Care.pdf. Accessed June 12, 2020.
3. Dietz JH Jr. Rehabilitation of the cancer patient. *Med Clin North Am.* 1969;53(3):607–624.
4. American Physical Therapy Association. Physical therapy documentation of patient/client management. https://www.apta.org/your-practice/documentation. Accessed June 18, 2020.
5. Warshauer J, Geiser MB. *Be Sherlock Holmes: Discover Your Documentation Gaps to Audit Proof Your Charts.* Lecture presented at American Physical Therapy Association Combined Sections Meeting, New Orleans, LA; February 22, 2018.
6. Cella D, Hahn EA, Jensen SE, et al. Types of patient-reported outcomes. In: *Patient-Reported Outcomes in Performance Measurement.* RTI Press; September 2015 https://www.ncbi.nlm.nih.gov/books/NBK424381/.
7. Inscore E, Litterini A. APTA oncology EDGE task force report summaries. Academy of Oncologic Physical Therapy. https://oncologypt.org/wp-content/uploads/2020/03/EDGE-Annotated-Bibliography-8.19-update-1.pdf. August 2019. Accessed January 3, 2021.
8. Jette A, Haley S, Coster W, Sheng Ni P. *AM-PAC^TM Short Forms for Inpatient and Outpatient Settings: Instruction Manual.* Version 4. CREcare LLC; 2014.
9. Karnofsky DA, Burchenal JH. The clinical evaluation of chemotherapeutic agents in cancer. In: MacLeod CM, ed. *Evaluation of Chemotherapeutic Agents.* Columbia University Press; 1949:191–205.
10. Extermann M, Hurria A. Comprehensive geriatric assessment for older patients with cancer. *J Clin Oncol.* 2007;25(14):1824–1831.
11. Krebber AMH, Buffart LM, Kleijn G, et al. Prevalence of depression in cancer patients: a meta-analysis of diagnostic interviews and self-report instruments. *Psycho-Oncology.* 2014;23:121–130.
12. Armstrong GT, Reddick WE, Petersen RC, et al. Evaluation of memory impairment in aging adult survivors of childhood acute lymphoblastic leukemia treated with cranial radiotherapy. *J Natl Cancer Inst.* 2019;105(12):899–907.
13. American Physical Therapy Association. Outcomes measurement. https://www.apta.org/your-practice/outcomes-measurement. Accessed September 10, 2020.
14. Andrus B, Gawenda R. Farewell, 97001: How to use the new PT and OT evaluation codes. WebPT. https://www.webpt.com/blog/post/farewell-97001-how-to-use-the-new-pt-and-ot-evaluation-codes/. October 12, 2016. Accessed June 18, 2020.
15. Centers for Medicare and Medicaid Services. 2017 Annual update to the therapy code list. https://www.cms.gov/outreach-and-education/medicare-learning-network-mln/mlnmattersarticles/downloads/mm9782.pdf. Accessed August 4, 2020.
16. American Physical Therapy Association. Physical therapy evaluation reference table; 2020. https://www.apta.org/your-practice/payment/coding-billing/tiered-evaluation-codes/tiered-codes-evaluation-table. Accessed August 21, 2020.
17. Daulong M. *Defensible Documentation Part 1: Balancing Offense and Defense.* Prerecorded Webinar from American Physical Therapy Learning Center. https://learningcenter.apta.org/student/MyCourse.aspx?id=8bdd0076-c8c4-419d-bf01-fd0b188c2bbb. Accessed March 14, 2022.
18. Centers for Medicare and Medicaid Services. Physical, occupational, and speech therapy services. https://www.cms.gov/Research-Statistics-Data-and-Systems/Monitoring-Programs/Medical-Review/Downloads/TherapyCapSlidesv10_09052012.pdf. Accessed June 18, 2020.
19. Web PT. Physical therapists' guide to CPT Codes. https://www.webpt.com/cpt-codes/. Accessed September 30, 2020.
20. Mckee K. CPTeach: Can PTs bill for patient education? WebPT. https://www.webpt.com/blog/post/cpteach-can-pts-bill-for-patient-education/. July 31, 2018. Accessed September 21, 2020.
21. Gawenda R. Most commonly used NCCI edits for PT, OT, and SLP private practice settings. Version 25.1 correct coding initiative (CCI) edits current as of April 2019. WebPT. https://www.webpt.com/resources/download/most-commonly-used-ncci-edits-for-pt-ot-and-slp-private-practice-settings/. Accessed September 21, 2020.
22. Tunis SR, Whyte JJ, Bridger P. Decision memo for pelvic floor electrical stimulation for urinary incontinence. Centers for Medicare and Medicaid Services. https://www.cms.gov/medicare-coverage-database/details/nca-decision-memo.aspx?NCAId=61&fromdb=true. October 5, 2000. Accessed August 28, 2020.
23. Centers for Medicare and Medicaid. 2020 Annual update to the therapy code list. https://www.cms.gov/Outreach-and-Education/Medicare-Learning-Network-MLN/MLNMattersArticles/Downloads/MM11501.pdf. January 28, 2020. Accessed September 21, 2020.
24. Centers for Medicare and Medicaid Services. IOM Chapter 15, 220.2 Part D. https://www.cms.gov/Regulations-and-Guidance/Guidance/Manuals/downloads/bp102c15.pdf. July 12, 2019. Accessed August 20, 2020.
25. Stout NL, Binkley JM, Schmitz KH, et al. A prospective surveillance model for rehabilitation for women with breast cancer. *Cancer.* 2012;118:2191–2200.
26. Silver JK, Raj VS, Fu JB, Wisotzky EM, Smith SR, Kirch RA. Cancer rehabilitation and palliative care: critical components in the delivery of high-quality oncology services. *Support Care Cancer.* 2015;23(12):3633–3643.
27. Silver JK, Baima J. Cancer prehabilitation: an opportunity to decrease treatment-related morbidity, increase cancer treatment options, and improve physical and psychological health outcomes. *Am J PMR.* 2013;92(8):715–727.
28. Andrus B. 5 Things you need to know about medicare audits. WebPT. https://www.webpt.com/blog/post/5-things-you-need-know-about-medicare-audits/. July 16, 2014. Accessed August 4, 2020.
29. Brandt K. CMS's 2017 Medicare Fee-For-Service improper payment rate is below 10 percent for the first time since 2013. Centers for Medicate & Medicaid Services. http:www.cms.gov/blog/cmss-2017-medicare-fee-service-improper-payment-rate-below-10percent-first-time-2013. November 15, 2017. Accessed August 28, 2020.
30. Total Health Care. Fraud and abuse; 2020. https://thcmi.com/support/fraud-abuse/. Accessed September 29, 2020.

35

Research and Scholarship

LAURA GILCHRIST, PT, PhD

Introduction

As so expertly addressed in each chapter of this book, further research is needed to improve the care of the millions of persons living with and beyond cancer (PLWBCs). While some research exists and forms the basis of evidence-based practice guidelines, many more clinically important questions need to be asked and answered. Further exploration of the best diagnostic tests, critical prognostic factors, and most effective and efficient rehabilitation interventions needs to occur. It is sometimes easy to become frustrated when evidence for a specific question does not exist, but if a clinical question is important to practice, there is much that a clinician can do to expand the critically needed research in the area of oncology rehabilitation (Onc R).

However, as much as a clinician may want to add to the research base for Onc R, often a lack of time, confidence, and skills for conducting research can thwart this effort. In addition, once the initial enthusiasm of developing a novel question has receded, the need for funding and multiple levels of approvals can overwhelm the limited energy that clinicians can muster to even get a project going. While the conduct of even a small trial can be daunting, the efforts can pay great dividends by improving patient care and advancing a clinician's career. In the end, even the initial steps in considering the need for a research project prompts a clinician to be a better consumer of current literature, thereby improving one's clinical knowledge for evaluating and treating future patients.

This chapter will serve as a call for Onc R clinicians to become active participants in the creation of new knowledge in Onc R critically needed to provide the best care for PLWBCs. In each of the previous chapters, authors have identified key areas where further research is required. This chapter will describe a number of ways that clinicians can start pursuing clinically relevant research to help address these questions. Whether it is by publishing a case report, participating in the recruitment for a clinical trial, or conducting an independent research study, each clinician can play a role in expanding the evidence base for this growing population.

State of the Literature and Clinical Practice

Each and every day in Onc R practice, clinicians encounter a lot of questions. With each person they treat, they are often asking if the intervention they chose is the most effective or efficient for the individual or condition. The clinician may also wonder if their examination is correctly identifying the individual's underlying issue or accurately tracks their progress.

Three questions need to be answered before starting down the path of developing a research study. The following are not simple yes/no questions, yet they get at the clinician's underlying motivation and the need for research on this topic.

First, **is this issue important**? Would the answer to this question be useful in daily clinical practice for the Onc R clinician and/or for others? The reason for these questions is two-fold. To start a research study on a topic, the researcher needs to believe an issue is important. The path toward a research study is long but rewarding and internal motivation is needed to drive the project forward and disseminate the research. The importance of the issue to the clinician's population will assist in preparing a case to present to any administrators that need to approve time and resources to allow for pursuit of this project. Additionally, once the research is completed, the clinician will want an audience for the work. If other healthcare professionals will also be interested in the answer to this question, journal editors will be more inclined to publish the work.

Secondly, **has this question already been answered?** Or will the question be answered in the near future? This second question should drive the clinician back to Chapter 3 where the literature was searched to find answers to clinical questions. Perhaps a case report exists on this exact question. If the issue is rare, it may be decided that the question is answered sufficiently, and no further research is needed. But if this issue is central to clinical practice, it may be decided that a larger clinical study is required to better answer the question. If a provider is going to take the time (and money) to design a well-constructed study, it is important to know if there is an on-going clinical trial that will answer the same question more quickly. Clinical trials in the United States (US) are registered at clinicaltrials.gov.

The third question, **are sufficient resources available to take on a research study** or even a case report? Sometimes there is motivation and an important question to be answered, but both time and resources are critical. The resources needed include time to devote to the project, institutional resources (described below), and administrative support. Depending on the scope of the project to be tackled, funding may be necessary. This will require a dive into the institution's available resources. If the institution does not have sufficient resources, such as an Institutional Review Board (IRB) or statistical support, is there an opportunity to partner with another person who does have access to those resources? If the plan is to start a new research project, this chapter will describe the breadth of resources needed to pursue that research question.

The Research Journey

The Research Team

Most projects, both big and small, require a team effort. It is rare that a research project can be accomplished completely by one person alone. Even a case report may need a few levels of approvals, and while a smaller group may be required, a team will make that project flow more smoothly. A key first step is to review the listing of individuals below and determine who on the team will serve in each role. One person may serve in multiple roles, but it is helpful to determine roles during the initial phases of project development.

- **Principal Investigator (PI):** This individual is in charge of the overall project. They are the person listed on any regulatory documents and, if grant funding is needed, they are the person in charge of obtaining and managing the funding.
- **Co-Investigators:** These are other individuals involved in determining the research question, methodology, carrying out the research plan, analyzing the data, and disseminating the findings (e.g., preparing the manuscript). They should bring complementary expertise to the project. For example, if preparing a study on the impact of a new medical treatment on neuropathy, inclusion of a co-investigator who has expertise in that particular medical treatment may be helpful. Typically, the co-investigators will be authors on publications from the project.
- **Research Methodologist and Statistician:** If the project to be completed is a research study, reflecting on the research design and analysis up front is important. See Table 35.1 for categories of research methods. If the clinician and the co-investigators are not experienced with study design and statistical analysis, it will be important to consult with a person/people with expertise in these areas before starting the project. It is important

TABLE 35.1	Oncology Rehabilitation Research Study Types			
Study Design	**Description**	**Best for**	**Example**	
Case Report	Detailed report of the examination, assessment, intervention, and follow-up of an individual patient	Novel clinical situations or novel interventions	Multimodal rehabilitation following gliosarcoma resection: a case report[1]	
Case Series	Detailed report of a small group of cases involving similar patients potentially given similar interventions	Novel interventions and/or clinical situations	Balance and physical functioning in patients after head and neck cancer post-neck dissection surgery: a case series[2]	
Retrospective Cohort	Observational study of patients treated in the past for a particular condition or with a particular intervention	Detailing outcomes with historical data available	Effect of physical condition on outcomes in transplant patients: a retrospective data analysis[3]	
Prospective Cohort	Observational study of patients treated for a particular condition or with a particular intervention enrolled prior to or at the beginning of intervention	Determining risk factors or prognostic markers for outcomes	Physical performance following hematopoietic stem cell transplantation: a prospective observational study[4]	
Case Control Cohorts	Observational study detailing outcomes of two or more groups where the grouping was not set by the investigator	Rare diseases or comparisons of new interventions to previous standard of care	Improving body function and minimizing activity limitations in pediatric leukemia survivors: the lasting impact of the Stoplight Program[5]	
Clinical Trials	Scientific experiment that randomly allocates subjects to a group, where the different groups receive different interventions	Determining effectiveness of interventions	Effectiveness of four types of bandages and kinesio-tape for treating breast-cancer-related lymphoedema: a randomized, single-blind, clinical trial[6]	

Created by Laura Gilchrist. Printed with permission.

to develop a robust methodology that will provide the highest level of evidence possible within the constraints of the clinical environment. This person will also be able to assist in determining the appropriate number of subjects needed for the study design. The investigator's institution may provide this support, or it may be beneficial to partner with an academic institution to find this support. In the event that financial support is a limitation, grant funding may be pursued to assist in engaging with these important professionals. Depending on the level of involvement, these team members may be authors on resulting publications as well.

Study Personnel and Processes

Study personnel can vary substantially depending on the type of research project being considered. If the project is to be a case report or case series, no other personnel may be needed other than the clinician's own effort and some support from the administration at the institution. At times, the co-investigators may be able to take on all of these roles, but with larger trials additional personnel may be needed. If the goal is to complete an observational or experimental study, assistance from trained assessors, records

abstractors, and/or medical records departments may be needed. Trained assessors, who administer the measures of interest, are needed for both prospective cohort studies and randomized controlled trials. The reliability of assessors and outcome instruments needs to be established prior to the initiation of the project. In addition, with trials that require informed consent from participants, tracking and maintaining a file of consent forms will need to be managed. In larger trials, this role is typically fulfilled by a trial coordinator. Personnel for all phases of study implementation need to be accounted for, and sometimes division of labor amongst the study group can decrease the risk of bias. See Table 35.2 for a worksheet that provides an overview of the key steps for completing a research project. It will need to be determined which individuals on the team are responsible for each of the following roles:

- **Recruitment:** Advertising or providing information about the study to potential participants. For prospective study designs only.
- **Informed Consent:** Use of an approved method to provide study information to potential participants, allow for questions about the study to be answered, and determine understanding of study procedures prior to enrolling the participant into the study. The forms used to document informed consent are different than a *Consent to Treat* form typically used in clinical care.

TABLE 35.2   Worksheet for Research Projects

Research Task	Questions to Consider	Personal Resources	Institutional Resources
Determining Need for Research	Is the research question of importance to the researcher and other clinicians? Has this question been answered sufficiently? Is it of interest to other clinicians?	Personal time and motivation Ability to access and assess the literature	Institutional librarians Colleague and administrator discussions
Draft Research Concept	Determine if a case report, observational study, or experimental trial is most appropriate Write a concept justification as to why this study is needed Create a research protocol after consulting with experts in study design and statistical analysis	Consider personal bandwidth to take on new project Consider needed connections within the institution or need to partner with an academic institution	Consider institutional resources needed for the particular project: Institutional Review Board (IRB) Statisticians Administrative support Internal or external grant funding Discuss the project concept with department administration
Prepare Study Protocol and Other Documents	Prepare IRB required forms including: IRB Application Consent Forms HIPAA Forms	Time	Consult with the IRB on questions
Obtain Grant Funding (if needed)	Determine which granting agency and program best fits the scope and intent of the project	Time	Consult with the research department or partner institution for assistance with preparing the grant documents
Complete Study as Designed	Carry out the detailed research plan Consider weekly, bi-weekly, or monthly meetings with the research team to maintain momentum and problem solve issues Maintain all study-related documents in a secure manner as approved by IRB Report any adverse events to the IRB	Management skills	Dedicated study team
Data Analysis	Ensure accurate entry of data into records prior to data analysis	Attention to detail in following data analysis plan	Statistical assistance
Dissemination	Prepare: Institutional presentations Professional conference presentations Manuscript(s)	Blocks of time for preparing the results and writing	Trusted colleagues willing to preview the results and provide feedback Consult with journal editor for questions on submissions

HIPAA, Health Insurance Portability and Protection Act. Created by Laura Gilchrist. Printed with permission.

- **Assessment:** Depending on study design, collection of diagnostic, examination, and outcome measures at one or more time points within the trial. It is best if this person is different from the individual(s) providing the study intervention and be blinded to the participant's study group (if applicable).
- **Intervention:** Provides the appropriate intervention, if applicable, to the appropriate patient. The intervention may be highly standardized in a randomized controlled trial or may be individually tailored in an observational study design. This person ideally would be blinded to all assessment-related data.
- **Data Analysis and Manuscript Preparation:** While the statistician can assist in the study analysis, all members of the team should play a role in the interpretation of the data and preparation of the manuscript. Even if the writing is completed by one primary team member, all authors on the study should understand the study methods and results and review the manuscript prior to submission for publication.

For all team members, it is important to mitigate the potential impact of conflicts of interest throughout the research process. For example, if the investigator has developed a new intervention for a specific population, the investigator may have a vested interest in the outcome, and it is best for this person to not act as an outcome assessor for the trial. An example would be if a clinician had developed a new garment for the management of cancer-related lymphedema, it would be best if they did not measure the outcomes of a trial designed to test its effectiveness. Likewise, having the same individual provide an experimental intervention to some members of a group but not others, and then assessing both groups for outcome can introduce bias (unintentional or not) to the study. The more the intervention and assessment portions of the study can be separated and blinded to one another, the less chance for introducing bias into the study design.

Institutional Review Board

An IRB is an accredited entity at institutions tasked with protecting the rights and welfare of human subjects participating in research activities. Most commonly, the IRB will be housed within an academic or clinical institution where the research will take place. If the clinician's clinic or institution does not have an IRB, this does not exempt that individual's project from IRB review. In this case, an outside IRB should be used to review the research proposal. In some cases of multi-centered research projects, a central IRB may be used. If an individual is acting as a site investigator for such a trial, they should ask the study's primary investigator if their site is covered by the central IRB review. If so, confirmation with the local IRB of the adequacy of the central review is also needed. See Box 35.1 for common roles of the IRB.

When determining if a project requires IRB approval it is important to decide if the project to be undertaken constitutes research. Department of Health and Human Services regulation 45 CFR 46.102(d) defines research as a *"systematic investigation, including research development, testing and evaluation, designed to develop or contribute to generalizable knowledge."* Therefore, if there is intention to provide this data outside of the clinician's institution in order to allow others to generalize it to other settings or situations, then the project may be considered research. Some types of projects that do not meet this definition include:

- Case studies.
- Small case series (3 subjects or less).
- Quality improvement projects that do not use research methodologies.
- Innovative clinical care.

• BOX 35.1   Common Roles of the IRB

Roles of the IRB are to determine if[7]:
Risks to human research subjects are minimized
Risks to human research subjects are reasonable in relation to the anticipated benefits
Monitoring occurs to ensure the safety of research subjects
Selection of human subjects for research participation is equitable
Research subjects are informed of the risks and benefits of participation in planned research
Provisions are in place to protect the privacy of research subjects and maintain data confidentiality
Appropriate safeguards are included to protect the subjects potentially vulnerable to coercion (e.g., children, prisoners, or economically or educationally disadvantaged persons)
Informed consent of research participants is obtained in advance of trial entry and is appropriately documented

IRB, Institutional Review Board.

It is important to work with the IRB early to determine if the potential project constitutes human subjects research. See Box 35.2 for considerations on working with the IRB. If the project does not meet the definition of human subjects research, submission for IRB review is not needed. All other projects need to be reviewed, which will then fall under one of three categories—exempt, expedited, or full.[8] (See the Department of HHS website https://www.hhs.gov/ohrp/ for further detailed instructions.)

1. **Exempt:** The research poses minimal risk to participants and falls into one of the following categories: education research, surveys, public observations, benign behavioral observations, analysis of previously collected information, federal demonstration projects, and taste/food evaluation. Review is often completed by a manager or administrator within the IRB to assure that the study is appropriately included in this category.
2. **Expedited:** The research poses minimal risk and utilizes noninvasive procedures, small samples of blood or other excreted substances, clinically collected data, and/or uses approved or exempted medical devices. Review in this category is often completed by one or a select few IRB members but does not require convening of the full IRB committee.

• BOX 35.2   Institutional Support for Successful Research

Institutions with an IRB or a research department have prioritized successful research as a component of their goal and mission—*they want to help researchers be successful.* Many IRBs offer periodic training and mentoring in navigating the research process. As every proposed study will go through the IRB office, they informally develop a wide and diverse network of researchers and may be able to help connect the researcher with statisticians, grant writers, or other expert professionals to help them to be successful. As might be expected, the IRB staff members may be able to help provide advice and consultations but will not complete the IRB application for the researcher. The process of developing the IRB application can be quite helpful as it requires the investigator to describe the aims and research protocol, and often leads to helpful changes to the research plan.

IRB, Institutional Review Board.

3. **Full:** The research involves more than minimal risk or involves one of the following groups or subjects: vulnerable populations, sensitive topics, genetic testing, or complex research design requiring the expertise of multiple IRB members. Due to the increased risk as compared to the exempt or expedited categories, this category requires the review of the entire committee. This process may take several months, especially if the IRB only convenes periodically.

Even if it is believed that a research study will fall into the exempt category, it is still a requirement to submit the proposed project for review. This will provide assurances that the study was correctly categorized as exempt and provide proper IRB documentation for future journal publication.

Prior to submitting a research protocol, investigators and key members of the research team will need to complete any required training on the protection of human subjects. Such training is offered by the Collaborative Institutional Training Initiative (CITI) (www.citiprogram.org). This training involves standardized online education and certification for a variety of different types of human research. While some institutions may be a member of the CITI program and therefore sponsor the training, independent investigators can also use this site as a source for online training at a nominal fee.

Required Forms for Institutional Review Board Submission

In addition to demonstrating an understanding of human subject protections, the IRB will typically require several different documents in order to review a research project. Many IRBs will already have templates or fillable forms for these items, therefore a meeting with the IRB representative before going too far into the study planning process saves time and energy. The four most common forms are: IRB Application, Research Protocol, Informed Consent and Assent, and a HIPAA Authorization Form.

1. **IRB Application:** An institution-specific document that details the risks of the research, the protections in place, and the roles of various members of the research team.
2. **Research Protocol:** A detailed accounting of the relevant background and research plan. This document will help the IRB assess the risks and benefits of the research. The research plan needs to include information about recruitment, informed consenting procedures, enrollment, assessment, intervention (if any), and data analysis. As a part of the protocol, data collection forms are typically included for IRB review.
3. **Informed Consent and Assent** (if needed): Adults participating in research may be required to sign a form indicating their consent to participate in the research project. The signing of the form is only a part of the consenting process, which involves informing the potential participant about the research plans during recruitment, their rights as a participant, ensuring adequate knowledge of the participant, and adequate time to have any questions answered. If children are involved in the research, assent also needs to be obtained and varies depending on the age of the participant. An assent is a shortened version of the consent process where the aims of the study and the research procedures are described in child-friendly terms. The assent process allows the child to be included in determining involvement in a developmentally appropriate manner. If the study only entails review of medical/rehabilitation records, a waiver for informed consent is possible. A consultation with IRB personnel will help to determine if a waiver of consent is possible for any project.

4. **HIPAA Authorization Form:** HIPAA refers to the Health Insurance Portability and Accountability Act. This is a form that participants sign that indicates what exact types of protected health information will be asked and/or extracted from the medical record for research purposes.

Once an IRB review approval is obtained, it is important for investigators to keep detailed records of their recruitment and enrollment, as this will need to be reported to the IRB on a yearly basis as a part of continuing review. For interventional studies, a study safety committee may need to be formed as a part of monitoring the on-going safety of the research participants. Injuries or other adverse events that may occur during the research processes need to be reported to the IRB. If changes need to be made to the research procedures during the conduct of the study, updated documents will need to be submitted to the IRB for review prior to instituting the change. Upon completion of an IRB approved research study, a closure report will be required to provide the IRB with a brief summary of the outcomes, any adverse events or protocol deviations, and how many subjects ultimately participated in the study.

Deciding on the Research Study Type

Case Report or Case Series

Case reports and small case series (up to 3 subjects) are helpful for detailing novel conditions, assessments, or interventions. In the best scenario, they help to move the practice of rehabilitation forward and inspire new research areas. This avenue of research is often the beginning point for novice researchers, as it follows many of the same principles of clinical practice and does not usually require an extensive outlay in terms of time and budget. These types of observational studies can identify novel issues for a field but have the disadvantage of having selection bias and inability to generalize the findings to larger populations. If a clinician's focus is on disseminating the findings, it should be ensured that the topic is novel as many journals will not publish case reports where a substantial body of evidence is already present. In order to assist clinicians to write and successfully disseminate case reports, the American Physical Therapy Association has published a user friendly and easy to read book entitled *Writing Case Reports: A How-to Manual for Clinicians* which is in its third edition.[9]

Once it has been established that a patient case is novel, either in terms of clinical diagnosis/presentation or intervention, a case report may be the best initial step. Ensuring adequate documentation of the clinical processes is especially important, as in most case reports, the clinical record is the main source of data. If a clinician encounters a unique clinical situation that may make an especially interesting case report, it is critical to record the details of the case and utilize valid, reliable, sensitive outcome measures to help quantify clinical gains or remaining deficits. When preparing the description of the case, it is important to consider likely journals for publication. Once a few journals are identified that may be a good fit for a case, it is helpful to review a number of previously published case reports and the particular format required by that journal prior to writing the paper. A common set of headings includes: abstract, introduction (including a brief statement of the interesting aspect of the case), case description, and discussion. The case description includes a description of relevant patient information, the result of medical and/or rehabilitation examinations, plan of care, and outcomes.

While the other parts of the case report are typically familiar to many clinicians, the format of the discussion may be more

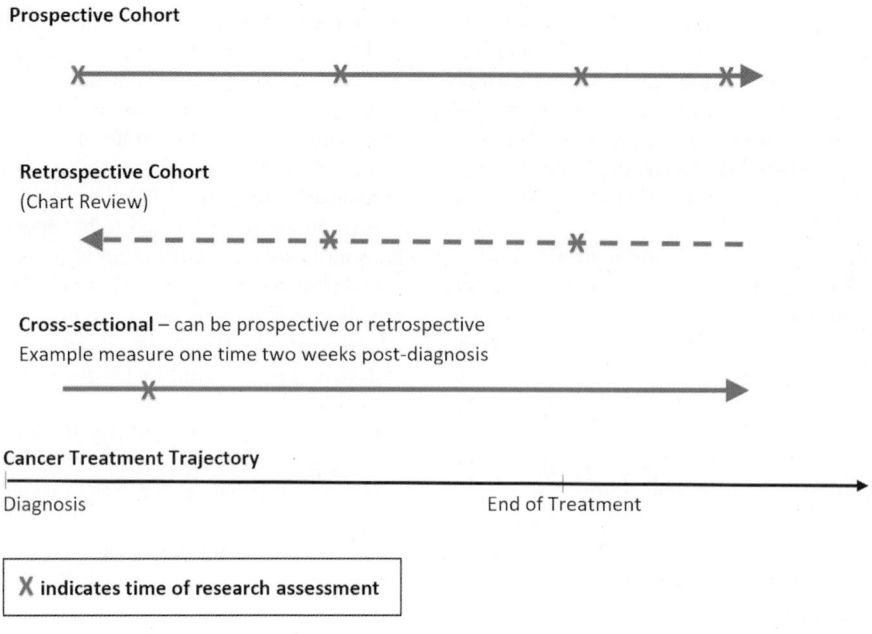

Prospective Cohort

Retrospective Cohort
(Chart Review)

Cross-sectional – can be prospective or retrospective
Example measure one time two weeks post-diagnosis

Cancer Treatment Trajectory

Diagnosis   End of Treatment

X indicates time of research assessment

• **Fig. 35.1** Observational Study Designs Created by Laura Gilchrist. Printed with permission.

challenging. The first part of the discussion should include a clear and concise description of the novelty of the case and how it relates to previously published literature. This typically expands on the information presented in the introduction. How this case then supports or detracts from current understanding of the condition, the assessments required, or appropriate interventions should be described. At the end of the discussion, the author can make recommendations for clinicians and researchers interested in the condition.

A case series is similar to a case report, and only typically differs in the number of patients described and the formatting of the case presentations. In the case series, the cases may be presented serially or as a small group in the assessment, intervention, and outcomes sections. If a case series reports on up to three patients, they are typically handled by IRB committees in the same manner as case reports. For case series of four or more patients, an IRB review is typically needed. It is sometimes difficult to differentiate case series from observational cohort studies (described in the next section), but in general a case series typically has a small number of participants and all participants are assessed using the same methods and/or have intervention plans that are alike.

For case reports and case series, a signed HIPAA authorization should be obtained from the participant or their authorized representative for the use of their protected health information. An exception to this rule may occur when the author of a case report or case series believes that the information is not identifiable. Even in this case, it may be best to consult with the IRB or the institution's privacy officer to ensure compliance with all needed policies. Even if an institution's IRB does not require a separate consent or authorization, many journals require that patient consent be obtained prior to publication.

Observational Studies

Observational studies are descriptive in nature and helpful to investigate particular issues in rehabilitation such as the incidence of a specific impairment or diagnosis, functional outcomes

in a specific population, and risk factors for an event of interest (Figure 35.1). For example, if a clinician wanted to understand the occurrence of chemotherapy-induced polyneuropathy (CIPN) in a particular population, an observational study design would be appropriate. There are many different approaches to an observational study, depending on how many times data would need to be obtained and whether this information would be obtained prospectively or retrospectively. Another consideration is if any sub-populations exist that could be examined. Sometimes, it may be useful to simply describe the incidence in a general population such as persons diagnosed with breast cancer, which would be considered a single group design. Other times, it may be beneficial to compare the outcome of interest across different groups, such as patients receiving taxanes versus patients receiving platinum-based therapy and therefore a two-group design can account for this difference in treatment. The difference between an observational and experimental study when there are two or more groups is that in an observational study the investigator does not manipulate the group assignment, and instead just describes the groups that already exist. In the experimental study design, described in more detail below, the investigator assigns the patients to different groups. There are multiple types of observational studies including: retrospective cohort and cross-sectional studies, prospective cohort and cross-sectional studies, and case control studies.

Retrospective cohort and cross-sectional studies: Chart review studies of interesting populations or intervention programs fall under the category of *retrospective cohort studies*. In essence, this involves looking back at a group of patients who have already received treatment and gathering their outcomes at one or more points during their care. If the outcomes are only reported at one point of the patient care trajectory for all subjects, it would be a *retrospective cross-sectional study* design. Some of the benefits of the retrospective approach are the relatively low cost of performing the study and the ease of obtaining the outcomes through abstraction of medical records. However, the results of retrospective studies can be biased by clinicians only recording relevant information for patients with the condition, making it difficult to generalize. For example, if a clinician reports on the prevalence of neuropathy for patients treated for cancer who were referred to therapy after a fall, this would not provide a good estimate of the overall incidence of neuropathy in the cancer population as a substantial portion of the cancer population would not be included. Likewise, the outcome of interest may not be captured in a standardized manner across all subjects. This can easily occur when many different measures can be used to assess the same impairment or activity limitation.

Prospective cohort and cross-sectional studies: *Prospective cohort studies* can mitigate some of the problems with the retrospective study design. A prospective study model sets the expectations for what will be measured at specific time points before the patients begin treatment. In this way the outcomes to be measured are predetermined, so that even in cases where the subject might not have been tested for a specific outcome as a part of typical clinical care, they will be assessed if enrolled in the prospective observational study. By predetermining what measure(s) would be used at certain points in the treatment trajectory, the incidence of a specific issue can be described. These types of studies have less potential for bias and are therefore more generalizable. The issues with this type of study design are the higher cost of providing these measures for all participants (and not only for those where it is clinically indicated) as well as attrition due to subjects relocating or becoming disinterested. Once again, it is also possible to complete a *prospective cross-sectional* observational study, measuring the cohort at only one point in the care trajectory, thereby reducing some of the cost and attrition issues.

Case control studies: A last option in the observational cohort model of studies is the addition of different groups. When considering the previously discussed question of comparing CIPN in patients receiving taxanes- versus platinum-based treatments, a researcher could set up a study, either prospectively or retrospectively, to compare the incidence and type of CIPN developed in each group. In this example, the researcher might study CIPN symptoms in women treated for breast cancer with taxanes and compare them with women who did not receive taxane-based chemotherapy. In essence, two side-by-side observational cohort studies are being run at the same time. This may allow for comparison across groups. If the second group chosen does not receive the treatment or intervention of interest but is otherwise similar in important characteristics (e.g., age, sex, condition), then this two-cohort study would be referred to as a *case-control study* design. Observational cohort studies can be very powerful if well designed and executed. They are a critical trial design for instances when it would be ethically problematic to withhold treatment or randomly assign treatment to a group of patients.

Experimental Study Designs

If the intent of the study is to examine the effect of an intervention on a population with a specific condition, and the investigator intends to determine who will and will not get that intervention, this would fall under an experimental trial design. It differs from the observational studies in that the investigator is manipulating the variable of interest—specifically who will get the treatment being investigated. This type of study design can remove some of the biases of the observational cohort designs if careful planning is in place.

Two major sources of bias that can be addressed by careful study planning are allocation of patients and the assessor's knowledge of the group to which the participant is assigned. In a study where there are treatment and control groups, random assignment of the participants to one of the two groups removes some bias that could occur when participants are allowed to choose their intervention. There are a number of different methods to create a random allocation system for a study, all based on using chance to determine which participants will be in the intervention and control groups.[10] The systems can be as simple as putting each group assignment into a separate sealed envelope, mixing up the envelopes and randomly picking one for the participant. They can also be more complex, such as stratified randomization procedures where another variable of interest (e.g., smokers vs. nonsmokers) are equally distributed across the two groups. For experimental studies, these are important issues that would benefit from consultation with experts in trial design during the protocol development phase of study planning.

The second source of bias comes from assessors or participants knowing the group to which they are assigned. If the participant or assessor knows the group assignment, they may either consciously or unconsciously bias the results of the assessment. For example, if a researcher is testing a new intervention for CIPN-related pain, and the individual knows that they received the experimental intervention, they may report improved pain scores because they expect the intervention to work. Likewise, if the assessor knows that an individual received the experimental treatment, their expectations for that person's performance may be different and this could unconsciously influence the outcome measurement. Blinding both the assessor and the research participant to their group is the most effective way to mitigate this issue. In rehabilitation, at times it is difficult to create placebo interventions that keep participants from understanding if they are receiving the experimental intervention. Again, careful consideration of this issue with experts in rehabilitation clinical trial design will assist the novice investigator in developing a high-quality trial.

Developing high-quality clinical trials in rehabilitation is a challenge, as some of the issues faced by rehabilitation are different that typical medical trials. For example, in a medical trial, a placebo medication can be given instead of an experimental drug. This can effectively blind the participant to their group assignment. Other issues more common in rehabilitation trials than medical trials are the wide variety and mixed use of interventions as well as the complexity of forming homogenous patient groups.[11] In the near future, recommendations on the best formats for constructing, conducting, and reporting rehabilitation clinical trials will be identified by a multi-national working group. This group is formulating Randomized Controlled Trial Rehabilitation Checklists (RCTRACK) to assist in the development and review of high-quality clinical trials in rehabilitation.[11] As these new tools are published, investigators can use them to develop clinical trials to better impact the Onc R evidence base.

It may be useful for a novice investigator to pair up with an experienced investigator who understands the intricacies of rehabilitation trial design. There are multiple clinical trial designs that can mitigate the loss of treatment to the control group and it is beyond the scope of this chapter to review each trial type. Multiple texts are available that delve deeply into the design and analysis of research studies that may assist clinicians in the development and dissemination of clinically based research (e.g., see Foundations of Clinical Research, 4th edition[12]). It is important that, no matter the trial design, sufficient follow-up is included to demonstrate not only short-term but also lasting impacts of interventions.

Participating in Multi-Site or Consortium Studies

One way to become involved in clinical research without independently taking on a full observational study or clinical trial is to participate in a multi-site or consortium investigation. Because of the rarity of some oncologic conditions, investigators may need to enroll subjects for a particular study at a number of different clinical sites. Participation in this type of study may allow for faster investigation of a particular issue and is helpful in demonstrating the generalizability of a finding. Not only will the novice researcher be assisting in developing the evidence-base, but they will gain supported experience in the conduct of clinically relevant research. Often, this type of participation is acknowledged in publications, but any expectations about authorship on manuscripts should be discussed prior to participating in the study to prevent misunderstandings. Typically, contributing data to a study alone does not warrant authorship on resulting manuscripts. Consortium-based trials can be multi-disciplinary and often the planning groups welcome the input of Onc R clinicians on measuring function-related outcomes. A good first step is investigating the existing oncology- or rehabilitation-related consortium groups that the reader's institution participates in and then attending meetings (if possible). Examples include the Children's Oncology Group (https://childrensoncologygroup.org/) for pediatric cancer trials and the SWOG (Southwest Oncology Group) Cancer Research Network (https://www.swog.org/) for adult cancer diagnoses. Current oncology consortium groups are mainly focused on the medical treatment of individuals with cancer. Development of multi-site consortiums for clinical trials in rehabilitation is in its infancy and Onc R would benefit greatly from such groups.

Prior to participating in a consortium or multi-site research study, issues of IRB approval and data use agreements need to be addressed. Clinicians should work with their institutions' research offices and IRBs to obtain the appropriate clearances and create any of the agreements necessary. In addition, there can sometimes be payment-related issues either in salary support or case-wise reimbursement. Working with grant administrators on this compensation is key to appropriate payment for the investigator's time and effort. This planning can still take some significant time prior to initiating data collection. The PIs for the study should be able to assist with the needed documents.

Funding for Clinical Research

Many of the study designs that have been discussed take significant time and resources, and therefore funding may be necessary. Case studies, case series, and retrospective cross-sectional or cohort studies can sometimes be completed without funding, depending on administrative support and how many nonworking hours the investigator(s) are willing to spend on the project. Other study types typically need either internal or external funding. Many hospital and health networks have existing internal grant programs that fund small clinical studies. Often, these funds are insufficient alone to support a larger clinical project, but offer the limited resources needed to support pilot studies that demonstrate feasibility and suggest possible outcomes. As noted previously, this funding may also support paying a statistician to assist in completing relevant analyses. Small pilot studies most often do not have large enough sample sizes to yield statistically significant results but can point to trends in the data that may be promising and lead to larger trials. Professional associations and foundations also can serve as a source of funding for smaller projects.

Larger projects, such as randomized clinical trials may need greater funding support. Some oncology-specific foundations, such as the American Cancer Society or the Susan G. Komen Foundation, can provide support for these larger trials. Grants are also available through state and federal programs such as the Centers for Disease Control and Prevention (CDC), National Institutes of Health (NIH), and the Department of Defense (DOD). Prior to applying, the specific requirements for each specific foundation or agency should be well understood as funders may have requirements for the training and length of employment for their specific mechanism. Clinicians should consult with their institution's research department to gain assistance in finding the right match between the project and funding sources.

Development of a grant for any of the internal or external funding sources takes significant time and resources. Personnel within an institution's research department may be available to assist with the development of the project from the concept to funding, and even may aid with data analysis and manuscript preparation. Before spending significant time writing the grant, investigators are advised to check out the resources available to them from their institutional research department. Many healthcare systems have significant supports in place to aide clinicians in pursuing research. In addition, institutional signatures will be required for most grants and allowing for sufficient time to get any scientific and administrative reviews completed prior to submission is important in developing a timeline. Likewise, grant-writing is a skill that takes time to develop. If possible, a novice researcher should team up with an experienced investigator or at least develop a mentoring relationship to gain feedback on drafts of the proposal. The researchers should be sure to clearly understand the criteria that the application will be judged against, as even small deficits can limit the ability to gain funding.

Lastly, most external grants are not funded the first time they are submitted. This may be a shock to new investigators. Oftentimes investigators are only allowed a set number of submissions for any specific project, so it is important to always put the best effort forward. However, expect to receive significant feedback from the first review that should be addressed on re-submission.

Implementing the Research Study

Once the planning and funding phases are complete, and IRB approval has been secured, the study can be implemented. All of the meticulous planning will be worthwhile, as the investigators know exactly what to do when and whom to report it to. A few notes of warning are warranted on this phase of the project. Keep track of all of the participants that are approached for recruiting, in a confidential manner, as this information will be needed to report back to the IRB. Carefully follow the procedures that have been established and described to the IRB. If processes need to be changed or if there are any adverse events, it is critical to notify the IRB and gain approvals before changes are made to the study. If any financial support is provided to individuals participating in the study, this should be provided and tracked according to institutional protocols. Finally, tracking the progress in the study and storing data safely and securely is critical for the eventual reporting on the study to the IRB and for disseminating the findings.

Disseminating the Research

The study is complete, the investigators have collaborated with appropriate individuals to analyze the data, and the investigators are now ready to present the data to others. There are many routes to disseminate the findings both within and outside of an institution. Within the investigator's institution, presentation of the information at department meetings, grand rounds, and institutional research conferences will provide valuable initial feedback useful for wider dissemination of the project. Questions asked by peers may help to identify the best format to present the data or may clarify where additional description is needed. Major limitations of the data may be brought forward, and then this can be included in the discussion of the project's contribution to the science of rehabilitation.

Conference Presentations

State, national, and international conferences are a great next step in sharing the results. Typically, an abstract describing the study in a small number of words (often 250–300) is submitted months before the conference. These abstracts are reviewed by peers, and then a decision will be made inviting the researchers to present the data. Investigators will often be asked if there is a preference to present a poster or platform. Posters have the advantage of more informal interaction with people interested in the topic. Typically, the information on the study is put into one poster-sized slide and either printed or presented in an electronic format. The conference planning committee will often provide the particular format or template needed. The investigator's institution may also have a ready-made slide template for use. Platforms are a more formal presentation of the study, using multiple slides. Here, the investigators will stand in front of an audience to present the work. Even in this format, the time allotted is typically short (less than 15 minutes generally), and concise presentation of the study design, results, and discussion is needed. While a formal question and answer session is typical, there is usually opportunity for more informal discussion after the presentation during the conference.

One point that should be checked before presenting the information at any conference is the novelty of the data being presented. Some conferences will only accept data that has not been previously presented at any conference while others allow for the re-presentation of information from other conferences. Likewise, if data is being presented which has been previously submitted for publication in a journal, it is important that it is allowable to present the data publicly to other scientists and clinicians. These issues are typically laid out in "embargo" policies for journals that speak to the investigators' ability to publicly share their data with other scientists and the media while a manuscript is under review or awaiting publication.

Publications

While dissemination within an investigator's own institution and at conferences can be important, widespread dissemination can occur when the work is published in a research journal. Determining the most appropriate journal is important. First, target audience should be determined—medical providers, multi-disciplinary rehabilitation providers, or a discipline's professionals (e.g., physical therapists). Most journals will have a mission statement, and the match of the study with their stated purpose may determine if the manuscript is ultimately accepted. By reading through the guidelines for authors from a journal, the investigator can also learn about the specific format needed for the paper and references. This will save time in the preparation of the manuscript. Researchers should target a credible journal that will provide them with important peer-reviewed feedback on their manuscript (Box 35.3).

• BOX 35.3   Reputable Journals and Conferences

Disseminating research in a reputable forum is an important step in the research process. New investigators should beware of "predatory" journals and conferences that promote poor quality science. Recently, a consensus definition for predatory journals was determined that describe the indicators of such journals[13]:

- *Prioritization of journal self-interest at the expense of scholarship, often in the form of excessive publication fees.*
- *Provide false or misleading information on journal metrics and processes.*
- *Deviate from best editorial and publication practices including peer review mechanisms.*
- *Lack of transparency in their processes.*
- *Use of aggressive and indiscriminate solicitation practices.*

A number of different checklists are available to assist researchers in finding reputable journals and conferences. The website thinkchecksubmit.org offers information about deceptive publication and conference practices developed by a coalition of organizations interested in ethical research dissemination. Collaborating with a medical or research librarian can be helpful to vet any potential journals that are being considered.

Most journals will define manuscript types—such as perspective article, systematic review, and original research. If the author is unsure of the appropriate heading for the manuscript, it is appropriate to send such a question to the editor or managing editor of the journal. Knowing the article type will also provide clarity as to the appropriate headings for the manuscript. Descriptions of what should be included and the appropriate length for each section is also often provided in the *Instructions to Authors* which may be located on the front page of a journal's website. Overall length of the manuscript and the number of allowed figures and tables is often described as well. Authors must carefully review all instructions prior to submission to avoid delays in the peer review process.

Once a draft of the paper has been written, it is suggested to have a trusted colleague review it for content and clarity. By this time, the authors know this project better than anyone, and things that are obvious to them may not be clear to others. Ultimately, the authors want the journal's reviewers to have a clear view of the research conducted, so the importance of this pre-review process cannot be understated. Also, it is important to remember that almost every study has limitations in the ability to generalize the findings to other populations. Just because a study has limitations that are acknowledged in the discussion section does not make it unworthy of publication. Most manuscripts require many drafts and revisions before they are ready for submission.

Once the manuscript has been refined and meets the criteria and format of the journal, it is time to submit the files. Almost all journals have an electronic submission system. After following the instructions on the journal's webpage, the author can then upload the files and ultimately submit the manuscript for review. If there are co-authors, they may need to also submit some forms and acknowledge their authorship. One last issue is selecting the type of access that is desired for the manuscript. Typical access usually means that readers need to have a subscription to that journal or pay a fee to access the paper. This can limit how widely the work is disseminated. Free and open access help to improve dissemination. Free access typically indicates that the material can be opened and read by the public free of charge, whereas open access indicates the additional ability to re-use the content within the article without restriction. Some federal granting agencies may mandate open access as a part of their funding expectations. There may be charges for free or open access to the article. Authors should carefully select the journal for submission as some journals require page charges, even for closed access articles, that can be quite costly. Importantly, it is important that the chosen journal uses a peer-review mechanism, as this is an indicator of journal quality. In this phase of the research process, investigators will want to choose reputable journals and conferences to disseminate their work. Box 35.3 provides resources on determining the credibility of such venues.

Once the manuscript is in the hands of a journal, it will be passed along to the editor or one of the editorial board members. This person will review the fit of the manuscript with the mission of the journal. If they feel that the manuscript does not fit within their scope, they may decline it immediately. Sometimes, they may suggest another publication more suited for the paper. If the paper passes this first level of review, it is then put through a peer-review process. Either in a blinded or nonblinded manner, the paper will be read by experts in the area and feedback is generated on the study design and clarity of the resulting manuscript. This process can take a few weeks to a few months. Most times, manuscripts will receive a decision of accept, decline, or revisions needed. If revisions are requested, it is expected that the revised manuscript be returned to the journal within a specified timeframe. A letter that addresses each one of the reviewers' concerns and details the changes made to manuscript is expected. Highlighting the specific changes to the manuscript made in response to the reviewers' comments is also needed. The decision letter should make clear the expectations for submitting the needed revisions to the journal. See Box 35.4 for the importance of resilience of the researcher, especially in the dissemination phase.

After the manuscript is accepted, the last hurdle is to review the draft of the manuscript that will be published in the journal. The journal will send the author a "proof" for review. It is important to look at all parts of the proof for formatting errors. This is not a time to revise the paper other than minor formatting issues. If major errors are found in the substance of the manuscript, it will be necessary to contact the editor to determine the next steps. Oftentimes, the proof is in a PDF format where annotations can be made

directly on the copy. Generally, there is only a short timeframe to return this version of the manuscript to the publisher (sometimes only a day or two). At this point, the paper may be *published ahead of print* on the journal's website. There still may be a delay between this initial proof and the publishing of the paper in an issue of the journal. More journals are turning to online only publications, and a lack of space within a paper publication is no longer the impediment to gaining wide dissemination of a project as it once was.

After publication of the data in a manuscript, there are still two tasks to finish. First, the investigator will want to make sure that they close the study with their IRB as long as there is no further need to access the data for additional publications. Secondly, it is time to celebrate with the team! The process of tackling a research question, developing a study, implementing the research plan, and disseminating the findings is at times long and arduous. It often takes extra time and effort in an already busy clinic schedule. Celebrating the accomplishment is an important step for all involved. Maybe during that celebration, the next research idea will be generated!

Conclusion

Completing a research study takes time, dedication, patience, and a growth mindset. Taking sufficient time up front to gather needed resources and develop the best methodology for the specific research question will smooth the journey. Ultimately, knowing that one's efforts helped to improve the care of those facing cancer can provide the motivation needed to see a study to completion.

Case Study

The clinic where you work has developed a new intervention program to address balance and falls in adults with cancer. Patients are brought into the rehabilitation program after their cancer treatment is complete and are put through a 6-week standardized program of education, strengthening exercise, and balance training. You think that this is a novel program that seems to be having good outcomes, and you want to share this work with others.

First Question: Is This a Research Study?

You could gather outcomes data on your program and share within your institution as a part of a quality improvement project. If you decide to share this information outside of your institution, to allow others to generalize this information and use it in their populations, this becomes a research project. Likewise, if you decide that only part of your population will gain access to this program in order to determine its effectiveness, again this would qualify as a research study.

Second Question: What Type of Study Design Would Work Best?

If this was a rare population or you have few participants, then a case report or case series might be the best first step. But since you have several patients who are participating in the program, an observational or experimental design might be best. If you have the time, support, and experience necessary to set up an experimental trial, a small clinical trial may be best to see if this new program is better than the typical standard of care. However, if you have already started the program and have difficulty keeping one set of patients from accessing it, an observational study of the

---

• BOX 35.4 Resilience of a Researcher

A key skill of any researcher is to have determination, professional confidence, and fortitude to navigate a project until the end. Two areas that clinicians have voiced challenges with include the IRB and the peer review process. Within both of these processes, a project is exposed to the scrutiny of content experts which is often intimidating. Any feedback that is received may feel very personal as the researcher has vested their time and knowledge into this labor of love! If negative feedback or a rejection is received, the researcher should employ the same self-reflection skills that they employ daily as a rehabilitation professional. Sometimes the feedback may seem curt or harsh, but it should be realized that the peer reviewer has dedicated their time and expertise to trying to make *you* a better author and researcher. Regardless of whether a project is eventually accepted in a particular journal or another venue for dissemination is pursued, a "growth mindset" is an important way to approach any feedback. One approach that has been helpful for many is to initially put the feedback aside for a few days after receiving a rejection, so that the critiques of the work can be more fully appreciated after the initial disappointment passes. After reading the feedback, the researcher should talk to peers and colleagues who can provide guidance, advice, or even just a forum to have a constructive conversation on the next steps for this important work.

IRB, Institutional Review Board.

program outcomes may be best. If program outcomes were already in place and regularly measured, a retrospective study detailing the program outcomes may yield data in a relatively quick fashion without the need of prospective informed consent, as this activity was completed during routine patient care. Otherwise, development of a prospective cohort study may be the best route. Depending on the case mix for the program, you may choose to keep all participants as one group or if you have two or more major groups, such as persons diagnosed with breast cancer and prostate cancer, you may complete a multi-cohort study where outcomes across the different groups are compared.

Whichever path you choose, ensure that you have reached out to the appropriate people in your institution to gather help with research design, administrative approvals, and protect your subjects through IRB approvals of the research protocol and informed consenting procedures.

Review Questions

Reader can find the correct answers and rationale in the back of the book.

1. A clinician has recently developed a research study that describes the short-term outcomes of a clinical program instituted at their clinic 5 years ago. They will report the post-intervention outcomes that were collected as a part of that program. Which of the following is a BEST descriptor of the study type?
   A. Prospective observational cohort
   B. Case controlled trial
   C. Retrospective observational cohort
   D. Experimental clinical trial

2. Which of the following is NOT true about the role of the IRB?
   A. The IRB does not need to review observational studies
   B. The IRB should review experimental research projects
   C. The IRB does not need to review case reports
   D. The IRB does not need to review quality improvement projects

3. Which of the following would be the MOST LIKELY study type for a manuscript entitled "Association between body mass and cancer-related fatigue in patients treated for colorectal cancer"?
   A. Case-control study
   B. Longitudinal cohort study
   C. Cross-sectional cohort study
   D. Experimental study

4. A clinician sees a patient with a rare cancer diagnosis, cannot find literature on the outcomes for patients with this condition, and would like to complete research to inform the practice for this condition. The MOST appropriate first study design would be:
   A. Case study
   B. Case-control study
   C. Multi-site observational study
   D. Multi-site clinical trial

5. Which of the following is NOT a responsibility of the IRB?
   A. Assessment of the risk and benefits of a research project
   B. Determination of sufficient information to be provided to potential participants
   C. Review of adverse events
   D. Administration of HIPPA consent forms

6. A co-investigator should be able to fulfill all of the roles listed below EXCEPT:
   A. Review of the research manuscript
   B. Provide identical expertise as the Principal Investigator
   C. Be aware of all research protections
   D. Assist in the development of research methodology

7. Which of the following documents are typically NOT included in a submission of an experimental research project to the IRB?
   A. Research protocol
   B. Names of all potential research participants
   C. Informed consent procedures
   D. HIPAA assurances form

8. Which of the following is the BEST descriptive term for a formal presentation of research data using multiple slides at a research conference?
   A. Platform presentation
   B. Poster presentation
   C. Plenary presentation
   D. Educational presentation

9. Which of the following is the best descriptor of a "proof" that is used in the clinical research process?
   A. A rationale for the proposed research project
   B. An analysis plan for an experimental study
   C. An accepted version of a research manuscript put into the publication format
   D. A manuscript draft to be submitted for peer review

10. Which of the following are NOT necessary to complete a clinical research project?
    A. Persistence
    B. Attention to procedures and detail
    C. Time
    D. A postprofessional doctoral degree

References

1. van Rij S, Andrews A, Freund J, Bailey S. Multimodal rehabilitation following gliosarcoma resection: a case report. *Rehabil Oncol.* 2021;39(1):56–63.
2. Tan CJ, Timon C, Stassen LFA, et al. Balance and physical functioning in patients after head and neck cancer post-neck dissection surgery: a case series. *Rehabil Oncol.* 2021;39(1):48–55.
3. Andres K, Wayman B, Rodriguez T, et al. Effect of physical condition on outcomes in transplant patients: a retrospective data analysis. *Rehabil Oncol.* 2020;38(3):116–121.
4. Rindflesch AB, Hake MP, Spiten MA, et al. Physical performance following hematopoietic stem cell transplantation: a prospective observational study. *Rehabil Oncol.* 2020;38(3):122–126.
5. Tanner LR, Hooke MC. Improving body function and minimizing activity limitations in pediatric leukemia survivors: the

lasting impact of the Stoplight Program. *Pediatr Blood Cancer.* 2019;66(5):e27596.

6. Torres-Lacomba M, Navarro-Brazález B, Prieto-Gómez V, Ferrandez JC, Bouchet JY, Romay-Barrero H. Effectiveness of four types of bandages and kinesio-tape for treating breast-cancer-related lymphoedema: a randomized, single-blind, clinical trial. *Clin Rehabil.* 2020;34(9):1230–1241.

7. OHRP, Department of Health and Human Service. 45 CFR 46. https://www.hhs.gov/ohrp/regulations-and-policy/regulations/45-cfr-46/index.html. March 10, 2021. Accessed April 10, 2021.

8. OHRP, Department of Health and Human Service. Expedited review: categories of research that may be reviewed through an expedited review procedure (1998). https://www.hhs.gov/ohrp/regulations-and-policy/guidance/categories-of-research-expedited-review-procedure-1998/index.html. November 9, 1998. Accessed April 1, 2021.

9. McEwen I. *Writing Case Reports: A How-to Manual for Clinicians.* 3rd ed. American Physical Therapy Association; 2009. ISBN 978-1-931369-62-6.

10. Kim J, Shin W. How to do random allocation (randomization). *Clin Orthop Surg.* 2014;6(1):103–109.

11. Negrini S, Armijo-Olivo S, Patrini M, et al. The randomized controlled trials rehabilitation checklist methodology of development of a reporting guideline specific to rehabilitation. *Am J Phys Med Rehabil.* 2020;99(3):210–215.

12. Portney L. *Foundations of Clinical Research.* 4th ed. F.A. Davis; 2020.

13. Grudniewicz A, Moher D, Cobey KD, et al. Predatory journals: no definition, no defence. *Nature.* 2019;576(7786):210–212.

Answer Key

Chapter 1

1. B: Limitless replicative potential
Rationale: Increase in mutations is from the uncontrolled replication stage.

2. A: Immune, endocrine
Rationale: The characteristics are genomic mutations and tumor promoting inflammation while the two emerging hallmarks deal with cellular energy metabolism avoiding immune destruction.

3. B: Secondary tumor
Rationale: The tumor that invaded surrounding tissue is the primary tumor. A second primary is a new cancer unrelated to the primary. There is no such thing as a tertiary tumor.

4. C: Moderately differentiated/moderate grade
Rationale: Gx is undetermined grade. G1 is well differentiated, G3 is poorly differentiated.

5. D: Large tumor with 4–9 lymph nodes involved and distant metastases
Rationale: Since there is metastasis (M1), A and B could not be correct. T4 designates a larger tumor size so D is the only correct answer.

6. D: TP53—Pancreatic cancer
Rationale: Pancreatic cancer risks increase with *BRCA1/ BRCA2* genetic mutations.

7. B: Individuals with a diagnosis of a primary cancer will only develop metastasis within 1–10 years of the initial diagnosis
Rationale: Individuals with a diagnosis of a primary cancer may experience cancer metastasis multiple years following their initial diagnosis.

8. B: Hyperplasia
Rationale: *Dysplasia* is defined as the presence of abnormal cells within a tissue or organ. Dysplasia is not cancer, but it may sometimes become cancer. Dysplasia can be mild, moderate, or severe, depending on how abnormal the cells look under a microscope and how much of the tissue or organ is affected. *Hyperplasia* is an increase in the number of cells in an organ or tissue that appear normal under a microscope. Although they are not cancer, they may become cancer. *Metaplasia* is the next step where a change of cells to a form that does not normally occur in the tissue in which it is found. Finally *neoplasia* is defined as abnormal and uncontrolled cell growth.

9. C: Genetic makeup
Rationale: Lifestyle behaviors as described in A, B, and D are all risk factors that we have control over and therefore can modify these lifestyle factors to decrease the risk of cancer.

10. C: Insomnia
Rationale: Insomnia can be related to medications, stress, psychosocial issues, and many other diseases so is not a common sign or symptom of cancer.

Chapter 2

1. D: Quaternary
Rationale: Education to prevent aggressive surgery and services is a form of "do no harm" or preventing over-medicalization.

2. D: 90%
Rationale: 90% of women diagnosed with breast cancer will have one or more adverse treatment effects at 6 months and 62% at 6 years.

3. B: Sustaining
Rationale: *Seasons of Survivorship* include *acute* survivorship, adding *transitional* survivorship (the period immediately following intense treatment including careful observation), and expanding *extended* survivorship.

4. A: Teach-Back Method
Rationale: Ensuring understanding of the educational components delivered can be aided by techniques such as the *Teach-Back Method* (i.e., asking the patient to reiterate in their own words the information learned).

5. B: CoC
Rationale: Please see Table 2.8 for definition. CARF is for rehabilitation accreditation. NAPBC accredits breast cancer centers and the NCPF is a forum for research and resources.

6. B: Impairment directed care, uncomplicated
Rationale: Impairment directed care, uncomplicated is defined as: Persons requiring this level of care are experiencing cancer-related adverse events and impairments that are challenging function. These can include radiation-induced fibrosis, axillary web syndrome, contractures from graft-versus-host disease, etc. Specialized training by the clinician is necessary to treat in this level.

7. A: Determining baseline function and monitoring potential toxicities from cancer treatment, then providing preventive and early intervention as needed.
Rationale: The Prospective Surveillance Model (PSM) is a comprehensive model of care that begins with an initial evaluation at the time of diagnosis to determine functional status before any cancer treatment. Although originally created for persons with breast cancer, the PSM has the potential to be developed for persons diagnosed with any cancer. This model includes a prehabilitation assessment by an Onc R clinician before surgery for breast cancer and then every 3 months for the first year.

8. **B:** Activity limitations and participation

   Rationale: Learning and applying knowledge is activity limitations and participation and is related to the body function—"mental", the body structure—"nervous system", the environmental factors—"products and technology", and personal factors—"lifestyle habits."

9. **C:** Environmental factors

   Rationale: Support and relationships are part of environmental factors while life events are part of personal factors, mobility is part of activity limitations and participation.

10. **B:** Supportive

    Rationale: See Table 2.1 as palliative is defined as emphasizes the maintenance of QOL in the setting of terminal illness/disease and restorative is defined as addresses the functional impairments of each PLWBC and aims to restore maximal function with minimal residual effects of treatment or disease and preventative is defined as focuses on reducing the chance of developing impairments. This phase can be started acutely after diagnosis, and continued through treatment (e.g., surgery, radiation therapy, systemic therapy).

Chapter 3

1. **A:** Patient population, intervention/treatment, comparison and outcome of interest

   Rationale: To pose a clear clinical question, four components, often referred to as PICO, need to be identified. These components include (1) patient population, (2) intervention/treatment, (3) comparison, and (4) outcome of interest.

2. **D:** Early active range of motion

   Rationale: Now apply a PICO to a clinical scenario to a woman who is currently receiving radiation for her breast cancer diagnosis. She has been referred to rehabilitation due to complaints of difficulty reaching overhead on her affected shoulder. The clinician wants to know if active shoulder flexion range of motion on the affected side will improve her self-reported upper extremity function using the disabilities of arm, shoulder and hand (DASH) while the woman is receiving radiation treatment compared to usual care which is rest. The following is how the clinician would apply the PICO to this clinical scenario: the "P" = the woman with breast cancer, the "I" = active shoulder flexion range of motion on the affected side, the "C" = usual care (rest), and the "O" = patient-reported function on the DASH.

3. **A:** Rehabilitation oncology

   Rationale: Membership in the APTA's Academy of Oncologic Physical Therapy will include access to the Academy's journal *Rehabilitation Oncology*, which allows for full-text access of articles including archives. *Rehabilitation Oncology* is an indexed resource for the dissemination of peer-reviewed research-based evidence related to oncologic physical therapy and cancer rehabilitation.

4. **D:** Case study

   Rationale: A variety of study designs exist, and it is vital to understand the differences between these designs as well as how they relate to the quality of evidence. One way to compare and contrast the different types of study designs used in evidence-based practice is understanding the levels of evidence pyramid (Figure 3.1). This pyramid provides a way to visualize the quality of evidence based on the study design. For example, the top of the pyramid (meta-analyses) means that it is both the highest level of evidence and typically the least common, whereas as you go down the pyramid, the amount of evidence will increase as the quality of evidence decreases (see Figure 3.1).

5. **C:** Gender

   Rationale: When examining differences between group means, data that is parametric would be characterized as ratio or interval whereas nonparametric data would be nominal or ordinal. Figure 3.2 shows the characteristics and examples of measurement scales in which gender is classified as a nominal variable.

6. **A:** *P*-value

   Rationale: *P*-values help determine the reliability by which the null hypothesis can be rejected and consequently the strength of the observed result, *P*-values do not provide evidence about the accuracy of the result. To address this, confidence intervals are calculated around the point estimate of the result to offer a range of values within which the true value is assured to exist with a specified level of confidence. An effect size demonstrates the magnitude of differences between groups, where larger effect sizes indicate a greater difference between groups. Responsiveness includes the minimal important change (MIC) (also known as minimal clinically important difference or MCID), which is the smallest change in a score that would likely be important from the patient's perspective.

7. **A:** Confidence interval

   Rationale: *P*-values help determine the reliability by which the null hypothesis can be rejected and consequently the strength of the observed result, *P*-values do not provide evidence about the accuracy of the result. To address this, confidence intervals are calculated around the point estimate of the result to offer a range of values within which the true value is assured to exist with a specified level of confidence. An effect size demonstrates the magnitude of differences between groups, where larger effect sizes indicate a greater difference between groups. Responsiveness includes the minimal important change (MIC) (also known as minimal clinically important difference or MCID), which is the smallest change in a score that would likely be important from the patient's perspective.

8. **B:** 0.6

   Rationale: Effect sizes have been operationally described and interpreted in the following ranges by Cohen: <0.2 = trivial effect, 0.2–0.5 = small effect, 0.5–0.8 = moderate effect, >0.8 = large effect. An ES of 0.6 would be considered a moderate effect.

9. **D:** 0.8

   Rationale: Intraclass correlation coefficient (ICC) is used to estimate stability in test-retest reliability because it considers measurement errors. intraclass correlation coefficient values greater than 0.90 are suggestive of excellent reliability, whereas values less than 0.50, between 0.50 and 0.75, and between 0.75 and 0.90 are suggestive of poor, moderate, and good reliability, respectively.

10. **B:** Criterion-related

    Rationale: While there are several different types of validity, for this chapter we will focus on content, criterion-related, and construct validity. These three forms of validity are important in determining the usefulness and limitations of specific outcomes and tests. Content validity is how a measure reproduces the proposed domain or area of content. Criterion-related validity is used to establish the precision of a measure or test by comparing it with the gold standard, or criterion measure, that reflects the variable being tested. Concurrent validity deals with present time and when being established, test developers examine the correlation between a new instrument and an accepted measure of the construct.

Chapter 4

1. A: The transcription complex E2F, which is required for progression from G1 to S phase of the cell cycle, is inactivated by binding with the retinoblastoma gene protein.
   Rationale: When Rb is hyperphosphorylated, it releases transcription factor E2F which binds at regulatory regions and facilitates transcription of genes that encode proteins that are needed by the cell during the S phase. Answer B is incorrect. Answer C, *p53* gene prevents cells with DNA damage from proceeding to S phase. Answer D is incorrect as *p53* gene activates apoptosis in cells detected to have oncogenic changes.

2. C: Activation of telomerase enzyme
   Rationale: Activation of telomerase enzyme (Answer C) is a fundamental process in tumorigenesis. Answers A, B, and D would all have anti-tumorigenesis effects.

3. C: Increasing levels of genomic instability in the tumor.
   Rationale: Genomic instability (Answer C) is a driving force in cancer initiation and progression. Answers A and B would have anti-tumorigenic effects. Answer D is also incorrect.

4. C: Driver mutations are essential for tumor transformation/growth
   Rationale: Answer C correctly describes the role of driver mutations. Answer A is incorrect as passenger mutations account for the largest number of mutations identified in any tumor. Answer B is incorrect as it is driver mutations that confer a growth advantage to a cell through the alteration of fundamental processes. Answer D is incorrect as passenger mutations are acquired over many years.

5. B: Prevents apoptosis
   Rationale: Overexpression of *BCL-2* prevents apoptosis (Answer B). Overexpression of *BCL-2*, therefore, does not result in cell death (Answer A), is not involved with telomere shortening (Answer C), and is not involved in epigenetic regulation (Answer D).

6. A: Diagnostic medical sonography
   Rationale: Diagnostic medical sonography (DMS or ultrasound) uses high-frequency sound waves to produce medical images of soft-tissue structures. It is referred to as nonionizing because this type of imaging has less energy when compared to ionizing radiation, and it cannot remove electrons from an atom. This makes nonionizing radiation less harmful. Computed tomography, general radiography, and fluoroscopy utilize X-rays, which is a type of ionizing radiation. Ionizing radiation is high energy, and has the ability to cause damage to cells by removing an electron from an atom.

7. D: Positron emission tomography
   Rationale: Positron emission tomography (PET) utilizes a radionuclide which is absorbed by areas in the body which may have an accelerated glucose metabolism. This increased use of sugar is an indicator of a functional change in the cells, such as malignancy. These functional changes may be visible on PET before any physical abnormality is visible on other imaging modalities, or before the patient exhibits any symptoms.

8. C: Her risk of breast carcinoma is increased
   Rationale: Smoking with long-term hormone replacement therapy (HRT) has increased her risk significantly

9. C: Decrease in induction of apoptosis of damaged cells.
   Rationale: The main function of wild type p53 is inducing apoptosis to the damaged cells.

10. A: Actively cycling normal cells are destroyed by the drug.
    Rationale: Adverse effects of chemotherapy. The drugs inhibit the DNA replication of normal and cancer cells. The goal of chemotherapy is to eliminate/destroy cancer cells.

Chapter 5

1. C: Always have a myelosuppressive effect
   Rationale: All patients who receive systemic chemotherapy treatment will undergo myelosuppression—all of them. Going into nadir with blood count values is a vital part of ensuring effective treatment directed toward cancer cells in the body. Only some systemic chemotherapy drugs are directly cardiotoxic, and only some systemic chemotherapy drugs work during the mitotic phase of the cell cycle. Targeted therapy drugs are in a whole separate category of chemotherapy drugs.

2. A: Locally invasive in the tissue of origin and into regional lymph nodes
   Rationale: The term "invasive" refers to a "local" spread of cells within the local region of the body. This includes the tissue of origin as well as regional lymph nodes. Once cancer cells move to distal sites—bone, brain, liver, lungs—then the correct term to use is "metastasis."

3. B: As a first line of treatment for curative intent
   Rationale: Induction chemotherapy is prescribed to patients for curative intent and is given as a first line of treatment prior to surgery and radiation.

4. C: To treat high grade aggressive lesions to induce a pathological complete response
   Rationale: Neoadjuvant chemotherapy is prescribed in cases with high grade, aggressive lesions to induce a pathological complete response. It is also prescribed to shrink large tumors with significant depth of invasion.

5. B: Cells are poorly differentiated and have high mitotic counts
   Rationale: Grade III is a high grade, aggressive tumor, and this means that the cell shapes are very distorted: poorly differentiated—to the point of amorphic, and it also means that there is a very high proportion of nuclei dividing within the cancer cells. The higher the nucleus division count, the more aggressively and fast the tumor is growing.

6. B: Slow release opioids
   Rationale: Slow release opioids—these are needed to control tumor-related pain that is constant by releasing medication into the patient's body slowly over time.

7. D: Soft tissue, organ surfaces, nerves, bones, and lympho-vascular structures
Rationale: Radiation therapy affects all body tissues within the treatment field including soft tissues, organ surfaces, nerves, bones, and lympho-vascular structures.

8. B: Can occur after an allogeneic transplant and will affect connective tissues
Rationale: In GvHD, the transplanted bone marrow or stem cells identify the cells in the recipient's body as a foreign substance and generate an immune response toward the body's cells. GvHD develops in connective tissues in the body, affecting skin, liver, or the gastrointestinal tract.

9. C: Targeted chemotherapy
Rationale: The overexpression of the HER2 receptor has resulted in the development of HER2-targeted therapies to directly inhibit the receptors, including trastuzumab (Herceptin), which has substantially improved patient survival.

10. B: One of the advantages of proton therapy is that it has almost no exit dose
Rationale: Proton beam therapy uses protons to deliver a very precise dose that does not have a substantial exit dose, unlike some other external beam therapies. It is useful where precision is needed such as in brain tumors.

Chapter 6

1. B: Full agonist
Rationale: Full agonists and partial agonists bind to the same receptor, but while a full agonist produces the maximal response, a partial agonist produces a more limited response. Antagonists do not produce a response when they bind to a receptor. They prevent receptor activation and block the effects of agonists. A physiologic antagonist causes a physiologic effect opposite to that induced by the agonist.

2. C: Cisplatin
Rationale: Cisplatin is a platinum analog, which is analogous to alkylating agents. It is used in the treatment of several different types of cancer, including testicular cancer. A common adverse effect of cisplatin therapy is polyneuropathy, which can cause symptoms such as numbness, weakness, burning, or tingling.

3. D: Inhibit topoisomerase
Rationale: Irinotecan is a topoisomerase inhibitor that is often used in the treatment of colorectal cancer. Its use is limited by severe gastrointestinal toxicity that can lead to potentially life-threatening diarrhea. The delayed form of diarrhea may occur about 2 to 10 days after treatment. It can be treated with loperamide. Patients with conditions such as Gilbert's syndrome are highly susceptible to irinotecan toxicity.

4. B: Communicate with the physician to see if any colony stimulating factors are being provided
Rationale: Colony stimulating factors are known to cause bone pain and this may have been administered concurrently with his chemotherapy. Aspirin is not an appropriate recommendation as there is not enough information to determine that the patient does not have thrombocytopenia which may be exacerbated by aspirin. The other two recommendations are not appropriate clinical choices.

5. B: Drowsiness
Rationale: While all of these options would impact rehabilitation, these medications used to address nausea and vomiting cause drowsiness.

6. A: She should have an exercise test and have close monitoring of vital signs for cardiotoxicity
Rationale: AC-T chemotherapy includes doxorubicin, an anthracycline, which is known to cause cardiotoxicity. Although most patients are asymptomatic at rest, close monitoring should be provided and an exercise test would be warranted to assure the patient's exercise regimen is safe. Exercise is still important, even with cardiotoxicity, but may need to be dosed down by a professional prior to performance. Many patients experience pancytopenia with chemotherapy and exercising in large groups may increase the risk of community-acquired infections. Although the patient may experience some weakness or balance issues, there is not clear evidence that a walker is warranted.

7. C: Age-related changes
Rationale: Platinum agents are neurotoxic and hemotoxic. White blood cells may be affected, allowing for opportunistic infections to emerge. The neurotoxicity due to cisplatin may affect the vestibular system nerves and peripheral nerves, further contributing to his balance disorders. Due to the rapid onset of symptoms, age-related changes are not likely to be the cause of his symptoms.

8. A: Explain that different chemotherapy medications have different effects on cancer cells to be more effective
Rationale: Answering the patient directly to explain the overall aim of combination therapy is accurate and does not provide too much information. The question should not be ignored or deferred. If the clinician provides too much detailed information, it increases the risk of contradicting the information that the physician provided or increasing the patient's anxiety at this time.

9. C: A detailed chemotherapeutic history should be obtained to allow the clinician to screen for any chemotherapy-induced adverse effects
Rationale: It is critical to have a thorough chemotherapeutic history to determine what medications the patient received as each drug has its own adverse effects on body systems. As there are a number of internet-based resources to look up drug effects and uses, memorization may not be the best use of the clinician's time, especially as medications are often changing. Finally, much of this information may be gathered from the patient's medical record and calling a physician every time may be damaging to the relationship with the Onc R clinician, although this may be needed in some cases.

10. A: The student is right, targeted therapies affect cancer cells through the same mechanisms as many traditional chemotherapy agents
Rationale: Chemotherapy is usually cytotoxic to most cells while targeted therapy uses small molecules or enables the person's own immune system to treat the cancer. Targeted therapies still do have adverse effects. Hormone therapy is often considered a type of targeted therapy for hormone-dependent cancers.

Chapter 7

1. D: Should consult the multidisciplinary team for safety guidance
Rationale: D is the correct answer. Once diagnosed with bone metastases, the PLWC should have a thorough work up and guidance from oncologist or orthopedic specialist

regarding a weight bearing status and any further restrictions or treatment plan. Once this is complete, a referral to physical therapy is appropriate; see Tables 7.11 and 7.12, and 7.15 for the exercise guidelines outlined in this chapter.

2. B: Imaging and clinical features
Rationale: B is the correct answer. The SINS and Mirels scale use radiologic information regarding depth of metastases in the structure of the bone, that is, percentage of collapse in vertebral body, spinal alignment or type of lesion. Both scales also use clinical features such as pain with worsened pain as a higher score than pain-free.

3. D: Pre-existing connective tissue disorders (scleroderma, lupus or Marfan syndrome)
Rationale: D is the correct answer. Radiation fibrosis is correlated with pre-existing connective tissue disorders that predispose the PLWC to have more fibrosis as well as larger radiation field size such as in Hodgkin lymphoma, a longer course of therapy (increased total radiation dose) as well as previous or concurrent chemotherapy not neo-adjuvant.

4. D: Risk of falls
Rationale: D is the correct answer. Basal et al. showed that one in three AI users experienced a fall. Chemotherapy side effects include hand and foot syndrome and CIPN. Myasthenia gravis is a secondary neuromuscular junction disorder often caused by the immune response to a cancerous tumor.

5. C: Are clinician rated tools and have considerable bias
Rationale: C is the correct answer. The Karnofsky and ECOG scale are regularly used to determine treatment decision and frailty is often underdiagnosed due to inconsistency in rating the PLWC comprehensive medical and functional status. A better alternative would be a comprehensive geriatric assessment, one example given in the text being the Fried frailty phenotype.

6. C: Treated with exercise and nutritional support
Rationale: C is the correct answer. Exercise in a PLWC that has cachexia may improve metabolism, function and reduce muscle mass loss. Without the necessary energy intake to balance physical activity, cachexia can worsen. Nutritional strategies such as use of appetite stimulants and use of high calorie, small, frequent meals or oral supplements can be utilized. Cachexia is common in older cancer survivors and is determined by use of DEXA scan not plain radiographs. The Fried frailty phenotype does not diagnose cachexia.

7. D: Radiation therapy
Rationale: D is the correct answer. Radiation therapy can greater effect body mechanics than any of the other options listed due to its adverse tissue and bony effects such as radiation fibrosis.

8. A: None, monitor for pain
Rationale: A is the correct answer. See Table 7.11. If the metastasis in the bony cortex is 0% to 25% involved, they are recommended to monitor pain, maintain full weight bearing and have no activity restrictions. Always consult with an oncologist for restrictions individual to each PLWC.

9. B: Restricted ROM in capsular pattern
Rationale: B is the correct answer. Capsular patterns are normal with adhesive capsulitis and are not a red flag. A, C and D are red flags and warrant referral back to physician or in the case of D an emergency.

10. C: Lymphedema
Rationale: C is the correct answer. Lymphedema is not caused by postural changes, otherwise lymphedema may cause postural changes given the weight of the swelling, however, A, B, and D all contribute most to postural changes from cancer treatments.

Chapter 8

1. B: Peripheral nervous system
Rationale: Cranial nerves are a part of the peripheral nervous system.

2. B: Tingling in toes and fingers
Rationale: Platinum-based chemo has an increased likelihood of CIPN due to being a neurotoxic chemo.

3. A: Coasting
Rationale: Coasting is a phenomenon that can be defined as neuropathy that worsens or develops once chemotherapy treatment is completed.

4. A: Paclitaxel (Taxol)
Rationale: Paclitaxel (Taxol) is the Taxane class of chemo which is neurotoxic.

5. A: Perception
Rationale: Perception is how sensory information is processed and integrated. It can be tested by identification of objects from sensory information, by the ability to recognize objects, and sounds, and by the intactness of perceptual fields.

6. D: FACT-GOG NTX/13:
Rationale: This a specific scale for QOL and looks at CIPN in detail.

7. C: Stomach
Rationale: Based on the tables in the text stomach is not a common cancer to have a brain or spinal metastasis.

8. C: Decreased cadence
Rationale: This is based off the article by Marshall et al., decreased cadence has been demonstrated in patients who have been diagnosed with CIPN.

9. A: Ankle strategy
Rationale: Ankle strategy is utilized when the patient experiences a small perturbation and is most difficult for patients with CIPN to elicit.

10. A: Sensory nerves
Rationale: Sensory nerves have been shown to be most affected by chemo due to the damage to the dorsal root ganglion which is the sensory relay system.

Chapter 9

1. D: Systemic chemotherapy
Rationale: Research shows that taxane-based chemotherapy is a risk factor for clinical lymphedema. Age and biomarkers are additional considerations.

2. B: At prehabilitation at the time of her initial diagnosis
Rationale: The prospective surveillance model of care is best initiated at the time of initial diagnosis to gather pretreatment volumetric and objective measures.

3. A: Subclinical lymphedema in her left upper extremity
Rationale: The measurement parameter for subclinical lymphedema is >3% and <10% volume increase in the affected extremity. Postsurgical edema would mostly be located in the breast/lateral chest area. The increased

volume measured in this case is in the patient's upper extremity which indicates a mild lymphatic component in addition to the normal, expected postsurgical edema presentation.

4. C: Her cellulitis infection

Rationale: All of these comorbidities play into risk stratification for this patient; however research shows that the most significant of these is her cellulitis infection because of the lymphatic system's immunological role in the body. The infection would have increased immunological stress and compromise to an already compromised system.

5. B: The timing is just right for considering a lympho-venous anastomosis (LVA) surgery

Rationale: Evidence-based research demonstrates that performing LVA surgery either prophylactically at the time of axillary dissection, or within the first 3 months postsurgery provides promising results in reducing risk of progression of subclinical lymphedema to clinical lymphedema.

6. C: Marjolin's ulcer

Rationale: The location of this wound is important in clinical reasoning. It is located in prior burned tissue, which raises suspicion for a Marjolin's ulcer. A venous would is more likely on the medial aspect of the lower leg. A pressure injury is unlikely based on both location and her mobility level. The wound presentation also provides cues. Hypergranulation and rolled edges are consistent with a Marjolin's ulcer. The irregular edges do not match the commonly symmetrical shape of arterial ulcers.

7. B: Biopsy followed by wound excision

Rationale: Any time cancer is suspected in a wound, a biopsy must be performed. There is sufficient reason to suspect a Marjolin's ulcer, therefore a biopsy is of utmost importance to confirm or rule out the presence of cancer.

8. C: Hydrofiber

Rationale: There is moderate, clear drainage, therefore drainage must be absorbed to promote a moist wound environment. The first 2 choices are not appropriate. A hydrogel will donate additional moisture that is not needed while a thin film will not absorb any drainage. A superabsorbent dressing is indicated in the presence of large amounts of drainage. Of all the dressings listed, a hydrofiber is the most appropriate for moderate amounts of drainage.

9. B: Inflammatory

Rationale: All of the listed medications are anti-inflammatory medications and therefore directly affect the inflammatory phase of wound healing.

10. A: Vitamin A

Rationale: While the other vitamins are important for wound healing and skin health, vitamin A is the only one that can mitigate the effects of corticosteroids, one of the patient's medications.

Chapter 10

1. C: Atrial fibrillation

Rationale: Atrial fibrillation is frequently observed in patients being treated for cancer and can lead to increased morbidity and mortality in this population.

2. D: High risk

Rationale: According to the Wells scoring system, the individual receives a point for active cancer, recent immobilization/major surgery within 4 weeks, and tenderness along the posterior calf. Three points put this patient in the high-risk category for developing a DVT.

3. C: Hemoglobin

Rationale: Hemoglobin is vital in transporting oxygen from the lungs to the tissues throughout the body. When hemoglobin is low, an individual is likely to experience shortness of breath, tachycardia, reduced activity tolerance, and endurance.

4. B: Quantify the intensity of a particular activity

Rationale: METS are a means of consistent and objective data that quantify the level of energy expenditure of an individual's experience for a particular activity. The Ainsworth compendium has quantified these activities based on MET level.

5. A: Stop activity and call the physician

Rationale: Contraindications to exercise testing include: irregular rhythm, hypotension with increasing workload, symptoms such as severe shortness of breath and dizziness. These symptoms are not a typical response expected with exercise and require further medical assessment.

6. A: Shortness of breath

Rationale: Shortness of breath is the most appropriate answer as this is a possible side effect of both chemotherapy and radiation therapy. Dry cough would be a more common side effect of pulmonary toxicity; whereas, heart palpitations and fluid retention are more common to cardiac toxicity.

7. D: Nonconcurrent mediastinal radiation

Rationale: Nonconcurrent mediastinal radiation is the least likely intervention to result in cardiotoxicity as this intervention is specifically targeted to the region of the radiation field. Chemotherapy interventions have evidence of systemic side effects with specific evidence of cardiotoxicity as a side effect.

8. B: Pursed lip breathing can be a useful adjunct to reduce stress and promote relaxation

Rationale: Energy conservation techniques include pursed lip breathing, relaxation techniques, allowing increased time for activities with rest following, and completing activities throughout the day as energy allows. Pursed lip breathing, prioritizing activities, advanced planning to streamline activities, pacing activities to minimize sympathetic responses and positioning of the body to decrease the work of breathing are elements of a good energy conservation program.

9. D: Workload is at 60% of the heart rate range

Rationale: The Borg scale starts at a 6 (resting) and increases to 20 (maximum exertion). When dosing an exercise, an RPE value of 12 to 14 would suggest a moderate level of activity and corresponds to 60% of the HR range; whereas a value of 16 would correspond to 85% of the HR range. An RPE of 13 suggests the patient is working just above his 60% HR range.

10. A: It is an independent predictor of mortality in heart disease

Rationale: Dyspnea is an independent predictor of mortality. It is a subjective measure and is the most prevalent symptom among individuals with cardiac and respiratory disease and can be brought on or exacerbated during the course of medical treatments for cancer. The Total

Dyspnea Scale for Cancer objectively measures the severity of dyspnea.

Chapter 11

1. C: Having the PLWBC complete the Multidimensional Fatigue Symptom Inventory
Rationale: Objective measurement is the key to ruling out A, as that is subjective measurement. While the Modified Brief Fatigue Inventory and Visual Analog Scale are more objective, evidence from the EDGE Taskforce recommends the Multidimensional Fatigue Symptom Inventory as the preferred assessment of fatigue for the oncologic GI population.

2. C: Six-minute walk test
Rationale: Answers A and B are sound assessments for cardiopulmonary fitness, though lack the functional component of the correct answer, C, the six-minute walk test. Answer D does not assess for cardiopulmonary fitness, rather is it an assessment of balance and transfer/gait performance.

3. C: Use of the Applied Wound Management tool and the National Wound Assessment Form
Rationale: Evidence supports the use of the Applied Wound Management tool and the National Wound Assessment Form for objective wound assessment.

4. C: Registered dietitian/registered dietitian nutritionist
Rationale: Referral to registered dietitian/registered dietitian nutritionist in cases where the needs are beyond the skills of the PT where collaboration is needed to address the suspected malnutrition.

5. B: Consider the patient's treatment plan and implement palliative therapeutic goals.
Rationale: As noted in the section on ascites relating to cancer diagnosis, the average survival after diagnosis of cancer related ascites was 5.7 months. Only 11% of person's diagnosed with ascites related to their cancer diagnosis survive longer than 6 months, therefore it is appropriate to consider shifting toward palliative therapeutic goals.

6. B: Refer back to oncologist for antioxidant supplementation
Rationale: There are many interventions that may benefit PLWCs who have symptoms of chemo-induced polyneuropathy long term such as A, C, D. This is well known by the oncologist at this time and are referring to you secondary to the need for these alternative interventions.

7. A: Clinical Test of Sensory Integration and Balance (CTSIB)
Rationale: Evidence supports use of Clinical Test of Sensory Integration and Balance over the other options for this question.

8. A: Apply abdominal binder by rolling left and right, carefully bend both lower extremities until feet are flat on the surface of the bed, perform a modified log roll to one side (head of bed elevated to comfort), advance lower extremities toward the edge and off of the side of the bed as upper extremities push down with same-side elbow and alternate-side hand across body, ensure both feet are flat on the floor before preparing to exit the bed.
Rationale: Performing a log roll allows for proper protection of the abdominal incision and surgical intervention site. Utilizing the lower extremities as a pendulum and having the head of the bed elevated allows for minimal activation of abdominal muscles.

9. B: Lifting his 4-year-old granddaughter for a hug
Rationale: Typical precautions include limited lifting (<5–10 lb) and no strenuous activity. The average 4-year-old is going to weigh well over this threshold.

10. D: Supine trunk strengthening program
Rationale: At this phase of healing, supine position has low tolerance and can result in tension on the incision if not performed corrected. He would benefit from early trunk strengthening but in upright postures such as sitting/standing.

Chapter 12

1. B: PFM atrophy as a result of androgen-deprivation therapy
Rationale: PFM strength is an active continence mechanism while the other options affect structure and are therefore passive mechanisms

2. A: Cerebrovascular accident due to thrombus formation
Rationale: Functional UI is an involuntary loss of urine due to gross or fine motor limitations from musculoskeletal or neurological impairments or cognitive deficits rather than a defect in the genitourinary system itself.

3. D: Constipation from abdominal surgery for tumor resection
Rationale: Constipation is a major contributor to UI and therefore management of constipation is a required component of reducing or resolving urinary incontinence.

4. C: Radiation cystitis from treatment for endometrial cancer
Rationale: While the symptoms of radiation cystitis may present the same as an infection (urinary urgency, frequency, incontinence, and bladder pain or dysuria), fibrosis of the bladder does not increase the risk of developing an infection and symptoms will not improve with antimicrobial treatment.

5. B: A man who has received chemotherapy will not be able to father a child of his own unless he banks his sperm prior to treatment.
Rationale: Spermatogenesis and sperm health are generally thought to be restored by 2 years after completion of treatment, with no documented increase in birth defects after this time.

6. A: Recurrent urinary tract infections and kidney stones due to methotrexate resulting in PFM overactivity
Rationale: Recurrent UTIs often result in PFM overactivity which is more associated with urinary urgency/frequency, urge UI, difficulty starting the flow of urine, interrupted urine flow, and/or urinary retention. In some cases, however, PFM overactivity results in a functional muscle weakness and therefore can contribute to SUI; normalizing PFM activity can serve to improve muscle strength.

7. C: PFM weakness due to chronic cough
Rationale: PFM weakness is associated with SUI rather than retention. Chronic cough is a risk factor for weak PFM, but conversely, it could make the muscles overactive which could then be a cause of urinary retention.

8. D: He has other risk factors and his cancer history is likely not relevant to his erectile dysfunction
Rationale: In this case, obesity, hypertension, diabetic peripheral neuropathy, and total hip replacement are the more likely causes of his erectile dysfunction.

9. C: CIPN from oxaliplatin
Rationale: CIPN will affect efferent and afferent pelvic nerve function resulting in PFM weakness and

decreased sensation and therefore anorgasmia rather than dyspareunia.

10. A: Altered gait mechanics from surgery resulting in pelvic asymmetry and altered lumbopelvic muscle length-tension relationships

Rationale: Testicular and groin pain is often due to impingement of the neurovasculature in the inguinal canal that passes through the abdominal wall and over the superior pubic ramus. These nerves originate from the lumbar spine. It is also due to abnormal tension in the urogenital triangle muscles, which attach to the ischiopubic ramus, the ischial tuberosity, perineal body, and to the penis itself.

Chapter 13

1. C: Hypocalcemia and hyperphosphatemia both occurring on the second day following treatment

Rationale: Tumor lysis syndrome occurs within the first 3 days prior to treatment and up to 7 days after the initiation of treatment. Although elevated creatinine is a sign of tumor lysis syndrome, there needs to be two or more metabolic abnormalities both occurring within 24 hours of each other in order to finalize a diagnosis. See the section on tumor lysis syndrome in Chapter 13 for more information.

2. A: T cells

Rationale: Androgen deprivation therapy has effects on the production of multiple cells, such as T cells, cytokines, and B cells. However, the treatment of estrogen positive breast cancers leads to a reduction in T-cells (CD4). Review the hormone therapy section for more information.

3. D: Post-transplant lymphoproliferative disorder (PTLD)

Rationale: Post-transplant lymphoproliferative disease (PTLD) is a malignancy seen after allogeneic transplant. Persons typically have fever, weight loss, night sweats, adenopathy, unexplained hematologic abnormalities, or symptoms of infiltration of extra lymphatic tissue. A positive PET scan with the presence of a mass and elevated serum markers are suggestive of PTLD. See the section on post-transplant lymphoproliferative disorder for more information.

4. B: Chronic inflammation increases a person's lymphoproliferative malignancy risk

Rationale: Autoimmunity leads to chronic inflammation, which can increase the risk for developing malignancy. Cancer leads to preneoplasia rheumatoid arthritis symptoms. Review the Autoimmune Disease section of Chapter 13 for more information—specifically, Figure 13.4 and Table 13.6 for the cyclic effects of cancer and autoimmunity.

5. D: Type IV

Rationale: Steven-Johnson syndrome is a Type IV hypersensitivity reaction. These symptoms of immune reactions have a long latency period after a seemingly uncomplicated treatment. If not recognized early, this can become life-threatening. See section on Hypersensitivity Reactions for more information, specifically Table 13.7.

6. A: Light aerobic exercise with focus on sit to/from transfers in order to assist with proximal muscle strengthening

Rationale: Although all options are good treatment session ideas, choice A is the *best* option. Steroid myopathy is commonly seen in this population due to long term use of corticosteroids. Focusing on sit to stand transfers can assist in addressing proximal hip girdle weakness. In addition, light aerobic exercise can assist with cancer-related fatigue and generalized deconditioning from inactivity. See Stem Cell Transplant Section for more information.

7. C: Hematopoietic stem cell—common lymphoid progenitor—T lymphocyte

Rationale: A common lymphoid progenitor cell is the cell intermediary between a hematopoietic stem cell and a T lymphocyte. Refer Figure 13.1 to review the stem cell-derived cell lineages of the major immune system cells. For application, consider the importance of full engraftment of hematopoietic stem cells after bone marrow transplantation so that the derivation of a complete cell lineage occurs in the recipient, including healthy T lymphocytes.

8. B: Chemotherapy administered through a central line for hematologic malignancy

Rationale: Option B describes an infusion method where the primary objective is the systemic delivery of a cancer therapeutic. Immune cells that circulate in the blood and lymph will be exposed to chemotherapy delivered intravenously. Options C and D treat tumors more locally. Option A describes the delivery of chemotherapy intrathecally via the cerebrospinal fluid (CSF) to a tumor in the central nervous system (CNS). Chemotherapy in the CSF does not conduct with systemic circulation due to the blood-brain barrier; therefore, systemic immunosuppression is less likely with Option A.

9. D: Palpable lymph node

Rationale: A palpable lymph node (Option D) may be present in persons living with cancer, but is not one of the screening criteria for systemic inflammatory response syndrome or sepsis. Options A, B, and C are concerning for the presence of a systemic inflammatory response. Refer to Table 13.8 and Table 13.9 for more information.

10. D: The innate immune system serves critical functions of first line defense, regulation of inflammation, and activation and instruction of the adaptive immune system responses.

Rationale: This question requires one to differentiate between the primary roles of the innate and adaptive immune system components. Option D is the only option that correctly describes the role of one of these systems. Review the sections on Innate and Adaptive Immunity at the beginning of Chapter 13 for more information.

Chapter 14

1. D: Spiritual

Rationale: The fourth area is financial.

2. B: Anxiety

Rationale: See Table 14.3.

3. A: Depression

Rationale: See Table 14.2.

4. C: 25%

Rationale: The evidence states that one quarter of all healthcare professions working in this field are at risk for compassion fatigue.

5. A: Distress

Rationale: The NCCN determined that the sixth vital sign was distress. Refer to the Distress Thermometer for clarification and its use as a measurement tool for distress.

6. B: Distress

Rationale: The NCCN defines distress as a multifactorial unpleasant emotional experience of a psychological (cognitive, behavioral, emotional) social, and/or spiritual nature that may interfere with the ability to cope effectively with cancer, its physical symptoms and its treatment. This scenario describes a patient in distress.

7. B: Redirect to the present moment by saying: I know this can be scary but tell me something that makes you feel encouraged today

Rationale: If a person begins to talk about their fears for the future, the PLWBC can be redirected to the present moment in a nonjudgmental way. Useful phrasing may include, "I know this can be scary but tell me about something in the present moment that makes you feel encouraged."

8. C: 24%

Rationale: A systematic review and meta-analysis of breast cancer survivors found that the presence of depression/anxiety was associated with a 24%/17% higher risk of cancer recurrence, 30%/13% increase risk of all-cause mortality, and 29%/0% increase risk of breast cancer-specific mortality.

9. C: This is really hard but I will get there

Rationale: See Table 14.4.

10. B: Combined effects of the caregiver's continuous visualizing of client's traumatic images added to the effects of burnout causing caregiver debilitation

Rationale: Compassion fatigue is that stress on a clinician or caregiver as a result of helping another person but it is not referring to the person that is suffering from the disease and being cared for.

Chapter 15

1. B: Were taking tamoxifen (Soltamox)

Rationale: Tamoxifen is a hormone therapy after surgery and radiation and will not cause lymphedema.

2. D: Pancreas

Rationale: The lung is the fourth most common site for metastasis. Pancreas is not a site of metastasis.

3. B: ER-PR-HER2-

Rationale: Triple negative means that the tumor is not expressing estrogen or progesterone receptors and that HER2 is not overexpressing.

4. A: Increased fatigue

Rationale: Fatigue is treated by an Onc R clinician. The other three areas of concern should prompt a patient to contact their physician immediately.

5. D: Strength at a 4/5

Rationale: Strength at that level is good post surgery or even during chemo or radiation but the challenges of the shoulder complex lie in the mechanical changes that have occurred.

6. B: Prominence of lateral and superior borders

Rationale: Because of the potential for nerve damage and muscular weakness, winging of the scapula is a concern. The medial and inferior borders will be prominent in that case, not the lateral and superior.

7. B: Radiation

Rationale: See Table 15.7 for common adverse effects.

8. A: Stacked DIEP flap surgery

Rationale: See Table 15.5 autologous reconstruction options.

9. D: Luminal A

Rationale: See Table 15.4 female breast cancer subtypes.

10. C: Decreased estrogen levels

Rationale: See Table 15.3 established risk factors for male breast cancer.

Chapter 16

1. A: Low back pain with sciatica in a man with a history of prostate cancer

Rationale: Low back pain with sciatica following prostate cancer could indicate progression, metastasis, and/or recurrence. B and C are common responses to these surgeries given visceral ligamentous attachments. D is one of the top reasons for PFPT Onc R referral.

2. C: Encourage her to follow up with her oncologist as soon as possible as Tamoxifen is a risk factor for endometrial cancer and she is reporting red flags

Rationale: While this could be part of the GSM brought on by breast cancer treatment, she is reporting several red flags, though not emergent.

3. C: Contact the referring physician to discuss concern for testicular cancer screening

Rationale: The patient's height, age, and race are risk factors for testicular cancer and groin pain and infertility are red flags.

4. D: Vaginal discharge or bleeding with foul odor

Rationale: Overactive bladder and/or pelvic pain are common reasons for referral to PFPT and are not in and of themselves a red flag as an abuse history and childbearing could contribute to this. However, new onset of these symptoms or lack of response to standard therapy may warrant follow up with a physician. B and C are risk factors and not red flags, though add context to her other symptoms. Vaginal discharge and bleeding, particularly with a foul odor, would be a red flag for referral back to the physician, if not for cancer at least to rule out infection or other pathology.

5. A: Lower risk of developing cancer

Rationale: The LGBTQIA+ community is disproportionately affected by anal, breast, cervical, colorectal, endometrial, lung, and prostate cancers.

6. A: Bridging with hip adductor ball squeeze

Rationale: The hip adductors can create overflow into the PFM and shortening of the perineal muscles in the irradiated field. Anterior hip flexibility, posture, and gluteal function will all benefit both hip recovery as well as PFM function for bladder control.

7. D: A home exercise program of 10 PFM contractions held for 10 seconds performed three times a day

Rationale: It can be harmful to prescribe Kegels without first assessing PFM length-strength balance and coordination. Postural retraining and core muscle synergistic function are safest and may have greater benefit.

8. A: Cancer history is an absolute contraindication for modality use

Rationale: Modalities may be used for palliative care or at a site distal from a cancer mass for a PWC. Surface EMG is never contraindicated. Modalities may be used without restriction after 5-years post treatment.

9. B: Dilation should be gentle, progressive, and discontinued if bleeding greater than spotting occurs

Rationale: There is no evidence to support improved outcomes, but perhaps poorer adherence, if dilation starts during radiation. Dilator therapy may be discontinued after 1 to 2 years. It is important to maintain vaginal dimensions for medical surveillance of recurrence.

10. A: All persons should perform Kegels daily to prevent or correct pelvic floor dysfunction

Rationale: Kegels are often over-prescribed and can exacerbate a GU/GYN complaint if the PFM are already overactive or fibrosed or if the person is not properly isolating and recruiting the PFM and instead using compensatory mechanisms.

Chapter 17

1. B: Pelvic radiation disease

Rationale: PRD is defined as any acute or long-term adverse effects arising in noncancerous tissues that start from RTx for tumors in the pelvis. The symptoms listed above impact the urinary, GI, and integumentary/musculoskeletal system. Adverse effects can affect these systems and the neurological, lymphatic, or cardiovascular as they are present in the pelvis.

2. D: Mucositis pathway

Rationale: Anti-metabolite systemic chemotherapies are utilized in most chemotherapy regimens for CRC. The primary clinical pathway based on the adverse effects is related to the mucosal lining of the GI and GU systems.

3. A: Abdominal crunches

Rationale: Early functional mobility, breathing and transverse abdominus activation is encouraged to initiate postural strength and function. Avoiding increased abdominal pressure with activities such as crunches, sit-ups, or Valsalva maneuver should be avoided with an ostomy present to reduce risk of herniation.

4. B: Prone press ups

Rationale: Direct pressure onto the ostomy can result in discomfort and excessive pressure directly on the bowel should be avoided. Additionally, prone press ups result in an over-extension stretch of the ostomy site and can increase the fascial tension around the ostomy.

5. A: Liver

Rationale: The liver is the most common site for CRC metastasis. Symptoms from liver cirrhosis include weight loss, dark urine, loss of appetite, nausea, fatigue, fever, jaundice, itchy skin, abdominal pain/discomfort, ascites, and ankle swelling.

6. C: Lung cancer

Rationale: While breast and prostate cancer are the leading diagnosis for each sex, they are not the leading causes of deaths. Lung cancer is second for diagnosis for both sex but first for deaths. Cervical cancer is high in both diagnosis and deaths world-wide but falls behind CRC.

7. A: Metastases to the peritoneum

Rationale: Colon cancer demographics, prognosis, and treatment vary based on the sidedness of the cancer, right to left. While left-sided colon cancers have a tendency to metastasize to the liver and lung, right-sided cancers metastasize to the peritoneum more often.

8. B: Gluteus medius

Rationale: Radiation impacts a lot of pelvic musculature including hip flexors, rotators, and adductors which dose concentrated to impact the central portion of the pelvic. Gluteus medius is superficial and protected by the ilium and has minimal if any radiation exposure.

9. D: Neurological system

Rationale: While the neurological system is significantly impacted by chemotherapy, there is not a large surgical impact and those does not need to be a focus of an Onc R evaluation.

10. B: Chemotherapy-induced peripheral neuropathy

Rationale: FOLFOX regimen includes leucovorin calcium (folinic acid), fluorouracil, oxaliplatin. Oxaliplatin is a known neurotoxic agent. Chemotherapy-induced diarrhea is more frequently experienced from florouricil versus constipation, Hand-foot syndrome is primarily seen in with capecitabine. While malnourishment is common , it is not a dominant adverse effect specific to FOLFOX.

Chapter 18

1. D: Decreased cardiopulmonary endurance

Rationale: Surgical resection of Stage I non-small cell cancer is considered curative and therefore it cannot be assumed that she had chemotherapy or radiation. The three tests performed are assessing functional lower body strength, transitional movements, and balance/fall risk with the 5XSTS, aerobic capacity and endurance with the 6MWT, and balance, sit to stand, mobility, and fall risk with the TUG. All three tests demonstrated impairments compared to age-related norms, but her TUG was below the high fall risk cut-off, indicating that her chief complaint is most likely impacted by decreased endurance which could also impact her lower body strength during functional activities.

2. A: Fatigue

Rationale: Screening for other treatment-related impairments is important during an evaluation and while all answers result from radiation therapy the adverse effect that is most likely to occur during the early part of radiation is fatigue.

3. C: Side bending toward the operative side

Rationale: Patients will often side bend toward the pain to relieve any tension on the drain site and decrease/inhibit rib expansion.

4. A: Immunotherapy-induced anemia

Rationale: Immunotherapy empowers the patient's immune system to fight cancer cells and are less likely to affect noncancerous cells.

5. B: Passive range of motion to improve pain

Rationale: Keeping a patient engaged in their life and self-care while maximizing their mobility should be the focus of treatment in palliative care and early in hospice. Teaching family members passive treatments, that are not considered skilled services, can be utilized later in hospice care to improve patient comfort.

6. D: Improving nutritional status and exercise capacity

Rationale: Pulmonary rehabilitation is safe to begin as early as 6 weeks after thoracic surgery and is comprised of individualized exercise prescription to enhance recovery and maximize exercise capacity.

7. B: Smoking at least 30 pack years
Rationale: Qualifications for a yearly low dose CT scan are: age 55–74, smoking at least 30 pack-years, or quitting <15 years ago.

8. C: Adaptive shortening of neck extensors and pectoralis major
Rationale: A common postural abnormality of individuals with COPD is increased thoracic kyphosis which would lead to adaptive shortening of neck extensors and pectoralis major.

9. C: Low-to-moderate intensity short duration functional exercises against body weight resistance
Rationale: The major concern is that Bob is demonstrating symptoms of lung cancer with possible metastasis to the bone. Low to moderate intensity exercises will help to improve his functional status and his fatigue in the long term, but it needs to be short duration to conserve needed energy for daily tasks. Making the exercises without resistance and against body weight will protect from increased pressure through bones that may have metastatic lesions.

10. D: Red flags: night pain, constant pain, cough, age greater than 50 years, smoking history—refer to PCP due to concern for metastatic lung cancer and initiate treatment with gentle exercise and pain modulation
Rationale: Patients with metastatic cancer are safe to perform gentle exercise against their own body weight or with no resistance and there is no contraindication to addressing his pain. Optimizing his aerobic capacity and functional status prior to treatment could have a positive impact on the treatment options that he is eligible for.

Chapter 19

1. A: Anterior neck soft tissue mobilization
Rationale: The patient presents with impaired cervical range of motion potentially due to acute effects of radiation therapy. At this time, soft tissue mobilization to anterior neck soft tissues would be contraindicated due to impaired skin integrity and breakdown (moist desquamation). Cervical lateral flexion active range of motion does not maximally elongate anterior neck soft tissues and would be appropriate to maintain neck mobility while protecting tissue at the anterior neck. Patient presents with a chief complaint of fatigue during the course of his radiation therapy consistent with cancer-related fatigue. Treatment options may include a combination of resistance and aerobic exercise. The patient did not present with any contraindications to resistance exercise or aerobic exercise as evidenced by an unremarkable musculoskeletal systems review except for impaired cervical AROM and no adverse events during Six Minute Walk Test.

2. B: Excessive scapular abduction during active shoulder abduction range of motion
Rationale: The spinal accessory nerve innervates the SCM and trapezius muscles. Therefore, patients with spinal accessory nerve palsy may present with SCM and trapezius muscle weakness and atrophy. During shoulder abduction, the trapezius muscle helps stabilize the scapula against the thoracic wall and works with the serratus anterior muscle to produce scapular upward rotation during arm elevation. Patients with spinal accessory nerve palsy will demonstrate excessive scapular abduction during active shoulder abduction range of motion due to the inability of the trapezius muscle to counteract the pull of the serratus anterior during shoulder abduction. Due its anatomical orientation, the trapezius muscle contributes to scapular elevation (upper fibers) and adduction (middle and lower fibers). Since spinal accessory nerve palsy is a neuromuscular disorder, patients will present with impaired shoulder abduction AROM and normal shoulder abduction PROM.

3. C: Normal physical examination, pain in jaw that is worse taking first few bites of food
Rationale: First bite syndrome refers to pain that occurs in the jaw/parotid gland region after initial bite of food and tends to diminish with subsequent bites. Swelling or sensory deficits in the facial region, and jaw mobility restrictions are not findings associated with first bite syndrome since pain is believed to be due to damage to sympathetic innervation.

4. C: Masseter hypertonicity
Rationale: Trismus is defined as any restriction to mouth opening (<35 mm) due to intra-articular or extra-articular temporomandibular joint (TMJ) problems. Trismus is a joint hypomobility disorder and not characterized by sensory deficits. A risk factor for developing trismus is greater radiation dosage to muscles of mastication that may cause radiation-induced dystonia or hypertonicity of muscles of mastication. Other causes of trismus may include tumor infiltrating muscles of mastication causing the reflexive spasm, destruction of temporomandibular joint surfaces due to tumor infiltration, damage to the trigeminal nerve causing abnormal activity and spasm, scarring after surgical approaches, and jaw pain and the adaptive protective mechanisms. A S-curve deviation during mandibular opening occurs due to hypermobility or articular disc disorder.

5. A: Adhesive capsulitis
Rationale: The patient presented with clinical findings consistent with adhesive capsulitis (shoulder pain and mobility deficits) as evidenced by the presence of shoulder pain and equal restriction of both active and passive shoulder range of motion in multiple directions (flexion and external rotation). He presented with scapular dyskinesis or a compensatory scapular movement pattern during shoulder abduction AROM. Excessive scapular elevation was noted during shoulder abduction AROM which occurs to increase the overall amount of shoulder motion (motion of the humerus in respect to the trunk) since glenohumeral joint motion (motion of the humerus in respect to the scapula) is limited in patients with adhesive capsulitis.

6. D: Standing biceps curls resistance exercise with manual assistance as needed to stabilize scapula
Rationale: He presented with clinical findings consistent with spinal accessory nerve palsy including decreased shoulder abduction AROM, trapezius muscle weakness, scapular dyskinesis, and positive scapular flip sign. Neuromuscular control and resistance exercise have been shown to reduce shoulder pain and disability in patients with SANP. Standing biceps curls with manual assistance to stabilize the scapula would be most appropriate because no trapezius muscle recovery is evident and the exercises do not target events trapezius muscle. Overhead

press resistance exercise would not be appropriate due to the patient only being able to his raise arm to 88 degrees of abduction. Prone shoulder horizontal abduction while maintaining glenohumeral external rotation would not be an appropriate resistance exercise at this time due to that exercise being testing position for middle trapezius muscle and the patient presented with 0/5 middle trapezius MMT. Standing shoulder abduction AROM would not be the best exercise at this time due to the patient presenting with no signs of trapezius muscle recovery and scapular dyskinesis during shoulder abduction AROM.

7. C: Cervical static active stretching: hold 30 seconds, 3 repetitions, 3 times per day
Rationale: The patient presented with neck rotation and extension passive mobility deficits likely due to radiation fibrosis evident by the anterolateral soft tissues of neck being firm to the touch. Exercises are recommended to improve soft tissue flexibility and address the patient's chief complaint of tightness when looking over her shoulder when driving and would include stretching. Cervical static active stretching would likely be most effective as compared to cervical dynamic stretching because patient had low irritability and total end range time was greater (270 seconds per day [30 seconds × 3 repetitions × 3 times per day] compared to 120 seconds per day [5 seconds × 8 repetitions × 3 times per day]).

8. A: Radiation-associated neck extensor muscle weakness
Rationale: This patient presented with reduced cervical extension AROM as compared to PROM indicating neck extensor muscle weakness which was contributing to her flexed and forward head posture and difficulty performing overhead work. Her neck pain was likely occurring due to prolonged tension being placed on the cervical extensors with a flexed and forward head posture and muscle overload due to demands of her daily activities. These findings are consistent with dropped head syndrome, which is believed to be due to radiation-induced damage to the spinal cord, nerves, and muscle.

9. A: Carotid artery disease
Rationale: Contraindications for head and neck compression include acute infection and vascular abnormalities. As this patient is a 67-year-old male with history of hypertension and radiation to neck region, he has increased risk for carotid artery stenosis. He did not present with any signs of acute infection (cellulitis) as evidenced by no redness or warmth to touch. Furthermore, he did not present with clinical findings suggesting a deep vein thrombosis of the subclavian vein extending to superior vena cava. Edema presentation was localized to the submental and anterior neck regions consistent with head and neck lymphedema and no dilation of collateral veins was noted. Radiation-related soft tissue fibrosis is not a contraindication for head and neck compression.

10. B: Difficulty breathing and swallowing
Rationale: Lymphedema associated with HNC can be external or internal. External lymphedema refers to swelling underneath the skin in the head and neck region. Patients with external lymphedema may report discomfort, tenderness, throbbing, pressure, heaviness, numbness, warmth, tightness, stiffness, firmness, difficulty moving the head or neck, and body image issues. Internal lymphedema refers to swelling that occurs inside the head and neck (i.e., arytenoid space, aryepiglottic folds, epiglottis, arytenoids, and base of tongue) and may contribute to difficulty breathing, voice problems, and trouble swallowing.

Chapter 20

1. B: His alignment of his pelvis is off causing increased pain in his back and hips
Rationale: Signs of aseptic loosening include: feeling unstable, increased pain at the bone/prosthetic articulation and signs of fracture or bone loss on imaging. His images were clear, and he was having more global pain versus focused pain at the prosthetic articulation. Bone sarcomas can usually be seen on X-ray as they cause osteolysis of the bone. His images were clear. Neuropathic pain does not cause global pain up into the spine.

2. C: Refer her to a lymphedema specialist for assessment
Rationale: While she had edema and swelling and symptoms in her left arm, they are not consistent with symptoms of cardiomyopathy, which has swelling of the lower extremities, and symptoms of fainting, fatigue, and changes in heart rhythm. Onset of lymphedema can take place any time after surgery and other treatment interventions.

3. B: He has outgrown his prosthetic socket and needs to be measured for a new one
Rationale: While difficulty with function can occur with neuropathic pain, those are not consistent with pain that goes away when the prosthetic is taken off. Weakness in his hips might contribute to functional limitations, but again would not relieve his pain if his prosthetic is taken off. If he had an infection in his limb, he would have other signs and symptoms such as edema, fever, and severe pain. As a growing young man, he might be experiencing growth spurts, weight gain, or leg length differences that are causing him to have pain in his residual limb when wearing his prosthetic.

4. A: Scar releases, with manual therapy, fascial releases, and modalities such as the low level laser and 6D fascial release system
Rationale: Scar releases with manual fascial releases and modalities is the best choice for starting her treatment sessions. Scars can impair muscle function, alignment, balance, and cause significant pain and restrictions. High velocity, low amplitude mobilizations are grade 5 mobilizations and should not be used. Aquatic therapy for back decompression and balance retraining is a great treatment option but should be used later on in her plan of care.

5. B: Check his strength, leg length, scar mobility, and look for compensation patterns
Rationale: Compensation patterns can be exhausting as they can change motor patterns, inhibit muscles, and can cause balance issues. A leg length difference and muscle weakness can contribute to his feeling of being off balance. While educating patients is highly valued and may need to be addressed at some point, the initial evaluation is not the optimal time to start addressing this. While the nerve assessments are a part of the systems review, they are not necessary at this time, and nothing indicates that he had a stroke. He does not note dizziness with his feeling off balance, so vestibular assessments would not be a high priority to screen.

6. D: Tingling and numbness, sensations of itching, sharp/shooting pain, feeling like the limb is still present

Rationale: After the limb is amputated, the nerves that are trying to regenerate have no place to go. The axons can become trapped in the scar tissue and create significant pain or phantom sensations.

7. A: Holding their breath while trying to recruit their core, over recruiting their hip flexors to compensate for abdominal weakness, using a posterior pelvic tilt while trying to engage the transverse abdominis

Rationale: Compensation patterns are often used as substitutions for areas that exhibit weakness or loss of function. Releasing the fascial restriction and avoiding compensation patterns can restore function and reduce pain, fatigue, and spasms.

8. C: Phantom limb and neuropathic pain

Rationale: Target muscle reinnervation is a surgical procedure that finds the nerve responsible for phantom limb pain, locates another nerve close by and has it donate a motor point to give to the hypersensitive nerve. This allows the nerve to heal.

9. B: Left and right discrimination, explicit motor imagery, mirror therapy to help with phantom limb pain

Rationale: Graded motor imagery is three sequential phases that help retrain the brain to recognize between the right and lift sides of the body with all of its individual parts and uses repetitive training to help improve speed and accuracy. Then it assists with concentrated and explicit motor imagery where the PLWBC is taught how to think through all of the different parts of a task and mentally perform the task in their mind in an organized fashion. The final phase includes mirror therapy that helps the PLWBC perceive their lost limb as being present by presenting an image of it using mirrors and the intact extremity.

10. A: Osteoinduction, osteoconduction, osseous integration

Rationale: The goals for an endoprosthesis are osteoinduction (stimulation of new cell growth), osteoconduction (cells starting to form new bone), and osseous integration (the bone grafts integrating through a creeping phenomenon in which the allograft, composite, and residual bone grow together and intertwine).

Chapter 21

1. B: Education about performing a walking program during admission.

Rationale: A walking program is important due to the required long-term hospital stay during induction chemotherapy to avoid deconditioning.

2. C: Continue with exercise intervention but omit resistance exercise.

Rationale: Platelets are too low for resistance exercise to be safe.

3. B: Never

Rationale: Neutropenic fever is an oncologic emergency, and you would not continue your session.

4. A: Referral to outpatient physical therapy

Rationale: All the above interventions are good, but for a full recovery from deconditioning after a long hospital stay, continuing his rehabilitation in the outpatient setting after discharge from the hospital would give him the most benefit.

5. B: Diffuse large B-cell lymphomas

Rationale: DLBCL is the most common form of NHL.

6. C: CHOP and R-CHOP

Rationale: CHOP and R-CHOP are the most common chemotherapy regimens for NHL.

7. C: Onc R clinicians need to avoid movements that place excessively high loads on fragile skeletal sites such as hyperflexion, hyperextension, or trunk rotation.

Rationale: Due to possible pathological fracture at the spine and possible cord compression.

8. D: Pain

Rationale: Bone lesions are often very painful. The others are less likely given his clinical presentation.

9. A: Spinal cord compression

Rationale: Due to bone lesions in his spine, spinal cord compression must be considered.

10. D: Calcium, renal failure, anemia, and bone lesions

Rationale: CRAB refers to calcium, renal failure, anemia, and bone lesions.

Chapter 22

1. C: Counselor

Rationale: A counselor would be the first indicated referral due to the history of anxiety and depression and the current significant worries reported. A dietician could be beneficial but there is potential that this pain experience is from mental health issues. A massage therapist could also be helpful for calming the sympathetic nervous system response, but there are some deeper issues regarding the situation that would benefit from a counselor first. A group fitness class is extremely important given the reported history; however, he is not yet ready for that level of engaged activity. A return to group fitness activities would be a good therapy goal.

2. B: Occasional "slouching" in chair causing decreased lumbar lordosis

Rationale: Due to excessive stress, this PLWBC needs to create opportunities to find restful positioning. Given the situation, excessive emphasis on ergonomics could be increasing shear forces. Along with a stressful work environment, this could lead to excessive lumbosacral muscle tension. Variable lumbosacral positioning can allow for improved circulation and decreased stress to remain in each position.

3. A: Work on skills toward playing baseball again.

Rationale: While strengthening, working on flexibility, and mobilizing tissues may benefit this PLWBC, his return to playing baseball would likely be a meaningful activity that would strengthen, improve flexibility, and move tissues with improved self-efficacy.

4. D: Pain neuroscience education

Rationale: All of these activities can be helpful for phantom limb pain, but knowledge of the pain issue is a priority for this PLWBC to improve their functional understanding.

5. A: Inflammatory response

Rationale: Nerve, skin, and bone/soft tissue related to answers B, C, and D are all potential structural issues related to the presented issue of pain. While these do have physiologic components, the inflammatory response is the only nonstructural contributor listed. However, it is important to note that an inflammatory response does have structural effect.

6. B: Peripheral nerve demyelination

Rationale: While there may be poor vasculature, axonal degeneration, and lumbar stenosis, these would more likely lead to a sensory loss versus peripheral nerve demyelination which can create significant sensitivity despite intact sensory integrity.

7. A: Allodynia

Rationale: Allodynia is a painful experience that should not normally be painful. Hyperalgesia is something that is normally painful but presents as excessively painful. Laterality is the discrimination between right and left, which may exist in this PLWBC but is not presented as such in this case. Cortical mapping is relevant but would not be directly related to the sensitivity and withdrawal.

8. A: Age-related demyelination

Rationale: Glial cells have a relationship to the central nervous system and chronic stress can play a role in how they are used. Age-related demyelination likely has a role in the falls that she has experienced but it is not likely to be a strong contributor as the other answers.

9. C: Forward rounding posture to disguise the lack of breast tissue

Rationale: While the other answers may be contributors, the most likely behavioral contributor presented would be that of disguising of postmastectomy changes as it would require static slump positioning. This can be quite aggravating to the sciatic nerves.

10. C: Counselor

Rationale: While all these providers may be able to help this person with these issues, a counselor is likely best equipped to improve the underlying psychological influences for the postural behavior.

Chapter 23

1. B: There is muscle protein synthesis activated by resistance training

Rationale: Sarcomeres are increased in a parallel fashion, a mechanical stretch increases insulin-like growth factor and phosphatidic acid, thus muscle protein synthesis is the correct answer as it is activated by resistance training.

2. C: Cachexia

Rationale: The loss in adipose tissue is only seen in cachexia, not sarcopenia.

3. C: Secondary prevention

Rationale: This exercise is a form of prehabilitation to improve function before the treatment of radiation begins which is classified as secondary prevention.

4. A: Primordial prevention

Rationale: Working to create opportunities for healthy lifestyles within a community is primordial prevention.

5. A: 2MWT

Rationale: Only A, B, and C are tests for functional endurance. Due to the potential discomfort from not only the surgery but the radiation to the pelvis and hip flexor muscles, the step test could be too uncomfortable, the 6MWT may be too long due to comfort so the 2MWT would be the best initial test to complete.

6. D: Rate of perceived stability

Rationale: A, B, and C are measures of intensity for functional endurance.

7. C: 52-year-old female with Stage IIIA, post mastectomy and radiation with CRF

Rationale: Although all patients B, C, D could be prescribed a HIIT program, it would be most effective for a person with CRF. HIIT would be most effective in eliminating CRF. Cardiotoxicity needs a strategic exercise program for endurance and if a person has CIPN the initial E/PA program needs to focus on deceasing the CIPN for safety.

8. C: Ambulation

Rationale: Functional performance includes CV fitness, strength and balance but not ambulation. That is functional mobility.

9. C: Complete Body Program

Rationale: She needs to work her entire body in order to decrease the fatigue and improve her lymphatic circulation, including aerobic, resistance and flexibility to the entire body. HIIT will be too challenging until she improves her overall status. Only working her UE has been unsuccessful and Yoga does not include enough aerobic challenge.

10. A: HIIT

Rationale: She is already walking and is motivated to get strong enough to ride her horses. She needs to be challenged. Although the complete body workout could also be sufficient, she is a good candidate for increased challenge that will allow her to achieve her goal of returning to horseback riding, which simulates HIIT.

Chapter 24

1. D: Discuss symptoms and lab oratory value changes with the physician prior to initiating evaluation.

Rationale: Hyperkalemia, flank pain, and dysuria can all be signs of tumor lysis syndrome, most commonly seen after chemotherapy and in leukemia treatment. If this is indeed tumor lysis syndrome, it would be considered a medical emergency.

2. A: Return later to provide education on specific goals of therapy post-ostomy as it has been shown to reduce the length of stay.

Rationale: Research shows positive outcomes with inpatient exercise therapy in regards to length of stay, which is beneficial to both the patient and the medical system.

3. B: Discuss the lack of progress and pain barrier with the interdisciplinary team with recommendation to support palliative goals.

Rationale: Progress toward goals can be achieved with the help of the interdisciplinary team to assist with modifying achievable goals at the end of life.

4. C: Suggest interval training ambulation with symptom-limited intensity and vital monitoring throughout.

Rationale: When platelet levels are between 10,000 and 20,000 uL, there is a risk of bleeding from high exertional blood pressure with aggressive exercise or with resistance training.

5. D: Arrange your session around nursing availability in order to clamp the ventriculostomy for mobility.

Rationale: Research has demonstrated that therapy interventions in patients with a ventriculostomy was both safe and feasible with bedside nursing assistance as a key component.

6. A: AMPAC 6-clicks

Rationale: The five times sit to stand and TUG test are predictive of fall risk while the 6-minute walk test helps determine endurance. AMPAC 6-clicks is specific to help predict destination of discharge.

7. C: Encourage her to speak with her physician about the side effects of corticosteroids.

Rationale: Corticosteroids can result in hypertension, weight gain, and difficulty with blood glucose regulation, so referring her back to the physician to review this and rule out other possible causes is the best course of action.

8. B: Decreased bilateral lower extremity sensation

Rationale: Dyspnea with exertion and decreased endurance are more likely related to the acute onset of pneumonia, with neuropathy a common long-term side effect of cisplatin.

9. B: Inpatient rehabilitation to train the PWC and family on transfer techniques

Rationale: Given the rapid and sudden decline in functional status, the poor prognosis, and the palliative treatment offered, the patient and his caregiver will benefit most from comprehensive training to maximize mobility and opportunity to travel for palliative radiation.

10. A: Sustained clonus with rapid manual stretch of the ankle

Rationale: Sustained clonus is an indicator or an upper motor neuron lesion. While lung cancer is one of the most common cancer diagnoses seen in the emergency center, the patient's clonus is a more unexpected and concerning finding that warrants careful examination.

Chapter 25

1. A: Ankle range of motion

Rationale: Children who receive vincristine become less able to detect light touch, pinprick sensations, vibration, and differences in temperature when hot or cold objects are applied to the skin. The Onc R plan of care should include fine motor, balance, range of motion (ROM), especially of ankle dorsiflexion due to ankle ROM deficits and gait deviations associated with vincristine use.

2. D: Squamous cell carcinoma

Rationale: Important risk factors for a second cancer included radiation therapy and doxorubicin. Patients who received radiation therapy to lungs due to metastasis have an increased risk of developing breast cancer. Leukemias and solid tumors are the most commonly diagnosed secondary cancers.

3. C: Seizures

Rationale: While HSCTs can be curative for a variety of conditions there are transplant related morbidity and mortality, risks. After HSCT children are at risk for acute complications within the first 90 days such as infection from myelosuppression, veno-occlusive disease (VOD), mucositis, and acute graft versus host disease (aGvHD).

4. A: Diverse treatment schedules

Rationale: Diverse treatment schedules facilitate adherence, compliance, and access to therapy. Coordinating therapy appointments with clinic visits will also aid in attendance compliance and in decreasing some burden on caregivers. Open, busy treatment areas increase infection risk, restricted support groups may deter social interactions and familial bonding and rigid work schedules may result in reduced expansion/growth of the program.

5. B: 6 Minute walk test

Rationale: Some tools for assessing fatigue include PedsQL Multidimensional Fatigue Scale, Childhood Cancer Fatigue Scale (CCFS), Fatigue Scale for a child (FS-C), Fatigue Scale for adolescents (FS-A), Timed Up and Go (TUG), 6 Minute walk test (6MWT) and 30 second walk test.

6. A: Acute respiratory distress and sepsis

Rationale: Wosten-van Asperen et al. performed a meta-analysis of children with cancer in the pediatric ICU (PICU). They found that 40% of children with cancer required at least one PICU admission often for acute respiratory distress (ARD) and sepsis. Mortality was found to be 28%, which is five times higher than typical PICU rates; further increased mortality in children requiring continuous renal replacement therapy (CRRT), mechanical ventilation or inotropic support.

7. B: Be addressed by both physical and psychological approaches.

Rationale: Onc R clinicians must acknowledge and attempt to address pain with both physical and psychological approaches through conventional, integrative, and newer approaches in chronic pain management.

8. C: Myopathy in the proximal muscle groups

Rationale: High dose steroids during induction, and throughout treatment, lead to myopathy causing weakness in the proximal muscle groups in the lower and upper extremities.

9. B: Three years

Rationale: Survivors of pediatric malignant brain tumors or ALL have demonstrated increased risk for cognitive difficulties with nonverbal abilities being most impaired such as short-term memory, processing speed, visual-motor integration, sequencing ability, attention and concentration. Younger children who received high doses of cranial radiation demonstrated decreased IQ, working memory, and processing speeds 3 years postradiation than older children and children of all ages that receive focal, proton radiation.

10. D: Long bones and spinal vertebrae

Rationale: Long bones and spinal vertebrae are often where the largest decrease in bone mineral density (BMD) is observed, resulting in osteoporosis. There are some reports of increased incidence of vertebral fractures in the first year of treatment.

Chapter 26

1. D: Oxaliplatin

Rationale: Patients with exposure to platinum-based chemotherapies, including oxaliplatin, have a higher risk of developing chemotherapy-induced polyneuropathy (CIPN).

2. B: Fullerton Advanced Balance (FAB) Scale

Rationale: Per the APTA Oncology EDGE Task Force resource, the Fullerton Advanced Balance (FAB) Scale is Highly Recommended for the assessment of balance in adult cancer survivors.

3. C: Interview the client to better understand their daily routine as well as barriers and supports to participation

Rationale: To support the client in their daily life participation you must first develop an understanding of what is important to them in their daily life, what makes participating difficulty, and who/what helps them participate in daily life. This information is critical to informing your treatment approach and goal development.

4. D: If she endorses any of the above

Rationale: There are several indicators that an individual may benefit from seeing a clinical psychologist; clinical-level distress, that is persistent and/or leading to significant functional impairment is an important consideration, but where resources permit AYAs can also gain significant benefit from having a consultation with a clinical psychologist to equip them with adaptive coping strategies.

5. B: Ice pack to the great toe following activity

Rationale: Exposure to platinum-based chemotherapy can induce Raynaud phenomenon-type symptoms of cold sensitivity. Physical therapists should assess for increased cold sensitivity prior to application of any cryotherapy for patients with a history of platinum-based chemotherapy.

6. B: Connect them with relevant resources, such as the Sam Fund

Rationale: The Sam Fund provides financial resources for AYAs with cancer whereas First Descents is an outdoor activity program. Emphasizing job skills or applications may increase the client's stress level and may be setting unrealistic expectations for the client.

7. D: Option A followed by C

Rationale: Young men can often "downplay" their distress, which can lead to under-reporting and also internalizing emotions. Depression can also often manifest differently in young men than young women—for example, appearing more bored, disengaged, frustrated, or angry rather than appearing sad and downcast per se. As a result, it is important to develop different, creative strategies to explore and make space for young male survivors to identify distress, in an empowering and nonpathologizing way (i.e., normalizing how common it can be to experience different kinds of distress and emotional reactions in survivorship).

8. A: Assessing for the presence of axillary web syndrome

Rationale: Both younger age and history of axillary lymph node dissection put this patient at higher risk for axillary web syndrome. While all the other tests should be a part of the assessment, screening for axillary web syndrome is unique to this patient's history and is a critical part of determining interventions and outcomes.

9. D: Rearrange the location of essential cooking items in her kitchen so she can easily reach them

Rationale: To maximize the client's ability to participate in cooking/meal preparation the therapist and client need to work together to adapt the environment to support participation given her current physical limitations. While having others help her is a reasonable option as well, this would not necessarily support her independence in the activity, as asked in the question.

10. A: Current mood and coping strategies, social supports and networks, and occupational/financial status

Rationale: While all the listed issues are important (e.g., diet, exercise, leisure) the most critical issues to explore in terms of broader well-being and mental health would be her mood and coping at the outset. Mood and general coping strategies are critical to ensure before a young person has the capacity to engage well with activities of daily living, exercise, a good diet, and hobbies. Social supports and networks are also critical to supporting good mental health, and research shows that occupational/financial status is linked to young people's mental health and levels of stress.

Chapter 27

1. B: Assess treadmill tolerance for walking in clinic and progressive walking program, increasing by 5 minutes in duration each day

Rationale: Walking programs as a component of the HEP are appropriate for many PLWCs because they do not require equipment, are straightforward to instruct the PLWC in performing and progressing, and are easy to track on a HEP log. The other exercises are appropriate and address the cardiovascular component of exercise, though do not specifically target the goal of improving functional walking capacity.

2. B: Wall washing (shoulder flexion, scaption, and horizontal/abduction with a towel on the wall and against gravity)

Rationale: Wall washing exercise is the most functional exercise listed and can address strength, ROM, and endurance deficits relative to how this exercise is prescribed.

3. B: Circumferential bilateral upper extremity lymphedema measurement

Rationale: It is principally important to obtain baseline circumferential measurements of the upper extremities in order to identify the onset of lymphedema at its earliest point.

4. D: Two Minute Walk Test

Rationale: The Two Minute Walk Test is the superior test to have the PLWC perform because it correlates with the 6 minute walk test, yet minimizes the impact of time on your limited window in which to screen and educate the PLWC. Minimizing the screening time, maximizes the time to provide education.

5. B: Band resistance exercises for the upper back musculature

Rationale: All of the exercises listed are appropriate for a HEP, however the impaired trunk strength and resulting poor posturing will be best remedied with resistance exercises to the upper back musculature. Resistance bands are helpful for compliance as they can be sent home with the PLWC.

6. C: The licensed medical social worker

Rationale: The skills and expertise of a licensed medical social worker are the best suited to address the concerns of coping and support. The nurse navigator is a good choice as a resource, though would also need to refer to the social worker for management.

7. A: Six Minute Walk Test

Rationale: Radiation therapy can cause the adverse effect of fatigue and may manifest as reduced function and/or functional walking capacity. It is therefore important to obtain a baseline distance for the Six Minute Walk Test.

8. C: Registered dietician nutritionist

Rationale: The skills and expertise of a registered dietician nutritionist are the best suited to address the concerns of malnutrition. The nurse navigator is a good choice as a resource, though would also need to refer to the registered dietician nutritionist for management.

9. D: Multimodal

Rationale: Multimodal prehabilitation programs have been correlated more frequently to positive post-treatment outcomes.

10. A: Head and neck

Rationale: Breast, colorectal and prostate cancers are among the most prevalent diagnoses in the prehabilitation literature, head and neck cancers are among the least.

Chapter 28

1. D: High intensity strengthening

Rationale: Based on Dietz' taxonomy of Onc R services, this patient will benefit from supportive services that focus on accommodating his current circumstance of receiving palliative treatments. "Supportive rehabilitation promotes accommodation of disabilities, teaches compensatory strategies, and provides ongoing therapy during disease recurrence or temporization efforts."

2. C: FACIT- F

Rationale: The FACIT-F has 13 questions that provides the most comprehensive assessment of fatigue-related symptoms. The NCCN Distress Thermometer and Problem List only asks for a yes/no response to the presence of fatigue while the remaining tools do not address fatigue at all.

3. B: AML

Rationale: "Alkylating chemotherapy regimens used to treat Hodgkin's lymphoma are attributed to an increase in AML development later in life." AML is most likely to occur within the first 10 years following Hodgkin Lymphoma diagnosis.

4. B: Doxorubicin and radiation

Rationale: "Childhood cancer survivors at the highest risk for cardiotoxic long-term and late effects include individuals who are female, were diagnosed and treated <7 years old, received chest radiotherapy, completed high doses of anthracyclines, and had higher body fat. The increase in cardiovascular risk is 4 to 6 times higher in childhood and young adult cancer survivors when compared to noncancer peers. This risk is increased in survivors of lymphoma, those receiving mediastinal RTx, or those receiving anthracycline chemotherapy. Anthracycline chemotherapy can result in acute cardiac complications during infusion as well as long-term cardiac damage resulting in heart failure. Coupled with cardiovascular risk, this population is at a ninefold risk for cerebrovascular accidents in adulthood." Also, per Landier, bleomycin has a predominant negative impact on pulmonary function.

5. C: Long-term effects begin during cancer treatment and late effects arise months to years following completion of cancer treatment

Rationale: Long-term adverse effects begin during cancer treatment and extend beyond the treatment window; whereas, late effects occur months to years following completion of cancer related medical treatment.

6. B: Letrozole

Rationale: Postmenopausal women on aromatase inhibitors (AIs) for breast cancer are at increased risk for arthralgias and ostealgia.

7. A: Removal of 7 lymph nodes, radiation therapy, local burn

Rationale: Causative factors of lymphedema can include the number of lymph nodes resected, field extent and dosage of RTx delivered, and the effects of increased fluid volume during chemotherapy infusion. Scar tissue leads to physical changes in the layers of skin and connective tissue where the lymphatic vessels are located.

8. C: Complete decongestive therapy

Rationale: Ultrasound, moist hot packs, and joint manipulation (vs. mobilization) are all contraindicated. Lymph volume reduction and improved range of motion need to be achieved before strengthening can be optimized.

9. C: Cyclophosphamide

Rationale: Cardiovascular toxicity is a late adverse effect notably observed following the use of chemotherapy drugs (anthracycline-based agents such as doxorubicin), hormone suppression drugs (AIs), and radiation therapy. Surgical intervention causes scar tissue that can lead to musculoskeletal deficits with reproducible pain. Cyclophosphamide is more closely identified with the late effects of infertility and increased risk of lymphoma or leukemia due to bone marrow damage.

10. C: Rehabilitation in reverse

Rationale: "Rehabilitation in reverse allows clinicians to provide education and skilled care that anticipates progressive decline; this may include the use of assistive devices, caregiver training, and modifications to an exercise program that may focus on mobility and comfort more than progress."

Chapter 29

1. A: Rehabilitation light—anticipate functional decline, procures needed equipment beforehand, teaches family positioning and safe patient handling before physical decline

Rationale: Rehabilitation light includes reducing the dosage, frequency, or intensity of rehabilitation services while the provided definition for rehabilitation light is more likely rehabilitation in reverse.

2. B: He is eligible for skilled PT/OT which would be covered by Medicare Part B for therapy services

Rationale: Palliative care is a consultative service that does not prompt a change in insurance coverage. Patients with palliative care are not necessarily imminently dying. This patient would be eligible for skilled PT under Medicare Part B as long as the services are skilled and medically necessary.

3. A: Medicare will pay for maintenance services when they require the skill of a licensed therapist/assistant

Rationale: According to the *Jimmo vs. Sebelius* settlement, even in the absence of expectation for improvement, if skilled services are medically necessary to maintain or slow the decline of a condition, they are eligible for payment. Medicare will not pay for maintenance services for a therapist when the task does not require the skill of a therapist. Limb swelling is closely associated with comfort and quality of life and if not addressed, it could cause more discomfort or reduced quality of life. A decision to be admitted to hospice is only determined by the patient's physicians if the patient has an expectation of less than 6 months to live.

4. A: This patient is right, hospice and palliative care are the same things

Rationale: Hospice is different from palliative care. The goal of palliative care is to coordinate a team for expert, proactive symptom management to optimize quality of life for anyone with a life-threatening or chronic illness. Although more often used in advanced stages of diseases, it is appropriate at any stage of a disease process.

5. C: Serves as a resource person for other therapists who also care for patients with palliative diagnoses during challenging situations

Rationale: There are multiple benefits to designating a lead therapist for the PC team as the go-between between the PC professionals and the rehabilitation team.

6. C: In order to optimize insurance reimbursement, a patient should always have a minimum of 5 visits per week

Rationale: Rehabilitation light often entails a decreased frequency or intensity of visits as excessive rehabilitation may overtax the person's body systems and worsen quality of life.

7. B: Skilled maintenance is needed when tasks are to complex or unsafe for caregivers to perform

Rationale: Skilled maintenance must be medically necessary and cannot be performed by laypersons or other healthcare providers without the skillset of rehabilitation professionals.

8. A: Contact the patient's doctor or cancer center to begin to address her financial toxicity

Rationale: Although all of the activities are important and within a therapist's scope of practice, the highest priority would be addressing the patient's immediate and emergent financial distress and would require a quick referral to appropriate resources. If this is not completed, the patient's cancer treatment may be disrupted or ceased, which could be life threatening.

9. A: FACT-G

Rationale: FACT-G is a measure of quality of life that is completed by the patient. Timed up and go is a physical measure of standing and gait speed. LEFS is a questionnaire that focuses specifically on lower extremity functioning. Dynamometry is a measure of handgrip strength.

10. B: Emotional and psychosocial distress

Rationale: As the patient's pain is not provoked or alleviated by musculoskeletal testing, it is not likely to be from a musculoskeletal origin. The patient has several areas of concern for psychosocial and emotional distress that may be acting as pain amplifiers or components of the patient's total pain according to Saunders.

Chapter 30

1. B: A referral to a dietitian is warranted to address decreased food intake. A referral back to the primary care physician is warranted to address anxiety and concerns for decreased energy.

Rationale: A referral to RDN is warranted due to decreased food intake and risk for malnutrition. An RDN can help curb adverse effects of chemotherapy, such as changes in taste. An RDN may suggest using plastic utensils instead of metal or seasoning food with tart flavors, such as lemon, to curb metallic taste. A referral to the PCP is warranted to address anxiety and concerns for decreased energy. It is imperative that the PCP is informed of all herbal supplements and vitamins that the patient is taking because of possible drug interactions, such reduced efficacy or adverse reactions to cancer meditations. The PCP will also assist PLWBC with sleep solutions and appropriate, individualized plan to control anxiety.

2. B: Work on positioning techniques and use of wedges to improve ease of breathing in his bed.

Rationale: Assessment of sleeping positions and appropriate modifications is a beneficial component of a rehabilitation treatment session, ensuring maximal comfort, prevention of pressure sores, and allowance for adequate breathing and pain reduction.

3. A: Educate on the importance of informing oncologists of all supplements he is consuming as there is a potential for interaction with chemotherapeutic agents. Discuss the importance of a patient-specific exercise program, nutritious diet, and adequate sleep for improved immunity.

Rationale: It is imperative that the oncologist is informed of all herbal supplements and vitamins that the patient is taking because of possible drug interactions, such as reduced efficacy or adverse actions to cancer meditations. The APTA supports the therapists' role in the promotion of health and wellness and states that identifying contributing lifestyle factors such as weight, exercise, and stress reduction are integral.

4. A: Educate on the importance of informing oncologists of all supplements he is consuming as there is a potential for interaction with chemotherapeutic agents. Educate on CRF and the evidence for a patient-specific exercise prescription to improve energy levels.

Rationale: It is imperative that the oncologist is informed of all herbal supplements and vitamins that the patient is taking because of possible drug interactions, such as reduced efficacy or adverse actions to cancer meditations. The APTA supports the therapists' role in the promotion of health and wellness and states that "identifying contributing lifestyle factors such as weight, exercise, and stress reduction are integral.

5. A: Encourage him to talk to his doctor. Provide resources for mediation and support groups.

Rationale: The PCP will also assist PLWBC with an appropriate, individualized plan to control anxiety. Social support groups and the use of CAM therapies may reduce anxiety in the PLWBC.

6. B: The therapist should encourage smoking cessation and provide the patient with resources.

Rationale: Tobacco causes a variety of other health consequences that can affect health and ability to heal from cancer diagnosis and treatment including decreased immune system, bone density, wound healing, and increased risk of developing type 2 diabetes, cardiovascular disease, and chronic obstructive pulmonary disease (COPD).

7. B: Complete Malnutrition Screening Tool. If the score is over 2, refer to RDN. Provide the patient with information on healthy diet guidelines and exercise

Rationale: The patient may be at risk for malnutrition. Overweight and obesity can coincide with malnutrition. The MST is a quick screening tool that will determine if a RDN referral is warranted. An MST score of 2 or above indicates that the PLWBC is at risk for malnutrition. Early intervention by an RDN can prevent malnutrition and improve the patient's outcome.

8. A: Explain that watching the screen 30 minutes before bed reduces sleep quality. Educate on sleep hygiene techniques and specific relaxation techniques to assist with falling asleep. Refer to the physician to address anxiety and to ensure there are no premorbid or underlying sleep issues.
Rationale: It is recommended to avoid loud noise or screens before bed. Screens should be turned off 30 minutes before bed as blue light disrupts sleep quality. CAM therapies may reduce stress-related symptoms in PLWBC. A referral to the physician is warranted to determine if trouble sleeping is due to anxiety, adverse effects or meditication, or another health condition and create an appropriate treatment plan.

9. C: A referral to the medical doctor as postmenopausal bleeding is a concern for uterine cancer
Rationale: Postmenopausal bleeding is a sign of possible uterine cancer and the patient should be referred to a physician for appropriate screening to rule out disease.

10. B: The therapist should encourage the patient to reduce alcohol consumption to 0-1 drinks per day and provide the patient with resources.
Rationale: Research indicates the amount of alcohol consumed over time, not the type of alcohol is linked to an increased risk of cancer. The more alcohol consumed the higher the risk.

Chapter 31

1. A: Integrating concepts of quality and accountability within the context of cost and patient-centered outcomes
Rationale: Value-based care is described as assuring quality within the context of costs with an emphasis on both short-term and long-term outcomes.

2. D: Ensuring that a clinician does not take any leaves of absence
Rationale: A career ladder is a commitment to the team members' professional growth and providing continuous improvement to quality care. Employees may still need to take leaves of absence for family or health events to address their personal life factors.

3. B: Facilitating a journal club with team members to review new literature and identifying ways to implement these new findings into routine clinical practice.
Rationale: Knowledge translation includes incorporating evidence-based rehabilitation clinical assessment tools into routine practice as well as including rehabilitation professionals in shared decision-making.

4. C: Acute care hospitalizations are covered under a DRG where the hospital gets a lump sum based on the patient's diagnosis and length of stay
Rationale: Under Medicare Part A for acute hospitalizations, the payment methodology is a DRG where the hospital will receive a lump sum based on estimated costs and length of stay of the hospitalization.

5. C: Fixed costs
Rationale: Fixed costs are the relatively stable costs that re-occur on an ongoing basis and generally include salaries, benefits, rent, utilities, insurance, etc.

6. C: Admit to IPR for a short stay of family training before home
Rationale: Although discharge home is this patient's ultimate goal, she also aims to be out and about and in order to do this, she and her family will need training in

equipment and safe handling that can be taught in the inpatient rehabilitation setting. Currently, inpatient hospice and a LTACH are too intensive and unnecessary and are not within the patient's remaining life goals.

7. B: An early step in the development process, driving all aspects of the organization, such as the funding process and direction for marketing
Rationale: Clarifying the mission early in the planning process provides the foundation for relationship building, development of referral, design and structure of services and policies, communications and marketing with consumers, as well as funding, measurement of outcomes and more. The mission is the guiding light of the program, and the gauge for determining whether a program is successful in meeting the "big picture" mission.

8. B: Recognizing the existing inequities within the current healthcare system and consciously creating opportunities to proactively address these inequities
Rationale: Research cited in the chapter clearly identified numerous levels of health disparity in access and provision of cancer rehabilitation (and cancer treatment in general). Minorities, members of the LBGTQIA+ community, and socioeconomic barriers impact prevention strategies, early diagnosis and treatment, proactive reporting of symptoms, and advocating for education.

9. B: Offering career mentorship, clinical career ladders, and ongoing financial support for lifelong learning in the field
Rationale: Achievement of the highest level of credential validates a certain level of skill set knowledge; yet the functionality of a team is a better predictor of effective communication, efficient operations, and staff retention. Skills sets are absolutely important and can be readily built between mentors and mentees. Having a shared vision, positive attitude, and a commitment to learning and the team are intrinsic satisfiers. Research findings report that teammates feel most valued when they are actively engaged in the process and have a voice in the workplace and have opportunity to grow within the workplace.

10. C: With enough searching and investigation, the team members will be able to find another program that is an exact fit for their program to emulate it to grow their program
Rationale: Services for varying points in oncology rehabilitation vary greatly and each program is unique but founded in common cancer rehabilitation principles. For example, providing rehabilitation services during acute treatment may focus on fundamentals of function and support for balance such as utilization of an assistive device, basic ADL support and pacing training as well as sleep and breathing hygiene. Post-treatment survivorship programming would include management of lymphedema, self-examination and cancer prevention strategies and coaching.

Chapter 32

1. C: Developing services based on equality as everyone benefits from the same support
Rationale: Health **equity** involves developing services where everyone receives the support required for optimal health and functioning. If the development of services is approached from **equality**, this assumes everyone benefits from the same support, and results in many not getting the same access to and benefit from health services due to the impact of

unearned disadvantages like race, gender, socioeconomic status, and many other systemic barriers and factors.

2. D: Women receive more and better medical treatment for pain control than men and have better clinical outcomes, because they engage in greater self-advocacy

Rationale: Women are generally under-treated for pain management even when they are engaged in self-advocacy as compared to men. All the other examples have been documented in research and illustrate how the barriers contributing to the prevalence of cancer-related disability are magnified within populations that are historically marginalized, like black, indigenous, and people of color (BIPOC).

3. C: We work to primarily elevate the "expert" role of oncology clinicians so that we can have the positions of power to aid persons impacted by cancer

Rationale: When engaging in justice-centered advocacy, the aim is to elevate the contributions, needs, and experiences of persons impacted by cancer and not the "expert" role of the oncology clinician. Elevating the position of power and the "expert" role of oncology clinicians directly minimizes, weakens, or even replaces a person's and community's strengths, resources, and unique traditional strategies that positively contribute to heath and function.

4. B: The risk of contributing to health disparities is lower when engaging in professional-oriented advocacy.

Rationale: The risk of contributing to disparities is **higher** when engaging in professional-oriented advocacy, as the efforts are led by clinicians with the emphasis on providing opportunities for the clinicians rather than on the direction and needs of those that experience the impact of health disparities.

5. B: A lack of self-advocacy behaviors is likely to be the only reason why there are poorer clinical outcomes for persons so coaching persons to be better self-advocates will always mitigate health inequities and result in increased access to and benefits from services.

Rationale: A lack of self-advocacy is unlikely to be the only reason why some people have poorer clinical outcomes due to the impact of various contributors including availability of resources in communities, impact of racism and discrimination within systems, and ineffective and discriminatory responses by clinicians when a person attempts to self-advocate.

6. B: Financial planning

Rationale: Parikh et al. proposed a three-pronged approach in which a quality-of-life focused pathway within an institution can be implemented. To drive an effective quality of life initiative, they recommend focusing on three key areas: clinical practice, messaging, and research.

7. D: Specific to Onc R services, it is not the role of the PN to support timely referrals to Onc R services to prevent or minimize functional decline.

Rationale: To support timely referrals to Onc R services to prevent or minimize functional decline is one of the potential roles of the PN within an oncology rehabilitation service delivery model, whether the PN is a healthcare professional or lay person.

8. C: Decreased competence related to clinical skills and patient care

Rationale: The knowledge and skills related to policy making and legislative advocacy contribute to enhanced competence related to clinical skills and patient care as they serve to strengthen professional identity and the ability to communicate confidently, effectively, and relevantly within a variety of contexts and cultures.

9. B: Emphasize that all communities should communicate, act, and mobilize in the same way

Rationale: A key element for successful social mobilization is to recognize that not all communities will communicate, act, and mobilize in the same way so a range of different methods should be employed. Furthermore, the biopsychosocial understanding of how a community interacts with its social, economic, and political environment acknowledges that social mobilization efforts will vary across cultures, countries, and contexts.

10. D: Facilitate meetings with private insurance on behalf of clinicians and voice concerns/requests directly to the insurer

Rationale: The APTA's mission, vision and goals for 2020 and beyond are to transform society by optimizing movement to improve the human experience. The mission statement is to build a community that advances the profession of physical therapy to improve the health of society. Unlike larger organizations that are focused on breast cancer research or the American Cancer Society, the APTA relies on its membership to finance its activities and is not set up as a charity foundation that can help pay medical bills or cover the cost of care. It also is not designed to offer legal resources but can offer professional guidance, but rather are focused on the practice of physical therapy as a necessary field of medicine.

Chapter 33

1. D: No conflict exists if it is disclosed.

Rationale: This question tests the reader's understanding of the criteria for what constitutes a conflict of interest. In this instance, the specific context is that of the interaction of a private business interest and a clinical setting with the potential for personal financial gain. The incorrect choices all describe legitimate areas where a conflict of interest would arise. However, the presence of a clinician who acts in a role that supports a private enterprise is not, in itself, a conflict of interest so long as that relationship is explicitly disclosed.

2. D: Arranging a meeting with your Director of Procurement at your hospital so that they can start to have you selling these garments to your patients as a certified vendor of their company, where you will also receive a commission

Rationale: This question again tests the reader's understanding of the criteria for what constitutes a conflict of interest, however asking the reader to apply the criteria of conflict of interests (COI) in a real-world scenario. In this instance, the question seeks to test the reader's understanding of the specific mechanics of a relationship that would result in a COI. Choice D is the correct answer because it is the only choice that explicitly places the therapist in a position to act as an agent of a private company whose goals may run counter to that of the clinic and its patients. All other choices display details where the clinician can fill their role in their clinic as well as in this company while avoiding COI.

3. C: Disclose all pertinent information regarding the relationship to your patients using this device as well as your employer and surrender the relationship.

Rationale: This question seeks to assess the reader's understanding of how to resolve a conflict of interest and apply that understanding to a behavior. Choices A, B and D fail to fully resolve the presence of a conflict of interest while also presenting the stakeholders with a pathway to resolve the conflict maximizing efficacy and ethics.

4. C: You perform a chart review prior to seeing a patient to ascertain any precautions that must be observed
Rationale: This question again tests the reader's understanding of the criteria for what constitutes the ethical principle of nonmaleficence applied to a real-world scenario. Choice C is the correct answer because it is the only choice that explicitly describes behaviors that avoid harming the patient.

5. B: Overutilization of services
Rationale: This question tests the reader's understanding of the ethical dilemmas in the context of a real-world scenario, while identifying the specific ethical dilemma of utilization of services in a clinical vignette.

6. A: He is disadvantaged geographically
Rationale: This question tests the reader's knowledge of factors that influence healthcare disparities and applying them. In this instance, the vignette identifies a patient whose limitations to accessing their needed services is related to living in a rural area implying few provider choices and a long distance to travel to access providers.

7. B: It would be unethical on the grounds of maintaining professional competence
Rationale: This question tests the reader's understanding of the ethical dilemmas and applying it in the context of a real-world scenario. The vignette describes a circumstance where the therapist is being asked to provide a service that is outside of their professional duties and education. This falls under acting in accordance to one's professional competence.

8. D: A physician's bias to use a less effective treatment because the patient has run out of money
Rationale: This question tests the reader's knowledge of the definition of financial toxicity and their ability to apply it. Financial toxicity is defined as "negative impacts on a patient's health and care as a result of increasing financial burden of their care." Choice D best describes a scenario where a detrimental impact on their care is elicited as a result of financial limitations.

9. D: Having medical coverage through a federal program such as Medicare
Rationale: This question tests the reader's knowledge of factors that influence healthcare disparities. In this instance, all choices except choice D describe a defined factor that leads to disparities in healthcare.

10. B: Providing a pamphlet on financial resources supporting cancer treatments and how to qualify
Rationale: This question tests the reader's knowledge of the principle of financial rehabilitation. In this instance, all choices except choice B describe a defined strategy that can serve to prepare the PLWC for the financial demands associated with cancer treatment.

Chapter 34

1. C: Complex
Rationale: The clinical presentation is only considered unstable when a patient has sudden and unpredictable fluctuations in vital signs or symptoms that are progressing without clear cause. Fluctuations in presentation related to the cancer diagnosis or cancer treatment fit best into the category of *evolving clinical presentation*.

2. D: Pt will be able to don her socks with the use of a sock aid modified independent in 1 week.
Rationale: Goal D is functional because it involves an activity limitation or participation restriction. The other three are focusing on impairments without a clear impact on function.

3. B: Gait Training
Rationale: *Gait Training* is to be used when the physical therapist is instructing a patient on how to use a new assistive device or proper sequencing with stairs in respect to a new injury. For example, training a patient to use crutches with partial weight bearing after a recent tibial bone biopsy. In the inpatient setting, this code can be used when the physical therapist is progressing the total distance a patient ambulates. *Neuromuscular Re-education* should be used with ambulation training when the focus is on training neuromuscular activation, balance response, coordination, or postural control. *Therapeutic Exercise* and *Therapeutic Activity* do not generally have relation to improving gait.

4. D: Objective tests will assure that an audit or denial will never occur
Rationale: Although objective tests help to defend and justify the Onc R services, there are many possible reasons for an audit or denial.

5. C: Performed
Rationale: Performed is not a descriptive word that indicates skill as a patient can perform a home exercise program without the skill of a licensed provider.

6. D: Describing the PWC prior level of function and current limitations
Rationale: Clinical documentation must clearly state the innovative, skilled, and medically necessary services. An important component to this is detailing the patient's abilities before the onset of this condition and what impairments, functional limitations, or participation restrictions are now present.

7. D: On visit two when the patient's status has not appreciably changed
Rationale: All options demonstrate a possible change in the functional status of the patient that could affect their prognosis, therefore it is appropriate to bill a re-evaluation code.

8. C: Patient's history, examination, clinical presentation, clinical decision making
Rationale: The patient's history, examination, clinical presentation, and clinical decision making are the four factors in determining an appropriate initial evaluation code.

9. B: Z48.3 Aftercare following surgery for neoplasm
Rationale: Z48.3 highlights that this is a component of aftercare, which is appropriate for rehabilitation to treat. The Onc R clinicians are not treating the cancer itself, therefore C59.919 is not appropriate. 97162 and 97140 are procedural CPT codes to bill for interventions, not diagnostic codes.

10. B: Providing skilled maintenance care to maintain or slow the decline of a condition
Rationale: According to the *Jimmo vs. Sebelius* settlement, skilled maintenance is a covered service as long as the

clinical documentation can justify the medical necessity and that the services required the skills of the licensed professional providing it.

Chapter 35

1. C: Retrospective observational cohort

Rationale: As the clinician did not determine who will and will not receive the intervention, this is an observational study design. As the outcomes that are to be reported on were collected in the past, this is a retrospective study design.

2. A: The IRB does not need to review observational studies.

Rationale: The IRB only reviews projects that are considered to be research. Both case reports and quality improvement projects do not fall under the classification of research.

3. C: Cross-sectional cohort study

Rationale: The title of the project implies an observational study that assesses one cohort of patients (patients treated for colorectal cancer) at one time point.

4. A: Case study

Rationale: In cases of rare conditions where little literature exists, the most expedient method for informing others about care of this population would be a case study. Gathering the numbers of subjects needed for other study types would take considerable time and effort and a case study would add to the evidence base for this population.

5. D: Administration of HIPPA consent forms.

Rationale: While the IRB reviews the scope and conduct of research at institutions to ensure patient safety and regulatory compliance, they do not conduct the components of a research project.

6. B: Provide identical expertise as the Principal Investigator.

Rationale: Co-investors typically provide complimentary expertise to the Principal Investigator and assist in the development and conduct of the research.

7. B: Names of all potential research participants

Rationale: In order to assure protection of the research subjects, the IRB will review the research protocol, procedures, and informed consenting forms which includes assurances about HIPAA protections.

8. A: Platform presentation

Rationale: A platform presentation allows researchers to give a short talk on their research findings using multiple slides while poster presentations only use one slide in a more informal format. Plenary presentations may or may not be research based and are longer-format than research study presentations. Educational sessions typically include research information from multiple studies to synthesize information in a specific area.

9. C: An accepted version of a research manuscript put into the publication format.

Rationale: A proof is an accepted version of a research manuscript used to proofread the final version of the paper prior to publishing in the journal.

10. D: A postprofessional doctoral degree

Rationale: Research can be accomplished by clinicians at any level of training if given the appropriate support.

Index

Page numbers followed by 'f' indicate figures, 't' indicate tables, 'b' indicate boxes.